Volume II

GIBBON'S
Surgery of the Chest
FOURTH EDITION

DAVID C. SABISTON, Jr., M.D.,

James B. Duke Professor and
Chairman, Department of Surgery
Duke University School of Medicine
Durham, North Carolina

FRANK C. SPENCER, M.D.

George David Stewart Professor and
Chairman, Department of Surgery
New York University School of Medicine
New York, New York

1983   W. B. SAUNDERS COMPANY
PHILADELPHIA/LONDON/TORONTO/MEXICO CITY/RIO DE JANEIRO/SYDNEY/TOKYO

W. B. Saunders Company: West Washington Square
                           Philadelphia, PA 19105

                           1 St. Anne's Road
                           Eastbourne, East Sussex BN21 3UN, England

                           1 Goldthorne Avenue
                           Toronto, Ontario M8Z 5T9, Canada

                           Apartado 26370—Cedro 512
                           Mexico 4, D.F., Mexico

                           Rua Coronel Cabrita, 8
                           Sao Cristovao Caixa Postal 21176
                           Rio de Janeiro, Brazil

                           9 Waltham Street
                           Artarmon, N.S.W. 2064, Australia

                           Ichibancho, Central Bldg., 22-1 Ichibancho
                           Chiyoda-Ku, Tokyo 102, Japan

Library of Congress Cataloging in Publication Data

Surgery of the chest.

Gibbon's Surgery of the chest.

Includes index.

1. Chest–Surgery.   I. Gibbon, John Heysham.
   II. Sabiston, David C., 1924–   .   III. Spencer, Frank
   Cole.   IV. Title. [DNLM: 1. Thoracic surgery. WF 980
   G439]

RD536.G48 1983   617'.54059   81–48401

ISBN 0–7216–7873–4   AACR2

Listed here is the latest translated edition of this book together
with the language of the translation and the publisher.

Spanish (*3rd Edition,* Vols. I & II)—Salvat Editores S.A.,
                           Barcelona, Spain

                                          Volume I   ISBN 0-7216-7879-3
                                          Volume II   ISBN 0-7216-7880-7
Gibbon's Surgery of the Chest   Complete Set   ISBN 0-7216-7873-4

Last digit is the print number: 9   8   7   6   5   4   3   2   1

Contributors

Robert W. Anderson, M.D.
Professor of Surgery, University of Minnesota Medical School. Director of Cardiovascular and Thoracic Surgery, University of Minnesota Hospital, Minneapolis, Minnesota.
Shock and Circulatory Collapse

Henry T. Bahnson, M.D.
George V. Foster Professor and Chairman of Surgery, University of Pittsburgh School of Medicine. Chief of Surgery, Presbyterian-University Hospital; Attending Surgeon, Children's Hospital of Pittsburgh, Pittsburgh, Pennsylvania.
The Aorta

Lionel M. Bargeron, Jr., M.D.
Professor of Pediatrics, University of Alabama in Birmingham School of Medicine, Birmingham, Alabama.
Surgical Treatment of Ventricular Septal Defect

William A. Baumgartner, M.D.
Assistant Professor of Surgery, Johns Hopkins University School of Medicine. Attending Cardiac Surgeon, Cardiac Surgical Service, Johns Hopkins Hospital, Baltimore, Maryland.
Heart and Lung Transplantation

Harvey W. Bender, Jr., M.D.
Professor of Surgery, Vanderbilt University School of Medicine. Attending Physician, Vanderbilt University Hospital, Nashville, Tennessee.
Major Anomalies of Pulmonary and Thoracic Systemic Veins

William N. Bernhard, M.D.
Associate Professor, Department of Anesthesiology, New York University School of Medicine. Medical Director, Respiratory Care Department, New York University Hospital, and New York University–Bellevue Respiratory Therapy Program; Staff Anesthesiologist, New York University Hospital and Bellevue Hospital Center, New York, New York.
Tracheal Intubation and Assisted Ventilation

Richard J. Bing, M.D.
Professor of Medicine, University of Southern California School of Medicine. Director of Cardiology and Intramural Medicine, Huntington Memorial Hospital, Pasadena, California.
Special Diagnostic Procedures in Cardiac Surgery

Arthur D. Boyd, M.D.
Professor of Surgery, New York University School of Medicine. Attending Surgeon, New York University Hospital, Bellevue Hospital, and Veterans Administration Hospital, New York, New York.
Endoscopy: Bronchoscopy and Esophagoscopy; Tracheal Intubation and Assisted Ventilation

Henry Buchwald, M.D., Ph.D.
Professor of Surgery and Biomedical Engineering, University of Minnesota Medical School. Attending Surgeon, University of Minnesota Hospital, Minneapolis, Minnesota.
Partial Ileal Bypass for Control of Hyperlipidemia and Atherosclerosis

William A. Check, Ph.D.
Editorial Consultant, Emory University School of Medicine, Atlanta, Georgia.
Infection, Thrombosis, and Emboli Associated with Intracardiac Prostheses

Denton A. Cooley, M.D.
Clinical Professor of Surgery, University of Texas Medical School at Houston. Surgeon-in-Chief, Texas Heart Institute of St. Luke's Episcopal Hospital and Texas Children's Hospital, Houston, Texas.
Congenital Aortic Stenosis

James L. Cox, M.D.
Chief, Division of Cardiothoracic Surgery, Washington University School of Medicine, St. Louis, Missouri.
The Surgical Management of Cardiac Arrhythmias

Fred A. Crawford, Jr., M.D.
Professor of Surgery and Chief, Division of Cardiothoracic Surgery, Medical University of South Carolina. Attending Surgeon, Medical University Hospital and Charleston Veterans Administration Hospital, Charleston, South Carolina.
Thoracic Incisions

Ivan K. Crosby, M.D., B.S.
Professor of Surgery, University of Virginia School of Medicine. Attending Surgeon, University of Virginia Hospital, Charlottesville, Virginia.
Acquired Disease of the Aortic Valve

Alfred T. Culliford, M.D.
Associate Professor of Surgery, New York University Medical School. Attending Cardiovascular and Thoracic Surgeon, New York University Medical Center, Bellevue Hospital, Manhattan Veterans Administration Hospital and St. Vincent's Hospital and Medical Center, New York, New York.
Postoperative Care

Gordon K. Danielson, M.D.
Professor of Surgery, Mayo Medical School. Consultant in Thoracic and Cardiovascular Surgery, Mayo Clinic, St. Marys Hospital, and Rochester Methodist Hospital, Rochester, Minnesota.
Atrioventricular Canal; Ebstein's Anomaly

Michael E. DeBakey, M.D.
Distinguished Service Professor and Chairman, Cora and Webb Mading Department of Surgery, Baylor College of Medicine. Director, National Heart and Blood Vessel Research and Demonstration Center, Baylor College of Medicine, Houston, Texas.
Aneurysms of the Sinuses of Valsalva

Aart Brutel de la Rivière, M.D.
Assistant Professor of Thoracic Surgery, University Hospital, State University at Leiden. Attending Thoracic Surgeon, University Hospital, State University at Leiden, Leiden, The Netherlands.
Univentricular Heart

Tom R. DeMeester, M.D., F.A.C.S.
Professor of Thoracic and Cardiovascular Surgery, University of Chicago, Pritzker School of Medicine. Chief, Section of Thoracic Surgery, University of Chicago Hospitals and Clinics, Chicago, Illinois.
The Pleura

William C. DeVries, M.D.
Chairman, Division of Cardiovascular and Thoracic Surgery, University of Utah Medical Center, Salt Lake City, Utah.
The Total Artificial Heart

Eugene Dong, M.D., J.D.
Associate Professor of Cardiovascular Surgery, Stanford University School of Medicine, Stanford, California.
Heart and Lung Transplantation

Donald B. Doty, M.D.
Professor, Department of Surgery, Division of Thoracic and Cardiovascular Surgery, The University of Iowa College of Medicine. Surgeon, Division of Thoracic and Cardiovascular Surgery, The University of Iowa Hospitals, Iowa City, Iowa.
Thoracic Surgery in Infants

John J. Downes, M.D.

Professor of Anesthesia and Pediatrics, University of Pennsylvania School of Medicine. Anesthesiologist-in-Chief and Director, Department of Anesthesia and Critical Care, The Children's Hospital of Philadelphia, Philadelphia, Pennsylvania.
Respiratory Support in Infants

Paul A. Ebert, M.D.

Professor and Chairman, Department of Surgery, University of California, San Francisco, School of Medicine. Chairman, Department of Surgery, University of California Hospitals, San Francisco, California.
The Pericardium

L. Henry Edmunds, Jr., M.D.

W. M. Measey Professor of Surgery and Chief of Cardiothoracic Surgery, University of Pennsylvania School of Medicine. Chief of Cardiothoracic Surgery, Hospital of the University of Pennsylvania and Children's Hospital of Philadelphia, Philadelphia, Pennsylvania.
Respiratory Support in Infants

Jesse E. Edwards, M.D.

Professor of Pathology, Graduate School, University of Minnesota, Minneapolis. Pathologist and Director, Program of Research and Training in Cardiovascular Pathology, United Hospitals, St. Paul, Minnesota.
Pathology of Coronary Atherosclerosis

F. Henry Ellis, Jr., M.D., Ph.D.

Clinical Professor of Surgery, Harvard Medical School. Chief, Department of Thoracic and Cardiovascular Surgery, Lahey Clinic Medical Center, Burlington, and New England Deaconess Hospital, Boston, Massachusetts.
Disorders of the Esophagus in the Adult; The Nissen Fundoplication

Thomas B. Ferguson, M.D.

Professor of Clinical Cardiothoracic Surgery; Washington University School of Medicine. Attending Thoracic Surgeon, Barnes Hospital and St. Louis Children's Hospital, St. Louis, Missouri.
Congenital Lesions of the Lungs and Emphysema

Robert M. Freedom, M.D., F.R.C.P. (C), F.A.C.C.

Professor of Paediatrics and Pathology, The University of Toronto Faculty of Medicine. Senior Staff Cardiologist and Director, Cardiovascular Pathology Registry, The Hospital for Sick Children, Toronto, Canada.
The Mustard Procedure

James C. A. Fuchs, M.D.

Professor of Surgery and Assistant Professor of Pharmacology, Duke University Mecical Center. Chief of Surgery, Veterans Administration Medical Center; Attending Surgeon, Duke University Medical Center, Durham, North Carolina.
Dietary and Pharmacologic Management of Atherosclerosis

Julian A. Gold, M.D., F.A.C.A.

Assistant Professor, Department of Anesthesiology, New York University School of Medicine. Assistant Attending Cardiac Anesthesiologist, New York University Hospital, Bellevue Hospital Center, and Manhattan Veterans Administration Hospital Center, New York, New York.
Anesthesia for Thoracic Surgery

Larry Goodman, M.D.

Assistant Professor of Internal Medicine and Assistant Dean of Curriculum, Rush Medical College. Attending Physician, Section of Infectious Diseases, Rush-Presbyterian-St. Luke's Medical Center, Chicago, Illinois.
The Use of Antibiotics in Cardiac and Thoracic Surgery

Vincent L. Gott, M.D.

Professor of Surgery, Johns Hopkins University School of Medicine. Staff Cardiac Surgeon, The Johns Hopkins Hospital, Baltimore, Maryland.
Heparinized Shunts for Thoracic Vascular Operations

George E. Green, M.D.
Professor of Surgery, Health Sciences Center, State University of New York at Stony Brook. Chief, Division of Cardiothoracic Surgery, Long Island Jewish-Hillside Medicine Center, New York, New York.
Internal Mammary–Coronary Artery Anastomosis for Myocardial Ischemia

Lazar J. Greenfield, M.D.
Stuart McGuire Professor of Surgery and Chairman, Department of Surgery, Medical College of Virginia, Virginia Commonwealth University. Chief of Surgery, Medical College of Virginia Hospitals, Richmond, Virginia.
Benign Tumors of the Lung and Bronchi

Hermes C. Grillo, M.D.
Professor of Surgery, Harvard Medical School. Chief of General Thoracic Surgery, Massachusetts General Hospital, Boston, Massachusetts.
Congenital Lesions, Neoplasms, and Injuries of the Trachea

Grady L. Hallman, M.D.
Clinical Professor of Cardiac and Thoracic Surgery, The University of Texas Medical School at Houston; Clinical Professor of Cardiothoracic Surgery, The University of Texas Health Science Center at San Antonio. Consultant, Cardiovascular Surgery, St. Luke's Episcopal Hospital and Texas Children's Hospital; Senior Consultant in Surgery, Texas Heart Institute, Houston, Texas.
Congenital Aortic Stenosis

John W. Hammon, Jr., M.D.
Assistant Professor of Surgery, Vanderbilt University Medical Center. Consultant, Nashville Veterans Hospital. Attending Surgeon, Vanderbilt University Hospital, Nashville, Tennessee.
Major Anomalies of Pulmonary and Thoracic Systemic Veins

Alden H. Harken, M.D.
Associate Professor of Surgery, University of Pennsylvania School of Medicine. Attending Surgeon, Hospital of the University of Pennsylvania and Children's Hospital of Philadelphia, Philadelphia, Pennsylvania.
Left Ventricular Aneurysm

Charles R. Hatcher, Jr., M.D.
Professor of Surgery and Chief of Cardiothoracic Surgery, Emory University School of Medicine. Attending Surgeon, Emory University Hospital, Crawford W. Long Memorial Hospital, and Grady Memorial Hospital, Atlanta, Georgia.
Infection, Thrombosis, and Emboli Associated with Intracardiac Prostheses

Brack G. Hattler, Jr., M.D., Ph.D.
Attending Physician, Porter Memorial Hospital and Swedish Medical Center, Denver, Colorado.
Tumors of the Heart

Lucius D. Hill, M.D.
Clinical Professor of Surgery, University of Washington School of Medicine. Head, Section of General, Thoracoesophageal, and Vascular Surgery, Virginia Mason Medical Center, Seattle, Washington.
The Hill Repair; Paraesophageal Hernia

R. Maurice Hood, M.D.
Professor of Clinical Surgery, New York University School of Medicine. Attending Surgeon, Bellevue Hospital, Veterans Administration Medical Center, and New York University Hospital, New York, New York.
Trauma to the Chest

John M. Jackson, M.D.
Assistant Professor of Anesthesiology, New York University Medical Center. Attending Anesthesiologist, New York University Medical Center, New York, New York.
Anesthesia for Thoracic Surgery

Ellis L. Jones, M.D.
Associate Professor, Department of Surgery, Emory University School of Medicine. Attending Surgeon, Emory University Hospital, Crawford W. Long Memorial Hospital, Henrietta Egleston Hospital for Children, and Grady Memorial Hospital, Atlanta, Georgia.
Infection, Thrombosis, and Emboli Associated with Intracardiac Prostheses

Siavosh Khonsari, M.B., B.Ch., F.R.C.S. (C)
Associate Professor of Cardiopulmonary Surgery, The Oregon Health Sciences University. Chief of Cardiopulmonary Surgery, Veterans Administration Hospital; Attending Cardiac Surgeon, The Oregon Health Sciences University, Portland, Oregon.
Acquired Disease of the Tricuspid Valve

James W. Kilman, M.D.
Professor of Surgery, Ohio State University College of Medicine. Chairman, Department of Thoracic Surgery, Columbus Children's Hospital; Attending Surgeon, University Hospital, Grant Hospital, and St. Anthony Hospital, Columbus, Ohio.
Congenital Mitral Stenosis

James K. Kirklin, M.D.
Assistant Professor of Surgery, University of Alabama in Birmingham School of Medicine and Medical Center, Birmingham, Alabama.
Cardiopulmonary Bypass for Cardiac Surgery; Surgical Treatment of Ventricular Septal Defect

John W. Kirklin, M.D.
Faye Fletcher Kerner Professor and Director, Division of Cardiothoracic Surgery, Department of Surgery, University of Alabama in Birmingham School of Medicine and Medical Center, Birmingham, Alabama.
Cardiopulmonary Bypass for Cardiac Surgery; Surgical Treatment of Ventricular Septal Defect

C. Frederick Kittle, M.D., LL.D.
Professor of Surgery, Rush Medical College. Senior Attending Surgeon and Director, Section of Thoracic Surgery, Rush-Presbyterian-St. Luke's Medical Center, Chicago, Illinois.
The Use of Antibiotics in Cardiac and Thoracic Surgery

Fred H. Kohanna, M.D.
Surgical Resident, Beth Israel Hospital, Boston, Massachusetts.
Thromboembolic Complications of Cardiac and Vascular Prostheses

John M. Kratz, M.D.
Assistant Professor of Surgery, Medical University of South Carolina. Attending Thoracic Surgeon, Medical University of South Carolina, Charleston Veterans Administration Medical Center, and Charleston Memorial Hospital, Charleston, South Carolina.
Thoracic Incisions

Edwin Lafontaine, M.D., F.R.C.S.(C)
Chief Resident, Section of Thoracic Surgery, University of Chicago Hospitals and Clinics, Chicago, Illinois.
The Pleura

William A. Lell, M.D.
Professor and Vice Chairman, Director, Cardiovascular Division, Department of Anesthesiology, University of Alabama in Birmingham School of Medicine and Medical Center, Birmingham, Alabama.
Cardiopulmonary Bypass for Cardiac Surgery

Stuart Levin, M.D.
Professor of Medicine, Rush Medical College. Chief, Section of Infectious Diseases, Associate Chairman, Department of Medicine; and Senior Attending Physician, Rush-Presbyterian-St. Luke's Medical Center, Chicago, Illinois.
The Use of Antibiotics in Cardiac and Thoracic Surgery

Floyd D. Loop, M.D.
Chairman, Department of Thoracic and Cardiovascular Surgery, The Cleveland Clinic Foundation, Cleveland, Ohio.
Repeat Coronary Artery Bypass Grafting for Myocardial Ischemia

James E. Lowe, M.D.
Assistant Professor of Surgery and Pathology and Established Investigator, American Heart Association, Duke University Medical Center, Durham, North Carolina.
Bronchoplastic Techniques in the Surgical Management of Benign and Malignant Pulmonary Lesions; Congenital Malformations of the Coronary Circulation; Prinzmetal's Variant Angina and Other Syndromes Associated with Coronary Artery Spasm

Philip D. Lumb, M.D., B.S.
Assistant Professor of Anesthesiology and Surgery, Duke University Medical Center. Attending Physician, Duke University Medical Center; Director, SICU Duke University Hospital (South); Co-Director SICU Duke University Hospital (North); Director, Postanesthesia Recovery Room; Chairman, Surgical Intensive Care Committee and Respiratory Therapy Advisory Committee, Duke University Medical Center, Durham, North Carolina.
Perioperative Pulmonary Physiology

James R. Malm, M.D.
Professor of Clinical Surgery, Columbia University College of Physicians and Surgeons. Chief of Thoracic and Cardiovascular Surgery, Columbia-Presbyterian Medical Center, New York, New York.
Pulmonary Atresia with Intact Ventricular Septum; Univentricular Heart

James B. D. Mark, M.D.
Johnson and Johnson Professor of Surgery and Head, Division of Thoracic Surgery, Stanford University School of Medicine. Chief of Thoracic Surgery, Stanford University Hospital, Stanford, California.
Surgical Management of Metastatic Neoplasms to the Lungs

Dwight C. McGoon, M.D.
Professor of Surgery, Mayo Medical School, Rochester, Minnesota.
Atrioventricular Canal; Truncus Arteriosus

Kathleen W. McNicholas, M.D.
Attending Physician, Pediatric Cardiothoracic Surgery, Deborah Heart and Lung Center, Browns Mills, New Jersey.
Pulmonary Atresia with Intact Ventricular Septum

Gordon F. Moor, M.D.
Attending Surgeon, Watson Clinic, Lakeland, Florida.
The Surgical Treatment of Pulmonary Tuberculosis

Richard B. Moore, M.D.
Associate Professor, Surgical Sciences, University of Minnesota Medical School and University of Minnesota Hospital, Minneapolis, Minnesota.
Partial Ileal Bypass for Control of Hyperlipidemia and Atherosclerosis

William H. Muller, Jr., B.S., M.D.
Vice President for Health Affairs, University of Virginia Medical Center. Attending Surgeon, University of Virginia Hospital, Charlottesville, Virginia.
Acquired Disease of the Aortic Valve

Eldred D. Mundth, M.D.
Professor of Surgery and Chairman, Department of Cardiothoracic Surgery, Hahnemann Medical College and Hospital, Philadelphia, Pennsylvania.
Assisted Circulation

Hassan Najafi, M.D.
Professor of Surgery, Rush Medical College. Professor and Chairman, and Senior Attending Surgeon, Cardiovascular-Thoracic Surgery, Rush-Presbyterian-St. Luke's Medical Center, Chicago, Illinois.
Aortic Dissection

George P. Noon, M.D.
Professor of Surgery, Baylor College of Medicine. Associate, Surgery Service, The Methodist Hospital, St. Luke's Episcopal Hospital, Texas Children's Hospital, and Ben Taub General Hospital, Houston, Texas.
Aneurysms of the Sinuses of Valsalva

David D. Oakes, M.D.
> Assistant Professor of Surgery, Stanford University School of Medicine. Chief, General and Thoracic Surgery, Santa Clara Valley Medical Center, San Jose, California.
> *Diaphragmatic Pacing*

C. Warren Olanow, M.D., F.R.C.P.(C)
> Assistant Professor of Medicine, Duke University Medical Center, Durham, North Carolina.
> *The Surgical Management of Myasthenia Gravis*

H. Newland Oldham, Jr., M.D.
> Professor of Surgery, Duke University Medical Center, Durham, North Carolina.
> *Cardiopulmonary Arrest and Resuscitation; The Mediastinum*

Mark B. Orringer, M.D.
> Professor of Surgery, Section of Thoracic Surgery, University of Michigan Medical School and University Hospital, Ann Arbor, Michigan.
> *Short Esophagus and Peptic Stricture*

Albert D. Pacifico, M.D.
> Professor of Surgery, Department of Surgery, University of Alabama in Birmingham School of Medicine, Birmingham, Alabama.
> *Surgical Treatment of Ventricular Septal Defect*

Donald L. Paulson, M.D., Ph.D.
> Clinical Professor, The University of Texas Health Science Center at Dallas Southwestern Medical School. Attending Thoracic Surgeon, Baylor University Medical Center; Senior Consulting Thoracic Surgeon, Parkland Memorial Hospital, Dallas, Texas.
> *Superior Sulcus Carcinoma*

Robert H. Peter, M.D.
> Professor of Medicine and Associate Director, Cardiovascular Laboratory, Duke University Medical Center, Durham, North Carolina.
> *Coronary Arteriography*

Marvin Pomerantz, M.D.
> Associate Clinical Professor of Surgery, University of Colorado School of Medicine. Staff Physician, Porter Memorial Hospital, Denver, Colorado.
> *The Diaphragm*

R. W. Postlethwait, M.D.
> Professor of Surgery, Duke University Medical Center. Chief of Staff, Durham Veterans Administration Medical Center, Durham, North Carolina.
> *Hiatal Hernia, Reflux, and Dysphagia After Vagotomy*

Francisco J. Puga, M.D.
> Assistant Professor of Surgery, Mayo Graduate School of Medicine. Staff Thoracic and Cardiovascular Surgeon, St. Marys Hospital and Rochester Methodist Hospital, Rochester, Minnesota.
> *Atrioventricular Canal*

Judson G. Randolph, M.D.
> Professor of Surgery, George Washington University School of Medicine. Surgeon-in-Chief, Children's Hospital National Medical Center, Washington, D.C.
> *Surgical Problems of the Esophagus in Infants and Children*

J. Scott Rankin, M.D.
> Assistant Professor of Surgery and Physiology, Duke University Medical Center. Attending Surgeon, Duke University Hospital, Durham, North Carolina.
> *Physiology of the Coronary Circulation and Intraoperative Myocardial Protection*

Mark M. Ravitch, M.D.
> Professor of Surgery, University of Pittsburgh School of Medicine. Surgeon-in-Chief, Montefiore Hospital, Pittsburgh, Pennsylvania.
> *Disorders of the Sternum and the Thoracic Wall*

Maruf A. Razzuk, M.D.
Associate Clinical Professor, University of Texas Health Science Center at Dallas. Attending Physician, Baylor University Medical Center and Parkland Memorial Hospital, Dallas, Texas.
Thoracic Outlet Syndrome

Bruce A. Reitz, M.D.
Professor of Surgery, Johns Hopkins University School of Medicine. Cardiac Surgeon-in-Charge, The Johns Hopkins Hospital, Baltimore, Maryland.
Heart and Lung Transplantation

Erwin Robin, M.D.
Assistant Professor of Medicine, Wayne State University School of Medicine. Chief, Section of Cardiology, Hutzel Hospital, Detroit, Michigan.
Special Diagnostic Procedures in Cardiac Surgery

David C. Sabiston, Jr., M.D.
James B. Duke Professor and Chairman, Department of Surgery, Duke University Medical Center, Durham, North Carolina.
The Mediastinum; Carcinoma of the Lung; Bronchoplastic Techniques in the Surgical Management of Benign and Malignant Pulmonary Lesions; Pulmonary Embolism; Tetralogy of Fallot; Physiology of the Coronary Circulation and Intraoperative Myocardial Protection; Congenital Malformations of the Coronary Circulation; Tumors of the Heart

Robert M. Sade, M.D.
Professor of Surgery, Medical University of South Carolina. Attending Surgeon, Medical University Hospital, Charleston, South Carolina.
Tricuspid Atresia

Edwin W. Salzman, A.B., M.A., M.D.
Professor of Surgery, Harvard Medical School. Attending Surgeon, Beth Israel Hospital, Boston, Massachusetts.
Thromboembolic Complications of Cardiac and Vascular Prostheses

Stephen W. Schwarzmann, M.D.
Associate Professor of Medicine, Infectious Diseases, Emory University School of Medicine. Attending Physician, Infectious Diseases, Emory University Hospital, Atlanta, Georgia.
Infection, Thrombosis, and Emboli Associated with Intracardiac Prostheses

Åke Senning, M.D.
Professor of Surgery, University of Zurich. Attending Surgeon, Surgical Clinic A, University Hospital, Zurich, Switzerland.
The Senning Procedure

Richard J. Shemin, M.D.
Assistant Professor of Surgery, Harvard Medical School. Attending Cardiovascular and Thoracic Surgeon, Brigham and Women's Hospital, Boston, Massachusetts.
Postoperative Care

Norman E. Shumway, M.D., Ph.D.
Professor of Cardiovascular Surgery, Stanford University School of Medicine. Chairman, Department of Cardiovascular Surgery, and Cardiovascular Surgeon, Stanford University Hospital, Stanford, California.
Heart and Lung Transplantation

David B. Skinner, M.D.
Dallas B. Phemister Professor of Surgery, University of Chicago Pritzker School of Medicine. Chairman, Department of Surgery, University of Chicago Medical Center, Chicago, Illinois.
Esophageal Hiatal Hernia: Clinical Manifestations and Diagnosis; The Belsey Mark IV Anti-Reflux Repair

Frank C. Spencer, M.D.
George David Stewart Professor of Surgery and Chairman, Department of Surgery, New York University Medical Center, New York, New York.
Endoscopy: Bronchoscopy and Esophagoscopy; Tracheal Intubation and Assisted Ventrilation; Atrial Septal Defect, Anomalous Pulmonary Veins, and Atrioventricular Canal; Acquired Disease of the Mitral Valve; Bypass Grafting for Coronary Artery Disease

Albert Starr, M.D.
Professor and Chief of Cardiopulmonary Surgery, The Oregon Health Sciences University, Portland, Oregon.
Acquired Disease of the Tricuspid Valve

Timothy Takaro, M.D.
Clinical Professor of Surgery, Duke University Medical Center, Durham. Chief, Surgical Service, Veterans Administration Medical Center, Asheville, North Carolina.
Lung Infections and Diffuse Interstitial Diseases of the Lungs

Stephen J. Thomas, M.D.
Associate Professor of Anesthesiology, New York University School of Medicine. Director of Cardiac Anesthesia, New York University Medical Center, New York, New York.
Anesthesia for Thoracic Surgery

George A. Trusler, M.D., B.Sc. (Med), M.S. (Tor.), F.R.C.S. (C), F.A.C.S. (C)
Associate Professor of Surgery, The University of Toronto Faculty of Medicine. Head, Division of Cardiovascular Surgery, The Hospital for Sick Children, Toronto, Canada.
The Mustard Procedure

G. Frank O. Tyers, M.D., F.R.C.S. (C), F.A.C.S.
Professor and Head, Division of Cardiovascular and Thoracic Surgery, The University of British Columbia Faculty of Medicine. Head, Division of Cardiovascular and Thoracic Surgery, Vancouver General Hospital and Health Sciences Centre Hospital, University of British Columbia, Vancouver, British Columbia, Canada.
Cardiac Pacemakers and Cardiac Conduction System Abnormalities

Harold C. Urschel, Jr., M.D.
Clinical Professor of Thoracic and Cardiovascular Surgery, University of Texas Health Science Center of Dallas. Attending Surgeon, Baylor University Medical Center and Parkland Memorial Hospital, Dallas, Texas.
Thoracic Outlet Syndrome

Richard L. Varco, M.D., Ph.D.
Regents' Professor of Surgery, University of Minnesota Hospitals, Minneapolis, Minnesota.
Partial Ileal Bypass for Control of Hyperlipidemia and Atherosclerosis

Nicolas Velasco, M.D.
Instructor of Surgery, University of Chile. Attending Surgeon, Hospital Jose J. Aguirre, Santiago, Chile.
The Hill Repair; Paraesophageal Hernia

Marc S. Visner, M.D.
Instructor in Surgery, University of Minnesota Medical School. Fellow, Department of Surgery, University of Minnesota Hospitals, Minneapolis, Minnesota.
Shock and Circulatory Collapse

Zeev Vlodaver, M.D.
Director, Section of Noninvasive Cardiology, Unity Medical Center, Fridley, Minnesota.
Pathology of Coronary Atherosclerosis

Andrew S. Wechsler, M.D.
Professor of General and Thoracic Surgery, Duke University School of Medicine. Surgeon, Duke University Hospital; Chief, Cardiac Surgery Section, Durham Veterans Administration Hospital, Durham, North Carolina.
The Surgical Management of Myasthenia Gravis

Samuel A. Wells, Jr., M.D.
Professor of Surgery, Washington University School of Medicine. Surgeon-in-Chief, Barnes Hospital, St. Louis, Missouri.
Immunologic Aspects of Pulmonary Neoplasms

Walter G. Wolfe, M.D.
Professor of Surgery, Duke University Medical Center, Durham, North Carolina.
Preoperative Assessment of Pulmonary Function: Quantitative Evaluation of Ventilation and Blood-Gas Exchange; Pulmonary Embolism

Magdi Yacoub, M.D.
Senior Lecturer and Recognised Teacher in Surgery, London University. Consultant Cardiac Surgeon, Harefield Hospital and National Heart Hospital; Honorary Consultant Royal Free Hospital, London, England.
Anatomic Correction of Transposition of the Great Arteries at the Arterial Level

W. Glenn Young, Jr., M.D.
Professor of Surgery, Duke University Medical Center, Durham, North Carolina.
The Surgical Treatment of Pulmonary Tuberculosis

Preface

Since the third edition of this text was published in 1976, it is astonishing to review the progress made in a wide variety of cardiothoracic disorders. Many significant changes have occurred that influence the daily practice of both cardiac and thoracic surgery. Being committed to a thoroughly updated text, the editors have placed maximal emphasis on a complete assessment of these advances and their specific application. This is evidenced by the number of new authors and of new subjects not covered in the previous edition.

In recent years, a distinctive trend in all disciplines of surgery has been toward a more thorough integration of the fundamental medical sciences, including physiology, biochemistry, pharmacology, immunology, pathology, and genetics, into everyday clinical practice. These changes have brought clearly into focus that the discriminating student, resident, and practicing cardiothoracic surgeon insist on these features if a text is to meet current standards of acceptance. An example of a field in which tremendous strides and indeed an entirely new dimension of thinking have occurred is that represented by intraoperative protection of the myocardium. In the present edition, this subject is reviewed in considerable detail, particularly in view of its major role in improvement of long-term postoperative results. Other new sections representing significant progress in the past 5 years include such subjects as surgical management of cardiac dysrhythmias, myasthenia gravis, the anatomic correction of transposition of the great arteries, repeat coronary artery bypass procedures for myocardial ischemia, and the emerging field of variant angina with its associated components of spasm as well as vascular lesions. Other additions include the sections on "Surgical Management of Metastatic Neoplasms to the Lung," "Bronchoplastic Techniques in the Surgical Management of Benign and Malignant Pulmonary Lesions," "Paraesophageal Hernia," and a completely updated chapter on the "Total Artificial Heart." As in any text, succeeding editions include new authors to assure fresh, vibrant, and fully contemporary contributions. Thus, in the present edition, more than half of the authors are new and are making contributions for the first time.

The editors hold a strong conviction concerning the importance of illustrations. The total number of illustrations in this edition is greatly increased over the previous one, and a number of former figures have been replaced with selections of better quality. Experience has emphasized repeatedly that readers both appreciate and utilize appropriate illustrations, and in each instance the figures in the present edition have been selected from among the very best in the literature. When such were not available, they have been specially drawn. Attention has also been directed toward a complete update of the bibliography to provide the reader with the most current sources. Similarly, the annotated references have been expanded and updated, allowing the reader to be aware of those contributions in the literature considered the most significant as well as providing a summary of their contents.

It is apparent that the text is the product of much hard work by many authors, and the editors wish to express their sincere thanks to each contributor. We are especially indebted to Mr. Carroll C. Cann of the W. B. Saunders Company, who has allowed a number of changes to be made at the last minute, a difficult feature in modern publishing, in order to assure that the latest information be included in this edition. The medical profession has long been accustomed to the high quality of the work characteristic of Saunders. Once again, unfailing attention to every detail and maintenance of their traditional standards are apparent in this edition and are gratefully acknowledged.

DAVID C. SABISTON, JR.
FRANK C. SPENCER

Acknowledgments

The fourth edition of *Surgery of the Chest* is composed of the contributions of a number of outstanding authorities in the field. Each has provided a section carefully balanced in the pathogenesis, diagnosis, and management of every topic, with appropriate attention to both the basic science and clinical balance. Our special thanks are due Ms. Carolyn Naylor and Ms. Karen McFadden of the W. B. Saunders staff who have been totally cooperative in all requests, including those of the most exacting detail.

Our gratitude is also extended to Mr. Robert C. Butler and his colleagues in the Production Department of Saunders who have maintained and expanded the high quality of reproduction and have reduced to a remarkable minimum the time required for publication, especially in view of the high quality of the finished product. To Ms. Margaret Shaw we are especially indebted for the special attention to the illustrations, particularly in view of the expanded number in this edition.

Finally, as in previous editions, the editors acknowledge their deepest appreciation and recognition to Ms. Kathryn Slaughter. She has reviewed each contribution in the most minute detail from inception to the finishing touches. Her standards of editorial perfection have served as a stimulus to each of us in seeking the very best in accuracy, expression, style, and content. As in other editions, her loyalty and enthusiasm for the entire process are gratefully acknowledged.

DAVID C. SABISTON, JR.
FRANK C. SPENCER

Contents

Chapter 24

Disorders of the Esophagus in the Adult

F. Henry Ellis, Jr.

Esophageal surgery is chiefly a twentieth-century development. It became possible only after the development of techniques that permitted safe access to intrathoracic structures. Subsequent advances required better understanding of the function of the esophagus, made possible by the development of techniques that permitted measurement of normal and abnormal esophageal behavior.

Chief among these techniques is esophageal manometry, perfected largely in the laboratories of Ingelfinger (1958) in Boston and Code and associates (1958) at the Mayo Clinic. For the first time, the surgeon was provided with the information necessary to direct operative management of esophageal problems along physiologic lines. Before this time, the esophagus had been considered basically a conduit to allow ingested material to reach the stomach, and operations on it were based on anatomy. In this chapter, emphasis will be placed on the physiology of the esophagus under normal and abnormal conditions, and discussions of surgical management will stress restoration of normal physiology.

HISTORICAL ASPECTS

Because of the inaccessibility of the intrathoracic portion of the esophagus, surgery was first confined to its cervical and intra-abdominal portions. The first operations on the esophagus were probably for the purpose of draining cervical abscesses resulting from foreign body perforation or for the removal of foreign bodies. The first recorded operation for removal of a foreign body from the cervical portion of the esophagus was performed by Goursand of France in 1738, and following it, a number of case reports of successful operations emanated from the continent and Great Britain. David Cheever of Boston is said to have performed the first successful esophagotomy in the United States in 1864. A pharyngoesophageal diverticulum was first successfully resected by Wheeler of Dublin in 1886. Billroth (1871) thought that localized carcinomas of the cervical esophagus were resectable, and his assistant Czerny first successfully resected and reconstructed the cervical esophagus in a patient with carcinoma as early as 1877. Carcinoma of the cardia was first attacked surgically by von Mikulicz in 1898.

Although his patient died, his efforts were finally brought to fruition by Voelcker, who successfully resected a malignant lesion of the cardia in 1908.

Surgery for esophageal achalasia was initiated by von Mikulicz (1903), who performed retrograde dilation of the esophagogastric junction through a gastrotomy. This initial surgical effort was followed by a series of abdominal procedures on the lower esophagus and cardia designed to facilitate gastric emptying. These included the Wendel cardioplasty (1910) and the Heyerovsky (1911) and Backer-Gröndahl (1916) esophagogastrostomies, which found considerable favor in Germany. It was not until Barrett and Franklin's paper in 1949, however, that the surgical world was alerted to the fact that such destructive procedures, although relieving esophageal obstruction, led inevitably to severe reflux esophagitis.

Heller's classic contribution to the surgical management of esophageal achalasia was reported in 1913 but was not widely practiced in his home country. Although originally a double myotomy, the Heller procedure was later modified in a number of ways but chiefly by the performance of a single myotomy across the esophagogastric junction (de Bruïne-Groeneveldt, 1918). Modifications of the single myotomy procedure are currently widely used when surgery is performed for esophageal achalasia.

Even though the intrathoracic portion of the esophagus remained out of the surgeon's reach for many years, a variety of ingenious reconstructive techniques were devised, primarily for the management of esophageal strictures secondary to ingestion of caustic materials. Some of these are still in use in modified form today. In 1905, Beck and Carrell, American surgeons, suggested a technique of antethoracic reconstruction of the esophagus using a tube of greater curvature of the stomach, a procedure first successfully performed by Jianu of Hungary in 1912. In 1907, Roux proposed using an isolated limb of jejunum for this purpose, and Lexer modified this procedure in 1908. His modification, which was basically an esophagodermatojejunogastric reconstruction, was the most common type of reconstructive procedure used at the time of Ochsner and Owens' exhaustive review of the subject in 1934.

A transpleural esophagectomy with staged reconstruction was not performed until 1913. The first one was performed by Torek, who, paradoxically, never performed a successful similar procedure afterward. Not until 1933 was a successful one-stage esophagogastrectomy and esophagogastrostomy for carcinoma of the cardia reported (Ohsawa, 1933). In 1937, Marshall (1938) of the Lahey Clinic was the first to perform such an operation successfully in the United States. His technique was followed the next year by the frequently discussed operation of Adams and Phemister (1938). Subsequent advances in esophageal resection have been concerned primarily with modifications in technique and have included in recent years a better understanding of the physiologic consequences of such procedures.

ANATOMY

Gross Anatomy

The esophagus is a tubular structure extending from the pharynx at the level of the sixth cervical vertebra to the stomach, which it joins within the peritoneal cavity opposite the body of the eleventh thoracic vertebra (Fig. 24–1). It measures approximately 24 cm. in length in the adult. At its upper end, the entrance to the esophagus is guarded by the upper esophageal sphincter (UES), which is composed primarily of the cricopharyngeus muscle. This muscle runs transversely across the posterior wall of the esophagus,

connecting the two lateral borders of the cricoid cartilage (Zaino *et al.*, 1970) (Fig. 24–2). This muscle is bordered superiorly by the oblique fibers of the inferior pharyngeal constrictor muscle, which pass upward and backward from their origin on the thyroid cartilage and insert into a median raphe. Inferiorly, the cricopharyngeus muscle blends into the circular and longitudinal muscle fibers of the upper esophagus, which lies in the midline immediately posterior to the trachea before its entry into the thorax. There, it curves slightly to the left behind the great vessels and returns to the midline at the level of the aortic arch. It then inclines to the right as it continues in the posterior mediastinum. Ultimately, it crosses the thoracic aorta to the left of the midline and angles anteriorly to pass through the diaphragmatic hiatus, which is a noose of fibers made up predominantly of the right crus of the diaphgram, with varying contribution from the left crus. Other variations occur in the structure of the diaphragmatic hiatus; in the most common variation, the noose of muscular tissue receives equal contributions from both right and left diaphragmatic crura (Carey and Hollingshead, 1955).

There is an intra-abdominal esophageal segment of variable length before the organ joins the stomach. External identification of the esophagogastric junction may be difficult. Perhaps the best landmark is a sling of gastric muscle fibers (collar of Helvetius). This is a structure difficult, if not impossible, to identify, except at autopsy (Fig. 24–3). From a practical standpoint,

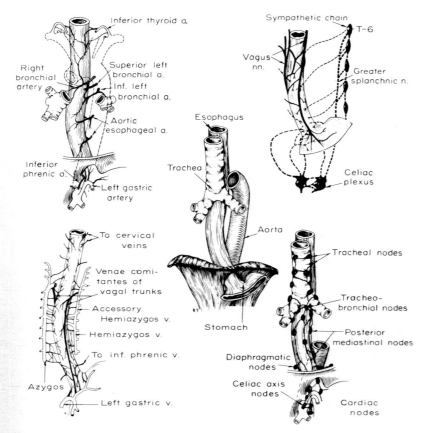

Figure 24–1. Anatomy of the human esophagus. Arterial supply *(upper left)*; venous drainage *(lower left)*; innervation *(upper right)*; lymph nodes *(lower right)*. (From Ellis, F. H., Jr.: The esophagus. *In* Christopher's Textbook of Surgery. 8th Ed. Edited by L. Davis. Philadelphia, W. B. Saunders Company, 1964, p. 593.)

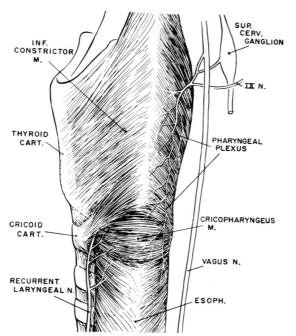

Figure 24–2. Anatomy of the pharynx and upper esophagus, posterolateral view. (From Ellis, F. H., Jr.: Upper esophageal sphincter in health and disease. Surg. Clin. North Am., *51*:554, 1971.)

the esophagogastric junction can best be described as that point where the esophageal tube meets the gastric pouch. In the past, much emphasis has been placed on the cardiac incisura or the angle of His between the esophagus and the stomach. This emphasis is highly

misleading, for the angle is not a constant finding, and many patients do not exhibit it at all. The phreno-esophageal ligament or membrane, first described by Laimer in 1883, helps to hold the distal esophagus loosely in place. Composed of mature collagenous fibers, this structure is a continuation of the transverse fascia of the abdominal parietes. It receives contributions from the endothoracic fascia and pleura above and the peritoneum below, and the fibers themselves fan out to insert into the lower 2 to 3 cm. of the esophagus in the region of the lower esophageal sphincter.

Histology

Histologically, the esophageal wall is composed of an inner circular layer of muscle and an outer longitudinal layer without a surrounding serosal covering (Higgs *et al.*, 1965b). The muscle layers consist of both striated and smooth muscle. Striated muscle composes the upper fifth of the organ, caudad to which is a middle zone where striated muscle and circular muscle are mixed. In the lower three fifths to one third of the esophagus, smooth muscle predominates. The transition zone occurs at a more cephalad level in the circular layer than in the longitudinal layer. With few exceptions (Pera *et al.*, 1975), no evidence for an anatomic sphincter at the lower end of the esophagus has been presented.

The mucous membrane of the esophageal lining is composed of stratified squamous epithelium. Occasionally, ectopic islands of gastric mucosa have been

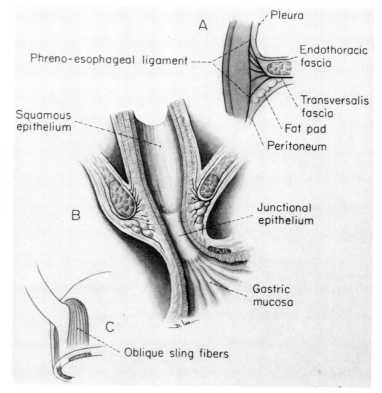

Figure 24–3. Gross anatomy of the region of the esophagogastric junction. *A*, Details of origin and insertion of phrenoesophageal membrane. *B*, Cross-section of distal esophagus and proximal stomach. *C*, Oblique gastric sling fibers. (From Payne, W. S., and Ellis, F. H., Jr.: Esophagus and diaphragmatic hernias. *In* Principles of Surgery. Edited by S. I. Schwartz. New York, McGraw-Hill, 1969, p. 870. Copyright 1969 by McGraw-Hill, Inc.)

identified, usually in the middle or upper portions of the esophagus. A prominent submucosa contains mucous glands, blood vessels, Meissner's plexus of nerves, and a rich network of lymphatic vessels. Transition from a squamous layer to a layer of junctional columnar epithelium occurs 1 to 2 cm. cephalad to the esophagogastric junction. The squamocolumnar junction is not well defined, since it is serrated in character. This junctional epithelium merges gradually with typical gastric mucosa distally in the stomach.

Vascular Supply

The blood supply is provided in the cervical portion of the esophagus by the inferior thyroid arteries and in the thoracic portion by branches from the aorta and by esophageal branches of the bronchial arteries (Swigert *et al.*, 1950). Supplemental vessels come from arteries on the abdominal side of the diaphragm as well as from branches of the intercostal arteries. The venous drainage is more complex (Butler, 1951). Subepithelial venous channels course longitudinally to empty above into the hypopharyngeal veins and below into the gastric veins. These channels also penetrate the esophageal muscle, from which they receive branches. They leave the esophagus to form a periesophageal plexus; the longest trunks of this plexus accompany the vagus nerves. Venous drainage from the cervical portion of the esophagus is into the inferior thyroid and vertebral veins. Drainage from the thoracic portion is into the azygos and hemiazygos veins, and from the abdominal portion, into the left gastric vein.

Lymphatic Drainage

The lymph vessels run longitudinally in the wall of the esophagus before penetrating the muscle layers to reach regional lymph nodes. Leaving the esophagus, these channels drain into the nearest group of nodes. Within the thorax these nodes are usually identified by their location as tracheal, tracheobronchial, posterior mediastinal, and diaphragmatic. In the upper esophagus, lymphatic channels drain into the cervical nodes, and in the lower esophagus, into gastric and celiac nodes.

Innervation

The esophagus is innervated by both the parasympathetic and the sympathetic systems. In the neck, the parasympathetic supply is mediated through branches of the recurrent laryngeal nerves and by branches from the ninth and tenth cranial nerves and the cranial root of the eleventh nerve. The vagus nerves lie on either side of the esophagus for most of their course, forming a plexus about it. As the hiatus is approached, two major trunks emerge, the left one coming to lie an-

teriorly and the right one posteriorly. The vagal plexus is joined by mediastinal branches of the thoracic sympathetic chain of the splanchnic nerves. The cervical esophagus receives its sympathetic supply from the pharyngeal plexus; lower down, it is supplied by fibers from the superior and inferior cervical sympathetic ganglia. Below the diaphragm, the esophagus receives fibers from the left greater splanchnic nerves, from the celiac plexus, and from plexuses around the left gastric and inferior phrenic arteries. The vagal trunk sends branches directly to the voluntary muscles of the esophagus and to the smooth muscle by parasympathetic preganglionic fibers. There they synapse with the myenteric plexus of Auerbach (located between the inner circular and outer longitudinal layers) as well as with the plexuses of Meissner. Some unmyelinated fibers from the vagi pass directly to the muscular fibers of the muscularis mucosa. Afferent fibers are carried through both vagal and sympathetic nerves and do not synapse with the ganglion cells in the enteric plexuses. Terminal sensory nerve elements rising from widely branching filaments form a rich intramucosal network and communicate with the myenteric plexuses.

PHYSIOLOGY

Although the esophagus was long considered an inert organ acting as a passive conduit for ingested

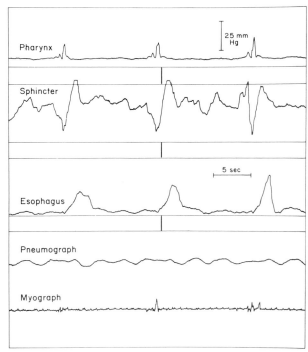

Figure 24–4. Deglutitive pressures at the pharyngoesophageal junction. Note relaxation of pressure in sphincter as pressure in pharynx increases. Sphincteric contraction follows relaxation to initiate esophageal peristalsis. (From Ellis, F. H., Jr.: The esophagus: Physiology. *In* Davis-Christopher Textbook of Surgery. 12th Ed. Edited by D. C. Sabiston, Jr. Philadelphia, W. B. Saunders Company, 1981, p. 797.)

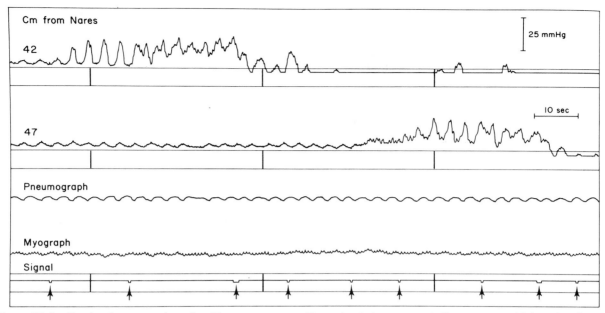

Figure 24–5. Resting lower esophageal sphincter pressures. Upward-pointing arrows indicate 1-cm. withdrawals of recording catheter. (From Ellis, F. H., Jr.: The esophagus: Physiology. *In* Davis-Christopher Textbook of Surgery. 12th Ed. Edited by D. C. Sabiston, Jr. Philadelphia, W. B. Saunders Company, 1981, p. 798.)

material, advances in radiographic techniques, and particularly the introduction of techniques for measuring intraluminal pressures, have disclosed that the esophagus is an active organ with a finely tuned, coordinated mechanism designed to propel ingested material from the pharynx to the stomach. At either end of this organ is a sphincter mechanism designed to prevent regurgitation of luminal contents from one portion of the gastrointestinal tract to another (Code and Schlegel, 1967).

At the upper end of the esophagus, resting pressures disclose a zone of increased pressure approximately 3 cm. in length that relaxes promptly with swallowing and contracts thereafter as a wave of high pressure passes through it. Resting pressures of the upper esophageal sphincter (UES) vary from 25 to 100 mm. Hg, with an average of 56 mm. Hg (Fig. 24–4). Contractions of this sphincter are in peristaltic sequence with those of the pharynx above and those of the esophagus below, and the primary peristaltic wave of the esophagus is thus initiated. This wave of positive pressure sweeps in an orderly peristaltic fashion down the body of the esophagus. The intensity of pressure so generated reaches between 40 and 80 mm. Hg, and pressure is somewhat more forceful in the lower esophagus than in the upper esophagus. Resting pressures in the intrathoracic portion of the esophagus are normally less than atmospheric, reflecting negative intrathoracic pressure at the lower end of the esophagus. Straddling the hiatus is another high-pressure zone, measuring 3 to 5 cm. in length and with pressures ranging from 10 to 18 mm. Hg. This zone is more or less equally divided into intra-abdominal and intrathoracic portions (Fig. 24–5). In response to a swal-

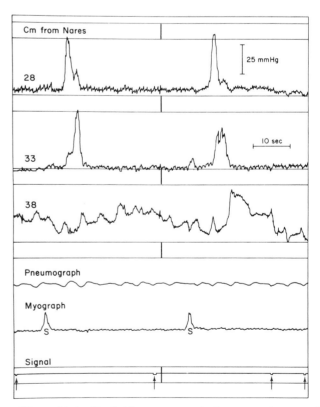

Figure 24–6. Deglutitive pressures in lower esophagus and sphincter. Sphincteric relaxation anticipates arrival of peristaltic wave (S = swallow). Upward-pointing arrows indicate 1-cm. withdrawal of recording catheter. (From Ellis, F. H., Jr.: The esophagus: Physiology. *In* Davis-Christopher Textbook of Surgery. 12th Ed. Edited by D. C. Sabiston, Jr. Philadelphia, W. B. Saunders Company, 1981, p. 798.)

lowing effort, relaxation of this zone of increased pressure can be identified manometrically. Sphincteric contraction follows relaxation, and thus, the esophagus is emptied of ingested material and of any material that might have refluxed during a period of sphincteric relaxation (Fig. 24–6).

The competence mechanism at the lower end of the esophagus is an important one, although its nature remains controversial. Factors that have been suggested as important include the diaphragm, a valve flap mechanism, the gastric sling fibers, and the oblique angle of entry of the esophagus into the stomach, as well as the mucosal rosette at the esophagogastric junction. Although an anatomic sphincter cannot usually be demonstrated, a physiologic mechanism at the lower esophagus clearly exists and normally prevents gastroesophageal reflux. This physiologic sphincter, perhaps aided by prominent folds of mucosa at the esophagogastric junction, constitutes the main antireflux mechanism.

A consensus exists that intrinsic lower esophageal sphincter (LES) tone is the major mechanism that prevents gastroesophageal reflux (Cohen and Harris, 1971; Pope, 1967). However, other studies have failed to corroborate a close correlation between the level of LES pressure and the presence or absence of reflux, a difference probably accounted for by variables in patient selection for manometry (Dodds *et al.*, 1981).

TABLE 24–1. REGULATION OF LOWER ESOPHAGEAL PRESSURE*

INCREASE	DECREASE
Hormones	
Gastrin	Secretin
Motilin	Cholecystokinin
Substance P	Glucagon
Vasopressin	Gastric inhibitory polypeptides
	Vasoactive intestinal polypeptides
	Progestational agents
Drugs	
α-Adrenergic agonist	α-Adrenergic antagonist
Norepinephrine	Phentolamine
Phenylephrine	β-Adrenergic agonist
Cholinergic	Isoproterenol
Bethanechol	Anticholinergic
Methacholine	Atropine
Anticholinesterase	Theophylline
Edrophonium	
Betazole	
Metoclopramide	
Miscellaneous	
Prostaglandin F_{2a}	Prostaglandins E_1, E_2, A_2
Protein meal	Nicotine
Gastric alkalinization	Ethanol
	Fat meal
	Chocolate
	Gastric acidification

*Modified from Castell, D. O.: The lower esophageal sphincter: Physiologic and clinical aspects. Ann. Intern. Med.,*83*:390, 1975.

Esophageal peristalsis is primarily under vagal control (Diamant and El-Sharkawy, 1977). The region of the lower esophageal sphincter is well supplied with adrenergic and cholinergic nerves. Both α-adrenergic and β-adrenergic receptors are present in abundance, with the former mediating contraction and the latter relaxation, a characteristic of circular muscle sphincters. The vagus nerve exerts a predominantly inhibitory influence on the sphincter (Tuch and Cohen, 1973). However, sphincteric relaxation has been identified in the dog even after complete denervation, suggesting a certain degree of autonomy of the lower sphincter (Mann *et al.*, 1968). Another important characteristic of the lower sphincter, which appears to be under vagal control, is its adaptive response to an increase in intragastric pressure. This consists of a rise in sphincteric pressure equal to or in excess of the increase in intragastric pressure caused by abdominal compression (Crispin *et al.*, 1967; Lind *et al.*, 1966).

Not only is lower esophageal sphincteric pressure under nervous control, but also its resting tone has been shown to respond to the gastrointestinal hormones and a variety of other agents (Table 24–1).

DIAGNOSTIC TECHNIQUES

Accurate diagnosis of esophageal disease requires a variety of diagnostic techniques, many of them only recently developed. These include various radiographic techniques, endoscopy, and measurement of the intraluminal pressures of the esophagus, as well as the determination of potential difference and pH changes at different intraluminal sites.

Radiologic Techniques

Proper radiographic examination of the esophagus requires a fluoroscopic device that amplifies the image electronically. Television display of the image permits it to be recorded on magnetic tapes, which allow repeated review of the study. Cinefluorography is extremely useful, particularly in studies of abnormalities of the pharynx and of the upper esophagus, in which events occur extremely rapidly. In addition, cinefluorography is an important tool in teaching and research, especially when combined with other techniques, such as manometry and the measurement of electrical activity of the mucous membrane and muscularis. The best contrast medium is a water suspension of barium sulfate, although a water-soluble contrast medium is advisable when perforation is suspected.

Radiographic studies are not the best way to identify the presence or absence of pathologic reflux, since about 25 per cent of patients undergoing the usual radiographic tests for reflux will exhibit its presence for no apparent reason (Linsman, 1965). Radiographic studies do, however, play a role in screening out patients in whom no reflux can be demonstrated despite the performance of abnormal maneuvers, such as abdominal compression, the Valsalva test, and so forth. A serious question arises, of course, as to whether gastroesophageal reflux is of any significance if it must be provoked by an event not usually occurring in ordinary life. Other more sensitive tests must be used to confirm a suspected diagnosis of gastroesophageal reflux.

Endoscopy

Endoscopy permits direct visualization and instrumentation of the interior of the esophagus and of the esophagogastric junction. It provides confirmation of information obtainable by radiographic or physiologic studies. It also provides pathologic verification of the nature of intraluminal esophageal pathology either by biopsy of the lesion or from cytologic study of smears and washings. In addition, it is useful in localizing the site of upper gastrointestinal bleeding.

The introduction of the flexible fiberscope has greatly simplified endoscopic examination of the esophagus. The original esophagoscopes were rigid instruments, which were difficult and sometimes dangerous to use. Currently, the rigid instrument is usually reserved for the removal of foreign bodies. Esophageal perforation, particularly in the cervical region, occurred in approximately 1 per cent of examinations performed with the rigid esophagoscope (Wychulis *et al.*, 1969a). This complication is far less frequent with the fiberoptic instrument because of its flexibility. Endoscopic studies constitute an important facet of the preoperative evaluation of any patient with esophageal disease.

Physiologic Studies

Manometry. The measurement of intraluminal pressures within the esophagus has become an important and reliable diagnostic technique in the evaluation of esophageal disease, particularly esophageal disease characterized by abnormalities of esophageal motility. Manometric studies are performed using saline-filled polyethylene or polyvinylchloride tubes with open-end or lateral orifices. The customary assembly consists of three or four tubes with orifices spaced 5 cm. apart connected to external strain-gauge manometers. Currently, the use of a constantly infused system, first suggested by Pope (1967), is most widely employed, for it has been proved to be more accurate and reproducible than other methods. The pressure changes are recorded graphically by an appropriate recorder.

Before performance of a test, the catheter assembly is either swallowed or passed through a nostril into the stomach. The assembly is then withdrawn at 1-cm. intervals while a continuous pressure recording is obtained with the patient in the supine position. Resting pressures are thus recorded, and the assembly is reinserted. Deglutitory responses of the esophagus are measured after each 1-cm. withdrawal of the assembly. The third aspect of this study concerns the adaptive response of the lower esophageal sphincter (Lind *et al.*, 1966). The assembly is inserted so that the distal unit lies in the stomach, the middle unit lies in the high-pressure zone, and the proximal unit lies in the body of the esophagus. Pressures in these three locations are measured before and after increasing intragastric pressure by manual compression on the abdominal wall or by the Valsalva maneuver and straight leg raising.

pH Reflux Test. The pH reflux test is an extremely sensitive measure of the presence or absence of gastroesophageal reflux, exceeding in sensitivity both manometry and cinefluorography. In this test, 200 to 300 ml. of 0.1 normal hydrochloric acid is injected into the stomach, a pH electrode is placed 5 cm. above the esophagogastric junction, and the pH is recorded at this point while the patient performs deep breathing and Valsalva, Müller, and coughing maneuvers in various positions. A fall in pH to below 4.0 is indicative of the existence of gastroesophageal reflux. This test is usually considered the most sensitive method for measuring gastroesophageal reflux (Skinner and Booth, 1970). The introduction by Johnson and De Meester (1974) of the technique of 24-hour pH monitoring of the distal esophagus has added a new dimension to the diagnosis of esophageal conditions. This technique is particularly useful in patients with complicated diagnostic problems.

Acid Cleaning Test. This test is used in patients with documented evidence of gastroesophageal reflux and measures the ability of the esophagus to clear regurgitated gastric contents. A prolonged acid clearance test is considered an abnormal finding and indicates a potentially bad prognosis in terms of the development of esophagitis and its complications.

Miscellaneous Studies. ACID PERFUSION TEST. The acid perfusion test was developed by Bernstein and Baker (1958) as a means of differentiating pain of esophageal origin from that of angina pectoris. Although possibly a useful screening test in patients with bizarre retrosternal or upper abdominal pain, its high incidence of false-negative and false-positive results detracts from its usefulness.

POTENTIAL DIFFERENCE DETERMINATION. Measurement of the potential difference (PD) between the inside and the outside of the stomach and of the esophagus has been found useful in identifying the squamocolumnar mucosal junction. In some laboratories, this measurement is an integral part of the routine diagnostic esophageal motility test (Helm *et al.*, 1965). In the normal individual, a sharp change in the measured PD is detected as the measuring unit is withdrawn from the stomach to the esophagus, and the site of change from gastric glandular mucosa to squamous esophageal epithelium is thus identified. When combined with manometry, this test may be useful in diagnosing a sliding esophageal hiatal hernia. However, when columnar epithelium lines the lower esophagus (Barrett esophagus), the change in PD does not accurately define the esophagogastric junction.

SCANNING TECHNIQUES. The use of radioactive scanning in the diagnosis of esophageal disease is relatively new. Technetium-99m (^{99m}Tc) scanning has been used to identify mucosal changes in patients with a Barrett esophagus and to diagnose tumors of the esophagus. Malmud and associates (1976) suggested that technetium scanning is a safe and sensitive noninvasive method of detecting and quantitating gastroesophageal reflux.

ESOPHAGEAL MOTILITY DISTURBANCES

The development of techniques for measuring intraluminal pressures within the esophagus, as described in the preceding section, now permits classification of many conditions of the esophagus according to their specific abnormal motility patterns. It is therefore possible not only for heretofore undiagnosable symptoms to be explained by distinct disease entities but also for surgical therapy to be directed along proper physiologic lines. It is useful in discussing these motility abnormalities to suggest a classification of esophageal motility disturbances (Table 24–2). The discussion of these abnormalities is simplified by separating the organ into (1) the upper sphincter and (2) the body of the esophagus and lower sphincter.

TABLE 24–2. ESOPHAGEAL MOTILITY DISTURBANCES

UPPER ESOPHAGEAL SPHINCTER
  Central nervous system disease
    Cerebrovascular accident
    Parkinson's disease
    Bulbar poliomyelitis
    Multiple sclerosis
    Amyotrophic lateral sclerosis
  Muscular diseases
    Muscular dystrophy (myotoxic, oculopharyngeal)
    Inflammatory (dermatomyositis, hypothyroidism)
    Myasthenia gravis
  Miscellaneous conditions
    Radical oropharyngeal surgery
    Cricopharyngeal "spasm"
    Premature contraction (pharyngoesophageal diverticulum)

BODY OF ESOPHAGUS AND LOWER ESOPHAGEAL SPHINCTER
  Achalasia
  Diffuse spasm
  Hypotensive lower esophageal sphincter
    Idiopathic
    Hiatal hernia
    Postoperative
    Scleroderma
  Miscellaneous conditions
    Dermatomyositis
    Myasthenia gravis
    Muscular dystrophy
    Cerebrovascular accident
    Parkinson's disease
    Amyotrophic lateral sclerosis
    Diabetic neuropathy
    Alcoholic neuropathy

Upper Esophageal Sphincter

Oropharyngeal dysphagia or cervical esophageal dysphagia is a symptom complex characterized by hesitation in the initiation of swallowing, sticking of food or liquids in the throat, and postdeglutitive cough and aspiration. A variety of diseases may be responsible for oropharyngeal dysphagia (Table 24–2). Abnormalities of sphincteric relaxation are said to characterize central nervous system lesions, whereas the muscle diseases interfere with effective pharyngeal contraction (Fischer et al., 1965). Cricopharyngeal myotomy has occasionally been used with success in such instances (Hurwitz and Duranceau, 1978). Difficulty in swallowing has also been reported after extensive operations on the oropharynx, presumably because of impaired function of the cricopharyngeal muscle. Cricopharyngeal myotomy has been suggested as a means of avoiding this complication (Mladick et al., 1971).

Spasm of the UES is another possible cause of oropharyngeal dysphagia, and hypertension of the UES has been reported in patients with globus sensation in the throat (Watson and Sullivan, 1974), some of whom may have radiographic evidence of "hypopharyngeal bar" (Fig. 24–7).

Pharyngoesophageal Diverticulum

A pharyngoesophageal diverticulum is the most common diverticulum of the esophagus. First described by Ludlow in 1767, the condition has been well recognized for many years. After Ludlow's description, von Ziemssen in 1875 collected 22 cases from the literature and added five of his own.

The condition usually occurs in elderly patients and is manifested by a false diverticulum, the esophageal mucosa presenting between the oblique fibers of the inferior constrictor muscle of the pharynx and the transverse fibers of the cricopharyngeus muscle. The radiographic appearance of a pharyngoesophageal diverticulum is diagnostic (Fig. 24–8). In some series, the incidence of coexisting hiatal hernia has been high, and the resulting gastroesophageal reflux has been said to be associated with high pressures in the upper sphincter. An etiologic relationship between the two has been suggested (Hunt et al., 1970; Smiley et al., 1970). Ellis and Crozier (1981), however, have shown that UES pressures are low in patients with upper esophageal pouches.

Cricopharyngeal spasm (Lahey, 1946) and cricopharyngeal achalasia (Sutherland, 1962) have been postulated as possible causes of upper esophageal pouches, but esophageal motility studies have failed to confirm these theories. Instead, incoordination of relaxation and contraction has been identified in patients with pharyngoesophageal diverticulum (Ellis and Crozier, 1981; Ellis et al., 1969; Lichter, 1978). This may be significant etiologically and is in keeping with earlier reported radiographic findings, suggesting that such patients may exhibit premature contraction of the

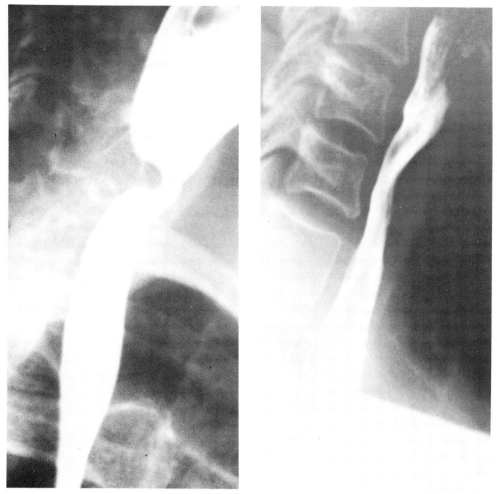

Figure 24–7. Lateral roentgenograms in a patient with hypertension of the upper esophageal sphincter before *(left)* and after *(right)* cricopharyngeal myotomy. (From Ellis, F. H., Jr.: The esophagus. *In* Practice of Surgery. Edited by H. S. Goldsmith. Hagerstown, Maryland, Harper and Row Publishers, 1979, p. 20.)

sphincter (Ardran and Kemp, 1961). As illustrated in Figure 24–9, this incoordination is characterized by an abnormal temporal relationship between pharyngeal contraction and cricopharyngeal sphincteric relaxation and contraction. In patients with such abnormalities, sphincteric contraction occurs before completion of contraction of the pharynx.

Single-stage resection has for many years been the preferred method of treatment. Since the pouch usually presents to the left, it is exposed through either a left vertical or a curved transverse cervical incision (Fig. 24–10, *top*). The diverticulum is reached by retracting the thyroid gland and larynx medially and by retracting the carotid sheath and sternocleidomastoid muscle laterally. The mucosal sac is dissected carefully up to its neck so that the surrounding ring of the muscular defect is clearly defined. A curved clamp is placed across the neck of the sac at a right angle to the long axis of the esophagus, and the sac is amputated flush with the esophagus. Interrupted fine silk sutures are placed in the mucosa as it is being incised (Fig.

24–10, *middle*). Alternatively, the diverticulum can be excised with a mechanical stapler (Hoehn and Payne, 1969). The suture line is then covered by the adjacent musculature of the pharynx and the upper esophagus using interrupted sutures (Fig. 24–10, *bottom*). A small Penrose drain is placed near the site of repair in the retrovisceral space and brought to the outside through the lower end of the incision. The operation carries minimal risk even in debilitated and elderly patients, and recurrences are rare (3 per cent [Welsh and Payne, 1973]). To prevent recurrences, concomitant cricopharyngeal myotomy should be performed (Belsey, 1966; Cross *et al.*, 1961).

Cricopharyngeal myotomy alone usually suffices for all but the larger diverticula (4 cm. or larger in diameter), and it is a simpler yet equally effective approach (Ellis and Crozier, 1981; Ellis *et al.*, 1969) (Fig. 24–11). The exposure is the same as for diverticulectomy. After the diverticulum is freed to its neck, the transverse fibers of the cricopharyngeus muscle bordering the inferior margin of the neck of the diver-

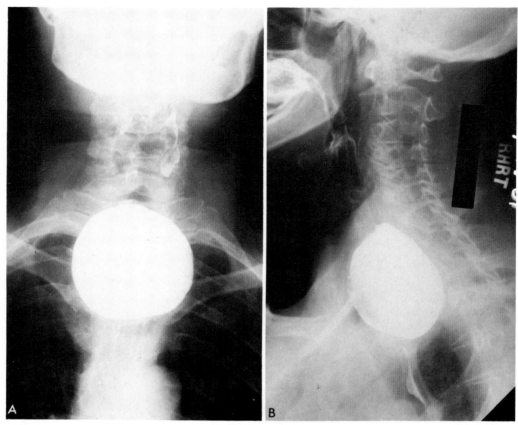

Figure 24–8. Posteroanterior (*A*) and lateral (*B*) esophagograms of a patient with typical pharyngoesophageal diverticulum. From Payne, W. S., and Clagett, O. T.: Pharyngeal and esophageal diverticula. *In* Current Problems in Surgery. Edited by M. Ravitch. Chicago, Year Book Medical Publishers, Inc., 1965.)

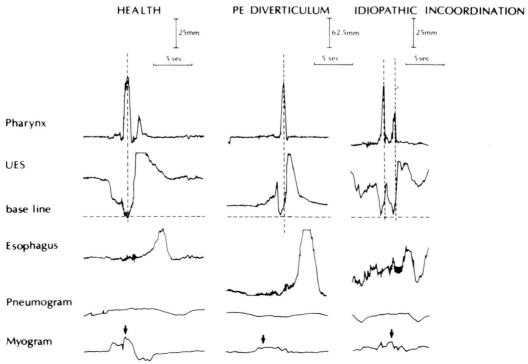

Figure 24–9. Deglutitive responses of the upper esophageal sphincter (UES) in health *(left)*, pharyngoesophageal diverticulum *(middle)*, and idiopathic incoordination *(right)*. Vertical dotted line is drawn through the point of peak pharyngeal contraction. Only in health *(left)* does it coincide with the maximal point of relaxation of the UES (downward) = swallow). (From Ellis, F. H., Jr., and Crozier, R. E.: Cervical esophageal dysphagia: Indications for and results of cricopharyngeal myotomy. Ann. Surg., *194*:283, 1981.)

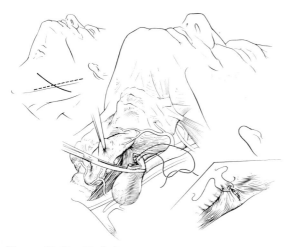

Figure 24–10. Technique of one-stage pharyngoesophageal diverticulectomy. *Top,* Surgical incision employed when neck is explored from the left. *Middle,* Exposure obtained during removal of diverticulum. The curved clamp has been placed across the neck of the sac, and the sac is being amputated and the esophageal mucosa closed with the use of "cut and sew" technique. *Bottom,* Layer closure of esophagus is completed with approximation of musculofascial tissue. (From Ellis, F. H., Jr.: The esophagus. *In* Christopher's Textbook of Surgery. 8th Ed. Edited by L. Davis. Philadelphia, W. B. Saunders Company, 1964, p. 602.)

ticulum are identified and incised vertically. The incision is carried down to the mucosa and extended caudally onto the esophagus; the length of the incision averages 3 cm. After the muscular incision is completed, the mucosal layer is freed of its encircling muscle for about half of its circumference to permit it to pout through the incision.

Body of Esophagus and Lower Sphincter

Motility disturbances of the body of the esophagus and of its lower sphincter are listed in Table 24–2. Diffuse spasm of the esophagus is characterized by hypermotility, hypotensive LES by hypomotility, and achalasia by some of both characteristics. In addition, there is a miscellaneous group of conditions about which less is known and for which the treatment is uncertain.

Achalasia

Esophageal achalasia is a disease of unknown etiology characterized by absence of peristalsis in the body of the esophagus, a high resting pressure at the

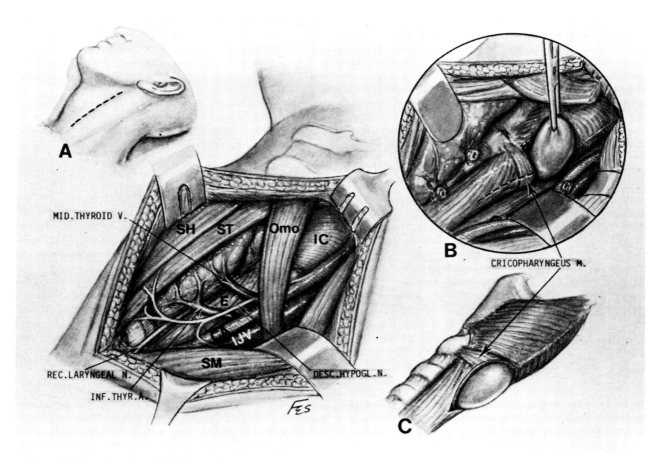

Figure 24–11. Operative field for performance of cricopharyngeal myotomy is displayed in middle drawing. *A,* Incision. *B,* Omohyoid, middle thyroid vein, and inferior thyroid artery have been divided, thyroid and trachea retracted, and diverticulum freed. Dotted line indicates site of proposed myotomy. *C,* Appearance of completed myotomy. (SH = sternohyoid; ST = sternothyroid; Omo = omohyoid, IC = inferior pharyngeal constrictor muscle; E = esophagus; CA = carotid artery; SM = sternocleidomastoid muscle; IJV = internal jugular vein.) (From Ellis, F. H., Jr., and Crozier, R. E.: Cervical esophageal dysphagia: Indications for and results of cricopharyngeal myotomy. Ann. Surg., *194*:284, 1981.)

lower esophageal sphincter, and failure of the lower esophageal sphincter to relax in response to swallowing. It was first described in 1674 by Thomas Willis, whose patient successfully treated himself for many years by bougienage. A variety of causes for the disease have been proposed, including weakness of the esophagus; spasm of the esophagus; mechanical factors, such as external compression or trauma; and congenital factors. Now, however, it is generally agreed that it has a neurogenic basis. This theory is supported by pathologic evidence in the form of absence of or diminution in number of the ganglion cells of Auerbach's plexus, a finding first reported by Rake in 1926. This abnormality is demonstrable at all levels of the thoracic esophagus, although it is more prominent in the body of the organ than at its lower end (Cassella et al., 1964).

The cause of these changes is unknown, and it is not understood whether they represent a primary or secondary manifestation of the disease. That the primary site of the disorder may be in the extra-esophageal nerve supply, in the vagus nerve itself, or in its central nuclei has been suggested by pathologic studies of biopsy and autopsy material (Cassella et al., 1964, 1965) and by experiments involving selective destruction of the motor nuclei of the vagus nerve in the cat and in the dog (Higgs et al., 1965a). Support for this concept has been provided by others (Lise et al., 1972). It has been suggested that a neurotropic virus of marked specificity may be involved, attacking the neurons in both the brain and the esophageal wall and traveling along the vagi between these points (Smith, 1970).

Other evidence for an extraesophageal site of denervation in achalasia has been provided by studies using cholinesterase inhibitor. These studies show a normal response of the sphincter, indicating local release of acetylcholine, a finding that supports preganglionic and not postganglionic denervation (Cohen et al., 1972; Misiewicz et al., 1969). The recent finding of supersensitivity of the lower sphincter to endogenous and exogenous gastrin provides further suggestive evidence in favor of denervation (Cohen and Guelrud, 1971). In addition, other evidence of vagal dysfunction in patients with achalasia includes the presence of abnormalities of gastric secretion that can be demonstrated in nearly half of the patients studied (Woolam et al., 1967).

In Brazil and other South American countries where the leishmanial forms of Trypanosoma cruzi exist, changes in Auerbach's plexus have been demonstrated in patients with Chagas' disease, who appear to have an esophageal condition indistinguishable from achalasia (Atias et al., 1963).

Symptomatology. Whatever the cause of esophageal achalasia may be, its clinical manifestations are well recognized. Obstruction to swallowing is the most common and usually the earliest symptom of the disease, occurring in nearly all patients. Often, the patient finds that food passes more readily when it is warm. Not infrequently, solid food passes more readily than liquids, particularly cold liquids in the early stages of the disease. This contrasts with the dysphagia experienced by patients with carcinoma or stricture.

Regurgitation is the second most common symptom, occurring in 70 per cent of patients. It is particularly noticeable at night, when nocturnal regurgitation may give rise to aspiration and respiratory symptoms. Pain is infrequent, being present in a little more than one fourth of patients. When present, it is usually an early symptom, and it may be difficult to distinguish the pain of achalasia from the pain of diffuse esophageal spasm. When achalasia of the esophagus is of long standing, loss of weight almost invariably occurs.

A familial incidence of achalasia is not demonstrable. It is commonly encountered in young and middle-aged adults. The highest incidence at the time of treatment is in patients between the ages of 30 and 60, although it may occur in children. It is a relatively uncommon disease, occurring at an annual incidence of 0.6 per 100,000 population, with equal frequency in the two sexes (Earlam et al., 1969). The disease is progressive, usually exhibiting progressive dilatation of the esophagus, yet the progression is not nearly as predictable as might be expected, for the duration of symptoms does not always correlate with the size of the esophagus. The most serious potential complication of untreated achalasia is the development of carcinoma of the esophagus, which usually occurs in the middle portion of the esophagus (Just-Viera et al., 1967). The incidence of esophageal carcinoma in patients with achalasia has been estimated at 41 cases per year per 100,000 population; this is approximately ten times the incidence of the disease in the white male population (Wychulis et al., 1971).

Diagnosis. The earliest radiographic evidence of esophageal achalasia is that of obstruction at the esophagogastric junction with proximal dilatation. As the disease progresses, the classic radiographic signs develop (Fig. 24–12). The esophagus is dilated, and the lower portion of the lumen appears conical and narrowed for a short distance, with a beak-like extension directed into the narrowed segment. Although esophageal achalasia in its more advanced forms has radiographic characteristics that distinguish it from carcinoma, it may not be differentiated easily in its early stages. Esophagoscopy is essential at this stage to distinguish early achalasia from carcinoma or benign esophageal stricture.

Confirmation of the clinical diagnosis of esophageal achalasia can be provided by studies of esophageal motility (Fig. 24–13). When constantly infused catheters are used, resting lower sphincteric pressures are found to be two or more times the level found in normal individuals. This elevated pressure has been related to the supersensitivity of the sphincter to endogenous gastrin (Cohen and Guelrud, 1971; Cohen et al., 1971). Resting pressures in the body of the esophagus are usually elevated over those of fundic pressures as a result of dilatation and retention, whereas pressures in the upper sphincter are usually in the normal range.

Abnormal function of the lower esophageal

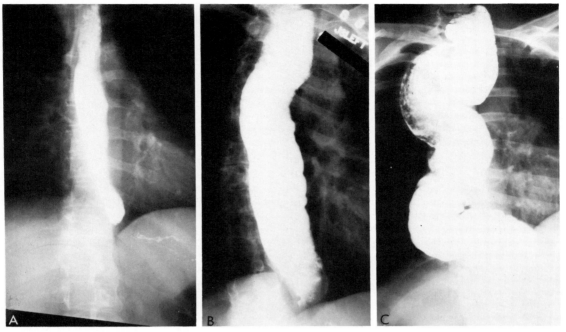

Figure 24–12. Roentgenographic appearance of (*A*) mild, (*B*) moderate, and (*C*) severe achalasia of the esophagus.

sphincter consists of failure of relaxation. In particular, the upper segment of the sphincter fails to relax completely in response to swallowing, and this is accompanied by premature restoration of tone in the sphincter with evidence of premature contraction. All of these abnormalities combine to limit the period during which the esophagus is capable of emptying (Butin *et al.,* 1953). Thus, both relaxation and contraction of the achalasic sphincter are abnormal. In addition, peristalsis does not occur in the body of the esophagus. Swallowing is followed by a modest elevation of pressure, which is simultaneous throughout the organ. The amplitude is usually less than in health.

The term "vigorous achalasia" has been applied to patients who have an abnormal achalasic pattern of contractions but in whom the strength of the contractions is equal to or exceeds that seen in health. These contractions are nearly always repetitive and resemble in some respects the findings in patients with diffuse spasm. Sphincteric relaxation is rarely seen in vigorous achalasia, whereas the sphincter relaxes normally in diffuse spasm (Sanderson *et al.,* 1967).

Treatment. In the past, medical efforts to relieve the symptoms of patients with achalasia by reducing or eliminating the distal esophageal obstruction have been unsuccessful. Although pharmacologic agents

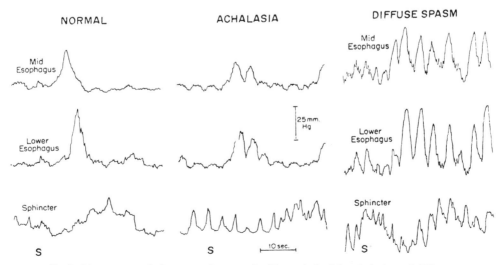

Deglutitive pressures in lower esophagus and sphincter in health, achalasia, and diffuse spasm.

Figure 24–13. Deglutitive pressures in lower esophagus and sphincter in health, achalasia, and diffuse spasm. (From Ellis, F. H., Jr.: The esophagus. *In* Practice of Surgery. Edited by H. S. Goldsmith. Hagerstown, Maryland, Harper and Row Publishers, 1979, p. 27.)

may be developed in the future that will be effective in reducing or eliminating the hypersensitivity of the achalasic sphincter to gastrin and thus relieve the distal esophageal obstruction, current therapeutic efforts are designed to weaken the sphincter by mechanical or surgical methods, since no effective method is currently available to restore peristalsis to the body of the esophagus.

The use of dilation in the treatment of esophageal achalasia has a long and successful history. Only by employing forceful dilation can success be achieved. Forceful dilation may be accomplished in a variety of ways by employing mechanical, pneumatic, or hydrostatic dilators. Two thirds to three fourths of patients treated with forceful dilation have been reported to have had good to excellent results (Okike *et al.*, 1979; Vantrappen and Hellemans, 1980). Significant complications occur in about 5 per cent of patients, many of whom require surgical intervention because of inadvertent rupture of the distal esophagus. Although clearly a valuable form of treatment of esophageal achalasia, this therapy is not without complications and often must be repeated to be effective.

Since the results of surgical treatment with the modified Heller myotomy have proved to be superior to forceful dilation, it should be the treatment of choice in this disease in all but patients in whom operation is contraindicated. The treatment has been shown to be more effective if performed early in the course of the disease before the development of marked esophageal dilatation with elongation and tortuosity. Surgical therapy is clearly the treatment of choice in children and in patients with the vigorous form of the condition, since forceful dilation has been unsuccessful in most such individuals.

A variety of surgical efforts to relieve the distal esophageal obstruction in patients with achalasia have been proposed, most of which involve destruction of the lower esophageal sphincter (Backer-Gröndahl, 1916; Heyerovsky, 1913; Wendel, 1910). Many of these procedures were popular until it was shown that severe reflux esophagitis almost invariably followed their performance (Barrett and Franklin, 1949). Fortunately, operations of this type are seldom used today, for they are obviously contraindicated. Current surgical therapy stems historically from the double cardiomyotomy first performed by Heller in 1913. The technique later underwent many modifications, the most important of which was restriction of the procedure to one myotomy (De Bruïne-Groeneveldt, 1918) and more recently to a myotomy that is primarily restricted to the distal esophagus (Ellis *et al.*, 1967).

Results of surgery are closely dependent on the technique used, especially with regard to the avoidance of postoperative reflux esophagitis. A thoracotomy is the preferred approach because it provides the

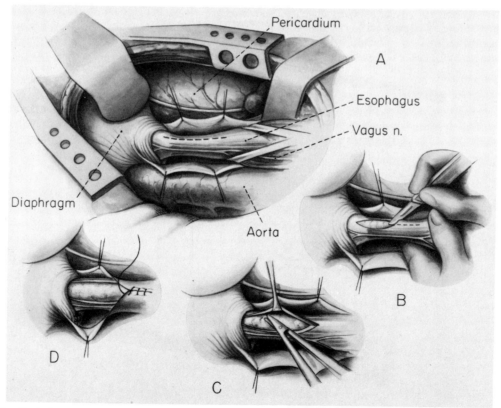

Figure 24–14. Technique of esophagomyotomy. *A,* Operative exposure—dotted line indicates line of incision. *B,* Beginning the incision. *C,* Dissection of muscle from mucosa. *D,* Restoration of esophagogastric junction to intra-abdominal position with suture narrowing of esophageal hiatus if necessary. (From Ellis, F. H., Jr., Kiser, J. C., Schlegel, J. F., *et al.*: Esophagomyotomy for esophageal achalasia: Experimental, clinical, and manometric aspects. Ann.Surg., *166*:646, 1967.)

most direct access to the distal esophagus (Fig. 24–14A). The distal esophagus is mobilized without dividing its hiatal attachments, with care being taken to preserve the vagus nerves. By gentle elevation of the distal esophagus, a longitudinal myotomy is begun on the left anterolateral surface of the organ (Fig. 24–14B). The incision is deepened through the encircling muscles of the lower end of the esophagus down to the mucosa and is extended distally just across the esophagogastric junction to ensure complete division of the distal esophageal musculature. An incision through the gastric musculature is a limited one, always less than 1 cm., and is usually only a few millimeters in length. The incision is then extended proximally onto the dilated, thick-walled portion of the esophagus in order to ensure total division of the circular muscle. The incision varies in length, depending on the anatomic circumstances of the particular patient, but it is usually between 5 and 7 cm. long. After the myotomy is completed, the muscle wall is dissected laterally from the mucosa so that approximately half of the circumference of the esophageal mucosa is freed, permitting it to pout freely through the incision (Fig. 24–14C). This maneuver is performed to minimize the possibility of reapproximation of the incised esophageal wall by scar in the postoperative period. It may occasionally be necessary to narrow the esophageal hiatus (Fig. 24–14D) or to repair a small coexisting diaphragmatic hernia. However, if care is taken not to disturb the supporting structures of the distal esophagus at the diaphragm, ancillary maneuvers in the region of the hiatus should rarely be necessary.

Fear of postoperative reflux esophagitis has led some to combine an antireflux procedure with myotomy (Mansour et al., 1976; Peyton et al., 1974). Not only does this unnecessarily complicate the surgical approach, but also it has potential inherent dangers, since an overly zealous wrap of the distal esophagus in an aperistaltic organ can lead to postoperative dysphagia.

Although the reported results of the Heller operation vary considerably in the literature, reflux esophagitis being reported in 1 to 30 per cent of patients so treated, the results of employing the technique as described are extremely satisfactory. Approximately 94 per cent of patients are improved, and demonstrable reflux esophagitis occurs in no more than 3 per cent (Ellis and Olsen, 1969; Ellis et al., 1980; Okike et al., 1979).

Diffuse Spasm of the Esophagus

Diffuse spasm of the esophagus occurs less frequently than esophageal achalasia and differs from it in that deglutition induces normal sphincteric relaxation. Esophageal motility studies demonstrate high-amplitude, nonperistaltic, often repetitive contractions in the body of the esophagus in response to swallowing. LES pressures may be normal or elevated, and, as mentioned, sphincteric relaxation occurs normally in response to swallowing (Code et al., 1960; Creamer et al., 1958) (Fig. 24–13). There is very little evidence, if any, to suggest that the condition is related to esophageal achalasia, although cases of vigorous achalasia may pose a problem in diagnosis since they possess some of the characteristics of diffuse esophageal spasm.

Differentiation of diffuse spasm of the esophagus from esophageal achalasia and from vigorous achalasia can usually be made on clinical grounds (Olsen and Creamer, 1957). Pain is far more pronounced in diffuse spasm than in other conditions, and dysphagia occurs intermittently or not at all. The pain is typically substernal, often radiating through to the back, up to the neck and ears, or even into the arms, suggesting angina pectoris. It varies from a sensation of discomfort beneath the lower sternum to severe colicky pain. Although it may be provoked by eating, the pain usually comes on spontaneously and even awakens the patient at night. Patients so afflicted tend to be high-strung and nervous, and the diagnosis of psychoneurosis is often entertained.

Although esophageal radiography will show normal findings in about half of patients suffering from these disorders, their appearance can occasionally explain the use of such terms as pseudodiverticulosis, functional diverticula, segmental spasm, curling or corkscrew esophagus, and idiopathic muscular hypertrophy of the esophagus (Fig. 24–15). A small diaphragmatic hernia or epiphrenic diverticulum frequently coexists.

The use of an extended esophagomyotomy for the treatment of patients with "diffuse nodular myomatosis of the esophagus" was suggested in 1950 by Lortat-Jacob. A similar approach was undertaken at the Mayo Clinic in 1956 in an effort to control the symptoms in carefully selected patients with hypermotility disorders of the esophagus (Ellis et al., 1960).In many respects, the operation resembles that used for achalasia. However, the lower esophageal sphincter is spared if it is normotensive, and the proximal limit of the esophageal muscular incision varies, depending on the preoperative estimate of the extent of the disease as defined by esophageal manometry. The incision may extend to the aortic arch or higher (Fig. 24–16). An associated diaphragmatic hernia is repaired concomitantly, and the diverticulum, if present, is excised.

Surgical treatment is less effective for hypermotility disorders of the esophagus than it is for esophageal achalasia, only approximately two thirds to three fourths of the patients so treated being benefited (Ellis et al., 1964; Ferguson et al., 1969). In a series of 11 patients with diffuse spasm of the esophagus reported by Leonardi and associates (1977) in which greater efforts to spare the lower esophageal sphincter were taken, the improvement rate was 91 per cent. Patients should be selected carefully for this operation. The ideal candidate is an emotionally stable individual with serious disability from the disease but without evidence of associated gastrointestinal problems. Evidence of the severity of the disease should be demon-

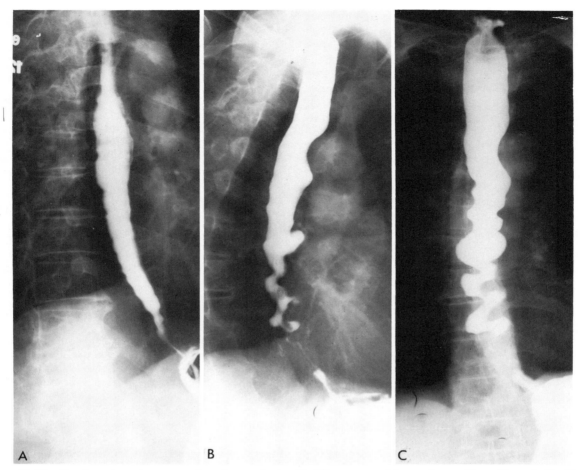

Figure 24–15. Esophageal roentgenograms from three patients with diffuse spasm of the esophagus. (From Olsen, A. M., Harrington, S. W., Moersch, A. J., and Andersen, H. A.: The treatment of cardiospasm: Analysis of a twelve-year experience. J. Thorac. Cardiovasc. Surg., *22*:166, 1951.)

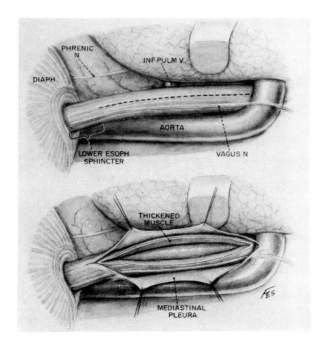

Figure 24–16. Technique of extended esophagomyotomy. Note that the incision spares the LES. (From Leonardi, H. K., Shea, J. A., Crozier, R. E., *et al.*: Diffuse spasm of the esophagus: Clinical, manometric, and surgical considerations. J. Thorac. Cardiovasc. Surg., *74*:739, 1977.)

strable in the form of a markedly abnormal esophageal motility pattern. Ideally, this evidence should be associated with radiographic evidence of esophageal spasm.

Epiphrenic Diverticulum

It is important to emphasize the high incidence of diverticula of the lower esophagus in patients with esophageal motility abnormalities, particularly those abnormalities characterized by hypermotility. Rarely are symptoms related to the diverticulum, and if diverticulectomy alone is performed, symptoms may persist. For this reason, any patient with an epiphrenic diverticulum should undergo esophageal manometry to ascertain the nature of the underlying motility disturbance. Such a disturbance should be treated concomitantly by a long esophagomyotomy (Debas et al., 1980). The preoperative and postoperative esophageal radiographs of such a patient are shown in Figure 24–17.

Hypotensive LES

In the past, reflux was thought to occur mainly in patients with a sliding esophageal hiatal hernia, but it is now clear that it may occur in many other conditions (Table 24–2) and that it represents a physiologic rather than an anatomic abnormality. The concept has been advanced that LES incompetence may be due to a diminished release of endogenous gastrin. Lipshutz and associates (1973) have shown that the lower esophageal sphincter in patients with reflux responds normally to stimulants that act directly on the muscle and to exogenous pentagastrin, but it responds abnormally to stimuli that release endogenous gastrin from the antrum. Others, however, have found no correlation between the level of endogenous gastrin and lower sphincter pressure (Hollenbeck et al., 1974).

Reflux secondary to a hypotensive LES may occur without any anatomic abnormality (Cohen and Harris, 1971; Hiebert, 1970). In infants, the term "chalasia" has been applied to the presence of free regurgitation, and it has been shown that sphincteric tone is low in infants and young children (Gryboski, 1965). Usually, but not always, sphincteric tone approaches normal as the child grows and develops, and abnormal reflux ceases.

The relationship between a sliding esophageal hiatal hernia and gastroesophageal reflux has been

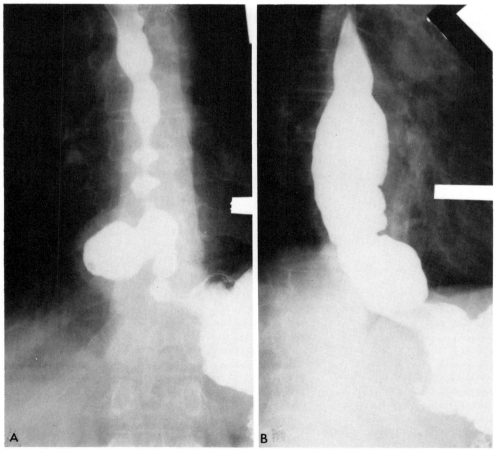

Figure 24–17. Esophageal roentgenograms (A) before and (B) after excision of epiphrenic diverticulum and long esophagomyotomy in a patient with diffuse esophageal spasm. (From Ellis, F. H., Jr.: The esophagus. In Christopher's Textbook of Surgery. 8th Ed. Edited by L. Davis. Philadelphia, W. B. Saunders Company, 1964, p. 603.)

emphasized for many years, yet only a minority of patients with this anatomic abnormality have reflux. Cohen and Harris (1970) have emphasized that it is the level of pressure at the LES, not the hernia, that is important in the cause of reflux. Some have even considered the hernia to be the result rather than the cause of reflux secondary to an incompetent sphincter (Johnson, 1966). Destructive operations on the cardia obviously lead to a reduction in sphincteric pressure and to free gastroesophageal reflux. Reflux has been demonstrated after subtotal gastrectomy, which has been attributed to the lowering of sphincteric tone by a reduction of endogenous gastrin (Windsor, 1964). Vagotomy, although sometimes resulting in obstructive symptoms, may lessen the tone of the lower sphincter and lead to reflux (Crispin et al., 1967).

Perhaps the most common systemic disease resulting in hypotension of the lower esophageal sphincter is scleroderma. When the esophagus is involved, the characteristic changes are fragmentation and homogenization of the submucosal connective tissue elements coupled with atrophy of the smooth muscle. Motor failure of the esophagus is a characteristic manometric finding and may often precede the development of systemic symptoms. Symptoms, when they develop, are the result of the involvement of the LES with loss of gastroesophageal competence (Garrett et al., 1971).

Hypotension of the LES has also been described in patients with pernicious anemia (Farrell and Castell, 1972). In this condition, the lower esophageal sphincter fails to respond normally to a variety of stimulants. This suggests that the musculature of the LES is defective in this disease. Smoking has also been shown to reduce the resting tone of the LES (Stanciu and Bennett, 1972), as has the ingestion of a number of different foods, notably fat (Babka and Castell, 1973). A number of hormones have been shown to reduce the level of pressure in the lower sphincter, particularly secretin and glucagon (Thomas and Earlam, 1973).

Regardless of the cause of hypotension of the LES, the symptoms are the same. They consist of substernal pain, heartburn, and regurgitation with accentuation of the symptoms with bending and recumbency. Nocturnal regurgitation with aspiration may occasionally be a complication. Major complications are the development of severe ulcerative esophagitis with bleeding or stricture formation or both. To avoid these complications, early diagnosis and treatment are advisable.

The diagnosis of hypotension of the LES is made manometrically and confirmed by endoscopic evidence of esophagitis both macroscopically and histologically and by objective evidence of reflux as demonstrated by cinefluorography or by the pH reflux test. Initial treatment should be medical therapy to reduce reflux or to minimize the damaging effects of regurgitating acid gastric juice. This includes dietary and pharmacologic means to lower the level of gastric acidity coupled with measures to minimize reflux, such as antacids, weight reduction, avoidance of constricting garments, and elevation of the head of the bed at night.

When medical measures fail, one or the other of the so-called sphincter-enhancing operations may be employed. These include posterior gastropexy (Hill), Mark IV (Belsey), and fundoplication (Nissen) procedures, which will be described in Chapter 25. All of these operations partially encircle varying lengths and amounts of the distal esophagus with adjacent gastric fundus and are accompanied by an increase in sphincteric pressure and by relief of gastroesophageal reflux.

Miscellaneous Conditions

As indicated in Table 24–2, a variety of miscellaneous conditions may affect the motility of the body of the esophagus and its lower sphincter. Although dysphagia may occur in most of the collagen diseases, as discussed earlier, it is encountered most frequently in dermatomyositis; an incidence of 60 per cent has been reported in one series (Donoghue et al., 1960). The motility abnormalities that occur in the body of the esophagus resemble those seen in scleroderma, although the integrity of the lower esophageal sphincter is usually preserved.

As is true of the upper esophageal sphincter, neuromuscular disorders may have an adverse effect on the function of the body of the esophagus and its lower sphincter. The most striking abnormalities are seen in patients with disorders that are primarily myotonic in origin, such as myasthenia gravis and myotonia dystrophica (Fischer et al., 1965). Rarely do esophageal motility studies give normal results in such patients. The amplitude of the peristaltic waves is decreased in myasthenia gravis, and the waves disappear in the lower esophagus during repetitive swallowing. Motor failure of the esophagus also occurs in myotonia dystrophica, a condition in which both smooth and striated muscles are affected.

A variety of nonspecific abnormalities, usually involving changes in peristalsis, may be seen in patients with central and peripheral neurologic disorders. An increase in the number of simultaneous waves may occur, or esophageal spasm may be demonstrated. Some of these changes are seen in patients with hemiplegia or Parkinson's disease. In amyotrophic lateral sclerosis, the most common finding is feeble peristaltic contractions in place of the vigorous contractions seen normally (Smith et al., 1957). Contractions are simultaneous and may be repetitive. Sphincteric changes are relatively less common. In multiple sclerosis, a variety of abnormalities may be noted, including poor relaxation of the gastroesophageal sphincter, simultaneous deglutition waves, incoordination of the swallowing complex, and diffuse spasm of the esophagus. Some patients with diabetic neuropathy of long standing have been found to have a decreased amplitude of peristaltic contractions throughout the esophagus and to have lowered sphincteric pressures (Silber, 1969). Neuropathy associated with alcoholism has also been implicated in esophageal dysfunction. Lack of primary peristalsis in the distal one third of the esophagus is the most common abnormality (Winship *et al.*, 1968). The term "presbyesophagus" has been used to describe abnormalities of esophageal motility in the aged. Studies in men aged 71 to 87 years, however, suggest that, with the exception of a reduction in amplitude of peristaltic contractions, elderly individuals exhibit abnormal esophageal motor function no more often than do healthy young subjects (Hollis and Castell, 1974).

STRICTURES

Caustic Strictures

Strictures resulting from the ingestion of solid or liquid caustics are most frequently encountered in children who have accidentally swallowed the material or in adults who have ingested the material for suicidal purposes (Leape *et al.*, 1971). The chemicals most commonly implicated in corrosive burns of the esophagus include alkaline caustics, acids or acid-like corrosives, and household bleaches. Lye, in the broad sense of the term, includes strong alkalis, most commonly sodium or potassium hydroxide. Most of the household cleaning agents, such as Dran-O, Liquid Plumr, and Easy-Off, contain one of these corrosive agents. Burns from the ingestion of such agents may involve the oral pharynx, larynx, esophagus, and stomach; 25 to 50 per cent of patients with oral burns have an esophageal injury. Successful management involves prompt recognition and early treatment.

Symptoms range from minimal to those of profound shock. If there is an associated burn of the larynx, dyspnea may be present. Prompt identification of the etiologic agent with early administration of an appropriate neutralizing agent and accurate assessment of the extent of the injury are important. Early esophagoscopy (within 12 to 48 hours) is indicated (except in very young children, in whom the risk of perforation is high) to determine whether or not an esophageal injury has occurred and, if it has, its extent. The administration of corticosteroids has been said to lessen the degree of stricture formation (Haller and Bachman, 1964), although the evidence is not conclusive. In one series, strictures developed in 83 per cent of those not treated with either steroids or antibiotics but in only 13 per cent of those in whom both were used (Campbell *et al.*, 1977). Such therapy associated with antibiotics is initiated promptly and is continued for 3 to 6 weeks. Subsequent management depends to a great extent on the severity of the esophageal injury. In the absence of obvious contraindications, clear liquids can be given orally and the diet can be progressively increased as tolerated. Radiographic examination of the esophagus at 10- to 14-day intervals determines whether or not a stricture is developing (Fig. 24–18). Stricture formation is a rela-

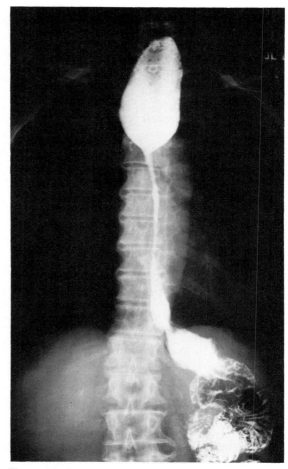

Figure 24–18. Roentgenographic examination of a patient with an extensive lye stricture of the esophagus. (From Rosenow, E. C., III, and Bernatz, P. E.: Chemical burns of the esophagus. *In* The Esophagus. Edited by W. S. Payne and A. M. Olsen. Philadelphia, Lea & Febiger, 1974, p. 143.)

tively late development in 5 to 10 per cent of patients (Borja *et al.*, 1969).

Bougienage is probably best deferred until after the first 3 to 4 weeks and should never be instituted unless stricture formation has been identified. The more severe the burn, the sooner the onset of stricture. Most patients with evidence of stricture can be managed satisfactorily by a graduated program of esophageal dilation performed at regular intervals.

Unfortunately, despite all appropriate measures, it is sometimes not possible to maintain an esophageal lumen. In such instances, gastrostomy with retrograde dilations is an alternative therapeutic approach. In some instances, nothing short of esophageal replacement will suffice to restore the swallowing mechanism. This can be accomplished best by a colon interposition procedure, the new esophagus being fashioned by a segment of colon, preferably the left, placed substernally between the pharynx above and the stomach below. The results are generally good, with a low operative risk. Other alternatives include gastric transposition and use of the Gavriliu gastric tube. If the proximal extent of the burn so dictates, the proximal anastomosis may have to be performed to the pharynx and extensive oropharyngeal reconstruction may be necessary. When lesser amounts of the esophagus are involved, the site of the stricture may be approached transthoracically and either resected or bypassed with a segment of jejunum or colon.

Caustic esophageal stricture is a precancerous lesion. In patients followed for at least 24 years, the risk of cancer of the esophagus developing was said to be increased a thousandfold (Kiviranta, 1952). Cancers engrafted on an esophagus injured by caustic agents account for 1 to 4 per cent of all cancers of the esophagus, and the average interval from injury to its development is about 40 years (Hopkins and Postlethwait, 1981).

Reflux Esophagitis and Stricture

The most common type of esophageal stricture is that secondary to the reflux of acid or alkaline secretions into the esophagus caused by esophagogastric incompetence as a result of a hypotensive lower esophageal sphincter. Although reflux of acid peptic juices is a far more common event, the marked sensitivity of the esophageal mucosa to the damaging effects of both acid and alkaline secretions has repeatedly been identified. The combination of both acid and alkaline reflux has been said to be particularly deleterious to the esophageal mucosa (Gillison et al., 1972). Regardless of the nature of the damaging agent, the disease is characterized pathologically by a pattern of alternating destruction and healing. It is a continuous process that may stop at any stage or may progress finally to severe fibrosis and the formation of a stricture with resulting dysphagia.

Although the extent of inflammation and esophageal scarring that may result from esophageal reflux varies widely, strictures of the esophagus secondary to reflux are basically of three types: (1) those occurring at the esophagogastric junction, (2) those occurring at a high level in the esophagus at the squamocolumnar junction but well above the true esophagogastric junction, and (3) long strictures involving the distal third or half of the esophagus. This division into three distinct types has clinical significance because treatment varies according to type.

Low Strictures. Strictures that occur at the esophagogastric junction are the most common and are frequently associated with organic shortening of the esophagus due to extensive fibrous tissue replacement of the organ (Fig. 24–19*A*). As a result, restoring the esophagogastric junction to its normal intraabdominal position may be difficult, even with extensive mobilization of the intrathoracic esophagus. In some instances, the degree of shortening may be such that normal anatomy cannot be restored. Although many have debated the existence of shortening of the esophagus, few with extensive experience in the field would deny its occasional occurrence. That it is an acquired condition and not congenital, except in the most exceptional circumstances, is generally agreed.

High Strictures. Strictures that occur at a higher level, often at the level of the aortic arch, are associat-

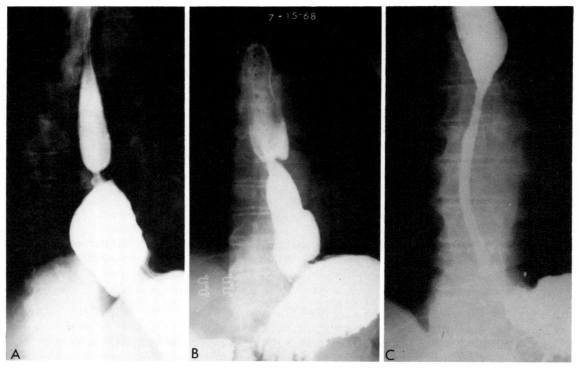

Figure 24–19. Roentgenograms of the esophagus in three patients with strictures of different anatomic varieties. *A*, Short esophagus and hiatus hernia with stricture. *B*, High esophageal stricture in a patient with a columnar lined lower esophagus. *C*, Long esophageal stricture characteristic of hyperemesis.

ed with a Barrett esophagus (columnar epithelium–lined lower esophagus) (Allison and Johnstone, 1953; Barrett, 1950) (Fig. 24–19*B*). In such strictures, the esophagus itself is usually of normal length, but there is hypotension of the lower sphincter, usually associated with a small sliding esophageal hiatal hernia. This is also usually an acquired condition in which the squamous epithelium has been eroded by the damaging effects of gastroesophageal reflux and has subsequently been replaced by columnar junctional epithelium (Bremner *et al.*, 1970). Parietal cells have been identified in the columnar epithelium–lined portion of the esophagus in some instances (Burgess *et al.*, 1971).

This is a rare condition, but its true incidence is probably much higher than has been reported, since it is difficult to diagnose. Esophageal radiographs are not always diagnostic, and esophagoscopic biopsies above and below the stricture are required for confirmation. Only recently has the premalignant character of the columnar epithelium–lined lower esophagus been appreciated. The malignancy is invariably an adenocarcinoma developing in the columnar epithelium–lined portion of the esophagus cephalad to the esophagogastric junction (Hawe *et al.*, 1973). Approximately 8.5 per cent of patients with a Barrett esophagus are said to develop carcinoma (Naef *et al.*, 1975).

Long Strictures. By far the rarest type of stricture secondary to reflux is a long stricture involving the distal half or one third of the esophagus. Common causes for such a stricture are postpartum vomiting, postoperative nasogastric suction, and vomiting secondary to an obstructing duodenal ulcer. The length of the strictured segment resembles, radiographically, the length of the segment in patients with strictures due to the ingestion of corrosive agents (Fig. 24–19*C*).

Treatment

Bougienage. Because of the complexity of surgical management, the initial treatment of choice in patients with dysphagia due to esophageal strictures resulting from reflux is that of peroral bougienage. When properly performed and combined with intensive medical treatment to neutralize the regurgitating material, such treatment may be successful in controlling a stricture for many years. This approach is particularly applicable to individuals who are poor surgical risks. When aggressively pursued, such a program has reportedly been successful in 65 to 95 per cent of patients (Buchin and Spiro, 1981; Jones and Smith, 1981). These findings support a continuing aggressive effort to manage symptomatic esophageal strictures by bougienage before undertaking complicated surgical therapy. Although peroral dilation is almost always possible, there are some advanced cases in which a retrograde approach is required through a gastrostomy. Such a technique permits retrograde passage of a catheter to which appropriately sized dilators may be attached, and these can then be pulled through the stricture (Kongtahworn and Rossi, 1972).

TABLE 24–3. SURGERY FOR SHORT ESOPHAGUS WITH STRICTURE

Resection
  Esophagogastrectomy with
    Esophagogastrostomy
    Interposition of jejunum or colon
    Esophagogastrostomy and antrectomy with Roux-en-Y
    gastroenterostomy
Local Plastic and Bypass Procedures
  Thal fundoplasty
  Thal fundoplasty plus Nissen fundoplication
  Nissen fundoplication alone
  Gavriliu tube
  Collis gastroplasty
Esophageal Lengthening plus Antireflux Procedures
  Collis-Belsey procedure
  Collis-Nissen procedure

Surgery. The surgical management of esophageal stricture will be discussed in detail in Chapter 25. Only a brief overview of the subject is presented here. As indicated by the variety of procedures listed in Table 24–3, surgeons are still seeking the ideal operation for the undilatable esophageal stricture. Although high strictures associated with a Barrett esophagus can usually be managed by intraoperative dilation and an antireflux procedure (Hill *et al.*, 1970), strictures occurring at the esophagogastric junction in a shortened esophagus present a difficult surgical problem. Simple resection and esophagogastrostomy lead to recurrent reflux, so alternate procedures were developed, including interposition of colon or jejunum (Fig. 24–20, *left*), esophagogastrostomy coupled with antrectomy and Roux-en-Y esophagojejunostomy (Payne *et al.*, 1964) (Fig. 24–20, *middle*), and use of the Gavriliu tube (Heimlich, 1972) (Fig. 24–20, *right*).

Because of the increased risk associated with resective procedures, the trend is now toward the use of more conservative surgical measures. Simple fundoplication around the strictured area has been advocated (Pennell, 1981) but has not had wide acceptance (Leonardi *et al.*, 1981; Mansour *et al.*, 1981). Although originally proposed as a panacea for many esophageal problems (Thal, 1968), the Thal fundoplasty was found useful in the management of strictures only when combined with a Nissen fundoplication (Maher *et al.*, 1981). This operation also exposes the patient to the potential hazards of a supradiaphragmatic wrap.

Credit for introducing an esophageal lengthening procedure for patients with a shortened esophagus belongs to Collis (1957), who described the operation of gastroplasty, in which esophageal length is restored by creating a tube from the lesser curvature of the stomach in continuity with the distal esophagus (Fig. 24–21). This operation was modified by Pearson (Pearson *et al.*, 1971), who incorporated a Belsey Mark IV antireflux maneuver around the lengthened esophagus at the level of the hiatus (Fig. 24–22). Although this approach to a difficult problem has been widely adopted, some (Ellis *et al.*, 1978; Orringer and Sloan, 1977) have contended that combining the Collis gastroplasty with a Nissen fundoplication provides better reflux control.

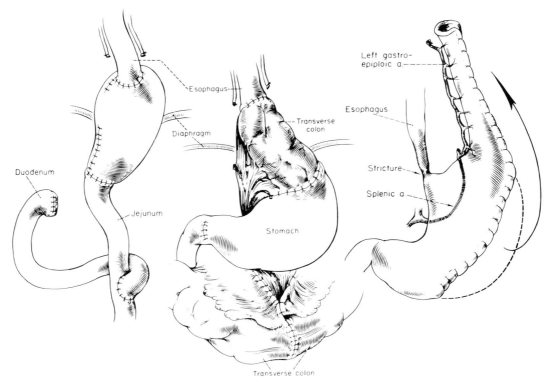

Figure 24–20. Operative procedures for management of short esophagus with stricture. *Left,* Esophagogastrectomy with Roux-en-Y esophagojejunostomy. *Middle,* Esophagogastrectomy colon interposition and pyloroplasty. *Right,* Gastric tube of Gavriliu. (From Payne, W. S., and Ellis, F. H., Jr.: Esophagus and diaphragmatic hernias. *In* Principles of Surgery. Edited by S. I. Schwartz. New York, McGraw-Hill, Inc., 1969, p. 886.)

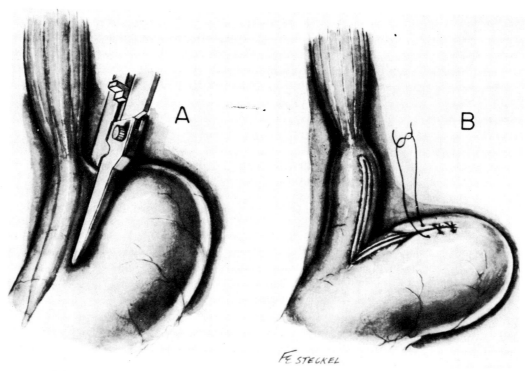

Figure 24–21. Technique of Collis gastroplasty. (From Ellis, F. H., Jr., Leonardi, H. K., Dabuzhsky, L., *et al.*: Surgery for short esophagus with stricture: An experimental and clinical manometric study. Ann. Surg., *188*:345, 1978.)

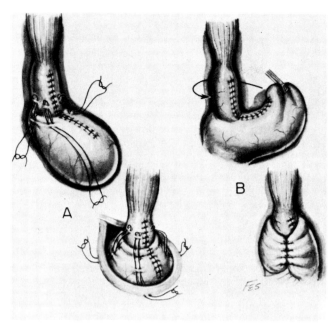

Figure 24–22. Techniques employed in performance of (*A*) Collis-Belsey procedure and (*B*) Collis-Nissen procedure. (From Ellis, F. H., Jr., Leonardi, H. K., Dabuzhsky, L., *et al.*: Surgery for short esophagus with stricture: An experimental and clinical manometric study. Ann. Surg., *188*:345, 1978.)

TUMORS

Benign Tumors and Cysts

In contrast to those in other organs, benign tumors of the esophagus are far less common than their malignant counterparts, constituting less than 10 per cent of neoplasms of the esophagus. In general, they occur at a younger age than carcinoma, and their symptoms, if present, are usually of longer duration than when the organ is involved by a malignant process.

Leiomyoma

The most common benign tumor of the esophagus is a leiomyoma, constituting two thirds of the benign lesions of the esophagus. They occur more frequently in men than in women. Although the tumors may occur anywhere in the esophagus, they are more commonly encountered in its lower third. By 1978, 838 esophageal leiomyomas had been reported (Seremetis *et al.*, 1975). Symptoms depend largely on the size of the lesion; those less than 5 cm. in diameter rarely give rise to symptoms. When they occur, symptoms consist primarily of dysphagia and a retrosternal feeling of pressure or of fullness. Esophageal leiomyomas are usually solitary, although rare instances of multiple tumors have been reported. Since the lesion is intramural with an overlying intact mucosa, bleeding is an exceedingly rare symptom.

The radiographic appearance of a leiomyoma is typical and consists of a filling defect on esophagog-

raphy with an intact esophageal mucosa (Schatzki and Hawes, 1950). The mass itself is usually ovoid with a sharply demarcated outline (Fig. 24–23). Endoscopy may be deceiving because of the intact overlying mucosa. Usually, however, a filling defect in the esophageal wall is identifiable endoscopically. Only large encircling tumors, which are rare, cause obstruction to the passage of the endoscope. If a leiomyoma is suspected, the endoscopist should not perform a biopsy, since it will complicate a subsequent surgical procedure. Histologically, the lesion consists of interlacing bundles of smooth muscle with eccentrically placed nuclei.

Symptomatic leiomyomas are treated surgically. They are approached through either a right or a left thoracotomy, depending on the location of the tumor, and can usually be enucleated through a longitudinal incision in the muscular wall of the esophagus without injuring the intact mucosa. However, those patients in whom the leiomyoma involves the esophagogastric junction may pose a more complicated technical prob-

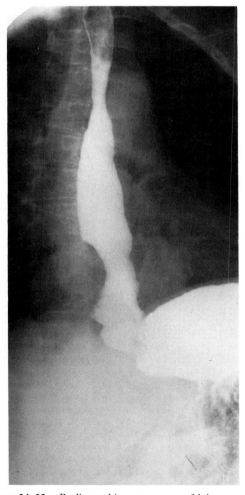

Figure 24–23. Radiographic appearance of leiomyoma of the lower esophagus. (From Andersen, H. A., and Pluth, J. R.: Benign tumors, cysts, and duplications of the esophagus. *In* The Esophagus. Edited by W. S. Payne and A. M. Olsen. Philadelphia, Lea & Febiger, 1974, p. 228.)

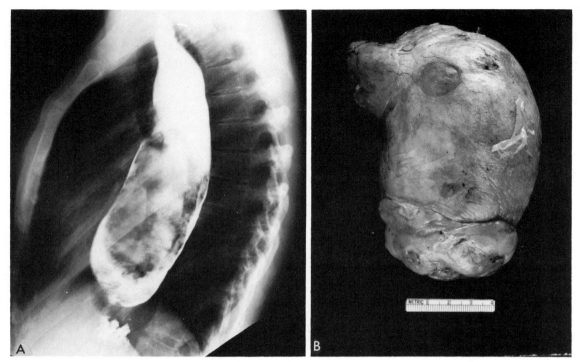

Figure 24–24. Large pedunculated fibrolipoma originating in the upper thoracic esophagus and extending to the lower esophagus. *A*, Esophageal roentgenogram. *B*, Gross appearance of specimen. (From Bernatz, P. E., Smith, J. L., Ellis, F. H., Jr., *et al.*: Benign, pedunculated, intraluminal tumors of the esophagus. J. Thorac. Cardiovasc. Surg., *35*:507, 1958.)

lem since such lesions often encircle the bowel, making enucleation of the tumor impossible. A limited esophagogastrectomy may be required for removal. Gastroesophageal competence should be restored by one of the plication procedures.

Pedunculated Intraluminal Tumors

A variety of polypoid intraesophageal tumors have been described, including mucosal polyps, chondromas, lipomas, fibrolipomas, and myxofibromas. The most common histologic finding is a mixture of loose fibrous tissue with myxomatous fatty changes, best termed a fibrolipoma (Bernatz *et al.*, 1958). Dysphagia is the usual symptom and is sometimes associated with regurgitation and weight loss. The most dramatic presentation, but a rare one, involves regurgitation of the tumor through the mouth. Radiographic examination is not always diagnostic, since the esophagus is sometimes so large that the tumor is obscured and the findings are confused with those of esophageal achalasia (Fig. 24–24*A*). Even esophagoscopy may be inconclusive because of the normal mucosal covering of the tumor.

Surgical removal is the treatment of choice for pedunculated intraluminal tumors, although some have been removed by means of a snare introduced through the esophagoscope. The site of origin of the tumor must be determined preoperatively to select the proper surgical approach. This may be either through a cervical incision or through a high thoracic incision and should be on the side opposite the origin of the tumor so that the pedicle can readily be seen after a

longitudinal incision through the esophageal wall. The tumor is identified and removed from the esophagus, the pedicle is divided, and the defect in the esophageal wall is closed in two layers.

Cysts and Duplications of the Esophagus

Esophageal cysts are the second most common benign neoplasms of the esophageal wall. They represent an embryonal rest, are intramural in location, and may be lined with either simple columnar ciliated epithelium or stratified squamous epithelium. The common location is in the wall of the upper thoracic esophagus in the region of the tracheal bifurcation. Radiographically, their appearance is identical to that of a leiomyoma, and surgical excision is conducted in the same fashion as for a leiomyoma.

An esophageal duplication is a less common abnormality and consists of a tubular structure composed of muscular and submucosal layers with a squamous epithelial lining. It may extend the entire length of the normal esophagus, running parallel to it, and the muscular layers of the two may intermingle. The common association of vertebral abnormalities with cysts and duplications has been noted repeatedly, the abnormality sometimes being called the "split notochord syndrome" (Tarnay *et al.*, 1970).

Treatment of these lesions is surgical excision. The cystic lesions, like leiomyomas, can usually be enucleated easily. Excision of esophageal duplication is more difficult because of the intimate association with the esophageal wall. Since the mucosa is not involved, however, esophageal duplications can usually be removed without necessitating esophageal resection.

Miscellaneous Benign Tumors

A number of other benign tumors have been described and are mentioned here only for the sake of completeness. These include squamous papilloma, granular cell myoblastoma, and hemangioma. Other benign lesions of the esophagus are lymphangiomas, neurofibromas, rhabdomyomas, osteochondromas, giant cell tumors, hamartomas, fibromas and lipomas, amyloid tumors, and eosinophilic granulomas.

Malignant Tumors

Carcinoma of the esophagus is predominantly a disease of men between the ages of 50 and 70. The incidence varies throughout the world, being 3.5 per 100,000 among white men and 13.3 per 100,000 among black men in the United States (Garfinkel *et al.*, 1980) and 130 per 100,000 in parts of the Honan province of North China (Day, 1975). The reason for the high incidence of esophageal carcinoma in China, Japan, Kazakhstan, Iran, Brittany, and among the native Bantu of South Africa is not clear (Doll *et al.*, 1966).

Epidemiologic surveys have revealed that two risk factors, smoking and high consumption of alcoholic beverages, predominate in patients with this disease (Wynder and Bross, 1961). The ingestion of nitrosamines has also been shown to be highly carcinogenic for the esophagus and may explain the high incidence of this condition among the South African Bantu (McGlashan *et al.*, 1968). Reference has already been made to such predisposing lesions as esophageal achalasia, the columnar epithelium–lined lower esophagus, and corrosive lye strictures. An increased incidence has also been reported in patients with the Paterson-Kelly syndrome (Wynder *et al.*, 1957), as discussed later, and in patients with tylosis (Shine and Allison, 1966).

Pathology

Squamous cell carcinoma is the most common malignant tumor of the body of the esophagus, accounting for more than 95 per cent of all esophageal malignancies in some series. Primary adenocarcinoma is extremely rare, accounting for less than 1 per cent (Raphael *et al.*, 1966) to 7 per cent of esophageal malignancies (Cederqvist *et al.*, 1980). By far the most common glandular tumor of the esophagus is an adenocarcinoma arising in the columnar epithelium of a Barrett esophagus (Hawe *et al.*, 1973), accounting for 86 per cent of all adenocarcinomas of the esophagus in one series (Haggitt *et al.*, 1978). Tumors similar in microscopic appearance to those arising in salivary glands represent less than one fifth of all glandular tumors of the esophagus. These mucoepidermoid and adenoid cystic carcinomas arise from the ducts of the submucosal glands. They are rare, only 27 cases

having been reported by 1980 (Bell-Thomson *et al.*, 1980).

Most malignant lesions are ulcerating and encircle the esophageal lumen. Only rarely are they polypoid. The most common polypoid malignant lesion of the esophagus is a carcinosarcoma, which has a somewhat more favorable prognosis than squamous cell carcinoma (Stener *et al.*, 1967). An even rarer polypoid lesion is a pseudosarcoma (Nichols *et al.*, 1979). Another rare sarcomatous lesion of the esophagus is a leiomyosarcoma, which tends to ulcerate, in contrast to a benign leiomyoma. Primary malignant melanoma of the esophagus has been reported (Kreuser, 1979), as have fibrosarcoma, rhabdomyosarcoma, plasmacytoma, and lymphosarcoma.

The indolent biologic behavior of verrucous squamous cell carcinoma makes it more susceptible to cure than other esophageal malignancies (Meyerowitz and Shea, 1971). The oat cell carcinoma is extremely rare (Reid *et al.*, 1980). It is considered to be a true apudoma arising from the argyrophilic Kulchitsky cells in the surface epithelium. Finally, the esophagus may be involved by primary tumors elsewhere in the body either by direct extension or by blood-borne metastases.

Malignant lesions involving the esophagogastric junction are almost invariably adenocarcinomas of gastric origin and constitute approximately half of the malignant tumors of the esophagus (Gunnlaugsson *et al.*, 1970) (Fig. 24–25). Fewer than 10 per cent of esophageal malignancies arise in the cervical region; all others arise in the intrathoracic body of the esophagus.

Although malignant tumors of the esophagus also spread by direct extension and by vascular invasion,

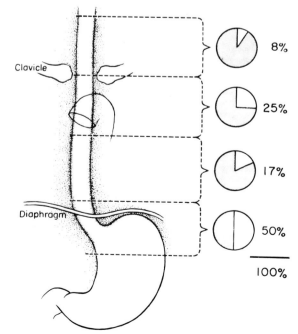

Figure 24–25. Distribution of carcinoma of the esophagus and esophagogastric junction according to anatomic location.

the sites of nodal metastases are important in deciding therapy. Cervical esophageal carcinoma disseminates through the lymphatic vessels to cervical nodes, particularly the anterior jugular and supraclavicular nodes. Those carcinomas arising in the thoracic esophagus spread early to the local and mediastinal glands and to the supraclavicular nodes and, occasionally, to the subdiaphragmatic nodes. Those occurring at the esophagogastric junction may involve local mediastinal as well as subdiaphragmatic nodes and nodes in the hilum of the spleen. Metastases through the bloodstream may produce liver, lung, or bone implants. Even though lymph node involvement does not occur, many tumors may show extensive local infiltration of vital structures with distal spread precluding curative resection.

Clinical Manifestations

The most common symptom of esophageal carcinoma is dysphagia. Initially, it is noted with the ingestion of solid foods, but ultimately, even swallowing liquids and saliva becomes difficult. Weight loss and weakness are the inevitable consequences. Aspiration pneumonitis is not infrequent as obstructive symptoms progress. Depending on the location of the tumor and the involvement of adjacent structures, recurrent nerve involvement or pulmonary symptoms resulting from compression or invasion of the trachea or of the bronchi may occur. Unfortunately, symptoms are rare until the tumor has totally encircled the esophagus, at which time the tumor may already be relatively far advanced. Early diagnosis is important, therefore, and anyone more than 40 years of age with complaints of either painful swallowing or of obstruc-

tion to swallowing should undergo appropriate diagnostic studies, including esophagoscopy, to exclude a malignant lesion.

Esophageal roentgenography will provide the diagnosis with a high degree of accuracy. The usual finding is that of an irregular, ragged mucosal pattern with anular luminal narrowing. Unlike benign obstructive lesions, carcinoma is usually not associated with marked proximal dilatation of the esophagus (Fig. 24–26).

The diagnosis should be confirmed by esophagoscopy in all patients not only to establish a tissue diagnosis but also to determine the anatomic limits of the lesion. Lesions involving the upper portion of the esophagus in the region of the tracheal carina require bronchoscopy to determine the presence or absence of malignant involvement of the tracheobronchial tree. In addition to biopsies of the suspected lesion, cytologic study of smears from such a lesion is valuable. Other studies, such as esophageal motility, are rarely of use except to exclude one of the more common motility disturbances.

Treatment

Controversy persists concerning the proper role of radiation therapy in the management of carcinoma of the esophagus. Some consider surgical therapy so unlikely to result in cure that irradiation is used for all patients. Others prefer a combination of radiation therapy and resection, and still others, having no confidence in preoperative irradiation, employ surgical therapy alone. Chemotherapy, whether used alone or in combination with other modalities, plays little role in the treatment of esophageal cancer (Priestman,

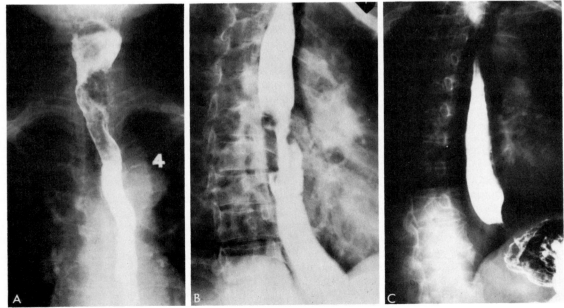

Figure 24–26. Radiographic examination of the esophagus after ingestion of contrast medium demonstrates typical abnormalities of carcinoma involving (*A*) the cervical esophagus, (*B*) the thoracic esophagus, and (*C*) the esophagogastric junction. (From Sanderson, D. R., and Bernatz, P. E.: Malignant tumors of the esophagus and cardia of the stomach. *In* The Esophagus. Edited by W. S. Payne and A. M. Olsen. Philadelphia, Lea & Febiger, 1974, p. 243.)

1976), although clinical trials of chemotherapy combined with preoperative irradiation and resection are currently under way.

Radiotherapy. Treatment of esophageal carcinoma by irradiation alone may be radical or palliative. If palliative, a dosage in the range of 20 to 30 Gy. (2000 to 3000 rads) over a 2-week period may provide temporary alleviation of such distressing symptoms as pain, hemorrhage, and dysphagia with relatively little morbidity.

Radical treatment for cure necessitates a dosage of between 50 and 60 Gy. (5000 to 6000 rads) delivered over a period of 4 or more weeks. This form of treatment is not without risk, for such complications as radiation pneumonitis and postradiation stricture are relatively common. Unusual complications include tracheoesophageal fistula, radiation myelitis, hemorrhage, and constrictive pericarditis. Pearson (1977) is the strongest proponent for irradiation as the primary form of therapy, and his updated results in 288 patients with a 5-year survival rate of 17 per cent are the best that radical radiotherapy has produced. It is not clear why no one else has been able to achieve comparable results, although patient selection may play a role. In an extensive review of the literature of the 25 years ending in 1979, Earlam and Cunha-Melo (1980) reported an overall survival rate of only 6 per cent after radiotherapy. If radiotherapy has a role in the treatment of esophageal malignancies, controversy would be least when it is applied to the cervical region of the esophagus.

Preoperative Irradiation. Combined irradiation and surgical resection have been found by some to be preferable to resection alone. Randomized selection of patients for alternative modes of treatment has not been employed, so that firm conclusions regarding combined therapy cannot be made. Nakayama (1964) reported improved results by employing a 3-day course of irradiation with a dose of 24 Gy. (2400 rads) followed by resection a week later. Although the 3-year survival rate using this combined method of treatment far surpassed that of resection alone in his experience, others have had less success with its use (Groves and Rodriguez-Antunez, 1973). Another combined technique involves the preoperative administration of 40 to 70 Gy. (4000 to 7000 rads) over a period of 4 to 7 weeks, followed a month or so later by resection. Such an approach has been used with success by both Akakura and associates (1970) in Japan and Parker and Gregorie (1976) in the United States. In a separate report of Parker's data by Marks and associates (1976), a somewhat different picture emerges. Of all patients selected for this form of therapy, only 41 per cent completed it. The hospital mortality rate was 18 per cent, and only 6 per cent of the patients lived 5 years. In the absence of more compelling evidence, the added time, expense, and mortality of combined therapy are hard to justify, although it may increase the resectability rate in selected patients.

Surgery. Over the years, a wide variety of resective techniques have been employed in the management of carcinoma of the esophagus, both as staged operations and as definitive procedures. These include esophagogastrectomy with esophagogastrostomy or interposition of the small or large bowel or a revascularized intestinal autograft and the use of a Gavriliu gastric tube. Resection has also been combined with such staged reconstructive plastic procedures as the Wookey operation for cervical esophageal cancers and the formation of anterior thoracic skin tubes to reconstruct alimentary tract continuity. Many of these procedures are now of historic interest only. Emphasis here is placed on those operations most commonly used now.

ESOPHAGOGASTRECTOMY WITH ESOPHAGOGASTROSTOMY. Because of its low hospital mortality rate and the fact that the operation need not be staged, esophagogastrectomy with esophagogastrostomy is now widely used in the surgical treatment of lesions at all levels of the esophagus. It is particularly appropriate for malignancies of the lower esophagus and esophagogastric junction, and left thoracotomy provides satisfactory exposure for performance of resection and intrathoracic anastomosis. For lesions requiring an anastomosis at or proximal to the aortic arch, a combined abdominal and right thoracic approach is employed (Fig. 24–27). When resection is performed for cervical esophageal cancer, a similar approach may be used, permitting elevation of the freed stomach into the neck with primary cervical esophagogastrostomy, or a thoracotomy may be avoided by freeing the esophagus by blunt dissection from the neck and abdomen, resecting it, and elevating the freed stomach through the posterior mediastinum into the neck, where an esophagogastrostomy is done (Orringer and Sloan, 1978) (Fig. 24–28).

Regardless of the extent of the resection and the location of the anastomosis, careful mobilization of the stomach is essential so that its blood supply may be preserved. The short gastric vessels are divided. The stomach is freed from the omentum and mesocolon, with care being taken to preserve the right gastroepi-

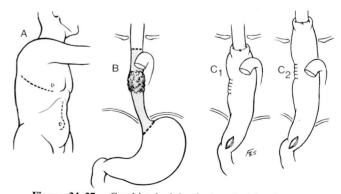

Figure 24–27. Combined abdominal and right thoracotomy (*A*) is used for esophageal lesions requiring a supra-aortic anastomosis (*B*). This may be done in the chest (*C₁*). If submucosal spread is great, a cervical anastomosis through a third incision may be performed (*C₂*). (From Ellis, F. H., Jr.: Esophagogastrectomy for carcinoma: Technical considerations based on anatomic location of lesion. Surg. Clin. North Am., *60*:273, 1980.)

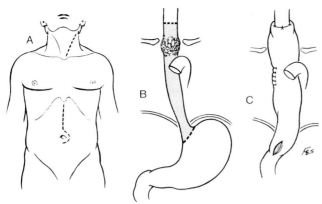

Figure 24–28. For esophagectomy without thoracotomy, the patient is in the supine position, and an upper midline incision (broken lines) is made (*A*). *B*, The extent of resection (shaded area) is shown. *C*, Completed anastomosis is pictured (From Ellis, F. H., Jr.: Esophagogastrectomy for carcinoma: Technical considerations based on anatomic location of lesion. Surg. Clin. North Am., *60*:275, 1980.)

ploic artery (Fig. 24–29*A*). If local extension of the malignancy so demands, the spleen and a portion of the pancreas can be included in the resected specimen (Fig. 24–29*B*). The left gastric artery is divided at its origin from the celiac axis, and if necessary, the duodenum is kocherized to permit further mobilization of the stomach (Fig. 24–30). When feasible, an extramucosal pyloromyotomy is performed to minimize the postvagotomy effect. The stomach is divided at an appropriate level by a stapling device of proper size (Fig. 24–31), and an end-to-side anastomosis between the stomach and the esophagus is performed without using clamps and while avoiding any tension. A number of anastomotic techniques can be used. A classic two-layer anastomosis with an inner layer of running catgut and an outer layer of interrupted silk sutures has proved satisfactory in my hands (Fig. 24–32). The completed anastomosis is surrounded by adjacent fundus, as in an "inkwell" or posterior invagination procedure. This protects the suture line

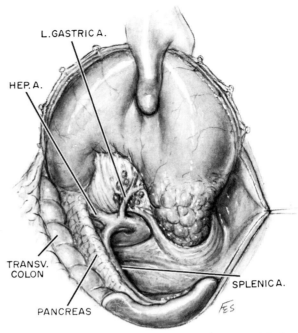

Figure 24–30. The left gastric artery is exposed before its division. (From Ellis, F. H., Jr.: Carcinoma of the distal esophagus and esophagogastric junction. *In* Modern Technics in Surgery: Cardiac/Thoracic Surgery. Edited by L. H. Cohn. Mount Kisco, New York, Futura Publishing Company, 1979, p. 13–5.)

but probably has little effect on providing competence.

Intercostal tube drainage and nasogastric tube drainage are employed to provide gastric decompression. The tubes are left in place for 4 or 5 days and removed after a contrast radiographic study confirms the integrity of the anastomosis, and oral feedings are begun.

ESOPHAGOGASTRECTOMY WITH COLON INTERPOSITION. Of the other varieties of esophageal reconstruction, the interposed colon is perhaps most widely

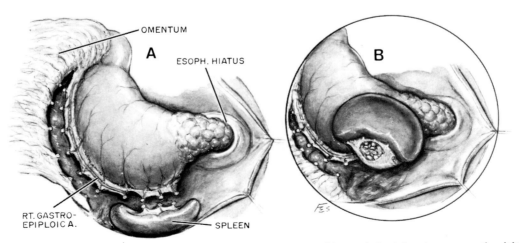

Figure 24–29. *A,* The stomach is freed from the spleen and the omentum, with care being taken to preserve the right gastroepiploic artery. *B,* Splenectomy can be incorporated with resection if tumor extension or nodal metastases or both so dictate. (From Ellis, F. H., Jr.: Carcinoma of the distal esophagus and esophagogastric junction. *In* Modern Technics in Surgery: Cardiac/Thoracic Surgery. Edited by L. H. Cohn. Mount Kisco, New York, Futura Publishing Company, 1979, p. 13–4.)

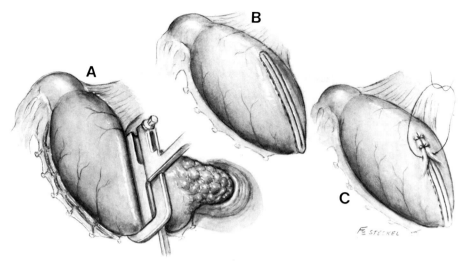

Figure 24–31. *A,* A TA-90 stapler is used to transect the stomach below the growth. *B,* Appearance of transected stomach after stapler has been activated. *C,* Interrupted silk sutures are placed over the stapled edge of the stomach. (From Ellis, F. H., Jr.: Carcinoma of the distal esophagus and esophagogastric junction. *In* Modern Technics in Surgery: Cardiac/Thoracic Surgery. Edited by L. H. Cohn. Mount Kisco, New York, Futura Publishing Company, 1979, p. 13–5.)

used as an alternative to esophagogastrostomy (Wilkins and Burke, 1974). Its use, however, is now more limited than heretofore because of the hospital mortality rate and because the procedure usually needs to be staged. However, when insufficient stomach remains after resection, it provides a viable alternative to esophagogastrostomy.

At the first stage, the abdomen is opened and searched for metastatic disease. If none is found, a Stamm gastrostomy and gastric drainage are performed. Total thoracic esophagectomy is performed through the right chest, the patient is repositioned to permit exposure of the cervical esophagus through a left cervical incision, and a temporary cervical esophagostomy is performed (Fig. 24–33*A,B*). At a later date,

after the patient's nutrition has been re-established and the integrity of the colon has been ascertained by barium enema study and, if desired, its vascular supply studied by arteriography, suitable colon preparation is initiated and the interposition procedure undertaken. Our preference is to place the left colon in an antiperistaltic fashion. Its blood supply is constant, and the caliber of the sigmoid is closer to that of the esophagus than other portions of the colon. The left colon is mobilized to receive its arterial supply from the middle colic artery. The colon is mobilized after reopening the abdominal incision, and its vascular supply is divided in such a way as to preserve the vascular arcade. Suitable points for division of the colon are selected, and the isolated colon is then

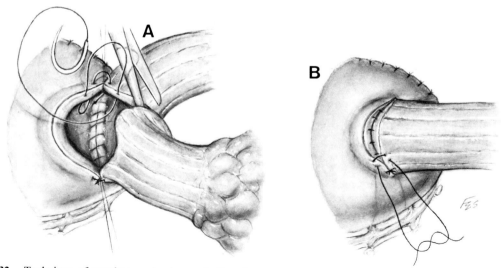

Figure 24–32. Technique of esophagogastrostomy. *A,* Running catgut mucosal stitch. *B,* Layer of interrupted silk sutures before invagination of anastomosis. (From Ellis, F. H., Jr.: Carcinoma of the distal esophagus and esophagogastric junction. *In* Modern Technics in Surgery: Cardiac/Thoracic Surgery. Edited by L. H. Cohn. Mount Kisco, New York, Futura Publishing Company, 1979, p. 13–7.)

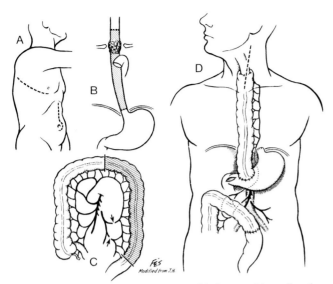

Figure 24–33. Esophagectomy with interposition of antiperistaltic segment of the left colon. *A,* Incisions used in performance of esophagectomy, cervical esophagostomy, pyloromyotomy, and gastrostomy. *B,* Extent of esophageal resection (shaded area). *C,* Preparation of segment of the left colon (shaded area) for interposition based on middle colic artery (note sites of vascular interruption that maintain the integrity of the vascular arcade). *D,* Completed operation. (From Ellis, F. H., Jr.: Esophagogastrectomy for carcinoma: Technical considerations based on anatomic location of lesion. Surg. Clin. North Am., *60*:277, 1980.)

passed behind the stomach and retrieved through the lesser sac before fashioning a substernal tunnel by blunt resection after reopening the cervical incision. The colon is then carefully advanced through the substernal tunnel, where an end-to-end esophagocolostomy is performed (Fig. 24–33*C,D*). The divided transverse colon is then sutured end to side to the antrum. A colocolostomy restores colonic integrity, and the operative area is reperitonealized. Postoperative management is similar to that after esophagogastrectomy.

PALLIATIVE PROCEDURES. Unfortunately, even with careful preoperative evaluation, certain tumors cannot be removed successfully because of local extension to vital structures. In these instances, a palliative procedure is indicated. A variety of plastic tubes are available that can be passed through the lesion transorally and retrieved during operation via gastrotomy and firmly fixed in place. The Celestin tube is widely preferred (Fig. 24–34); it is associated with an operative mortality of approximately 10 per cent but also with worthwhile palliation of dysphagia in 75 per cent of patients (Sanfelippo and Bernatz, 1973). For nonresectable lesions of the cardia, an alternative palliative procedure is a side-to-side bypass technique, which joins the freed fundus of the stomach to the esophagus proximal to the growth (Kwun and Kirschner, 1981). Interest in a tube similar to the Souttar push-through type is being rekindled, and if the patient is determined preoperatively to have an inoperable lesion, serious consideration should be given to the use of such tubes. The plastic Proctor-Livingston tube has been widely used abroad (Proctor,

1980), and in the United States, Boyce (1973) has written enthusiastically about the results of palliative permanent transoral plastic intubation for inoperable carcinoma of the esophagus. The use of this technique has its greatest application for lesions below the cervical esophagus and especially for those complicated by esophagorespiratory fistulas.

A feeding gastrostomy as a palliative procedure is mentioned only to condemn its use. It provides no symptomatic palliation. It does not restore the swallowing mechanism and is not without mortality and morbidity. The gastrostomy should be employed only as a temporary measure either between the stages of a colon interposition or to maintain adequate nutrition in the patient undergoing radiation therapy before the temporary beneficial effects from this form of treatment become manifest.

RESULTS OF RESECTION. The role of surgery in treating cancer of the esophagus has been challenged on the basis of low resectability and high mortality rates. Although some recent surveys certainly have been discouraging, reporting resectability rates of 40 to 50 per cent, hospital mortality rates of 13 to 30 per cent, and 5-year survival rates of only 4 to 12 per cent, they are based for the most part on outdated information and do not reflect current practices. The recent report of Wu and Huang (1979) from the People's Republic of China is more representative, for in the recent experience of a number of Chinese hospitals, the resectability rate was 80 per cent, the hospital mortality rate was 3 to 5 per cent, and the 5-year survival rate was approximately 30 per cent. My experience at the Lahey Clinic reflects these improved results. The published operability rate for all patients seen with carcinoma of the esophagus or cardia was 81 per cent (Ellis and Gibb, 1979). Between January 1970 and July 1981, 127 patients were operated on, 113 of whom underwent resection (89 per cent) (Ellis, 1981). Two deaths within 30 days of operation account for a hospital mortality rate of 1.8 per cent. The average survival was 20.8 months, although tumor was

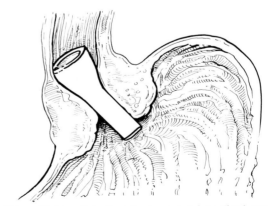

Figure 24–34. Celestin tube impacted into distal esophageal neoplasm provides a satisfactory channel for swallowing in patients with nonresectable lesions. (From Sanderson, D. R., and Bernatz, P. E.: Malignant tumors of the esophagus and cardia of the stomach. *In* The Esophagus. Edited by W. S. Payne and A. M. Olsen. Philadelphia, Lea & Febiger, 1974, p. 250.)

left behind in 15 per cent of patients. Most important, over 90 per cent of the patients had successful and permanent relief of dysphagia. Survival at 4 years was 52 per cent for patients with Stage I and II disease and 11 per cent for patients with Stage III disease.

Survival rates for patients with adenocarcinoma are not as good as those for patients with squamous cell cancer, the most favorable results being obtained with squamous carcinoma of the lower esophagus and esophagogastric junction. For these patients, the 5-year survival rate was 45 per cent in the absence of nodal involvement in a large series reported from the Mayo Clinic (Gunnlaugsson et al., 1970). The adverse influence of nodal metastases on survival further emphasizes the need for early detection. That cures are possible with early detection is evidenced by the report from the People's Republic of China (Coordinating Group for Research on Esophageal Cancer, 1976) from the Linhsien County of the Honan Province, where the incidence of cancer of the esophagus is so high that widespread screening techniques are employed. The resectability rate in 170 patients with early carcinoma of the esophagus was 100 per cent, and the 5-year survival rate was 90 per cent.

PERFORATION OF THE ESOPHAGUS

Despite modern forms of therapy, esophageal perforation or rupture continues to be associated with a high mortality and morbidity. Prompt recognition and proper treatment may avert death or minimize a prolonged and difficult convalescence.

Etiology and Mechanism

Until the introduction of the flexible esophagoscope, most esophageal perforations were the result of esophageal instrumentation either by the rigid esophagoscope or by bougienage, the incidence approximating 0.4 per cent (Wychulis et al., 1969a and b). Other possible causes include blunt or penetrating trauma or the accidental ingestion of foreign bodies. Of special interest is spontaneous rupture of the esophagus (Boerhaave's syndrome), a consequence of the strain of emesis with or without predisposing esophageal disease. A variety of conditions have also been implicated in noninstrumental perforation of the esophagus, including stress associated with neurologic disease or after operations or burns remote from the esophagus and a postoperative leak developing in association with intrathoracic esophageal anastomoses.

Perforations by instruments or foreign bodies can occur at any level of the esophagus. However, the sites of normal narrowing are the ones most frequently involved. The narrowest of these is the esophageal introitus, and here occur most perforations that follow instrumentation. The impingement of the rigid esophagoscope on the bodies of hyperextended cervical vertebrae may result in a crushing effect on the mucosa, particularly in the presence of hypertrophic bony

spurs. The second most common site for instrumental and foreign body perforations is the lower esophagus immediately above the point where the esophagus narrows to pass through the diaphragmatic hiatus. The incidence of perforation at this level is further contributed to by the increased occurrence of disease and by the frequent need for endoscopic manipulations in this region. Perforations of the middle third and abdominal parts of the esophagus occur infrequently.

The mechanism of postemetic perforation of the lower esophagus has evoked considerable interest. It occurs as a longitudinal through-and-through split of all esophageal layers in the distal esophagus just above the diaphragm. Apparently, the sudden onset of pressure in the lower esophagus, rather than the amount of pressure by itself, may be a critical factor in such injuries. The fact that most postemetic perforations occur in adults rather than in children may be explained by the higher incidence of predisposing factors in adults and by the fact that the strength of the esophagus is greater in infants than in adults.

Pathophysiology

The consequences of esophageal perforation are the result of contamination of periesophageal spaces with corrosive digestive fluids, food, and bacteria, which leads to diffuse cellulitis with localized or extensive suppuration. Anatomic considerations are important both in the evolution of signs and symptoms and in treatment. The majority of cervical esophageal perforations occur posteriorly and result in suppuration, first in the retrovisceral space and then extending along fascial planes into the mediastinum. Perforations of the anterior wall of the cervical esophagus and those involving the lateral pharyngeal spaces and pyriform fossae enter the pretracheal space, which communicates with the mediastinum by way of the fascial attachment to the pericardium. The manifestations of perforation depend on the relation of the esophagus to the contiguous spaces. The upper two thirds of the thoracic esophagus is in close proximity to the right pleural cavity. In its lower third, the esophagus lies adjacent to the left pleural space. In rare cases, the intra-abdominal or subphrenic esophagus may be perforated, leading to peritonitis and intra-abdominal abscess.

Clinical Manifestations

The symptoms of esophageal perforation depend to a large degree on the site of perforation and the extent of the inflammatory reaction. Pain, fever, and dysphagia are the most frequent early complaints. Cervical tenderness and pain on swallowing and flexion of the neck are early and common features of cervical esophageal perforation. Cervical crepitation may be minimal but is an almost constant finding. Dyspnea is usually related to pleural space involvement with or without pneumothorax.

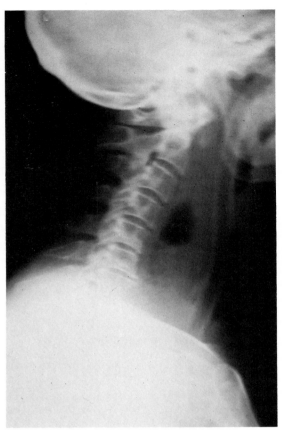

Figure 24–35. Instrumental perforation of cervical esophagus. Note retrovisceral abscess with air fluid level and anterior displacement of airway. (From Payne, W. S., and Olsen, A. M.: The Esophagus. Philadelphia, Lea & Febiger, 1974, p. 175.)

The physical findings with thoracic esophageal perforation are usually limited to the thorax; cervical crepitation may be a feature, but usually no cervical tenderness is present. Auscultation over the heart may elicit signs of mediastinal emphysema (Hamman's sign). Cardiorespiratory embarrassment with shock and cyanosis is more commonly seen in the early stages of thoracic and subphrenic esophageal perforations, but it may not be apparent until a late stage.

Radiographic studies are of great assistance in diagnosis. Anteroposterior and lateral views of the cervical spine often demonstrate pathognomonic signs of cervical perforation (Fig. 24–35). Anterior displacement of the trachea, widening of the retrovisceral space, air in tissue spaces, and, occasionally, widening of the superior mediastinum are seen. The last is a common sign in perforation of the cervical or upper thoracic part of the esophagus. Mediastinal emphysema and pleural effusion with or without pneumothorax may be present with thoracic or subphrenic esophageal injuries. Studies with an opaque medium are occasionally indicated to localize the site or sites of perforation and to detect associated abnormalities. The medium should be nonirritating and, preferably, absorbable. Endoscopic procedures are rarely indicated in the diagnosis of esophageal perforations, except when a foreign body is present.

Treatment

Adequate drainage and prevention of continued contamination are the major goals of therapy of esophageal perforation. Thus, conservative treatment with parenteral antibiotics plus parenteral fluid and electrolyte correction and support is only rarely appropriate, although the selective conservative management of contained perforation has its advocates (Cameron *et al.*, 1979).

Simple surgical exploration with drainage of the retrovisceral space or, on rare occasions, of the pretracheal space is the treatment of choice for cervical esophageal perforation (Fig. 24–36). Suppuration extending as low as the fourth vertebra can be evacuated effectively by this procedure. Because it is rarely possible to identify a reparable laceration in such cases, the accepted treatment is drainage of the retrovisceral and contiguous spaces with postoperative parenteral administration of appropriate antibiotics and fluids.

Instrumental perforations of the thoracic and subphrenic parts of the esophagus are often large and require surgical exploration, repair, and drainage. The upper two thirds of the esophagus is best approached transpleurally through a right midthoracotomy and the lower third through a lower left thoracotomy. The rare subphrenic lacerations are best explored transabdominally. Gastric decompression either by nasogastric tube or, rarely, by gastrostomy is indicated. On occasion, resection of the perforation and of the associated esophageal lesion is required.

Postemetic perforations of the esophagus involve the distal thoracic and, occasionally, the abdominal segments of the esophagus. These major linear tears require early surgical intervention with debridement, closure of the laceration by sutures, and appropriate drainage, as suggested by Barrett (1947). Covering the suture line by a flap of adjacent pleura helps to reduce the mortality rate (Michel *et al.*, 1981). Some means of continuous gastric decompression during healing is essential with the addition of parenteral antibiotics and fluids postoperatively.

Particularly difficult to manage are those thoracic esophageal perforations diagnosed more than 18 to 24 hours after they occur or those in which a fistula with acute suppuration develops after initial repair. The mortality rate is 50 per cent or higher in patients with esophageal perforations treated more than 24 hours after injury (Sawyers *et al.*, 1975).

Various solutions have been proposed for the management of these desperately ill patients. These include primary esophagogastrectomy, use of a fundic patch to cover the defect (Thal, 1968), and the use of a T tube (Abbott *et al.*, 1970). Johnson and associates (1956) have suggested total esophageal exclusion by creation of a cervical esophagostomy. The thoracic esophagus is closed proximal and distal to the perforation. Pleural drainage is instituted, and gastric decompression and subsequent alimentation are accomplished by gastrostomy. Esophageal replacement is performed later by colon interposition. A modification

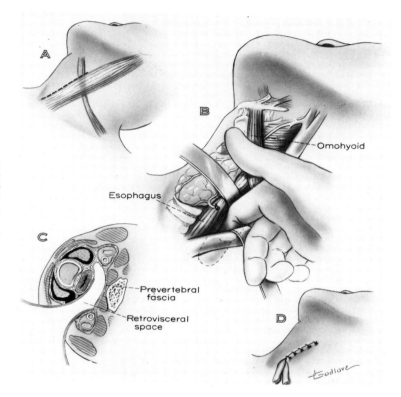

Figure 24–36. Technique of cervical mediastinotomy. *A,* Site of incision (dotted line). *B,* Retrovisceral space is reached by retracting the sternocleidomastoid muscle and cervical vessels laterally and the trachea and thyroid medially. *C,* Cross-section of access route to retrovisceral space. *D,* Completed procedure with drains in place. (From Payne, W. S., and Larson, R. H.: Acute mediastinitis. Surg. Clin. North Am., *49*:1005, 1969.)

of this procedure by Urschel and associates (1974) requires temporary diversion of the cervical esophageal stoma and temporary occlusion of the distal esophagus. This permits recovery and later restoration of normal esophageal function without the need for esophageal replacement. Direct closure of the defect has been advocated even in delayed cases (Finley *et al.,* 1980).

A leaking intrathoracic esophageal anastomosis is invariably fatal unless properly treated. If the leaking anastomosis is recognized early, it is sometimes possible to repair or to reconstruct it. If not, the mediastinal inflammation may be so great and the patient's condition so precarious that aggressive measures may be inadvisable, and simple pleural drainage alone may be permissible. Such an approach may lead to a well-drained esophagopleural cutaneous fistula, with ultimate healing promoted by adequate nutrition provided by hyperalimentation.

Results

The results of treatment of cervical esophageal perforation, regardless of cause, have been excellent with early cervical exploration and drainage. Even in major injuries with marked contamination and delayed treatment, the results of surgical management have been satisfactory. Although the incidence of complications, secondary procedures, prolonged hospitalization, and late sequelae has been greater in this latter group, the mortality has been negligible. The results of treatment for perforations involving the thoracic and subphrenic esophagus have been less satisfactory; hospital mortality rates from 10 to 30 per cent have

been reported. Delay in diagnosis appears to be a major factor contributing to morbidity and mortality.

MISCELLANEOUS ESOPHAGEAL CONDITIONS

Esophageal Webs and Rings

Esophageal webs and rings may be encountered at different levels of the esophagus and cause dysphagia if the esophageal lumen is sufficiently narrowed. Although webs have been described in the midportion of the esophagus, they are extremely unusual. It is likely that what in the past has been considered a mid-esophageal web may actually represent a Barrett esophagus with a stricture at the level of the esophageal change from squamous epithelium to the columnar epithelium–lined lower esophagus.

Esophageal webs that occur in the cervical esophagus constitute a distinct clinical entity. In 1919, Paterson and Kelly independently described a clinical state (the Paterson-Kelly syndrome) with which the names of Plummer and Vinson later became associated in the United States. This syndrome consists of dysphagia, glossitis, and anemia, and although it may occur in men, most patients are postmenopausal women. The typical patient is a middle-aged edentulous woman with atrophic oral mucosa, spoon-shaped fingers with brittle nails, and a long-standing history of anemia and dysphagia. The cause of the dysphagia is usually a fibrous web partially obstructing the esophageal lumen a few millimeters below the esophageal introitus. Because of the common finding of iron-deficiency anemia, the term "sideropenic dysphagia" has been used by some authors to describe the condition. This condition is more common in the Scandinavian countries than in the United States. A dietary deficiency has been established as the cause, and the condition responds well to iron therapy and to forceful dilation of the stricture. As previously mentioned, the condition is a premalignant one; in approximately 10 per cent of affected persons, carcinoma of the oral cavity, hypopharynx, or esophagus develops.

This syndrome covers a broad spectrum of clinical entities, and not all patients exhibit hypochromic anemia nor do they necessarily show evidence of malnutrition. Conversely, not all patients with the other clinical features of the Paterson-Kelly syndrome are found to have esophageal webs. Furthermore, some younger patients with esophageal webs who lack the clinical stigmas of the classic syndrome may have a congenital lesion, although congenital strictures of the esophagus are exceedingly rare. All patients should be studied endoscopically to exclude the existence of a malignant lesion. In the typical patient, endoscopy will reveal a fibrous web partially obstructing the esophageal lumen in an eccentric fashion a few millimeters below the cricopharyngeus muscle. Treatment by dilating the esophagus with a size 45 to 50 Fr. bougie is usually successful.

The most common site of an esophageal ring is the lower esophagus; this was described by Schatzki and Gary (1953) in the course of roentgenographic examination of patients with esophageal hiatal hernia. The nature and cause of the lower esophageal ring remain controversial, but its clinical significance is clear. Dysphagia is a prominent symptom when the lumen of the esophagus is reduced to less than 13 mm. and is rare when the lumen is larger than 20 mm. Lower esophageal ring is usually present only in patients with a hiatal hernia, and its reported incidence varies from 15 to 27 per cent of hernia patients. The cause of the condition remains obscure, but most now believe it to be related in some way to reflux esophagitis, although endoscopic examination may fail to reveal any evidence of superficial inflammation. Biopsy specimens, however, uniformly show evidence of submucosal fibrosis, indicating that it may well represent the end result of healing of a previously existing inflammatory lesion at the lower end of the esophagus (Eckardt *et al.*, 1972, 1980).

In a study of 100 anatomic specimens, a lower esophageal ring was found in 14 of the specimens, and the rings proved to be of two types (Goyal *et al.*, 1971). The more common type was a mucosal ring located at the esophagogastric junction; other rings occurred at a higher level and consisted of thickening of the circular muscle of the esophagus at the level of the upper attachment of the phrenoesophageal membrane in the region corresponding to the lower esophageal sphincter. Roentgenographically, the ring may be demonstrated by distending the esophagus with contrast medium above and below the web (Fig. 24–37).

Treatment depends on the severity of the symptoms, and when symptoms are severe, simple bougie-

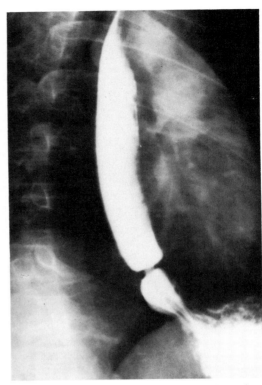

Figure 24–37. Esophageal roentgenogram of a patient with a small diaphragmatic hernia and a typical Schatzki ring.

nage or pneumatic dilation has occasionally been found useful. Since some patients with a lower esophageal ring also have an incompetent lower esophageal sphincter with gastroesophageal reflux that requires correction, the ring may be managed surgically at the time of correction of the existing hiatal hernia. Such treatment consists of either excision or incision of the ring at the time of repair of the hiatal hernia and correction of the incompetent sphincter, although symptomatic occurrences develop frequently (Ottinger and Wilkins, 1980).

Mallory-Weiss Syndrome

Spontaneous rupture of the esophagus (Boerhaave's syndrome) and esophagogastric mucosal lacerations (Mallory-Weiss syndrome [Mallory and Weiss, 1929]) are believed to have a similar cause. A sudden increase in intra-abdominal pressure, the result of an explosive vomiting effort, is the usual initiating mechanism. A history of prolonged retching or vomiting, often, but not always, associated with alcoholism, is characteristic.

The upper part of the stomach is usually involved, and the greater curvature portion of the cardia is the site most commonly affected. The lesion initially exhibits evidence of an acute laceration, but subsequent peptic digestion may occur, and the clinical symptoms that result from this consist of painless gastrointestinal bleeding, usually manifested as hematemesis or, less commonly, melena. A definitive diagnosis depends on objective demonstration of the mucosal laceration by endoscopic visualization of the esophagogastric junctional area (Michel et al., 1980). Both radiography and selective celiac angiography are less definitive diagnostic techniques. Surgical exploration is the best means of establishing a definitive diagnosis.

The initial management is based on routine supportive measures, and not infrequently, the hemorrhage subsides spontaneously and recovery follows without recurrence. If bleeding persists, surgery is indicated and necessitates the use of specific maneuvers designed to demonstrate and to treat the lesion of Mallory-Weiss syndrome. An upper abdominal incision providing adequate exposure for a generous proximal transverse gastrotomy is essential to permit adequate intraluminal inspection of the cardia.

After manual evacuation of clots and the insertion of proper retractors for exposure, the lacerated area should be repaired with sutures. A suture line of running, locked, absorbable suture material usually provides adequate repair of the acute mucosal laceration and controls hemorrhage. Large bleeding vessels in the base of an actively bleeding inflammatory ulceration should be ligated with nonabsorbable sutures. After closure of the gastrotomy, a nasogastric tube should be left in place to maintain gastric decompression and to monitor for postoperative bleeding. Surgical treatment of Mallory-Weiss syndrome is highly effective, and recurrence is extremely rare.

Unusual Diverticula and Acquired Fistulas

Most esophageal diverticula are associated with motility disturbances of the esophagus. Occasionally, however, a diverticulum may develop in the midthoracic esophagus. Rarely do such diverticula produce symptoms. They are usually the result of granulomatous infections of the mediastinal lymph nodes, particularly those lymph nodes in the subcarinal and parabronchial regions, although some have been associated with an underlying motility disorder (Kaye, 1974). These diverticula are characteristically traction diverticula and rarely require surgical treatment unless complications develop.

More uncommon even than midesophageal traction diverticula are examples of a condition termed "intramural diverticulosis of the esophagus," first reported by Mendl and associates in 1960. Radiographs of the esophagus demonstrate multiple tiny outpouchings along the course of the esophagus, and the most common symptom described by patients with such findings is dysphagia. The condition is often secondary to other esophageal disease, such as esophageal web, reflux esophagitis, and disturbances in esophageal motility. Some evidence has been presented that chronic infection of esophageal submucosal glands may be the predominant cause (Hammon et al., 1974). Therapy should be directed toward relieving the underlying cause. Roentgenographically, the appearance is usually confused with inflammatory lesions of the esophagus, particularly monilial esophagitis.

Occasionally, a fistulous communication between the esophagus and the lower respiratory tract may develop and require treatment (Wychulis et al., 1966). Other potential sites of fistulous communication include the aorta, heart, and vena cava. The most common cause of acquired fistula is carcinoma, and the fistula usually represents a preterminal event in the course of incurable carcinoma of the esophagus, lung, or neck structures.

A fistula between the esophagus and the tracheobronchial tree typically produces symptoms of coughing on eating or drinking, although it may rarely present more subtly with pulmonary symptoms alone. Many of these fistulas, if benign, will close spontaneously, provided the esophagus is not obstructed distally, yet surgical therapy is sometimes required. The basic goals of such therapy include division of the fistulous tract, suture closure of the defects in the esophagus and in the respiratory tree, and interposition of viable tissue to prevent recurrence. Attention must also be paid to correcting distal esophageal obstruction and to providing adequate drainage of the chest. Rarely, an esophagopleural fistula occurs as a complication of radical pneumonectomy, particularly on the right side, and may be a late complication of such a surgical procedure (Benjamin et al., 1969).

Inflammatory Lesions of the Esophagus

Increasing numbers of cases of esophageal moniliasis are now being reported, undoubtedly as a result of the increasingly widespread use of immunosuppressive therapy, steroids, and antibiotics. The symptoms are those of painful dysphagia, and the radiographic features include an irregular, ragged mucosal pattern with numerous small indentations and protrusions, sometimes referred to as a "cobblestone" esophagus (Goldberg and Dodds, 1968). Treatment should be devoted to supportive measures and to correction of the underlying predisposing factors with discontinuation of immunosuppressive steroids or antibiotics. If the infection does not subside spontaneously, oral use of nystatin has been reported to be successful (Kantrowitz et al., 1969).

Other infections that, in the past, were occasionally reported as involving the esophagus include tuberculosis and syphilis. Although cases of Crohn's disease of the esophagus have been difficult to document, some probable examples of this condition have been reported in the literature (Miller et al., 1977). Since the esophagus, like the skin, is covered with squamous epithelium, it is not surprising that certain dermatologic disorders are associated with esophageal manifestations, particularly pemphigoid vulgaris, bullous pemphigoid, or benign mucosal pemphigoid.

Extrinsic Compression of the Esophagus

Among the many varieties of anomalies of the aortic arch system that either completely or partially encircle the trachea and esophagus, the most common type is the aberrant right subclavian artery arising as the fourth branch of the aorta. Since this artery only partially encircles the esophagus, it is usually asymptomatic, although, rarely, it may give rise to symptoms of esophageal obstruction ("dysphagia lusoria"). A double aortic arch, which completely encircles both the trachea and the esophagus, is more likely to be symptomatic, although the symptoms of this anomaly are more commonly respiratory than esophageal in origin. Another vascular lesion, which may compress the esophagus and produce dysphagia, is an aneurysm of the descending aorta, and cases of marked tortuosity of the distal thoracic aorta have been reported as causing lower esophageal obstruction. Rarely, dysphagia may result from giant enlargement of the left atrium, as seen in patients with severe mitral insufficiency, and dysphagia has occasionally been reported in a patient with an enlarged left ventricle resulting from compression between the enlarged cardiac chamber anteriorly and a tortuous thoracic aorta posteriorly.

Although idiopathic mediastinal fibrosis usually presents with symptoms of superior vena caval obstruction, other structures may also be involved, including the esophagus, which may be compressed thereby. Other unusual causes of extrinsic esophageal compression include hypertrophic spurs of the cervical spine, which may project anteriorly sufficiently to compromise the lumen of the esophagus, and carcinoma of the bronchus, which, on rare occasions, may cause symptoms of dysphagia before respiratory symptoms are noted by the patient. Obviously, almost any tumor of the midmediastinum can cause dysphagia. Enlargement of the thyroid either because of an adenomatous goiter or because of carcinoma, if of sufficient size, may displace or even surround the esophagus and cause obstruction. Lymphoma, particularly Hodgkin's disease, may either invade the esophagus or compress its wall, and metastatic tumors to lymph nodes may lead to dysphagia for similar reasons. Treatment in all of these instances is directed toward removal of the cause of the compression. Such therapy is most useful in compression by vascular lesions. Secondary involvement of the esophagus by malignant processes — primary, in the thorax, or metastatic — is clearly less amenable to medical or surgical treatment.

Postvagotomy Dysphagia

Dysphagia may follow truncal vagotomy, and although the procedure is performed less frequently now than previously, it is discussed here for the sake of completeness. It is a rare complication, occurring only nine times in 1298 patients undergoing transabdominal vagotomy at the Mayo Clinic (Andersen *et al.*, 1966). The symptoms appear 1 to 2 weeks after operation and usually disappear in a few days or weeks. Most are the result of periesophageal inflam-

mation and fibrosis. Only rarely can a motility disorder be identified.

SELECTED REFERENCES

Code, C. F., and Schlegel, J. F.: Motor action of the esophagus and its sphincters. *In* Handbook of Physiology. Edited by W. Heidel. Baltimore, Williams and Wilkins Company, 1967, pp. 1821–1839.

This superb summary by two of the pioneers in the field of esophageal manometry provides the reader with information necessary for a basic understanding of the normal function of the esophagus and its sphincters.

Dodds, W. J., Hogan, W. J., Helm, J. E., *et al.*: Pathogenesis of reflux esophagitis. Gastroenterology, *81*:376, 1981.

An up-to-date summary of current knowledge concerning the complexities governing gastroesophageal competence and reflux.

Ellis, F. H., Jr., and Olsen, A. M.: Achalasia of the Esophagus. Philadelphia, W. B. Saunders Company, 1969.

This monograph represents a summary of all aspects of this interesting disease. Emphasis is placed on the surgical management of esophageal achalasia, which the authors prefer to forceful dilation as primary therapy.

Fischer, R. A., Ellison, G. W., Thayer, W. R., *et al.*: Esophageal motility in neuromuscular disorders. Ann. Intern. Med., *63*:229, 1965.

A good summary of what little is known of this complex and ill-defined subject.

Hacker, V., and Lotheissen, G.: Chirurgie der Speiseröhre. Band XXXIV. Neue Deutsche Chirurgie. Stuttgart, Enke, 1926.

This book is probably the best historical summary of early efforts to treat esophageal disease by surgical techniques. As so often happens in medicine, what now seems new and innovative was thought of and done before and unfortunately forgotten until modern advances permitted its reintroduction under more favorable circumstances.

Payne, W. S., and Clagett, O. T.: Pharyngeal and esophageal diverticula. Curr. Probl. Surg., 1–31, April 1965.

Diverticula of the esophagus are well covered in this brief but complete survey of this subject. Only cricopharyngeal myotomy is omitted, but enthusiasm for the use of this technique in the management of pharyngeal pouches is of more recent origin.

Payne, W. S., and Olsen, A. M.: The Esophagus. Philadelphia, Lea & Febiger, 1974.

Those interested in the esophagus have long awaited a modern summary of diagnosis and treatment of diseases of this organ. This monograph, based on the extensive experience of the Mayo Clinic, more than fulfills this need.

Postlethwait, R. W.: Surgery of the Esophagus. New York, Appleton-Century-Crofts, 1979.

A new, updated, and totally rewritten edition of Postlethwait and Sealy's early esophageal monograph. The current edition is exhaustive in its coverage of esophageal surgery and has an excellent bibliography.

REFERENCES

Abbott, O. A., Mansour, K. A., Logan, W. D., Jr., *et al.*: Atraumatic so-called "spontaneous" rupture of the esophagus: A review of 47 personal cases with comments on a new method of surgical therapy. J. Thorac. Cardiovasc. Surg., *59*:67, 1970.

Adams, W. E., and Phemister, D. B.: Carcinoma of lower thoracic esophagus: Report of successful resection and esophagogastrostomy. J. Thorac. Cardiovasc. Surg., *7*:621, 1938.

Akakura, I., Nakamura, Y., Kakegawa, T., *et al.*: Surgery of carcinoma of the esophagus with preoperative radiation. Chest, *57*:47, 1970.

Allison, P. R., and Johnstone, A. S.: Oesophagus lined with gastric mucous membrane. Thorax, *8*:87, 1953.

Andersen, H. A., Schlegel, J. F., and Olsen, A. M.: Postvagotomy dysphagia. Gastrointest. Endosc., *12*:13, 1966.

Ardran, G. M., and Kemp, F. H.: The radiography of the lower lateral food channels. J. Laryngol. Otol., *75*:358, 1961.

Atias, A., Neghme, A., Aguirre-Mackay, L., *et al.*: Megaesophagus, megacolon, and Chagas' disease in Chile. Gastroenterology, *44*:433, 1963.

Babka, J. C., and Castell, D. O.: On the genesis of heartburn: The effect of specific foods on the lower esophageal sphincter. Am. J. Dig. Dis., *18*:391, 1973.

Backer-Gröndahl, N.: Cardiaplastik ved Cardiospasmus. Forhandlingar Nord. Kirurg. Forenings, *11*:236, 1916.

Barrett, N. R.: Chronic peptic ulcer of the oesophagus and "oesophagitis." Br. J. Surg., *38*:175, 1950.

Barrett, N. R.: Report of case of spontaneous perforation of oesophagus successfully treated by operation. Br. J. Surg., *35*:216, 1947.

Barrett, N. R., and Franklin, R. H.: Concerning unfavorable late results of certain operations performed in treatment of cardiospasm. Br. J. Surg., *37*:194, 1949.

Beck, C., and Carrell, A.: Demonstration of specimens illustrating a method of formation of prethoracic esophagus. Ill. Med. J., *7*:463, 1905.

Bell-Thomson, J., Haggitt, R. C., and Ellis, F. H., Jr.: Mucoepidermoid and adenoid cystic carcinomas of the esophagus. J. Thorac. Cardiovasc. Surg., *79*:438, 1980.

Belsey, R.: Functional disease of the esophagus. J. Thorac. Cardiovasc. Surg., *52*:164, 1966.

Benjamin, I., Olsen, A. M., and Ellis, F. H., Jr.: Esophagopleural fistula: A rare postpneumonectomy complication. Ann. Thorac. Surg., *7*:139, 1969.

Bernatz, P. E., Smith, J. L., Ellis, F. H., Jr., *et al.*: Benign, pedunculated, intraluminal tumors of the esophagus. J. Thorac. Cardiovasc. Surg., *35*:503, 1958.

Bernstein, L. M., and Baker, L. A.: A clinical test for esophagitis. Gastroenterology, *34*:760, 1958.

Billroth, T.: Ueber die Resection des Oesophagus. Arch. Klin. Chir., *13*:65, 1871.

Borja, A. R., Ransdell, H. T., Jr., Thomas, T. V., *et al.*: Lye injuries of the esophagus. Analysis of ninety cases of lye ingestion. J. Thorac. Cardiovasc. Surg., *57*:533, 1969.

Boyce, H. W., Jr.: Nonsurgical measures to relieve distresses of late esophageal carcinoma. Geriatrics, *28*:97, 1973.

Bremner, C. G., Lynch, V. P., and Ellis, F. H., Jr.: Barrett's esophagus: Congenital or acquired? An experimental study of esophageal mucosal regeneration in the dog. Surgery, *68*:209, 1970.

Buchin, P. J., and Spiro, H. M.: Therapy of esophageal stricture: A review of 84 patients, J. Clin. Gastroenterol., *3*:121, 1981.

Burgess, J. N., Payne, W. S., Andersen, H. A., *et al.*: Barrett esophagus: The columnar-epithelial-lined lower esophagus. Mayo Clin. Proc., *46*:728, 1971.

Butin, J. W., Olsen, A. M., Moersch, H. J., *et al.*: A study of esophageal pressures in normal persons and patients with cardiospasm. Gastroenterology, *23*:278, 1953.

Butler, H.: Veins of oesophagus. Thorax, *6*:276, 1951.

Cameron, J. L., Kieffer, R. F., Hendrix, T. R., *et al.*: Selective nonoperative management of contained intrathoracic esophageal disruptions. Ann. Thorac. Surg., *27*:404, 1979.

Campbell, G. S., Burnett, H. F., Ransom, J. M., *et al.*: Treatment of corrosive burns of the esophagus. Arch. Surg., *112*:495, 1977.

Carey, J. M., and Hollingshead, W. H.: Anatomic study of esophageal hiatus. Surg. Gynecol. Obstet., *100*:196, 1955.

Cassella, R. R., Brown, A. L., Jr., Sayre, G. P., *et al.*: Achalasia of

the esophagus: Pathologic and etiologic considerations. Ann. Surg., *160*:474, 1964.

Cassella, R. R., Ellis, F. H., Jr., Brown, A. L., Jr., *et al.*: Fine-structure changes in achalasia of the esophagus. I. Vagus nerves. Am. J. Pathol., *46*:279, 1965.

Cederqvist, C., Nielsen, J., Berthelsen, A., *et al.*: Adenocarcinoma of the oesophagus. Acta Chir. Scand., *146*:411, 1980.

Cheever, D. W.: Cited by Meade, R. H.: A History of Thoracic Surgery. Springfield, Illinois, Charles C Thomas, 1961, p. 571.

Code, C. F., and Schlegel, J. F.: Motor action of the esophagus and its sphincters. *In* Handbook of Physiology. Edited by W. Heidel. Baltimore, Williams and Wilkins Company, 1967, pp. 1821–1839.

Code, C. F., Creamer, B., Schlegel, J. F., *et al.*: an Atlas of Esophageal Motility in Health and Disease. Springfield, Illinois, Charles C Thomas, 1958, pp. 1–134.

Code, C. F., Schlegel, J. F., Kelley, M. L., Jr., *et al.*: Hypertensive gastroesophageal sphincter. Mayo Clin. Proc., *35*:391, 1960.

Cohen, B. R., and Guelrud, M.: "Cardiospasm" in achalasia: Demonstration of supersensitivity of the lower esophageal sphincter. Gastroenterology, *60*:769, 1971.

Cohen, S., and Harris, L. D.: Lower esophageal sphincter pressure as an index of lower esophageal sphincter strength. Gastroenterology, *58*:157, 1970.

Cohen, S., and Harris, L. D.: Does hiatus hernia affect competence of the gastroesophageal sphincter? N. Engl. J. Med., *284*:1053, 1971.

Cohen, S., Fischer, R., and Tuch, A.: The site of denervation in achalasia. Gut, *13*:556, 1972.

Cohen, S., Lipshutz, W., and Hughes, W.: Role of gastrin supersensitivity in the pathogenesis of lower esophageal sphincter hypertension in achalasia. J. Clin. Invest., *50*:1241, 1971.

Collis, J. L.: An operation for hiatus hernia with short esophagus. J. Thorac. Cardiovasc. Surg., *34*:768, 1957.

Coordinating Group for Research on Esophageal Cancer, Linhsien County, Honan: Early diagnosis and surgical treatment of esophageal cancer under rural conditions. Chin. Med. J., *2*:113, 1976.

Creamer, B., Donoghue, F. E., and Code, C. F.: Pattern of esophageal motility in diffuse spasm. Gastroenterology, *34*:782, 1958.

Crispin, J. S., McIver, D. K., and Lind, J. F.: Manometric study of the effect of vagotomy on the gastroesophageal sphincter. Can. J. Surg., *10*:299, 1967.

Cross, F. S., Johnson, G. F., and Gerein, A. N.: Esophageal diverticula: Associated neuromuscular changes in the esophagus. Arch. Surg., *83*:525, 1961.

Czerny, V.: Neue Operationen: Vorläufige Mittheilung. Zentralbl. Cir., *4*:433, 1877.

Day, N. E.: Some aspects of the epidemiology of esophageal cancer. Cancer Res., *35*:3304, 1975.

Debas, H. T., Payne, W. S., Cameron, A. J., *et al.*: Physiopathology of lower esophageal diverticulum and its implications for treatment. Surg. Gynecol. Obstet., *151*:593, 1980.

De Bruïne-Groeneveldt, J. R.: Over cardiospasmus. Ned. Tijdschr. Geneeskd., *62*(Sec. 2):1281, 1918.

Diamant, N. E., and El-Sharkawy, T. Y.: Neural control of esophageal peristalsis. A conceptual analysis. Gastroenterology, *72*:546, 1977.

Dodds, W. J., Hogan, W. J., Helm, J. E., *et al.*: Pathogenesis of reflux esophagitis. Gastroenterology, *81*:376, 1981.

Doll, R., Payne, P., and Waterhouse, J. (Eds.): Cancer Incidence in Five Continents: A Technical Report. Vol. 1. New York, Springer-Verlag, 1966, pp. 1–241.

Donoghue, F. E., Winkelmann, R. K., and Moersch, H. J.: Esophageal defects in dermatomyositis. Ann. Otol. Rhinol. Laryngol., *69*:1139, 1960.

Earlam, R., and Cunha-Melo, J. R.: Oesophageal squamous cell carcinoma. II. A critical review of radiotherapy. Br. J. Surg., *67*:457, 1980.

Earlam, R. J., Ellis, F. H., Jr., and Nobrega, F. T.: Achalasia of the esophagus in a small urban community. Mayo Clin. Proc., *44*:478, 1969.

Eckardt, V. F., Dagradi, A. E., Stempien, S. J., et al.: The esophagogastric (Schatzki) ring and reflux esophagitis. Am. J. Gastroenterol., 58:525, 1972.

Eckardt, V. F., Adami, B., Hücker, H., et al.: The esophagogastric junction in patients with asymptomatic lower esophageal mucosal rings. Gastroenterology, 79:426, 1980.

Ellis, F. H., Jr.: Unpublished data, 1981.

Ellis, F. H., Jr., and Crozier, R. E.: Cervical esophageal dysphagia: Indications for and results of cricopharyngeal myotomy. Ann. Surg., 194:279, 1981.

Ellis, F. H., Jr., and Gibb, S. P.: Esophagogastrectomy for carcinoma: Current hospital mortality and morbidity rates. Ann. Surg., 190:699, 1979.

Ellis, F. H.,Jr., and Olsen, A. M.: Achalasia of the Esophagus. Philadelphia, W. B. Saunders Company, 1969, p. 196.

Ellis, F. H., Jr., Code, C. F., and Olsen, A. M.: Long esophagomyotomy for diffuse spasm of the esophagus and hypertensive gastroesophageal sphincter. Surgery, 48:155, 1960.

Ellis, F. H., Jr., Gibb, S. P., and Crozier, R. E.: Esophagomyotomy for achalasia of the esophagus. Ann. Surg., 192:157, 1980.

Ellis, F. H., Jr., Kiser, J. C., Schlegel, J. F., et al.: Esophagomyotomy for esophageal achalasia: Experimental, clinical, and manometric aspects. Ann. Surg., 166:640, 1967.

Ellis, F. H., Jr., Leonardi, H. K., Dabuzhsky, L., et al.: Surgery for short esophagus with stricture: An experimental and clinical manometric study. Ann. Surg., 188:341, 1978.

Ellis, F. H., Jr., Schlegel, J. F., Code, C. F., et al.: Surgical treatment of esophageal hypermotility disturbances. J.A.M.A., 188:862, 1964.

Ellis, F. H., Jr., Schlegel, J. F., Lynch, V. P., et al.: Cricopharyngeal myotomy for pharyngo-esophageal diverticulum. Ann. Surg., 170:340, 1969.

Farrell, R. L., and Castell, D. O.: The abnormal lower esophageal sphincter in pernicious anemia. (Abstract.) Clin. Res., 20:453, 1972.

Ferguson, T. B., Woodbury, J. D., Roper, C. L., et al.: Giant muscular hypertrophy of the esophagus. Ann. Thorac. Surg., 8:209, 1969.

Finley, R. J., Pearson, F. G., Weisel, R. D., et al.: The management of nonmalignant intrathoracic esophageal perforations. Ann. Thorac. Surg., 30:575, 1980.

Fischer, R. A., Ellison, G. W., Thayer, W. R., et al.: Esophageal motility in neuromuscular disorders. Ann. Intern. Med., 63:229, 1965.

Garfinkel, L., Poindexter, C. E., and Silverberg, E.: Cancer in black Americans. CA., 30:39, 1980.

Garrett, J. M., Winkelmann, R. K., Schlegel, J. F., et al.: Esophageal deterioration in scleroderma. Mayo Clin. Proc., 46:92, 1971.

Gillison, E. W., DeCastro, V. A., Nyhus, L. M., et al.: The significance of bile in reflux esophagitis. Surg. Gynecol. Obstet., 134:419, 1972.

Goldberg, H. I., and Dodds, W. J.: Cobblestone esophagus due to monilial infection. Am. J. Roentgenol. Radium Ther. Nucl. Med., 104:608, 1968.

Goursand: Cited by Meade, R. H.: A History of Thoracic Surgery. Springfield, Illinois, Charles C Thomas, 1961, p. 567.

Goyal, R. K., Bauer, J. L., and Spiro, H. M.: The nature and location of the lower esophageal ring. N. Engl. J. Med., 284:1175, 1971.

Groves, L. K., and Rodriguez-Antunez, A.: Treatment of carcinoma of the esophagus and gastric cardia with concentrated preoperative irradiation followed by early operation. Ann. Thorac. Surg., 15:333, 1973.

Gryboski, J. D.: The swallowing mechanism of the neonate. I. Esophageal and gastric motility. Pediatrics, 35:445, 1965.

Gunnlaugsson, G. H., Wychulis, A. R., Roland, C., et al.: Analysis of the records of 1,657 patients with carcinoma of the esophagus and cardia of the stomach. Surg. Gynecol. Obstet., 130:997, 1970.

Hacker, V., and Lotheissen, G.: Chirurgie der Speiseröhre. Band XXXIV. Neue Deutsche Chirurgie. Stuttgart, Enke, 1926.

Haggitt, R. C., Tryzelaar, J., Ellis, F. H., Jr., et al: Adenocarcinoma complicating columnar epithelium-lined (Barrett's) esophagus. Am. J. Clin. Pathol., 70:1, 1978.

Haller, J. A., Jr., and Bachman, K.: The comparative effect of current therapy on experimental caustic burns of the esophagus. Pediatrics, 34:236, 1964.

Hammon, J. W., Jr., Rice, R. P., Postlethwait, R. W., et al.: Esophageal intramural diverticulosis: A clinical and pathological survey. Ann. Thorac. Surg., 17:260, 1974.

Hawe, A., Payne, W. S., Weiland, L. H., et al.: Adenocarcinoma in the columnar epithelial lined lower (Barrett) oesophagus. Thorax, 28:511, 1973.

Heimlich, H. J.: Esophagoplasty with reversed gastric tube: Review of fifty-three cases. Am. J. Surg., 123:80, 1972.

Heller, E.: Extramukose Cardiaplastik beim chronischen Cardiospasmus mit Dilatation des Oesophagus. Mitt. Grenzgeb. Med. Chir., 27:141, 1913.

Helm, W. J., Schlegel, J. F., Code, C. F., et al.: Identification of the gastroesophageal mucosal junction by transmucosal potential in healthy subjects and patients with hiatal hernia. Gastroenterology, 48:25, 1965.

Heyerovsky, H.: Casuistik und Therapie der idiopathischen Dilatation der Speiseröhre: Oesophagogastroanastomose. Arch. Klin. Chir., 100:703, 1913.

Heyerovsky, H.: Discussion. Vierter Sitzungstag. Part I. Protokolle, Discussionen und kleine Mittheilung. Verh. Dtsch. Ges. Chir., 40:286, 1911.

Hiebert, C. A.: Primary incompetence of the gastric cardia. Am. J. Surg., 119:365, 1970.

Higgs, B., Kerr, F. W., and Ellis, F. H., Jr.: The experimental production of esophageal achalasia by electrolytic lesions in the medulla. J. Thorac. Cardiovasc. Surg., 50:613, 1965a.

Higgs, B., Shorter, R. G., and Ellis, F. H., Jr.: A study of the anatomy of the human esophagus with special reference to the gastroesophageal sphincter. J. Surg. Res., 5:503, 1965b.

Hill, L. D., Gelfand, M., and Bauermeister, D.: Simplified management of reflux esophagitis with stricture. Ann. Surg., 172:638, 1970.

Hoehn, J. G., and Payne, W. S.: Resection of pharyngoesophageal diverticulum using stapling device. Mayo Clin. Proc., 44:738, 1969.

Hollenbeck, J. I., Maher, J.W., Wickbom, G., et al.: Effect of feeding on the canine lower esophageal sphincter. Surg. Forum, 25:346, 1974.

Hollis, J. B., and Castell, D. O.: Esophageal junction in elderly man: A new look at "presbyesophagus." Ann. Intern. Med., 80:371, 1974.

Hopkins, R. A., and Postlethwait, R. W.: Caustic burns and carcinoma of the esophagus. Ann. Surg., 194:146, 1981.

Hunt, P. S., Connell, A. M., and Smiley, T. B.: The cricopharyngeal sphincter in gastric reflux. Gut, 11:303, 1970.

Hurwitz, A. L., and Duranceau, A.: Upper-esophageal sphincter dysfunction: Pathogenesis and treatment. Am. J. Dig. Dis., 23:275, 1978.

Ingelfinger, F. J.: Esophageal motility. Physiol. Rev., 38:533, 1958.

Jianu, A.: Gastrotomie und Oesophagoplastik. Dtsch. Z. Chir., 118:383, 1912.

Johnson, H. D.: Active and passive opening of the cardia and its relation to the pathogenesis of hiatus hernia. Gut, 7:392, 1966.

Johnson, J., Schwegman, C. W., and Kirby, C. K.: Esophageal exclusion for persistent fistula following spontaneous rupture of the esophagus. J. Thorac. Cardiovasc. Surg., 32:827, 1956.

Johnson, L. F., and De Meester, T. R.: Twenty-four–hour pH monitoring of the distal esophagus: A quantitative measure of gastroesophageal reflux. Am. J. Gastroenterol., 62:325, 1974.

Jones, D. B., and Smith, P. M.: Conservative management of benign oesophageal strictures. Endoscopy, 13:55, 1981.

Just-Viera, J. O., Morris, J. D., and Haight, C.: Achalasia and esophageal carcinoma. Ann. Thorac. Surg., 3:526, 1967.

Kantrowitz, P. A., Fleischli, D. J., and Butler, W. T.: Successful treatment of chronic esophageal moniliasis with a viscous suspension of nystatin. Gastroenterology, 57:424, 1969.

Kaye, M. D.: Oesophageal motor dysfunction in patients with diverticula of the mid-thoracic oesophagus. Thorax 29:666, 1974.

Kelly, A. B.: Spasm at entrance to oesophagus. J. Laryngol. Otol., 34:285, 1919.

Kiviranta, U. K.: Corrosion carcinoma of esophagus: 381 cases of corrosion and 9 cases of corrosion carcinoma. Acta Otolaryngol., 42:89, 1952.

Kongtahworn, C., and Rossi, N. P.: Dilatation for severe esophageal stricture. Ann. Thorac. Surg., 14:678, 1972.

Kreuser, E. D.: Primary malignant melanoma of the esophagus. Virchows Arch. (Pathol. Anat.), 385:49, 1979.

Kwun, K.-B., and Kirschner, P. A.: Palliative side-to-side oesophagogastrostomy for unresectable carcinoma of the oesophagus and cardia. Thorax, 36:441, 1981.

Lahey, F. H.: Pharyngoesophageal diverticulum: Its management and complications. Ann. Surg., 124:617, 1946.

Laimer, E.: Beitrag zur Anatomie des Oesophagus. Med. Jahrbücher, 1883, pp. 333–388.

Leape, L. L., Ashcraft, K. W., Scarpelli, D. G., et al.: Hazard to health — liquid lye. N. Engl. J. Med., 284:578, 1971.

Leonardi, H. K., Crozier, R. E., and Ellis, F. H., Jr.: Reoperation for complications of the Nissen fundoplication. J. Thorac. Cardiovasc. Surg., 81:50, 1981.

Leonardi, H. K., Shea, J. A., Crozier, R. E., et al.: Diffuse spasm of the esophagus: Clinical, manometric, and surgical considerations. J. Thorac. Cardiovasc. Surg., 74:736, 1977.

Lexer, E. B.: Oesophagoplastik: Verein für wissentschaftliche Heilkunde in Königsberg. Dtsch. Med. Wochenschr., 34:574, 1908.

Lichter, I.: Motor disorder in pharyngoesophageal pouch. J. Thorac. Cardiovasc. Surg., 76:272, 1978.

Lind, J. F., Warrian, W. G., and Wankling, W. J.: Responses of the gastroesophageal junctional zone to increases in abdominal pressure. Can. J. Surg., 9:32, 1966.

Linsman, J. F.: Gastroesophageal reflux elicited while drinking water (water siphonage test): Its clinical correlation with pyrosis. Am. J. Roentgenol. Radium Ther. Nucl. Med., 94:325, 1965.

Lipshutz, W. H., Gaskins, R. D., Lukash, W. M., et al.: Pathogenesis of lower-esophageal-sphincter incompetence. N. Engl. J. Med., 289:182, 1973.

Lise, M., Perrino, G., Cordioli, G. P., et al.: The autonomic nervous system in esophageal achalasia. Chir. Gastroenterol., 6:103, 1972.

Lortat-Jacob, J. L.: La myomatose nodulaire diffuse de l'oesophage. Acquis. Méd. Récent., 1950, pp. 103–111.

Ludlow, A.: Obstructed deglutition from a preternatural dilatation of and bag formed in the pharynx. Medical Observations and Inquiries by a Society of Physicians in London, 3:85, 1762–1767.

Maher, J. W., Hocking, M. P., and Woodward, E. R.: Long-term follow-up of the combined fundic patch fundoplication for treatment of longitudinal peptic strictures of the esophagus. Ann. Surg., 194:64, 1981.

Mallory, G. K., and Weiss, S.: Hemorrhages from lacerations of cardiac orifice of stomach due to vomiting. Am. J. Med. Sci., 178:506, 1929.

Malmud, L. S., Fisher, R. S., Lobis, I., et al.: Quantitation of gastroesophageal (GE) reflux before and after therapy using the GE scintiscan. (Abstract.) J. Nucl. Med., 17:559, 1976.

Mann, C. V., Code, C. F., Schlegel, J. F., et al.: Intrinsic mechanisms controlling the mammalian gastro-oesophageal sphincter deprived of extrinsic nerve supply. Thorax, 23:634, 1968.

Mansour, K. A., Burton, H.G., Miller, J. I., et al.: Complications of intrathoracic Nissen fundoplication. Ann. Thorac. Surg., 32:173, 1981.

Mansour, K. A., Symbas, P. H., Jones, E. L., et al.: A combined surgical approach in the management of achalasia of the esophagus. Ann. Surg., 42:192, 1976.

Marks, R. D., Jr., Scruggs, H. J., and Wallace, K. M.: Preoperative radiation therapy for carcinoma of the esophagus. Cancer, 38:84, 1976.

Marshall, S. F.: Carcinoma of esophagus: Successful resection of lower end of esophagus with reestablishment of esophageal gastric continuity. Surg. Clin. North Am., 18:643, 1938.

McGlashan, N. D., Walters, C. L., and McLean, A. E.: Nitrosamines in African alcoholic spirits and oesophageal cancer. Lancet, 2:1071, 1968.

Mendl, K., McKay, J. M., and Tanner, C. H.: Intramural diverticulosis of the oesophagus and Rokitansky-Aschoff sinuses in the gall-bladder. Br. J. Radiol., 33:496, 1960.

Meyerowitz, B. R., and Shea, L. T.: The natural history of squamous verrucose carcinoma of the esophagus. J. Thorac. Cardiovasc. Surg., 61:646, 1971.

Michel, L., Grillo, H. C., and Malt, R. A.: Operative and nonoperative management of esophageal perforations. Ann. Surg., 194:57, 1981.

Michel, L., Serrano, A., and Malt, R. A.: Mallory-Weiss syndrome: Evolution of diagnostic and therapeutic patterns over two decades. Ann. Surg., 192:716, 1980.

Miller, L. J., Thistle, J. L., Payne, W. S., et al.: Crohn's disease involving the esophagus and colon: Case report. Mayo Clin. Proc., 52:35, 1977.

Misiewicz, J. J., Walter, S. L., Anthony, P. P., et al.: Achalasia of the cardia: Pharmacology and histopathology of isolated cardiac sphincteric muscle from patients with and without achalasia. Q. J. Med., 38:17, 1969.

Mladick, R. A., Horton, C. E., and Adamson, J. E.: Cricopharyngeal myotomy: Application and technique in major oral-pharyngeal resections. Arch. Surg., 102:1, 1971.

Naef, A. P., Savary, M., and Ozzella, L.: Columnar-lined lower esophagus: An acquired lesion with malignant predisposition. Report on 140 cases of Barrett's esophagus with 12 adenocarcinomas. J. Thorac. Cardiovasc. Surg., 70:826, 1975.

Nakayama, K.: Pre-operative irradiation in the treatment of patients with carcinoma of the oesophagus and of some other sites. Clin. Radiol., 15:232, 1964.

Nichols, T., Yokoo, H., Craig, R. M., et al.: Pseudosarcoma of the esophagus: Three new cases and review of the literature. Am. J. Gastroenterol., 72:615, 1979.

Ochsner, A., and Owens, N.: Anterothoracic oesophagoplasty for impermeable strictures of oesophagus. Ann. Surg., 100:1055, 1934.

Ohsawa, T.: The surgery of the oesophagus. Arch. Jpn. Chir., 10:605, 1933.

Okike, N., Payne, W. S., Neufeld, D. M., et al.: Esophagomyotomy versus forceful dilation for achalasia of the esophagus: Results in 899 patients. Ann. Thorac. Surg., 28:119, 1979.

Olsen, A. M., and Creamer, B.: Studies of oesophageal motility, with special reference to the differential diagnosis of diffuse spasm and achalasia (cardiospasm). Thorax, 12:279, 1957.

Orringer, M. B., and Sloan, H.: Complications and failings of the combined Collis-Belsey operation. J. Thorac. Cardiovasc. Surg., 74:726, 1977.

Orringer, M. B., and Sloan, H.: Esophagectomy without thoracotomy. J. Thorac. Cardiovasc. Surg., 76:643, 1978.

Ottinger, L. W., and Wilkins, E. W., Jr.: Late results in patients with Schatzki rings undergoing destruction of the ring and hiatus herniorrhaphy. Am. J. Surg., 139:591, 1980.

Parker, E. F., and Gregorie, H. B.: Carcinoma of the esophagus: Long term results. J.A.M.A., 235:1018, 1976.

Paterson, D. R.: Clinical type of dysphagia. J. Laryngol. Otol., 34:289, 1919.

Payne, W. S., and Clagett, O. T.: Pharyngeal and esophageal diverticula. Curr. Probl. Surg., 1–31, April 1965.

Payne, W. S., and Olsen, A. M.: The Esophagus. Philadelphia, Lea & Febiger, 1974.

Payne, W. S., Andersen, H. A., and Ellis, F. H., Jr.: Reappraisal of esophagogastrectomy and antral excision in the treatment of short esophagus. Surgery, 55:344, 1964.

Pearson, F. G., Langer, B., and Henderson, R. D.: Gastroplasty and Belsey hiatus hernia repair: An operation for the management of peptic stricture with acquired short esophagus. J. Thorac. Cardiovasc. Surg., 61:50, 1971.

Pearson, J. G.: The present status and future potential of radiotherapy in the management of esophageal cancer. Cancer, *39*(Suppl. 2):882, 1977.

Pennell, T. C.: Supradiaphragmatic correction of esophageal reflux strictures. Ann. Surg., *193*:655, 1981.

Pera, C., Suner, M., and Capdevila, J.: Anatomical demonstration of the lower esophageal sphincter: A biometrical analysis of 300 specimens. Bull. Soc. Int. Chir., *34*:285, 1975.

Peyton, M. D., Greenfield, L. J., and Elkins, R. C.: Combined myotomy and hiatal herniorrhaphy: A new approach to achalasia. Am. J. Surg., *128*:786, 1974.

Pope, C. E., II: A dynamic test of sphincter strength: Its application to the lower esophageal sphincter. Gastroenterology, *52*:779, 1967.

Postlethwait, R. W.: Surgery of the Esophagus. New York, Appleton-Century-Crofts, 1979.

Priestman, T. J.: Progress report: Cytotoxic therapy for gastrointestinal carcinoma. Gut, *17*:313, 1976.

Proctor, D. S. C.: Esophageal intubation for carcinoma of the esophagus. World J. Surg., *4*:451, 1980.

Rake, G. W.: Annular muscular hypertrophy of the oesophagus: Achalasia of the cardia without oesophageal dilatation. Guy's Hosp. Rep., *76*:145, 1926.

Raphael, H. A., Ellis, F. H., Jr., and Dockerty, M. B.: Primary adenocarcinoma of the esophagus: 18-year review and review of literature. Ann. Surg., *164*:785, 1966.

Reid, H. A., Richardson, W. W., and Corrin, B.: Oat cell carcinoma of the esophagus. Cancer, *45*:2342, 1980.

Roux, C.: L'oesophago-jéjuno-gastrostomose, nouvelle opération pour rétrécissement infanchissable de l'oesophage. Sem. Méd., *27*:37, 1907.

Sanderson, D. R., Ellis, F. H., Jr., Schlegel, J. F., et al.: Syndrome of vigorous achalasia: Clinical and physiologic observations. Chest, *52*:508, 1967.

Sanfelippo, P. M., and Bernatz, P. E.: Celestin-tube palliation for malignant esophageal obstruction. Surg. Clin. North Am., *53*:921, 1973.

Sawyers, J. L., Lane, C. E., Foster, J. H., et al.: Esophageal perforation: An increasing challenge. Ann. Thorac. Surg., *19*:233, 1975.

Schatzki, R., and Gary, J. E.: Dysphagia due to diaphragm-like localized narrowing in the lower esophagus ("lower esophageal ring"). Am. J. Roentgenol. Radium Ther. Nucl. Med., *70*:911, 1953.

Schatzki, R., and Hawes, L. E.: Tumors of esophagus below mucosa and their roentgenological differential diagnosis. Rev. Gastroenterol., *17*:991, 1950.

Seremetis, M. G., deGuzman, V. C., Lyons, W. S., et al.: Leiomyoma of the esophagus: A report of 19 surgical cases. Ann. Thorac. Surg., *16*:308, 1973.

Shine, I., and Allison, P. R.: Carcinoma of the oesophagus with tylosis (keratosis palmaris et plantaris). Lancet, *1*:951, 1966.

Silber, W.: Diabetes and oesophageal dysfunction. Br. Med. J., *3*:688, 1969.

Skinner, D. B., and Booth, D. J.: Assessment of distal esophageal function in patients with hiatal hernia and/or gastro-esophageal reflux. Ann. Surg., *172*:627, 1970.

Smiley, T. B., Caves, P. K., and Porter, D. C.: Relationship between posterior pharyngeal pouch and hiatus hernia. Thorax, *25*:725, 1970.

Smith, A. W., Mulder, D. W., and Code, C. F.: Esophageal motility in amyotrophic lateral sclerosis. Mayo Clin. Proc., *32*:438, 1957.

Smith, B.: The neurological lesion in achalasia of the cardia. Gut, *11*:388, 1970.

Stanciu, C., and Bennett, J. R.: Smoking and gastro-oesophageal reflux. Br. Med. J., *3*:793, 1972.

Stener, B., Kock, N. G., Pettersson, S., et al.: Carcinosarcoma of the esophagus. J. Thorac. Cardiovasc. Surg., *54*:746, 1967.

Sutherland, H. D.: Cricopharyngeal achalasia. J. Thorac. Cardiovasc. Surg., *43*:114, 1962.

Swigert, L. L., Siekert, R. G., Hanbley, W. C., et al.: Esophageal arteries: Anatomic study of 150 specimens. Surg. Gynecol. Obstet., *90*:234, 1950.

Tarnay, T. J., Chang, C. H., Migert, R. G., et al.: Esophageal duplication (foregut cyst) with spinal malformation. J. Thorac. Cardiovasc. Surg., *59*:293, 1970.

Thal, A. P.: A unified approach to surgical problems of the esophagogastric junction. Ann. Surg., *168*:542, 1968.

Thomas, P. A., and Earlam, R. J.: The action of gastrointestinal polypeptide hormones on the isolated perfused gastrooesophageal sphincter. Br. J. Surg., *60*:306, 1973.

Torek, F.: The first successful case of resection of the thoracic portion of the oesophagus for carcinoma. Surg. Gynecol. Obstet., *16*:614, 1913.

Tuch, A., and Cohen, S.: Lower esophageal sphincter relaxation: Studies on the neurogenic inhibitory mechanism. J. Clin. Invest., *52*:14, 1973.

Urschel, H. C., Jr., Razzuk, M. A., Wood, R. E., et al.: Improved management of esophageal perforation: Exclusion and diversion in continuity. Ann. Surg., *179*:587, 1974.

Vantrappen, G., and Hellemans, J.: Treatment of achalasia and related motor diseases. Gastroenterology, *79*:144, 1980.

Voelcker, F.: Ueber Exstirpation der Cardia wegen Carcinoms. Verh. Dtsch. Ges. Chir., *37*:126, 1908.

von Mikulicz, J.: Beiträge zur Technik der Operationen des Magencarcinoms. Arch. Klin. Chir., *57*:524, 1898.

von Mikulicz, J.: Small contributions to the surgery of the intestinal tract. 1. Cardiospasm and its treatment. 2. Peptic ulcer of the jejunum. 3. Operative treatment of severe forms of invagination of the intestine. 4. Operation on malignant growths of the large intestine. Boston Med. Surg. J., *148*:608, 1903.

von Ziemssen, H. (Ed.): Handbuch der Speciellen Pathologie und Therapie. Vol. I. Leipzig, F. C. W. Vogel, 1875, pp. 1–208.

Watson, W. C., and Sullivan, S. M.: Hypertonicity of the cricopharyngeal sphincter: A cause of globus sensation. Lancet, *2*:1417, 1974.

Welsh, G. F., and Payne, W. S.: The present status of one-stage pharyngo-esophageal diverticulectomy. Surg. Clin. North Am., *53*:953, 1973.

Wendel, W.: Zur Chirurgie des Oesophagus. Arch. Klin. Chir., *93*:311, 1910.

Wheeler, W. I.: Pharyngocele and dilatation of pharynx, with existing diverticulum at lower portion of pharynx lying posterior to the oesophagus, cured by pharyngectomy, being the first case of the kind recorded. Dublin J. Med. Sci., *82*:349, 1886.

Wilkins, E. W., Jr., and Burke, J. F.: Experience with the colon esophageal bypass. Presented before the New England Surgical Society, Sept. 27, 1974.

Willis, T.: Pharmaceutice rationalis: Sive diatriba de medicametorum: Operationibus in humano corpore. London, Hagae-Comitis, 1674.

Windsor, C. W.: Gastro-oesophageal reflux after partial gastrectomy. Br. Med. J., *2*:1233, 1964.

Winship, D. H., Caflisch, C. R., Zboralske, F. F., et al.: Deterioration of esophageal peristalsis in patients with alcoholic neuropathy. Gastroenterology, *55*:173, 1968.

Woolam, G. L., Maher, F. T., and Ellis, F. H., Jr.: Vagal nerve function in achalasia of the esophagus. Surg. Forum, *18*:362, 1967.

Wu, Y. K., and Huang, K. C.: Chinese experience in the surgical treatment of carcinoma of the esophagus. Ann. Surg., *190*:361, 1979.

Wychulis, A. R., Ellis, F. H., Jr., and Andersen, H. A.: Acquired nonmalignant esophagotracheobronchial fistula: Report of 36 cases. J.A.M.A., *196*:117, 1966.

Wychulis, A. R., Fontana, R. S., and Payne, W. S.: Instrumental perforations of the esophagus. Chest, *55*:184, 1969a.

Wychulis, A. R., Fontana, R. S., and Payne, W. S.: Noninstrumental perforations of the esophagus. Chest, *55*:190, 1969b.

Wychulis, A. R., Woolam, G. L., Andersen, H. A., et al.: Achalasia and carcinoma of the esophagus. J.A.M.A., *215*:1638, 1971.

Wynder, E. L., and Bross, I. J.: A study of etiological factors in cancer of the esophagus. Cancer, *14*:389, 1961.

Wynder, E. L., Hultbert, S., Jacobson, F., et al.: Environmental factors in cancer of the upper alimentary tract: Swedish study with special reference to Plummer-Vinson (Paterson-Kelly) syndrome. Cancer, *10*:470, 1957.

Zaino, C., Jacobsen, H. G., Lepow, H., et al.: The Pharyngoesophageal Sphincter. Springfield, Illinois, Charles C Thomas, 1970, pp. 1–209.

Chapter 25

Esophageal Hiatal Hernia
I   THE CONDITION: CLINICAL MANIFESTATIONS AND DIAGNOSIS

David B. Skinner

A small herniation of the gastric cardia upward through the esophageal hiatus of the diaphragm is a common finding on radiographic barium swallow examination and is of no clinical significance at all unless accompanied by an abnormal degree of gastroesophageal reflux. Any discussion of esophageal hiatal hernia must distinguish between the inconsequential anatomic defect and the physiologic abnormality that can cause symptoms and severe complications. The two conditions, hiatal hernia and gastroesophageal reflux, may occur together, but each may occur in the absence of the other, and therefore, they are discussed as separate entities (Hiebert and Belsey, 1961). The usual Type I axial or sliding hiatal hernia is very common and is estimated to occur in at least 10 per cent of North American adults examined by barium swallow. Pathologic reflux is much less common, estimated to be present consistently in only 5 per cent of those having a hiatal hernia. Among patients with symptomatic reflux, approximately four fifths have a coincidental Type I hiatal hernia, but one fifth have no demonstrable radiographic abnormality at the hiatus.

NORMAL ANATOMY AND HIATAL HERNIA

The esophagus begins at the cricopharyngeal sphincter muscle (cricopharyngeus) at the level of the sixth cervical vertebral body. The sphincter muscle arises and inserts on the back of the cricoid cartilage of the larynx and superiorly blends into the inferior constrictor fibers of the hypopharynx. Anatomically, the cricopharyngeus is about 1 cm. wide, but pressure recordings demonstrate a high-pressure zone usually extending over several centimeters. The upper esophagus passes through the thoracic inlet constrained by adjacent anatomic structures, including the trachea anteriorly, the great vessels of the aortic arch laterally, and the vertebral bodies posteriorly. The aortic arch indents the esophagus approximately 8 cm. below the cricopharyngeus, marking the junction of the upper and middle thirds of the esophagus. Below this, the esophagus normally dilates somewhat, as determined by radiographic or endoscopic inspection. This is because the right lateral aspect of the esophagus is covered by the parietal pleura of the right hemithorax, so that the esophagus is directly exposed to the less-than-atmospheric intrathoracic pressure. The midesophagus anteriorly passes from the tracheal bifurcation onto the surface of the pericardium. On the left lateral side the esophagus abuts the aorta and left pleura, and posteriorly, it is in contact with the azygos vein, the thoracic duct, and the vertebral bodies. In its lower third, the esophagus begins to deviate slightly toward the left and anterior to the aorta until it penetrates the diaphragm through the esophageal hiatus almost directly anterior to the aortic hiatus of the diaphragm. The average length of the esophagus in an adult is approximately 25 cm. The amount above the clavicles is approximately 4 cm. in a young adult but decreases with age owing to anterior bowing of the skeleton. The aortic impulse on the esophagus is noted approximately 8 to 9 cm. from the cricopharyngeus. The left atrial pulsation can be observed at the junction of the mid and lower esophagus, approximately 16 to 18 cm. from the cricopharyngeus. The esophagus enters the hiatal tunnel, and the most distal 3 to 4 cm. become intra-abdominal in a normal adult.

Throughout its length the esophagus consists of two muscular layers, an outer longitudinal layer and an inner zone of circular muscle fibers. The transition between longitudinal and circular fibers is not abrupt or anatomically distinct, for "bracket" longitudinal fibers appear to bind bands of circular muscle together. Some of these transitional fibers are oblique in orientation (Friedland et al., 1966; Higgs et al., 1965). In the adult, the esophagus has no true serosa or mesentery. However, in the embryo, there is a meso-esophagus during development of the foregut, and accordingly, the arterial and venous connections of the esophagus as well as lymphatic drainage proceed dorsally for the most part to the aorta, azygos vein, and thoracic duct, respectively. Although the esophagus does not have true serosal layer, adjacent structures perform a serosa-like function by serving as points of origin and insertion for longitudinal muscle fibers. The serosa-like attachments include the membranous portion of the trachea and pericardium anteriorly and the pleural surfaces where these are adjacent to the esophagus.

The mucosa of the esophagus is separated from the muscle layers by a loose submucosa. This permits considerable mobility of the mucosa relative to the muscle layers and helps account for the ability of the esophagus to make rapid changes in diameter and length during swallowing or vomiting. The submucosa includes a rich collateral blood supply that is sufficient to maintain the viability of the esophagus if the organ remains attached to nutrient arteries and veins at either its upper or lower end, even though all other segmental esophageal vessels are divided. The submucosa contains a rich lymphatic network. There is a well-developed layer of muscularis mucosae upon which the mucosa itself rests. In humans, the esophagus is lined throughout its intrathoracic length by stratified squamous epithelium. The distal 2 to 3 cm. of the esophagus is lined with the simple columnar epithelium of the gastric cardia type. Submucosal mucous glands may occur along the length of the esophagus but are noted particularly at the uppermost and lowermost ends. During fetal life, the esophagus is lined with glandular epithelium for a time. Rarely, in adults, rests of glandular epithelium may be found at various levels in the esophagus surrounded by otherwise normal squamous epithelium.

The arterial blood supply reaches the esophagus from varying sources at different levels. The intra-abdominal segment of the esophagus is nourished by an ascending branch of the left gastric artery at the top of the gastrohepatic omentum, and an ascending branch of the left inferior phrenic artery joins the esophagus on its left lateral aspect. The intrathoracic esophagus receives three or more direct branches from the aorta. Near the midesophagus there are usually common arterial branches providing both bronchial and esophageal arteries. The highest of these branches usually arises from the back of the aortic arch. The cervical esophagus receives blood supply from branches originating in the thyrocervical trunk of the subclavian arteries. As previously mentioned, the submucosal network of arterial collaterals is sufficient to maintain viability of the esophagus even when all the segmental thoracic branches and the arterial supply at either the upper or lower end are divided, provided the blood supply at one end of the esophagus remains intact. Venous drainage of the esophagus enters the coronary vein and paracardial venous plexus below the diaphragm. Segmental veins join the azygos system from the thoracic esophagus and the high intercostal veins in its upper portion. The lymphatic drainage is mainly posteriorly toward the thoracic duct through most of the length of the esophagus, although there are anterior lymphatic connections to the subcarinal lymph nodes from the midportion and to the cervical lymph node from the upper esophagus.

The esophageal muscle is innervated by the preganglionic fibers of the vagus nerve synapsing with the ganglion cells in the myenteric plexus of the esophagus. The upper esophagus receives this innervation from the recurrent branches of the vagus nerve after they have looped around the aortic arch or the subclavian artery. Sympathetic innervation occurs from the thoracic ganglion. Sensory innervation of the esophagus appears limited to fibers stimulated by muscular stretch or by temperature. These sensory fibers reach the central nervous system through the vagus nerves.

ANATOMY OF THE GASTROESOPHAGEAL JUNCTION

Understanding the anatomy of the esophageal hiatus is essential to the understanding of mechanisms of reflux and its correction. Posteriorly, the diaphragm muscle arises from the lumbar vertebral bodies and the arcuate ligament, crossing over the aorta as it enters the abdomen. The diaphragm muscle initially rises in a cephalad direction. One vertebral body higher than the aortic hiatus, the muscle splits to form the aperture of the esophageal hiatus. The columns of diaphragm muscle rising off the vertebral body and arcuate ligament form two distinct pillars, the right and left crura. Although the esophageal hiatus lies slightly to the left of the midline, the margins of the hiatus in most dissections prove to arise from muscle of the right crus (Collis et al., 1954). There is, however, a great deal of variability and interdigitation of fibers from both pleurae. The looping of muscle fibers around the esophageal hiatus as the muscle passes toward its insertion in the central tendon of the diaphragm provides the diaphragmatic tunnel through which the esophagus passes as it enters the abdomen. This sling of muscle around the distal esophagus is approximately 2 cm. in length. The muscle surrounding the esophagus in the diaphragmatic hiatus is innervated by the left phrenic nerve.

The hiatal aperture around the esophagus is closed by several layers that separate the thoracic and abdominal cavities. Most important of these is the phrenoesophageal membrane, which anchors the esophagus within the hiatus. This membrane consists primarily of an extension of the endoabdominal fascia off the underside of the diaphragmatic muscle (Bombeck et al., 1966). This fascia extends slightly cephalad to form a cone-like structure as it approaches the esophagus. It is usually joined by fibroelastic tissue of the endothoracic fascia coming off the superior surface of the diaphragm, but the thoracic contribution to the membrane is less in amount and importance. The phrenoesophageal membrane formed by the fusion of the two fascial layers inserts in a series of fibrous attachments that penetrate the esophageal muscle and blend into the submucosa of the esophagus approximately 3 to 4 cm. above the junction of the tubular esophagus with the stomach. The insertion of this membrane into the esophageal submucosa marks the point at which the esophagus becomes intra-abdominal. If one incises the layers of tissue anterior to the esophagus within the hiatus, the following layers are divided proceeding from the thoracic to abdominal direction: pleura, mediastinal fat, endothoracic fascia, endoabdominal fascia comprising the sheet of phreno-esophageal membrane, retroperitoneal fat, and peritoneum. In addition to the esophagus, the vagus nerves penetrate through the phrenoesophageal membrane on the wall of the esophagus. The hepatic branch of the right vagus nerve is given off just below the phrenoesophageal membrane, as is a major trunk of the left vagus nerve to the celiac plexus.

Discussion of the gastroesophageal junction requires precise definition of terms. Much confusion has resulted from at least three different definitions that have been used to describe the esophagogastric junction (EGJ). To the endoscopist and radiologist, the mucosal junction of squamous and columnar epithelium is often called the EGJ. This junction is irregular, the ora serrata, and somewhat variable in location. To define the esophagogastric junction as the mucosal junction ignores the fact that the most distal 2 to 3 cm. of tubular, muscular esophagus is normally lined by columnar epithelium. A second and more realistic physiologic definition of the esophagogastric junction is the point at which esophageal muscular peristalsis stops. The peristaltic wave of the esophagus sweeps distally, ending with the closed distal esophageal segment, often referred to as the distal sphincter, at the junction where the muscular tube of esophagus joins the gastric pouch. This lowest portion of the muscular esophageal tube is usually lined with gastric-type columnar epithelium, so that the muscular junction is distal to the mucosal junction. In normal persons, this definition of the EGJ is most useful when discussing esophageal physiology and mechanisms of reflux.

In disease states such as achalasia or scleroderma, the esophageal peristaltic pattern is disrupted, so that a third definition is necessary. In such cases, the esophagogastric junction is defined as the junction of the narrow-diameter esophageal swallowing tube with the large-diameter gastric pouch. Usually, this junction is 3 to 4 cm. below the insertion of the phrenoesophageal membrane and coincides with the location of the most distal esophageal muscle contraction following peristalsis. Again, this definition places the junction slightly more caudal than the normal squamocolumnar mucosal junction. When the stomach is greatly distended, such as after a large meal, this segment of intra-abdominal tubular esophagus is shortened or effaced by the radial pull of the distended stomach wall. For this reason, the length of the submerged segment of distal intra-abdominal esophagus seen by a radiologist during a barium swallow depends on the degree of gastric filling or retention. As will be discussed subsequently, the theories concerning control of reflux focus on the role of the distal esophageal muscle and the length of intra-abdominal tubular esophagus. Accordingly, the most useful definitions for discussion of the esophagogastric junction are the latter two, rather than confusing the readily visible squamocolumnar junction with the EGJ.

HIATAL HERNIA

Hiatal hernias are divided into two major types, each involving a different anatomic defect and having differing clinical significance (Fig. 25–1). The Type I axial or sliding hiatal hernia is common and without significance, unless accompanied by pathologic degrees of reflux. The abnormality is a slight dilatation in the diameter of the hiatal opening and a stretching or attenuation of the phrenoesophageal membrane. This permits a portion of the gastric cardia to slide upward into the hiatus. There is no defect or aperture in the endoabdominal fascia covering the hiatus and inserting into the esophagus, so that there is no true peritoneal hernia sac. In the great majority of patients in whom this type of hernia is seen on barium swallow examination, the insertion of the phrenoesophageal membrane into the esophagus is at a normal location 3 to 4 cm. above the junction, and there is no pathologic reflux. Another indication that the Type I hiatal hernia by itself is not a disease is the wide variability in in-

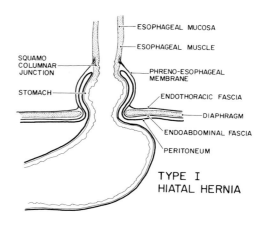

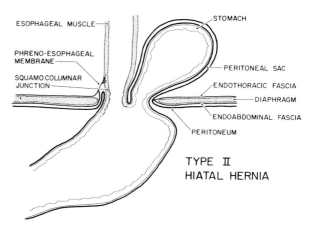

Figure 25–1. Diagrammatic representation of a Type I and Type II hiatal hernia. In the Type I hernia, the phrenoesophageal membrane is intact and there is no true peritoneal sac extending into the thorax. In the Type II hiatal hernia, there is a defect in the phrenoesophageal membrane, permitting a free peritoneal sac to enter the lower-pressure thoracic cavity. (From Skinner, D. B.: Hiatal hernia and gastroesophageal reflux. *In* Davis-Christopher Textbook of Surgery. 12th Ed. Edited by D. C. Sabiston, Jr. Philadelphia, W. B. Saunders Company, 1981.)

cidence when this condition is seen by radiologists. Some radiologists boast that a Type I hiatal hernia can be demonstrated with diligent effort, position, abdominal compression, and other maneuvers in up to 90 per cent of barium swallow examinations. It should be recalled that during the act of vomiting, the cardia of the stomach normally herniates somewhat through the hiatus as the esophagus shortens and gastric and abdominal wall muscles contract violently. It should be no surprise that a Type I hiatal hernia can be demonstrated by forceful maneuvers in normal people. The demonstration of this type of hiatal hernia under the artificial conditions of a stressful radiographic examination is of no importance at all and should be disregarded unless clear evidence of spontaneous gastroesophageal reflux is seen.

In some patients, a larger Type I hiatal hernia is seen that is easily demonstrated on radiographic study with the patient at rest. Such patients with a pouch of stomach greater than 3 cm. protruding through the hiatus under resting conditions seem to have a much higher association with abnormal degrees of gastroesophageal reflux (O'Sullivan et al., 1981). In such cases, the insertion of the phrenoesophageal membrane appears to be closer than normal to the gastroesophageal junction, as demonstrated by both manometric evaluation and surgical dissection. Whether this low insertion of the phrenoesophageal membrane is congenital or acquired in an individual case is uncertain. Some of these patients give a history of regurgitation and reflux since childhood, suggesting a congenital problem. Others clearly acquire the symptoms and evidence of reflux later in life.

The presence of the Type I hiatal hernia itself does not indicate loss of the intra-abdominal segment of esophagus. The abdominal portion of esophagus is defined by the insertion of the phrenoesophageal membrane into the esophageal submucosa. As long as this insertion remains 3 to 4 cm. above the junction of the tubular esophagus with the gastric pouch, the most distal esophagus remains within the abdominal pressure chamber, even when translocated cephalad through the hiatus. Increases in abdominal pressure will be transmitted through the hiatus to compress the esophagus below the phrenoesophageal membrane. The high association of reflux with a larger Type I hiatal hernia suggests that the intra-abdominal esophagus may be lost in some of these patients. It is conceivable that mild degrees of esophagitis, as can be caused by overeating, alcoholic indulgence, and heavy smoking, may lead to periesophageal inflammation and adhesions between the oblique entrance of the phrenoesophageal membrane into the esophageal wall, with effective fusion of these structures and loss of the intra-abdominal esophagus. Another theory would suggest that the build-up of fatty tissue at this critical junction may interfere with the transmission of abdominal pressures to the esophagus within a hiatal hernia pouch. In any case, it is only when pathologic reflux can be documented that a Type I hiatal hernia acquires clinical significance.

The second major type of hiatal hernia, the paraesophageal rolling or Type II hernia, is much less common but is a significant clinical problem in itself. In this type of hernia, there is a defect in the phrenoesophageal membrane, usually on the left ventral aspect of the hiatus, but also occasionally to the right and posteriorly. These defects allow protrusion of the peritoneum through the fascia in the manner of a true hernia sac. The adjacent stomach herniates through the defect in the fascia and enters the chest. Since the fascia no longer restrains the upward migration of the stomach and since intrathoracic pressure is less than abdominal pressure most of the time, the natural history of this defect is a progressive enlargement of the hernia. In advanced stages, the entire stomach may be herniated through the defect, so that the cardia, still fixed by a portion of the phrenoesophageal membrane, and the pylorus come to lie close together. This sets the stage for gastric volvulus, torsion, obstruction, strangulation, and intrathoracic gastric dilatation, any of which can be fatal (Fig. 25–2). For this reason, the Type II hiatal hernia is taken seriously as a defect requiring surgical correction, even if the patient is asymptomatic.

With enlargement of the Type II hernia, the phrenoesophageal membrane frequently becomes attenuated as well, owing to the constant tension placed upon it by the distortion of the stomach pulling on the cardia. When a patient has a herniation of the cardia well above the diaphragm in addition to a paraesophageal hernia sac, this type of hernia may be classified as a Type III or combined hiatal hernia with the clinical significance of the paraesophageal hernia as well as an increased incidence of reflux, which may accompany the larger Type I hernias. When other organs such as the colon or small intestine enter the paraesophageal hernia sac, the clinical implications are changed to reflect the possibility of obstruction or torsion of these other organs. This can be classified as a Type IV or multiorgan hiatal hernia.

NORMAL FUNCTION OF THE ESOPHAGUS AND CARDIA

The mechanisms by which the esophagus and cardia function normally to transport an ingested bolus and prevent reflux remain controversial in spite of an enormous amount of investigation. When two or more theories are supported by experimental and clinical evidence, both explanations are provided in this discussion.

The swallowing process begins with an upward and posterior thrust of the tongue and larynx, so that the laryngeal orifice is covered by the epiglottis, and the solid, liquid, or gas bolus being ingested is thrust back into the hypopharynx. As the pharyngeal constrictors contract, there is a coordinated relaxation or opening of the cricopharyngeus muscle, so that pharyngeal pressures exceed the cricopharyngeal sphincter pressure. The timing as well as amplitude of

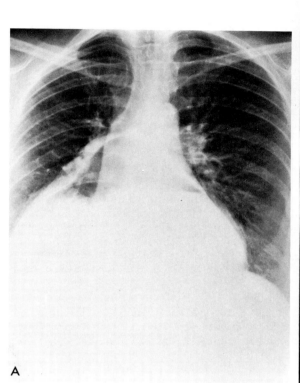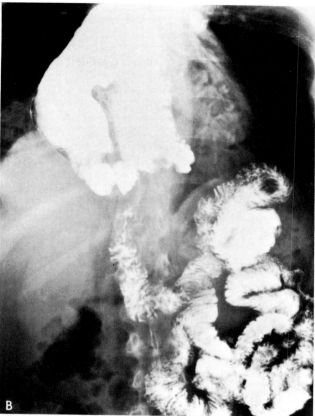

Figure 25–2. Typical radiographic appearance of a large Type II hiatal hernia. As in this case, there is often a loosening of the phrenoesophageal membrane as well, making it a combined sliding and paraesophageal, or Type III, hernia. (From Skinner, D. B.: Hiatal hernia and gastroesophageal reflux. *In* Davis-Christopher Texbook of Surgery. 12th Ed. Edited by D. C. Sabiston, Jr. Philadelphia, W. B. Saunders Company, 1981.)

the contraction and relaxation of the constrictors and cricopharyngeus is critical to smooth swallowing and can be disordered by neurologic damage in the brain stem or to the vagus and glossopharyngeal nerves, suggesting that the coordination is neurogenically controlled. As the cricopharyngeus relaxes and then contracts again, a progressive peristaltic wave is started down the esophagus, characterized by an initial phase of slight relaxation followed by a muscular contraction that normally ranges from 20 to 60 mm. Hg in pressure. This pressure wave proceeds down the esophagus in a coordinated manner, traveling caudally at the rate of 5 to 10 cm. per second. Intact innervation of the esophagus is essential for coordinated peristalsis, but it appears that the innervating fibers enter the esophageal wall much proximally to the level at which the contraction is occurring, since a lower thoracic vagal transection has no effect on the peristalsis of the distal esophagus. Transection and reanastomosis of the esophagus do not interfere with the progression of the peristaltic wave across the anastomotic line, provided that the innervation of the distal segment remains intact.

As the peristaltic wave reaches the distal esophagus, the high-pressure zone of the distal 3 to 4 cm. of

the esophagus relaxes to the level of resting gastric pressure. This segment contracts again as the bolus passes through the cardia, and the initial elevated resting pressure is restored. During the act of swallowing followed by primary peristalsis, the length of the esophagus shortens through longitudinal muscle contraction and is restored as the bolus passes distally in front of the contracting band of circular muscle.

Two theories accounting for the relaxation of the distal segment warrant consideration. One explanation is that the distal esophageal muscle segment undergoes an active phase of relaxation controlled by its innervation. The other explanation is that the resting pressure in the distal segment is reduced as the esophagus shortens through longitudinal muscle contraction and pulls upward on the phrenoesophageal membrane insertion. Since the membrane inserts from a lateral direction circumferentially, this has the physicial effect of tugging the lumen open and reducing pressure to that of the gastric cavity. The active phase would then be the contraction of the circular muscle as the bolus passes. Since there is anatomically no identifiable sphincter muscle in humans and subhuman primates and since the idea of one band of muscle maintaining a constant tonic contraction during rest without showing hypertrophy or different development from adjacent gastric or esophageal muscle seems improbable, the theory of passive relaxation and passive maintenance of tone in the distal esophagus by virtue of its intraabdominal location and small diameter relative to the stomach pouch is attractive. The explanation for failure of the distal segment to relax in achalasia can fit in with either theory. If active muscle relaxation is controlled by innervation, failure to relax would be expected in the denervated state of achalasia. Similarly, if the distal segment relaxation is passive and secondary to longitudinal muscle contraction against the phrenoesophageal membrane, the absence of peristalsis in achalasia could account for failure of the distal segment to relax.

Regardless of the precise mechanisms of peristalsis and distal segment relaxation, coordinated peristaltic clearing of the esophagus is an important aspect in the protection against the noxious effects of gastroesophageal reflux (Booth et al., 1968). Distention of the esophagus or irritation of the mucosa might trigger a coordinated peristaltic contraction not initiated by an act of swallowing. This is called secondary peristalsis and may be a factor in the ability of the esophagus to clear regurgitated material without the patient's awareness.

The mechanism by which the second function of the esophagus, the prevention of gastric reflux, works is controversial. The barrier preventing gastric reflux into the esophagus is identified by the resting high-pressure zone in the distal esophagus (Fyke et al., 1956). Many have accepted this as evidence for an active muscular sphincter, even though a distinct sphincter muscle cannot be identified anatomically. Discussion of the distal esophageal sphincter is widespread in publications. To understand the control of reflux, it is more useful to think of this high-pressure zone as a physiologic sphincter or barrier to reflux and to inquire into mechanisms by which this barrier can be augmented.

The barrier to reflux can be described in several terms. It rests in the most distal 3 to 4 cm. of the esophagus and is measured by a discrete zone of pressure elevated 8 to 20 mm. Hg higher than resting intragastric pressure. In normal people, the majority of this high-pressure zone (HPZ) is beneath the insertion of the phrenoesophageal membrane into the esophageal wall, as evidenced by the point of respiratory inversion on manometry studies. The high-pressure zone corresponds to the submerged or compressed segment of esophagus seen on barium swallow examinations to remain in a closed state after the peristaltic wave passes. Endoscopically, this barrier is seen as a segment of distal esophagus that remains closed even when air is insufflated into the thoracic esophagus. Often, the ora serrata or gastroesophageal mucosal junction is seen at the top of this closed segment.

Regardless of how the distal esophagus is described, this segment is responsible for the control of gastroesophageal reflux. At least two theories are supported by evidence concerning the function of the distal esophageal HPZ. The most widely accepted and classical theory is that the distal esophageal muscle is an intrinsic sphincter that maintains a closed tonic state of contraction during rest and actively relaxes during swallowing. This contraction is believed to be under neurologic and hormonal control (Cohen and Lipshutz, 1970). The second theory is that the distal esophageal HPZ is caused by the narrow-diameter distal esophageal tube entering abruptly into the larger digestive pouch within the common pressure chamber of the abdomen. According to the law of LaPlace, it takes more force to distend the smaller-diameter tube than the larger-diameter pouch, and hence, the observed high-pressure zone may represent these physical forces governing wall tension.

A number of hormones and chemicals influence foregut pressure, including that of the distal esophageal HPZ. Under the intrinsic muscle sphincter theory, these hormones work selectively on the sphincter muscle. Under the second theory, hormones causing a general relaxation or tightening of foregut muscle would have a magnified effect, since the pressures governed by the law of LaPlace are inversely related to the fourth power of the radius. A small change in radius of the distal esophagus would have a much greater effect on wall tension than a similar percentage change in radius would have on the larger-diameter gastric pouch.

Although the behavior of the distal esophageal segment meets the physiologic definition of a muscular sphincter, several observations point to physical forces being important. No anatomically identifiable sphincter muscle has been found in primates, and the electron microscopic and microscopic evaluation of human distal esophageal muscle does not show qualitative differences from adjacent midesophagus or gastric muscle. The first observations pointing toward physical forces accounting for the sphincter zone stem from the first antireflux repairs. In spite of the trauma caused by the surgical dissection and suturing, the pressure in the distal esophageal segment is increased immediately postoperatively. If the pressure is generated by an intrinsic muscle tone, the surgical trauma should cause interference with muscular function rather than strengthening it in the early stages after surgery. Additional observations indicate that a distal esophagus replaced by a small-diameter gastric tube can be effective in preventing reflux as long as there is a significant intra-abdominal segment of the gastric tube (Henderson, 1980). A high-pressure zone in a small-diameter swallowing tube replacing the esophagus can be found when the replacement organ is a gastric tube, jejunal segment, or colon interposition segment. When the distal esophagus is replaced by a gastric tube, this shows a similar pattern of increased or decreased pressure, depending on administration of specific hormones (Moossa, et al., 1977). Finally, an in vitro model demonstrates that competency of the cardia can be maintained when equalized intragastric and intra-abdominal pressures are applied to the outer surface of the esophagus, as is usual in the resting state. Under these circumstances, the control of reflux is directly proportional to the length of esophagus exposed to abdominal pressure, with a 3- to 4-cm. segment of abdominal esophagus being sufficient to prevent reflux when there is a 10 cm. H_2O abdomino-thoracic pressure difference (DeMeester et al., 1979). All these pieces of evidence point to the importance of the intra-abdominal segment of esophagus as a primary or at least important supplementary factor to whatever a specific muscle function of the distal esophagus contributes to control of reflux. Hence, two measurable parameters of distal esophageal function are related to control of reflux: (1) the pressure in the distal esophageal segment and (2) the length of distal esophageal segment exposed to abdominal pressure.

GASTROESOPHAGEAL REFLUX AND ESOPHAGITIS

With this understanding of the anatomy and the physiologic components preventing reflux, some of the factors leading to reflux and esophagitis can be identified. The frequent association between pathologic reflux and a Type I hiatal hernia points to alterations in the anatomy of the hiatus as contributing to reflux in some cases. A widening of the hiatus tends to put some lateral tension on the distal esophageal segment, increasing its diameter and reducing the pressure required to distend the esophagus. The presence of an axial hiatal hernia itself, however, does not cause reflux in the great majority of patients. Presumably, this is because the phrenoesophageal membrane insertion still leaves an adequate segment of distal esophagus exposed to abdominal pressure transmitted into the hernia pouch from below. Under these circumstances, the extrinsic pressure on the stomach and abdominal portion of esophagus remains similar, even though the cardia and distal esophagus are seen radiographically to be above the diaphragm.

Factors that lead to recurrent or chronic elevation of gastric pressure contribute to reflux. Physiologic reflux normally occurs after meals, when the stomach is full and contracting (DeMeester et al., 1976). Failure of gastric emptying, as in pyloric stenosis, or a mass in the stomach, duodenum, pancreas, or gallbladder that delays gastric emptying can be a cause of secondary gastroesophageal reflux. Obliteration of the muscle tone in the esophageal wall, as occurs in scleroderma, can be a cause of reflux. Overdistention of the distal esophageal segment, as created by a Heller esophago-cardiomyotomy or forceful balloon dilatation, may lead to secondary reflux. A low insertion of the phrenoesophageal membrane into the distal esophagus, whether congenital or acquired, reduces the abdominal segment and its role in the control of reflux and encourages pathologic degrees of regurgitation. It appears that a congenitally low insertion of the phrenoesophageal membrane is a common factor in severe reflux in children and young adults, who often recall that they had considerable regurgitation in early child-

hood. Obliteration of the angle of entry of the phrenoesophageal membrane into the esophagus with fusion of the membrane to the wall of the esophagus might occur in patients who have chronic low-grade esophagitis from heavy smoking or alcohol ingestion. Similarly, it can be envisioned that obese patients are more apt to have reflux because of the cuff of extraperitoneal fatty tissue around the cardia preventing full transmission of intra-abdominal pressure to the abdominal segment of esophagus. Undoubtedly, there are other presently unknown alterations in anatomy and control of foregut muscle tone that contribute to the problem.

From prolonged intraesophageal pH monitoring, it is known that reflux after meals is a normal event in healthy people. When reflux becomes prolonged or occurs throughout the day or at night, pathologic degrees of reflux are diagnosed. For esophagitis to develop as a complication of reflux, two factors must occur. The noxious gastric acid–peptic or pancreaticobiliary secretions must reach the esophagus with increased frequency, and the esophagus must be unable to clear the refluxed material back into the stomach. In normal individuals, acid in the esophagus is cleared by repeated peristaltic action, usually initiated by a swallow. In those with esophagitis, delay in or lack of clearing is frequently noted.

From prolonged pH monitoring, several patterns of reflux can be observed. In some patients, reflux occurs frequently during the day when they are in the upright position. These individuals often have the habit of snacking frequently and of swallowing air to initiate the peristalsis required to clear the refluxed material. These habits, in turn, lead to persistent volume of air and food in the stomach, contributing to gastric contraction and recurrent bouts of reflux. A recurring cycle of ingestion, reflux, air swallowing, reflux, and so on is created. These patients are often highly aware of their reflux condition. However, the frequency of swallowing encourages acid clearing from the esophagus, so that severe damage to the esophagus causing esophagitis is not a great risk.

In other patients, reflux occurs at night while they are supine. Since swallowing is infrequent at night and absent during sound sleep, regurgitation during the night may lead to prolonged contact of the refluxed material with the esophageal mucosa, permitting injury to the mucosa to occur without the patient's awareness of the problem. Comparison of patterns of reflux with degrees of esophagitis shows a strong correlation between esophagitis and nocturnal reflux. Patients with pure upright daytime reflux rarely have significant esophagitis. The most severe degrees of reflux, often leading to surgical management, usually occur both as daytime and nocturnal upright and supine reflux patterns.

When abnormal reflux occurs, the degree of damage to the esophagus may range from none, when the material is cleared rapidly, to a rapidly developing severe peptic stricture. It is useful to grade esophagitis by the degree of abnormality observed by the esophagoscopist. The absence of erythema or ulceration is graded as no esophagitis. Grade I is recorded when there is erythema of the mucosa without ulceration. In Grade 0 or Grade I, there may be microscopic changes of hypertrophy of the basal layer of the squamous epithelium and proximity of the rete pegs to the surface (Ismail-Beigi et al., 1970). However, these findings are nonspecific and may be caused by a variety of stimulants to the esophagus, and therefore, they should not be interpreted as diagnostic of reflux esophagitis. Grade II esophagitis is noted when frank ulcerations are seen. Repeated chronic ulcerations lead to some fibrosis and stiffness of the wall of the esophagus, recorded as Grade III esophagitis. When a frank stricture occurs that prevents the passage of the esophagoscope, a Grade IV esophagitis or stricture is recorded. Progression from no esophagitis to a frank stricture may occur very rapidly or may proceed slowly over a period of years. In some patients, the degree of esophagitis remains static for a long time. The earliest case of stricture that I have seen was in a 5-day-old infant; postoperative severe reflux esophagitis in a debilitated patient with a nasogastric tube may lead to stricture formation within 5 to 10 days. It is because of the uncertainty of time sequence in progression to stricture that surgical correction of reflux esophagitis is advocated when the ulcerative phase is observed.

When chronic reflux esophagitis causes ulcerations, observations indicate that healing occurs by upward migration of the acid-resistant columnar cells of the gastric cardia into the ulcerated area. When this progression becomes marked and the columnar-type epithelium extends more than 3 cm. into the tubular esophagus, the condition of "Barrett's esophagus," or esophagus lined with columnar epithelium, occurs (Barrett, 1957). In many cases, this appears to be an acquired condition associated with chronic reflux. In others, the presence of rests or islands of gastric epithelium in the esophagus or the presence of normal-appearing gastric fundic mucosa, including parietal cells, suggests that there may be some cases in which gastric epithelium in the esophagus occurs congenitally as well. An important factor in Barrett's epithelium is the propensity of this stimulated mucosa to proceed toward neoplasia (Berenson et al., 1978). For this reason, multiple biopsies must be taken at esophagoscopy and the finding of dysplasia accepted as evidence of progression toward neoplasia.

In addition to esophagitis, stricture, and Barrett's esophagus, reflux may cause acute hemorrhage from the esophagus and aspiration of regurgitated contents into the lung. Cases of acute hemorrhage from esophagitis are rare. When seen, the entire lower esophageal mucosa is observed to be weeping blood as if a split-thickness skin graft had been taken and the bleeding encouraged to persist by further washes of acid regurgitation over the raw mucosa. Although this type of frightening rapid bleeding from the surface is rare, chronic small amounts of bleeding sufficient to cause a guaiac-positive stool and mild anemia are a common problem with chronic ulcerative esophagitis. When the esophagus acquires a gastric mucosal lining, it is prone to deep penetrating ulcers on the gastric side of the squamocolumnar junction (Sandry, 1962). These may erode into adjacent structures, including the aorta and heart, and lead to massive hemorrhage.

In patients with reflux, the possibility of regurgitation into the hypopharynx and aspiration into the larynx is always present. However, frank documented aspiration causing pulmonary symptoms is shown conclusively in only about 8 per cent of patients having documented pathologic reflux (Skinner and Belsey, 1967; Pellegrini et al., 1979). These patients appear to share a disorder of esophageal motor function as well, which inhibits clearing of regurgitated material into the esophagus. Since respiratory disease and reflux are both common problems in the population, a cause-and-effect relationship must be established by appropriate testing before assuming that one condition causes the other.

CLINICAL PRESENTATION

The Type I sliding hiatal hernia rarely causes symptoms severe enough for a patient to seek medical advice. Only when pathologic reflux is associated with the hiatal hernia are specific symptoms encountered. The Type II paraesophageal hernia may cause symptoms in the absence of reflux. Such patients often present with complaints of early satiety, vomiting after a large meal, epigastric distress, dysphagia, and gurgling noises within the chest. All of these relate to the intrathoracic pouch of herniated stomach filling up rapidly and reaching capacity. Dysphagia appears to be caused by lateral compression of the esophagus by the adjacent herniated viscus. With a very large hernia, compression of the lung and occupation of a portion of the thoracic space may lead to cough following meals and occasional dyspnea.

Symptoms caused by reflux are a much more common clinical presentation. The classic symptoms are heartburn and regurgitation aggravated by postural changes such as stooping or lying flat. Heartburn is a term used by various patients to mean different things and is a nonspecific symptom. The heartburn typically caused by reflux is a burning or hot sensation beneath the lower sternum and in the epigastrium. In severe cases, this may progress upward toward the neck and even into the shoulder and upper arm. This type of heartburn is usually relieved by ingestion of food or antacids. It occurs most commonly after meals but may be nearly continuous in severe cases.

The regurgitation from reflux is of gastric contents. Patients will note that the regurgitated material is sour, burns, or tastes bitter. If undigested food is regurgitated, this is not coming from the stomach and cannot be diagnosed as gastroesophageal reflux.

Dysphagia is a common symptom with reflux. It can also be caused by a carcinoma. For this reason, the symptom of dysphagia, or difficulty in swallowing, must be taken seriously, and every patient should have an evaluation of the esophagus, including at least a barium swallow and flexible fiberoptic esophagoscopy. Dysphagia may occur with reflux in the absence of esophagitis. In these cases, the difficulty in swallowing can be attributed to a degree of esophageal spasm or inefficient motor contraction of the esophagus. When the esophagitis has extended to a frank stricture, the difficulty in swallowing will be noted for solid food but not for liquids. The ingestion of hot or cold beverages or alcohol may cause an increase in burning. Heartburn usually diminishes as the stricture increases to protect the esophagus from regurgitated material. The dysphagia caused by diffuse esophageal spasm differs from the dysphagia of a stricture. The former occurs equally with liquids or solids, is episodic, and tends to improve as a meal progresses. There are other atypical symptoms caused by reflux. The pattern of angina pectoris may be mimicked by esophageal spasm triggered by reflux. In these cases, the chest pain may be severe and may cause a systemic reaction that mimics an acute myocardial infarction. In severe cases, a patient is often admitted directly to the coronary care unit for the esophageal spasm disorder.

Referral of symptoms to the neck may occur from reflux. In these cases, the patient has difficulty in initiating the swallow or complains of a persistent sensation of a lump in the neck. This may be misdiagnosed as globus hystericus. In such patients, high reflux to the cervical esophagus with a secondary irritation and spasm of the cricopharyngeus is found.

Bleeding from reflux is rare, although occult blood in the stool is common with ulcerative esophagitis. When massive bleeding occurs, it is due either to the unusual cases of diffuse hemorrhagic esophagitis or to a penetrating ulcer in the gastric mucosa lining the distal esophagus. These patients may have massive life-threatening hemorrhage.

Aspiration caused by reflux most commonly presents as nocturnal cough associated with regurgitation of food in the mouth, often awakening the patient. Morning hoarseness is another symptom suggesting nocturnal aspiration. Aspiration is particularly suspected in patients whose cough occurs mainly at night and not during the daytime. Severe aspiration from reflux can lead to lung abscess, recurring pneumonia, or bronchiectasis. Asthma is occasionally suggested as being possibly caused by reflux. Cases in which this is truly documented are rare and controversial. However, a patient with an underlying asthmatic tendency may have more frequent attacks triggered by bouts of reflux. When any of the aforementioned symptoms bring a patient to see a physician, gastroesophageal reflux must be included in the differential diagnosis and objective tests used to confirm the correct diagnosis.

In children reflux may be less apparent symptomatically. This is because young children are not able to express an accurate description of their symptoms and are not familiar with terms such as heartburn.

Accordingly, in children, the disease may lead to complications such as failure to thrive, chronic anemia, and chronic aspiration without many complaints from the child. In these circumstances, objective means for diagnosing reflux are particularly important.

DIAGNOSIS OF REFLUX AND HIATAL HERNIA

In any patient suspected of having esophageal disease, a barium swallow is the first study indicated. The radiologist should be informed of the suspicion of an esophageal disorder so that attention will be paid to the important areas. Ordering an upper gastrointestinal radiograph frequently results in a cursory examination of the esophagus. The initial observation of the swallow should focus on the hypopharyngeal and cricopharyngeal swallowing mechanism and should exclude mechanical deformities above the aortic arch. The body of the esophagus is screened to rule out diverticula, extrinsic abnormalities, or mucosal abnormalities that might suggest neoplasia. The cardia is examined during and between swallows. During a swallow, the distal esophagus should open to permit passage of the bolus of barium. At the end of the swallow, the distal esophageal segment should remain closed. If free spontaneous gastroesophageal reflux is seen, this is highly significant, for we have always been able to confirm this with other more rigorous tests for reflux. Of the maneuvers that may be employed to stimulate reflux, the Müller maneuver, inhalation against a closed glottis, is most effective and significant. Some radiologists use a "water-sipping" test in which the patient is asked to swallow water with barium in the stomach and while the radiologist compresses the abdomen. This will elicit physiologic reflux in the great majority of normal people and has no clinical significance. It is helpful to have the radiographic study recorded on videotape so that it may be inspected repeatedly, as swallowing disorders or a brief spurt of reflux may be difficult to interpret accurately in the course of the examination. If a mechanical deformity such as stricture is seen, multiple views of this should be obtained in an effort to help decide whether it has the appearance of a neoplasm, an ulcerative benign stricture, or a motor disorder. However, the radiologist's opinion as to the etiology of the stricture cannot be accepted as diagnostic, and a tissue diagnosis is necessary in every case.

If the patient complains of dysphagia or the radiologist sees a mechanical abnormality in the esophagus, flexible fiberoptic endoscopy is performed. Even in cases of frank stricture, this examination should precede rigid esophagoscopy, because a diagnosis may be obtained by superficial biopsy or brushing and the discomfort and increased risk of rigid esophagoscopy may be avoided. When the clinical problem is reflux, evidence for ulceration and erythema is recorded. The location of the squamocolumnar junction is noted relative to the aortic arch pulsation and relative to the entrance of the tubular esophagus into the gastric pouch. The number, depth, and arrangements of ulcerations should be reported. If a patulous cardia is seen throughout the respiratory cycle, this may confirm other evidence that reflux is present. If the complaint is dysphagia or if a hiatal hernia is present, a J maneuver during gastroscopy provides a look at the cardia from below. Early carcinoma in this area is very difficult to visualize, and the retroflex maneuver with the gastroscope is most important. In every case, a full examination of the stomach and pylorus is made to exclude gastric factors that may be contributory to increased reflux. If a stricture or severe esophagitis is encountered, or if Barrett's epithelium is suspected, multiple biopsies should be taken. If these do not give an exact diagnosis, deeper biopsies and brushings on a subsequent rigid esophagoscopy may be necessary to exclude carcinoma as a cause of the stricture and dysphagia.

In some patients with stricture, it is wise to perform a series of dilatations after the initial endoscopy and then repeat the procedure at a later time to be certain of the diagnosis and the degree of improvement achieved by the dilatations. Bougienage is usually accomplished in these cases by employing the Maloney mercury-filled tapered dilators.

If reflux is suspected or a hiatal hernia is seen without reflux and if no free spontaneous reflux is seen by radiography, esophageal function tests may be necessary to make an exact diagnosis. When dysphagia is a prominent symptom, esophagoscopy and barium swallow often precede the esophageal function tests. When dysphagia is not a symptom and the barium swallow is not diagnostic, then esophageal function tests are performed first and may obviate the need for subsequent endoscopy.

A battery of esophageal function tests is commonly performed on an outpatient basis and provides most of the information necessary for a diagnosis, except in the more confusing cases (Skinner and Booth, 1970). The esophageal function tests frequently used include esophageal manometry, a standardized acid reflux test using the pH electrode in the esophagus, an acid clearing test, and the acid perfusion test (Fig. 25–3). In more difficult cases in which the diagnosis is still uncertain, prolonged 24-hour pH monitoring and prolonged esophageal manometry may provide essential additional information. The technique for each of these tests is described below.

Esophageal manometry may be performed with open-tipped fluid-infused catheters bonded together with the openings at different levels. Alternatively, pressure-sensitive transducers in a chain of three or more may be employed (Code *et al.*, 1958). Traditionally, manometry involves three recordings spaced 5 cm. apart. The catheter is placed into the stomach and its position confirmed by recording positive-pressure abdominal contractions with inspiration on all three channels. The catheter train is slowly pulled back across the gastroesophageal junction with recordings made at 0.5- or 1-cm. intervals. A distal esophageal high-pressure zone is identified. Its amplitude, quality

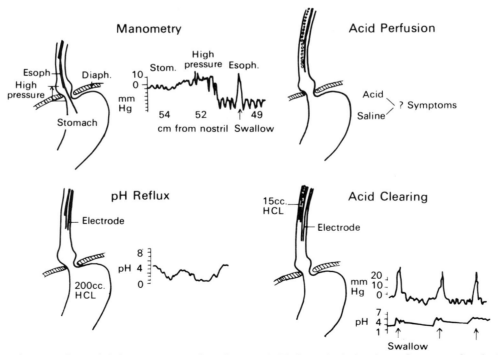

Figure 25–3. Placement for a triple-lumen manometric catheter and pH electrode during the performance of each of four esophageal function tests. Representative examples of the type of data obtained are illustrated (see text for details of technique and interpretation). (From Skinner, D. B., and Booth, D. J.: Assessment of distal esophageal function in patients with hiatal hernia and/or gastroesophageal reflux. Ann. Surg., *172*:627, 1970.)

of relaxation, and portion reflecting intra-abdominal location are noted (Fig. 25–4). In the body of the esophagus, the proportion of progressive peristaltic contractions, amplitude of contractions, and presence of any tertiary contractions are noted. In the upper esophagus, the resting tone and timing of relaxation of the cricopharyngeus relative to hypopharyngeal contraction are recorded. Information obtained from this test describes the characteristics of the high-pressure zone, including pressure and intra-abdominal length, and also reveals the presence of other esophageal motor abnormalities such as achalasia, spasm, or scleroderma.

After identification of the high-pressure zone, an acid load is placed in the stomach for a standard acid-reflux test (Kantrowitz et al., 1969). In an adult, this is usually 300 ml. of 0.1 normal HCl. The long intestinal pH electrode is positioned 5 cm. above the HPZ in the lower esophagus. A standardized series of respiratory and postural maneuvers is performed by the patient, including coughing, deep breathing, a Valsalva maneuver, and a Müller maneuver, in each of four body positions, supine, head down, right side down, and left side down. This test is standardized against results in a large number of normal volunteers. Three or more episodes of reflux measured by a drop of pH to less than 4 in the esophagus is an abnormal finding. In patients with severe reflux, it may not be possible to clear regurgitated acid from the esophagus.

With the pH probe still located 5 cm. above the high-pressure zone, a 15-ml. bolus of 0.1 normal HCl is placed in the midesophagus through the proximal tip of the manometry catheter. After flushing this through

with a small amount of water, the patient is asked to swallow at 30-second intervals. Normal individuals clear this amount of acid in 10 swallows or less and have a low incidence of esophagitis. Patients with reflux who cannot clear the acid have a high probability of esophagitis and require subsequent esophagoscopy for confirmation (Booth et al., 1968).

If symptoms are atypical, an acid perfusion test (Bernstein et al., 1962) is useful. The catheter remains positioned in the midesophagus, and the proximal end is led behind the patient. Two intravenous solution bottles joined by a Y connector are attached to the catheter. One bottle contains 0.1 normal HCl, and the other contains normal saline. One solution or the other is infused for approximately 10 minutes. The patient's spontaneous reaction to the infusion is recorded without coaching by the observer. If the infusion of the acid solution evokes the patient's own spontaneous symptoms, and these symptoms are not caused by saline, a positive acid perfusion test is recorded, indicating that the patient's symptoms can be reproduced by acid in the esophagus. This coupled with a positive acid reflux test provides a basis for diagnosing symptomatic reflux. Based on these tests, the great majority of cases of significant reflux, risk of esophagitis, and symptoms caused by reflux are diagnosed, and a variety of complicating conditions such as the motor disorders of the esophagus can be eliminated.

In patients who have undergone previous esophageal surgery, in those whose symptoms are complicated or overlap with other known conditions, and in patients suspected of having reflux-induced aspiration or angina-like pain, prolonged 24-hour pH monitoring in the esophagus is proving invaluable (Johnson and

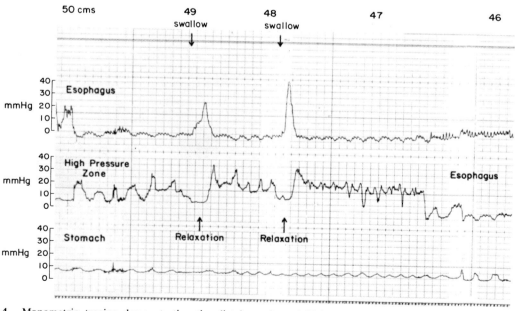

Figure 25–4. Manometric tracing demonstrating the distal esophageal high-pressure zone. Recordings are made from catheter lumens spaced 5 cm. apart. The catheter train is withdrawn from the stomach into the esophagus so that the proximal, middle, and distal recording channels pass sequentially through the high-pressure zone, which measures mm. Hg. Notice the relaxation with swallowing. (From Skinner, D. B.: Hiatal hernia and gastroesophageal reflux. *In* Davis-Christopher Textbook of Surgery. 12th Ed. Edited by D. C. Sabiston, Jr. Philadelphia, W. B. Saunders Company, 1981.)

DeMeester, 1974). Following a battery of standard esophageal function tests, the pH probe is left 5 cm. above the distal esophageal high-pressure zone. The probe is connected to a strip chart recorder through the pH meter. The patient is asked to record symptoms and activities during the ensuing 24 hours. During this time, the patient is instructed to eat normally but is restricted to a diet of fluids and food with a pH greater than 5. The number of bouts of reflux can be measured quantitatively based on their frequency and duration in both the supine and upright position. Alkaline reflux can be detected when the pH rises above 7. A scoring system is available based on known values in normal controls. By this method, patients can be categorized as normal or abnormal for both upright and supine reflux, disorders of acid clearing can be identified, and correlation of unusual symptoms with reflux may be observed. This test provides the most sensitive and quantitative method for evaluating possible gastroesophageal reflux.

SUMMARY

Based on an understanding of the normal and abnormal anatomy and pathophysiology of hiatal hernia and reflux, knowledge of a range of symptom complexes, and availability of a variety of tests of esophageal function, the clinician may quickly acquire all the information necessary to make a decision about treatment for reflux and hiatal hernia. As discussed in a subsequent section, the principal indication for hiatal hernia repair today is a paraesophageal Type II hiatal hernia, which should be repaired regardless of symptoms. There is no indication for the repair of a Type I axial hiatal hernia unless pathologic reflux causing symptoms and complications is present. When reflux is diagnosed as causing symptoms, medical therapy is initiated. Only in advanced cases with ulcerative esophagitis, stricture, bleeding observed to be coming from esophagitis, or documented aspiration shown to be caused by reflux or prolonged pH monitoring is anti-reflux surgery indicated. The several types of anti-reflux operations available and specific indications for each are discussed in subsequent sections of this chapter.

SELECTED REFERENCES

DeMeester, T. R., Johnson, L. F., Joseph, G. J., Toscano, M. S., Hall, A. W., and Skinner, D. B.: Patterns of gastroesophageal reflux in health and disease. Ann. Surg., *184*:459, 1976.

In this paper, the technique and interpretation for prolonged reflux monitoring are described. From analysis of a large number of patients studied, various patterns of abnormal reflux emerge. These, in turn, serve as the base for greater selectivity in treatment and identification of aberrant syndromes caused by reflux.

Payne, W. S., and Olsen, A. M. (Eds.): The Esophagus. Philadelphia, Lea & Febiger, 1974.

This monograph describes the extensive Mayo Clinic experience with esophageal diseases. The pioneering work of Code and asso-

ciates that set the stage for recurrent understanding of esophageal pathophysiology is especially well presented. The entire book is practical and readable. The first half is particularly relevant to problems of reflux and esophagitis.

Skinner, D. B., Belsey, R. H. R., Hendrix, T. R., and Zuidema, G. D. (Eds.): Gastroesophageal Reflux and Hiatal Hernia. Boston, Little, Brown and Company, 1972.

This monograph is devoted entirely to a discussion of hiatal hernia and reflux from anatomy, physiology, through various digestive studies, to therapy for reflux and its complications. With the exception of more recent data acquired from prolonged pH monitoring, it remains an excellent guide for the assessment and treatment of patients with symptomatic reflux.

REFERENCES

Barrett, N. R.: The lower esophagus lined by columnar epithelium. Surgery, *41*:881, 1957.

Berenson, M. M., Riddell, R. H., Skinner, D. B., and Freston, J. W.: Malignant transformation of esophageal columnar epithelium. Cancer, *41*:544, 1978.

Bernstein, L. M., Fruin, R. C., and Pacini, R.: Differentiation of esophageal pain from angina pectoris: Role of the esophageal acid perfusion test. Medicine, *41*:143, 1962.

Bombeck, C. T., Dillard, D. H., and Nyhus, L. M.: Muscular anatomy of the gastroesophageal junction and role of phrenoesophageal ligament. Autopsy study of sphincter mechanism. Ann. Surg., *164*:643, 1966.

Booth, D. J., Kemmerer, W. T., and Skinner, D. B.: Acid clearing from the distal esophagus. Arch. Surg., *96*:731, 1968.

Code, C. F., Creamer, B., Schlegel, J. F., et al.: An Atlas of Esophageal Motility in Health and Disease. Springfield, Illinois, Charles C Thomas, 1958, p. 104.

Cohen, S., and Lipshutz, W.: Hormonal control of lower esophageal sphincter competence: Interaction of gastrin and secretin. Gastroenterology, *58*:937, 1970.

Collis, J. L., Kelly, T. D., and Wiley, A. M.: Suturing of the crura of the diaphragm and the surgery of hiatus hernia. Thorax, *9*:175, 1954.

DeMeester, T. R., Wernly, J. A., Bryant, G. H., Little, A. G., and Skinner, D. B.: Clinical and in vitro analysis of determinants of gastroesophageal competence. Am. J. Surg., *137*:39, 1979.

DeMeester, T. R., Johnson, L. F., Joseph, G. J., Toscano, M. S., Hall, A. W., and Skinner, D. B.: Patterns of gastroesophageal reflux in health and disease. Ann. Surg., *184*:459, 1976.

Friedland, G. W., Melcher, D. H., Berridge, F. R., and Gresham, G. A.: Debatable points in the anatomy of the lower oesophagus. Thorax, *21*:487, 1966.

Fyke, F. E., Jr., Code, D. F., and Schlegel, J. F.: The gastroesophageal sphincter in healthy human beings. Gastroenterologia (Basel), *86*:135, 1956.

Henderson, R. D.: The Esophagus: Reflux Primary Motor Disorders. Baltimore, Williams and Wilkins Company, 1980, p. 127.

Hiebert, C. A., and Belsey, R.: Incompetency of the gastric cardia without radiologic evidence of hiatus hernia. J. Thorac. Cardiovasc. Surg., *42*:352, 1961.

Higgs, B., Shorter, R. G., and Ellis, F. H., Jr.: A study of the anatomy of the human esophagus with special reference to the gastro-oesophageal sphincter. J. Surg. Res., *5*:503, 1965.

Ismail-Beigi, F., Horton, P. F., and Pope, C. E., II: Histological consequences of gastroesophageal reflux in man. Gastroenterology, *58*:163, 1970.

Johnson, L. F., and DeMeester, T. R.: Twenty-four hour pH monitoring of the distal esophagus: A quantitative measure of gastroesophageal reflux. Am. J. Gastroenterol., *62*:325, 1974.

Kantrowitz, P. A., Corson, J. G., Fleischli, D. L., and Skinner, D. B.: Measurement of gastroesophageal reflux. Gastroenterology, *56*:666, 1969.

Moossa, A. R., Hall, A. W., Wood, R. A. B., Cooley, G. R., and Skinner, D. B.: Effect of pentagastrin infusion on gastroesophageal manometry and reflux status before and after esophagogastrectomy. Am. J. Surg., *133*:23, 1977.

O'Sullivan, G. C., DeMeester, T. R., Smith, R. B., Ryan, J. W., Johnson, L. F., and Skinner, D. B.: Twenty-four-hour pH monitoring of esophageal function. Arch. Surg., *116*:581, 1981.

Payne, W. S., and Olsen, A. M. (Eds.): The Esophagus. Philadelphia, Lea & Febiger, 1974.

Pellegrini, C. A., DeMeester, T. R., Johnson, L. F., and Skinner, D. B.: Gastroesophageal reflux and pulmonary aspiration. Incidence, functional abnormality, and results of surgical therapy. Surgery, *36*:110, 1979.

Sandry, R. J.: The pathology of chronic oesophagitis. Gut, *3*:189, 1962.

Skinner, D. B., and Belsey, R. H. R.: Surgical management of esophageal reflux and hiatus hernia: Long-term results with 1,030 patients. J. Thorac. Cardiovasc. Surg., *53*:33, 1967.

Skinner, D. B., and Booth, D. J.: Assessment of distal esophageal function in patients with hiatal hernia and/or gastroesophageal reflux. Ann. Surg., *172*:627, 1970.

Skinner, D. B., Belsey, R. H. R., Hendrix, T. R., and Zuidema, G. D. (Eds.): Gastroesophageal Reflux and Hiatal Hernia. Boston, Little, Brown and Company, 1972.

II THE BELSEY MARK IV ANTI-REFLUX REPAIR

David B. Skinner

In the early 1950s, gastroesophageal reflux and secondary esophagitis became recognized as a serious illness. Starting from methods employed for years to treat hiatal hernia, Ronald Belsey, in Bristol, England, developed by trial and error a specific anti-reflux operation that he called the Mark IV repair. This term recognized three preceding efforts to devise an anti-reflux repair that were unsuccessful. The first was similar to the repair described by Allison (1951), designed to correct reflux by shortening and reattaching the phrenoesophageal membrane. Allison's repair correctly recognized the importance of the intra-abdominal esophagus, but by circumferentially placing tension on the phrenoesophageal membrane, the esophageal diameter was widened, encouraging reflux. Allision recognized the high rate of persistent reflux following his repair in a long-term follow-up study (1973).

The Mark II repair of Belsey was a transitional procedure en route to the concept of a fundoplication of stomach around the esophagus. The Mark III operation was instructive in that three rows of plicating sutures were placed between the stomach and the esophagus, imbricating 5 to 6 cm. of esophagus into the stomach wall below the diaphragm. This effectively prevented reflux, but dysphagia was the common outcome. The Mark IV repair eliminated the third row of plicating sutures and achieved the proper balance between the creation of an intra-abdominal segment of esophagus constricted by the surrounding stomach so that reflux was prevented, but it did not make the submerged segment so long as to interfere with the transport of food across the barrier.

The Mark IV repair described in this section has stood the test of time as an effective anti-reflux operation with a low incidence of complications and recurrences (Skinner and Belsey, 1967). It incorporates those principles deemed to be important in the control of reflux that are discussed in detail in the preceding section. Specifically, the Mark IV operation restores a 3- to 4-cm. length of intra-abdominal esophagus, maintains a narrow diameter of the distal swallowing tube by compression by the adjacent gastric fundoplication, creates an abrupt change in diameter as the swallowing tube enters the gastric pouch, and leaves a portion of the circumference of the esophagus free posteriorly to dilate as necessary as a bolus of swallowed food passes (Fig. 25–5).

INDICATIONS FOR OPERATION

The anti-reflux operations, including the Mark IV, are specifically designed to prevent gastroesophageal reflux and can be expected only to relieve symptoms and complications caused by this disturbance. The first step in choosing an anti-reflux operation is to be absolutely certain that the symptoms are caused by reflux or its complications. Since the complaints caused by reflux may be numerous and overlap with a variety of other conditions, objective quantitation of

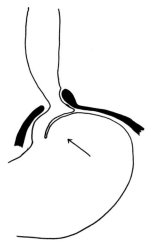

Figure 25–5. Principle of the Mark IV repair. The segment of lower esophagus restored to the abdomen is compressed by the positive intra-abdominal pressure against the posterior crural buttress.

reflux by esophageal function tests is often essential. The next step is to ascertain the degree of esophagitis. Esophagoscopy to grade the degree of esophagitis is a prerequisite to a decision about the necessity for surgery and the type of operation that may prove most effective (see preceding section for esophageal function tests and grading of esophagitis).

If no or minimal (Grade I) esophagitis is found, medical therapy is indicated. If a 6-month trial of medical treatment fails to bring symptoms under control, anti-reflux surgery may be considered for the relief of symptoms. A prolonged trial of medical treatment is necessary to allow for temporary stresses in the life of the patient that may aggravate symptoms and to allow for seasonal variations in acid peptic disorders. The demands of certain occupations that require stooping, bending, or lifting may make postural therapy ineffective and make the surgical relief of symptoms inevitable. However, when the indication for surgery is the relief of symptoms alone, the surgeon must be especially careful to ascertain that reflux is causing the symptoms and that other conditions such as duodenal ulcer, cholelithiasis, pancreatitis, gastric ulcer, and coronary artery disease have been excluded.

The customary indication for anti-reflux surgery is a complication of reflux, including ulcerative esophagitis, stricture, bleeding esophagitis, or repeated aspiration. When frank ulceration results from esophagitis, the virulence of the condition is established. The ulcer granulation tissue heals with the deposition of collagen in the submucosa. As the collagen contracts over time and the process of ulceration and healing is repeated or continuous, the outcome may be a stricture. This sequence of events is documented repeatedly and can occur with remarkable rapidity, e.g., in a matter of days in occasional patients. Since ulcerative esophagitis is a known precursor of stricture and since stricture is more difficult to treat and has a poorer long-term prognosis, anti-reflux surgery is recommended in patients with ulcerative esophagitis who do not have overriding medical contraindications. Patients who present with a stricture are candidates for surgical relief. Repeated dilatation of the stricture with medical treatment for reflux is an alternative method of management, but it usually proves ineffective and unacceptable to most patients who are otherwise healthy and vigorous.

Rapid bleeding from esophagitis is occasionally seen and is an indication for anti-reflux surgery in approximately 1 per cent of patients requiring operation. The bleeding is best handled acutely without operation by intravenous cimetidine and an iced milk antacid drip through a nasoesophageal tube while the patient sits upright. After the bleeding stops, which usually occurs within hours, the patient is evaluated and prepared for an elective anti-reflux operation to prevent a recurrence of this frightening complication.

Repeated aspiration of gastric contents into the lung is a serious complication of reflux and may occur in the absence of esophagitis or symptomatic heartburn. Any patient with morning hoarseness, chronic cough with recurring episodes of acute bronchitis or pneumonia, and a history of nocturnal cough often associated with a sour or brackish taste in the mouth should be suspected of having reflux-induced aspiration. Respiratory symptoms are common in the general population, as is reflux. The coexistence of the two conditions does not establish a cause-and-effect relationship. In these patients, continuous long-term pH monitoring is essential to establish that reflux is the cause of the respiratory disorder.

In children, the indications for anti-reflux surgery are less precise and more controversial. Frequent regurgitation and reflux are normal findings in children up to 12 to 18 months of age. After this time, nearly all children acquire competency of the cardia, and the need for anti-reflux surgery is rare during childhood and the teenage years. Since the natural history of frequent reflux in infancy and early childhood is progressive improvement, the decision as to whether to operate in a baby is difficult. Nevertheless, some young children do have progression of complicated reflux to a stricture, with weight loss, failure to thrive, aspiration, and occult bleeding with anemia. When reflux is clearly interfering with the well-being of the child, as documented by such complications, and the reflux does not respond readily to medical measures, including maintaining the child in a constant upright position with the so-called "chalasia chair," anti-reflux surgery may yield dramatic results.

Another indication for anti-reflux surgery is the condition called Barrett's esophagus (Barrett, 1953; Allison and Johnstone, 1953). It is normal for the distal 2 to 3 cm. of the tubular esophagus to be lined with columnar epithelium as the transition between the acid-sensitive squamous epithelium of the esophagus and the acid-producing gastric mucosa. In some patients, this columnar epithelium may extend farther up the esophagus, may be associated with a zone of ulcerative esophagitis between the columnar epithelium and squamous mucosa, and may undergo degeneration to atypia, intestinalization, dysplasia, and neoplasia (Berenson et al., 1978). Deep, penetrating, gastric-type ulcers may occur in the esophagus lined with this aberrant gastric mucosa. When this condition is diagnosed, the patient is said to have a Barrett's esophagus with or without a Barrett's ulcer. The diagnosis is often suspected by radiographic findings and confirmed by endoscopy with multiple biopsies. Because the dysplasia and neoplasia are multicentric and interspersed among islands of more normal-appearing columnar and goblet cell mucosa, a number of biopsies are essential to exclude malignant degeneration. Because of severe and long-standing reflux and the risk of neoplasia, some type of surgery is almost always indicated in a patient with Barrett's esophagus. The choice is between an esophageal resection and reconstruction or an anti-reflux repair. Whenever dysplasia or neoplasia is found in the biopsies, esophagectomy is recommended. In patients with no evidence of neoplastic degeneration, an anti-reflux repair is advocated, but the patient is advised that lifetime follow-up is necessary. It is not known whether and to what degree Barrett's epithelium may regress following a successful anti-reflux repair, and whether an anti-reflux repair will eliminate the risk of future malignant degeneration in the abnormal epithelium.

PREOPERATIVE PREPARATION

When the diagnosis of reflux is certain and ulcerative esophagitis is found, the indicated surgery is done promptly. When a stricture or severe esophagitis is encountered or when the patient has had recent severe hemorrhage from esophagitis or a recent bout of aspiration pneumonia, time devoted to preoperative preparation increases the safety of the operation and the likelihood of a successful long-term outcome. A reflux-induced stricture consists of two components, true fibrosis from collagen deposition during the healing process and a degree of esophageal muscle spasm, edema, and inflammation from the acute ulceration. The latter is reversible, and persistent efforts to treat and heal the esophagitis before surgery may convert a difficult stricture with a "short" esophagus into a straightforward problem that can be handled with an anti-reflux repair alone. Some patients with long-standing symptoms and a well-established stricture have too much fibrosis to enable the stricture to be reversed preoperatively. These patients often obtain a poor result from any type of anti-reflux surgery, including gastroplasty or fundic patch procedures, and require esophageal resection and reconstruction. The great majority of patients presenting with a stricture have the condition reversed by intensive in-hospital therapy with hourly antacids, cimetidine, and daily bougienage. Up to 2 weeks but often less time invested in such preoperative therapy converts a Grade III or IV esophagitis to a healing Grade II esophagitis. When this course is followed, it is rare to find the indurated, edematous mediastinum that was commonly encountered in the past, making dissection difficult, and a shortened esophageal tube that cannot be reduced beneath the diaphragm. When the esophagitis is reversed preoperatively, long-term recurrence rates are no greater than when anti-reflux surgery is performed in patients without severe esophagitis (i.e., 10 to 15 per cent).

When the indication for surgery is acute bleeding, the patient undergoes several days of intensive medical treatment to reverse the inflammation in the esophageal wall and mediastinum before the Mark IV operation is performed. When aspiration is an indication for surgery, several days of postural drainage, pulmonary physical therapy, and treatment with appropriate antibiotics are worthwhile prior to an anti-reflux repair.

CHOICE OF OPERATION

The surgeon who frequently operates for reflux and its complications is experienced with several types

of operations and chooses the one suited to the individual patient's requirements. Factors influencing the choice include whether a thoracic or abdominal approach is advantageous, whether the patient has had a previous anti-reflux repair, whether a resection or esophagomyotomy may be necessary, and the patient's body habitus. The Belsey Mark IV operation is performed only through a thoracotomy incision. The Hill anti-reflux operation is performed only through an abdominal approach. The Nissen fundoplication, Collis gastroplasty coupled with anti-reflux repair, and Thal gastric patch procedure plus anti-reflux repair may be performed through either a thoracic or abdominal approach, although many surgeons choose the chest exposure for the more complicated procedures. Esophageal resection and reconstruction are done through a thoracotomy or a thoracoabdominal approach.

In my practice, a thoracotomy approach is employed for patients with extensive esophagitis in whom more than the usual mobilization of the esophagus is anticipated and the possible need for a resection, gastroplasty, or fundic patch procedure is anticipated. A thoracotomy approach is advantageous for repeat anti-reflux operations, as a primary cause of failure of the previous operation is likely to be insufficient esophageal mobilization. A thoracic approach provides better exposure and less difficult operating conditions in an obese patient. This approach is used when other pulmonary or mediastinal disease is noted. We prefer the abdominal approach in patients undergoing their first anti-reflux repair in whom the esophagitis is under control and in whom obesity is not a major factor. The abdominal operation is also used in patients with other concurrent intra-abdominal disease requiring surgery.

Through the thoracic approach, the Belsey Mark IV or Nissen fundoplication is the usual anti-reflux repair. The degree of mobilization required for either is similar, and follow-up results offer little reason to choose one over the other. There are certain circumstances in which the Mark IV approach has advantages. These include patients with an esophageal motor disorder such as spasm, in whom the partial fundoplication is less likely to aggravate the esophageal obstruction than a full fundoplication. A modification of the Mark IV repair, in which the middle suture in each row is omitted, is used in conjunction with an esophagomyotomy in patients with standard or vigorous achalasia and following the resection and esophagomyotomy employed for epiphrenic diverticulum (Belsey, 1966).

Although some surgeons employ and advocate the Collis (1961) gastroplasty frequently, we find the need for this procedure to be rare if the patient is properly prepared for anti-reflux surgery. When the Collis maneuver is employed, it is coupled with either a Mark IV or a Nissen type of fundoplication, with the residual fundus being wrapped around the newly created distal esophageal tube (Pearson and Henderson, 1973; Henderson, 1977). The Thal gastric patch operation (Thal, 1968) is rarely indicated in our practice and is reserved for those cases in which entry is made into the esophagus in the course of intraoperative dilatation of a stricture. Esophagectomy and reconstruction, preferably by an isoperistaltic segment of left colon or jejunum, are reserved for those patients who have had multiple previous operations and in whom the esophagus is found to be mainly an unyielding fibrous tube (Belsey, 1965). Occasionally, sufficient damage occurs to the esophagus in the course of a reoperation for stricture that a resection is preferable to attempts at repairing the damage. Resection with colon or jejunal interposition is employed for specific indications in patients with a Barrett's esophagus.

THE MARK IV REPAIR

The Mark IV operation (Fig. 25–6) is a procedure of choice for the thoracic approach in anti-reflux surgery and is employed by many thoracic surgeons as their principal or best procedure for this condition. The operation is performed through a left sixth interspace thoracotomy. For optimal long-term results, it is important to minimize post-thoracotomy discomfort. To this end, the surgeon should not fracture ribs or the costal margin or use an incision larger than necessary. In children and young adults, the rib cage is sufficiently pliable that an intercostal incision without dividing a rib provides satisfactory exposure. In older patients, postoperative discomfort is minimized if a short segment of rib is resected underneath the paraspinal muscle mass behind the posterior angle of the rib. When this is done, the intercostal bundle is usually divided for hemostasis. The sixth interspace is chosen because it provides excellent exposure of the lower half of the esophagus and hiatus and causes less postoperative discomfort than does a lower interspace incision.

After the chest is opened, all lung adhesions are divided and the pulmonary ligament is incised. The dissection of the esophagus is begun just caudal to the inferior pulmonary vein. The pleura overlying the esophagus is incised, and the esophagus is dissected free from the aorta. Normally, two or three esophagobronchial arteries from the aorta are clamped and ligated in mobilizing the esophagus. Anteriorly, the esophagus is freed from the pericardium. The vagal nerve plexus is left on the esophageal muscle. The right pleural reflection is carefully dissected off the esophagus to avoid entry into the opposite pleural cavity, where blood may accumulate unnoticed during the operation. Once the esophagus is freed circumferentially, a tape is passed around the organ and used to elevate it. The dissection is carried cephalad well up under the arch of the aorta. The esophageal collateral blood supply in the submucosa is excellent, so that there is no concern about causing esophageal ischemia by this mobilization. The thoracic approach for an anti-reflux repair is often chosen because of the advantage of extensive esophageal mobilization, so that failure to perform this maneuver denies the patient the benefit of this approach.

After the proximal mobilization to the aortic arch is complete, the dissection is carried caudally. As the esophagus is elevated from its bed, the vagus nerves are easily palpable as two taut strings behind the esophagus. Posteriorly, the dissection is carried down to the crura of the diaphragm. The right pleural reflection is bluntly dissected and the pericardium mobilized off the right crus, so that the tendinous origin of the crus is prepared for suturing. Anteriorly, the dissection is extended down until the cuff of diaphragmatic muscle is cleared circumferentially.

Upward retraction of the esophagus places tension on the phrenoesophageal membrane, which becomes visible inserting into the wall of the esophagus as it enters the hiatus. Using scissors, an incision is made in the phrenoesophageal membrane directly anteriorly and at a right angle to the axis of the esophagus. The incision passes through the endothoracic and endoabdominal fascia and retroperitoneal fat, and finally, the peritoneal sac is entered. The cardia is freed completely from the hiatus, preserving only the vagal nerve branches on the wall of the gastroesophageal junction. The mobilization requires ligation and division of the esophageal branch of the left inferior phrenic artery running close to the left vagus nerve, and ligation and division of the ascending esophageal branch from the left gastric artery lying close to the right vagus nerve in the retroperitoneum. When the latter vessel is divided, the lesser peritoneal sac is opened, which completes the hiatal dissection. The fundus of the stomach is delivered up through the hiatus. The gastroesophageal junction anteriorly between the two vagus nerves is cleared of fibrofatty tissue to facilitate the repair. The stage is now set for the Mark IV reconstruction.

With the cardia retracted anteriorly, the decussation of the crura is visualized posteriorly. A 0 silk suture is placed through the tendinous portion of the right crus near its origin and through the left crus, catching a portion of the muscular cuff and piercing the endothoracic fascia immediately in front of the aorta. Two or three similar sutures are placed progressing anteriorly at 1-cm. intervals. An average anti-reflux repair requires three such sutures, but as many as six or seven may be needed if the hiatus is very large. These sutures are left in place and tied later, after the fundoplication is complete.

The first row of suturing for stomach plication to the esophagus is performed using 2-0 silk sutures placed first through the stomach and then obliquely through the esophageal wall 2 cm. above the gastroesophageal junction. The suture is reversed and passed back obliquely through the esophagus and through the gastric fundus. Three such mattress sutures are used. The first is placed near the left vagus nerve; the second (center) stitch is placed anterior midway between the vagus nerves, and the third stitch is placed adjacent to the right vagus nerve. An oblique stitch catching a deep bite of both longitudinal and circular muscle is important to prevent the esophageal sutures from cutting through.

For the final row of sutures, 0 silk on a large,

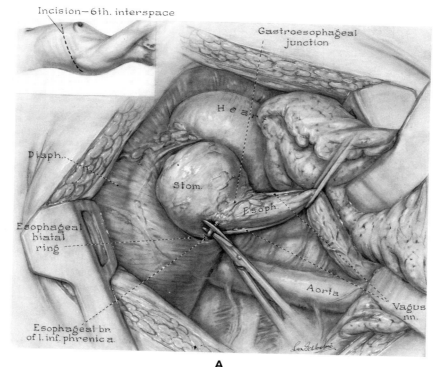

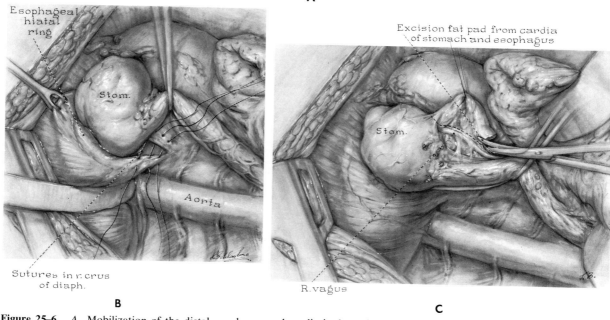

Figure 25–6. *A,* Mobilization of the distal esophagus and cardia is done through a left sixth interspace lateral thoracotomy. The esophagus with vagus nerves attached is completely freed up to the lung root. After the hernia sac is entered anteriorly, the entire circumference of the cardia is separated from its attachments. This requires division of branches from the left inferior phrenic artery laterally *(illustrated)* and left gastric artery posteriorly *(not shown)*. *B,* At the start of the repair, sutures are placed in two limbs of the right crus posteriorly, but these are not tied until the completion of the reconstruction. Tension on a clamp applied to the diaphragm anteriorly makes it easier to identify the strong tendinous tissue in the crus where the sutures should be placed. *C,* After complete mobilization of the esophagogastric junction, the pad of fibrofatty tissue at the cardia is excised anteriorly and laterally. The vagus nerves, which tend to be elevated off the esophagus during this dissection, are carefully preserved.

Illustration continued on following page

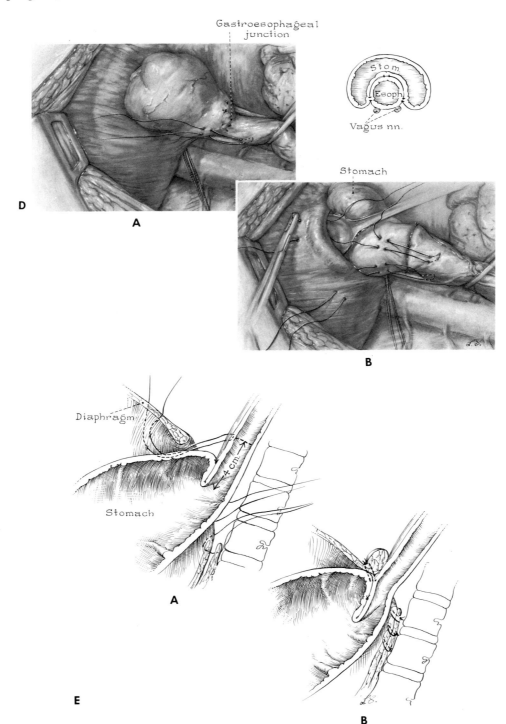

Figure 25–6. *Continued D,* (**A**) The reconstruction is started by placing the first of three mattress sutures between the fundus of the stomach and esophagus 2 cm. above the junction. The spacing of these sutures around the circumference of the esophagus is shown in the cross-sectional insert. (**B**) After completion of the first row of sutures, a second row of three mattress sutures is placed through the diaphragm, fundus, and esophagus. In the illustration, the first suture is in place, and the second is being passed through the diaphragm in the bowel of a spoon retractor, which is used to protect structures beneath the diaphragm. The posterior sutures in the crus are in place but have not been tied. *E,* Sagittal sections of the repair. (**A**) The sutures in the crus posteriorly have been placed but not yet tied. The first row of mattress sutures between the stomach and esophagus have been tied. One of the mattress sutures in the second row is illustrated. (**B**) The completed repair. The posterior sutures in the crus and second row of mattress sutures joining the diaphragm, stomach, and esophagus are tied after the reconstruction has been placed beneath the diaphragm. (From Belsey, R. H. R., and Skinner, D. B.: Surgical treatment: Thoracic approach. *In* Gastroesophageal Reflux and Hiatal Hernia. Edited by D. B. Skinner, R. H. R. Belsey, T. R. Hendrix, and G. D. Zuidema. Boston, Little, Brown and Company, 1972.)

curved needle is employed. A spoon inserted through the hiatus with the bowl on the underside of the diaphragm protects subdiaphragmatic organs. The needle is passed through the edge of the central tendon of the diaphragm into the bowl of the spoon and out through the hiatus. Next, the suture is passed through the fundus of the stomach and then an additional 2 cm. cephalad on the esophagus, taking an oblique bite. The suture is then reversed, passing back through the esophagus and the fundus of the stomach and out through the tendinous portion of the diaphragm. Three sutures are placed in this row, corresponding in location to the sutures in the first row. After all three sutures are in place, the reconstructed cardia is set below the diaphragm manually before any tension is placed on the sutures. After pulling each suture up snugly to hold the reconstruction beneath the diaphragm, the sutures are tied gently. At this point, the repair should lie easily below the diaphragm without apparent tension. The posterior crural sutures are now tied, with care being taken to leave an orifice through the hiatus that is sufficient to admit the operator's index finger easily or to pass a No. 60 bougie without obstruction at the cardia. The thoracotomy is closed with chest tube drainage.

POSTOPERATIVE CARE

A nasogastric tube is not used routinely. The chest tube is removed after 48 hours or when drainage falls below 200 ml. daily. Ambulation is started the evening of surgery, and liquids may be taken by mouth on the next day. When the patient is eating well, a postoperative barium swallow examination is performed to record the status of the repair. A satisfactory result should show the 4-cm. segment of intra-abdominal esophagus and the adjacent fundoplication (Fig. 25–7). The lumen of the esophagus opens fully as the barium bolus passes, but remains closed otherwise.

At the time of discharge, usually the seventh postoperative day, the patient is advised to chew food carefully and avoid large boluses. Certain sticky foods such as soft bread and pithy vegetables tend to pass slowly through the reconstruction and should be avoided during the first month. Normal physical activity is encouraged. Depending on the patient's employment, work can usually be resumed within 3 to 6 weeks.

FOLLOW-UP AND RESULTS

For the surgeon who is dedicated to perfecting the technique of anti-reflux surgery and anxious to determine long-term results, an ongoing follow-up program is essential. After the first 6 months of check-ups, patients are asked to return at yearly intervals. Provided the patient remains asymptomatic, a routine barium swallow and outpatient esophageal function tests

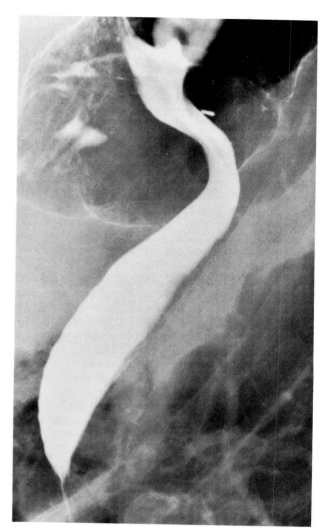

Figure 25–7. Postoperative barium swallow after Mark IV repair showing typical 4-cm. segment of intra-abdominal esophagus compressed by adjacent gastric fundus.

should be repeated at 2 years and 5 years following operation. Any patient who returns complaining of symptoms remotely related to reflux should be evaluated promptly by a barium swallow, esophageal function tests, and if these are positive, esophagoscopy. In this way, objective evidence of the results of surgery can be obtained in addition to assessing the patient's satisfaction with the operation. Based on a systematic follow-up approach in which more than 97 per cent of patients were accounted for, 83 per cent of patients were shown to be asymptomatic and had a satisfactory barium swallow 5 or more years after a Mark IV repair (Skinner and Belsey, 1967). In a subsequent study, recurrence of specific symptoms of reflux or a recurrent hiatal hernia were found in 15 per cent of 272 patients followed for more than 10 years, and 76 per cent remained relieved of all preoperative symptoms (Orringer et al., 1972). In a separate independent evaluation of the operation, 71 per cent of patients were found to be completely symptom-free after 10 years (Hiebert and O'Mara, 1979).

SELECTED REFERENCES

Hiebert, C. A., and O'Mara, C. S.: The Belsey operation for hiatal hernia: A twenty-year experience. Am. J. Surg., *137*:532, 1979.

Long-term results (10-year follow-up) are given from another excellent series of Mark IV operations verifying the original Belsey experience.

Orringer, M. B., Skinner, D. B., and Belsey, R. H. R.: Long-term results of the Mark IV operation for hiatal hernia and analyses of recurrences and their treatment. J. Thorac. Cardiovasc. Surg., *63*:25, 1972.

The long-term follow-up beyond 10 years for the Mark IV repair performed in Belsey's clinic is reported along with an analysis of types and causes of recurrences.

Pearson, F. G., and Henderson, R. D.: Experimental and clinical studies of gastroplasty in the management of acquired short esophagus. Surg. Gynecol. Obstet. *136*:737, 1973.

The rationale and use of the Collis gastroplasty coupled with a Mark IV type of reconstruction is presented and clinical results given.

Skinner, D. B., and Belsey, R. H. R.: Surgical management of esophageal reflux and hiatus hernia: Long-term results with 1,030 patients. J. Thorac. Cardiovasc. Surg., *53*:33, 1967.

This paper presents the first formal description of the Mark IV operation from Belsey's clinic, its indications, rationale, and results. Results from the early types of anti-reflux repairs are given. The use of the operation in children, Type II hiatal hernia, and stricture cases is analyzed.

REFERENCES

Allison, P. R.: Reflux esophagitis, sliding hiatal hernia, and the anatomy of repair. Surg. Gynecol. Obstet., *92*:419, 1951.
Allison, P. R.: Hiatus hernia: A 20-year retrospective survey. Ann. Surg., *178*:273, 1973.
Allison, P. R., and Johnstone, A. S.: The esophagus lined with gastric mucous membrane. Thorax, *8*:87, 1953.
Barrett, N. R.: Chronic peptic ulcer of the oesophagus lined with gastric mucous membrane. Thorax, *8*:87, 1953.
Belsey, R. H. R.: Functional disease of the esophagus. J. Thorac. Cardiovasc. Surg., *52*:164, 1966.
Belsey, R. H. R.: Reconstruction of esophagus with left colon. J. Thorac. Cardiovasc. Surg., *49*:33, 1965.
Belsey, R. H. R., and Skinner, D. B.: Surgical treatment: Thoracic approach. *In* Gastroesophageal Reflux and Hiatal Hernia. Edited by D. B. Skinner, R. H. R. Belsey, T. R. Hendrix, and G. D. Zuidema. Boston, Little, Brown and Company, 1972.
Berenson, M. M., Riddell, R. H., Skinner, D. B., and Freston, J. W.: Malignant transformation of esophageal columnar epithelium. Cancer, *41*:544, 1978.
Collis, J. L.: Gastroplasty. Thorax, *16*:197, 1961.
Henderson, R. D.: Reflux control following gastroplasty. Ann. Thorac. Surg., *24*:206, 1977.
Hiebert, C. A., and O'Mara, C. S.: The Belsey operation for hiatal hernia: A twenty-year experience. Am. J. Surg., *137*:532, 1979.
Orringer, M. B., Skinner, D. B., and Belsey, R. H. R.: Long-term results of the Mark IV operation for hiatal hernia and analyses of recurrences and their treatment. J. Thorac. Cardiovasc. Surg., *63*:25, 1972.
Pearson, F. G., and Henderson, R. D.: Experimental and clinical studies of gastroplasty in the management of acquired short esophagus. Surg. Gynecol. Obstet., *136*:737, 1973.
Skinner, D. B., and Belsey, R. H. R.: Surgical management of esophageal reflux and hiatus hernia: Long-term results with 1,030 patients. J. Thorac. Cardiovasc. Surg., *53*:33, 1967.
Thal, A. P.: A unified approach to surgical problems of the esophagogastric junction. Ann. Surg., *168*:542, 1968.

III   THE NISSEN FUNDOPLICATION

F. HENRY ELLIS, JR.

The chief physiologic abnormality responsible for gastroesophageal reflux is a hypotensive lower esophageal sphincter (LES), and operations designed to correct reflux must have as their goal restoration of normal function rather than normal anatomy. Since most patients with gastroesophageal reflux have a sliding esophageal hiatal hernia, it was natural that surgical emphasis in the past was on restoration of normal anatomy. Only after careful analysis of the long-term results of anatomically designed operations revealed a high percentage of unsatisfactory results (Allison, 1973) were surgical techniques modified.

Of the three most commonly used anti-reflux procedures, the Nissen fundoplication is the only one that was originally devised to restore normal function. The other two operations, the Hill posterior gastropexy and the Belsey Mark IV procedure, were originally devised with strictly anatomic goals in mind, although subsequently it was recognized that they also improved the function of the LES. Before discussing the technical aspects of the procedure itself and its results, it is pertinent to review some historical and experimental aspects of the development of the Nissen fundoplication.

HISTORICAL ASPECTS

In December 1955, Professor Rudolph Nissen, of Basel, Switzerland, operated on a 49-year-old woman who had a long history of gastroesophageal reflux without radiographic evidence of a hiatal hernia (Nissen, 1956). He employed a technique that he had used nearly 20 years before in attempting to minimize postoperative reflux after resection of a peptic ulcer in the region of the cardia (Nissen, 1937). This involved enveloping the lower esophagus with gastric fundus by suture approximation of anterior and posterior fundal folds anterior to the esophagus, in which a large intraesophageal bougie had been positioned. Since his original description, the Nissen fundoplication has undergone a variety of modifications designed to minimize complications and poor results. Nissen himself later combined the operation with anterior gastropexy (Nissen, 1961), only to discontinue that modification later (Nissen and Rossetti, 1965). The degree of the fundal wrap has been varied to encircle less than 360 degrees of the esophageal tube in order to avoid the gas bloat syndrome (Menguy, 1978; Guarner et al., 1980). Anchoring of the plication sutures to the preaortic fascia has been advocated as a means of preventing mediastinal migration of the wrap (Cordiano et al., 1976; Kaminski et al., 1977). Concomitant performance of parietal cell vagotomy has been advocated not only to reduce gastric acidity but also to simplify performance of the fundoplication (Jordan, 1978; Jones and Anders, 1979). Thus, the term Nissen fundoplication may be applied to a variety of procedures since so many modifications of this widely employed operation are currently in vogue.

EXPERIMENTAL BACKGROUND

Although the relevance of experimental studies on various fundoplication techniques to the clinical setting may be questioned because of differences between species, they may provide useful insights if properly interpreted. Bombeck and associates (1971) studied a variety of sphincter-enhancing procedures in dogs whose LES had been rendered incompetent by myectomy. Only the Nissen fundoplication was uniformly successful in preventing reflux, as assessed by cinefluorography. Butterfield's studies (1971) of cadaver specimens confirmed the superiority of the Nissen repair. A wrap greater than 270 degrees was found by Alday and Goldsmith (1973) in in vitro studies to fulfill best the criterion of establishing competence, and the human cadaver studies of Lortat-Jacob and coworkers (1961) concluded that at least 4 cm. of esophagus must be wrapped to achieve competence.

The animal experiments of Leonardi and colleagues (1977) are more relevant, for they were in vivo studies in the cat, whose esophagus is similar to that of man. In a comparison of the effectiveness of the Nissen, Hill, and Belsey procedures employing postoperative manometry and pH reflux testing, the Nissen fundoplication proved superior to the others in its ability to raise LES pressures and to prevent reflux. In another study involving variations on the technique of fundoplication, it was concluded that fundoplication optimally restores normal LES function when it encircles the esophagus completely over a length equivalent to the normal length of the high-pressure zone

(Leonardi and Ellis, 1977). The findings of Donahue and Bombeck (1977) that a loose, "floppy" wrap protects against gastric distention have also contributed to the development of the proper surgical technique of fundoplication.

The mechanism by which these anti-reflux operations succeed in restoring competence is not clearly understood. The postoperative increase in resting LES pressure is most readily explained by purely mechanical factors, as supported by the experimental studies of Condon and associates (1976). In addition to the mechanical effect of fundoplication in raising resting LES pressures, manometric studies have demonstrated a return to normal of the adaptive response of the LES to graded increases in intragastric pressure (Ellis et al., 1976). Furthermore, it has been shown that the subnormal response of the hypotensive LES to parenterally administered pentagastrin is restored to normal after clinical fundoplication (Lipshutz et al., 1974) and experimental fundoplication (Siewert et al., 1973). These findings, which document a restoration of the neural and hormonal response to the LES, require more than a mechanical explanation.

Lipshutz and associates (1974) suggested that these changes are the result of alteration in the length-tension characteristics of the LES muscle produced by surgical repair. They hypothesize that these anti-reflux procedures may place the LES muscle at its optimal degree of stretch and allow the LES to respond normally to both neural and hormonal stimulation. The explanation of Siewart and associates (1973, 1975) seems more logical. They demonstrated by in vitro studies that excised strips of smooth muscle from the LES and from adjacent gastric fundus exhibit a similar response to such stimuli as pentagastrin. These studies suggest that the normal physiologic response of the newly created high-pressure zone is restored after fundoplication because the smooth muscle of the gastric fundus composing the wrap responds to neurohumoral stimuli in a fashion similar to the smooth muscle of the normal LES. Further support for this concept is the demonstration that the bundles of both the superficial and deep muscle layers of the gastric fundus have a transverse orientation to the stomach axis, so that circularly arranged muscle fibers surround the LES after fundoplication (Liebermann-Meffert, 1975).

TECHNIQUE OF FUNDOPLICATION

Certain key points to the operation should be emphasized at the outset. Careful mobilization of the distal esophagus without injury to the vagus nerves is essential, so that 5 to 6 cm. lie loosely within the abdomen. The gastric fundus must be mobilized widely without injury to the spleen. If splenectomy is required, the complication rate is said to be tripled (Rogers et al., 1980). The fundoplication stitches must incorporate esophageal wall to maintain the position of the wrap, and the hiatus should be narrowed to prevent its mediastinal migration.

An abdominal approach is preferred, a thoracic incision being employed only in those patients who have had a previous thoracotomy or in whom shortening of the esophagus is suspected. The abdomen is entered through an upper midline incision, skirting to the left of the umbilicus (Fig. 25–8). The left lobe of the liver is mobilized to permit exposure of the esophagogastric junctional area. When a hiatus hernia is present, it is reduced, and the peritoneum and phrenoesophageal membrane overlying the esophagus are divided, allowing development of an adequate length of intra-abdominal esophagus to permit performance of the procedure. The gastrohepatic omentum is divided. The short gastric vessels are ligated and divided, as are the vessels between the posterior gastric wall and the posterior abdominal parietes, to mobilize the gastric fundus thoroughly (Fig. 25–9).

A Maloney dilator (40 French) is passed transorally by the anesthesiologist across the esophagogastric junction, and the gastric fundus is passed behind the mobilized esophagus from left to right, as illustrated in Figure 25–10A. The fundus is grasped with a Babcock clamp to the right of the esophagus and held in place as three or four seromuscular sutures of nonabsorbable material approximate the adjacent folds of gastric fundus anterior to the esophagus. These sutures incorporate a small portion of anterior esophageal wall, with care being taken to avoid the vagus nerves (Fig. 25–10B). The length of the wrap varies from 4 to 5 cm. in length. Additional sutures of finer material are placed between these heavy sutures to ensure security of the wrap (Fig. 25–10C). The position of the collar of the wrap around the esophagus is ensured by placement of several fine interrupted sutures between the seromuscular layer of the gastric

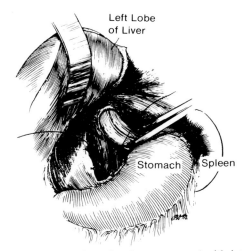

Figure 25–9. The hiatus has been narrowed with interrupted sutures after mobilization of the fundus and distal esophagus. (From Ellis, F. H., Jr., Garabedian, M., and Gibb, S. P.: Fundoplication for gastroesophageal reflux: Indications, surgical technique, and manometric results. Arch. Surg., *107*:187, 1973.)

fundus and the esophageal musculature. To prevent migration of the wrap into the thoracic cavity, the esophageal hiatus is narrowed posterior to the esophagus by two or three heavy sutures of nonabsorbable material in the diaphragmatic crura (Fig. 25–9). Only then is the large-bore, indwelling stent removed.

The postoperative management of patients after fundoplication is straightforward. Oral feedings are permitted when bowel sounds return. Early ambulation is encouraged, and dismissal from the hospital is usually possible within a week.

PATIENT SELECTION AND RESULTS OF OPERATION

Proper patient selection determines to a great extent the success of an operation. The Nissen fundoplication is no exception, for experience has shown that the procedure is not applicable to all patients. Needless to say, no patient should be considered for operation until a strict medical program has failed; operation is required in less than 10 per cent of patients with gastroesophageal reflux. Although some advocate performing a Nissen fundoplication around an esophagogastric peptic stricture (Harrison and Gompels, 1971; Safaie-Shirazi *et al.*, 1975), this approach has not been uniformly successful. Under such circumstances, I prefer to perform an esophageal lengthening procedure, such as the Collis gastroplasty, after intraoperative dilation of the stricture, so that the fundal wrap surrounds pliable tissue and restoration of competence is ensured. Even in the absence of a stricture, patients with esophageal shortening should not have a simple Nissen wrap left in the chest. Instead, the esophagus should be lengthened by a

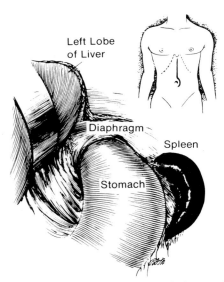

Figure 25–8. Incision and exposure of the esophagus and fundus in preparation for fundoplication. The left lobe of the liver has been mobilized to facilitate exposure. (From Ellis, F. H., Jr., Garabedian, M., and Gibb, S. P.: Fundoplication for gastroesophageal reflux: Indications, surgical technique, and manometric results. Arch. Surg., *107*:187, 1973. Copyright 1973, American Medical Association.)

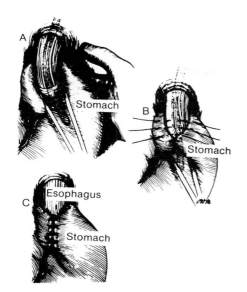

Figure 25–10. Technique of fundoplication. *A,* The mobilized fundus is passed posterior to the esophagus. Note the indwelling large-bore (40-French) Maloney dilator. *B,* Seromuscular sutures incorporating anterior esophageal wall approximate adjacent portions of the gastric fundus. Reinforcing fine nonabsorbable sutures have been placed and the dilator withdrawn. (From Ellis, F. H., Jr., Garabedian, M., and Gibb, S. P.: Fundoplication for gastroesophageal reflux: Indications, surgical technique, and manometric results. Arch. Surg., *107*:187, 1973.)

Collis gastroplasty and competence restored by wrapping the gastroplasty tube and leaving the Nissen wrap in the abdomen. A fundal wrap left within the chest may lead to notable complications (Mansour *et al.,* 1981). Patients who do not have normal peristalsis (those with achalasia or scleroderma, for example) are poor candidates for a 360-degree fundal wrap, because postoperative dysphagia is common in these patients. A wrap of less than 360 degrees should be performed in such individuals to prevent this complication.

The ideal candidate for the Nissen fundoplication is a patient whose condition is unresponsive to medical therapy, who does not have a stricture at the esophagogastric junction, and who has no evidence of esophageal shortening but in whom normal peristalsis can be demonstrated in the body of the esophagus. If these criteria for patient selection are followed, results of the Nissen fundoplication for gastroesophageal reflux secondary to a hypotensive LES should be excellent.

Rossetti and Hell (1977) have reported the largest series of patients with the Nissen fundoplication. Over a 20-year period, 1400 such patients were treated at the University of Basel, where the procedure was originated. Some of these patients underwent a modified fundoplication confined to the anterior wall of the fundus (Rossetti, 1968). Long-term follow-up of 590 patients with simple reflux esophagitis showed that 87.5 per cent were free of symptoms. The largest series reported in the United States is that of Polk (1978). Among 400 patients, the failure rate was only 4.5 per cent, with an average follow-up period of 3.8

years. Similarly favorable results have been reported by other surgeons from the United States (Battle *et al.,* 1973; Ellis *et al.,* 1976; Bushkin *et al.,* 1977) as well as from Belgium (Henrion, 1971), Great Britain (Shah and Daniel, 1972; Franklin *et al.,* 1973), France (Jacquemet *et al.,* 1972), and New Zealand (Morgan, 1971).

In addition to these excellent clinical results, objective confirmation of the effectiveness of the operative procedure in raising sphincter pressure and eliminating reflux has had ample documentation (Ellis *et al.,* 1976; Kaminski *et al.,* 1977; Bushkin *et al.,* 1977). Not only does the operation triple the amplitude of LES pressure, but also the length of the high-pressure zone is increased and the neurohumoral responsiveness of the LES is restored.

It is difficult to compare results of the Nissen fundoplication with those of other types of anti-reflux surgery, for usually the patients are not comparable. Unfortunately, only a few studies have been published in which the different operations were compared in a single institution, not necessarily in a randomized fashion. DeMeester and associates (1974) evaluated results after the Nissen, Belsey, and Hill procedures. The Nissen fundoplication was found to be superior to the other operations in restoring LES function and in preventing reflux. Nicholson and Nohl-Oser (1976), from Great Britain, have confirmed the superiority of the Nissen procedure over the Belsey Mark IV operation in preventing gastroesophageal reflux, as have Dilling and coworkers (1977). Sillin and colleagues (1979), in a comparative study of 207 patients undergoing anti-reflux surgery, found the failure rate to be 18 per cent with the Belsey Mark IV procedure and 13 per cent with the Hill posterior gastropexy but only 8 per cent with the Nissen fundoplication. In a similar study of 101 patients. Ferraris and Sube (1981) compared results after the Belsey, Hill, and Nissen procedures and found that the lowest recurrence rate was associated with the Nissen operation combined with posterior gastropexy.

Despite these many favorable reports of the results of the Nissen fundoplication, legitimate concern has been expressed regarding the ability of patients to belch and vomit postoperatively. In the original series of Woodward and associates (1971), the gas bloat syndrome was said to occur in 54 per cent of patients, but this dropped to 11 per cent with a longer follow-up period (Bushkin *et al.,* 1977). Others who have employed a loose wrap have encountered this syndrome rarely and usually only transiently (Ellis *et al.,* 1976; Polk, 1978). The reported incidence of recurrent reflux varies from 2 to 10 per cent (Woodward *et al.,* 1971; Polk, 1978). Permanent competence can be assured by employing a loose wrap.

In a review of fundoplication failures requiring reoperation, Leonardi and associates (1981) found that postoperative dysphagia was the most common cause. Although transient dysphagia may occur between 7 and 10 days after operation in 15 to 20 per cent of patients, only rarely is it severe and persistent. The most common cause of dysphagia in Leonardi's series was a previously undiagnosed motility disorder of the esophagus characterized by aperistalsis. The reason for dysphagia in most of the remaining patients was thought to be too tight a wrap. Another cause of postoperative dysphagia is gastric obstruction resulting from a "slipped Nissen" (Olson *et al.*, 1976). Although the fundal wrap may slip from its esophageal position to obstruct the stomach if fixation sutures are not used around the collar of the wrap, most examples of this syndrome are probably the result of improper placement of the wrap at the time of operation. Other complications that have occasionally occurred after a Nissen fundoplication include paraesophageal hernia (Balison *et al.*, 1973), gastric ulceration (Bushkin *et al.*, 1976; Bremner, 1979), and leaks and fistulous communication with other viscera (Ikard and Jacobs, 1974; Mullen *et al.*, 1975; Burnett *et al.*, 1977).

Because the operation of fundoplication is the most successful of the available anti-reflux procedures in terms of permanently preventing reflux and because complications are rare if the operation is properly performed on carefully selected patients, many surgeons consider it to be the operation of choice for all patients with gastroesophageal reflux who fail to respond to medical therapy. If patients are carefully selected to avoid those with an underlying motility disorder, stricture, or esophageal shortening, unsatisfactory results will be minimized. If the fundal wrap is loosely made around a large, indwelling stent, postoperative gas bloat, dysphagia, and disruption with recurrent reflux should be rare. The operation has rightly become the most widely used anti-reflux procedure throughout the world in the management of selected patients with reflux esophagitis.

SELECTED REFERENCES

Ellis, F. H., Jr., and Gibb, S. P.: Fundoplication for hypotensive lower esophageal sphincter. Hosp. Prac., *9*:80, 1974.

The technique of the Nissen fundoplication is clearly illustrated in this article through outstanding photographic and art work.

Fisher, R. S., Malmud, L. S., Lobis, I. F., *et al.*: Antireflux surgery for symptomatic gastroesophageal reflux: Mechanism of action. Am. J. Dig. Dis., *23*:152, 1978.

An objective analysis of the effects of the Nissen fundoplication on symptoms and manometrics is outlined here from the standpoint of the gastroenterologist.

Nissen, R.: Eine einfache Operation zur Beeinflussung der Refluxoesophagitis. Schweiz. Med. Wochenschr., *86*:590, 1956.

In this classic article, Professor Nissen describes the technique and rationale of the fundoplication procedure as first performed by him.

Skinner, D. B.: Complications of surgery for gastroesophageal reflux. World J. Surg., *1*:485, 1977.

This article presents clearly and concisely the types of complications that may follow all anti-reflux operations, including the Nissen fundoplication.

REFERENCES

Alday, E. S., and Goldsmith, H. S.: Efficacy of fundoplication in preventing gastric reflux. Am. J. Surg., *126*:322, 1973.

Allison, P. R.: Hiatal hernia: A 20-year retrospective study. Ann. Surg., *178*:273, 1973.

Balison. J. R., Macgregor, A. M., and Woodward, E. R.: Postoperative diaphragmatic herniation following transthoracic fundoplication: A note of warning. Arch. Surg., *106*:164, 1973.

Battle, W. S., Nyhus, L. M., and Bombeck, C. T.: Nissen fundoplication and esophagitis secondary to gastroesophageal reflux. Arch. Surg., *106*:588, 1973.

Bombeck, C. T., Coelho, R. G., Castro, V. A., *et al.*: An experimental comparison of procedures for the operative correction of gastroesophageal reflux. Bull. Soc. Int. Chir., *30*:435, 1971.

Bremner, C. G.: Gastric ulceration after a fundoplication operation for gastroesophageal reflux. Surg. Gynecol. Obstet., *148*:62, 1979.

Burnett, H. F., Read, R. C., Morris, W. D., *et al.*: Management of complications of fundoplication and Barrett's esophagus. Surgery, *82*:521, 1977.

Bushkin, F. L., Woodward, E. R., and O'Leary, J. P.: Occurrence of gastric ulcer after Nissen fundoplication. Am. Surg., *42*:821, 1976.

Bushkin, F. L., Neustein, C. L., Parker, T. H., *et al.*: Nissen fundoplication for reflux peptic esophagitis. Ann. Surg., *185*:672, 1977.

Butterfield, W. C.: Current hiatal hernia repairs: Similarities, mechanisms, and extended indications — an autopsy study. Surgery, *69*:910, 1971.

Condon, R. E., Kraus, M. A., and Wollheim, D.: Cause of increase in "lower esophageal sphincter" pressure after fundoplication. J. Surg. Res., *20*:445, 1976.

Cordiano, C., Rovere, G. Q., Agugiaro, S., *et al.*: Technical modification of the Nissen fundoplication procedure. Surg. Gynecol. Obstet., *143*:977, 1976.

DeMeester, T. R., Johnson, L. F., and Kent, A. H.: Evaluation of current operations for the prevention of gastroesophageal reflux. Am. Surg., *180*:511, 1974.

Dilling, E. W., Peyton, M. D., Cannon, S. P., *et al.*: Comparison of Nissen fundoplication and Belsey Mark IV in the management of gastroesophageal reflux. Am. J. Surg., *134*:730, 1977.

Donahue, P. E., and Bombeck, C. T.: The modified Nissen fundoplication — reflux prevention without gas bloat. Chir. Gastroenterol., *11*:15, 1977.

Ellis, F. H., Jr., and Gibb, S. P.: Fundoplication for hypotensive lower esophageal sphincter. Hosp. Prac., *9*:80, 1974.

Ellis, F. H., Jr., El-Kurd, M. F. A., and Gibb, S. P.: The effect of fundoplication on the lower esophageal sphincter. Surg. Gynecol. Obstet., *143*:1, 1976.

Ellis, F. H., Jr., Garabedian, M., and Gibbs, S. P.: Fundoplication for gastroesophageal reflux: Indications, surgical technique, and manometric results. Arch. Surg., *107*:187, 1973.

Ferraris, V. A., and Sube, J.: Retrospective study of the surgical management of reflux esophagitis. Surg. Gynecol. Obstet., *152*:17, 1981.

Fisher, R. S., Malmud, L. S., Lobis, I. F., *et al.*: Antireflux surgery for symptomatic gastroesophageal reflux: Mechanism of action. Am. J. Dig. Dis., *23*:152, 1978.

Franklin, R. H., Iweze, F. I., and Owen-Smith, M. S.: Fundoplication for hiatus hernia. Br. J. Surg., *60*:65, 1973.

Guarner, V., Martinez, N., and Gavino, J. F.: Ten year evaluation of posterior fundoplasty in the treatment of gastroesophageal reflux: Long-term and comparative study of 135 patients. Am. J. Surg., *139*:200, 1980.

Harrison, G. K., and Gompels, B. M.: Treatment of reflux strictures of the oesophagus by the Nissen-Rossetti operation. Thorax, *26*:77, 1971.

Henrion, C.: Cure de la hernie hiatale selon Nissen: Étude des résultats tardifs de 60 opérations. Acta Chir. Belg., *70*:497, 1971.

Ikard, R. W., and Jacobs, J. K.: Gastropericardial fistula and pericardial abscess: Unusual complications of subphrenic abscess following Nissen fundoplication. South. Med. J., *67*:17, 1974.

Jacquemet, L. R., Glanddier, G., Devif, J. J., et al.: Résultats d'une opération "type Nissen" dans le traitement du reflux gastroésophagien de l'adulte. Chirurgie, 98:128, 1972.

Jones, N. A., and Anders, C. J.: A new approach to the surgical treatment of reflux oesophagitis. Ann. R. Coll. Surg. Engl., 16:48, 1979.

Jordan, P. H., Jr.: Parietal cell vagotomy facilitates fundoplication in the treatment of reflux esophagitis. Surg. Gynceol. Obstet., 147:593, 1978.

Kaminski, D. L., Codd, J. E., and Sigmund, C. J.: Evaluation of the use of the median arcuate ligament in fundoplication for reflux esophagitis. Am. J. Surg., 134:724, 1977.

Leonardi, H. K., and Ellis F. H., Jr.: Experimental fundoplication: Comparison of results of different techniques. Surgery, 82:514, 1977.

Leonardi, H. K., Crozier, R. E., and Ellis, F. H., Jr.: Reoperation for complications of the Nissen fundoplication. J. Thorac. Cardiovasc. Surg., 81:50, 1981.

Leonardi, H. K., Lee, M. E., El-Kurd, M. F., et al.: An experimental study of the effectiveness of various anti-reflux operations. Ann. Thorac. Surg., 24:215, 1977.

Liebermann-Meffert, D.: Architecture of the musculature of the gastroesophageal junction and in the fundus. Chir. Gastroenterol., 9:425, 1975.

Lipshutz, W. H., Eckert, R. J., Gaskins, R. D., et al.: Normal lower-esophageal sphincter function after surgical treatment of gastroesophageal reflux. N. Engl. J. Med., 291:1107, 1974.

Lortat-Jacob, J. L., Maillard, J. N., and Fekete, F.: A procedure to prevent reflux after esophagogastric resection: Experience with 17 patients. Surgery, 50:600, 1961.

Mansour, K. A., Burton, H. G., Miller, J. I., Jr., et al.: Complications of intrathoracic Nissen fundoplication. Ann. Thorac. Surg., 32:173, 1981.

Menguy, R.: A modified fundoplication which preserves the ability to belch. Surgery, 84:301, 1978.

Morgan, A. G.: The place of fundoplication in the treatment of hiatal hernia. Aust. N.Z. J. Surg., 40:329, 1971.

Mullen, J. T., Burke, E. L., and Diamond, A. B.: Esophagogastric fistula: A complication of combined operations for esophageal disease. Arch. Surg., 110:826, 1975.

Nicholson, D. A., and Nohl-Oser, H. C.: Hiatus hernia: A comparison between two methods of fundoplication by evaluation of the long-term results. J. Thorac. Cardiovasc. Surg., 72:938, 1976.

Nissen, R.: Die transpleurale Resektion der Kardia. Dtsch. Z. Chir., 249:311, 1937.

Nissen, R.: Eine einfache Operation zur Beeinflussung der Refluxoesophagitis. Schweiz. Med. Wochenschr., 86:590, 1956.

Nissen, R.: Gastropexy and "fundoplication" in surgical treatment of hiatal hernia. Am. J. Dig. Dis., 6:954, 1961.

Nissen, R., and Rossetti, M.: Surgery of hiatal and other diaphragmatic hernias. J. Int. Coll. Surg., 43:663, 1965.

Olson, R. C., Lasser, R. B., and Ansel, H.: The "slipped Nissen." (Abstract.) Gastroenterology, 70:924, 1976.

Polk, H. C., Jr.: Indications for, technique of, and results of fundoplication for complicated reflux esophagitis. Am. Surg., 44:620, 1978.

Rogers, D. M., Herrington, J. L., Jr., and Morton, C.: Incidental splenectomy associated with Nissen fundoplication. Ann. Surg., 191:153, 1980.

Rossetti, M.: Zur Technik der Fundoplication. Acta Chir., 3: 229, 1968.

Rossetti, M., and Hell, K.: Fundoplication for the treatment of gastroesophageal reflux in hiatal hernia. World J. Surg., 1:439, 1977.

Safaie-Shirazi, S., Zike, W. L., and Mason, E. E.: Esophageal stricture secondary to reflux esophagitis. Arch. Surg., 110:629, 1975.

Shah, I. K., and Daniel, O.: The results of fundoplication for the relief of oesophageal reflux due to hiatus hernia. Br. J. Surg., 59:285, 1972.

Siewert, R., Jennewein, H. M., Waldeck, F., et al.: Experimentelle und klinische Untursuchungen zum Wirkungsmechanismus der Fundoplication. Langenbecks Arch. Chir., 333:519, 1973.

Siewert, R., Koch, A., Krtsch, H., et al.: The mechanism of action of fundoplication. (Abstract.) Bull. Soc. Int. Chir., 34:284, 1975.

Sillin, L. F., Condon, R. E., Wilson, S. D., et al.: Effective surgical therapy of esophagitis: Experience with Belsey, Hill, and Nissen operations. Arch. Surg., 114:536, 1979.

Skinner, D.B.: Complications of surgery for gastroesophageal reflux. World J. Surg., 1:485, 1977.

Woodward, E. R., Thomas, H. F., and McAlhany, J. C.: Comparison of crural repair and Nissen fundoplication in the treatment of esophageal hiatus hernia with peptic esophagitis. Ann. Surg., 173:782, 1971.

IV   THE HILL REPAIR

Lucius D. Hill

Nicolas Velasco

Wider use of sophisticated diagnostic tests has stimulated an increase in the recognition of gastroesophageal reflux (GER) with or without sliding hiatal hernia.

The etiology of GER still remains obscure, and, as in peptic ulcer disease, an imbalance between aggressive factors (reflux of acid, bile salts, pepsin, pancreatic enzymes) and factors that protect esophageal mucosa (saliva, esophageal clearance, esophageal motility, esophageal secretions, gastric emptying, duodenogastric reflux, and gastroesophageal sphincter tone) results in symptomatic GER. Of all these factors, the most fully studied is the lower esophageal sphincter (LES). A hypotensive sphincter is present in the majority of these patients (DeMeester et al., 1976). Once this barrier to reflux is opened, esophageal motility becomes an important factor in returning gastroduodenal material to the stomach. Prompt return of gastric juice to the stomach prevents long exposure of the esophageal mucosa to damage by enzymes and acid.

INDICATIONS FOR SURGICAL MANAGEMENT

Since GER is so common, the indications for surgery must be strict. The diagnosis of GER should be ruled out during the evaluation of other surgical problems of the upper gastrointestinal tract (e.g., peptic ulcer and gallbladder disease). Persistent GER after operation for other gastrointestinal abnormalities represents a surgical failure.

The indications for surgery are as follows:

1. *Failure of medical treatment.* The most common indication for surgery is intractability or recurrence of symptoms after at least 6 months of well-controlled medical treatment in patients with more than 1 year of incapacitating symptoms.

2. *Stricture.* This is a common and serious complication of GER. In our experience, 12.6 per cent of patients were operated on for stricture. Early diagnosis and treatment of symptomatic GER must be attempted to avoid this complication.

3. *Pulmonary complications.* Overflow of gastric contents into the tracheobronchial tree occurs with greater frequency than has been previously recognized. Occasionally, recurrent pneumonia or chronic obstructive pulmonary disease is the only symptom of underlying GER that has not been diagnosed.

4. *Esophagitis.* This is the result of continuous contact of gastroduodenal material with the esophageal mucosa. In our experience, esophagitis is the second most common indication for surgery. Attempts must be made to correct other problems that can provoke severe esophagitis (e.g., pyloric stenosis secondary to peptic ulcer, bile reflux after gastrectomy).

5. *Esophageal ulcerations.* These may vary from superficial and linear ulcers to profound ulcerations located at the squamocolumnar junction. Chronic anemia is often present, but severe hemorrhage is an uncommon complication of esophageal ulceration.

6. *Large symptomatic hiatal hernias.* A small number of patients require operation because displacement of the stomach through the hiatus causes pressure symptoms in the chest. Occasionally, ulceration of the stomach with severe bleeding may occur. Incarceration and obstruction or gangrene with perforation of the herniated stomach is an uncommon complication that requires immediate treatment.

7. *Coexisting surgical problems.* Upper gastrointestinal problems, especially duodenal ulcer and gallbladder disease, may accompany symptomatic GER. In our experience, 9 per cent of the patients had some other pathologic condition.

PREOPERATIVE EVALUATION

The most common method of evaluation of patients with GER is a barium upper gastrointestinal series. This study can detect (1) the presence of spontaneous or provoked reflux; (2) the presence of a sliding or paraesophageal hiatal hernia; (3) esophageal stenosis and its level and extension; (4) ulcers of the esophagus; and (5) other upper gastrointestinal problems such as peptic ulcer and carcinoma. Unfortunately, upper gastrointestinal series are insensitive, and the radiologic criteria for interpretation of reflux are variable. Sometimes, the ampullary zone of the esophagus is interpreted as being "a small sliding hiatal hernia." When spontaneous reflux is seen, it is generally associated with severe symptoms of GER. In older patients, radiologic diagnosis of hiatal hernia can be made up to 80 per cent of the time, but only 10 to 15 per cent of these patients complain of reflux symptoms. GER can also be detected without radiologic evidence of hiatal hernia. Radiologic diagnosis alone for identifying a "hiatal hernia" without awareness of simultaneous reflux may lead to poor surgical results, despite excellent radiologic postoperative controls.

Other more objective tests are available for determination of the status of the esophagus and lower esophageal sphincter and the presence or absence of reflux. These are manometry and lower esophageal sphincter pressure (LESP) measurements and distal esophageal pH studies (Behar *et al.,* 1976). These tests are important to establish a preoperative baseline in order to calculate LESP and pH changes with surgery. Manometric studies allow exclusion from surgery of patients with certain associated pathologic conditions such as scleroderma and provide information on motility of the esophagus, especially of the distal esophagus, which is altered in 20 per cent of patients with GER (Russell *et al.,* 1981b). In our laboratory, an LESP measurement below 10 mm. Hg generally indicates an incompetent sphincter, but there is considerable overlap in pressure values between normal and symptomatic patients, although the mean LESP of symptomatic patients is lower than that of normal controls. Sixty-five per cent of our patients going to surgery have an LESP below 10 mm. Hg. We have employed distal esophageal pH studies for the last 20 years. This has proved to be the most sensitive test in determining reflux, and 93 per cent of our patients have a positive reflux test before surgery.

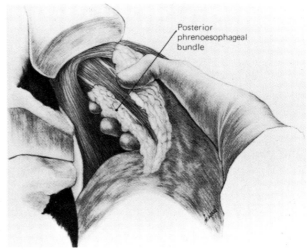

Figure 25–11. After the greater curvature is freed, the stomach can be rotated to visualize the posterior phrenoesophageal bundle, including the posterior seromuscular layer of the stomach. The anterior and posterior vagi are carefully identified. (From Hill, L. D.: Transabdominal hiatal herniorrhaphy with median arcuate ligament repair. Surgical Techniques Illustrated, *1*:59, 1976.)

Direct inspection of esophageal mucosa through a fiberoptic endoscope is of value before surgery. Diverse types of esophagitis, varying from erythema and edema to severe ulcerations and stenosis, can be seen. The endoscopic appearance does not always correlate with symptoms, however, and normal mucosa may appear in conjunction with severe symptoms, but the histology of adequate biopsies gives important information in these cases. The fiberoptic endoscope is also a valuable tool to rule out esophageal carcinoma.

Recently, newer techniques using radionuclides for determination of esophageal motility have been employed at our institution. This technique was proved to be highly sensitive in detecting esophageal motor abnormalities in patients with reflux who complained of dysphagia and who had normal manometric and radiologic studies. We have recently reported 52 per cent of esophageal motor disorders in GER with this technique before anti-reflux surgery (Russell *et al.*, 1981a).

Radionuclide studies have also been used at our institution in the detection of reflux, with sensitivity comparable to that of the pH probe. Using this technique, we have been able to detect reflux in 75 per cent of our patients. When only severely symptomatic

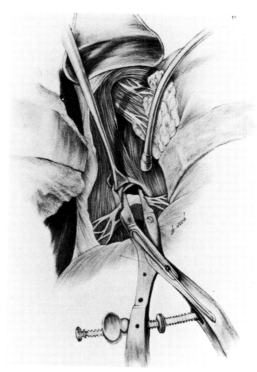

Figure 25–13. As the dilator is passed cephalad, little or no resistance is encountered if the instrument is in the correct plane. If resistance is met, the instrument must not be forced. The plane between the preaortic fascia and aorta is loose areolar tissue that separates easily. If any force is used, the aorta or celiac trunk may be damaged. (From Hill, L. D.: Surgical Techniques Illustrated, *1*:59, 1976.)

patients are considered, the diagnosis is made in 86 per cent of the patients, which is comparable to the 92 per cent diagnosis rate of the acid reflux test. Quantitation of reflux as well as time of exposure of the esophagus to gastric contents can also be obtained. It is also possible to obtain information about gastric emptying of solid and liquid meals with radionuclide studies, and this is important in patients going to surgery. We have found that 42 per cent of our patients have delayed gastric emptying of solids.

Radionuclide studies can already be done in most hospitals and have the advantage of avoiding the use of tubes as well as providing similar or greater accuracy than the studies currently in use. Combined studies of esophageal transit, reflux, and gastric emptying can be performed without additional difficulty.

RATIONALE FOR OPERATION

The main purpose of anti-reflux surgery is the development of a barrier to reflux of gastric contents into the esophagus. This can be accomplished with adequate calibration of the cardia. If a sliding hiatal hernia is present, replacement and anchoring of the displaced viscus to restore normal anatomy are necessary to prevent recurrence. A simple closure of the

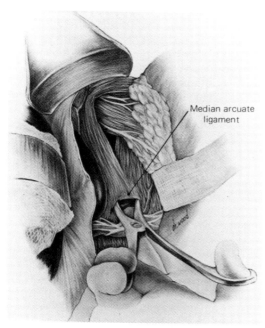

Median arcuate ligament

Figure 25–12. After dissecting the fibroareolar tissue off the celiac axis, the celiac ganglion is retracted caudally. Two diaphragmatic branches, one from each side of the celiac axis, go to the crura of the diaphragm. By staying in the midline, these two branches can be avoided. If one of them is inadvertently divided, marked bleeding may occur; the branch should be visualized and carefully sewn with an arterial suture without compromising the lumen of the celiac trunk. After the nerve and fibroareolar tissue are dissected from the celiac axis, the median arcuate ligament or aortic hiatus can be visualized readily. The median arcuate ligament is elevated from the celiac axis, and a Goodell cervical dilator placed beneath the median arcuate ligament is passed cephalad. (From Hill, L. D.: Surgical Techniques Illustrated, *1*:59, 1976.)

enlarged esophageal hiatus is not sufficient for correcting reflux and will not prevent persistent herniation.

TECHNIQUE

A midline incision is made and extended high up to the left of the xiphoid process, which may be removed to enhance exposure. Good exposure is the first step in performing successful surgery. For this purpose, an "upper hand" retractor (double-bladed) is invaluable. The abdomen is carefully explored, and the triangular ligament of the left lobe of the liver is divided and then retracted to the right. This allows a good exposure of the phrenoesophageal membrane, which is divided at its diaphragmatic origin to expose the esophageal hiatus and the underlying esophagus (Fig. 25–11). The hernia is then gently reduced. The lesser omentum is dissected, and attempts must be made to preserve the hepatic branch of the anterior vagus nerve. The esophagus is freed with careful dissection of the posterior aspect, and both vagus nerves are identified to prevent inadvertent damage with sutures.

The gastric fundus is partially mobilized from its diaphragmatic attachments, and, to gain mobility, two

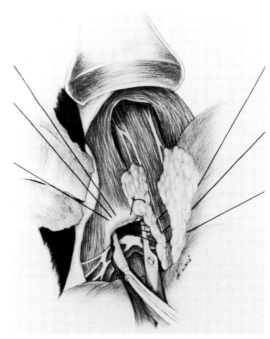

Figure 25–15. Four or more additional imbricating sutures are placed deeply through the anterior and posterior phrenoesophageal bundles, including the seromuscular layers of the stomach, and are carried beneath the median arcuate ligament. (From Hill, L. D.: Surgical Techniques Illustrated, *1*:59, 1976.)

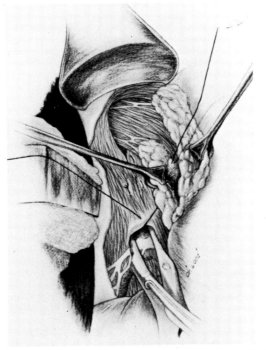

Figure 25–14. Following closure of the hiatus, Babcock clamps are placed on the anterior and posterior phrenoesophageal bundles to permit the posterior wall of the stomach, including the seromuscular layer, to be visualized. A fixation suture is placed through the posterior phrenoesophageal bundle and passed through the preaortic fascia. This fixation suture does not tighten the esophageal introitus. It is placed with the posterior vagus nerve in view to avoid damage to the vagus nerve. (From Hill, L. D.: Surgical Techniques Illustrated, *1*:59, 1976.)

or three short gastric vessels are divided carefully to prevent damage to the spleen. If gastric analysis has shown an elevated basal acid output or if the patient has known duodenal ulcer disease, a highly selective vagotomy should be performed.

The pylorus must be carefully checked to rule out any local pathology that could be responsible for the delayed gastric emptying that is commonly seen in these patients. If there is any doubt as to the patency of the pylorus or if the patient has delayed gastric emptying in a preoperative evaluation, a 3-cm. pyloromyotomy is performed.

The stomach is then retracted to the patient's left, and the preaortic fascia is exposed. The aorta and celiac axis are located by palpation, and immediately cephalad to the celiac trunk, the areolar tissue and nerve fibers are dissected to expose the inferior border of the median arcuate ligament (Fig. 25–12). Blunt dissection of the median arcuate ligament is carefully performed immediately cephalad to the celiac trunk, and a Goodell cervical dilator is then placed under the median arcuate ligament to protect the celiac axis (Fig. 25–13).

A variation of this technique may be employed by surgeons who do not wish to dissect the median arcuate ligament. Following palpation of the celiac trunk, Babcock clamps are placed on the preaortic fascia to elevate it off of the aorta, and then sutures are placed through the preaortic fascia. Another variation involves opening the esophageal hiatus and passing a finger down beneath the preaortic fascia. Then, sutures may be placed through the fascia, with care being taken to protect the aorta. The esophageal hiatus is closed posterior to the esophagus by loose approximation of both crura with heavy nonabsorbable sutures so that the tip of the index finger can be admitted alongside the esophagus into the posterior mediastinum.

Following closure of the hiatus, the anterior and posterior phrenoesophageal fascial bundles are exposed by rotation of the stomach and are picked up with Babcock clamps. A first nonabsorbable imbricating suture is then placed deep through the anterior and then the posterior bundles, right at the gastroesophageal junction (Fig 25–14). Four additional sutures are placed in a similar manner caudad to the initial suture and are brought through the median arcuate ligament (Fig. 25–15). The first two sutures are the most important in narrowing and calibration of the cardia to provide a barrier to reflux. The imbricating suture and the two immediately adjacent sutures are tied with a single throw and clamped to prevent slipping of the knots. This strengthens the sphincter mechanism and increases the pressure of the LES. This is checked with intraoperative manometry with a perfused catheter system. We have found that this method provides

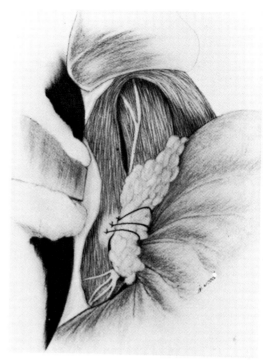

Figure 25–17. After the sutures are tied, the overall anatomy can be visualized. At least a 3-cm. length of abdominal esophagus can be seen. The esophagogastric junction is securely anchored to the preaortic fascia and median arcuate ligament. (From Hill, L. D.: Surgical Techniques Illustrated, *1*:59, 1976.)

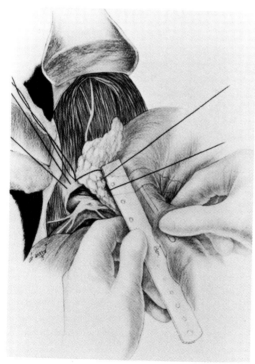

Figure 25–16. The first imbricating suture and the two immediately adjacent are tied. Measurement is taken of the lower esophageal sphincter pressure. If the suture has been properly placed, the tension it creates on the collar sling musculature tightens the esophageal opening so that the sphincter pressure registers at least 40 mm. Hg. This measurement is repeated three times, and the mean of the three measurements is obtained. If the mean pressure is less than 40 mm. Hg, an additional imbricating suture is placed to tighten the esophageal introitus and to raise the sphincter pressure. (From Hill, L. D.: Surgical Techniques Illustrated, *1*:59, 1976.)

an objective parameter of suture tension (Fig. 25–16). Pressure values no greater than 55 mm. Hg must be obtained to avoid dysphagia. Pressure values less than 35 mm. Hg may lead to recurrence of symptoms (Hill, 1978). If intraoperative manometry is not available, a 30-French bougie may be used to indicate the state of the lumen. When the desired suture tension has been achieved, the knots are firmly completed, and the remaining two sutures can be firmly secured (Fig. 25–17). The problem with the bougie method is that it is impossible to tell how tight the gastroesophageal junction is against the bougie. The nasogastric tube is removed on the third or fourth postoperative day, and the LESP is determined at this time. The range varies from 18 to 26 mm. Hg postoperatively.

POSTOPERATIVE FOLLOW-UP

As mentioned before, careful evaluation of symptoms is the best means of assessing postoperative results. A successful result is obtained when there is complete and permanent relief of all preoperative symptoms and no symptoms develop from the operative procedure.

Upper gastrointestinal radiologic series are useful to see if the hernia was successfully repaired, but they are not the best examination to rule out postoperative reflux. Postoperative pH studies and LESP measure-

TABLE 25–1. CLINICAL ASSESSMENT OF 169 PATIENTS AFTER OPERATION FOR REFLUX

	GROUP 1 (N = 76)	%	GROUP 2 (N = 93)	%
Excellent	36	47.4	58	62.3
Good	14	18.4	25	26.9
Fair	17	22.4	10	10.8
Poor	9	11.8	0	0

TABLE 25–3. pH STUDY (%)

	GROUP 1		GROUP 2	
	Preop.	*Postop.*	*Preop.*	*Postop.*
pH (+)	91.9	31.5	93.9	1.6
pH (−)	8.1	68.5	6.1	98.4

ments, as well as radionuclide studies, are of value in objectively determining the results of surgery. Long-term follow-up studies should be performed because abnormal pH or histologic studies have been observed postoperatively in some asymptomatic patients (Brand et al., 1979).

Since 1969, 639 patients have been operated on at our institution, the Virginia Mason Medical Center, for primary reflux with or without accompanying hiatal hernia. Four have been reoperated on in our service for recurrence of reflux. Of these, three are without symptoms and the remaining patient died 24 months after surgery from other causes but had had relief of symptoms of reflux.

In a recent review of results of primary repair in 169 patients, an objective questionnaire was completed by patients. According to the date of operation, these were divided into two groups: Group 1 — patients who had operations before changes in operative technique and the introduction of intraoperative manometry in 1973, and Group 2 — patients operated on after 1973 with use of intraoperative manometry. Both groups were matched according to sex and age and are comparable. Manometric and pH studies were performed before and after surgery. The mean follow-up for patients was 93 months for those in Group 1 and 49 months for patients in Group 2. The clinical assessment is shown in Table 25–1. The results were graded as follows: excellent — no symptoms; good — minimal symptoms that do not require any medication; fair — improved symptoms or symptoms derived from surgery that require occasional medication; poor — no improvement, requiring daily medication. Tables 25–2 and 25–3 show LESP measurements and pH studies performed before and after surgery. There is a significant improvement in clinical results and pH studies in patients operated on after 1973. However, LESP in both groups increased a mean of 7.7 and 6.8 mm. Hg, respectively.

RECURRENCE

Recurrence in repaired hiatal hernias has been reported with all techniques by several authors, but there are only a few reports concerned exclusively with recurrent hernia. In 1971, we reported 63 patients who had undergone prior repairs elsewhere. In the last 10 years, we have operated on 125 more patients. Some of these were reported previously (Hill et al., 1979). The most common types of operations done initially are shown in Table 25–4. Many patients had undergone multiple previous repairs. In these patients, surgery is often difficult, and dissection is hampered by adhesions and loss of normal tissue planes. Careful dissection is necessary to prevent inadvertent damage to the esophagus, stomach, and spleen. After reconstruction of the anatomy, two common problems with the previous repair are seen. One is the patulous cardia, which admits two to three fingers and allows free reflux, and the other is failure to anchor the stomach in its diaphragmatic position or sutures improperly placed or placed in tissues that will not hold properly. At operation, almost all patients had a median arcuate repair with careful cardial calibration. In these patients, the phrenoesophageal bundles may be inadequate, and sutures may lead to tear with leakage at the gastroesophageal junction with peritonitis. We had this problem in three patients. Now in these circumstances, we utilize small pledgets of Teflon soaked in providone-iodine (Betadine) through which the repair sutures are passed. This promotes fibrous ingrowth around the Teflon and prevents postoperative problems. If the bundles are completely destroyed, a collar of Teflon is fashioned around the lesser curvature of the LES to substitute for the bundles. The mortality rate in this group was 4.08 per cent, and the late follow-up is summarized in Table 25–5. As can be seen, the fair and poor results and mortality have significantly increased in this group. This emphasizes the fact that the optimal time to repair a hiatal hernia is at the first operation.

TABLE 25–2. LESP VALUE (%)

	GROUP 1		GROUP 2	
	Preop.	*Postop.*	*Preop.*	*Postop.*
Low (<11 mm. Hg)	74.2	27.8	57	10
Normal	25.8	72.2	43	90

TABLE 25–4. RECURRENT HIATAL HERNIA— MOST COMMON PREVIOUS OPERATIONS

Allison	29
Belsey	17
MAL	21
Nissen	31
Other or unknown	27
TOTAL	125

TABLE 25–5. RECURRENT HIATAL HERNIA—FOLLOW-UP RESULTS*

Excellent or Good	57.4%
Fair	21.3%
Poor	21.3%

*Mean follow-up—57.9 months (range—8 to 105 months)

ESOPHAGEAL STRICTURES

One of the most frequent complications of GER is stricture of the esophagus. This occurs most frequently at the squamocolumnar junction but not necessarily at the same level as the gastroesophageal junction. Careful evaluation of these patients with endoscopy, surgery, and motility studies reveals that the epithelium distal to the stricture is of the gastric type, but manometric studies show an esophageal motility pattern with a low LES at the cardioesophageal junction. A combined manometric and potential difference (PD) study reveals the LES at its normal location, whereas the change in the PD is always at the level of the stricture.

At the time of operation, the esophagus is rarely shortened, and a segment of intra-abdominal esophagus can be obtained. A median arcuate ligament repair with careful calibration of the cardia was peformed in all patients. In most cases, correction of reflux permits regression of the stricture in a few months, and only a few patients require further dilatation with a Hurst bougie. In those patients with high fibrous strictures, a median arcuate ligament repair with cardial calibration is performed, and a gastrostomy may be necessary for postoperative feeding and further retrograde dilatations.

In a follow-up of 79 patients operated on since 1969, with a mean follow-up period of 59 months, 67.1 per cent had excellent or good results and only 11.9 per cent did not improve with surgery. The operative mortality for this group was 3 per cent.

SELECTED REFERENCES

Behar, J., Biancani, P., and Sheahan, D. G.: Evaluation of esophageal tests in the diagnosis of reflux esophagitis. Gastroenterology, 71:9, 1976.

This article is an excellent study of the sensitivity and specificity of the most common test in use in the diagnosis of gastroesophageal reflux (GER). It is clearly demonstrated that one single study is of little value in the diagnosis of GER since a high incidence of positive results can be obtained in normal volunteers, but combinations of two tests allow separation of normal from symptomatic patients. The authors conclude that the most sensitive and specific test combination for the diagnosis of reflux esophagitis is esophageal biopsy with esophageal pH study after loading the stomach with HCl.

Brand, D. L., Eastwood, T. R., Martin, D., Carter, W., and Pope, C. E.: Esophageal symptoms, manometry, and histology before and after antireflux surgery. Gastroenterology, 76:1383, 1979.

This article emphasizes the importance of long-term follow-up in patients operated on for reflux. They controlled 13 patients for 69 months following anti-reflux surgery (Nissen) with clinical assessment, esophageal manometry, pH study, and suction biopsy of the esophagus. Despite a high incidence of patient satisfaction, half of the patients who had normal postoperative biopsy and negative pH studies were abnormal in the long-term follow-up.

DeMeester, T. R., and Johnson, L. F., et al.: Patterns of gastroesophageal reflux in health and disease. Ann. Surg., 184:459, 1976.

The authors carefully studied with 24-hour pH monitoring the incidence of GER in 15 normal volunteers and 100 symptomatic patients. They concluded that minimal reflux is physiologic, but patients with pathologic reflux all have a lower LES pressure (LESP). Patients with supine and upright reflux are at more risk of developing complications.

Hill, L. D.: Intraoperative measurement of lower esophageal sphincter pressure. J. Thorac. Cardiovasc. Surg., 75:378, 1978.

This study emphasizes that an objective method during surgery is of great value in obtaining successful postoperative results. This is the first study that measured the LESP during anesthesia in patients operated on for GER. Two hundred patients are included in this study, and LESP measurements were recorded before surgery, during operation, 3 to 4 days immediately after surgery, and 2 to 3 months after surgery. A mean LESP of 50 mm. Hg during operation allows a late LESP high enough to prevent postoperative reflux.

Hill, L. D., Ilves, R., Stevenson, J. K., and Pearson, J. M.: Reoperation for disruption and recurrence after Nissen fundoplication. Arch. Surg., 114:542, 1979.

This report deals with 25 unsuccessful Nissen operations. A method of classifying the type of failure is presented. Manometric studies document disordered motor activity in 10 of these patients, with return to normal activity after re-repair. With these difficult patients, intraoperative manometrics allowed a satisfactory anti-reflux barrier to be created with posterior gastropexy. Good to excellent results were achieved in 22 of 24 patients. A search of the world literature is presented with complications ranging from the well-known "gas bloat" syndrome to potentially lethal fistulas. This study emphasizes that there are basic flaws in the Nissen procedure that may lead to potentially lethal complications.

Russell, C. O. H., Pope, C. E., Gannan, R. M., Allen, F. D., Velasco, N., and Hill, L. D.: Does surgery correct esophageal motor dysfunction in gastroesophageal reflux? Ann. Surg., 194:290, 1981.

This is a careful evaluation of esophageal motor problems in patients with severe symptoms of gastroesophageal reflux. The radionuclide technique used in this study proved to be highly sensitive, finding 52 per cent of motor abnormalities in this type of patient, whereas conventional manometric study showed a motility disturbance in only . 18 per cent of the patients. However, after a successful correction of reflux (Hill repair) and disappearance of symptoms of dysphagia, the motor abnormalities persisted unchanged.

REFERENCES

Behar, J., Biancani, P., and Sheahan, D. G.: Evaluation of esophageal tests in the diagnosis of reflux esophagitis. Gastroenterology, 71:9, 1976.

Brand, D. L., Eastwood, T. R., Martin, D., Carter, W. B., and Pope, C. E.: Esophageal symptoms, manometry, and histology before and after antireflux surgery. Gastroenterology, 76:1383, 1979.

DeMeester, T. R., Johnson, L. F., Joseph, G. J., Toscano, M. S., Hall, A. W., and Skinner, D. B.: Patterns of gastroesophageal reflux in health and disease. Ann. Surg., *184*:459, 1976.

Fisher, R. S., and Cohen, S.: Gastroesophageal reflux. Med. Clin. North Am., *62*:3, 1978.

Hill, L. D.: Intraoperative measurement of lower esophageal sphincter pressure. J. Thorac. Cardiovasc. Surg., *75*:378, 1978.

Hill, L. D., Ilves, R., Stevenson, J. K., and Pearson, J. M.: Reoperation for disruption and recurrence after Nissen fundoplication. Arch. Surg., *114*:542, 1979.

McCallum, R. W., Berkowitz, D. M., and Lerner, E.: Gastric emptying in patients with gastroesophageal reflux. Gastroenterology, *80*:285, 1981.

Russell, C. O. H., Hill, L. D., Holmes, D. A., Gannan, R. M., and Pope, C. E.: Radionuclide transit: A sensitive screening test for esophageal dysfunction. Gastroenterology, *80*:887, 1981a.

Russell, C. O. H., Pope, C. E., Gannan, R. M., Allen, F. D., Velasco, N., and Hill, L. D.: Does surgery correct esophageal motor dysfunction in gastroesophageal reflux? Ann. Surg., *194*:290, 1981b.

Silverstein, B., and Pope, C. E.: Role of diagnostic test in esophageal evaluation. Am. J. Surg., *139*:744, 1980.

V PARAESOPHAGEAL HERNIA

Lucius D. Hill

Nicolas Velasco

Despite an increase in the diagnosis and treatment of gastroesophageal problems, major differences of opinion remain about the classification, pathophysiology, and management of hiatal hernia. There is agreement, however, that there are two major types of hernias that may occur at the esophageal hiatus — the *sliding* and the *paraesophageal* hiatal hernia. The first is a common problem involving incompetence of the lower esophageal sphincter allowing reflux of stomach or duodenal contents into the distal esophagus. The second is a rare entity, and the true paraesophageal hernia occurs secondary to deranged anatomic structures without reflux.

A third type of hernia is the combined or mixed paraesophageal and sliding hernia, in which both physiologic and anatomic problems are present. In an early stage, this mixed type appears to be a sliding hernia, because reflux is present and the gastroesophageal junction has lost its normal location. After some time, however, part of the fundus rolls into the thorax with the gastroesophageal junction, as in the paraesophageal hernia. The sliding type of hiatal hernia with gastroesophageal reflux is seen far more frequently than the paraesophageal hernia. The incidence of paraesophageal hernia is only 3 per cent in patients undergoing surgery for hiatal hernia. When one considers the large number of hiatal hernias of the sliding type that do not require surgery, it appears that paraesophageal hernia is a rare condition; actually, less than 2 per cent of herniations through the esophageal hiatus are of the paraesophageal type.

PATHOPHYSIOLOGY

A paraesophageal hernia may be present for years without serious symptoms or complications. In the classic type of paraesophageal hernia, the stomach rolls up alongside the esophagus and the esophagogastric junction and through the esophageal hiatus with no separate opening and no component of the diaphragm between the esophagus and the hernia sac. The etiology is still obscure. Its diagnosis in patients under 40 years of age is the exception. It is probable that the genesis of this condition is not different from that of hernias in other locations (e.g., inguinal, crural) and may be initiated by increased abdominal stress (obesity, distention) over weakened tissue. The greatly enlarged esophageal hiatus in some of these patients suggests a congenital origin.

The esophagus normally lies posteriorly in the esophageal hiatus, fixed in its normal location by the firm posterior phrenoesophageal membranes. This structure consists of fiberoelastic tissue extending from the esophageal wall into the rim of the hiatus as well as the preaortic fascia and median arcuate ligament. The anterior and lateral components of the phrenoesophageal fascial complex are attenuated and form the sac of the herniation. Careful dissection of the anatomy of this condition demonstrates that the phrenoesophageal ligament is intact posteriorly and the gastroesophageal junction lies in its normal location.

The essential difference between the paraesophageal hernia and the sliding hernia is this intact posterior fixation of the esophagus to the preaortic fascia and the median arcuate ligament in the paraesophageal hernia. In the true paraesophageal hernia, reflux does not occur and esophagitis is not part of the clinical picture. Symptoms of dysfunction of the lower esophageal sphincter are noted only in rare instances, and most of these cases are of the mixed type of hernia with both sliding and paraesophageal components. In the mixed hernia, the posterior part of the phrenoesophageal ligament is weak, and the gastroesophageal junction loses its normal angle and position and rolls into the posterior mediastinum. In such cases, gastroesophageal reflux may be part of the clinical picture.

That paraesophageal hernia is a separate entity from hernias with reflux and may occur with other abnormalities of the upper gastrointestinal tract is depicted in Figure 25–18. Note the dilated esophagus ending in a narrow segment and the tertiary contractions in the body of the esophagus typical of achalasia of the esophagus. The gastroesophageal junction lies below the diaphragm but alongside the esophagus in the posterior mediastinum. Part of the fundus and body of the stomach can be seen.

Normally, the defect alongside the esophagus and gastroesophageal junction enlarges anterior to the esophagus with time. The most mobile portion of the stomach tends to move up with the cardia maintained in its normal position by the posterior ligament. The greater curve and body of the stomach are the most mobile portions and migrate into the posterior mediastinum. Migration of these portions is associated with organoaxial rotation of the viscus. The entire first portion of the duodenum may eventually ascend into the thorax, but the stomach actually is not malrotated. This is clearly demonstrated when the hernia is reduced and the hiatus closed. The stomach then lies in its normal location, indicating that it was simply inverted in an opening in the diaphragm and not malrotated.

Figures 25–19 and 25–20 illustrate typical cases of paraesophageal hernia that may clarify the etiology of this entity.

Demonstration of a large typical paraesophageal hernia by conventional gastrointestinal radiograph is

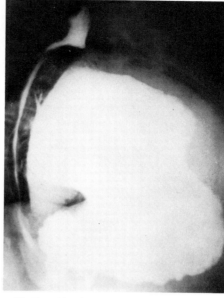

Figure 25–19. Classical paresophageal hernia. The hernia contains all the stomach except for the antrum in the posterior mediastinum behind the heart. The esophagus is in its normal location, with the gastroesophageal junction fixed below the diaphragm by a competent posterior phrenoesophageal ligament. (From Hill, L. D., and Tobias, J. A.: Paraesophageal hernia. Arch. Surg., 96:735, 1968.)

illustrated in Figure 25–19. All of the stomach except for a small part of the antrum and gastroesophageal junction is displaced into the posterior mediastinum. The entire stomach and first portion of the duodenum may be dislocated into the thorax, and occasionally, a portion of the colon and small bowel may be displaced into the thorax if the sac is large. The posteroanterior view of a large paraesophageal hernia containing all of the stomach except for a small part of the fundus and the gastroesophageal junction in the thorax is shown in Figure 25–20. As with any other true anatomic hernia, the paraesophageal hernia may be complicated by volvulus, obstruction, incarceration, gangrene, or perforation.

CLINICAL MANIFESTATIONS

Paraesophageal hernias often have few symptoms, run benign courses while enlarging with time, and remain undiagnosed for several years. Usually, the patient has a long history of postprandial distress and discomfort, accompanied by a sensation of nausea and substernal pressure after eating due to a dilated intrathoracic gastric segment and trapping of large volumes of gas and food. These symptoms may be relieved by belching or regurgitation. Occasionally, moderate symptoms of dysphagia may occur as a result of external compression of the esophagus by the herniated stomach. Symptoms of breathlessness and a sense of suffocation are due to mechanical impairment of ventilation. Pressure over the heart can produce pain that mimics the pain of angina. Chronic bleeding,

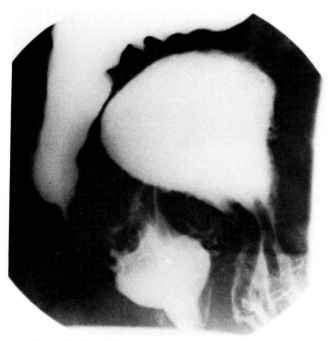

Figure 25–18. This radiograph shows part of the fundus and body of the stomach in the chest in a patient with a long history of dysphagia secondary to achalasia of the esophagus. The dilated esophagus ending in a narrow segment can be easily identified, and the gastroesophageal junction lies below the diaphragm.

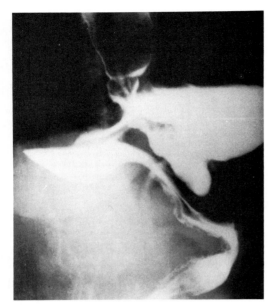 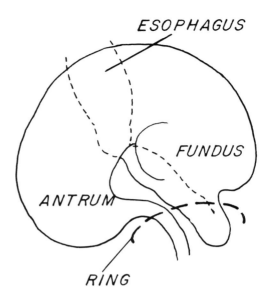

Figure 25–20. Posteroanterior view of gastrointestinal series. This shows paraesophageal hernia with the entire stomach, except for a very small portion of the fundus and the gastroesophageal junction in the thorax. (From Hill, L. D., and Tobias, J. A.: Paraesophageal hernia. Arch. Surg., *96*:735, 1968.)

sometimes with severe anemia of unexplained origin, produces lethargy and weakness. Heartburn is rarely seen in these patients because the gastroesophageal junction maintains its normal angle and intra-abdominal fixation without changes in the lower esophageal sphincter pressure. The patient often learns to live with these symptoms for several years before visiting the physician. Without treatment, probably a large number of patients will live without severe problems; however, about 25 per cent will die from a complication of this hernia.

The main complications of paraesophageal hernias are ulceration of the herniated stomach with acute bleeding, volvulus, obstruction with incarceration, and gangrene with perforation. When the patient develops one of these complications, the correct diagnosis is often difficult to establish, and sometimes he is treated for myocardial infarction or other thoracic problems. When obstruction by a volvulated stomach or incarceration is suspected, decompression through a nasogastric tube to relieve the obstruction and prevent strangulation is imperative. Decompression is usually accompanied by a rush of gas and large amounts of fluid, followed by relief of symptoms. When this procedure is not successful, the patient must be taken to the operating room for emergency surgery, which is associated with a high morbidity and mortality rate.

The most frequent origin of bleeding is from a gastric ulcer, which was present in over 30 per cent of our patients. Impairment of gastric emptying with retention of acid and food is probably the main cause of ulceration and acute bleeding, but occult and insidious bleeding secondary to trauma after repeated

episodes of incarceration and interference with vascular supply and lymph drainage is also frequent and may lead to congestive gastritis with multiple bleeding points. Bleeding from a paraesophageal hernia is a difficult problem to manage conservatively, and a surgical approach is often required within a few days as the only possibility of correcting the underlying problem.

Volvulus with incarceration and obstruction is another frequent complication. This occurs when the fundus, filled with food, becomes distended and prolapses from its intrathoracic position through the esophageal opening into the abdomen. Obstruction occurs at the level of the gastroesophageal junction and at the midgastric and duodenal levels (Fig. 25–21). It appears that as long as the paraesophageal hernia contains the entire stomach rolled up into the posterior mediastinum, obstruction does not occur, but when it does take place, both the antrum and the fundus become enormously dilated and distended, with marked engorgement of the stomach wall and marked vascular dilatation leading to bleeding. These patients often present with a high obstruction. Vomiting may be minimal since there is obstruction of the terminal esophagus causing regurgitation of saliva along with complete inability to swallow food or fluid. Other patients may present with early or profound shock, severe chest and abdominal pain, and, occasionally, hematemesis secondary to gastric bleeding. In these patients, the diagnosis must be made promptly to prevent gangrene and perforation with extravasation of large amounts of fluid to the mediastinum and abdominal cavity. Morbidity and mortality in perforated paraesophageal hernia is nearly 100 per cent.

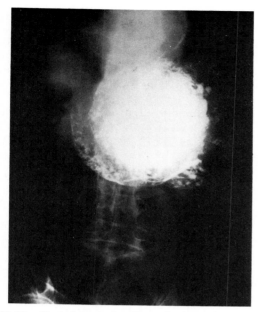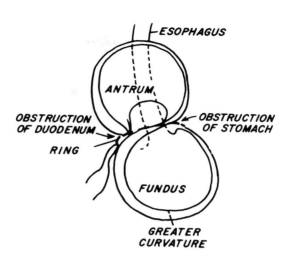

Figure 25–21. Gastrointestinal radiograph showing incarceration and obstruction in a paraesophageal hernia. The fundus has dropped out of the thorax, through the ring, and into the abdomen, leaving the antrum in the posterior mediastinum. Obstruction occurs both at the midgastric level and at the level of the duodenum. (From Hill, L. D., and Tobias, J. A.: Paraesophageal hernia. Arch. Surg., 96:735, 1968.)

DIAGNOSIS

In the mildly or moderately symptomatic patient with substernal discomfort and dyspnea after ingestion of a heavy meal, a careful clinical history together with a plain chest radiograph showing an air-fluid level behind the heart allows the diagnosis to be made. An upper gastrointestinal series is helpful in evaluating the part of the stomach involved in the hernia and also provides some information about gastric emptying. Occasionally, barium enema examination shows part of the transverse colon as part of the herniated viscus in the posterior mediastinum. Pressure and pH studies are performed, except in patients with incarceration; these test are usually normal. These studies clearly demonstrate that the gastroesophageal junction and the terminal esophagus lie in the normal position and are functioning properly.

TREATMENT

Because no effective medical treatment exists for the anatomic defect of paraesophageal hernia and because of its numerous and life-threatening complications, surgical repair is indicated. If the operation is performed properly, there should be few, if any, recurrences. Episodes of incarceration, bleeding, or obstruction are obviously indications for immediate surgery. In paraesophageal hernia, if the esophagus is in its normal location and if the lower esophageal sphincter functions properly and reflux does not occur, it is a technical mistake to free the esophagus from its posterior attachments and subject the patient to the risk of a sliding hernia, which may produce more

complications than the presenting paraesophageal hernia.

The paraesophageal hernia may be approached either transthoracically or transabdominally. The technique is essentially the same whichever route is used. When there are concomitant abdominal problems, such as cholelithiasis or duodenal ulcer, the abdominal approach is preferred. The hernia can then be carefully and easily reduced by slow manual retraction starting in the fundal portion of the stomach and ending in the abdominal cavity (Fig. 25–22). When the terminal esophagus is below the diaphragm with an intra-abdominal segment of esophagus firmly in place, the surgeon can be assured that a true paraesophageal hernia and not a combined sliding and paraesophageal hernia is being dealt with.

The large hernia sac that occupies the posterior mediastinum is readily removed by blunt and sharp dissection of the peritoneal lining of the sac to eliminate the possibility of recurrence or development of a mediastinal serous cyst.

With an obstructed or incarcerated hernia that cannot be decompressed before surgery, division of the esophageal hiatus is necessary to reduce the incarcerated viscus without perforation of the gastric wall. After division of the tight hiatal ring, the stomach can usually be reduced readily. Sometimes, a decompressing gastrotomy is a helpful procedure, and it can be used later as a gastrostomy to fix the stomach to the peritoneal wall, thus avoiding the use of a nasogastric tube after surgery.

Following reduction of the viscus and elimination of the hernia sac, the diaphragmatic opening is closed with interrupted heavy silk sutures (Fig. 25–23). Generally, the rim of the opening is composed of fascial

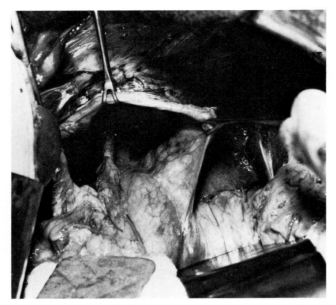

Figure 25–22. All the stomach reduced into the abdomen. The esophagus is firmly fixed in its normal location in the posterior aspect of the diaphragmatic opening by a competent posterior phrenoesophageal ligament. (From Hill, L. D., and Tobias, J. A.: Paraesophageal hernia. Arch. Surg., 96:735, 1968.)

tissue, which is strong and holds well. The opening is closed to the point at which the surgeon's index finger can be inserted alongside the esophagus to insure an adequate lumen. If a gastrostomy is not performed, two or three fixation sutures may be placed along the lesser curvature down to the preaortic fascia to pre-vent a sliding hernia later. With a mixed type of paraesophageal hernia in which an incompetent sphincter and reflux are found preoperatively, a formal repair of the herniated stomach as well as a posterior gastropexy with careful calibration of the cardia is necessary, using intraoperative manometry for proper evaluation of the sphincter pressure.

When hemorrhage is present, simple suturing of the bleeding ulcer is sufficient.

Restoring the stomach to the abdomen promotes adequate emptying with healing of the ulcer, but since the stomach is usually slow in resuming its peristaltic activity in these patients with symptoms of incarcera-tion and acute dilatation, intermittent nasogastric suc-tion for a week or more may be anticipated.

This simplified approach has yielded good results, with recurrence of symptoms in less than 2 per cent of patients.

We recently reviewed our experience with 19 patients with true paraesophageal hernias who were operated on over the past 8 years. The mean age for this group was 66 years (with a range of 46 to 86 years). Fifty-two per cent of these patients had the main complaint of epigastric fullness and substernal pressure and discomfort after eating, 21 per cent had simultaneous moderate to severe dysphagia, and 10 per cent presented with dysphagia as the main symptom. An acute episode of incarceration was present in four patients (21 per cent), one of whom had associated acute upper gastrointestinal bleeding. The overall incidence of anemia was 26 per cent, and four patients had associated severe respiratory

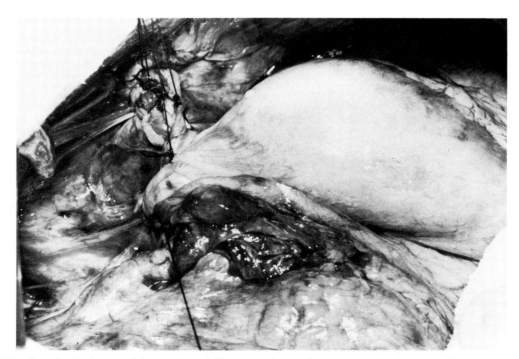

Figure 25–23. Completed closure of the esophageal hiatus anterior to the esophagus by interrupted heavy sutures. One or two additional anchoring sutures are placed along the lesser curvature to the preaortic fascia to prevent sliding of the gastroesophageal junction into the posterior mediastinum. (From Hill, L. D., and Tobias, J. A.: Paraesophageal hernia. Arch. Surg., 96:735, 1968.)

problems due to aspiration of fo   ings. There was no operative morta   tient needed a second operation for a s   oscess. No recurrence of symptoms due to the paraesophageal hernia was found in this group.

Because of the good results obtained with this simple procedure and because of the life-threatening complications to which the patient is exposed without appropriate treatment, surgery is indicated once the diagnosis is confirmed. The aim of treatment is restoration of the viscus to its normal location, with closure of the defect in the diaphragm and fixation of the stomach in the abdominal cavity.

No definitive anti-reflux procedure is necessary unless a mixed type of hernia with a hypotensive lower sphincter and reflux is found. In these patients, a careful cardial calibration anchoring the esophagus to the preaortic fascia is necessary along with the anatomic repair of the hiatus.

REFERENCES

Hill, L. D.: Incarcerated paraesophageal hernia: A surgical emergency. Am. J. Surg., *126*:286, 1973.
Hill, L. D., and Tobias, J. A.: Paraesophageal hernia. Arch. Surg., *96*:735, 1968.
Ozdemir, I. A., Burke, W. A., and Ikins, P. M.: Paraesophageal hernia: A life-threatening disease. Ann. Thorac. Surg., *16*:547, 1973.
Skinner, D. B., and Belsey, R. H. R.: Surgical management of esophageal reflux and hiatal hernia. J. Thorac. Cardiovasc. Surg., *53*:33, 1967.
Wichterman, K., Geha, A. S., Canow, C. E., and Bave, A. E.: Giant paraesophageal hernia with intrathoracic stomach and colon: The case for early elective repair. Surgery, *86*:497, 1979.

VI SHORT ESOPHAGUS AND PEPTIC STRICTURE

Mark B. Orringer

Peptic esophageal stricture is the end result of the inflammatory reaction produced in the esophagus by reflux from the stomach of both acid and alkaline secretions through an incompetent lower esophageal sphincter mechanism. That gastroesophageal reflux can occur independently of the presence of a hiatal hernia has been pointed out (see Section I of this chapter). Erosion of esophageal squamous epithelium by the chemical "burn" of gastric contents is associated with submucosal edema and inflammatory cellular infiltration, which may extend into the muscular layers of the esophageal wall and adjacent periesophageal tissues. The healing process results in varying degrees of fibrosis. Because acute reflux esophagitis tends to be cyclical, with periods of quiescence followed by recrudescence, repetitive bouts of acute inflammation and then healing may result in progressive mural fibrous infiltration beginning in the submucosa and ultimately involving the muscle and periesophageal tissues. As fibrous deposition continues, and contraction of collagen fibers within the stricture takes place, not only does circumferential narrowing reduce the size of the lumen, but also varying degrees of esophageal shortening develop as longitudinal contracture occurs.

HISTORICAL ASPECTS

The surgical approach to peptic esophageal strictures has progressively evolved toward conservative and nonresective techniques. In earlier years, the preoperative assessment of peptic esophageal strictures with radiographic studies, esophagoscopy, and biopsy and ease of dilatation dictated the choice of operation. Strictures that were difficult to dilate were considered irreversible and were treated with operations of relatively great magnitude. These included distal esophagectomy with esophagogastrostomy (Belsey, 1952; Dunlop, 1956; Tanner, 1955), jejunal interposition (Allison *et al.*, 1943; Allison, 1948; Merendino and Dillard, 1955; Barnes and Redo, 1957), colonic interposition (Popov, 1961; Neville and Clowes, 1963; Belsey, 1965), the reversed gastric tube (Heimlich, 1962), plastic procedures on the distal esophageal stenosis with attempts at establishing valvular competence (Thal *et al.*, 1965; Thal, 1968; Woodward, 1975), and resection of the stricture with esophagogastrostomy in combination with antrectomy, vagotomy, and Roux-en-Y gastroenterostomy (Ellis *et al.*, 1958; Payne, 1970).

Hayward (1961), of Australia, was the first to suggest that the majority of peptic strictures could be treated successfully with operative dilatation and an anti-reflux operation. Hill was the first to advocate use of this approach in the United States (Hill *et al.*, 1970), emphasizing the need to obtain adequate reflux control for this method to be successful. As will be discussed, recent surgical developments in this area have focused on techniques of obtaining the most reliable reflux control after dilatation of peptic strictures. These advances have been in part due to a greater insistence on objective evidence of reflux control permitted by refinements in techniques of esophageal manometry as well as documentation of abnormal reflux with the intraesophageal pH probe. Since the pioneering work in esophageal manometry by Ingelfinger (1958) and Code and associates (1958) and the introduction of the long gastrointestinal pH electrode to assess competency of the distal esophageal sphincter mechanism by Tuttle and Grossman (1958), esophageal function laboratories have become the hallmark of the modern esophageal surgeon. For just as the cardiac surgeon now relies upon physiologic catheterization data and the pulmonary surgeon utilizes pulmonary function tests as a gauge for predicting the safety of a pulmonary resection, the esophageal surgeon now has a reliable, objective means for documenting not only the preoperative functional abnormality, but also the results of operations on the esophagus. The precision in both diagnosis and treatment that has come to characterize the cardiac surgeon should now be expected of the esophageal surgeon as well.

ANATOMIC CONSIDERATIONS

Three general varieties of peptic esophageal strictures are encountered clinically. The majority are short, 1 to 2 cm. in length, and localized to the esophagogastric junction (Fig. 25–24). At the other

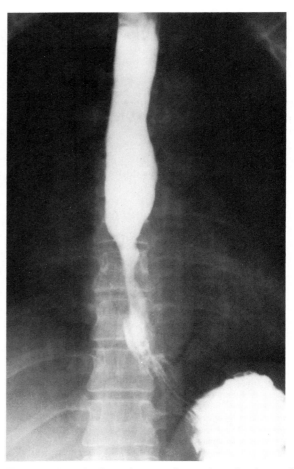

Figure 25–25. An 8-cm. long peptic esophageal stricture that followed severe protracted vomiting. There is an associated sliding hiatal hernia.

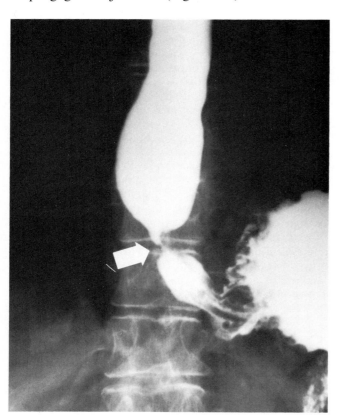

Figure 25–24. Esophagogram illustrating the most common type of peptic stricture. This high-grade stenosis (arrow) proximal to a small sliding hiatal hernia is less than 2 cm. in length and is localized to the esophagogastric junction.

extreme are the more extensive strictures that involve the distal half or third of the esophagus (Fig. 25–25). This type of stricture most commonly occurs after prolonged nasogastric intubation in a critically ill patient who is supine for many days and, occasionally, after severe protracted vomiting, as in hyperemesis gravidarum or in association with gastric outlet obstruction. Finally, localized strictures occurring in the mid or upper thoracic esophagus should suggest the possibility of a Barrett's esophagus (columnar epithelium–lined lower esophagus) (Figs. 25–26 and 25–27).

In the *Barrett's esophagus*, the stricture characteristically occurs at the squamocolumnar epithelial junction, which is in the mid or upper third of the organ in these patients. The esophagus distal to the stricture is lined by columnar or gastric-type epithelium, which may include acid-producing parietal cells, and a sliding hiatal hernia is generally present. Although originally thought to be a congenital abnormality, the columnar epithelium–lined esophagus is viewed by more modern concepts as an acquired condition that is a consequence of reflux esophagitis. After the normal esophageal epithelium is denuded by reflux esophagitis, the esophagus is re-epithelialized by the upward growth of gastric columnar epithelium, which

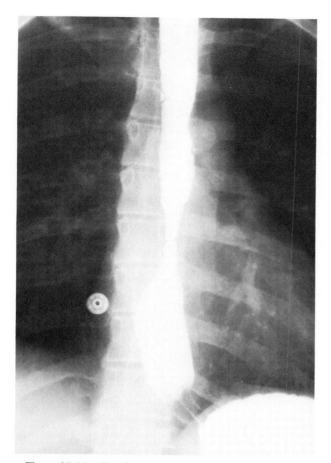

Figure 25–26. Esophagogram of a patient with long-standing dysphagia and a Barrett's esophagus. The mid-esophageal stricture suggested a Barrett's esophagus, and multiple biopsies distal to the stricture showed columnar epithelium. Normal squamous epithelium was found proximal to the stenosis. A sliding hiatal hernia was present.

esophageal strictures had columnar epithelium distal to the stenosis. Unfortunately, Barrett (1950) concluded that any portion of the swallowing passage lined by columnar epithelium is stomach. The term "short esophagus" thus arose, since many regarded the columnar epithelium–lined length of the esophagus below the stricture as stomach. The result of this erroneous belief that strictures always occur at the anatomic esophagogastric junction was a policy of treating high strictures by resection and esophageal replacement with intestine to provide the "missing" length of esophagus.

It has subsequently been recognized that columnar epithelium in the esophagus is generally an *acquired* lesion due to reflux esophagitis (Allison and Johnstone, 1953; Mossberg, 1966; Naef *et al.*, 1975). Furthermore, esophageal manometry has documented that there is in fact a distal esophageal sphincter mechanism, although a weak one, at the anatomic esophagogastric junction, well below the squamocolumnar epithelial junction. This has led Hill (Hill *et al.*, 1970) to dispute the existence of the "short esophagus" and to argue that the esophagogastric junction can nearly always be reduced below the diaphragmatic hiatus for his median arcuate ligament posterior gastropexy.

The majority of esophageal surgeons, however, believe that a true shortening of the distance between the esophageal introitus and the esophagogastric junction *does* occur as a result of fibrous contracture associated with reflux esophagitis, in a similar fashion to the well-recognized "shortening" that may follow a caustic esophageal injury. In addition, clinical observation suggests that *fibrosis need not be present for acquired esophageal shortening to occur*, since some degree of contraction of both the circular and longitudinal esophageal musculature may be induced by reflux esophagitis, rendering it more difficult to reduce the esophagogastric junction below the diaphragm without tension. Thus, the designation of "short esophagus" does not necessarily require that a stricture be present but may follow an assessment of the anatomy at the time of hiatal hernia repair, with particular attention to the degree of stretch on the distal esophagus that exists once the esophagogastric junction is reduced below the diaphragm. As will be pointed out, for practical purposes, the critical issue is not *whether* the esophagogastric junction can be reduced below the diaphragm, but rather, the degree of residual *tension* on the distal esophagus once the reduction is complete, for tension associated with a hiatal hernia repair is just as undesirable as it is when repairing abdominal wall hernias at other sites, and the implications for subsequent recurrence are the same.

has a more rapid growth rate than squamous epithelium. This pathologic entity is being reported with increasing frequency, and its true incidence has undoubtedly been underestimated in the past, since barium esophagograms may not be diagnostic, and biopsies both above and below the stricture are a prerequisite for establishing the diagnosis. The premalignant nature of the columnar epithelium–lined esophagus has only recently been appreciated, with adenocarcinomas developing within the columnar-lined region in at least 10 to 16 per cent of these patients (Fig. 25–28) (Adler, 1963; Naef *et al.*, 1975).

Controversy exists about the definition of the term "short esophagus," with some disputing that such an entity in association with gastroesophageal reflux even exists. According to Barrett (1950), peptic ulceration of the esophagus was first described by Albers in 1839, and Rokitansky later gave his support to the existence of this pathologic entity. In a review of the literature, Tileston (1906) reported 44 patients with peptic ulceration of the esophagus and clearly described stenosis associated with this condition. As "reflux esophagitis" was publicized by Allison (1948), it became apparent that many of these patients with

TREATMENT

The most important factor in the treatment of a benign peptic esophageal stricture is *prevention* – i.e., controlling gastroesophageal reflux *before* mural fibrosis occurs. This requires, however, that reflux esopha-

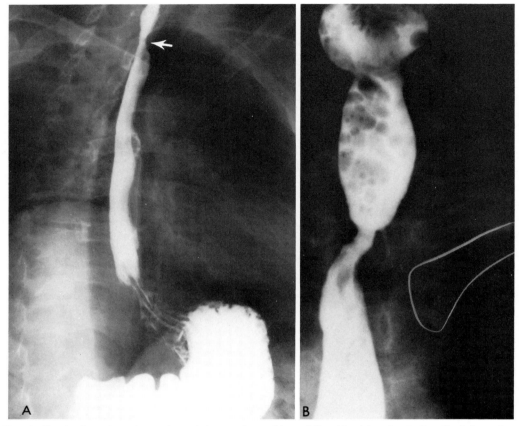

Figure 25–27. *A,* Cervicothoracic stricture (arrow) in a patient with a sliding hiatal hernia. *B,* Detail of the stricture, at level of clavicle (highlighted), initially thought to be secondary to carcinoma. Multiple esophageal biopsies at 5-cm. intervals distal to the stricture revealed columnar epithelium. Squamous epithelium was found proximal to this unusually high stenosis that occurred in this Barrett's esophagus.

gitis be diagnosed at a relatively early stage. Unfortunately, such diagnosis is hampered by two curious facets of this disease: first, the notoriously poor correlation between the patient's symptoms and the degree or extent of esophagitis present, and second, the inability of the most widely used study to evaluate the esophagus — the barium esophagogram — to detect esophagitis consistently and reliably before mural fibrosis has occurred. The endoscopic grading system for esophagitis proposed by Belsey provides a more objective and meaningful description of the gross pathologic changes seen than the more traditional designations of "mild," "moderate," or "severe" esophagitis, which have inherent wide variations in meaning between observers.

Endoscopic Grades of Esophagitis (Skinner and Belsey, 1967)

Grade I: Distal esophageal mucosal erythema (which may obscure the esophagogastric squamocolumnar epithelial junction).

Grade II: Mucosal erythema with superficial ulceration, typically linear and vertical and with an overlying fibrinous membranous exudate that is easily wiped away, leaving a bleeding surface

(often misinterpreted as "scope trauma" by the inexperienced endoscopist).

Grade III: Mucosal erythema with superficial ulceration and associated mural fibrosis — a dilatable "early" stricture.

Grade IV: Extensive ulceration and fibrous luminal stenosis — may represent irreversible panmural fibrosis.

Unfortunately, although the radiologist may infer the presence of early esophagitis on the basis of distal spasm or occasionally demonstrated superficial mucosal irregularity, he cannot *consistently* detect esophagitis until some degree of esophageal narrowing is seen on the barium swallow examination. At this point, the report of a "mild" esophageal stricture may imply that the process has been detected at a sufficiently early stage that conservative therapy is adequate. As is evident from the endoscopic grades of esophagitis, however, a "mild" radiographic stricture is an *advanced* stage of esophagitis, and appropriate therapy is long overdue.

Bougienage

The surgeon confronted with a distal esophageal stricture must answer two questions: Is the stricture

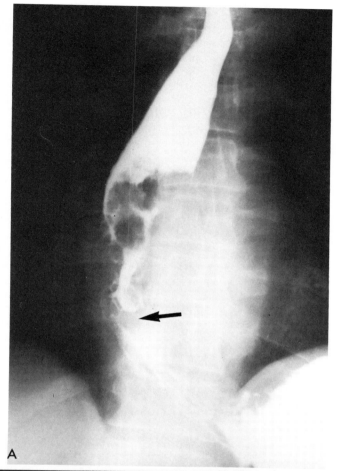

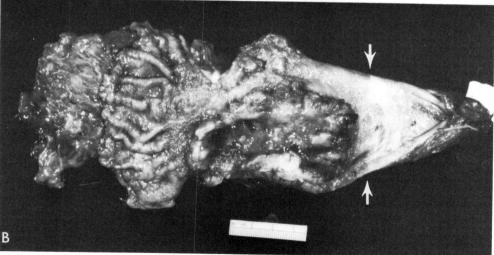

Figure 25–28. *A,* Adenocarcinoma arising in a Barrett's esophagus. Esophagogram showing an extensive tumor proximal to a sliding hiatal hernia (arrow indicates the esophagogastric junction). *B,* Resected specimen demonstrating the squamocolumnar epithelial junction (arrows) and the ulcerated adenocarcinoma arising in the columnar epithelium that lined the lower half of this Barrett's esophagus.

benign or malignant? If benign, can the stricture be dilated? Both of these questions are answered by esophagoscopy, which is a mandatory part of the evaluation of *every* stricture. Although this subject receives relatively little emphasis in the thoracic surgical literature, dilatation of an esophageal stricture is among the most dangerous of operations performed. Despite recent modern advances in flexible fiberoptic esophagogastroscopy, we believe that the *initial* endoscopic evaluation of a distal esophageal stricture should be performed with the rigid esophagoscope and with the patient under general anesthesia to optimize conditions for both the patient and the surgeon (Fig. 25–29). Neither the pliability nor the extent of the stenosis can be assessed adequately through a flexible fiberoptic esophagoscope. With the patient totally relaxed, the surgeon is able to devote his entire attention to the endoscopic field. If the stricture is mild, it can be dilated directly with the rigid esophagoscope. If the stenosis is of a higher grade, however, it is gently probed and evaluated with gum-tipped bougies passed under direct vision through the stenosis. The largest such dilator that will pass through most rigid esophagoscopes is a size 26 French. When a stricture is pliable and minimal resistance is encountered during dilatation, the esophagoscope is removed, and the dilatation is continued with Hurst-Maloney, mercury-filled, tapered rubber dilators passed "blindly" through the mouth. If, on the other hand, initial evaluation has revealed a *dense*, rigid stricture, "blind" passage of the Hurst-Maloney dilators is not

performed, because the bougie could "curl" proximal to the nonyielding stenosis and a perforation could occur. In such difficult cases, after removing the standard rigid esophagoscope, we replace it with a special-order 45-cm. long rigid esophagoscope (Pilling Company) that will accommodate up to a 50-French bougie (Fig. 29–30). This esophagoscope is introduced to the level of the stricture, and *under direct vision*, progressively larger dilators, beginning with a size 28 French, are passed through the stenosis. In our experience, virtually all strictures that can be dilated either directly per os or through the esophagoscope to the range of a 40-French bougie can be further dilated *intraoperatively* to the 56- to 60-French range (see discussion that follows). After dilating the stricture, both esophageal biopsies and brushings for cytologic evaluation are performed to exclude carcinoma. Rigid esophagoscopy permits a far more substantial biopsy to be performed than can be done through the flexible fiberoptic instrument. The combination of esophageal biopsy and brushings establishes the diagnosis of esophageal carcinoma in more than 95 per cent of patients with carcinoma, and if no evidence of neoplasm is found with these studies, the distal esophageal stricture can generally be assumed to be benign with a high degree of confidence.

As indicated previously, symptoms may correlate poorly with the degree of esophagitis present. Thus, some patients with severe reflux symptoms may have no more than Grade I esophagitis on endoscopic evaluation. Conversely, at least a quarter of the elder-

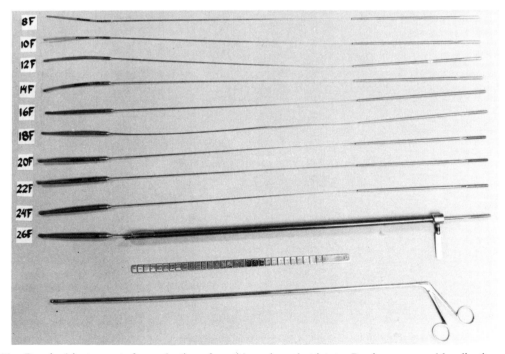

Figure 25–29. Required instruments for evaluation of peptic esophageal stricture. Precise, measured localization of the stricture in centimeters from the incisor teeth and adequate biopsies as well as brushings from the stricture are obtained. The gum-tipped Jackson dilators gently manipulated through the stenosis, permit evaluation of the extent and pliability of the obstruction. The 26-French dilator is the largest size that will pass through the standard 45-cm. rigid esophagoscope.

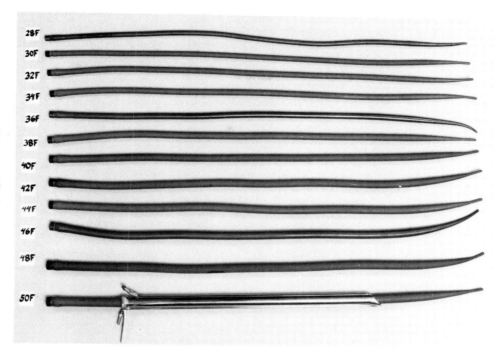

Figure 25–30. Tapered Hurst-Maloney esophageal dilators and 45-cm. Pilling esophagoscope, which accommodates up to a 50-French bougie, thus permitting progressive dilatation of severe peptic strictures under direct vision.

ly patients we treat for peptic strictures have had few, if any, esophageal symptoms prior to the onset of dysphagia from their esophageal stenoses. Thus, these patients have experienced the first three endoscopic grades of esophagitis without significant heartburn or regurgitation. In these patients, dilatation of the stricture relieves the only esophageal symptom—dysphagia—and the addition of a medical program for reflux control may constitute adequate therapy. Such patients generally accept intermittent outpatient esophageal bougienage as a welcomed alternative to impaired swallowing and between dilatations are quite comfortable and satisfied with their ability to eat. In contrast to these latter patients are others with high-grade peptic esophageal strictures who give a history of long-standing, severe reflux symptoms, which gradually subsided as dysphagia occurred. Dilatation of the stricture in these patients relieves the dysphagia but also permits return of significant regurgitation from the stomach into the esophagus. Thus, reflux symptoms again become prominent, and relief of the esophageal obstruction alone does not satisfy the patient.

Many physicians believe that esophageal bougienage in combination with a strict anti-reflux medical regimen is the treatment of choice for the patient with a peptic stricture. This belief is based on (1) the notoriously poorer operative results with reflux control in patients with strictures undergoing standard hiatal hernia repairs, and (2) the complexity of the operations involved in esophageal resection or reconstruction. Modern surgical advances, however, have resulted in a major change in the approach to peptic esophageal strictures, with the salvage of esophagi that in the past were routinely resected. Because of these developments and the fact that the patient with a peptic esophageal stricture, regardless of the severity

of his symptoms, has *advanced* reflux esophagitis, we recommend surgical control of reflux in all such patients who are relatively young and good candidates for operation.

Surgical Treatment

The presence of peptic stricture and esophageal shortening interferes with the success of standard anti-reflux operations in these patients. The incidence of recurrent hiatal hernia or reflux in patients with strictures undergoing the standard Belsey Mark IV operation, for example, is between 45 and 75 per cent (Orringer *et al.*, 1972; Donnelly and Deverall, 1973). The mural inflammation, esophagitis, and esophageal shortening that characterize peptic esophageal strictures prevent the *tension-free* reduction of the prerequisite 3- to 5-cm. segment of distal esophagus below the diaphragm, where the influence of positive intra-abdominal pressure transmitted to the esophagus by the partial fundoplication helps prevent reflux. Since the Belsey and Nissen fundoplications, as well as the Hill median arcuate ligament repair, all strive for an intra-abdominal location of the esophagogastric junction and all require sutures in the distal esophageal or periesophageal tissues, the long-term success of these anti-reflux procedures *must* be jeopardized if mural inflammation and esophageal shortening are present, because these factors necessitate not only suturing to inflamed tissues, but also fixing the esophagogastric junction below the diaphragm under tension. Mobilizing the short esophagus, if necessary to the level of the aortic arch, has been described as a means of enabling better reduction of the esophagogastric junction below the diaphragm. (Orringer *et al.*, 1972). The necessity for such a maneuver, however, implies that the surgeon is truly concerned about the degree of tension on the repaired esophagus and now suggests to us that an alternative operation is needed.

The realization that peptic stricture and esophageal shortening adversely affected the results of the Mark IV operation led to Belsey's recommendation for resection rather than hernia repair in patients with these conditions. However, distal esophagectomy with an intrathoracic esophagogastric anastomosis is a *poor* operation for the patient with reflux esophagitis, because the lower esophageal sphincter incompetence inherent in this technique is responsible for the development of reflux esophagitis in the residual esophagus in as many as 20 to 40 per cent of these patients. Various operations designed to prevent gastroesophageal reflux after an intrathoracic esophagogastric anastomosis have been reported (Okada *et al.*, 1974; Bombeck *et al.*, 1970; Demos and Biele, 1980), but none has been found to be reliable or has gained widespread acceptance. The alternative techniques of distal esophagectomy and reconstruction with either a jejunal or short-segment colonic interposition provide excellent relief of dysphagia and reflux symptoms in patients with peptic strictures. These are, of course, sizable and technically demanding operations, the need for which has been greatly diminished by the advent of newer, more conservative nonresective techniques.

In 1971, Pearson and associates reported success with the Collis gastroplasty operation (Collis, 1957, 1961) in combination with the Belsey hiatal hernia repair in patients with severe peptic esophagitis and secondary esophageal shortening. With elimination of reflux, sufficient resolution of the distal esophageal stenosis occurred to allow comfortable swallowing. In our experience, if at the initial endoscopic evaluation, it is ascertained that the stricture is benign and can be dilated per os to a size 40-French bougie, treatment with dilatation and a combined gastroplasty-fundoplication operation will most likely be possible, because virtually every stricture that can be dilated to this size per os will be amenable to later forceful intraoperative dilatation, performed with the surgeon's hand supporting the mobilized esophagus from without, and resection can be avoided. Alternatively, if passage of a 40-French dilator is not possible, a barium enema examination is performed to evaluate the suitability of the colon as an esophageal substitute, and the colon is prepared preoperatively in the event that intraoperative forceful dilatation of the stricture is unsuccessful and resection is required. The colon is also evaluated and prepared in patients with recurrent reflux esophagitis after multiple prior hiatal hernia repairs, because repetitive mobilization of the gastric fundus may result in questionable viability, which contraindicates construction of the Collis gastroplasty tube from the stomach.

The combined Collis-Belsey operation is performed through a left sixth or seventh intercostal space posterolateral thoracotomy rather than the thoracoabdominal incison described by Collis (Fig. 25–31). As in the routine Belsey Mark IV procedure, the fundus of the stomach is delivered into the chest through the hiatus without the routine use of a diaphragmatic counter incision. This necessitates division

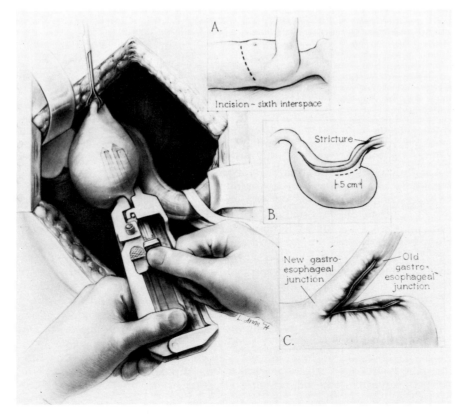

Figure 25–31. Collis gastroplasty using the GIA surgical stapler. *A,* The esophagus and fundus of the stomach are mobilized through a lateral thoracotomy in the sixth left intercostal space. *B,* A 56- or 58-French Hurst-Maloney dilator is passed through the esophageal stricture and displaced against the lesser curvature of the stomach as the stapler is applied. The knife assembly is advanced (main illustration), and the stapler is removed. *C,* The result if a 5-cm. long gastric tube extension of the esophagus. An additional 2 to 3 cm. of length can be gained by a second, partial application of the stapler. (From Orringer, M. B., and Sloan, H.: An improved technique for the combined Collis-Belsey approach to dilatable esophageal strictures. J. Thorac. Cardiovasc. Surg., *68*:298, 1974.)

and ligation of several of the short gastric vessels along the high greater curvature of the stomach. Great care must be taken to avoid undue tension on these vessels in order to prevent injury to the spleen. Furthermore, gentle but precise ligation is required, since these vessels readily retract beneath the diaphragm and may be a source of subsequent intra-abdominal hemorrhage. If adhesions from prior operations at the hiatus necessitate abdominal exposure, a 5- to 10- cm. peripheral diaphragmatic counter incision 2 to 3 cm. from the attachments of the diaphragm on the costal arch is made. Division of the costal arch is avoided if possible, as this is one of the most painful incisions both in the early postoperative period as well as later. Thus, a separate abdominal incision, if necessary, is far preferable to a thoracoabdominal incision.

The distal esophagus is mobilized and encircled with a rubber drain, and the fat pad at the cardia is excised. Progressively larger Hurst-Maloney tapered dilators, up to the range of a 56 to 58 French, are passed by the anesthetist per os and are guided across the esophagogastric junction by the surgeon, who supports the wall of the esophagus to avoid disruption. Considerable force may be required to achieve satisfactory intraoperative dilatation. With the 56- or 58-French intraesophageal dilator displaced against the lesser curvature of the stomach and the fundus retracted in the opposite direction, the GIA surgical stapler is applied to the stomach adjacent to the dilator and

parallel to the lesser curvature (Fig. 25–31). Use of the GIA surgical stapler for construction of the gastroplasty tube, instead of the originally described gastric clamps, greatly simplifies this portion of the operation and prevents gastrointestinal contamination of the field (Orringer and Sloan, 1974). After advancing the knife assembly, a 5-cm. long gastric tube extension of the esophagus is created and is mechanically sutured closed by two staggered rows of stainless steel staples. If there is a great deal of distal esophageal shortening and fibrosis, the stapler can be partially applied a second time to gain an additional 2 to 3 cm. of "esophageal" length. The staple suture line is then oversewn, and the dilator is removed. The standard posterior crural sutures of Number 1 silk are placed and left untied for the present.

Following intraoperative dilatation of the stricture and construction of the gastroplasty tube, Pearson advocated a standard Belsey repair around the "new" distal esophagus, i.e., the gastroplasty tube (Pearson et al., 1971) (Fig. 25–32). Two rows of sutures, each consisting of three horizontal mattress sutures of 2-0 silk, are placed in the newly created distal esophageal gastric tube. The first row is 2 cm. above the new esophagogastric junction, and the second is 2 cm. above the first and also passes through the diaphragm. After the stomach is secured below the diaphragm and the posterior crural sutures have been tied, a 4-cm. *tension-free* segment of intra-abdominal "esophagus"

Figure 25–32. Belsey reconstruction of the esophagogastric junction after constructing the Collis gastroplasty tube. Oversewing the staple suture line (main illustration). *A,* Placement of standard posterior crural sutures and the first row of three mattress sutures between the fundus of the stomach and the new distal "esophagus," 2 cm. above the new esophagogastric junction. *B,* Placement of the second row of mattress sutures through the diaphragm, fundus, and new distal "esophagus." *C,* The completed repair, showing a 4-cm. segment of intra-abdominal distal "esophagus."

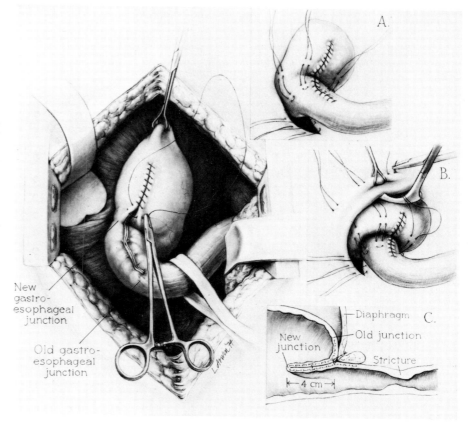

is produced (Fig. 25–32C). As the sutures of the Belsey reconstruction in this combined operation are taken in resilient, healthy stomach (gastroplasty tube), the need to suture to inflamed distal esophagus is totally eliminated. The combined Collis-Belsey operation is conceptually sound, lengthening the functional distal esophageal tube to avoid tension on the repair and providing a resilient gastric tube, rather than the inflamed esophagus, around which to perform the Belsey partial fundoplication. Pearson has reported excellent relief of both dysphagia and reflux symptoms following dilatation of peptic strictures and the Collis-Belsey operation in 25 of 33 patients so treated and followed for 5 to 12 years (Pearson and Henderson, 1976; Pearson, 1977).

However, after initial enthusiasm for the combined Collis-Belsey operation (Pearson and Henderson, 1973; Urschel et al., 1973; Orringer and Sloan, 1976), reports of unsatisfactory reflux control emerged from those who were assessing the objective results of operation with the intraesophageal pH electrode. Orringer and Sloan (1977) suggested that construction of the gastroplasty tube so reduces the amount of gastric fundus available for fundoplication that an adequate 240-degree Belsey wrap around the new distal esophagus may not be possible (Fig. 25–33). Thus, even with a 3- to 7-cm. intra-abdominal segment of functional distal esophagus, with an inadequate fundoplication, gastroesophageal reflux may not be prevented.

In an effort to improve reflux control after performance of the Collis gastroplasty, Henderson (1977) and Orringer and Sloan (1978) recommended use of a 360-degree Nissen-type fundoplication. After dilatation of the stricture and construction of a 5- to 8-cm. long gastroplasty tube, as described above, the 56- or 58-French esophageal dilator is removed and replaced with a 46-French Hurst-Maloney bougie. The elongated, narrowed gastric fundus is passed behind the gastroplasty tube (Fig. 25–34). With interrupted seromuscular 2-0 silk sutures placed approximately 1 cm. apart, a fundoplication 4 to 6 cm. long is begun (Fig. 25–35). Each suture passes through the gastric fundus, then through the gastroplasty tube or adjacent stomach, and finally through the gastric fundus again. The gastric wrap enfolds 3 to 4 cm. of the gastroplasty tube and the proximal 2 to 3 cm. of adjacent fundus of the stomach (Fig. 25–35A). The sutures are tied with the 46-French dilator still lying within the gastroplasty tube. The dilator is removed, and the suture line is oversewn with a 4-0 running polypropylene Lembert stitch through the seromuscular layers on each side. The fundoplication is reduced beneath the diaphragm, and the posterior crural sutures are tied so that the hiatus will admit one finger alongside the esophagus. Intraoperatively, silver clip markers are placed at the new esophagogastric junction (the apex of the gastroplasty tube) and at the edges of the diaphragmatic hiatus. On postoperative roentgenograms, the distance between these two rows of markers represents the 3- to 5-cm. tension-free intra-abdominal segment of functional esophagus, encircled completely by the gastric wrap (Fig. 25–36).

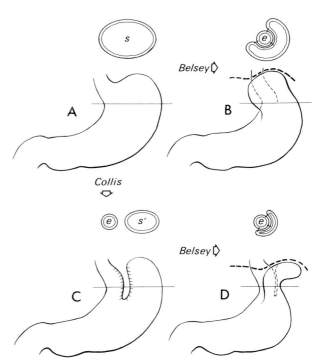

Figure 25–33. Limitation of fundoplication by Collis procedure. *A*, Cross section through gastric fundus in plane indicated shows area of stomach(s) available for standard Belsey Mark IV repair, with 240-degree fundoplication shown in *B*, *C*, The use of stomach in the Collis procedure to form the new distal esophagus (e) results in a smaller area of gastric fundus (s') available for the Belsey fundoplication. *D*, Only a limited 180-degree fundoplication is possible after the Collis maneuver, and the elongated, narrowed gastric fundus is angulated beneath the diaphragm (dotted line) as the second row of sutures of the Belsey repair are tied. (From Orringer, M. B., and Sloan, H.: Complications and failings of the combined Collis-Belsey operation. J. Thorac. Cardiovasc. Surg., *74*:726, 1977.)

We have found that more than 95 per cent of peptic strictures associated with reflux esophagitis are dilatable and will regress sufficiently to allow comfortable swallowing if adequate reflux control can be achieved, because the esophageal narrowing seen on the barium swallow examination generally is not totally the result of end-stage scarring and fibrosis. Rather, there is a significant acute inflammatory component — edema and round cell infiltrate — that is reversible. Only 4 of the last 80 peptic strictures that we have treated could not be dilated and required resection. Of our patients with strictures treated with dilatation and the combined Collis gastroplasty–fundoplication technique, 26 have had a Collis-Belsey repair and 30 have had the Collis-Nissen procedure. The proportion of moderate and severe strictures was approximately the same in both groups. Prior antireflux operations had been performed in 10 of the patients (38 per cent) who had the Collis-Belsey operation and 6 (20 per cent) of those who had the Collis-Nissen procedure.

The severity of a stricture is determined intraoperatively on the basis of the degree of resistance encountered during dilatation. A *mild* stricture is de-

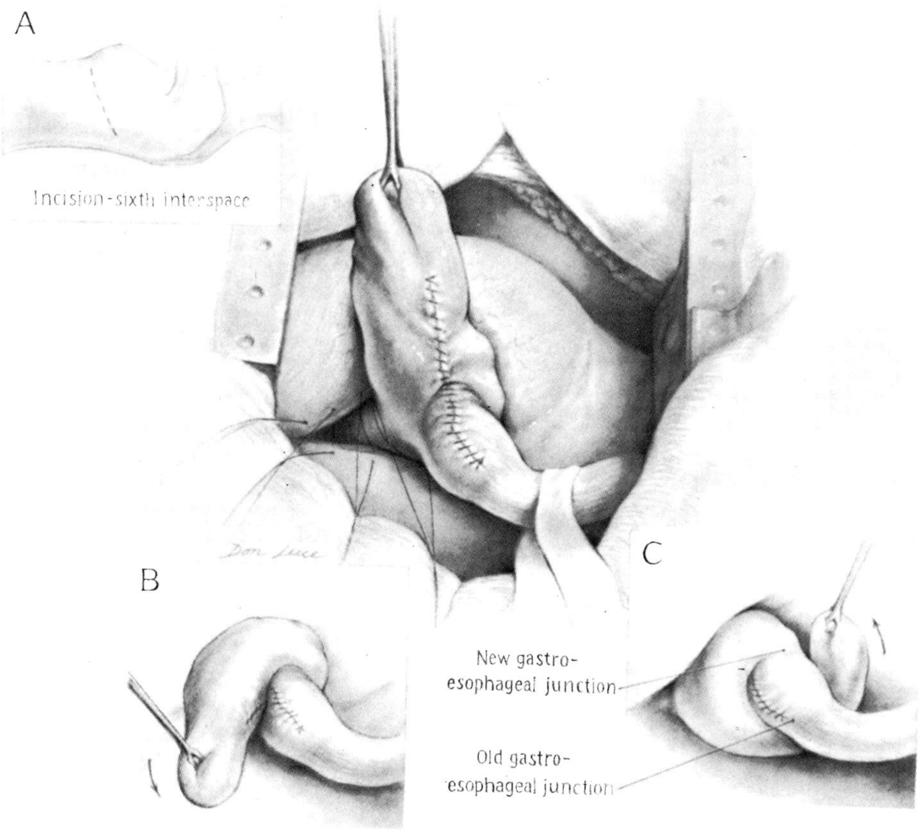

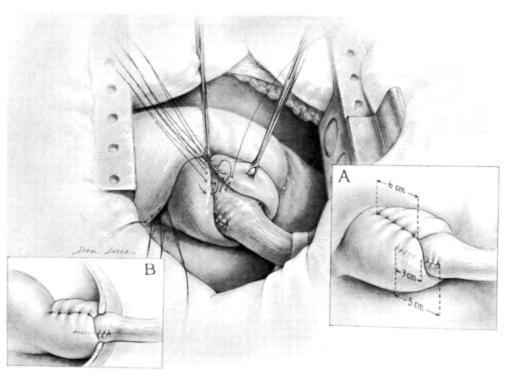

Figure 25–34. The main drawing illustrates the elongated, narrow gastric fundus available for the fundoplication after completion of the Collis procedure. *A* shows the placement of the incision through the left sixth intercostal space. *B* and *C* show the gastric fundus being wrapped around the gastroplasty tube and adjacent stomach. Note that the posterior crural sutures are left untied for the moment. (From Orringer, M. B., and Sloan, H.: Combined Collis-Nissen reconstruction of the esophagogastric junction. Ann. Thorac. Surg., *25*:16, 1978.)

Incision-sixth interspace

New gastro-esophageal junction

Old gastro-esophageal junction

6 cm

3 cm

5 cm

Figure 25–35. Placement of the seromuscular sutures from gastric fundus to gastroplasty tube and back to gastric fundus for the proximal three or four sutures, and from gastric fundus to anterior stomach wall and then gastric fundus for the distal three or four sutures. After these sutures are tied, the fundoplication includes the distal 3 to 4 cm. of gastroplasty tube and the proximal 3 to 4 cm. of stomach. *A,* The fundoplication, reduced in the abdomen, rests below the diaphragm without tension on the distal esophagus after the posterior crural sutures are tied *(B)*. (From Orringer, M. B., and Sloan, H.: Combined Collis-Nissen reconstruction of the esophagogastric junction. Ann. Thorac. Surg., *25*:16, 1978.)

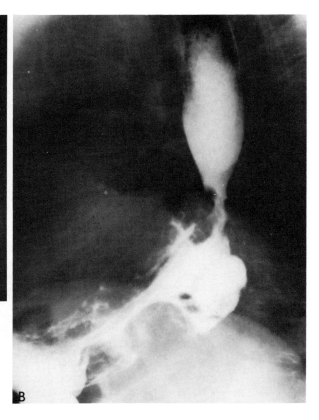

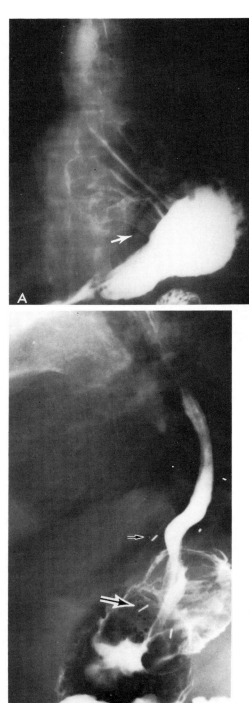

Figure 25–36. *A,* Posteroanterior esophagogram showing large sliding hiatal hernia with one half of stomach above the left hemidiaphragm (arrow). *B,* Lateral view shows the hernia, a proximal stricture, and esophageal dilatation from the obstruction. *C,* Postoperative appearance of the reconstructed distal esophagus following intraoperative dilatation of the stricture and a Collis-Nissen repair. The horizontal gastric folds in the fundoplication around the distal 5 to 7 cm. of the functional esophagus can be seen. Small arrow indicates silver clips marking the diaphragmatic hiatus. Large arrow indicates clips at the new esophagogastric junction. There is no evidence of esophageal stenosis, and the dilation proximal to the obstruction has resolved.

fined as one that is easily dilated during operation with minimal resistance; *moderate* strictures require some, but not excessive, forceful dilatation; and a *severe* stricture requires vigorous forceful dilatation and is generally associated with marked periesophagitis and mural thickening of the esophagus. In this regard, we have been impressed that neither the severity of the

stricture nor its ability to be dilated can be accurately predicted by its radiographic or endoscopic appearance, for once the esophagus has been mobilized and is supported from without by the surgeon's hand, manipulation of Hurst-Maloney dilators through the stricture is almost always possible. In the rare instance that antegrade dilatation is not possible, retrograde dilatation of severe strictures using Hegar dilators passed through a high gastrotomy may be performed (Herrington *et al.*, 1975).

Among our 56 patients with strictures treated with the combined Collis gastroplasty–fundoplication operation, there have been no postoperative deaths. The only major complication occurred in one patient whose stricture was disrupted during intraoperative dilatation. He developed an esophagopleural cutaneous fistula, which subsequently closed spontaneously and regressed. The incidence of unsatisfactory reflux control in our patients has been determined by regular postoperative evaluation with interview and the intraesophageal pH probe (Table 25–6). Manometric characteristics of the distal esophageal high-pressure zone (HPZ), as well as the degree of abnormal reflux present, as assessed by the standard acid reflux test, have been compared preoperatively and postoperatively. Distal esophageal sphincter (HPZ) pressure and length have increased from an average of 5.1 mm. Hg and 1.7 cm., respectively, preoperatively, to 9 mm. Hg and 2.9 cm. after the Collis-Belsey operation. After the Collis-Nissen procedure, HPZ pressures have increased from 4.8 mm. to 12 mm. Hg, and length has increased from 1.7 cm. to 4.3 cm. All of these patients with strictures have had markedly abnormal gastroesophageal reflux (3+) documented with the pH probe preoperatively. Postoperatively, 12 (46 per cent) of the patients who had the Collis-Belsey operation have demonstrated moderate to severe abnormal reflux after an average follow-up of 49 months. Six of these patients had measurable abnormal reflux at the time of their first postoperative evaluation at 4 to 12 months, suggesting that adequate reflux control was never achieved by the operation. Six have developed reflux after initial good control from 5 to 48 months (average 24 months) postoperatively. Of the 12 patients with unsatisfactory *objective* reflux control, two are asymp-

tomatic, four have mild symptoms, two are moderately symptomatic, and four have had severe reflux symptoms that necessitated additional anti-reflux operations. The remaining 54 per cent of these patients continue to do well after an average follow-up of 49 months. These are clearly unacceptable results. Reflux control has been far better with the Collis-Nissen combination, although these patients have been followed for only an average of 28 months. Two patients with strictures (7 per cent) have developed measurable abnormal reflux after initial good control for 1 year. One of these has no reflux symptoms; the other has moderately severe recurrent symptoms. The remaining 28 patients (93 per cent) have had no abnormal reflux detected from 1 to 36 months (average 28 months) postoperatively.

Patients undergoing intraoperative dilatation of strictures are dilated again postoperatively according to the severity of the stricture. Patients with mild strictures that are easily dilated during the operation are not dilated again unless dysphagia recurs. Those with moderate or severe strictures are calibrated at the bedside with a 50-French Hurst-Maloney dilator 1 week after operation, prior to discharge. If resistance to the passage of the dilator is encountered, outpatient dilatations are continued at 2- to 4-week intervals until little or no resistance is encountered or as dictated by the recurrence of dysphagia. Of our 30 patients who underwent the Collis-Nissen procedure, 22 (73 per cent) have required no further bougienage after the initial intraoperative dilatation. Approximately one half of these patients with severe strictures have required postoperative dilatations, but only two have needed it at regular intervals because of inadequate stricture regression. Postoperative barium esophagograms have shown varying degrees of stricture regression, but it is clear that symptomatic relief of dysphagia associated with a peptic stricture can be obtained

TABLE 25–6. RESULTS OF COLLIS GASTROPLASTY–FUNDOPLICATION OPERATIONS FOR PEPTIC STRICTURES

	COLLIS-BELSEY PROCEDURE—26 PATIENTS (AVERAGE FOLLOW-UP: 49 MOS.)	COLLIS-NISSEN PROCEDURE—30 PATIENTS (AVERAGE FOLLOW-UP: 28 MOS.)
OBJECTIVE REFLUX CONTROL (pH PROBE DETERMINATION*)		
Good (0–1+ Reflux)	14 (54%)	28 (93%)
Poor (2–3+ Reflux)	12 (46%)	2 (7%)
	26 (100%)	30 (100%)
SUBJECTIVE REFLUX CONTROL (REFLUX SYMPTOMS)		
None	17 (66%)	29 (97%)
Mild	4 (15%)	0 —
Moderate	1 (4%)	1 (3%)
Severe	4 (15%)	0 —
	26 (100%)	30 (100%)

*Reflux evaluated using the intraesophageal pH probe positioned 5 cm. above the lower esophageal sphincter after placing 300 ml. bolus of 0.1 normal hydrochloric acid in the stomach, as described by Kantrowitz, P. A., Corson, J. G., Fleischli, D. L., and Skinner, D. B.: Measurement of gastroesophageal reflux. Gastroenterology, 56:666, 1969.

even when some radiographic evidence of residual distal stenosis persists.

The combined Collis gastroplasty–fundoplication operation has also been used successfully in patients with scleroderma reflux esophagitis (Henderson and Pearson, 1973; Orringer *et al.*, 1976; Orringer and Orringer, 1981). This population is particularly prone to peptic esophageal strictures, since their combined esophageal problems of lower esophageal sphincter incompetence as well as impaired motility result in prolonged contact between refluxed gastric acid and the esophageal mucosa. Despite their systemic disease, gratifying palliation with relief of severe dysphagia and reflux symptoms can be achieved by dilating the strictures and controlling reflux with a gastroplasty-fundoplication procedure. In our operative experience with scleroderma reflux esophagitis in 37 patients, 16 (43 per cent) of whom have had peptic strictures, good to excellent relief from reflux symptoms has been obtained in 89 per cent. Despite their abnormal esophageal motility, significant problems with esophageal emptying through the reconstructed distal esophagus have not occurred in these scleroderma patients. Ten of the 16 strictures have totally regressed; five require intermittent dilatation.

The preliminary results of reflux control in patients with peptic strictures treated by the combined Collis gastroplasty–fundoplication operation are encouraging, but still lack the supporting data of adequate long-term follow-up. Technologic advances, however, particularly the availability of manometry and the intraesophageal pH probe to objectively document the results of our anti-reflux operations, have provided tools for more precise evaluation of our procedures. It is our belief that the intraesophageal pH probe is so superior to the barium swallow examination and esophagoscopy in determining abnormal reflux that it is virtually a mandatory tool in the armamentarium of any esophageal surgeon who claims to have an operation that controls reflux. It is only with insistence that an anti-reflux operation provide *objective* evidence of reflux control that the quality of our long-term operative results in this challenging area will improve.

Two additional nonresective operative techniques for managing peptic stricture and esophageal shortening should be mentioned. The fundic patch technique of Thal (Thal *et al.*, 1965) was originally described for use in patients with reflux strictures, and unfortunately, this procedure was subsequently applied to a variety of problems of the esophagogastric junction (hiatal hernia with reflux esophagitis, achalasia, and perforation) (Thal, 1968) with the mistaken notion that it could prevent gastroesophageal reflux. It was soon recognized that addition of a Nissen fundoplication to the Thal operation was required for reflux control (Thomas *et al.*, 1972; Woodward, 1975; Hollenbeck and Woodward, 1975) (Fig. 25–37). There are two primary objections to this approach: first, the necessity of intentionally incising and opening the most inflamed and diseased portion of the esophagus, to which the gastric fundus is then sutured with the

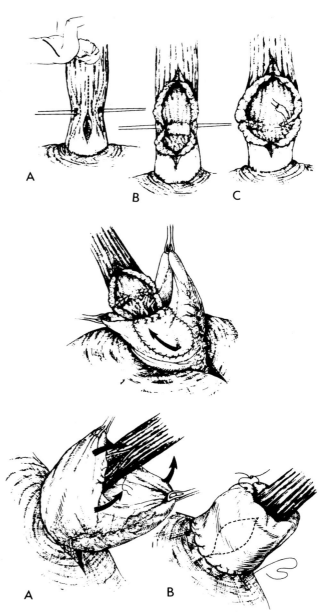

Figure 25–37. Combined Thal fundic patch operation and Nissen fundoplication for peptic esophageal stricture. *Upper panel: A,* Longitudinal incision of the stricture. *B,* The opened stricture. *C,* Transverse approximation of gastric fundus and esophagus, thus widening the stenotic area, but foreshortening the esophagus. *Middle panel:* The serosa of the gastric fundus is covered with a split-thickness skin graft and then rotated upward to fill the esophageal defect. *Lower panel: A,* The fundic patch is sutured into the esophageal defect. *B,* The fundus is wrapped around the lower esophagus and sutured to itself. (From Thomas, H. F., Clarke, J. M., Rayl, J. E., and Woodward, E. R.: Results of the combined fundic patch-fundoplication operation in the treatment of reflux esophagitis with stricture. Surg. Gynecol. Obstet., *135*:241, 1972. By permission of Surgery, Gynecology and Obstetrics.)

expectation that it will heal; and second, the need for an intrathoracic fundoplication, in effect, a man-made paraesophageal hiatal hernia. With this operation, not only have problems with suture line disruption been appreciable (Strug *et al.*, 1974), but also the mechanical complications of a paraesophageal hernia have

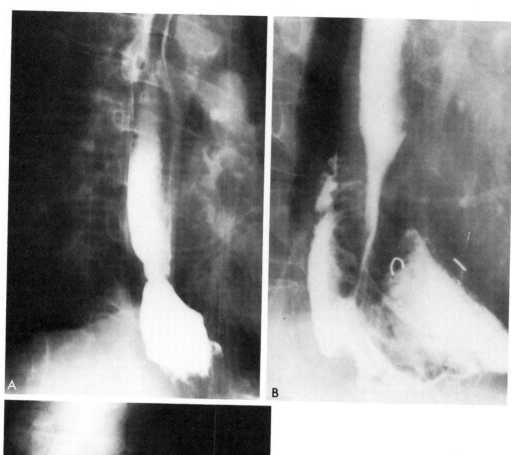

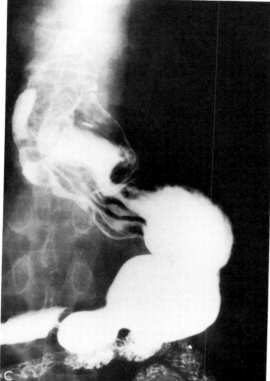

Figure 25–38. *A,* Preoperative esophagogram showing sliding hiatal hernia with mild proximal esophageal stenosis and esophageal shortening associated with reflux esophagitis. *B,* Postoperative appearance after Thal fundic patch and Nissen fundoplication. Distal esophagus is wrapped by the intrathoracic fundoplication. *C,* Postoperative esophagogram in the same patient showing intrathoracic fundic wrap. This patient was referred with recurrent bouts of chest pain related to intermittent distention of his intrathoracic stomach. His esophageal obstruction had been exchanged for this paraesophageal hiatal hernia and its attendant complications.

been well documented (Polk, 1976; Richardson and Polk, 1981) (Fig. 25–38). For the same reasons, although an intrathoracic fundoplication alone can provide a competent distal esophageal sphincter mechanism (Krupp and Rossetti, 1966; Safaie-Shirazi et al., 1974, 1975), the potential hazards of incarceration, strangulation, and bleeding from the intrathoracic stomach are quite real (Burnett et al., 1977; Rossman et al., 1979). We believe it is *always* preferable to restore the fundoplication to the abdomen whenever possible to avoid these complications, and we therefore favor the combined Collis gastroplasty–fundoplication technique when confronted with a dilatable peptic stricture and/or short esophagus.

In the rare instance in which a stricture proves to be nondilatable or attempts at dilatation result in esophageal disruption, resectional therapy and visceral esophageal substitution are required. Although jejunal interposition is an effective method of distal esophageal replacement, this technique has inherent difficulties with the delicate blood supply and length limitations of the jejunum. Colonic interposition with isoperistaltic left colon based on the ascending branch of the left colic artery is an excellent alternative that offers a more constant blood supply and greater length for esophageal reconstruction (Belsey, 1965). The relative ease of mobilization of the left and transverse colon through a left thoracoabdominal incision permits one-stage esophageal resection and replacement of either the distal or the entire thoracic esophagus (Orringer et al., 1977). The naturally alkaline mucous secretions of the colon resist acid regurgitation from the stomach. Despite these advantages, colonic interposition remains a formidable operation in elderly or nutritionally depleted patients with esophageal obstruction. Increasing experience with *total* thoracic esophagectomy and esophageal replacement using the stomach anastomosed to the cervical esophagus indicates that this may be the best option in patients requiring esophageal resection for benign disease. Not only is the early postoperative danger from an intrathoracic anastomotic leak eliminated with this approach, but also the troublesome gastroesophageal reflux associated with an intrathoracic esophagogastric anastomosis is virtually nonexistent when the entire stomach is mobilized into the chest for a cervical anastomosis (Orringer and Sloan, 1978).

SELECTED REFERENCES

Hayward, J.: The treatment of fibrous stricture of the oesophagus associated with hiatal hernia. Thorax, 16:45, 1961.

Based on his success with 14 patients with tough, fibrous strictures, this Australian surgeon was the first to express his view that resection of such stenoses is "seldom, if ever, needed and that good results can be obtained by repair of the hernia, dilatation of the stricture to the point of internal splitting at the time of operation, and post-operative dilatation by self bougienage. . . ." Although his contribution is seldom acknowledged, his conviction that fibrous tissue associated with reflux esophagitis will regress if the inflammatory stimulus can be eliminated is the foundation for the modern surgical approach to peptic esophageal strictures.

Henderson, R. D.: Reflux control following gastroplasty. Ann. Thorac. Surg., 24:206, 1977.

Liberalizing the use of the combined Collis gastroplasty–fundoplication operation for control of gastroesophageal reflux and its complications, the author reports his experience with 135 patients undergoing the Collis-Belsey procedure and with 78 patients undergoing a "new" combination — the Collis gastroplasty combined with a Nissen-type 360-degree fundoplication (Collis-Nissen procedure). Among the patients who underwent the Collis-Belsey procedure, 44.6 per cent had unsatisfactory reflux control (demonstrated in all radiographically and in 25.7 per cent symptomatically) after an average follow-up of 2.8 years. Among the patients who underwent the Collis-Nissen procedure, after an average follow-up of 10.7 months, there was no evidence of recurrent reflux. The superiority of a total fundoplication, as opposed to a partial Belsey fundoplication, after performance of the gastroplasty is stressed. The author's use of the combined Collis-Nissen procedure in *all* patients requiring surgical control of reflux (not only those with strictures and esophageal shortening) may unfairly "skew" his good results, since patients with "uncomplicated" reflux might be expected to do well after any of the standard hiatal hernia repairs. Long-term follow-up of these patients is obviously needed.

Hill, L. D., Gelfand, M., and Bauermeister, D.: Simplified management of reflux esophagitis with stricture. Ann. Surg., 172:638, 1970.

This is a report of a group of 36 patients with esophageal strictures treated by dilatation of the stricture and Hill's median arcuate ligament (posterior gastropexy) repair. Using intraesophageal pH and manometric studies, the authors demonstrated the existence of a lower esophageal sphincter well below the squamocolumnar epithelial junction in patients with a Barrett's esophagus, thus proving that these strictures did not, in fact, occur at the anatomic esophagogastric junction and that Barrett's concept of the "short esophagus" was incorrect. Good to excellent results were obtained in 85 per cent of the reported patients for varying periods of follow-up as long as 6 years. With this report, Hill became the first proponent in this country of the nonresective operative approach to peptic esophageal strictures.

Orringer, M. B., and Sloan, H.: Complications and failings of the combined Collis-Belsey operation. J. Thorac. Cardiovasc. Surg., 74:726, 1977.

This report reviews a series of 83 patients with "risk factors" predisposing to recurrent reflux after standard hiatal hernia repairs who underwent the Collis-Belsey procedure. Fifty-three per cent (44) of these patients had reflux esophagitis, and 30 per cent (25) had peptic strictures. There were two postoperative deaths. Complications included splenic injury (three patients); gastrocutaneous fistula (two patients); ischemic necrosis of the esophagus (two patients); and esophageal perforation (two patients). In addition to postoperative interviews and barium swallows, 77 patients were evaluated with esophageal manometry and acid reflux testing with the intraesophageal pH electrode. After an average follow-up of 12 months, 19 per cent had symptomatic reflux, but 30 per cent had moderate to severe reflux as demonstrated by pH reflux testing. It is suggested that construction of the gastroplasty tube so reduces the area of gastric fundus ordinarily available for the standard 240-degree Belsey fundoplication that an adequate Mark IV operation often cannot be achieved. Cautious, continued, *objective* assessment of the long-term results of the Collis-Belsey operation is urged.

Pearson, F. G., and Henderson, R. D.: Long-term follow-up of peptic strictures managed by dilatation, modified Collis gastroplasty, and Belsey hiatus hernia repair. Surgery, 80:396, 1976.

This report reviews results in 33 patients with peptic strictures operated on more than 5 years earlier. Among 26 patients followed 5 to 12 years since operation, 25 have had sustained excellent results, being able to eat a regular diet without dysphagia or reflux symptoms. There were no operative deaths in this series, and one esophageal perforation was sustained during dilatation. This experience provides convincing evidence that in patients with dilatable peptic strictures, dependable reflux control can be achieved with the combined Collis-Belsey procedure. However, although 24 of these patients had postoperative esophageal manometric studies, objective documentation of reflux control with the intraesophageal pH probe was not obtained.

Pearson, F. G., Langer, B., and Henderson, R. D.: Gastroplasty and Belsey hiatus hernia repair. J. Thorac. Cardiovasc. Surg., 61:50, 1971.

This is the initial description of the results of the combination of the esophageal-lengthening Collis gastroplasty and Belsey Mark IV hiatal hernia repair in patients with peptic strictures with acquired short esophagus. Utilizing this innovative and conceptually sound method for avoiding both tension on the hiatal hernia repair as well as the need to suture to the inflamed distal esophagus in patients with peptic esophagitis and stricture, the authors report complete subjective relief of reflux in 22 of 24 patients and completely normal subjective swallowing in 17 patients after follow-up ranging from 3 months to 5½ years. This pioneering work has been the dominant influence in the improved operative approach toward peptic strictures during the past decade.

Skinner, D. B., Belsey, R. H. R., Hendrix, T. R., and Zuidema, G. D. (Eds.): Gastroesophageal Reflux and Hiatal Hernia. Boston, Little, Brown and Company, 1972.

This concise, authoritative book has become a key reference for those wishing to understand the pathophysiology, diagnosis, and treatment of reflux and its complications. Written by nine authors, this text provides particularly strong sections on the pathophysiology of reflux esophagitis (Chapter 5); techniques of esophagoscopy (Chapter 8); management of esophageal strictures (Chapter 14); and current diagnostic tests used to evaluate normal and abnormal esophageal function (Chapter 7).

REFERENCES

Adler, R. H.: The lower esophagus lined by columnar epithelium: Its association with hiatal hernia, ulcer, stricture, and tumor. J. Thorac. Cardiovasc. Surg., 45:13, 1963.

Allison, P. R.: Peptic ulcer of oesophagus. Thorax, 3:30, 1948.

Allison, P. R., and Johnstone, A. S.: The esophagus lined with gastric mucous membrane. Thorax, 8:87, 1953.

Allison, P. R., Johnstone, A. S., and Royce, G. B.: Short esophagus with simple peptic ulceration. J. Thorac. Surg., 12:432, 1943.

Barnes, W. A., and Redo, S. F.: Evaluation of esophagojejunostomy in the treatment of lesions at the esophagogastric junction. Ann. Surg., 146:224, 1957.

Barrett, N. R.: Chronic peptic ulcer of the oesophagus and "oesophagitis." Br. J. Surg., 38:175, 1950.

Belsey, R.: Diaphragmatic hernia. In Modern Trends in Gastroenterology. New York, Hoeber, 1952, pp. 128–178.

Belsey, R. H.: Reconstruction of the esophagus with left colon. J. Thorac. Cardiovasc. Surg., 49:33, 1965.

Bombeck, C. T., Coelko, R. C. P., and Nyhus, L. M.: Prevention of gastroesophageal reflux after resection of the lower esophagus. Surg. Gynecol. Obstet., 130:1035, 1970.

Burnett, H. F., Read, R. C., Morris, W. D., and Campbell, G. S.: Management of complications of fundoplication and Barrett's esophagus. Ann. Surg., 82:521, 1977.

Clarke, J. M., and Woodward, E. R.: Transthoracic fundoplication for hiatal hernia and short esophagus in a 3-year-old child: Case report. Surgery, 64:858, 1968.

Code, C. F., Creamer, B., Schlegel, J. F., et al.: An Atlas of Esophageal Motility in Health and Disease. Springfield, Illinois, Charles C Thomas, 1958.

Collis, J. L.: An operation for hiatus hernia with short esophagus. Thorax, 12:181, 1957.

Collis, J. L.: Gastroplasty. Thorax, 16:197, 1961.

Demos, N., and Biele, R. M.: Intercostal pedicle method for control of postresection esophagitis. J. Thorac. Cardiovasc. Surg., 80:679, 1980.

Donnelly, R. J., Deverall, P. B., and Watson, D. A.: Hiatus hernia with and without stricture: Experience with the Belsey Mark IV repair. Ann. Thorac. Surg., 16:301, 1973.

Dunlop, E. E.: Problems in the treatment of reflux oesophagitis. Gastroenterologica, 86:287, 1956.

Ellis, F. H., Jr., Anderson, H. A., and Clagett, O. T.: Treatment of short esophagus with stricture by esophagogastrectomy and antral excision. Ann. Surg., 148:526, 1958.

Ellis, F. H., Jr., Leonardi, H. K., Dabuzhsky, L., et al.: Surgery for short esophagus with stricture: An experimental and clinical manometric study. Ann. Surg., 188:341, 1978.

Hayward, J.: The treatment of fibrous stricture of the esophagus associated with hiatus hernias. Thorax, 16:45, 1961.

Heimlich, H. J.: Peptic esophagitis with stricture treated by reconstruction of the esophagus with a reversed gastric tube. Surg. Gynecol. Obstet., 114:673, 1962.

Heimlich, H. J.: Esophagoplasty with reversed gastric tube. Am. J. Surg., 123:80, 1972.

Henderson, R. D.: Reflux control following gastroplasty. Ann. Thorac. Surg., 24:206, 1977.

Henderson, R. D., and Pearson, F. G.: Surgical management of esophageal scleroderma. J. Thorac. Cardiovasc. Surg., 66:686, 1973.

Herrington, J. L., Jr., Wright, R. S., Edwards, W. H., et al.: Conservative surgical treatment of reflux esophagitis and esophageal stricture. Ann. Surg., 181:552, 1975.

Hill, L. D., Gelfand, M., and Bauermeister, D.: Simplified management of reflux esophagitis with stricture. Ann. Surg., 172:638, 1970.

Hollenbeck, J. I., and Woodward, E. R.: Treatment of peptic esophageal stricture with combined fundic patch fundoplication. Ann. Surg., 182:472, 1975.

Ingelfinger, F. J.: Esophageal motility. Physiol. Rev., 38:533, 1958.

Krupp, S., and Rossetti, M.: Surgical treatment of hiatal hernia by fundoplication and gastropexy (Nissen repair). Ann. Surg., 164:927, 1966.

Merendino, K. A., and Dillard, D. H.: The concept of sphincter substitution by an interposed jejunal segment for anatomic and physiologic abnormalities at the esophagogastric junction. Ann. Surg., 142:486, 1955.

Mossberg, S. M.: The columnar lined esophagus (Barrett's syndrome): An acquired condition? Gastroenterology, 50:671, 1966.

Naef, A. P., and Savary, M.: Conservative operations for peptic esophagitis with stenosis in columnar-lined lower esophagus. Ann. Thorac. Surg., 13:543, 1972.

Naef, A. P., Savary, M., and Ozello, L.: Columnar-lined lower esophagus: An acquired lesion with malignant predisposition. J. Thorac. Cardiovasc. Surg., 70:826, 1975.

Neville, W. E., and Clowes, G. H. A., Jr.: Surgical treatment of the complications resulting from cardioesophageal incompetence. Dis. Chest., 43:572, 1963.

Okada, N., Kuriyama, T., Urmemoto, H., et al.: Esophageal surgery: A procedure for posterior invagination esophagogastrostomy in one stage without positional change. Ann. Surg., 179:27, 1974.

Orringer, M B., and Orringer, J. S.: Combined Collis-gastroplasty-fundoplication for scleroderma reflux esophagitis. Surgery, 90:624, 1981.

Orringer, M. B., and Sloan, H. E.: An improved technique for the combined Collis-Belsey approach to dilatable esophageal strictures. J. Thorac. Cardiovasc. Surg., 68:298, 1974.

Orringer, M. B., and Sloan, H. E.: Collis-Belsey reconstruction of the esophagogastric junction. J. Thorac. Cardiovasc. Surg., 71:295, 1976.

Orringer, M. B., and Sloan, H.: Complications and failings of the combined Collis-Belsey operation. J. Thorac. Cardiovasc. Surg., 74:726, 1977.

Orringer, M. B., and Sloan, H.: Combined Collis-Nissen reconstruction of the esophagogastric junction. Ann. Thorac. Surg., 25:16, 1978.

Orringer, M. B., and Sloan, H.: Esophagectomy without thoracotomy. J. Thorac. Cardiovasc. Surg., 76:643, 1978.

Orringer, M. B., Kirsh, M. M., and Sloan, H.: Esophageal reconstruction for benign disease. J. Thorac. Cardiovasc. Surg., 73:807, 1977.

Orringer, M. B., Skinner, D. B., and Belsey, R. H. R.: Long-term results of the Mark IV operation for hiatal hernia and analyses of recurrences and their treatment. J. Thorac. Cardiovasc. Surg., 63:25, 1972.

Orringer, M. B., Dabich, L., Zarafonetis, C. J. D., and Sloan, H.: Gastroesophageal reflux in esophageal scleroderma: Diagnosis and implications. Ann. Thorac. Surg., 22:120, 1976.

Payne, W. S.: Surgical treatment of reflux esophagitis and stricture associated with permanent incompetence of the cardia. Mayo Clin. Proc., 45:553, 1970.

Pearson, F. G.: Surgical management of acquired short esophagus with dilatable peptic stricture. World J. Surg., 1:463, 1977.

Pearson, F. G., and Henderson, R. D.: Experimental and clinical studies of gastroplasty in the management of acquired short esophagus. Surg. Gynecol. Obstet., 136:737, 1973.

Pearson, F. G., and Henderson, R. D.: Long-term follow-up of peptic strictures managed by dilatation, modified Collis gastroplasty, and Belsey hiatus hernia repair. Surgery, 80:396, 1976.

Pearson, F. G., Langer, B., and Henderson, R. D.: Gastroplasty and Belsey hiatal hernia repair. J. Thorac. Cardiovasc. Surg., 61:50, 1971.

Polk, H. C., Jr.: Fundoplication for reflux esophagitis: Misadventures with the choice of operation. Ann. Surg., 183:645, 1976.

Popov, V. I.: Reconstruction of the esophagus in cases of stricture. Arch. Surg., 82:226, 1961.

Richardson, J. D., and Polk, H. S., Jr.: Intrathoracic fundoplication for shortened esophagus: A treacherous solution to a challenging problem. Presented at the Society of the Alimentary Tract. New York, May 19–20, 1981.

Rossman, F., Brantigan, C. O., and Sawyer, R. B.: Obstructive complications of the Nissen fundoplication. Am. J. Surg., 138:860, 1979.

Safaie-Shirazi, S., Zike, W. L., and Masson, E. E.: Esophageal stricture secondary to reflux esophagitis. Arch. Surg., 110:629, 1975.

Safaie-Shirazi, S., Zike, W. L., Anuras, S., Condon, R. E., and Denbestein, L.: Nissen fundoplication without crural repair. Arch. Surg., 108:424, 1974.

Skinner, D. B., and Belsey, R. H. R.: Surgical management of esophageal reflux and hiatus hernia. J. Thorac. Cardiovasc. Surg., 53:33, 1967.

Skinner, D. B., Belsey, R. H. R., Hendrix, T. R., and Zuidema, G. D. (Eds.): Gastroesophageal Reflux and Hiatal Hernia. Boston, Little, Brown and Company, 1972.

Strug, B. S., Jordan, P. H., Jr., and Jordan, G. L., Jr.: Surgical management of benign esophageal strictures. Surg. Gynecol. Obstet., 138:74, 1974.

Tanner, N. C.: Treatment of oesophageal hiatus hernia. Lancet, 2:1050, 1955.

Thal, A. P.: A unified approach to surgical problems of the esophagogastric junction. Ann. Surg., 168:542, 1968.

Thal, A. P., Hatafuker, T., and Kurtzman, R.: New operation for distal esophageal stricture. Arch. Surg., 90:464, 1965.

Thomas, H. G., Clarke, J. M., Rayl, J. E., and Woodward, E. R.: Results of the combined fundic patch–fundoplication operation in the treatment of reflux esophagitis with stricture. Surg. Gynecol. Obstet., 135:241, 1972.

Tileston, W.: Peptic ulcer of the oesophagus. Am. J. Med. Sci., 132:240, 1906.

Toledo-Pereyra, L. H., Michel, H., Manifacio, G., and Humphrey, E. W.: Management of acid peptic esophageal strictures. J. Thorac. Cardiovasc. Surg., 72:518, 1976.

Tuttle, S. G., and Grossman, M. I.: Detection of gastroesophageal reflux by simultaneous measurement of intraluminal pressures on pH. Proc. Soc. Exp. Biol. Med., 98:225, 1958.

Urschel, H. C., Razzuk, M. A., Wood, R. E., Galbraith, N., and Paulson, D. L.: An improved surgical technique for the complicated hiatal hernia with gastroesophageal reflux. Ann. Thorac. Surg., 15:443, 1973.

Woodward, E. R.: Sliding esophageal hiatal hernia and reflux peptic esophagitis. Mayo Clin. Proc., 50:523, 1975.

VII HIATAL HERNIA, REFLUX, AND DYSPHAGIA AFTER VAGOTOMY

R. W. POSTLETHWAIT

After the descriptions by Dragstedt and Owens in 1943 of vagotomy for duodenal ulcer, the operation rapidly attained widespread application. Compared with resection of two thirds of the stomach, vagotomy offered lower immediate morbidity and mortality, as well as fewer late complications, including ulcer recurrence. The operative complications of vagotomy, mainly splenic injury and esophageal perforation, are well recognized. The complications of hiatal hernia (Fig. 25–39), reflux, and dysphagia after vagotomy are the subject of this section.

HIATAL HERNIA

Transthoracic vagotomy is seldom performed, except for recurrent ulcer following incomplete division of the vagus nerves. Truncal vagotomy through an abdominal incision is properly called a supradiaphragmatic vagotomy, however, because of the extent of the dissection above the diaphragm. After the peritoneum is divided anterior to the esophagus, the esophagus is dissected from its posterior attachments, mainly to the right crus, and elevated. A tape around the esophagus provides traction, and the lower part of the esophagus is mobilized into the mediastinum for 5 to 6 cm. This allows identification of the vagus nerves and any branches and permits an adequate segment of each nerve to be removed. In parietal cell vagotomy, dissection of the esophagus is more extensive.

This mobilization of the cardia and lower part of the esophagus effectively destroys the major anatomic structure anchoring the esophagus in position, the phrenoesophageal ligament. Exploration months or years later will most frequently show the cardia and

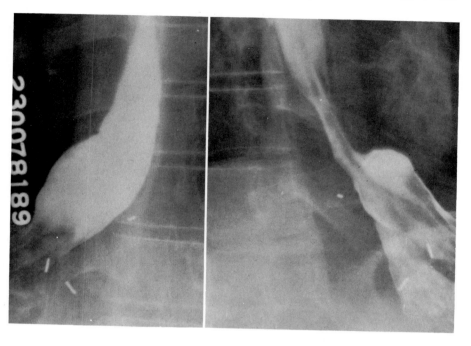

Figure 25–39. A 46-year-old man developed regurgitation when recumbent or bending 3 months after vagotomy. Hernia was demonstrated, as shown. The patient has done well with nonoperative treatment.

lower esophagus in normal position, secured by adhesions of variable extent. After operation, however, for a period of 5 days or more before adhesion formation, the cardia and esophagus are relatively mobile and free to migrate into the mediastinum (Fig. 25–40). Factors favoring this migration include abdominal distention, which increases the intra-abdominal pressure, the negative intrathoracic pressure, contraction of the longitudinal muscle of the esophagus, and pre-existing hiatal hernia.

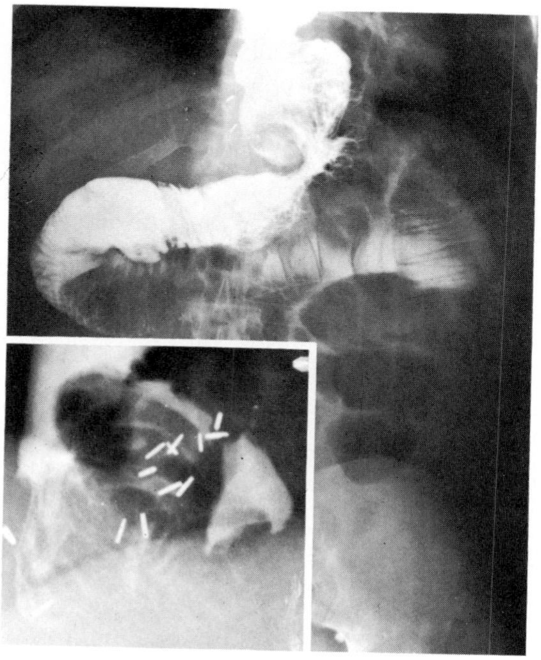

Incidence

In 1948, Beal reported the first hiatal hernia after transabdominal vagotomy, which later required transthoracic repair. Subsequent reports have consisted of only a few patients, usually those with severe symptoms or complications, but have not stated the total number of patients who had vagotomy, so that the incidence cannot be determined. Of 135 patients who did not have herniation preoperatively, we found, utilizing cineradiography, herniation in 11 per cent 6 months to 5 years after vagotomy. This high frequency is surprising, considering the thousands of vagotomies that have been performed. It is probable that many are not recognized, either because reflux is minimal or because of the reduction in acid pepsin production following the primary operation.

Of greater importance is the frequency of symptomatic reflux of gastric contents into the esophagus after vagotomy. In one series of 150 patients, 45 had regurgitation and heartburn after vagotomy, but the symptoms persisted in only 10 patients and were severe in only two (Williams and Woodward, 1967). In our 135 patients, nine had reflux, and two of these had symptoms that were minor.

Pathophysiology

The anatomic changes produced by vagotomy that were noted above are, at least in part, the basis for possible physiologic alterations, whether an actual hernia is demonstrable or not. That incompetence and

Figure 25–40. A 61-year-old man had truncal vagotomy and gastroenterostomy for obstruction due to ulcer. He became acutely ill on the tenth postoperative day, and his stomach was shown to be above the diaphragm. He underwent immediate operation with subsequent recovery.

reflux can occur in the absence of hiatal hernia is well known. Enlargement of the hiatus and cephalad displacement of the lower esophageal sphincter area, less than that required to permit radiographic demonstration of an actual hernia, might be expected to increase the tendency for reflux to occur.

Manometric studies after vagotomy have not been entirely in agreement. In dogs, a significant decline in pressure in the subhiatal portion of the sphincter was found, although coordination with swallowing was not affected (Elebute *et al.*, 1966). In another study, 10 patients showed no change in resting sphincter pressure after truncal vagotomy, but the response of the sphincter to abdominal compression was less than normal (Crispin *et al.*, 1967). This decrease of response with abdominal compression was confirmed in 26 patients who also had truncal vagotomy (Angorn *et al.*, 1977). In two other studies, a transient decrease of sphincter pressure was noted in one and no change in the other, but in both significant decrease after gastric resection was found (Mann and Hardcastle, 1967; Thomas and Earlam, 1972). Another interesting study showed no effect on the pressure and negative pH reflux tests in 12 patients. Subsequently, one patient developed symptomatic reflux and had a reduced high-pressure zone (Mazur *et al.*, 1973). An investigation of 80 patients after various types of vagotomy (33 were parietal cell vagotomies) showed no change in sphincter pressure or the incidence of reflux (Csendes *et al.*, 1979). Another study of 20 patients confirmed these findings (Oomen *et al.*, 1979). In dogs, truncal vagotomy resulted in a marked decrease in response to abdominal compression, which did not occur after parietal cell vagotomy (Khan, 1981).

Gastrin increases lower esophageal sphincter pressure, and one review suggests that the gastrin effect may be more important than the anatomic location of the sphincter (Cohen and Harris, 1972). Fasting gastrin decreases significantly after vagotomy and antrectomy but does not decrease after vagotomy and pyloroplasty (McGuigan and Trudeau, 1972). Selective vagotomy with drainage and parietal cell vagotomy are followed by increased gastrin, the increase being higher in patients who undergo the latter (Csendes *et al.*, 1979).

From the available evidence, the anatomic disturbance incident to the vagotomy is the major factor in hiatal hernia formation and may be most significant in the cause of reflux. A neurogenic basis does not appear feasible. Gastrin should theoretically prevent reflux rather than cause it, particularly after vagotomy and drainage.

Prevention

In every report of hiatal hernia following vagotomy, some form of repair of the hiatus is recommended as a preventive measure. Our preference is the Nissen fundoplication, with the Hill repair being a second choice. Mobilization of the esophagus is more extensive during parietal cell vagotomy, and the anatomy may be sufficiently altered to cause herniation. Experience is inadequate to determine this, but routine reconstruction may be advisable.

Demonstration of hiatal hernia preoperatively, or such a finding at operation, would indicate the necessity for repair whether or not symptoms are present.

Treatment

The radiographic or manometric demonstration of a hiatal hernia and reflux does not necessarily require operation (except, of course, in the case of paraesophageal hernia with the possibility of obstruction or strangulation). As indicated previously, many of these patients with slight or moderate degrees of reflux are asymptomatic. This may be due in part to the decreased acid level of the refluxed gastric content. Conversely, an extremely severe esophagitis may be caused by reflux of alkaline bile and pancreatic juice. Basically, therefore, the indications for operation are the same as those for any patient with hernia and reflux. The decision is based on the symptomatology, radiographic studies, and endoscopic findings.

The operation must be individualized for the patient. A transthoracic Belsey repair is technically easier for the surgeon and probably less disturbing for the patient. In addition, if the completeness of the vagotomy is in question, this can be corrected at the same time. If other factors, such as outlet obstruction, indicate the desirability of an abdominal approach, the transabdominal route should be employed. The adhesions subsequent to the previous operation can be anticipated to cause more difficult dissection, but a Nissen or Hill repair can usually be accomplished. A large tube such as a Maloney dilator placed in the esophagus will aid in identification of the proper planes for mobilization of the esophagus. Once the esophagus is elevated, the abdominal aspects of the crura will be exposed, thus permitting dissection inferior to the median arcuate ligament.

In an occasional patient with alkaline reflux esophagitis, conversion to a Roux-en-Y anastomosis to divert duodenal juices well down into the jejunum will produce relief (Mackman *et al.*, 1971). We have performed this procedure in severe patients, accompanied by an anti-reflux procedure when possible.

Results

Hiatal hernia repair after vagotomy is rarely identified separately in reports of results of hiatal hernia repair in general. One report of 10 patients who had had hiatal hernia repair for bilious vomiting after vagotomy noted good results (Turner, 1973).

DYSPHAGIA

In 1947, Moses described the first patient with dysphagia after vagotomy, manifested by achalasia-like changes that persisted for 5 weeks. That same year, Grimson and associates reported temporary difficulty in swallowing in 21 of 57 patients who had had vagotomy. Since then, dysphagia has frequently been described as a complication of vagotomy.

Incidence

The reported incidence of dysphagia after vagotomy ranges from 0 to 37 per cent. The wide differences are difficult to explain. An example is the review of 114 papers by Cox and associates (1969), who found the incidence of dysphagia to be 17.9 per cent in 262 patients after vagotomy and drainage and 0.7 per cent in 405 patients after vagotomy and antrectomy. They suggested that the difference is "probably related to the uncritical approval accorded by many authors" to the latter operation. In reviewing collected reports of a total of 5267 patients who had truncal vagotomy in which the authors specifically mentioned dysphagia, we found this complication occurred in 3.6 per cent.

In one series of 748 patients, the incidence of dysphagia was 9 per cent after selective vagotomy and drainage, 4 per cent after selective vagotomy and antrectomy, 6 per cent after parietal cell vagotomy and drainage, and 12 per cent after parietal cell vagotomy alone (Amdrup *et al.*, 1978). The authors emphasize that the dysphagia is nearly always relieved by 3 months.

Etiology

The cause of postvagotomy dysphagia can usually be attributed to one of the following:
1. An unrecognized preoperative esophageal disorder.
2. Temporary neurogenic or hormonal imbalance.
3. Transient periesophageal inflammatory reaction.
4. Periesophageal fibrosis.
5. Stricture of the esophagus.

In the average patient with duodenal ulcer and no esophageal symptoms, the focus of the radiologist is on the duodenum; cineradiographic studies are infrequently done, and manometric studies are not performed. A small hernia or a minor degree of esophageal spasm are readily overlooked.

Experimental studies in animals have not yielded consistent results, but division of the vagus nerves in the neck or as low as the hilum frequently produces spasm of the lower portion of the esophagus. Manometric studies in patients after vagotomy have been described previously. Of considerable interest are the manometric studies by Anderson and colleagues (1966) on 15 patients who had dysphagia after vagotomy. One group of these patients showed absence of relaxation of the sphincter area with swallowing and sometimes atonicity of a part of the esophagus, suggesting to them a disruption of the normal innervation. The other group had normal relaxation with swallowing and normal or increased tone of the esophageal musculature, indicating to them periesophageal edema or fibrosis at the hiatus causing mechanical obstruction. A neurogenic imbalance, such as altered gastrin secretion or response to gastrin, remains a possible cause of the dysphagia, but proof is not available at present.

Periesophageal inflammatory reaction, essentially edema due to the trauma of the vagotomy, probably occurs to a variable degree in most patients, but again, confirmation is lacking, because the dysphagia is transient and a second operation is rarely necessary to prove this. We have examined by careful cineradiographic study 15 patients within 10 days after vagotomy. Five showed narrowing of the lower part of the esophagus, and it was severe in one. None had dysphagia. The radiologist interpreted the narrowing as being due to spasm, but edema around the esophagus could not be excluded.

Inflammation, edema, hematoma, and possible infection around the esophagus would be expected occasionally to lead to fibrous tissue formation sufficient to compromise the esophageal lumen. The first reported patient had an extensive periesophageal mass of scar tissue requiring esophageal resection (Bruce and Small, 1959). Histologic study showed the outer muscle layer encased but uninvolved by the fibrous tissue. We know of eight other reported cases, including our own. The collar of scar tissue can usually be removed without disturbing the esophagus.

The possible development of reflux with or without hiatal hernia has already been discussed. Whether the reflux material is acid or alkaline, an esophagitis of sufficient severity to cause stricture may result. The sensitivity of the esophageal epithelium to acid-pepsin has long been known. Recent interest in alkaline gastritis and esophagitis has prompted additional studies, two of which are particularly interesting; both were based on back diffusion studies in animals. Briefly, with an acid pH, the conjugated bile salts caused the diffusion and mucosal injury; with a neutral or alkaline pH, the deconjugated bile salts were the cause (Kivilaakso *et al.*, 1980; Harmon *et al.*, 1981).

Another factor causing reflux, not peculiar to vagotomy, is a nasogastric tube. Studies of normal subjects have demonstrated the frequency of reflux around a nasogastric tube when the subjects were in the supine position (Nagler and Spiro, 1963). The exact mechanism is not understood, although it may be due to trapping of the refluxed juice in the esophagus.

Diagnosis and Treatment

The most common transient dysphagia after vagotomy has its onset any time from the first intake of food to the third, and rarely the fourth, week after vagotomy. The food lodges in the lower esophagus,

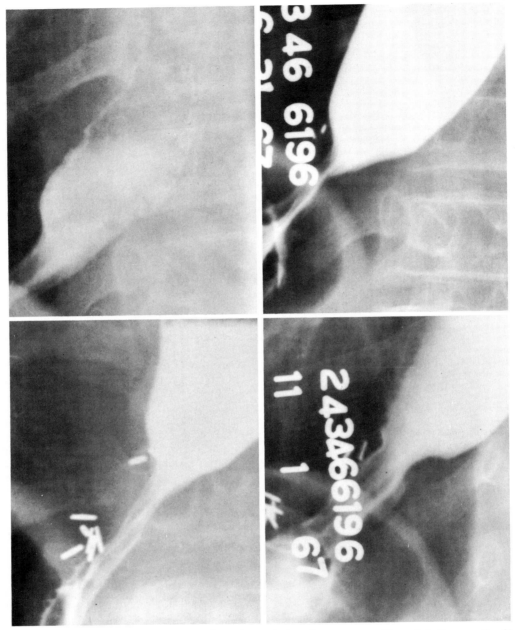

Figure 25–41. A 63-year-old male developed dysphagia on the tenth day after vagotomy. *Upper left,* Preoperative film. *Upper right,* Narrowing of esophagus when dysphagia developed. *Lower left,* Film after one dilatation. *Lower right,* Film 5 months later when patient was asymptomatic.

but the referral of the sensation may be to the epigastric, substernal, or even cervical region. As with any obstruction, retching, regurgitation, and excessive mucus may result. Pain is usually not prominent, although discomfort is present. Radiographically, the lower part of the esophagus is narrowed to a variable degree, sometimes tapered, and may not transmit the peristaltic wave. Esophagoscopy shows normal mucosa with narrowing of the lower portion, usually the distal few centimeters. After return to a liquid diet for a few days, soft and then solid food will be tolerated by most patients. If the dysphagia persists, dilatation will be necessary, and prompt relief usually follows one or two dilatations (Fig. 25–41).

Periesophageal fibrosis is manifested by a later onset of dysphagia, which is progressive in severity, and failure to respond to dilatation. Barium radiographic study shows the smooth narrowing, the extent, of course, depending on the periesophageal area involved. The firm stricture may be confirmed by endoscopy. As noted previously, Anderson and associates felt that manometric study might differentiate

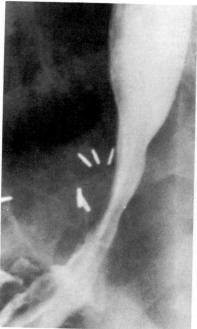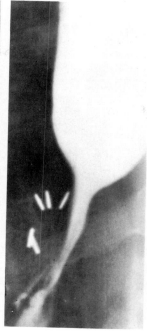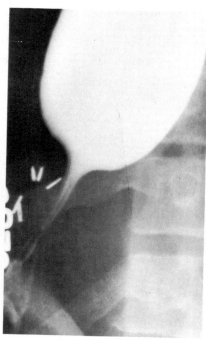

Figure 25–42. A 38-year-old man underwent vagotomy and gastroenterostomy. He returned after discharge, with dysphagia starting on the eleventh postoperative day. The film on the left was made prior to discharge when he was swallowing normally. The center film was made on readmission. The patient's condition did not improve with dilatations, and the stricture became more severe, as shown on the right. At operation, a collar of periesophageal fibrous tissue was found to be causing obstruction. The patient is now asymptomatic.

spasm and periesophageal fibrosis. If prompt response to dilatation is not obtained, operation will be necessary, with division or excision of the collar of fibrous tissue (Fig. 25–42). Resection was required in two reported patients.

The diagnosis of hiatal hernia, reflux, and stricture after vagotomy does not differ from that for the usual patient. Similarly, the decision regarding treatment is based on the same criteria.

SELECTED REFERENCES

Bruce, J., and Small, W. P.: Dysphagia following vagotomy. J. R. Coll. Surg. Edin., *4*:170, 1959.

This is the first complete report of the various causes of dysphagia after vagotomy, based on 116 operations. Patients were appropriately studied, and the symptoms and radiologic changes are recorded.

Cohen, S., and Harris, L. D.: The lower esophageal sphincter. Gastroenterology, *63*:1066, 1972.

An excellent review of lower esophageal sphincter studies that emphasizes the hormonal effects. Recent studies, including the authors', are discussed, and the role of gastrin is described.

Csendes, A., Oster, M., Moller, J. T., Flynn, J., Funch-Jensen, P., Overgaard, H., and Amdrup, E.: Gastroesophageal reflux in duodenal ulcer patients before and after vagotomy. Ann. Surg., *188*:803, 1978.

The authors' 80 patients were carefully studied with regard to reflux symptoms and manometric and acid secretory changes after selective or parietal cell vagotomy.

Mazur, J. M., Skinner, D. B., Jones, E. L., and Zuidema, G. D.: Effect of transabdominal vagotomy on the human gastroesophageal high-pressure zone. Surgery, *73*:818, 1973.

This is an example of a thorough follow-up study of 12 patients after truncal vagotomy. Manometry, acid reflux, and acid clearing were carefully documented.

REFERENCES

Amdrup, E., Andersen, D., and Hostrup, H.: The Aarhus County vagotomy trial. I. An interim report on primary results and incidence of sequelae following parietal cell vagotomy and selective gastric vagotomy in 748 patients. World J. Surg., *2*:85, 1978.

Anderson, H. A., Schlegel, J. F., and Olsen, A. M.: Postvagotomy dysphagia. Gastrointest. Endosc., *12*:13, 1966.

Angorn, I. B., Dimopoulos, G., Hegarty, M. M., and Moshal, M. G.: The effect of vagotomy on the lower oesophageal sphincter: A manometric study. Br. J. Surg., *64*:466, 1977.

Beal, J. M.: Diaphragmatic hernia following subdiaphragmatic vagotomy: A case report. Surgery, *24*:625, 1948.

Bruce, J., and Small, W. P.: Dysphagia following vagotomy. J. R. Coll. Surg. Edin., *4*:170, 1959.

Cohen, S., and Harris, L. D.: The lower esophageal sphincter. Gastroenterology, *63*:1066, 1972.

Cox, A. G., Spencer, J., and Tinker, J.: Clinical results reviewed. *In* After Vagotomy. Edited by J. A. Williams and A. G. Cox. New York, Appleton-Century-Crofts, 1969, pp. 119–130.

Crispin, J. S., McIver, D. K., and Lind, J. F.: Manometric study of the effect of vagotomy on the gastroesophageal sphincter. Can. J. Surg., *10*:299, 1967.

Csendes, A., Oster, M., Moller, J., Brandsborg, O., Brandsborg, M., and Amdrup, E.: The effect of extrinsic denervation of the lower part of the esophagus on resting and cholinergic stimulated gastroesophageal sphincter in man. Surg. Gynecol. Obstet., *148*:375, 1979.

Csendes, A., Oster, M., Moller, J. J., Flynn, J., Funch-Jensen, P., Overgaard, H., and Amdrup, E.: Gastroesophageal reflux in duodenal ulcer patients before and after vagotomy. Ann. Surg., *188*:803, 1978.

Dragstedt, L. R., and Owens, F. M.: Supra-diaphragmatic section of the vagus nerves in treatment of duodenal ulcer. Proc. Soc. Exper. Biol. Med., *53*:152, 1943.

Elebute, E., Kelly, M. L., and Schwartz, S. I.: Pressure effects of transabdominal supra-diaphragmatic vagotomy on the inferior esophageal sphincter of dogs. Surg. Gynecol. Obstet., *123*:326, 1966.

Grimson, K. S., Baylin, G. J., Taylor, H. M., Hesser, F. H., and Rundles, R. W.: Transthoracic vagotomy. The effects in 57 patients with peptic ulcer and the clinical limitations. J.A.M.A., *14*:925, 1947.

Harmon, J. W., Johnson, L. F., and Maydonovitch, C. L.: Effects of acid and bile salts on the rabbit esophageal mucosa. Digest. Dis. Sci., *26*:65, 1981.

Khan, T. A.: Effect of proximal selective vagotomy on the canine lower esophageal sphincter. Am. J. Surg., *141*:219, 1981.

Kivilaakso, E., Fromm, D., and Silen, W.: Effect of bile salts and related compounds on isolated esophageal mucosa. Surgery, *87*:280, 1980.

Mackman, S., Lemmer, K. E., and Morrissey, J. R.: Postoperative reflux alkali gastritis and esophagitis. Am. J. Surg., *121*:694, 1971.

Mann, C. V., and Hardcastle, J. D.: Effect of vagotomy and partial gastrectomy on gastro-esophageal sphincter pressures. J. R. Coll. Surg. Edin., *12*:326, 1967.

Mazur, J. M., Skinner, D. B., Jones, E. L., and Zuidema, G. D.: Effect of transabdominal vagotomy on the human gastroesophageal high-pressure zone. Surgery, *73*:818, 1973.

McGuigan, J. E., and Trudeau, W. L.: Serum gastrin levels before and after vagotomy and pyloroplasty or vagotomy and antrectomy. N. Engl. J. Med., *286*:184, 1972.

Moses, W. R.: Critique on vagotomy. N. Engl. J. Med., *237*:603, 1947.

Nagler, R., and Spiro, H. M.: Persistent gastroesophageal reflux induced during prolonged gastric intubation. N. Engl. J. Med., *269*:490, 1963.

Oomen, J. P. C. M., Wittebol, P., Geurts, W. J. C., and Akkermans, L. M. A.: Lower esophageal sphincter function after highly selective vagotomy. Arch. Surg., *114*:908, 1979.

Postlethwait, R. W., Seuk, K. K., and Dillon, M. L.: Esophageal complications of vagotomy. Surg. Gynecol. Obstet., *128*:481, 1969.

Thomas, P., and Earlam, R.: The gastroesophageal junction in duodenal ulcer after operation. Br. J. Surg., *59*:309, 1972.

Turner, F. P.: Postoperative bilious vomiting: Treatment by repair of hiatus hernia. Arch. Surg., *106*:685, 1973.

Williams, J. A., and Woodward, D. A. K.: The effect of subdiaphragmatic vagotomy on the function of the gastroesophageal sphincter. Surg. Clin. North Am., *47*:1341, 1967.

Chapter 26

The Diaphragm

I THE DIAPHRAGM

MARVIN POMERANTZ

HISTORICAL BACKGROUND

Ambrose Paré is credited with reporting the first case of a traumatic diaphragmatic hernia in 1579 (Sutton *et al.*, 1967). He reported two autopsy cases, one patient dying 3 days after injury with stomach herniated through the diaphragmatic hole and the other dying 8 months following injury with a large portion of the colon herniated into the thorax. According to Allison (1969), Petit (1674–1750) described cases of diaphragmatic hernia and differentiated the congenital from the acquired varieties. In 1769, Morgagni wrote a monograph on diaphragmatic hernia, describing those varieties of hernias passing through natural diaphragmatic openings. In 1853, Bowditch was the first to make an antemortem clinical diagnosis of a ruptured diaphragm and to emphasize the clinical criteria for making this diagnosis. In 1886, Riolfi repaired a laceration of the diaphragm through which omentum had prolapsed, and in 1888, Naumann operated on a patient who had stomach herniated into the left chest through a traumatic diaphragmatic hernia (Grage *et al.*, 1959). In the twentieth century, surgery on the diaphragm, including congenital and acquired lesions, has increased in frequency, and at present, these procedures, which were once rare, are now common.

ANATOMY

Development of the diaphragm takes place between the eighth and tenth weeks of intrauterine life. The central portion of the diaphragm, which attaches to the costal cartilages and sternum, develops from the septum transversum, and the muscular components develop as ingrowth from the cervical myotomes (Wills, 1954).

The diaphragm is a dome-shaped fibromuscular structure that separates the thoracic cavity from the abdominal cavity. The peripheral portion of the diaphragm consists of muscular fibers that take their origin from the circumference of the thoracic outlet. The muscular fibers arise from three areas: from the back of the xiphoid, from the lower six ribs and costal cartilages posteriorly, interdigitating with the transversus abdominis muscle, and from the lumbocostal arches and lumbar vertebrae. The muscular portions of the diaphragm converge and are inserted into a central tendon that is somewhat closer to the front than the back. Diaphragmatic muscle fibers vary in length. They are longest in the posterolateral portion, where the greatest muscular excursion takes place.

There are three major openings in the diaphragm allowing for passage of structures from the chest to the abdomen. These are the aortic, vena caval, and esophageal apertures. The aortic opening allows for passage of the aorta, azygos vein, and thoracic duct. Through the esophageal hiatus passes the esophagus and vagus nerves, and the vena caval opening transmits the vena cava.

Motor supply to the diaphragm is supplied by the phrenic nerves, arising primarily from the fourth cervical nerve but also from the third and fifth cervical nerves. The branch from the fifth nerve is not constant and is called the accesory phrenic nerve. The phrenic nerve passes from the neck anterior to the medial border of the scalenus anticus muscle, through the chest, entering the hila of the lungs to the diaphragm.

CONGENITAL DIAPHRAGMATIC HERNIA

There are three types of congenital diaphragmatic hernias: esophageal hiatal hernia, posterolateral (Bochdalek) hernia, and subcostosternal (Morgagni) hernia.

Esophageal hiatal hernia is a common finding in adults. Prior to 1951, only 93 accounts of hiatal hernia in infants and children had been reported (Cahill *et al.*, 1969). Since that time, the diagnosis has been made more frequently, and in symptomatic infants, it is associated with a high degree of morbidity. In reality, congenital esophageal hiatal hernia is a common defect in children, and its symptoms and morbidity are related to gastroesophageal reflux (Lilly and Randolph, 1968). Vomiting, respiratory complications, anemia, and failure to thrive are the four main diagnostic features. The diagnosis is easily confirmed by esophagography along with fluoroscopy revealing free reflux of gastric contents into the esophagus. The degree of stricture formation can also be ascertained during these studies. Esophagoscopy is not necessary for the diagnosis but is an excellent method for evaluating the presence and severity of esophagitis. Conserative management consists of maintaining the infant in the upright position, usually at an angle of 60 degrees for 24 hours a day (Cahill *et al.,* 1969; Lilly and Randolph, 1968). Thickened small feedings are an adjunct to conservative management, but anticholinergics are of little value. If medical management is unsuccessful, surgical repair should be performed. The type of repair is less important than the creation of a competent esophagogastric spincter, preventing the reflux of gastric contents into the esophagus. In some cases, stricture dilatation may be necessary. Pyloroplasty has been used to improve gastric emptying in selected cases.

Posterolateral (Bochdalek) diaphragmatic hernia is the result of a congenital diaphragmatic defect in the posterior costal part of the diaphragm in the region of the tenth and eleventh ribs. There is usually free communication between the thoracic and abdominal cavities. The defect is most commonly found on the left (90 per cent), but may occur on the right, where the liver often prevents detection (Gravier, 1974). The male-to-female ratio is 2:1 (Gravier, 1974). Owing to the negative intrathoracic pressure, herniation of abdominal contents through left-sided defects occurs with resultant collapse of the left lung, shifting of the mediastinum to the right, and compression of the right lung. Most often, these hernias are manifested by acute respiratory distress in the newborn. A second but less well-recognized group of patients with Bochdalek hernia survive beyond the neonatal period and usually present at a later time with "failure to thrive, intermittent vomiting, or progressive respiratory difficulty" (Saw *et al.,* 1973).

The diagnosis can often be made on clinical grounds by the presence of respiratory distress, absence of breath sounds on the left, and presence of bowel sounds over the left chest. Roentgenograms of the chest confirm the diagnosis. Obstruction and strangulation have been reported but are rare. Treatment consists of nasogastric decompression, replacement of fluids and electrolytes, correction of acid-base imbalance, respiratory support, and surgical correction. Repair is accomplished through a right thoracotomy for right-sided defects. For left-sided defects, an abdominal incision is preferred owing to the high incidence of malrotation and obstructing duodenal bands. In the neonate, operative mortality varies from 30 to 50 per cent (Saw *et al.,* 1973). Repairs performed in older infants are almost always successful. Closure of the defect can usually be accomplished by direct suture. Chest tubes to help with expansion of the lung are connected to underwater seal drainage. Long-term follow-up has shown residual pulmonary defects in those patients found to have hypoplastic lungs at the time of surgical repair (Saw *et al.,* 1973). Recently, vasodilator therapy with tolazoline has been used to treat the increased pulmonary vascular resistance found in many neonates with congenital diaphragmatic hernias (Shochat *et al.,* 1979; Bloss *et al.,* 1980). A good response to tolazoline has been associated with improved survival. Since tolazoline may be associated with hypotension, gastrointestinal bleeding, seizures, and thrombocytopenia, other pharmacologic agents, such as prostaglandin E, are now being tried. In addition to pharmacologic attempts to alter pulmonary vascular resistance, extracorporeal membrane oxygenation has been employed when the preceding methods have failed to produce a satisfactory result. Early reports with this technique are encouraging (Hardesty *et al.,* 1981).

Subcostosternal (retrosternal, Morgagni) hernias are located behind the sternum, either just to the right or the left (Fig. 26–1). They rarely produce symptoms in childhood. Most commonly, they produce symptoms after the age of 40 and may become symptomatic after increases in intra-abdominal pressure secondary to trauma or obesity. Most frequently, the transverse colon has herniated through the defect, which usually is associated with a sac of peritoneum. Diagnosis is often made on routine screening chest films by the presence of colon in one chest cavity. Symptoms are related to obstruction of the colon, which has herniated into the chest. Repair is reserved for symptomatic patients, and although it has been accomplished both transthoracically and transabdominally, the abdominal route is probably easier (Thomas, 1972). The anterior

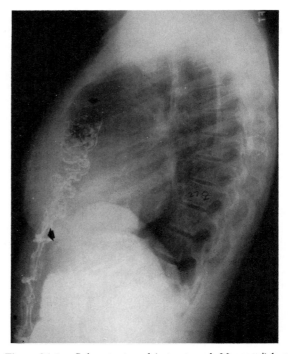

Figure 26–1. Subcostosternal (retrosternal, Morgagni) hernia, with colon herniated into the retrosternal space.

defect can usually be repaired by direct suture after the contents of the hernia sac have been reduced. If the defect cannot be closed directly, sutures may be placed so as to attach the margins to the costal margins or to the posterior aspect of the sternum.

TUMORS

The diaphragm is frequently involved by malignant tumor extending from neighboring structures. Metastatic spread commonly occurs from primary lung tumors but may come from the esophagus, stomach, gallbladder, liver, colon, or retroperitoneum. Primary tumors are rare lesions. They may be cysts, inflammatory lesions, or benign or malignant neoplasms.

Cystic lesions of the diaphragm are either acquired or congenital. Simple cysts (Fig. 26–2) and fibrous lined ones have been found (Clagett and Johnson, 1949), as well as cysts resulting from trauma with resultant hematoma formation and degeneration.

Although the diaphragm is commonly involved by inflammatory processes, it is rare for an inflammatory process to present as a primary intradiaphragmatic abscess. Hydatid disease, tuberculosis, and involvement with Echinococcus have all been reported (Anderson and Forrest, 1973). Echinococcal involvement of the diaphragm is usually secondary to liver or lung disease.

Benign tumors of the diaphragm may arise from any of the normal components of the diaphragm. Lipomas, fibromas, mesotheliomas, angiofibromas, neurofibromas, and neurilemmomas have been reported.

Malignant tumors are usually of fibrous tissue origin (Anderson and Forrest, 1973). Vascular or muscular tissue is the source of most of the remaining malignant tumors. According to Olafsson and associates, of the primary tumors of the diaphragm, malignant ones predominate in a 60:40 ratio. The majority of patients with malignant tumors have pleuritic chest pain or referred epigastric pain (Weiner and Chou, 1965). Trivedi (1958) reported three patients with neurogenic diaphragmatic tumors having pulmonary osteoarthropathy who were all cured after resection. Occasionally, a mass has been palpated through the ribs or in the abdomen.

Radiographic manifestation of diaphragmatic tumor consists of an enlarging mass on the diaphragmatic surface, usually remaining extrapleural (Anderson and Forrest, 1973). The site of the tumor can be further identified by artificial pneumothorax or pneumoperitoneum or CT scan.

Excision of the tumor is indicated whenever possible. Closure of the diaphragm by direct suture is preferable, but when this is impossible, replacement with prosthetic material can be utilized. In cases of inflammatory disease, treatment of the underlying condition is indicated.

EVENTRATION AND UNILATERAL PARALYSIS

There is considerable confusion in the literature regarding the differentiation of eventration and unilateral paralysis of the diaphragm. The causes of unilateral paralysis of the phrenic nerve include surgical section, birth trauma, viral infection, pulmonary or pleural infections, and invasion by malignant tumors (Fig. 26–3). In the case of unilateral paralysis, there is paradoxical movement of the diaphragm.

In 1954, Bingham reported his belief that eventration was due to an acquired phrenic nerve injury occurring at birth. Chin and Lynn (1956) felt that a true distinction should be made between acquired paralysis and true eventration. They stated that the diaphragm that showed paradoxical motion could not be classified as an eventration, the latter term being reserved for a true congenital maldevelopment. Thomas (1970) reviewed the subject of eventration and used Bisgard's definition (1947) as the currently accepted definition of eventration. This definition described eventration as "an abnormally high or elevated position of one leaf of the intact diaphragm as a result of paralysis, aplasia or atrophy of varying degrees of the muscle fibers." Thomas further classified eventration etiologically into two categories: congenital or nonparalytic and acquired or paralytic. Congenital eventrations were further divided into complete, partial, and bilateral. In the acquired form, the movement of the diaphragm, either paradoxical or not, is most likely to represent the stage of the acquired process. The differentiation of acquired eventration from "unilateral paralysis" may be very difficult, if not impossible. It is probably best to

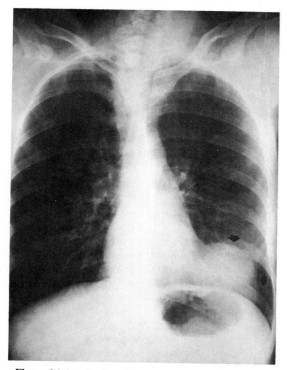

Figure 26–2. Benign simple cyst of the diaphragm.

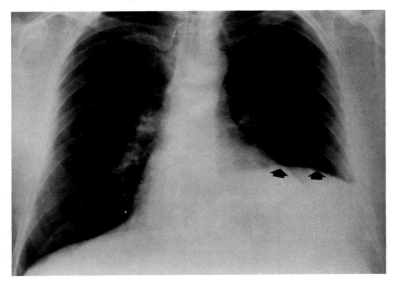

Figure 26–3. Unilateral paralysis of the left hemidiaphragm secondary to viral infection.

assume the last opinion, that of Thomas, dividing eventration into the congenital and acquired forms.

Eventration in adult life is more commonly found on the left side, but in infants it is more common on the right.

Most patients with eventration of the diaphragm are asymptomatic (Fig. 26–4). Symptomatic eventration is most commonly found in infants (Symbas *et al.*, 1977). Symptoms in infancy are usually those of respiratory insufficiency, which are believed to be due to a more mobile mediastinum. This more mobile mediastinum, with shifting, causes inadequate ventilation and torsion of the heart and great vessels. If respiratory symptoms do not occur in infancy, the individual is most likely to remain asymptomatic until the fifth or sixth decade. In addition to respiratory symptoms, other symptoms may simulate large diaphragmatic hernias with dysphagia, belching, heartburn, and epigastric pain (Symbas *et al.*, 1977). The diagnosis is usually made with the aid of posteroanterior and lateral chest films, fluoroscopy, and, occasionally, barium studies. Decreased perfusion of the lower lobe of the lung on the eventrated side may occur. Photoscanning and bronchospirometric studies have demonstrated 50 to 75 per cent ventilatory decreases on the involved side. Surgical repair in the symptomatic patient with unilateral eventration is best done through a posterolateral thoracotomy. For bilateral eventrations, the abdominal approach can be employed, or two separate thoracotomies may be performed 2 to 3 weeks apart (Thomas, 1970). Repair is accomplished by plication of the redundant attenuated diaphragm, with or without resection of some of the attenuated tissue. In addition, support can be increased by the addition of prosthetic material.

TRAUMATIC PERFORATION

Traumatic diaphragmatic hernias are produced either by blunt thoracoabdominal trauma or from penetrating wounds of the diaphragm. Automobile accidents are the usual cause of blunt traumatic diaphragmatic hernias. These injuries produce a sudden increase in the pleuroperitoneal pressure gradient. This results in an explosive bursting force, usually rupturing the left hemidiaphragm (90 per cent), the right one being protected by the cushioning effect of the liver (Pomerantz *et al.*, 1968). Other factors, such as muscle contraction or fixations, may also play a role. Associated injuries are common, with fractures, lacerated livers and spleens, and head injuries being most common (Pomerantz *et al.*, 1968; Hood, 1971).

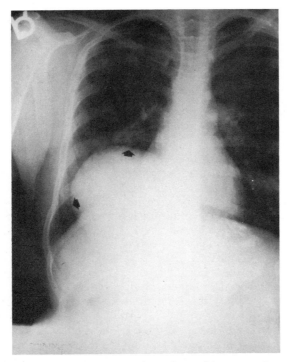

Figure 26–4. Asymptomatic patient with eventration of a large portion of the right hemidiaphragm.

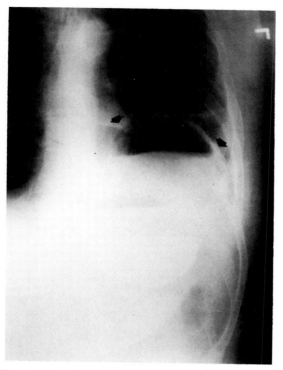

Figure 26–5. Blunt traumatic diaphragmatic hernia with stomach bubble in the left chest.

Symptoms of acute diaphragmatic rupture usually consist of respiratory distress, with dyspnea, cyanosis, and hypotension being the most common. In acute ruptures, mediastinal displacement is more abrupt and is greater than that observed with pleural effusions, producing more severe symptoms that would be expected in comparison with the reduction of respiratory volumes observed (Nano *et al.*, 1980). A ruptured diaphragm should be suspected if bowel sounds are heard on auscultation of the chest (Iuchtman *et al.*, 1977). The diagnosis in the acute phase is usually confirmed by roentgenograms of the chest (Fig. 26–5). Difficulty in inserting a nasogastric tube or, after passage of a nasogastric tube, finding it radiographically within the confines of the left chest is further confirmative evidence. If there is not immediate herniation of viscera into the left chest and no other significant injuries, the diagnosis may be overlooked initially. The patient then enters an "interval phase" in which he may be totally asymptomatic. However, a third phase of intestinal obstruction and strangulation later ensues, usually (85 per cent) within 3 years (Pomerantz *et al.*, 1968; Hood, 1971).

Symptoms of right-sided rupture are usually less severe and more vague, the diagnosis being confirmed by fluoroscopy, diagnostic pneumoperitoneum, and contrast studies to differentiate this entity from eventration.

Penetrating diaphragmatic injuries usually do not produce early symptoms unless the hole is large enough to permit immediate herniation of abdominal viscera.

Once the diagnosis is confirmed, repair should be carried out as soon as fluid, electrolyte, and metabolic defects are corrected. Since there is a high incidence of associated intra-abdominal injuries with blunt left diaphragmatic ruptures, those patients whose injuries are diagnosed acutely should undergo transabdominal exploration so that associated injuries can be corrected. If the diagnosis is delayed and there are no associated intra-abdominal injuries, repair is more easily accomplished by the transthoracic route. Regardless of the approach, direct closure of the defect is usually possible using heavy nonabsorbable sutures. If this can not be accomplished, closure with a prosthetic graft can be employed.

SELECTED REFERENCES

Anderson, L.S., and Forrest, J.V.: Tumors of the diaphragm. Roentgenol. Radium Ther. Nucl. Med., *119*:259, 1973.

This article presents a radiographic analysis of diaphragmatic tumors and a clear classification of diaphragmatic tumors into the following groups: (1) Primary benign neoplasms. (2) Primary malignant neoplasms. (3) Secondary malignant neoplasms. (4) Cysts. (5) Inflammatory lesions. (6) Endometriosis.

Iuchtman, M., Freire, E., and Jacob, E.T.: Acute diaphragmatic hernia caused by blunt trauma. Ann. Surg., *42*:460, 1977.

This paper reviews the etiology, incidence, and clinical picture of traumatic diaphragmatic hernia, as well as diagnostic aids. Also discussed is the surgical approach to repair.

Shochat, S.J., Naeye, R.L., Ford, W.D.A., Whitman, V., and Maisels, M.J.: Congenital diaphragmatic hernia—new concept in management. Ann. Surg., *190*:332, 1979.

A new concept for the pharmacologic management of the vasoconstrictive response noted in the pulmonary vascular bed of patients with congenital diaphragmatic hernias is presented. Treatment with tolazoline is introduced, and speculation is made concerning the use of other pharmacologic agents.

Thomas, T.V.: Congenital eventration of the diaphragm. Ann. Thorac. Surg., *10*:180, 1970.

This is a collective review outlining the etiology, symptoms, and therapy of diaphragmatic eventration. A classification separating congenital (nonparalytic) from acquired (paralytic) eventration is put forth.

Thomas, T.V.: Subcostosternal diaphragmatic hernia. J. Thorac. Cardiovasc. Surg., *63*:278, 1972.

This article reviews the anatomy and embryology of the diaphragm, pointing out how developmental abnormalities may result in congenital diaphragmatic hernias. The article emphasizes the late onset of symptoms, usually related to entrapment of the transverse colon in the retrosternal position.

REFERENCES

Allison, P.R.: *In* Gibbon's Surgery of the Chest. 2nd Ed. Philadelphia, W. B. Saunders Company, 1969, p. 243.

Anderson, L.S., and Forrest, J.V.: Tumors of the diaphragm. Am. J. Roentgenol. Radium Ther. Nucl. Med., *119*:259, 1973.

Bingham, J.A.W.: Two cases of unilateral paralysis of the diaphragm in the newborn treated surgically. Thorax, *9*:248, 1954.

Bisgard, J.D.: Congenital eventration of the diaphragm. J. Thorac. Surg., *16*:484, 1947.

Bloss, R.S., Turmen, T., Beardmore, H.E., and Aranda, J.V.: Tolazoline therapy for persistent pulmonary hypertension after congenital diaphragmatic hernia repair. J. Pediatr., *97*:984, 1980.

Bowditch, H.I.: Diaphragmatic hernia. Buffalo Med. J., *9*:1,65,94, 1853.

Cahill, J. L., Aberdeen, E., and Waterston, D.J.: Results of surgical treatment of esophageal hiatal hernia in infancy and childhood. Surgery, *66*:597, 1969.

Chin, E.F., and Lynn, R.B.: Surgery of eventration of the diaphragm. J. Thorac. Surg., *32*:6, 1956.

Clagett, O.T., and Johnson, M.A.: Tumors of the diaphragm. Am. J. Surg., *78*:526, 1949.

Grage, T.B., MacLean, L.D., and Cambell, G.S.: Traumatic rupture of the diaphragm, a report of 26 cases. Surgery, *46*:669, 1959.

Gravier, L: Congenital diaphragmatic hernia. South. Med. J., *67*:59, 1974.

Hardesty, R.L., Griffith, B.P., Debski, R.F., Joffries, M.R., and Borovetz, H.S.: Extracorporeal membrane oxygenation —successful treatment of persistent fetal circulation following repair of congenital diaphragmatic hernia. J. Thorac. Cardiovasc. Surg., *81*:556, 1981.

Hood, R. M.: Traumatic diaphragmatic hernia. Ann. Thorac. Surg., *12*:311, 1971.

Iuchtman, M., Freire, E., and Jacob, E.T.: Acute diaphragmatic hernia caused by blunt trauma. Ann. Surg., *42*:460, 1977.

Lilly, J.R., and Randolph, J.G.: Hiatal hernia and gastroesophageal reflux in infants and children. J. Thorac. Cardiovasc. Surg., *55*:42, 1968.

Limjoco, U.R., Langley, B.J., and Mendenhall, J.T.: Cystic hematoma of the diaphragm. Ann. Thorac. Surg., *6*:82, 1968.

Morgagni, G.B.: Seats and Causes of Diseases. Zellts 54, Monograph on Hernia of the Diaphragm, 1769.

Nano, M., DeiPoli, M., Mossetti, C., and Maggi, G.: Traumatic diaphragmatic hernias. Surg. Gynecol. Obstet., *151*:191, 1980.

Olafsson, G., Rausing, A., and Holen, O.: Primary tumors of the diaphragm. Chest, *59*:568, 1971.

Pomerantz, M., Rodgers, B.M., and Sabiston, D.C., Jr.: Traumatic diaphragmatic hernia. Surgery, *64*:529, 1968.

Saw, E.S., Arbegast, N.R., and Comer, T.P.: Congenital posterolateral diaphragmatic hernia in children. California Med., *119*:6, 1973.

Shochat, S.J., Naeye, R., Ford, W.D.A., Whitman, V., and Maisels, M.J.: Congenital diaphragmatic hernia — new concept in management. Ann. Surg., *190*:332, 1979.

Sutton, J.P., Carlisle, R.B., and Stephenson, S.E.: Traumatic diaphragmatic hernia. Ann. Thorac. Surg., *3*:136, 1967.

Symbas, P.N., Hatcher, C.R., and Waldo, W.: Diaphragmatic eventration in infancy and childhood. Ann. Thorac. Surg., *24*:113, 1977.

Thomas, T.V.: Congenital eventration of the diaphragm. Ann. Thorac. Surg., *10*:180, 1970.

Thomas, T.V.: Subcostosternal diaphragmatic hernia. J. Thorac. Cardiovasc. Surg., *63*:278, 1972.

Trivedi, S.A.: Neurolemmoma of the diaphragm causing severe hypertrophic pulmonary osteoarthropathy. Br. J. Tuberculosis, *52*:214, 1958.

Weiner, M.F., and Chou, W.H.: Primary tumors of the diaphragm. Arch. Surg., *90*:143, 1965.

Wells, L.J.: Development of human diaphragm and pleural sacs. Contrib. Embryol., *35*:107, 1954.

II   DIAPHRAGMATIC PACING

David D. Oakes

After more than 30 years of experimental and clinical research, an effective and reliable diaphragm pacer has been developed that permits long-term, intermittent ventilatory support by electrophrenic stimulation (Glenn, 1978; Glenn *et al.,* 1980a). Paralleling this development, however, have been striking advances in the technology of positive-pressure ventilation and dramatic changes in disease patterns (e.g., the virtual abolition of poliomyelitis as a significant clinical entity and the discovery that many cases of "sleep apnea" are caused by upper airway obstruction and can be cured by tracheostomy), which have markedly narrowed the patient population to which diaphragm pacing is applicable. This section discusses the historical development of diaphragm pacing, describes the components and function of the apparatus presently available, examines the selection of patients who might benefit from this technique, outlines operative and perioperative management, and analyzes the current capabilities and limitations of this mode of artificial ventilation.

HISTORICAL DEVELOPMENT

The first use of electricity to stimulate respiration in humans is credited to Christoph Hufeland, who, in 1783, proposed this technique for the treatment of asphyxia neonatorum (Schechter, 1970). That the resultant ventilatory activity was in fact secondary to phrenic nerve stimulation was supported by the work of Andrew Ure in 1818. Using the body of a criminal who had been dispatched on the gallows about 1 hour previously, he applied wires from a voltaic battery to incisions in the neck and beneath the fifth costal cartilage: "The result was prodigious: one saw instantly established in the cadaver the movements of a strong and laborious respiration; the chest rose and fell, the abdomen advanced and then collapsed, and the diaphragm widened and contracted as in natural respiration." In 1846, Hugo von Ziemssen reported that 2 hours of "faradization" of the phrenic nerves resulted in successful resuscitation of a 27-year-old woman who had been asphyxiated by charcoal fumes.

By 1872, Guillaume Duchenne de Boulogne, an early advocate of electrotherapy in resuscitation, proclaimed that that electrical stimulation of the phrenic nerves was "assuredly the best means of imitating natural respiration." In spite of these early successes, electrophrenic stimulation failed to become an integral part of the medical armamentarium, and by the early twentieth century, the technique had nearly disappeared from clinical practice (Schechter, 1970, 1978).

In 1937, Waud reported that rabbits rendered apneic by drugs could be successfully ventilated or even hyperventilated "for hours" by rhythmic stimulation of the phrenic nerves. Moreover, he observed that the technique obviated the circulatory changes that complicated positive-pressure ventilation.

In the 1940s Sarnoff and associates became interested in electrical stimulation of the phrenic nerves as a means of aiding respiration in victims of bulbar poliomyelitis (Sarnoff et al., 1948; Whittenberger et al., 1949). Their methods (directly implanting a wire electrode around the phrenic nerve, then passing it out through the skin, or stimulating the nerve transcutaneously using a metal thimble electrode) allowed stimulation to be continued for, at most, a few days. In a series of acute experiments, however, they defined the essential physiology of *electrophrenic respiration* in both nonhuman and human subjects; subsequent research has added little to our understanding of this technique. Their principal conclusions were: (1) Artificial respiration by phrenic nerve stimulation can be performed in man. (2) A smooth, gradual diaphragmatic contraction occurs when an increasing voltage is applied to the phrenic nerve. The diaphragm thus performs a motion closely resembling that which it performs during natural inspiration. (3) Respiratory minute volumes in excess of the patient's spontaneous minute volumes can readily be obtained with the submaximal stimulation of one phrenic nerve. (4) The depth of inspiration is proportional to the peak voltage applied to the phrenic nerve in man, as in the experimental animal. (5) Adequate oxygenation of the blood can be maintained by electrophrenic respiration in the absence of spontaneous respiration. (6) The human subject, like the experimental animal, completely relinquishes spontaneous control of respiration when electrophrenic respiration is induced. In at least one experiment, they demonstrated that "remote stimulation" of the phrenic nerve could be achieved using electromagnetic induction coils, obviating the necessity of having a lead wire emanate from the wound (Whittenberger et al., 1949). Although they were thus on the verge of developing a technique for long-term electrophrenic stimulation, they failed to follow up on this methodology — probably because the conquest of poliomyelitis robbed their research of its clinical relevance.

Beginning in the late 1950s and continuing to the present, Glenn and associates have actively pursued the development and clinical application of chronic diaphragm pacing using radiofrequency signals to stimulate phrenic nerves through the intact skin (Farmer et al., 1978; Glenn, 1978; Glenn et al., 1972, 1978a, 1978b, 1978c, 1980a, 1980b; Judson and Glenn, 1968; Kim et al., 1976; Oda et al., 1981; Sato et al., 1970; Tanae et al., 1973). It is largely through their efforts that the presently available apparatus has been developed. They have, moreover, defined the patient populations to whom chronic diaphragm pacing is applicable, established the safety of prolonged intermittent phrenic nerve stimulation, and investigated the mechanism of fatigue by which effective pacing is usually limited to less than 24 consecutive hours. Most of the following clinical experience is based on their research.

APPARATUS

The only commercially available diaphragm pacer is made by Avery Laboratory, located in Farmingdale, New York, and consists of four components (Fig. 26–6). Two of these components, the transmitter and the antenna, are extracorporeal; the other two, the receiver and the electrode assembly, are implanted.

The Transmitter. Coded radiofrequency signals are generated by an external transmitter. Unlike cardiac pacemakers, which produce a single impulse, the output signal of the diaphragm pacer is a train of pulses lasting between 1.20 and 1.45 seconds (0.5 to 0.8 second in infants). The duration of the pulse train defines the length of inspiration, and the number of pulse trains per minute establishes the respiratory rate. The individual pulses are separated by 50 milliseconds; this "pulse interval" is preset by the manufacturer and usually is not adjusted. (Shortening the pulse interval leads to more rapid fatigue of diaphragmatic response; lengthening it results in less effective contraction.) Pulses are of the same amplitude but differ in width such that each successive pulse

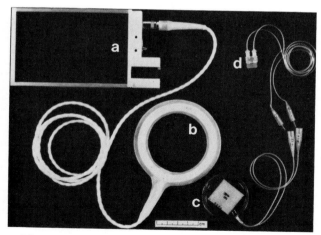

Figure 26–6. Radiofrequency diaphragm pacemaker: *a*, Transmitter. *b*, Antenna. *c*, Receiver. *d*, Bipolar electrode. This is the basic unit for peripheral nerve stimulation. (From Glenn, W. W. L.: Diaphragm pacing. *In* Gibbon's Surgery of the Chest, 3rd Ed. Edited by D. C. Sabiston, Jr. and F. C. Spencer. Philadelphia, W. B. Saunders Company, 1976.)

in the train is wider than its predecessor. The *width* of each radiofrequency pulse, after demodulation by the receiver, determines the *amplitude* of the current delivered to the phrenic nerve, which, in turn, determines the depth of inspiration (Fig. 26–7). The gradual increase in energy delivered during the pulse train is necessary to provide a smooth excursion of the diaphragm by progressively recruiting more and more nerve fibers. The contour of the pulse train is determined by the "slope control," which adjusts the amount by which the first stimulating pulse in the train differs from the last; the normal increase is one milliampere.

Recommended initial settings for adults are a respiratory rate of 12 breaths per minute, an inspiration time of 1.3 seconds (hence, an expiration time of 3.7 seconds), and a pulse interval of 50 milliseconds. The amplitude of the final signal is selected by gradually increasing the stimulus until diaphragmatic excursion is noted to be maximal when observed fluoroscopically. Fatigue is minimized by using an amplitude that produces slightly submaximal diaphragmatic con-

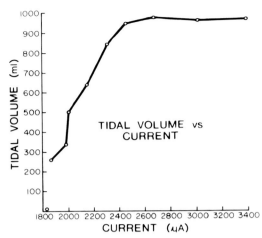

Figure 26–8. Influence of current amplitude on tidal volume. In the patient whose study is illustrated, the threshold (first contraction of the hemidiaphragm) occurred about 1800 microamperes, and the maximal contraction (hence, the maximal tidal volume) occurred at 2600 microamperes. Pacing should be carried out at or just below maximum tidal volume, at about 2500 microamperes in this patient. Use of higher current levels will accelerate nerve fatigue without adding appreciably to minute ventilation (From Glenn, W. W. L., Hogan, J. F., and Phelps, M. L.: Ventilatory support of the quadriplegic patient with respiratory paralysis by diaphragm pacing. Surg. Clin. North Am., *60*:1055, 1980.)

traction (Fig. 26–8). Subsequent adjustments are usually limited to changing the respiratory rate or the amplitude of the stimulus and are determined by monitoring the patient's arterial blood gases and tidal volumes.

The Antenna. The antenna transfers the radiofrequency signal from the transmitter across the intact skin to the subcutaneously implanted receiver. It is composed of several turns of wire wound concentrically in a flat plane with an outside diameter of 85 mm. It is connected to a flexible wire lead that plugs into the transmitter. To effect stimulation, the antenna is placed directly over the implanted receiver and secured in place with hypoallergenic tape. Because the intensity of the transmitted signal is determined by pulse width rather than amplitude, the antenna can be displaced up to 2.5 cm. from the center of the receiver without affecting operation.

The Receiver. The receiver is 44 mm. in diameter, 15 mm. thick, and weighs 30.5 gm. It has no intrinsic energy source, but rather consists of subminiature integrated circuitry that receives energy and stimulus information from the external transmitter by inductive electromagnetic coupling. The signal is demodulated into a unidirectional current, the amplitude of which varies directly with the width of the originally transmitted pulse. All components are hermetically sealed, encapsulated in an epoxy disc, and covered with medical-grade silicone rubber. Two flexible stainless steel lead wires terminate in female connectors that are attached to the electrode at the time of operation.

The Electrode. A bipolar electrode is formed by two platinum bands embedded in a cuff of silicone

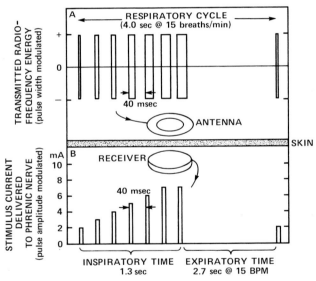

Figure 26–7. A schematic drawing of the electrical signals necessary to produce a single inspiration. For illustrative purposes the wave forms are not drawn to scale in time. *A,* The output of the transmitter is a train of biphasic pulses that vary progressively in width (within the range of 600 microseconds to 2.0 milliseconds) and that occur at intervals of 40 to 50 milliseconds. If the inspiration time is set at 1.3 seconds, each pulse train will therefore contain 26 to 32 impulses. This radiofrequency energy is broadcast via an external antenna to a subcutaneous receiver. *B,* The receiver modulates the signal and sends to the nerve a train of unidirectional impulses that vary in amplitude between 0 and 10.0 milliamperes. The amplitude of a given pulse is determined by the width of the corresponding biphasic signal. The contour of this final pulse train is determined by the "slope control." Usually, the first pulse is set at the threshold value (the amount of current necessary to produce the first evidence of diaphragmatic contraction) and the final pulse at the current needed to produce a slightly submaximal contraction. Alternatively, the final pulse is set for submaximal contraction, and the first pulse is arbitrarily set 1.0 milliampere less. In either case, a train of gradually increasing pulses is necessary to produce a smooth contraction of the diaphragm.

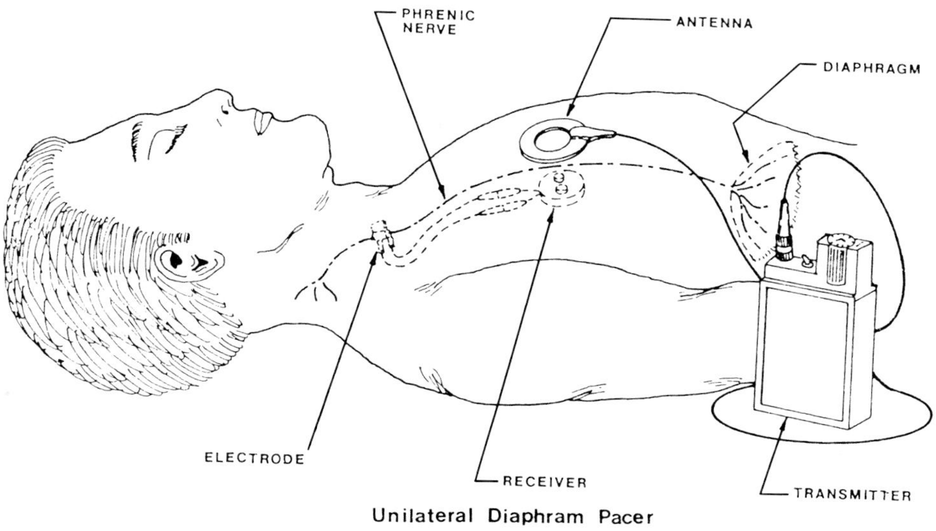

Figure 26-9. Schematic drawing illustrating the relationship of the four components of the diaphragm pacer. A bipolar electrode is shown. (From Avery Laboratories, Inc.: Diaphragm Pacer (product brochure 6011B-5/79). Farmingdale, New York, Avery Laboratories, Inc., May 1979.)

Unilateral Diaphram Pacer

rubber. Each band has an exposed area of 11.5 mm.^{2} The cuff is designed to fit loosely around a 1.5-cm. segment of phrenic nerve and to permit firm fixation to the adjacent tissues. Two flexible stainless steel lead wires, 40 cm. long, allow the platinum bands to be connected with the receiver. (More recently, a monopolar electrode has been developed that is placed under the nerve, rather than around it; when using this lead, a titanium disc indifferent electrode must be implanted elsewhere and connected to the anode.)

A diagram of the complete pacing system is shown in Figure 26-9.

PATIENT SELECTION AND RESULTS

General Considerations

Diaphragm pacing can support a patient's respiratory needs only if there is a viable phrenic nerve that can stimulate a normal diaphragm to contract, expanding lung parenchyma that is capable of satisfactory ventilation and alveolar-capillary gas exchange. Pacing is therefore contraindicated in cases of diaphragmatic paralysis resulting from (1) destruction of the anterior horn cells at the level of the third, fourth, or fifth cervical vertebrae, (2) damage to the peripheral axons of the phrenic nerve, (3) impaired diaphragmatic function secondary to atrophy, eventration, myositis, or muscular dystrophy, or (4) severe damage to the pulmonary parenchyma such that voluntary hyperventilation does not result in an improvement in arterial P_{O_2} or P_{CO_2} (Glenn, 1978).

Specific Indications

Central Alveolar Hypoventilation

Central alveolar hypoventilation occurs when the respiratory center fails to respond to hypercapnea by increasing minute ventilation. The carotid body may also be unresponsive to hypoxemia. Periodic apnea may occur, especially during sleep. Patients suffering from this syndrome develop polycythemia, pulmonary arterial hypertension, cor pulmonale, lethargy, somnolence, and, in many cases, sleep apnea. Although frequently idiopathic, the condition can occur secondary to encephalitis, tumor, or cerebral vascular accidents (Farmer et al., 1978; Glenn et al., 1978b, 1978c).

In 1968, Judson and Glenn reported the first clinical application of long-term diaphragm pacing in a 38-year-old male with chronic hypoventilation, possibly secondary to viral encephalitis. The patient presented with leukocytosis, polycythemia, pneumonia, cor pulmonale, and increasing lethargy. Cardiac catheterization revealed a pulmonary artery pressure of 60 mm. Hg. Chronic hypercapnea, hypoxemia, and respiratory acidosis were documented; during sleep, the arterial gas tensions deteriorated markedly. Inhalation of 7 per cent carbon dioxide did not stimulate an increase in minute ventilation. In May 1966, a bipolar electrode was placed around the left phrenic nerve in the neck and attached to a receiver in the pectoral area. Diaphragmatic excursion diminished markedly after 20 hours of continuous stimulation, but this "fatigue" disappeared completely after 35 hours without pacing. By September 1966, the patient tolerated 10 hours of pacing each night. During this time, arterial gas tensions showed consistent improvement during pacing (Fig. 26-10). After 10 months of pacing, polycythemia was ameliorated and cor pulmonale improved. The stimulation threshold remained constant, and diaphragmatic fatigue was always reversible, indicating that no significant permanent damage to the nerve had occurred. After 2 years of successful nocturnal pacing, the patient died from a myocardial infarction. Autopsy revealed perineural fibrosis at the level of electrode, but no histologic evidence of structural damage to the nerve per se (Kim et al., 1976) (Fig. 26-11).

By 1978, Glenn had utilized diaphragm pacing in

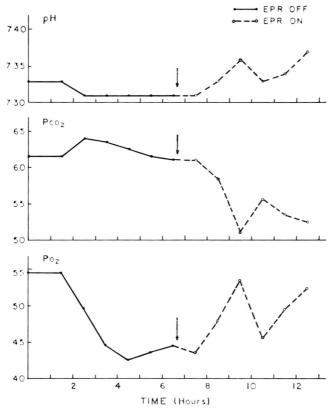

Figure 26–10. Beneficial effect of nocturnal diaphragm pacing in a patient with central alveolar hypoventilation. The patient was dozing or sleeping from the second to the twelfth hour. (EPR = electrophrenic respiration.) (From Judson, J. P., and Glenn, W. W. L.: Radiofrequency electrophrenic respiration: Long-term application to a patient with primary hypoventilation. J.A.M.A., *203*:1033, 1968.)

36 patients who met the following criteria for the diagnosis of central alveolar hypoventilation: (1) clinical features of hypoventilation, which usually included cyanosis, polycythemia, and cor pulmonale with right heart failure; (2) hypoxemia and hypercapnea, worsening during sleep; (3) hypoventilation during sleep, sometimes punctuated by periodic apnea; (4) near-normal tests of ventilatory capacity; (5) diminished ventilatory response to induced hypoxemia and hypercapnea; (6) either the absence of upper airway obstruction during a sleep study or the persistence of hypoventilation following relief of the obstruction (Glenn, 1978). (Many patients with "sleep apnea syndrome" have been found to develop severe upper airway obstruction during sleep. The condition may be *worsened* by diaphragm pacing, unless a tracheostomy is performed. Frequently tracheostomy alone, by eliminating the mechanical obstruction to ventilation, will completely correct nocturnal hypoventilation, thus obviating the need for diaphragm pacing [Glenn *et al.*, 1978c]). It is apparent that the diagnosis of central alveolar hypoventilation cannot be made without resort to the facilities of sophisticated pulmonary function and sleep-study laboratories.

Long-term ventilatory support was achieved in all but one of the 36 patients. Hypoxemia and hypercapnea were substantially lessened or eliminated by pacing. Hematocrit levels were reduced, and several patients had a documented fall in pulmonary arterial pressure. Although repeated electrical stimulation caused temporary nerve fatigue, it did not result in permanent damage. This is illustrated by the fact that xenon perfusion washout times were not significantly prolonged, even after years of nocturnal pacing (Fig. 26–12). Equally impressive is the stability of pacing thresholds over time (Fig. 26–13). These observations confirm the ability of the phrenic nerves to tolerate this type of long-term stimulation without appreciable structural or physiologic damage. Nerve dysfunction following implantation of a diaphragm pacer is therefore thought to result entirely from intraoperative damage to the nerve and perineural vessels or from subsequent fibrosis around the electrode cuff.

Because of partial paralysis of the accessory muscles of respiration, three of the 36 patients required simultaneous bilateral pacing. Most patients with central alveolar hypoventilation, however, are successfully managed with unilateral pacing; usually, the left side is chosen because operative damage to the phrenic nerve would lead to less disability than if ventilation of the right lung were compromised.

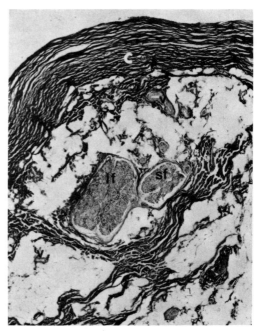

Figure 26–11. Transverse section of the phrenic nerve at the level of electrode showing thick capsular connective tissue (c) and microscopically unremarkable large (lf) and small fascicles (sf). Note the loose perineural fibroadipose tissue with several patent nutrient vessels (v). (Masson trichome stain, × 30.) The nerve had been stimulated intermittently for 26 months without apparent damage. (From Kim, J. H., Manuelidis, E. E., Glenn, W. W. L., and Kaneyuki, T.: Diaphragm pacing: Histopathological changes in the phrenic nerve following long-term electrical stimulation. J. Thorac. Cardiovasc. Surg., 72:602, 1976.)

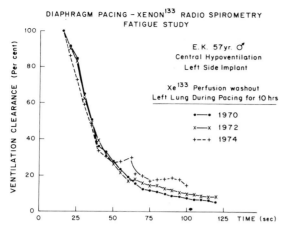

Figure 26–12. Xenon-133 radiospirometry during pacing of the left side of the diaphragm at 2-year intervals. Pacing was begun in this patient in 1968. Over the 5½ years, the nearly identical results probably indicate no change in nerve conduction or lung and diaphragm function. (From Glenn, W. W. L.: Diaphragm pacing. *In* Gibbons Surgery of the Chest. 3rd Ed. Edited by D. C. Sabiston, Jr. and F. C. Spencer. Philadelphia, W. B. Saunders Company, 1976.)

Quadriplegia

Proof that diaphragm pacing alone could provide total ventilatory support in man was dramatically provided by Glenn's group in 1971 when they successfully transferred a ventilator-dependent quadriplegic patient to full-time radiofrequency electrophrenic respiration (Glenn *et al.*, 1972). Since the patient's spinal cord injury was at the level of the first and second cervical segments, the lower motor neurons of the phrenic nerves were intact, but they were completely disconnected from the respiratory center. By forceful contraction of his neck muscles, the patient could breathe satisfactorily for a few minutes but was soon overcome by fatigue. Diaphragm pacing was consid-

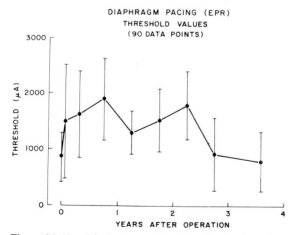

Figure 26–13. Diaphragm pacing. Threshold values. There is a significant rise during the first month, and no significant change thereafter, although the trend of the threshold values is downward. (From Glenn, W. W. L.: Diaphragm Pacing. *In* Gibbon's Surgery of the Chest. 3rd Ed. Edited by D. C. Sabiston, Jr. and F. C. Spencer. Phialdelphia, W. B. Saunders Company, 1976.)

ered the only means of freeing this patient, who was both intelligent and mentally alert, from permanent confinement in an intensive care unit. Between 5 and 6 months after injury, after first confirming that the phrenic nerves were viable by stimulating them transvenously, electrodes were placed in the cervical region. Early trials of stimulation resulted in rapid fatigue of the diaphragm, presumably because of disuse atrophy. To strengthen the diaphragm, the nerves were stimulated intermittently each day for gradually lengthening periods. Three months of diaphragm "conditioning" were necessary before positive-pressure ventilation could be completely discontinued. Thereafter, the nerves were stimulated alternately for 12 hours each to prevent fatigue. Initially, ventilation was adequate in the supine position but not in the sitting position. Only after 9 months of pacing could the patient sit for 10 hours a day supported by electrophrenic respiration alone. Even at that time, ventilation was better in the recumbent position. The patient's tracheostomy tube was eventually removed and the stoma plugged, except for endotracheal suctioning. He was discharged to his home and assumed limited business activities. That diaphragm pacing can be achieved without mechanical or electrical damage to the phrenic nerve is indicated by the fact that after more than 2 years, the threshold current required for diaphragmatic contraction did not increase, but actually declined.

Glenn's most recent report reviews his experience with diaphragm pacing in 20 quadriplegic patients (Glenn *et al.*, 1980a). Full-time ventilatory support was achieved in eight patients, and part-time support in an additonal eight. Even part-time pacing was felt to simplify nursing care and to play an important role in the rehabilitation of these patients. Similar results have been reported from other centers that specialize in the treatment of spinal cord injury (Oakes *et al.*, 1980).

Diaphragm pacing in quadriplegic patients requires consideration of factors not usually relevant to patients with central alveolar hypoventilation:

1. The injury or lesion that produced quadriplegia must be localized to the first or second cervical segments of the spinal cord. If the third, fourth, or fifth segments are also involved, some of the anterior horn cells may be destroyed, and the surviving neurons may be inadequate to elicit satisfactory diaphragm function. In all cases, therefore, permanent electrodes should not be implanted until nerve viability has been demonstrated, either by a transcutaneous technique or by direct stimulation of the nerve at the time of operation.

2. Since few spinal cord injuries are complete, recovery of spontaneous ventilatory function may occur. Diaphragm pacing should therefore be delayed until several months after injury to be certain that it is really necessary.

3. Disuse atrophy of the diaphragm requires slow and gradual conditioning before diaphragm pacing can be expected to provide satisfactory ventilation.

4. Additional conditioning and other mechanical aids such as abdominal binders may be needed before the patient can be adequately paced in the sitting position.

5. Fatigue of the diaphragm requires that pacing be interrupted periodically to permit recovery of the neuromuscular junction. Total ventilatory support is therefore possible only if both phrenic nerves are viable and can be stimulated for alternating periods.

6. Diaphragm pacing is indicated only in the long-term rehabilitation of these patients. During the first few months after injury, quadriplegic patients should be supported by conventional positive-pressure ventilation. Comatose patients with no potential for meaningful rehabilitation should not be considered for diaphragm pacing.

Chronic Obstructive Pulmonary Disease

Most patients with chronic obstructive pulmonary disease develop respiratory failure secondary to irreversible destruction of pulmonary parenchyma and, hence, would not be aided by diaphragm pacing. Even with voluntary hyperventilation, they may be unable to improve their arterial blood gases. Moreover, their diaphragms may contribute very little to ventilatory mechanics because they are frequently flattened by chronic hyperexpansion of the lungs and may have very limited excursion.

Glenn and colleagues have, however, reported one patient in whom central alveolar hypoventilation was superimposed on chronic obstructive lung disease (Glenn *et al.*, 1978a). The patient presented with repeated episodes of respiratory and ventricular failure. Not only did he fail to respond to hypercarbia, he seemed insensitive to dangerously low levels of arterial Po_2. Low-flow oxygen therapy (FI_{O_2} of 0.24 via Ventimask) led to CO_2 retention (Pco_2 of 58 mm. Hg, rising to 70 mm. Hg) even in the face of an arterial Po_2 of only 32 mm. Hg! He was polycythemic (hematocrit 60 per cent) and manifested chronic hypoxia, hypercarbia, and respiratory acidosis. He experienced frequent episodes of congestive heart failure.

Diaphragm pacing was considered in order to allow oxygen administration without inducing respiratory arrest ("pacer-protected oxygenation"). The decision to attempt pacing was based on four factors: (1) rapid, progressive deterioration of ventilation, (2) intolerance to even 24 per cent oxygen, (3) the presence of a domed diaphragm that descended 4 cm. during voluntary inspiration, and (4) the patient's ability to improve his arterial blood gases during voluntary hyperventilation. In August 1974, a pacer was implanted on the left side. Nocturnal pacing was begun 2 weeks later for 10 to 12 hours, during which time the patient received supplemental oxygen through nasal prongs at a rate of 2 to 4 liters per minute. The efficacy of this therapeutic approach is illustrated in Figure 26–14. At last report (Glenn *et al.*, 1978a), the patient had tolerated 42 months of pacer-protected nocturnal oxygenation without complications. During the 42

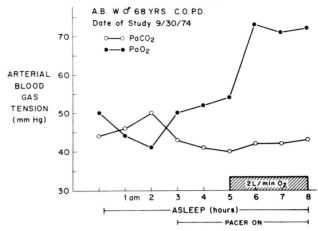

Figure 26–14.   Nocturnal blood gas study made on September 30, 1974. After the patient fell asleep, the arterial PO_2 level decreased and the arterial PCO_2 level increased owing to hypoventilation. Pacing of the left hemidiaphragm increased ventilation and resulted in a modest rise in arterial PO_2 and a fall in arterial PCO_2. The addition of oxygen (2 L. per minute) in the inspired air caused a further rise in oxygen without an appreciable change in the carbon dioxide level. It should be noted that on this admission, the patient was not in respiratory failure, as evidenced by the lack of carbon dioxide retention during the administration of oxygen without pacing demonstrated several nights later. (From Glenn, W. W. L., Gee, J. B. L., and Schachter, E. N.: Diaphragm pacing: Application to a patient with chronic obstructive pulmonary disease. J. Thorac. Cardiovasc. Surg., 75:273, 1978.)

months, he had required only four hospital admissions, compared with seven in the year prior to pacing. His hematocrit declined. Pacing ameliorated his insomnia and daytime somnolence. Moreover, several days of pacer malfunction led to a recurrence of somnolence, cyanosis, and coma — all of which responded to replacement of the pacemaker receiver.

Glenn stresses that the majority of patients with chronic obstructive pulmonary disease do not require pacing, since they are either in stable condition or can be safely oxygenated. If pacing is to be considered, the following criteria should be applied: (1) no significant upper airway obstruction, (2) presence of hemodynamically compromising hypoxemia, (3) intolerance of controlled oxygen therapy, (4) adequate expiratory flow, and (5) adequate diaphragmatic function. The rarity with which these criteria are met is indicated by the fact that no other patient has yet been reported to have received pacer-protected nocturnal oxygenation!

SPECIAL CONSIDERATIONS

Infants

Central alveolar hypoventilation, usually idiopathic, occasionally occurs in the newborn. These patients can be supported by diaphragm pacing, but simultaneous bilateral stimulation is necessary to achieve satisfactory ventilation. Although one infant was paced continuously for 142 days before succumbing to an overwhelming bronchopneumonia (Radecki and Tomatis, 1976), diaphragm fatigue usually intervenes after a few hours; hence, the infants are only intermittently freed from positive-pressure ventilation. Because their necks are short, infants require transthoracic placement of the phrenic nerve electrodes. The receivers are placed subcutaneously in the lateral aspect of the midabdomen bilaterally. It has not yet been determined at what age unilateral pacing will suffice in the growing child.

Pathologic Lesions of the Brain Stem

Glenn and associates (1980b) have described 13 patients who survived brain stem disruption secondary to stroke, tumor, or inflammation. These patients subsequently faced three life-threatening respiratory complications; central alveolar hypoventilation, upper airway obstruction, and aspiration pneumonia. All were treated by diaphragm pacing and tracheostomy (for central alveolar hypoventilation and upper airway obstruction, respectively). Aspiration was managed by

gastrostomy in 10 patients and by surgical closure of the larynx in three. Six patients died after discharge, but six are reported to be leading "productive lives" in spite of severe paresis or ataxia. It remains to be seen how useful diaphragm pacing will ultimately prove to be in the management of patients with this type of brain stem injury.

OPERATIVE TECHNIQUE

Cervical Electrode (Glenn, 1978; Glenn *et al.*, 1980a)

Through a transverse incision about 2 cm. above the clavicle, the prescalene fascia is exposed by splitting the sternocleidomastoid muscle and retracting the internal jugular vein medially and the scalene fat pad laterally (Fig. 26–15). The phrenic nerve lies just beneath the prescalene fascia and crosses the anterior scalene muscle obliquely, coursing downward from a posterolateral to an anteromedial position. It is located using a bipolar nerve probe. In about the midportion of the anterior scalene muscle, the nerve is

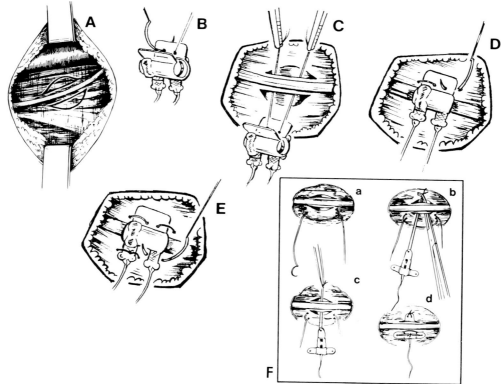

Figure 26–15. Operative technique. *A,* Through a transverse cervical incision the phrenic nerve is exposed as it overlies the scalenus anticus muscle. The internal jugular vein is retracted medially and the scalene fat pad laterally. (Exposure of the right phrenic nerve is depicted.) *B,* Traction sutures are passed through one horn of the silicone cuff that encloses the bipolar electrode. *C,* A 1.5-cm. segment of nerve is isolated, taking care to preserve 2 to 3 mm. of perineural tissue in all directions. The cuff electrode is then passed gently around the nerve. The red thread marker must be cephalad to assure cathodal stimulation. *D* and *E,* The cuff is anchored securely to the adjacent tissues, carefully avoiding distortion of the nerve. *F,* A similar technique is used to implant a monopolar electrode. Note that the nerve rests in a groove in the electrode cuff, rather than being encircled by it. An indifferent electrode is implanted near the receiver. (Adapted from Glenn, W. W. L.: Diaphragm pacing: Present status. PACE, *1*:357, 1978; Avery Laboratories, Inc.: Diaphragm Pacer [product brochure 6025B-11/79]. Avery Laboratories, Inc., Farmingdale, New York, May 1979.)

isolated by making 1.5-cm. parallel incisions that are kept 2 to 3 mm. from the nerve in order to preserve the perineural blood supply. The electrode cuff is then carefully inserted around the nerve (bipolar) or beneath the nerve (monopolar) and secured to the surrounding structures as shown in Figure 26–15, taking great care to avoid twisting or kinking. The bipolar cuff contains a red thread that must be placed cephalad to assure cathodal stimulation. The lead wires are then passed through a subcutaneous tunnel to join those from the receiver. The receiver is placed in a subcutaneous pocket (a) over the upper chest in the midclavicular line (for quadriplegics), (b) over the lower chest wall in the midaxillary line (for patients with central alveolar hypoventilation), or (c) over the lateral abdomen (for infants and children). Regardless of location, the subcutaneous pocket should be fashioned so that no part of the apparatus lies directly under the incision. The copper coil of the receiver should always face outward toward the undersurface of the skin. If bilateral units are implanted, the receivers must be separated by at least 15 cm. to avoid cross interference. Before terminating the operation, the ability of the system to produce a diaphragmatic contraction should be demonstrated using a sterile antenna. Thresholds are characteristically high in the early postoperative period. Pacing should therefore be delayed for 12 to 14 days to allow time for wound healing and for the subsidence of perineural edema.

Intrathoracic Electrodes

Intrathoracic placement of the cuff electrode is necessary in infants and may be desirable in some adults, because accessory fibers sometimes join the phrenic nerve as it courses through the thoracic inlet. The technique is similar to cervical implantation in that 2 to 3 mm. of pleura or pericardium are left on either side of the nerve to preserve perineural vessels (Fig. 26–16). Meticulous handling of the nerve and firm fixation of the cuff without twisting or angulation are as important here as in the neck. The leads are mated to a subcutaneous receiver. When placed intrathoracically, monopolar electrodes should be placed high in the mediastinum (5 to 10 cm. above the heart) to prevent the theoretical risk of cardiac arrhythmias.

SUMMARY

Safe and reliable diaphragm pacing is now possible using externally generated radiofrequency energy to activate permanently implanted subcutaneous electrodes. The major limitation of the present system is that ventilation usually becomes progressively less adequate after more than 20 to 24 hours of continuous pacing. Fatigue apparently arises from changes at the neuromuscular junction (Sato *et al.,* 1970) and can be delayed but not prevented by altering the level of current, stimulation wave form, electrode design, impulse frequency, and rate of pulse train repetition (Oda

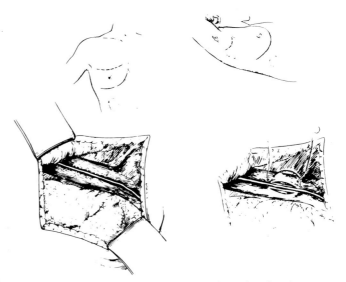

Figure 26–16. Transthoracic approach to the phrenic nerve. The mediastinum is exposed through an incision either in the second interspace anteriorly or through the third interspace in the axilla. The electrode cuff is inserted and secured as illustrated in Figure 26–15. If the nerve is isolated high in the mediastinum (5 to 10 cm. above the heart), either a bipolar or a monopolar electrode may be employed. Nearer the heart, a bipolar electrode is recommended. (From Glenn, W. W. L., Hogan, J. F., and Phelps, M. L.: Ventilatory support of the quadriplegic patient with respiratory paralysis by diaphragm pacing. Surg. Clin. North Am., *60:*1055, 1980.)

et al., 1981; Tanae *et al.,* 1973). If pacing is stopped when fatigue intervenes, the phenomenon is completely reversible. Indefinite pacing is possible for up to 12 hours if periods of stimulation are alternated with similar periods of rest.

Diaphragm pacing is applicable to a highly selected population of patients. It has proved useful in the management of patients with documented central alveolar hypoventilation, but only after sophisticated studies have ruled out significant upper airway obstruction. It has aided the long-term rehabilitation of certain quadriplegics with lesions high in the spinal cord (first and second cervical segments). By creating negative intrathoracic pressure and permitting utilization of the upper airways, diaphragm pacing closely mimics the normal physiology of ventilation. It remains to be seen, however, whether or not this will have significant long-term advantages over positive-pressure ventilation delivered by the more sophisticated and compact units that are now becoming available. Given the rigorous criteria by which candidates for diaphragm pacing must be selected and the necessity of close and indefinite follow-up, application of the technique should probably be limited to centers with special interest and expertise in the diagnosis and management of patients with central alveolar hypoventilation or respiratory insufficiency secondary to spinal cord injury.

Perhaps the greatest contribution of diaphragm pacing to medical science is the demonstration that peripheral nerves can be intermittently stimulated for months and years by artificial impulses without apparent structural or physiologic damage. As Glenn has speculated: "If the diaphragm can be paced indefinitely . . . artificial control of other body parts innervated by viable nervous tissue can be expected and may eventually become even more commonplace than cardiac pacing."

SELECTED REFERENCES

Note: The first two annotated references plus the product brochure "Diaphragm Pacing," available from Avery Laboratories, Inc., 145 Rome Street, Farmingdale, New York, 11735, should be considered *absolutely required reading* for anyone contemplating the use of one of these devices.

Glenn, W. W. L.: Diaphragm pacing: Present status. PACE, *1*:357, 1978.

In this comprehensive review article, Dr. Glenn summarizes his personal experience with diaphragm pacing in 50 patients. He enumerates the indications and contraindications for diaphragm pacing and tabulates the preoperative screening tests that should be performed. Documentation of phrenic nerve viability is obviously of cardinal importance. He stresses the need to rule out upper airway obstruction as a cause of sleep apnea in patients with central alveolar hypoventilation; this requires an overnight sleep study with appropriate monitoring. He briefly reviews the operative technique and strongly recommends that bilateral units be implanted at separate operations. He discusses pacing schedules and the need for diaphragm "conditioning" in quadriplegic patients. After presenting his results with diaphragm pacing in three categories of disease (central alveolar hypoventilation, quadriplegia, and chronic obstructive pulmonary disease), he lists six reasons that the technique may fail: (1) Poor selection of cases. (2) Iatrogenic injury to the phrenic nerve. (3) Improper use of the pacemaker. (4) Unrecognized upper airway obstruction. (5) Defective apparatus. (6) Further deterioration of ventilatory function secondary to depressant drugs, debilitating illnesses, pulmonary infection, or pulmonary edema. He emphasizes that when pulmonary function is acutely compromised, one cannot rely upon diaphragm pacing but must reinstitute mechanical ventilation.

Glenn, W. W. L., Hogan, J. F., and Phelps, M. L.: Ventilatory support of the quadriplegic patient with respiratory paralysis by diaphragm pacing. Surg. Clin. North Am., *60*:1055, 1980.

Twenty quadriplegic patients, aged 3 to 71 years (average 32 years), received diaphragm pacers at Yale University School of Medicine. Long-term ventilatory support was achieved by pacing in 18 patients. The two failures were predicted by poor phrenic nerve function at the time of operation. Of 16 patients with complete quadriplegia, eight were paced full-time, some for up to 10 years; the other eight tolerated only part-time support. There were 10 deaths, three of which were pacer-related: One death occurred during weaning from the pacer, and the other two deaths occurred during mechanical ventilation after prolonged bilateral pacing had produced irreversible diaphragmatic fatigue. In addition to a detailed description of the operative technique for both cervical and thoracic implantations, the article provides a revision of the recommended electrical parameters: pulse interval — 50 to 60 milliseconds, inspiration duration — 1.3 seconds, respiratory rate — 10 to 12 breaths per minute, and a current amplitude of just maximal or slightly submaximal. The authors emphasize that one should never use supramaximal current, a pulse interval less than 40 milliseconds, or a respiratory rate greater than 16 breaths per minute (except in infants). In Table IV, Dr. Glenn lists nine "concerns and caveats" in diaphragm pacing. These include the need to individualize pacing schedules, the need for a fail-safe alarm for quadriplegic patients, the observation that irreparable damage may occur to the nerve and diaphragm if pacing is continued in the face of diaphragmatic fatigue, and, the most important warning, "Even with parameters adjusted so that the electrical charge to the tissue is the lowest that is

possible without jeopardizing ventilation, electrical pacing of a hemidiaphragm must never be carried out beyond 16 hours."

Oakes, D. D., Wilmot, C. B., Halverson, D., and Hamilton, R. D.: Neurogenic respiratory failure: A 5-year experience using implantable phrenic nerve stimulators. Ann. Thorac. Surg., *30*:118, 1980.

Twenty phrenic nerve stimulators were implanted in 11 patients over a 5-year period. Ten patients had traumatic spinal cord lesions; one had a demyelinating disease. The only complications were one stimulator malfunction and one pneumothorax. Three patients became completely independent of their ventilators; four others were felt to have gained some long-term benefit in terms of simplified nursing care, enhanced mobility, and a more physiologic mechanism of ventilation. The authors conclude that complete ventilator independence should not be the sole criterion of success of diaphragm pacing in quadriplegic patients. They stress that phrenic nerve stimulation is not designed to supplant tracheostomy and positive-pressure ventilation in the initial management of patients with post-traumatic respiratory failure. Rather, its role is in the long-term rehabilitation of these patients. The technique should not be considered until several months have passed to be certain that recovery of spontaneous ventilatory ability will not occur. Likewise, it is not applicable to comatose patients for whom meaningful rehabilitation is not possible.

Schechter, D. C.: Application of electrotherapy to non-cardiac thoracic disorders, Bull. N.Y. Acad. Med., 46:932, 1970.
Schechter, D. C.: Flashbacks: Phrenic electrostimulation. PACE, *1*:393, 1978.

In 1783, the Reverend John Wesley submitted to electrotherapy for acute bronchopneumonia, and his reaction was that "God so blessed this that I had no more fever or cramp and no more load or tightness across my breast." Dr. Schechter describes the subsequent uses of electricity in medicine: To treat asthma, kyphoscoliosis, tuberculosis, laryngitides, and "many other intractable ailments." "Electromuscular gymnastics" strengthened the chest wall, improving both breathing and appetite! Ciniselli (1870) reported 23 patients whose aneurysms of the descending thoracic aorta were treated by percutaneous "galvano-puncturing." Six patients survived . . . briefly! The history of phrenic nerve stimulation and electrophrenic respiration constitutes the latter portion of the first article and the body of the second. Dr. Schechter's lucid reviews make fascinating reading for anyone interested in the history of medicine.

REFERENCES

Avery Laboratories, Inc.: Diaphragm Pacing (product brochure). Farmingdale, New York, May 1979.
Farmer, W. C., Glenn, W. W. L., and Gee, J. B.: Alveolar hypoventilation syndrome: Studies of ventilatory control in patients selected for diaphragm pacing. Am. J. Med., 64:39, 1978.
Glenn, W. W. L.: Diaphragm pacing: Present status. PACE, *1*:357, 1978.
Glenn, W. W. L., Gee, J. B. L., and Schachter, E. N.: Diaphragm pacing: Application to a patient with chronic obstructive pulmonary disease. J. Thorac. Cardiovasc. Surg., 75:273, 1978a.
Glenn, W. W. L., Hogan, J. F., and Phelps, M. L.: Ventilatory support of the quadriplegic patient with respiratory paralysis by diaphragm pacing. Surg. Clin. North Am., *60*:1055, 1980a.
Glenn, W. W. L., Phelps, M., and Gersten, L. M.: Diaphragm pacing in the management of central alveolar hypoventilation. *In* Sleep Apnea Syndromes. Edited by C. Guilleminault and W. C. Dement. New York, Alan R. Liss, 1978b, pp. 333–345.
Glenn, W. W. L., Haak, B., Sasaki, C., and Kirchner, J.: Characteristics and surgical management of respiratory complications accompanying pathologic lesions of the brain stem. Ann. Surg., *191*:655, 1980b.
Glenn, W. W. L., Gee, J. B. L., Cole, D. R., Farmer, W. C., Shaw,

R. K., and Beckman, C. B.: Combined central alveolar hypoventilation and upper airway obstruction: Treatment by tracheostomy and diaphragm pacing. Am. J. Med., *64*:50, 1978c.

Glenn, W. W. L., Holcomb, W. G., McLaughlin, A. J., Hare, J. M., Hogan, J. F., and Yasuda, R.: Total ventilatory support in a quadriplegic patient with radiofrequency electrophrenic respiration. N. Engl. J. Med., *286*:513, 1972.

Judson, J. P., and Glenn, W. W. L.: Radiofrequency electrophrenic respiration: Long-term application to a patient with primary hypoventilation. J.A.M.A., *203*:1033, 1968.

Kim, J. H., Manuelidis, E. E., Glenn, W. W. L., and Kaneyuki, T.: Diaphragm pacing: Histopathological changes in the phrenic nerve following long-term electrical stimulation. J. Thorac. Cardiovasc. Surg., *72*:602, 1976.

Oakes, D. D., Wilmot, C. B., Halverson, D., and Hamilton, R. D.: Neurogenic respiratory failure: A 5-year experience using implantable phrenic nerve stimulators. Ann. Thorac. Surg., *30*:118, 1980.

Oda, T., Glenn, W. W. L., Fukuda, Y., Hogan, J. F., and Gorfien, J.: Evaluation of electrical parameters for diaphragm pacing: An experimental study. J. Surg. Res., *30*:142, 1981.

Radecki, L. L., and Tomatis, L. A.: Continuous bilateral electrophrenic pacing in an infant with total diaphragmatic paralysis. J. Pediatr., *88*:969, 1976.

Sarnoff, S. J., Hardenbergh, E., and Whittenberger, J. L.: Electrophrenic respiration. Am. J. Physiol., *155*:1, 1948.

Sato, G., Glenn, W. W. L., Holcomb, W. G., and Wuench, D.: Further experience with electrical stimulation of the phrenic nerve: Electrically induced fatigue. Surgery, *68*:817, 1970.

Schechter, D. C.: Application of electrotherapy to non-cardiac thoracic disorders. Bull. N.Y. Acad. Med., *46*:932, 1970.

Schechter, D. C.: Flashbacks: Phrenic electrostimulation. PACE, *1*:393, 1978.

Tanae, H., Holcomb, W. G., Yasuda, R., Hogan, J. F., and Glenn, W. W. L.: Electrical nerve fatigue: Advantages of an alternating bidirectional waveform. J. Surg. Res., *15*:14, 1973.

Waud, R. A.: Production of artificial respiration by rhythmic stimulation of the phrenic nerves. Nature, *140*:849, 1937.

Whittenberger J. C., Sarnoff, S. J., and Hardenbergh, E.: Electrophrenic respiration: II. Its use in man. J. Clin. Invest., *28*:124, 1949.

Chapter 27

The Surgical Management of Myasthenia Gravis

C. Warren Olanow

Andrew S. Wechsler

Myasthenia gravis is a disorder of neuromuscular transmission characterized by weakness and fatigue of voluntary muscles. It is now reasonably established to be due to an autoimmune attack directed against the postsynaptic nicotinic acetylcholine receptors of voluntary muscles. Many detailed accounts of the clinical picture have been recorded prior to this century. The similarity of the clinical features of myasthenia gravis to those resulting from curare poisoning and the beneficial effect of prostigmine, demonstrated by Mary Walker in 1934, focused attention on impaired neuromuscular transmission as the basis of the disorder.

Interactions between quanta of acetylcholine released from the presynaptic terminal at the neuromuscular junction and acetylcholine receptors on the postsynaptic membrane determine the likelihood of muscular contraction. The excess number of potential interactions beyond that necessary to provide for maximal muscle contraction is referred to as the "safety factor" for neuromuscular transmission. Elmqvist and associates (1964) demonstrated that patients with myasthenia gravis had reduced miniature end-plate potential amplitudes, reflecting fewer interactions between acetylcholine (ACh) and acetylcholine receptors (AChR) and hence a diminished safety factor. Initially, this was thought to be due to inadequate release of ACh. More recent studies using specific neurotoxins (prepared from snake venom) have demonstrated a reduction in the number of acetylcholine receptors in patients with myasthenia gravis, as has been suggested by histologic and electron microscopic studies. In 1960, Simpson proposed that myasthenia gravis was due to an autoimmune disorder. The recognition by Patrick and Lindstrom in 1973 of an experimental allergic myasthenia gravis following immunization of rabbits with purified acetylcholine receptor and the detection of specific AChR antibodies in 90 per cent of patients with myasthenia gravis support this hypothesis.

A relationship between myasthenia gravis and the thymus gland has been appreciated since at least 1901. In 1912, Sauerbruch removed an enlarged thymus gland from a patient with myasthenia gravis who subsequently improved. In 1939, Blalock removed an enlarged thymus from a young woman with generalized myasthenia gravis. Encouraged by her response, in 1941, he made the important demonstration that removal of nontumorous thymus glands could lead to clinical improvement in patients with myasthenia gravis. His success stimulated subsequent investigators to examine the role of thymectomy in the treatment of myasthenia gravis. Although the role of the thymus gland in myasthenia gravis is incompletely defined, there are numerous reports suggesting that thymectomy is an effective therapy. Recent studies in our clinic have demonstrated that the use of thymectomy as the sole method of treatment results in dramatic clinical improvement in many patients, suggesting that a specific thymic factor contributes to the development of clinical weakness in myasthenia gravis.

CLINICAL FEATURES

Myasthenia gravis has a prevalence in the population of 1:75,000. There is a biphasic mode of distribution, with a tendency for populations of young women and elderly men to be affected. Females are involved twice as often as males, and in younger patients this ratio is increased to 4.5:1. The mean age of onset of symptoms is 26 years. Males tend to be affected at a later age and to have a higher incidence of thymoma. A genetic predisposition to develop myasthenia gravis is suggested by a high incidence of specific HLA antigens.

Weakness and fatigue with activity are the hallmarks of myasthenia gravis (Fig. 27–1). Virtually any muscle group in the body may be involved, and fluctuation in strength from day to day and even from hour to hour is common. Individual muscle groups may be selectively involved. Weakness tends to be more pronounced as the day progresses and following exercise. It may develop gradually or rapidly, and recovery may be total or incomplete. The ocular muscles are the most frequently affected muscle group and are the presenting feature in 50 to 60 per cent of myasthenia gravis patients, and they are ultimately involved in 90 per cent of patients. This is most often

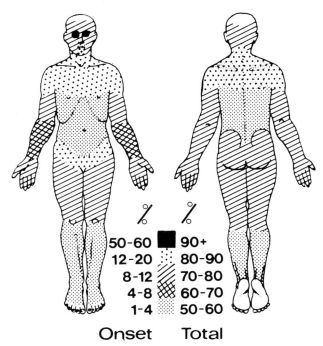

Figure 27–1. Involvement of muscle groups in patients with myasthenia gravis at time of onset (left column) and during course of illness (right column). (From Simpson, J. A.: *In* Myasthenia gravis and myasthenic syndromes. Disorders of Voluntary Muscle. 4th Ed. Edited by J. N. Walton. Edinburgh, Churchill Livingstone, 1978, pp. 585–624.)

manifested by ptosis and diplopia and may be exaggerated by repetitive testing or sustained exercise. Ptosis may fluctuate during the course of the examination, and Cogan's sign (a downward fall of the levator palpebrae superioris after upward gaze) may be demonstrated. Weakness of the orbicularis oculi is a frequent accompanying feature of ocular muscle involvement. Other cranial nerves may also be affected, leading to potentially fatal complications such as dysphagia and respiratory distress. Impaired chewing, dysarthria, and nasal speech are particularly common in patients with late-onset myasthenia gravis. Facial weakness with a transverse smile and involuntary grimace may develop. The tongue may become atrophic with a characteristic triple furrow. Weakness of the flexor or extensor muscles of the neck may require patients to support their heads with their hands.

In the extremities, there is generally symmetric weakness, involving proximal muscles more than distal groups and the arms more than the legs. There is considerable variation in this pattern, and in a specific patient, there may be asymmetric involvement, with any muscle group or even an isolated muscle being affected. The deep tendon reflexes tend to be preserved but may temporarily disappear with repetitive stimulation. The results of sensory examination are within normal limits, although patients may complain

of nonspecific sensations. Autonomic system involvement with pupillary changes, bladder disturbances, and increased sweating have all been described but are uncommon.

The onset of symptoms may be insidious or sudden, spontaneous or precipitated by emotional stress, exercise, allergies, vaccinations, or pregnancy. Myasthenia gravis may also become manifest as prolonged weakness following the use of relaxant drugs and anesthesia during surgery. Symptoms may remain confined to the ocular muscles, but more than 80 per cent of patients develop generalized weakness within 1 year of the onset of ocular disturbances. Grading systems to monitor clinical status are handicapped by difficulty in quantifying muscular strength and the variation that occurs in myasthenic patients, particularly after exposure to heat, exercise, stress, and drugs that interfere with neuromuscular transmission. The most widely used scale is the Osserman classification, which is presented in Table 27–1. This is a clinical classification that is limited by its failure to consider dependency on medication or to reflect subtle clinical improvement, creating difficulty in monitoring response to treatment.

The incidence of spontaneous remission, without drug or other therapy, is not known but is thought to be uncommon and short-lasting and to occur in patients with primarily ocular involvement. The ultimate course cannot be predicted with certainty, and many variations, including spontaneous remission in patients with long-standing disease or sudden deterioration in patients who have been asymptomatic for many years, have been recorded. A fixed myopathy late in the course of the disorder with permanent muscle weakness has been described. We have been concerned that this may be due to chronic anticholinesterase administration, but it has also been recorded in patients who have not received such medication.

A transient neonatal myasthenia gravis has been reported in infants of mothers with myasthenia gravis. Symptoms usually include diffuse weakness, impaired crying and sucking, poor swallowing, and, occasionally, feeble respiration. Symptoms are self-limited and generally resolve within 6 weeks. There are no clinical consequences as long as the initial symptoms are recognized and dealt with appropriately. Passive transfer of immunoglobulin across the placenta (presumably anti-AChR antibodies) is thought to be responsible. Interestingly, there is little correlation between the clinical status of the infant and that of the mother, despite comparable AChR antibody titers, supporting the hypothesis that host factors contribute to the development of clinical weakness.

A congenital myasthenia gravis that is more common in males has been described; it is often familial, but the mother is usually unaffected. The clinical configuration is usually not severe, and improvement occurs after 6 to 10 years of symptoms. Drugs and thymectomy are generally not effective. It has been

TABLE 27–1. MODIFIED CLINICAL CLASSIFICATION OF PATIENTS WITH MYASTHENIA GRAVIS

Group I *Ocular Myasthenia*
Involvement of ocular muscles only, with ptosis and diplopia.
Very mild. No mortality.

Group II
A. *Mild Generalized*
Slow onset, frequently ocular, gradually spreading to skeletal and bulbar muscles.
Respiratory system not involved. Response to drug therapy is good. Low mortality rate.

B. *Moderate Generalized*
Gradual onset with frequent ocular presentations, progressing to more severe generalized involvement of the skeletal and bulbar muscles. Dysarthria, dysphagia, and difficult mastication more prevalent than in mild generalized myasthenia gravis. Respiratory muscles not involved. Response to drug therapy is less satisfactory; patients' activities are restricted, but mortality rate is low.

C. *Severe Generalized*
1. *Acute fulminating.* Rapid onset of severe bulbar and skeletal muscle weakness with early involvement of respiratory muscles. Progress normally complete within 6 months. Percentage of thymomas is highest in this group. Response to drug therapy is less satisfactory, and patients' activities are restricted, but mortality rate is low.
2. *Late severe.* Severe myasthenia gravis develops at least 2 years after most of Group I or Group II symptoms. Progression of myasthenia gravis may be either gradual or sudden. Second highest percentage of thymomas occurs in this group. Response to drug therapy is poor, and prognosis is poor.

postulated that a delay in the maturation of the neuromuscular apparatus results in a prolonged reduction of the safety factor for neuromuscular transmission. Another congenital myasthenic syndrome, due to a reduction of acetylcholinesterase in the subneural apparatus of the end-plate, has also been described. These patients do not have AChR antibodies and do not respond to anticholinesterase medications.

The myasthenic or Eaton-Lambert syndrome consists of weakness and fatigability of proximal muscles, particularly in the lower extremities. Ocular and bulbar involvement is mild or absent. Deep tendon reflexes tend to be depressed or absent, and there is a characteristic electrophysiologic abnormality on the electromyogram. This syndrome is usually seen in association with an underlying oat cell carcinoma of the lung and may antedate recognition of the tumor. Less frequently, it occurs with other chronic disease states. The condition is due to the release of decreased quanta of acetylcholine from nerve endings. Anticholinesterase drugs are much less effective than they are in myasthenia gravis. Agents that facilitate the release of acetylcholine from the presynaptic nerve terminal, such as guanidine, calcium, or 4-aminopyridine, may be helpful.

In general, the diagnosis of myasthenia gravis is not difficult to make if it is considered. Hysteria, thyroid disease, neuromyopathies, and other myasthenic conditions are occasionally mistaken for myasthenia gravis, but a Tensilon test, single-fiber electromyography, and determination of acetylcholine receptor antibody levels (see discussion that follows) allow a definitive diagnosis to be made in the vast majority of cases.

Associated Conditions

A number of conditions have been associated with myasthenia gravis. Many of these, such as rheumatoid arthritis, systemic lupus erythematosus, polymyositis, Sjögren's syndrome, and ulcerative colitis, are thought to be autoimmune in nature. An association with vitamin B_{12} deficiency, thyroid disorders, diabetes mellitus, parathyroid disease, adrenal disorders, and vitiligo has been described as part of a polyglandular failure syndrome. These may be genetically predetermined, based on their linkage with histocompatibility antigens, particularly HLA-A1, -B8, and -Dw3. These may constitute genetic risk factors for autoimmune diseases whereby a specific exposure triggers an abnormal immune response in a patient with a given haplotype. This theory is supported by studies of monozygotic twins in which only one has been affected.

Thyroid dysfunction has been reported in 5 per cent of patients with myasthenia gravis, and the overall incidence may be much higher. At times, it may be difficult to distinguish features of thyroid disease from those of myasthenia gravis, as each can cause proximal muscle weakness and ocular disturbances. It would appear that these conditions are distinct, however, because it has been demonstrated that increased quantities of thyroid hormone per se do not result in myasthenia gravis and that the relationship is more likely to be immunologic or genetic than hormonal. All forms of thyroid disease, including goiter, myxedema, Graves' disease, and Hashimoto's thyroiditis, have been associated with myasthenia gravis.

Thymic Abnormalities

Disorders of the thymus gland are found in 75 to 85 per cent of patients with myasthenia gravis, and new staining techniques suggest that this incidence may be even higher. Ten to 15 per cent of patients with myasthenia gravis have thymomas. In most instances, these are benign, well-defined, encapsulated lesions that may be cystic or calcified. They are generally composed of epithelial or lymphoid cells. On the other hand, two thirds of thymomas have no association with myasthenia gravis and contain mainly spindle cells. Malignancy is usually defined by tumor infiltration into surrounding tissue such as pleura and pericardium rather than by changes in the histologic pattern. As many as 43 per cent of thymomas were malignant in one series. By contrast, in our experience, malignancy is a rare occurrence, perhaps reflecting our tendency to perform thymectomy earlier in the course of myasthenia gravis. Thymomas have not been described in children, are generally not seen before the age of 30 years, and are more common in male patients. A high-quality CT scan of the mediastinum can detect virtually all thymomas (Fig. 27–2). We have had an occasional false-positive CT scan but have not failed to recognize a thymoma by computed tomography in our study, in which all patients with myasthenia gravis undergo thymectomy, regardless of the interpretation of the CT scan.

Lymphoid hyperplasia of both the cortex and medulla is found in the thymus gland of most young patients with myasthenia gravis. There may be an increase in the number of germinal centers, but this is not unique to myasthenia gravis, and its significance is uncertain. Attempts to relate the numbers of ger-minal centers to the duration and severity of the disease and the response to treatment have been inconclusive. The T-cell composition of the thymus gland, in terms of both numbers and subsets, is generally normal. In contrast, there is an increased number of B cells in the thymus gland of patients with myasthenia gravis.

Patients with late-onset myasthenia gravis (after the age of 55 years) most often have an atrophic involuted thymus gland. Occasionally, these can be recognized on CT scan by the existence of relatively low density (presumably fat) throughout the anterior mediastinum punctuated by dots of high density (presumably thymic tissue). There is evidence to suggest that an atrophic thymus gland may still be immunologically active, with thymic cells identified within the anterior mediastinal fat. This is an important consideration with respect to the role of thymectomy in these patients. They have a relative lymphopenia in the peripheral blood consisting primarily of a reduction in T lymphocytes and 3A1+ and OKT4 T-cell subsets. These changes are rapidly reversed following the removal of the "involuted" thymus gland.

DIAGNOSTIC STUDIES

Pharmacologic Agents

Anticholinesterase agents block the hydrolysis of ACh in the synaptic cleft, prolonging its action and increasing the likelihood of an interaction between ACh and the postsynaptic AChR. As a consequence, there is an increase in the miniature end-plate potential and in the safety factor for neuromuscular transmission. These agents may reverse or improve the clinical and electrical abnormalities in myasthenia gravis. The most widely used anticholinesterase agent for diagnosis is edrophonium (Tensilon). This is a short-acting drug that improves clinical and/or electrical abnormalities in 95 per cent of patients with myasthenia gravis. Its use is widespread, and prior to more sophisticated laboratory evaluations, a positive response was central to the definition of myasthenia gravis. The response in individual patients varies from dramatic improvement, confirming the diagnosis, to subtle or no change. The ocular muscles are least sensitive to this drug, making it occasionally difficult to diagnose cases of myasthenia gravis confined to the ocular muscles. However, failure to respond to edrophonium does not exclude myasthenia gravis. It is recommended that the test be performed at the end of the day or after exercise, when the patient's weakness is maximal.

Two to 10 mg. of edrophonium are administered intravenously. The initial 2 mg. may detect hypersensitivity, so that the possibility of enhancing cholinergic weakness in patients receiving anticholinesterase medications may be avoided. Facilities to treat anaphylactic and respiratory complications should be available. A positive response generally develops within 30 to 60 seconds and lasts for approximately 1

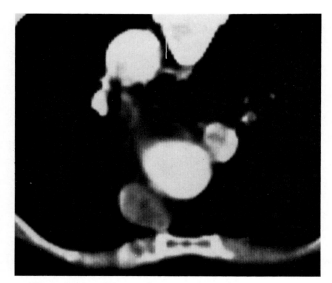

Figure 27–2. CT scan from a patient with a thymoma. The anterior mediastinal mass is easily visualized. With increasing experience, this test has become progressively more helpful in separating patients with thymomas from those with normal thymus glands and has even been able to identify islands of functioning thymus tissue within generally atrophic glands.

to 5 minutes. It has been our practice to perform the edrophonium test in a triple-blind fashion with saline and nicotinic acid as control agents. Edrophonium generally causes a light-headed, hot sensation associated with lacrimation and flushing that patients may learn to recognize. Nicotinic acid reproduces some of these features without influencing neuromuscular transmission and thus serves as a suitable control substance.

Long-lasting anticholinesterase agents may be used when responses are too transient to record by standard bedside techniques. These agents have a longer latency and duration. Neostigmine may be used in a dosage of 1.5 mg. administered intramuscularly. Improvement is seen within 10 to 30 minutes and lasts up to 4 hours. When the response is still equivocal, a long-term trial of oral anticholinesterase agents over several weeks can be considered.

Patients with myasthenia gravis are highly sensitive to the neuromuscular blocking effect of curare and curare-like drugs. This heightened sensitivity has been used in the past as a test to confirm the diagnosis. One tenth of a curarizing dose may cause the patient to become significantly weak. An anesthetist must be present at this test because of the risk of respiratory decompensation, and consequently, this test is rarely used today.

An abnormal "dual response" following administration of decamethonium has been described, consisting of brief depolarization following a longer period of curare-like competitive block. Although interesting pharmacologically, this test is no longer employed in practice.

Electrophysiologic Studies

The hallmark of myasthenia gravis is failure of neuromuscular transmission. This is characterized electrically by a reduction in the amplitude of the miniature end-plate potential. In 1895, Jolly recognized that faradic stimulation of a peripheral nerve resulted in muscle fatigue. He recognized that in patients with myasthenia gravis, supramaximal repetitive stimulation of the nerve led to a gradual decrease of the evoked action potential without a change in antidromic conduction. The Jolly test consists of repetitive stimulation of a peripheral nerve. In normal patients, the safety margin is of such a magnitude that repeated stimulations can be tolerated to a rate of 40 to 50 per second. In patients with myasthenia gravis, abnormal diminution begins to occur at stimulation rates of 2 to 3 per second, particularly if these are performed following tetanic contractions of muscle or the administration of regional curare. This test has the advantage of being simple and inexpensive, but unfortunately, it is not particularly sensitive. Changes are not detected in more than 50 per cent of patients with myasthenia gravis, particularly in the early stages.

The development of single-fiber electromyography has provided a much more sensitive method of detecting impaired neuromuscular transmission. A single-fiber needle electrode is placed between two muscle fibers innervated by the same motor unit. The variability in the latency between the two action potentials is referred to as jitter (Fig. 27–3). The variability of neuromuscular transmission in myasthenia gravis leads to increased jitter or blocking of one of the action potentials in severe cases. Jitter measurements are abnormal in 95 per cent of patients with myasthenia gravis if multiple muscle groups are studied. In patients with purely ocular symptoms, the frontalis or levator palpebrae superioris muscle should be examined. Jitter measurements must be analyzed in light of the clinical picture, as abnormalities can be seen in disorders other than myasthenia gravis. Since jitter is a function of the amplitude of the miniature end-plate potential, this test can be used to monitor the clinical course of patients with myasthenia gravis. Although it has the advantage of being sensitive in the early detection of myasthenia gravis, it requires expensive complex machinery and neurophysiologic expertise.

Stapedial reflex decay has recently been used as a diagnostic study in myasthenia gravis. Preliminary results indicate a high sensitivity in patients with ocular dysfunction, but results are less encouraging in patients with generalized weakness.

TABLE 27–2. DRUGS THAT INTERFERE WITH NEUROMUSCULAR TRANSMISSION UNDER EXPERIMENTAL CONDITIONS

Antibiotics
  Amikacin
  Paramycin
  Polymyxin A
  Sisomicin
  Viomycin

Antiarrhythmic
  Ajmaline

Antirheumatic
  Colchicine

Anticonvulsant
  Ethosuximide

Psychotropic
  Amitriptyline
  Amphetamines
  Droperidol
  Haloperidol
  Imipramine
  Paraldehyde
  Trichloroethanol

Others
  Amantadine
  Diphenhydramine
  Emetine
  Pindolol
  Sotalol

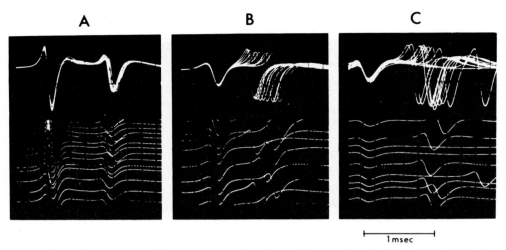

Figure 27–3. Electromyographic jitter recordings; traces are superimposed on top line. *A,* Normal jitter. Note the constant latency between the two muscle action potentials. *B,* Increased jitter but without impulse blocking in a patient with myasthenia gravis. *C,* Increased jitter with occasional blocking in a patient with severe myasthenia gravis. (From Stalberg, E., Trontel, J. V., and Schwartz, M.S.: Single muscle fiber recording of jitter phenomenon in patients with myasthenia gravis and in members of their families. Ann. N.Y. Acad. Sci., *274*:189, 1976.)

Serum Antibodies

A number of nonspecific antibodies have been described in patients with myasthenia gravis. These include antistriational, antinuclear, antithyroid, antigastric, antispermatogenic, and antineuronal antibodies.

The isolation of specific neurotoxins from the venom of elapid snakes such as cobras and kraits allowed the recognition of specific serum antiacetylcholine receptor antibodies. Alpha-bungarotoxin, a specific neurotoxin from the banded krait, has been found to bind specifically and irreversibly to the active site of the AChR. This toxin can be used to measure the number of receptors, to purify receptors, and to assay for serum acetylcholine receptor antibody. The assay consists of the reaction between test serum and AChR antigen derived from human muscle that has been incubated with ^{125}I-labeled alpha-bungarotoxin. If serum AChR antibodies are present, they bind to the AChR and form a complex with the ^{125}I-labeled alpha-bungarotoxin, which is bound to a neighboring site on the receptor. Antihuman globulin then precipitates this complex, and the radioactivity in the precipitant allows for an estimation of the quantitative AChR antibody level. Serum AChR antibodies are present in 90 per cent of patients with myasthenia gravis. These antibodies are highly specific for myasthenia gravis and have been found otherwise only following administration of penicillamine or inoculation with snake venom, but in no other disease state. Furthermore, AChR released from damaged muscle does not evoke the development of AChR antibodies. AChR antibody levels do not directly correlate with the clinical status of patients with myasthenia gravis, but patients with purely ocular disease tend to have the lowest antibody titers.

PATHOGENESIS

Considerable evidence has accumulated since the original hypothesis by Simpson (1960) to support the concept that myasthenia gravis is an autoimmune disorder involving the postsynaptic nicotinic AChR. Histologically, the postsynaptic membrane is simplified and disorganized (Fig. 27–4). Alpha-bungarotoxin binding studies have demonstrated quantitative reduction in the amount of AChR correlating with the reduction in the amplitude of the miniature end-plate action potential and the clinical severity of the condition. The detection of specific AChR antibodies in the serum of approximately 90 per cent of patients with myasthenia gravis has focused attention on this antibody in the pathogenesis of myasthenia gravis. It has been postulated that these antibodies induce clinical weakness by reducing the number of functioning AChR, thus impairing neuromuscular transmission. Mechanisms proposed include (1) accelerated degradation of AChR on the postsynaptic membrane; (2) immunopharmacologic blockade in which the antibody hinders interactions between ACh and the AChR; (3) modulation or accelerated internalization with intracellular degradation of the AChR–AChR antibody complex; (4) reduced synthesis of AChR.

Passive transfer of serum and, more specifically, IgG from patients with myasthenia gravis to experimental animals can induce a myasthenic syndrome characterized by clinical, electrical, and pharmacologic features similar to that of human myasthenia gravis. This syndrome may also be caused by specific monoclonal AChR antibodies. Passive transfer among animal species has been demonstrated. Furthermore, IgG from patients with myasthenia gravis accelerates the degradation of AChR in myotube tissue culture. In human myasthenia gravis, plasmapheresis and ste-

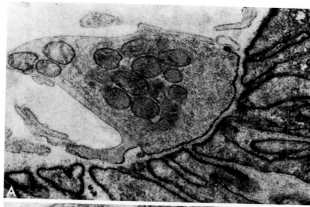

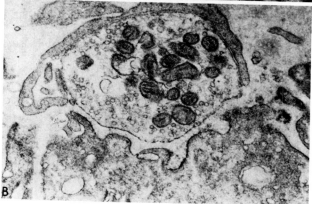

Figure 27–4. Neuromuscular junction with acetylcholine receptors stained by peroxidase-labeled alpha-bungarotoxin technique. *A*, Normal neuromuscular junction with normal quantity of acetylcholine receptors. *B*, Neuromuscular junction in patient with moderately severe myasthenia gravis. Note the disorganization and destruction of the postsynaptic membrane, with reduction in staining for acetylcholine receptor. (Courtesy of A. G. Engel.)

roids lead to clinical benefit in association with a reduction in the serum AChR antibody titer. The removal of thoracic duct lymph containing immunoglobulin also results in clinical improvement, and the readministration of this material results in rapid clinical deterioration. These observations support the hypothesis that AChR antibodies contribute to and may be the major mechanism responsible for receptor damage in myasthenia gravis.

Nevertheless, it is by no means clear that the AChR antibody is the sole factor responsible for clinical weakness. In studies at Duke University in which all patients were treated with thymectomy as the sole means of therapy and in which all drugs, including anticholinesterase agents, were avoided, dramatic clinical benefit was seen in the majority of patients without a reduction in the AChR antibody titer. There was no direct correlation between the serum AChR antibody level and the clinical status of individual patients. We hypothesized that a thymic factor was essential to the development of clinical weakness in myasthenia gravis. This is supported by the development of transient neonatal myasthenia

gravis in the infant of an asymptomatic thymectomized mother, with comparable levels and bioactivity of AChR antibody in each. Although steroids and plasmapheresis provide dramatic clinical improvement in many patients, the corresponding reduction in AChR antibody titer may be an independent phenomenon. It is presumptive to assume that this reduction is essential for clinical improvement, and clearly, more than AChR antibodies are removed by plasmapheresis. Furthermore, the reduction in the AChR antibody titer following plasmapheresis is often short-lived, whereas clinical benefit may persist for weeks or months.

Different AChR antibodies that react to different sites on the AChR have been identified, and it is possible that the current techniques fail to identify the specific subset that would better correlate with the clinical status of patients with myasthenia gravis. It must also be remembered that serum AChR antibody titers may not accurately reflect antibody activity at the neuromuscular junction. Still, in our drug-free group, no patient converted to a negative antibody titer following thymectomy, despite clinical improvement, and when antibody titers did fall, they did so gradually over a period of years rather than in direct correlation with the clinical status.

In an elegant series of experiments, Engel and coworkers (1977) demonstrated deposits of IgG and C3 complement on segments of the postsynaptic membrane in the distribution of the AChR and on fragments of degenerating junctional folds in the synaptic space (Fig. 27–5). More severely affected myasthenic patients bind relatively smaller amounts of IgG and C3 complement, presumably because there are fewer residual acetylcholine receptors. The presence of C3 complement indicates activation of the complement reaction. Subsequent activation of the major or alternate pathway could then set the stage for a complement-mediated lysis of the membrane.

More recently, Sahashi and associates (1980), using an immunoperoxidase method, demonstrated the presence of the C9 terminal and lytic complement component at the postsynaptic junctional folds and in debris within the synaptic clefts in the same basic distribution as C3 complement. Once again, there was an inverse relationship between the structural integrity of the junctional folds and the abundance of C9. The areas of involvement were discrete and widely separated, supporting the concept of an autoimmune attack. C3 complement does not necessarily result in membrane damage and may be found over long portions of junctional membrane. Activation to C9, however, leads to irreversible damage to the membrane. Demonstration of C9 over only short portions of junctional folds and in abundance in the degenerated material of the synaptic cleft supports the role of the complement-mediated lysis as the mechanism of membrane damage in myasthenia gravis. This differs from other conditions such as Duchenne's muscular dystrophy in which degeneration of junctional folds occurs in the absence of IgG or C9 complement. It is possible

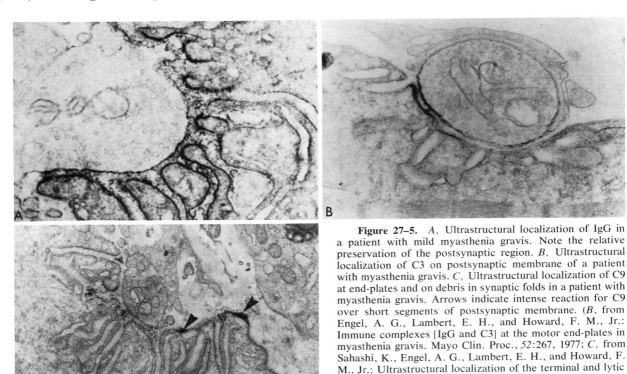

Figure 27–5. *A,* Ultrastructural localization of IgG in a patient with mild myasthenia gravis. Note the relative preservation of the postsynaptic region. *B,* Ultrastructural localization of C3 on postsynaptic membrane of a patient with myasthenia gravis. *C,* Ultrastructural localization of C9 at end-plates and on debris in synaptic folds in a patient with myasthenia gravis. Arrows indicate intense reaction for C9 over short segments of postsynaptic membrane. (*B,* from Engel, A. G., Lambert, E. H., and Howard, F. M., Jr.: Immune complexes [IgG and C3] at the motor end-plates in myasthenia gravis. Mayo Clin. Proc., *52:*267, 1977; *C,* from Sahashi, K., Engel, A. G., Lambert, E. H., and Howard, F. M., Jr.: Ultrastructural localization of the terminal and lytic 9th complement component [C9] at the motor end-plate in myasthenia gravis. J. Neuropathol. Exp. Neurol., *39:*160, 1980.)

that the AChR antibody marks the receptor for complement-mediated lysis, and some current evidence suggests that the thymus gland may activate the alternate complement pathway, facilitating this reaction.

Although most attention has been focused on humoral immune mechanisms, cell-mediated immune mechanisms have not been excluded from playing a role in the pathogenesis of myasthenia gravis. Studies in our laboratories have demonstrated a reduction in the number of peripheral blood T cells in patients with late-onset myasthenia gravis. This reduction consists primarily of T-cell subsets 3A1 and OKT4, and these changes normalize rapidly following thymectomy. Lymphocyte transformation has been described in several laboratories following exposure of peripheral blood and thymic lymphocytes to purified AChR antigen. This stimulation index has also been reported to be reduced following thymectomy. Alterations in mixed lymphocyte reactions and autologous lymphocyte reactions have been observed and are currently being studied. Although not a consistent finding, lymphorrhages, which are small groups of lymphocytes within muscle, are occasionally detected. All of these changes suggest that a cell-mediated mechanism plays some role in the pathogenesis of myasthenia gravis, but its importance has not yet been defined. The possibility of multiple mechanisms and heterogeneous patient populations must be considered.

Experimental Allergic Myasthenia Gravis

Using snake venom such as alpha-bungarotoxin, Patrick and Lindstrom (1973) were able to isolate AChR from homogenized muscle. Purified receptor was then injected into rabbits in an effort to provoke specific AChR antibodies. Several weeks following this immunization, the rabbits became weak and died. The weakness had clinical, electrical, and pharmacologic features resembling those seen in human myasthenia gravis, and this disorder is now known as experimental autoimmune myasthenia gravis. It is thought to be the result of AChR antibodies generated by immunization with AChR cross-reacting with the rabbits' own AChR, leading to impaired neuromuscular transmission. Histologic changes seen at the neuromuscular junction are similar to those seen in human patients, and passive transfer of serum or lymphocytes from these animals can induce the disease when injected into normal animals. An acute state occurs approximately 1 week after immunization and is characterized by severe muscle weakness and a cellular invasion of the neuromuscular junction with breakdown of the postsynaptic membrane and AChR. Approximately 3 weeks following immunization, a chronic stage develops in association with a rising AChR antibody titer. The postsynaptic membrane becomes decreased in area and simplified, with a consequent reduction in the total number of acetyl-choline receptors. The chronic phase of experimental autoimmune myasthenia gravis is virtually identical to that in the human disorder, but the experimental autoimmune condition differs from human myasthenia gravis in that the acute transient phase is not seen in human patients. This may reflect a differing nature of the immunizing event, with the human patient not being exposed to a massive bolus of antigen at one time, or differences in host response. It has also been suggested that the acute phase may be related to the adjuvant rather than the AChR.

Significantly, experimental autoimmune myas-thenia gravis will not develop in animals who have been thymectomized prior to immunization. This sug-gests that a thymic factor may be essential to the development of clinical weakness in this condition. Furthermore, C3 complement deficiency also atten-uates the clinical and electrical features of experimen-tal autoimmune myasthenia gravis, supporting the hypothesis that complement-mediated lysis may be the mechanism leading to membrane damage.

Role of the Thymus Gland

A relationship between the thymus gland and myasthenia gravis has been appreciated since the beginning of this century. Seventy to 80 per cent of patients with myasthenia gravis have pathologic changes in their thymus gland, and for 50 years thymectomy has been known to influence the clinical course of myasthenia gravis. It is therefore not sur-prising that thymic factors have been suggested to play a role in the pathogenesis of myasthenia gravis. The exact role that the thymus gland plays, however, remains to be defined. There are cells within the thymus gland (myoid cells) that have a striking simi-larity to embryonic muscle cells. These cells contain AChR on their surface and react with AChR antibod-ies. The thymic cells in culture can produce AChR antibody, and radiated thymic cells that have been thus rendered functionally inactive can augment the production of AChR antibody from peripheral lym-phocytes. It is also known that the thymus gland plays a major part in lymphocyte maturation and is capable of influencing virtually all humoral and cellular im-mune reactions. It has been proposed that an initiating event, possibly of a viral nature, induces a "thymitis." Because of the unique location of myoid cells in immediate proximity to maturing lymphocytes, an autoimmune reaction may develop directed against the AChR on myoid cells that later cross-reacts with AChR at the neuromuscular junction. The altered thymus gland might also generate a population of killer T cells, which destroy the neuromuscular junc-tion, or a population of helper cells, which stimulate the production of AChR antibody by peripheral lym-phocytes. More recently, it has been suggested that thymic factors may also play a role in activating the complement pathway leading to membrane lysis. The

association of myasthenia gravis with other autoim-mune disorders, particularly the polyglandular failure syndrome, suggests that the immunologic attack may be more widely directed than to the AChR alone in some patients. The relationship with HLA antigens in some patients with myasthenia gravis also suggests that there is a genetically predisposed population of patients whose immunologic tolerance may be altered in such a manner that a specific exposure results in altered immunologic responses.

The mechanism whereby thymectomy leads to clinical benefit has not yet been elucidated. It has been demonstrated that thymectomy influences cell-mediated immunity and peripheral T-cell counts in patients with late-onset myasthenia gravis, but the clinical relevance of this is not established. Thymec-tomy may serve to remove a source of (1) AChR antigen, (2) AChR antibody production, (3) sensitized killer T cells directed against the neuromuscular junc-tion, (4) sensitized helper T cells that facilitate the production of AChR antibody by peripheral lympho-cytes, and (5) a putative thymic factor that may activate the complement pathway leading to comple-ment-mediated lysis at antibody-labeled receptor sites. It is also possible that thymectomy acts by multiple or unknown mechanisms.

Failure of thymectomy to induce clinical remis-sion might be due to (1) incomplete thymectomy, (2) permanent irreparable damage to the neuromuscular junction, (3) a thymic influence exerted by extrathymic populations of lymphocytes within the spleen, lymph nodes, and so on that are unaffected by thymectomy, (4) the influence of long-lived peripheral T cells, and (5) heterogeneous disease mechanisms, whereby the thymic influence differs in individual patients.

TREATMENT

Numerous methods of treatment have been em-ployed in the management of myasthenia gravis. Var-iations in the natural history and the lack of prospec-tive control studies of the different treatment modalities prevent an absolute determination of the preferred form of treatment for a given patient at the present time. Furthermore, it has been suggested that the natural history of myasthenia gravis as it is seen today follows a more benign course than that seen in previous decades. Improvement in supportive meas-ures and surgical technique may contribute to the improved patient statistics, independent of the specific therapy chosen. The large number of variables to be controlled and physician bias favoring one form of therapy over another make it unlikely that a controlled study can be effected, and at least for the present, some judgment is required in instituting therapy.

We have favored total thymectomy performed as early as possible after the development of generalized weakness. Drugs are avoided and employed only when necessary rather than as a routine part of treatment. All patients are managed according to a prospective standardized treatment protocol to minimize variables and to avoid a physician bias. In our practice, after a mean follow-up of 25.5 months, 87 per cent of patients were free from generalized weakness, and 61 per cent required no medication. Our protocol does not compare thymectomy with other forms of treatment, but the excellent results and the possibility of avoiding additional medications lead us to favor this form of treatment in patients with generalized myasthenia gravis. Prior to a more detailed discussion of thymectomy, we will consider the advantages and disadvantages of the major forms of treatment currently being employed. In each instance, drugs that interfere with neuromuscular transmission (Table 27–2) should be avoided or used with caution, as they may lead to a deterioration in the myasthenic status.

Medical Treatment

Anticholinesterase Agents. Anticholinesterase agents have been a standard form of medical treatment for myasthenia gravis since their introduction in the mid 1930s. They act by preventing the hydrolysis of acetylcholine and increase the likelihood of interactions between acetylcholine and the acetylcholine receptor. The safety margin for neuromuscular transmission is thereby increased, providing temporary improvement in the clinical and electrical features of myasthenia gravis. These agents may result in marked improvement with restoration of muscle strength. It should be emphasized, however, that this response is only symptomatic and that these drugs in and of themselves do not lead to remission. Side effects of anticholinesterase drugs include abdominal colic, diarrhea, nausea, salivation, and lacrimation as a result of smooth muscle and glandular stimulation. These symptoms may be controlled by atropine; this is not recommended, however, because the symptoms may forewarn the patient and physician of developing "cholinergic crisis." Cholinergic crisis is the result of excessive stimulation of acetylcholine receptors with prolonged depolarization of receptors and consequent muscle weakness not directly related to myasthenia gravis. Cholinergic weakness can be differentiated from myasthenic weakness by administration of a test dose of Tensilon, as symptoms will fail to respond or will deteriorate following the administration of additional anticholinesterase medication. Treatment consists of discontinuation of anticholinesterase agents and appropriate support measures.

Neostigmine (Prostigmin) and pyridostigmine (Mestinon) are the most commonly employed anticholinesterase agents. Neostigmine is available in 15-mg. tablets, which are usually administered every 4 hours, or more frequently as required. There is usually a 30-minute delay before maximal efficacy, and the optimal dosage is determined by trial and error. It must be recalled that parenteral administration of 0.5 mg. is equivalent to 15 mg. orally. Pyridostigmine is the more popular medication because it is felt to have a smoother effect and to be longer-acting, with a less abrupt loss of efficacy. Sixty milligrams of pyridostigmine is equivalent to 15 mg. of neostigmine, and the time span of 180 mg. is available for more prolonged use, such as at night.

Despite the popularity of these agents, we have preferred not to employ them whenever possible. The symptomatic benefits that they provide may delay the introduction of early thymectomy, which we believe to be the preferred form of therapy. These agents increase bronchial and oropharyngeal secretions, which may lead to respiratory complications, particularly at the time of surgery. Furthermore, following thymectomy, there appears to be an increased sensitivity to anticholinesterase medications, which may lead to cholinergic weakness, complicating the postoperative management. We have thus avoided anticholinesterase agents in our thymectomy patients without an evident loss of clinical efficacy and with what appears to be a smoother operative and postoperative course (see discussion that follows).

Evidence in experimental animals indicates that chronic exposure to anticholinesterase agents independently leads to acetylcholine receptor damage and electron microscopic alterations identical to those seen in myasthenia gravis. Although there is no proof that a similar phenomenon occurs in human patients, there has been the concern that long-term employment of these agents may lead to a fixed myopathic state unrelated to the myasthenia.

Corticosteroids. There have been many studies demonstrating the beneficial effect of corticosteroids in patients with myasthenia gravis. The clinical response may be dramatic with total remission of symptoms, but it is important to appreciate that the introduction of steroids may be associated with a transient clinical deterioration (usually between the fourth and eighth days), and it is recommended that they be started in the hospital setting, where provisions for respiratory assistance are available. Prednisone has been most widely employed, beginning with a dosage of 60 to 80 mg. per day. Once an adequate response is obtained, patients are changed to an alternate-day dosage schedule, and the medication is gradually tapered as clinically appropriate. When an alternate-day dosage of 60 mg. of prednisone has been reached, it is recommended that reductions in dosage should not exceed 5 mg. every other day, no more frequently than once every other month, to minimize the risk of inducing myasthenic crisis.

Although many use steroids as a primary mode of therapy, particularly for patients with late-onset myasthenia gravis, we have preferred to employ them only in patients who cannot or will not undergo a thymectomy or in patients who have had a clinically unsatisfactory response to thymectomy. We have also used corticosteroids in a low-dose alternate-day schedule for patients with ocular myasthenia gravis or with residual ocular dysfunction following thymectomy. Corticosteroids have been employed to prepare patients for thymectomy, but the same can now be accomplished with plasmapheresis without the risk of clinical deterioration and the difficulty in withdrawing steroid medication.

The mechanism of action of corticosteroids is not understood. Most attention has focused on immunosuppression. Several groups have reported a reduction in the acetylcholine receptor antibody titer that correlates with clinical improvement in patients with myasthenia gravis, raising the possibility that suppression of immunoglobulin is responsible for clinical benefit. However, studies of thymectomy as the sole treatment modality have failed to confirm a direct correlation between the clinical status of patients with myasthenia gravis and the acetylcholine receptor antibody titer. Although these studies suggest that an essential thymic factor contributes to the development of clinical weakness, the possibility exists that steroids and thymectomy act by different mechanisms. Steroids may have a thymolytic effect, although it is noteworthy that they may be effective in patients who have already undergone thymectomy. A direct effect on neuromuscular transmission has also been suggested by the transient deterioration during the off day reported by patients on an alternate-day steroid schedule.

Once steroids have been initiated, they may be difficult to discontinue. Although the dosage may be substantially reduced, in many patients steroids have to be maintained indefinitely. Aside from the risk of clinical deterioration related to dosage change, there are many side effects associated with sustained administration of steroids. These include cataracts, psychosis, gastrointestinal bleeding, carbohydrate intolerance, hypertension, obesity, osteoporosis, growth failure in the juvenile population, and decreased resistance to infection. In one large series, as many as 50 per cent of patients developed cushingoid features. Although the benefit of the steroids is not questioned, prospective control studies demonstrating that they are superior to other forms of therapy such as thymectomy do not exist, and we have preferred to employ these drugs only when necessary rather than on a routine basis in an effort to avoid these potential complications.

Plasmapheresis. Plasmapheresis is a technique that permits the selective removal of plasma or plasma components by a centrifugal method. The remaining red cells are then suspended in a solution such as lactated Ringer's solution and reintroduced to the patient. The procedure, which is easy to accomplish, produces a rapid transient clinical improvement in patients with myasthenia gravis and has proved to be a valuable tool. We have employed plasmapheresis primarily to optimize the medical status of patients prior to surgical thymectomy. One to 3 liters of plasma is removed per run on an alternate-day basis until the maximal clinical benefit has been obtained (usually four to six runs). This clinical improvement facilitates the perioperative period while avoiding the need for additional medications. Aside from occasional hypotension during the first or second run, plasmapheresis is generally well tolerated. Hypocalcemia and hypoalbuminemia may result from repeated runs and need

to be identified and treated appropriately. We do not perform surgical intervention within 48 hours of the last run of plasmapheresis to minimize the risk of bleeding and infection due to removal of clotting factors or immunoglobulins.

Plasmapheresis has been used in some centers as a primary therapeutic modality. Because plasmapheresis produces only temporary clinical benefit, immunosuppressive drugs must be employed as well to obtain a stable clinical improvement, and it has not been established to date that plasmapheresis increases the likelihood of clinical remission compared with the use of immunosuppressive drugs alone. We have employed this form of treatment only in patients whose symptoms are refractory to thymectomy or who have experienced acute deterioration following thymectomy.

The mechanism of action of plasmapheresis is presumably related to the removal of a specific plasma factor. The serum acetylcholine receptor antibody has been implicated, as levels are dramatically reduced at the time of plasmapheresis in conjunction with clinical improvement. Clinical benefit, however, may persist for substantially longer periods of time than the acetylcholine receptor antibody remains depressed, and some patients respond to plasmapheresis who have no detectable serum antiacetylcholine receptor antibodies. It must be emphasized that more than serum immunoglobulins are removed at the time of plasmapheresis, and it is possible that it is the removal of an additional factor(s) that contributes to the improvement following plasmapheresis.

Immunosuppressive Agents. The evidence supporting an immunologic basis for myasthenia gravis and the response to plasmapheresis and thoracic duct drainage have fostered an interest in immunosuppressive drugs. In general, these have been employed in patients who are refractory to more conventional therapies such as thymectomy or steroids. Azathioprine has been most widely employed in a dose of 1.5 to 3 mg./kg. There is a latency period of 6 to 12 weeks prior to onset of benefit, and maximal effect may not be obtained for 1 year or longer. European physicians have a wide experience with this drug and report favorable responses in the majority of their patients, although serious complications such as marrow suppression, gastrointestinal bleeding, decreased resistance to infection, and death have all been reported. The possibility of delayed side effects such as the development of malignancies must also be considered. Generally, the medication is well tolerated, although severe nausea, vomiting, and diarrhea have restricted its employment in some patients. More potent cytotoxic drugs, such as cyclophosphamide, have not been widely studied, but there are occasional reports of benefit.

Immunosuppressant drugs may be more effective when combined with plasmapheresis, as described in the previous section. Antilymphocyte serum, antithymocyte serum, and splenic radiation have all been tried and have been reported to have some effectiveness in refractory cases of myasthenia gravis. Clearer delineation of the humoral and/or cellular immune mechanism directed against the acetylcholine receptor may allow for more specific immunosuppression. Trials of monoclonal antibodies directed against the putative etiologic agents may be seen in the near future.

Surgical Treatment

Thymectomy

Evidence suggesting the central role of the thymus gland in myasthenia gravis combined with the deficiencies of medical management has resulted in the increasing application of thymectomy in the management of myasthenia gravis. At Duke University Medical Center, thymectomy is employed as the primary mode of therapy for myasthenia gravis. Patients with myasthenia gravis are considered for thymectomy as soon as possible after the development of generalized weakness. Plasmapheresis is used to optimize medical status prior to thymectomy if patients exhibit significant weakness. Patients referred on anticholinesterase agents have these agents slowly withdrawn during plasmapheresis. It is rare to identify patients that cannot be withdrawn from anticholinesterase agents with plasmapheresis, and as a result, patients come to the operating suite without these supportive pharmacologic agents and consequently have a less complex perioperative course.

Patients receiving corticosteroids are maintained on them throughout the perioperative period to prevent adrenal insufficiency. Thereafter, attempts are made to gradually lower the dosage as tolerated.

Thymectomy should be performed in an institution with an experienced treatment team. There must be a close working relationship between the neurologist, the anesthesiologist, the surgeon, and the intensive care unit personnel. When thymectomy is performed under these conditions, the operative mortality should be below 1 per cent and should occur only in high-risk patients with profound clinical weakness. Preoperative sedation may be given, but doses should be less than in patients without myasthenia gravis. Atropine is avoided. Most anesthesiologists use short-acting barbiturates for induction of anesthesia and maintain anesthesia with an inhalation agent. Succinyl chloride and curare are rarely necessary and are best avoided. Patients who have experienced significant respiratory difficulty or profound weakness prior to operation are generally managed with nasotracheal intubation, as it is more comfortable if ventilator support is required. When early extubation is anticipated, orotracheal intubation is employed, which has the advantages of speed and avoidance of nasal mucosal trauma.

Surgical Anatomy of the Thymus Gland. Knowledge of the surgical anatomy of the thymus gland begins with an understanding of its embryonic differentiation. Human thymic primordium arises primarily from the third branchial pouch in close association with the inferior parathyroid gland, which affixes to the posterior side of the thyroid gland, whereas the thymus descends into the thorax. A portion of the thymic primordium may also develop from the fourth branchial pouch in association with the superior parathyroid gland. In the branchial complex stage, the pharyngobranchial duct closes and the communication

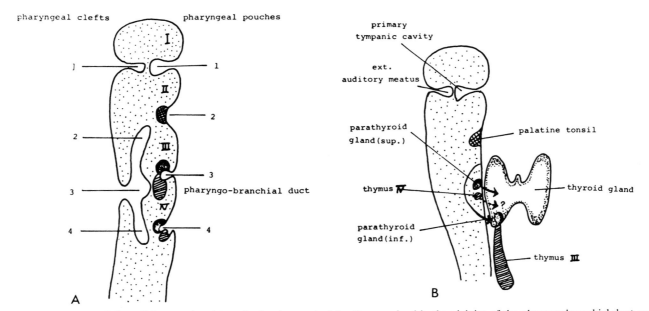

Figure 27–6. *A,* Primordial stage showing early development of the thymus gland in the vicinity of the pharyngobranchial duct and from the third branchial pouch. *B,* Definitive form demonstrating later embryonic development of the thymus gland. By this stage, the close association of the thymus gland to the thyroid gland superiorly is demonstrated as well as the overlapping anatomic areas for location of the parathyroid gland. Some minor controversy still exists regarding some contribution to thymic development from the fourth branchial pouch. (From Langman, J.: Medical Embryology. Baltimore, Williams and Wilkins Co., 1969.)

between the pharynx and the thymus is loosened. Ultimately, the lobes of the thymus separate from the parathyroid glands and descend into the thorax. Controversy remains regarding ectopic portions of the thymus gland found in the neck, cephalad to the main body of the thymus gland. It has been suggested that this thymic tissue may derive from the fourth branchial pouch along with parathyroid tissue. An alternative postulate suggests that this thymic tissue originates from the third branchial pouch but breaks off during its descent into the thorax. This complex migratory pattern of the thymus gland is thought to be responsible for the finding of ectopic thymic tissue in such locations as the left main bronchus, the lung parenchyma, the posterior mediastinum, and the lung hilum. This is shown in Figure 27–6A, which illustrates the branchial complex stage in which thymus is identified in close approximation to the cervical sinus and originating from the third branchial cleft prior to its descent into the thorax and prior to the formation of the gland from ectodermal cells surrounding the cervical sinus. In the definitive form stage (Fig. 27–6B), a separation of thymic tissue has occurred following migration of the thymic tissue from the third branchial cleft inferiorly, and residual thymus is identified superiorly in proximity to the superior parathyroid gland.

After the thymus gland has migrated into the inferior mediastinum, it relates to the major mediastinal structures, as illustrated in Figure 27–7. It overlies the pericardium and great vessels at the base of the heart and is in close proximity to the left innominate vein. The thymus gland has an H-shaped configuration, with variable fusion of the right and left lobes at about the midportion of the gland. The superior poles of the gland are thinner than the inferior poles. The uppermost portion of the gland attenuates into the thyrothymic ligament, which connects the thymus gland to the thyroid gland. There are many variations in the regional anatomy of the thymus gland. It may lie posterior or anterior to the left innominate vein, and the superior pole of the gland may extend along the pretracheal fascia into the root of the neck. At the lateral extent of the gland, there is a fine capsule that separates it from the pleura and the parapleural mediastinal fat that lies in close proximity to the phrenic nerve. The arterial supply to the thymus gland comes from the internal mammary arteries via their pericardiophrenic branches. Venous drainage is through one or two large veins that drain into the anterior aspect of the left innominate vein. When the thymus gland lies posterior to the left innominate vein, drainage may be into the posterior portion of that vein. The thymus gland is largest relative to body size within the first or second year of life, when it may attain as much as 50 per cent of its ultimate weight. The mass of the gland is usually greatest at the time of puberty and weighs 25 to 50 grams. After puberty, there is gradual replacement of the densely packed lymphocyte architecture of the gland by adipose tissue, and in late life, thymic remnants may be detectable only microscopically. Normally, there is a distinct thymic capsule that allows its separation from surrounding mediastinal and cervical structures.

Some representative anatomic thymus configurations are shown in Figure 27–8. Of greatest variability are the degree of fusion and the extent of upper pole development.

Surgical Technique. A variety of surgical techniques are available for the performance of thymectomy. The particular choice of technique varies as dictated by the personal preference of the surgeon and his beliefs concerning the pathogenesis of myasthenia and the role of thymectomy in the treatment of myasthenia gravis. Thymic tissue has been documented to be a normal component of perithymic fat, and if a diligent search for such tissue is made, it can be found about 75 per cent of the time. Thymic tissue is frequently located in multiple sites within the anterior mediastinum, and for this reason, we prefer the median sternotomy approach for thymectomy, since it allows the most complete approach for total removal of thymic tissue. Surgical approaches for thymectomy include the following:

1. Transcervical thymectomy.
2. Median sternotomy.
3. Partial median sternotomy.
4. Median sternotomy plus cervical incision.
5. Upper median sternotomy combined with transsternal sternotomy.

The technique of cervical thymectomy was ini-

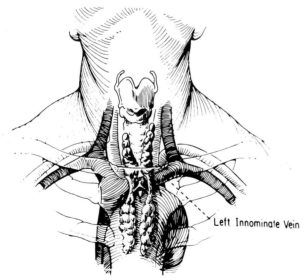

Left Innominate Vein

Figure 27–7. Location of the "normal" thymus gland in relation to other major intrathoracic structures. Of particular importance is the relationship of the thymus gland to the innominate vein. The draining veins from the thymus to the innominate vein are occasionally inconstant and may be a source of bleeding if not identified and carefully ligated. Occasionally, the thymus gland will run behind the innominate vein in close proximity to the innominate artery. Variable amounts of thymic fusion make the innominate vein more or less visible in the course of the dissection. (From Kark, A. E., and Kirschner, P. A.: Total thymectomy by the transcervical approach. Br. J. Surg., *58:*321, 1971.)

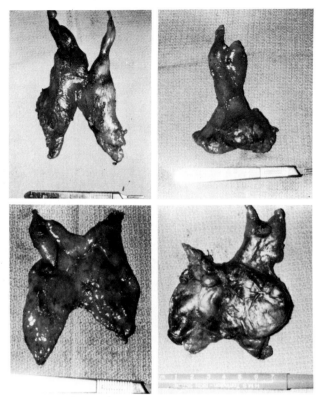

Figure 27–8. Operative specimens showing the broad range of anatomic variation in the normal thymus gland. The figure at the upper left represents the generally described "H" configuration. Other figures illustrate greater fusion between the right and left portions of the gland, disproportionate development of the lower poles compared with the upper poles of the gland, and disproportionate development of one upper pole as compared with the other. The number of upper poles is variable, and careful anatomic dissection is required for complete removal of the gland.

By traction on the upper pole of the gland, it is possible to continue mobilization, and the arterial supply to the gland is then divided using electrocautery. Resection is generally limited to that portion of the gland enclosed within the thymic capsule. If the wound is dry, drainage is generally not necessary. Inadvertent pleural entry can be treated by hyperinflation of the lungs as the deep tissue planes are closed. If the wound is not entirely free from bleeding at termination of the procedure, a small drainage catheter can be introduced into the superior mediastinum for several hours to a day to collect any residual blood. Advocates of this procedure generally cite remission rates for their patients comparable to those using the transsternal approach, although patients are usually pre-selected and the studies are neither standardized nor controlled. Further residual mediastinal thymic tissue has been found in up to 60 per cent of patients following transcervical sternotomy. Recently, recurrent myasthenia associated with significant amounts of residual thymic tissue and even thymomas have been reported following transcervical thymectomy. Although it is an aesthetically pleasing and technically feasible procedure, transcervical thymectomy achieves a less complete thymectomy than transsternal thymectomy. Although the importance of total thymectomy is unknown, there is concern that incomplete removal of the thymus may be associated with a higher recurrence rate of myasthenia gravis.

The initial concern with median sternotomy for thymectomy is related to impaired pulmonary me-

tially described by Crotti in 1938, was reintroduced by Crile, and was extended by Kark and Kirschner. The technique is favored by some surgeons because of the cosmetic incision, low morbidity, and minimal hospital stay. It has been advocated to be particularly useful in patients with significant respiratory distress and in whom no tracheostomy has been performed. When cervical thymectomy is performed, the patient is prepared and draped for a median sternotomy in the event of the occurrence of an intrathoracic complication requiring exploration or an unanticipated problem in removing the gland. The procedure is initiated by making a curvilinear incision about 2 cm. above the supersternal notch and then extending this incision to the level of the strap muscles. After retraction of the strap muscles, the cervical fascia covering the thymus gland is entered, and the manubrium can be elevated anteriorly. Special retractors have been devised that allow anterior traction to be placed on the sternum to facilitate the dissection. The thymus is mobilized from the innominate vein, and its venous attachment is divided between silver clips (Fig. 27–9).

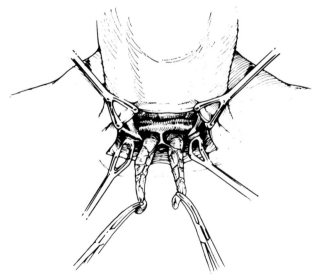

Figure 27–9. Transcervical thymectomy. The patient's head is at the upper portion of the picture and the figure illustrates the surgeon's view following retraction of the upper poles of the thymus gland to expose the venous drainage into the innominate vein. The use of specially constructed sternal retractors facilitates this procedure that generally results in removal of a good operative specimen as defined by the capsule of the gland. Thymic tissue in the mediastinum is more difficult to visualize and remove using this technique. (From Kark, A. E., and Kirschner, P. A.: Total thymectomy of the transcervical approach. Br. J. Surg., 58:321, 1971.)

chanics following a major chest incision. Splinting of the chest, damage to the phrenic nerves, mediastinal infection, a higher pain medication requirement, a cosmetically less appealing incision, and postoperative pulmonary complications such as atelectasis and pneumonia have all been cited as drawbacks to the transsternal approach. Several factors have changed this situation. Patients are referred for thymectomy earlier in the course of their disease and tend to be less ill. Medical status can usually be improved by plasmapheresis prior to thymectomy, so that even patients experiencing respiratory difficulty come to thymectomy with good ventilatory potential. The better clinical state of patients prior to thymectomy has allowed early mobilization and has reduced the incidence of pulmonary complications following the procedure. For patients requiring tracheostomy, an incision can be employed that is anatomically separated from the tracheostomy stoma and that minimizes the risk of contamination and mediastinal sepsis.

Figure 27–10 is a composite drawing constructed from the work of Jaretski and associates (1977), who performed careful anatomic and histologic examination of the mediastinal and cervical regions at the time of thymectomy. The normal location of the thymus gland is illustrated, along with the variety of other locations for thymic tissue that were noted. The wide range of locations of thymic tissue in the mediastinum emphasizes the need for good exposure of both the mediastinal contents and the cervical extent of the

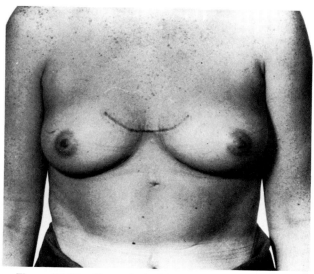

Figure 27–11. Cosmetic incision for median sternotomy in young women. The incision can be placed just on the superior surface of the breast as shown here, or it can be placed entirely in the inframammary region. In either case, the incision leaves an extremely acceptable scar, and the resulting dissection allows excellent visualization of both the intrathoracic and cervical thymus gland.

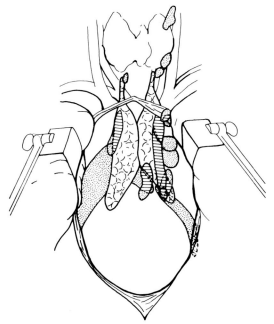

Figure 27–10. "Classic" location of the thymus gland. Based on the work of Jaretski and associates (1977) the location of other thymic tissue is shown in the stippled or lined areas. Of particular importance is the location of thymic tissue deep in the lateral mediastinum and also superiorly in relationship to the thyroid gland and frequently not in continuity with the remainder of the thymus gland.

thymus gland if thymectomy is to be attempted. Such exposure can be obtained with a median sternotomy. In men, a short vertical skin incision can be made and can be mobilized adequately cephalad and caudad to allow median sternotomy, sternal separation, and adequate cervical exposure by skin retraction. In women, a median sternotomy with excellent exposure of the superior extent of the thymus gland and the lower cervical region can be obtained utilizing supramammary or inframammary incisions that leave a cosmetically excellent scar. In these approaches, a curvilinear incision is made just over the breast and extended inferiorly in the midline (supramammary incision) or beneath the breasts (inframammary incision).

Using skin hooks and electrocautery, it is possible to establish a bloodless plane of dissection that allows elevation of the anterior chest wall to well above the suprasternal notch superiorly and to the xiphoid inferiorly. The sternotomy is then performed using a saw and taking care to remain in the midline of the sternum. This approach affords an excellent visualization of the thymus gland and its vascular attachments and is a cosmetically acceptable incision (Fig. 27–11). It also allows for extensive removal of perithymic tissue and mediastinal fat.

The pleural reflections onto the thymus gland are gently pushed to the sides by blunt dissection. A plane is then established between the inferior aspect of the thymus gland and the anterior aspect of the pericardium. Starting in the midline and working toward the pleural spaces, each lobe of the inferior thymus gland is freed from its superficial pericardial attachments.

As the gland gradually assumes form, gentle traction separates it from the pleura. Efforts are made not to enter the pleural space, but if this should occur, it is not a significant complication. As the dissection proceeds cephalad, the thymus gland is retracted superiorly to identify the thymic vein or veins on the posterior surface of the gland as they enter the left innominate vein. These are divided between silver clips, and the gland is separated from the innominate vein. Each of the superior poles of the thymus gland is then dissected from the surrounding fascial tissue until it is identified as an attenuated fibrous cord. Both fibrous cords are transected and the thymus removed. This technique is illustrated in Figure 27–12.

Placement of a warm cotton pad in the anterior mediastinum for a few moments will generally result in excellent hemostasis, following which a No. 28 chest tube is positioned in the mediastinum and the sternum reapproximated. If the pleural space has been entered, the tip of the chest tube may be advanced into that pleural space, but a separate pleural drainage catheter is almost never necessary. Postoperative bleeding is usually minimal, and the tube can be removed several hours following the operation. The sternotomy wound is closed in layers, with a subcuticular skin closure.

Modification of Thymectomy for Thymoma. When the thymus gland appears unusually firm or is adherent to any of the surrounding structures, the surgeon should be highly suspicious that a thymoma is present. This may not have been appreciated in the preoperative assessment, even if computed tomographic scanning of the mediastinum was performed. If a thymoma is present, infiltration into surrounding structures must be searched for carefully, since this is the major criterion for malignancy. Since there may be recurrences even after removal of a benign thymoma, a complete and careful dissection of the tumor mass is required. Care should be taken to avoid injury to the phrenic nerve; however, if it is incorporated within the tumor mass and complete resection is otherwise possible, it may be sacrificed. Extensive involvement of the left innominate vein or of the internal surface of the pericardium is an ominous prognostic sign, and complete resection may not be possible. If a malignancy is suspected, however, an aggressive attempt

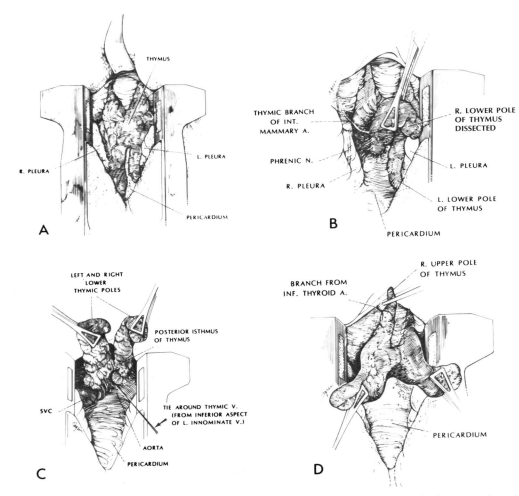

Figure 27–12. Procedure for removal of the thymus gland using a median sternotomy. *A–D*, The key steps for safe and complete removal of the thymus gland, as described in the text. (From Wilkins, E. W.: *In* Modern Techniques in Surgery. Cardiac/Thoracic Surgery. Edited by L. H. Cohn. Mt. Kisco, New York, Futura Publishing Co., 1979.)

at tumor removal is warranted, and removal of a portion of the pericardium, the left innominate vein, one of the phrenic nerves, and the pleural reflections should be performed. Total surgical extirpation offers the best chance for long-term cure in cases of malignant thymoma. If tumor removal is impossible, radiation therapy is generally employed, and the field can be better defined by marking the peripheral extent of tumor involvement with surgical clips. Frozen tissue biopsies are of little help in diagnosing malignant thymomas since the determination of malignancy is primarily from the biologic behavior of the tumor. Biopsy may, however, disclose the presence of cell types other than thymomas.

Postoperative Care. Following thymectomy, the patient is returned to the intensive care unit for observation by the physician and nursing team. The effects of the anesthetic agents are allowed to dissipate while the patient is supported with a ventilator, usually employing intermittent mandatory ventilation at low rate settings. The decision of when to extubate the patient is based largely on his or her preoperative condition. In patients with disease of relatively short duration and mild symptoms, extubation is considered several hours following operation. Patients with more severe myasthenia gravis may require intubation for longer periods of time. Extubation is performed when the patient is alert and demonstrates a satisfactory vital capacity. The patient should be able to generate inspiratory negative pressure greater than 20 cm. H_2O. Following extubation, frequent measurements of vital capacity should be performed using a bedside digital spirometer. Patients must be watched carefully, as deterioration of ventilatory status may occur several days postoperatively. Preoperative preparation reduces the likelihood of prolonged intubation or subsequent ventilatory deterioration. The patient may be ambulated the morning following surgery and, in most cases, is prepared for discharge within a few days.

Results of Thymectomy. Improvement following thymectomy has been reported in 57 to 86 per cent of patients and permanent remission in 20 to 36 per cent of patients. This clinical improvement may be delayed from 3 to 5 years from the time of operation. Analysis of these data is hampered by differences in patients selected for operation, timing of thymectomy, choice of route, underlying pathologic conditions, and perioperative care. Furthermore, it is known that even without treatment, spontaneous remission may occasionally occur. There are no prospective controlled studies that allow comparison of the results of thymectomy versus medical therapy versus the natural history of myasthenia gravis in a given population. Nonetheless, in reviewing most published articles, it has not been possible to find any reported series in which patients treated medically fared better than those treated surgically. A retrospective, controlled, matched, computerized study (Fig. 27–13) favored thymectomy over medical therapy with respect to remission and survival (Buckingham *et al.*, 1976). It is difficult to determine which patients with delayed improvement following thymectomy might have experi-

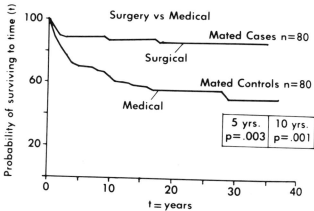

Figure 27–13. A matched, computerized, retrospective analysis of medical versus surgical management in myasthenia gravis. This work performed at the Mayo Clinic provides the longest comparative follow-up for patients treated both medically and surgically in which the patients were matched for severity of disease as well as for their personal characteristics. The improved survival in the surgical group of patients was statistically significant at both 5 and 10 years, and this difference was maintained with additional passage of time. (From Buckingham, J. M., Howard, F. M., Bernatz, P. E., *et al.*: The value of thymectomy in myasthenia gravis: A computer-assisted matched study. Ann. Surg., *184*:453, 1976.)

enced spontaneous remission without therapy. Although the data are confusing, it is the impression of most groups that the greatest chance for permanent remission is seen following thymectomy. In general, patients with nonthymomatous myasthenia gravis have better remission rates and long-term survivals than those with thymomatous myasthenia gravis (Papatestas *et al.*, 1971).

Only 10 per cent of patients with a noninvasive thymoma are reported to have remission. When the tumor is invasive, remission is less likely, and more than 50 per cent of patients die within 5 years. Most of these deaths occur in the first year following surgery and are related to myasthenic complications. Since the primary feature of malignancy in thymoma is local invasion, the argument for early thymectomy has been advanced in an attempt to perform thymectomy prior to the infiltration of surrounding tissues. Such an approach may result in a lesser percentage of malignant thymomas. The present ability to perform thymectomy safely and to potentially avoid long-term drug side effects leads many authorities to consider thymectomy as the treatment of choice for myasthenia gravis.

Five years ago, a prospective management plan for patients with myasthenia gravis was established at Duke University Medical Center. All patients with evidence of generalized myasthenia gravis, regardless of severity, underwent thymectomy, with preoperative plasmapheresis being employed to optimize medical status if necessary. Efforts were made to employ thymectomy as the sole treatment modality and to use medications only if necessary rather than by routine. The results have been most gratifying and are indicated in Table 27–3. Thymectomy was not withheld because of age, and good results were obtained in all

TABLE 27–3. CLINICAL STATUS OF PATIENTS HAVING THYMECTOMY FOR TREATMENT OF MYASTHENIA GRAVIS IN THE DUKE MEDICAL CENTER SERIES

| Clinical State | BEFORE THYMECTOMY | | CLINICAL STATE AFTER THYMECTOMY | | | | | |
	No. of Patients	No. Receiving Medication	Normal	I	IIA	IIB	IIC	Died
IIA	28	21	24	4				
IIB	9	8	4	2	3			
IIC	10	10	2	3	3	1		1
Number of patients receiving anti-myasthenia drugs after thymectomy according to post-thymectomy clinical state			1	1	3	1		

age groups with all types of thymic pathology. Residual myasthenic symptoms have largely been confined to the ocular muscles. Forty-six of 47 patients were improved following thymectomy in comparison with their pre-thymectomy, pre-plasmapheresis state (mean follow-up 25.5 months). Thirty patients were functionally intact and free of generalized weakness at normal levels of activity. Nine patients had only residual ocular dysfunction. Thus, 83 per cent of patients were free of significant generalized weakness. The majority of these patients require no medication. It is of interest that prior to thymectomy, AChR antibody titers generally correlated with the severity of the myasthenia. Postoperatively, there was no direct relationship between AChR antibody titer and clinical status, as AChR antibody levels did not change significantly, but there was dramatic clinical improvement in the patients.

There has not been a prospective randomized study that compares the effects of thymectomy with the effects of other forms of management for myasthenia gravis. The Duke Medical Center Study is unique in its utilization of thymectomy as the primary mode of therapy for all patients once they entered the program. It is difficult to contrast these results with

other thymectomy series, since in some institutions thymectomy is employed only when medical management for treatment of myasthenia gravis has failed or when patients are suspected of having a thymoma. Because of the strict treatment protocol in the Duke series, no physician bias as to which patient should undergo thymectomy entered into the treatment decision. Rather than pursuing medical management, every effort was made to avoid the use of antimyasthenic medications. Optimization of clinical state was by plasmapheresis without immunosuppression rather than with drug therapy when necessary. All thymectomies were performed in a standardized manner, were radical in nature, and were performed by the same surgeon. This approach demonstrated that in the majority of patients, thymectomy alone could result in dramatic and sustained clinical improvement without the need for additional medications. Moreover, reduction in the acetylcholine receptor antibody titer was not essential for clinical improvement. These observations support the hypothesis that a factor elaborated by or in the thymus gland plays a role in acetylcholine receptor destruction. Further studies to identify, isolate, and characterize a putative thymic factor are necessary, because the identification of such

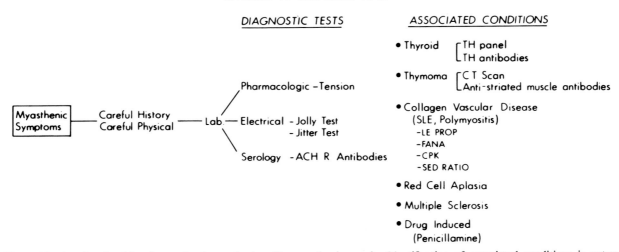

Figure 27–14. An algorithm for evaluating patients with myasthenia gravis. Identification of associated conditions is extremely important for optimal management of patients with myasthenia gravis.

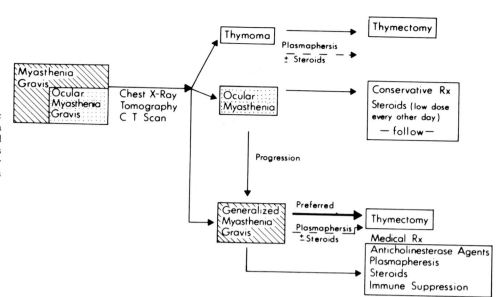

Figure 27–15. Therapeutic phase in treatment of myasthenia gravis. The decision that isolated ocular myasthenia gravis exists is made only if careful single-fiber testing of peripheral muscles is entirely normal.

a "thymic factor" could allow for the development of special techniques to provide for its removal or neutralization.

Because data continue to emerge relating the effects of thymectomy to the course of myasthenia gravis, it seems particularly important that a thymectomy that is as complete as possible be performed. Assessment of long-term data should not be confused by uncertainty regarding the presence of residual thymic tissue.

Algorithms for Management of Patients with Myasthenia Gravis

Because of success with the ongoing treatment plans discussed in this chapter, a summary for the diagnosis and management of patients with myasthenia gravis is provided here.

As outlined in Figure 27–14, when a patient with myasthenic symptoms is seen, the first portion of the evaluation is a diagnostic phase, starting with a careful history and physical examination. One of the primary goals at this time is to determine whether the patient has myasthenia gravis or weakness associated with another clinical condition. The diagnosis of true myasthenia gravis is made by a combination of history, physical examination, and appropriate laboratory tests. The response to Tensilon, the Jolly and jitter test, and determination of the level of the acetylcholine receptor antibodies usually identify the disease correctly in more than 95 per cent of instances. The patient is then subgrouped according to functional classification, and careful distinction is made as to whether or not the patient has ocular or generalized myasthenia gravis. Many patients who seek the atten-

tion of a physician because of ocular symptoms, in fact, have generalized myasthenia gravis but are unaware of it. Since the treatment method for each type differs at this time, it is extremely important to make this differentiation. A variety of laboratory tests are designed to determine whether or not there are associated conditions in addition to the clinical myasthenia gravis, and when present, these are specifically treated. Radiographic studies are used to detect the presence of a thymoma.

Once the diagnosis of generalized myasthenia has been made, the therapeutic phase is entered, as is demonstrated in Figure 27–15. In patients who are thought to have isolated ocular myasthenia, a conservative treatment program is initiated, generally employing low-dose corticosteroids on an alternate-day schedule. These patients are followed carefully, since the majority develop generalized weakness and are then treated similarly to patients who initially present with generalized myasthenia gravis. In our clinic, the primary treatment mode is thymectomy. For patients who are weak or who become weak when pharmacologic treatment is withdrawn, plasmapheresis is employed to prepare the patient for thymectomy. If the patient's general condition is good, if weakness is not severe, and if there are no other contraindications, thymectomy is then performed as the primary means of treatment. For those few patients with specific contraindications or reluctance to accept operation, medical therapy is employed.

Using this overall treatment plan, the systemic complications of pharmacologic management of myasthenia gravis can be avoided or minimized. Thymectomy as the primary therapy for myasthenia gravis yields remission in the majority of patients and allows for reduced pharmacologic requirements in those patients with residual symptoms after thymectomy.

SELECTED REFERENCES

Blalock, A., Mason, M. F., Morgan, H. J., and Riven, S. S.: Myasthenia gravis and tumors of the thymic region. Ann. Surg., *110*:544, 1939.

In this paper, Blalock reports the first successful removal of a thymic tumor for the treatment of myasthenia gravis. He uses this case as the impetus for reviewing the literature and provides an excellent summary of the rationale for surgical extirpation of the thymus gland in the treatment of myasthenia gravis. The comments from the audience at the end of the manuscript are well worth reading.

Drachman, D. B.: Myasthenia gravis. N. Engl. J. Med., *298*:136, 186, 1978.

This is a broad review of myasthenia gravis in which the disease process is discussed from the basic concepts of neuromuscular transmission to specific therapy. It serves as a good source of reference for the reader interested in pursuing certain areas of the subject in greater depth. It differs somewhat from the views presented in this chapter in that treatment is more dependent on medical therapy and indications for thymectomy are more conservative.

Jaretzki, A., Bethea, M., Wolff, M., Olarte, M., Lovelace, R. E., Penn, A. S., and Rowland, L.: A rational approach to total thymectomy in the treatment of myasthenia gravis. Ann. Thorac. Surg., *24*:120, 1977.

This is an important article for those interested in the surgical technique of thymectomy. The authors explore the completeness of thymectomy performed by transcervical, median sternotomy, and combined transcervical and median sternotomy routes in a group of their own patients. There are extremely well done anatomic drawings showing some of the atypical thymus gland locations encountered in the course of their clinical experience. There is also an excellent discussion that includes comments by proponents of other techniques of thymectomy and the rationale behind their arguments.

Lindstrom, J. M., Lennon, V. A., Seybold, M. E., et al.: Experimental autoimmune myasthenia gravis and myasthenia gravis: Biochemical and immuno-chemical aspects. Ann. N.Y. Acad. Sci., *274*:254, 1976.

This is an extremely well-presented and comprehensive review of experimental work dealing with immune mechanisms in myasthenia gravis. It provides an excellent background for the understanding of current therapies designed to interfere with humoral and cell-mediated immunity.

Olanow, C. W., Wechsler, A. S., and Roses, A. D.: A prospective study of thymectomy and serum acetylcholine receptor antibodies in myasthenia gravis. Ann. Surg., *196*:113, 1982.

This study, performed at Duke University Medical Center, is unique in that every patient admitted with the diagnosis of myasthenia gravis was treated in accordance with a strict clinical protocol. For most patients, thymectomy was used as the primary, and frequently the only, means of therapy. Very high remission rates were reported, with minimal reliance on drug therapy.

REFERENCES

Abdou, N. I., Lisak, R. P., Sweiman, B., et al.: The thymus in myasthenia gravis: Evidence for altered cell populations. N. Engl. J. Med., *291*:1271, 1974.

Abramsky, O., Aharonov, A., Teitelbaum, D., et al.: Myasthenia gravis and acetylcholine receptor: Effect of steroids in clinical course and cellular immune response to acetylcholine receptor. Arch. Neurol., *32*:684, 1975.

Appel, S. H., Almon, R. R., and Levy, N.: Acetylcholine receptor antibodies in myasthenia gravis. N. Engl. J. Med., *293*:760, 1975.

Argov, Z., and Mastaglia, F. L.: Disorders of neuro-muscular transmission caused by drugs. N. Engl. J. Med., *301*:409, 1979.

Blalock, A., Mason, M. F., Morgan, H. J., and Riven, S. S.: Myasthenia gravis and tumors of the thymic region. Ann. Surg., *110*:544, 1939.

Buckingham, J. M., Howard, F. M., Bernatz, P. E., et al.: The value of thymectomy in myasthenia gravis: A computer-assisted matched study. Ann. Surg., *184*:453, 1976.

Castleman, B.: The pathology of the thymus gland in myasthenia gravis. Ann. N.Y. Acad. Sci., *135*:496, 1966.

Chang, C. C., Chen, T. F., and Chuang, S.-T.: Influence of chronic neostigmine treatment on the number of acetylcholine receptors and the release of acetylcholine from the rat diaphragm. J. Physiol., *230*:613, 1973.

Dau, P. C., Lindstrom, J. M., Cassel, C. K., et al.: Plasmapheresis and immunosuppressive drug therapy in myasthenia gravis. N. Engl. J. Med., *297*:1134, 1977.

Drachman, D. B.: Myasthenia gravis. N. Engl. J. Med., *298*:136, 186, 1978.

Drachman, D. B., Kao, I., Pestronk, A., et al.: Myasthenia gravis as a receptor disorder. Ann. N.Y. Acad. Sci., *274*:226, 1976.

Early thymectomy for myasthenia gravis. (Editorial.) Br. Med. J., *3*:262, 1975.

Elmqvist, D., Hofmann, W. W., Kugelberg, J., et al.: An electrophysiological investigation of neuromuscular transmission in myasthenia gravis. J. Physiol., *174*:417, 1964.

Emeryk, B., and Strugalska, M. H.: Evaluation of results of thymectomy in myasthenia gravis. J. Neurol., *211*:155, 1976.

Engel, A. G., Lambert, E. H., and Howard, F. M., Jr.: Immune complexes (IgG and C3) at the motor end-plate in myasthenia gravis. Mayo Clin. Proc., *52*:267, 1977.

Frambrough, D. M., Drachman, D. B., and Satyamurti, S.: Neuromuscular junction in myasthenia gravis: Decreased acetylcholine receptors. Science, *182*:293, 1973.

Genkins, G., Papatestas, A. E., Horowitz, S. H., et al.: Studies in myasthenia gravis. Early thymectomy: Electrophysiologic and pathologic correlations. Am. J. Med., *58*:517, 1975.

Goldman, A. J., Hermann, C., Jr., Keesey, J. C., et al.: Myasthenia gravis and invasive thymoma: A 20-year experience. Neurology, *25*:1021, 1975.

Jaretzki, A., Bethea, M., Wolff, M., Olarte, M., Lovelace, R. E., Penn, A. S., and Rowland, L.: A rational approach to total thymectomy in the treatment of myasthenia gravis. Ann. Thorac. Surg., *24*:120, 1977.

Koelle, G. B.: Anticholinesterase agents. *In* The Pharmacological Basis of Therapeutics. 5th Ed. Edited by L. S. Goodman and A. Gilman. New York, Macmillan Company, 1975, pp. 445–466.

Langman, J.: Medical Embryology. Baltimore, Williams and Wilkins Co., 1969.

Legg, M. A., and Brady, W. J.: Pathology and clinical behavior of thymomas: A survey of 51 cases. Cancer, *18*:1131, 1965.

Lindstrom, J. M., Lennon, V. A., Seybold, M. E., et al.: Experimental autoimmune myasthenia gravis and myasthenia gravis: Biochemical and immuno-chemical aspects. Ann. N.Y. Acad. Sci., *274*:254, 1976.

Matell, G., Bergstrom, K., Franksson, C., et al.: Effects of some immuno-suppressive procedures on myasthenia gravis. Ann. N.Y. Acad. Sci., *274*:659, 1976.

Mittag, T., Kornfeld, P., Tormay, A., et al.: Detection of antiacetylcholine receptor factors in serum and thymus from patients with myasthenia gravis. N. Engl. J. Med., *294*:691, 1976.

Mulder, D. G., Hermann, C., and Buckberg, G. D.: Effect of thymectomy in patients with myasthenia gravis: A sixteen year experience. Am. J. Surg., *128*:202, 1974.

Namba, T., Brown, S. B., and Grob, D.: Neonatal myasthenia gravis: Report of two cases and review of the literature. Pediatrics, *45*:488, 1970.

Olanow, C. W., and Roses, A. D.: The pathogenesis of myasthenia gravis. A hypothesis. Med. Hypotheses, 7:957, 1981.

Olanow, C. W., Wechsler, A. S., and Roses, A. D.: A prospective study of thymectomy and serum acetylcholine receptor antibodies in myasthenia gravis. Ann. Surg., 196:113, 1982.

Papatestas, A. E., Genkins, G., Horowitz, S. H., et al.: Thymectomy in myasthenia gravis: Pathologic, clinical, and electrophysiologic correlations. Ann. N.Y. Acad. Sci., 274:555, 1976.

Papatestas, A. E., Genkins, G., Kornfeld, P., et al.: Transcervical thymectomy in myasthenia gravis. Surg. Gynecol. Obstet., 140:535, 1975.

Papatestas, A. E., Alpert, L. I., Osserman, K. E., et al.: Studies in myasthenia gravis. Effects of thymectomy: Results on 185 patients with nonthymomatous and thymomatous myasthenia gravis, 1941–1969. Am. J. Med., 50:465, 1971.

Patrick, J., and Lindstrom, J.: Autoimmune response to acetylcholine receptor. Science, 180:871, 1973.

Pinching, A. J., Peters, D. K., and Newsom, D. J.: Remission of myasthenia gravis following plasma-exchange. Lancet, 2:1373, 1976.

Roses, A. D., Olanow, C. W., McAdams, M. W., and Lane, R. J. M.: There is no direct correlation between serum antiacetylcholine receptor and antibody levels and the clinical status of individual patients with myasthenia gravis. Neurology, 31:220, 1981.

Rowland, L. P.: Controversies about the treatment of myasthenia gravis. J. Neurol. Neurosurg. Psych., 43:644, 1980.

Sahashi, K., Engel, A. G., Lambert, E. H., and Howard, F. M., Jr.: Ultrastructural localization of the terminal and lytic 9th complement component (C9) at the motor end-plate in myasthenia gravis. J. Neuropathol. Exp. Neurol., 39:160, 1980.

Simpson, J. A.: Myasthenia gravis: A new hypothesis. Scott. Med. J., 5:419, 1960.

Simpson, J. A.: Myasthenia gravis and myasthenic syndromes. In Disorders of Voluntary Muscle. 4th Ed. Edited by J. N. Walton, Edinburgh, Churchill Livingstone, 1978, pp. 585–624.

Stalberg, E., Trontel, J. V., and Schwartz, M. S.: Single muscle fiber recording of jitter phenomenon in patients with myasthenia gravis and in members of their families. Ann. N.Y. Acad. Sci., 274:189, 1976.

van der Geld, H. W. R., and Strauss, A. J. L.: Myasthenia gravis: Immunological relationship between striated muscle and thymus. Lancet, 1:57, 1966.

Wechsler, A. S., and Olanow, C. W.: Myasthenia gravis. Surg. Clin. North Am., 60:946, 1980.

Chapter 28

Special Diagnostic Procedures in Cardiac Surgery

ERWIN ROBIN

RICHARD J. BING

RIGHT HEART CATHETERIZATION

In the past two decades, right heart catheterization has become widely used in the detection of intra- and extracardiac lesions. It has proved its value in the field of cardiovascular research, contributing to the understanding of the physiology of the circulation and the metabolism of the heart.

Historical Note

In 1861, Chauveau and Marey (Forssmann, 1929) measured intracardiac pressures in animals by inserting catheters via the arteries and veins into the heart, and Claude Bernard (Buzzi, 1959) repeated these experiments in 1879. Bleichroeder (1912) passed ureteral catheters into the arteries and veins of man and dog in 1905. Forssmann, in 1929, was the first to insert a ureteral catheter into a vein of his own forearm and to advance the tip of the catheter under fluoroscopic control into the right atrium. In 1930, Klein applied the Fick principle to determine the cardiac output by obtaining mixed venous blood from the right atrium and arterial blood from a peripheral artery. Right heart catheterization was introduced into clinical medicine in 1941 by Cournand and Ranges and was further developed and applied by Bing and associates (1947), Cournand and coworkers (1945), Dexter and colleagues (1947), Richards (1945), and others.

Technique

The technique of right heart catheterization has been described repeatedly (Bing, 1952; Cournand *et al.*, 1945; Wood, 1953). Under sterile conditions, a plastic radiopaque catheter is inserted through a peripheral vein into the right atrium. In infants and small children the saphenous vein is usually utilized. In newborns, because of the small caliber of the saphenous vein, the superficial femoral or the umbilical vein can be used (Fig. 28–1*A*). In older children and adults the median cubital or basilic vein is preferred (Fig. 28–1*B*). The catheter is frequently flushed with a saline solution containing heparin, and when pressures are to

be recorded, it is connected to a three-way stopcock and a pressure gauge.

Catheters are available in different sizes and models, depending on the procedure or the caliber of the vessel (Fig. 28–2). Pressures are best recorded with open-end catheters, such as the Cournand and the Goodale-Lubin catheters. During the course of angiography, closed-end catheters, such as the Lehman ventriculography or NIH catheter, are used to prevent recoil and intramural injection of contrast material. If additional stiffness is required, an appropriately designed stylet may be introduced in the catheter lumen.

Preparation of the Patient

In adults it is usually not necessary to administer sedatives. However, if it is needed, small amounts of a narcotic or barbiturate may be used. Children, as a rule, need sedation. Moffitt and associates (1961) and Smith and coworkers (1958) reported that the intramuscular injection of a combination of 6.25 mg. of promethazine (Phenergan), 6.25 mg. of chlorpromazine (Thorazine), and 25 mg. of meperidine hydrochloride (Demerol) per ml. of mixture provides good sedation. The dose varies according to the age, weight, and condition of the patient. Noncyanotic children receive 1 ml. per 20 pounds of body weight. Cyanotic children should receive a smaller dose.

Taylor and Stoelting (1959) recommended a combination of meperidine hydrochloride (1 mg. per pound of body weight) and secobarbital (Seconal) (3 to 5 mg. per pound). Eggers and associates (1959) reported a series of 67 children managed under general anesthesia. The inhalation of gases influences the analysis of oxygen and carbon dioxide in the blood and renders the whole procedure hazardous.

Newborns rarely need sedation. However, if it is needed, oral chloral hydrate may be administered in a dose of 10 to 15 mg. per pound of body weight.

Sedation should be given 30 minutes to 1 hour before catheterization. The patient should be fasted 3 to 6 hours prior to the study. Cyanotic children, because of the high viscosity of their blood, should receive fluids 2 to 3 hours before the procedure.

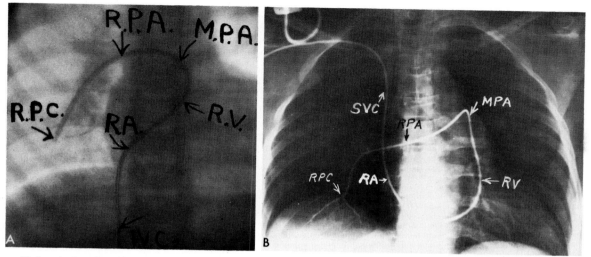

Figure 28–1. *A*, A catheter has been introduced into the right saphenous vein and guided through the inferior vena cava (I.V.C.), right atrium (R.A.), right ventricle (R.V.), main pulmonary artery (M.P.A.), and right pulmonary artery (R.P.A.) to the right pulmonary capillary position (R.P.C.). *B*, A catheter has been introduced into a right antecubital vein and passed through the superior vena cava (SVC), right atrium (RA), right ventricle (RV), main pulmonary artery (MPA), right pulmonary artery (RPA) to the right pulmonary capillary position (RPC).

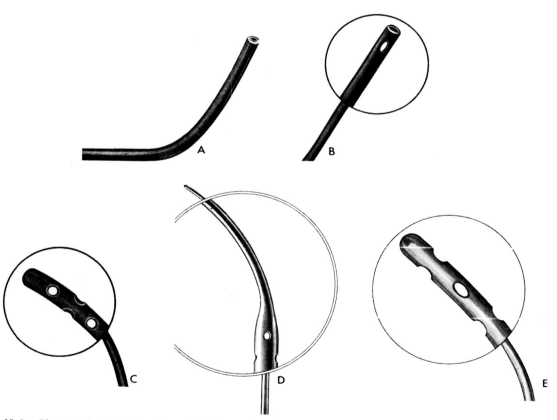

Figure 28–2. Photograph of catheter tips used during cardiac catheterization. *Above*, Open-end catheter tips. *A*, Cournand catheter tip. *B*, Goodale-Lubin catheter tip with two laterally opposed eyes close to the distal tip. *Below*, Closed-end catheter tips. *C*, NIH catheter tip with six round openings arranged in three laterally opposed pairs within the first cm. of the tip. *D*, Lehman ventriculography catheter tip with four eyes arranged in two laterally opposed pairs 4 cm. from the distal tip. *E*, Shirey transvalvular retrograde catheter with a tapered flexible tip containing six holes arranged in two laterally opposed pairs. (Reproduced with permission from U.S. Catheter and Instrument Corporation.)

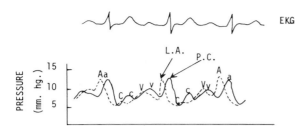

Figure 28–3. Simultaneous left atrial (L.A.) and pulmonary capillary (P.C.) pressures. The left atrial pressure was obtained by means of the transseptal technique. Both curves are similar in their contour and amplitude. The pulmonary capillary pressure is slightly delayed.

Indications

The chief indications for right heart catheterization are congenital or acquired defects and valvular abnormalities that involve the lesser circulation and the right side of the heart. There are no absolute contraindications to right heart catheterization. However, an increased risk is expected in cyanotic children or in patients with severe pulmonary hypertension (Schafer *et al.*, 1956).

Recording of Pressures

The importance of the zero or reference level has been pointed out by Rokseth and colleagues (1960). Usually in adults this level corresponds to the fourth intercostal space in the anterior axillary line at a point 10 cm. anterior to the back of the patient in the supine position.

Pulmonary Wedge Pressure

Several investigators have shown that the pulmonary wedge pressure resembles the left atrial pressure (Calazel *et al.*, 1951; Björk *et al.*, 1953; Connolly *et al.*, 1954; Shaffer and Silber, 1956) (Fig. 28–3). The pressure curve may be similar to the left atrial pressure curve even in the presence of slightly or moderately increased pulmonary resistance. The first wave, the "a" wave, corresponds to atrial systole; and the second wave, the "v" wave, corresponds to the passive atrial filling against a closed mitral valve. Abnormalities of the mitral valve may be reflected in an elevation and alteration of the pulmonary capillary

pressure (Gorlin *et al.*, 1952; Owen and Wood, 1955). However, it has been shown by Samet and coworkers (1959) that wide variations occur in the pulmonary artery pressure and that a tight mitral stenosis may exist with a normal pulmonary wedge pressure.

In infants and children, the pulmonary capillary pressure may be 5 to 10 mm. Hg higher than the left atrial mean pressure (Nadas, 1963); in adults, it may be up to one-third higher than a simultaneously recorded left atrial pressure. Incomplete wedging or wedging of the catheter tip into the wall of a sharply angulated tortuous pulmonary artery is a common cause of an unsatisfactory pulmonary capillary pressure tracing (Bell *et al.*, 1962).

Pulmonary Artery Pressure

The pulmonary artery pressure ranges from 15 to 30 mm. Hg systolic and 5 to 15 mm. Hg diastolic, with a mean of 10 to 20 mm. Hg (Table 28–1).

Pulmonary hypertension can be classified as hyperkinetic and obstructive types. The former type is due to a marked increase in pulmonary blood flow at the atrial, ventricular, or pulmonary level.

In childhood, pulmonary hypertension rarely occurs in cases of uncomplicated atrial septal defect. Bedford and Sellors (1960) reported that 4.8 per cent of their patients under 20 years of age had pulmonary hypertension and 40 per cent had it after 40 years of age. Nadas and associates (1960) indicated that one would not expect a significant rise in pulmonary artery pressure up to 20 years of age.

Ventricular septal defect and patent ductus arteriosus are more often associated with pulmonary hypertension. In the pediatric age groups, 70 to 80 per cent of the patients with ventricular septal defect have normal pulmonary artery pressure; 10 to 20 per cent have moderate pulmonary artery hypertension; and about 10 per cent have severe pulmonary artery hypertension (Arcilla *et al.*, 1963; Kidd, 1965; Lucas *et al.*, 1961). Nadas and colleagues (1960) reported that there was no significant increase in pulmonary artery pressure up to 13 years of age. This is to be contrasted with the report of Wood (1958), who recorded the presence of severe pulmonary artery hypertension in 16 per cent of the patients with ventricular septal defect at the average age of 23 years.

The incidence of pulmonary hypertension associated with patent ductus arteriosus alone is unknown.

TABLE 28–1. NORMAL PRESSURES OBTAINED BY RIGHT HEART CATHETERIZATION

	Systolic	PRESSURES (MM. HG) Diastolic	Mean
Right atrium	3 to 7	−2 to 2	−2 to 7
Right ventricle	15 to 30	0 to 7	
Pulmonary artery	15 to 30	5 to 15	10 to 20
Pulmonary capillary			5 to 12

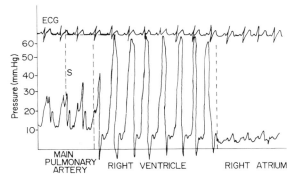

Figure 28–4. Pulmonic valvular stenosis. Pressure tracing obtained during pullback from main pulmonary artery to right atrium. There is a 34 mm. Hg systolic gradient (S) between the main pulmonary artery and the right ventricle.

It was present in all 10 cases catheterized by Ziegler (1952) and in 11 per cent of 168 children studied by Keith and associates (1967). It tends to progress between infancy and childhood (Nadas *et al.*, 1960).

Obstructive pulmonary hypertension may be the end result of the hyperkinetic type. In this case, the pulmonary blood flow may be normal or even decreased. Other causes are multiple pulmonary emboli, pulmonary parenchymal disease, left heart failure with chronically elevated pulmonary capillary pressure, mitral valve disease, or pulmonary vasculitis.

Right Ventricular Pressure

A maximum systolic gradient of 10 mm. Hg between the main pulmonary artery and the right ventricle is considered normal.

In pulmonic valvular stenosis, the systolic gradient between the pulmonary trunk and the outflow tract of the right ventricle is abrupt (Fig. 28–4); in infundibular stenosis, on the other hand, distinctive gradients in pressures may be found between the infundibular chamber and the right ventricle (Fig. 28–5).

In a series of 198 cases of isolated pulmonic stenosis operated on by Brock (1961), there were 17 instances (9 per cent) of infundibular stenosis or of

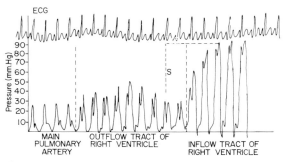

Figure 28–5. Pulmonic infundibular stenosis. Pressure tracing obtained during pullback from a case of tetralogy of Fallot. There is a 38 mm. Hg systolic gradient (S) between the outflow tract (infundibulum) and the inflow tract of the right ventricle.

combined valvular and infundibular stenosis; the remaining cases (91 per cent) were purely valvular. In contrast, in the tetralogy of Fallot, pulmonary stenosis is infundibular in 43 per cent of cases, valvular in 35 per cent, and combined valvular and infundibular in 22 per cent (Brock, 1957). Isolated infundibular stenosis can develop late in the course of large ventricular septal defects (Gasul *et al.*, 1957).

Right Atrial Pressure

The right atrial pressure curve consists of three waves, "a," "c," and "v," each of which is followed by a descent, "x," "x¹," and "y." The "a" wave is produced by the atrial systole and the "c" wave by transmission during the ventricular systole of the rising pressure in the ventricle through the closed tricuspid valve. The "v" wave results from the inflow of blood into the atrium during atrial diastole. A tracing illustrating these waves is included in the discussion of left atrial pressure (see Fig. 28–10).

In tricuspid stenosis and atresia, if atrial fibrillation is absent, there is a prominent or giant "a" wave; if the valve is incompetent, there is often ventricularization of the curve. The "x¹" descent has been replaced by a single positive wave (the "v" wave or regurgitant wave), sustained throughout the ventricular systole.

Right-sided heart failure may be reflected in an increase in the right atrial pressure. It should be remembered that elevated pressures in the right side of the heart may be due to myocardial failure as well as to mechanical obstruction in the left side of the heart.

Swan-Ganz Catheterization Technique

In the last two decades, hemodynamic measurements from the right heart, pulmonary circulation, and left heart have been reported in patients with acute myocardial infarction. These data have been valuable in understanding the extent of altered cardiovascular function, classifying the severity of the disease, measuring the response to treatment, and predicting the prognosis of the patient. To obviate the logistical problems of transferring ill patients to the cardiac catheterization laboratory, Swan and associates (1970) developed a flexible catheter with a small balloon at its tip. The catheter is inserted into an antecubital vein and advanced 35 to 40 cm. from the antecubital fossa. Inflation of the balloon with air allows the catheter to be passed with ease from the right atrium and ventricle to the pulmonary artery. This technique can be performed at the bedside without fluoroscopy. The position of the catheter tip is verified by electrocardiographic and pressure monitoring (Figs. 28–6 and 28–7). Following recording of a pulmonary artery pressure, the catheter is advanced until a pulmonary wedge pressure is observed. The balloon is deflated, and the pulmonary artery pressure reappears. The diastolic

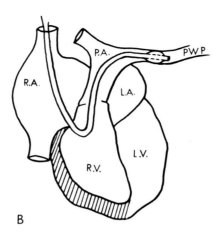

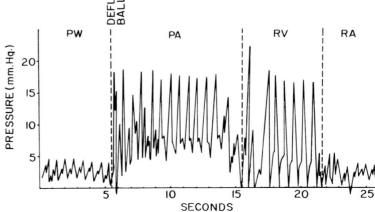

Figure 28–6. A Swan-Ganz catheter has been passed from a right antecubital vein to the left pulmonary artery. *A,* With the balloon deflated a pulmonary artery pressure (PAP) is recorded. *B,* With the balloon inflated a pulmonary wedge pressure (PWP) is recorded.

pressure of the pulmonary artery and the pulmonary wedge pressure can be used as indicators of left ventricular filling pressure (Kaltman *et al.*, 1966; Hunt *et al.*, 1970; Forrester *et al.*, 1972). The catheter was further modified so that accurate measurements of cardiac output could be performed by the thermodilution technique (Forrester *et al.*, 1971).

Sampling of Blood for Determination of Oxygen and Calculation of Flow

Many methods have been designed to identify, localize, and quantify shunts. Lesions that consist of shunting or backflow can be recognized by means of dye dilutions, nitrous oxide, radioactive krypton, hydrogen ion, and ascorbic acid.

Shunts can also be diagnosed by oxygen analysis of blood drawn from the cardiac chambers and the great veins and arteries. Normally, there is a great variability in the oxygen of blood withdrawn from the right atrium because of laminar flow from the superior and inferior venae cavae and coronary sinus. Truly mixed venous blood is found only in the pulmonary artery (Dexter *et al.*, 1947). (See Table 28–2.)

Multiple samples of blood should be obtained in rapid succession, beginning at the pulmonary wedge

position and ending at the vena cava. At least two samples should be obtained in the right ventricle: one in the outflow tract and the other in the main cavity. In the right atrium at least three samples should be drawn: one near the inferior vena cava, one in the middle of the atrium near the lateral wall, and the third just below the superior vena cava.

Flows are calculated according to the Fick principle (Bing *et al.*, 1947):

1. Systemic flow (S.F.) (L./min.)
$$= \frac{O_2 \text{ consumption (ml./min.)}}{\text{systemic A-V difference} \times 10}, \text{ where}$$

   A (vol. %) = peripheral arterial blood
   V (vol. %) = mixed venous blood
2. Pulmonary flow (P.F.) (L./min.)
$$= \frac{O_2 \text{ consumption (ml./min.)}}{\text{pulmonary A-V difference} \times 10}, \text{ where}$$

   A (vol. %) = pulmonary vein blood
   V (vol. %) = pulmonary artery blood

If pulmonary flow is more than systemic flow, there is a left-to-right shunt. If the systemic flow is greater than the pulmonary flow, there is a right-to-left shunt.

If bidirectional shunting is present, the "effective

Figure 28–7. Pressure tracing obtained during pullback from the left pulmonary artery (PA) to the right atrium (RA) with a Swan-Ganz catheter. A left pulmonary wedge pressure (PW) is obtained with inflation of the balloon. With the balloon deflated a left pulmonary artery pressure (PA) is recorded.

TABLE 28-2. SIGNIFICANT DIFFERENCES IN OXYGEN SATURATION AND CONTENT

	O_2 SATURATION DIFFERENCE (%) (Rudolph and Cayler, 1958)	O_2 CONTENT DIFFERENCE (VOL. %) (Dexter et al., 1947)	TYPE OF DEFECT*
SVC-RA	9.0	2.0	ASD
RA-RV	5.0	1.0	VSD
RV-PA	3.0	0.5	PDA

Left-to-right shunts less than 20 per cent of the pulmonary flow are not detectable by the conventional blood oxygen saturation methods.

*ASD = atrial septal defect; VSD = ventricular septal defect; PDA = patent ductus arteriosus.

pulmonary blood flow" must be calculated first. The "effective pulmonary blood flow" is the volume of mixed blood that, after returning to the right atrium, is aerated in the pulmonary capillaries (Bing *et al.*, 1947):

3. Effective pulmonary flow (E.F.) =

$$\frac{O_2 \text{ consumption (ml./min.)}}{\substack{\text{pulmonary venous } O_2 \text{ content (vol. \%) -} \\ \text{mixed venous } O_2 \text{ content (vol. \%)} \times 10}}$$

Then a. left-to-right shunt = P.F. − E.F. (L./min.)
b. right-to-left shunt = S.F. − E.F. (L./min.)

Figure 28–8 illustrates the use of these formulae in the calculation of various shunts and flows.

At the level of a left-to-right shunt and downstream to it, the oxygen saturation of blood is higher than in the chamber immediately upstream. The pulmonary flow also exceeds the systemic flow. In contrast, in right-to-left shunts the pulmonary flow is less than the systemic flow; the oxygen saturation is normal in the pulmonary veins and decreased in the peripheral arterial blood. In many cases, a bidirectional shunt is present. This results in a left-to-right shunt

and a diminished oxygen saturation in the peripheral arterial blood.

Observation of the Position and Mobility of the Catheter

The position and the mobility of the catheter are important in the recognition of abnormal communications between the cardiac chambers and the great vessels. If abnormal channels are encountered, serial blood samples should be drawn, and continuous pressure should be recorded.

The tip of the catheter may pass over to the left side of the heart through a septal defect, although a patent foramen ovale sometimes permits entrance into the left atrium. In endocardial cushion defects, either partial or complete, the position of the catheter is lower than in septum secundum defects. If the tip of the catheter is manipulated into the left ventricle, one may obtain, on withdrawal, an abrupt pressure change from the left ventricular to the right atrial form.

If an anomalous pulmonary vein is intubated, the shaft of the catheter will take an abnormal position in relation to the cardiac silhouette. However, distinction between an atrial septal defect and an anomalous pulmonary vein cannot be made from the position of the catheter alone.

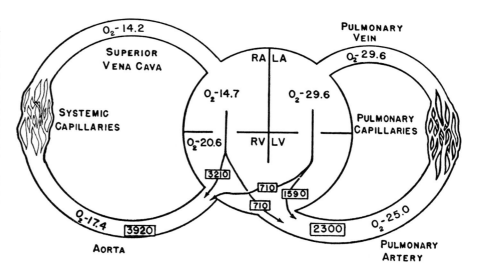

Figure 28–8. The circulation of a specific malformation is diagrammed (transposition of the aorta and overriding of the pulmonary artery). It is used as an example to illustrate the value of the calculation of flows and shunt. O_2 indicates oxygen content of the blood in volumes per cent. Oxygen content of the blood in pulmonary vein was calculated on the assumption that the blood was 96 per cent saturated. Figures in boxes give volume of blood flow in milliliters per minute per square meter of body surface. It may be seen that the large volume of the right atrial blood flows directly from the right ventricle into the aorta and only a small volume of blood passes into the pulmonary artery. This latter represents the effective pulmonary blood flow.

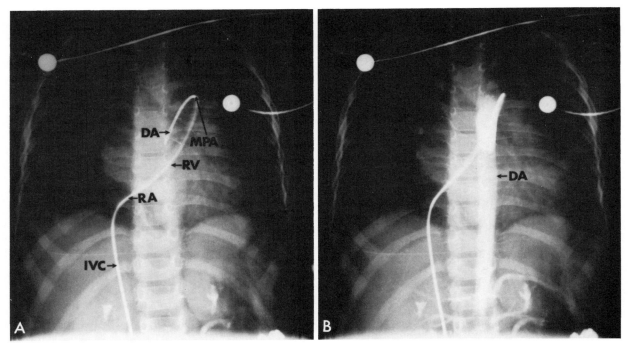

Figure 28–9. Patent ductus arteriosus. *A,* A catheter has been passed from the inferior vena cava (IVC) to the right atrium (RA), right ventricle (RV), and main pulmonary artery (MPA) to the descending thoracic aorta (DA) via a patent ductus arteriosus (*B*).

Often the catheter may be threaded through the patent ductus arteriosus into the aorta (Fig. 28–9). In the tetralogy of Fallot, aortic transposition, or ventricular defects in the membranous part of the septum, the aorta may be intubated directly from the right ventricle.

LEFT HEART CATHETERIZATION

In many instances, the principal cardiac lesions, especially those located on the left side of the heart, are difficult to evaluate by right heart catheterization. The development of left heart catheterization has made it possible to assess more accurately the size and location of left-to-right shunts and to evaluate lesions of the mitral and aortic valves. In addition, aortic valvular stenosis can be differentiated from supravalvular, subvalvular, and idiopathic hypertrophic subaortic stenosis; selective angiocardiography of the left heart chambers and the aorta can be performed, and postoperative results can be evaluated.

Pressure Relationship of the Left Heart

The diagnostic value of left heart catheterization is to a large extent based on the pressure relationships among the left atrium, the left ventricle, and the aorta (Table 28–3). The components of the normal left atrial pressure tracing are shown in Figure 28–10. Over 50 per cent of normal subjects show a prominent "v" wave, which ranges between 5 and 15 mm. Hg, while in the remainder, a prominent "a" wave with a height of between 3 and 7 mm. Hg is observed. In atrial fibrillation, the "a" wave is absent, whereas in atrioventricular block, giant "a" waves may be present. Nodal rhythm generally causes superimposition of the "a" wave on the "c" wave and replacement of the normal "x" descent (Braunwald, 1960).

Heart failure or valvular disease modifies normal pressure tracings by changes in contour or height. In congestive heart failure, there is an elevation of the left ventricular end-diastolic pressure and a rise in left atrial pressure. In mitral stenosis, there is usually an increase in the left atrial pressure and a prolongation of

TABLE 28–3.   NORMAL PRESSURES RECORDED DURING LEFT HEART
CATHETERIZATION

| | PRESSURES (MM. HG) | | |
	Systolic	*Diastolic*	*Mean*
Left atrium			4 to 12
Left ventricle	100 to 140	4 to 12	
Aorta	100 to 140	60 to 90	70 to 90

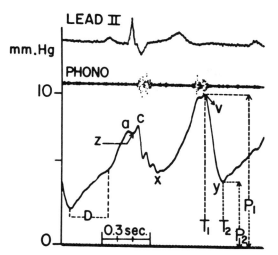

Figure 28–10. The normal left atrial pressure tracing. The "a" wave represents atrial systole and follows the P wave of the electrocardiogram; atrial pressure then declines to the "z" point. Following the QRS of the electrocardiogram, left ventricular contraction occurs, resulting in closure and bulging of the mitral valve into the atrium. This rise in atrial pressure produces the "c" wave. During left ventricular ejection the mitral valve ring descends, causing an abrupt fall in left atrial pressure, the "x" descent. With continued left atrial filling, the atrial volume and pressure rise, resulting in the "v" wave. The peak of this wave corresponds to the opening of the mitral valve. The "y" descent follows as a result of rapid filling of the ventricle, the so-called diastolic inflow phase. P_1 is the pressure peak of the "v" wave, and P_2 is the pressure termination of the "y" descent; $T_2 - T_1$ refers to the time interval for this pressure drop. D (the period of diastasis) is the fourth rise in left atrial pressure, which occurs during the period of slow left ventricular filling prior to left atrial contraction. (From Morrow, A. G., Braunwald, E., Haller, J. A., and Sharp, E. H.: The left atrial pressure in mitral valve disease. A correlation of pressures obtained by transbronchial puncture of the valvular lesion. Circulation, *16*:399, 1957.)

pressure (LAMP). In patients in whom mitral commissurotomy was indicated, the ratio $\frac{Ry}{LAMP}$ was less than 4. A ratio greater than 4 suggested mitral insufficiency as the predominant lesion. These investigators concluded that, regardless of the method employed, when mitral stenosis is the predominant lesion, the severity of the accompanying mitral regurgitation cannot be detected.

In mitral stenosis, the decrease in the left atrial pressure and the increase in the left ventricular pressure after the onset of its diastolic rise are such that the mitral diastolic gradient declines exponentially with respect to time. Consequently, logarithmic plotting of the gradient results in a straight line. The mitral diastolic gradient half-time is defined as the time required for the gradient to fall to half of its initial value from the beginning of the left ventricular filling (Fig. 28–12).

Libanoff and Rodbard (1968) found a good correlation between the mitral diastolic gradient and the severity of mitral stenosis. In mild mitral stenosis the half-time was approximately 100 msec., in moderate stenosis it was about 200 msec., and it was 300 msec. or longer in severe stenosis. Coexistent mitral regurgitation did not invalidate the results of the test. In addition, Libanoff and Rodbard (1966) proposed the formula for the index (see below). This index ranged from 0.4 to 0.8 in normal subjects, from 0.6 to 2.0 in patients with predominant mitral regurgitation, and from 5.7 to 10 in cases of mitral stenosis.

Although pressure contours are of value in the evaluation of patients with mitral disease, the most important criterion of the severity of mitral stenosis is

the "y" descent, indicating resistance to flow across the mitral valve (Fig. 28–11). Diastasis is usually absent in patients with mitral stenosis, unless the left atrioventricular diastolic gradient falls to zero.

The degree of mitral valvular obstruction has been expressed by the $\frac{Ry}{V}$ ratio, where Ry is the rate of descent in mm. Hg per second (determined by dividing the difference in pressure at the height of the "v" wave, and that at the termination of the "y" descent, by the time in seconds $\left(\frac{P_1 - P_2}{T_2 - T_1}\right)$ and $\dot{V}$ is the height of the "v" wave (P_1) in mm. Hg above the sternal angle (see also Fig. 28–10). This $\frac{Ry}{V}$ ratio has proved useful in distinguishing mitral stenosis from mitral insufficiency. In patients with pure mitral stenosis, the ratio is commonly 0.6 to 1.0; in pure mitral incompetence or left ventricular failure, the ratio ranges between 2 and 6 (Owen and Wood, 1955).

However, because the height of the "v" wave varies according to respiration and the length of preceding diastole, Morrow and coworkers (1957) related the rate of the "y" descent (Ry) to the left atrial mean

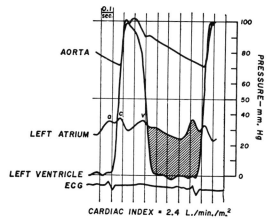

Figure 28–11. Simultaneously recorded left atrial, left ventricular, and aortic pressure tracings of a 49-year-old man with pure mitral stenosis. Note the elevated left atrial pressure and prolongation of the "y" descent, indicating resistance to flow across the mitral valve. The rise in atrial pressure during the period of slow left ventricular filling is also absent. The mitral diastolic gradient in this patient was 28 mm. Hg to maintain an output of 2.4 liters per min. per square meter. This pressure gradient, as shown by the cross lines, persists throughout diastole. (From Fox, I. J., Coolidge, S. W., Connolly, D. C., and Wood, E. H.: Left atrial and ventricular pulses in mitral valvular disease. Proc. Staff Meet. Mayo Clin., *31*:127, 1956.)

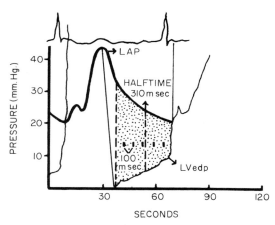

Figure 28–12. Simultaneous left atrial (LAP) and ventricular diastolic pressures recorded in a patient with severe mitral stenosis. The diastolic pressure gradient starting at the beginning of the rise in ventricular pressure is measured at 100 msec. intervals (short vertical lines). The shaded area demonstrates the changing atrioventricular pressure gradient. (LVedp = left ventricular end-diastolic pressure.)

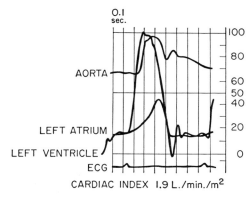

Figure 28–13. Simultaneously recorded left atrial, left ventricular, and aortic pressure tracings of a 24-year-old man with pure mitral insufficiency. The "a" wave is absent because of atrial fibrillation. Note the tall "v" wave (regurgitant wave) occurring in late ventricular systole and the steep "y" descent indicating little or no resistance to flow across the valve. Diastasis is present in mitral regurgitation. (From Fox, I. J., Coolidge, J. W., Connolly, D. C., and Wood, E. H.: Left atrial and ventricular pulses in mitral valve disease. Proc. Staff Meet. Mayo Clin., *31*:130, 1956.)

the left atrioventricular diastolic pressure gradient across the mitral valve at rest and during exercise. Normally this gradient is 1 mm. Hg or less, whereas in mitral stenosis gradients of 5 to 30 mm. Hg at rest have been found. The gradient rises significantly with exercise (Friedberg, 1966). Following successful mitral commissurotomy, a marked reduction or abolition of the mitral gradient is observed (Braunwald *et al.*, 1955).

It should be emphasized that the mere presence of a mitral diastolic gradient does not always indicate mitral stenosis. It may result from obstructive hypertrophy of the anterior papillary muscles, myxoma of the left atrium, anomalous myocardial hypertrophy adjacent to the mitral valve, or generalized obstructive left ventricular hypertrophy (Davis and Andrus, 1954; Litwak *et al.*, 1960; Lurie *et al.*, 1959.)

In mitral insufficiency, the characteristic features are a tall "v" wave (the so-called regurgitant wave) and a steep "y" descent, indicating little or no resistance to flow across the valve (Fig. 28–13). In these patients, unlike patients with mitral stenosis, there is a normal rise in left atrial pressure during the period of slow left ventricular filling (diastasis). The left ventricular tracing also shows an abrupt fall in pressure following ventricular systole (Braunwald, 1960).

In combined lesions of the mitral valve, the pressure tracing is a combination of the findings described in mitral insufficiency and stenosis, the gradations depending on the severity of each.

The normal left ventricular pressure in man is 120 mm. Hg (100 to 140) systolic and 4 to 12 mm. Hg diastolic. In infants, the systemic arterial pressure averages 60 to 70 mm. Hg. There is a difference of

10 to 15 mm. Hg between the central systolic aortic pressure and the peripheral systolic pressure, the latter being higher. Supravalvular aortic stenosis is characterized by an abrupt fall in pressure as the catheter passes the site of a narrowing above the aortic valve (Fig. 28–14) (Morrow *et al.*, 1959). In congenital or acquired valvular aortic stenosis, the systolic gradient between the aorta and the left ventricle is considered mild if it is below 50 mm. Hg, moderate between 50 and 100 mm. Hg, and severe above 100 mm. Hg (Fig. 28–15). In discrete subaortic stenosis, Morrow and associates (1958) demonstrated that the systolic pressure gradient shows a progressive fall between the left ventricle and the aorta similar to that described in isolated pulmonic infundibular stenosis. In idiopathic hypertrophic subaortic stenosis, the site of obstruction has been localized to the left ventricular outflow tract (Fig. 28–16) (Braunwald *et al.*, 1960). The ascending limb of the left ventricular pressure tracing, recorded proximal to the obstruction, generally exhibits a notch at a level that corresponds to the peak pressure distal to the obstruction (Fig. 28–16). Administration of digitalis, amyl nitrite, nitroglycerin, or isoproterenol or a Valsalva maneuver increases the systolic gradient (Figs. 28–17 and 28–18), whereas methoxamine and beta-adrenergic blocking agents, such as propranolol, tend to decrease the systolic gradient (Fig. 28–19). Brockenbrough and coworkers (1962) have also described a fall in the peripheral pulse pressure following the normal beat that succeeds a ventricular premature contraction (Fig. 28–20). This contrasts with patients with discrete supravalvular, valvular, or subvalvular stenosis, in whom a widened pulse pressure occurs

$$\text{Mitral stenosis index} = \frac{\text{mitral diastolic gradient half-time (msec.)} \times 100}{\text{cardiac index (L./min./m.}^2\text{)}}$$

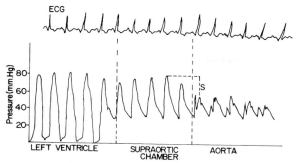

Figure 28–14. Supravalvular aortic stenosis. Pressure tracing obtained during pullback from left ventricle to ascending aorta. There is a 22 mm. Hg systolic gradient (S) within the ascending aorta.

after the first normal beat following a premature ventricular contraction (Fig. 28–21). Braunwald and colleagues (1964) have summarized the concept of idiopathic hypertrophic subaortic stenosis.

In aortic insufficiency, left ventricular diastolic pressure exceeds left atrial pressure in mid-diastole and continues to rise, so that the aortic and ventricular diastolic pressures are about equal at the onset of systole (Wright *et al.*, 1956). The aortic pressure contour also exhibits a low diastolic pressure and a wide pulse pressure, whereas peripheral arterial tracings show an abrupt rise in systolic pressure followed by an abrupt fall in late systole preceding the dicrotic notch (Wright and Wood, 1958). In patients with aortic insufficiency and aortic stenosis, a combination of these signs is seen, and the brachial artery pulse pressure exhibits the so-called "pulsus bisferiens."

However, even with the most refined analytic techniques, the clinical examination of patients with valvular heart disease remains, in the opinion of this group, the most significant part of the diagnostic evaluation.

Methods of Left Heart Catheterization

During the past 15 years, numerous methods of catheterizing the left heart have been employed clini-

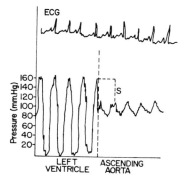

Figure 28–15. Aortic valvular stenosis. Pressure tracing obtained during pullback from left ventricle to ascending aorta. There is a 45 mm. Hg systolic gradient (S) between the left ventricle and the ascending aorta.

cally (Morrow *et al.*, 1960). These have included the transbronchial technique (Facquet *et al.*, 1952; Morrow *et al.*, 1957; Scott *et al.*, 1960), the posterior percutaneous left atrial puncture technique (Björk *et al.*, 1953; Fisher, 1955, 1959; Kent *et al.*, 1955), the suprasternal left atrial puncture technique (Radner, 1955; Fox, 1959), and the anterior left ventricular approach technique (Nunez and Ponsdomenech, 1951; Brock *et al.*, 1956; Fleming *et al.*, 1957, 1958; Morrow *et al.*, 1957).

Because of their relative ease and low morbidity, the transseptal left heart and the retrograde aortic left heart catheterization techniques are widely used at the present time, and they will be discussed in greater detail.

Transseptal Left Heart Catheterization. As noted previously, a cardiac catheter, when introduced from the saphenous or superficial femoral vein, can be passed through a patent foramen ovale or atrial septal defect (Cournand *et al.*, 1947). The relative ease with which this can be done suggested that the intact atrial septum could be traversed with an appropriately curved needle in the region of the fossa ovalis (Ross *et al.*, 1959, 1960). In experimental studies in dogs, Ross (1959) showed that the procedure was technically feasible. Clinical trials by Cope (1959) and Ross and associates (1959, 1960) were then undertaken.

When the transseptal technique was first applied to man, the saphenous vein had to be surgically exposed and ultimately sacrificed (Ross *et al.*, 1960). Furthermore, the polyethylene catheter used in intubating the left ventricle was not radiopaque; thus, the position of the catheter tip had to be monitored by pressure recordings alone. Finally, contrast material could not be injected with sufficient rapidity to obtain angiograms of high quality. Therefore, an improved technique of transseptal left heart catheterization was introduced by Brockenbrough and coworkers (1962).

The femoral vein is punctured according to the technique described by Seldinger (1953). Following puncture of the femoral vein just below the inguinal ligament, a guide wire is inserted through a needle in the inferior vena cava. The needle is withdrawn, and a right heart catheter is passed over the guide wire and inserted in the femoral vein and inferior vena cava. The guide wire is then removed, and a stylet is introduced in the catheter to keep the end of the catheter straight. Both are advanced to the right atrium, where the stylet is removed, and the right heart catheterization is performed in the usual manner.

When the right heart catheterization is completed, the spring wire is reinserted into the catheter. The catheter is removed, and the left heart catheter is inserted (Fig. 28–22*A*). The latter is advanced to the right atrium with a straight stylet (Fig. 28–22*B*), which is then withdrawn and replaced by the transseptal needle (Fig. 28–22*C*). The catheter and needle are rotated in a posteromedial direction to puncture the lower one third of the atrial septum or higher beneath the ledge of the limbus fossa (Bloomfield and Sinclair-

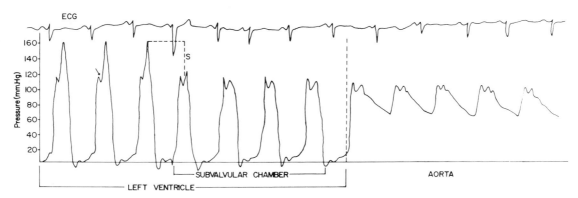

Figure 28-16. Subaortic hypertrophic stenosis. Pressure tracing obtained during pullback from left ventricle to ascending aorta. There is a 45 mm. Hg systolic gradient (S) within the left ventricular chamber. The arrow denotes the notch on the ascending limb of the left ventricular pressure curve that corresponds to the peak systolic pressure distal to the obstruction.

Smith, 1965) (Fig. 28-23). The location of the needle is confirmed by pressure and blood sampling. The needle is withdrawn, and the catheter is advanced across the mitral valve into the left ventricle (Fig. 28-24). The ventricle pressure can be checked, and a pullback across the mitral valve is recorded. Furthermore, selective left ventricular angiography can be performed (Beuren and Apitz, 1963; Braunwald *et al.*, 1962).

Transseptal left heart catheterization should not be performed in patients with large right atria, rotational anomalies of the heart or great vessels, severe scoliosis, or marked aortic root dilatation, patients on anticoagulants, or patients with recent systemic arterial embolization (Ross, 1966).

Complications of the transseptal approach include puncture of the aorta or the free wall of the right atrium with subsequent hemopericardium and cardiac tamponade (Androuny *et al.*, 1963; Russell *et al.*, 1964); left atrial mural thrombus (Pinkerson *et al.*, 1963); broken needle with embolization to the liver (Susmano and Carleton, 1964); coronary artery embolization or thrombophlebitis with resultant pulmonary embolism (Androuny *et al.*, 1963); and persistent

puncture defect with a left-to-right shunt (Ross *et al.*, 1963).

The main advantage of the transseptal left heart catheterization is that it can be combined easily with right heart catheterization through a single venous approach. Furthermore, in some cases of severe aortic stenosis, this technique permits intubation of the left ventricle when the aortic valve cannot be crossed in a retrograde fashion.

Retrograde Left Heart Catheterization. Retrograde aortic catheterization was reported by Zimmerman and associates in 1950. The procedure was successful in 11 patients with aortic insufficiency but was unsuccessful in those patients with normal aortic valves because of the short ejection periods of the left ventricle. In 1957, Priotin and coworkers, employing Seldinger's technique (1953), described a method for catheterizing the left ventricle through a percutaneous femoral artery approach. They found that the aortic valve was freely traversed in normal individuals and in patients with aortic insufficiency. In the presence of severe aortic stenosis, however, the catheter usually was diverted from entering the left ventricle.

In Priotin's method, a spring guide is passed 6 to 8 cm. beyond an indwelling femoral arterial needle. The needle is then withdrawn from the artery, leaving the

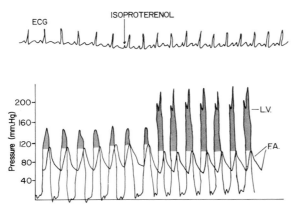

Figure 28-17. Effect of intravenous isoproterenol on the systolic gradient (shaded area) between the left ventricle (L.V.) and the femoral artery (F.A.) in subaortic hypertrophic stenosis. The baseline systolic gradient (shaded area) is about 40 mm. Hg. During infusion of isoproterenol it increases to 90 mm. Hg (shaded area).

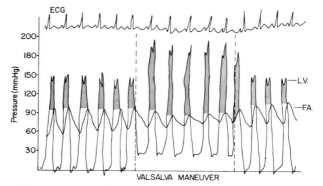

Figure 28-18. Effect of Valsalva maneuver on the systolic gradient (shaded area) between the left ventricle (L.V.) and the femoral artery (F.A.) in subaortic hypertrophic stenosis. The baseline systolic gradiant (shaded area) is about 60 mm. Hg. During the maneuver it is increased to 110 mm. Hg (shaded area).

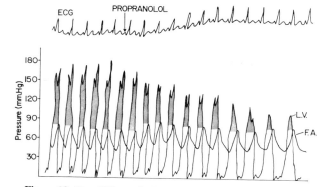

Figure 28-19. Effect of a beta-adrenergic blocking agent (propranolol) on the systolic gradient (shaded area) between the left ventricle (L.V.) and the femoral artery (F.A.) in subaortic hypertrophic stenosis. The baseline systolic gradient (shaded area) is about 80 mm. Hg. During infusion of propranolol it decreases to about 20 mm. Hg (shaded area).

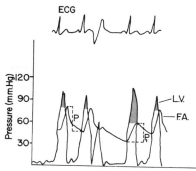

Figure 28-20. Effect of a post-premature contraction on pulse pressure of the femoral artery (F.A.) in subaortic hypertrophic stenosis. The baseline pulse pressure (P) in the femoral artery (F.A.) is about 35 mm. Hg. During the post-premature contraction, pulse pressure (P₁) in the femoral artery (F.A.) is about 25 mm. Hg. Shaded area represents the systolic gradient between the left ventricle (L.V.) and the femoral artery (F.A.).

spring guide in place. A catheter, curved near its tip, is passed over the guide percutaneously into the femoral artery so that a few centimeters of the guide remain distal to the catheter tip. The catheter and the guide are then advanced under fluoroscopic control until the ascending aorta is reached: Instead of the Seldinger spring guide, a long flexible coil spring with an inner wire stiffener has been employed as a guide (Dotter, 1960). The guide wire has been sealed with Teflon tubing to avoid arterial injury and breakage (Cope, 1962).

Littman and associates (1960) described a flexible loop catheter, which, except in cases of severe aortic stenosis, readily enters the left ventricle.

Grundemann and coworkers (1960) inserted a radiopaque catheter in the brachial artery through an arteriotomy incision. The catheter is passed to the ascending aorta and across the aortic valve into the left ventricle. Following the procedure, the arteriotomy site is closed with atraumatic silk sutures. By this technique Grundemann reached the left ventricle in 66 per cent of patients with severe aortic stenosis and in 77 per cent of patients with minimal or no aortic stenosis. Hildner and colleagues (1966) reviewed their experience of the transbrachial approach in 600 consecutive adult cases. The left ventricle was intubated in 96 per cent of the cases. The failure rate of 4 per cent was due to tortuous or aberrant great arteries, dilated aortas, calcified aortic valves, and local arteriospasm. In 216 cases of significant aortic stenosis, the left ventricle was entered in 98 per cent of the cases. In the presence of aortic obstruction, the chances of failure are decreased considerably if the right arm is employed, because anatomically the catheter passes more easily through the innominate than through the subclavian artery in the ascending aorta. Complications include hematoma, aortic perforation due to injudicious forcing of the tip of the guide wire, and ventricular arrhythmias. In one third of the patients in Voci and Hamer's series (1960), brachial artery thrombosis was reported. However, owing to

the well-developed collateral circulation, there were no untoward effects.

Using a specially designed catheter (see Fig. 28-2), Shirey and Sones (1966) described a technique for transbrachial retrograde catheterization of the aorta, left ventricle, and left atrium. They reported a 90 per cent overall successful selective catheterization of the left atrium. With a predominantly stenotic mitral valve, the left atrium was entered in 84 per cent of the cases. With mitral insufficiency, catheterization of the left atrium was successful in 97 per cent of the cases. Hemopericardium was a complication in two patients, and ventricular fibrillation and tachycardia occurred in six of 315 studies.

The main advantage of retrograde left heart catheterization techniques is their simplicity and relative safety. They are, by far, the most widely used techniques in the study of the left heart and aorta; they also permit visualization of the coronary vascular bed.

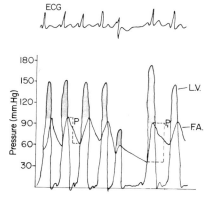

Figure 28-21. Effect of a post-premature contraction on pulse pressure (P) of the femoral artery (F.A.) in valvular aortic stenosis. The baseline pulse pressure (P) of the femoral artery (F.A.) is about 35 mm. Hg. During post-premature contraction, pulse pressure (P₁) of the femoral artery (F.A.) is about 55 mm. Hg. Shaded area represents the systolic gradient between the left ventricle (L.V.) and the femoral artery (F.A.).

Complications of Cardiac Catheterization

The reader is referred to a survey of complications of cardiac catheterization published by the American Heart Association (Braunwald and Swan, 1968).

Transient arrhythmias occur during every procedure. Conduction defects, knotted catheters, pyrogenic reactions, air emboli, venous or arterial spasm, thrombophlebitis, and perforation of the atria, ventricles, and coronary sinus with subsequent hemopericardium and cardiac tamponade have been reported. An increased risk is expected in cyanotic children and in patients with severe pulmonary hypertension. (See also the discussion of contrast materials under Angiocardiography, p. 895.)

INDICATOR-DILUTION TECHNIQUES

Dye-Dilution Method

Practical methods for direct, continuous recording of time-concentration curves of indicator dyes in the whole blood were introduced in 1950 by Freidlich, Heimbecker, and Bing and by Nicholson and Wood.

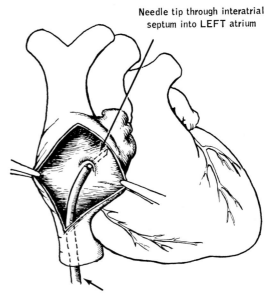

Needle tip through interatrial septum into LEFT atrium

Catheter in RIGHT atrium

Figure 28–23. This diagram shows the position of the cardiac catheter and transseptal needle following puncture of the interatrial septum. (From Braunwald, E.: Methods for the study of the circulation in man. *In* Clinical Cardiopulmonary Physiology. 2nd Ed. Edited by B. L. Gordon. New York, Grune & Stratton, 1960.)

Since then, the technique has become a valuable tool in diagnostic cardiology.

The direct recording of the peripheral arterial dye-dilution curve yields much information about the circulation in a relatively short time. Thus, it is possible to estimate the cardiac output, the fastest and the mean circulation time, and the blood volume between the points of injection and sampling and to determine the presence of shunts or valvular insufficiency (Wood *et al.*, 1957).

The usefulness of the technique is increased when it is employed in conjunction with right and left heart catheterization. Selective injection and selective sam-

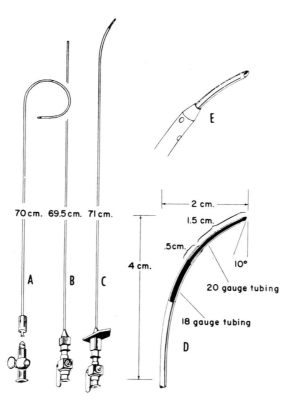

Figure 28–22. Diagram of the equipment employed in transseptal left heart catheterization. *A,* Transseptal catheter. *B,* Transseptal stylet. *C,* Transseptal needle. *D,* Detail of transseptal needle tip. *E,* Transseptal catheter tip with protruding tip. (From Brockenbrough, E. C., Braunwald, E., and Ross, J.: Transseptal left heart catheterization — a review of 450 studies and description of an improved technique. Circulation, *25*:15, 1962.)

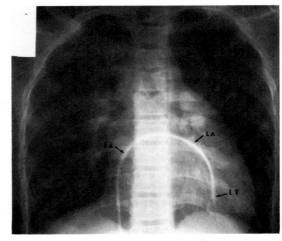

Figure 28–24. This radiographic film shows the radiopaque catheter transversing the right atrium (RA), the interatrial septum, left atrium (LA), and mitral valve into the left ventricle (LV).

pling have made possible the localization of the sites of intra- and extracardiac shunts as well as the establishment of the direction of shunts. Methods for localizing incompetent valves and estimating their degree of regurgitant flow have also been described. The residual volume of the right ventricle has been estimated by injecting dye into the right ventricle and recording the resulting dilution curve from the pulmonary artery (Bing *et al.,* 1951; Freis *et al.,* 1960).

The indicator-dilution techniques, helpful as they are as diagnostic aids, have definite limitations, particularly when they are used for quantitative studies, as pointed out in a review by Dow (1956). This is especially the case at very low flows, because of the large area under the curve and its prolonged downslope. This applies also to measurements of central volume when that volume is greatly increased. Equally important, the presence of high flow may lead to a considerable error because of the small area under the curve. At high flows, an error can be introduced because of the lag of the recording system; under these conditions, the peak of the dye concentration is often obscured. When a continuously recording densitometer is used, the flow through the sampling system must be controlled critically to avoid distortion. In the interpretation of dye-dilution curves, adequate mixing of the indicator with the blood is assumed; mixing, however, may be inadequate, particularly when injection and sampling sites are too close together. It is important to keep these limitations of this technique in mind when interpreting quantitative results obtained with this method.

The Normal Dye-Dilution Curve. The concentration of dye in the blood is measured by recording the change in optical density of the blood by photoelectric means (decrease in the transmission of light) as the blood is drawn through a cuvette at a constant rate (Gilford *et al.,* 1953). Arterial sampling after rapid injection of a known amount of nondiffusable dye into the venous side of the circulation (i.e., pulmonary artery, right ventricle or atrium, or any vein) reveals a sudden appearance of the dye a few seconds after the injection. The concentration of the dye rises rapidly to a peak and then falls to a point above the base line. A smaller, blunter peak of recirculating dye is recorded. The final dye concentration represents a state of equilibrium of dye concentration in the vascular system (Fig. 28–25).

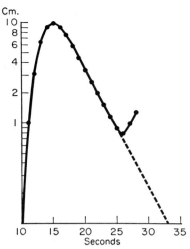

Figure 28–26. Semilogarithmic replot of the normal dye-dilution curve, showing the straight line assumed by the downslope and the extrapolation of the theoretic disappearance time.

In 1897, Stewart recognized that the time-course of the downstream concentration of an injected indicator was related to the flow of the volume of blood that diluted it. Moore and associates (1929) and Hamilton and coworkers (1932), using interrupted sampling and rapid injection of dye, showed that when the downslope of the initial appearance curve was replotted on semilogarithmic paper, it assumed a straight line (Fig. 28–26). The extrapolation of that line by zero (or nearly zero, since the zero point is approached asymptotically) separated the area under the curve due to the first circulation of the indicator from the area due to recirculation (Fig. 28–26).

It is convenient to plot, at one-second intervals, only the downslope of the continuously recorded dilution curve on semilogarithmic paper, expressed as centimeters of deflection from the base (Fig. 28–26). The straight-line downslope is extrapolated to the base and replotted on the recorded curve from the beginning of recirculation to the theoretic disappearance time, which is taken as the point where the extrapolated line comes within 0.1 cm. of the extended base line (see Fig. 28–25). The area under the curve is then determined by planimetry. The mean height is determined by dividing the area, in square centimeters, by the length of the base, in centimeters, from the time of first appearance of dye to the theoretic disappearance time.

To three aliquots of a blood sample taken from the patient prior to the procedure, dye* is added to make concentrations of 1.5, 3.0., and 6.0 mg. per liter. Each aliquot and an aliquot of undyed blood are then drawn through the cuvette at the same rate at which blood was sampled from the patient during the recording of the dye-dilution curve, and the deflections are recorded with the same settings on the amplifier as were used

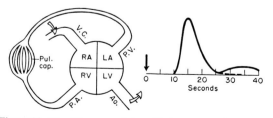

Figure 28–25. The normal dye-dilution curve with the replot to theoretic disappearance time (V.C. = venae cavae; P.V. = pulmonary vein; P.A. = pulmonary artery; Ao. = aorta; RA = right atrium; RV = right ventricle; LA = left atrium; LV = left ventricle; Pul. Cap. = pulmonary capillaries).

---

*Cardio-Green is used exclusively (Fox and Wood, 1957). The standard dose used for adults is 5 mg.

in recording the curve from the patient. The heights of the deflections, in centimeters, using the height of the deflection of the undyed sample as zero, are then plotted against the concentration of dye in milligrams per liter on linear paper. The straight line so obtained serves as a check on the linearity of the recording apparatus. From this line the mean concentration of the dye-dilution curve is read from its mean height.

The cardiac output is determined from the Stewart-Hamilton formula (Kinsman *et al.*, 1929):

$$F = \frac{60\ I}{CT}$$

where F = cardiac output in liters per minute, I = the amount of dye injected expressed in milligrams, 60 = number of seconds per minute, C = mean concentration of dye in milligrams per liter, and T = time in seconds from the first appearance of the dye to the theoretic disappearance.

The mean circulation time is the time that the mean dye particle takes to arrive at the sampling site from the injection site. This time may be calculated by multiplying each concentration value by its time value at one-second intervals, beginning from the midpoint of injection as time zero. The sum of all these products divided by the sum of the concentrations represents the mean circulation time (Hamilton *et al.*, 1932).

The product of the mean circulation time and the flow (cardiac output) represents the blood volume between the point of injection and sampling, including the volume of the cardiac chambers and pulmonary circulation and all temporally equivalent venous and arterial samples (Dow, 1956; Hamilton *et al.*, 1932). Therefore, in the case of peripheral venous injection, this volume includes all the venous blood, from all venous channels, that will arrive at the heart at the same time as the injected dye. It also includes the volume of all the arterial blood in all the arteries to that point in each artery at which sampling would have given a dye-dilution curve with the same mean circulation time as the one actually recorded.

Abnormal Dye-Dilution Curves. INCREASED CENTRAL BLOOD VOLUME. The dye-dilution curve in congestive heart failure and in other conditions that increase central blood volume resembles the normal, except that the appearance time is later, the peak concentration is lower, and the slope of the disappearance curve is not so steep (Figs. 28–27 and 28–28).

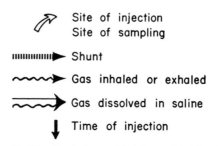

Figure 28–27. Symbols used in Figures 28–28 to 28–43.

- ↗ Site of injection
- ↗ Site of sampling
- ⅢⅢⅢⅢ▶ Shunt
- ⌇⌇⌇▶ Gas inhaled or exhaled
- ⌇▶ Gas dissolved in saline
- ↓ Time of injection

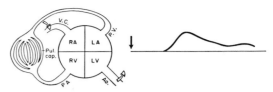

Figure 28–28. The altered dye curve produced by dilution of the dye by an increased central blood volume.

When a stenotic valve is present between the points of injection and sampling, a similar type of curve is obtained only after a significant increase in central blood volume has occurred.

RIGHT-TO-LEFT SHUNTS. The detection of a right-to-left shunt by the indicator-dilution technique is based on the early appearance of a portion of the dye on the left side of the circulation following its rapid injection on the right. This is due to bypassing of the pulmonary circulation by a portion of the dye. The curve recorded from a peripheral artery shows an early appearance time with a large or small peak, depending on the size of the shunt, and the recording of a secondary peak, representing the dye that has traversed the normal circulation (Fig. 28–29a). The significant finding in right-to-left shunts, therefore, is the modification of the upslope of the indicator-dilution curve. The site of the right-to-left shunt may be localized by selective multiple injections; injection upstream to the shunt shows the modified slope, whereas injection downstream to the shunt shows a normal type of curve since the shunt has been bypassed (Swan *et al.*, 1953) (Fig. 28–29b).

LEFT-TO-RIGHT SHUNTS. The detection of left-to-right shunts depends on the characteristic alteration of the downslope of the peripheral dye-dilution curve that takes place because some of the dye recirculates rapidly through the lung (Fig. 28–30a). Consequently,

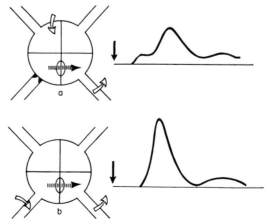

Figure 28–29. *a*, Ventricular septal defect with a right-to-left shunt. Diagrammatic representation of the dye curve showing the early appearance time of the shunted dye, which modifies the upslope of the curve. This modified upslope is produced by the portion of the dye that circulates through the abnormal pathway. *b*, When dye is injected downstream to the right-to-left shunt, a normal curve is produced as shown in the diagrammatic representation.

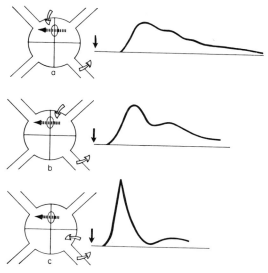

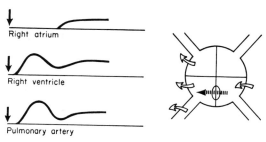

Figure 28-31. Ventricular septal defect with a left-to-right shunt. Injection of dye into the left ventricle results in early appearance of dye in the right ventricle and in the pulmonary artery but not in the right atrium. The shunt is thus localized at the ventricular level.

Figure 28-30. *a*, Atrial septal defect with a left-to-right shunt. The downslope of the dye curve is altered by the recirculation through the lungs of left-to-right shunted dye. Note the normal appearance time and the low peak concentration. *b*, Injection proximal to or at the site of the left-to-right shunt causes an altered downslope. *c*, Injection of dye downstream to the shunt results in a normal dye curve.

the appearance time and the upslope of the curve will be normal, but the peak will be low. The downslope is prolonged by the appearance of the abnormally recirculated dye, and there may be a hump or secondary peak in the downslope, depending on the size of the shunt. The changes in the downslope can be differentiated from normal recirculation because they occur faster and are usually more marked. Since this method frequently misses small left-to-right shunts and since the site of the shunt cannot be localized, injections often are made into the left side of the heart.

Localization of Left-to-Right Shunts. This can be accomplished by several methods:

Dye is injected into the left atrium, the left ventricle, or the aorta, and sampling is from a peripheral artery. Injection upstream to the site of the shunt gives the altered curve just described for left-to-right shunts (Fig. 28-30*b*). Injection downstream to the defect results in the normal dye curve (Fig. 28-30*c*) (Braunwald *et al.*, 1957).

Dye may be injected into the left atrium or left ventricle or at the root of the aorta, with sampling by catheter from the pulmonary artery, the right atrium, or the superior or inferior vena cava. For example, in the presence of a ventricular septal defect with a left-to-right shunt, injection of the dye into the left atrium or left ventricle results in early appearance of dye in the right ventricle or the pulmonary artery but not in the right atrium (Fig. 28-31). Detection of left-to-right shunts by the method described here may be difficult because of laminar flow. Consequently, the catheter should be placed as close as possible to the outflow tract of the chamber from which samples are to be taken (Wood *et al.*, 1957).

Peripheral venous injection of dye with sampling

through a right heart catheter has been described (Braunwald *et al.*, 1959) (Fig. 28-32). This results in a normal curve if the tip of the catheter is placed upstream to the shunt. When the tip is downstream to the shunt, recirculating dye will modify the downslope of the curve (Fig. 28-32).

In the fourth method, dye is injected into a branch of the right or left pulmonary artery instead of the left atrium, and sampling is by catheter from the main pulmonary artery, the right ventricle, the right atrium, and the vena cava in turn. The dye will appear rapidly in the chamber or chambers downstream to the left-to-right shunt (Swan *et al.*, 1958) (Fig. 28-33).

Quantification of Left-to-Right Shunts. The altered downslope of the dye curve in left-to-right shunts is not logarithmic. Therefore, in the presence of a left-to-right shunt, it is difficult to calculate the area under the curve by the Stewart-Hamilton method. An empiric method has been presented for the quantification of such curves, which relies on the assumption that the area under the initial portion of a dye-dilution curve (from appearance time to the time of peak concentration or the "forward triangle") bears a constant relationship to the area under the entire curve, whether or not the downslope is altered (Wood *et al.*, 1957) (Fig. 28-34). Although the validity of this method has been doubted (Dow, 1955), the method seems to work empirically. It is possible to measure the pulmonary flow and the left-to-right shunt by injecting

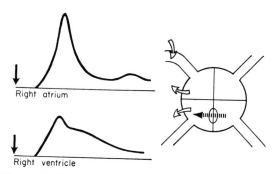

Figure 28-32. Ventricular septal defect with left-to-right shunt. Peripheral venous injection of the dye with sampling upstream to, and at the site of, a left-to-right shunt localizes the shunt to the chamber in which an altered downslope first appears.

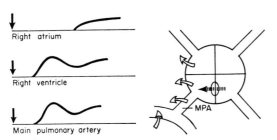

Figure 28–33. Ventricular septal defect with left-to-right shunt. Dye injected into the distal pulmonary artery appears early in the right ventricle and in the pulmonary artery but not in the right atrium.

dye into a distal pulmonary artery and sampling simultaneously from the main pulmonary artery and a peripheral artery. From the curve recorded at the peripheral artery, the total pulmonary flow is calculated. From the "forward triangle" portion of the curve recorded at the pulmonary artery, the flow of the left-to-right shunt is calculated. The pulmonary flow minus the shunt is the systemic flow.*

BIDIRECTIONAL SHUNTS. Bidirectional shunts may be demonstrated by combining arterial and venous sampling and injection techniques as just described.

Diagnosis of Anomalous Pulmonary Venous Drainage. The diagnosis of anomalous pulmonary venous drainage is especially important, since 15 to 20 per cent of interatrial septal defects are complicated by this condition. The appearance of the catheter in the lung fields from the right atrium permits no conclusions. It is not surprising that injection of dye into the pulmonary vein so entered gives a dilution curve from the peripheral artery that in all details resembles that recorded after injection into the atrium into which the pulmonary vein drains (Wood *et al.*, 1957) (Fig. 28–35). On the other hand, if the pulmonary vein is not entered during right heart catheterization and an atrial septal defect is suspected, dye should be injected into several lobar branches of both the left and right pulmonary arteries. Thus, injection of dye into a lobe of the lung that drains into the right atrium gives a curve with a late appearance time, a low peak concentration, and a prolonged downslope (Fig. 28–36*a*). The injection of dye into a portion of the lung that drains normally into the left atrium produces a curve with an

earlier appearance time and a higher peak concentration, but still with an altered downslope due to the left-to-right shunt from the interatrial septal defect (Fig. 28–36*b*). It should be remembered, however, that most of the blood in a left-to-right shunt due to an atrial septal defect is from the right lung (Swan *et al.*, 1956).

Diagnosis of Valvular Regurgitation by Dye-Dilution Techniques. The dye-dilution curve inscribed in the presence of valvular insufficiency is similar to that seen in left-to-right shunts. There is a prolongation of the downslope of the curve when dye is injected upstream to the chamber with the regurgitant valve and sampling is from a peripheral artery (Fig. 28–37). The peak concentration is lower, and the build-up time from appearance to peak concentration is prolonged. The regurgitant valve may be localized by selective injection of dye with peripheral arterial sampling. Injection at any site upstream to the insufficient valve gives a curve with the characteristic modification of the downslope. However, if a competent valve is interposed between the site of injection and the incompetent valve, a normal dilution curve results (Wood *et al.*, 1957) (Fig. 28–37).

Several methods have been proposed for the quantification of the regurgitant flow. One of these methods is based on the comparison of a series of normal curves with those obtained from patients with insufficient valves (Korner and Shillingford, 1955). The value and accuracy of this method are not yet proved. The second method is the injection of dye immediately downstream to a suspected incompetent valve and sampling immediately upstream to it. This method assumes adequate mixing of the dye with the blood at the site of injection; the tip of the catheter at the upstream site should be placed in such a manner that it lies in the regurgitant stream. The method is thus subject to technical difficulties (Wood *et al.*, 1957). In a third method, proposed by Lange and Hecht in 1958, which applies only when a regurgitant valve is on the left side of the heart, sampling is simultaneously from the pulmonary artery and a peripheral artery. The dye is injected into either the right atrium or one of the venae cavae. The flow through the incompetent valve, as measured at the peripheral artery, consists of the forward flow into the systemic circulation plus the regurgitant stream. The flow, as

---

*The calculations are as follows: The pulmonic flow =

$60 \times \dfrac{I}{A_{SA_{PA}}}$, where I is the amount of dye injected in milligrams and $A_{SA_{PA}}$ is the area of the curve recorded at a peripheral artery (calculated by the empiric formula: $A_{SA_{PA}} = 2.7 \times BT \times Cp$, where BT = time appearance to peak concentration, Cp = peak concentration in milligrams per liter, and 2.7 is a proportionality factor).

The left-to-right shunt is expressed as a fraction:

$$F_{L-R} = \frac{A_{PA_{PA}}}{A_{SA_{PA}}} \times 100$$

where F_{L-R} is the left-to-right shunt and $A_{PA_{PA}}$ is the area calculated for the curve recorded at the main pulmonary artery by the same method. Systemic flow = pulmonic flow $\times (1 - F_{L-R})$.

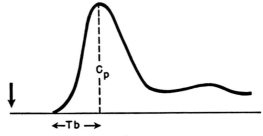

Figure 28–34. The "forward triangle" is demonstrated. *Tb* is the time from the appearance of the dye to the peak concentration of the dye. *Cp* is the peak concentration of the dye in milligrams per liter.

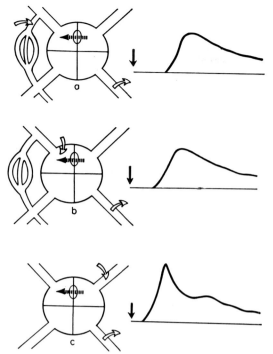

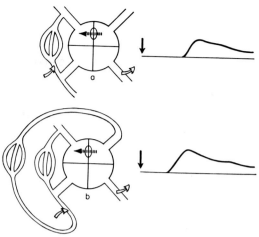

Figure 28–36. Anomalous pulmonary venous drainage and atrial septal defect with left-to-right shunt. *a,* Dye injected into an artery of a lobe of a lung, which drains into the right atrium or one of its tributaries, appears late in a peripheral artery. There is a low peak concentration because of greater dilution, and the downslope is prolonged by the left-to-right shunt through the interatrial septal defect. *b,* Dye injected into a lobar artery, which drains normally, appears at a normal time; thus, the curve is different in contour from that obtained from an anomalously draining lobe.

Figure 28–35. Anomalous pulmonary venous drainage and atrial septal defect with left-to-right shunt, *a* and *b.* It can be seen that the diagrammatic representations of the dye curves produced by injection of dye into either the anomalously draining pulmonary vein or the right atrium are similar to each other. In *c,* the curve from a normally draining pulmonary vein is not similar, showing only the effect of interatrial septal defect.

measured by the curve from the pulmonary artery, represents only the systemic flow. Consequently, the dye curve from the peripheral artery has a normal appearance time and a prolonged descent, whereas the dye curve from the pulmonary artery is normal (Fig. 28–38).

Other Methods for the Diagnosis and Localization of Shunts

Included among the substances that may be used as indicators for the detection of shunts are nitrous oxide, hydrogen, sodium ascorbate, krypton[85], and ^{131}I-tagged albumin. Except for ^{131}I-tagged albumin, most of these substances are not true indicators, such as tricarbocyanine (Cardio-Green), since they diffuse freely into the extracellular and often the intracellular spaces. Also, the gaseous substances are exhaled by the lung.

Oxygen Analysis. As noted previously (see Sampling of Blood for Determination of Blood Oxygen and Calculation of Flow, p. 874), analysis of oxygen content of the blood may be used in the detection and quantification of shunts.

Determination of oxygen content can be accomplished by the manometric method of Van Slyke and Neill (1924) or by spectrophotometry (Hickam and Frazer, 1949; Holling *et al.*, 1955). These methods are

time-consuming, and in infants multiple sampling may constitute a considerable loss of blood.

By use of either transmission (Harned *et al.*, 1952) or reflection (Rodrigo, 1953) methods, direct analysis of blood oxygen content can be obtained rapidly by flow through cuvettes connected directly to a catheter.

Oxygen tension (Po$_2$) may be continually monitored using a platinum electrode (Bargeron *et al.*, 1961; Clark *et al.*, 1958).

A fiberoptic catheter developed by Polanyi and Hehir (1960) incorporates instantaneous and continuous measurement of oxygen saturation without withdrawal of blood samples. The same instrument can also be used in the determination of cardiac output (Hugenholtz *et al.*, 1965).

The Nitrous Oxide Technique for the Detection of Left-to-Right Shunts. This test, introduced in 1958 by Morrow, Sanders, and Braunwald and modified by Sanders and Morrow that same year, is based on the

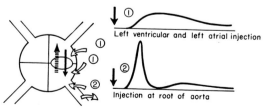

Figure 28–37. Mitral insufficiency. Dye injected into either the left atrium or the left ventricle in the presence of mitral insufficiency is diluted in increasing volumes of blood as the dye is washed back and forth through the incompetent valve. Note the normal appearance time, the prolonged upslope, the low peak concentration, and the prolonged downslope. However, injection at the roof of the aorta with a competent aortic valve results in a normal curve.

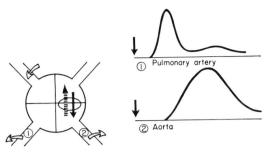

Figure 28-38. The quantification of mitral insufficiency. Simultaneous sampling from the pulmonary artery and a peripheral artery after injection of dye into the venae cavae reveals grossly different curves owing to the regurgitant valve on the left side of the heart. The area under the curve from the pulmonary artery represents systemic flow, whereas the area under the curve from a peripheral artery represents systemic flow plus regurgitant flow across the mitral valve.

fact that during the first minute of inhalation of nitrous oxide, the arteriovenous difference is relatively large owing to the avid tissue uptake of the gas. The patient breathes a mixture of 50 per cent nitrous oxide with 21 per cent oxygen for a period of 30 seconds. From the tenth to the thirtieth seconds, integrated simultaneous samples are drawn from a peripheral artery and from the pulmonary artery, the right ventricle, or the right atrium. The nitrous oxide content of the blood is analyzed in a Van Slyke manometric apparatus, and an arbitrary ratio is determined between the nitrous oxide content of the right heart blood and the arterial blood (Fig. 28-39). A value of 15 per cent or less demonstrates the absence of a shunt, whereas a value over 20 per cent is diagnostic of a left-to-right shunt. The test should be repeated when the ratio lies between 15 and 20 per cent. The tests may be repeated several times during a catheterization to permit selective sampling. Prior to the performance of each test, a blood blank is

drawn. In some cases, as in patients with prolonged circulation time or impairment of pulmonary diffusion, it may be necessary to begin sampling later or to prolong sampling. The relative flow of the shunt may be quantified (Fig. 28-39).

The quantification, as given, also applies to the use of krypton[85] to detect left-to-right shunts, which will be described. The chief advantages of the nitrous oxide test are simplicity and accuracy in localizing the site of the shunt. The chief disadvantage is that the results of the tests are not immediately available to the operator because of time-consuming analysis.

The Use of Radioactive Krypton. Krypton[85] also may be used for the detection of left-to-right shunts, as reported by Sanders and Morrow in 1959. When the gas is inhaled, blood samples collected simultaneously from the right side of the circulation and from a peripheral artery are rapidly analyzed by a Geiger-Mueller tube. During the first 30 to 60 seconds of gas inhalation, krypton[85] appears in the pulmonary veins and the left cardiac chambers. It diffuses freely in the interstitial and cellular compartments, so that its concentration in venous blood returning to the heart is low. Thus, in the presence of a left-to-right shunt, the concentration of krypton[85] in the right cardiac chambers and the ratio of the concentration of the gas in the right heart to systemic arterial blood are increased (Braunwald *et al.*, 1962; Singleton *et al.*, 1965) (Fig. 28-40).

Instead of being inhaled, the gas also may be dissolved in saline and injected into the left atrium, the left ventricle, and the aorta (Long *et al.*, 1960) (Fig. 28-41). The patient's expired air is then directed across a thin-window Geiger-Mueller tube placed in the line of expired air in a closed breathing circuit. The output of the tube is integrated by a count rate meter and recorded. This method depends on the fact that the gas is exhaled by the lungs during the first circulation. The

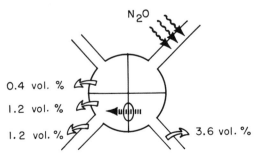

Figure 28-39. Ventricular septal defect with left-to-right shunt. When nitrous oxide is inhaled, there is normally a large arteriovenous difference in the first half minute: $\dfrac{N_2O_{RA}}{N_2O_A} = \dfrac{0.4}{3.6} \times 100$ $= 11\% =$ less than 15%, revealing the absence of a left-to-right shunt at the atrial level. However, in the presence of an interventricular septal defect with left-to-right shunts: $\dfrac{N_2O_{RA}}{N_2O_A} \times 100 = \dfrac{N_2O_{PA}}{N_2O_A} \times 100$ $= \dfrac{1.2}{3.6} \times 100 = 33\% =$ greater than 20%, indicating the presence of a left-to-right shunt at the ventricular level. Furthermore, the ratio of pulmonary to systemic flow $= \dfrac{100\% = 11\%}{100\% - \dfrac{N_2O_{PA}}{N_2O_A}} \times 100 = \dfrac{89}{67} = 1.33.$

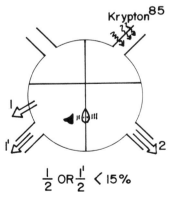

Figure 28-40. Localization of ventricular septal defect with left-to-right shunt with krypton[85]. Inhaled krypton[85] appears rapidly in the left cardiac chambers. It diffuses freely in the interstitial and cellular compartments so that its concentration in venous blood returning to the heart is low. Thus, in the presence of a left-to-right shunt at the ventricular level there will be an increase in the concentration of krypton[85] in the right ventricle and the pulmonary artery. As a result, the ratio of the concentration of the gas in the right heart to systemic arterial blood is increased. Normally, this ratio is less than 15 per cent.

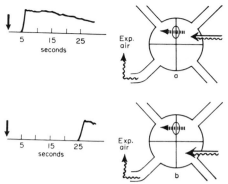

Figure 28–41. Localization of atrial septal defect with left-to-right shunt with krypton[85]. A rapid appearance time (1 to 8 seconds) of krypton[85] in the expired air after a solution of the gas is injected into the left atrium indicates the presence of a left-to-right shunt at the atrial level but does not rule out a left-to-right shunt at the ventricular level.

appearance time in the expired air is much more rapid than usual (1 to 8 seconds) when the gas is injected upstream to a left-to-right shunt (Fig. 28–41).

If krypton[85] dissolved in saline is injected in the right side of the circulation, the finding of a significant amount of radioactivity in a peripheral arterial sample indicates the presence of a right-to-left shunt downstream to the site of the injection, since 95 per cent of the gas is exhaled by the lungs during its first circulation (Fig. 28–42). These tests are technically simple, and the results are immediately available. They are more sensitive in the detection of small left-to-right shunts than in the analysis of the oxygen content of blood, and they can be used in locating the site of entry of a shunt.

The Hydrogen Ion Electrode. Clark and associates (1959, 1960) have described potentiometric electrodes for intravascular use. The presence of dissolved hydrogen in the blood changes the potential difference between a platinized platinum electrode in the blood and a silver reference electrode placed on the skin with suitable contact. The electrodes are connected directly to the D.C. input of a recording amplifier. One silver reference electrode may be used with several platinum electrodes.

For the detection of left-to-right shunts, the pa-

tient is given a breath of hydrogen, the timing of the breath being recorded from a platinum electrode at the tip of a nasal catheter (Fig. 28–43). A left-to-right shunt results in an early deflection recorded by a suitably placed right heart electrode (Fig. 28–43). For the detection of right-to-left shunts, an arterial electrode is used. Hydrogen, dissolved in saline by being bubbled through the solution, is injected into a peripheral vein. Since the hydrogen is exhaled almost completely by the lungs during its first circulation, the appearance of a deflection on the left side of the circulation indicates a right-to-left shunt. Blood sampling is not necessary, and multiple simultaneous recordings from different sites can be obtained easily. However, hydrogen is an explosive gas; furthermore, quantification of shunts has not yet been achieved.

Sodium ascorbate also produces a potential in the presence of a platinum electrode and is used to test the electrodes *in situ* before hydrogen is administered. Therefore, in the future, sodium ascorbate may be of value in the detection of shunts without blood sampling.

MEASUREMENTS OF CARDIAC VOLUMES

There are well-established techniques for determining cardiac volumes. When such measurements are combined with those of pressures and flows, the severity of the mechanical defects in patients with valvular and congenital heart disease and the status of left ventricular myocardial performance can be determined. With advances in cardiac surgery, these quantitative methods have become increasingly important in evaluating patients as candidates for surgery and for assessing the physiologic effects of surgery.

The thermodilution technique was introduced by Fegler (1954) in order to measure cardiac output. The indicator may be warmer or colder than circulating blood, but usually cold saline or blood is injected. The detector is a thermistor-tipped catheter. Repeated measurements may be made without withdrawal of blood. The catheter is placed beyond the aortic or pulmonic valve. A bolus of ice-cold blood or saline is injected via a second catheter into the ventricle during diastole. As the cold solution is injected into the heart,

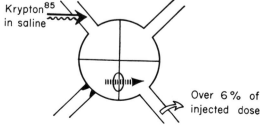

Figure 28–42. Ventricular septal defect with right-to-left shunt localized with krypton[85]. Since 95 per cent of the krypton[85] injected into the venous side of the circulation is excreted by the lungs during its first passage through the pulmonary circulation, the finding of a significant amount of radioactivity in the blood sampled from a peripheral artery indicates a right-to-left shunt.

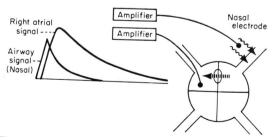

Figure 28–43. Detection of atrial septal defect with a left-to-right shunt with hydrogen. The early appearance in the right atrium of a change in potential caused by inhaled hydrogen indicates the presence of an interatrial septal defect with a left-to-right shunt. The inhalation of hydrogen is timed by an electrode placed in the nose as shown in the diagram.

the thermistor temperature drops and then progressively rises as the cold solution is marked out of the ventricle (Fig. 28–44). Recirculation is negligible. Cardiac output may be calculated by the Stewart-Hamilton method (Lüthy and Galletti, 1966).

The thermodilution technique yields the ventricular end-diastolic volume for a single cardiac cycle. *In vitro* studies show good correlation between calculated and directly measured volumes if the pulse is less than 100 beats/min. and the end-diastolic volume is less than 300 ml. (Salgado and Galletti, 1966).

Other indicators such as dye (Bing *et al.*, 1951) and isotopes (Folse and Braunwald, 1962) may be used for the measurements of ventricular volume. The optical density changes associated with the washout of opaque media from the ventricle may be quantitated by analysis of the cineangiocardiogram (Wood, 1962). A fiberoptic catheter system with a 95 per cent response in 0.1 second allows measurements of cardiac output and ventricular volume with indocyanine green as the indicator (Hugenholtz *et al.*, 1968; Wagner *et al.*, 1968). The volume of one or both ventricles may be derived from washout curves obtained by precordial counting of the passage of a radioactive gamma-emitting tracer through the heart and the lungs (Folse and Braunwald, 1962).

Left ventricular volumes have been measured by angiocardiography (Arvidsson, 1961; Chapman *et al.*, 1958; Dodge *et al.*, 1962). The left ventricle is treated as an ellipsoid, and its end-systolic and end-diastolic surface areas are measured on the film in two planes, with correction for magnification. Single-plane angiocardiography has also been used (Greene *et al.*, 1967; Sandler and Dodge, 1968). Right ventricular volume is not directly determinable by radiologic techniques because of the shape of the right ventricle (Reedy and Chapman, 1963). By the washout methods the ejection fraction of the left ventricle is 0.3 to 0.4, and by radiologic techniques the ejection fraction is 0.5 to 0.7. Although incomplete mixing tends to cause overestimation of the ventricular end-diastolic volume (Rapa-

port *et al.*, 1966; Carleton *et al.*, 1966; Bartle and Sanmarco, 1966), the dilution technique avoids the hemodynamic effects of opaque media and provides a rapid assessment of relative changes in right (Rapaport *et al.*, 1966) and left ventricular volumes during selected interventions. The stroke volume obtained by radiologic methods agrees well with indicator-dilution and Fick determinations (Dodge *et al.*, 1962).

The opacified left atrium is also represented as an ellipsoid so that left atrial volume can be calculated (Hawley *et al.*, 1966). By this method, regurgitant left atrial flow has been noted to equal or surpass effective left ventricular stroke volume (Hawley *et al.*, 1966).

Some of the parameters obtained from the measurements of left ventricular volumes are summarized in Table 28–4.

Intracardiac Phonocardiography

Soulié and associates (Feruglio, 1959) and Yamakawa and coworkers (1954) were the first to attempt direct recordings of intracardiac sounds. Further experiences with intracardiac phonocardiography were presented in 1957 by Soulié and associates, Moscovitz and coworkers, and Wallace and associates.

For intracardiac phonocardiography, Lewis and associates (1959) used underwater barium titanate microphones attached to the end of a specially designed sound catheter feeding into a transistor amplifier. The recordings were made on a regular phonochannel. Luisada and Liu (1957) recorded intracardiac sounds transmitted by a column of 5 per cent glucose or saline solution within a regular catheter connected to a pressure transducer.

The origin of heart sounds and murmurs can be localized quite sharply, since they can be recorded only in certain parts of the chambers (Lewis *et al.*, 1959). Sounds are transmitted downstream, and the amplitude and frequency diminish when the catheter is moved farther downstream. Sounds from other

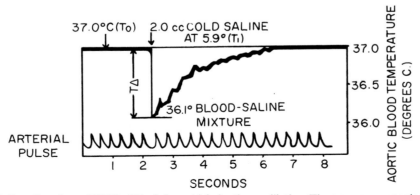

Figure 28–44. End-diastolic volume (EDV) of the left ventricle by thermodilution. The curve was recorded from the aorta following the injection of cold normal saline solution into the left ventricle during diastole.

$$EDV = \frac{\text{Amount of cold shared by the injectate and blood}}{\Delta T \text{ (change in the temperature of aortic blood during the first systole following injection)}}$$

$$EDV = \frac{(37.0° - 5.9°) \times 2.0 \text{ cc.}}{(37.0° - 36.1°)} = 69.0 \text{ cc.}$$

TABLE 28–4. VALUES OBTAINED FROM MEASUREMENTS OF LEFT VENTRICULAR VOLUMES

PARAMETER	FORMULAE	NORMAL VALUES
End-Diastolic Volume (EDV)		70-85 ml./m.²
End-Systolic Volume (ESV)		25-30 ml./m.²
Stroke Volume (SV)	EDV − ESV	45-55 ml./m.²
Ejection Fraction (EF)	$\dfrac{EDV - ESV}{EDV}$	0.65–0.75
Stroke Work (SW)	SV × Asm*	50-80 Gm.-M./m.²
Function Index	$\dfrac{SW}{EDV}$	1.0 Gm.-M./ml.
Effective Stroke Volume (SVe)		45-55 ml./m.²
Regurgitant Volume (V_R)	SV − SVe	0 ml./m.²
Regurgitant Fraction	$\dfrac{V_R}{SV}$	0

*Asm (mm. Hg.) = mean aortic systolic pressure.

chambers may be recorded if the catheter impinges against the muscular wall.

The first and second sounds are recorded throughout the heart, but the first sound reaches its maximal intensity in the ventricles and the second sound in the pulmonary artery and aorta. If a third heart sound is present, its greatest intensity is in the ventricles. The fourth heart sound is present in all patients with normal sinus rhythm; it is best recorded from the atrium, but it also can be recorded from the ventricles. A systolic murmur is observed routinely in the pulmonary artery.

Lewis and associates (1959) presented a series of 74 children, of whom 63 had congenital heart disease. Adults with a normal cardiovascular status had no abnormal murmurs; in children a faint systolic murmur was recorded on occasion in the ventricle or aorta. Striking results were obtained in children with congenital heart disease: In patent ductus arteriosus, the murmur was localized to the pulmonary artery, and in pulmonic stenosis, to the pulmonary artery just downstream to the valve. In ventricular septal defect with a left-to-right shunt, the murmur was recorded with the right ventricle. In atrial septal defects, the systolic murmur was found to arise in the pulmonary artery. A series of 160 patients was reported by Feruglio (1959) with similar results.

Left-sided sounds and murmurs can be studied by retrograde techniques (Segal *et al.*, 1964) or by transseptal left heart techniques (Forman *et al.*, 1962).

The murmur of aortic stenosis originates at the level of the valve and travels distally, diminishing in intensity as the catheter is passed into the left ventricle. In aortic insufficiency, the murmur appears in the left ventricular cavity and radiates toward the apex.

The murmur of mitral stenosis is best recorded in the inflow tract of the left ventricle and that of mitral insufficiency in the left atrium.

Intracardiac Electrocardiography

Intracardiac electrocardiography is the study of electrical potentials as obtained from the endocardial surface of the heart. During the performance of cardiac catheterization, a small electrode attached to the catheter serves as the exploring electrode.

The first studies of intracardiac electrocardiograms obtained in man were reported by Lenegre and Maurice (1945). The normal intracardiac electrocardiogram was further described by others, including Hecht (1946), Battro and Bidoggia (1947), Sodi-Pallares and associates (1947), Duchosal and coworkers (1948), Levine and colleagues (1949), Kossman and associates (1950), and Zimmerman and Hellerstein (1951).

Intracardiac electrocardiography has been useful for the following reasons:

1. Better understanding of the genesis of the electrocardiogram. For instance, the finding of a negative curve in the left ventricular cavity throughout ventricular depolarization supports the concept that the activation wave spreads from the endocardium to the epicardium. On the other hand, the curve recorded from the right ventricular cavity shows an initial small positive wave that corresponds to initial septal activation from left to right followed by a persistent negative deflection conforming to the concept of activation from endocardium to epicardium.

2. Precise location of the various cardiac chambers and vessels in complicated malformations (Watson, 1964). This is accomplished by the analysis of the shape and voltage of the P waves and QRS complexes as recorded in the cardiac chambers and vessels. The superior vena caval and atrial electrocardiograms consist of relatively large P waves, generally inverted in the superior vena cava and high in the right atrium, diphasic in midatrium, and positive in the lower portion of the atrium. In contrast to the large P waves, the QRS voltage within the superior vena cava and right atrium is small. The ventricular electrocardiogram demonstrates isoelectric or relatively small P waves, whereas the QRS complex is large. The electrocardiogram recorded from the pulmonary artery resembles the atrial electrocardiogram in that the QRS voltage is small, but differs in that the P waves are of similar magnitude to those observed within the ventricle (Fig. 28–45).

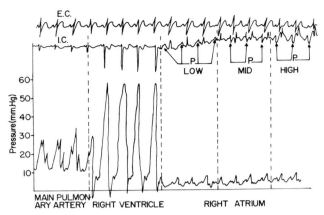

Figure 28–45. Intracardiac electrocardiography. Tracings from pulmonary artery to right atrium obtained from a 5-year-old patient with pulmonic valvular stenosis. E.C. is lead II of the external electrocardiogram. The intracardiac electrocardiogram (I.C.) reflects the course of the catheter. The pressure gradients coincide with the changing pattern of the intracardiac complexes. Furthermore, the morphology of the P wave changes depending on the atrial site from which it originates.

3. Diagnosis of Ebstein's anomaly. This is accomplished by recording simultaneously intracavitary pressures and electrocardiographic patterns proximal to the tricuspid valve (Fig. 28–46). The following findings are diagnostic: typical right ventricular intracavitary curves with simultaneously recorded atrial pressure curves, and the production of intracavitary right ventricular monophasic waves by pressure of the catheter tip in the distal portion of the low-pressure chamber (Hernandez et al., 1958).

4. Improved definition of atrial activity in cases of arrhythmias (Nutter and Kelser, 1965; Vogel et al., 1964).

BUNDLE OF HIS ELECTROCARDIOGRAPHY

Bundle of His electrocardiography (BHE) is a useful procedure in the evaluation of arrhythmias and conduction disorders. The His bundle electrograms in the isolated perfused animal heart were described by Alanis and associates (1958) and those in man by Scherlag and coworkers (1969).

The technique consists of passing a bipolar electrode catheter through a femoral vein (Scherlag et al., 1969) or through an antecubital vein (Narula, 1972) to the right atrium. The tip of the catheter lies in close proximity to the tricuspid valve. The signals from the catheter are then amplified, filtered, and recorded. Multiple surface EKG leads should be simultaneously recorded with the BHE. The procedure is simple and safe, the morbidity being that of right heart catheterization.

The relationship of the BHE to the conduction system of the heart and to the surface EKG is shown in Figure 28–47.

Analysis of the BHE reveals three distinct spikes. The first spike (A) is a local bipolar electrogram

recorded from the low right atrium close to the atrial septum. The second spike (H) reflects His bundle depolarization. The third spike (V) represents ventricular depolarization.

Recording of the BHE enables the breakdown of the PR interval into three components: (1) The P-A interval is an approximation of intra-atrial conduction time and is measured from the onset of the P wave on the surface EKG to the first deflection of the "A" spike on the BHE. (2) The A-H interval represents the conduction time through the A-V node. This is measured from the first high-frequency deflection of the "A" spike to the first high-frequency deflection of the "H" spike. (3) The H-V interval represents the conduction time through the His-Purkinje system and is measured from the onset of "H" spike to the earliest appearance of ventricular activation recorded on either the BHE ("V" spike) or any of the multiple surface EKG leads. Normal conduction time values are shown in Figure 28–47.

Stressing the conduction system with atrial pacing may demonstrate conduction disorders not apparent during sinus rhythm. During rapid atrial pacing, the normal response is an increase in A-H with H-V remaining constant (Damato et al., 1969). At a critical paced rate, Wenckebach periods are noted proximal to the His bundle. The increase in A-H and the development of Wenckebach periods are physiologic. The development of a block distal to the "H" spike (absent "V" spike) suggests disease in the His-Purkinje system (Rosen et al., 1971).

In patients with first-degree atrioventricular block and narrow QRS, the conduction delay (generally atrionodal) results in a prolongation of A-H. In patients with bundle-branch block, H-V may be prolonged enough to reflect itself as a first-degree atrioventricular block (Rosen et al., 1971). In these cases, H-V prolongation reflects conduction delay in the functioning bundle branch and is a manifestation of bilateral bundle-branch disease.

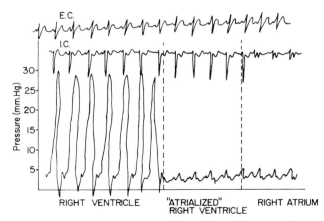

Figure 28–46. Intracardiac electrocardiography. Tracings obtained during pullback from right ventricle to right atrium from a patient with Ebstein's anomaly. E.C. is lead II of the external electrocardiogram. There is a change from right ventricular to atrial pressure, but the intracardiac electrocardiogram (I.C.) maintains its right ventricular morphology.

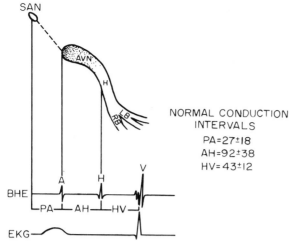

NORMAL CONDUCTION
INTERVALS
PA=27±18
AH=92±38
HV=43±12

Figure 28–47. Diagram showing the relationship of the conduction system of the heart and the surface electrocardiogram (EKG) to the bundle of His electrogram (BHE) (SAN = sinoatrial node; AVN = atrioventricular node; H = bundle of His; RB = right bundle; LB = left bundle). (From Rosen, K.M.: Catheter recording of His bundle electrograms. Mod. Concepts Cardiovasc. Dis., *42*:23, 1973.)

In patients with second- and third-degree block, three sites of block may be delineated (Damato *et al.*, 1969; Narula *et al.*, 1971): (1) The block may be proximal to the His bundle, in which P waves are not followed by conducted "H" spikes. (2) The block may be in the His bundle. Two "H" spikes can be recorded, one proximal to ("H_1") and the other distal to ("H_2") the area of the block. (3) The block may be distal to the His bundle, in which P waves are conducted to the His bundle but "H" spikes are not followed by conducted QRS complexes (absent "V" spikes). This is also a form of bilateral bundle-branch block.

Second-degree atrioventricular block can be divided into two types (Damato *et al.*, 1969; Narula *et al.*, 1970): (1) Type I block (Mobitz I, Wenckebach phenomenon) is characterized by prolongation of conduction intervals prior to the dropped beat. This occurs most commonly in the A-V node. (2) Type II block (Mobitz II) is characterized by fixed conduction intervals prior to the dropped beat. This usually reflects bilateral bundle-branch disease.

In acute inferior wall myocardial infarction, complete atrioventricular block is usually proximal to the His bundle, reflecting occlusion of the right coronary artery proximal to the origin of the A-V node artery (Rosen *et al.*, 1970). In acute anteroseptal infarction, the block is distal to the His bundle, reflecting septal injury and bilateral bundle-branch block (Rosen *et al.*, 1970). In complete congenital heart block, the block is proximal to the His bundle, reflecting disruption of conduction tissue in the A-V junction (Rosen *et al.*, 1971).

Symptoms of dizziness, confusion, and syncope may accompany atrioventricular block at any site. However, they are more common in patients with a block distal to the His bundle. Patients with markedly

prolonged H-V and without any manifest symptoms of block should be followed closely for the development of atrioventricular block. It should be emphasized that the decision for pacemaker implantation is based primarily on clinical symptoms.

Calculation of Valve Areas

In order to calculate the surface area of the valves, Gorlin and Gorlin (1951) derived the following general equation:

$$A = \frac{F}{C \times 44.5 \sqrt{P_1 - P_2}}, \text{ where}$$

A (cm.²) = orifice area
F (ml./sec.) = flow through orifice
44.5 = constant related to gravity acceleration
$P_1 - P_2$ (mm. Hg) = pressure gradient across the orifice
P_1 = pressure proximal to orifice
P_2 = pressure distal to orifice

Mitral Valve Area
Using the foregoing formula, the mitral valve area can be calculated as follows:

$$MVA = \frac{MVF = \dfrac{CO}{DFP}}{31 \sqrt{LAm - LVmd}}, \text{ where}$$

MVA (cm.²) = mitral valve area
MVF (ml./sec.) = mitral valve flow
CO (ml./min.) = cardiac output
DFP (sec./min.) = diastolic filling time
LAm (mm. Hg) = left atrial mean pressure
LVmd (mm. Hg) = left ventricular mean diastolic pressure (This may be assumed to be 5 mm. Hg in most cases.)

Although in the majority of cases there is a good correlation between the calculated and the actually measured surface area of the mitral valve (Gorlin and Gorlin, 1951), the following factors may introduce errors in the calculations:

1. The presence of mitral insufficiency.
2. Small pressure gradients across the mitral valve.
3. Left ventricular failure introduces some inaccuracy if the left ventricular mean diastolic pressure is assumed.
4. Changes in flow and in pressure gradients between measurements.

The average effective surface area of the normal mitral valve is about 4 to 5 cm.² The surface area of the mitral valve can be narrowed down to 2.5 cm.² without the presence of significant symptoms. Between 2.5 cm.² and 2.0 cm.², the narrowing produces symptoms on severe exertion only. Between 2.0 cm.² and 1.5

cm.², symptoms are present with moderate exertion. Below 1.5 cm.², minimal exercise may provoke severe symptoms.

Aortic Valve Area

The formula to calculate the effective aortic valve surface area is as follows:

$$AVA = \frac{AVF = \dfrac{CO}{SEP}}{C \times 44.5 \sqrt{LVsm - Asm}}, \text{ where}$$

AVA (cm.²) = aortic valve area
AVF (ml./sec.) = aortic valve flow
CO (ml./min.) = cardiac output
SEP (sec./min.) = systolic ejection period
C = empiral constant = 1.0
44.5 = gravity acceleration factor
LVsm (mm. Hg) = left ventricular mean systolic pressure
Asm (mm. Hg) = aortic mean systolic pressure

Calculations of the aortic valve surface area are not accurate in the presence of aortic insufficiency.

The normal effective surface area of the aortic valve is about 3 to 4 cm.². Usually the symptoms of angina and syncope do not appear until the aortic valve area measures between 0.5 to 0.7 cm.².

Calculation of Resistance

Vascular resistance can be defined as an impedance to blood flow. This can be translated in a simplified form of Poiseuille's equation:

$$\text{Resistance (R)} = \frac{\text{pressure gradient}}{\text{flow}}$$

The result can be expressed in simple units (R). However, one can express resistance in fundamental units of force as follows:

$$\begin{aligned}\text{Resistance (dynes} &= \text{sec./cm.}^5) = \\ \frac{\text{pressure gradient (mm. Hg)} &\times 1332\,\text{dynes/cm.}^2}{\text{blood flow (cm.}^3\text{/sec.)}}\end{aligned}$$

Each unit of resistance (R) can be converted into dynes-sec./cm.⁵ by multiplying by 80.*

In order to compare data obtained from infants, children, and adults, resistance should be related to flow index (L./min./m.²).

Thus, the formula for systemic resistance is as follows:

$$SVR = \frac{AOm - RAm \times 80}{SBF}, \text{ where}$$

SVR (dynes-sec./cm.⁵) = systemic vascular resistance

---

*$\dfrac{1332\,\text{dynes/cm.}^2 \times 60\,\text{sec.}}{1000\,\text{cm.}^3}$

AOm (mm. Hg) = mean aortic pressure
RAm (mm. Hg) = mean right atrial pressure
SBF (L./min. or L./min./m.²) = systemic blood flow.

Pulmonary vascular resistance can be calculated as follows:

$$PVR = \frac{PAm - LAm \times 80}{PBF}, \text{ where}$$

PVR (dynes-sec./cm.⁵) = pulmonary vascular resistance
PAm (mm. Hg) = mean pulmonary artery pressure
LAm (mm. Hg) = mean left atrial pressure
PBF (L./min. or L./min./m.²) = pulmonary blood flow.

Normal value for pulmonary vascular resistance is one to three units (80 to 240 dynes-sec./cm.⁵).

As described previously (see Pulmonary Artery Pressure, p. 872), pulmonary hypertension can be classified as hyperkinetic and obstructive types. In the hyperkinetic type, the pulmonary artery pressure may be high in spite of a normal and fixed pulmonary arterial resistance. In contrast, in the obstructive type, the pulmonary arterial resistance is usually elevated.

MYOCARDIAL WALL TENSION AND MYOCARDIAL OXYGEN CONSUMPTION

Five determinants of myocardial oxygen consumption (MVO_2) have been recognized (Graham et al., 1968). They are (1) myocardial tension development, (2) myocardial contractility, (3) pressure-volume work and kinetic energy, (4) basal myocardial metabolism, and (5) myocardial activation. The first two factors are by far the most important ones.

The importance of myocardial wall tension in determining MVO_2 was first suggested by Rohde (1912). Shortly thereafter, Evans and Matsuoka (1914) concluded from studies on the Starling heart-lung preparation that an increase in cardiac work resulting from an elevation of arterial pressure augmented MVO_2 to a much greater degree than a similar increment in work resulting from an increase in stroke volume. The relation of MVO_2 to derivatives of developed tension was also explored by using such parameters as the tension-time index (TTI) (Sarnoff et al., 1958) or the index of cardiac effort (Katz and Feinberg, 1958).

$$\text{TTI} = \text{Asm} \times \text{SEP, where}$$

TTI = tension-time index (mm. Hg sec./min.)
Asm = mean systolic aortic pressure (mm. Hg)
SEP* = systolic ejection time (sec./min.)

---

*SEP = systolic ejection period (sec./beat) × heart rate (beat/min.)

Index of cardiac effort=
Heart rate (beat/min.) × mean aortic pressure (mm. Hg)

Despite the good correlations between MVO₂ and these parameters, it was recognized that according to the law of LaPlace, the myocardial wall tension needed to produce a given ventricular pressure was increased as the volume of the ventricle enlarged. Thus,

$$T = \frac{Pr}{2h}, \text{ where}$$

T = intramyocardial tension
r = radius of ventricular chamber
h = ventricular thickness

More recent studies have confirmed that tension rather than developed pressure is the more definitive determinant of myocardial oxygen consumption (Sonnenblick *et al.*, 1968).

FIRST TIME DERIVATIVE OF THE VENTRICULAR PRESSURE (dp/dt)

The first time derivative of the ventricular pressure is the rate of change of pressure with respect to time and is usually expressed as dp/dt. Its maximum value, achieved during early ventricular systole, is designated as peak dp/dt (Fig. 28–48).

The first requirement for an accurate measurement of the peak dp/dt is the faithful recording of the ventricular pressure through a catheter-tipped micromanometer (Laurens *et al.*, 1959; Yanof *et al.*, 1963). A conventional catheter connected to an external transducer is generally unsatisfactory unless the natural frequency response of the system equals or exceeds 30 cycles per second (Nobel, 1953). The dp/dt curve is generated by coupling a differentiator to the pressure course.

Peak dp/dt of the left ventricle is greater than that of the right ventricle in normal subjects. In Gleason and Braunwald's series (1962), left ventricular peak dp/dt ranged between 841 and 1969 mm. Hg/sec. Right

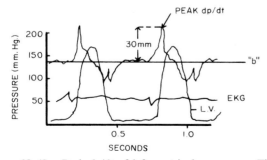

Figure 28–48. Peak dp/dt of left ventricular pressure. The left ventricular pressure curve (L.V.) and its dp/dt curve are recorded simultaneously. Height of the peak dp/dt curve = 30 mm. Calibration factor = 54 mm. Hg/sec. of deflection of dp/dt for the differentiator used in this case. Peak dp/dt = 30 × 54 = 1620 mm. Hg/sec.

ventricular peak dp/dt ranged between 223 and 296 mm. Hg/sec.

The peak dp/dt has been used in the assessment of myocardial function because of its increase following inotropic intervention (Mason and Braunwald, 1963; Gleason and Braunwald, 1962) and diminution in conductions associated with depressed myocardial contractility (Wiggers, 1952). However, augmented preload (elevated end-diastolic volume and pressure) (Wallace *et al.*, 1963) and afterload (increased aortic diastolic pressure) (Mason, 1969) both increase peak dp/dt. Tachycardia is also associated with an increase in peak dp/dt (Gleason and Braunwald, 1962). Thus, several parameters have been derived from dp/dt in order to eliminate the effects of the preload and afterload (Reeves *et al.*, 1960; Siegel and Sonnenblick, 1964; Mason *et al.*, 1965; Veragut and Krayenbuhl, 1965; Mason *et al.*, 1967; Frank and Levinson, 1968; Braunwald *et al.*, 1969).

ANGIOCARDIOGRAPHY

Contrast Materials

The most commonly used preparations in angiocardiography are sodium and methylglucamine diatrizoate (Hypaque 75 per cent or 90 per cent, Renovist 69 per cent), sodium acetrizoate (Urokon 70 per cent), sodium iothalamate (Angio-Conray 80 per cent), iodopyracet (Diodrast 70 per cent), and sodium iodomethamate (Neo-Iopax 75 per cent).

Contrast media have a direct myocardial depressant effect (Mason *et al.*, 1968). Because of their hypertonicity (greater than 1500 mOsm./liter), injection of large quantities of contrast medium has been shown to cause a temporary increase in cardiac output, blood volume, left ventricular end-diastolic and pulmonary artery pressures (Brown *et al.*, 1965). In addition, an increase in heart rate and a decrease in systemic arterial pressure have been observed (Edwards and Biguria, 1934). In normal patients and in patients with mitral valve disease, there is a rise in left atrial pressure, the increase being more marked in the latter group (Rahimtoola *et al.*, 1966).

All iodinated contrast substances are capable of producing reactions. A previous allergic history or pre-existing cerebral and renal disease should prompt carefully evaluation of the indications to perform angiocardiography. Reactions are also related to the quantity, concentration, and duration of action of the material used. In 1957, Abrams reported 29 deaths in a series of 1705 thoracic aortographies. The majority of these deaths were due to cerebral damage. However, renal complications and cardiorespiratory disturbances also were noted. This study further indicated that when 70 per cent contrast media are employed, the mortality is eight times greater than when a concentration of 30 per cent is used.

Owing to systemic arterial vasodilation, a feeling of heat and a flushing of the skin are almost universal.

TABLE 28-5. SELECTIVE ANGIOCARDIOGRAPHY

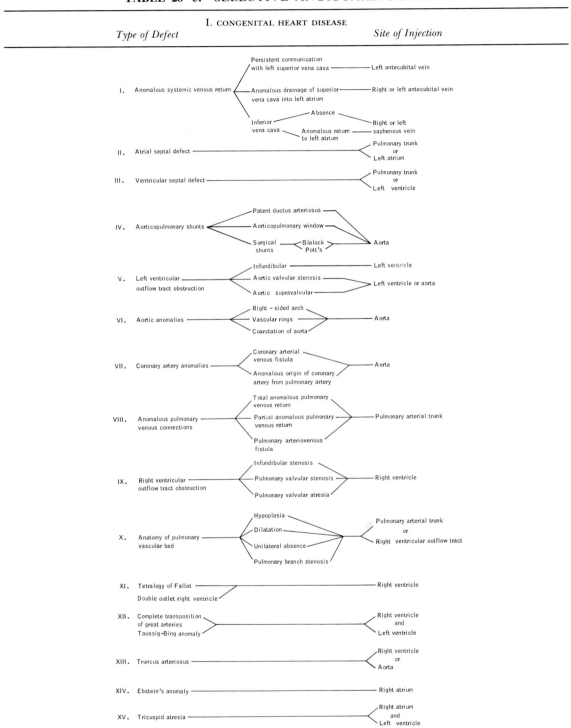

Osmotic red cell agglutination can occur in cyanotic children (Read, 1959).

Electrocardiographic changes are frequently noted. They may consist of premature atrial, nodal, and ventricular systoles. Occasionally these arrhythmias may persist for a long period of time (Zinn et al., 1951). T waves may become flat or even inverted (Horger et al., 1951).

The occurrence of arrhythmias may lead to temporary mitral insufficiency. A diagnosis of true mitral insufficiency is justified only if the contrast material appears in the left atrium in the absence of bradycardia or ventricular arrhythmias (Björk and Lodin, 1959). The same reservations also must be made in the case of aortic insufficiency.

Selective Angiocardiography

Until 1947, peripheral intravenous angiocardiography was the most commonly used method. This technique afforded good visualization of the right heart chambers. However, a considerable degree of dilution occurred in the pulmonary vascular bed. As a result, the left cardiac chambers and aorta were ill defined.

In 1947, Chavez and colleagues reported the first selective angiocardiography in which radiopaque substances were deliberately injected through a catheter in the right ventricle. Jonsson and associates developed the method further and proposed selective visualization of the cardiac chambers and great vessels. These workers are credited with the term "selective angiocardiography."

The advantages of selective angiocardiography are the injection of small quantities of less diluted radiopaque materials, the injection of a radiopaque medium in the chamber of interest, so that surrounding structures are not superimposed on each other, and the detection of shunts by a sensitive and precise method.

Delivery of contrast material should be as rapid as possible. This is accomplished by choosing a catheter with a large lumen. Because of the possibility of recoil, the catheter should have a closed end with laterally placed holes (Rodriguez-Alvarez and Martinez de Rodriguez, 1975). Injection of radiopaque material is performed either by hand or by a power injector, the latter being five times more efficient (Klatte et al., 1959).

To study anatomic or physiologic changes, films must be taken in rapid sequence. This is made possible by rapid film changers or by image intensifiers with cinecamera attachments.

Single-plane or biplane rapid film changers can take from one to six frames per second. These machines use either precut film loaded in a cassette or roll films (Scott and Moore, 1949). This technique provides excellent anatomic details. However, the amount of radiation used is high, and the injection of contrast material cannot be monitored.

Cineangiocardiography permits recording of the passage of contrast medium by means of x-ray motion picture photography. This is made possible by the development of amplification and an intensification fluoroscopy, whereby the ordinary fluoroscopic image is converted into an electron image (Campbell et al., 1960). The electron image is then reconverted into a light image of much increased brightness that can be viewed by mirror optics, photographed by a cinecamera, or monitored by television. The signal can also be relayed to a video recorder for immediate replay. This method permits motion pictures from 7½ to 60 frames per second using a 16- or 35-mm. movie camera. Thus, cardiac anatomy, as well as the direction of blood flow, can be studied while keeping the dose of radiation low. In addition, single-plane and biplane cineangiocardiographic techniques have been used in the evaluation of cardiac function (see Measurements of Cardiac Volumes, p. 889).

Complications occurring during the course of angiocardiography are related to the radiopaque media (see Contrast Materials, p. 895) and to the pressure generated by the injector. Before pressure injection, the tip of the catheter should be free in the cardiac chamber away from the myocardial wall. The position of the catheter tip can be ascertained by the injection of small quantities of contrast material under low pressure. Myocardial extravasation of radiopaque medium occurs in about 5 per cent of cases (Bookstein and Sigmann, 1963). However, the majority of cases are asymptomatic. Occasionally, perforation of the atria or ventricles occurs, resulting in cardiac tamponade (Levin et al., 1965; Popper et al., 1967). Myocardial infarction and ventricular fibrillation (Rowe and Zarnstorff, 1965) have also been observed.

Tables 28–5 and 28–6 summarize some of the types of congenital and acquired cardiac anomalies

TABLE 28–6. SELECTIVE ANGIOCARDIOGRAPHY

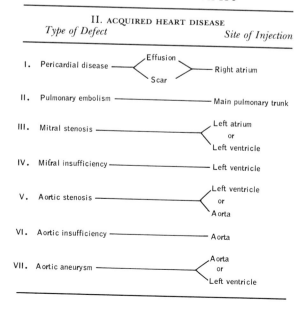

| II. ACQUIRED HEART DISEASE | |
Type of Defect	Site of Injection
I. Pericardial disease	Effusion / Scar — Right atrium
II. Pulmonary embolism	Main pulmonary trunk
III. Mitral stenosis	Left atrium or Left ventricle
IV. Mitral insufficiency	Left ventricle
V. Aortic stenosis	Left ventricle or Aorta
VI. Aortic insufficiency	Aorta
VII. Aortic aneurysm	Aorta or Left ventricle

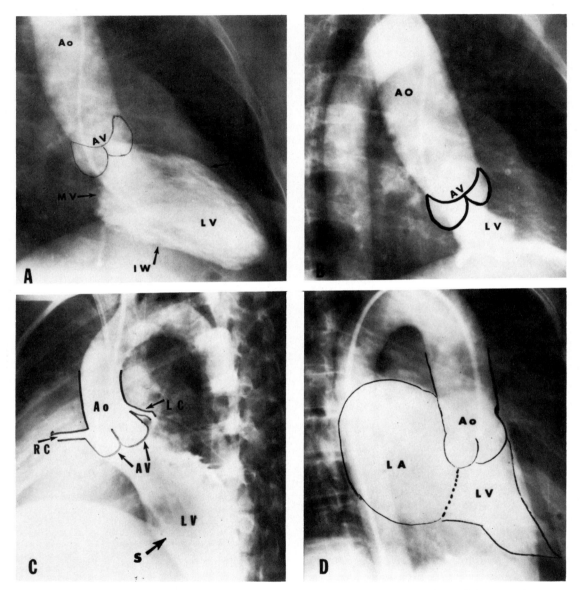

Figure 28–49. Left-ventriculography. *A*, Normal left ventriculogram in diastole (right anterior oblique projection). *B*, Normal left ventriculogram in systole (right anterior oblique projection). *C*, Normal left ventriculogram (left anterior oblique projection). *D*, Left ventriculogram demonstrating mitral insufficiency (right anterior oblique projection). (LV = left ventricle; LA = left atrium; Ao = aorta; MV = mitral valve; AV = aortic valve; IW = inferior wall; S = septum; RC = right coronary artery; LC = left coronary artery.)

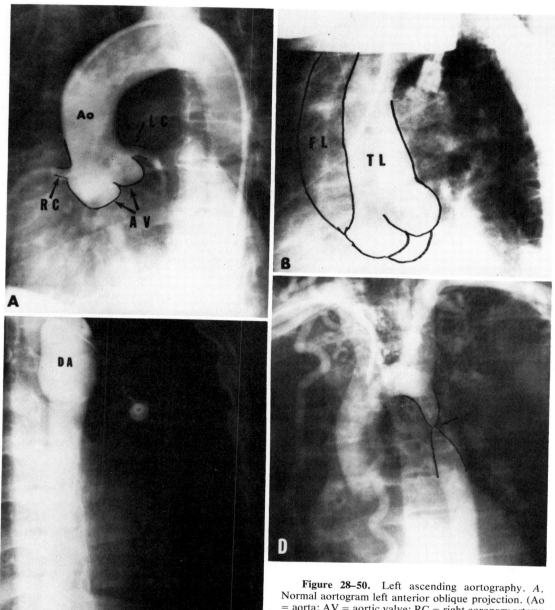

Figure 28–50. Left ascending aortography. *A,* Normal aortogram left anterior oblique projection. (Ao = aorta; AV = aortic valve; RC = right coronary artery; LC = left coronary artery.) *B,* Dissecting aneurysm of ascending aorta (FL = false lumen; TL = true lumen). *C,* Traumatic aneurysm of the descending thoracic aorta (DA). *D,* Adult type of coarctation of the aorta.

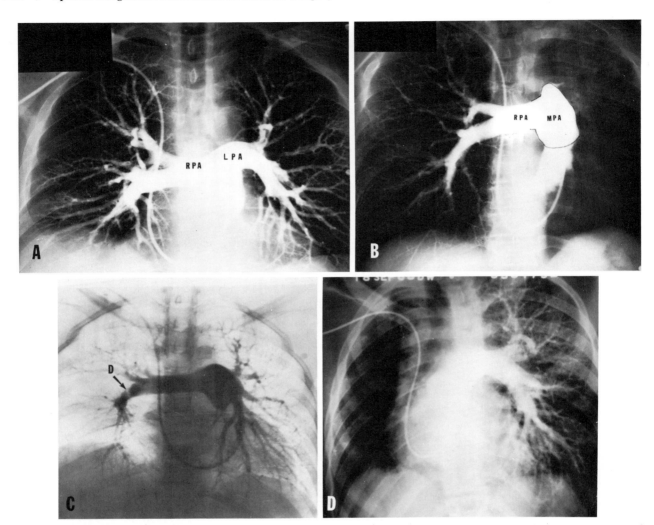

Figure 28–51. Pulmonary arteriography. *A*, Normal pulmonary arteriogram. *B*, Massive embolus to left pulmonary artery. *C*, Defect (D) in right pulmonary artery due to an embolus. *D*, Congenital absence of the right pulmonary artery. (RPA = right pulmonary artery; LPA = left pulmonary artery; MPA = main pulmonary artery.)

that can be identified by the selective injection of contrast medium.

The indications for angiocardiography depend on the nature of the malformation. The need for it is particularly great in complicated anomalies, since data obtained from cardiac catheterization may be misleading. Anatomic demonstration of a defect by properly obtained selective angiocardiograms is superior or at least complementary to results obtained from catheterization.

Using selective angiocardiography, the following can be accomplished:

1. Assessment of the position and size of the cardiac chambers in relation to each other and to the great veins and arteries.

2. Precise localization of intracardiac and extracardiac defects, including shunts.

3. Assessment of the location, anatomy, and motion of the cardiac valves.

4. Rough estimation of the degree of valvular insufficiency.

5. Visualization of the coronary vascular tree.

Examples of selective angiocardiograms are shown in Figures 28–49 to 28–51.

VENTRICULAR ASYNERGY

Myocardial ischemia or scarring frequently results in an uncoordinated and disrupted contraction and, hence, in reduced (hypokinesia), absent (akinesia), or paradoxical systolic ventricular motion (dyskinesia) (Herman *et al.*, 1967).

Assessment of regional left ventricular wall motion is made by visual inspection of the cineventriculogram. The normal pattern of left ventricular contraction is a uniform and almost concentric inward movement of all points along the endocardial surface during systole. The term "asynergy" has been used to indicate a disturbance of the normal contraction pattern (Harrison, 1965). The Ad Hoc Committee for Grading of Coronary Artery Disease of the American

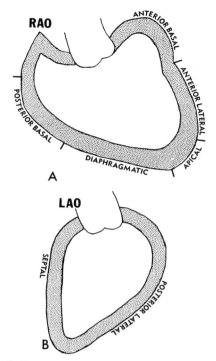

Heart Association has recommended that five right anterior oblique and two left anterior oblique left ventricular segments be defined and characterized as to wall motion (Fig. 28–52). Five basic types of surgery have been defined (Herman *et al.*, 1967). However, a majority of cardiologists adhere to a simplified classification (Fig. 28–53).

Localized contractile abnormalities may be due to chronically ischemic, viable myocardium. Inotropic agents (Horn *et al.*, 1974), post-extrasystole potentiation (Dyke *et al.*, 1974), and nitrates (Helfant *et al.*, 1974) have been used to identify these segments with potentially reversible contraction abnormalities. A significant correlation has been observed between pharmacologic responsiveness and improvement in segmental contraction following coronary artery surgery (Helfant *et al.*, 1974).

MISCELLANEOUS USAGE OF CARDIAC CATHETERS

In addition to hemodynamic measurements and performance of angiographic studies, specialized catheters have been devised to fulfill various functions. These include:

1. Endomycardial biopsy for the diagnosis of cardiomyopathies (Olsen, 1977; Sakakibara and Konno, 1962) and of acute rejection following cardiac transplantation (Caves *et al.*, 1974).

Figure 28–52. *A* and *B*, Left ventricular wall silhouette in the right anterior oblique (RAO) and left anterior oblique (LAO) veins using the nomenclature suggested by the American Heart Association.

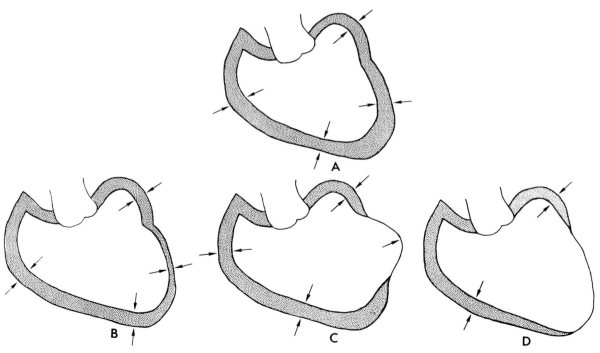

Figure 28–53. *A–D*, Basic types of ventricular asynergy.

2. Retrieval of foreign bodies from the right heart (Curry, 1970; Massumi and Rose, 1967).

3. Closure of atrial septal defects (King *et al.*, 1976).

4. Closure of patent ductus arteriosus (Kitamura *et al.*, 1976).

5. Dilation of coronary arterial stenosis (Güntzig *et al.*, 1979).

SELECTED REFERENCES

Beckman, C. H., and Dooley, B.: Complications of left heart angiography, a study of 1,000 consecutive cases. Circulation, *41*:825, 1970.

A study of 1,000 consecutive left-heart cineangiocardiograms is presented. Major problems were associated with the procedure in 3.1 per cent of the cases. Most cardiac complications resulted from open-end catheter angiography, especially through transseptal catheters.

Braunwald, E., and Swan, H. J. C. (Eds.): Cooperative study on cardiac catheterization. Circulation, *37*(Suppl. 3):80, 1968.

This monograph is the latest study in the assessment of the risks of various cardiac catheterization methods in a total of 12,367 procedures carried out over a period of two years.

Braunwald, E., Lambrew, C. T., Morrow, A. G., Pierce, G. E., Rockoff, S. D., and Ross, J., Jr.: Idiopathic hypertrophic subaortic stenosis. Circulation, *30*(Suppl. 4):3, 1964.

This classic monograph represents the primary source of information about this most fascinating disease.

Braunwald, E., Moscovitz, H. L., Amram, S. S., Lasser, R. P., Sapin, S. O., Himmelstein, A., Ravitch, M. M., and Gordon, A. J.: The hemodynamics of the left side of the heart as studied by simultaneous left atrial, left ventricular and aortic pressure. Particular reference to mitral stenosis. Circulation, *12*:69, 1955.

In six patients without mitral stenosis and in patients with mitral stenosis, the hemodynamics of the left heart were studied at operation by means of simultaneous needle puncture of the left atrium, left ventricle, and aorta.

Brockenbrough, E. C., Braunwald, E., and Ross, J., Jr.: Transseptal left heart catheterization — a review of 450 studies and description of an improved technic. Circulation, *25*:15, 1962.

The technique of transseptal left heart catheterization is described. This method was applied in 450 studies. The left atrium was intubated in all but two patients. The left ventricle was entered in 95 per cent of the cases. The only serious complication was accidental puncture of the aorta in three patients.

Hildner, F. J., Drake, E. H., Gale, H. H., and Ormond, R. S.: Transbrachial retrograde left heart catheterization. Evaluation of 600 consecutive cases in adults. Am. J. Cardiol., *18*:52, 1966.

The transbrachial retrograde arterial approach was used in 600 consecutive adult cases. The left ventricle was intubated in 96 per cent of the cases. The failure rate of 4 per cent was due to tortuous or aberrant great arteries, tortuous aortas, calcified valves, and local arteriospasm. In 216 cases of significant aortic stenosis, the left ventricle was entered in 98 per cent of cases.

Leonard, J. J., and Kroetz, F. W.: Lessons learned through intracardiac phonocardiography. Mod. Concepts Cardiovasc. Dis., *35*:69, 1966.

A summary of the current concepts of the origin of cardiac sounds and murmurs as obtained by intracardiac phonocardiography is presented. Sounds and murmurs related to congenital anomalies such as atrial and ventricular septal defects, patent ductus arteriopulmonic stenosis, and acquired defects of the mitral, aortic, and tricuspid valves are discussed.

Rosen, K. M.: Catheter recording of His bundle electrograms. Mod. Concepts Cardiovasc. Dis., *62*:23, 1973.

A description of the indications and information obtained by the technique of His bundle electrocardiography.

Rudolph, A. M., and Cayler, G. G.: Cardiac catheterization in infants and children. Pediatr. Clin. North Am., *5*:907, 1958.

An excellent and concise report on the different cardiac catheterization techniques and their application to the evaluation of heart disease in infants and children.

Shirey, E. K., and Sones, F. M., Jr.: Retrograde transaortic and mitral valve catheterization. Physiologic and morphologic evaluation of aortic and mitral valve lesions. Am. J. Cardiol., *18*:745, 1966.

The retrograde method of left atrial catheterization using the right brachial arterial approach is discussed. This technique was used in 310 patients for a total of 315 studies. The left atrium was intubated in 285 studies. In 84 per cent of cases of mitral stenosis, the left atrium was successfully catheterized. Ventricular fibrillation occurred in five cases.

Sonnenblick, E. H., and Skelton, C. L.: Oxygen consumption of the heart: Physiological principles and clinical implications. Mod. Concepts Cardiovasc. Dis., *60*:9, 1971.

A report of the factors that are the main determinants of myocardial oxygen consumption.

Yang, S. S., Bentivoglio, L. C., Maranhao, V., and Goldberg, H.: From Cardiac Catheterization Data to Hemodynamic Parameters. Philadelphia, F. A. Davis Company, 1972.

An excellent review of the interpretation of hemodynamic data obtained from cardiac catheterization and noninvasive techniques.

REFERENCES

Abrams, H. L.: Radiologic aspects of operable heart disease. III. The hazards of retrograde aortography: A survey. Radiology, *68*:812, 1957.

Alanis, J., Gonzalez, H., and Lopez, E.: The electrical activity of the bundle of His. J. Physiol. (Lond.), *142*:127, 1958.

Androuny, Z. A., Southerland, D. W., Griswold, H. E., and Ritzman, L. W.: Complications with transseptal left heart catheterization. Am. Heart J., *65*:327, 1963.

Arcilla, R. A., Agutsson, M. M., Bicoff, J. P., Lynfeld, J., Weinberg, M., Jr., Fell, H. G., and Gasul, B. M.: Further observations on the natural history of isolated ventricular septal defect in infancy and childhood. Circulation, *28*:560, 1963.

Arvidsson, H.: Angiocardiographic determination of left ventricular volume. Acta Radiol., *56*:321, 1961.

Bargeron, L., Clark, L. C., and Lyons, C.: Use of an electrode for continuously recording intracardiac PO_2 changes in cardiac catheterizations. Circulation, *24*:881, 1961.

Bartle, S. H., and Sanmarco, M. E.: Measurement of left ventricle volume by biplane angiocardiography and indicator-washout techniques. A comparison in the canine heart. Circ. Res., *19*:295, 1966.

Battro, A., and Bidoggia, H.: Endocardiac electrocardiogram obtained by heart catheterization in man. Am. Heart J., *33*:604, 1947.

Beckman, C. H., and Dooley, B.: Complications of left heart angiography, a study of 1,000 consecutive cases. Circulation, 41:825, 1970.

Bedford, D. E., and Sellors, T. H.: Atrial septal defects. In Modern Trends in Cardiology. London, Butterworth, 1960, p. 138.

Bell, L. A. L., Haynes, W. F., Jr., Shimomura, S., and Dallas, D. P.: Influence of catheter tip position on pulmonary wedge pressures. Circ. Res., 10:215, 1962.

Beuren, A. J., and Apitz, J.: Left ventricular angiography by transseptal puncture of the left atrium. Circulation, 28:209, 1963.

Bing, R. J.: Catheterization of the heart. Adv. Intern. Med., 5:59, 1952.

Bing, R. J., Cohen, A., and Blümchen, G.: Tobacco alkaloids and circulation. In Tobacco Alkaloids and Related Compounds. Proceedings of the 4th International Symposium. New York, Pergamon Press, 1965, p. 241.

Bing, R. J., Heimbecker, R., and Falholt, W.: An estimation of the residual volume of blood in the right ventricle of normal and diseased human hearts in vivo. Am. Heart J., 42:483, 1951.

Bing, R. J., Vandam, L. D., and Gray, F. D., Jr.: Physiological studies in congenital heart disease: results of preoperative studies in patients with tetralogy of Fallot. Bull. Johns Hopkins Hosp., 80:121, 1947.

Bing, R. J., Vandam, L. D., and Gray, F. D., Jr.: Physiological studies in congenital heart disease: procedures. Bull. Johns Hopkins Hosp., 80:107, 1947.

Björk, V. O., and Lodin, H.: Evaluation of mitral stenosis with selective left ventricular angiocardiography. J. Thorac. Cardiovasc. Surg., 40:17, 1960.

Björk, V. O., and Lodin, H.: Left heart catheterization with selective left atrial and ventricular angiocardiography in the diagnosis of mitral and aortic valvular disease. Prog. Cardiovasc. Dis., 2:116, 1959.

Björk, V. O., Lodin, H., and Malers, E.: The evaluation of the degree of mitral insufficiency by selective left ventricular angiocardiography. Am. Heart J., 60:691, 1960.

Björk, V. O., Malmström, G., and Uggla, L. G.: Left auricular pressure measurements in man. Ann. Surg., 138:718, 1953.

Bleichroeder, F.: Intra arterielle Therapie. Berl. Klin. Wochenschr., 2:1503, 1912.

Bloomfield, D. A., and Sinclair-Smith, B. C.: The limbic ledge. A landmark for transseptal left heart catheterization. Circulation, 31:103, 1965.

Boettcher, D., Corsini, G., Daniels, C., Cowan, C., and Bing, R. J.: The determination of myocardial blood flow in the anesthetized dog after a bolus of 84 Rb. J. Nucl. Med., 20:83, 1969.

Bookstein, J. J., and Sigmann, J. M.: Intramural deposition of contrast agent during selective angiography. Radiology, 81:932, 1963.

Braunwald, E.: Methods for study of the circulation in man (cardiac catheterization, indicator-dilution curves and recorded techniques). In Clinical Cardiopulmonary Physiology. 2nd Ed. Edited by B. L. Gordon. New York, Grune & Stratton, Inc., 1960, p. 145.

Braunwald, E., and Swan, H. J. C. (Eds.): Cooperative study on cardiac catheterization. Circulation, 37 (Suppl. 3):80, 1968.

Braunwald, E., Brockenbrough, E. C., Talbert, J. L., Folse, J. R., and Rockoff, S. D.: Selective left heart angiography by the transseptal route. Am. J. Med., 33:213, 1962.

Braunwald, E., Goldblatt, A., Long, R. T. L., and Morrow, A. G.: The krypton inhalation test for the detection of left to right shunts. Br. Heart J., 24:47, 1962.

Braunwald, E., Lambrew, C. T., Morrow, A. G., Pierce, G. E., Rockoff, S. D., and Ross, J., Jr.: Idiopathic hypertrophic subaortic stenosis. Circulation, 30 (Suppl. 4):3, 1964.

Braunwald, E., Morrow, A. G., Cornell, W. P., Augen, M. M., and Hilbish, T.: Idiopathic hypertrophic subaortic stenosis. Clinical hemodynamic and angiographic manifestations. Am. J. Med., 29:940, 1960.

Braunwald, E., Moscovitz, H. L., Amram, S. S., Lasser, R. P., Sapin, S. O., Himmelstein, A., Ravitch, M. M., and Gordon, A. J.: The hemodynamics of the left side of the heart as studied by simultaneous left atrial, left ventricular, and aortic pressures.

Particular reference to mitral stenosis. Circulation, 12:69, 1955.

Braunwald, E., Pfaff, W. W., Long, R. T. L., and Morrow, A. G.: A simplified indicator-dilution technique for the localization of left-to-right circulatory shunts. An experimental and clinical study of intravenous injection and right heart sampling. Circulation, 20:875, 1959.

Braunwald, E., Ross, J., Jr., Gault, J. H., Mason, D. T., Mills, C., Gabe, L. T., and Epstein, S. E.: Assessment of cardiac function. Ann. Intern. Med., 70:369, 1969.

Braunwald, E., Tanenbaum, H. L., and Morrow, A. G.: Dye-dilution curves from left heart and aorta for localization of left-to-right shunts and detection of valvular insufficiency. Proc. Soc. Exper. Biol. Med., 94:510, 1957.

Brock, R., Anatomy of Congenital Pulmonic Stenosis. New York, Paul B. Hoeber, 1957.

Brock, R.: The surgical treatment of pulmonary stenosis. Br. Heart J., 23:337, 1961.

Brock, R., Milstein, B. B., and Ross, D. N.: Percutaneous left ventricular puncture in the assessment of aortic stenosis. Thorax, 11:163, 1956.

Brockenbrough, E. C., and Braunwald, E.: A new technique for left ventricular angiocardiography and transseptal left heart catheterization. Am. J. Cardiol., 6:1062, 1960.

Brockenbrough, E. C., Braunwald, E., and Morrow, A. G.: A hemodynamic technique for the detection of hypertrophic subaortic stenosis. Circulation, 23:189, 1961.

Brockenbrough, E. C., Braunwald, E., and Ross, J., Jr.: Transseptal left heart catheterization — A review of 450 studies and description of an improved technic. Circulation, 25:15, 1962.

Brown, R., Rahimtoola, S. H., Davis, G. D., and Swan, H. J. C.: The effect of angiographic contrast medium on circulatory dynamics in man. Cardiac output during angiocardiography. Circulation, 31:234, 1965.

Buzzi, A.: Claude Bernard on cardiac catheterization. Am. J. Cardiol., 4:405, 1959.

Calazel, P., Gerard, R., Daley, R., Draper, A., Foster, J., and Bing, R. J.: Physiological studies on congenital heart disease. XI. A comparison of the right and left auricular, capillary and pulmonary artery pressures in nine patients with auricular septal defect. Bull. Johns Hopkins Hosp., 88:20, 1951.

Campbell, J. A., Klatte, E. C., and Shalkowski, R. A.: Factors influencing image quality in cineroentgenography. Am. J. Roentgenol., 83:345, 1960.

Carleton, R. A., Bowyer, A. F., and Graettinger, J. S.: Overestimation of left ventricular volume by the indicator dilution technique. Circ. Res., 18:248, 1966.

Caves, P. K., Stinson, E. B., Bellingham, M. D., et al.: Serial transvenous biopsy of the transplanted human heart: Improved management of acute rejection episodes. Lancet, 1:821, 1974.

Caves, P. K., Schulz, W. P., Dong, E., Jr., Stinson, E. B., and Shumway, N. E.: New instrument for transvenous cardiac biopsy. Am. J. Cardiol., 33:264, 1974.

Chapman, C. B., Baker, O., Reynolds, J., and Bonte, F. J.: Use of biplane cinefluorography for measurement of ventricular volume. Circulation, 18:1105, 1958.

Chavez, I., Dorbecker, N., and Celis, A.: Direct intracardial angiocardiography: Its diagnostic value. Am. Heart J., 33:560, 1947.

Clark, L. C., and Bargeron, L. M., Jr.: Detection and direct recording of left-to-right shunts with the hydrogen electrode catheter. Surgery, 46:797, 1959.

Clark, L. C., Bargeron, L. M., Jr., Lyons, C., Bradley, M. N., and McArthur, K. T.: Detection of right-to-left shunts with an arterial potentiometric electrode. Circulation, 22:949, 1960.

Clark, L. C., Kaplan, S., Matthews, E. C., Edwards, F. K., and Helmworth, J. A.: Monitor and control of blood oxygen tension and Ph during total body perfusions. J. Thorac. Surg., 36:488, 1958.

Connolly, D. C., Kirklin, J. W., and Wood, E. H.: The relationship between pulmonary artery wedge pressure and left atrial pressure in man. Circ. Res., 2:434, 1954.

Cope, C.: Intravascular breakage of Seldinger spring guide wires. J.A.M.A., 180:1061, 1962.

Cope, C.: Technique for transseptal catheterization of left atrium. Preliminary report. J. Thorac. Surg., *37*:482, 1959.

Cournand, A., Motley, H. L., Himmelstein, A., Dresdale, D., and Baldwin, J.: Recording of blood pressure from the left auricle and the pulmonary veins in human subjects with interauricular septal defect. Am. J. Physiol., *150*:267, 1947.

Cournand, A., and Ranges, H. A.: Catheterization of the right auricle in man. Proc. Soc. Exper. Biol. Med., *46*:462, 1941.

Cournand, A., Riley, R. L., Breed, E. S., Baldwin, E. de F., and Richards, D. W., Jr.: Measurement of cardiac output in man using the technique of catheterization of the right auricle or ventricle. J. Clin. Invest., *24*:106, 1945.

Curry, J. L.: Recovery of detached catheter fragments. J.A.M.A., *211*:2156, 1970.

Damato, A. N., Lau, S. H., Helfant, R., Stein, E., Patton, R. D., Scherlag, B. J., and Berkowitz, W. D.: A study of heart block in man using His bundle recordings. Circulation, *39*:297, 1969.

Davis, F. W., Jr., and Andrus, E. C.: Mitral stenosis in facsimile. N. Engl. J. Med., *251*:297, 1954.

Dexter, L., Haynes, F. W., Burwell, C. S., Eppinger, E. C., Siebel, R. E., and Evans, J. M.: Studies of congenital heart disease. I. Technique of venous catheterization as a diagnostic procedure. J. Clin. Invest., *26*:554, 1947.

Dexter, L., Haynes, F. W., Burwell, C. S., Eppinger, E. C., Sogerson, R. P., and Evans, J. M.: Studies of congenital heart disease. II. The pressure and oxygen content of blood in the right auricle, right ventricle and pulmonary artery in control patients with observation on the oxygen saturation and source of pulmonary "capillary" blood. J. Clin. Invest., *26*:554, 1947.

Dodge, H. T., Hay, R. E., and Sandler, H.: An angiocardiographic method for directly determining left ventricular stroke volume in man. Circ. Res., *11*:739, 1962.

Dotter, C. T.: Left ventricle and systemic arterial catheterization: A simple percutaneous method using a spring guide. Am. J. Roentgenol., *6*:969, 1960.

Dow, P.: Dimensional relationships in dye-dilution curves from humans and dogs, with an empirical formula for certain troublesome curves. J. Appl. Physiol., *7*:399, 1955.

Dow, P.: Estimations of cardiac output and central blood volume by dye-dilution. Physiol. Rev., *36*:77, 1956.

Duchosal, P. W., Ferrero, C., Doret, J. P., Andereggen, P., and Rilliet, B.: Les potentiels intra-cardiaques récueillis par cathétérisme chez l'homme. Cardiologia, *13*:113, 1948.

Dyke, S. M., Cohn, P. F., Gorlin, R., and Sonnenblick, E. M.: Detection of residual myocardial functions in coronary artery disease using post-extrasystolic potentiation. Circulation, *50*:694, 1974.

Edwards, E. A., and Biguria, F. A.: A comparison of Skiodan and Diodrast as vasographic media: With special reference to their effect on blood pressure. N. Engl. J. Med., *211*:589, 1934.

Eggers, G. W. N., Jr., Stoeckle, H. G. E., Jr., and Allen, C. R., Jr.: General anesthesia for cardiac catheterization. Anesthesiology, *20*:817, 1959.

Enson, Y., Briscoe, W. A., Polanyi, M. L., and Cournand, A.: In vivo studies with an intravascular and intracardiac reflection oximeter. J. Appl. Physiol., *17*:552, 1962.

Evans, C. L., and Matsuoka, Y.: Effect of various mechanical conditions on the gaseous metabolism and efficiency of the mammalian heart. J. Physiol., *49*:328, 1914.

Facquet, J., Lemoine, J. M., Alhomme, P., and Lefebvre, J.: La mesure de la pression auriculaire gauche par voie transbronchique. Arch. Mal. Coeur, *45*:741, 1952.

Fegler, G.: Measurement of cardiac output in anesthetized animals by a thermo-dilution method. Q. J. Exper. Physiol., *39*:153, 1954.

Feruglio, G. A.: Intracardiac phonocardiography: A valuable diagnostic technique in congenital and acquired heart disease. Am. Heart J., *58*:827, 1959.

Fisher, D. L.: The use of pressure recordings obtained at transthoracic left heart catheterization in the diagnosis of valvular heart disease. J. Thorac. Surg., *30*:379, 1955.

Fisher, D. L.: Catheterization of left heart. *In* Intravascular Catheterization. Edited by H. Zimmerman. Springfield, Illinois, Charles C Thomas, 1959.

Fleming, H. A., Hancock, E. W., Milstein, B. B., and Ross, D. H.: Percutaneous left ventricular puncture with catheterization of aorta. Thorax, *13*:97, 1958.

Fleming, P., and Gibson, R.: Percutaneous left ventricular puncture in the assessment of aortic stenosis. Thorax, *12*:37, 1957.

Folse, R., and Braunwald, E.: Determination of fraction of left ventricular volume ejected per beat and clinical observations with a precordial dilution technique. Circulation, *25*:674, 1962.

Forman, J., Laurens, P., and Serville, M.: Catheterization of the left cavities with micromanometry by transseptal route. Arch. Mal. Coeur, *55*:601, 1962.

Forrester, J. S., Diamond, G., McHugh, T. J., and Swan, H. J. C.: Filling pressures in the right and left sides of the heart in acute myocardial infarction. N. Engl. J. Med., *285*:190, 1971.

Forrester, J. S., Ganz, W., Diamond, G., McHugh, T., Chonette, D. W., and Swan, H. J. C.: Thermodilution cardiac output determination with a single flow-directed catheter. Am. Heart J., *83*:306, 1972.

Forssmann, W.: Die Sondierung des Rechten Herzens. Klin. Wochenschr., *8*:2085, 1929.

Fox, I. J., and Wood, E. H.: Applications of dilution curves recorded from the right side of the heart or venous circulation with the aid of a new indicator dye. Proc. Staff Meet. Mayo Clinic, *32*:541, 1957.

Fox, S. M.: Pretrachial left heart catheterization: Difficult technique with some advantages. Circulation, *20*:696, 1959.

Frank, M. J., and Levinson, G. E.: An index of the contractile state of the myocardium in man. J. Clin. Invest., *47*:1615, 1968.

Freidlich, A., Heimbecker, R., and Bing, R. J.: A device for continuous recording of concentration of Evans blue dye in whole blood and its application to determination of cardiac output. J. Appl. Physiol., *3*:12, 1950.

Freis, E. D., Rivara, G. L., and Gilmore, B. L.: Estimation of residual and end-diastolic volumes of the right ventricle of men without heart disease, using the dye-dilution method. Am. Heart J., *60*:898, 1960.

Friedberg, C. K.: Diseases of the Heart. 3rd Ed. Philadelphia, W. B. Saunders Company, 1966.

Gasul, B. M., Dillon, R. J., Vrla, V., and Hart, G.: Ventricular septal defects. Their natural transformation in those with infundibular stenosis or with the cyanotic or non-cyanotic type of tetralogy of Fallot. J.A.M.A., *164*:847, 1957.

Gilford, S. R., Gregg, D. E., Shadle, O. W., Ferguson, T. B., and Marzetta, L. A.: An improved cuvette densitometer for cardiac output determination by the dye-dilution method. Rev. Sci. Instrum., *24*:696, 1953.

Gleason, W. L., and Braunwald, E.: Studies on the first derivative of the ventricular pressure pulse in man. J. Clin. Invest., *41*:80, 1962.

Gorlin, R., and Gorlin, S. G.: Hydraulic formula for calculations of the area of the stenotic mitral valve, other cardiac valves and central circulatory shunts. Am. Heart J., *41*:1, 1951.

Gorlin, R., Lewis, B. M., Haynes, F. W., and Dexter, L.: Studies of the circulatory dynamics at rest in mitral valvular regurgitation with and without stenosis. Am. Heart J., *43*:357, 1952.

Graham, T. P., Jr., Covell, J. W., Sonnenblick, E. H., Ross, J., Jr., and Braunwald, E.: The control of myocardial oxygen consumption: Relative influence of contractile state and tension development. J. Clin. Invest., *47*:375, 1968.

Greene, D. G., Carlisle, R., Grant, C., and Bunnell, I. L.: Estimation left ventricular volume by one-plane cineangiography. Circulation, *35*:61, 1967.

Gross, R. E., and Longino, L. A.: The patent ductus arteriosus: Observations from 412 surgically treated cases. Circulation, *3*:125, 1951.

Grundemann, A. M., Bosch, C., Schwantje, E. J. M., Reijns, G. A., and Verheught, A. P. M.: Retrograde catheterization of the left ventricle in aortic stenosis. Am. J. Cardiol., *6*:915, 1960.

Güntzig, A. R., Senning, A., and Siegenthaler, W. E.: Nonoperative dilatation of coronary artery stenosis. Percutaneous transluminal coronary angioplasty. N. Engl. J. Med., *301*:61, 1979.

Hamilton, W. F., Moore, J. W., Kinsman, J. M., and Spurling, R. G.: Studies on the circulation. IV. Further analysis of the injection method, and of changes in hemodynamics under physiological and pathological conditions. Am. J. Physiol., 99:534, 1932.

Harned, H. S., Lurie, P. R., Croethers, C. H., and Whittmore, R.: Use of the whole blood oximeter during cardiac catheterization. J. Lab Clin. Med., 40:445, 1952.

Harrison, T. R.: Some unanswered questions concerning enlargement and failure of the heart. Am. Heart J., 69:100, 1965.

Hawley, R. R., Dodge, H. T., and Graham, T. P.: Left atrial volume and its changes in heart disease. Circulation, 34:989, 1966.

Hecht, H. H.: Potential variations of the right auricular and ventricular cavities in man. Am. Heart J., 32:39, 1946.

Helfant, R. H., Pine, R., Meister, S. G., Feldman, M. S., Trout, R. G., and Banks, V. S.: Nitroglycerin to unmask reversible asynergy: Correlation with post-coronary bypass ventriculography. Circulation, 50:108, 1974.

Herman, M. V., Heinke, R. A., Klein, M. D., and Gorlin, R.: Localized disorders in myocardial contractions. N. Engl. J. Med., 277:222, 1967.

Hernandez, F. A., Rockkind, R., and Cooper, H. R.: The intracavitary electrocardiogram in the diagnosis of Ebstein's anomaly. Am. J. Cardiol., 1:181, 1958.

Hickam, J. B., and Frazer, R.: Spectrophotometric determination of blood oxygen. J. Biol. Chem., 180:457, 1949.

Hildner, F. J., Drake, E. H., Gale, H. H., and Ormond, R. S.: Transbrachial retrograde left heart catheterization. Evaluation of 600 consecutive cases in adults. Am. J. Cardiol., 18:52, 1966.

Holling, H. E., MacDonald, I., O'Holloran, J. A., and Venner, A.: Reliability of a spectrophotometric method of estimating blood oxygen. J. Appl. Physiol., 8:249, 1955.

Horger, E. L., Dotter, C. T., and Steinberg, E.: Electrocardiographic changes during angiocardiography. Am. Heart J., 41:651, 1951.

Horn, R. R., Teicholz, L. E., Cohn, P. E., Herman, M. V., and Gorlin, R.: Augmentation of left ventricular contraction pattern in coronary artery disease by inotropic catecholamine: The epinephrine ventriculogram. Circulation, 49:1063, 1974.

Hugenholtz, P. G., Gamble, W. J., Monroe, R. G., and Polanyi, M.: The use of fiberoptics in clinical cardiac catheterization. II. In vivo dye dilution curves. Circulation, 31:344, 1965.

Hugenholtz, P. G., Wagner, H. R., and Sandler, H.: The in vivo determination of left ventricular volume: Comparison of the fiberoptic-indicator dilution and the angiocardiographic methods. Circulation, 37:489, 1968.

Hunt, D., Pombo, J., Potanin, C., Russell, R. O., Jr., and Rackley, C. E.: Intravascular monitoring in acute myocardial infarction. Am. J. Cardiol., 25:104, 1970.

Jonsson, G., Broden, B., and Karwen, J.: Selective angiocardiography. Acta Radiol., 32:486, 1949.

Kaltman, A. J., Herbert, W. H., Conroy, R. J., and Kossman, C. E.: Gradient in pressure across the pulmonary vascular bed during diastole. Circulation, 34:377, 1966.

Katz, L. H., and Feinberg, H.: The relation of cardiac efforts to myocardial oxygen consumption and coronary flow. Circ. Res., 6:656, 1958.

Keith, J. O., Rowe, R. D., and Vlad, P.: Heart Disease in Infancy and Childhood. New York, The Macmillan Co., 1967.

Kent, E. M., Ford, W. B., Fisher, D. L., and Childs, T. B.: The estimation of the severity of mitral regurgitation. Ann. Surg., 141:47, 1955.

Kidd, L.: The hemodynamics in ventricular septal defect in childhood. Am. Heart J., 70:732, 1965.

King, T. D., Thompson, S. L., Steiner, C., and Milles, N. L.: Secundum atrial septal defect. Nonoperative closure during cardiac catheterization. J.A.M.A., 233:2506, 1976.

Kinsman, J. M., Moore, J. W., and Hamilton, W. F.: Studies on the circulation. I. Injection method: Physical and mathematical considerations. Am. J. Physiol., 89:322, 1929.

Kitamura, S., Sato, K., Naito, J., Shimizu, J., Fujino, M., Oyama, C., Nabano, S., and Kawashima, Y.: Plug closure of patent ductus arteriosus by transfemoral catheter method. A comparative study with surgery and a new technical modification. Chest, 70:631, 1976.

Klatte, E. C., Campbell, J. A., and Lurie, P. R.: Technical factors in selective cinecardioangiography. Radiology, 73:539, 1959.

Klein, O.: Zur Bestimmung des Zirkulatorischen Minutenvolumens beim Menschen nach dem Fickschen Prinzip. München. Med. Wochenschr., 77:1311, 1930.

Korner, P. I., and Shillingford, J. P.: The quantitative estimation of valvular incompetence by dye-dilution curves. Clin. Sci., 14:553, 1955.

Kossman, C. E., Berger, A. R., Rader, B., Brumlik, J., Briller, S. A., and Donnelly, J. H.: Intracardiac and intravascular potentials resulting from electrical activity of the normal human heart. Circulation, 2:10, 1950.

Lange, R. L., and Hecht, H. H.: Quantitation of valvular regurgitation from multiple indicator-dilution curves. Circulation, 18:623, 1958.

Laurens, P., Bouchajd, F., Brial, E., Cornu, C., Baculard, P., and Soulie, P.: Bruite et pressions cardiovasculaires enregistrés in situ à l'aide d'un micromanomètre. Arch. Mal. Coeur, 52:121, 1959.

Lenegre, J., and Maurice, P.: De quelques résultats obtenus par la derivation directe intracavitaire des courants électriques de l'oreillette et du ventricule droits. Arch. Mal. Coeur., 38:298, 1945.

Leonard, J. J., and Kroetz, F. W.: Lessons learned through intracardiac phonocardiography. Mod. Concepts Cardiovasc. Dis., 35:69, 1966.

Levin, A. R., Spach, M. S., Anderson, P. A. W., and Capp, M. P.: Cardiac perforation following left ventricular cineangiocardiography. Circulation, 32:593, 1965.

Levine, H. D., Hellems, H. K., Dexter, L., and Tucker, A. S.: Studies in intracardiac electrocardiography in man. II. The potential variations in the right ventricle. Am. Heart J., 37:46, 1949.

Levine, H. D., Hellems, H. K., Wittenberg, M. H., and Dexter, L.: Studies in intracardiac electrocardiography in man. I. The potential variations in the right atrium. Am. Heart J., 37:46, 1949.

Lewis, D. H., Deitz, G. W., Wallace, J. D., and Brown, J. R., Jr.: Intracardiac phonocardiography. Prog. Cardiovasc. Dis., 2:85, 1959–1960.

Lewis, D. H., Ertugrul, A. E., Deitz, G. W., Wallace, J. D., Brown, J. R., Jr., and Moghadam, A. N.: Intracardiac phonocardiography in the diagnosis of congenital heart disease. Pediatrics, 23:837, 1959.

Libanoff, A. J., and Rodbard, S.: Evaluation of the severity of mitral stenosis and regurgitation. Circulation, 33:218, 1966.

Libanoff, A. J., and Rodbard, S.: Atrioventricular pressure half-time. Measure of mitral valve orifice area. Circulation, 38:144, 1968.

Lind, J., Boesen, I. B., and Wegelius, C.: Selective angiocardiography in congenital heart disease. Prog. Cardiovasc. Dis., 2:293, 1959.

Littman, D., Starobin, O. E., Hall, J. H., Matthews, R. J., and Williams, J. A.: A new method of left ventricular catheterization. Circulation 21:1150, 1960.

Litwak, R. S., Bernstein, W. H., and Samet, P.: Problems in the interpretation of left atrial left ventricular mean diastolic gradients. Am. J. Cardiol., 6:1023, 1960.

Long, R. T. L., Braunwald, E., and Morrow, A. G.: Intracardiac injection of radioactive krypton[85]. Clinical applications of new methods for characterization of circulatory shunts. Circulation, 21:1126, 1960.

Looney, W. B.: Late clinical changes following the internal deposition of radioactive materials. Ann. Intern. Med., 42:378, 1955.

Lucas, R. V., Jr., Adams, P., Jr., Anderson, R. C., Meyne, N. G., Lillihei, C. W., and Varco, R. L.: The natural history of isolated ventricular septal defect. A serial physiological study. Circulation, 24:1372, 1961.

Luchsinger, P. C., Seipp, H. W., Jr., and Patel, D. J.: Relationship of pulmonary artery wedge pressures to left atrial pressures in man. Circ. Res., 11:315, 1962.

Luisada, A. A., and Liu, C. K.: Simple methods for recording intracardiac electrocardiograms and phonocardiograms during left or right heart catheterization. Am. Heart J., 54:531, 1957.

Lurie, P. R., Shumacker, H. B., Jr., Schulz, D. M., Klatte, E. C., and Grajo, M. Z.: Obstructive hypertrophy in congenital heart disease: Definition, classification, and surgical importance. Circulation, 20:732, 1959.

Lüthy, E., and Galletti, P. M.: In vivo evaluation of the thermodilution technique for measuring cardiac output. Helv. Physiol. Pharmacol. Acta, 24:15, 1966.

Mason, D. T.: Usefulness and limitations of the rate of rise of intraventricular pressure (dp/dt) in the evaluation of myocardial contractility in man. Am. J. Cardiol., 23:516, 1969.

Mason, D. T., and Braunwald, E.: Studies of digitalis. IX. Effects of ouabain on the nonfailing human heart. J. Clin. Invest., 42:1105, 1963.

Mason, D. T., Sonnenblick, E. H., Covell, J. W., Ross, J., Jr., and Braunwald, E.: Assessment of myocardial contractility in man: Relationship between the rate of pressure rise and developed pressure throughout isometric left ventricular contraction. Circulation, 36(Suppl. 2):183, 1967.

Mason, D. T., Sonnenblick, E. H., Ross, J., Jr., Covell, J. W., and Braunwald, E.: Time to peak dp/dt: A useful measurement for evaluating the contractile state of the human heart. Circulation, 32(Suppl. 2):145, 1965.

Mason, D. T., Spann, J. F., Jr., Beiser, G. D., and Gold, H.: Effects of angiographic dye on isometric contraction and force-velocity characteristics of cat papillary muscle (Abstract). Clin. Res., 16:239, 1968.

Massumi, R. A., and Rose, A. M.: A traumatic nonsurgical technique for removal of broken catheters from cardiac cavities. N. Engl. J. Med., 277:195, 1967.

Moffit, E. A., Dawson, B., and O'Neill, N. C.: Anesthesia for pediatric cardiac catheterization and angiography. Anesth. Analg., 40:483, 1961.

Moore, J. W., Kinsman, J. M., Hamilton, W. F., and Spruling, R. G.: Studies on the circulation. II. Cardiac output determinations: Comparison of the injection method with the direct Fick procedure. Am. J. Physiol., 89:331, 1929.

Morrow, A. G., Braunwald, E., Haller, J. A., and Sharp, E. H.: Left atrial pressure pulse in mitral valve disease. A correlation of pressures obtained by transbronchial puncture with the valvular lesion. Circulation, 16:399, 1957.

Morrow, A. G., Braunwald, E., Haller, J. A., Jr., and Sharp, E. H.: Left heart catheterization by the transbronchial route: Technique and applications in physiologic and diagnostic investigations. Circulation, 16:1033, 1957.

Morrow, A. G., Braunwald, E., and Ross, J., Jr.: Left heart catheterization. An appraisal of techniques and their applications in cardiovascular disease. Arch. Intern. Med., 105:645, 1960.

Morrow, A. G., Sanders, R. J., and Braunwald, E.: The nitrous oxide test. An improved method for the detection of left-to-right shunts. Circulation, 17:284, 1958.

Morrow, A. G., Sharp, E. H., and Braunwald, E.: Congenital aortic stenosis: Clinical and hemodynamic findings, surgical technique, and results of operation. Circulation, 18:1091, 1958.

Morrow, A. G., Waldhausen, J. A., Peters, R. L., Bloodwell, R. D., and Braunwald, E.: Supravalvular aortic stenosis, clinical hemodynamics and pathological observations. Circulation, 20:1003, 1959.

Moscovitz, H. L., Donoso, E., and Gelb, I. J.: The demonstration of flow murmurs by intracardiac phonocardiography. Clin. Res. Proc., 5:162, 1957.

Nadas, A. S.: Pediatric Cardiology. Philadelphia, W. B. Saunders Company, 1963.

Nadas, A. S., Rudolph, A. M., and Gross, R. E.: Pulmonary hypertension in congenital heart disease. Circulation, 22:1041, 1960.

Narula, O. S.: Recording of His bundle electrograms via the arm veins (Abstract). Circulation, 46(Suppl. 2):197, 1972.

Narula, O. S., and Samet, P.: Wenckebach and Mobitz II A-V block due to block within the His bundle and bundle branches. Circulation, 41:947, 1970.

Narula, O. S., Schenlag, B. J., Samet, P., and Javier, R. P.: Atrioventricular block: Localization and classification by His bundle recordings. Am. J. Med., 50:146, 1971.

Nicholson, J. W., III, and Wood, E. H.: Estimation of cardiac output and blood volume by continuous recording of Evans blue time-concentration curves in man employing an oximeter (Abstract). Am. J. Physiol., 163:738, 1950.

Nobel, F. W.: Electrical Methods of Blood-pressure Recordings. Springfield, Illinois, Charles C Thomas, 1953.

Nunez, V. B., and Ponsdomenech, E. R.: Heart puncture cardioangiography: Clinical and electrocardiographic results. Am. Heart J., 41:855, 1951.

Nutter, D. O., and Kelser, G. A.: The percutaneous intracavitary electrocardiogram in the diagnosis of arrhythmias. Ann. Intern. Med., 62:706, 1965.

Olsen, E. G. H.: Myocardial biopsies. In Recent Advances in Cardiology. Edited by J. Hamer. Edinburgh and London, Churchill Livingston, 1977, p. 349.

Owen, S. G., and Wood, P.: A new method of determining the degree or absence of mitral obstruction: An analysis of the diastolic part of indirect left atrial pressure tracings. Br. Heart J., 17:41, 1955.

Pinkerson, A. L., Kelser, G. A., Jr., and Adkins, P. C.: Left atrial thrombosis 2° to transseptal left heart catheterization. N. Engl. J. Med., 268:367, 1963.

Polanyi, M. L., and Hehir, R. M.: New reflection oximeter. Rev. Instrum., 31:401, 1960.

Popper, R. W., Schumacher, D., and Quinn, C. H.: Cardiac tamponade due to hypertonic contrast medium in the pericardial sac following cineangiography. Circulation, 35:933, 1967.

Priotin, J. B., Thévenet, A., Pelissier, M., Peuch, P., Latous, H., and Pourquier, J.: Cardiographie ventriculaire gauche par cathétérisme retrograde percutane femoral. Presse Méd., 65:1948, 1957.

Radner, S.: Extended suprasternal puncture technique. Acta Med. Scand., 151:223, 1955.

Rahimtoola, S. H., Duffy, J. P., and Swan, H. J. C.: Hemodynamic changes associated with injection of angiographic contrast medium in assessment of valvular lesions. Circulation, 33:52, 1966.

Rapaport, E., Wong, M., Escobar, E. E., and Martinez, G.: The effect of upright posture on right ventricular volume in patients with and without heart failure. Am. Heart J., 71:146, 1966.

Read, R. C.: Cause of death in cardioangiography. J. Thorac. Cardiovasc. Surg., 38:685, 1959.

Reedy, T., and Chapman, C. B.: Measurement of right ventricular volume by cineangiofluorography. Am. Heart J., 66:221, 1963.

Reeves, T. J., Hefner, L. L., Jones, W. B., Coghlan, C., Prieto, G., and Corroll, J.: The hemodynamic determinants of the rate of change in pressure in the left ventricle during isometric contraction. Am. Heart J., 60:745, 1960.

Richards, D. W., Jr.: Cardiac output by catheterization technique in various clinical conditions. Fed. Proc., 4:215, 1945.

Rodrigo, J. A.: Determination of the oxygen saturation of blood in vitro by using reflected light. Am. Heart J., 45:809, 1953.

Rodriguez-Alvarez, A., and Martinez de Rodriguez, G.: Studies in angiocardiography. The problems involved in the rapid, selective and safe injections of radiopaque materials. Development of a special catheter for selective angiocardiography. Am. Heart J., 53:841, 1957.

Rohde, E.: Über den Einfluss mechanischen Bedingungen auf die Tatigkeit und den Sauerstoffverbrauch des Warmnluterherzens. Arch. Exp. Pathol. Pharmakol., 68:401, 1912.

Rokseth, R., Helle, I., Marstrander, F., and Storstein, O.: Reference level in pressure recordings during right heart catheterization. Scand. J. Clin. Lab. Invest., 12:116, 1960.

Rosen, K. M.: Catheter recording of His bundle electrograms. Mod. Concepts Cardiovasc. Dis., 62:23, 1973.

Rosen, K. M., Loeb, H. S., Chuquimia, R., Sinno, M. Z., Rahimtoola, S. H., and Gunnar, R. M.: Site of heart block in acute myocardial infarction. Circulation, 42:925, 1970.

Rosen, K. M., Rahimtoola, S. H., Chuquimia, R., Loeb, H. S., and Gunnar, R. M.: Electrophysiological significance of first degree atrioventricular block with intraventricular conduction disturbance. Circulation, 43:491, 1971.

Ross, J., Jr.: Considerations regarding the technique for transseptal left heart catheterization. Circulation, 34:391, 1966.

Ross, J. Jr.: Transseptal left heart catheterization: A new method of left atrial puncture. Ann. Surg., 37:482, 1959.

Ross, J., Jr., Braunwald, E., Mason, T., Braunwald, N. S., and

Morrow, A. G.: Interatrial communication and left atrial hypertension. A cause of continuous murmur. Circulation, 28:853, 1963.

Ross, J., Jr., Braunwald, E., and Morrow, A. G.: Left heart catheterization by the transseptal route. A description of the technique and its applications. Circulation, 22:927, 1960.

Ross, J., Jr., Braunwald, E., and Morrow, A. G.: Transseptal left atrium puncture: New technique for measurement of left atrial pressure in man. Am. J. Cardiol., 3:653, 1959.

Rowe, G. G., and Zarnstorff, W. C.: Ventricular fibrillation during selective angiocardiography. J.A.M.A., 192:105, 1965.

Rudolph, A. M., and Cayler, G. G.: Cardiac catheterization in infants and children. Pediatr. Clin. North Am., 5:907, 1958.

Russell, R. O., Caroll, J. F., and Hood, W. G., Jr.: Cardiac tamponade. A complication of the transseptal technique of left heart catheterization resulting in a fatality. Am. J. Cardiol., 13:558, 1964.

Sakakibara, S., and Konno, S.: Endomyocardial biopsy. Jpn. Heart J., 3:537, 1962.

Salgado, C. R., and Galletti, P. M.: In vitro evaluation of thermodilution technique for the measurement of ventricular stroke volume and end-diastolic volume. Cardiologica, 49:65, 1966.

Samet, P., Litwak, R. S., Bernstein, W. H., Fierer, E. M., and Silverman, L. M.: Clinical and physiologic relationships in mitral valve disease. Circulation, 19:517, 1959.

Sanders, R. J., and Morrow, A. G.: The diagnosis of circulatory shunts by the nitrous oxide test. Improvements in technique and methods for quantification of shunts. Circulation, 188:56, 1958.

Sanders, R. J., and Morrow, A. G.: The identification and quantification of left-to-right circulation shunts. A new diagnostic method utilizing the inhalation of a radioactive gas, krypton[85] Am. J. Med., 26:508, 1959.

Sandler, H., and Dodge, H. T.: The use of single plane angiocardiograms for the calculation of left ventricular volume in man. Am. Heart J., 75:325, 1968.

Sarnoff, S. J., Braunwald, E., Welch, G. H., Jr., et al.: Hemodynamic determinants of oxygen consumption of the heart with special reference to the tension-time index. Am. J. Physiol., 192:148, 1958.

Schafer, H., Blain, J. M., Ceballos, R., and Bing, R. J.: Essential pulmonary hypertension. A report of clinical physiologic studies in three patients, with death following catheterization of the heart. Ann. Intern. Med., 44:505, 1956.

Scherlag, B. J., Lau, S. H., Helfant, R. H., Berkowitz, W. D., Stein, E., and Damato, A. N.: Catheter technique for recording His bundle activity in man. Circulation, 35:13, 1969.

Scott, S. M., Fish, R. G., and Takaro, T.: A double needle technique for transbronchial left heart catheterization. Circulation, 22:976, 1960.

Scott, W. G., and Moore, S.: Rapid serialization of x-ray exposures by the radiography utilizing roll of film nine and one-half inches wide. Radiology, 53:846, 1949.

Scott, W. G., and Moore, S.: The development of the tautography and the advantages of automatization in cardiovascular angiography. Am. J. Roentgenol., 62:33, 1949.

Segal, B. L., Novack, P., and Kasparian, H.: Intracardiac phonocardiography. Am. J. Cardiol., 13:188, 1964.

Seldinger, S. I.: Catheter replacement of the needle in percutaneous arteriography: New technique. Acta Radiol., 39:368, 1953.

Shaffer, A. B., and Silber, E. N.: Factors influencing the character of the pulmonary arterial wedge pressure. Am. Heart J., 5:522, 1956.

Shirey, E. K., and Sones, F. M., Jr.: Retrograde transaortic and mitral valve catheterization. Physiologic and morphologic evaluation of aortic and mitral valve lesions. Am. J. Cardiol., 18:745, 1966.

Siegel, J. H., and Sonnenblick, E. H.: Quantification of myocardial contractility and prediction of myocardial failure. Arch. Surg., 89:1026, 1964.

Singleton, R. T., Donald, D. H., and Scherlis, L.: Krypton[85] in the detection of intracardiac left-to-right shunts. Circulation, 32:134, 1965.

Smith, C., Rowe, R. D., and Vlad, P.: Sedation of children for cardiac catheterization with an ataractic mixture. Can. Anaesth. Soc. J., 5:35, 1958.

Sodi-Pallares, D., Vizcaino, M., Soberon, J., and Cabrera, E.: Comparative study of the intracavitary potential in man and in dog. Am. Heart J., 33:819, 1947.

Sonnenblick, E. H., and Skelton, C. L.: Oxygen consumption of the heart: Physiological principles and clinical implications. Mod. Concepts Cardiovasc. Dis., 60:9, 1971.

Sonnenblick, E. H., Ross, J., Jr., and Braunwald, E.: Oxygen consumption of the heart: Newer concepts of its multifactoral determination. Am. J. Cardiol., 22:328, 1968.

Soulié, P., Laurens, P., Bouchard, F., Cornu, C., and Brial, E.: Enregistrement des pressions et des bruits intracardiaques à l'aide d'un micromanomètre. Bull. Mém. Soc. Méd. Hôp. Paris, 22:713, 1957.

Stewart, G. N.: Researches on the circulation time and on the influences which affect it. IV. The output of the heart. J. Physiol., 22:11, 1897.

Susmano, A., and Carleton, R. A.: Transseptal catheterization of the left atrium. Report of an unusual complication. N. Engl. J. Med., 270:897, 1964.

Swan, H. J. C., Burchell, H. B., Linder, E., Birkhead, N. C., and Wood, E. H.: Symposium on diagnostic applications of indicator-dilution curves recorded from left and right sides of the heart. Part II. Proc. Staff Meet. Mayo Clin., 33:581, 1958.

Swan, H. J. C., Ganz, W., Forrester, J., Marcus, H., Diamond, G., and Chonnette, D.: Catheterization of the heart in man with use of a flow-directed balloon-tipped catheter. N. Engl. J. Med., 283:447, 1970.

Swan, H. J. C., Hetzel, P. S., Burchell, H. B., and Wood, E. H.: Relative contribution of blood from each lung to the left-to-right shunt in atrial septal defects. Circulation, 14:200, 1956.

Swan, H. J. C., Zapata-Diaz, J., and Wood, E. H.: Dye-dilution curves in cyanotic congenital heart disease. Circulation, 8:70, 1953.

Taylor, C., and Stoelting, V. K.: The anesthetic management of small children undergoing cardiac catheterization and angiocardiography. Anesth. Analg., 38:441, 1959.

Van Slyke, D. D., and Neill, J. M.: Determination of gases in blood and other solutions by vacuum extraction and manometric measurement. J. Biol. Chem., 61:523, 1924.

Veragut, U. P., and Krayenbuhl, H. P.: Estimation and quantification of myocardial contractility in the closed-chest dog. Cardiologia, 47:96, 1965.

Voci, G., and Hamer, N. A. J.: Retrograde arterial catheterization of the left ventricle. Am. J. Cardiol., 5:492, 1960.

Vogel, J. H. K., Tabari, K., Averill, K. H., and Blount, S. G., Jr.: A simple technique for identifying P waves in complex arrhythmias. Am. Heart J., 67:158, 1964.

Wagner, H. R., Gamble, W. J., Albers, W. H., and Hugenholtz, P. G.: Fiberoptic-dye dilution method for measurement of cardiac output. Circulation, 37:694, 1968.

Wallace, A. G., Skinner, N. S., Jr., and Mitchell, J.: Hemodynamic determinants of the maximal rate of rise of left ventricular pressure. Am. J. Physiol., 205:30, 1963.

Wallace, J. O., Brown, J. R., Lewis, D. H., and Deitz, G. W.: Acoustic mapping within the heart. J. Acoust. Soc. Am., 29:9, 1957.

Watson, H.: Electrode catheters and the diagnostic application of intracardiac electrography in small children. Circulation, 29:284, 1964.

Wiggers, C. J.: Dynamics of ventricular contraction under abnormal conditions. Circulation, 5:321, 1952.

Wood, E. H.: Diagnostic applications of indicator-dilution techniques in congenital heart disease. Circ. Res., 10:531, 1962.

Wood, E. H.: Special techniques of value in the cardiac catheterization laboratory. Proc. Staff Meet. Mayo Clin., 28:58, 1953.

Wood, E. H., Swan, H. J. C., Fox, I. J., et al.: Symposium on diagnostic applications of indicator-dilution techniques. Proc. Staff Meet. Mayo Clin. 32:463, 1957.

Wood, P.: The Eisenmenger syndrome. II. Br. Med. J., 2:755, 1958.

Wright, J. L., Toscano-Barboza, E., and Brandenburg, R. O.: Left ventricular and aortic pressure pulses in aortic valvular disease. Proc. Staff Meet. Mayo Clin., *31*:120, 1956

Wright, J. L., and Wood, E. H.: Value of central and peripheral intraarterial pressure and pulse contours in cardiovascular diagnosis. J. Minnesota Med., *41*:215, 1958.

Yamakawa, K., Shionoya, Y., Kitamura, K., Nagai, T., Yamomoto, T., and Ohta, S.: Intracardiac phonocardiography. Am. Heart J., *47*:424, 1954.

Yang, S. S., Bentivoglio, L. C., Maranhao, V., and Goldberg, H.: From Cardiac Catheterization Data to Hemodynamic Parameters. Philadelphia, F. A. Davis, Co., 1972.

Yanof, H. M., Rosen, A. L., McDonald, N. M., and McDonald, D. A.: Critical study of the response of manometers to forced oscillations. Phys. Med. Biol., *8*:407, 1963.

Ziegler, R. F.: The importance of patent ductus arteriosus in infants. Am. Heart J., *43*:1, 1952.

Zimmerman, H. A., and Hellerstein, H. K.: Cavity potentials of the human ventricles. Circulation, *3*:95, 1951.

Zimmerman, H. A., Scott, R. W., and Becker, N. O.: Catheterization of the left side of the heart in man. Circulation, *1*:357, 1950.

Zinn, W. J., Levinson, D. C., Johns, V., and Griffith, J. C.: The effect of angiocardiography on the heart as measured by electrocardiographic alterations. Circulation, *3*:658, 1951.

Chapter 29

Cardiopulmonary Bypass for Cardiac Surgery

John W. Kirklin

James K. Kirklin

William A. Lell

Cardiopulmonary bypass is a technique by which the pumping action of the heart and the gas exchange functions of the lung are temporarily replaced by a mechanical device, the pump-oxygenator, attached to the vascular system of the patient. Although by present techniques some temporary organ and system dysfunction follows its use, cardiopulmonary bypass has become an indispensable technique for most kinds of cardiac surgery. It has also been used in series with the patient's own heart and lung for partial temporary cardiopulmonary bypass in patients with severe but potentially reversible respiratory distress, for patients undergoing operations on the thoracic aorta, and for a few other purposes, but we shall not discuss these in this chapter.

PRINCIPLES OF USE FOR CARDIAC SURGERY

An arterial cannula is inserted into the aorta or one of its major branches for the input of arterialized blood from the pump-oxygenator. One or more venous cannulae are inserted into the right atrium or its large venous tributaries for draining all the patient's venous blood into the pump-oxygenator. Since bronchial arterial and aortopulmonary collateral flow enters the heart by way of the pulmonary veins and coronary blood flow enters the heart through the coronary sinus and thebesian veins, an intracardiac vent or sucker is usually needed to remove this blood and return it to the venous side of the pump-oxygenator.

Normal individuals under anesthesia have a cardiac index (systemic perfusion rate) of about 2.5 liters/min./M.^{2} The arterial perfusion rate from the pump-oxygenator to the patient at normothermia should be similar; in practice, flows of 2 to 2.5 liters/min./M.^{2} are used. Optimal arterial oxygen and carbon dioxide levels are maintained by current oxygenators. Yet it is an illusion to believe that during cardiopulmonary bypass the patient is in a near-normal state physiologically, and appropriate deviations from this so-called "high-flow, normothermic" technique are at least as well tolerated as is that technique. Furthermore, efforts to maintain so-called

normal arterial perfusion flow rates, pressures, temperature, coronary perfusion, and so on often compromise the cardiac operation that is the reason for the patient's being on cardiopulmonary bypass.

The availability of additional modalities such as hypothermia and the tolerance of the patient to certain abnormalities such as hemodilution and temporary cardiac ischemia allow the surgical team to use cardiopulmonary bypass as a flexible surgical tool whose purpose is to prevent as much as possible damage to organs and subsystems of the patient and to facilitate the cardiac surgery.

HISTORICAL NOTE

The historical aspects of cardiopulmonary bypass for cardiac surgery are not easily described, for it is almost impossible to know who first had the idea of diverting the circulation to an oxygenator outside the body and pumping it back to the patient's arterial system in order to allow surgery within the heart.

References to extracorporeal gas exchange in blood go back to the last part of the nineteenth century. Thus, Frey and Gruber worked with an "oxygenator" in 1885. Subsequently, scores of laboratory studies with oxygenators and pumps were reported. However, serious consideration of the use of pump-oxygenators for cardiac surgery had to await the development of modern anesthesia and modern surgical methods and, particularly, scientific developments such as the discovery and use of heparin, plastic material, and the like. Without doubt, Gibbon, with his pioneering experimental work at the Massachusetts General Hospital in Boston in the late 1930s (Gibbon, 1939), was a major contributor to the advancement of cardiopulmonary bypass from the mere idea to successful laboratory work and then successful clinical application. Gibbon's work was interrupted by World War II, but when he came to Jefferson Medical School in Philadelphia after his military service, he resumed his work with cardiopulmonary bypass, its pathophysiology, and the equipment required for it. Most of the medical and surgical world took little note of his work and, in fact, considered it unlikely to lead to any useful knowledge. However, he persevered. As a result, the first successful operation in which the patient was totally supported by cardiopulmonary bypass was done by Gibbon, when he repaired an atrial septal defect in a young woman using a pump-oxygenator in 1953 (Gibbon, 1954). Unfortunately, his subsequent four patients died from a variety of problems, and he became discouraged about the method (Gibbon, 1955).

Meanwhile, in the late 1940s, a few others began to work with pump-oxygenators for cardiopulmonary bypass. Among these were Dennis at the University of Minnesota. His laboratory studies led him to make what may have been the first attempt to use a pump-oxygenator for clinical cardiac surgery in 1951 (Dennis *et al.*, 1951). He and Varco operated on a patient thought to have an atrial septal defect and felt that they had done a satisfactory repair, but the patient died. Autopsy showed that the lesion was, in fact, a partial atrioventricular canal defect, and misinterpretation of the anatomy was a major factor in the patient's death. In Stockholm, Sweden, Bjork (1948) and Senning (1952) also worked with cardiopulmonary bypass in the late 1940s and early 1950s. Related to this is Crafoord's early use of this method for removal of an atrial myxoma (Crafoord *et al.*, 1957).

After Dennis' unsuccessful effort, Lillehei and colleagues at the University of Minnesota began working in the laboratory with controlled cross-circulation, using another intact subject as the "oxygenator" (Cohen and Lillehei, 1954). Their experimental studies led them to adopt the "azygos flow principle" (Andreasen and Watson, 1952), which was that only very small perfusion flow rates were needed. In April 1954, they began a spectacular series of operations for congenital heart disease using "controlled cross-circulation" and usually the mother as the "oxygenator" (Warden *et al.*, 1954). Although this particular technique ultimately was abandoned, the work of Lillehei and colleagues brought into being the modern era of open heart surgery (Lillehei *et al.*, 1955).

We began experimental work at the Mayo Clinic in Rochester, Minnesota, in the early 1950s (Donald *et al.*, 1955; Jones *et al.*, 1955) with pump-oxygenators, which led to our first use of cardiopulmonary bypass with a pump-oxygenator in March 1955 in successfully repairing a ventricular septal defect. We then began the world's first series of intracardiac operations using a pump-oxygenator (Kirklin *et al.*, 1955).

Quickly, the field of intracardiac surgery using a pump-oxygenator for cardiopulmonary bypass began to expand, and today it is practiced in all parts of the world.

INTRODUCTION

The temporary provision of arterial blood flow by means of a *pump-oxygenator* is an abnormal situation, in which most if not all of the body's physiologic processes are affected. When essentially all systemic venous blood returns to the pump-oxygenator instead of the heart, the situation is termed *total cardiopulmonary bypass (CPB)*. When some systemic venous blood returns to the heart and is ejected into the aorta, the situation is termed *partial cardiopulmonary bypass*.

In contrast to the situation in intact man, a number of physiologic variables are directly under external control during CPB. These include *total systemic blood flow* ("cardiac output"), *input pressure wave form, systemic venous pressure, pulmonary venous pressure, hematocrit of the initial perfusate* and *its chemical composition, arterial oxygen* and *carbon dioxide* (and *nitrogen*) *levels,* and *temperature* of the perfusate and patient. Decisions should therefore be made concerning all of these matters. Unfortunately, at times no formal decision is made, and a situation is merely accepted rather than decided upon.

Another group of variables is determined in part by the externally controlled variables and in part by the patient. These include *systemic vascular resistance, total-body oxygen consumption, mixed venous oxygen levels, lactic acidemia* and *pH, regional* and *organ blood flow,* and *regional* and *organ function.*

A number of undesirable *side effects* occur to a greater or lesser degree with CPB. These include *blood coagulation abnormalities, changes in red blood cells* and *plasma proteins* produced by their passage through the extracorporeal system, *gaseous* and *particulate emboli,* and *liberation* or *production* of a wide variety of *vasoactive* and otherwise *biologically active substances* by contact of blood with foreign surfaces.

SURGICAL TECHNIQUES

Arterial Cannulation. Usually, the ascending aorta is cannulated directly when using cardiopulmonary bypass for cardiac surgery (exceptions, in whom the femoral artery is cannulated, include, for example, patients undergoing resection of aneurysms of the ascending aorta and those undergoing closure of a previously constructed descending aorta–left pulmonary artery or Potts anastomosis). The hemodynamic advantages of entrance of the arterial inflow into the ascending aorta as opposed to the femoral artery have been argued. Most studies indicate that regional blood flow, including cerebral blood flow, is the same, no matter which site is chosen (Camishion *et al.*, 1963; Lees *et al.*, 1971; Schenk *et al.*, 1963). One study found left carotid blood flow to be greater with femoral cannulation than with several types of cannulation of the ascending aorta (Magilligan *et al.*, 1972). We believe the experimental conditions in that study were different from clinical conditions since (1) the researchers used a relatively small arterial cannula and thus had a relatively powerful jet effect, and (2) the tip of their cannula was in each instance near or downstream from the takeoff of the head vessels. The aortic

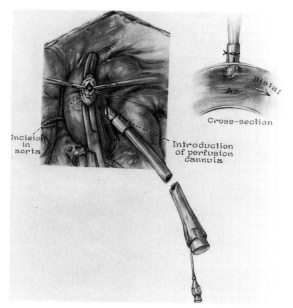

Figure 29–1. Insertion of arterial cannula into ascending aorta. Note that the cannula has been fitted with a small plastic collar so that only a short length of cannula is inserted into the aorta.

TABLE 29–1. ARTERIAL CANNULAE FLOW CHART: PRESSURE GRADIENT IN MILLIMETERS OF MERCURY (mm. Hg.)

		FLOW IN LITERS PER MINUTE							
		0.5	1.0	1.5	2.0	2.5	3.0	3.5	4.0
Cannula Size in French Scale	10	60	175	350					
	12	40	100	225	325				
	14	25	60	140	240	350			
	16		25	50	90	150	200	260	
	18		20	40	60	80	120	150	200
	20			25	40	60	80	100	120
	22			25	40	50	60	75	90
	24				40	50	60	70	80

cannula should be inserted as proximal to the takeoff of the innominate artery as is surgically acceptable, and only a short length of cannula is introduced, so that its tip cannot by chance actually enter a brachiocephalic vessel or lie near its orifice.

We generally place two concentric purse-string sutures of 2-0 silk in the aortic adventitia and media at the proposed site of cannulation. The aorta is then incised as by a stab wound within the purse-string stitch, and the arterial cannula is directly inserted. Alternatively, this portion of the aorta is exteriorized with a side-biting clamp, such as the Derra or Cooley clamp, the exteriorized portion of the aorta incised, and a tapered plastic cannula inserted as the clamp is removed (Fig. 29–1). The ends of the inner purse-string stitch have previously been threaded through a long narrow rubber tube, and the tube is tucked down snugly and secured as a tourniquet and then tied to the cannula. After the cannula is connected to the arterial lines in such a way as to exclude or remove any air bubbles, the line and cannula are secured so that the end of the cannula lies freely within the aortic lumen and the beveled end faces downstream, the surgical field is uncluttered, and the line from the pump-oxygenator is free from kinks.

As the cannula is removed after bypass, the outer purse-string suture is crossed by the assistant for hemostasis, and the surgeon ties the inner one. The outer purse-string suture is then tied by the assistant. Rarely is anything further required to establish hemostasis.

The tapered plastic cannula* is fitted for each

patient with a small collar adjusted so that just the right short length of cannula is beyond the collar. The cannula is inserted up to the collar. A size of cannula across which the pressure gradient, at the highest flow rate that will be used, is less than 100 mm. Hg is selected (Table 29–1). We use this relatively low gradient in order to minimize the turbulence as blood leaves the cannula tip and to keep the arterial line pressure (as measured by the arterial line manometer on the pump-oxygenator) less than about 250 mm. Hg to minimize the chance for blowouts of the line or its connectors.

Venous Cannulation. Usually, the venae cavae or the right atrium is cannulated to provide for the return of systemic venous blood to the pump-oxygenator. A Tygon tube fitted with a metal basket at the end serves well as a venous cannula in adults and large children. For smaller patients, its relatively large wall thickness–to–lumen ratio is unfavorable and the thin-walled Rygg right-angled cannulae* are preferred. In either case, cannulae with relatively large internal diameters are used, their exact size being determined by the maximal perfusion flow rate to be used for that patient (Table 29–2). This is to assure as low a venous pressure as is possible during bypass. When two or more venous cannulae are used, they are joined to the large single venous line to the pump-oxygenator by a Y connector fitted with a Luer lock adapter. Through this, air is aspirated separately from each venous line before bypass is established.

When both venae cavae are to be cannulated, we insert the cannula for the inferior vena cava through a stab wound in the center of a previously placed purse-string suture in the anterior aspect of the right atrium a little cephalad of the orifice of the inferior vena cava (Fig. 29–2). The cannula is advanced about

*THI Aortic Perfusion Cannula, Med-Science Electronics, Inc., St. Louis, Missouri.

*Manufactured by Polystan, distributed by Sherwood Medical Industries, Inc., St. Louis, Missouri.

TABLE 29–2.   VENOUS CANNULAE CHART

TOTAL FLOW (LITERS/MIN.)	SINGLE TYGON CANNULA	TWO TYGON CANNULAE	DOUBLE RYGG CANNULAE
<0.7	—	—	4 mm.
0.7 –0.9	3/16 in.	—	4 mm.
0.91–1.75	4/16 in.	3/16 in.	5 mm.
1.76–2.2	4/16 in.	4/16 in.	6 mm.
2.21–2.8	5/16 in.	4/16 in.	6 mm.
2.81–3.2	5/16 in.	5/16 in.	6 mm.
3.21–3.7	6/16 in.	5/16 in.	7 mm.
>3.7	7/16 in.	6/16 in.	7 mm.

1 to 2 cm. into the inferior vena cava. The cannula for the superior vena cava is placed through the right atrial appendage, around which a purse-string suture has been placed. When a persistent left superior vena cava is also present, we cannulate it unless it is very small, although we know that some surgeons do not do so. For this, usually a Tygon cannula is inserted into the right atrium through the atrial appendage (the superior vena cava is cannulated through a lateral atrial stab wound in such circumstances) and passed into the

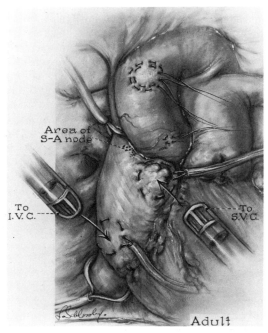

Figure 29–2. Purse-string sutures are in position on the ascending aorta for insertion of arterial cannula and for later insertion of needle vent, around the right atrial appendage for insertion of superior vena caval (SVC) cannula, and low on the right atrium for insertion of inferior vena caval (IVC) cannula. Note the area of the sinoatrial (SA) node, which must be avoided in placing purse-string sutures and cannulating.

coronary sinus and then into the left superior vena cava. In some patients, we cannulate the left superior vena cava directly with a Rygg cannula.

In patients undergoing isolated aortic valve replacement, a single venous cannula is placed in the right atrium through the atrial appendage. When the Kyoto-Barratt-Boyes technique of profound hypothermia (Hikasa *et al.,* 1967; Barratt-Boyes *et al.,* 1971), limited cardiopulmonary bypass, and total circulatory arrest is used (in infants less than about 3 months of age, or in older infants with three venae cavae), a single venous cannula is inserted into the right atrium.

For the operation of interatrial transposition of venous return (Mustard's operation), the superior vena cava and inferior vena cava are cannulated directly. The inferior vena caval cannula is inserted through a stab wound in the right atrium at the caval-atrial junction. The superior caval cannulation is through a silk purse-string suture placed as a narrow ellipse, rather than a circle, whose long axis is parallel to that of the cava. We use a similar superior vena caval cannulation for repair of the sinus venosus type of atrial septal defect.

Intracardiac Suction Devices. Suction lines are required to aspirate blood from the opened heart and return it to the pump oxygenator as part of the venous return, and to decompress the heart (particularly the left side) when needed. Therefore, just after establishing cardiopulmonary bypass for most operations, a Tygon tube (2/16- or 3/16-inch internal diameter, depending on the amount of anticipated intracardiac return) or a Rygg right-angled catheter (4- or 5-mm. internal diameter) is inserted into the left atrium. We insert this through a small stab wound, protected by a purse-string suture, in the right side of the left atrium or in the anterior wall of the superior pulmonary vein near the left atrium (Fig. 29–3). For some operations (primarily aortic valve replacement), the venting catheter is advanced through the mitral valve into the left ventricle. Gentle suction is applied to the vent, ideally by a regulated vacuum system but in practice by a well-controlled occlusive pump.

For aspirating blood from the opened heart, a special sucker is used that has a guard over the tip to minimize the tendency of leaflet and other intracardiac tissue to be drawn up into the sucker. This is used as a sump drain and therefore functions best when positioned in a pool of blood in a dependent portion of the opened heart. The sucker is attached to one of the intracardiac return lines, again activated by a well-controlled occlusive pump.

A suction line is also used for evacuating air from the cardiac chambers and ascending aorta just before the termination of cardiopulmonary bypass. For this, one of the suction lines referred to above is attached to a 15- or 18-gauge needle, which is inserted into a cardiac chamber or the aorta for this purpose.

The intracardiac suction system is recognized to be the most traumatic to blood of any part of the apparatus for cardiopulmonary bypass (Osborn *et al.,*

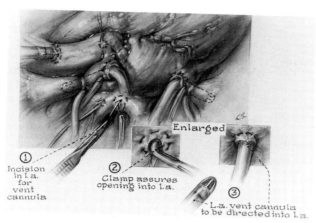

Figure 29–3. Insertion of left atrial (l.a.) vent catheter. *(1)* A stab incision is made in the center of the previously placed purse-string suture. *(2)* A clamp enlarges the incision. Care must be taken that the incision goes through the endocardium and that the clamp penetrates into the atrium as it is spread. *(3)* The vent cannula is inserted.

1962). The trauma can be minimized if the pumps or other activating mechanisms are run so that only the exact amount of suction required is exerted. The blood returned by the suction devices usually has more debris than that returning through the venous lines, and, therefore, an efficient minipore filter is interposed between the suction line and the oxygenator.

EXTERNALLY CONTROLLED VARIABLES DURING CARDIOPULMONARY BYPASS

Total Systemic Blood Flow (Perfusion Flow Rate). During total CPB, the systemic blood flow ($\dot{Q}$) is under the control of the perfusionist. This can be set at an arbitrary level or may be determined by the venous return from the patient ("pump back all that is received"). We believe it is rational to set it at an arbitrary flow rate.

The *optimal flow rate* during CPB is still being debated. A few facts are clear. Acidosis with increased lactic acid production, low oxygen consumption, and the other features of cardiogenic shock result from normothermic CPB at flows of less than about 1.6 L./min./M.² (or less than about 50 ml./kg./min.) (Diesh *et al.,* 1957). Animal experiments and our clinical data (Levin *et al.,* 1960; Moffitt *et al.,* 1962) and experience indicate that, at normothermia, flows over about 1.8 L./min./M.² are quite acceptable with regard to total-body oxygen consumption, but that flows of 2.2 to 2.5 L./min./M.² are more securely adequate. During hypothermic perfusions, "adequate" or "acceptable" flow rates are somewhat lower (Fig. 29–4).

The best criterion of "acceptability" or "adequacy" of flow rate at any temperature is the survival of the subject without structural or functional evidence of organ or system damage. Just as in total circulatory arrest, this is no doubt a probability phenomenon, with no precise predictors or criteria of adequacy other

than this. We believe survival without damage is most likely to occur when the entire microcirculation is perfused at flows that maintain near-normal tissue oxygen levels. In man on bypass, this probably pertains when whole-body oxygen consumption ($\dot{V}O_2$) is near (± 85 per cent of) the asymptote of the temperature-specific curve relating flow to $\dot{V}O_2$ (represented by the x's in Figure 29–4).

As might be expected, high flow is achieved at the expense of some loss of safety and convenience in other variables. Blood trauma in the oxygenator is probably greater when high blood flows pass through it, and with a bubble oxygenator, the risks of gaseous emboli are also greater. The pressure gradients across the arterial cannula are greater at high flows. This increases cavitation, and thus blood trauma, and the risk of bubbles forming as blood emerges from the cannula.

In clinical practice, when body temperature is at 28° C. or above, we usually choose a flow of 2.5 L./min./M.² for infants and children less than about 4 years of age, and one of 2.2 L./min./M.² for older patients. For very large adults with a body surface area of 2.0 M.² or more, we usually select a flow of 1.8 to 2.0 L./min./M.², in order to avoid the disadvantage of high flows through the oxygenator. Lower flows are chosen when body temperature is lower (see Fig. 29–4).

Temperature of the Perfusate and the Patient. Since the introduction by Ivan Brown of an efficient heat exchanger for extracorporeal circulation (Brown *et al.,* 1958), the temperature of the perfusate and, secondarily, that of the patient have been under the control of the perfusionist. This has come to be one of the most important decisions to be made about CPB for each patient. The potential surgical flexibility of CPB is achieved only when it is combined with hypothermia.

In deciding on the temperature of the patient

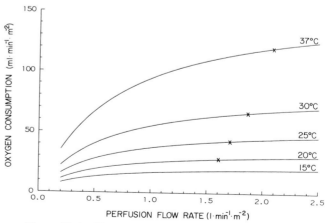

Figure 29–4. Nomogram of an equation, expressing the relation of oxygen consumption ($\dot{V}O_2$) to perfusion flow rate ($\dot{Q}$) and temperature (T). The small x's represent the perfusion flow rates used by us at these temperatures. The equation is:
$$1/\dot{V}O_2 = 0.168 \cdot 10^{-0.387 \cdot T} + 0.0378 \cdot \dot{Q}^{-1} \cdot 10^{-0.0253 \cdot T}$$

during CPB, several facts need to be considered. Somewhat lower CPB flow rates can be used at low temperatures. Because of the coronary collateral circulation, some of the perfusate reaches the heart and affects its temperature, even when the aorta is cross-clamped. Thus, after cold cardioplegia, the heart has a tendency to return to the temperature of the body around it. The patient's body temperature is related to the "safe" total circulatory arrest time that is available. If the nasopharyngeal temperature is, for example, 28° C., 10 to 15 minutes of circulatory arrest are available for repair of a split arterial pump tube or electrical or mechanical pump-oxygenator failure or to improve surgical exposure. Another fact to be considered is that longer rewarming times are required when hypothermia is profound.

At the University of Alabama at Birmingham (UAB) we use profound hypothermia (20° to 25° C.) in nearly all CPB procedures. We do this partly for reasons concerned with myocardial preservation and partly for the flexibility of profound hypothermia with regard to low flow and total circulatory arrest.

Arterial Input Pressure Wave Form. The most commonly used type of arterial pump is the roller pump (originally used by DeBakey for blood transfusion [DeBakey, 1934]). It generates a relatively *nonpulsatile flow*, and the relatively narrow orifice of the arterial cannula tends to depulse the inflow still further.

A *pulsatile arterial input* can be achieved in several ways. When the atrial pressures, and thus ventricular filling pressures, are increased by increasing the patient's blood volume (with no tapes around the caval cannulae, arterial inflow to the patient is temporarily increased over venous return from the patient; or venous return is temporarily reduced below arterial input by partially occluding the venous line), and cardiac function is good, left ventricular ejection augments systemic blood flow and produces a pulsatile arterial blood flow; in other words, pulsation is achieved by substituting partial CPB. We use this during cooling and rewarming whenever possible. A pulsatile wave form can also be produced by using intra-aortic balloon pulsation during bypass (Pappas *et al.*, 1975). A third method is the use of a pulsatile type of arterial pump.

The effect on the patient of using a system that results in a *pulsatile* (vs. a nonpulsatile) *arterial wave form* during CPB has been controversial since clinical CPB began.

Systemic Venous Pressure. Systemic venous pressure in the patient during cardiopulmonary bypass is determined by the cannulation methods used (Kirklin and Theye, 1962), since

$$\bar{P}v_{sys} = f \frac{\dot{Q}, \text{ viscosity, venous line suction}}{\text{Cannula size, venous line size}} \quad (1)$$

where $\bar{P}v_{sys}$ = the mean systemic venous pressure, and $\dot{Q}$ = the systemic blood flow. The cross-sectional area of the single or multiple venous cannulae and

their length and, to a lesser extent (because it usually has a large diameter), that of the venous line to the pump-oxygenator are the fixed factors determining venous pressure during total CPB. For this reason, we use the largest venous cannulae that are compatible with the clinical situation. When smaller cannulae must be used, the other variables in equation 1 can be manipulated (for example, the systemic blood flow may be reduced) to assure an acceptable venous pressure.

There is no apparent physiologic advantage in having a central venous pressure above zero during cardiopulmonary bypass. Raising the venous pressure requires more intravascular volume and often an additional priming volume. We prefer to keep the venous pressure close to zero, and certainly not above 10 mm. Hg, in order to minimize increases in extracellular fluid.

Pulmonary Venous (Left Atrial) Pressure. Ideally, this should be at zero during total cardiopulmonary bypass, and certainly not above 10 mm. Hg. Undue elevations are dangerous, because they tend to produce increased extravascular lung water and eventually pulmonary edema, according to Starling's law of transcapillary fluid exchange:

$$p_c - p_t = \pi_c - \pi_t \quad (2)$$

where p_c = "effective" blood pressure within the capillary; p_t = "tissue turgor pressure" (interstitial fluid pressure); π_c = osmotic pressure of the plasma (colloid) inside the capillary; and π_t = osmotic pressure of the extracellular fluid (tissue colloid osmotic pressure). The increase in extracellular lung water is related to the duration of elevation of pulmonary venous or pulmonary capillary pressure, other things being equal.

Hematocrit of the Mixed Patient and Pump-Oxygenator Blood Volume. This is determined by the composition and amounts of blood and fluids infused before and during CPB, the blood loss, and the amount and composition of the initial (priming) volume of the pump-oxygenator. The hematocrit is also affected by patient interactions, primarily transcapillary movement of fluid from the intravascular to the interstitial space and into urine volume.

In intact man at 37° C., the normal hematocrit of 0.40 to 0.50 is optimal for oxygen transport (Chien, 1972). This provides sufficient oxygen delivery to maintain normal mitochondrial P_{O_2} levels of about 0.05 to 1.0 mm. Hg and average intracellular P_{O_2} levels of about 5 mm. Hg, these being reflected in normal oxygen levels ($P\bar{v}_{O_2}$ of about 40 mm. Hg, $S\bar{v}_{O_2}$ of about 75 per cent) in mixed venous blood. The normal hematocrit is optimal rheologically in intact man as well (Chien, 1972). When the hematocrit is abnormally high, oxygen content is high, but the increased viscosity tends to decrease blood flow. Thus, the rate of oxygen transport varies directly with hematocrit (because oxygen content varies directly with hematocrit, assuming normal red cell hemoglobin concentrations and adequate oxygenation) and inversely with the blood's (apparent) viscosity (which is also determined primarily by hematocrit). Hypothermia increases the blood's (apparent) viscosity, so that at low temperatures, a lower hematocrit is more appropriate than that at 37° C.

A hematocrit *less* than "normal" appears desirable during hypothermic CPB because of its association with lower apparent blood viscosity and low shear rates, thus presumably resulting in better perfusion of the microcirculation. Thus, a hematocrit of about 0.25 is desirable during moderately hypothermic perfusions, and one of about 0.20 during profoundly hypothermic CPB. During rewarming, a higher hematocrit (≥ 0.30) is desirable because of the increased oxygen demands, and the higher apparent viscosity at these higher hematocrits is quite appropriate during normothermia. In fact, the body's autoregulatory mechanisms, including its capacity to recover from transient abnormalities in oxygen delivery, are so well developed that a considerable range (± 0.05) of hematocrits around the desirable point are quite acceptable. This is fortunate, for otherwise the need for homologous blood, with its own economic and medical disadvantages, in the priming volume would be increased. Since at our institution essentially all of our CPB procedures are done with profound hypothermia (20° to 25° C.), we accept an initial hematocrit of 0.20 to 0.25. Thus, we calculate the mixed patient-machine hematocrit that will result if the pump-oxygenator is primed with an asanguineous solution, using equations (3) and (4).

where Hct_{p-m} = hematocrit of combined patient-machine blood volume, and BV = blood volume. Therefore, when no blood is in the priming volume:

$$Hct_{p-m} = \frac{[\text{Body Weight (kg.)} \cdot f \cdot 1000] [Hct_p]}{[\text{Body weight (kg.)} \cdot f \cdot 1000] + \text{machine BV}}$$

(4)

where f = 0.08 in infants and children (≤ 12 years), and f = 0.065 in older patients (> 12 years).* If the calculated hematocrit is in the desired range, the clear priming solution is used. About 20 per cent of the priming solution is 5 per cent dextrose and 80 per cent balanced salt solution with enough concentrated human albumin added to make it colloidally iso-osmotic. If the calculated hematocrit is too low, an appropriate amount of blood is added.

"Banked blood" less than about 48 hours old is used, but we accept older blood for adults when necessary. The blood has, of course, been rendered Ca^{++}-free by the anticoagulant solution and is acidotic,

---

*These are average values and provide a method of estimating blood volume. More complex regression equations are available for more precise estimates.

TABLE 29–3. ADDITIVES TO A UNIT OF CPD BLOOD FOR THE PUMP-OXYGENATOR

CPD Blood	500 ml.
Heparin	3 ml. (3000 units — mean 6 units/ml. of blood)
$NaHCO_3$ (8.4%)	10 ml.
$CaCl_2$ (10%)	5 ml. (added last)
	568 ml.

so that additions of heparin, calcium, and buffer are made (Table 29–3).

Albumin Concentration in the Mixed Patient and Pump-Oxygenator Blood Volume. This is also affected by the amount of hemodilution. Theoretically, according to equation 2, a reduction of albumin, and thus of the colloidal osmotic pressure of the plasma, accentuates movement of fluid out of the vascular space into the interstitial space, and we believe that this does occur. Cohn and colleagues showed that the extracellular fluid volume increases more rapidly when hemodilution is used than when it is not. We have felt that during long periods of cardiopulmonary bypass with hemodilution, more volume additions are required when albumin is not added to produce more or less normal colloidal osmotic pressure than when it is. This is presumably the result of transcapillary fluid loss (and, to some extent, urinary losses). However, the adaptiveness of the patient allows these transient abnormalities to be well tolerated in most cases.

We add enough concentrated serum albumin to the balanced salt solution in the priming volume to make it approximately colloidally iso-osmotic. We believe this to be particularly important in infants.

Glucose Concentration. At UAB, where no mannitol is used in the priming solution, the glucose concentration (350 mg. per cent) is deliberately raised to promote osmotic diuresis during and for a few hours after operation and to provide a source of energy.

Ionic Composition of the Perfusate. The perfusate should have an ionic composition similar to that of plasma. Thus, our vehicle for hemodilution is a balanced salt solution with a relatively normal pH.

Arterial Oxygen Levels. With present-day bubble and membrane oxygenators, maintenance of an arterial oxygen pressure (Pa_{O_2}) of about 250 mm. Hg is easily accomplished and can be considered optimal. A higher Pa_{O_2} is unnecessary and theoretically subjects the patient to the risk of oxygen toxicity and bubble formation. A Pa_{O_2} lower than about 85 mm. Hg results in a rather rapidly declining arterial oxygen content (according to the oxygen dissociation curve of the blood) and a corresponding reduction of tissue and mixed

---

$$Hct_{p-m} = \frac{\text{Patient red cell volume (ml.)} + \text{machine red blood cell volume (ml.)}}{\text{patient BV} + \text{machine BV (ml.)}}$$

(3)

venous oxygen levels. Shepard (1973) showed in dogs that when during normothermic CPB arterial oxygen saturation fell below 65 per cent, total-body oxygen consumption fell. This indicates hypoxic cell damage.

The temperature of the patient, related as it is to whole-body oxygen consumption ($\dot{V}_{O_2}$), affects arterial oxygen levels with any given oxygenator at any given blood and gas flow rate. A reduction of the patient's body temperature reduces $\dot{V}_{O_2}$ and increases $P\bar{v}_{O_2}$, both resulting, in this setting, in increased Pa_{O_2}. During rewarming by perfusion from the pump-oxygenator, increasing $\dot{V}_{O_2}$, due presumably in part to the oxygen debt that has accumulated, results in relatively low mixed venous oxygen levels and relatively high $\dot{V}_{O_2}$ (Theye and Kirklin, 1963; Theye et al., 1962a, 1962b). This period, then, determines the requirements on the oxygenator with regard to oxygen transfer capacity for any given patient (Levin et al., 1960; Theye et al., 1962a, 1962b).

Arterial Carbon Dioxide Pressure. We believe that an arterial carbon dioxide pressure (Pa_{CO_2}) between 30 and 40 mm. Hg (measured at 37° C.) is desirable during CPB. As in the lungs of intact man, this is determined by the ratio of gas flow to blood flow in the oxygenator (Hallowell *et al.*, 1967), higher ratios resulting in lower Pa_{CO_2}. Present-day bubble and membrane oxygenators ventilated appropriately give a Pa_{CO_2} within this range.

Optimal Pa_{CO_2} during profound hypothermia is controversial, in part because of the effect of Pa_{CO_2} on arterial pH. Reeves (1976a, 1976b), Rahn and colleagues (1975), and Swan (1974) have emphasized that at low temperatures *neutrality* is associated with a higher pH than at normothermia because of the change in the dissociation constant of water. They argue that during CPB, when the perfusate temperature and the patient's nasopharyngeal temperature are 20° C., the Pa_{CO_2} measured at 37° C. should be 30 to 40 mm. Hg, which indicates a Pa_{CO_2} of about 14 to 20 mm. Hg at 20° C. (by the Reeves correction [Reeves, 1976a, 1976b]) and that pH measured at 37° C. should be about 7.38, which indicates a pH of about 7.6 at 20° C. (by the Rosenthal correction [Rosenthal, 1948]). When CO_2 has been added to the ventilatory mixture during cooling for profound hypothermia (in the belief that brain cooling would be more rapid because of the assumed increase in cerebral blood flow), too acidotic a milieu develops, according to this concept. Instead, Rahn and associates (1975) believe that *relative* hyperventilation should be practiced

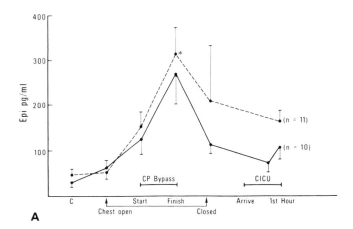

A

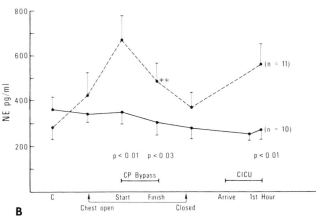

B

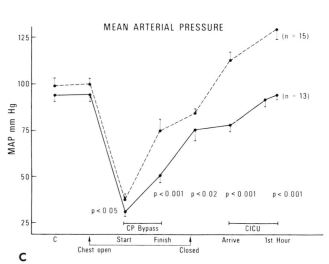

C

Figure 29–5. Studies in patients undergoing CPB for coronary artery bypass grafting at various stages of the operation and early postoperative period. *A*, Plasma epinephrine levels (mean ± standard error) in patients who were normotensive early postoperatively (solid line) and those who were hypertensive (dotted line). *B*, Plasma norepinephrine levels (solid and dotted lines represent same as in *A*,). *C*, Mean arterial blood pressure (solid and dotted lines represent same as in *A*).

during hypothermic CPB, so that Pa_{CO_2} will be below 40 mm. Hg and the milieu alkalotic. This can be accomplished by maintaining the ratio of gas flow to blood flow constant during cooling and *not* adding CO_2 to the ventilatory mixture. CO_2 production falls as the patient cools, and relative hyperventilation results. At UAB, these principles are followed.

PATIENT RESPONSES TO CARDIOPULMONARY BYPASS

The patient response to CPB involves the entire body, is complex, and almost defies complete description because of gaps in our knowledge. Part of this is in response to the damaging effects of cardiopulmonary bypass and is described later under that heading. Part of the response becomes apparent only in the postoperative period. Here we describe some of the easily categorized responses during operation.

Systemic Vascular Resistance. At the onset of normothermic or moderately hypothermic CPB, systemic vascular resistance usually falls abruptly. After that, it gradually rises throughout the period of CPB. There is considerable variation from patient to patient in the systemic vascular resistance, and thus in the systemic arterial blood pressure, during perfusion. Patients with coronary artery disease tend particularly to develop a high systemic vascular resistance during CPB (Wallach *et al.*, 1980). When profound hyperthermia is produced during CPB, systemic vascular resistance usually falls more than during normothermic or moderately hypothermic bypass.

The advisability of pharmacologically manipulating the systemic vascular resistance during CPB has been extensively debated. Some evidence indicates that cerebral blood flow is lower than is desirable when mean arterial blood pressure during normothermic or moderately hypothermic CPB falls below about 55 mm. Hg. Therefore, when it is lower than that for more than a few minutes during rewarming, we generally pharmacologically increase systemic vascular resistance and thus arterial blood pressure. This, in turn, provides more adequate coronary blood flow. Increasing the perfusion flow rate above the usual values during rewarming is quite ineffective in increasing arterial pressure. When systemic vascular resistance during this phase of CPB becomes so high that mean arterial blood pressure rises above 100 mm. Hg, we believe it prudent to reduce it pharmacologically below that level.

Total-Body Oxygen Consumption. Although total-body oxygen consumption ($\dot{V}o_2$) is to a great extent determined by the perfusion flow rate and the patient's temperature during CPB, the patient's biologic response is also a factor. Its exact nature has not been completely determined.

Mixed Venous Oxygen Levels. Although mixed venous oxygen levels are related to the controlled variables of perfusion flow rate, the hemoglobin concentration of the perfusate, and the arterial oxygen tension, they are also related to the patient's response in terms of $\dot{V}o_2$. In addition, they are related to some partially controlled variables that probably affect $\dot{V}o_2$, such as 2,3-DPG levels in the red blood cells and pH. These former interrelations are expressed by the Fick equation.

When most of the microcirculation is known to be perfused, mixed venous oxygen levels reflect some sort of mean value for tissue oxygen levels. Thus, the assumption can be made that when mixed venous oxygen levels during CPB are relatively normal ($P\bar{v}_{O_2}$ of 30 to 40 mm. Hg, $S\bar{v}_{O_2}$ of 60 to 70 per cent and total-body oxygen consumption is relatively normal, tissue oxygen levels are relatively normal and the whole-body perfusion is meeting the patient's metabolic demands.

Metabolic Acidosis. Metabolic acidosis, primarily from lactic acidemia, is well known to complicate many situations characterized by acute reductions of systemic blood flow rate, including CPB. There is always a steady and significant increase in blood lactate concentration during an operation with CPB, but when the recommended criteria are followed in setting perfusion flow rates, this concentration never exceeds 5 mmol./L. in our experience (Harris *et al.*, 1970).

Catecholamine Response. The response of circulating epinephrine (released primarily from the adrenal medulla), norepinephrine (which overflows into the bloodstream from generalized sympathetic nervous system discharge), and dopamine to CPB has been studied by many groups, with somewhat conflicting results (Harris, 1973; Hine *et al.*, 1976; Philbin *et al.*, 1979; Turley *et al.*, 1979; Tan *et al.*, 1976). Recent studies at UAB suggest that investigations that failed to show increases probably suffered from methodological problems.

Wallach and colleagues (1980) at UAB have recently studied these responses in a group of patients undergoing coronary artery bypass grafting. The responses are probably similar in all patients undergoing CPB. With the onset of CPB, plasma epinephrine levels increased in all patients and began to decline after bypass (Fig. 29-5A). Persisting elevation 1 hour after operation occurred only in patients with postoperative hypertension. In contrast, norepinephrine levels did not rise in patients who remained normotensive postoperatively but did increase in those with postoperative hypertension at the start of operation, to reach a peak at the start of CPB (Fig. 29-5B). It remained elevated at 1 hour postoperatively in this group. These patients showed blood pressure responses typical for patients undergoing CPB, with a striking fall at the onset of CPB from reduced systemic arteriolar resistance (Fig. 29-C). Mean blood pressure 1 hour after operation correlated positively and significantly with both plasma epinephrine and norepinephrine levels.

The sympathetic-adrenal system discharge during, and in some patients after, CPB is presumably related to the damaging effects of CPB. Part of the catecholamine increase, particularly that of norepinephrine, is due to the fact that during CPB blood does not pass through the lungs, where the norepinephrine is largely inactivated (Reves *et al.*, 1982).

THE DAMAGING EFFECTS OF CARDIOPULMONARY BYPASS

"*Safe*" CPB is characterized by the absence of structural or functional damage after the perfusion. Paradoxically, detailed information about these parameters is currently more complete following profound hypothermic circulation arrest procedures than following conventional CPB. We do know, of course, that thousands of patients have no apparent ill effects from CPB, but few specific studies of organ function have been made. Walker and colleagues (unpublished data) at UAB have found no change in the intelligence quotient and Intellectual Performance Tests before and 1 week after coronary artery bypass grafting using CPB. In general, however, the conclusion that CPB is "safe" has not been rigorously supported.

The apparent safety of CPB is clearly constrained by some incremental risk factors. One is the *duration of perfusion*; in adults, the probability of structural or functional damage seems to increase as the perfusion extends beyond 3 hours. Another is the *age of the patient*, with damage seeming to increase in patients under 6 months of age and even more so in those under 3 months old (Kirklin, 1979); this is probably also true in the elderly. These two risk factors probably interact, for in small infants, CPB may produce damage after 1 or 2 hours rather than after 3. Other factors include the *perfusion flow rate*, the *composition of the perfusate*, the *oxygenating surface*, and the *temperature of the patient*. These, and no doubt other variables, relate to and interact with the duration of perfusion and the age of the patient and influence the probability of absence of functional or structural damage. All these factors must determine the probability of "safe CPB" in a continuously variable way, as is described by the logistic equation, but unfortunately, in contrast to total circulatory arrest, we do not have the data even to estimate the nomograms of the equations describing these curves.

As a substitute for these more desirable analyses, we can define only the "adequacy" of certain parameters (such as perfusion flow rate and total-body oxygen consumption) and, for the moment, assume that this improves the probability of safe CPB. We can also describe some of the damaging effects of CPB about which we have knowledge and begin to relate these to hospital morbidity and mortality and to the presence or absence of temporary or permanent functional and structural damage. In this way, we can learn to understand better the abnormal state of CPB and to increase its safety in circumstances currently associated with increased risk. Most such studies of the ill effects of cardiopulmonary bypass merely document that these effects exist without elucidating the basic mechanisms involved. As a result, both prevention and treatment remain largely empirical.

During clinical cardiopulmonary bypass, the most obvious possible mechanisms for damage are *exposure of blood to various abnormal events* and *altered arterial blood flow patterns*. The complexity of the situation is aggravated by the interactions between these. We believe the first of these, the exposure of blood to abnormal events, is the most generalized and the most powerful in its effects on the patient, and it is therefore the one that we will discuss.

The damage is manifested after CPB by an abnormal tendency to bleed externally and also into tissues; a diffuse or whole-body "inflammatory reaction," characterized by increased capillary permeability with consequent transcapillary plasma loss, increased interstitial fluid, leukocytosis, and fever; peripheral and perhaps central vasoconstriction, which persists for a variable time after CPB and results in both hemodynamic and metabolic problems; and breakdown of red blood cells, resulting in hemoglobinemia, hemoglobinuria, and anemia. This results in variable organ dysfunction and has been referred to as a "postperfusion syndrome" or "postpump syndrome." The fact that most patients convalesce normally after CPB attests only to the patient's ability to compensate for these damaging phenomena and not to their absence. The uncommon occurrence of such changes as severe pulmonary edema without elevated left atrial pressure, severe bleeding diatheses, and transient subtle neurologic changes occasionally brings these abnormalities of CPB forcefully to our attention. Much of the current residual morbidity and mortality from open heart operations is secondary to these poorly understood changes produced by CPB.

Exposure of Blood to Abnormal Events

Blood is a complex substance containing formed elements (red blood cells, white blood cells, and platelets) and unformed elements. Among the latter, the plasma proteins are particularly vulnerable. They can be divided into those with *primarily osmotic effects* (albumin), those that are *carrier vehicles* for other blood borne substances (albumin, lipoproteins, immunoglobulins), and those that are part of the *humoral amplification systems** (coagulation, fibrinolytic, complement, and kallikrein-bradykinin cascades).

Blood's nonphysiologic experiences during CPB include *exposure to unphysiologic* (i.e., nonendothelial) *surfaces, exposure to shear stresses,* and *incorporation of abnormal substances* such as bubbles, fibrin particles, and aggregates of platelets. Again, the effects of these result from their interaction.

Humoral amplification systems are those in which a small stimulus results in a self-perpetuating and ever-widening response in the system. Generally, in intact man, these are triggered and are active in a localized area, such as a burn, an area of peritonitis, or a wound. CPB is perhaps the only situation in which the whole body is exposed directly to the results of activation of these substances. In hemodialysis, in which the blood is returned to a large vein, only the heart and lungs are exposed directly.

Exposure of Blood to Unphysiologic Surfaces

The damage produced by contact of blood with a nonendothelial surface is, other things being equal, greater the larger the proportion of blood in the boundary layer where surface effects occur. Thus, the most critical surfaces are those of the oxygenating area, where a relatively large proportion of blood is deliberately maneuvered into the boundary layer for gas exchange. In bubble, disc, and screen oxygenators, the unphysiologic surface is gas (generally 100 per cent O_2). In membrane oxygenators, the surface is generally the membrane. However, studies (Ward *et al.*, 1974) have shown that microbubbles of air have a strong tendency to cling to the membrane surface, so that the unphysiologic surface is more complex than expected. Next are the unphysiologic surfaces of the heat exchanger, where a large proportion of blood is present in the boundary layer for heat exchange, and those of the various defoaming, debubbling, and filtering devices. The proportion of blood in the boundary layer is quite small in the reservoirs, tubes, and cannula, and thus, these surfaces should be expected to be the least critical.

The unphysiologic surfaces have direct and indirect effects on *platelets,* which result in platelet clumps that may embolize, a reduction in the number of platelets, and a reduction simultaneously in their important adhesive and aggregating properties (as measured by their response to adenosine diphosphate [ADP], epinephrine, or collagen). Platelet thrombi have been demonstrated in membrane oxygenators by Edmunds and colleagues (1978). Many studies have documented the reduction in the number of circulating platelets after CPB. For example, Kalter and colleagues (1979), using a bubble oxygenator, observed a decrease from a mean preoxygenation platelet count of 222,100 mm.[3] to a postoxygenation one of 85,000 mm.[3]. Han and associates (1980) report a platelet count of 210,950 mm.[3] before bypass and one of 138,000 mm.[3] after it. The decrease did not correlate with the duration of CPB. These and other workers (Addonizio *et al.*, 1979c; Friedenberg *et al.*, 1978) have shown a significant deterioration in function in the platelets that remain, as demonstrated by a decrease in platelet aggregation in response to ADP (Bharadwaj and Chong, 1980).

Platelets are apparently not reduced in either number or function by shear stresses per se (Addonizio *et al.*, 1979a; Solen *et al.*, 1978; Tamari *et al.*, 1975). Indeed, there is no evidence to indicate that platelets are destroyed in any important quantity during CPB. Rather, the decrease in their number is due to clumping on the foreign surfaces in response to the "invasion" of the body's integrity and to the finite number of replacement platelets that are available. This unwanted stimulation of clumping on foreign surfaces apparently also depletes granule-stored aggregating protein in the surviving platelets, which also adversely affects their adhesiveness (Addonizio *et al.*, 1980). The severe reduction in the number of normally functioning platelets is probably the most important factor in the postoperative bleeding diathesis produced by CPB.

Prevention of platelet damage and depletion could theoretically be accomplished by reducing the platelet-stimulating properties of the nonbiologic surface or by making the platelets reversibly nonfunctional during CPB so that they do not adhere and aggregate. Addonizio and colleagues (1979a) have shown that the former can to some extent be accomplished by "coating" the membrane oxygenator surfaces with albumin. They and others have also conducted investigations suggesting the feasibility and usefulness of rendering the platelets reversibly nonfunctional by infusing prostaglandins (prostaglandin E_1 and prostacyclins) during CPB (Addonizio *et al.*, 1979a, 1979b, 1979c; Addonizio *et al.*, 1978).

Exposure of the blood to unphysiologic surfaces probably has some effect on *leukocytes,* but shear stresses probably have the most important effect.

Damage to erythrocytes, either from direct cell fragmentation or from alterations of the cellular membrane and later cell fragmentation, results in liberation of hemoglobin into the plasma. This is generally estimated by measuring serum hemoglobin levels. The damage is produced mainly by shear forces (see following discussion), but also to some extent by exposure of blood in the boundary layer to nonbiologic surfaces (Solen *et al.*, 1978).

The *carrier proteins* are significantly damaged by exposure of blood to nonbiologic surfaces. Lee and colleagues (1961) showed many years ago that protein denaturation occurred in oxygenators, with the lipoproteins liberating free fat in the process. Fat microemboli result. During CPB for cardiac surgery, the large globules of free fat seen on the surface of the intracardiac or intrapericardial blood pool result from this change. Because of protein denaturation, plasma viscosity is increased, which, no doubt, has other widespread effects. The denatured proteins are also believed to increase the clumping of red cells, which makes them more likely to be traumatized by shear forces.

The carrier gamma globulins are denatured at the foreign interface, especially when it is a blood-gas interface (Pruit *et al.*, 1971; Scott, 1970). The magnitude of this is related to the proportion of the plasma in the boundary layer and also to the concentration of gamma globulin. The latter argues for hemodilution during CPB. This denaturation seems to be less in the presence of albumin. In addition to the mechanical effects, denaturation of gamma globulins may contribute to the humoral and cellular immune defects that seem to be present after CPB.

Damage to the *proteins* that are *part of the humoral amplification* systems has more complex and widespread results, involving all four components of the systems. No doubt, the protein called *Hageman factor* (Factor XII) is activated (denatured or uncoiled) almost immediately after the start of CPB by the massive contact of blood in the boundary layers with nonbiologic surfaces (Feijen, 1977; Verska, 1977). (Most of the evidence for this is indirect. It includes the demonstration of fibrinopeptide A, a product of fibrinogen activation, during CPB [Davies *et al.*, 1980] and the demonstration of the presence of bradykinin and plasmin during CPB, both of which are by-products of the activation of Hageman factor.) This initiates the *cascade of the coagulation humoral amplification system* and may initiate the cascades of the other three amplification systems. Thus, even in the presence of "adequate" heparin levels during cardiopulmonary bypass, microcoagulation is continuing, generating fibrin and consuming the coagulation factors to a varying degree (Davies *et al.*, 1980; Kalter *et al.*, 1979). The demonstrated reduction of essentially all of these (except the Hageman factor) is believed to be a result of this consumption, rather than of denaturation at contact with nonendothelial surfaces. The relative degree to which various nonbiologic surfaces, including an air-blood interface, activate the coagulation cascade has not been determined in detail. Microcoagulation and consumption of coagulation factors are further aggravated by the previously described platelet adhesion, aggregation, and granule release.

The *fibrinolytic cascade,* a second humoral amplification system, is probably activated to some degree in all operations in which CPB is used (and perhaps in many in which it is not). Thus, many studies have shown an important incidence of fibrinolysis following CPB. For example, hyperfibrinolysis has been shown to be present in 159 (20 per cent) of 774 patients undergoing coronary artery bypass grafting (Lambert *et al.*, 1979). Naturally occurring plasminogen (which normally is incorporated within thrombi) can be transformed into the active fibrinolytic agent plasmin, and measurable blood plasmin levels have been demonstrated in patients shortly after initiation of CPB (Backmann *et al.*, 1975). This is believed to be in response to the disseminated microcoagulation mentioned previously. Since the conversion of plasminogen to plasmin is facilitated by kallikrein, which also results from the activation of Hageman factor, the fibrinolytic cascade may be initiated also by the activation of Factor XII. Furthermore, since plasmin also serves as an activator of complement, prekallikrein, and possibly Hageman factor, the widespread activation of plasminogen into plasmin (which in intact man is usually a circumscribed and localized phenomenon) may initiate the cascades of all the humoral amplification systems. Again, as an example of the possibly powerful effects of what in intact man are localized events occurring systemically during CPB, breakdown products of fibrinogen (produced by the coagulation cascade), when acted upon by plasmin, have been shown experimentally to produce important pulmonary dysfunction.

A *third humoral amplification system* involves *complement,* a group of circulating glycoproteins that function as a part of the body's response to various kinds of injury, such as traumatic, immunologic, or foreign-body insult. The final product of complement activation is a complex of glycoproteins (called C5 to C9) that forms on antibody at immunoglobulin-coated membranes and aids in membrane lysis and phagocytosis. The complement cascade, once activated, also results in the production of powerful *anaphylatoxins* (Hugli, 1978) (called C3a and C5a), which increase vascular permeability, cause smooth muscle contraction, mediate leukocyte chemotaxis, and facilitate leukocyte aggregation and enzyme release (Grant *et al.*, 1975; Goldstein *et al.*, 1973). The usefulness of all this as a response to localized injury is obvious, but the problems of a whole-body response to the generalized injury of cardiopulmonary bypass are also obvious. Complement activation occurs either via the classical pathway or via the so-called alternative pathway. The complement system can be activated upon contact of blood with nonbiologic surfaces, perhaps by way of Hageman factor (Factor XII), but other substances such as thrombin and plasmin can also activate it.

Complement activation during cardiopulmonary bypass was reported by Hairston and associates (1969) and by Parker and colleagues (1972) from UAB. Recent studies at UAB by Chenoweth and coworkers (1981) and Stewart and colleagues (unpublished data) have demonstrated C3a, a complement breakdown product, in blood shortly after commencing CPB for cardiac surgery, with the continuing production of this breakdown product of complement being directly related to body temperature and perfusion flow rate. Complement activation has also been demonstrated to occur during hemodialysis (Craddock *et al.*, 1977a, 1977b), seeming to result from exposure of blood to the cellophane dialysis membrane (Aljama *et al.*, 1978). Complement activation in this setting is via the alternative pathway with depletion of C3 but not C1 (Craddock *et al.*, 1977a, 1977b). During cardiopulmonary bypass with a membrane oxygenator, activation probably is also via the alternative pathway, whereas with the bubble oxygenator, it probably proceeds by the classical pathway, with depletion of C1 (Clark *et al.*, 1979).

The adverse effects of complement activation are twofold, one being the depletion of a component (complement) necessary for normal immune response, and the other being the adverse effects of the intravascular production of the anaphylatoxins (C3a and C5a). Hairston and associates (1969) showed a decreased ability of postbypass serum to inhibit the growth of certain bacteria and related this in part to complement depletion. The adverse effects of the anaphylatoxins have already been described in general. In this regard, pulmonary sequestration of polymorphonuclear leukocytes and neutropenia have been shown to develop during hemodialysis and to be temporally related to complement activation (Craddock *et al.*, 1977b). Similar observations have been made during CPB (Stewart *et al.*, unpublished data; Wilson, 1972). That these changes are functionally significant is evident from the increased alvelolar-arterial oxygen difference that develops with them during hemodialysis (Craddock *et al.*, 1977a). This all suggests that *leukocyte-mediated pulmonary endothelial injury* (see following discussion) is one of the mediators of the adverse effects of cardiopulmonary bypass on pulmonary function. Similar sequestrations may take place in other organs during CPB.

That important complement activation is dependent on a large proportion of blood in the boundary layer (such as in an oxygenator or hemodialysis coil) is evident from the demonstration by Birek and colleagues (1976) in sheep that venovenous bypass produced no adverse effects on white blood cells, platelets, or pulmonary artery pressure. Adding an oxygenator to the circuit resulted in a decrease in circulating white blood cells and in platelets (presumably from pulmonary sequestration) and a marked rise in pulmonary artery pressure. Fountain and associates (1980) showed that infusion of complement-activated plasma produced the same result.

The shear stresses of CPB are quite damaging to leukocytes, and we have already seen that the exposure to nonphysiologic surfaces has profound effects on platelets. Complement activation can be hypothesized to interact with these effects and compound them. The anaphylatoxin C5a is a stimulus to polymorphonuclear aggregation, which, with the shear stress damage, results in pulmonary sequestration of leukocytes. These shear-stressed, damaged leukocytes have unstable lysosomes (Martin, 1979), and the release of these against the pulmonary basement membrane and endothelial cells can be presumed to be damaging. Wilson (1972) has demonstrated in biopsies of human lung taken after CPB increased numbers of polymorphonuclear leukocytes adherent to pulmonary endothelium. The leukocytes have lucent cytoplasmic areas consistent with loss of lysosomal contents. Adjacent to these leukocytes are areas of endothelial and alveolar Type I cell swelling. This, as well as relative pulmonary ischemia, may result in a decrease of pulmonary *surfactant* and a strong tendency toward atelectasis (Panossian *et al.*, 1969). Tsiao and coworkers (1973) have reported similar findings in the lung and also in heart and skeletal muscle.

With regard to the interactions affecting platelets, their injury at surfaces causes them to aggregate and release vasoactive substances, a trend that is aggravated by activated complement. Aggregates of activated platelets in the lungs also give rise to pulmonary endothelial injury (Jorgensen *et al.*, 1970), which is expected to result in increased pulmonary artery pressure and pulmonary dysfunction.

A fourth humoral amplification system involves *kallikrein* and *bradykinin*. Contact activation of the Hageman factor initiates the kallikrein-bradykinin cascade, resulting in the production of bradykinin. Bradykinin increases vascular permeability, dilates arterioles, initiates smooth muscle contraction, and elicits pain. Kallikrein activates Hageman factor and activates plasminogen to form plasmin, demonstrating again the complex interactions between the various reactions of blood to a nonphysiologic experience.

Several studies using appropriate methodology have shown important amounts of bradykinin to be present during CPB (Ellison *et al.*, 1980; Friedli *et al.*, 1973; Pang *et al.*, 1979). Hypothermia itself apparently results in bradykinin production. Apparently, immaturity, such as is present in young infants, results in less effective means of bradykinin elimination (Friedli *et al.*, 1973). Exclusion of the pulmonary circulation probably also reduces the patient's ability to cope with circulating bradykinin, since the lungs are the main site of bradykinin elimination.

Nagaoka and Katori (1975) demonstrated a reduction in peripheral resistance and in fluid requirement during CPB with the administration of Trasylol. This agent is known to neutralize the kallikrein-bradykinin system.

Incorporation of Abnormal Substances

In normal intact man, blood circulates in an endothelium-lined closed system, protected against abnormal intrusions. During intracardiac operations with CPB, blood inadvertently has incorporated into it micro- and macro-bubbles of air, bits of fibrin and tissue debris, defoaming agents, and so forth. Shed blood that has made contact with injured tissues contains thromboplastinogen, a coagulation activator, and its aspiration by the pump-oxygenator sucker system must contribute to intravascular coagulation.

THE PUMP-OXYGENATOR

The apparatus available for CPB changes continually, but some general points are important.

A *venous* reservoir is generally used and is positioned to provide adequate siphonage from gravity (Paneth *et al.*, 1947). Such a reservoir allows for the escape of any air returning with the venous blood and for the storage of excess volume. Bubble oxygenators can act as a venous reservoir. A venous pump, instead of gravity drainage, can be used to move blood directly from the venae cavae into the oxygenator, but such a system requires precise control.

Bubble oxygenators are the most commonly used, and at present, we use them exclusively. They have a built-in medium-porosity mesh filter. *Membrane oxygenators* probably reduce blood trauma and should not produce emboli. They make control of Pa_{O_2} and Pa_{CO_2} during hypothermia easier. However, no clear-cut advantage of membrane over bubble oxygenators has been demonstrated, even in children (Sade *et al.*, 1980). Perhaps this is in part due to platelet adhesion in spite of the absence of a blood-gas interface (Sade *et al.*, 1980).

An efficient *heat exchanger* is necessary. This may be located within the oxygenator or freestanding. The former type tends to be less efficient.

The *arterial pump* is most commonly a roller pump. It should be adjusted before each perfusion so as to be slightly nonocclusive. The pump tubing should be Silastic or latex, for neither will become stiff at low temperatures. Other plastic tubing stiffens at low temperatures, and the recoil and thus the stroke volume of the pump and perfusion flow rate are reduced during hypothermia. The arterial pump should be calibrated at frequent intervals so that the perfusion flow rate can be accurately established.

The *arterial line pressure* in the pump-oxygenator must be continuously monitored. When this pressure becomes greater than 250 to 300 mm. Hg, the risk of disruption of the arterial line and of cavitation in the region of the arterial cannula increases. These risks are prevented by a properly positioned, adequately sized cannula.

An *arterial bubble trap* may be used as a safety device to remove air that has inadvertently entered the arterial line.

A *low-porosity arterial filter* can be used. A randomized study by Walker and colleagues (unpublished data) at UAB failed to demonstrate beneficial effects from such a filter.

The CPB circuit should contain at least two *cardiotomy suction lines* for return of blood from the opened heart. This blood contains particulate matter and air and must be passed through a low-porosity filter and defoamed in a separate chamber open to air before it is returned to the circuit. If this blood remains long in the pericardial space, it is a potent source of hemolysis. This part of the extracorporeal apparatus is the most damaging to blood. Ideally, these lines should be activated by a continuously and rapidly variable high-capacity vacuum system, but this has proved impractical, and roller pumps are therefore used. With this system, when the end of the line is blocked, the suction rapidly increases, and this may damage either the tissue or the blood. This necessitates constant supervision of the open heart roller pump rates.

The pump-oxygenator should be designed to *minimize priming volume*. This is most critical in infants, in whom the priming volume can be greatly in excess of blood volume. Nearly all infant circuits are less than optimal in this regard (Turina *et al.*, 1972).

SELECTED REFERENCES

Barratt-Boyes, B. G., Simpson, M., and Neutze, J. M.: Intracardiac surgery in neonates and infants using deep hypothermia with surface cooling and limited cardiopulmonary bypass. Circulation, *43, 44*(Suppl. 1):25, 1971.

The idea that hypothermia might permit surgeons to operate on the "bloodless heart" was suggested originally by Bigelow (Bigelow, W. G., Lindsay, W. K., and Greenwood, W. F.: Hypothermia: Its possible role in cardiac surgery: An investigation of factors governing survival in dogs at low body temperatures. Ann. Surg., *132*:849, 1950). A combined technique of hypothermia and cardiopulmonary bypass had been used by a number of groups, but a special way of using this combination for intracardiac surgery in infants was described by the Kyoto University group (Hikasa, Y., Shirotani, H., Satomura, K., Muraoka, R., Abe, K., Tsushimi, K., Yokota, Y., Miki, S., Kawai, J., Mori, A., Okamoto, Y., Koie, H., Ban, T., Kanzaki, Y., Yokota, M., Mori, C., Kamiya, T., Tamura, T., Nishii, A., and Asawa, Y.: Open heart surgery in infants with an aid of hypothermic anesthesia. Arch. Jap. Chir., *36*:495, 1967). However, this paper by Barratt-Boyes and colleagues really provided the

impetus for the present trend of primary intracardiac repair of nearly all malformations in infancy. The details of the technique of inducing deep hypothermia with surface cooling and limited cardiopulmonary bypass are described. Their clinical experience included nine babies operated on for ventricular septal defect or partial atrioventricular canal with no deaths, six babies operated on for total anomalous pulmonary venous connection with two deaths, and 15 babies operated on for tetralogy of Fallot or transposition of the great arteries with two deaths. All were younger than 20 months of age.

Chenoweth, D. E., Cooper, S. W., Hugli, T. E., Stewart, R. W., Blackstone, E. H., and Kirklin, J. W.: Complement activation during cardiopulmonary bypass: Evidence for generation of C3a and C5a anaphylatoxins. N. Engl. J. Med., *304*:497, 1981.

Cardiopulmonary bypass has become a very safe clinical tool for most good-risk patients. For example, coronary artery bypass grafting can be done with a hospital mortality of less than 1 per cent. Nevertheless, in seriously ill patients, particularly those who are very young or very old, cardiopulmonary bypass still contributes to morbidity and mortality. The damaging effects of cardiopulmonary bypass have been known for a long time, but new and powerful research tools can now be applied to the solution of these problems. This paper reports the production of anaphylatoxins, C3a and C5a, as products of complement degradation during cardiopulmonary bypass. This is the result of the exposure of blood to foreign surfaces. This study suggests a possible way in which future research may determine the causes of the unfavorable responses to cardiopulmonary bypass and methods for their prevention.

Gibbon, J. H.: Application of a mechanical heart and lung apparatus to cardiac surgery. Minn. Med., *37*:171, 1954.

In this classic paper, the originator of cardiopulmonary bypass describes the application of the heart-lung machine to cardiac surgery. This was based on basic experimental studies in dogs (Gibbon, J. H.: The maintenance of life during experimental occlusion of the pulmonary artery followed by survival. Surg. Gynecol. Obstet., *69*:602, 1939). In this paper, the author discusses the basic mechanical and physiologic problems of heart and lung machines as well as the use of intracardiac suction and left ventricular venting as methods for keeping a blood-free operating field and preventing air emboli. The problems of hemolysis and adequate blood flow to the tissues are presented. In this paper, he also describes the first patient successfully operated on with a pump-oxygenator. Dr. Gibbon concludes, "It seems to me that there will always be a place for an extracorporeal blood circuit because it permits a longer safe interval for opening the heart than can ever be obtained by any of the hypothermia methods."

Kirklin, J. W., DuShane, J. W., Patrick, R. T., Donald, D. E., Hetzel, P. S., Harshbarger, H. G., and Wood, E. H.: Intracardiac surgery with the aid of a mechanical pump-oxygenator (Gibbon type): Report of eight cases. Proc. Staff Meet. Mayo Clin., *30*:201, 1955.

This paper is the first to report a series of patients successfully undergoing intracardiac repair using a totally nonvital pump-oxygenator. At the time that this work was done, it was widely predicted that nonvital pump oxygenators could never be used for this work, and that hypothermia alone or cross-circulation (see Lillehei *et al.*) would be needed. Four patients had ventricular septal defect, and two died postoperatively. Two had atrioventricular canal, and one died. One had tetralogy of Fallot, and he died postoperatively. One 2-year-old child survived after repair of an atrial septal defect.

Lillehei, C. W., Cohen, M., Warden, H. E., and Varco, R. L.: The direct-vision intracardiac correction of congenital anomalies by controlled cross circulation. Surgery, *38*:11, 1955.

This paper describes the first series of successful intracardiac operations with cardiopulmonary bypass. The experimental and physiologic bases for the controlled cross circulation with another human being as the oxygenator (which was used in these cases and later discarded) are discussed. Certain technical considerations in intracardiac surgery are described in detail. Thirty-two patients are reviewed in the study. Twenty-two had repair of ventricular septal defect with four deaths (18 per cent mortality), six patients had tetralogy of Fallot with three deaths (50 per cent mortality), two had common atrioventricular canal with one death, and two had pulmonic stenosis with one death. This surgical group later was the first to introduce the disposable bubble-type oxygenator (Lillehei, C. W., DeWall, R. A., Read, R. C., Warden, H. E., and Varco, R. L.: Direct vision intracardiac surgery in man using a simple, disposable artificial oxygenator. Dis. Chest, 29:1, 1956), a variant of which is used by most surgeons today.

REFERENCES

Addonizio, V. P., Jr., Macarak, E. J., Nicolaou, K. C., Edmunds, L. H., Jr., and Colman, R. W.: Effects of prostacyclin and albumin on platelet loss during in vitro simulation of extracorporeal circulation. J. Am. Soc. Hematol., 53:1033, 1979a.

Addonizio, V. P., Jr., Macarak, E. J., Niewiarowski, S., Colman, R. W., and Edmunds, L. H., Jr.: Preservation of human platelets with prostaglandin E$_1$ during in vitro simulation of cardiopulmonary bypass. Circ. Res., 44:350, 1979b.

Addonizio, V. P., Jr., Smith, J. B., Strauss, J. F., III, Colman, R. W., and Edmunds, L. H., Jr.: Thromboxane synthesis and platelet secretion during cardiopulmonary bypass with bubble oxygenator. J. Thorac. Cardiovasc. Surg., 79:91, 1980.

Addonizio, V. P., Jr., Strauss, J. F., III, Colman, R. W., and Edmunds, L. H., Jr.: Effects of prostaglandin E$_1$ on platelet loss during in vivo and in vitro extracorporeal circulation with a bubble oxygenator. J. Thorac. Cardiovasc. Surg., 77:119, 1979c.

Addonizio, V. P., Jr., Strauss, J. F., III, Macarak, E. J., Colman, R. W., and Edmunds, L. H., Jr.: Preservation of platelet number and function with prostaglandin E$_1$ during total cardiopulmonary bypass in rhesus monkeys. Surgery, 83:619, 1978.

Aljama, P., Bird, P. A. E., Ward, M. K., Feest, T. G., Walker, W., Tanboga, H., Sussman, M., and Kerr, D. N. S.: Haemodialysis-induced leucopenia and activation of complement: Effects of different membranes. Proc. Eur. Dial. Transplant Assoc., 15:144, 1978.

Andreasen, A. T., and Watson, F.: Experimental cardiovascular surgery, "the azygos factor." Br. J. Surg., 39:548, 1952.

Backmann, F., McKenna, R., Cole, E. R., and Najafi, H.: The hemostatic mechanism after open-heart surgery. I. Studies on plasma coagulation factors and fibrinolysis in 512 patients after extracorporeal circulation. J. Thorac. Cardiovasc. Surg., 70:76, 1975.

Barratt-Boyes, B. G., Simpson, M., and Neutze, J. M.: Intracardiac surgery in neonates and infants using deep hypothermia with surface cooling and limited cardiopulmonary bypass. Circulation 43, 44(Suppl. 1):25, 1971.

Bharadwaj, B. B., and Chong, G.: Effects of extracorporeal circulation on structure, function, and population distribution of canine blood platelets. Presented at the Combined Meeting of the Royal Australasian College of Surgeons and Royal Australasian College of Physicians, Sydney, Australia, February 24–29, 1980.

Birek, A., Duffin, J., Glynn, M. F. X., and Cooper, J. D.: The effect of sulfinpyrazone on platelet and pulmonary responses to onset of membrane oxygenator perfusion. Trans. Am. Soc. Artif. Intern. Organs, 22:94, 1976.

Bjork, V. O.: Brain perfusions in dogs with artifically oxygenated blood. Acta Chir. Scand., 96(Suppl. 137):1, 1948.

Brown, I. W., Smith, W. W., and Emmons, W. O.: An efficient blood heat exchanger for use with extracorporeal circulation. Surgery, 44:372, 1958.

Camishion, R. C., Scicchitano, C. P., Trotta, R., and Gibbon, J. H., Jr.: Blood flow through superior mesenteric artery during retrograde perfusion. Surgery, 54:651, 1963.

Chenoweth, D. E., Cooper, W. W., Hugli, T. E., Stewart, R. W., Blackstone, E. H., and Kirklin, J. W.: Complement activation during cardiopulmonary bypass: Evidence for generation of C3a and C5a anaphylatoxins. N. Engl. J. Med., 304:497, 1981.

Chien, S.: Present state of blood rheology. In Hemodilution: Theoretical Basis and Clinical Application. Edited by K. Messmer and H. Schmid-Schonbein. New York and Basel, Karger, 1972, pp. 1–45.

Clark, R. E., Beauchamp, R. A., Magrath, R. A., Brooks, J. D., Ferguson, T. B., and Weldon, C. S.: Comparison of bubble and membrane oxygenators in short and long perfusions. J. Thorac. Cardiovasc. Surg., 78:655, 1979.

Cohen, M., and Lillehei, C. W.: A quantitative study of the "azygos factor" during vena caval occlusion in the dog. Surg. Gynecol. Obstet., 98:225, 1954.

Cohn, L. H., Angell, W. W., and Shumway, N. E.: Body fluid shifts after cardiopulmonary bypass. 1. Effects of congestive heart failure and hemodilution. J. Thorac. Cardiovasc. Surg., 62:423, 1971.

Craddock, P. R., Fehr, J., Brigham, K. L., Kronenberg, R. S., and Jacob, H. S.: Complement and leukocyte-mediated pulmonary dysfunction in hemodialysis. N. Engl. J. Med., 296:769, 1977a.

Craddock, P. R., Fehr, J., Dalmasso, A. P., Brigham, K. L., and Jacob, H. S.: Pulmonary vascular leukostasis resulting from complement activation by dialyzer cellophane membranes. J. Clin. Invest., 59:879, 1977b.

Crafoord, C., Norberg, B., and Senning, Å.: Clinical studies in extracorporeal circulation with a heart-lung machine. Acta Chir. Scand., 112:200, 1957.

Davies, G. C., Sobel, M., and Salzman, E. W.: Elevated plasma fibrinopeptide A and thromboxane B$_2$ levels during cardiopulmonary bypass. Circulation, 61:808, 1980.

DeBakey, M. D.: Simple continuous flow blood transfusion instrument. New Orleans Med. Surg. J., 87:386, 1934.

Dennis, C., Spreng, D. S., Jr., Nelson, G. E., Karlson, K. E., Nelson, R. M., Thomas, J. V., Eder, W. P., and Varco, R. L.: Development of a pump-oxygenator to replace the heart and lungs; an apparatus applicable to human patients, and application to one case. Ann. Surg., 134:709, 1951.

Diesh, G., Flynn, P. J., Marable, S. A., Mulder, D. G., Schmutzer, K. J., Longmire, W. P., Jr., and Maloney, J. V., Jr.: Comparison of low (azygos) flow and high flow principles of extracorporeal circulation employing a bubble oxygenator. Surgery, 42:67, 1957.

Donald, D. E., Harshbarger, H. G., Hetzel, P. S., Patrick, R. T., Wood, E. H., and Kirklin, J. W.: Experiences with a heart-lung bypass (Gibbon type) in the experimental laboratory: Preliminary report. Proc. Staff Meet. Mayo Clin., 30:113, 1955.

Edmunds, L. H., Jr., Saxena, N. C., Hillyer, P., and Wilson, T. J.: Relationship between platelet count and cardiotomy suction return. Ann. Thorac. Surg., 25:306, 1978.

Ellison, N., Behar, M., MacVaugh, H., III, and Marshall, B. E.: Bradykinin, plasma protein fraction and hypotension. Ann. Thorac. Surg., 29:15, 1980.

Feijen, J.: Thrombogenesis caused by blood–foreign surface interaction. In Artificial Organs. Edited by R. M. Kenedi, J. M. Courtney, J. D. S. Gaylor, and T. Gilchrist. Baltimore, University Park Press, 1977, pp. 235–247.

Fountain, S. W., Martin, B. A., Musclow, C. E., and Cooper, J. D.: Pulmonary leukostasis and its relationship to pulmonary dysfunction in sheep and rabbits. Circ. Res., 46:175, 1980.

Frey, M. V., and Gruber, M.: Untersuchungen über den Stoffwechsel isolierter Organe. Ein Respirations-Apparat fur isolierte Organe. Arch. Physiol., 9:519, 1885.

Friedenberg, W. R., Myers, W. O., Plotka, E. D., Beathard, J. N., Kummer, D. J., Gatlin, P. F., Stoiber, D. L., Ray, J. F., III, and Sautter, R. D.: Platelet dysfunction associated with cardiopulmonary bypass. Ann. Thorac. Surg., 25:298, 1978.

Friedli, B., Kent, G., and Olley, P. M.: Inactivation of bradykinin in the pulmonary vascular bed of newborn and fetal lambs. Circ. Res., 33:421, 1973.

Gibbon, J. H., Jr.: The maintenance of life during experimental occlusion of the pulmonary artery followed by survival. Surg. Gynecol. Obstet., *69*:602, 1939.

Gibbon, J. H., Jr.: Application of a mechanical heart and lung apparatus to cardiac surgery. Minn. Med., *37*:171, 1954.

Gibbon, J. H., Jr.: Personal communication, 1955.

Goldstein, I. M., Brai, M., Osler, A. G., and Weissman, G.: Lysosomal enzyme release from human leukocytes: Mediation by the alternate pathway of complement activation. J. Immunol., *111*:33, 1973.

Grant, J. A., Dupree, E., Goldman, A. S., Schultz, D. R., and Jackson, A. L.: Complement-mediated release of histamine from human leukocytes. J. Immunol., *114*:1101, 1975.

Hairston, P., Manos, J. P., Graber, C. D., and Lee, W. H., Jr.: Depression of immunologic surveillance by pump-oxygenator perfusion. J. Surg. Res., *9*:587, 1969.

Hallowell, P., Austen, W. G., and Laver, M. B.: Influence of oxygen flow rate on arterial oxygenation and acid-base balance during cardiopulmonary bypass with use of a disc oxygenator. Circulation, *35*(Suppl. 1):199, 1967.

Han, P., Turpie, A. G. G., Butt, R., LeBlanc, P., Genton, E., and Gunstensen, S.: The use of β-thromboglobulin release to assess platelet damage during cardiopulmonary bypass. Presented at the Combined Meeting of the Royal Australasian College of Surgeons and Royal Australasian College of Physicians, Sydney, Australia, February 24–29, 1980.

Harris, E. A.: Metabolic aspects of profound hypothermia. *In* Heart Disease in Infancy. Edited by B. G. Barratt-Boyes, J. M. Neutze, and E. A. Harris. Edinburgh, Churchill Livingstone, 1973, p. 65.

Harris, E. A., Seelye, E. R., and Barratt-Boyes, B. G.: Respiratory and metabolic acid-base changes during cardiopulmonary bypass in man. Br. J. Anaesth., *42*:912, 1970.

Hikasa, Y., Shirotani, H., Satomura, K., Muraoka, R., Abe, K., Tsushimi, K., Yokota, Y., Miki, S., Kawai, J., Mori, A., Okamoto, Y., Koie, H., Ban, T., Kanzaki, Y., Yokota, M., Mori, C., Kamiya, T., Tamura, T., Nishii, A., and Asawa, Y.: Open heart surgery in infants with the aid of hypothermic anesthesia. Arch. Jpn. Chir., *36*:495, 1967.

Hine, I. P., Wood, W. G., Mainwaring-Buton, R. W., Butler, M. J., Irving, M. H., and Booker, B.: The adrenergic response to surgery involving cardiopulmonary bypass, as measured by plasma and urinary catecholamine concentrations. Br. J. Anaesth., *48*:355, 1976.

Hugli, T.: Chemical aspects of the serum anaphylatoxins. Contemp. Top. Mol. Immunol., *7*:181, 1978.

Jones, R. E., Donald, D. E., Swan, H. J. C., Harshbarger, H. G., Kirklin, J. W., and Wood, E. H.: Apparatus of the Gibbon type of mechanical bypass of the heart and lungs: Preliminary report. Proc. Staff Meet. Mayo Clin., *30*:105, 1955.

Jorgensen, L., Hovig, T., Towsell, H. C., and Mustard, J. F.: Adenosine diphosphate–induced platelet aggregation and vascular injury in swine and rabbit. Am. J. Pathol., *61*:161, 1970.

Kalter, R. D., Saul, C. M., Wetstein, L., Soriano, C., and Reiss, R. F.: Cardiopulmonary bypass. Associated hemostatic abnormalities. J. Thorac. Cardiovasc. Surg., *77*:428, 1979.

Kirklin, J. W.: A letter to Helen. J. Thorac. Cardiovasc. Surg., *78*:643, 1979.

Kirklin, J. W., and Theye, R. A.: Whole-body perfusion from a pump oxygenator for open intracardiac surgery. *In* Surgery of the Chest. Edited by J. H. Gibbon, Jr.: Philadelphia, W. B. Saunders Company, 1962, pp. 694–707.

Kirklin, J. W., DuShane, J. W., Patrick, R. T., Donald, D. E., Hetzel, P. S., Harshbarger, H. G., and Wood, E. H.: Intracardiac surgery with the aid of a mechanical pump-oxygenator system (Gibbon type): Report of eight cases. Proc. Staff Meet. Mayo Clin., *30*:201, 1955.

Lambert, C. J., Marengo-Rowe, A. J., Leveson, J. E., Green, R. H., Theile, P. P., Geisler, G. F., Adam, M., and Mitchel, B. F.: The treatment of postperfusion bleeding using epsilon-aminocaproic acid, cryoprecipitate, fresh-frozen plasma, and protamine sulfate. Ann. Thorac. Surg., *28*:440, 1979.

Lee, W. H., Jr., Krumbhoar, D., Fonkalsrud, E. W., Schjeide, O. A., and Maloney, J. V., Jr.: Denaturation of plasma proteins as a cause of morbidity and death after intracardiac operations. Surgery, *50*:29, 1961.

Lees, M. H., Herr, R. H., Hill, J. D., Morgan, C. L., Ochsner, A. J., III, Thomas, C., and Van Fleet, D. C.: Distribution of systemic blood flow of the rhesus monkey during cardiopulmonary bypass. J. Thorac. Cardiovasc. Surg., *61*:570, 1971.

Levin, M. B., Theye, R. A., Fowler, W. S., and Kirklin, J. W.: Performance of the stationary vertical-screen oxygenator (Mayo-Gibbon). J. Thorac. Cardiovasc. Surg., *39*:417, 1960.

Lillehei, C. W., Cohen, M., Warden, H. E., and Varco, R. L.: The direct-vision intracardiac correction of congenital anomalies by controlled cross circulation. Surgery, *38*:11, 1955.

Magilligan, D. J., Jr., Eastland, M. W., Lell, W. A., DeWeese, J. A., and Mahoney, E. B.: Decreased carotid flow with ascending aortic cannulation. Circulation, *45, 46*(Suppl. 1):130, 1972.

Martin, R. R.: Alterations in leukocyte structure and function due to mechanical trauma. *In* Quantitative Cardiovascular Studies: Clinical and Research Applications of Engineering Principles. Edited by N. H. C. Hwang, D. R. Gross, and D. J. Patel. Baltimore, University Park Press, 1979, pp. 419–454.

Moffitt, E. A., Kirklin, J. W., and Theye, R. A.: Physiologic studies during whole-body perfusion in tetralogy of Fallot. J. Thorac. Cardiovasc. Surg., *44*:180, 1962.

Nagaoka, H., and Katori, M.: Inhibition of kinin formation by a kallikrein inhibitor during extracorporeal circulation in open-heart surgery. Circulation, *52*:325, 1975.

Osborn, J. J., Cohn, K., Hait, M., Russi, M., Salel, A., Harkins, G., and Gerbode, F.: Hemolysis during perfusion: Sources and means of reduction. J. Thorac. Cardiovasc. Surg., *43*:459, 1962.

Paneth, M., Sellers, R., Gott, V. L., Weirich, W. L., Allen, P., Read, R. C., and Lillehei, C. W.: Physiologic studies upon prolonged cardiopulmonary bypass with the pump-oxygenator with particular reference to (1) acid-base balance, (2) siphon canal drainage. J. Thorac. Surg., *34*:570, 1947.

Pang, L. M., Stalcup, S. A., Lipset, J. S., Hayes, C. J., Bowman, F. O., Jr., and Mellins, R. B.: Increased circulating bradykinin during hypothermia and cardiopulmonary bypass in children. Circulation, *60*:1503, 1979.

Panossian, A., Hagstrom, J. W. C., Nehlsen, S. L., and Veith, F. J.: Secondary nature of surfactant changes in postperfusion pulmonary damage. J. Thorac. Cardiovasc. Surg., *57*:628, 1969.

Pappas, G., Winter, S. D., Kopriva, C. J., and Steele, P.: Improvement of myocardial and other vital organ functions and metabolism using a simple method of pulsatile flow (IABP) during clinical CPB. Surgery, *77*:34, 1975.

Parker, D. J., Cantrell, J. W., Karp, R. B., Stroud, R. M., and Digerness, S. B.: Changes in serum complement and immunoglobulins following cardiopulmonary bypass. Surgery, *71*:824, 1972.

Philbin, D. M., Levine, F. H., Emerson, C. W., Buckley, M. J., Coggins, C. H., Moss, J., and Slater, E.: The renin-catecholamine vasopressor response to cardiopulmonary bypass with pulsatile flow. (Abstract.) Circulation, *59,60*(Suppl. 2):34, 1979.

Pruitt, K. M., Stroud, R. M., and Scott, J. W.: Blood damage in the heart-lung machine (35651). Proc. Soc. Exp. Biol. Med., *137*:714, 1971.

Rahn, H., Reeves, R. B., and Howell, B. J.: Hydrogen ion regulation, temperature, and evolution. Am. Rev. Respir. Dis., *112*:165, 1975.

Reeves, R. B.: Temperature-induced changes in blood acid-base status: pH and PCO_2 in a binary buffer. J. Appl. Physiol., *40*:752, 1976a.

Reeves, R. B.: Temperature-induced changes in blood acid-base status: Donnan rCl and red cell volume. J. Appl. Physiol., *40*:762, 1976b.

Reves, J. G., Karp, R. B., Buttner, E. E., Tosone, S., Smith, L. R., Samuelson, P. N., Kreusch, G. R., and Oparil, S.: Neural and adrenomedullary catecholamine release in response to cardiopulmonary bypass in man. Circulation, *66*:49, 1982.

Rosenthal, T. B.: The effect of temperature on the pH of blood and plasma in vitro. J. Biol. Chem., *173*:23, 1948.

Sade, R. H., Bartles, D. M., Dearing, J. P., Campbell, L. J., and

Loadholt, C. B.: A prospective randomized study of membrane vs. bubble oxygenators in children. Ann. Thorac. Surg., *29*:502, 1980.

Schenk, W. G., Jr., Pollock, L. A., Kjarstansson, K. B., and Delin, N. A.: Influence of aortic perfusion on regional blood flow. Arch. Surg., *87*:1059, 1963.

Scott, J.: Mechanism of gamma globulin denaturation. Doctoral Dissertation, University of Alabama at Birmingham, 1970.

Senning, Å.: Ventricular fibrillation during extracorporeal circulation: Used as a method to prevent air-embolisms and to facilitate intracardiac operations. Acta Chir. Scand., *171*(Suppl.):1, 1952.

Shepard, R. B.: Whole body oxygen consumption during hypoxic hypoxemia and cardiopulmonary bypass circulation. Proceedings of the Tenth International Symposium on Space Technology and Science, Tokyo, 1973, pp. 1307–1318.

Solen, K. A., Whiffen, J. D., and Lightfoot, E. N.: The effect of shear, specific surface, and air interface on the development of blood emboli and hemolysis. J. Biomed Mater. Res., *12*:381, 1978.

Stewart, R. W., Blackstone, E. H., Kirklin, J. W., and Pacifico, A. D.: Clinical experiences in profound hypothermia and total circulatory arrest. (Unpublished data.)

Swan, H.: Thermoregulation and Bioenergetics: Patterns for Vertebrate Survival. New York, American Elsevier Publishers Inc., 1974, pp. 183–187.

Tamari, Y., Aledort, L., Puszkin, E., Degnan, T. J., Wagner, N., Kaplitt, M. J., and Peirce, E. C., II: Functional changes in platelets during extracorporeal circulation. Ann. Thorac. Surg., *19*:639, 1975.

Tan, C. K., Glisson, S. N., El-Etr, A. A., and Ramakrishnaiah, K. B.: Levels of circulating norepinephrine and epinephrine before, during, and after cardiopulmonary bypass in man. J. Thorac. Cardiovasc. Surg., *71*:928, 1976.

Taylor, K. M., Bain, W. H., Maxted, K. J., Hutton, M. M., McNab, W. Y., and Caves, P. K.: Comparative studies of pulsatile and nonpulsatile flow during cardiopulmonary bypass. I. Pulsatile system employed and its hematologic effects. J. Thorac. Cardiovasc. Surg., *75*:569, 1978.

Theye, R. A., and Kirklin, J. W.: Vertical film oxygenator performance at 30°C and oxygen levels during rewarming. Surgery, *54*:569, 1963.

Theye, R. A., Donald, D. E., and Jones, R. E.: The effect of geometry and filming surface on the priming volume of the vertical-film oxygenator. J. Thorac. Surg., *43*:473, 1962a.

Theye, R. A., Kirklin, J. W., and Fowler, W. S.: Performance and film volume of sheet and screen vertical-film oxygenators. J. Thorac. Cardiovasc. Surg., *43*:481, 1962b.

Tsiao, C., Lin, C. Y., Glgov, S., and Replogle, R. L.: Disseminated leukocyte injury during open-heart surgery. Arch. Pathol., *95*:357, 1973.

Turina, M., Housman, L. B., Intaglietta, M., Schauble, J., and Braunwald, N. S.: An automatic cardiopulmonary bypass unit for use in infants. J. Thorac. Cardiovasc. Surg., *63*:263, 1972.

Turley, K., Graham, B., Roizen, M., and Ebert, P. A.: Catecholamine response to deep hypothermia and total circulatory arrest. (Abstract.) Circulation, *59, 60*(Suppl 2):169, 1979.

Verska, J. J.: Control of heparinization by activated clotting time during bypass with improved postoperative hemostasis. Ann. Thorac. Surg., *24*:170, 1977.

Walker, D. R., Blackstone, E. H., Kirklin, J. W., Karp, R. B., Kouchoukos, N. T., Pacifico, A. D., Shealy, A., Roe, C. R., and Bradley, E. L.: The effect of micropore filtration of the arterial return during cardiopulmonary bypass: A randomized clinical study. (Unpublished data.)

Wallach, R., Karp, R. B., Reves, J. G., Oparil, S., Smith, L. R., and James, T. N.: Pathogenesis of paroxysmal hypertension developing during and after coronary artery bypass surgery: A study of hemodynamic and humoral factors. Am. J. Cardiol., *46*:559, 1980.

Ward, C. A., Ruegsegger, B., Stanga, D., and Zingg, W.: Reduction in platelet adhesion to biomaterials by removal of gas nuclei. Trans. Am. Soc. Artif. Intern. Organs, *20*:77, 1974.

Warden, H. E., Cohen, M., Read, R. C., and Lillehei, C. W.: Controlled cross circulation for open intracardiac surgery. J. Thorac. Surg., *28*:331, 1954.

Wilson, J. W.: Pulmonary morphologic changes due to extracorporeal circulation: A model for 'the shock lung' at cellular level in humans. *In* Shock in Low- and High-Flow States. Proceedings of a Symposium at Brook Lodge, Augusta, Michigan. Edited by B. K. Forscher, R. C. Lillehei, and S. S. Stubbs. Amsterdam, Excerpta Medica, 1972, pp. 160–171.

Chapter 30

The Aorta

I HISTORICAL BACKGROUND

Henry T. Bahnson

Modern, definitive treatment of diseases of the aorta and adjacent vessels began with the successful ligation of a patent ductus arteriosus by Gross in 1938 and was soon followed by excision and anastomosis of coarctation of the aorta. In 1944, Blalock and Park described experimental methods for the treatment of coarctation by anastomosis of the left subclavian artery to the distal aorta. In the following year (1945), Crafoord and Nylin, and Gross independently, described excision and primary anastomosis of the aorta, the method that is used today whenever possible. Clinical use was thus made of techniques of suturing and handling of arteries that had been carefully studied by Carrel and Guthrie shortly after the turn of the century (Guthrie, 1959). The next important milestone was the use of aortic homografts to replace deficiencies following excision of coarctation (Gross *et al.*, 1949), another technique that Carrel and Guthrie (1906) had demonstrated to be feasible.

With improvement of instruments for performing vascular anastomoses, and particularly with increasing familiarity with great vessels, attacks were made upon aortic aneurysms. Blakemore (1947) and Cooley and DeBakey (1952) excised aneurysms of the innominate artery, suturing the mouth of this vessel in the aorta. DuBost (1952) used a homograft in replacing abdominal aortic aneurysms. In 1953, I described excision of saccular aneurysms of all areas of the aorta, and DeBakey and Cooley described excision of thoracic aneurysms with homograft replacement. When the frequency of late degeneration of homografts became evident, an intense search for a durable aortic prosthesis culminated in the development of Dacron and Teflon prostheses by 1956 and 1957. Many people have contributed to improvements in technique, as well as to the development of prosthetic aortic materials and methods for maintaining the circulation by cardiopulmonary bypass while the aorta is occluded or excised, so that now all areas of the aorta are susceptible to surgical attack.

For references see page 990.

II AORTOGRAPHY

Henry T. Bahnson

Development of methods of opacification of the aorta and its branches leading to the exact radiologic diagnosis and localization of arterial and aortic lesions has paralleled advances in vascular surgery. Each endeavor has been stimulated by the other in this progress. Clinically useful contrast studies of the great vessels of the thorax were first described by Robb and Steinberg (1939) with their technique of angiocardiography by venous injection. The technique is still occasionally useful, especially if visualization of great veins or pulmonary arteries is desired or if catheterization of an artery is to be avoided. It is now usually performed with selective injection by means of a catheter.

Aortography with access via a catheter through a peripheral artery is the mainstay of radiologic diagnosis of aortic disease. Arterial injection was first performed successfully in man in 1936 by Nuvoli by injection through a large-bore needle through the sternum into the ascending aorta (Abrams, 1971). Such direct injections also have been made through the carotid artery, through the suprasternal notch, and directly into the aneurysm. Better control was obtained by inserting a ureteral-type catheter through a radial artery and guiding the tip into the ascending aorta under fluoroscopic control, as introduced by Radner (1948). Percutaneous insertion of the catheter into the femoral artery and retrograde passage, as described by Peirce (1951), simplified the technique.

Seldinger (1953) described a method by which larger catheters could be inserted percutaneously. In the Seldinger technique, which has become a standard means of vascular access, needle puncture of the artery is followed by passage of a small wire and removal of the needle. The wire remaining in the artery acts as a guide over which a large-bore, plastic, radiopaque catheter is passed, which then can be positioned in the aorta as desired. Injection generally is made into the ascending aorta so that the entire aorta is visualized but, more importantly, so that the entire bolus of contrast material does not go to the brain through a carotid or vertebral artery or to the spinal cord through an intercostal artery. In some instances, injection may be made into an aneurysm or in the region of a patent ductus arteriosus if demonstration of the latter is required. Access is most commonly percutaneously through a femoral artery, but it may be from above in an axillary artery.

Retrograde injection into the brachial artery has been used effectively in infants and young children (Keith *et al.*, 1958). Rapid injection allows visualization of the distal aortic arch and demonstration of coarctation or a patent ductus arteriosus. This technique has limited but important use in small children in heart failure but is not so satisfactory in older children.

Less invasive studies may give preliminary or supportive information. Useful sonographic study is limited to the ascending aorta because of interference elsewhere by air in the lungs. Computed tomography with contrast enhancement will be of increasing value with further development and use, but it does not yet match aortography in providing useful information to the surgeon.

Contrast Material

Numerous radiopaque materials have been used, most containing iodine and all possessing varying degrees of toxicity, particularly to neurologic tissue. Several compounds have been found to be less toxic than the original 70 per cent Diodrast (iodopyracet) used by Robb and Steinberg, but other important considerations are the density of roentgen rays and the viscosity of the solution of adequately dense material. The most satisfactory materials presently available are probably sodium diatrizoate (Hypaque) in a 50 to 75 per cent solution (Abrams, 1971) and meglumine diatrizoate (Renografin) in a 60 to 76 per cent solution.

Radiographic technique may be of many types, including a single film accurately timed after the injection, repeated rapid direct exposure, which makes accurate timing less critical, and cineangiography, in which moving pictures are taken of the fluoroscopic screen. The last gives better demonstration of the course of the circulation and rapidly changing events, but resolution of each individual frame of the film is less satisfactory than the detail that can be obtained with direct exposure of roentgenograms, a circumstance that in large measure is compensated for by the continuous action.

For references see page 990.

III   AORTIC GRAFTS AND PROSTHESES

Henry T. Bahnson

Replacement of the human aorta was first accomplished by Gross and associates (1949) in the treatment of coarctation of the aorta, employing a technique for procurement and preservation of vessels that Carrel had used at the beginning of the century for peripheral arteries. Special precautions were taken to obtain the graft aseptically very soon after death, and it could be demonstrated by culture methods that the tissue was viable for as long as 37 days if stored in a balanced salt solution at 1° to 4°C. (Peirce *et al.*, 1949). It soon became apparent, however, that implanted homografts did not persist as living structures, that the cells died, and that only the collagen and elastic framework persisted. Schuster and Gross (1961), after a 12-year follow-up of homograft replacement of the aorta, found homografts to be satisfactory replacements, since they saw no aneurysmal distention or occlusion. Calcification does appear in many cases, however. Freeze-drying allowed longer storage, and any of several methods of sterilization of grafts, which did not need to be procured aseptically, allowed easier, wider use of homografts, but for replacement of major vessels they became of historical interest only when synthetic prostheses of porous fabrics were developed.

Voorhees and colleagues (1952) used porous fabric tubes of Vinyon N for replacement of abdominal aortic aneurysms. A number of synthetic materials were used subsequently, both experimentally and clinically, including nylon, Orlon, Dacron, and Teflon in various patterns of knit and weave. Basic qualities of flexibility, porosity, and durability were recognized early. An important contribution was made by Edwards and Tapp (1955), who introduced a permanent circular crimp into the construction of a tubular graft, a significant factor when a prosthesis must bend, as in the aortic arch, to avoid kinking.

Porosity of the prosthesis is worthy of consideration. Porous fabrics require clotting to fill the interstices, and they are usually preclotted before being exposed to full arterial pressure. When fabrics were used initially for arterial replacement, it was thought that an ingrowth of blood vessels through the interstices would improve incorporation into the body. In a study of porosity, Harrison and Davalos (1961) demonstrated that in the replacement of the canine aorta, thrombosis occurred less frequently with prostheses of greater porosity. With larger interstices, there was less resistance to ingrowth of fibrous tissue from the outer covering to replace the inner fibrin lining, resulting in better attachment of the inner lining to prevent dissection or dislodgment. Earlier healing of the prosthesis occurred with increased porosity. The pseudointima that forms, first from clot on the wall, followed by fibrin and flattened cells on the surface, probably never completely heals (Berger *et al.*, 1972), and in actual practice, the amount of bleeding through the interstices at the time of implantation has proved to be a more important consideration than the ingrowth of tissue that might derive from greater porosity.

If tightness and low porosity are desired, a woven prosthesis can be made less porous than a knitted one because of technical factors involved in its manufacture. This is of critical importance in aortic replacement if a pump bypass requiring heparinization is used. The clotting that normally occurs to seal the small interstices of fabric prostheses will not occur with heparin, and alarming and even fatal hemorrhage has occurred. For this reason, Teflon and Dacron woven prostheses may actually be filled in order to reduce porosity to a minimum. A velour prosthesis allows adequate porosity, but the loops of uncut pile provide a trellis that entraps and clots blood and creates a framework to hold the pseudointima as it forms. Of the three types of fabric — woven, knitted, and velour — ingrowth of tissue and incorporation into tissues of the body are greatest with velour and least with tightly woven prostheses.

Dacron and Teflon are the materials most commonly used. Teflon is remarkably inert chemically, so much so that there is insufficient reaction to the material for its firm incorporation into the body. Dacron maintains its strength well and is relatively inert in the body but is well incorporated into the tissues. It is the material most commonly used currently. With finer thread and thinner fabrics, a tighter weave or knit can be obtained, but durability is forfeited and late rupture has been reported, mostly with the extra-lightweight fabric. In the thoracic aorta, durability is a more important factor because of the greater stress on the central aorta, and conversely, significant narrowing and occlusion are less of a concern because of larger diameter and more rapid flow. None of the prostheses developed has been totally free of deterioration. Berger and Sauvage (1981) reported a 3 per cent deterioration of prostheses available before 1974 in a review and discussion of the state of the art, published from a symposium at the National Institutes of Health (Sawyer and Kaplitt, 1978).

For references see page 990.

IV   ANOMALIES OF THE AORTIC ARCH

HENRY T. BAHNSON

Constriction by an abnormality of the aortic arch must be considered in patients, particularly infants, who present evidence of tracheal or esophageal obstruction. Many anomalies of the aortic arch, of its branches, and of the great veins in the superior mediastinum are of no clinical significance, and, in fact, most of the reported cases were discovered incidentally. In 1946, Gross and Ware, however, clearly demonstrated that embarrassing and sometimes fatal obstruction of the trachea and esophagus may arise from a double aortic arch, a right aortic arch with a ligamentum arteriosum completing a ring about the trachea, or an anomalous innominate, left common carotid, or subclavian artery (Gross, 1953).

EMBRYOLOGY

In order to understand the variations that might be encountered, it is helpful to review the embryology of the aortic arch system (Barry, 1951; Bahnson, 1952). During the first 3 weeks of embryonic life, six aortic arches join the ventral aortic sac and the dorsal paired aortas around the interposed pharynx. Only the third, from which the carotid arteries form, the fourth, which becomes the normal adult aortic arch, and the sixth, from which the pulmonary arteries derive, need to be considered (Edwards, 1977). The aorta caudal to the branchial arches becomes fused as an unpaired dorsal aorta. Figure 30–1A shows diagrammatically the approximate configuration of the aortic arches in the 12-mm. embryo. The embryonic subclavian artery is the seventh cervical segmental

artery, which supplies the limb bud. As the heart and aortic sac move caudad and the cranial portion of the embryo elongates, the subclavian artery migrates craniad on the aorta. Normally, the most caudal segment of the right fourth arch becomes obliterated as the left fourth arch takes over the majority of the cardiac output. Most of the right third arch persists as the proximal part of the carotid artery. It ultimately arises from the fourth arch, which persists as the innominate and subclavian arteries. The left fourth arch persists as the definitive aorta, and the left carotid and subclavian arteries arise independently. In rare instances, the left subclavian artery may ascend to the third arch and a left innominate artery results.

If the right aortic arch persists and the left arch becomes obliterated, the mirror image of the arrangement just described may occur, resulting in a right

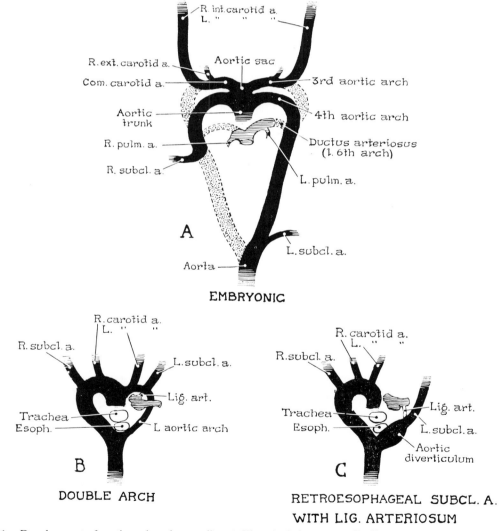

Figure 30–1. Development of aortic arch and anomalies. *A,* The stippled areas usually disappear. Normally, only the left fourth arch persists in its entirety. *B,* Both fourth arches persist in the double aortic arch. *C,* When the right fourth arch persists and the left fourth arch disappears, the left subclavian artery is retroesophageal. A ligamentum arteriosum may join this to the pulmonary artery, completing the ring. (From Bahnson, H. T., and Blalock, A.: Aortic vascular rings encountered in surgical treatment of congenital pulmonic stenosis. Ann. Surg., *131*:356, 1950.)

aortic arch. If the proximal rather than the distal part of the right fourth arch becomes obliterated, the right subclavian artery arises from the unpaired aorta and courses behind the esophagus to reach the right arm, resulting in a retroesophageal subclavian artery. In rare instances, the vessel may go between the trachea and the esophagus or anterior to the trachea. A short segment of the distal end of the right fourth arch may persist as an aortic diverticulum, the diverticulum of Kommerell, from which the subclavian artery arises.

The ductus arteriosus usually connects the main or the left pulmonary artery (derived from the sixth arch) with the left aortic arch. When the proximal left fourth arch becomes obliterated, the ductus arteriosus is connected with the most distal portion of the left dorsal aorta along with the subclavian artery (Fig. 30–1C). If the arch becomes obliterated distal to the ductus arteriosus, this relationship is lost.

When both aortic arches persist, a complete aortic ring is formed about the trachea and esophagus (Fig. 30–1B). In such instances, the brachiocephalic vessels usually arise from the arches independently, although double aortic arch with an innominate artery has been described.

PATHOLOGIC ANATOMY

A vascular ring about the trachea and esophagus may be composed of any of the several remnants of the aortic arch system. Conversely, obliteration may occur at any point in the system, and almost every possible resulting anomaly has been reported, many of them rare and of little clinical importance (Edwards, 1977). A double aortic arch results when neither of the aortic arches regresses. In such cases, the ascending aorta bifurcates, with one branch going to the right and behind the trachea and esophagus and the other to the left in front of the trachea. Both limbs join behind to complete a ring about the trachea and esophagus (Fig. 30–2). In most instances, the descending aorta is on the left side, although a right descending aorta may occur with the aorta lying to the right of the vertebral column. Regardless of the side of the descending aorta, the smaller of the two arches is usually to the left and anterior, an important consideration in selecting the side of surgical approach.

If the left fourth aortic arch, rather than the right, disappears in the embryo, the subject is born with a right aortic arch, which ascends, passes to the right of the trachea and esophagus, and descends usually on the left, but occasionally on the right, of the vertebral column. Such an arch in itself rarely causes symptoms, although there may be some tracheal or right bronchial compression. In many such cases, the ligamentum arteriosum courses from the pulmonary artery and joins the innominate artery* at its bifurcation into the carotid and subclavian arteries. In some instances, however, the ligamentum passes from the pulmonary artery to the left of the trachea and esophagus and to the distal end of the right aortic arch, thus completing a ring about the trachea and esophagus (Fig. 30–3). This ring may be small enough to compress and interfere with the function of the trachea and esophagus. A mirror-image defect occurs, but rarely, that is a left arch and a right ductus, subclavian artery, and descending aorta (Park et al., 1976).

_____

*The innominate artery arises as the first vessel off the aortic arch, regardless of the side of the arch, and, hence, in this case supplies the left arm and the left common carotid.

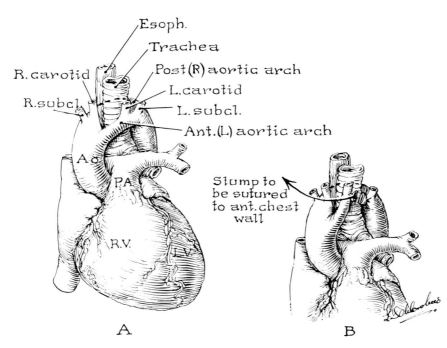

A

B

Figure 30–2. Double aortic arch. _A,_ The larger channel is usually the posterior one and on the right. Branches of the arch arise independently. In almost all instances, the descending thoracic aorta is on the left, as shown. _B,_ The point of division of the smaller arch is selected to preserve the circulation to the branches. The left common carotid artery is then tacked to the anterior chest wall to further relieve tracheal compression.

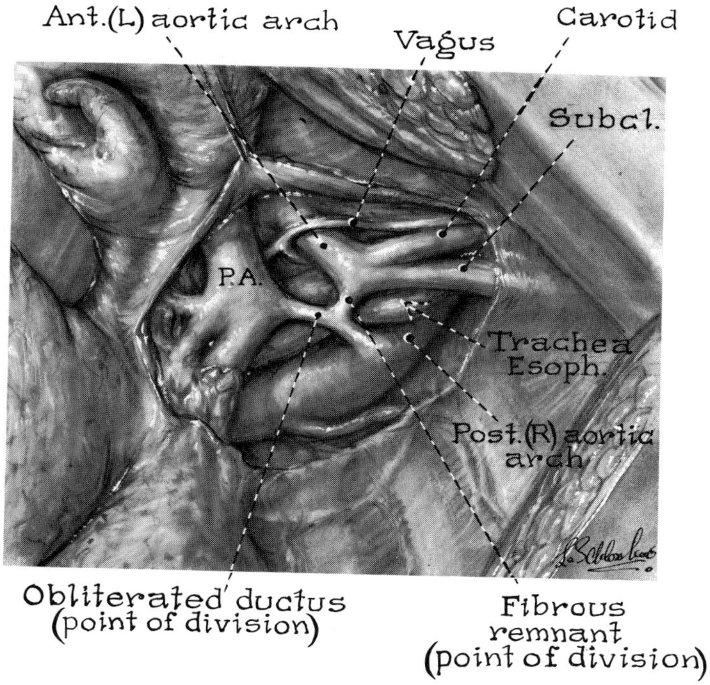

Figure 30–3. Tracheal ring completed by obliterated remnant of distal left arch and ligamentum arteriosum. After complete exposure of the vascular components, the proper point of division of the ligaments can easily be determined.

Of the anomalies of the branches of the aortic arch, that of the right subclavian is the most easily recognized and best understood. If in the development of the aortic arch system the proximal portion of the right fourth arch disappears instead of the distal portion and before the subclavian artery has established its origin on the proximal segment, the right subclavian artery will arise as the last branch of the aortic arch and course behind the esophagus (or in rare instances between the esophagus and trachea or in front of the trachea) to supply the right arm. This anomaly was clearly recognized by Bayford in 1794 and has long been known to cause "dysphagia lusoria."

Although the innominate artery normally arises to the left of the trachea, in some instances it arises farther along the arch than normal and must wind across the trachea in reaching the apex of the right chest. If the vessel is lax, no symptoms are caused, but when it is tight, there may be constriction of the trachea. Similarly, if the left common carotid arises from the aortic arch more to the right than usual, it may wind across the anterior surface of the trachea as it courses upward and to the left and may cause tracheal compression.

Virtually all possible combinations of anomalies have been reported. Most common have been double aortic arch, right aortic arch with constricting left ligamentum arteriosum, and anomalous origin of the right subclavian artery.

CLINICAL PICTURE

Why some children with aortic arch anomalies remain asymptomatic and others are severely bothered is an unanswered question. Symptoms are those of tracheal obstruction, often with stridor and even a crowing type of respiration, frequent respiratory infections with secretions that cannot adequately be cleared, and a wheeze, which often may be heard without the stethoscope. There may be difficulty in swallowing, and in some instances, this is the presenting complaint. Respiratory distress is frequently worse after eating or drinking, and aspiration pneumonia is often seen because of esophageal obstruction. The infant appears to get some relief by lying in a position of hyperextension, and this is frequently the preferred position. Respiratory obstruction may be exaggerated if the neck is flexed forcibly.

Symptoms may be alarming with any of the compressing anomalies, but they are usually more prominent with the double aortic arch or a right arch with a ring completed by the ligamentum arteriosum. When difficulty occurs with these anomalies, it is almost always evident in infancy or early childhood, many patients being under 6 months of age. These infants often have severe respiratory distress and have an element of tracheomalacia at the site of compression. Few older patients have symptoms or require treatment. The anomalous right subclavian artery causes difficulty principally in swallowing, there usually being little or no respiratory distress except that occasioned by dysphagia and aspiration after eating.

Clinically important anomalies of the aortic arch system are not common, but over 300 cases have been reported (Richardson et al., 1981).

DIAGNOSIS

Consideration of the possibility of an aortic arch anomaly is the most important step in diagnosing the

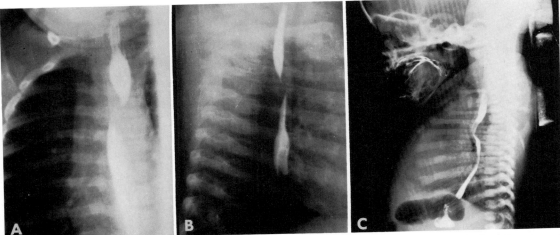

Figure 30–4. Roentgenograms of vascular ring. *A,* Double aortic arch. The location and direction of esophageal compression suggest a larger posterior arch coursing from above downward but with anterior compression as well. *B,* Obstruction by remnant of left fourth arch and obliterated ductus, as shown in Figure 30–3. *C,* The large posterior arch is pulled forward, compressing the trachea and esophagus.

condition. Roentgenograms may show pneumonitis and, in some instances, the outline of the trachea and its compression. Barium swallow shows the posterior compression of the esophagus (Fig. 30–4), and by careful examination of the films and the direction and level of the compression, the exact anomaly can often be determined (Neuhauser, 1946; Shuford and Sybers, 1974). The combination of anterior tracheal compression and posterior esophageal compression justifies an almost certain diagnosis of a vascular ring. The relative sizes of the right and left arches can be estimated by the size of the indentation on barium swallow. Angiography may demonstrate the anomaly but is usually not necessary. A tracheogram with Lipiodol instillation may clearly identify the tracheal compression, but the resulting pulmonary irritation contraindicates its use. The level and obliquity of the tracheal and esophageal compression usually allow identification of the type of vessel when obstruction is due to anomalous arteries from the aortic arch.

SURGICAL TREATMENT

Division of the constricting ring or displacement of an aberrant vessel has much to offer these patients in providing more room for the trachea and esophagus and in relieving their obstruction. Adequate exposure is an absolute necessity, and this usually is obtained through the left chest. The arch and the vessels arising from it, the ductus, and the fibrous tissue attached to the vascular ring must be clearly exposed. Removal of the thymus often helps.

Once adequate exposure is obtained, selection of the proper component for division usually is not difficult. In the case of the right aortic arch with a ligamentum arteriosum completing the vascular ring, simple division of the ligamentum arteriosum and mobilization of the arch should relieve the constriction. Full mobilization of the arch with division of all ligamentous structures is crucial, however, because simply dividing the ligamentum has been found to be inadequate. When a double arch is present, the side and position of the smaller arch must be determined. The small arch, usually the anterior one and on the left, is divided in a manner that does not interfere with circulation to the common carotid arteries. This usually means division of the arch between the left common carotid and left subclavian arteries. The adjacent and possibly constricting fibrous tissue must be divided, and if the divided arch and carotid in any way compress the trachea, the arch could be tacked with multiple stitches through the adventitia to the posterior surface of the sternum or chest wall in order to hold the vessel away from the trachea. Although theoretically the smaller arch can be divided at any site and circulation will continue into the branches through the distal or proximal opening, in some instances the distal end of the smaller arch is narrowed, and circulation to the carotid through this opening may be curtailed.

The subclavian artery, if it is causing compression, arises as the last branch of the aortic arch; by dissecting in the posterior mediastinum, it can be mobilized behind the aorta. Usually, it can be divided with impunity, and in cases of an aberrant retroesophageal left subclavian artery, freeing the artery from its bed and doubly ligating and dividing it is all that is required. Collateral circulation is usually adequate through the second and third portions of the subclavian artery to maintain adequate circulation to the arm. In other patients or in those with aneurysm of the anomalous subclavian artery, a carotid-subclavian bypass may be indicated. In such a case, surgical approach may be better through a median sternotomy, an exception to the usual choice of a left thoracotomy. In cases of compression by an anomalous innominate or carotid artery, the continuity of the artery must be maintained. Hence, proper treatment is complete mobilization of the artery, division of any constricting fibrous tissue about it, and suturing of the vessel away from the trachea and against the back wall of the sternum by multiple fine sutures through the adventitia.

After operation in patients in whom there has been some tracheal compression, particular care must be taken to provide an atmosphere with high humidity; there must also be close supervision of tracheobronchial secretions. Not infrequently, because of the tracheal manipulation and pre-existing obstruction, there may be respiratory obstruction and even stridor for the first few postoperative days. In babies with tracheomalacia, assisted ventilation may be required for a longer period.

RESULTS OF TREATMENT

Relief of the tracheal and esophageal obstruction is usually associated with dramatic clinical improvement, often evident immediately after operation. In some instances, there is deformity of the trachea, which may persist. No long-term follow-up of such cases is yet available, but it is likely that relief of the compression will allow the trachea to grow in a normal fashion. Persisting deformity of the tracheal cartilage is more common in patients with a double arch or a right arch with a ligamentum arteriosum.

Published mortality rates with surgical treatment have averaged 6 per cent (Richardson *et al.*, 1981.)

For references see page 990.

V   PATENT DUCTUS ARTERIOSUS

Henry T. Bahnson

With the ligation of a patent ductus arteriosus by Gross in 1938, surgeons first entered the field of congenital heart disease, and treatment of the patent ductus is representative of the rapid advance made in thoracic surgery in the last 40 years. Four decades ago, ligation of the ductus arteriosus was a *pièce de résistance* performed by few surgeons in the country. It is now considered one of the simplest operations, which some surgeons perform in the nursery when needed in premature infants. Interruption of a ductus is one of the most satisfactory and curative operations in the field of surgery of the heart and great vessels.

PATHOLOGIC ANATOMY

In the majority of typical cases, the only discernible abnormality is the presence of the duct joining the main, or left, pulmonary artery with the lesser curvature of the aortic arch opposite the left subclavian artery, the channel conducting an aortic-pulmonary shunt of blood. The diameter may vary from several millimeters to 1 or 2 cm. It is variable in length, with some large ductus being almost flush aortic-pulmonary connections. An aberrant position of the ductus is extremely rare; it is almost always on the left, even in the presence of a right aortic arch where it joins the pulmonary artery and distal innominate artery. The channel, a structure present during fetal life, normally closes soon after birth. Christie (1930) studied 558 infants and found that the ductus was open 2 weeks after birth in 65 per cent but that this rapidly decreased so that only 2 per cent were open after 32 weeks and 1 per cent at 1 year. Many of these were small openings and functionally unimportant.

In most cases of patent ductus arteriosus, there are no secondary changes, but as in other conditions in which there is a large left-to-right shunt, pulmonary vascular resistance may increase and pulmonary hypertension will result.

CLINICAL FINDINGS

The symptoms of patients with patent ductus arteriosus vary widely from none to severe cardiac failure, the variation depending on age, the size of the aortic-pulmonary shunt, and other undetermined factors. Some children grow normally, have no shortness of breath or other limitation of activity, and lead a fairly normal life. A significant number of children are retarded in physical growth, in some instances strikingly. In many cases, particularly if the ductus is a moderately large one, the additional burden on the heart becomes apparent as the patient ages and is evident in loss of energy, shortness of breath, and fatigue. A typical ductus without superimposed pulmonary hypertension or an additional cardiac defect rarely causes cardiac failure, but cardiac failure may be a problem, particularly in infants with a large ductus in whom there is pulmonary hypertension and often a high pulmonary blood flow.

Subacute bacterial endarteritis at the site of the ductus is a less frequent and less distressing problem now than it was prior to the use of antibiotics. Endarteritis occurs most commonly in young adults but rather infrequently in children and is manifested by fever, weight loss, anemia, and positive blood cultures.

That the typical patent ductus arteriosus appears to be an innocuous lesion in many children may lead to the assumption that the condition is compatible with a long life and little or no disability, but such is not usually the case. Keys and Shapiro (1943) found that those who are alive at 17 years of age with a patent ductus arteriosus have a subsequent life expectancy of about one-half that of the normal population.

The heart is usually normal in size or only slightly enlarged. In the presence of a large ductus, it may be overactive. There may be a normal systolic pressure with a low diastolic level because of the leakage into the pulmonary circuit, and this may be accompanied by peripheral signs similar to those of aortic insufficiency. The murmur is a characteristic one and allows an accurate diagnosis of the condition in about 95 per cent of cases. In the typical case, it is a continuous murmur, often rumbling in systole, sometimes obscuring the pulmonary second sound, heard most prominently in the left second to third intercostal space, and frequently associated with a thrill. The pulmonary second sound may be accentuated. The rumbling systolic phase, the banging second sound, and the continuous murmur give the impression of machinery, the name usually applied to it. Transmission of the murmur depends largely on its intensity, the systolic phase usually being transmitted more widely than the diastolic one. If the channel is small, only a systolic murmur may be heard, although the flow and turbulence are probably continuous. If the shunt of blood through the ductus is extremely large, there may be a rumbling diastolic flow murmur at the apex of the heart suggestive of relative mitral stenosis; there may be other murmurs due to a large blood flow through the active heart. When pulmonary hypertension occurs, the diastolic element may be short. Characteristically, the pulmonary second sound is loud, indicative of the hypertension. In the extreme case with pulmonary hypertension, reversed flow occurs, with pulmonary blood entering the aorta and causing cyanosis of the toes in contrast to fingers of normal color. This late and irreversible stage is rarely seen in children but results from progressive pulmonary vascular changes.

Roentgenologic studies show the heart to be of normal size or slightly enlarged. When enlargement is significant, it is apt to be predominantly of the left atrium and left ventricle. The region of the left pulmonary artery is often full along the upper left contour of the heart. The lung fields show increased vascularity, and there may be a hilar dance, although this is not so striking in patients with a ductus as in those with a left-to-right intracardiac shunt. These changes are not specific for the patent ductus, because the picture may be similar to that of other shunts, notably a ventricular septal defect. Although it often cannot be determined by routine radiologic methods, the ascending aorta characteristically is larger in the patient with a patent ductus (by virtue of the flow through it) than in one with a ventricular septal defect.

Tissue in the wall of the fetal ductus is sensitive to oxygen, contracting when the oxygen level is high. At birth, with the onset of ventilation and a drop in pulmonary vascular resistance, flow through the ductus reverses from the right to left of fetal life to left to right, and the ductus is bathed in more oxygenated blood. The ductus constricts, and anatomic closure follows. Prostaglandin E_1 dilates the ductus and has been used in infants to preserve patency in those cases when the ductus compensates for diminished pulmonary blood flow. Conversely, indomethacin, an inhibitor of prostaglandin E_1, has been used to block vasodilation of the duct and to enhance closure (Heymann and Rudolph, 1981).

In premature infants, there is a high incidence of patency of the ductus, probably related to immaturity of the contractile tissue that initiates the process of closure and to continuing hypoxia of respiratory distress. In the newborn infant with the respiratory distress syndrome, the presence of an appropriate murmur, bounding femoral pulses, unusual vascularity of the lung fields, and greater-than-usual right ventricular hypertrophy on the electrocardiogram should indicate the use of pharmacologic agents, and if this is not effective, surgical closure should follow (Horsley *et al.*, 1973). Operative closure of the ductus, even in a 1-kg. infant, is well tolerated. That this is only one of many important facets in the sophisticated care of these sick infants is emphasized by reports that advocate ligation of the ductus in the neonatal intensive care unit (Oxnard *et al.*, 1977). We have preferred to move the baby to the operating room, rather than vice versa.

DIAGNOSIS

In 95 per cent of cases, the diagnosis can be made easily and simply, largely on the basis of the characteristic continuous murmur. The murmur may be simulated by a venous hum, although a hum is usually more prominent over the right upper chest, is less intense with the patient supine, and may be obliterated by compression of the jugular vein in the neck. Arteriovenous fistulas of the lung cause a similar murmur, although this is usually high-pitched and is transmitted more widely for its intensity, and the lesion frequently can be seen in the lung field on a plain roentgenogram.

The diagnosis can be sufficiently certain and other abnormalities excluded on the basis of the murmur, roentgenogram, and electrocardiogram, so that one might proceed with operation in the majority of typical cases. In others, there may still be uncertainty after use of the noninvasive diagnostic methods. Cardiac catheterization, and especially its associated cineangiocardiography, should establish the diagnosis in almost all instances with demonstration of a right-to-left shunt into the pulmonary artery and opacification of the channel or passage of a catheter through it. A more proximally located aortopulmonary window may be hardest to differentiate, but it is relatively uncommon.

SELECTION OF PATIENTS FOR OPERATION

Establishment of the diagnosis in a child is sufficient indication for interruption of an uncomplicated patent ductus arteriosus. The operative risk should be little more than that of the anesthesia, and the cure is complete. Clatworthy and McDonald (1958) emphasized that the operative mortality and morbidity in infants and young children is no greater than that in older children with symptoms when the diagnosis is established or in asymptomatic patients before the age of 5. There is little advantage in postponing operation.

A difficult problem arises in the patient, usually an adult or older child, with pulmonary hypertension and a reverse ductus. When pulmonary hypertension is striking, in the presence of a reversed shunt, there may be such severe pulmonary vascular changes and increased pulmonary vascular resistance that the patient will not tolerate the stresses of the postoperative period. Cyanosis of the toes or electrocardiographic evidence of significant right ventricular hypertrophy suggests that an irreversible condition has developed. Ellis and associates (1956) presented a good analysis of the problem and concluded that if the shunt is predominantly left to right but nearly balanced, operation is probably indicated but involves considerable risk. Indications are clearer for operation when the shunt is only left to right without right to left. When flow is predominantly right to left, there is great operative risk and little chance of benefit from the operative closure. Several studies have shown a decrease in pulmonary artery pressure and pulmonary vascular resistance after interruption of a ductus with pulmonary hypertension, but in follow-up of 68 patients after closure of a ventricular septal defect, DuShane and Kirklin (1973) found that of those patients operated on after age 2 with moderately or severely elevated pulmonary vascular resistance, over half had persistence of the high pulmonary resistance. When operated on before age 2, over 90 per cent had a favorable result. These observations are probably applicable to patent ductus arteriosus and emphasize the need for early operation when pulmonary artery pressure and resistance are high. The condition is more apt to be reversible in young children than in adults. A current review of pulmonary vascular disease with congenital heart lesions was published by Hoffman and colleagues (1981).

In some cases, as in the tetralogy of Fallot, the ductus is a compensating structure. The ductus must not be interrupted in such situations unless the condition for which it is compensating can be corrected.

SURGICAL TREATMENT

Whether the ductus is surgically exposed from an anterolateral or a posterolateal incision is largely a matter of personal preference. Mobilization of the aorta may be accomplished more easily through a posterolateral fourth interspace incision. Exposure is more time-consuming and the position is more embarrassing to ventilation, however, so that we have used this only for the uncommon patient with a mycotic aneurysm involving the ductus or the patient with an extremely large main pulmonary artery, which might obscure exposure of the ductus from in front.

We prefer to make an incision through the third interspace, going below the breast in females (Fig. 30–5A). The incision must extend well around laterally, with division of almost the entire intercostal muscle bundle, separating the serratus and dividing the anterior edge of the latissimus dorsi so that good exposure is obtained well up into the axilla. In our experience, this has given wide and ample exposure of the ductus, adjacent aorta, and pulmonary artery. An incision is made overlying the pulmonary artery between the phrenic and vagus nerves. If the ductus is not readily seen, it may be found by tracing the recurrent branch of the vagus nerve around the ductus and the aorta. There is usually a small lappet of pericardium extending over the ductus, which should be elevated, and the ductus should be bared of its adventitia and freed of attachments.

Sharp dissection under direct vision is preferable to blunt, tearing dissection. The angle between the distal pulmonary artery and the ductus is particularly susceptible to injury. Attachments between the pericardium, pulmonary artery, and lesser curvature of the aortic arch should be exposed and divided. After the ductus is mobilized as much as possible and the adjacent pulmonary artery and aorta freed, a right-angled clamp may be placed around the ductus and umbilical tape passed. This clamp is probably more safely passed behind the ductus from the caudal, distal, aortic side. Slight traction may be applied on the tape, and the ductus can be freed posteriorly, thus obtaining additional length.

There is room for personal preference also in the method of interruption of the ductus (Ekström, 1952). Most would agree that, theoretically, closure of any large artery can best be accomplished by division of the artery. In actual practice, however, multiple suture ligation of the ductus with occlusion over the entire length of the ductus has given excellent results (Scott, 1950). Ligation with multiple transfixing sutures was championed by Blalock (1946) at a time when division was associated with considerably greater risk than at present. The method is safe and satisfactory.

If ligation is to be done, purse-string sutures are placed at the aortic and pulmonary ends and tied snugly, nearly obliterating the flow through the ductus (Fig. 30–5B). Two mattress sutures are then placed between these, and the ductus is obliterated over a centimeter or more of length.

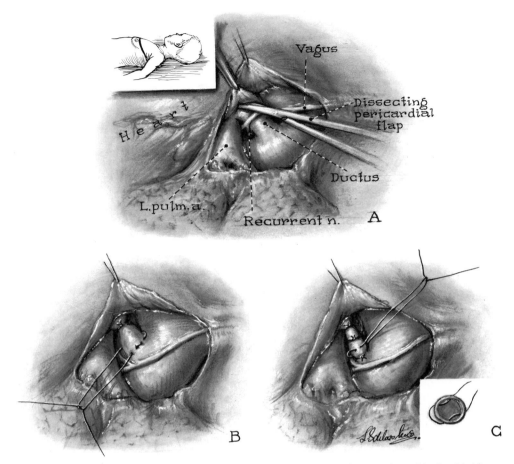

Figure 30–5. Operative treatment of ductus arteriosus by ligation. *A,* The incision is anterolateral in the third interspace. In females, the incision circles beneath the breast. Elevation of the pericardial lappet exposes the ductus. *B,* Purse-string sutures, which do not enter the lumen, are placed at either end, followed by perforating mattress sutures between (*C*). The ductus should be obliterated over an 8- to 10-mm. distance.

Increased experience with the great vessels, particularly the development of finer clamps for occluding vessels, has greatly reduced the risk of division of the ductus. This procedure is probably practiced more widely than ligation. After the ductus is mobilized as much as possible, fine vascular clamps, such as the multitooth Potts ductus clamp, are placed on the aortic-pulmonary ends with sufficient room in between for division and closure (Fig. 30–6*A*). When the ductus is divided, the occluding clamps must be held against the pulmonary artery and the aorta, thus lessening the danger of their being pulled off and at the same time giving greater exposure for suture closure. A satisfactory method is to suture adjacent to the clamp with a mattress suture and continue back over the free edge with an over-and-over whip suture (Fig. 30–6*B*). Suturing the lappet of pericardium across the pulmonary end of the divided ductus to tissue posterior, between the pulmonary artery and aorta, separates the two ends more completely.

If the ductus is unusually large, greater than 1.5 cm. in diameter, simple ligation is dangerous because of the possibility of the suture tearing through the wall. In such patients, division of the ductus is advocated. When the ductus is extremely short and large, additional length for closure can be gained by clamping the ductus at the pulmonary end and then cross-clamping the aorta just above and below the ductus. The ductus is then divided with sufficient cuff on the pulmonary end for closure, and the tangential opening in the aorta is closed while the aorta is collapsed. The safe occlusion time of the aorta is unknown and unpredictable, but 15 minutes' occlusion is probably safe, and this should be ample to allow closure.

Convalescence should be smooth in the patient with the typical ductus. When cardiac failure, pulmonary hypertension, or endarteritis on the ductus is present, recovery may be slower.

RESULTS OF OPERATION

Few operations in cardiac surgery are more satisfyingly curative. The work of the heart is immediately lowered as the burden of the excessive shunt is removed. In 689 cases of all types of patent ductus arteriosus at the Johns Hopkins Hospital, both typical and atypical, with and without cardiac failure, and

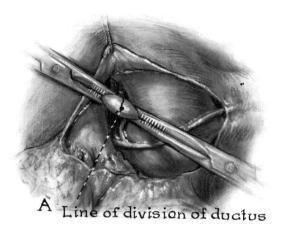 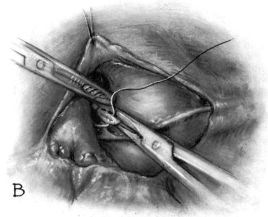

A Line of division of ductus B

Figure 30–6. Treatment of ductus arteriosus by division. *A,* The anterolateral third interspace incision is used for exposure, as for ligation. A thin occluding clamp is placed on either end and the ductus is divided. Pressing the clamp against the pulmonary artery or aorta after division reduces the likelihood of slipping. *B,* Suture of the ductus is by a continuous mattress suture down adjacent to the clamp, followed by a whip stitch back up over the free edge. Suture of the pulmonary artery end is easier from the patient's right side.

with additional defects in a number of cases, the mortality was 2.6 per cent. Gross (1953) reported that in his experience in patients who had no failure or infection prior to operation, the mortality was less than 0.5 per cent. In a collective review of 3986 cases, the operative mortality was 2 per cent with ligation and 2.1 per cent with division in children, and 4.3 and 5.2 per cent, respectively, in adults (Waterman *et al.,* 1956). With modern anesthetic and surgical techniques, the risk should be significantly lower.

Long-term evaluation of patients who have been operated on clearly demonstrates the value of occlusion of the ductus. In view of the low risk, prophylac-

tic occlusion seems indicated in all children and young adults, even in the absence of symptoms. There is even greater reason for operation in most of the patients who are symptomatic. When balanced against the likelihood of complications and a shortened life expectancy, the low operative risk indicates to most cardiologists and surgeons that the ductus should be interrupted in asymptomatic children and young adults. In symptomatic patients, the interruption may be urgent and necessary for the control of cardiac failure.

For references see page 990.

VI   AORTOPULMONARY WINDOW

Henry T. Bahnson

Aortopulmonary window (or aortopulmonary fenestration, fistula, or septal defect) resembles patent ductus arteriosus in its functional and clinical manifestations. In fact, differential diagnosis is difficult, and many cases have been discovered at the time of evaluation or operation for patent ductus arteriosus or ventricular septal defect, the two commonly confused conditions.

PATHOLOGIC ANATOMY

Between the fifth and eighth weeks of fetal life, the aortic septum divides the truncus arteriosus into the aorta and the pulmonary artery. At the same time, the cardiac chambers are developing. The bulbus

cordis connects the right ventricle to the pulmonary artery, and the ventricular septum separates the left ventricle and permits its attachment to the aorta. Ultimately, the aortic septum from above fuses with the ventricular septum from below. Failure of development of the various septa may result in an aortopulmonary window, a ventricular septal defect, or, if there is complete failure in development, a truncus arteriosus.

The typical fistula is anatomically located just above the aortic valve (Fig. 30–7) and varies in size from a few millimeters to several centimeters. Although in many instances the aorta and pulmonary artery are separate between the heart and the region of the window, in some cases the defect is located immediately adjacent to the coronary arteries and

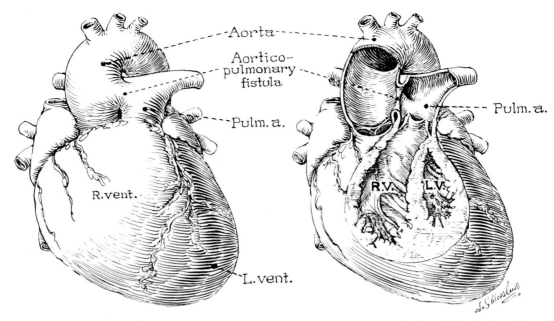

Figure 30–7. Aorticopulmonary window similar to that shown treated in Figure 30–8. The size of the fistula and its relation to the semilunar valves are variable. (From Scott, H. W., Jr., and Sabiston, D. C., Jr.: Surgical treatment for congenital aorticopulmonary fistula. Experimental and clinical aspects. J. Thorac. Surg., *25*:26, 1953.)

valves, and the condition may be indistinguishable externally from a truncus arteriosus, in which the aortic and pulmonary valves are part of a single opening. Richardson and associates (1979) have emphasized that the aortic septum develops near the connection of the right pulmonary artery to the arch system. As a consequence, the right pulmonary artery might arise at the site of the window or even from the aorta itself, if the septum forms to the left of the pulmonary artery.

CLINICAL PICTURE

This condition is practically indistinguishable from a large patent ductus arteriosus without special studies. Cardiac enlargement is almost always present, along with physical underdevelopment. The murmur produced varies from a continuous to a soft systolic one, and in some instances, there is no murmur at all. The murmur has been described as more superficial than that of patent ductus and may be loudest along the left sternal border in the third and fourth interspaces. As in patent ductus arteriosus with pulmonary hypertension, the pressure in the two vessels may be essentially equal, so that there is not a continuous murmur. The pulmonary second sound is usually loud, and there may be a diastolic murmur of pulmonary insufficiency. A wide pulse pressure may be noted. Increased pulmonary vascularity, often with dilatation of the main pulmonary artery, is similar to that seen roentgenologically in patent ductus arteriosus, as is the electrocardiographic evidence of left ventricular hypertrophy or both left and right hypertrophy in the

presence of pulmonary hypertension. Echocardiography will show the defect between the pulmonary artery and aorta.

Cardiac catheterization should demonstrate pulmonary hypertension and the left-to-right shunt into the pulmonary artery. Passage of a catheter into the aorta from the pulmonary artery close to the heart may be helpful, but the best differentiation from patent ductus, truncus arteriosus, and ventricular septal defect is by cineangiography. Even then an exact diagnosis cannot always be expected, and exploratory thoracotomy may be necessary with the realization that one may have to treat a patent ductus, truncus arteriosus, ventricular septal defect, or aortopulmonary window.

Evaluation of the pulmonary vascular resistance is of great importance. Considerations in selection of patients for operation are similar to those given in the preceding section on patent ductus, the operative risk being a bit greater for aortopulmonary window.

SURGICAL TREATMENT

Aortopulmonary windows have been treated by ligation, by simple clamping and division, and by division and suture during caval occlusion with hypothermia or during cardiopulmonary bypass. In cases in which the defect is small or in which there is no significant pulmonary hypertension and there is room between the defect and the cardiac valves to allow mobilization, clamping and division may be used. In most cases, however, the conditions are not favorable for clamping. The vessels are large and tense with

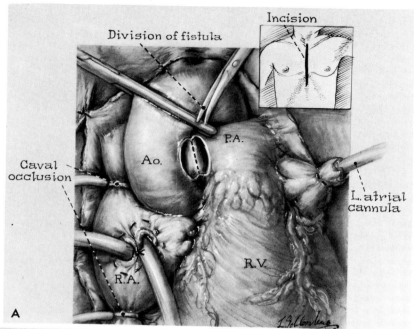

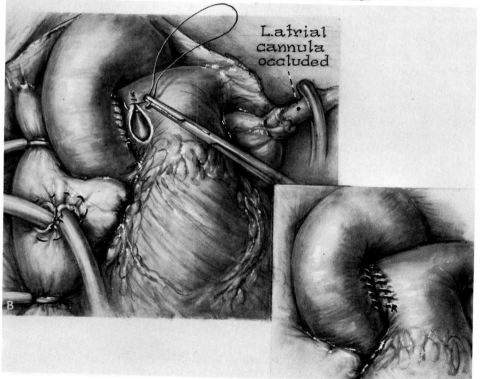

Figure 30–8. Closure of aorticopulmonary window during cardiopulmonary bypass. *A,* The aorta is occluded while the fistula is divided and the aortic end closed. The cannula in the left atrium through the appendage helps keep the operative area free of blood; this is clamped after closure of the aortic opening is completed and air is evacuated from the left side. *B,* The aorta is unclamped and coronary circulation is restored while the pulmonary opening is closed.

pulmonary hypertension; the right pulmonary artery seems to arise almost from the back wall of the fistula; and the vessels are easily torn during mobilization or attempted occlusion. In such instances, the use of cardiopulmonary bypass converts a difficult and hazardous procedure into a relatively straightforward and easy one (Cooley *et al.,* 1957).

A midline sternal splitting incision provides good exposure and permits treatment of intracardiac defects if such are present (Fig. 30–8). Although the exposure is not ideal, a large patent ductus arteriosus also can be treated from this incision. The site and size of the fistula should be determined as accurately as possible, although in some instances differentiation from a truncus arteriosus is not possible on external examination. A finger may be passed through the right auricular appendage and the right ventricle and pulmonary valve palpated in order to identify the presence of any portion of the aortopulmonary septum. Once cardiopulmonary bypass is begun (see Chapter 29), the left side of the heart can be kept empty by a cannula placed into the left atrium. The aorta is clamped distal to the fistula, and an incision is made along the anterior surface of the defect. Then, under direct vision, the pulmonary artery and aorta are separated and the aortic opening closed. Following this, the cannula in the left atrium is clamped, the left side is allowed to fill to evacuate air, and the flow through the ascending aorta and coronary arteries is resumed. The pulmonary artery can then be reconstructed while the heart receives blood and beats. The 5- to 15-minute period of cardiac ischemia should be well tolerated in the usual case, especially if the body is cooled to 30°C. When the right pulmonary artery arises at the window, transaortic repair with a patch may be preferable (Richardson *et al.*, 1979).

RESULTS OF OPERATION

Aortopulmonary window is not a common condition. Pulmonary hypertension has been present in almost all instances. Decrease in heart size and relief of cardiac failure are usually impressive. In most instances, the pulmonary arterial pressure falls and approaches the normal level. Whether the pulmonary vascular bed will return to normal in the majority of cases is not known, but considerations are probably similar to those in patent ductus arteriosus. Operation should be done at as early an age as possible.

For references see page 990.

VII   COARCTATION OF THE AORTA

Henry T. Bahnson

Coarctation of the aorta is an important congenital cardiovascular defect that occurs in a significant number of persons. It shortens life if untreated, but it can be corrected to render the patient functionally normal.

PATHOLOGIC ANATOMY

Coarctation most commonly occurs in the region of the aortic isthmus just distal to the left subclavian artery. It occurs less frequently in the aortic arch itself, and in occasional cases, the constriction is in the midthoracic aorta at the level of the diaphragm or below in the region of the renal arteries (Bahnson *et al.*, 1949). In rare instances, the coarctation may be multiple.

Coarctation in the aortic arch or isthmus can be helpfully classified as preductal or postductal (Fig. 30–9). In the preductal type, formerly called infantile because of its association with early death, the pulmonary artery communicates through a ductus, often a large one, with the distal aorta, and there are usually additional major intracardiac defects, most commonly a ventricular septal defect but, in a significant number of cases, transposition of the great vessels, atrial septal defect, and other anomalies. The coarctation then separates the flow from the left ventricle to the head and arms and the flow from the pulmonary artery and right ventricle to the caudal half of the body through the ductus. This type of coarctation often involves the distal aortic arch along with the isthmus and tends to be more elongated or diffuse. It is generally discovered in infancy because of the striking disturbance of the circulation by the aortic obstruction in addition to the cardiac defect. Cardiac failure usually occurs, is intractable, and results in death unless correction is possible.

Interrupted aorta, or aortic atresia, is a severe form of coarctation of the aorta usually but not always associated with persistence of the ductus arteriosus.

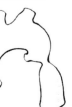

POSTDUCTAL

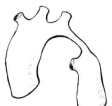

PREDUCTAL

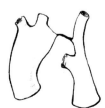

INTERRUPTED AORTA

Figure 30–9. Sketches of representative types of coarctation of the aorta.

Although most cases have been found at autopsy in newborn infants, a few patients have survived to reach adulthood.

In the typical uncomplicated, postductal type of coarctation, formerly called adult, there is a localized constriction just distal to the ductus or ligamentum arteriosum. The aortic valve is bicuspid in 25 to 40 per cent of the cases, but other cardiac defects are uncommon. Most patients with this type of anomaly survive to adult life. Although the typical postductal coarctation is usually localized to the region of the ligamentum arteriosum, it may involve the mouth of the left subclavian artery, may be more elongated and diffuse, or may be associated with a hypoplastic distal aortic arch.

In patients who survive beyond infancy, a number of additional features are often noted, the most striking being development of collateral circulation, as demonstrated by Bramwell and Jones (1941). Arteries connecting the upper and lower parts of the body, notably the internal mammary, subscapular, and lateral thoracic arteries, become dilated. These communicate with the intercostal arteries, which may be greatly dilated, thin-walled, friable, and subject to dangerous aneurysm formation. Immediately distal to the coarctation, there is often poststenotic dilatation of the thoracic aorta, which has as much the appearance of a congenital dilatation as a functional one caused by flow through the stenotic area. There is an increased incidence of cystic medial necrosis of the ascending aorta in association with coarctation.

The etiology is unknown, although the most widely mentioned cause is in connection with the obliterative process, which causes disappearance of the aortic arches and possible closure of the ductus arteriosus. In the unusual type of coarctation that occurs in the midthoracic aorta, there appears to be a more diffuse inflammatory process, also of unknown etiology.

CLINICAL PICTURE

Most children with uncomplicated coarctation are asymptomatic, and their condition is discovered because of a murmur or the presence of arterial hypertension discovered during a routine examination. Symptoms are more common in the adult. Headache, dyspnea, palpitation, vertigo, throbbing in the head, visual troubles, precordial pain, or symptoms of cardiac decompensation, all related to hypertension of the upper part of the body, may drive the patient to seek medical aid. General weakness is a common complaint. In a number of instances, weakness and fatigue of the legs and even intermittent claudication are present, but conversely, it is striking how many patients have no difficulty with the lower extremities, some even being unusually athletic before the condition is recognized.

Diagnosis is made simply and easily in almost all cases by finding a difference in arterial pulsations and blood pressure in the upper and lower extremities. A comparison of radial and femoral pulsations should be part of every complete physical examination and, of course, is essential in any patient with hypertension or in one who has complaints such as those just listed. Normally, the pulses in the radial and the femoral arteries are synchronous, but in the presence of coarctation, there is a noticeable delay in the femoral pulse. Blood pressures and pulses in both upper extremities should be compared with the same measurement in the legs, because, in rare cases, the orifice of one subclavian artery, usually the left, may be involved in the coarctation, giving rise to a low blood pressure in that arm. Indeed, either subclavian artery may arise below the coarctation. A case has been described in which both subclavian arteries arose from the region of the coarctation and were hypoplastic. Consequently, there was no brachial hypertension. In such patients, observation of collateral circulation is most important in the diagnosis.

In addition to the pathognomonic pulse and pressure gradient, there are often pulsations in the neck and supraclavicular areas due to hypertension. A systolic murmur is often heard over the base of the heart or in the mid-back around the sixth or seventh dorsal vertebra. Diastolic murmurs may be heard in either place. Posteriorly, a diastolic murmur probably represents flow through the narrowed area or through the dilated intercostal arteries. Wells and associates (1949) found diastolic sounds posteriorly in all 15 patients with coarctation of the aorta examined by phonocardiography. These sounds were a continuation of those noted during systole. A diastolic murmur anteriorly should also be carefully sought, since, when present, it may indicate a patent ductus arteriosus or aortic regurgitation due to a bicuspid aortic valve or dilatation of the proximal aorta.

Except in young children, enlarged collateral vessels may often be felt over the back adjacent to the scapula, and in some cases, a murmur may even be heard over them. In 1933, Sir Thomas Lewis pointed out that, in the proper light, pulsations can be seen in these vessels, and he carefully mapped the circulation in this condition. The subscapular artery is often enlarged as well and can be felt by compressing the subscapular tissue between the thumb and index finger. Collateral circulation should always be looked for, because the disparity between pressure and pulse characteristic of coarctation may also be caused by terminal aortic thrombosis or other types of aortic obstruction.

The heart may show some increase in size, particularly of the left ventricle, but when it is unduly large, other anomalies must be considered. The upper mediastinum is often widened because of the enlarged left subclavian artery. Prominence of the left subclavian artery and the proximal and distal aorta is responsible for a characteristic notch in the upper left mediastinal shadow on roentgenography, giving the appearance of the number 3, the upper convexity being the proximal aorta, the notch being the coarc-

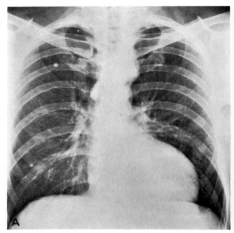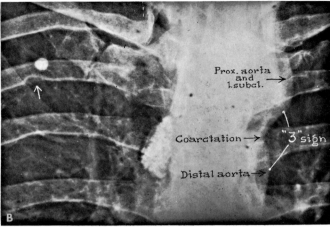

Figure 30–10. Radiologic signs, which are diagnostic but not always present in coarctation, include notching of the ribs and the "3" sign caused by the dilated proximal segment and the left subclavian artery, by the constricted area, and by poststenotic dilatation. *A,* Note the rounded lower left cardiac border, indicating left ventricular enlargement. *B,* Enlargement of part of *A,* showing notching of rib (adjacent to calcified lesion) and "3" sign.

tation, and the lower convexity being the poststenotic dilatation (Fig. 30–10*A*). Notching of the ribs, as first noted by Railsbach and Dock (1929), remains one of the most characteristic radiologic features and is caused by dilatation, elongation, and tortuosity of the intercostal vessels serving as collaterals between the subclavian arteries above and the aorta below the narrowing (Fig. 30–10*B*). Notching is seldom seen before the age of 12 to 14 years. When present in the uncomplicated case, it is most noticeable in the third to the seventh ribs and is bilaterally symmetric. If the distribution is more prominent in other areas or is asymmetric, an atypical coarctation or involvement of the mouth of the subclavian artery must be considered. When a subclavian artery arises from the aorta below the coarctation, notching will be present only on the contralateral side.

The electrocardiogram may vary from normal to that of a striking left ventricular hypertrophy, depending on the severity of the coarctation and the degree of hypertension. This examination is especially important in older patients, in whom changes associated with myocardial damage presage a greater operative risk.

All the signs mentioned point to an obstruction to blood flow in the aorta between the origin of the vessels to the head and arms and those to the lower extremities. In the majority of cases beyond infancy, it would be correct to assume that the coarctation is at the junction of the arch and the descending aorta. There is an occasional patient, however, with constriction distal to the usual site. It is important to identify these patients prior to thoracotomy, since successful treatment of such a lesion often requires an aortic replacement and the area may not be readily accessible from the usual thoracotomy incision.

A satisfactory aortogram demonstrates the lesion in the unusual site, but this examination is unnecessary in most instances of typical coarctation. If one is aware of the possibility of the unusual coarctation, there are several features that suggest the use of aortography. A diffuse murmur heard low in the back is unusual in the typical case and suggests an atypical site in the back or abdomen. Notching that is most prominent in the lower ribs or the absence of notching in patients with other signs of significant aortic obstruction, such as definite hypertension or the brachial-femoral pressure gradient, is suggestive. When the coarctation is in the abdominal aorta, pulsations in the upper abdominal aorta may be palpable. If the possibility is kept in mind, one may safely reserve aortography for patients presenting any or all the atypical signs mentioned.

Coarctation in either the preductal or postductal site is an important cause of cardiac failure in infants. Such children with cardiac failure are irritable and dyspneic, fail to grow and eat normally, and may have cyanosis. The baby may look quite sick, with tachypnea, tachycardia, rales over the lungs, hepatomegaly, and an overactive heart. The diagnosis may be difficult to make in sick infants, and the discrepancy in the pulses of the upper and lower extremities may not be readily apparent. Examination should be repeated until the diagnosis is clarified, although in doubtful cases an aortogram may be used to demonstrate the coarctation.

PROGNOSIS

In a review of 108 infants by Glass and associates (1960), 90 per cent of the fatalities in infants under 1 year of age were due to preductal coarctation, usually in association with cardiac defects. It is important to define whether the principal problem in such patients is due to obstruction of coarctation or to the cardiac defect, the latter often being associated with increased pulmonary blood flow. Many infants with postductal coarctation can be tided over the failure with non-operative treatment, and they may improve, presumably as collateral channels develop (Gross, 1953). In others, this is not possible, and surgical relief is necessary.

Adults with typical postductal coarctation have an abbreviated life expectancy. Abbott (1928), in her 142 postmortem cases, found the average age of patients to be 32 years. Reifenstein and colleagues (1947) reviewed a large group of patients and found that 61 per cent died at or before 40 years of age. About one fourth of the patients lived far into adult life with no incapacity; about one fourth died from bacterial endocarditis or aortitis; about one fourth died suddenly from rupture of the aorta (the aorta being susceptible both proximal and distal to the coarctation); and about one fourth died because of the hypertensive state with cardiac failure or cerebral hemorrhage. It is evident that although some subjects may live a normal life and be unhindered by coarctation, in most instances the defect is a hazardous one.

PATHOLOGIC PHYSIOLOGY

Physiologic studies have been concerned primarily with the cause of hypertension above coarctation of the aorta. Scott and Bahnson (1951) produced coarctation experimentally in dogs, with a resultant carotid hypertension and discrepancy in femoral and carotid arterial pressures similar to that seen in clinical cases. In such animals, transplantation of a kidney to the neck and removal of the contralateral kidney caused a prompt fall in carotid pressure, although the gradient between carotid and femoral pressures remained. Elevated plasma renin activity with coarctation has been found by some, but not all, investigators (Parker et al., 1980), and although difficult to substantiate in the compensated state, the mechanism of hypertension probably involves renal ischemia or hypotension.

SELECTION OF PATIENTS FOR OPERATION

Almost all patients with coarctation of the aorta should be operated on at an appropriate time unless there are significant contraindications. There are degrees of coarctation, and in some patients in whom only a slight discrepancy in pressure exists between the upper and lower extremities, suggesting less total obstruction, it may be difficult to be sure that the obstruction is not more complete and that it is not simply compensated by adequate collateral circulation. Probably the most satisfactory age for operation is between 4 and 12 years. Although technically easy in younger children, the operation is apt to be more permanently beneficial if the aorta is allowed to approach its adult size. With increasing age beyond the optimum, the operation is of greater magnitude, the

aorta is more sclerotic, less elastic, and more difficult to approximate and suture, and aneurysms of the intercostal arteries are found more frequently. Hypertension also is more apt to be of a fixed nature and to respond less satisfactorily to the relief of the aortic obstruction.

Operation is clearly indicated in some patients above and below the optimum age. As Gross (1953) emphasized, during the first few months of life many babies have cardiac embarrassment from uncomplicated coarctation of the aorta, but the majority of them can be tided over by nonoperative means. Once compensation is gained, they often survive to later childhood without difficulty. On the other hand, there are a significant number of infants who will not survive unless surgical help can be given. In such infants, the operative risk is undoubtedly high. However, Glass and coworkers (1960) recommended that babies with symptoms in the first month of life should be operated on promptly, unless they show dramatic response during a 12-hour trial of treatment with digitalis, and that babies over 1 month of age who respond to digitalis may be kept on this medication until adequate compensation has taken place and operation can be performed at the optimum age. When a ventricular septal defect is present with coarctation, the left-to-right shunt is aggravated by increased systemic resistance from the coarctation. If the coarctation is repaired, and even if the pulmonary artery is not banded, the child may improve sufficiently so that repair of the ventricular defect may be deferred. In some patients, the defect will close spontaneously (Neches et al., 1977).

At the other end of the age scale, some persons are unaware of coarctation of the aorta until well into adult life. Beyond the age of 30, there is some increase in the operative risk, and although modern statistics are not available, this almost surely rises with increased age. Of 51 patients older than 30 years treated by Blalock and staff, there was a 10 per cent hospital mortality rate as compared to a rate of 7 per cent for patients in the 4- to 15-year-old age group (Eifrig, 1960). It should be emphasized, however, that there is no more specific treatment for arterial hypertension than excision of a coarctation of the aorta, and the operation should be seriously considered at any age. Successful results have been obtained in patients in their fifth and sixth decades.

Certain conditions greatly increase the operative risk (Shumacker et al., 1968). Mild to moderate aortic insufficiency may be present, due either to rheumatic heart disease or to a congenitally bicuspid valve. In a few instances, the valve as well as the coarctation has been surgically treated. The risk is greater when there are significant cardiac abnormalities: mitral disease from rheumatic fever, septal defects, or myocardial damage. In almost all such cases, the burden on the heart would be decreased if the hypertension due to coarctation could be relieved, but the risk may be prohibitive and operation inadvisable.

SURGICAL TREATMENT

Blalock and Park (1944) reported an experimental operation designed to bypass coarctation of the aorta by anastomosing the left subclavian artery to the distal aorta. This method was not attempted on a patient until Crafoord and Nylin (1945) and Gross and Hufnagel (1945) independently resected the involved area and performed end-to-end anastomosis of the divided aorta. This operation quickly became the standard one. Use of the subclavian artery is rarely, if ever, indicated, as sacrifice of a large number of collaterals is required.

The operation is performed with the patient in the lateral position (Fig. 30–11). Almost the entire length of the left fifth rib is removed, as suggested by Crafoord, and the chest is entered through the bed of this rib. If the entire rib from neck to cartilage is removed, good exposure can be obtained and the removal of segments of other ribs is not necessary. The coaractation and the arrangement of the aorta and the vessels should be inspected before the pleura is opened, because often a good view is obtained before the tissues are stained. A long incision is made in the pleura over the coarctation, the adjacent subclavian above and the aorta below, and the pleural flaps are held back with sutures. The easier dissection is done first, namely, mobilizing the left subclavian artery and the adjacent aorta, the coarctation, and the ligamentum arteriosum or the ductus. Considerable mobility of the aorta is often obtained when the ductus or ligament is divided, so that division of this as soon as possible is helpful. If there are large intercostal arteries adjacent to the coarctation, mobilization of the aorta a short distance below may help to avoid injury to these thin-walled and sometimes troublesome collaterals.

Once this area is mobilized, the intercostal arteries can be visualized from both sides and isolated more carefully. Great care must be exercised in dissection about the intercostal arteries, for they are friable and easily torn from the wall of the aorta. There are few places where it is easier to stay out of difficulty than to get out of difficulty than in this portion of the operation for coarctation. It is preferable to divide none of these collateral vessels, but although this is usually feasible, one or two of the upper ones may need to be severed. As soon as tapes can be placed around the aorta, it can be pulled up slightly away from the vertebral column and better visualization of the posterior aspect obtained.

In most patients with an uncomplicated postductal coarctation, the constricted segment is short, but in some instances there is a narrow proximal aortic segment and in others a long area of marked constriction. It must be emphasized that in order to obtain relief of hypertension, all the coarctation must be removed. It is tempting to remove only a short segment and thus avoid tension in performing the anastomosis. If in doing this an anastomosis smaller than the diameter of the distal aortic arch is obtained or, when the ends cannot be approximated, if insufficient length is removed to relieve the constriction, some form of aortoplasty or aortic replacement must be used.

That only 14 prostheses were used in the first 275 cases treated by Blalock and staff may not be representative of the actual need in modern practice. In

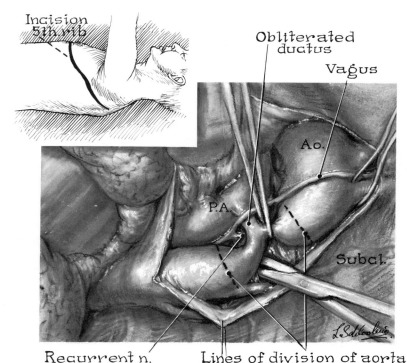

Figure 30–11. Operative exposure for resection of coarctation of the aorta is through the bed of the fifth rib. The entire rib is removed from neck to cartilage. The constricted segment is usually held medially by an obliterated ductus, division of which allows considerable mobility. The coarctation is held forward to facilitate dissection posteriorly. Large intercostal arteries must be carefully avoided. Division of the aorta should be through a point of normal diameter.

some of the early operations, the left subclavian artery was used, and in a few other early cases, a compromise in the direction of a small anastomosis was made. Increased confidence through the years has led to the greater use of prostheses. Such procedures have been used in 2 to 40 per cent of cases, depending on the inclination of the surgeon and the age range of his patients. Less elasticity of the aorta and greater frequency of aneurysms (often of the distal aorta or adjacent intercostal arteries) and arteriosclerotic lesions in the adult require more frequent use of complicated reconstruction. In occasional cases, constriction of the mouth of the left subclavian or damage to the artery may require a prosthesis with a side arm. However, a prosthesis is rarely needed in young children, because the aorta can be mobilized and is elastic enough to allow approximation of the two ends.

Various types of anastomoses may be performed. We prefer a single row of continuous 5-0 Polydek

through all layers, the intima being everted with a mattress suture (Fig. 30–12). In the usual case, this gives a smooth approximation of the intima of the two vessels. An overhand, noneverting suture works satisfactorily, particularly if the anastomosis is begun with eversion and efforts are made to continue the everting. In view of experimental work showing that a continuous suture may prevent growth of the anastomosis (Sauvage and Harkins, 1952), we interrupt the suture frequently on the anterior row or, especially in children, in whom growth is important, perform the entire anterior portion with interrupted sutures. It is often helpful to place much of the posterior row of an everting mattress suture before the vessels are closely approximated and the posterior suture line is pulled up, as described by Blalock (1946) (Fig. 30–12A).

Any one of a number of instruments may be used to occlude the aorta proximally and distally. It is advantageous to allow flow to continue through the

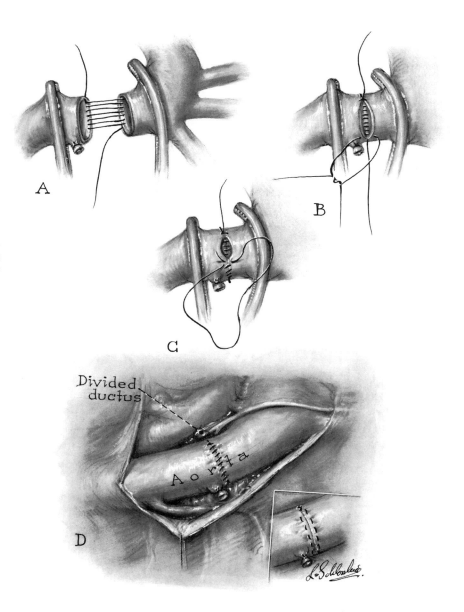

Figure 30–12. *A–D,* Anastomosis following excision of coarctation. An everting mattress suture is placed over about one third of the posterior row before the vessels are approximated and the suture pulled up. The anastomosis is completed with a continuous over-and-over suture. Insert in *D* shows the everting mattress suture sometimes used. In young children, the entire anterior row is formed with interrupted sutures.

left subclavian artery and its branches, which serve as collaterals, but this may not be possible if the anastomosis must be made to the distal portion of the aortic arch in order to obtain an unrestricted lumen, which is the ideal goal of the operation. Small clamps may be used to temporarily occlude the preserved intercostals when the aorta is opened. Following completion of the anastomosis, the distal clamp is removed and any necessary sutures placed in order to obtain a tight anastomosis. The proximal clamp should be released slowly and blood given intravenously during this time. In some patients, a too rapid release of the clamp may lead to profound hypotension.

Interruption of the aorta is especially hazardous, and only a few survivors have been reported, the first being by Tyson and associates (1970). Although a few patients have lived to adulthood, this is more commonly a condition of infancy, and repair is more complicated (Bailey et al., 1981).

RESULTS OF OPERATION

In 1601 cases collected from around the world, the average mortality rate was 8.6 per cent (Rumel et al., 1957). It was 6.8 per cent between the ages of 4 and 15 years and significantly higher below the age of 3 or over the age of 30. In the patients who survived, satisfactory relief of hypertension was obtained in 95.2 per cent, and entirely normal readings were present in 72 per cent. The incidence of persistent hypertension increased progressively with the age of the patient. Maron and coworkers (1973), in an 11- to 25-year follow-up of many of the first patients treated by Blalock and associates, found a higher incidence of hypertension and cardiovascular disease in a fraction of their patients studied more intensively and emphasized the need for early diagnosis and treatment as well as continued follow-up.

Other follow-up now extends for 36 years, with satisfactory results (Bergdahl et al., 1980). Recent reports reflect the larger number of operations now being done during infancy, when the need and risk are greater. Most of the deaths occur in patients less than 6 months of age (Berman et al., 1980). Also reflecting the earlier age at operation are reports of recoarctation due to insufficient resection, residual ductal or fibrous tissue, thrombosis, or failure to grow because of scarring or a constricting continuous suture (Iberra-Perez et al., 1969).

One complication, which appears to be an unfortunate by-product of the relief of hypertension, has been a necrotizing arteritis. Although rare, this has occasionally been fatal. Examination shows the arteritis to be limited to the lower part of the body. Most of the clinical manifestations have been in the abdomen, causing abdominal pain and, in some instances, resulting in gangrene of the intestine. This is probably the most severe form of a condition affecting about one third of young patients operated on for resection of the coarctation, in whom blood pressure may rise to a higher level after operation than it was before — a "paradoxical hypertension." Abdominal symptoms are often noted in this group of patients and occur in one fourth to one half of them (Tawes et al., 1970). The cause of this complication is unknown, although it is recognized that there is increased sympathetic nerve activity following resection of coarctation (Goodall and Sealy, 1969) and elevated plasma renin activity (Rocchini et al., 1976). Sympathicolytic drugs are indicated in such cases (Sealy et al., 1957).

For unknown reasons, the blood pressure does not always reach its final level immediately after operation. In the majority of patients, the pressure is normal at the time of discharge from the hospital, but it commonly remains elevated for 10 to 14 days and occasionally for several months.

A rare and distressing complication has been paraplegia or weakness of the lower part of the body after operation, reported by Brewer and associates (1972) to occur with an incidence of 0.41 per cent in review of 12,532 cases. This appears to result from inadequate circulation through the anterior spinal artery. Explanations proposed, but not verified, include interruption of important intercostal or collateral arteries, inadequate collateral flow during aortic clamping and resulting distal hypotension, and a reflow phenomenon after relief of the coarctation. No specific means of preventing the complication has been established.

For references see page 990.

VIII ANEURYSMS OF THE SINUSES OF VALSALVA

MICHAEL E. DEBAKEY

GEORGE P. NOON

There are normally three aortic sinuses of Valsalva: the right, the left, and the noncoronary, each named according to its relation to the aortic valve leaflets and the coronary ostia. Originating proximally at the aortic anulus, the sinuses extend distally as dilated pouches in the aorta to a point usually just beyond the coronary ostia. Abnormalities of the sinuses of Valsalva may be congenital or acquired.

James Hope (1831) is credited with being the first to describe an aneurysm of a sinus of Valsalva, which had ruptured into the right ventricle. Nine years later, Thurnam (1840) reported this case and added five cases of his own. In the ensuing 125 years (Kwittken et al., 1965), fewer than 200 cases had been found. In 1965, we reported two cases of variations of this unusual entity (DeBakey et al., 1965). Two years later, we reviewed the records of 35 cases of abnormal sinuses of Valsalva referred for cardiac evaluation and suggested, as a more logical method than the previously used classification by cause, a classification based on pathologic anatomy (DeBakey et al., 1967).

Brown and coworkers (1955) attempted surgical repair of an aneurysm of a sinus of Valsalva in 1953. Four years later, Lillehei and associates (1957) performed the first reported successful operative repair of an aneurysm of a sinus of Valsalva. Both congenital and acquired abnormalities of the sinuses of Valsalva are now corrected surgically with considerable success as a result of subsequent refinements in extracorporeal cardiopulmonary assistance, operative techniques, and patient care.

ANATOMIC AND HISTOLOGIC CONSIDERATIONS

Congenital aneurysms of the sinuses of Valsalva are confined to one aortic sinus and consist of a localized diverticular outpouching of the coronary sinus, which eventually protrudes into a cardiac chamber or the myocardium. The aneurysm usually ruptures into a cardiac chamber and produces an aorto-intracardiac fistula. These aneurysms may or may not be associated with cardiovascular anomalies. The most common associated congenital anomaly is ventricular septal defect. Aortic valvular insufficiency occurs from distortion or fibrosis of the aortic valve.

The cause of congenital aneurysms is controversial. Abbott (1936) attributed them to defective development of the distal bulbar system, resulting in weakness at the point of fusion with the aorticopulmonary septum. This would explain abnormalities of the right and noncoronary sinus but not of the left. Edwards and Burchell (1957) beautifully demonstrated separation between the aortic media and the anulus fibrosus of the aortic valve, which results in a weakness and subsequent formation of an aneurysm. This weakness could account for aneurysms in all three sinuses.

Sakakibara and Konno (1963) classified congenital aneurysms according to their location on the coronary sinuses, their site of projection into the ventricle or atrium, and the presence of associated ventricular septal defect. Six main types and 16 subtypes have been recognized.

In contrast to congenital aneurysms, acquired aneurysms usually involve more than one sinus of Valsalva, and the ascending aorta as well. Acquired aneurysms result from infection, such as syphilis or bacterial and fungal endocarditis, as well as from cystic medial necrosis and collagen and connective disorders. The last two conditions may cause an aneurysm by enlargement, dissection, or both. Rarely, an aneurysm, with or without a fistula, results from blunt, penetrating trauma. Aortic valvular insufficiency is commonly associated with these aneurysms because of valvular or anular distortion. Rupture is usually extracardiac rather than intracardiac.

CLINICAL CONSIDERATIONS

Congenital aneurysms of the sinuses of Valsalva are not common. The reported incidence is highest in Japan, where they represent about 3.5 per cent of all congenital cardiovascular disorders operated on (Taguchi et al., 1969). These aneurysms generally enlarge until they rupture into the ventricle or atrium during the fourth decade of life. Until then, they are usually asymptomatic. The aneurysm is detected early only if the diagnosis is established during evaluation for other congenital cardiovascular defects, if the aneurysm produces symptoms by distortion and impairment of function of intracardiac structures, or if bacterial endocarditis develops. The most common cause of death is congestive heart failure, which develops after intracardiac rupture. Sawyers and associates (1957) reported the average age of death in their patients with congenital aneurysms of sinuses of Valsalva to be 33.5 years. The mean survival time after rupture in their series was about 1 year, if two patients who lived 10 and 15 years were excluded. Bacterial endocarditis is the second most common cause of death.

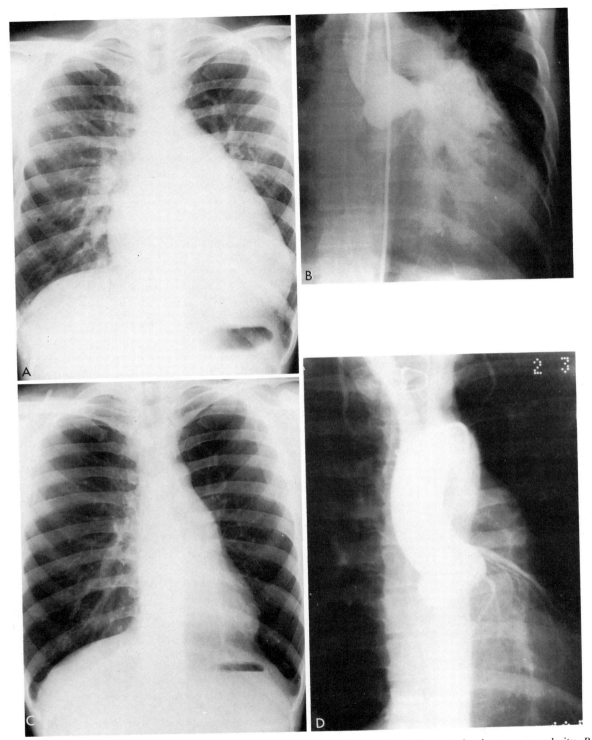

Figure 30–13. *A*, Posteroanterior roentgenogram of the chest shows cardiomegaly and increased pulmonary vascularity. *B*, Aortic root injection with radiopaque medium demonstrates aneurysm of the right coronary sinus with fistula to the right ventricle immediately below the pulmonary valve. *C*, After operation, cardiac size and pulmonary vascularity decreased. *D*, The aortic root injection with radiopaque medium shows absence of the left-to-right shunt 2 years after operation.

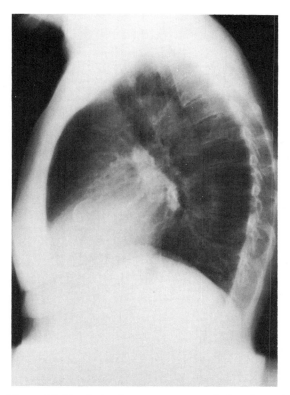

Figure 30–14. Lateral roentgenogram of the chest shows calcification of an aneurysm of the right coronary sinus.

Intracardiac rupture of the aneurysm usually causes abrupt onset of symptoms. Pain is common and most often is precordial or upper abdominal. The patient also has dyspnea, tachycardia, and increasing manifestations of congestive heart failure. Results of physical examination before rupture are usually normal. Parasternal systolic murmur can occasionally be heard. After rupture, a murmur develops, which is continuous and is best heard over the sternum or left sternal border in the second, third, and fourth intercostal spaces. Aortic valvular insufficiency often develops because of valvular distortion or fibrosis. The murmur that is heard after rupture might be confused with the murmurs of patent ductus arteriosus, aorticopulmonary window, aortic valvular disease, coronary arteriovenous fistula, and ventricular septal defect. Acute onset of the foregoing symptoms in a previously asymptomatic patient in the fourth decade of life, however, is highly suggestive of aneurysm of sinus of Valsalva.

Rarely can the radiographic diagnosis be made from plain roentgenograms. The sinuses are within the cardiac silhouette, which usually appears normal until ruptured, after which signs of a left-to-right shunt with cardiac enlargement and increased pulmonary vascularity develop (Fig. 30–13A). Aortic valvular insufficiency, if present, produces left ventricular enlargement.

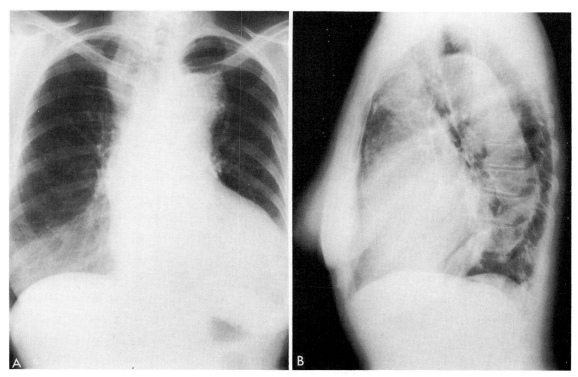

Figure 30–15. Posteroanterior (A) and lateral (B) roentgenograms of the chest show diffuse aortic calcification in a patient with aneurysms of all three sinuses of Valsalva extending into the ascending aorta.

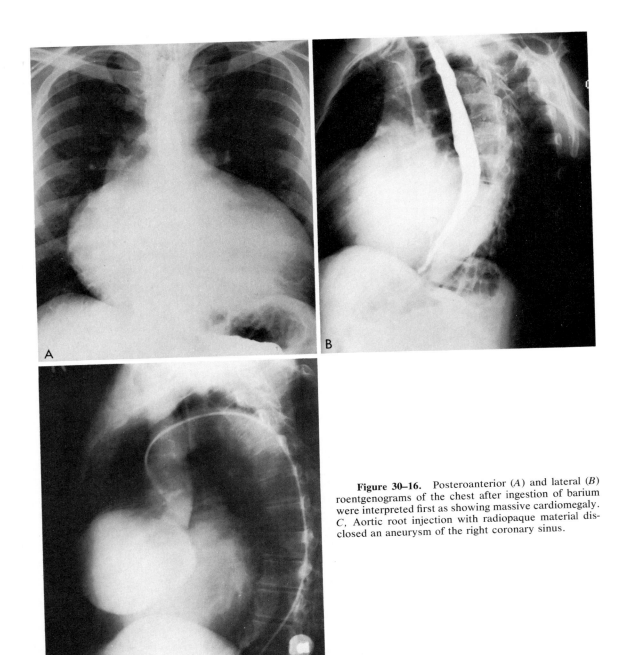

Figure 30–16. Posteroanterior (*A*) and lateral (*B*) roentgenograms of the chest after ingestion of barium were interpreted first as showing massive cardiomegaly. *C*, Aortic root injection with radiopaque material disclosed an aneurysm of the right coronary sinus.

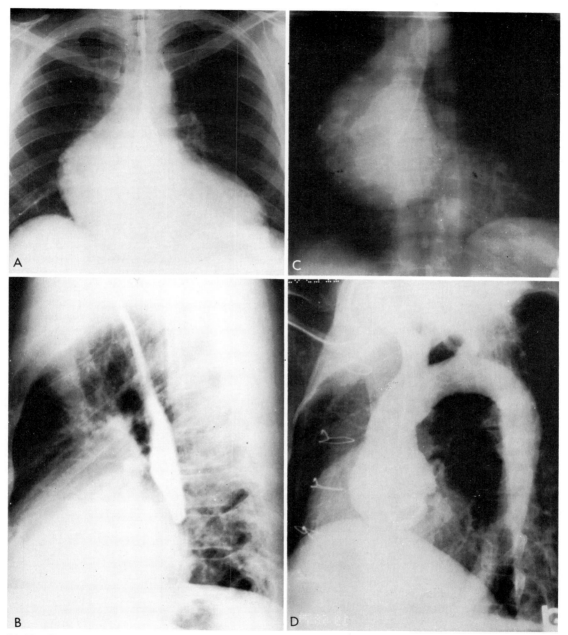

Figure 30–17. Posteroanterior (*A*) and lateral (*B*) roentgenograms of the chest of a patient with aneurysms of all three sinuses of Valsalva and the ascending aorta show increased cardiothoracic ratio with prominence of the right border of the heart, first interpreted as right atrial enlargement. *C,* Aortic root injection with radiopaque material shows large aneurysms of all three sinuses of Valsalva with extension into the ascending aorta. *D,* Aortic valve in place with Dacron graft replacement of excised segment of an ascending aorta 1 year after operation.

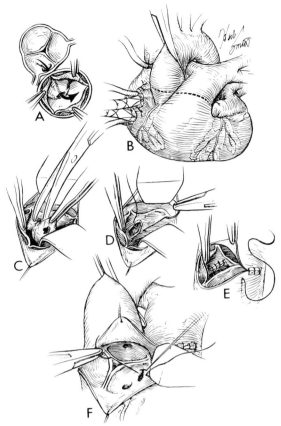

Figure 30–18. Operative technique for repair of aneurysm of the right coronary sinus with fistula into the right ventricle (*A*). *B*, Transverse incision is made in the pulmonary artery. *C*, The pulmonary valve is elevated, and the aneurysm is exposed and excised. *D*, The fistula is closed with suture. *E*, The pulmonary arteriotomy is repaired. *F*, The fistula is closed with suture in the aortic sinus of Valsalva.

Electrocardiographic tracings yield nonspecific information, which is usually within normal limits until rupture occurs. Signs of hypertrophy of the chamber and strain develop. Arrhythmias, which result from pressure of the aneurysm on the conducting system, are rarely a presenting symptom.

Echocardiography is a useful noninvasive method for obtaining suggestive evidence of the presence of or identifying intact or ruptured aneurysms of the sinuses of Valsalva.

The diagnosis can be established only by cardiac catheterization and aortography. Associated cardiac disease is also identified in this way. Before rupture, the aneurysm is visualized as a diverticulum of the sinus. Cardiac function is normal unless the patient has aortic valvular insufficiency or pulmonary outflow obstruction produced by distortion by the aneurysm. After rupture, an intracardiac fistula develops primarily into the right ventricle or atrium. Aortography shows a jet of contrast medium from the aneurysm entering the appropriate cardiac chamber. A left-to-right shunt is produced with increase of oxygen. Congestive heart failure usually develops.

Acquired aneurysms of the sinuses of Valsalva occur in a small percentage of patients with aneurysms of the ascending aorta. They are found usually in men over the age of 30 years.

Acquired aneurysms may be asymptomatic, or they may produce a wide variety of symptoms, depending on the size and involvement of cardiac structures. Cardiac symptoms result primarily from aortic valvular insufficiency due to a deformed aortic valve, anulus, or both. Patients with aneurysms due to infection may seek medical advice during the acute or chronic stages. Bacterial or fungal endocarditis produces an aneurysm of the sinus of Valsalva by erosion of the sinus and formation of an abscess. Endocarditis may develop in normal, diseased, or prosthetic valves. Syphilitic infection is usually manifested by aortic valvular insufficiency and deteriorating congestive heart failure. Patients with cystic medial necrosis and collagen and connective tissue disorders may be asymptomatic or may have evidence of progressive aortic valvular insufficiency or acute onset of dissection.

These aneurysms are rarely detected on physical examination. An occasional case has been encountered in which the patient has a large aneurysm that deforms or erodes through the sternum or anterior wall of the chest and produces visible, palpable pulsation. On physical examination, the usual findings are aortic valvular insufficiency secondary to valvular

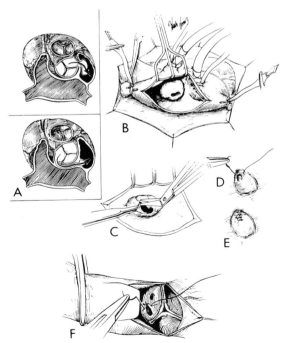

Figure 30–19. *A*, Aneurysms of the left and right coronary sinus with protrusion and fistular formation into the right atrium. *B*, The aneurysm is exposed in the right atrium. *C*, The aneurysm is excised. *D* and *E*, The fistulous tract is closed with suture. *F*, The sinus of Valsalva aneurysm is closed through the aortotomy.

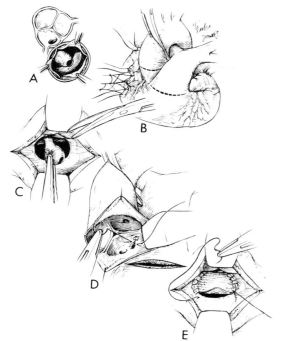

Figure 30–20. *A*, Aneurysm of the right coronary sinus with fistular formation into the right ventricle through an associated ventricular septal defect. *B*, The aneurysm and fistulous tract are exposed through an aortotomy and a transverse right ventriculotomy. *C*, The aneurysm is excised. *D*, The origin of the aneurysm in the sinus of Valsalva is closed with suture. *E*, The associated ventricular septal defect is closed with a Dacron patch.

mined. Coronary arteriography should be performed on these patients to determine whether they have coronary abnormalities. Atherosclerosis would be the primary disease, since most of these patients are in the age group in which atherosclerosis is common.

TREATMENT

The primary treatment of congenital aneurysms of the sinuses of Valsalva is surgical closure of the defect and resection or obliteration of the aneurysm, fistulous tract, or both. Some have advised not operating on patients with asymptomatic congenital aneurysms because they believe that sudden death is rare in the natural history of the disease. Intracardiac rupture, which eventually occurs, will produce symptoms, at which time repair can be effected. The operation is performed with use of total cardiopulmonary bypass. Repair is usually accomplished by a combined approach through the aorta and the chamber of intracardiac protrusion or rupture. The windsock-like deformity produced by the aneurysm, fistula, or both, is resected and obliterated via the cardiac chamber involved. The defect in the sinus is closed through the aorta to avoid injuring the aortic valve; the valve

dysfunction from distortion by fibrosis, and prolapse from dissection, destruction, or enlargement of the aortic anulus. Fistulas rarely develop in acquired aneurysms of the sinuses of Valsalva and usually are the result of penetrating trauma.

The electrocardiographic tracing is normal or may indicate nonspecific abnormalities related to the aortic valvular insufficiency producing left ventricular hypertrophy or strain.

Plain roentgenograms of the chest show varying degrees of abnormality, depending on the size and location of the aneurysm. Calcification in the wall of the aneurysm is common when the aneurysm is due to syphilis (Figs. 30–14 and 30–15), but it is also noted in some patients with atherosclerotic aneurysms. Aneurysms confined to one or more sinuses may produce no demonstrable radiographic abnormalities because of their location within the cardiac silhouette. When they enlarge, they may be suggestive of cardiac chamber enlargement, primarily of the right atrium (Fig. 30–16). Because acquired aneurysms usually involve multiple sinuses and a portion of the ascending aorta, they appear as fusiform or saccular aneurysms of the ascending aorta (Fig. 30–17).

The diagnosis is established by cardiac catheterization and aortography. Associated cardiac disease is identified, and the extent of the aneurysm is deter-

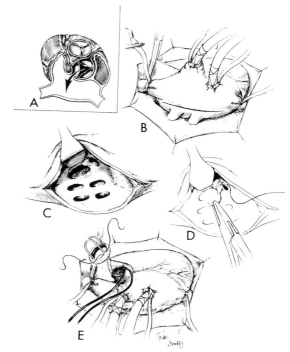

Figure 30–21. *A*, Aneurysm of the fistulous tract of the left coronary sinus into the left atrium. *B*, The left atrium is exposed, and an incision is made into the left atrium below the right inner atrial groove. *C*, The fistulous tract is identified and (*D*) closed with suture. *E*, Because of associated aortic valvular insufficiency, the valve is replaced. Right and left coronary arterial perfusion is used.

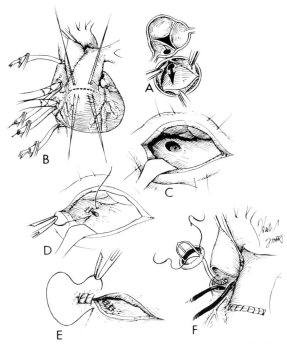

Figure 30–22. Operative technique for repair of (*A*) fistula between the right coronary sinus and the right ventricle associated with aortic incompetence. *B* and *C*, Fistula is exposed through a right ventriculotomy. *D*, Fistula is closed with suture. *E*, Right ventriculotomy is repaired. *F*, Aortic valve is replaced with prosthetic caged ball valve.

can also be reconstructed or replaced simultaneously if required (Figs. 30–18 and 30–19).

Sakakibara and Konno (1968) analyzed and classified the anatomic variations when ventricular septal defect is associated with the aneurysm. Repair is performed through the aorta and right ventricle; the aneurysm is resected or obliterated, and the ventricular septal defect is closed primarily or with a patch graft (Fig. 30–20). The aortic valve is reconstructed or replaced, when necessary, to relieve aortic insufficiency (Figs. 30–21 and 30–22).

Since acquired aneurysms rarely involve intracardiac structures except the aortic valve, they can be repaired through the aorta alone with use of total cardiopulmonary bypass. The method of repair depends on the size and location of the aneurysm. Reconstruction or replacement of the aortic valve is often necessary because of valvular or anular deformity. Small or localized aneurysms may be obliterated or resected and replaced with a woven Dacron patch graft (Fig. 30–23). Involvement of several sinuses and the ascending aorta will require resection of the sinuses and ascending aorta and replacement with a woven Dacron graft. Reimplantation of the coronary ostia into the graft and replacement of the aortic valve may also be required (Fig. 30–24). If the patient has associated atherosclerotic occlusive disease of the coronary arteries, bypass grafts to the diseased coronary arteries can be performed concomitantly.

Results of operative correction of congenital and acquired aneurysms of the sinuses of Valsalva have been gratifying. Mortality and morbidity rates have been steadily reduced as experience has been gained in patient care, cardiac and vascular surgery, and extracorporeal circulatory support. The operative mortality rate for congenital aneurysms is less than 5 per cent, and for acquired aneurysms, less than 10 per cent. Evaluation after surgical correction has shown that congenital aneurysms rarely recur. The most common postoperative complication is residual aortic valvular insufficiency. In patients who have repair of acquired aneurysms, rarely does an aneurysm develop later in a noninvolved sinus. Recurrent or residual endocarditis is an occasional postoperative complication in patients operated on with infection. Aortic valvular insufficiency may result from persistent or subsequent involvement of the valve or anulus. Careful evaluation of the aortic valve is important during repair of both congenital and acquired aneurysms. Valvular replacement should be seriously considered if there is any question regarding valvular function in order to avoid postoperative aortic insufficiency and subsequent reoperation.

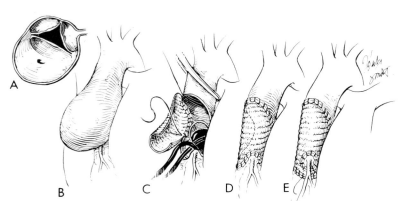

Figure 30–23. *A* and *B*, Aneurysm of the sinus of Valsalva with aortic valvular incompetence and method of repair. *C*, The aortic valve is replaced with a prosthetic caged ball valve, and Dacron patch angioplasty of the aortic root are performed. *D*, The patch graft angioplasty is tailored around the coronary ostia and (*E*) the coronary ostium is reimplanted into the Dacron graft.

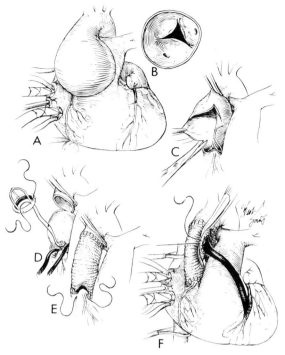

Figure 30–24. Operative technique for repair of (A and B) aneurysms of all three coronary sinuses and aortic valvular incompetence. C, The aneurysm is opened and partially excised. D, The aortic valve is replaced with a caged ball valve prosthesis. E, The ascending aorta and sinuses are replaced with a woven Dacron graft down to the aortic anulus and tailored around the coronary ostia. F, When associated atherosclerotic coronary arterial disease is present, bypass graft from the ascending aorta to the coronary artery is performed.

SELECTED REFERENCES

DeBakey, M. E., Diethrich, E. B., Liddicoat, J. E., Kinard, S. A., and Garrett, H. E.: Abnormalities of the sinuses of Valsalva. J. Thorac. Cardiovasc. Surg., *54*:312, 1967.

This article presents a review of the records of 35 patients with abnormal sinuses of Valsalva referred for cardiac evaluation. The cases were classified into three groups according to the pathologic anatomy: aneurysm, aneurysm with fistula, and fistula. Common clinical manifestations included dyspnea, fatigue, widened pulse pressure, left ventricular hypertrophy, and diastolic murmur of aortic insufficiency. Diagnosis was made by cardiac catheterization and aortic root injection. Treatment for those with aneurysm consisted of excision and primary repair of the aortic root or Dacron graft replacement; for those with aneurysm and fistula, excision of the aneurysm and suture closure of the fistula; and for those with fistula, suture closure of the fistula. There were three operative deaths and three late deaths; the remaining patients were all leading normal lives.

Edwards, J. E., and Burchell, H. B.: The pathological anatomy of deficiencies between the aortic root and the heart, including aortic sinus aneurysms. Thorax, *12*:125, 1957.

This article contains a discussion of the anatomy of coronary sinuses and a pathologic description of the defects between the aortic root and the heart observed by the authors. The defects were secondary to deficiency of the normal continuity between the aortic media and the heart, which may represent failure of union or secondary separation.

Sakakibara, S., and Konno, S.: Congenital aneurysm of the sinus of Valsalva. Am. J. Cardiol., *12*:100, 1963.
Sakakibara, S., and Konno, S.: Congenital aneurysm of the sinus of Valsalva. Anatomy and classification. Am. Heart J., *63*:405, 1962.

These authors classify congenital aneurysms of the sinus of Valsalva morphologically into four basic types, which are derived from the site of origin on the coronary sinuses. These basic types are further classified according to the site of intracardiac protrusion, presence of associated ventricular septal defect, and stage of development of the aneurysm. Schematic drawings of the surgical repair of Types I, II, and IV are included.

REFERENCES

Abbott, M. E.: Atlas of Congenital Heart Disease. New York, American Heart Association, 1936.

Brown, J. W., Heath, D., and Whitaker, W.: Cardioaortic fistula; a case diagnosed in life and treated surgically. Circulation, *12*:819, 1955.

DeBakey, M. E., and Lawrie, G. M.: Aneurysm of sinus of Valsalva with coronary atherosclerosis: Successful surgical correction. Ann. Surg., *189*:303, 1979.

DeBakey, M. E., Howell, J. F., Garrett, H. E., *et al.*: Sinus of Valsalva aneurysms and fistulas; report of two cases. Cardiovasc. Res. Cen. Bull., *3*:72, 1965.

DeBakey, M. E., Diethrich, E. B., Liddicoat, J. E., *et al.*: Abnormalities of the sinuses of Valsalva. J. Thorac. Cardiovasc. Surg., *54*:312, 1967.

Edwards, J. E., and Burchell, H. B.: The pathological anatomy of deficiencies between the aortic root and the heart, including aortic sinus aneurysms. Thorax, *12*:125, 1957.

Engel, P. J., Held, J. S., van der Bel-Kahn, J., and Spitz, H.: Echocardiographic diagnosis of congenital sinus of Valsalva aneurysm with dissection of the interventricular septum. Circulation, *63*:705, 1981.

Haaz, W. S., Kotler, M. N., Mintz, G. S., Parry, W., and Spitzer, S.: Ruptured sinus of Valsalva aneurysm: Diagnosis by echocardiography. Chest, *78*:761, 1980.

Hope, J.: A Treatise on Diseases of the Heart and Great Vessels. London, W. Kidd, 1831.

Kwittken, J., Christopoulos, P., Dua, N. K., *et al.*: Congenital and acquired aortic sinus aneurysms: a case report of each with histologic study. Arch. Intern. Med., *115*:684, 1965.

Lillehei, C. W., Stanley, P., and Varco, R. L.: Surgical treatment of ruptured aneurysms of the sinus of Valsalva. Ann. Surg., *146*:459, 1957.

Nakamura, K., Suzuki, S., and Satomi, G.: Detection of ruptured aneurysm of sinus of Valsalva by contrast two-dimensional echocardiography. Br. Heart J., *45*:219, 1981.

Sakakibara, S., and Konno, S.: Congenital aneurysm of the sinus of Valsalva. Anatomy and classification. Am. Heart J., *63*:405, 1962.

Sakakibara, S., and Konno, S.: Congenital aneurysm of the sinus of Valsalva. Am. J. Cardiol., *12*:100, 1963.

Sakakibara, S., and Konno, S.: Congenital aneurysm of the sinus of Valsalva associated with ventricular septal defect. Anatomical aspects. Am. Heart J., *75*:595, 1968.

Sawyers, J. L., Adams, J. E., and Scott, H. W., Jr.: Surgical treatment for aneurysms of the aortic sinuses with aorticoatrial fistula. Surgery, *41*:26, 1957.

Taguchi, K., Sasaki, N., Matsuura, Y., *et al.*: Surgical correction of aneurysm of the sinus of Valsalva. A report of forty-five consecutive patients, including eight with total replacement of the aortic valve. Am. J. Cardiol., *23*:180, 1969.

Thurnam, J.: On aneurisms, and especially spontaneous varicose aneurisms of ascending aorta and sinus of Valsalva, with cases. Medico-chir. Trans., *23*:323, 1840.

IX   AORTIC DISSECTION

HASSAN NAJAFI

INCIDENCE, ETIOLOGY, AND PATHOGENESIS

Dissection is the most common acute catastrophe involving the thoracic aorta. It occurs with greater frequency than rupture of atherosclerotic thoracic or abdominal aortic aneurysms. The peak incidence of aortic dissection is in the 40- to 60-year-old age group, with predominance in males. It occurs rarely in persons under the age of 40, except in those with a familial predisposition (Hanley and Bennett-Jones, 1967). The exact cause of spontaneous aortic dissection is usually unknown, and specific histologic abnormalities are rare, even at the entrance site into the dissecting process (Roberts, 1981). It is known, however, that about 70 per cent of patients with aortic dissection have or have had hypertension, and at necropsy, about 90 per cent have left ventricular hypertrophy (Edwards, 1973; Hirst et al., 1958). Often, aortic dissection represents the patient's first serious illness. It is likely that the higher the systemic blood pressure, the greater the likelihood of aortic dissection (Burchell, 1955; Roberts, 1975). For example, in the presence of coarctation of the aorta, acute dissection occurs more frequently proximal than distal to the coarctation (Abbott, 1928); it also occurs more often in patients with accelerated or malignant hypertension than in those with benign elevation of blood pressure. Reduction of blood pressure clearly reduces the incidence of aortic dissection (Reifenstein et al., 1947). Despite its being the common denominator in aortic dissection, systemic hypertension cannot be viewed as the sole cause of aortic disruption.

Pregnancy is often listed as a cause of aortic dissection (Schnitker and Bayer, 1944), but the number of patients reported is small, and even among them, little information is available on the presence or absence of hypertension. Marfan's syndrome, idiopathic cystic medionecrosis, bicuspid aortic valve, and coarctation are associated with an increased incidence of aortic dissection. Nonpenetrating trauma is a well-recognized although rare cause of aortic dissection, and the tear occurs in the region of the aortic isthmus (Parmley et al., 1958).

In recent years, iatrogenic aortic dissections have become more frequent and better recognized. They may be secondary to cannulation, such as occurs with retrograde arterial perfusion during cardiopulmonary bypass (Najafi, 1979), or attendant to intra-aortic balloon counterpulsation (Isner et al., 1980) or may arise from the aortic incision used for aortic valve replacement and/or aortocoronary bypass grafting (Muna et al., 1977; Nicholson et al., 1978).

After the intima tears and the dissecting hematoma forms, a second set of forces result in the extension of the dissection. These include blood pressure, ejection velocity, turbulence, and steepness of the pulse wave (dp/dt_{max}). Based on experimental evidence, it appears that the steepness of the pulse wave is the most important of the forces propagating the dissecting process. It involves the pulsatile nature of the blood flow in the large arteries. This is known because (1) the aorta is remarkably resistant to static pressure, (2) the static pressure provides no pressure gradients as driving forces to induce shear stress on the aortic tissues, (3) experimental models (i.e., aortas made of Tygon tubing with rubber cement linings or dog aortas) dissect only when flow is pulsatile and not when it is nonpulsatile (Prokop et al., 1970), and (4) in turkeys, protection from aortic rupture can be accomplished with propranolol, a beta-adrenergic blocking agent, administered in a dosage that does not affect mean aortic pressure but does alter the quality of pulsatile blood flow (Prokop et al., 1970). Propranolol exerts its main effect directly on the myocardium and decreases the steepness of the pulse wave.

The discouraging feature is the obscure pathogenesis of the lesion. A critical appraisal of the literature substantiates that medial elastic tissue lesions of the "mucoid cyst and cystic" types are not common causes of aortic dissection. Such lesions are found most commonly associated with Marfan's syndrome, which constitutes less than 3 per cent of the total patient population with acute aortic dissection (Hirst et al., 1958). Therefore, it seems advisable to abandon the term idiopathic cystic medionecrosis in favor of one that designates the defective component(s) of the dissected vessel wall.

ANATOMIC CONSIDERATIONS

All dissections are characterized by longitudinal separation of the aortic media initiated by a transverse intimal and medial aortic tear (Hirst et al., 1958). In approximately two thirds of the patients, the tear is located about 2 cm. distal to the aortic valve (Edwards, 1973; Hirst et al., 1958; Kouchoukos et al., 1980). The second most common site of a primary tear is in the most proximal portion of the descending aorta and accounts for nearly one fourth of the patients. In 10 per cent of patients, the intimal laceration is located in the aortic arch. The entrance tear is usually incomplete, and very rarely, the entire circumference of the aorta is lacerated (Murray and Edwards, 1973). A re-entry tear is identified far less frequently (15 per cent), with half occurring in the aorta and the other half in the peripheral arteries.

Once blood under pressure enters the media, the

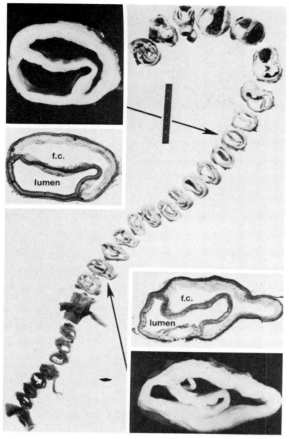

Figure 30–25. Dissection involving the entire length of the aorta in a 66-year-old woman. She suffered this serious complication 3 days after a seemingly uneventful aortic valve replacement (f.c. = false channel). (From Roberts, W. C.: Aortic dissection: Anatomy, consequences, and causes. Am. Heart J., *101*:212, 1981.)

time required for dissection of the entire aorta appears to be a few seconds. This is in keeping with the observation made on retrograde aortic dissection during cardiopulmonary bypass and the virtually instantaneous death of many patients who suffer aortic dissection. The plane of separation is in the outer half of the aortic media. Consequently, the wall of the false channel is exceedingly thin and therefore vulnerable to rupture. Two days after the onset of dissection, necrosis of the aortic wall may develop, causing further predisposition to rupture. In one series of dissections, aortic wall necrosis was observed histologically in 21 of 34 necropsies (62 per cent) (Barsky and Rosen, 1978).

The course of the dissecting process is fairly characteristic. When dissection begins in the ascending aorta, the tear usually involves the right lateral aortic wall, and thereafter, dissection courses distally along the greater curvature of the ascending, transverse, and descending aorta. Since the brachiocephalic arteries arise from the greater curvature of the arch, dissection of these arteries is common. Regardless of the location of the primary intimal tear, the descending aorta is the most commonly involved

segment, since almost all ascending aortic dissections extend down into the descending aorta; rarely, however, descending aortic dissections extend retrograde into the ascending aorta. Dissections limited to the ascending aorta are quite uncommon (Fig. 30–25).

CLINICAL MANIFESTATIONS AND DIAGNOSIS

Clinically, aortic dissection has a myriad of variations, depending on the location, extent, and progression of the dissecting process, the anatomy of the arterial disruption, and the resultant pathophysiology (Table 30–1). The symptoms and signs occur first in the chest and then extend more or less rapidly to other regions such as the legs, abdomen, groin, and lower extremities. This sequence of manifestations is a reflection of the progress of the disease and the consequent ischemic effects on the organs supplied by the branches of the aorta that may become involved in the dissecting process. The most common and striking symptom is the sudden onset of severe pain in the chest or epigastrium that may extend along the course of the ribs to the back and up into the neck and shoulders or down into the abdomen. In some instances, this may be associated with loss of consciousness. Initially, shock may occur and is usually out of proportion to the decrease in systolic pressure. There may be associated cyanosis, tachypnea, and tachycardia. A very small number of patients may not experience any pain with onset of the dissection. Neurologic complications, particularly hemiplegia or paraplegia, are not uncommon, whereas in some patients abdominal symptoms may be predominant, resulting in confusion with acute abdominal conditions caused by other etiologic mechanisms. Disruption of one or both renal arteries may lead to Goldblatt hypertension and/or acute renal insufficiency. Abrupt interference with peripheral arterial flow into the lower extremities may erroneously be attributed to acute arterial embolism. A new aortic diastolic murmur constitutes the most significant diagnostic clue and is present in one fourth to one half of the patients. Approximately two thirds of the patients are hypertensive, and occasionally, ecchymosis is observed in the lower part of the back, chest, or the abdomen.

TABLE 30–1. COMPLICATIONS OF AORTIC DISSECTION

Aortic rupture, leading to hemopericardium, hemothorax, hemoperitoneum, mediastinal or retroperitoneal hematoma

Obstruction, occlusion, or separation of one or more aortic branches, causing myocardial infarction, stroke, paraplegia, intestinal, renal, or leg ischemia

Aortic regurgitation, leading to acute left heart failure

Aortic obstruction, by either the protruding false lumen hematoma or intussusception of circumferentially torn inner dissected layers

These characteristic manifestations should suggest the diagnosis of aortic dissection. Confusion with myocardial infarction is resolved in most instances by electrocardiographic examination, showing either a normal pattern or evidence only of left ventricular hypertrophy.

When correlated with an appropriate history and physical findings, a plain chest roentgenogram may be suggestive of the diagnosis. The roentgenographic manifestations can be summarized as (1) a change in the configuration of the aorta on successive films, (2) displacement of an intimal calcification, (3) a localized hump in the aortic arch, (4) disparity in the size of the ascending versus the descending aorta, and (5) a left pleural effusion. Prior films, when available for comparison, can be very useful. In a series from the Mayo Clinic, however, about 20 per cent of the patients had negative films or had findings of cardiac enlargement or congestive heart failure (Earnest et al., 1979). Furthermore, similar findings on the chest films of patients without an event in their history suggesting dissection are less reliable, because these signs can be associated with other disease processes such as aneurysmal dilatation and/or tortuosity of the aorta, as seen in elderly hypertensive patients. Once the patient is stable, retrograde aortic angiography should be performed as soon as possible to establish the diagnosis and to assess the possible need for surgery. Deformity of the true aortic lumen and opacification of the false channel are the most common angiographic abnormalities (Fig. 30–26). Abdominal aortographic examinations are often helpful in dem-

onstrating the extent of the dissection and involvement of the major visceral branches (Fig. 30–27). Aortic wall thickening as an isolated abnormality is an unreliable sign of aortic dissection.

In a small percentage of patients with dissection, particularly that confined to the arch, the aortogram may be interpreted as being normal (Najafi et al., 1972). A typical history together with the pathognomonic finding of a definitely new aortic regurgitant murmur in a patient suffering from left heart failure dictates the need for an emergency operation in spite of a seemingly normal aortogram. Recently, computed tomography (CT) has added a new dimension to the diagnosis of aortic dissection. Conventional CT scanning with intravenous injection of contrast medium can establish the diagnosis of aortic dissection by demonstrating (1) double channels with an intimal flap or (2) displaced intimal calcifications if one channel is thrombosed. Dynamic computed tomography following the injection of a bolus of contrast medium shows the relative rate of filling of the true and false channels and demonstrates the intimal flap with optimal clarity. It can be easily repeated to assess the progress of the lesion and, in some patients, constitutes a safe screening procedure. Intimal flaps missed by conventional aortography have been clearly identified by computed tomography. Pitfalls in CT examination include the finite section thickness and failure to delineate the entire abdominal aorta. The major advantage of this study, however, is its noninvasive nature; hence, it can be used to distinguish myocardial infarction from dissection in patients with chest pain. If dissection is

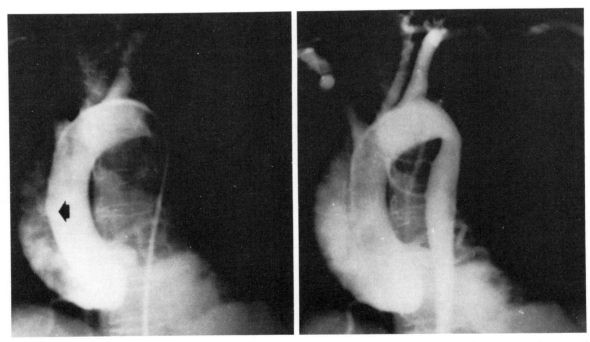

Figure 30–26. Retrograde aortic root injection of contrast medium demonstrates aortic regurgitation secondary to dissection originating in the proximal ascending aorta. The arrow points to the partition between the true lumen (medial) and false channel (lateral). The picture on the right shows the characteristically narrow true lumen in the descending aorta. The distal false channel has not as yet opacified. (From SESATS Thoracic Surgical Syllabus. Dubuque, Iowa, Kendall-Hunter Publishing Company, 1980, p. 63.)

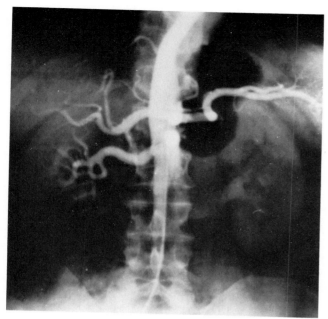

Figure 30–27. The abdominal aortogram in the patient whose thoracic aortogram is shown in Figure 30–26 demonstrates right renal artery flow from the true lumen while the left renal artery arising from the false channel remains obscure.

detected, aortography may or may not be requested, depending on the patient's condition and age and the plan of treatment. Computed tomography is superior to plain chest films for follow-up studies because the latter usually do not delineate the medial border of the aorta. Moreover, with chest films, the apparent position of the lateral border is strongly influenced by slight changes in rotation of the patient, whereas CT images, being cross-sectional, are unaffected by rotation (Godwin *et al.*, 1980).

PATHOPHYSIOLOGIC CONSIDERATIONS AND PROGNOSIS

Death occurs in 90 per cent of untreated patients and is more common when there is no re-entry site. Aortic rupture (usually near the site of entrance tear) is the most common cause of death (Hirst *et al.*, 1958). The most frequent site of rupture is the ascending aorta, and the bleeding is always into the pericardial cavity. Descending aortic dissections rupture into the left pleural space, and occasionally, the abdominal aorta is the site of rupture, with bleeding into the peritoneal cavity or the retroperitoneal space. Extension of the dissection into a main coronary artery (more often the right) may cause myocardial ischemia or infarction, which may be fatal. Another consequence of dissection involving the aortic root is the loss of commissural support of the aortic cusps, leading to acute aortic regurgitation. Occasionally, the extension of blood into the myocardium may result in the development of an aortoatrial or aortic–right ventricular fistula or a high degree of atrial ventricular block (Perryman and Gay, 1972; Thiene *et al.*, 1979).

Involvement of the aortic arch branches may produce arm or cerebral ischemia. Dissection of the visceral branches may result in renal failure, systemic hypertension, and intestinal ischemia or infarction. Iliac occlusion may lead to acute arterial insufficiency of the lower extremities.

Aortic obstruction or occlusion can be caused either by the protruding false lumen hematoma or by intussusception of circumferentially torn inner dissected layers. About 10 per cent of all acute aortic dissections heal spontaneously. Nearly all have an identifiable re-entry site, usually in the abdominal aorta or one of the iliac arteries (Hirst *et al.*, 1958). The proximal intimal tear under these circumstances most commonly is located near the aortic isthmus, and therefore, the brachiocephalic and coronary arteries are often spared.

In contrast to its inappropriate use in most aortic dissections, the term aneurysm is usually appropriate in chronic dissections, since the false channel is often large and contains laminated thrombi. Occasionally, the false channel is completely filled by a thrombus. The chance for survival after dissection is proportional to the distance of the entrance tear from the aortic valve. Consequently, few patients with healed aortic dissection have an intimal tear in the ascending aorta. Once healing has occurred, however, in general, the longer the false channel, the longer the survival (Roberts, 1981).

CLASSIFICATION

The literature contains five different but closely related classifications for this disease entity. (1) The first classification was described by DeBakey and associates (1965), who defined three types based on where the process originates and how far it extends. In Types I and II, the intimal tear is located in the ascending aorta. Type I dissections extend beyond the descending aorta, whereas Type II dissections are confined to the ascending aorta. Type III dissections originate in the proximal descending aorta and often propagate antegrade into the distal aorta or, very rarely, retrograde into the arch and ascending aorta. (2) Since Type I and II dissections behave similarly in many respects, some investigators refer to them collectively as anterior dissections (Najafi *et al.*, 1972). In this simple classification, Type III is called a posterior dissection. (3) In 1970, Daily and associates proposed a categorization based on the extent of the aortic involvement rather than the site of the primary intimal tear. They classified all dissections involving the ascending aorta as Type A dissections and those involving only the descending thoracic aorta as Type B dissections. In Type A, the primary tear may be located anywhere along the course of the aorta, but in Type B, the site or origin of the dissection is in the aorta just distal to the origin of the left subclavian artery. (4) Ascending versus descending, and (5) proximal versus distal aortic dissections in reality are the same as anterior and posterior dissections.

The detailed classification described by DeBakey and colleagues is somewhat complicated from the standpoint of clinical decision-making. Simple categorization into A and B types or anterior versus posterior dissections have practical advantages in terms of treatment plans and operative approach. Dissection is considered to be acute if it is less than 2 weeks old, with the time of initial dissection being defined by the acute onset of pain.

TREATMENT

Medical Therapy

Introduction of surgical therapy for acute dissection by DeBakey and associates in 1955 represented a landmark in the treatment of this disease with such a high mortality rate. Medical therapy as a prelude to a surgical approach in some patients and as definitive therapy in others was first advocated by Wheat and coworkers in 1965. Their report led to widespread application of medical therapy for acute and long-term treatment of aortic dissection. Subsequently, however, some investigators expressed reservations about medical therapy, particularly for ascending aortic dissection (Attar et al., 1971; Austen and DeSanctis, 1965). Current management of aortic dissection depends primarily on the site of origin and particularly on the extent of the dissecting process. As defined initially by Wheat and colleagues (1965), there are two major objectives of medical therapy. The first is to lower arterial blood pressure; this is important because two thirds of the patients with aortic dissection are severely hypertensive. Reducing arterial blood pressure clearly diminishes the force exerted against the damaged aortic wall. The second objective is to reduce the velocity with which the contracting left ventricle ejects blood. In mathematical calculations and experimental models of aortic dissection, Prokop and coworkers (1970) have demonstrated that cardiac ejection velocity constitutes a major shearing force that tends to initiate and propagate dissection. Reducing the ejection velocity with medication is the rationale for medical treatment of normotensive patients with dissection.

Medical therapy should be instituted immediately. The patient is admitted into the intensive care unit, where vital signs can be continuously monitored. An intra-arterial cannula permits precise blood pressure control during administrationn of potent hypotensive agents. A Swan-Ganz catheter is also recommended to determine cardiac filling pressures. The route of drug administration should be parenteral, because in acutely ill patients, gastrointestinal absorption is unreliable and the need for immediate drug effect is often urgent. Furthermore, surgery may be imminent for many. The pain of aortic dissection is often difficult to manage with opiates and usually subsides once the progression of the disease is halted. The systolic pressure is reduced to the lowest level commensurate with sustaining adequate cerebral, cardiac, and renal function. Elderly patients usually require a higher perfusion pressure. Therapy aimed toward reducing ejection velocity is begun in all patients, including those who are pain-free or normotensive.

The drugs presently used are listed in Table 30–2 (Doroghazi et al., 1981). The most effective agent for immediate reduction of blood pressure is sodium ni-

TABLE 30–2. AGENTS USED IN MANAGING ACUTE AORTIC DISSECTION*

DRUG	DOSAGE	EFFECT ON BLOOD PRESSURE	EFFECT ON EJECTION VELOCITY	SIDE EFFECTS AND COMPLICATIONS	COMMENTS
Sodium nitroprusside	50–100 mg. in 500 ml. D₅W infused initially at 25–50 µg./min.; not more than 1 mg./kg. should be given in the first 3 hours and 0.2–0.3 mg./kg./hr. thereafter	Marked reduction	Increase	Cyanide and thiocyanate toxicity; methemoglobinemia; hypotension; nausea; somnolence; tachycardia; increased ejection velocity	Powerful hypotensive agent; very short duration of action; light sensitive; requires intensive monitoring
Trimethaphan	500 mg.–2 gm. in 500 ml. of D₅W infused initially at 1 mg./min.	Marked reduction	Decrease	Hypotension; respiratory arrest; somnolence; signs of sympathetic blockade; tachyphylaxis develops rapidly	Requires intensive monitoring
Propranolol	0.5 mg. IV, following by incremental doses of 1 mg. every 5 min. until adequate effect is achieved or a total dose of 0.15 mg./kg. has been given	Modest reduction	Decrease	Bradycardia; bronchospasm; congestive heart failure	
Reserpine	0.5–2 mg. IM every 4–8 hours	Modest to marked reduction	Decrease	Depression; somnolence; acute gastric ulceration	Antacids and cimetidine should be given concomitantly

*Doroghazi, R. M., et al.: Medical therapy for aortic dissections. J. Cardiovasc. Med., 6:187, 1981.

troprusside, and if it is ineffective or poorly tolerated, trimethaphan is the agent of choice. Trimethaphan reduces ejection velocity and is therefore especially useful for therapy when propranolol is contraindicated. The hypotensive effect of sodium nitroprusside and trimethaphan can be blunted by fluid retention; therefore, concomitant administration of diuretics is often necessary. In patients with refractory hypertension, the possibility of dissection of one or both renal arteries setting the stage for the Goldblatt phenomenon must be considered. Beta-adrenergic blockade with propranolol is the therapy of choice to reduce ejection velocity. Administered intravenously, it has minimal hypotensive effect, and a heart rate of 50 to 60 beats per minute indicates an optimal effect. Reserpine is another drug that lowers both blood pressure and ejection velocity acutely and can be used when propranolol is contraindicated.

Medical therapy is considered by many as the treatment of choice for uncomplicated posterior or Type B dissection. Medical therapy is also employed by some for uncomplicated but stable anterior or Type A dissection if the patient is a poor surgical candidate. It should also be considered for dissections originating in the aortic arch, because of exceedingly high surgical mortality, although there has been recent success with total arch reconstruction or a lesser procedure of reinforcing the arch with Dacron wrapping (Griepp et al., 1975; Kolff et al., 1977).

If long-term medical treatment is selected, oral administration of drugs that both control blood pressure and diminish ejection velocity is begun, and a diuretic is usually added to avoid water retention (Harris et al., 1967). Systolic blood pressure is maintained at approximately 130 mm. Hg or less if this can be tolerated by the patient. Unfortunately, data concerning long-term prognosis of patients with aortic dissection treated medically are scarce, and comparative studies of medical versus surgical therapy based on control matching of patient populations are unavailable.

Surgical Therapy

There is now a consensus among surgeons that all acute dissections involving the ascending aorta are best treated by operation to relieve or prevent aortic regurgitation and rupture into the heart or the pericardium (Appelbaum et al., 1976; Collins and Cohn, 1973; Crawford et al., 1979; DeBakey et al., 1965; Kouchoukos et al., 1980; Miller et al., 1979; Najafi et al., 1972). It is also agreed that acute dissection arising in and involving the descending thoracic aorta and associated with progressive extension, occlusion of vital arteries, significant aortic dilatation, and rupture should be treated by operation. Patients with any form of aortic dissection (acute or chronic) complicating Marfan's syndrome are candidates for surgical treatment because of a high incidence of recurrent dissection and rupture.

Chronic aortic dissection is arbitrarily defined as dissection occurring more than 2 weeks before presentation. It is noteworthy that patients with chronic disease have already survived the initial phase of dissection during which 75 per cent of patients die, and therefore, a more conservative approach may be appropriate. It should also be mentioned that patients treated surgically for chronic dissection tend to have excellent early and late survival in most series (Doroghazi et al. 1980; Miller et al., 1979). Some patients require surgical repair of early or late anatomic complications of their dissections. The most common complications are fusiform or saccular aneurysms and severe aortic regurgitation.

Immediate operation provides the most satisfactory results for acute aortic dissection complicated by aortic insufficiency. There is some controversy concerning the method utilized to restore aortic valve competence. Some consider valve replacement mandatory, whereas others have reported excellent results with reconstructive surgery (Collins and Cohn, 1973; Meng et al., 1981; Najafi et al., 1972, 1975). The current trend favors primary repair by graft replacement of a segment of the ascending aorta. In the Stanford series of 32 patients with acute Type A or anterior dissection associated with aortic regurgitation who survived simple graft replacement of the ascending aorta, only two subsequently required valve replacement. In our series of 19 patients with severe aortic regurgitation secondary to anterior dissection, valve competence was restored either by primary repair or segmental graft replacement of the ascending aorta in 17 patients. Only one patient suffered recurrent dissection and required aortic valve replacement 8 years after primary repair (Meng et al., 1981). Valve replacement should be considered for Marfan's syndrome and those with aneurysm of the sinuses of Valsalva. In chronic dissection associated with aortic regurgitation, the necessity for replacement of the aortic valve is somewhat greater, with approximately one third of these patients requiring such an additional procedure. In certain instances of extremely precarious aortic tissue down to the anulus, it may be advisable to insert a composite graft and valve prosthesis and reimplant the coronary orifices into the graft (Bentall and DeBono, 1968; Najafi, 1973; Weldon et al., 1979). In general, because of the tendency of the condition to progress rapidly toward death, surgical treatment should be applied as soon as possible. If the indication for operation is congestive heart failure caused by severe aortic insufficiency, it is not essential to insist on delineating the type of dissection, since the operative approach and technique utilized are not dependent on precise determination of the extent of the process or the site of the intimal tear. The exception is when involvement of certain vital arteries pose a more acute problem, involvement of such as both renal vessels, causing anuria.

Earlier, medical treatment, which yielded a higher survival rate, was considered to be preferable by some in patients with uncomplicated descending aortic dissection (Wheat *et al.,* 1965; Wheat and Palmer, 1968). More recently, however, a combination of medical and surgical treatment has become popular for these patients (Appelbaum *et al.,* 1976; Attar *et al.,* 1971; Reul *et al.,* 1975; Wolfe and Moran, 1977). This approach has been justified on the basis of a steady decline in operative mortality and a 60 per cent 3-year cumulative survival rate in contrast to a rate of 30 per cent in medically treated patients (Reul *et al.,* 1975; Wolfe and Moran, 1977). Since dissection remains uncomplicated for several hours and the operative risk under such circumstances is relatively low, it may be argued that the management of choice is immediate surgery for all acute and uncomplicated posterior dissections. Furthermore, it has been estimated that between 15 and 25 per cent of such patients initially treated successfully with hypotensive agents will eventually require operation (Wheat, 1973; Wheat and Shumacker, 1976), and the operative risk associated with elective repair of posterior dissection in the chronic phase is not substantially lower than that in the acute phase (Appelbaum *et al.,* 1976; Reul *et al.,* 1975; Rosenberg and Mulder, 1972). In general, however, such procedures should be reserved for patients with otherwise normal cardiac, renal, and pulmonary function, because long-term survival in uncomplicated descending aortic dissection is influenced as much by advanced age and arteriosclerosis as by late complications of the dissection itself.

Although most commonly operations for dissection are done on the thoracic aorta, in some patients the abdominal aorta becomes the pathologic focal point threatening the patient's life. It is under these circumstances that resection of the distal abdominal aorta with the re-entry procedure may be the appropriate therapy (Fig. 30–28). The concept of the re-entry procedure was described in detail by DeBakey and associates (1955). The impetus for the procedure was derived from the recognition that spontaneous re-entry played an important role in stabilizing the dissecting process and allowing the patient to survive. Abdominal surgical procedures have an occasional application in descending aortic dissection. The indications for such an approach include considerable dilatation of the abdominal aortic false lumen, retroperitoneal rupture, visceral artery compromise, and iliac artery obstruction threatening the integrity of the involved extremity. Insertion of a graft assures stable re-entry and eliminates the distal aneurysmal false channels. In 1976, Hunter and colleagues reported on five patients who had abdominal surgery for thoracic aortic dissection. All had an aortic bifurcation graft with re-entry of the false lumen established at the level of the renal arteries. Two patients subsequently underwent thoracic aortic procedures to control intrathoracic progression of the disease.

Operative Technique

Anterior or Type A dissections are approached by a median sternotomy. Low-pressure cardiopulmo-

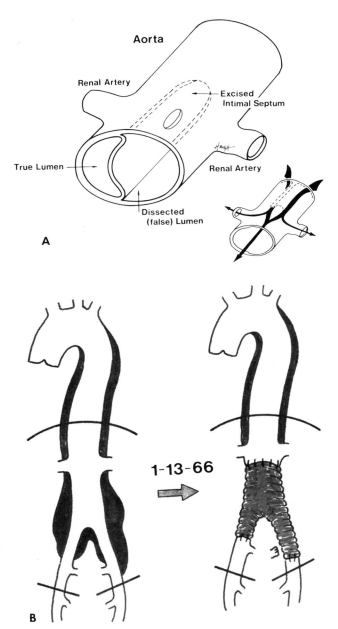

Figure 30–28. *A,* Diagram of aorta divided distal to renal arteries. Excision of a generous tongue of intima or partition allows for both proximal lumina to provide flow into the renal arteries and the distal vessels. *B,* Aortic continuity is restored by insertion of a bifurcation graft anastomosed proximally to the composite lumen and distally to the right common and left external iliac arteries. (From Hunter, J. A., *et al.*: Abdominal aortic resection in thoracic dissection. Arch. Surg., *111*:1259, 1976.)

nary bypass with moderate systemic hypothermia and hemodilution is utilized. During aortic cross-clamping, myocardial preservation is achieved by continuous profound topical hypothermia and by perfusion or infusion of hypothermic potassium cardioplegia solution into the coronary arteries. The initial incision in the aorta is a transverse aortotomy immediately superior to the aortic valve. This incision usually coincides with the level of the intimal tear. Vertical

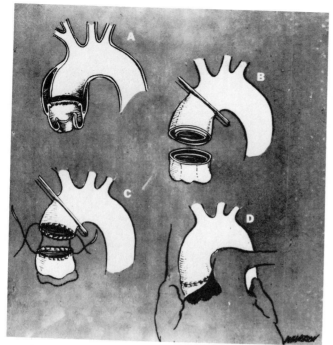

Figure 30–29. Schematic drawing of an anterior dissection demonstrating the technique of primary repair of the dissected layers and restoration of aortic valve competence. The latter is accomplished by elevating the prolapsed aortic cusps to their original position.

aortotomy should be avoided, since in some patients, particularly in the earlier stage of the disease, it is possible to avoid graft replacement of the ascending aorta. Often, it is necessary to transect the descending aorta completely at the level of the initial aortotomy. The aortic anulus is of normal size in most of these patients, and acute regurgitation is caused by downward displacement of normal aortic cusps into the left ventricle. Aortic valve competence, therefore, is restored by elevating the prolapsed cusps to their original positions by reapproximating the dissected layers (Spencer and Blake, 1962) (Fig. 30–29). The repair is performed with simple sutures, passing the needle from outside into the aortic lumen and taking somewhat deeper sutures in the inner dissected layers. These maneuvers result in eversion of the intima so that, subsequently, when the aorta is reanastomosed or a graft is used to replace the ascending aorta, the second suture line excludes the first suture line and reinforces the intima. This reduces the possibility of recurrence of dissection. Insertion of carefully tailored pieces of Teflon felt within the dissected layers, as advocated by Collins and Cohn (1973), adds additional support to the repair and is likely to reduce the possibility of proximal aortic dilatation. The method described is particularly applicable in the earlier stages of dissection when there is minimal anatomic disruption and distortion of the aorta at the site of the intimal tear. The procedure is designed to restore mural integrity, permitting normal blood flow into the true lumen, and by obliterating the false lumen, it prevents

further progression of the dissecting process. In many patients, it is necessary to resect the segment of the ascending aorta containing the intimal tear and to restore the aortic continuity with a tubular woven Dacron graft. The proximal anastomosis under these circumstances is generally just above the aortic valve commissures. Occasionally, it is necessary to extend reconstruction to the transverse aortic arch, which, of necessity, would require reimplantation of the brachiocephalic arteries. Coronary ostial implantation or coronary bypass grafting may be necessary in certain patients. It is encouraging that local procedures on the aortic root in patients with dissection extending from the aortic valve distally to the iliac arteries is effective in stabilizing the disease process. Figure 30–30 shows an aortogram obtained 7 years postoperatively in a patient in whom an acute anterior dissection extending into the left iliac artery was treated by insertion of a short tube graft to replace the proximal portion of the ascending aorta. Thirteen years postoperatively, the patient remains asymptomatic and is fully employed. Stepwise illustrations of the surgical correction of dissection of the ascending aorta with aortic insufficiency are depicted in Figure 30–31 (Wolfe, 1980). These illustrations include the use of specially placed sutures to correct aortic insufficiency in the majority of patients and the insertion of a prosthetic valve for those patients in whom this technique is not feasible.

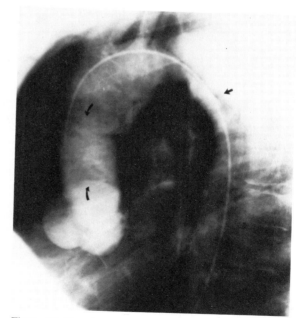

Figure 30–30. Aortogram obtained 7 years after partial replacement of the ascending aorta for dissection extending from the aortic valve to the left common iliac artery. The patient had presented with acute aortic regurgitation and a pulseless left lower extremity. The study shows a competent aortic valve and a satisfactory reconstructed ascending aorta. The curved arrows point to the extent of the tubular graft. The straight arrow points to the partition between the true lumen (containing the catheter) and the false channel, as the dissecting process has remained stabilized.

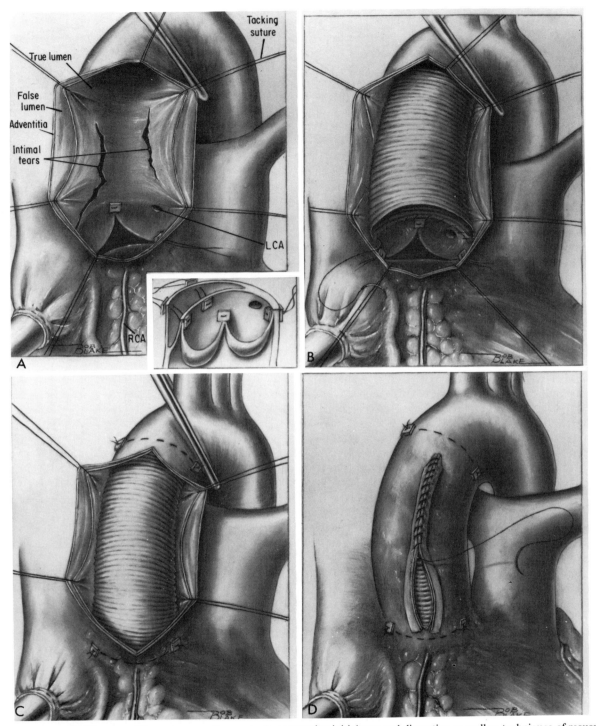

Figure 30–31. *A,* Diagram of the open ascending aorta demonstrating initial tear and dissection as well as techniques of resuspension of the aortic valve. *B,* Suturing of the woven Dacron graft inside the aorta. *C,* The graft sutured within the ascending aorta. *D,* Closure of the adventitia over the Dacron graft. (From Wolfe, W. G.: Acute ascending aortic dissection. Ann. Surg., *192*:658, 1980.)

An important aspect of the operation on the ascending aorta under these circumstances pertains to the site of arterial cannulation. In patients with anterior dissection and a second tear distally (re-entry), there is a hazard of retrograde perfusion of the false lumen. Undoubtedly, this has contributed to the death of some patients treated surgically. Fortunately, in our experience, as in many reported by others, retrograde perfusion through a femoral artery has been successful in most instances. This in part relates to the absence of a second intimal tear distally. In patients with anterior dissection and unilateral iliac occlusion, one can be reasonably sure that a second tear does not exist, and therefore, the contralateral femoral artery can safely be cannulated for arterial inflow. Some have advocated cannulation of the aortic arch under these circumstances. We have not tested the effectiveness of this method and hesitate to believe that it would be superior to femoral artery cannulation.

Posterior or Type B dissections are approached through a left posterolateral thoracotomy. A conservative resection of the descending aorta, containing the intimal tear, if possible, is performed, and then a tubular Dacron graft is inserted to restore aortic continuity. This can be accomplished with simple aortic cross-clamping without using any adjuncts to avoid distal ischemia or provide proximal decompression. If this is considered inadvisable, femoro-femoral bypass using a pump-oxygenator or left atrial–femoral bypass using only a pump can be employed to prevent left ventricular strain and to establish distal perfusion. The same principles apply to those lesions that involve both the thoracic and the abdominal aorta, including the segments from which brachiocephalic arteries or the visceral branches arise. The only contraindications to surgical management are complications that predictably preclude postoperative rehabilitation, such as massive stroke, extensive bowel infarction, bilateral renal infarctions, and paraplegia. In the absence of these serious complications, salvage rates exceeding 80 per cent can be expected.

Complications

Potential postoperative complications are numerous and include hemorrhage, renal insufficiency, pulmonary insufficiency, low cardiac output syndrome, perioperative myocardial infarction, bowel necrosis, cerebral vascular accident, and paraplegia. Pulmonary insufficiency of such gravity to require tracheostomy and particularly paraplegia occur more frequently in operations on the descending thoracic aorta. Fortunately, infection is rare following operation for aortic dissection.

RESULTS OF MEDICAL AND/OR SURGICAL TREATMENT OF AORTIC DISSECTION

In 1976, Appelbaum and associates reported a series of 108 patients with ascending and descending aortic dissection seen between 1966 and 1973. Seventy-eight patients had acute dissection and 30 had chronic dissection. The age and incidence of hypertension (49 years and 32 per cent, respectively) were signficantly lower in the 56 patients in whom dissection originated in the ascending aorta than in the 52 patients in whom the dissection occurred in the descending aorta (60 years and 71 per cent, respectively). The mortality rate in medically treated patients with acute ascending aortic dissection was 88 per cent, whereas it was 24 per cent in similar patients treated surgically. Fifteen patients (54 per cent) with ascending aortic dissection associated with significant aortic

regurgitation did not have aortic valve replacement, and only two subsequently (53 and 92 months later) required replacement of the aortic valve. Although the initial mortality rates in patients with acute descending aortic dissection treated medically and surgically were similar, the long-term survival rate was higher in the surgically treated group. Appelbaum and colleagues concluded that immediate surgical treatment is indicated for patients with acute ascending aortic dissection. Patients with acute descending aortic dissection could be treated medically initially, followed by elective operation. In 1979, Miller and associates reported an unselected consecutive series of 125 patients who had undergone operative repair for acute and chronic dissections with a tubular graft interposition over a 16-year span. Patients were classified according to whether the ascending aorta was involved (Type A with involvement; Type B without involvement), irrespective of the site of intimal tear, and according to the age of the dissection. Fifty-three patients had acute Type A, 29 had chronic type A, 20 had acute type B, and 23 had chronic Type B dissections. Fourteen per cent (17 of 125) had ruptured. Concomitant aortic valve replacement was performed in only 11 per cent of acute Type A dissections and in 38 per cent of chronic Type A dissections. The follow-up averaged 4 years and extended to 13.7 years. Operative mortality was 34 per cent (18 of 53) for acute Type A dissection, 14 per cent (4 of 29) for chronic Type A dissection, 45 per cent (9 of 20) for acute Type B dissection, and 22 per cent (5 of 23) for chronic Type B dissection. During the most recent 5-year interval, these figures have decreased to 27 per cent, 8 per cent, 20 per cent, and 20 per cent, respectively. Operative survivors generally experienced satisfactory functional results. Late attrition rate averaged 8 per cent per year, with 61 per cent of all late deaths having been related to cardiac or cerebral causes. Overall actuarial survival for the entire series was 54 per cent ± 5 per cent at 5 years and 26 per cent ± 7 per cent at 7 years. For the 89 patients who survived the operation, these figures were 76 per cent ± 5 per cent and 37 per cent ± 10 per cent, respectively. No significant difference in long-term survival rates was evident among the various subgroups. Whether the primary intimal tear had been resected or concomitant aortic valve replacement had been performed had no statistically significant influence on operative mortality, functional result, necessity for reoperation, or late attrition. The results of this analysis again support immediate operative treatment for patients with acute Type A or anterior dissections. In addition, surgical treatment of patients with symptomatic or enlarging chronic Type A and chronic Type B dissections provided satisfactory rehabilitation and long-term survival.

The most recent significant report is the review of the results of medical and surgical therapy in 184 patients with aortic dissections seen at Massachusetts General Hospital (Doroghazi *et al.*, 1980). The average follow-up was longer than 4 years, and information was available on 98 per cent of the patients. Most patients with acute and chronic proximal or anterior dissections were treated surgically. Of 78 patients with acute distal dissections, 35 were treated medically and 43 surgically. Hospital survival was 80 per cent in the medically treated group as compared with 51 per cent in the surgically treated group. The substantial number of the late deaths, 27 per cent in the surgically treated patients and 47 per cent in the medically treated patients, occurred as a result of problems unrelated to aortic dissection. In particular, patients with uncomplicated posterior or Type B dissection demonstrated excellent early and late survival when treated by definitive medical therapy.

SELECTED REFERENCES

Doroghazi, R. M., Slater, E. E., DeSanctis, R. W., Rosenthal, S. V., Austen, W. G., and Buckley, M. J.: Long-term survival for 184 patients with treated aortic dissection. (Abstract.) Am. J. Cardiol., 45:489, 1980.
Doroghazi, R. M., Slater, E. E., and DeSanctis, R. W.: Medical therapy for aortic dissections. J. Cardiovasc. Med., 6:187, 1981.

In the first article, the authors addressed the general issue of medical and surgical treatment of aortic dissection based on the review of the records of 184 patients. The second is a fine description of medical therapy of aortic dissection with proper prospective and appropriate reference to the currently acceptable surgical indications.

Hirst, A. E., Jr., Johns, V. J., Jr., and Kime, S. W., Jr.: Dissecting aneurysm of the aorta: A review of 505 cases. Medicine, 37:217, 1958.

This is the classic reference on the natural history of this disorder with appropriate emphasis on the pathologic and other basic aspects of the aortic dissection. Anyone interested in this lesion must read this review, because it is the most comprehensive and original publication of the largest series of aortic dissection.

Miller, D. C., Stinson, E. B., Oyer, P. E., Rossiter, S. J., Reitz, B. A., Griepp, R. B., and Shumway, N. E.: Operative treatment of aortic dissections. Experience with 125 patients over a sixteen-year period. J. Thorac. Cardiovasc. Surg., 78:365, 1979.

This is an excellent clinical review of a large and consecutive series of patients with acute and chronic aortic dissection managed surgically. The clinical descriptions are clear, the surgical techniques are sound, and the statistical analysis of early mortality and late results admirable.

Roberts, W. C.: Aortic dissection: Anatomy, consequences, and causes. Am. Heart J., 101:195, 1981.

This is an outstanding article on fundamental aspects of aortic dissection. The expertise of the author and his vast experience as a meticulous pathologist are evident as the reader gains a much better understanding of anatomic and pathologic features of this disease entity. In many respects, this is a unique reference, complemented by superb and appropriate photographs.

REFERENCES

Abbott, M. E.: Coarctation of the aorta of the adult type. II. A statistical study and historical retrospect of 200 recorded cases, with autopsy, of stenosis or obliteration of the descending arch in subjects above the age of two years. Am. Heart J., 3:392, 574, 1928.
Appelbaum, A., Karp, R. B., and Kirklin, J. W.: Ascending vs. descending aortic dissections. Ann. Surg., 183:296, 1976.
Attar, S., Fardin, R., Ayella, R., and McLaughlin, J. S.: Medical versus surgical treatment of acute dissecting aneurysm. Arch. Surg., 103:568, 1971.
Austen, W. G., and DeSanctis, R. W.: Surgical treatment of dissecting aneurysm of the thoracic aorta. N. Engl. J. Med., 272:1314, 1965.
Barsky, S. H., and Rosen, S.: Aortic infarction following dissecting aortic aneurysm. Circulation, 58:876, 1978.
Bentall, H., and DeBono, A.: A technique for complete replacement of the ascending aorta. Thorax, 23:338, 1968.
Burchell, H. B.: Aortic dissection (dissecting hematoma; dissecting aneurysm of the aorta). Circulation, 12:1068, 1955.
Collins, J. J., and Cohn, L. H.: Reconstruction of the aortic valve. Correcting valve incompetence due to acute dissecting aneurysm. Arch. Surg., 106:35, 1973.
Crawford, E. S., Palamara, A. E., Saleh, S. A., and Roehm, J. O. F., Jr.: Aortic aneurysm: Current status of surgical treatment. Surg. Clin. North Am., 59:597, 1979.
Daily, P. O., Trueblood, H. W., Stinson, E. B., Wuerflein, R. D., and Shumway, N. E.: Management of acute aortic dissections. Ann. Thorac. Surg., 10:237, 1970.
DeBakey, M. E., Cooley, D. A., and Creech, O., Jr.: Surgical considerations of dissecting aneurysm of the aorta. Ann. Surg., 142:586, 1955.
DeBakey, M. E., Henly, W. S., Cooley, D. A., Morris, G. C., Crawford, E. S., and Beall, A. C., Jr.: Surgical management of dissecting aneurysms of the aorta. J. Thorac. Cardiovasc. Surg., 49:130, 1965.
Doroghazi, R. M., Slater, E. E., and DeSanctis, R. W.: Medical therapy for aortic dissections. J. Cardiovasc. Med., 6:187, 1981.
Doroghazi, R. M., Slater, E. E., DeSanctis, R. W., Rosenthal, S. V., Austen, W. G., and Buckley, M. J.: Long-term survival for 184 patients with treated aortic dissection. (Abstract). Am. J. Cardiol., 45:489, 1980.
Earnest, F., IV, Muhm, J. R., and Sheedy, P. F.: Roentgenographic findings in thoracic aortic dissection. Mayo Clin. Proc., 54:43, 1979.
Edwards, J. E.: Aneurysms of the thoracic aorta complicating coarctation. Circulation, 48:195, 1973.
Godwin, J. D., Herfkens, R. L., Oldbrand, C. G., Federle, M. P., and Lipton, M. J.: Evaluation of dissections and aneurysms of the thoracic aorta by conventional and dynamic CT scanning. Radiology, 136:125, 1980.
Griepp, R. B., Stinson, E. B., Hollingsworth, J. F., and Buehler, D.: Prosthetic replacement of the aortic arch. J. Thorac. Cardiovasc. Surg., 70:1051, 1975.
Hanley, W. B., and Bennett-Jones, N.: Familial dissecting aortic aneurysm: A report of three cases within two generations. Br. Heart J., 29:852, 1967.
Harris, P. D., Malm, J. R., Bigger, J. T., Jr., and Bowman, F. O., Jr.: Follow-up studies of acute dissecting aortic aneurysms managed with antihypertensive agents. Circulation, 35,36(Suppl. 1):183, 1967.
Hirst, A. E., Jr., Johns, V. J., Jr., and Kime, S. W., Jr.: Dissecting aneurysm of the aorta: A review of 505 cases. Medicine, 37:217, 1958.
Hunter, J. A., Dye, W. S., Javid, H., Najafi, H., Goldin, M. D., and Serry, C.: Abdominal aortic resection in thoracic dissection. Arch. Surg., 111:1258, 1976.
Isner, J. M., Cohen, S. R., Virmani, R., Lawrinson, W., and Roberts, W. C.: Complications of the intraaortic balloon counterpulsation device: Clinical and morphologic observations in 45 necropsy patients. Am. J. Cardiol., 45:260, 1980.
Kolff, J., Bates, R. J., Balderman, S. C., Shenkoya, K., and Anagnostopoulos, C. E.: Acute aortic arch dissection: Re-evaluation of the indications for medical and surgical therapy. Am. J. Cardiol., 39:727, 1977.
Kouchoukos, N. T., Karp, R. B., Blackstone, E. H., Kirklin, J. W., Pacifico, A. D., and Zorn, G. L.: Replacement of the ascending aorta and aortic valve with a composite graft: Results in 86 patients. Ann. Surg., 192:403, 1980.

Meng, R. L., Najafi, H., Javid, H., Hunter, J. A., and Goldin, M. D.: Acute ascending aortic dissection — surgical management. Circulation, 64(Suppl. 2):231, 1981.

Miller, D. C., Stinson, E. B., Oyer, P. E., Rossiter, S. J., Reitz, B. A., Griepp, R. B., and Shumway, N. E.: Operative treatment of aortic dissections. Experience with 125 patients over a sixteen-year period. J. Thorac. Cardiovasc. Surg., 78:365, 1979.

Muna, W. F., Spray, T. L., Morrow, A. G., and Roberts, W. C.: Aortic dissection after aortic valve replacement in patients with valvular aortic stenosis. J. Thorac. Cardiovasc. Surg., 74:65, 1977.

Murray, C. A., and Edwards, J. E.: Spontaneous laceration of the ascending aorta. Circulation, 47:848, 1973.

Najafi, H.: Aneurysm of the cystic medionecrotic aortic root — a modified surgical approach. J. Thorac. Cardiovasc. Surg., 66:71, 1973.

Najafi, H.: Vascular complications of extracorporeal circulation. In Complications of Intrathoracic Surgery. Edited by A. R. Cordell and R. G. Ellison. Boston, Little, Brown and Co., 1979, pp. 78–83.

Najafi, H., Dye, W. S., Javid, H., Hunter, J. A., Goldin, M. D., and Julian, O. C.: Acute aortic regurgitation secondary to aortic dissection: Surgical management without valve replacement. Ann. Thorac. Surg., 14:474, 1972.

Najafi, H., Dye, W. S., Javid, H., Hunter, J. A., Goldin, M. D., and Serry, C.: Aortic insufficiency secondary to aortic root aneurysm and/or dissection. Arch. Surg., 110:1401, 1975.

Nicholson, W. J., Crawley, I. S., Logue, R. B., Dorney, E. R., Cobbs, B. W., and Hatcher, C. R., Jr.: Aortic root dissection complicating coronary bypass surgery. Am. J. Cardiol., 41:103, 1978.

Parmley, L. F., Mattingly, T. M., Manion, W. C., and Jahnke, E. J., Jr.: Nonpenetrating traumatic injury of aorta. Circulation, 17:1086, 1958.

Perryman, R. A., and Gay, W. A.: Rupture of dissecting thoracic aortic aneurysm into the right ventricle. Am. J. Cardiol., 30:277, 1972.

Prokop, E. K., Wheat, M. W., Jr., and Palmer, R. F.: Hydrodynamic forces in dissecting aneurysms. Circ. Res., 27:131, 1970.

Reifenstein, G. H., Levine, S. A., and Gross, R. E.: Coarctation of the aorta. A review of 104 autopsied cases of "adult type," 2 years of age or older. Am. Heart J., 33:146, 1947.

Reul, G. J., Jr., Cooley, D. A., Hallman, G. H., Reddy, S. B., Kyger, E. R., and Wukasch, D. C.: Dissecting aneurysm of the descending aorta. Improved surgical results in 91 patients. Arch. Surg., 110:632, 1975.

Roberts, W. C.: The hypertensive diseases. Evidence that systemic hypertension is a greater risk factor to the development of other cardiovascular disease than previously suspected. Am. J. Med., 59:523, 1975.

Roberts, W. C.: Aortic dissection: Anatomy, consequences, and causes. Am. Heart J., 101:195, 1981.

Rosenberg, H. L., and Mulder, D. G.: Dissecting thoracic aneurysms. Arch. Surg., 105:19, 1972.

Schnitker, M. A., and Bayer, C. A.: Dissecting aneurysm of the aorta in young individuals, particularly in association with pregnancy. With report of a case. Ann. Intern. Med., 20:486, 1944.

Spencer, F. C., and Blake, H.: A report of the successful surgical treatment of aortic regurgitation for a dissecting aortic aneurysm in a patient with Marfan's syndrome. J. Thorac. Cardiovasc. Surg., 44:238, 1962.

Thiene, G., Rossi, L., and Becker, A. E.: The atrioventricular conduction system in dissecting aneurysm of the aorta. Am. Heart J., 98:447, 1979.

Weldon, C. S., Connors, J. P., and Martz, M. N.: Use of saphenous vein to extend and relocate coronary arteries: Clinical experience during extensive reconstructive operations of the aortic root. Arch. Surg., 114:1330, 1979.

Wheat, M. W., Jr.: Treatment of dissecting aneurysms of the aorta. Current status. Prog. Cardiovasc. Dis., 16:87, 1973.

Wheat, M. W., Jr., and Palmer, R. F.: Dissecting aneurysms of the aorta: Present status of drug versus surgical therapy. Prog. Cardiovasc. Dis., 11:198, 1968.

Wheat, M. W., Jr., and Shumacker, H. B., Jr.: Dissecting aneurysm. Problems of management. Chest, 70:650, 1976.

Wheat, M. W., Jr., Palmer, R. F., Bartley, T. B., and Seelman, R. C.: Treatment of dissecting aneurysms of the aorta without surgery. J. Thorac. Cardiovasc. Surg., 50:364, 1965.

Wolfe, W. G., and Moran, J. F.: The evolution of medical and surgical management of acute aortic dissection. (Editorial.) Circulation, 56:503, 1977.

Wolfe, W. G.: Acute ascending aortic dissection. Ann. Surg., 192:658, 1980.

X   THORACIC ANEURYSMS

Henry T. Bahnson

The intrathoracic aorta and great vessels arising from the arch may be involved with aneurysms from a variety of causes. These aneurysms present many different pictures and may severely tax the surgeon's ability. They may be caused by syphilis, bacterial infection, congenital abnormalities, cystic medial necrosis, trauma, or arteriosclerosis, or they may be of the dissecting type. Of these, syphilis was the most common cause before venereal disease was able to be controlled or satisfactorily treated. Now, arteriosclerosis heads the list. Excisional therapy, begun in 1952, has made surgical treatment of aortic aneurysm much more satisfactory than the palliative procedures that were formerly used, such as wiring, wrapping with cellophane, and endoaneurysmorrhaphy.

PATHOLOGIC ANATOMY

Syphilis. Syphilis produces periarteritis and mesarteritis of the aorta, causing destruction and scarring of the media with subsequent dilatation. The aorta may be diffusely involved, the changes being most striking near the heart and usually becoming less prominent at the level of the diaphragm. Syphilitic aneurysms occur less frequently in the areas of the aorta farther removed from the heart. This is in striking contrast to arteriosclerotic aneurysms, which characteristically are more common in the terminal aorta than in the intrathoracic portion. Cranley and associates (1954) found that 89 per cent of 189 syphilitic aneurysms were in the thoracic aorta, 78 per cent being in the ascending aorta or arch; only two aneurysms occurred below the renal arteries. With the diffuse aortitis of syphilis, a fusiform aneurysm may occur. On the other hand, saccular aneurysms are more commonly due to syphilis than to other causes, and it would appear that some aneurysms represent blowouts from local gummatous lesions, a point well recognized by Tuffier in 1902. In many instances, except for the localized saccular blowout, the remaining aorta may be of nearly normal diameter, although it may show histologic evidence of syphilis, and if the point of great weakness can be excised, the remaining aorta may function satisfactorily for years (Fig. 30–32). The innominate artery is frequently involved with fusiform dilatation or even a saccular aneurysm; the other branches of the aortic arch are less frequently affected. The duration of disease from chancre to onset of complications of aortitis was 10 to 20 years in the majority of cases when it could be determined in Kampmeier's series (1938).

Bacterial Infection. Bacterial infection, usually secondary to endocarditis, may cause a mycotic aneurysm. This is apt to be a localized, saccular lesion in a patient with an otherwise normal aorta.

Cystic Medial Necrosis. Cystic medial necrosis, described by Gsell (1928) and Erdheim (1929), may be seen in aneurysms of several types. It is the cause of aneurysm in a fairly specific clinical entity, occurring predominantly in young men and involving the ascending aorta from the region of the valve to the innominate artery (Bahnson and Nelson, 1956). There are necrosis and disappearance of muscle cells in the elastic laminae, and there are often cystic spaces filled with a mucoid material. Similar histologic changes may be found throughout the body to a lesser extent, but in most instances, histologic changes are strikingly

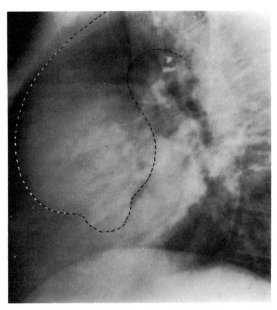

Figure 30–33. Retouched angiocardiogram demonstrating localized aneurysm due to cystic medial necrosis arising just above the sinuses of Valsalva. Note the normal size of the valve ring and sinus of Valsalva and of the aortic arch at the level of the innominate artery.

limited to the ascending aorta. The resulting aneurysm is fusiform, all areas of the circumference being nearly equally affected. Dissection and separation of the layers of the aorta are common, often localized to the ascending aorta but in some instances extending up into the innominate artery and aortic arch. Perhaps as a result of the dissection, pericarditis is frequently seen, particularly adjacent to the aneurysm. In spite of the pericarditis, the aneurysm may be mobilized more readily from adjacent structures than can those due to syphilis or trauma. The dilatation frequently extends to the aortic valve but often not into the sinus of Valsalva (Fig. 30–33). Because of the dilation, aortic insufficiency may result, the leaflets usually being unaffected.

Localized fusiform aneurysms of the ascending aorta occur with cystic medial necrosis in the absence of other stigmata of Marfan's syndrome. Usually, in Marfan's syndrome, in which there are skeletal defects, dislocated lenses of the eye, arachnodactyly, and a generalized defect of the connective tissue, there is a diffuse dilatation of the ascending aorta, often with aortic dissection. In such cases, the dilatation usually extends into the sinuses of Valsalva.

Cystic medial necrosis is often found in cases of dissecting aneurysm of the aorta, although involvement is not so severe as that in fusiform aneurysms due to this condition. The cause of cystic medial necrosis is unknown, but a similar histologic picture may be seen in patients with presumed congenital aneurysms and in experimental animals given beta-aminonitrile (Bean and Ponseti, 1955).

Congenital Aneurysms. Congenital aneurysms have been described most commonly in the region of

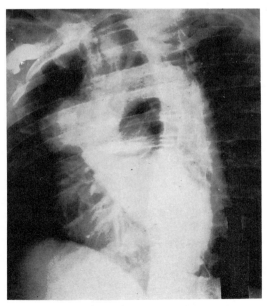

Figure 30–32. Angiocardiogram showing localized saccular aneurysm of the ascending aorta with essentially normal aortic diameter elsewhere. (From Bahnson, H. T.: Considerations in the excision of aortic aneurysms. Ann. Surg., *138*:377, 1953.)

the aortic isthmus, usually in association with other congenital defects — often coarctation of the aorta. The congenital origin is assumed in the absence of other etiologic agents. The histologic picture is usually similar to that of cystic medial necrosis, occurring in a well-localized area. Similar histologic changes are often seen in the immediate vicinity of coarctation of the aorta. Most of the reported aneurysms of this type have been in adults.

Traumatic Aneurysms. Traumatic aneurysms occur as a result of sudden deceleration and are being seen with increasing frequency. The aorta is most susceptible to tear at two places: immediately adjacent to the heart at the origin of the aorta and posteriorly just distal to the left subclavian artery, where the aorta becomes fixed in the region of the vertebral column. Much less commonly, a tear may occur in the aortic arch, near the origin of the innominate or left carotid artery. A tear in the ascending aorta usually results in sudden death, with few persons living to develop an aneurysm. In an appreciable number of individuals with rupture distal to the aortic arch, the intima and media may be transected, but if the adventitia is intact, a pulsating hematoma forms, which later results in a false aneurysm. The aortic tear is a circumferential one, and either part or all of the circumference of the aorta may be involved. The resulting hematoma may prevent hemorrhage for hours or weeks if sudden death does not occur, but exsanguinating hemorrhage may result from delayed rupture. Survival longer than this is associated with the formation of a false aneurysm.

Arteriosclerosis. Arteriosclerosis may cause a thoracic aortic aneurysm, although more commonly aneurysms from this cause are localized to the terminal aorta. Once considered rare as a cause of thoracic aneurysms at a time when syphilis was the most common cause, arteriosclerosis has acquired greater frequency and importance with our aging population. Usually fusiform, these aneurysms are more common in the lower thoracic aorta, seldom occurring in the arch or the ascending aorta.

In rare instances, large aneurysms involving the entire thoracic aorta from the left subclavian artery to the diaphragm may be seen in patients in the third and fourth decades in whom no cause is obvious other than arteriosclerosis. It is possible that in these cases the arteriosclerosis is secondary to another undisclosed etiology.

Dissecting Aneurysm of the Aorta. Dissecting aneurysm of the aorta is a specific clinical and pathologic entity, although the word dissection is often used in speaking of aneurysms of other types to designate further rupture and enlargement of the aneurysm. Aortic dissection is discussed in detail in the preceding section of this chapter.

CLINICAL PICTURE

Symptoms of aortic aneurysm usually occur because of pressure or obstruction of adjacent structures. Pain commonly accompanies the development of dissecting aneurysm, and in addition, pain may occur in some patients in whom there is no explanation other than aortitis. Aneurysm of the ascending aorta causes symptoms less frequently, and there may be none until the aneurysm actually erodes through the ribs and the sternum and forms a pulsating, palpable tumor. In the early stage, it may obstruct the superior vena cava or an innominate vein and produce venous distention over the upper extremities and neck. Tracheal or bronchial obstruction, often caused by aneurysms of the arch, leads to a wheeze, the characteristic brassy cough, and pneumonitis secondary to obstruction. The recurrent and even the phrenic nerves may be paralyzed because of pressure from an expanding lesion. Innominate aneurysms are apt to produce symptoms from the expanding mass, which may cause Horner's syndrome or venous obstruction. The mass may resemble carcinoma of the thyroid if it is clotted and firm. Aneurysms occurring posteriorly in the thoracic aorta more frequently are painful, presumably from pressure on the spinal nerves and erosion of the vertebral column. Esophageal obstruction is uncommon.

Aortic insufficiency from simple dilatation without significant abnormality of the leaflets may result from aneurysms involving the ascending aorta, particularly fusiform ones in which the first portion of the aorta is dilated. This is especially true in patients with cystic medial necrosis. In rare instances, cardiac failure has occurred as the result of pressure from an aneurysm on the pulmonary artery or even the outflow tract of the right ventricle.

Prognosis for patients with thoracic aortic aneurysm is not easily determined. Early reports such as Kampmeier's (1938) included a high percentage of syphilitic aneurysms, which are uncommon today. Saccular syphilitic aneurysms generally pose a greater threat of enlargement and rupture than do those of arteriosclerotic origin.

Joyce and associates (1964) followed 91 per cent of 107 cases of untreated thoracic aortic aneurysms for 5 years. Etiologies of the aneurysms closely approximated those seen in clinical practice today. Large size of the aneurysm, the presence of symptoms, and associated cardiovascular disease were important determinants of a poor prognosis. Only half of the patients survived for 5 years. Pressler and McNamara (1980) determined the history of 90 patients with arteriosclerotic aneurysms. Forty-two per cent of the patients had pain in the back or chest when first seen, and 50 per cent were asymptomatic. The aneurysm was discovered at autopsy in 8 per cent. Rupture of the aneurysm accounted for 44 per cent of the deaths. Cardiovascular disease was the second leading cause of death, in 33 per cent of the patients. The surgical mortality rate for elective resection of arteriosclerotic aneurysm was significantly less than the risk of late rupture.

The clinical manifestations of dissecting aneurysm may differ from those of other types of aneurysm. In fact, the possible involvement of the entire aorta may give protean manifestations and direct attention to the abdomen or chest. The most common picture is that of sudden onset of epigastric or precordial pain radiating to the shoulders, neck, or abdomen. A variety of abdominal, neurologic, and peripheral signs may appear, depending on the degree of interference with blood supply to various organs and areas. The condition is mistaken most commonly for myocardial infarction.

DIAGNOSIS

In some cases, the diagnosis can be made on the basis of a history of respiratory obstruction, possibly with findings of thoracic pulsation, tracheal tug, or brassy cough. In most instances, however, the diagnosis is a radiologic one based on the discovery of a mass contiguous with a part of the aortic shadow. The aorta can be seen surprisingly well in most normal chests if both posteroanterior and lateral roentgenograms are made. Confirmation of the diagnosis and determination of the extent of the aneurysm, the presence of clot, and the involvement of displacement of adjacent structures can be made by angiocardiography or direct aortography. Contrast visualization is desirable if surgery is contemplated.

Differentiation from solid mediastinal tumors may be difficult. Pulsation may be a misleading sign, since many aortic aneurysms have sufficient scarring about them to limit pulsation, whereas a solid tumor without inflammation sitting on a normally pulsating aorta may give the fluoroscopic appearance of expansile pulsation.

Rupture of the aorta is a recognized result of severe trauma to the chest, and this should be suspected in the pre-aneurysmal stage when there is a combination of severe injury to the chest and radiographic evidence of widening of the mediastrinum, displacement of the trachea or left main bronchus, blurring of the normally sharp aortic shadow and of the space between the aorta and pulmonary artery, or opacification of the medial aspect of the left upper chest (March and Sturm, 1976). The diagnosis may be established by aortography, and successful repair of acute rupture may be done (Clarke *et al.*, 1967).

SURGICAL THERAPY

Excision is the standard of therapy for aortic aneurysms, and other methods used in the past are almost purely of historical interest; these methods included wiring, endoaneurysmorrhaphy, and wrap-

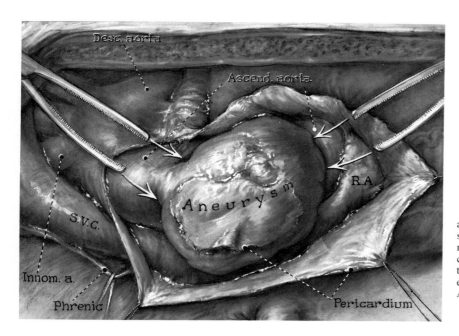

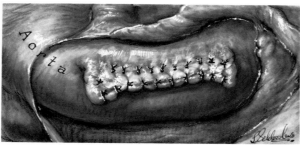

Figure 30–34. Excision of saccular aneurysm of the ascending aorta such as that shown in Figure 30–32. The adjacent aorta is mobilized and the base of the aneurysm clamped. The adjacent aorta is often essentially normal. (From Bahnson, H. T.: Considerations in the excision of aortic aneurysms. Ann. Surg., *138*:377, 1953.)

ping with fibrogenic or reinforcing materials. Excision of the aneurysm alone may be satisfactory when it is saccular and the adjacent aorta is not badly diseased, but in most cases, the aneurysm and the adjacent aorta must be excised and the segment replaced. The problems encountered and the operative techniques, risks, and results differ strikingly in the diferent portions of the intrathoracic aorta.

The manner of excision depends on the location of the aneurysm and whether it is saccular or fusiform. In all cases, the adjacent aorta should be mobilized before the aneurysm, since the more normal aorta is, in most instances, relatively free of or loosely attached to adjacent structures, often in contrast to the aneurysm itself. The neck of a saccular aneurysm can be occluded and divided and the opening closed with multiple figure-of-eight sutures (Fig. 30–34). The thickened, fibrous neck of saccular aneurysms facilitates clamping the neck, and the tissue is usually adequate for suture closure. Caution is necessary in clamping the mouth of the sac to be sure that it does not contain a clot or a calcified rim, which might be broken off to form an embolus. This usually can be detected by gentle palpation. In the area distal to the aortic arch, it is simpler to occlude the aorta briefly above and below the aneurysm, incise the neck, and then reconstruct the aortic continuity (Fig. 30–35). On inspection of the opened aneurysm, it is easy to detect the edge of the aneurysm if it is a saccular one and to determine whether the lumen can be reconstructed with relatively normal adjacent aorta.

For most aneurysms, however, the aorta must be occluded. When this occurs, both the heart and distal organs are damaged. A brief insult may be tolerated, but usually one must decrease the load on the heart and provide protection for the body.

Aneurysms of the Ascending Aorta

Aneurysms of the ascending aorta are now most commonly caused by cystic medial necrosis, with or without the other stigmata of Marfan's syndrome, or by dissection of the aorta (dissecting hematoma), with or without cystic medial necrosis. Replacement of the ascending aorta requires cardiopulmonary bypass and interruption of circulation to the heart. The heart can best be protected during this interruption by moderate general cooling of the body and perfusion of the coronary arteries with cold (4°C.) cardioplegic solution containing added potassium. In many instances, the aneurysm is limited to the ascending aorta, and only this portion must be replaced. Lesser degrees of dilatation or dissection may extend into the aortic arch, but replacement of the arch adds greatly to the complexity and risk of the operation, and often control of the diameter at the distal anastomosis proximal to the innominate artery serves to halt progression of the disease.

Controversy is more commonly encountered with regard to the origin of the ascending aorta. The aortic

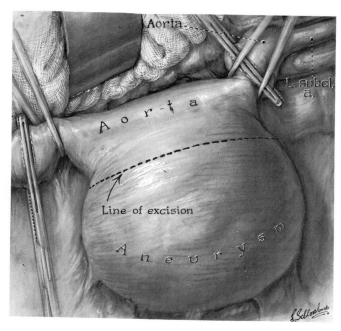

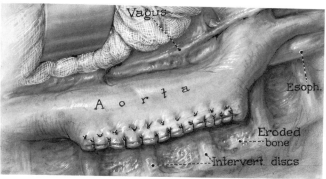

Figure 30–35. Aneurysm of upper thoracic aorta treated by proximal and distal aortic occlusion, excision, and aortic reconstruction. Such aneurysms frequently erode the vertebral column. In the case of a saccular aneurysm, the border between satisfactory aortic wall and aneurysm can be seen readily once the aneurysm is opened. (From Bahnson, H. T.: Considerations in the excision of aortic aneurysms. Ann. Surg., *138*:377, 1953.)

valve is often involved, usually with regurgitation, and there may be dilatation of the sinuses of Valsalva, where the coronary arteries arise. In some instances, only the ascending aorta distal to the sinus ridge is significantly involved, and if the sinuses of Valsalva are only minimally dilated, the proximal anastomosis may be done to the region of the sinus ridge (Fig. 30–36). In doing so, the aortic regurgitation may be improved or controlled. Resuspension of a commissure dropped by the dissecting hematoma may correct regurgitation. The aortic leaflets in themselves are often normal, and making a bicuspid valve by excision of the noncoronary sinus may be satisfactory. In the presence of moderate or severe aortic regurgitation, however, aortic valve replacement is required. Our preference at present is for the Bjork-Shiley tilting disc.

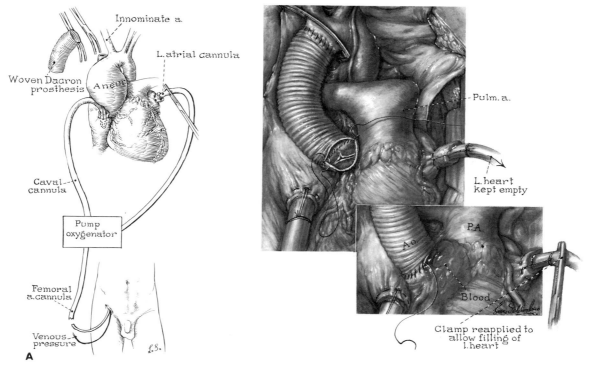

Figure 30–36. Excision of fusiform aneurysm of the ascending aorta. *A*, Plan of bypass. *B*, During cardioplegia and cold arrest of the heart, the woven prosthesis is sutured in place. The wall of the aneurysm may be preserved and wrapped around the prosthesis.

If the sinuses of Valsalva are not significantly aneurysmal or if the coronary arteries arise low on the sinus, the coronary arteries may be preserved, possibly in a tongue of aortic wall, and the prosthesis anastomosed to this (Fig. 30–36) (Miller *et al.*, 1980). In most cases of Marfan's syndrome, the dilatation extends into the sinuses of Valsalva and the coronary arteries arise high on the sinuses. When this occurs, a composite valve-containing tubular prosthesis should be used after excision of the aortic valve, as described by Bentall and DeBono (1968), and the coronary arteries are transposed to the prostheses with a button of adjacent aortic wall (Kouchoukos *et al.*, 1980) (Fig. 30–37) or possibly with a vein graft (Fig. 30–38).

There is sufficient variation in the pathologic anatomy to allow selection among the several techniques available (Campbell *et al.*, 1978). The wall of the aneurysm may be preserved to wrap around the prosthesis or the anastomoses, because bleeding has been a major complication. This must be done cautiously to avoid kinking and compression of either the prosthesis or the coronary arteries by hematoma between the two layers. The recent operative mortality rate has been below 5 per cent (Kouchoukos *et al.*, 1980; Miller *et al.*, 1980).

Aneurysms of the Aortic Arch

Aneurysms of the aortic arch were first excised in 1952, but the risk of surgical treatment has been almost prohibitive unil recently. Better methods of diagnosis, preoperative evaluation, anesthesia, and intraoperative support and new concepts of surgical technique have greatly reduced the risk. Earlier techniques involved temporary or permanent bypass or a replacement graft to the brachiocephalic vessels and to the distal aorta. Cardiopulmonary bypass and perfusion of the vessels to the head were added, along with hypothermia, but the techniques were complicated, the procedures were long, and persistent bleeding was a major complication. Crawford and Vaccaro's recent synthesis of techniques involves a median sternotomy, cardiopulmonary bypass, and profound hypothermia (Crawford and Vaccaro, 1981). Once the patient is cooled, the brachiocephalic vessels are occluded, flow from the machine to the femoral artery is reduced to a minimal level to keep the aorta softly filled, and the aneurysm is opened. Prosthetic reconstruction is performed from inside the opened aneurysm, and the great vessels are similarly sutured to a window made in the prosthesis (Fig. 30–39). Steps are taken to avoid embolism of air or debris from the aorta. After the appropriate connections are completed and during rewarming, the sac of the aneurysm may be sutured around the prosthesis to control hemorrhage.

Whether or not the innominate and left common carotid arteries must be occluded is an important determinant of the risk of excision of arch aneurysms. Using the technique outlined, Crawford and Vaccaro (1981) reported that 19 of 20 patients survived replacement of the transverse aortic arch.

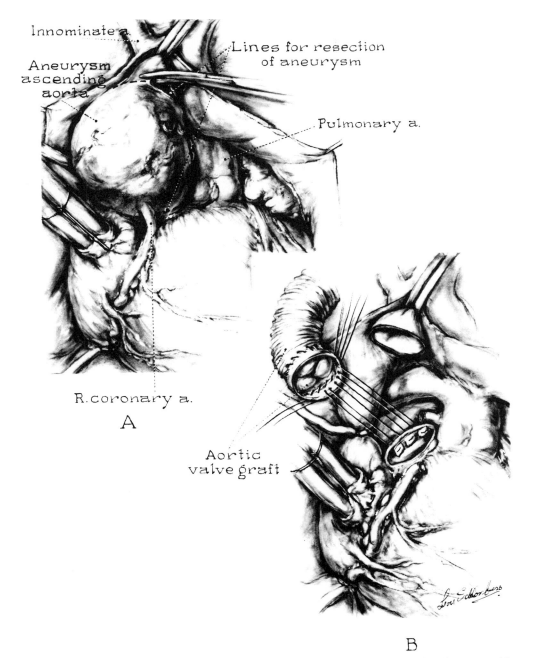

Innominate a.

Lines for resection
of aneurysm

Aneurysm
ascending
aorta

Pulmonary a.

R. coronary a.

A

Aortic
valve graft

B

Figure 30–37. *A* and *B*, Excision of aneurysm of the ascending aorta and the aortic valve and replacement with a composite valve and conduit. Coronary arteries must then be implanted as in Figure 30–38. Use of a tissue valve obviates the use of long-term anticoagulation. (From Campbell, C. D.: Aortic Aneurysm: Surgical Therapy. Mount Kisco, New York, Futura Publishing Co., 1981.)

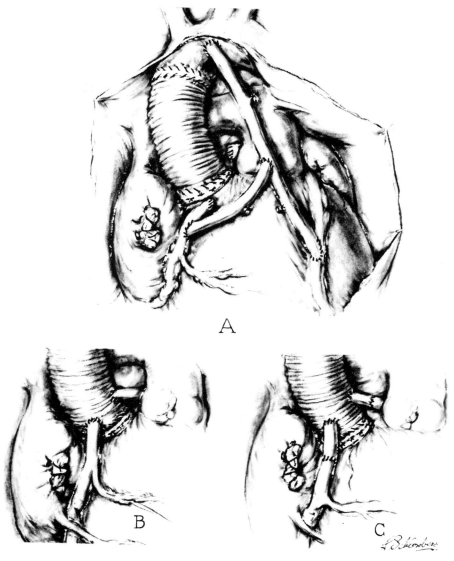

A

B

C

Figure 30–38. Options for reconstruction of coronary circulation after replacement of aortic valve and ascending aorta as a composite prosthesis. *A*, Saphenous vein bypass graft. *B*, Direct implantation, usually with a button of aortic wall. *C*, Interposed saphenous vein graft. (From Campbell, C. D.: Aortic Aneurysm: Surgical Therapy. Mount Kisco, New York, Futura Publishing Co., 1981.)

Aneurysms of the Descending Thoracic Aorta

Aneurysms of the descending thoracic aorta, sometimes involving the adjacent left subclavian artery, can be treated much more easily than those of the aortic arch. Traumatic aneurysms in this region are especially important because of their frequency and curability. The proximal descending thoracic aorta is most commonly involved, and exposure is best obtained through the bed of the resected fifth rib or through the adjacent fourth interspace. The seventh interspace may be better suited for more distally located aneurysms, and in some instances in which the aneurysm is large and extensive, both spaces may be entered.

The lung is frequently adherent to the aneurysm, especially if there has been recent enlargement. It can usually be dissected from the aneurysm, and often this is required in order to gain exposure. If possible, however, it should be done only after proximal and distal control of the aorta has been obtained.

Control of the afterload on the heart and protection of the spinal cord and abdominal viscera are prime considerations, just as is the case with the more proximal aorta. In the thoracic aorta, the limit of safe occlusion time is determined less by possible damage to the heart than by tolerable limits of ischemia of the abdominal viscera and the spinal cord, which receives important tributaries from the intercostal arteries in this region. An arteria magna arises from a segment varying between the eighth thoracic and fourth lumbar vertebrae, division of which is hazardous (Adams and van Geertruyden, 1956). Identification of this artery is difficult, if even possible, by clinical means, and hence, if an aneurysm in this region must be excised, only those intercostal arteries that must be removed with the aneurysm should be ligated.

A number of techniques have been developed to

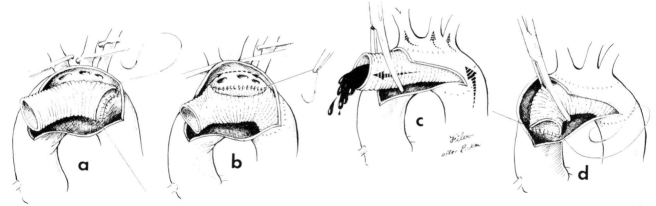

Figure 30–39. Replacement of the aortic arch as described by Crawford and associates (1981). Under deep hypothermia and low-level perfusion with cardiopulmonary bypass, the prosthesis is sutured to the aorta from inside the aneurysm (*a*), as are the mouths of the great vessels (*b*), and then the ascending aorta (*c* and *d*).

provide protection, including hypothermia, femoral artery–to–femoral vein bypass with a pump-oxygenator, complete cardiopulmonary bypass, left atrial–to–femoral artery bypass with a pump, and ventricular or aortic–to–distal aorta or femoral bypass. Of these, left atrial–to–femoral artery bypass

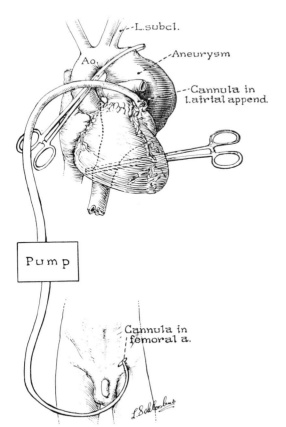

Figure 30–40. Plan of left atrial–to–femoral artery bypass for excision of aneurysm of the thoracic aorta.

has been the most satisfactory in our experience (Fig. 30–40). This technique requires heparinization, but it also allows scavenging and return of shed blood. Alternatively, a shunt treated with anticoagulants, as described by Gott, may be used (see the following section of this chapter).

An interesting and promising recent development has been the demonstration, originally advocated by Crawford and Rubio in 1973, that results are as good or better with simple clamping of the aorta without shunt or bypass than with use of the latter methods. Benefits from this simplified technique include shortening of the steps of the operation and avoidance of heparin and extracorporeal circulation. Damage appears to occur as much from shock before or after the period of occlusion as from the occlusion itself. Intercostal arteries should be ligated from inside the aneurysm, thus preserving intercostal collateral circulation. An effort should be made to preserve the intercostal arteries by techniques such as a patch graft, replacement of the anterior wall of the aorta when possible, or reattachment of large or multiple intercostal arteries. Sewing the prosthesis to the proximal and distal aorta from inside the opened aneurysm, as first used on the abdominal aorta by Creech, eliminates dissection about the aneurysm, and the aortic wall can be wrapped around the prosthesis after removal of clots (Fig. 30–41). There is increasing evidence from other experienced surgeons that excision without adjuncts to avoid ischemia is preferable (Najafi *et al.*, 1980). Nevertheless, the surgeon who treats thoracic aneurysms less frequently will probably continue to want the security of some type of bypass. Perhaps this is advisable when the aorta must be occluded for longer than 30 to 40 minutes. Regardless of this, other principles presented by Crawford and associates should be followed. No technique has been shown to prevent completely the dreaded complication of paraplegia.

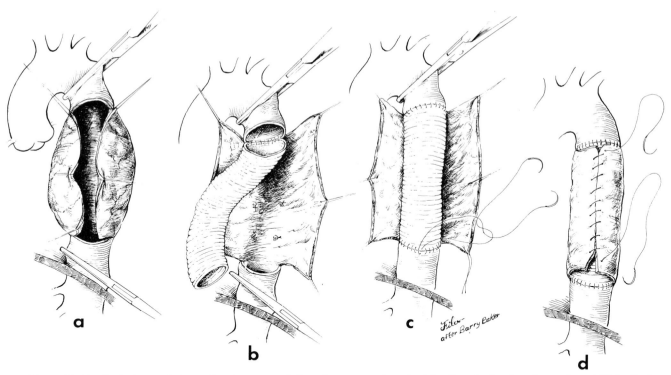

Figure 30–41. Inclusion technique of replacement of thoracic aorta as described by Crawford and and associates (1981). During aortic occlusion, the aneurysm is longitudinally opened, and the prosthesis is sutured from inside (*a–c*). Part of the aneurysmal wall may be wrapped around the prosthesis for hemostasis (*d*).

Reconstruction of aortic continuity in the absence of heparin might be accomplished with a knitted Dacron tubular prosthesis. When heparin is used, a more tightly woven fabric is required. Nonabsorbable synthetic sutures, such as coated Dacron, are recommended.

Recent mortality rates have been reported to range from 0 to 15 per cent. Crawford and associates (1981) reported a 9 per cent mortality rate for their last 112 patients, with an actuarial 5-year survival rate of 58 per cent.

For references see page 990.

XI   HEPARINIZED SHUNTS FOR THORACIC VASCULAR OPERATIONS

VINCENT L. GOTT

There has been general agreement for a number of years that some type of temporary vascular bypass is required for major surgical procedures involving the thoracic aorta. Aneurysms of the ascending aorta or proximal arch of the aorta require total cardiopulmonary bypass. For the resection of segments of the distal arch of the aorta or the descending thoracic aorta, there are several different bypass techniques that are available. From a historical standpoint, the most common bypass technique that was used for aneurysms of the descending thoracic aorta during the 1960s and early 1970s was the technique of left atrial–femoral

artery bypass. This technique utilizes a pump to transfer approximately one half of the cardiac output from the left atrium to the femoral artery during the time that the descending thoracic aorta is cross-clamped. A second technique, which became popular about 10 years ago, was the use of femoral vein–femoral artery bypass with an interposed pump-oxygenator. This latter technique has the advantage of not requiring cardiac cannulation, but it does require the use of a heart-lung machine. Both of these bypass techniques do require systemic heparinization.

Because of problems with generalized bleeding

from a large operative field in a heparinized patient, the concept of using a simple temporary shunt around a thoracic aneurysm has considerable appeal. This technique has the advantage of eliminating not only the need for systemic heparinization, but also the need for an interposed blood pump. Actually, some of the earliest resections of aneurysms of the descending thoracic aorta were performed with either a temporary internal plastic shunt (Johnson *et al.*, 1955) or a temporary external shunt (Stranahan *et al.*, 1955; Chamberlain *et al.*, 1956). With the availability of suitable blood pumps, the simple tube-shunt techniques were virtually abandoned for the technique of left atrial–femoral artery bypass.

The introduction of polymers with wall-bonded heparin (Gott *et al.*, 1963) allowed for the reintroduction of a temporary tube-shunt system that can be employed in a safe manner. The first bypass shunts with wall-bonded heparin (Valiathan *et al.*, 1968) utilized a polyvinyl tubing with a graphite surface that was subsequently immersed in benzalkonium chloride (a cationic surfactant) and then in heparin. The graphite, with its absorptive properties, firmly bonded the positively charged surfactant, and then, with immersion in heparin, there was a strong electrochemical bond because heparin has a high negative charge. This surface permitted the bonding of heparin to the polyvinyl shunt and thus eliminated the necessity for systemic heparinization for those patients with aneurysms of the descending thoracic aorta. The graphite-benzalkonium-heparin (GBH)–coated shunts were utilized initially as a bypass conduit for patients with thoracic aneurysms. Subsequently, an improved heparinized surface was developed by polymer chemists at the Battelle Columbus Laboratories, and this coating is called the TDMAC-heparin surface (Grode *et al.*, 1969). With this newer heparinized surface, the graphite-benzalkonium portion of the coating was replaced with the cationic surfactant TDMAC (tridodecylmethylammonium chloride). TDMAC is combined with a solvent, so that when the plastic device is immersed in this solution, the solvent etches the surface of the plastic, allowing the TDMAC to be embedded in the wall. When the device is then immersed in heparin, the anticoagulant is firmly bound to the positively charged TDMAC radicals.

This latter heparinizing system has several distinct advantages over the GBH surface. First, with the elimination of graphite, the heparinized surface is completely transparent and can be clamped with a crushing metal clamp without fear of damage. In addition, greater quantities of heparin can be more firmly bound to the underlying polymer by the interposed TDMAC coating. Extensive studies, performed over several years by the Battelle chemists on this TDMAC-heparin surface, have demonstrated very firm bonding of high concentrations of heparin to the polymer (10 μg./cm.^{2}).

An aortic bypass shunt made of polyvinyl chloride and tapered at each end to facilitate proximal and distal cannulation has been designed* (Fig. 30–42). The central portion of this unitized shunt has a larger diameter to reduce the overall resistance to blood flow. This shunt is then coated with the transparent TDMAC-heparin coating, and after sterilization with ethylene oxide, it has an indefinite shelf life from the standpoint of deterioration of the wall-bonded heparin.

Several excellent hemodynamic studies have been done on the use of the tapered heparinized shunt. One study (Frantz *et al.*, 1981) demonstrated that in adult sheep the mean left ventricular pressure rose by 64 ± 15 mm. Hg when the descending thoracic aorta was cross-clamped. At the same time, the mean femoral artery pressure was only 28 ± 4 mm. Hg. With the

---

*Available from Sherwood Medical Industries, Inc., 1831 Olive Street, St. Louis, Missouri 63103.

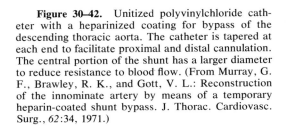

Figure 30–42. Unitized polyvinylchloride catheter with a heparinized coating for bypass of the descending thoracic aorta. The catheter is tapered at each end to facilitate proximal and distal cannulation. The central portion of the shunt has a larger diameter to reduce resistance to blood flow. (From Murray, G. F., Brawley, R. K., and Gott, V. L.: Reconstruction of the innominate artery by means of a temporary heparin-coated shunt bypass. J. Thorac. Cardiovasc. Surg., *62*:34, 1971.)

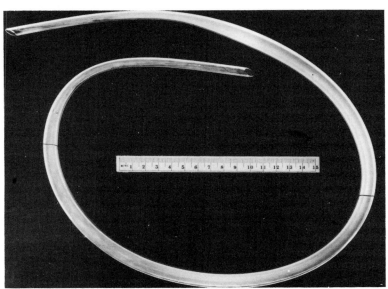

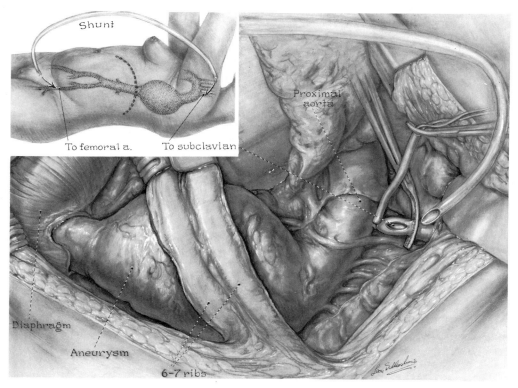

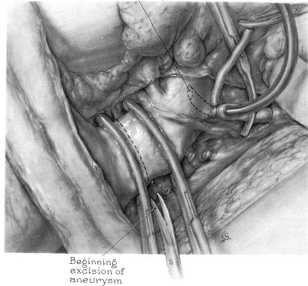

Figure 30–43. One type of surgical approach employing the heparinized shunt during the resection of a large arteriosclerotic aneurysm of the descending thoracic aorta. *A,* Excellent exposure obtained through the bed of the fifth rib with a second incision through the seventh interspace. In this patient, the proximal cannulation is being performed through the left subclavian artery, and the distal cannulation is being done through the left common femoral artery. *B,* The aorta is prepared for proximal transection. *C,* Placement of the prosthetic graft with the heparinized shunt in position. (From Valiathan, M. S., *et al.:* Resection of aneurysms of the descending thoracic aorta using a GBH-coated shunt bypass. J. Surg. Res., *8:*197, 1968.)

cross clamp on the descending thoracic aorta, the left ventricular end-diastolic pressure rose to an average of 31 ± 8 mm. Hg, with the mean left atrial pressure rising by 6 ± mm. Hg and V waves developing in the left atrium. At the same time, the left ventricle showed evidence of cardiac decompensation, with ventricular fibrillation frequently occurring after 15 to 20 minutes. With the insertion of the tapered heparinized shunt from the apex of the left ventricle to the left common iliac artery, the mean left ventricular pressure rose only by 23 ± 9 mm. Hg; the mean femoral artery pressure was 62 ± 15 mm. Hg, and the left ventricular end-diastolic pressure and mean left atrial pressure were within normal range. Shunt flow averaged 1.6 ± 0.49 L./min., which was approximately one third of the cardiac output. In these animals with left ventricular–common iliac bypass, the overall cardiac output was essentially normal. This technique of placing a vascular shunt between the left ventricular apex and the common iliac artery was first suggested by English, of Guy's Hospital, London, in 1965. These original shunts were constructed of simple polymer tubing without wall-bonded heparin. In 1976, Murray and Young first utilized the heparinized shunt as a left ventricular–common iliac conduit. Murray, likewise, has demonstrated that even though there is no valve in the tapered shunt, the reverse flow in the shunt is less than 10 per cent of the forward flow.

Finally, it should be emphasized that a number of thoracic aneurysms have been resected with simple cross-clamping and no protective shunting. It appears that cross-clamping of the thoracic aorta is tolerated reasonably well for periods up to 30 minutes, but cross-clamping beyond this time carries a fairly high risk of spinal cord injury. A recent excellent study (Katz et al., 1981) has very clearly demonstrated the importance of some type of shunt bypass when the thoracic aorta is cross-clamped for more than 30 minutes. In this study, 35 patients had undergone resection of a portion of the descending thoracic aorta for acute trauma. In 15 patients, no shunt was utilized, and there was no paresis or paralysis in patients with the cross clamp placed for less than 30 minutes. However, five of seven patients (71 per cent) with cross-clamping times of 32 to 53 minutes did show evidence of spinal cord injury. Twenty additional patients had either a simple tube shunt or femorofemoral bypass, and only three of these patients demonstrated paresis or paralysis in the postoperative period. The cross-clamping times for these three patients were 34, 40, and 82 minutes. This study clearly demonstrated that if the time that the thoracic aorta is cross-clamped exceeds 30 minutes, then some type of shunt or pump bypass should be utilized.

HEPARINIZED SHUNTS FOR ANEURYSMS OF THE DESCENDING THORACIC AORTA

Selection of Patients

Heparinized shunts for temporary bypass of the descending thoracic aorta appear to be quite satisfactory for any patient with a nonrupturing atherosclerotic aneurysm within any portion of the descending thoracic aorta. The ideal patient for shunt bypass has an aneurysm that commences just distal to the left subclavian artery and terminates several centimeters above the diaphragm. This type of aneurysm then permits easy cannulation of the subclavian artery proximally. However, if the aneurysm involves the distal arch of the aorta, the shunt can be used with proximal cannulation in the ascending aorta or with proximal cannulation in the left ventricular apex, as reintroduced by Murray and Young (1976).

Heparinized shunts have been used successfully in patients with a rupturing atherosclerotic aneurysm of the descending thoracic aorta. However, in my opinion, femoral vein–femoral artery bypass with a pump-oxygenator is preferable for these patients since this system allows the retrieval of free blood from the chest cavity by means of a cardiotomy sucker system. If a pump-oxygenator system is not available for the patient with a rupturing atherosclerotic aneurysm of the descending thoracic aorta, the heparinized shunt bypass combined with an autotransfusion system can be a satisfactory alternative.

Surgical Technique

There are currently several different methods for bypassing aneurysms of the descending thoracic aorta with the heparinized shunt. The original technique that was first introduced in 1968 (Valiathan et al., 1968) utilized a cannulation approach (Fig. 30–43). This particular bypass technique works well when the proximal portion of the aneurysm is 3 or 4 cm. distal to the left subclavian artery. Ordinarily, a thoracotomy is made through the fourth interspace or through the bed of the fifth rib. In the case depicted in Figure 30–43, because the aneurysm extended to the diaphragm, a second incision was made in the seventh interspace to facilitate cross-clamping of the aorta below the aneurysm. Ordinarily, for the more standard sized aneurysms of the descending thoracic aorta, the total procedure can be performed through the bed of the fifth rib. After the thoracotomy is completed, the aorta is encircled with umbilical tapes above and below the aneurysm at the sites for eventual application of the vascular clamps.

In addition, the distal cannulation site most commonly selected is the left common femoral artery (Fig. 30–43). It is possible, of course, to use the left common iliac site, or in the case of a smaller aneurysm that does not extend to the diaphragm, the distal cannulation site may be placed in the descending thoracic aorta just above the diaphragm.

If the aneurysm involves the aorta at the take-off site of the left subclavian artery, then the proximal cannulation site can be placed in the distal transverse arch or in the ascending aorta. If the ascending aorta is used, then ordinarily the thoracotomy incision is extended across the sternum into the right chest. My preference for the latter type of aneurysm, though, is

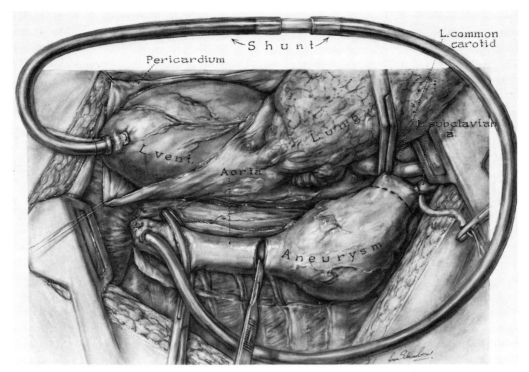

Figure 30–44. The newer cannulation technique utilizing the heparin-coated shunt for resection of a thoracic aneurysm. The use of the left ventricle–to–aorta or iliac artery shunting technique has been popularized by Murray and Young (1976). The procedure is performed through the bed of the fifth rib. The shunt has been divided to facilitate cannulation of the left ventricular apex proximally and the descending thoracic aorta distally.

to utilize the ventricular apex, popularized by Murray and Young (1976). This technique (Fig. 30–44) has the advantage of not requiring extensive dissection either in the transverse arch or in the area of the ascending aorta, which can be difficult through a left thoracotomy. Most cardiac surgeons are quite familiar with the placement of left ventricular vents in the apex, and the proximal end of the shunt is placed in a similar manner. As mentioned previously, the hemodynamic parameters determined by Murray with this type of cannulation were quite satisfactory, and there was a less than 10 per cent reversal of flow, even though there is no valve in the shunt.

Although the TDMAC-heparin surface has an indefinite shelf life from the standpoint of its anticoagulant properties, it is advisable to moisten the surface of the catheter in heparinized saline prior to use (100 mg. of heparin in 100 ml. of saline). I prefer to cut the shunt in two, perform the proximal cannulation initially, followed by the distal cannulation, and then re-establish continuity using a highly polished stainless steel connector. The aneurysm is then isolated with vascular clamps, and resection of the aneurysm and insertion of a prosthetic graft can be performed without haste. A woven Dacron prosthesis is preferred, but a preclotted, knitted Dacron graft can be used since systemic heparinization is not employed. The aortic anastomoses are ordinarily performed with 3-0 monofilament polypropylene suture material. After

the graft is in place and the clamps have been removed, the heparinized shunt is removed and the cannulation sites are repaired.

Results

A number of reports have appeared during the past 10 years from several different institutions on the use of the heparinized shunt for aneurysms of the decending thoracic aorta. Because this is not a particularly common cardiovascular problem, no one institution has obtained a large experience. One of the best reports in the literature was a survey of the experience of the members of the Samson Thoracic Surgery Society regarding repair of aneurysms of the descending aorta (Lawrence et al., 1977). In this report, there were 29 patients who had shunt bypass of nontraumatic thoracic aneurysms with four deaths (13.8 per cent), and there was no incidence of paraplegia. In the same report, there were 127 patients who had bypass of thoracic aneurysms using a pump system with systemic heparinization. There were 28 deaths (22 per cent) and no instances of paraplegia in this group. There were a total of 14 patients who had resection of thoracic aneurysms without any type of shunt protection, and there were two deaths (14.3 per cent) and one instance of paraplegia (7.1 per cent). It was interesting, too, that 9 of 61 respondents did 82 per cent of the operations and that the 17 other surgeons who did the remaining operations performed an average of only 3.5 operations per decade. These data point out that the average cardiothoracic surgeon deals with the problem of thoracic aneurysm rather infrequently, and therefore, a technique that protects the spinal cord should be utilized so that resection and repair can be performed in a careful and unhurried manner.

At the Johns Hopkins Hospital, 26 patients have had resection of nontraumatic aneurysms of the descending thoracic aorta using the heparinized shunt. All 10 patients who had elective resection of an atherosclerotic aneurysm of the descending aorta survived with satisfactory long-term results. Of the three patients who were operated on in our institution with acute rupturing atherosclerotic aneurysms of the descending thoracic aorta, only one has survived. Although the results in these critically ill patients might not have been improved using femoral vein–femoral artery bypass, we currently favor this approach for rupturing thoracic aneurysms because of the availability of a cardiotomy suction unit in combination with the pump-oxygenator. The operative results with resection for Type III dissections of the descending thoracic aorta have not been as good, particularly in those individuals with acute dissections. Five of eight patients operated on for a chronic Type III dissection survived. On the other hand, only one of five patients with an acute Type III dissection survived. Two of these five patients had a rupturing process at the time of surgery, and the remaining three patients all had preoperative leg ischemia and/or bowel necrosis secondary to the dissecting process. None of these latter three patients survived. In this series of 26 patients with nontraumatic aneurysms, there were two instances of paraplegia, both in patients with rupturing atherosclerotic aneurysms. Both patients had long segments of descending thoracic aorta resected; one patient survived and the other died of a myocardial infarction 3 weeks postoperatively.

Other excellent reports with the heparinized shunt for aneurysms of the descending thoracic aorta include a series of 39 patients from Duke University (Wolfe et al., 1977). Thirty-four of these patients (87 per cent) survived. The proximal end of the shunt was placed in the subclavian artery in 17 patients, in the left ventricle in 10, and in the ascending or transverse aortic arch in 12. These authors feel that if a choice exists for the site of proximal insertion of the shunt, it should be placed distal to the aortic valve, since they found somewhat better hemodynamics than with the proximal cannulation in the left ventricular apex.

Frantz and associates (1981) reported the excellent clinical experience from the University of North Carolina. These investigators have utilized the ventriculo-iliac bypass technique with the heparinized shunt in 33 patients. As indicated earlier, these authors found excellent hemodynamic parameters with the use of the ventriculo-iliac bypass. There were only six deaths in this group of 33 patients, with three occurring among six patients who were being operated on for dissection of the thoracic aorta. There was one incident of a patient who was rendered paraplegic after resection of a long segment of thoracic aorta from the left subclavian artery to the diaphragm.

HEPARINIZED SHUNTS FOR TRAUMA OF THE THORACIC AORTA

Selection of Patients

Most patients sustaining major trauma to the thoracic aorta do not survive long enough to reach the operating room. This is particularly true for patients with penetrating wounds of the thoracic aorta. If the patient is alive on arrival at the hospital after a penetrating injury of the aorta, it is imperative that he be moved quickly to the operating suite. Occasionally, a patient with this type of injury can be stabilized briefly prior to the operative procedure, and in this case, an aortogram should then be obtained. Sometimes, it is not possible to set up a heart-lung machine for immediate bypass to the aorta. In many instances, a heart-lung machine is not even available at the hospital. For these patients, the use of the temporary shunt may permit immediate surgical intervention with successful correction of an otherwise hopeless clinical problem.

A relatively common injury of the aorta occurs as the result of an automobile collision in which there is near transection of the descending thoracic aorta at the level of the ligamentum ductus. In these patients with a blunt injury of the aorta, there is frequently more time available to prepare for surgery than in those patients with a penetrating injury of this vessel. These patients, however, frequently have associated head and soft tissue injuries, which contraindicate systemic heparinization. For these patients, the use of the heparinized shunt appears to have considerable value.

Surgical Technique

The same shunting techniques that were described previously for resection of thoracic aortic aneurysms can, of course, be utilized for traumatic injuries of the aorta. The real advantage of the heparinized shunt in such cases is that it can be used in hospitals in which there is no pump-oxygenator or when the urgency of the procedure dictates that the surgeon proceed quickly and not wait for the availability of the pump team. A case of this type has been previously reported from our institution (DeMeester et al., 1973) and is depicted in Figure 30–45. This patient was admitted at 2:00 A.M. with a gunshot wound of the left chest. The wound of entrance was located over the second rib near the midclavicular line, with

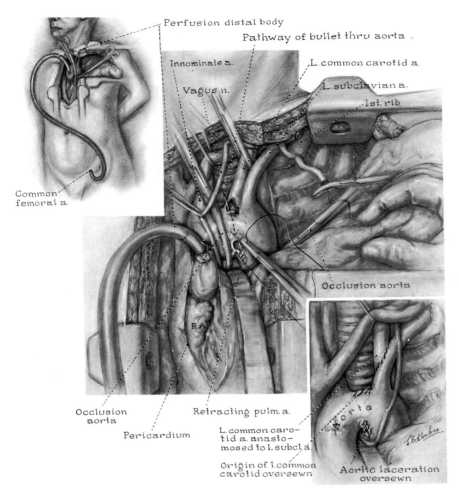

Figure 30–45. The operative approach for a through-and-through gunshot wound of the arch of the aorta using a heparinized shunt. The wound has been isolated by cross-clamping the arch of the aorta just distal to the innominate artery and also clamping the proximal descending thoracic aorta, the left carotid artery, and the left subclavian artery. During the operative repair, blood is being shunted to the lower portion of the body through the heparinized shunt from the ascending aorta to the common femoral artery. (From De-Meester, T. R., *et al.*: Repair of a through-and-through gunshot wound of the aortic arch using a heparinized shunt. Ann. Thorac. Surg., *16*:193, 1973.)

no wound of exit (skin). The left carotid pulse was absent, and a progressive right-sided hemiparesis (face and trunk) was observed. The peripheral systolic blood pressure was 65 mm. Hg. A chest roentgenogram showed a widened superior mediastinum with extension of the opacification into the left chest. A metallic foreign body could be seen in the vicinity of the great vessels.

The patient was taken directly to the operating room, and a median sternotomy was made. Massive bleeding occurred from the anterior mediastinal hematoma. Cardiac massage was performed while the descending thoracic aorta was exposed and cross-clamped distal to the innominate artery. A left anterior thoracotomy incision was made in the third intercostal space, and the descending thoracic aorta was isolated and cross-clamped. The heparinized shunt was then inserted between the ascending aorta and the left femoral artery for perfusion of the distal aorta, as depicted in Figure 30–45. After this, the aortic arch was dissected out to localize the injury. This injury consisted of an evulsion of the left carotid artery at its origin and a linear laceration on the underside of the aortic arch (wound of exit) just above the left pulmonary artery. The bullet was found resting be-

tween the latter two structures. Retrograde bleeding from the left subclavian artery and the avulsed left carotid artery was controlled by cross-clamping these vessels, and the linear laceration on the underside of the aortic arch was then closed. The avulsed orifice of the left carotid artery on the arch was oversewn. The distal left carotid artery was then anastomosed end-to-side to the left subclavian artery. During the repair, the patient suffered two cardiac arrests and both times responded to massage and intracardiac epinephrine. Neurologic examination on the first postoperative day confirmed the presence of a right-sided hemiparesis, but at the time of discharge, the patient had begun to demonstrate return of function of his right arm. With continued physical therapy he regained total function of his right arm except for fine movement of the right hand.

In addition to the use of the heparinized shunt bypass for acute penetrating injuries of the thoracic aorta, as in the foregoing case, this bypass technique should have considerable application to patients sustaining blunt trauma of the descending thoracic aorta. In patients with trauma to the descending thoracic aorta, there is frequently extensive mediastinal hematoma, and thus, it is simpler in these patients to perform proximal cannulation of the shunt in the apex of the left ventricle, as depicted in Figure 30–44.

Results

As indicated earlier, most patients with major trauma to the thoracic aorta do not survive long enough to reach a hospital for definitive repair. Therefore, there have not been any reports from any one institution with a large number of patients operated on using the heparinized shunt for traumatic lesions of the thoracic aorta. There have been a number of reports of small groups of these patients who have been sucessfully treated in this manner. Again, one of the best reports on this topic is the summary of the experience of the members of the Samson Society of Thoracic Surgeons (Lawrence et al., 1977). In that paper, the authors reported their own personal experience with 16 traumatic aneurysms of the thoracic aorta treated with the use of the heparinized shunt with only two deaths (12 per cent) and one case of paraplegia (6 per cent). In addition, they summarized the experience of the 26 respondents to a questionnaire. These 26 surgeons had utilized the heparinized shunt in 39 patients with trauma of the thoracic aorta, with no deaths and no paraplegia. On the other hand, their experience with pump bypass and systemic heparinization for traumatic injury of the thoracic aorta totaled 134 cases, with 11 deaths (8 per cent) and three instances of paraplegia (2 per cent).

At our institution, we have had a total of nine patients with trauma to the thoracic aorta who had surgical repair using the heparinized shunt. Five patients were operated on for acute traumatic damage, and four patients had surgery for chronic traumatic problems. There were no deaths in this group of trauma patients treated at our institution and no instances of paraplegia.

HEPARINIZED SHUNTS FOR SURGERY OF THE INNOMINATE ARTERY

Selection of Patients

Vascular reconstruction for innominate artery lesions has become possible only during the past 25 years. Successful excision of a saccular aneurysm in the innominate artery with preservation of arterial continuity was first reported in 1953 (Bahnson, 1953). In addition, a 10-year experience with reconstruction for arteriosclerotic occlusive disease of the innominate artery has been reported (Crawford et al., 1969).

Provision for perfusion of the central nervous system must be considered in the surgical correction of any innominate artery lesion. The common technique used in the past for repair of traumatic lesions or aneurysms of the innominate artery employed cardiopulmonary bypass with perfusion of the cerebral

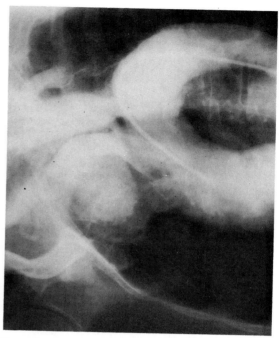

Figure 30–46. Thoracic aortogram demonstrating a luetic aneurysm of the innominate artery. (From Murray, G. F., Brawley, R. K., and Gott, V. L.: Reconstruction of the innominate artery by means of a temporary heparin-coated shunt bypass. J. Thorac. Cardiovasc. Surg., 62:34, 1971.)

vessels. Although this technique of innominate artery bypass is perfectly satisfactory from the standpoint of supporting the cerebral circulation, the overall procedure can be simplified considerably by using the heparinized shunt (Murray et al., 1971).

It is true that a number of operative procedures have been performed on the innominate artery with simple occlusion of this vessel during the operative procedure. Catlin (1960) reported a patient who survived bilateral carotid artery ligation. On the other hand, the reported incidence of hemiplegia following ligation of the common carotid artery ranges from 25 to 70 per cent (Watson and Silverstone, 1939). Similarly, the ability of patients to tolerate periods of innominate artery occlusion is inconsistent (DeBakey and Crawford, 1957; Kirby and Johnson, 1953).

Surgical Technique

A thoracic aortogram of a patient with a large syphilitic aneurysm of the innominate artery is shown in Figure 30–46. The surgical approach for the resection of this aneurysm is depicted in Figure 30–47. We favor the use of the sternal split incision, because this gives the best exposure for this region and the procedure can be done with minimal morbidity. At the time this patient underwent surgery, a GBH-coated shunt was used. Currently, a double-tapered shunt with smaller cannulating tips (7 mm. O.D.) is available

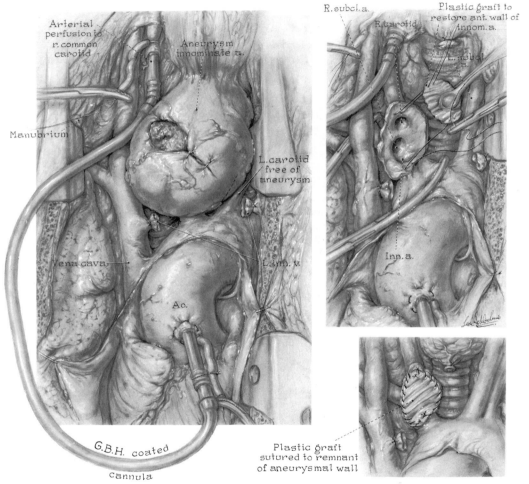

Figure 30–47. Bypass of the luetic aneurysm shown in Figure 30–46 with a GBH-coated shunt. *Top inset,* Excision of the aneurysmal sac demonstrating the narrow neck of the aneurysm arising from the confluence of the subclavian, carotid, and innominate arteries. *Bottom inset,* Repair with a woven Dacron fabric roof. (From Murray, G. F., Brawley, R. K., and Gott, V. L.: Reconstruction of the innominate artery by means of a temporary heparin-coated shunt bypass. J. Thorac. Cardiovasc. Surg., *62*:34, 1971.)

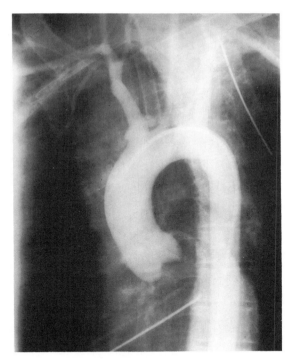

Figure 30–48. Thoracic aortogram of a patient who sustained blunt trauma to the chest. Disruption of the innominate artery near its origin and of the left subclavian artery in its second portion can be seen. (From Murray, G. F., Brawley, R. K., and Gott, V. L.: Reconstruction of the innominate artery by means of a temporary heparin-coated shunt bypass. J. Thorac. Cardiovasc. Surg., 62:34, 1971.)

for these patients undergoing innominate artery surgery. The proximal cannulation is accomplished through a double purse-string suture in the ascending aorta, and the distal tip of the cannula is placed into the right common carotid artery. This then allows the base of the innominate artery to be cross-clamped and the large aneurysm to be resected. In this case, the back wall of the artery appeared normal, and a patch graft was applied. This patient had an entirely uneventful postoperative course and did well for a number of years until lost to follow-up.

A second example of the application of the heparinized shunt for innominate artery surgery is in the patient whose arteriogram is presented in Figure 30–48. This was a 47-year-old man who was brought to our hospital after an automobile accident. He had suffered severe head injuries with a scleral rupture of his left globe and, in addition, had a flail right chest with associated hemopneumothorax. X-ray films of the skull and facial bones demonstrated multiple facial fractures. A retrograde aortogram revealed avulsion injuries of the innominate and left subclavian arteries (Fig. 30–48).

This patient was taken to the operating room 5 hours after admission, and through a median sternotomy incision, the ascending aorta and great vessels were exposed (Fig. 30–49). A GBH-coated shunt was

placed between the proximal aorta and the right common carotid artery to bypass the innominate artery injury. A partial occluding clamp was placed across the arch of the aorta, sparing the left carotid artery. The innominate artery was occluded distally and the false aneurysm entered. A complete avulsion of the innominate artery from the aortic arch was found. The defect in the aorta was oversewn, and the vessel was reconstructed with a Dacron prosthesis, as depicted in the illustration. A complete circumferential tear in the left subclavian artery just distal to the vertebral artery was repaired through a separate supraclavicular incision. The scleral rupture was repaired, and exploratory laparotomy revealed bleeding from a small mesenteric vessel. This patient had a difficult postoperative course, but subsequently, he did improve. However, several months after discharge from the hospital, he became jaundiced and had evidence of homologous serum hepatitis. His condition then deteriorated, and death was precipitated by pneumonia 10 months after surgery.

It is this type of patient with an avulsion injury of the innominate artery and multiple head and abdominal injuries who will not tolerate systemic heparinization for total cardiopulmonary bypass, and the use of the heparinized shunt may therefore be a determining factor in achieving successful results.

Results

There has not been widespread use of the heparinized shunts for innominate artery operations to date, but in the few reported cases, the results have been quite favorable. We have now had a total of seven patients who have undergone innominate artery surgery utilizing the heparinized shunt. In addition to the two patients depicted, we have had four patients who have undergone innominate artery endarterectomy for arteriosclerotic disease with excellent results and an additional patient who had a successful repair of a penetrating injury of the innominate artery.

OTHER SURGICAL APPLICATIONS FOR HEPARINIZED VASCULAR SHUNTS

Although the primary application of this type of heparinized shunt has been in patients with either aneurysms or trauma involving the descending thoracic aorta or in patients requiring an operative procedure on the innominate artery, there have been reports of other vascular procedures with this bypass system. Murray (1974) has reported the use of the heparin-coated shunt in two patients with atypical coarctation of the aorta. In both of these patients, coarctation of the aorta occurred proximal to or involved the left subclavian artery. At the time of cross-clamping of the aorta for the coarctation repair, there was inadequate collateral flow to the distal aorta, with

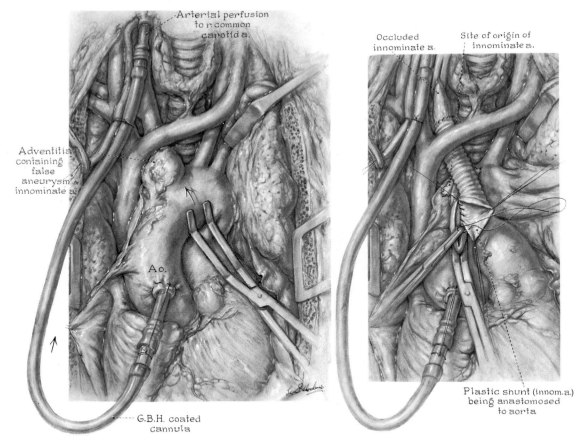

Figure 30–49. Bypass of the traumatic aneurysm shown in Figure 30–48 with a GBH-coated shunt. Entry into the false aneurysm revealed complete avulsion of the innominate artery from the arch. As depicted, the defect in the aorta was oversewn and the innominate artery was reconstructed with a Dacron prosthesis. (From Murray, G. F., Brawley, R. K., and Gott, V. L.: Reconstruction of the innominate artery by means of a temporary heparin-coated shunt bypass. J. Thorac. Cardiovasc. Surg., 62:34, 1971.)

a virtual collapse of this vessel beyond the vascular clamps. In both cases, bypass was established with the heparinized shunt and a satisfactory repair of the coarctation was achieved. This type of heparinized shunt has also been utilized for the resection of an aneurysm of the upper aspect of the abdominal aorta (Edwards, 1973). The aneurysm in this patient was secondary to an earlier gunshot wound, and the operating surgeon reported that the procedure was considerably simplified using this heparinized shunt bypass.

An additional nonthoracic application of the heparinized shunt has been in carotid endarterectomy. Standard carotid artery plastic shunts have been prepared with the TDMAC-heparin coating, and this obviates the need for systemic heparinization. In these patients, of course, the operative field is much smaller than in patients undergoing resection of a thoracic aneurysm, and the advantage of eliminating systemic heparinization would not be as great as in the thoracic cases.

SELECTED REFERENCES

Frantz, P. T., Murray, G. F., Shallal, J. A., and Lucas, C. L.: Clinical and experimental evaluation of left ventriculoiliac shunt bypass during repair of lesions of the descending thoracic aorta. Ann. Thorac. Surg., 31:551, 1981.

This paper reports the most thorough hemodynamic evaluation of the heparinized shunt to date. The studies were performed in adult sheep using left ventriculoiliac shunt bypass, and when compared with control animals with total occlusion of the thoracic aorta, aortic pressures above and below the clamped aorta returned almost to normal with the use of the interposed shunt. No significant changes occurred in cardiac output, left ventricular end-diastolic pressure, or left atrial pressure with the use of the shunt and a cross-clamped thoracic aorta. In addition, reversed flow through the shunt was less than 10 per cent, in spite of the fact that there is no valve in the shunt.

Gott, V. L., Whiffen, J. D., and Dutton, R. C.: Heparin bonding on colloidal graphite surfaces. Science, 142:1297, 1963.

This is the first report of a surface that appears to have significant thromboresistance. Both *in vitro* and *in vivo* studies demonstrated that a surface coated with graphite, benzalkonium, and heparin is superior to plain polymer and silicone surfaces. The *in vitro* studies were performed using standard Lee-White clotting times, and the *in vivo* studies were done using small conduits placed in the canine vena cava.

Grode, G. A., Anderson, S. J., Grotta, H. M., and Falb, R. D.: Nonthrombogenic materials via a simple coating process. Trans. Am. Soc. Artif. Intern. Organs, 15:1, 1969.

This important article presents an improved method for heparinizing the surface of polymers using the cationic surfactant tridodecylmethylammonium chloride (TDMAC) as the bonding substance for the heparin. The TDMAC-heparin coating allows for the bonding of a greater quantity of heparin than does the GBH coating, and the surface is transparent and has excellent mechanical durability.

Murray, G. F., and Young, W. G.: Thoracic aneurysmectomy utilizing direct left ventriculo-femoral shunt (TDMAC-heparin) bypass. Ann. Thorac. Surg., *21*:26, 1976.

In this paper, the authors describe the first reported use of the heparinized shunt with proximal cannulation in the left ventricular apex and distal cannulation in the femoral artery. They report successful use of this technique in two patients with traumatic aneurysms of the descending thoracic aorta. This particular shunting technique has now become a popular method of bypassing the thoracic aorta, and for some patients, it is simpler than cannulating the arch of the aorta or the left subclavian artery. This technique of left ventriculofemoral shunting was first described by English (1965) and employed a non–heparin-coated shunt for the resection of a coarctation of the aorta.

Valiathan, M. S., Weldon, C. S., Bender, H. W., Jr., Topaz, S. T., and Gott, V. L.: Resection of aneurysms of the descending thoracic aorta using a GBH-coated shunt bypass. J. Surg. Res., *8*:197, 1968.

This is the first report of the use of a shunt with wall-bonded heparin for the resection of aneurysms of the descending aorta. Four patients had elective resection of an aneurysm of the descending thoracic aorta, and all four of these patients made an excellent recovery. Two patients were operated on with rupturing aneurysms of the descending aorta, and long-term survival was not achieved in these two patients.

REFERENCES

Bahnson, H. T.: Definitive treatment of saccular aneurysms of the aorta with excision of sac and aortic suture. Surg. Gynecol. Obstet., *96*:383, 1953.

Catlin, D.: A case of carcinoma of the larynx surviving bilateral carotid artery ligation. Ann. Surg., *153*:809, 1960.

Chamberlain, J. M., Klopstock, R., Parnassa, P., Grant, A. R., and Cincotti, J. J.: The use of shunts in surgery of the thoracic aorta. J. Thorac. Surg., *31*:251, 1956.

Crawford, E. S., DeBakey, M. E., Morris, G. C., Jr., and Howell, J. F.: Surgical treatment of occlusion of the innominate, common carotid and subclavian arteries: A 10 year experience. Surgery, *65*:17, 1969.

DeBakey, M. E., and Crawford, E. S.: Resection and homograft replacement of innominate and carotid arteries with use of shunt to maintain circulation. Surg. Gynecol. Obstet., *105*:129, 1957.

DeMeester, T. R., Cameron, J. L., and Gott, V. L.: Repair of a through-and-through gunshot wound of the aortic arch using a heparinized shunt. Ann. Thorac. Surg., *16*:193, 1973.

Edwards, W. S.: Personal communication, 1973.

English, T. A. H.: Direct left ventriculofemoral bypass during resection of coarctation of the aorta with anomalous subclavian arteries. Thorax, *20*:36, 1965.

Frantz, P. T., Murray, G. F., Shallal, J. A., and Lucas, C. L.: Clinical and experimental evaluation of left ventriculoiliac shunt bypass during repair of lesions of the descending thoracic aorta. Ann. Thorac. Surg., *31*:551, 1981.

Gott, V. L., Whiffen, J. D., and Dutton, R. C.: Heparin bonding on colloidal graphite surfaces. Science, *142*:1297, 1963.

Grode, G. A., Anderson, S. J., Grotta, H. M., and Falb, R. D.: Nonthrombogenic materials via a simple coating process. Trans. Am. Soc. Artif. Intern. Organs, *15*:1, 1969.

Johnson, J., Kirby, C. K., and Lehr, H. B.: A method of maintaining adequate blood flow through the thoracic aorta while inserting an aorta graft to replace an aortic aneurysm. Surgery, *37*:54, 1955.

Katz, N. M., Blackstone, E. H., Kirklin, J. W., and Karp, R. B.: Incremental risk factors for spinal cord injury following operation for acute traumatic aortic transection. J. Thorac. Cardiovasc. Surg., *81*:669, 1981.

Kirby, C. K., and Johnson, J.: Innominate artery aneurysm treated by resection and end-to-end anastomosis. Surgery, *33*:562, 1953.

Lawrence, G. H., Hessel, E. A., Sauvage, L. R., and Krause, A. H.: Results of the use of the TDMAC-heparin shunt in the surgery of aneurysms of the descending thoracic aorta. J. Thorac. Cardiovasc. Surg., *73*:393, 1977.

Murray, G. F.: Atypical proximal coarctation of the aorta: Reconstruction by means of a heparin-coated temporary shunt bypass. Ann. Surg., *180*:309, 1974.

Murray, G. F., and Young, W. G., Jr.: Thoracic aneurysmectomy utilizing direct left ventriculofemoral shunt (TDMAC-heparin) bypass. Ann. Thorac. Surg., *21*:26, 1976.

Murray, G. F., Brawley, R. K., and Gott, V. L.: Reconstruction of the innominate artery by means of a temporary heparin-coated shunt bypass. J. Thorac. Cardiovasc. Surg., *62*:34, 1971.

Stranahan, A., Alley, R. D., Sewell, W. H., and Kausel, H. W.: Aortic arch resection and grafting for aneurysm employing an external shunt. J. Thorac. Surg., *29*:54, 1955.

Valiathan, M. S., Weldon, C. S., Bender, H. W., Jr., Topaz, S. T., and Gott, V. L.: Resection of aneurysms of the descending thoracic aorta using a GBH-coated shunt bypass. J. Surg. Res., *8*:197, 1968.

Watson, W. L., and Silverstone, S. M.: Ligature of the common carotid artery in cancer of the head and neck. Ann. Surg., *109*:1, 1939.

Wolfe, W. G., Kleinman, L. H., Wechsler, A. S., and Sabiston, D. C., Jr.: Heparin-coated shunts for lesions of the descending thoracic aorta: Experimental and clinical observations. Arch. Surg., *112*:1481, 1977.

XII OCCLUSIVE DISEASE OF BRANCHES OF THE AORTA

Henry T. Bahnson

That obstruction of arteries at their point of origin from the aortic arch can cause circulatory disturbances in the head or arms has long been recognized, having been described by Broadbent in 1875. Takayasu (1908) reported a syndrome of occlusion of the principal vessels arising from the aortic arch, and Shimizu and Sano (1951) recognized its appearance most commonly in young women and termed the condition "pulseless disease." Interest in the condition was heightened by demonstration that the obstructive process, more commonly due to arteriosclerosis, is often segmental and localized and, as with other similarly localized lesions in the abdominal and peripheral arterial system, amenable to surgical attack.

PATHOLOGIC ANATOMY

There are a number of causes of obstruction of the branches of the aortic arch. Many cases of localized obstruction are undoubtedly due to atherosclerosis localized, as often happens, to a vessel just beyond its branching. Syphilis has been present in a number of the reported cases. The syndrome of multiple occlusions of the arch vessels occurring in young women, frequently reported in the Orient and first described by Takayasu (1908), may represent a specific entity and a different one from the many cases that have been treated recently by surgery and that appear to be caused by atherosclerosis. Tuberculosis, collagen vascular disease, periarteritis nodosa, thromboangiitis obliterans, rheumatic fever, and trauma have all been implicated.

The extent of the obstruction is variable, but it is usually localized to the first few centimeters of the innominate, carotid, subclavian, or vertebral arteries and almost never extends beyond the bifurcation of the common carotid artery or the supraclavicular portion of the subclavian artery. The vessel beyond is usually grossly uninvolved and widely patent.

The more striking symptoms are similar to those of occlusive disease at the bifurcation of the common carotid artery, and the two conditions are often considered together. In almost all instances, carotid obstruction is due to atherosclerosis.

CLINICAL PICTURE

Clinical manifestations depend on the site and extent of the occlusive process and the adequacy of collateral circulation. "Cerebral intermittent claudication" (Hunt, 1914) nicely describes the transient ischemic attack in relation to the well-recognized disease of the lower extremities. Symptoms of inadequate cerebral circulation include unilateral impairment of motor or sensory function, sometimes with both modalities involved, syncope, headache, disorders of speech, and impairment of vision. In more severe cases, convulsions and paralysis may occur. An important feature of the cerebral manifestations, at least in regard to prognosis and the hope of surgical treatment, is their intermittent and transient nature, resulting from a precariously balanced cerebral circulation, which becomes inadequate with a minor fall in blood pressure, changes in posture, or perhaps temporary spasm of the artery. Symptoms of arterial insufficiency in the upper extremities are usually mild but may consist of weakness, easy fatigability, and occasional intermittent weakness and discomfort on exertion equivalent to intermittent claudication of the lower extremities. Pulses are diminished or absent distal to the obstruction. Because surgical treatment is more effective before complete occlusion and thrombosis of the internal carotid occur, it is important to recognize premonitory symptoms in the early stage of the condition.

Obstruction of the vertebral artery may cause an unsteady gait, dizziness, and signs of cerebellar dysfunction in addition to those of inadequate cerebral circulation because of disturbance of the basilar arterial supply (Cate and Scott, 1959; DeBakey et al., 1959). Reivich and colleagues (1961) have shown that similar symptoms may arise from obstruction of the proximal subclavian artery, in which case blood flow may be retrograde in the vertebral artery, establishing collateral flow to the upper extremity but removing it from the brain—a "subclavian steal."

DIAGNOSIS

The symptoms described, with diminished or absent pulses in the carotid or brachial arteries, allow the diagnosis to be made in most instances much more readily than in cases of obstruction of the internal carotid artery, in which one cannot with certainty feel the distal pulse. Obstruction of the vertebral artery is more difficult to diagnose. Aortography is desirable in instances when the diagnosis is suggested and to establish the extent of disease. This can best be done with a rapid injection of contrast material into the ascending aorta, so that all branches may be visual-

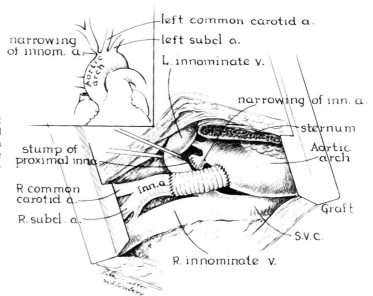

Figure 30–50. Occlusive disease of innominate and left common carotid arteries. The replacement is anastomosed to the ascending aorta during partial occlusion of this area and then to the distal innominate artery. Treatment of the innominate obstruction gave over 20 years' relief of symptoms.

ized. Since the occlusive points are often multiple, it is advisable to visualize the innominate, left common carotid, left subclavian, and vertebral arteries.

SURGICAL TREATMENT

Several methods of surgical treatment are available, including thromboendarterectomy, excision with replacement, and bypass. There are indications for the use of each of these.

Thromboendarterectomy. Thromboendarterectomy is probably best used for lesions of the vertebral artery. Because of the small size of the vertebral artery, it is advisable to make an incision opposite its mouth in the subclavian artery and then to remove the plaque, beginning at the orifice, and core it out. Although endarterectomy may be useful for many short, localized obstructions, it is often unsatisfactory for occlusion of the origin of the brachiocephalic arteries from the arch because of involvement of the adjacent aorta. In such cases, a bypass is preferable.

Graft Replacement. Graft replacement is also best suited to localized obstruction of only one vessel and must be used instead of endarterectomy when the vessel is narrowed. Narrowing is usually a result of arteritis rather than sclerosis and thrombosis; the latter may consist of a nearly normal-sized artery filled with clot (Fig. 30–50). In most instances, the replacement should be anastomosed to the aorta at a site slightly removed from the normal origin of the vessel to be replaced in order to avoid the involved area; a distal end-to-end anastomosis is then performed.

Bypass Replacement. Bypass replacement may be used in almost all instances and is particularly helpful when there is widespread occlusion or when there are long areas of stenosis. A bifurcation prosthesis may be sutured to the ascending aorta during partial occlusion of the aorta and a distal limb then sutured to the side of the subclavian, carotid, or vertebral artery (Fig. 30–51). Bypass replacement is less likely to produce injury or interference with established collateral vessels and has great breadth of application, since additional limbs may be attached to a bypass prosthesis.

If all vessels from the aortic arch, and the arch itself, need to be exposed, the best approach is probably through a median sternotomy. Splitting the entire

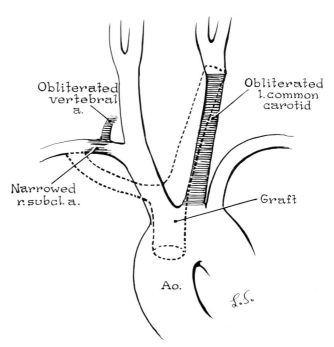

Figure 30–51. Schematic drawing of treatment of occlusion of the left common carotid artery and stenosis of proximal right subclavian artery with bypass bifurcation prosthesis. The thrombosed right vertebral artery was not treated.

sternum gives unusually good exposure for midline disease and is less disadvantageous to the patient than partial sternotomy with entrance into the pleural cavity through one of the upper intercostal spaces. If only the first portion of the arch is to be exposed, an upper sternotomy and entry into the right pleura through the second interspace are preferred. The distal portion of the aortic arch, left common carotid artery, and left subclavian artery can best be exposed through a left anterolateral second interspace incision. When a bypass is to extend into the neck, the ascending aorta may be exposed through a second right interspace incision and the distal carotid or subclavian artery through a short incision in the neck. Exposure of the subclavian artery and the vertebral artery at its origin may be obtained through a short collar incision on the involved side and a split of the upper sternum with entrance into the pleural cavity through the third interspace, as described by Shumacker (1948).

Use of an extrathoracic bypass reduces the morbidity of a transthoracic procedure, and recent results have been better with this approach. Such a bypass may be carotid-subclavian, subclavian-subclavian, axillary-axillary, or even femoroaxillary (Maggisaro and Provan, 1981).

RESULTS OF OPERATION

Reported results of surgical treatment have been almost invariably good. The requirements for successful treatment are a proximal source of blood under adequate pressure, which is always available in the aorta, and a vessel distal to which anastomosis can be made. Since the disease is usually limited to the first portion of the vessels arising from the arch and almost never extends beyond the first branches of these vessels, circulation to the distal arterial tree can be established in almost all instances. Late results have yet to be determined, but our first patient, one of the first of this type to be treated in 1953, lived for 20 years with relief of his symptoms. More important is the determination that symptoms are due to the obstruction and that relief is needed.

SELECTED REFERENCES

Crawford, E. S. (Ed.): Progress in treatment of aortic aneurysms. World J. Surg., 4:501, 1980.

This issue of the World Journal of Surgery includes a collection of articles that give an update on aortic aneurysms and their treatment.

Crisler, C., and Bahnson, H. T.: Aneurysms of the aorta. Curr. Probl. Surg., 1–64, December 1972.

This is a review of aneurysms in all areas of the aorta. Techniques of the authors as well as those reported are described, and the results of many workers' studies are summarized.

Gross, R. E.: The Surgery of Infancy and Childhood: Its Principles and Practice. Philadelphia, W. B. Saunders Company, 1953, p. 106.

Although old, this is the classic text on children's surgery by the author who figured prominently in the development of surgical treatment of congenital defects discussed in this chapter. An excellent reference of early personal experience.

Shumacker, H. B., Jr., King, H., Nahrwald, D. L., and Waldhausen, J. A.: Coarctation of the aorta. Curr. Probl. Surg., 1–64, February 1968.

This is a comprehensive review of the condition, including all but the most recent references at the time.

REFERENCES

Abbott, M. E.: Coarctation of the aorta of the adult type. Am. Heart J., 3:574, 1928.

Abrams, H. L.: Angiography. 2nd Ed. Boston, Little, Brown and Co., 1971.

Adams, H. D., and van Geertruyden, H.: Neurologic complications of aortic surgery. Ann. Surg., 144:574, 1956.

Bahnson, H. T.: Coarctation of the aorta and anomalies of the aortic arch. Surg. Clin. North Am., 32:1313, 1952.

Bahnson, H. T.: Considerations in the excision of aortic aneurysms. Ann. Surg., 138:377, 1953a.

Bahnson, H. T.: Definitive treatment of saccular aneurysms of the aorta with excision of sac and aortic suture. Surg. Gynecol. Obstet., 96:382, 1953b.

Bahnson, H. T., and Blalock, A.: Aortic vascular rings encountered in surgical treatment of congenital pulmonic stenosis. Ann. Surg., 131:356, 1950.

Bahnson, H. T., and Nelson, A. R.: Cystic medial necrosis as a cause of localized aortic aneurysms amenable to surgical treatment. Ann. Surg., 144:519, 1956.

Bahnson, H. T., and Spencer, F. C.: Excision of aneurysm of the ascending aorta with prosthetic replacement during cardiopulmonary bypass. Ann. Surg., 151:879, 1960.

Bahnson, H. T., Cooley, R. N., and Sloan, R. D.: Coarctation of the aorta at unusual sites. Am. Heart J., 38:905, 1949.

Bailey, L. L., Jacobson, J. G., Doroshow, R. W., Merritt, W. H., and Perry, E. L.: Anatomic correction of interrupted aortic arch complex in neonates. Surgery, 89:553, 1981.

Barry, A.: The aortic arch derivatives in the human adult. Anat. Rec., 111:221, 1951.

Bean, W. B., and Ponseti, I. V.: Dissecting aneurysm produced by diet. Circulation, 12:185, 1955.

Bentall, H., and DeBono, A.: A technique for complete replacement of the ascending aorta. Thorax, 23:338, 1968.

Bergdahl, L., Jonasson, R., and Bjork, V. O.: Late results of operation in children with coarctation of the aorta. Scand. J. Thorac. Cardiovasc. Surg., 14:83, 1980.

Berger, K., and Sauvage, L. R.: Late fiber deterioration in Dacron arterial grafts. Ann. Surg., 193:477, 1981.

Berger, K., Sauvage, L. R., Rao, A. M., and Wood, S. J.: Healing of arterial prostheses in man: Its incompleteness. Ann. Surg., 175:118, 1972.

Berman, L. B., Neches, W. H., Patnode, R. E., Fricker, F. J., Mathews, R. A., and Park, S. C.: Coarctation of the aorta in children. Am. J. Dis. Child., 134:464, 1980.

Blakemore, A. H.: The surgical aspects of aneurysm of the aorta. Trans. South. Surg. Assoc., 59:27, 1947.

Blalock, A.: Operative closure of the patent ductus arteriosus. Surg. Gynecol. Obstet., 82:113, 1946.

Blalock, A., and Park, E. A.: The surgical treatment of experimental coarctation (atresia) of the aorta. Ann. Surg., 119:445, 1944.

Bramwell, C., and Jones, A. M.: Coarctation of the aorta: The collateral circulation. Br. Heart J., 3:205, 1941.

Brewer, L. A., III, Fosburg, R. G., Mulder, G. A., and Verska, J. J.: Spinal cord complications following surgery for coarctation of the aorta. A study of 66 cases. J. Thorac. Cardiovasc. Surg., 64:368, 1972.

Campbell, C. D.: Aortic Aneurysm: Surgical Therapy. Mount Kisco, New York, Futura Publishing Co., 1981.

Campbell, C. D., Hardesty, R. L., Siewers, R. D., Lerberg, D. L., Peel, R. L., and Bahnson, H. T.: Selected therapy for ascending aortic aneurysms. Arch. Surg., 113:1324, 1978.

Carrel, A., and Guthrie, C. C.: Uniterminal and biterminal venous transplantations. Surg. Gynecol. Obstet., 2:266, 1906.

Cate, W. R., Jr., and Scott, H. W., Jr.: Cerebral ischemia of central origin: Relief by subclavian-vertebral artery thromboendarterectomy. Surgery, 45:19, 1959.

Christie, A.: Normal closing time of the foramen ovale and the ductus arteriosus: Anatomical and statistical study. Am. J. Dis. Child., 40:323, 1930.

Clarke, C. P., Brandt, P. W. T., Cole, D. S., and Barrett-Boyes, B. G.: Traumatic rupture of the thoracic aorta: Diagnosis and treatment. Br. J. Surg., 54:353, 1967.

Clatworthy, H. W., Jr., and McDonald, V. G., Jr.: Optimum age for surgical closure of patent ductus arteriosus. J.A.M.A., 167:444, 1958.

Cooley, D. A., and DeBakey, M. E.: Surgical considerations of intrathoracic aneurysms of the aorta and great vessels. Ann. Surg., 135:660, 1952.

Cooley, D. A., McNamara, D. G., and Latson, J. R.: Aorticopulmonary septal defect: Diagnosis and surgical treatment. Surgery, 42:101, 1957.

Crafoord, C., and Nylin, G.: Congenital coarctation of the aorta and its surgical treatment. J. Thorac. Surg., 14:347, 1945.

Crawford, E. S. (Ed.): Progress in the treatment of aortic aneurysms. World J. Surg., 4:501, 1980.

Crawford, E. S., and Rubio, P. A.: Reappraisal of adjustments to avoid ischemia in the treatment of aneurysms of descending thoracic aorta. J. Thorac. Cardiovasc. Surg., 66:693, 1973.

Crawford, E. S., and Vaccaro, P. S.: Aneurysms of the transverse aortic arch. In Aneurysms, Diagnosis and Treatment. Edited by J. J. Bergan and J. S. T. Yao. New York, Grune and Stratton, 1981, p. 131.

Crawford, E. S., DeBakey, M. E., and Cooley, D. A.: Clinical use of synthetic arterial substitutes in three hundred seventeen patients. Arch. Surg., 76:261, 1958.

Crawford, E. S., Walker, H. S. J., III, Galeh, S. A., and Normann, N. A.: Graft replacement of aneurysms in descending thoracic aorta: Results without bypass or shunting. Surgery, 89:73, 1981.

Crisler, C., and Bahnson, H. T.: Aneurysms of the aorta. Curr. Probl. Surg., 1–64, December 1972.

DeBakey, M. E., and Cooley, D. A.: Successful resection of aneurysms of thoracic aorta and replacement by graft. J.A.M.A., 152:673, 1953.

DeBakey, M. E., Crawford, E. S., Cooley, D. A., and Morris, G. C., Jr.: Surgical considerations of occlusive disease of innominate, carotid, subclavian, and vertebral arteries. Ann. Surg., 149:690, 1959.

DuBost, C.: Resection of an aneurysm of the abdominal aorta. Arch. Surg., 64:405, 1952.

DuShane, J. W., and Kirklin, J. W.: Late results of the repair of ventricular septal defect on pulmonary vascular disease. In Advances in Cardiovascular Surgery. Edited by J. W. Kirklin. New York, Grune and Stratton, 1973, pp. 9–16.

Edwards, J. E.: Anomalies of the aortic arch system. Birth Defects, 13:47, 1977.

Edwards, W. S., and Tapp, J. S.: Chemically treated nylon tubes as arterial grafts. Surgery, 38:61, 1955.

Eifrig, D. E.: Review of cases of coarctation treated at the Johns Hopkins Hospital. Personal communication, 1960.

Ekström, G.: The surgical treatment of patent ductus arteriosus. A clinical study of 290 cases. Acta Chir Scand. (Suppl.), 169, 1952.

Ellis, F. H., Jr., Kirklin, J. W., Callahan, J. A., and Wood, E. H.: Patent ductus with pulmonary hypertension. J. Thorac. Surg., 31:268, 1956.

Erdheim, J.: Medionecrosis aortae idiopathica. Virchows Arch. Pathol. Anat., 273:454, 1929.

Glass, I. H., Mustard, W. T., and Keith, J. D.: Coarctation of the aorta in infants. A review of twelve years' experience. Pediatrics, 26:109, 1960.

Goodall, M. C., and Sealy, W. C.: Increased sympathetic nerve activity following resection of coarctation of the thoracic aorta. Circulation, 39:345, 1969.

Gross, R. E.; Surgical correction for coarctation of the aorta. Surgery, 18:673, 1945.

Gross, R. E.: The Surgery of Infancy and Childhood: Its Principles and Practice. Philadelphia, W. B. Saunders Company, 1953, p. 806.

Gross, R. E., and Hubbard, J. P.: Surgical ligation of a patent ductus arteriosus. Report of first successful case. J.A.M.A., 112:729, 1939.

Gross, R. E., and Hufnagel, C. A.: Coarctation of the aorta. Experimental studies regarding its surgical correction. N. Engl. J. Med., 233:287, 1945.

Gross, R. E., and Ware, P. F.: Surgical significance of aortic arch anomalies. Surg. Gynecol. Obstet., 83:435, 1946.

Gross, R. E., Hurwitt, E. S., Bill, A. H., Jr., and Peirce, E. C., II: Methods for preservation and transplantation of arterial grafts: Observations on arterial grafts in dogs: Report of transplantation of preserved arterial grafts in nine human cases. Surg. Gynecol. Obstet., 88:689, 1949.

Gsell, O.: Wandnekrosen der Aorta als selbständige Erkrankung und ihre Beziehung zur Spontanruptur. Virchows Arch. Pathol. Anat., 270:1, 1928.

Guthrie, C. C.: Blood Vessel Surgery and Its Application. The Contributions of Dr. C. C. Guthrie to Vascular Surgery by Samuel P. Harbison, M.D. and Bernard Fisher, M.D., Pittsburgh, University of Pittsburgh Press, 1959.

Harrison, J. H., and Davalos, P. A.: Influence of porosity on synthetic grafts. Fate in animals. Arch. Surg., 82:8, 1961.

Heymann, M. A., and Rudolph, A. M.: Neonatal manipulation: Patent ductus arteriosus. Cardiovasc. Clin., 11:301, 1981.

Hoffman, J. I. E., Rudolph, A. M., and Heymann, M. A.: Pulmonary vascular disease with congenital heart lesions: Pathological features and causes. Circulation, 64:873, 1981.

Horsley, B. L., Lerberg, D. B., Allen, A. C., Zuberbuhler, J. A., and Bahnson, H. T.: Respiratory distress from patent ductus arteriosus in the premature newborn. Ann. Surg., 177:806, 1973.

Hunt, J. R.; The role of the carotid arteries in the causation of vascular lesions of the brain, with remarks on certain special features of the symptomatology. Am. J. Med. Sci., 147:704, 1914.

Iberra-Perez, C., Castaneda, A. R., Varco, R. L., and Lillehei, C. W.: Recoarctation of the aorta. Nineteen-year clinical experience. Am. J. Cardiol., 23:778, 1969.

Joyce, L. W., Fairbairn, J. F,. Kincaid, O. W., and Juergens, J. L.: Aneurysms of the thoracic aorta. A clinical study with special reference to prognosis. Circulation, 29:176, 1964.

Kampmeier, R. H.: Saccular aneurysm of the thoracic aorta: A clinical study of 633 cases. Ann. Intern. Med., 12:624, 1938.

Keith, J. D., Rowe, R. D., and Vlad, P.: Heart Disease in Infancy and Childhood. New York, The Macmillan Co., 1958.

Keys, A., and Shapiro, M. J.: Patency of the ductus arteriosus in adults. Am. Heart J., 25:158, 1943.

Kouchoukos, N. T., Karp, R. B., Blackstone, E. H., Kirklin, J. W., Pacifico, A. D., and Zorn, G. L.: Replacement of the ascending aorta and aortic valve with a composite graft. Results in 86 patients. Ann. Surg., 192:403, 1980.

Lewis, T.: Material relating to coarctation of the aorta of the adult type. Heart, 16:205, 1933.

Maggisaro, R., and Provan, J. L.: Surgical management of chronic occlusive disease of the aortic arch vessels and vertebral arteries. Can. Med. Assoc. J., 124:972, 1981.

Maron, B. J., Humphries, J. O., Rowe, R. D., and Mellits, E. D.: Prognosis of surgically corrected coarctation of the aorta. A 20 year postoperative appraisal. Circulation, 47:119, 1973.

Marsh, D. G., and Sturm, J. T.: Traumatic aortic rupture: Roentgenographic indications for angiography. Ann. Thorac. Surg., 21:337, 1976.

Miller, D. C., Stinson, E. B., Oyer, P. E., Moreno-Cabral, R. J., Reitz, B. A., Rossiter, S. J., and Shumway, N. E.: Concomitant resection of ascending aortic aneurysms and replacement of the aortic valve. Operative and long-term results with ''conventional'' techniques in ninety patients. J. Thorac. Cardiovasc. Surg., 79:388, 1980.

Najafi, H., Javid, H., Hunter, J. A., Serry, C., and Monson, D. O.: An update on treatment of aneurysms of the descending thoracic aorta. World J. Surg., 4:553, 1980.

Neches, W. H., Park, S. C., Lenox, C. C., Zuberbuhler, J. R., Siewers, R. D., and Hardesty, R. L.: Coarctation of the aorta with ventricular septal defect. Circulation, 55:189, 1977.

Neuhauser, E. B. D.: The roentgen diagnosis of double aortic arch and other anomalies of the great vessels. Am. J. Roentgenol., 56:1, 1946.

Oxnard, S. C., McGough, E. C., Jung, A. L., and Ruttenberg, H. D.: Ligation of the patent ductus arteriosus in the newborn intensive care unit. Ann. Thorac. Surg., 23:564, 1977.

Park, S. C., Siewers, R. D., Neches, W. H., Lenox, C. C., and Zuberbuhler, J. R.: Left aortic arch with right descending aorta and right ligamentum arteriosum. J. Thorac. Cardiovasc. Surg., 71:779, 1976.

Parker, F. B., Jr., Farrell, B., Streeten, D. H., Blackman, M. S., Sondheimer, H. M., and Anderson, G. H., Jr.: Hypertensive mechanisms in coarctation of the aorta. Further studies of the renin angiotensin system. J. Thorac. Cardiovasc. Surg., 80:568, 1980.

Peirce, E. C., II: Percutaneous femoral artery catheterization in man with special reference to aortography. Surg. Gynecol. Obstet., 93:56, 1951.

Peirce, E. C., II, Gross, R. E., Bill, A. H., Jr., and Merrill, K., Jr.: Tissue-culture evaluation of the viability of blood vessels stored by refrigeration. Ann. Surg., 129:333, 1949.

Pressler, V., and McNamara, J. J.: Thoracic aortic aneurysms — natural history and treatment. J. Thorac. Cardiovasc. Surg., 79:489, 1980.

Radner, S.: Thoracal aortography by catheterization from the radial artery. Acta Radiol., 29:178, 1948.

Railsbach, O. C., and Dock, W.: Erosion of the ribs due to stenosis of the isthmus (coarctation) of the aorta. Radiology, 12:58, 1929.

Reifenstein, G. H., Levine, S. A., and Gross, R. E.: Coarctation of the aorta. Am. Heart J., 33:146, 1947.

Reivich, M., Holling, H. E., Roberts, B., and Toole, J. F.: Reversal of blood flow through the vertebral artery and its effect on cerebral circulation. N. Engl. J. Med., 265:878, 1961.

Richardson, J. V., Doty, D. G., Rossi, N. P., and Ehrenhaft, J. L.: The spectrum of anomalies of aortopulmonary septation. J. Thorac. Cardiovasc. Surg., 78:21, 1979.

Richardson, J. V., Doty, D. G., Rossi, N. P., and Ehrenhaft, J. L.: Operation for aortic arch anomalies. Ann. Thorac. Surg., 31:426, 1981.

Robb, G. P., and Steinberg, I.: Visualization of the chambers of the heart, the pulmonary circulation, and the great vessels in man. Am. J. Roentgenol., 41:1, 1939.

Rocchini, A. P., Rosenthal, A., Barger, A. C., Castaneda, A. R., and Nadas, A. S.: Pathogenesis of paradoxical hypertension after coarctation resection. Circulation, 54:382, 1976.

Rumel, W. R., Bailey, C. P., Samson, P. C., Waterman, D. H., and Bing, R. J.: Surgical treatment of coarctation of the aorta. Report of the section on cardiovascular surgery. Am. Coll. Chest Physicians. J.A.M.A., 164:5, 1957.

Sauvage, L. R., and Harkins, H. N.: Growth of vascular anastomosis: An experimental study of the influence of suture type and suture method with a note on certain mechanical factors involved. Bull. Johns Hopkins Hosp., 91:276, 1952.

Sawyer, P. N., and Kaplitt, M. S.: Vascular Grafts. First Vascular Graft Symposium, National Institutes of Health, 1976. New York, Appleton-Century-Crofts, 1978.

Schuster, S. R., and Gross, R. E.: Surgery for coarctation of the aorta: A review of 500 cases. J. Thorac. Cardiovasc. Surg., 43:54, 1961.

Scott, H. W., Jr.: Closure of patent ductus arteriosus by suture-ligation technique. Surg. Gynecol. Obstet., 90:91, 1950.

Scott, H. W., Jr., and Bahnson, H. T.: Evidence for a renal factor in the hypertension of experimental coarctation of the aorta. Surgery, 30:206, 1951.

Scott, H. W., Jr., and Sabiston, D. C., Jr.: Surgical treatment for congenital aorticopulmonary fistula. Experimental and clinical aspects. J. Thorac. Surg., 25:26, 1953.

Sealy, W. C., Harris, J. S., Young, W. G., Jr., and Callaway, H. A., Jr.: Paradoxical hypertension following resection of coarctation of the aorta. Surgery, 42:135, 1957.

Seldinger, S. I.: Catheter replacement of the needle in percutaneous arteriography: A new technique. Acta Radiol., 39:368, 1953.

Shimizu, K., and Sano, J.: Pulseless disease. J. Neuropathol. Clin. Neurol., 1:37, 1951.

Shuford, W. H., and Sybers, R. G.: The aortic arch and its malformations with emphasis on angiographic features. Springfield, Illinois, Charles C Thomas, 1974.

Shumacker, H. B.: Operative exposure of the blood vessels in the superior-anterior mediastinum. Ann. Surg., 127:464, 1948.

Shumacker, H. B., Jr., King, H., Nahrwald, D. L., and Waldhausen, J. A.: Coarctation of the aorta. Curr. Probl. Surg., 1–64, February 1968.

Takayasu, M.: Case of queer changes in central blood vessels of retina. Acta Soc. Ophthalmol. Jpn., 12:554, 1908.

Tawes, R. L., Jr., Bull, J. C., and Roe, B. B.: Hypertension and abdominal pain after resection of aortic coarctation. Ann. Surg., 171:409, 1970.

Tuffier, T.: Intervention chirurgicale directe dans un anéurisme de la crosse de l'aorta. Ligature du sac. Bull. Soc. Chir. Paris, 28:326, 1902.

Tyson, K. R., Harris, L. S., and Nghiem, Q. X.: Repair of aortic arch interruption in the neonate. Surgery, 67:1006, 1970.

Voorhees, A. B., Jr., Jaretzki, A., II, and Blakemore, A. H.: The use of tubes constructed from Vinyon "N" cloth in bridging arterial defects. Ann. Surg., 135:332, 1952.

Waterman, D. H., Samson, P. C., and Bailey, C. P.: The surgery of patent ductus arteriosus. A report of the section on cardiovascular surgery. Dis. Chest, 29:102, 1956.

Wells, B. G., Rappaport, M. B., and Sprague, H. B.: Sounds and murmurs in coarctation of the aorta. A study of auscultation and phonocardiography. Am. Heart J., 38:69, 1949.

Chapter 31

The Pericardium

PAUL A. EBERT

HISTORICAL ASPECTS

The pericardium was described by Hippocrates (460 B.C.) as "a smooth tunic which envelops the heart and contains a small amount of fluid resembling urine." Galen (130 A.D.) observed pericardial effusion in a monkey and scirrhous thickening of the pericardium in a cock and surmised that the same conditions might occur in man.

Richard Lower (1631–1691) should receive credit for the first satisfactory account of pericardial disease in man. He accurately described cardiac tamponade: "It sometimes happens that a profuse effusion oppresses and inundates the heart. This envelope becomes filled in hydrops of the heart; the walls of the heart are compressed by the fluid settling everywhere so that they cannot dilate sufficiently to receive blood, then the pulse becomes exceedingly small, until finally it becomes utterly suppressed by the great inundation of fluid, whence succeed syncope and death itself."

In 1649, J. Riolan suggested performing a pericardiotomy for an effusion compressing the heart by trephining the sternum, a technique not adopted until two centuries later. Vieussens reported cases in 1679 and 1715 and insisted that pericardial adhesions were inflammatory and not congenital in origin.

Lancisi (1728) correlated the clinical picture of constrictive pericarditis with the necropsy findings. Morgagni (1761) reported seven cases of constrictive pericarditis and recognized the danger of cardiac compression by describing the heart as "so constricted and confined that it could not receive a proper quantity of blood to pass on." He also recognized that most of these cases were incommoded little or not at all even shortly before death. Senac (1749) recognized clinical symptoms of "hydropsia pericardii." Laennec (1819) further emphasized the few symptoms often associated with pericardial constriction and noted the "bread and butter" appearance of the pericardial and epicardial surfaces in pericarditis.

Romero (1819), through an approach in the fifth interspace on the left, incised the pericardium in three patients, two of whom recovered. Schuh (1840) performed a blind insertion of a trocar into the pericardial sac for relief of effusion. Karanaeff (1840) performed pericardiocentesis for hemorrhagic effusion accompanying an outbreak of scurvy. Seven of his 30 patients survived.

Cheevers (1842), under the title of "Observations on the Diseases of the Orifice and Valves of the Aorta," presented a clear clinical picture of chronic constrictive pericarditis. Chevers concluded that "the principal cause of dangerous symptoms appears to rise from the occurrence of gradual contraction in the layer of adhesive matter which has been deposited around the heart, compressing its muscular tissue and embarrassing its systolic and diastolic movements, but more particularly the latter." Wilkes (1870) observed in constrictive pericarditis that "the predominant thickening was in front so as to involve the right ventricle and auricle." Kussmaul (1873) presented the first critical exposition of the paradoxical pulse and the rise in venous pressure on inspiration in constrictive pericarditis. In 1877, Cohnheim performed classic experiments to show that as oil was injected into the pericardial sac, the venous pressure rose and the arterial pressure fell, with a diminution in cardiac output. Rose (1884) described the deleterious effects of an effusion or hemorrhage upon the heart and presented the term "herz tamponade."

In 1896, Pick presented a paper entitled "Concerning Chronic Pericarditis Running Its Course Under the Guise of Cirrhosis of the Liver (pericarditis pseudocirrhosis of the liver) with Observations on the Frosted Liver." Weill (1895) and Délorme (1898) proposed the excision of the thickened fibrous pericardium in constrictive pericarditis. Pericardial resection was introduced independently by Rehn and by Sauerbruch in 1913. Schmieden and Fischer (1926) reported seven cases of pericardial resection with pertinent descriptions of the operative technique. Many English and American authors have contributed to our understanding and treatment of pericardial disease, including the internists Wood (1956) and White (1951). Sellors (1946) considered tuberculosis the primary agent in constrictive pericarditis; Churchill (1929) performed the first successful pericardiectomy for constrictive pericarditis in this country; Beck (1937) was a pioneer in the experimental production of pericarditis; Blalock and Levy (1937), Burwell and Blalock (1938), Bloomfield and associates (1946), and McKusick (1952) have clarified both the clinical and the physiologic picture of pericardial disease. Mannix and Dennis (1955) and Blakemore and coworkers (1960) extended the usefulness of pericardiectomy by advocating its early application to chronic, massive effusions producing symptoms of cardiac compression and to a relapsing type of chronic pericarditis with effusion.

Parsons and Holman (1951 and 1955) and Isaacs

and colleagues (1952) performed classic experimental studies that clarified the physiologic effects of segmental compressions of the heart. Bigelow and associates (1956), Schumacker and Roshe (1960), and Fitzpatrick and coworkers (1962) have emphasized the necessity of radical pericardiectomy as the only means by which recurrence of pericardial constriction requiring secondary operations can be avoided.

Fowler (1970) re-emphasized the importance of understanding the hemodynamics of cardiac tamponade and constrictive pericarditis in order to provide the proper treatment. Bush and associates (1977) identified occult constrictive pericardial disease as that which impaired cardiac performance without actual adherence to the epicardium. Advancements in the diagnosis and management of the disease processes of the pericardium continue to improve the prognosis.

FUNCTIONS OF THE PERICARDIUM

The pericardium is presumed to serve a useful purpose since it is present in most mammals. Yet there is little, if any, disability noted after operative removal of the pericardium or in patients with congenital absence of the structure. The pericardium provides a smooth serous sac with secreted fluid that allows the heart a frictionless chamber in which to function. The pericardium is a strong fibrous sac that provides a restraining influence over overdilatation of the heart, a condition that might lead to the destruction of myocardial cells and the degeneration of cardiac musculature. Enlargement of the heart over a period of time results in stretching and enlargement of the pericardial sac, but sudden changes in heart size are restricted by this structure. This restraining influence also tends to support the heart and limit its displacement with changes in body position. It prevents kinking and torsion of the great vessels and vena cava.

The unusual strength of the pericardium has made it an excellent tissue to use to close intracardiac defects, reconstruct the pulmonary artery and right ventricular outflow, and serve as a material to reconstruct the major veins. The strength of this tissue protects the heart from extension of infection from neighboring structures, such as the lungs, mediastinal glands, and esophagus and from infradiaphragmatic abscesses, which frequently rupture into the pleural spaces.

It is clear that the pericardium does limit cardiac dimensions and prevent acute distention. The pericardium appears to contribute more to prevention of right heart distention in patients with existing severe left ventricular disease. In some of these instances, right ventricular performance may be impaired by bulging of the ventricular septum into the right ventricle in a setting in which the pericardium limits outward distention of the right ventricular wall. In some settings dilatation of the left ventricle, because of its larger mass, increases intrapericardial pressure and thus limits right ventricular filling. Thus, the pericardium

can evoke reciprocal shifts of the Frank-Starling curves of the two ventricles. The pericardium may play a more major role in cardiac performance in patients with the acute development of left ventricular or right ventricular failure.

CONGENITAL PERICARDIAL DEFECTS

Congenital Absence

Congenital absence of the entire pericardium has been reported, but more commonly small segments may be missing. Absence of small portions of the pericardium on the left side is most often seen. This results from a defect that occurs during the fifth week of fetal life. It has been postulated that premature obliterations of the left duct of Cuvier produce deficiency of the blood supply to the pleuropericardial membrane, resulting in failure of formation or incomplete formation. No clinical symptoms are known to result from congenital absence of the pericardium. Ronka and Tessmer (1944) studied 74 recorded clinical cases; all patients were found to have led active, strenuous lives, and in no instance was the defect associated with symptoms or related ultimately to the cause of death. Studies in the experimental animal have substantiated the clinical impression, as complete excision of the pericardium in the adult results in no obvious deleterious effects. Beck and Moore (1925) showed that vigorous swimming for 30 to 60 minutes was tolerated without signs of fatigue or abnormal cardiac rhythm. If an animal is subjected to acute hydremic plethora by intravenous infusion of blood and salt solution (Holman and Beck, 1925) and the pericardium is incised widely, marked dilatation of the heart occurs, the pulse rate doubles, and the cardiac output is temporarily greatly increased. Barnard (1898) found that without its pericardium, the heart ruptures under an intracardiac pressure of 1 atm., whereas with an intact pericardium, 1.75 atm. of pressure is required to rupture the heart.

Cysts

The pericardium has been postulated to form from a series of disconnected lacunae that appear early in fetal life (Lambert, 1940). For a brief period, these lacunae remain as individual spaces in the mesenchyme, but they eventually coalesce to form the pericardial coelom. Occasionally, the communication with the pericardium in such cysts persists and is called a diverticulum. If one or any of these lacunar cavities fail to fuse, it may either atrophy or persist as a separate pericardial space or cyst. In general, these cysts do not cause symptoms and are usually discovered on routine chest x-ray or at necropsy (Craddock, 1950). A mass lying anteriorly in the chest in either cardiophrenic sulcus is the classic description of a pericardial coelomic cyst given by radiologists (Bates and Leaver, 1951). Exploratory thoracotomy is usually recommended to establish a definitive diagnosis. Pericardial cysts can be confused radiographically with lung tumors, thymomas, and other mediastinal lesions.

Occasionally, a pericardial cyst can be incapacitating and life-threatening. Shidler and Holman (1952) reported such a case in an infant with marked respiratory distress requiring oxygen for the first 3 months of life. Marked dyspnea, fluctuating cyanosis, wheezing, and difficulty in swallowing were the symptoms. Two operations were required to remove this intrapericardial ''spring-water'' cyst, located between the aorta and superior vena cava. A similar case in an adult had been reported by Lam in 1947. This patient was incapacitated by dyspnea, fatigue, and angina and was bedridden for a year. A large cyst was present in the anterior chest in close association with the pericardium. Recovery followed removal of the cyst.

Diverticula

The literature reflects the considerable difficulty in defining the difference between pericardial cysts and diverticula. The latter are described as protrusions of the pericardial sac at points of weakness. The diverticula vary greatly from 0.5 to 12 cm. in size and occur more frequently on the right side. These lesions may be confused on routine roentgenograms of the chest with aneurysm of the ascending aorta or dermoid cysts of the mediastinum. These lesions, by definition, communicate with the pericardial sac. Areas of congenital weakness, such as the point at which the fibrous pericardial layer passes out along the great vessels, are common locations for diverticula. The structure may not have a normal absorptive surface, but communication with the pericardium prevents fluid accumulation. However, mechanical kinking of the communicating isthmus can result in distention of the diverticulum either by fluid being formed by its own membrane or by pericardial fluid being forced into the sac by the massaging action of the heart beat. It is conceivable that after the communicating tract is kinked, atrophy of the tract would occur and the lesion would, by definition, be considered a cyst. These diverticula are rarely symptomatic, and excision is advised to establish a definitive diagnosis.

ACQUIRED PERICARDIAL DEFECTS

Neoplasms

Primary neoplasms of the pericardium are extremely rare. Benign tumors, such as lipomas, lobulated fibrous polyps, and hemangiomas, have been reported. Several instances of primary mesotheliomas have been described, which apparently arise from the lining endothelium. Sarcomas and teratomas occasionally arise from the pericardium, and successful removal of these lesions has rarely been reported. The pericardium is commonly infiltrated by primary myocardial tumors and by infiltrating lung cancer.

Cardiac Tamponade

In cardiac tamponade, the heart is limited during diastole by increased pressure from the pericardium or from fluid or blood filling the pericardial space. Systolic contraction is rarely limited, but during diastole the filling of the ventricles requires a greater venous pressure owing to the force applied against the heart surface. Tamponade may occur following penetrating injuries to the heart in which blood escapes into the pericardial sac. If the blood or fluid cannot escape through the laceration in the pericardium, tamponade ensues. In acute injuries, a relatively small amount of blood, 150 to 250 ml., may be sufficient to cause tamponade, whereas in cases of chronic effusion, the pericardium becomes stretched over a period of time and may have the capacity to contain several liters of fluid with minimal cardiodynamic effects. The fluid or blood around the heart ultimately stretches the pericardium to a critical point. Prior to this, cardiac output is minimally reduced, but when this stage is reached, the addition of a small volume may reduce cardiac output and death may ensue. Treatment may be equally dramatic with removal of a small volume of blood or fluid, allowing a return of blood pressure and cardiac output to near normal ranges.

As pressure in the pericardial sac increases, diastolic filling pressure rises and the stroke volume is reduced. Compensatory mechanisms attempt to maintain circulatory dynamics. Increased sympathetic activity causes vasoconstriction, which tends to maintain systemic arterial pressure. The heart rate increases, and systolic ejection becomes more vigorous. These increase the ejection fraction so that a greater portion of blood present in the heart at the end of diastole is expelled. Venous pressure rises as a result of compression of the heart during diastole. No gradients have been demonstrated between the great veins and the right atrium during experimental cardiac tamponade. Coronary blood flow may be affected because of the reduction of cardiac output and of the pressure gradient between the aorta and coronary circulation. Myocardial failure can result from reduced coronary flow.

In acute cardiac tamponade, clinical shock is evident. The patient has cool and moist skin, heart sounds are distant, pulse is rapid, and blood pressure may be normal or low. The striking clinical manifestation is venous distention at a time when other signs suggest peripheral circulatory failure similar to that in hemorrhagic shock. Cyanosis may be present as a result of venous stasis. Martin and Schenk (1960) have emphasized the importance of using the venous pressure, rather than the arterial pressure, as a guide to treatment, since the latter may be artificially maintained by an elevated peripheral resistance.

Treatment of acute tamponade must not be delayed, as it is a life-threatening situation. Venous pressure should be obtained immediately in any patient suspected of having cardiac tamponade. Further elevation of venous pressure by infusion of blood or colloid solution will temporarily improve cardiac output by increasing diastolic filling pressure. Pericardial aspiration should be performed with an electrocardiogram lead attached to the needle to identify contact with the heart surface and may be a lifesaving procedure (Fig. 31–1). Repeated aspirations have been successful in treating traumatic tamponade, but the patient requires careful observation of arterial and venous pressures by skilled personnel. Thoracotomy with direct repair of the cardiac injury is preferable to repeated pericardial aspirations. Aspiration of a few milliliters of blood may restore cardiac output and reduce venous pressure, but since reaccumulation of such a small volume can cause such marked hemodynamic consequences, early operative treatment should be instituted in most cases. In some cases of chronic effusion, a small plastic catheter may be passed percutaneously into the pericardial sac. Pericardiotomy is often indicated in chronic effusion and may be necessary as an emergency procedure if repeated aspirations do not relieve the tamponade.

Hydropneumopericardium

Brichteau (1844) reported a case of air in the pericardium. This rare phenomenon was reviewed by Shackelford (1931), and 77 cases were recorded in the world literature at that time. The characteristic signs are precordial tympany and metallic splashing sounds that may be heard several feet away and may keep the patient awake. A chest film is conclusive. It should be noted that small amounts of air in or about the pericardial sac are common findings after severe chest trauma.

In general, the prognosis is good if the disease is limited to a pneumopericardium, since air itself is not

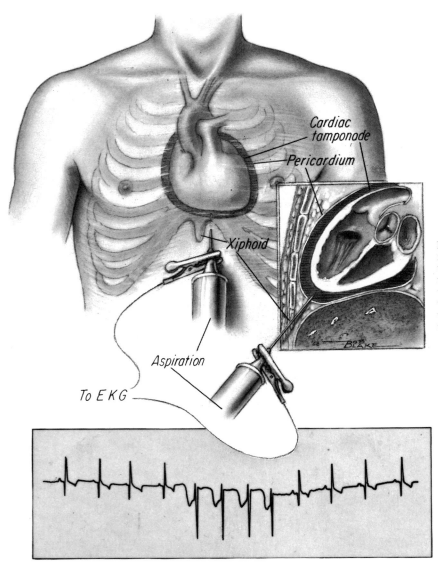

Figure 31–1. The needle is inserted to the left of the xiphoid and directed toward the midscapular area. The electrocardiogram is attached to the needle, and the negative deflection of the QRS complex represents contact with the heart surface. The needle is slowly withdrawn, and the electrocardiogram reverts to normal when the needle loses contact with the myocardium.

deleterious. If infection is present, the organisms must be identified by pericardial aspiration and the proper systemic antibiotics administered. Pericardiotomy is indicated if prompt improvement is not obtained with systemic antibiotics.

Acute Necrosis of Pericardial Fat

Precordial or pleuritic pain in the left lower chest associated with a soft-tissue mass that cannot be distinguished from the pericardium on a chest film is the classic description of acute necrosis of pericardial fat. Histologic study of the excised tissue reveals the necrosis to be due to a vascular accident with extravasation of blood, formation of a hematoma, and intravascular thrombosis. Surgical removal provides prompt relief (Chester and Tully, 1959; Jackson *et al.*, 1957).

Pericarditis

Pericarditis occurs as a primary disease process without systemic illness, as a secondary manifestation of a systemic disease, and as the only area of involvement of a normally systemic disease process. It has been given many names, such as acute, chronic, dry, fibrinous, transudative, hemorrhagic, exudative, or purulent. In its simplest and most common form, pericarditis is an acute, self-limiting inflammation, due probably to a diversity of etiologic agents, among which viruses are included. Coxsackie viruses A and B and influenza viruses A and B have been identified by culture and neutralization tests from pericardial fluid (Gillett, 1959). This disease may occur in any age group but is often seen in young, otherwise healthy individuals.

Nonspecific Pericarditis. Nonspecific pericarditis, or so-called "benign pericarditis," is seen preceded by an upper respiratory tract infection. The symptoms are not always specific, but findings of fever, usually about 38.3°C. (101°F.) but sometimes as high as 40° to 40.5°C. (104° to 105°F.), substernal or precordial pain, and a pericardial friction rub are classic. All degrees of severity are found. Frequently the disease is minimal, and symptoms may persist for weeks before medical advice is sought. Shortness of breath, grunting respirations, dry cough, and orthopnea with a tendency to lean forward are characteristic symptoms. The pain may be sharp or dull with radiation to the right or left shoulder, arm, or back. It can be accentuated by coughing, respiration, or activity, exaggerated by lying down, or relieved by sitting up. Leukocytosis, with a predominant lymphocyte increase, is usually present. A chest x-ray may show mild cardiac enlargement due to pericardial effusion. These symptoms at times may be difficult to separate from pain due to myocardial ischemia. Marked S-T segment elevation of the electrocardiogram, with absence of Q waves in the presence of a pericardial friction rub, is strongly suggestive of pericarditis. Arrhythmias are uncommon, usually atrial in origin, and more frequent in patients having pre-existing heart disease.

Laparotomy has been performed unnecesarily for abdominal symptoms, including epigastric pain, cramps, distention, and vomiting, that simulated acute abdominal catastrophe (Powers *et al.*, 1955). This has been ascribed to peritoneal serositis, a local manifestation of a more generalized polyserositis.

The diagnosis of nonspecific pericarditis is usually made by excluding the more specific forms, such as rheumatic, purulent, and traumatic. The disease process is usually self-limiting, and complications are extremely rare, although recurrences have been noted. Infrequently, pericardial effusion occurs, and cardiac tamponade may result. There have been isolated reports of constrictive pericarditis developing after the inflammatory process had subsided (Krook, 1954). It is likely that many cases of constrictive pericarditis in which the etiology remains obscure are a result of benign idiopathic pericarditis, which may have been present with few, if any, symptoms.

Treatment is usually supportive, consisting of bed rest for 2 to 3 weeks and analgesics. Salicylates have been quite successful in relieving pain, although morphine may be required. In occasional patients not responding to supportive treatment, steroids have been used to control the inflammatory process. Relief of symptoms is prompt, but routine use is discouraged since the disease may recur when the steroids are withdrawn. A distressing factor of this disease is that pain, fever, friction rub, and even pericardial effusion frequently recede only to recur in a short period of time. These remissions and exacerbations may continue, with the whole attack lasting several months. Heart failure is an infrequent finding, but when present, digitalis is indicated. Arrhythmias, such as ectopic ventricular activity, can be controlled with quinidine or lidocaine. Atrial fibrillation occasionally develops, but spontaneous reversal to sinus rhythm may occur after the inflammatory process subsides.

Pericarditis may occur as a result of many systemic diseases. When pericardial effusion or inflammation accompanies rheumatic arthralgia, the prognosis is worse. It frequently accompanies other collagen diseases, such as scleroderma, rheumatic fever, and lupus erythematosus. Sarcoidosis commonly involves the pericardium and heart but is rarely responsible for isolated pericarditis. It may be a manifestation of tertiary syphilis. Hypersensitivity states, such as serum sickness, autoimmune reactions, and various drug reactions, result in either pericarditis or effusion.

Less than 2 per cent of patients with amebic abscesses in the liver develop pericarditis. It is thought to result from direct extension of the abscess, usually from the left lobe of the liver. Rupture of the abscess into the pericardium is accompanied by severe pain, dyspnea, and collapse. Cardiac tamponade associated with suppurative pericarditis requires immediate pericardial aspiration. Echinococcus cysts are extremely rare in the pericardium. The majority are primary in the heart and rupture into the pericardium. Rupture may cause only a localized reaction about the contents of the cyst, or rapid multiplication can occur, with involvement of the entire pericardial sac. It is rare for hepatic hydatid cysts to rupture into the pericardial sac.

Cholesterol Pericarditis. In cholesterol pericarditis, the pericardial fluid has a characteristic "gold paint" color. Diagnosis is usually confirmed by pericardial aspiration and demonstration of cholesterol crystals. Hypothyroidism is frequently present, and in many instances, the pericarditis disappears with administration of thyroid extract (Brawley *et al.,* 1966). Cholesterol turnover in the pericardium has been shown to be about 12 times longer in this disease (Doherty and Jenkins, 1966). If effusion persists, pericardiectomy is indicated (Creech *et al.,* 1955).

Acute Pyogenic Pericarditis. Acute pyogenic pericarditis can occur as a result of direct contamination of the pericardium following a penetrating injury. It may also result from septicemia or pyemia or follow the bacteremia of osteomyelitis or pneumonia. Hepatic or subphrenic abscesses can rupture into the pericardial sac, or acute pyogenic pericarditis may be a complication of an operation of the heart, lungs, or esophagus.

Severe chest pain and fever are the usual clinical signs. It is difficult to differentiate pyogenic pericarditis from the more common benign form in the early stages. A pericardial effusion can occur more rapidly, and cardiac tamponade must be expected since the fluid accumulates quickly from the severely inflamed pericardium.

In the past, the most common cause of acute pyogenic pericarditis was pneumococcus, usually associated with pneumonia. Currently, in children, the more common cause is staphylococcus (Weir and Joffe, 1977), and in adults, it is either staphylococcus or gram-negative bacteria (Klacsmann *et al.,* 1977). The diagnosis is confirmed by pericardial aspiration, with the finding of organisms on smear and subsequent culture. Treatment with systemic antibiotics is indicated, and open drainage usually results in a more rapid convalescence. Systemic antibiotics penetrate the pericardium with difficulty, and it is usually preferable to make a small subxiphoid incision and place a drainage catheter behind the heart with a second catheter placed on the anterior surface of the heart. Thus, irrigation of the posterior catheter results in drainage out of the anterior catheter, and the purulent material can be more easily evacuated. Drainage usually results in rapid cessation of fever and symptoms.

Tuberculous Pericarditis. Tuberculous pericarditis is usually considered to be secondary to tuberculosis elsewhere, the disease spreading to the pericardial sac by direct extension from the pleura or lung, from mediastinal lymph nodes, or through the blood or lymphatics. The onset of clinical symptoms may be so insidious that the patient cannot date the inception.

Usually the patient is not known to have pulmonary tuberculosis, and pericarditis is not suspected from the early nonspecific symptoms. Tuberculous pericarditis can be accompanied by malaise, fever, sweats, pleural pain, cough, and a pericardial friction rub. In this situation, the diagnosis of pericarditis is more evident. Pericardial effusion develops slowly, allowing distention of the pericardium to occur without cardiac tamponade. The fluid may be clear, straw-colored, or sanguineous. Early pericardiocentesis may establish the diagnosis by the finding of acid-fast bacilli in the fluid. In some cases, the skin test may be negative even though acid-fast bacilli are present in the pericardium and should not be used to exclude the diagnosis. Occasionally, the large cardiac area must be differentiated from cardiac dilatation. If the patient is not treated, the course may be prolonged, with progressive emaciation, toxemia, and death. Untreated patients may die from cardiac failure, but the more common cause is widespread tuberculosis (Carroll, 1951).

Early treatment of tuberculous pericarditis is important because the fibrous scarring prevents effective concentrations of antituberculosis drugs from reaching the tubercle bacilli. The fibrotic process of healing, beneficial in pulmonary tuberculosis, is associated with the threat of pericardial contracture and constriction. There seems to be a direct relationship between the development of pericardial constriction and the length of time the disease had been present prior to the institution of treatment. Wood (1956) emphasized that pericardial constriction was the rule if treatment was delayed more than 4 months from the recognized onset of the disease. This again emphasizes the value of pericardial aspiration in determining specific causes of pericardial effusion.

Treatment with antituberculosis drugs should be started as soon as the diagnosis is established. In some cases, confirmation of the diagnosis of tuberculous pericarditis by laboratory techniques can be most difficult, and if the clinical picture is convincing, it is probably best to administer antituberculosis therapy even though the diagnosis is not confirmed. Use of a single drug is ineffectual, and only combination therapy should be undertaken. In most patients who are treated promptly, clinical signs of improvement appear in 2 to 3 weeks. Increased heart size, elevated venous pressure, and the quantity of effusion disappear more slowly, usually requiring 2 months before significant changes are noted.

It is predictable that a significant number of patients with massive effusion due to tuberculous pericarditis will suffer the effects of pericardial constriction (Sellors, 1946). As the fluid is absorbed, it becomes more viscid and is more irritating to the surrounding structures. It is postulated that the fluid then gravitates toward the diaphragmatic pericardium, since the majority of these patients are ambulatory. This area is subjected to longer periods of irritation and thus to a greater deposition of fibrous tissue. At operation, the diaphragmatic surface of the heart is found to have a thicker, more fibrous, and more calcified pericardial covering. The anterior pericardium over the right side of the heart also is found to be more severely involved. This is ascribed to the more forceful pulsations of the left ventricle, which displace the exudate during the preconstrictive period into the less active and quieter areas over the right ventricle. This concept is questioned since the great vessels and atria have minimal movement and yet are rarely heavily calcified.

No concrete statement can be made concerning the stage in tuberculous pericarditis in which surgical therapy is best undertaken. It is futile to operate on febrile, acutely ill, toxic patients with active tuberculous pericarditis. However, it is also equally unwise to await a period of relative inactivity, a time when the operation is most difficult. Although some believe that these patients should not be operated on until the disease has been present for 2 years or longer (Sellors, 1956), this seems to lead to prolonged and needless suffering and probably to deaths that could have been prevented. The period in the early phase when the patient is clinically well appears to be the optimal time for surgery. These patients should receive antituberculosis therapy with two drugs; the addition of a third approximately 10 days prior to the operation is common practice.

Chronic Pericardial Effusion. The patient with a large heart shadow on the chest film presents the differential diagnosis of heart failure with marked cardiomegaly or chronic pericardial effusion. Physical findings of heart murmurs, gallop rhythm, or vigorous precordial pulsations are suggestive of myocardial disease. Distant heart sounds, absence of murmurs, and shifting intensity of heart sounds are more likely seen in pericardial effusion; a pericardial splash or friction rub is rarely heard.

The electrocardiogram in effusion may show low voltage, S-T segment elevation, and electrical alternans of the QRS complex. These QRS complexes are regular in time but alternate in height or direction of the major deflection. This is not affected by respiration. The explanation for this electrical alternans is that the heart, floating freely in abundant fluid, is no longer under normal mediastinal and pulmonary restraints; a periodic rotary oscillation can be established similar to that of the pendulum of a clock. S-T segment elevation is seen in acute tamponade and results from compression and consequent myocardial ischemia.

Various diagnostic techniques have been used to differentiate effusion from cardiomegaly. Wood (1951) used cardiac catheterization and pressure measurements to identify cardiac failure. Soulen and associates (1966) have had good results using echocardiography, and this seems to be the best current technique. Turner and coworkers (1966) used an intravenous carbon dioxide injection with the patient lying on his left side and differentiated the right atrial wall and pericardium. Routine angiocardiography similarly outlines the heart in reference to the cardiac silhouette

(Holman and Steinberg, 1958). Pericardiocentesis, using the electrocardiogram to identify contact with the heart, is the most direct means of confirming the diagnosis (see Fig. 31–1). Fluid removed should be examined for bacteria and fungi; cytologic studies should be performed and serology and cell counts taken.

Repeated pericardiocentesis may provide temporary relief from effusion, but surgical therapy offers the best prognosis. The creation of a window between the pericardial sac and the pleural space to drain fluid into the pleural space for absorption has produced good results (Effler and Proudfit, 1957). However, whenever resection of the pericardium can be accomplished at a comparable risk, it should be employed, since relief of effusion is most certain.

Most surgeons prefer to resect the pericardium in cases of chronic effusion, with the view that this is a more definitive procedure than the creation of a simple pleuropericardial window. The chance of recurrence is less, and the possibility of developing constrictive pericarditis is practically eliminated. Operative resection can be performed with ease in this situation, and fluid formed by the pericardial remnant drains into either pleural space. Excellent results have been reported in children with chronic effusion and tamponade treated with pericardiectomy (Shumacker and Harris, 1956; Roshe and Shumacker, 1959).

Bloody pericardial effusion commonly occurs in uremia and in patients receiving chronic hemodialysis. This effusion has not responded well to aspiration, and repeated aspirations are contraindicated since these patients may be prone to profuse bleeding from injury by the needle. Even though the uremic patient may be desperately ill, excellent response to creation of a simple pleuropericardial window has been noted. This should be performed early after diagnosis, as tamponade and death are common from intrapericardial bleeding.

The diagnosis of chronic low-grade tamponade in the first several days after open heart surgery may be elusive. A persistent elevation of venous pressure, often about 15 to 20 cm. H_2O, is the most uniform finding. Differential diagnosis includes heart failure, hypervolemia, and pulmonary embolism. There are no certain diagnostic techniques for excluding the diagnosis, such as pericardial scan, ultrasound, or echocardiography. A high degree of clinical suspicion accompanied by these diagnostic techniques can usually identify intrapericardial fluid accumulations. Pericardial aspiration has been advocated by Borkon and associates (1981), and the role of anticoagulants and the postpericardiotomy syndrome as causes of pericardial effusion has been emphasized by Ofori-Krakye and coworkers (1981). A diagnostic subxiphoid exploration of the pericardial cavity is the most certain way to confirm the diagnosis, and placement of drainage catheters into the pericardial space will resolve the diagnostic dilemma and result in rapid clearing of the effusion.

Chronic Constrictive Pericarditis. Constrictive pericarditis is the end stage of a chronic inflammatory process that produces a fibrous, thickened, constricting pericardium surrounding the heart with a limitation of diastolic ventricular filling. As the encompassing scar shrinks, the heart is compressed further, especially the right heart and great veins. This thickened and scarred pericardium is densely adherent to the heart, thus limiting systolic ejection as well as restricting diastolic filling. This results in an elevated venous pressure and a reduced cardiac output, usually with a low systemic blood pressure. The elevation in venous pressure is of particular interest since further elevation by infusion of blood or plasma results in no change in cardiac output. Similar observations have been noted when paracentesis or phlebotomies were performed. In these instances, venous pressure was reduced with no change in cardiac output. Obviously, these measures cannot be carried to extremes since reduction of venous pressure below a critical value lowers cardiac output. However, in contradistinction to acute cardiac tamponade, raising venous pressure does not result in an increase in cardiac output. This is due to more rigid restriction of diastolic filling imposed by the fibrous or calcified pericardium as compared with that imposed by fluid or blood.

The reduced cardiac output results in less effective perfusion of the liver and kidney. The tendency toward salt and water accumulation accounts for an expansion of blood volume and further increases venous pressure. Thus, the kidney actually worsens the condition, increasing venous pressure and blood volume even though these measures will not increase cardiac output. Ganglionic blocking agents may reduce venous pressure 35 to 50 per cent without effecting a change in cardiac output (Lange, 1967). Such patients may undergo diuresis with reduction of venous pressure and diastolic pressure in both the left and right heart while still maintaining an adequate cardiac output. These considerations suggest that some of the secondary manifestations of constrictive pericarditis can be improved by means that do not attack the primary disorder.

Patients complain of weakness, easy fatigability, and shortness of breath with exertion that clears with rest. Ascites formation without peripheral edema is a common finding. In fact, the ascites can be profound, with no evidence of pedal edema, despite a venous pressure of 30 to 45 cm. of water. Syncopal attacks may occur in association with activity and are thought to be due to the inability of the heart to increase its output to meet demands. Abdominal pain and tenderness may accompany liver enlargement. The feeling of fullness is due at first to the liver and then to ascites formation. The ascites becomes excessive, with no evidence of peripheral edema, the opposite being true in congestive heart failure.

Physical findings vary considerably, depending on the stage of the disease. The patient may present a grotesque appearance with a puffy face and protuberant abdomen, although dyspnea may be present only with exercise. The heart is quiet, the apex beat may not be felt, and there is no right ventricular lift. A distinct diastolic shock may be palpated at the time of rapid filling, with an elevated venous pressure. A rapid diastolic heart sound, coinciding with the rapid filling, has been described (Potain, 1856; Mounsey, 1955). Murmurs are usually absent. The liver is usually enlarged and is tender, and ascites may be present. Pedal edema, if present, is not marked. The disease is found more commonly in younger patients, 25 to 45 years old.

The hepatojugular reflex is prominent, and venous pressure momentarily increases during inspiration in patients with constrictive pericarditis (Kussmaul, 1873). Atrial fibrillation is present in about one third of the patients. The peripheral pulse may be paradoxical, disappearing during inspiration, even though cardiac rate and the apical pulse remain unchanged. Explanations of the mechanisms of the paradoxical pulse are that blood is sequestered in the pulmonary bed during inspiration (Hitzig, 1942) or that the thickened pericardium anchors the heart rigidly to the diaphragm. As the latter descends in inspiration, it further tenses the pericardium, which interferes with ventricular filling (Lower, 1669; Wood, 1956). Arterial blood pressure is usually low with a narrowed pulse pressure. Arm-to-tongue circulation time is prolonged.

The heart is usually normal or mildly enlarged on chest x-ray. Calcium deposits may be seen more commonly on the lateral film (Fig. 31–2). The superior vena cava may be prominent. The pulsation of the heart is diminished on fluoroscopic examination. The electrocardiogram shows a low voltage in the QRS complexes, the reason for which is not clear. T waves are flat and often inverted. The P wave may be broadened and bifid, with the second wave taller than the first. The serum proteins may be low because of a loss of protein throughout the gastrointestinal tract. The increased portal pressure may cause an increase in lymph production and an increased rate of thoracic duct flow (Wilkinson et al., 1965). Lymphatic dilatation causes chylous effusions in the chest and abdomen. Intestinal lymphangiectasis is thought to result from increased pressure in the capillaries and lymphatics. The resulting congestion of the intestinal wall and the mucosal surface of the small bowel results in diminished absorption of ingested protein accompanied by an actual loss of protein from the congested lymphatics. Studies of thoracic duct lymph showed an increased production with a low protein content. Fat transport is reduced after ingestion. The loss of protein, especially albumin, probably results from the increased intestinal capillary pressure, which causes increased lymph production and secondary dilation of the lymphatics. Fat and protein are lost by transudation under high pressure or by rupture of these dilated lymphatics. This process is reversed following relief of pericardial constriction.

Establishing the diagnosis in constrictive pericarditis is not always simple, the entity often being confused with hepatic cirrhosis or cardiac disease. Various forms of familial and acquired myocardio-

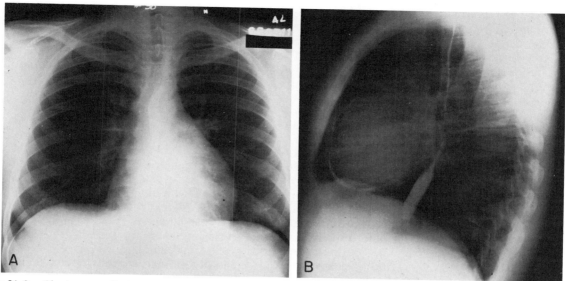

Figure 31–2. Chest x-rays of a 45-year-old man with calcific constrictive pericarditis. The rim of calcium is clearly visible encircling the heart on the lateral film (*B*) but is not identifiable on the anterior view (*A*).

pathy are easily confused clinically with constrictive pericarditis. Catheterization of the heart has been the most satisfactory technique for differentiating between myocardial and pericardial disease. In constrictive pericarditis, the diastolic pressure in the right ventricle rises rapidly during early filling with a plateau effect and a small A wave (Fig. 31–3). The systolic pulmonary artery pressure is not above 45 mm. Hg. Right atrial pressure is always markedly elevated. The left ventricular end-diastolic pressure is not much greater than the right (average 4 mm. Hg), whereas in myocardiopathies, it was usually much greater, with an average of 17 mm. Hg (Conti and Friesinger, 1967). Angiocardiography is helpful in outlining the thickness of the atrial wall, the stiffness of the atrium, and the quality of atrial contraction. In constrictive pericarditis, the thin atrial wall is fixed to the scarred pericardium and contracts poorly, whereas atrial activity is usually vigorous in myocardial disease. In approximately three fourths of the patients the correct diagnosis is

obtained by these techniques. In a certain number the diagnosis remains elusive and can be accurately defined only by pericardial biopsy. This can be followed by an immediate extension of the thoracotomy or by a sternal splitting approach if pericardial constriction is confirmed.

In many patients the cause of constrictive pericarditis is unknown. It can follow suppurative pericarditis. In the past, tuberculosis was a common cause, but any type of infectious process may initiate dense pericardial scarring. Hemopericardium resulting from a penetrating injury has been a rare cause of chronic pericardial constriction (McKusick *et al.,* 1955). Blunt trauma to the chest, such as a kick, auto accident, or athletic injury that results in hemopericardium, may precipitate chronic scarring. The time interval between injury and pericardial disease may be considerable (Schneider and Rivier, 1960). The process may be quite rapid, as in the case of a 25-year-old man who was stabbed in the chest with a penknife. Pericardiocentesis with removal of 200 ml. of blood was required to control tamponade, but no subsequent aspirations were necessary. Pericardial calcification and symptoms of constrictive heart disease were present 4 months later, and pericardiectomy was performed.

Pericardial constriction has been reported after cardiac surgery, but the incidence is low, probably less than 1 per cent. In some instances, the constriction has occurred within 2 weeks after operation, suggesting an acute inflammatory response with immediate adherence of the pericardium to the heart. Similarly, constrictive pericarditis occurs after Dressler's syndrome following myocardial infarction.

TECHNIQUE OF PERICARDIAL ASPIRATION

Pericardial aspiration can be a lifesaving therapeutic technique for cardiac tamponade or a diagnostic

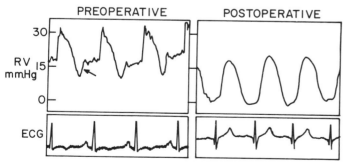

Figure 31–3. The right ventricular pressure tracing of a patient with constrictive pericarditis. The early rapid diastolic pressure elevation (*arrow*) with a plateau throughout the remainder of diastole is characteristic. Atrial contraction results in minimal pressure change in late diastole. The right ventricular pressure is normal at the time of catheterization 6 months after pericardiectomy.

tool for pericarditis or effusion. Serous fluid is usually found in nonspecific pericarditis. Characteristic gold-colored, thick fluid can be obtained in cholesterol pericarditis or in pericardial effusion following myocardial infarction. Frank pus or cloudy, milky fluid may be aspirated in pyogenic pericarditis. Blood or serosanguineous fluid may be seen in cases of neoplasm and also of idiopathic pericarditis. Blood aspirated from the pericardial sac does not clot because it has been rapidly defibrinated by the movement of the heart. Aspiration of blood that subsequently clots usually means that it was obtained from a heart chamber.

Pericardial aspiration is performed routinely by either the left parasternal approach (in the fourth and fifth intercostal spaces) or the subxiphoid route under local anesthesia. A long needle (12 to 18 cm.) is attached to a stopcock and syringe and inserted just beneath the xiphoid process. A precordial electrocardiogram lead is attached to the needle by a small clip (see Fig. 31–1). The needle is inserted at a 45-degree angle directed posteriorly toward a point midway between the scapulas. The needle should be advanced until fluid is encountered or the electrocardiogram shows contact with the heart surface. This is easily detected by the marked negative deflection seen on the electrocardiogram (see Fig. 31–1). If the needle is in contact with the heart, it should be withdrawn slowly to a point just proximal to cardiac contact, which should place the needle tip in the pericardium. Fluid aspirated should be saved for bacteriologic and cytologic examinations. The protein content should be

determined. If a large volume of fluid is removed, the insertion of 100 to 200 ml. of air into the pericardial sac is helpful in determining the thickness of the pericardium (Fig. 31–4). Immediate x-ray studies following air injection reveal not only the pericardial thickness but also the size of the heart and any masses projecting into the pericardial space.

There are certain complications that must be considered in needle aspiration in either the parasternal or the subxiphoid approach: laceration of the heart or a coronary artery, laceration of the internal mammary artery, penetration and possible contamination of the pleural cavity in purulent pericarditis, laceration or puncture of the lung with resultant pneumothorax, aspiration of blood from the intracardiac chambers, and, rarely, a shock-like reaction to the penetration of the pericardium by the needle. In addition, in the subxiphoid approach, perforation of abdominal organs and laceration of the liver may occur. Such complications are unusual, however.

In large effusions or cardiac tamponade from penetration of the heart, a larger bore, thin-walled needle can be positioned in the pericardial space and a polyethylene catheter passed through the needle into the pericardial sac. A reasonable estimate of continued bleeding into the pericardial sac can be obtained since the blood rarely clots in the catheter because of the defibrinating effect of the heart. These catheters can be left in place for several hours without fear of infection and may alleviate the necessity for repeated pericardiocentesis.

Some surgeons prefer open pericardiocentesis. In

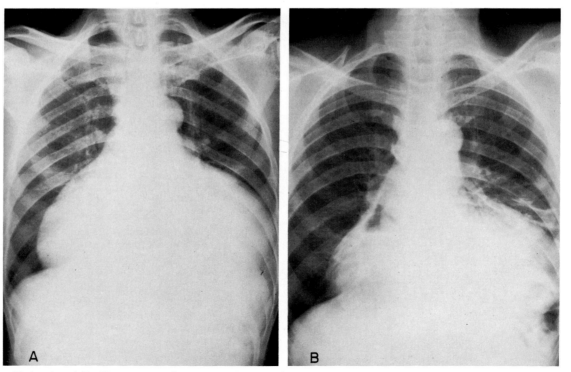

Figure 31–4. *A* and *B,* Chest x-rays of a 48-year-old man with massive pericardial effusion. 1500 ml. of fluid was removed by pericardiocentesis and a small quantity of air injected into the pericardial sac. X-ray *B* shows the thin line of pericardium that is not adherent to the heart. An additional liter of fluid was removed after film *B* was taken.

this procedure, the pericardium is exposed under local anesthesia through a small incision in the fourth or fifth interspace 1 cm. to the left of the sternum. The needle is then passed through the pericardium under direct vision. A similar approach can be made by a small subxiphoid incision, bluntly freeing the diaphragm from the anterior abdominal wall. Thus, the pericardium can be exposed superiorly to the diaphragm without entering either the abdominal or the thoracic cavity. Direct aspiration of the pericardial sac can be accomplished.

Unfortunately, pericardiocentesis may result occasionally in sudden death due to laceration of a coronary artery or to ventricular fibrillation. Pericardial tapping must be considered a serious procedure and must be performed with care. The use of the electrocardiogram to detect contact with the heart markedly reduces the chance of myocardial or coronary artery injury and has significantly reduced the hazards of this procedure.

PERICARDIOTOMY

Open drainage of the pericardium is usually performed in cases of purulent pericarditis in which adequate drainage of pus is as important as in any type of purulent collection. Repeated needle aspiration of thick purulent material often is unsatisfactory in controlling infection. Originally, pericardiotomy was done by trephining an opening 2 to 3 cm. in diameter in the sternum, but this is now obsolete.

A subxiphoid approach by an incision just to the left of the xiphoid process is carried through the rectus muscles to the transversus abdominis fibers. The dissection remains above this muscle and proceeds superiorly beneath the costal margin so as to enter the pericardial sac without encountering peritoneum, diaphragm, or pleura. Excellent drainage is obtained through this approach, since the most dependent area of the pericardial sac is opened.

The anterior approach is most commonly used when the cartilages of the fifth and sixth ribs are resected. The entire cartilage between rib and sternum must be resected in order to avoid chondritis. Some advocate excision of the seventh cartilage to obtain more dependent drainage. The mammary artery is divided, and the pleura is displaced laterally. A section of exposed pericardium is excised and sent for histologic examination and culture.

For best drainage, two catheters should be placed in the pericardium — one anterior and one posterior to the heart. By this method, the posterior catheter may be irrigated, and the fluid rising can exit via the anterior catheter. In this way, the thick pus and loculations are more apt to be broken down and a more complete drainage of the pericardial space accomplished.

PERICARDIAL BIOPSY

Biopsy of the pericardium is frequently the best approach in establishing an exact and early diagnosis (Effler and Proudfit, 1957). Under general anesthesia, the pericardium is exposed through the fourth left interspace. A round segment of pericardium is excised for examination. Pericardial fluid may be examined microscopically and bacteriologically. In the case of chronic pericardial fluid, the defect may be drained into the pleural space, from which it may be evacuated by an indwelling catheter. In some instances, the catheter can be left directly in the pericardial space for drainage of the chronic effusion. This is most useful when the effusion is likely to be self-limiting, as in nonmalignant conditions.

An alternate method of pericardial biopsy is to resect the fifth costal cartilage on the left. All cartilage is removed and the pericardium exposed through the bed of the cartilage (Fig. 31–5). This technique is preferred when the differential diagnosis is between constrictive pericarditis and myocardiopathy, since the pleural space need not be entered. If constrictive pericarditis is present, the incision may be closed and a median sternotomy approach used, or the transverse incision can be extended to a left anterior thoracotomy

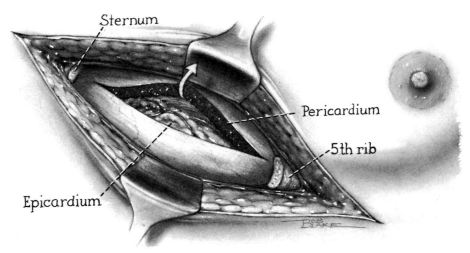

Figure 31–5. The left fifth costal cartilage is resected and the pericardium exposed. A section of pericardium can be excised for histologic examination. The surface of the heart must be identified, since a thick granular layer, loosely attached to the pericardium and more firmly adherent to the epicardium, can be present.

Sternum

Pericardium

5th rib

Epicardium

and the sternum transected to gain exposure to the right ventricle and atrium.

PERICARDIECTOMY

By definition, constrictive pericarditis is a mechanical limitation of cardiac filling. Taking into account that myocardial atrophy may result from long-standing constrictive pericarditis, excision of the constricting tissue should offer definite improvement. Surgical results have to be evaluated in reference to the period of time in which the operation was performed (Kloster *et al.,* 1965). Operative removal of the pericardium from the anterior and posterior surfaces of the heart is much more extensive than the original surgical procedures. Pericardial resections formerly were inadequate and the clinical results disappointing (Shumacker and Roshe, 1960). Operative mortality has been lowered by improved anesthesia, blood replacement, antibiotics, and management of cardiac arrhythmias.

Preoperative Preparation

Pericardiectomy is usually not performed as an emergency operation, although there have been instances in which very ill patients benefited by emergency resection (Bigelow *et al.,* 1956). The patients usually are hospitalized and brought into a better nutritional and cardiovascular state while diagnostic studies are being performed. Vigorous efforts to correct ascites and cardiac failure should be made by salt restriction, control of arrhythmias, and adequate digitalization. Antituberculosis therapy should be instituted in any suspected case of tuberculous pericarditis.

Operative Technique

If the diagnosis of constrictive pericarditis has been assured by preoperative studies, a definitive surgical approach should be undertaken. If the diagnosis remains elusive, open pericardial biopsy through a small left anterior incision with resection of either the fourth or fifth costal cartilage should be performed initially (Fig. 31–5). This incision can be closed and the median sternal splitting approach used, or the incision can be extended into a bilateral thoracotomy with the sternum divided. The unilateral left anterior transpleural approach is adequate for limited decortications but not for the more radical pericardiectomy preferred by Holman and Willett (1949), Johnson and Kirby (1951), Bigelow and associates (1956), and Shumacker and Roshe (1960). Inadequate exposure does not allow complete removal of the pericardium and does not permit the operator to handle effectively any emergency, such as penetration of the thin-walled right ventricle or right atrium. The extent of pericardial resection should be determined by the operative findings, but most errors have been made by removal of insufficient pericardium.

A median sternotomy incision is frequently employed (Holman and Willett, 1949). This incision gives good exposure of the left ventricle, even though the area posterior to the left phrenic nerve is difficult to visualize. Exposure of the right heart and great vessels is excellent. Laceration of the thin-walled right ventricle commonly occurs. This complication is dangerous only if the exposure is inadequate to simply suture the elevated pericardial flap back to the right ventricle and thus effectively close the hole.

A vertical skin incision is made from the manubrium to below the xiphoid. The sternum is divided by use of an electric bone saw. The two edges are separated and the mediastinum exposed. On initial examination, it may appear that the heart is not beating because of the thickness and immobility of the diseased pericardium. The pleura is freed laterally and the thymus elevated off the pericardium. The pericardium is continuously incised longitudinally just anterior to the left heart border (Fig. 31–6). When cardiac musculature is identified, a plane is selected just exterior to the muscle for the mobilization of the pericardium. The correct plane of dissection is anterior to the epicardium, removing the organized pericardial exudate and the pericardium. This plane may initially be difficult to find. Bleeding usually indicates that one has dissected too deeply through the epicardium into the myocardium. If the correct plane can be followed, blood loss may be surprisingly small. Care is taken to avoid injury to the coronary vessels, since many of the arrhythmias encountered at the time of operation may be due to small infarcts created by injury to coronary vessels. Bleeding from the heart muscle should be controlled by very finely placed sutures. The dissection is carried laterally over the left ventricle and apex. It may be of importance to free the left ventricle first so that pulmonary congestion does not occur when the right ventricular output increases. The heart is elevated to the right so that the posterior surface of the left ventricle can be freed and the pericardium excised (Fig. 31–7). The phrenic nerve should be mobilized from the pericardium to avoid damage to this structure and to allow resection of the left posterior pericardium.

Caution is observed in excising the pericardium from the thin-walled right ventricle and right atrium. The resection is continued laterally to include the great veins and superiorly onto the aorta and pulmonary artery (Fig. 31–8). The unusually thickened pericardium, extending from the inferior vena cava to the diaphragm and the apex of the heart, is excised (Fig. 31–9). Pockets of localized pus may be encountered between the epicardium and the thickened pericardium. Emphasis has been placed on the fact that the epicardial lining of such pockets should be removed to lessen the chance of subsequent scarring (Churchill, 1936). Oozing from the heart surface usually ceases with gentle pressure. Overzealous suturing of bleeders on the heart surface should be discouraged to lessen

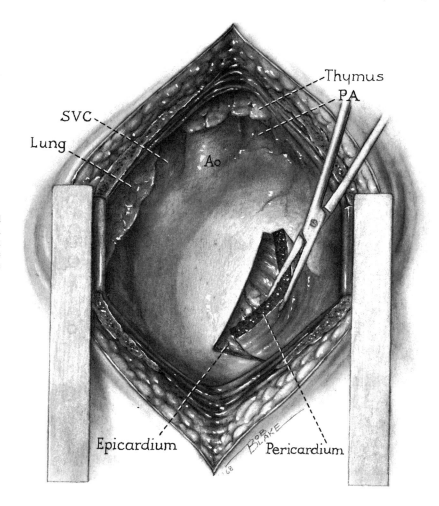

Figure 31–6. The pericardium is exposed through a midline sternal splitting incision. A longitudinal incision is made in the pericardium and a plane of dissection established so that the thickened pericardium can be removed from the left ventricle.

the chance of injuring coronary vessels. The large area of denuded tissue resulting from the pericardiotomy can cause an outpouring of fluid. The pleura is opened widely into both pleural spaces, and catheter drainage of each is instituted, using gentle suction in the usual water-seal technique. Hemostasis is again checked to be certain that the accumulation of blood about the heart is kept at a minimum; this reduces the chance of recurrent fibrosis or of the formation of narrow bands that can again compress the heart. The edges of the sternum are approximated with encircling, interrupted stainless steel wire sutures. The fascia, subcutaneous tissues, and skin are closed with interrupted silk sutures. Cardiopulmonary bypass has been employed to facilitate removal of the thickened pericardium because of the ability to control hemorrhage in manipulation of the heart. Bleeding is increased, however, from the required use of heparin, so bypass should be used only when simpler measures are inadequate.

Arrhythmias can be a cause of concern during the course of operation because of manipulation of the heart and the small areas of infarction that can result from injury to small coronary vessels. Usually the patients have been receiving digitalis; this reduces the likelihood of a rapid ventricular response to atrial arrhythmias, such as fibrillation and flutter. Ectopic

ventricular activity is best controlled by a slow intravenous drip of 0.1 per cent solution of lidocaine hydrochloride. This will usually control ectopic ventricular beats without depressing myocardial function. Care must be taken not to overtransfuse these patients during the operation or in the early postoperative period, since the thin-walled right ventricle can overdilate.

Postoperative Care

Although the hemodynamic improvements from pericardiectomy are dramatic, cardiac function may not return to normal owing to chronic myocardial injury from the pericardial constriction. Measurement of ventricular filling pressures is useful to prevent overdistention of the thin-walled right and left ventricles. Myocardial stimulants may be needed if cardiac contractility decreases. A slow infusion of dopamine is preferable since it is an agent that is least likely to produce ventricular irritability. Antibiotics are usually administered, and if tuberculosis is suspected, chemotherapy should be continued for several months until the culture reports on the pericardial material are returned. Daily maintenance fluid is kept at a low level

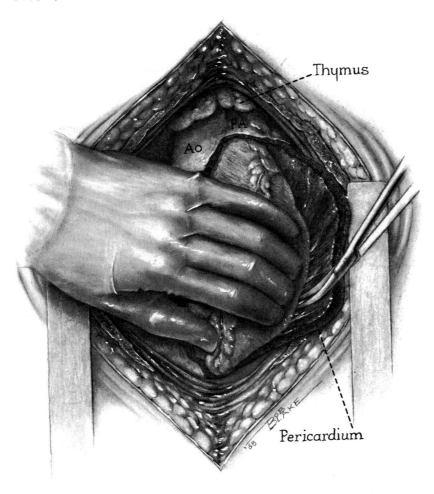

Thymus

PA

Ao

Pericardium

Figure 31–7. The heart is held to the right so that the posterior left ventricle can be freed. The phrenic nerve must be isolated to avoid injuring this structure. The large pericardial flap will be excised.

until the cardiac status is stable and renal function is established. Digitalis may be necessary for several months postoperatively to help strengthen the damaged myocardium. Ambulation and exercise are gradually increased, depending on symptoms, but should be limited for at least the first month. Ascites and edema as well as hepatic enlargement usually subside after surgery.

Some surgeons have felt it unnecessary to free the vena cava and right atrium, contending that only liberation of the ventricles was important, but failure to completely liberate the right heart has necessitated subsequent operations. Constriction of the great veins as they enter the heart has been shown at cardiac catheterization after incomplete excision of the pericardium. Operative removal of the remaining pericardium over the right atrium and great veins lowered venous pressure and cured the patient's ascites.

It has been shown with animals that in experimentally produced generalized pericardial constriction, removal of the scar over the right heart resulted in the disappearance of the high venous pressure and ascites, but the animals died in congestive heart failure (Isaacs *et al.*, 1952). In other animals, the scar was removed from the left heart with no reduction in venous pressure or loss of ascites. Thus, a complete pericardiectomy is necessary before failure to relieve a high

venous pressure or to clear ascites is blamed on myocardial atrophy. Similarly, emphasis has also been placed on the importance of removing the pericardium from the right heart and vena cava in order to relieve ascites and venous hypertension (Parsons and Holman, 1951, 1955).

POSTPERICARDIOTOMY SYNDROME

An unusual syndrome, which may be characterized by fever, pericardial pain, pleural pain, pulmonary infiltrates, arthralgias, dyspnea, pericardial effusion, pleural effusion, pericardial friction rub, or any combination of these signs and symptoms, occurs in approximately 10 to 40 per cent of patients undergoing cardiac surgery. The actual incidence is probably higher, since mild cases remain unrecognized. The sedimentation rate is elevated, leukocytosis with an increase in lymphocytes is usually present, and occasionally the electrocardiogram shows changes of pericarditis. The syndrome must be differentiated from such postoperative conditions as incisional pain, myocardial infarction, pulmonary embolus, bacterial endocarditis, pneumonia, and atelectasis.

This syndrome was first depicted by Cox (1928) and Koucky and Milles (1935). It was initially de-

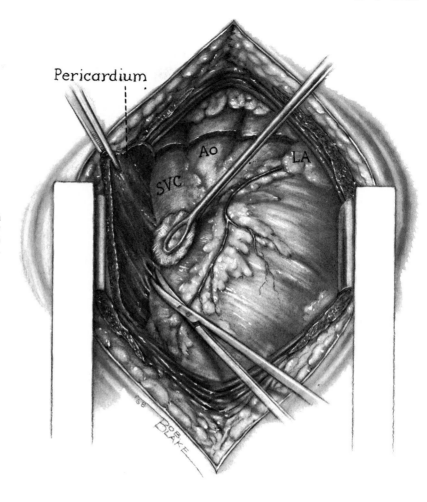

Figure 31–8. The pericardium is freed from the right atrium and venae cavae. These very thin-walled structures are easily torn, and adequate exposure is mandatory for this part of the dissection.

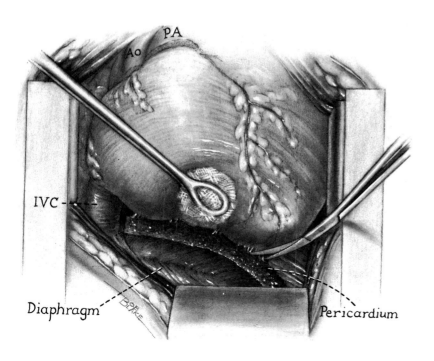

Figure 31–9. The very thickened pericardium attached between the apex of the heart and the diaphragm must be excised to prevent recurrent adherent bands and inferior vena caval obstruction.

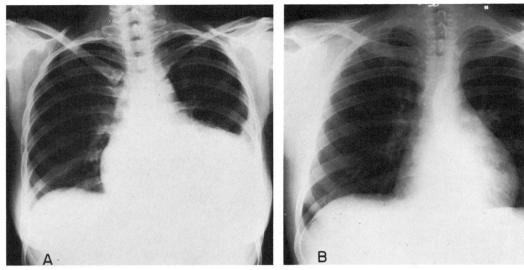

Figure 31–10. *A,* Chest x-ray of a 40-year-old woman 10 days after open heart surgery. She had fever, pericardial friction rub, and a left pleural effusion. *B,* After 4 days' treatment with steroids and salicylates, the pleural effusion cleared, and the symptoms of postpericardiotomy syndrome did not return.

scribed following wounds of the heart and was referred to as "polyserositis." It was called the "postcommissurotomy syndrome" in the early fifties because of its being observed following mitral commissurotomy. At this time, it was postulated to be due to a reactivation of rheumatic fever. The syndrome was observed after a pericardiotomy and termed the "postpericardiotomy syndrome" (Dresdale *et al.,* 1956). Since then, it has been reported after minor violation of the pericardium, such as following percutaneous left ventricular puncture (Peter *et al.,* 1966).

The precise etiology of this syndrome remains unknown. A common factor seems to be trauma and residual blood in the pericardial sac. Experimentally, it may be produced following injection of autogenous blood or fat into the pericardial space (Ehrenhaft and Taber, 1952). Autoantibodies have been demonstrated in rheumatic fever and in the postcommissurotomy syndrome (Kaplan, 1960). An antiheart antibody can be measured, and the serum concentration varies with the severity of the clinical symptoms (Engle *et al.,* 1974). Whether this antibody is causative or simply registers the state of the disease is unknown.

Treatment is directly related to the severity of the syndrome. The course is variable and often self-limiting, requiring no therapy. In severe cases, accumulation of fluid in serous cavities may compromise cardiac or pulmonary function (Fig. 31–10). Salicylates and rest provide dramatic improvement in most cases. Salicylates should be given every 4 hours until improvement is noted. In severe cases, fluid balance and nutrition must be maintained, and complete bed rest is indicated. Corticosteroids usually produce improvement within 72 hours. After this short course of steroids, salicylates may be adequate to control symptoms. Prolonged use of steroids should be avoided, as rebound may occur with cessation of treatment. If this occurs, the patient should be maintained on the lowest

steroid dose that will control symptoms; the drug should gradually be withdrawn after 5 to 7 days. A low serum albumin, associated with poor nutrition as a factor in the development of clinical symptoms, has been described (Aronstam and Cox, 1966). Administration of albumin intravenously and reversal of the negative nitrogen balance resulted in clinical improvement. If collections of fluid persist, pericardiocentesis or thoracentesis may be necessary for precise diagnosis or for the relief of dyspnea.

Misdiagnosis with resulting failure to treat a specific infection, delay in recuperation with prolongation of hospitalization, and recurrences are always dangers in this syndrome. The recurrences are usually associated with withdrawal of therapy, commonly steroids, although recurrences may appear several years after the first episode. Postpericardiotomy syndrome usually does not play a role in the ultimate prognosis for the patient, even though the convalescent period can be prolonged. Persistent recurrent effusion is uncommon, but relief can be obtained with pericardiectomy.

SELECTED REFERENCES

Engle, M. A., McCabe, J. C., Ebert, P. A., and Zabriskie, J.: The postpericardiotomy syndrome and antiheart antibodies. Circulation *49*:401, 1974.

This article describes the clinical course and possible etiologies of the postpericardiotomy syndrome. The immunologic significance of this rather common complication of cardiac surgery is emphasized. The findings of a heart reactive antibody that closely correlates with the clinical symptoms and the use of this as a diagnostic test in patients having persistent pain and fever after thoracotomy are demonstrated. The level of antibody is directly related to the clinical symptoms and could be used to predict recurrences.

Issacs, J. P., Carter, B. N., II, and Haller, J. A., Jr.: Experimental pericarditis: The pathologic physiology of constrictive pericarditis. Bull. Johns Hopkins Hosp., *90*:259, 1952.

This represents one of the few well-detailed experimental studies in which constrictive pericarditis was produced. It emphasized the minimal effect of constriction about the atrium in elevating venous pressure. The authors showed that all the systemic manifestations of constrictive pericarditis occurred when the constrictive component was present over the ventricles. In addition, the importance of removing the pericardium from the left ventricle before the right at surgery was demonstrated by the occurrence of pulmonary edema when left ventricular restriction was not relieved. The effect on the myocardium of constrictive pericarditis was emphasized by seeing the marked change in the elasticity of the ventricle after removal of the constrictive scar. There was an excellent review of the hemodynamics associated with constrictive pericarditis and the effects on the systemic organs.

Kloster, F. E., Crislip, R. L., Bristow, J. D., Herr, R. H., Ritzmann, L. W., and Griswold, H. E.: Hemodynamic studies following pericardiectomy for constrictive pericarditis. Circulation, 32:415, 1965.

This report very nicely shows the hemodynamic improvements in patients after relief of constrictive pericarditis. Improvements in serum proteins and other blood components are emphasized. There are ventricular tracings in the article that demonstrate the effects of constrictive pericarditis on ventricular performance. The article gives a detailed discussion of pressure changes and hemodynamic patterns of patients with constrictive pericardial disease and emphasizes the diagnostic difficulty often encountered in distinguishing constrictive pericarditis from restrictive myocardial disease.

REFERENCES

Aronstam, E. M., and Cox, W. A.: A new concept of the pleuropericardial syndrome. Postpericardiotomy or postcardiotomy syndrome. J. Thorac. Cardiovasc. Surg., 51:341, 1966.

Barnard, H. L.: The functions of the pericardium. J. Physiol., 22:42, 1898.

Bates, J. C., and Leaver, F. Y.: Pericardial celomic cysts: Presentation of 5 new cases and 5 similar cases illustrating difficulty of diagnosis. Radiology, 57:330, 1951.

Beck, C. S.: Acute and chronic compression of the heart. Am. Heart J., 14:515, 1937.

Beck, C. S., and Griswold, R. A.: Pericardiectomy in the treatment of the Pick syndrome: Experimental and clinical observations. Arch. Surg., 21:1064, 1930.

Beck, C. S., and Moore, R. L.: The significance of the pericardium in relation to surgery of the heart. Arch. Surg., 11:550, 1925.

Bigelow, W. G., Dolan, F. G., Wilson, D. R., and Gunton, R. W.: The surgical treatment of chronic constrictive pericarditis. Can. Med. Assoc. J., 75:814, 1956.

Blakemore, W. S., Zinsser, H. F., Kirby, C. K., Whitaker, W. B., and Johnson, J.: Pericardiectomy for relapsing pericarditis and chronic constrictive pericarditis. J. Thorac. Cardiovasc. Surg., 39:26, 1960.

Blalock, A., and Levy, S. E.: Tuberculous pericarditis. J. Thorac. Surg., 7:132, 1937.

Bloomfield, R. A., Lauson, H. D., Cournand, A., Breed, E. S., and Richards, D. W., Jr.: Recording of right heart pressures in normal subjects and in various types of cardio-circulatory disease. J. Clin. Invest., 25:639, 1946.

Borkon, A. M., Schaff, H. V., et al.: Diagnosis and management of postoperative pericardial effusions and late cardiac tamponade following open-heart surgery. Ann. Thorac. Surg., 31:512, 1981.

Brawley, R. K., Vasko, J. S., and Morrow, A. G.: Cholesterol pericarditis. Am. J. Med., 41:235, 1966.

Bricheteau, I.: Observations d'hydropneumopéricarde. Arch. Gén. Méd., 4s, 4:334, 1844.

Burwell, C. S., and Blalock, A.: Chronic constrictive pericarditis: Physiologic and pathologic considerations. J.A.M.A., 110:265, 1938.

Bush, C. A., Stand, J. M., et al.: Occult constrictive pericardial disease. Circulation, 56:924, 1977.

Carroll, D.: Streptomycin in the treatment of tuberculous pericarditis. Bull. Johns Hopkins Hosp., 88:425, 1951.

Chester, M. H., and Tully, J. B.: Acute pericardial fat necrosis. J. Thorac. Surg., 38:62, 1959.

Chevers, N.: Observations on the disease of the orifice and valves of the aorta. Guy's Hosp. Rep., 7:387, 1842.

Churchill, E. D.: Decortication of heart (Délorme) for adhesive pericarditis. Arch. Surg., 19:1457, 1929.

Churchill, E. D.: Pericardial resection in chronic constrictive pericarditis. Ann. Surg., 104:516, 1936.

Cohnheim, J.: Lectures on general pathology. New Syndenham Soc., 1:21, 1889.

Conti, C. R., and Friesinger, G. C.: Chronic constrictive pericarditis. Clinical and laboratory findings in 11 cases. Johns Hopkins Med. J., 120:262, 1967.

Cox, W. M.: Wounds of the heart. Arch. Surg., 17:484, 1928.

Craddock, W. L.: Cysts of the pericardium. Am. Heart J., 40:619, 1950.

Creech, O., Hicks, W. M., Snyder, H. B., and Erickson, E. E.: Cholesterol pericarditis: Successful treatment by pericardiectomy. Circulation, 12:193, 1955.

Délorme, E.: Sur un traitement chirurgical de la symphyse cardo-péricardique. Gaz. Hop., 71:1150, 1898.

Doherty, J. E., and Jenkins, B. J.: Radiocarbon cholesterol turnover in cholesterol pericarditis. Am. J. Med., 41:322, 1966.

Dresdale, D. T., Ropstein, C. B., Gusman, S. J., and Greene, M. A.: Postpericardiotomy syndrome in patients with rheumatic heart disease. Am. J. Med., 21:57, 1956.

Effler, D. B., and Proudfit, W. L.: Pericardial biopsy: Role in diagnosis and treatment of chronic pericarditis. Am. Rev. Tuberc., 75:469, 1957.

Ehrenhaft, J L., and Taber, R. E.: Hemopericardium and constrictive pericarditis. J. Thorac. Surg., 24:355, 1952.

Engle, M. A., McCabe, J. C., Ebert, P. A., and Zabriskie, J.: The postpericardiotomy syndrome and antiheart antibodies. Circulation, 49:401, 1974.

Fitzpatrick, D. P., Wyso, E. M., Bosher, L. H., and Richardson, D. W.: Restoration of normal intracardiac pressures after extensive pericardiectomy for constrictive pericarditis. Circulation, 25:484, 1962.

Fowler, N. O.: Physiology of cardiac tamponade and pulsus paradoxus. Mod. Concepts Cardiovasc. Dis., 47:109, 1978.

Gillett, R. L.: Acute benign pericarditis and the Coxsackie viruses. N. Engl. J. Med., 261:838, 1959.

Hitzig, W. M.: On mechanisms of inspiratory filling of the cervical veins and pulsus paradoxus in venous hypertension. J. Mt. Sinai Hosp., 8:625, 1942.

Holman, C. W., and Steinberg, I.: The role of angiocardiography in the surgical treatment of massive pericardial effusions. Surg. Gynecol. Obstet., 107:639, 1958.

Holman, E., and Beck, C. S.: The physiological response of the circulatory system to experimental alterations. II. The effect of variations in total blood volume. J. Exper. Med., 42:681, 1925.

Holman, E., and Willett, F.: The surgical correction of constrictive pericarditis. Surg. Gynecol. Obstet., 89:129, 1949.

Holman, E., and Willett, F.: Results of radical pericardiectomy for constrictive pericarditis. J.A.M.A., 157:789, 1955.

Isaacs, J. P., Carter, B. N., II, and Haller, J. A., Jr.: Experimental pericarditis: The pathologic physiology of constrictive pericarditis. Bull. Johns Hopkins Hosp., 90:259, 1952.

Jackson, R. C., Clagett, O. T., and McDonald, J. R.: Pericardial fat necrosis. J. Thorac. Surg., 33:723, 1957.

Johnson, J., and Kirby, C. K.: A new incision for pericardiectomy. Ann. Surg., 133:540, 1951.

Kaplan, M. H.: The concept of autoantibodies in rheumatic fever and in the postcommissurotomy state. Ann. N.Y. Acad. Sci., 86:974, 1960.

Karanaeff: Paracentese des Brustkastens und des Pericardiums. Med. Z., 9:251, 1840.

Klacsmann, P. G., Bulkley, B. H., and Hutchins, G. M.: The changed spectrum of purulent pericarditis. Am. J. Med., 63:666, 1977.

Kloster, F. E., Crislip, R. L., Bristow, J. D., Herr, R. H., Ritzman, L. W., and Griswold, H. E.: Hemodynamic studies following pericardiectomy for constrictive pericarditis. Circulation, 32:415, 1965.

Koucky, J. D., and Milles, G.: Stab wounds of the heart. Arch. Intern. Med., 56:281, 1935.

Krook, H.: Acute non-specific pericarditis: Study in 24 cases including descriptions of 2 with later development into constrictive pericarditis. Acta Med. Scand., 148:201, 1954.

Kussmaul, A.: Ueber schwielige Mediastino-Perikarditis und den paradoxen Puls. Berl. Klin. Wochenschr., 10:433, 445, 461, 1873.

Laennec, R. T. H.: Traité d'Auscultation Médicale et des Maladies du Poumon et du Coeur. Paris, Brosson & J. S. Chaude, 1819.

Lam, C. R.: Pericardial celomic cyst. Radiology, 48:239, 1947.

Lambert, A. V.: Etiology of thin-walled thoracic cysts. J. Thorac. Surg., 10:1, 1940.

Lange, R. L.: Treatment of chronic constrictive pericarditis. Mod. Treat., 4:162, 1967.

Lower, R.: Tractatus de Corde (London, 1669). *Cited in* Major, R. H.: Classic Descriptions of Disease. Springfield, Illinois, Charles C Thomas, 1932, p. 630.

Mannix, E. P., Jr., and Dennis, C.: The surgical treatment of chronic pericardial effusion and cardiac tamponade. J. Thorac. Surg., 29:381, 1955.

Martin, A.: Acute non-specific pericarditis. A description of nineteen cases. Br. Med. J., 2:279, 1966.

Martin, J. W., and Schenk, W. G., Jr.: Pericardial tamponade: Newer dynamic concepts. Am. J. Surg., 99:782, 1960.

McKusick, V. A.: Chronic constrictive pericarditis: Some clinical and laboratory observations. Bull. Johns Hopkins Hosp., 90:3, 1952.

McKusick, V. A., and Cochran, T. H.: Constrictive endocarditis. Bull. Johns Hopkins Hosp., 90:90, 1952.

McKusick, V. A., Kay, J. H., and Isaacs, J. P.: Constrictive pericarditis following traumatic hemopericardium. Ann. Surg., 142:97, 1955.

Morgagni, G. B.: De Sedibus et Causis Morborum per Anatomen Indagatis. Venetiis, typ. Remondiniana, 1761.

Mounsey, P.: The early diastolic sound of constrictive pericarditis. Br. Heart J., 17:143, 1955.

Ofori-Krakye, S. K., Tyberg, T. L., et al.: Late cardiac tamponade after open heart surgery: Incidence, role of anticoagulants in its pathogenesis and its relationship to the postpericardiotomy syndrome. Circulation, 63:1323, 1981.

Parsons, H. G., and Holman, E.: Experimental Ascites. Surg. Forum (1950). Philadelphia, W. B. Saunders Company, 1951, p. 251.

Parsons, H. G., and Holman, E.: Experimental segmental pericarditis. Arch. Surg., 70:479, 1955.

Peter, R. H., Whalen, R. E., Orgain, E. S., and McIntosh, H. D.: Postpericardiotomy syndrome as a complication of percutaneous left ventricular puncture. Am. J. Cardiol., 17:718, 1966.

Pick, F.: Ueber chronische, unter dem Bilde der Lebercirrhose verlaufende Pericarditis (pericarditische Pseudolebercirrhose) nebst Bemerkungen ueber Zuckergussleber (Curshmann). Z. Klin. Med., 29:385, 1896.

Potain, P. C.: Adhérence général du péricarde. Bull. Soc. Anat. Paris, Aug. 29, 1856.

Powers, P. P., Read, J. L., and Porter, R. R.: Acute idiopathic pericarditis simulating acute abdominal disease. J.A.M.A. 157:224, 1955.

Rehn, I.: Zur experimentellen Pathologie des Herzbeutels. Verh. Dtsch. Ges. Chir., 42:339, 1913.

Riolan, J.: Encheiridium Anatomicum et Pathologicum Lugduni Batavorum. Ex Officina Adriani Wyngaerden, 1649, p. 206.

Romero, *cited by* Baizeau: Mémoire sur le fonction du péricarde au point de vue chirurgical. Gaz. Med. Chir., 1868, p. 565.

Ronka, E. K. F., and Tessmer, C. F.: Congenital absence of pericardium: Report of case. Am. J. Pathol., 20:137, 1944.

Rose, E.: Herz Tamponade (Ein Beitrag zur Herzchirurgie). Dtsch. Z. Chir., 20:329, 1884.

Roshe, J., and Shumacker, H. B., Jr.: Pericardiectomy for chronic cardiac tamponade in children. Surgery, 46:1152, 1959.

Sauerbruch, F.: Die Chirurgie der Brustorgane, Vol. II (Berlin, 1925).

Schmieden, V., and Fischer, H.: Die Herzbeutelentzundung und ihre Folgezustande. Ergeb. Chir. Orthop., 19:98, 1926.

Schneider, S., and Rivier, J. L.: Hemopéricarde traumatique et péricarde calleux. Rev. Méd. Suisse Romande, 80:171, 1960.

Sellors, T. H.: Constrictive pericarditis. (Hunterian lecture abridged). Br. J. Surg., 33:215, 1946.

Sellors, T. H.: General observations on constrictive pericarditis with special reference to results of surgery. Minerva Cardioangiol. Europea, 4:489, 1956.

Senac, J. B.: Traité de la Structure du Coeur, de son Action, et de ses Maladies. v. 1. Paris, chez Briasson, 1749, p. 2.

Shackelford, R. T.: Hydropneumopericardium; Report of case with summary of the literature. J.A.M.A., 96:187, 1931.

Shidler, F. P., and Holman, E.: Mediastinal tumors: Presentation of 34 cases. Stanford Med. Bull., 10:217, 1952.

Schumacker, H. B., Jr., and Harris, J.: Pericardiectomy for chronic idiopathic pericarditis with massive effusion and cardiac tamponade. Surg. Gynecol. Obstet., 103:535, 1956.

Shumacker, H. B., Jr., and Roshe, J.: Pericardiectomy. J. Cardiovasc. Surg., 1:65, 1960.

Soulen, R. L., Lapayowker, M. S., and Gimenz, J. L.: Echocardiography in the diagnosis of pericardial effusion. Radiology, 86:1047, 1966.

Turner, A. F., Meyers, H. I., Jacobson, G., and Lo, W.: Carbon dioxide cineangiocardiography in the diagnosis of pericardial disease. Am. J. Roentgenol., 97:342, 1966.

Vieussens, R.: Traité Nouveau de la Structure et des Causes du Mouvement Naturel de Coeur. Toulouse, J. Guillemette, 1715.

Weill, E.: Traité Clinique des Maladies du Coeur chez les Enfants. Paris, O. Doin Co., 1895.

Weir, E. K., and Joffe, H. S.: Purulent pericarditis in children: An analysis of 28 cases. Thorax, 32:438, 1977.

White, P. D.: Chronic constrictive pericarditis (Pick's disease) treated by pericardial resection. Lancet, 2:597, 1935.

White, P. D.: Heart Disease. 4th Ed. New York, The Macmillan Co., 1951.

Wilkinson, P., Pinto, B., and Senior, J. R.: Reversible protein-losing enteropathy with intestinal lymphangiectasia secondary to chronic constrictive pericarditis. N. Engl. J. Med., 273:1178, 1965.

Wood, P.: Diagnosis of pericardial effusion by means of cardiac catheterization. Br. Heart J., 13:574, 1951.

Wood, P.: Diseases of the Heart and Circulation. 2nd Ed. Philadelphia, J. B. Lippincott Co., 1956.

Chapter 32

Atrial Septal Defect, Anomalous Pulmonary Veins, and Atrioventricular Canal

FRANK C. SPENCER

Defects in the atrial septum range from the simple, uncomplicated ostium secundum defect to the more complex ostium primum and atrioventricular canal, representing different degrees of severity of embryologic malformation of the atrial and ventricular septa. Partial anomalous drainage of the pulmonary veins is present in 10 to 15 per cent of secundum defects and is virtually always present with the sinus venosus defect. As the physiologic burden with a secundum defect and partial anomalous drainage of pulmonary veins is identical, consisting of a left-to-right shunt, these two abnormalities are considered together in the following section. In subsequent sections, the more severe abnormalities — total anomalous drainage of the pulmonary veins, ostium primum defect, and atrioventricular canal — are considered. In the last two malformations, mitral and tricuspid insufficiencies are usually present in addition to the left-to-right shunt.

ATRIAL SEPTAL DEFECT AND PARTIAL ANOMALOUS DRAINAGE OF PULMONARY VEINS

Historical Considerations

Several ingenious operative approaches developed between 1947 and 1955, before extracorporeal circulation became clinically possible, are now only of historical interest. The modern era of extracorporeal circulation actually began in 1953, when the first successful intracardiac operation in man was done by Gibbon to close an atrial septal defect (Gibbon, 1954).

Similarly, little could be done with anomalous drainage of pulmonary veins until extracorporeal circulation was possible. The abnormality was well recognized, and a few isolated closed heart operations were successful, including that reported by Muller (1951) in which an anomalous left pulmonary vein was connected to the left atrium. Between 1952 and 1955, temporary occlusion of the venae cavae for 10 to 12 minutes during hypothermia at 28° to 30°C. was used to correct certain abnormalities. Such operations, of course, were hampered by the sharp limita-tion in time and the uncertainties about the exact diagnosis (Spencer and Bahnson, 1959). Widespread, safe surgical therapy promptly became possible with the development of extracorporeal circulation.

Pathologic Features

Secundum-type atrial defects are among the most common cardiac malformations, representing 10 to 15 per cent of all patients with congenital heart disease. Females are affected about twice as frequently as males. No etiologic factors are known.

Atrial defects vary widely in size and location. Most are 2 to 3 cm. in diameter, ranging from as small as 1 cm. to virtual absence of the atrial septum. Occasionally, the atrial septum is fenestrated with multiple defects. A foramen ovale is a normal opening, not an abnormality, as it occurs in 15 to 25 per cent of adult hearts. With its slit-like construction, it is normally sealed, unless there is a marked rise in right atrial pressure.

Most secundum defects are in the mid-portion of the septum. *Low* defects may involve the orifice of the inferior vena cava, requiring caution at operation to avoid constriction of the caval orifice. In 5 to 10 per cent of patients, a *high* defect occurs at the junction of the superior vena cava and the right atrium, termed a sinus venosus defect because of its embryologic origin. Anomalous drainage of the pulmonary veins from the right upper lobe into the superior vena cava occurs in almost all such patients. Hence, this is the most common variety of atrial septal defect associated with anomalous pulmonary veins.

Less frequently, veins enter directly into the posterior wall of the right atrium, anterior to the margin of the atrial septal defect. The rarest abnormality is entry of the pulmonary veins into the inferior vena cava. A variant of this unusual anomaly, associated with other malformations, has been termed the "scimitar" syndrome, emphasizing the radiologic appearance produced by the shadow of the anomalous pulmonary vein parallel to the right border of the heart. There is usually an associated hypoplasia of the right lung and anomalous origin of the pulmonary arteries from the aorta. Because the amount of blood shunted through the hypoplastic lung is small, the physiologic disturbance is not severe.

Partial anomalous drainage of pulmonary veins usually involves the veins of only one lung, but a few unusual examples of partial drainage of pulmonary veins from both lungs have been reported. In addition, anomalous pulmonary veins rarely are found entering the right atrium with an intact atrial septum. One of the most detailed reports of the variety of pathologic patterns that occurs with anomalous pulmonary veins was published by Blake and associates (1965), an analysis of 113 patients from the Armed Forces Institute of Pathology. Twenty-seven patterns were found. This fact emphasizes the importance of routinely identifying the location of all pulmonary veins at the time of operation.

In a small percentage of patients with a secundum defect, mitral stenosis is also present, a combination termed Lutembacher's syndrome. With restriction of flow of blood into the left ventricle because of the mitral stenosis, an enormous left-to-right shunt is present, with massive dilatation of the pulmonary arteries. Craig and Selzer (1968) pointed out that the combination of lesions represented a true susceptibility of patients with secundum defects to rheumatic fever, because the frequency of the syndrome was far greater than would occur from random association. Mitral stenosis also is virtually never found with other congenital lesions, such as ventricular septal defect or mitral insufficiency.

Finally, mitral insufficiency rarely occurs in association with a secundum defect. It is usually unsuspected because of the absence of findings, but in a few instances, closure of the atrial septal defect without recognizing the mitral insufficiency produced fatal pulmonary congestion similar to that resulting from closure of a primum defect without correction of the associated mitral insufficiency.

This rare syndrome can either be recognized on a preoperative ventriculogram or detected at operation by routine measurement of left atrial pressure following closure of the secundum defect.

Although sufficient data are not available, probably the mitral insufficiency in such patients could be corrected by a type of Carpentier ring valvuloplasty, as described in Chapter 46 on mitral valve disease.

Pathophysiology

An atrial septal defect results in a shunt of oxygenated blood from the left atrium to the right atrium because the left ventricle is a thicker muscle than the right ventricle. The difference in thickness is reflected by a difference in distensibility of the two ventricles, as a result of which, with an intact atrial septum, normal mean left atrial pressure is near 8 to 10 mm. Hg, whereas normal mean right atrial pressure is seldom above 4 to 5 mm. Hg. During the first 2 years of life, the right ventricle is similar to the left. Thus,

only a small shunt may exist across an atrial septal defect, increasing in magnitude with growth of the child. Hence, an atrial septal defect may be first recognized in children over 2 to 3 years of age.

Rudolph (1974) offered an alternative explanation for infants in whom catheterization a few hours after birth shows a large shunt at the atrial level, suggesting that differences in the vascular resistance in the pulmonary and systemic circulations may be as important as the difference in distensibility of the two ventricles.

Depending on both the size of the defect and the difference in distensibility between the two ventricles, the size of the shunt varies from as little as 1 L./min. to as great as 20 L./min. Usually, the pulmonary blood flow is two to three times greater than the systemic blood flow. Fortunately, there is a reciprocal decrease in pulmonary vascular resistance with the increased pulmonary blood flow, so that pulmonary hypertension is rare. It is rare in childhood but does develop in 15 to 20 per cent of adults. One of the enigmas of the pathophysiology of congenital heart disease is the frequency of development of a progressive increase in pulmonary vascular resistance, ultimately to a lethal degree, with an untreated ventricular septal defect or aortopulmonary window, whereas with an atrial septal defect, even with a large shunt, such an increase in pulmonary vascular resistance virtually never develops in the first several years of life.

Because the intracardiac shunt causes a reduction in systemic blood flow, there may be retardation of growth and development, producing a so-called gracile habitus. In adults, the cardiac index is usually near the lower limits of normal (2.5 L./M.²/min.). In a group of 128 adult patients studied by Craig and Selzer (1968), only nine had a cardiac index less than 2.0. A slight decrease in arterial oxygen saturation is frequent, probably from mixing of oxygenated and unoxygenated blood in the atria. In this group, they found that 51 had an arterial oxygen saturation of 90 to 94 per cent, and 17 had saturations less than 90 per cent. Severe hypoxia appears only when there is a marked increase in pulmonary vascular resistance.

The handicap from a pulmonary blood flow two to three times greater than normal is surprisingly well tolerated in most children. Most are asymptomatic; a few have dyspnea on extreme exertion. There may be some increase in susceptibility to pneumonia, as well as an increased susceptibility to rheumatic fever. Fortunately, bacterial endocarditis is almost unknown. With the benign course of atrial defects in childhood in many patients, the natural question was whether such a course would continue in adult life. In the same report on 128 patients over 18 years of age, Craig and Selzer found the majority had dyspnea on exertion but were not seriously limited. Overt cardiac failure, with or without chronic atrial fibrillation, occurred in only a small percentage, most of whom were over 40 years of age. The most alarming finding, however, was an increase in pulmonary vascular resistance above the upper limits of normal (400 dynes/sec./cm.⁻⁵) in 13 per cent of patients. This was a very grave finding, representing a catastrophe, because the development of a major increase in pulmonary vascular resistance changed an atrial septal defect from an easily curable lesion to an inevitably lethal one. The pattern of development of an increase in pulmonary vascular resistance was accordingly studied in some detail in the 18 patients in whom it occurred. It could not be correlated with age or with the degree of increase in pulmonary blood flow. Hence, it was not a "wear and tear" phenomenon. Apparently, an individual susceptibility of unknown type was the basic factor. The increased resistance occurred in about one third of patients before 20 years of age, in another one third in the third and fourth decades, and in the remainder after 40 years of age. In a few patients studied with serial catheterizations, the rise in pulmonary vascular resistance, once it began, continued at a rapid rate. In two patients, it continued despite surgical closure of the defect.

This unpredictability of the development of an increase in pulmonary vascular resistance, although it never occurs in the majority of patients, constitutes sufficient reason in itself to routinely close atrial septal defects in all patients whenever they are diagnosed, even though the majority are asymptomatic.

Also in 1968, Gault and associates reported studies in 62 patients over 40 years of age. In contrast to the younger group reported by Craig and Selzer, most were symptomatic, with 45 per cent classified as Class III or Class IV cardiac patients. Seventy per cent had an increase in pulmonary vascular resistance, a frequency identical to that found by Craig and Selzer.

Craig and Selzer commented on the rarity of a patient over 50 years of age with an atrial septal defect. Statistical analyses indicate that this low frequency is far less than would occur in the normal population, implying that most patients have succumbed to either cardiac failure or pulmonary hypertension before the sixth decade. The average life expectancy of all patients with atrial septal defects has been estimated to be near 40 years. Fifteen to 20 per cent of patients die from pulmonary hypertension. The others die from cardiac failure 15 to 20 years earlier than the normal population.

Clinical Features

When symptoms are present, the most common are exertional dyspnea, fatigue, and palpitations. In a 1966 study of 275 patients who were operated on, Sellers and colleagues found that 113 were asymptomatic. As mentioned earlier, dyspnea is much more frequent in adults, resulting from either pulmonary hypertension or cardiac failure. Atrial arrhythmias become more frequent in the fourth decade, probably from hypertrophy of the right atrium, and may precipitate or intensify symptoms of congestive failure. As with atrial fibrillation developing with chronic mitral stenosis, such arrhythmias may be permanent, remaining even after closure of the septal defect. Cyanosis appears only in the small percentage of patients in whom pulmonary vascular resistance has increased sufficiently to produce a large right-to-left shunt.

On physical examination, a soft, systolic murmur in the left second or third intercostal space near the sternum is the most common finding. The murmur arises from the increased flow of blood through the pulmonic valve. Wide, fixed splitting of the second sound is another important auscultatory finding.

On the chest roentgenogram, slight to moderate cardiac enlargement from dilatation of the right ventricle may be evident. Enlargement of the pulmonary artery is frequent. The electrocardiogram usually shows typical abnormalities, including right ventricular hypertrophy with a right axis deviation and conduction abnormalities.

The diagnosis can be readily confirmed by cardiac catheterization, which demonstrates that blood in the right atrium has a greater degree of oxygen saturation than blood in the venae cavae. The presence of anomalous pulmonary veins can be recognized if the cardiac catheter enters a pulmonary vein directly from the superior vena cava. If the pulmonary vein is entered from the right atrium, however, the diagnosis is uncertain, because the catheter may have traversed an atrial septal defect. Fortunately, precise delineation of the pulmonary veins can be done with selective angiography. In addition, their location should be checked routinely at operation. In most patients, the systolic right ventricular pressure is between 30 and 40 mm. Hg. With large shunts, a gradient of 20 to 40 mm. Hg may be found across the normal pulmonic valve because of the increased flow of blood.

Surgical Treatment

Indications and Contraindications. Operation is usually recommended if cardiac catheterization reveals an increase in pulmonary blood flow more than one and one half times greater than systemic blood flow. Because children with a shunt of this size are almost always asymptomatic, the decision for operation is based entirely on the findings at catheterization. The ideal time for operation is near the age of 5 or 6, before the child starts school, in order to avoid the psychologic school handicap of having a "heart problem."

The only contraindication to operation is a marked increase in pulmonary vascular resistance, which, fortunately, is now virtually never seen. If the pulmonary vascular resistance has increased to more than 50 per cent of systemic resistance, the risk of operation may be as great as 50 per cent, and surviving patients may show little benefit. As the progressive nature of the increasing pulmonary vascular resistance is well documented, however, such patients should be operated on, because operation is their only chance for long-term survival.

Age per se is not a contraindication, for several reports in the past decade have demonstrated the benefit of operations in patients with congestive failure in their fifth and sixth decades (Yalav *et al.*, 1971). In 1969, Hanlon and coworkers described experiences with 56 patients over 60 years of age. In a discussion of this report, Ellis reported 155 patients over 45 years of age, 21 of whom had had thromboembolic complications. In 1968, Gault and associates described a 7 per cent mortality rate in 31 patients over 40 years old, 45 per cent of whom were functional Class III or IV before operation.

Technique of Operation. All patients are operated on with extracorporeal circulation. The technique for extracorporeal circulation currently used at New York University is described in Chapter 46. A median sternotomy incision is employed, except in females. In female patients, for cosmetic reasons, a right thoracotomy in the fourth intercostal space gives satisfactory exposure if the patient is positioned properly in an anterolateral position, turned about 60 degrees from the horizontal plane. Brom (1980) has described a submammary incision used in Holland for over a decade for cosmetic purposes that gives satisfactory results. If there is any uncertainty about the diagnosis, certainly a median sternotomy should be employed, because the ability to treat previously unrecognized cardiac pathology is significantly hampered if operation is performed through a right anterolateral incision.

Once the pericardial cavity has been opened, the atrium is explored with a finger introduced through the atrial appendage. Seven or eight anatomic features should be routinely identified: the size and location of the atrial septal defect and its relation to the orifices of the superior and inferior venae cavae; the point of entry of the right and left pulmonary veins; the size and location of the coronary sinus ostium (a large ostium indicates a left superior vena cava); the presence of any mitral or tricuspid insufficiency; and the ventricular septum, which normally bulges in systole, unless a septal defect is present.

The superior vena cava is carefully inspected for anomalous pulmonary veins entering the cava directly. Absence of the left innominate vein usually indicates the presence of a left superior vena cava. A left superior vena cava is an important anomaly to recognize, as it can be simply managed at operation by a variety of methods. If it is not recognized, the operative field is, of course, flooded with blood. It can be detected by any of three methods: noting an enlarged coronary sinus on palpation, noting the absence of a left innominate vein, or elevating the heart and noting the left superior vena cava entering the coronary sinus just above the left atrial appendage.

Once cardiopulmonary bypass has been established, the temperature is lowered to 25°C., and the heart is arrested by infusion of cold blood with potassium, using the technique described under open mitral commissurotomy in Chapter 46. Topical hypothermia is also briefly used to lower the myocardial temperature to below 20°C. With the aorta clamped and the heart arrested and cooled, the right atrium is opened widely and the intracardiac structures are identified, confirming the location of the structures previously palpated. Ventilation of the lungs is stopped. A crucial point is to *avoid* aspirating intracardiac blood from the left of the septal defect, which will introduce air into the left atrium. If for any reason this is done

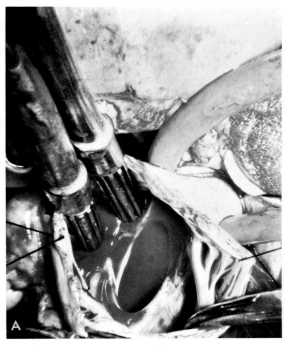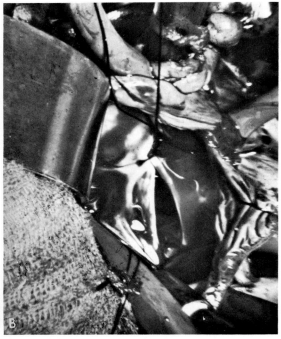

Figure 32–1. *A,* An atrial septal defect located in the midportion of the atrial septum. *B,* Such defects can usually be closed by direct suture. A suture has been inserted at the top margin of the defect and will be continued caudad to approximate the two edges. Care is taken as the final sutures are inserted to avoid trapping air in the left atrial cavity.

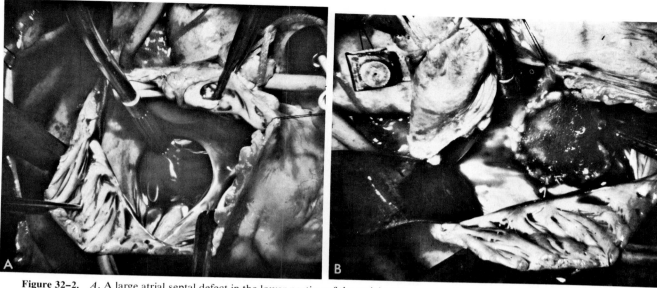

Figure 32–2. *A*, A large atrial septal defect in the lower portion of the atrial septum, extending to the orifice of the inferior vena cava. The patient, an adult, had gradually developed increasing congestive failure. *B*, A Teflon felt patch has been attached with circumferential sutures to close the defect.

because of uncertainty of pathology in the left side of the heart, the danger of fatal trapping of air is significant. Maneuvers for removal of air similar to those used after replacement of the mitral valve should then be employed. If the left atrium remains filled with blood during the procedure, these measures are unnecessary. The reason that introduction of air into the left atrium may be disastrous is because blood from the aorta may drain from the aortic valve into the left ventricle and into the left atrium, with air rising from the left atrium into the aorta, much as air enters a bottle filled with fluid when the bottle is turned upside down and fluid poured out. This insidious accumulation of air in the aorta can easily be fatal if not prevented or treated.

Once the margins of the defect have been identified, closure can be done with a continuous suture, usually 3-0 Prolene in 70 to 80 per cent of patients (Fig. 32–1). If the lower margin of the defect is missing, the defect ending on the inferior atrial wall near the vena cava, one or two purse-string sutures may be inserted and tied to be certain that the orifice of the inferior vena cava is not constricted. These sutures are placed well away from the coronary sinus and the AV node.

Complete heart block can occur in adult patients, probably from traction or stretching in the region of the coronary sinus (Fig. 32–2). In older patients, especially those with a large defect, perhaps a patch of pericardium inserted with a circumferential suture, rather than a direct suture, may be preferable, as tissues in the adult are less elastic than those in the child (Fig. 32–2). After all sutures have been placed, but before they are tightened, the atrium is allowed to fill with blood and the lungs are gently ventilated, causing red blood to spurt from the left atrium through the defect and mix with the darker blood in the right

atrium. The sutures are then tied while partially covered with blood. This is a very valuable method for being certain that all air has been removed from the left atrium.

The aortic occlusion clamp may be released at this time, venting the aorta as an additional precaution to be certain that air has not inadvertently risen into the aorta. Our preference is to induce ventricular fibrillation before the aorta is unclamped and leave the heart fibrillating after unclamping the aorta until the right atriotomy has been sutured. Fibrillation is used to prevent contraction of the heart during suturing of the right atrium because of the rare possibility that contraction of the right ventricle, with a competent tricuspid valve, might propel air through the pulmonary circulation into the left heart and produce air embolism.

Once the incisions have been sutured, bypass is slowed and stopped. Left and right atrial pressures are routinely checked for reasons described earlier. The correction of all left-to-right shunts can be confirmed by aspirating blood from the superior and inferior venae cavae and pulmonary artery, confirming that oxygen saturation from all three areas is similar.

In patients with anomalous drainage of both right pulmonary veins into the right atrium, a patch of pericardium or knitted Dacron should be used to close the defect, bringing the suture line onto the right atrial wall in front of the point of entry of the pulmonary veins, so that the veins enter the left atrium normally. This is preferable to the older technique of directly suturing the margin of the defect to the atrial wall anterior to the point of entry of the pulmonary veins (Fig. 32–3).

When a sinus venosus defect is present—the combination of a high atrial septal defect and anomalous pulmonary veins entering the superior vena cava

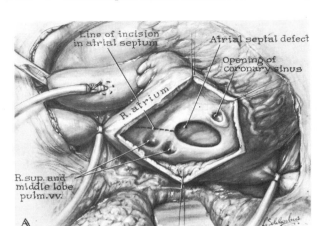

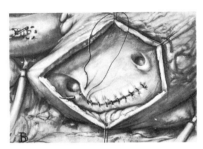

Figure 32–3. Atrial septal defect with anomalous drainage of pulmonary veins into the right atrium. In this patient, enlargement of the septal defect was necessary to permit shifting of the atrial septum to divert the anomalous pulmonary veins into the left atrium. A prosthetic patch could also have been used. The operation illustrated was performed under hypothermia in 1958. (From Bahnson, H. T., Spencer, F. C., and Neill, C. A.: Surgical treatment of 35 cases of drainage of pulmonary veins to the right side of the heart. J. Thorac. Surg., *36*:787, 1958.)

— certain guidelines are crucial. Repair is safe and effective when properly done, but a number of serious or lethal disasters can occur, such as thrombosis of the superior vena cava or thrombosis of the pulmonary veins. The first principle is to dissect the extrapericardial superior vena cava superiorly above the point of entry of the azygos vein and encircle it at this point. For embryologic reasons, anomalous pulmonary veins entering the superior vena cava above the point of entry of the azygos vein are virtually unknown.

Second, the right pleural cavity should be opened to facilitate identification of the right pulmonary veins when the cava is opened by the simple introduction of a curved clamp into the ostium of the veins, and noting that the clamp enters the veins coming from the lung.

Third, the cardiac incision should begin in the right atrium and be extended up the *right* anterolateral wall of the superior vena cava to remain well away from the area of the sinus node. The incision should be extended superiorly to the highest point of entry of the anomalous veins. If the superior caval cannula has been snared above the azygos vein, occluding the azygos vein as well, exposure is excellent. However, if this has not been done, it may be impossible to

expose the orifice of the anomalous veins because of blood flowing from the superior cava when the caval cannula is retracted.

Once adequate exposure has been obtained, a patch of pericardium can be inserted with a continuous suture of 4-0 Prolene, sewing around the point of entry of the pulmonary veins and the atrial defect so that the pulmonary veins are diverted into the left atrium (Fig. 32–4). The sutures should be placed in the superficial portion of the posterior caval wall to avoid injury to the sinus node. Usually, the reconstruction can be done without significant stenosis of the superior cava. If stenosis does occur, the superior vena cava can be widened by the application of another patch, usually of pericardium. Proper correction of the abnormality without stenosis can be confirmed by measuring pressures in the superior vena cava, pulmonary veins, and right atrium after completion of the procedure.

In the rare patient with a single atrium resulting from absence of the atrial septum, additional anomalies are common. The most frequent is a cleft in the mitral valve. Occasionally, a left superior vena cava enters the left atrium directly, rather than through the coronary sinus. This requires construction of an intracardiac tunnel to adequately drain the left superior vena cava into the right atrium, unless it is so small that it can be safely ligated.

In the majority of patients, convalescence following operation is uneventful. Atrial fibrillation is the most frequent postoperative arrhythmia, occurring most commonly in adult patients.

In 1969, Hawe and associates analyzed results following repair in 546 patients at the Mayo Clinic, particularly observing the occurrence of emboli some time after operation. Atrial fibrillation was present before operation in only 33 patients, but 50 per cent of patients over 40 years of age had atrial fibrillation. Quite striking was the fact that 35 of the 546 patients had an embolic episode some time after operation, as late as 10 years afterward in some patients. These usually occurred in older patients with atrial fibrillation, indicating that long-term anticoagulation should perhaps be considered in such patients. Amputation of the left atrial appendage is another possible form of preventive treatment. At New York University, for uncertain reasons, this has not been recognized as a significant problem.

The risk of operation if pulmonary vascular resistance is normal is surprisingly small. A number of reports between 1966 and 1970 described experiences with more than 100 patients, with the mortality rate varying from 0 to 2 per cent (Stansel *et al.*, 1971). In my experience with secundum defects, no deaths have been seen in children in the past 20 years. One death occurred about 10 years ago in a 65-year-old adult from massive neurologic injury, probably air embolism.

Fortunately, even in patients over 40 years of age with pulmonary hypertension or cardiac failure, significant benefits usually result. In 1968, Gault and

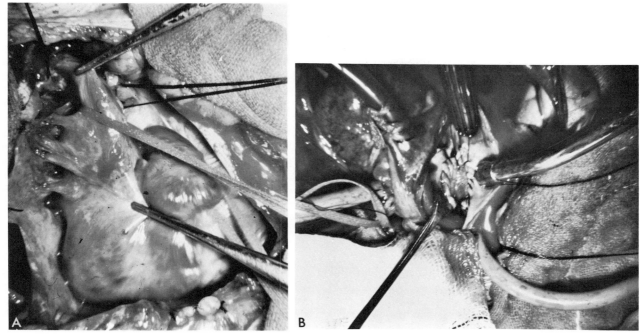

Figure 32–4. *A,* Three anomalous pulmonary veins entering the superior vena cava near its juncture with the right atrium. This anomalous drainage is frequently encountered with the sinus venosus type of atrial septal defect. *B,* A pericardial patch has been applied to close the atrial septal defect in such a manner that the anomalous veins entering the superior vena cava are diverted into the left atrium. The cannula in the superior vena cava has been retracted upward, illustrating that insertion of the patch has not significantly narrowed the diameter of the superior vena cava.

associates reported that operations performed on 62 patients over 40 years of age resulted in substantial improvement in the majority. Similarly, in 1967, Coles and colleagues described the late findings in 10 of 12 adults with pulmonary hypertension who survived operation. Almost all showed marked clinical improvement. Studies 4 years after operation found a late regression in pulmonary vascular resistance to about two thirds of the preoperative value.

OSTIUM PRIMUM DEFECTS

Ostium primum defects are unusual, representing about 5 per cent of all atrial septal defects. They result from arrested development of the endocardial cushions that normally meet with the atrial and ventricular septa during embryonic life to form the four chambers of the heart. Primum defects are found in 20 to 30 per cent of children with mongolism, but other than this unusual association, no etiologic factors are known.

Atrioventricularis communis, discussed in a subsequent section, is a more severe malformation caused by a similar but more extensive arrest in development of the endocardial cushions. The abnormally long and narrow aortic vestibule, where, during embryonic development, the aortic infundibulum joins the left ventricle, indicates the diffuse extent of the arrest in development (Gerbode *et al.,* 1967). Because of the embryonic origin of these malformations, synonyms for ostium primum defects and atrioventricularis com-

munis are endocardial cushion defects, partial or complete, or atrioventricular canal, partial or complete.

The two significant defects are a cleft in the anterior leaflet of the mitral valve and a low, crescent-shaped defect in the atrial septum, the inferior border of which is the top of the ventricular septum. The sickle-shaped superior border of an ostium primum defect can be recognized easily on digital palpation, differentiating it from the more common low secundum defect.

Even in the unusual clinical circumstance in which the presence of an ostium primum defect was not suspected before operation, the diagnosis can be readily made by this characteristic finding on palpation.

There is considerable variation in the degree of mitral regurgitation present, although a cleft of varying extent is found in the aortic leaflet of the mitral valve in the majority of patients. The reason for this variation, even though a cleft is almost always present, is uncertain. It is probably related to the fortuitous attachment of the chordae tendineae. Associated defects in the tricuspid valve are present in nearly half of the patients, although, fortunately, the degree of tricuspid insufficiency is clinically insignificant and does not require surgical treatment.

The chordae tendineae are usually normally attached along the margins of the two halves of the cleft aortic leaflet of the mitral valve. These are valuable guidelines during repair. In some patients, however, there are anomalous chordae, attached either to the cleft margin or directly to the ventricular septum, that may partly obstruct the left ventricular outflow tract.

There is also considerable variation in the size and shape of the cleft in the aortic leaflet. In some patients, it resembles a triangle, resulting from absence of tissue, rather than a simple cleft. As a result of these pathologic variations, there is a corresponding wide range in the severity of mitral insufficiency, absent in some patients but severe in others. Associated abnormalities also occur frequently, being found in 40 of 232 patients described by McMullan and associates (1973). The most common of these were a secundum defect, pulmonic stenosis, and anomalous venae cavae.

Pathophysiology

The two physiologic abnormalities are a left-to-right shunt at the atrial level combined with mitral insufficiency. When mitral insufficiency is small, the disability is identical to that of a secundum defect. When insufficiency is severe, cardiac failure and pulmonary hypertension develop at a much earlier age than in secundum defects. In the previously quoted series by McMullan and coworkers (1973), catheterization data were described in 74 patients. The ratio of pulmonary flow to systemic flow was 2.7, ranging from 1.3 to 5.6. Pulmonary resistance averaged 2.7 units per square meter, ranging from 0.5 to 7.5. Systemic pulmonary artery pressure greater than 30 mm. Hg was found in 36 patients.

With the described range in degree of mitral insufficiency, there is a corresponding wide range in symptoms. With severe mitral insufficiency, exertional dyspnea is common, with other symptoms of pulmonary congestion if cardiac failure is more severe. In a series of 30 patients described by Braunwald and Morrow (1966), as well as in 48 patients reported by Ellis and associates, 30 to 50 per cent were asymptomatic.

On physical examination, the dominant finding is a loud systolic murmur along the left sternal border as well as at the cardiac apex, warning that some abnormality other than a simple secundum defect is present. The pulmonic second sound is increased in intensity and widely split. If cardiac failure is present, there may be signs of pulmonary and hepatic congestion.

The findings on the chest roentgenogram are variable. Enlargement of the pulmonary artery is the most frequent abnormality. With severe abnormalities, there is corresponding enlargement of the right ventricle. However, if mitral insufficiency is dominant, there is preponderant enlargement of the left ventricle.

The electrocardiogram almost always shows a left axis deviation and may provide the first clue on clinical evaluation to the correct diagnosis. There are varying degrees of right and left ventricular hypertrophy. Conduction defects, with prolongation of the P-R interval, are frequent. The electrocardiographic abnormalities are due primarily to the conduction defect and not to the associated left ventricular hypertrophy.

The most characteristic finding is on the vectorcardiogram, in which the frontal plane is characteristically inscribed in a counterclockwise loop, an occurrence regularly associated with ostium primum defects and virtually confirming the diagnosis. On cardiac catheterization, the left-to-right shunt at the atrial level can be readily demonstrated. The degree of mitral insufficiency is best evaluated by left ventricular angiography. Normally, the diagnosis can be established with reasonable certainty from the clinical picture, the changes on the electrocardiogram and vectorcardiogram, and the findings on cardiac catheterization.

Surgical Treatment

In most patients, operation should be performed once the diagnosis has been established, if the child is older than 3 or 4 years. Operation can be performed in younger children — or infants — if there is significant cardiac failure and pulmonary hypertension. Fortunately, there has been a great reduction in mortality in operations with infants and children less than 2 years of age in recent years. Earlier, the mortality rate was as high as 27 per cent in patients operated on under 1 year of age, as compared with a mortality rate of 2 per cent in patients operated on between the ages of 6 and 19 (McMullan *et al.*, 1973).

As the course of the disease progresses rapidly, with eventual congestive heart failure and pulmonary hypertension, there is little advantage in postponing operation beyond 4 to 5 years of age, even in the absence of symptoms. Rarely, an adult is seen in the third, fourth, or fifth decade with a history of little disability. In such patients, mitral insufficiency is minimal, and the clinical course has resembled that of a secundum defect (Fig. 32–5).

Technique of Operation. The four principal objectives are repair of the mitral insufficiency, avoidance of heart block, closure of the atrial septal defect, and prevention of air embolism (Fig. 32–6). A median sternotomy is preferable. Although a right anterior thoracotomy in the fourth intercostal space provides good exposure, it is much less satisfactory for prevention of air embolism. Palpation of the intracardiac chambers through the right atrial appendage will readily confirm the diagnosis, with note being taken of the characteristic upper curved margin of the septal defect, as described earlier. The degree of mitral insufficiency can be estimated by noting the vigor of the regurgitant jet.

At present, with the safety and simplicity of potassium cardioplegia, there is a choice in operative approach between performing the entire procedure during cardiac arrest with induced potassium cardioplegia or performing part of the procedure with ventricular fibrillation and then completing it with potassium cardioplegia. Our preference is for the latter

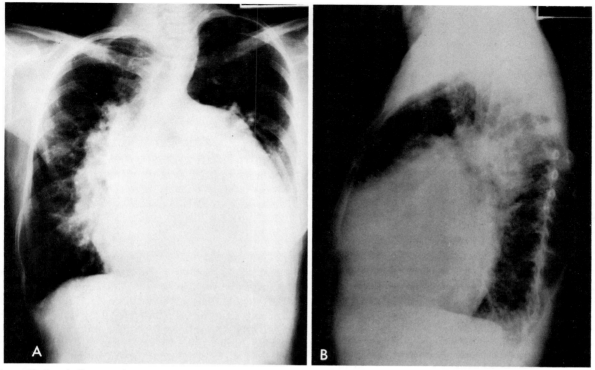

Figure 32–5. *A*, Preoperative chest roentgenogram of a 45-year-old woman with massive cardiomegaly from a large atrial septal defect, operated on with blood cardioplegia. Recovery was uneventful. *B*, Preoperative lateral chest roentgenogram of the patient described in *A*.

technique, which provides greater protection from the production of heart block for the reasons described in the following paragraphs.

Once bypass has been started, ventricular fibrillation is induced before the atrium is opened to prevent air embolism. The right atrium is opened widely, and appropriate retractors are inserted. A left ventricular vent is inserted at this time to aspirate intracardiac blood. The intracardiac anatomy is carefully examined, noting the size of the septal defect, the extent of the cleft of the mitral valve, the presence of abnormal chordae that might obstruct the aortic outflow tract, any abnormalities in the tricuspid valve, and the presence of any ventricular septal defect.

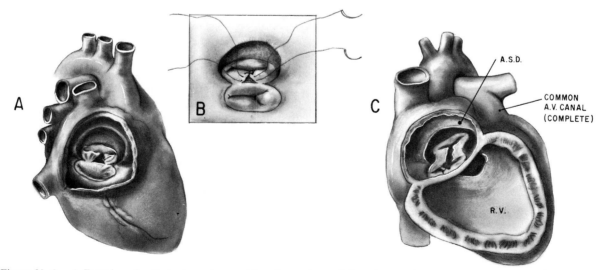

Figure 32–6. *A*, Drawing of pathologic anatomy with ostium primum defect that consists of a low atrial septal defect, ending on the ventricular septum, with a cleft of the mitral valve. *B*, The insert shows repair of the cleft mitral valve with interrupted sutures, after which the atrial septal defect can be closed. *C*, The extensive malformation present with atrioventricularis communis. There is extensive deformity of the mitral and tricuspid valves, with a large cleft between the two valves, creating both mitral and tricuspid insufficiency. In addition, there are atrial and ventricular septal defects. These may vary from a small defect to virtually complete absence of the ventricular septum. (From Schwartz, S. I. (Ed.): Principles of Surgery, 2nd Ed. New York, McGraw-Hill Book Co., 1974.)

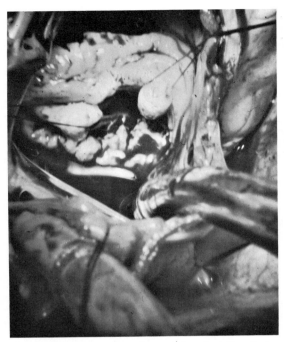

Figure 32–7. Operative photograph of cleft mitral valve through an incision in the atrial septum. Sutures have been placed in the margins of the cleft valve. The ventricular septum is visible in the midportion of the field, with the orifice of the tricuspid valve at the superior part of the field.

The cleft in the mitral valve is repaired first, using figure-of-eight sutures of Teflon or Dacron (Fig. 32–7). As the edges of the cleft are rolled and thickened, the margins should be stretched to permit insertion of the sutures precisely in the free margin to prevent abnormal shortening of the reconstructed leaflet. The sutures are inserted from the ventricular septum medially out to near the area of the insertion of the chordae tendineae on the margin of the mitral valve centrally. There is little risk of producing mitral stenosis. The usual error is inadequate correction of the mitral insufficiency.

For the last 3 years, we have found the selective induction of mitral insufficiency by manipulating a catheter retrograde from the aorta across the aortic valve to be a useful guide in assessing residual mitral insufficiency after suture of the cleft. This is described in detail in Chapter 46 in the discussion of mitral commissurotomy.

Division of abnormal chordae has been recommended by some. We remain uncertain about the value and safety of this maneuver, having had one patient in whom division of an abnormal chorda was associated with significant postoperative mitral insufficiency.

The use of the retrograde catheter has demonstrated that residual insufficiency is often diffuse, centrally located, and not amenable to correction by further suturing of the cleft mitral valve. Perhaps the anuloplasty technique of Carpentier with the Carpentier ring would be useful in these circumstances,

although we have not had experience with this. The advantage of recognizing the extent of any residual mitral insufficiency following suturing of the cleft is obvious, if additional valvuloplasty maneuvers can be performed.

Following repair of the mitral valve cleft, the atrial defect is closed with a patch, usually pericardium, although knitted Dacron seems to give equally good results. The atrioventricular conduction bundle is along the posterior border of the septal defect, originating at the AV node near the coronary sinus ostium and traveling downward to the ventricular septum. It is very susceptible to injury but, fortunately, can be protected with proper precautions (Gerbode *et al.*, 1967). A bundle of His detector has been used periodically by some groups but has never been found feasible for routine clinical use.

The importance of precise surgical technique is evidenced by the reported variation in frequency of heart block, ranging from as high as 20 per cent in operations performed over 20 years ago to as low as 1 to 2 per cent in recent reports. In our experience, an important guide in avoiding heart block is to defibrillate the heart after the sutures have been inserted along the posterior rim of the defect, to be certain that the conduction is intact. Our preference is to place a series of interrupted sutures superficially to the *left* of the rim of the defect, directly in the anulus of the mitral valve. This is precisely done, making traction on the mitral valve by encircling appropriate chordae tendineae to stretch the mitral valve and define the anulus exactly. The heart is then defibrillated and the electrocardiogram observed to confirm adequacy of conduction. Once this has been done, the heart can be arrested by the induction of potassium cardioplegia and the operative procedure can be completed. The previously placed sutures are threaded through the pericardial patch, which is then tied in position.

Once the sutures near the conduction bundle have been tied, the remaining margins of the patch can be easily attached with a continuous suture of 4-0 Prolene. Any defect in the tricuspid valve is usually left alone, as it is not amenable to simple repair and has not been found to be clinically significant.

Prevention of air embolism is a critical feature of the operation, because air can be expelled by the functioning left ventricle once the mitral valve has been made competent by repair of the cleft. This is one of the obvious attractions of routine potassium cardioplegia with cardiac arrest. When the heart is defibrillated to monitor the electrocardiogram, the mitral valve is carefully kept incompetent to prevent any expulsion of air from the left ventricle into the aorta. The heart is then arrested. When the aorta is unclamped, following closure of the different cardiac incisions, air is removed from the atria, from the ventricle through the left ventricular vent, and from the aorta through a vent, vigorously ventilating the lungs and massaging the cardiac chambers with the heart fibrillating. After all of this is done, the heart is then defibrillated, maintaining gentle suction on a catheter in the aortic root until bypass is stopped. With this technique, neurologic injury has not occurred in our experience in the past several years.

Following cessation of cardiopulmonary bypass, the left atrial pressure should be measured, noting the contour as well as the absolute level. Although not diagnostic, the contour of the left atrial pressure provides some indication of any residual mitral insufficiency. A similar abnormal contour, however, can result simply from cardiac failure. Theoretically, severe mitral insufficiency and inadequate cardiac output could necessitate prosthetic replacement of the mitral valve at the time of operation. In our experience, however, replacement with a prosthetic valve has never been found necessary at the initial operation.

A pacemaker wire is routinely left in the right ventricle and right atrium for a few days after operation because of the frequency of transitory conduction defects, probably from edema near the conduction bundle.

Postoperative Considerations

Postoperative recovery is usually uneventful if the hazards described earlier are avoided. A permanent heart block, fortunately virtually unknown in our experience, should be treated by implantation of a pacemaker before discharge from the hospital because of the risk of sudden death in such cases. Most patients have a mild residual systolic murmur, often of no hemodynamic significance. A loud apical systolic murmur warns that significant mitral insufficiency may be present on subsequent left ventricular angiography.

The risk of operation is now small, in the range of 1 to 3 per cent. Ten years ago, McMullan and associates (1973) at the Mayo Clinic reported a series of 232 patients with an operative mortality of 5.6 per cent, and only 2 per cent in patients over 6 years of age. By contrast, in a series of 100 patients operated on in France reported by Lévy in 1974, the overall mortality was 16 per cent, decreasing to 5 per cent during the last 4 years. These discrepancies in mortality clearly indicate the importance of precise technical details during operation.

In 1978 Losay and colleagues reported experiences at the Children's Hospital in Boston over a period of 20 years (1955 to 1975) with the operative repair of 92 patients. The results were not as good as those reported from the Mayo Clinic. The in-hospital mortality rate was 10 per cent, and the late mortality rate was 5 per cent. The mortality rate for elective operations, however, was 4 per cent, two of 54 patients. Complete heart block developed in six patients; it was transient in five patients, but the sixth required a permanent pacemaker. Mitral valve replacement was performed at the initial operation in four patients, something I have fortunately never found necessary. Subsequently, seven patients required

mitral valve replacement in the next several years because of severe mitral insufficiency. Hence, a total of 11 patients in the group (12 per cent) required mitral valve replacement either at the initial or subsequent operation. Complete heart block developed in 16 per cent of patients; it was transient in five patients, present in five who died in the immediate postoperative course, and necessitated a permanent pacemaker in five others. Two of these did not develop complete heart block until 1 to 10 years after operation, indicating the need for careful monitoring on a long-term basis.

Functional results in most patients are very good. The majority of patients become asymptomatic, often with a significant decrease in heart size. An apical systolic murmur remains in over one half of the patients and is apparently of little clinical significance. To date, there have been a few patients reported who subsequently developed severe mitral insufficiency, probably from turbulent flow of blood from the residual mild mitral insufficiency. In the Mayo Clinic series cited previously, the long-term survival calculated by the actuarial method was 96 per cent and 94 per cent at 5 and 15 years, respectively, in the 219 patients surviving operation. There were eight late cardiac deaths; in seven other patients, late prosthetic replacement of the mitral valve was necessary.

The unusual syndrome of severe hemolytic anemia following operation, described by Neill in 1964, has not been seen in our experience in over 15 years. This has been simply avoided in almost all centers by a precise operative technique that prevents the development of localized mitral insufficiency.

ATRIOVENTRICULARIS COMMUNIS

As described earlier, this defect results from a more severe arrest in the development of the endocardial cushions than that which produces an ostium primum defect. With atrioventricularis communis, a complete cleft divides both mitral and tricuspid valves, producing varying degrees of a common valve anteriorly and posteriorly. The atrial septal defect is similar to that with an ostium primum defect. Beneath the abnormal atrioventricular valve, there is a ventricular septal defect, ranging from a small opening to a large one that extends into the muscular septum. Abnormal chordae tendineae are common.

The classic pathologic studies by Rastelli and associates (1965, 1966, 1968) identified three distinct anatomic types. In type A, the most common, the anterior common leaflet is divided in the mitral and tricuspid portions with chordae from the rim of the ventricular septal defect attached to the margins. In Type B, occurring rarely, there is a divided anterior common leaflet, not attached to the septum, but both mitral and tricuspid components are attached medially to an abnormal papillary muscle. In Type C, the anterior common leaflet is undivided and free-floating, with virtually no chordae attaching it to the septum.

Obviously, the physiologic handicap with atrio-ventricularis communis is far more severe than with zn ostium primum defect, with the left-to-right shunt at both the ventricular and atrial levels. Cardiac failure occurs at an early age, often in infancy, and pulmonary hypertension develops very early in life. Differentiation from an ostium primum defect is primarily by angiography, with demonstration of a shunt at both the ventricular and atrial levels.

Surgical Treatment

The technique of operation has advanced greatly in the last several years. At one time, several experienced surgeons felt that infants with this abnormality could be treated only by prosthetic valve replacement. Rastelli and coworkers at the Mayo Clinic developed a successful operative technique based on their precise, elegant anatomic studies (1968). Their procedure was described in detail in the report by McMullan and associates in 1972. This report showed an astonishing reduction in mortality, describing operations on 27 patients with only two deaths, neither related to technical factors. Replacement of the mitral valve was not necessary in anyone. Some mitral regurgitation often remained but was neither severe nor progressive. All but two of the surviving patients were asymptomatic.

The technique of reconstruction varies with the type of deformity present and cannot be described in great detail here. The original references, listed in the bibliography, should be consulted in detail because of the complexity of this malformation.

In brief, the cleft mitral valve is first reconstructed, much as with a primum defect. A large prosthetic patch is then attached to the ventricular septum, placing sutures to the right of the crest of the septum to avoid heart block. The mitral and tricuspid valves are then reattached at approximately the level where they normally would have been attached to the ventricular septum. Finally, the atrial septal defect is closed by attaching the prosthetic patch with a circumferential suture. Fortunately, reconstruction of the tricuspid valve has not been found to be necessary. The illustrations in the 1972 publication by McMullan and coworkers are excellent and describe the technique well.

A dramatic advance in the treatment of this severe condition has been the successful operation on infants in the first few months of life, using techniques of deep hypothermia with circulatory arrest (Alfieri and Subramanian, 1975). Previously, infants with severe cardiac failure usually died before 1 year of age.

In 1977, Mair and McGoon reported operation on eight infants less than 1 year of age, with one operative death and one late death. In 1978, Berger and associates reported experiences with operation on 27 patients less than 2 years of age. There were eight deaths among 11 patients operated on before 1975, but only three deaths among the 16 patients operated on after that time. This striking decrease in mortality clearly illustrates the importance of operative technique and myocardial preservation at the time of operation. Both of these reports indicate that operation should be performed in the first or second year of life if there is severe cardiac failure or pulmonary hypertension, rather than attempting palliative procedures such as banding of the pulmonary artery.

Another report indicating the progressive advances in surgical therapy was published by Mills and colleagues in 1976 and described eight consecutive patients with the Type C atrioventricular canal, all of whom survived operation; on repeat catheterization, seven of the eight patients had a definite decrease in mitral insufficiency.

TOTAL ANOMALOUS DRAINAGE OF PULMONARY VEINS

This severe anomaly, with drainage of all of the pulmonary veins into the right side of the heart, is one of the most lethal congenital defects, often leading to death in the first few months of life unless operation is performed.

The classification suggested by Darling and associates (1957), based on the point of emptying of the pulmonary veins, is generally used. Four different types were described: supracardiac (55 per cent of cases), paracardiac (30 per cent), infracardiac (12 per cent), and mixed (3 per cent). In the supracardiac type, the most common pattern is entry of the anomalous veins into an anomalous left vertical vein, which in turn drains into the left innominate vein. A less frequent supracardiac type is direct entry of the common anomalous venous trunk into the posterior aspect of the right superior vena cava.

With paracardiac drainage, the veins may enter the right atrium directly or, less frequently, drain into the coronary sinus. With infracardiac drainage, the pulmonary veins enter a common channel that travels caudad through the diaphragm to connect with the inferior vena cava through a hepatic vein or the portal vein. This particular anomaly is fatal within the first few weeks or months of life without operation because the hepatic and portal venous channels progressively fibrose and become obliterated.

In a series of 62 patients reported by Cooley and associates in 1966, drainage was into a left superior vena cava in 28, into the right superior vena cava in seven, into the right atrium in eight, into the coronary sinus in 12, and into the portal vein in three. Multiple points of drainage were present in four patients.

Pathophysiology

Life is possible with total anomalous pulmonary venous drainage only as long as an atrial septal defect, often only a foramen ovale, is present, because this is the only point of entry of oxygenated blood into the systemic circulation. The complete admixture of pulmonary venous blood with systemic venous blood results in cyanosis of varying degree, principally determined from the pulmonary blood flow and the size of the atrial septal defect. As complete mixing of oxygenated blood occurs in the right atrium, the findings on cardiac catheterization are unique and distinctive. Oxygen saturations of blood withdrawn from the right atrium, right ventricle, pulmonary artery, and femoral artery are identical.

A particularly severe physiologic handicap is pulmonary venous hypertension, resulting from constriction of the point of entry of the anomalous pulmonary veins into the systemic venous system. This apparently initiates development of serious pulmonary hypertension. Conversely, if an adequate communication exists between the anomalous pulmonary veins and the systemic circulation, and a large atrial septal defect is present, patients may do surprisingly well for a long time without developing pulmonary hypertension. The disability resembles a large atrial septal defect. This fortunate situation occurs only in about 20 per cent of patients. In the majority, severe pulmonary hypertension develops early, with half of the patients dying within the first 3 months of life and most of the remainder within the first year. Cardiac failure develops with great rapidity, often with severe cyanosis.

The influence of age on prognosis is well illustrated in the report from the Mayo Clinic by Gomes and colleagues (1970) of 59 patients undergoing operative repair. The mortality rate for patients under 1 year of age was 47 per cent but was only 7 per cent in older patients. Fortunately, this high mortality rate in infants has decreased markedly in recent years.

Clinical Features

The clinical findings are a seriously ill infant with congestive failure, cyanosis, and rapidly progressing cardiac enlargement. A murmur may or may not be present. The chest roentgenogram may be diagnostic if there is drainage into a dilated anomalous left vertical vein, creating a characteristic double contour termed a "snowman" (Fig. 32–8). If pulmonary venous obstruction is severe, diffuse bead-like pulmonary congestion can be seen.

Total anomalous drainage of pulmonary veins is probably the fourth most common cause of cyanotic congenital heart disease in infants, the other three being tetralogy of Fallot, transposition, and tricuspid atresia. The usual differential diagnosis is between anomalous drainage of pulmonary veins and transposition, because both conditions produce cardiac enlargement and cardiac failure. Diagnosis can usually be readily established by cardiac catheterization.

In the fortunate minority of patients with an adequate pulmonary blood flow without pulmonary hypertension, the clinical findings may simply be a mild degree of cyanosis with enlargement of the right side of the heart. Again, the diagnosis is readily made by cardiac catheterization.

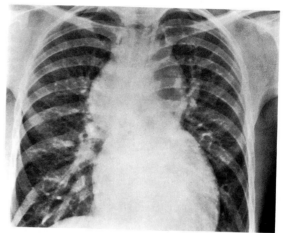

Figure 32–8. Chest roentgenogram of a 24-year-old patient with total anomalous drainage of the pulmonary veins into a left vertical vein. The mediastinal shadow is composed of the dilated left vertical vein and the large superior vena cava. This roentgenographic appearance is frequently referred to as a "snowman" effect.

Treatment

As stated earlier, nearly half of the infants with this abnormality die within the first 3 months of life unless surgical correction is possible. A decade ago, the surgical mortality in most centers approached 90 per cent in the first few months of life. Great advances have been made, however, with the development of techniques for intracardiac surgery in infants, using the combination of hypothermia and circulatory arrest, developed to an excellent degree by Barratt-Boyes and associates in New Zealand (1973).

In 1980, Turley and associates reported detailed experiences with 22 infants undergoing correction of total anomalous pulmonary veins between 1975 and 1978. Six were operated on within the first 4 days of life, all of whom survived. Six others were operated on between 5 and 30 days of age, and 10 additional patients between 1 and 12 months of age. Nineteen of the 22 survived, an 87 per cent survival rate. Two deaths occurred subsequently from progressive fibrosis of the pulmonary veins proximal to the site of atrial anastomosis.

Earlier, in 1978, Katz and coworkers collected experiences from the University of Alabama in Birmingham, Children's Hospital Medical Center in Boston, and the Great Lane Hospital in Auckland, New Zealand. Total experiences included 51 patients, 23 operated on within the first months of life, with a 22 per cent mortality rate, and the others operated on between 1 and 12 months of age. There were two deaths among 21 patients operated on between 1 and 6 months of age, a 10 per cent mortality rate, and no deaths in the seven operated on between 6 and 12 months of age.

The data in these two reports clearly indicate that total correction is usually the procedure of choice, performed even in the first week or month of life. A two-stage repair was believed to be indicated only in those patients with infracardiac connections. The phenomenon of late stenosis of the ostia of the pulmonary veins, separate from the site of anastomosis, was also noted.

These results with infants are especially impressive, because earlier studies by Kirklin and associates (Parr *et al.*, 1974) specifically found abnormalities in left ventricular function in a series of nine infants studied following operation. The improved results may possibly be related to improved myocardial preservation.

With the supracardiac type of malformation, the basic operation is the creation of a large side-to-side anastomosis between the common pulmonary venous trunk behind the heart and the left atrium. An adequate anastomosis is crucial to prevent pulmonary consolidation, the most common cause of death. This was emphasized in a report by Roe (1970), who used a left posterolateral thoracotomy to facilitate the construction of a very large anastomosis. Most operations are performed through a sternotomy, but regardless of the type of approach employed, the adequacy of the anastomosis should be confirmed by demonstrating that there is no longer a residual gradient between the pulmonary veins and the left atrium. The atrial septal defect is subsequently closed and the anomalous communication with the systemic venous circulation ligated (Figs. 32–9 and 32–10).

Although meaningful data are not available, a palliative procedure may be considered in infants in whom a complete repair does not seem feasible, enlarging the atrial septal defect as well as creating an anastomosis between the left atrium and the anomalous pulmonary veins. Leaving the atrial septal defect

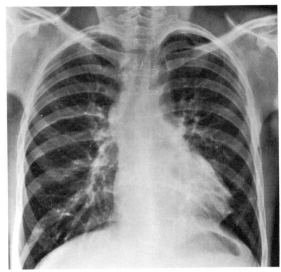

Figure 32–10. Postoperative roentgenogram 5 weeks following correction of the anomalous drainage of the pulmonary veins. The patient is the same one seen in Figure 32–8. The dilated superior vena cava has already decreased to virtually normal size. During extracorporeal circulation the anomalous pulmonary veins were anastomosed to the left atrium, following which the anomalous left vertical vein was ligated.

open might avoid severe pulmonary congestion, the most common cause of postoperative death. If such a palliative operation were chosen, simply enlarging the atrial septal defect might well be inadequate, because the pulmonary hypertension results from restricted drainage of the pulmonary veins into the systemic circulation. Hence, an anastomosis must be created between the anomalous veins and the left atrium as well. If the anastomosis appears too small, the anomalous entry of the pulmonary veins into the systemic venous circulation could be left intact. With the impressive results from total corrective operation in infancy cited earlier by Turley and associates (1980) and by Katz and coworkers (1978), it is probable that a palliative operation will rarely be indicated.

With the paracardiac type of malformation, in which the anomalous veins enter the right atrium or the coronary sinus, surgical reconstruction is much simpler (Fig. 32–11). If the pulmonary veins enter the right atrium directly, a prosthetic patch can be used to close the septal defect, so that the pulmonary veins drain directly into the left atrium. If the veins enter the coronary sinus, the septum between the coronary sinus and the atrial septal defect can be excised, after which the common opening thus created can be closed with a prosthetic patch, diverting coronary sinus blood as well as the blood draining from the pulmonary veins into the left atrium. The small amount of unoxygenated blood entering the systemic circulation from the coronary venous drainage is physiologically insignificant. Care is naturally taken to avoid injury of the AV node located at the medial and inferior margin of the coronary sinus ostium.

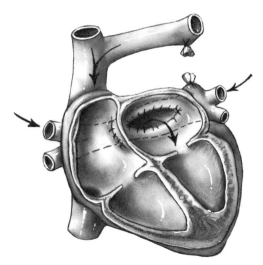

Figure 32–9. The operation performed for total anomalous pulmonary venous drainage is diagrammatically shown. It consists of an anastomosis between the anomalous pulmonary veins and the left atrium, followed by ligation of the anomalous left vertical vein and closure of the atrial septal defect. (From Schwartz, S. I., (Ed.): Principles of Surgery, 2nd Ed. New York, McGraw-Hill Book Co., 1974.)

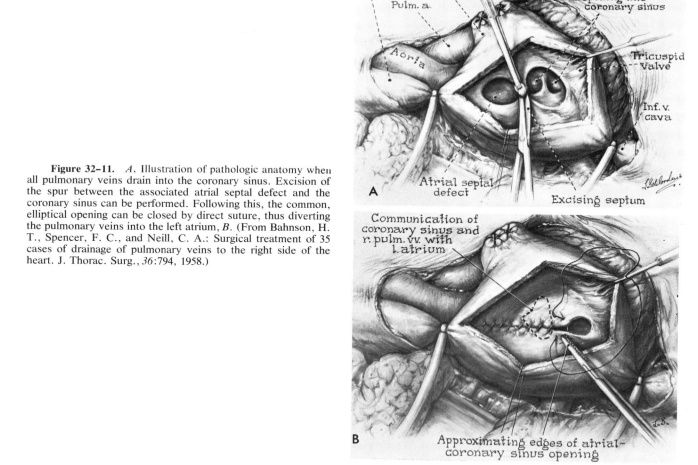

Figure 32–11. *A*, Illustration of pathologic anatomy when all pulmonary veins drain into the coronary sinus. Excision of the spur between the associated atrial septal defect and the coronary sinus can be performed. Following this, the common, elliptical opening can be closed by direct suture, thus diverting the pulmonary veins into the left atrium, *B*. (From Bahnson, H. T., Spencer, F. C., and Neill, C. A.: Surgical treatment of 35 cases of drainage of pulmonary veins to the right side of the heart. J. Thorac. Surg., *36*:794, 1958.)

A method for the correction of the unusual situation in which anomalous pulmonary veins directly enter the inferior vena cava from the right lung was described in a report of six cases by Murphy and colleagues in 1971.

Patients surviving the immediate postoperative course usually obtain an excellent result. The data described in the Mayo Clinic report by Gomes and associates (1970) indicate that the long-term outlook is excellent.

SELECTED REFERENCES

Berger, T. J., Kirklin, J. W., Blackstone, E. H., Pacifico, A. D., and Kouchoukos, N. T.: Primary repair of complete atrioventricular canal in patients less than two years old. Am. J. Cardiol., *41*:906, 1978.

This report describes impressive results with 27 patients less than 2 years of age for repair of a complete atrioventricular canal. Operative mortality was 19 per cent in the 16 patients operated on after January 1975, reflecting the great decrease in mortality with present techniques of open cardiac surgery in infancy.

Katz, N. M., Kirklin, J. W., and Pacifico, A. D.: Concepts and practices in surgery for total anomalous pulmonary venous connection. Ann. Thorac. Surg., *25*:479, 1978.

Previously, operations for total anomalous pulmonary veins in the first few months of life had a very high mortality. This paper summarizes experiences from three large medical centers, involving a total of 51 patients operated on in the first year of life with 14 deaths, a vast improvement over results previously obtained.

Turley, K., Wilson, J. M., and Ebert, P. A.: Atrial repairs of infant complex congenital heart lesions. Emphasis on the first three months of life. Arch. Surg., *115*:1335, 1980.

A dramatic development in recent years has been the efficacy of intracardiac operations performed during infancy with the combination of hypothermia and either circulatory arrest or low rates of perfusion. This remarkable paper describes 106 patients, 70 operated on in the first 3 months of life and 16 less than 1 week old. The overall survival rate was 95 per cent, a remarkable achievement for what was virtually a hopeless problem 8 to 10 years ago.

Turley, K., Tucker, W. Y., Ullyot, D. J., and Ebert, P. A.: Total anomalous pulmonary venous connection in infancy: Influence of age and type of lesion. Am. J. Cardiol., *45*:92, 1980.

This report describes 22 infants operated on in the first year of life, 12 in the first month and six in the first 4 days. Nineteen of the 22 survived, a remarkable achievement, especially considering the fact that in the past, the mortality rate in infants operated on before the first month of life approached 80 to 90 per cent.

REFERENCES

Alfieri, O., and Subramanian, S.: Successful repair of complete atrioventricular canal with undivided anterior common leaflet in a 6-month-old infant. Ann. Thorac. Surg., 19:1, 1975.

Bahnson, H. T., Spencer, F. C., and Neill, C. A.: Surgical treatment of 35 cases of drainage of pulmonary veins to the right side of the heart. J. Thorac. Surg., 36:787, 1958.

Barratt-Boyes, B. G.: Primary definitive intracardiac operations in infants: Total anomalous pulmonary venous connection. *In* Advances in Cardiovascular Surgery. Edited by J. W. Kirklin. New York, Grune and Stratton, 1973, p. 127.

Berger, T. J., Kirklin, J. W., Blackstone, E. H., Pacifico, A. D., and Kouchoukos, N. T.: Primary repair of complete atrioventricular canal in patients less than two years old. Am. J. Cardiol., 41:906, 1978.

Blake, H. A., Hall, R. C., and Manion, W. C.: Anomalous pulmonary venous return. Circulation, 32:406, 1965.

Braunwald, N. S., and Morrow, A. G.: Incomplete persistent atrioventricular canal. J. Thorac. Cardiovasc. Surg., 51:71, 1966.

Brom, A. G.: Submammarian incision. (Letter.) J. Thorac. Cardiovasc. Surg., 80:464, 1980.

Coles, J., Sears, G., and MacDonald, C.: Atrial septal defect complicated by pulmonary hypertension — a long-term follow-up. Ann. Surg., 166:495, 1967.

Cooley, D. A., Hallman, G. L., and Leachman, R. D.: Total anomalous pulmonary venous drainage. J. Thorac. Cardiovasc. Surg., 51:88, 1966.

Craig, R. J., and Selzer, A.: Natural history and prognosis of atrial septal defect. Circulation, 37:805, 1968.

Darling, R. C., Rothney, W. B., and Craig, J. M.: Total pulmonary venous drainage into the right side of the heart: Report of 17 autopsied cases not associated with other major cardiovascular anomalies. Lab. Invest., 6:44, 1957.

de la Rivière, A. B., Brom, G. H. M., and Brom, A. G.: Horizontal submammary skin incision for median sternotomy. Ann. Thorac. Surg., 32:101, 1981.

Gault, J. H., Morrow, A. G., Gay, W. A., Jr., and Ross, J., Jr.: Atrial septal defect in patients over the age of forty years: Clinical and hemodynamic studies and effects of operation. Circulation, 37:261, 1968.

Gerbode, F., Sanchez, P. A., Arguero, R., Kerth, W. J., Hill, J. D., deVries, P. A., Selzer, A., and Robinson, S. J.: Endocardial cushion defects. Ann. Surg., 166:486, 1967.

Gibbon, J. H., Jr.: Application of a mechanical heart and lung apparatus to cardiac surgery. Minnesota Med., 37:171, 1954.

Gomes, M. M. R., Feldt, R. H., McGoon, D. C., and Danielson, G. K.: Total anomalous pulmonary venous connection. J. Thorac. Cardiovasc. Surg., 60:1, 1970.

Hanlon, C. R., Barner, H. B., Willman, V. L., Mudd, J. G., and Kasier, G. C.: Atrial septal defect: Results of repair in adults. Arch. Surg., 49:275, 1969.

Hawe, A., Rastelli, G. C., Brandenburg, R. O., and McGoon, D. C.: Embolic complications following repair of atrial septal defects. Circulation, 39(Suppl. 1):185, 1969.

Katz, N. M., Kirklin, J. W., and Pacifico, A. D.: Concepts and practices in surgery for total anomalous pulmonary venous connection. Ann. Thorac. Surg., 25:479, 1978.

Lévy, S., Blondeau, P., and Dubost, C.: Long-term follow-up after

surgical correction of the partial form of common atrioventricular canal (ostium primum). J. Thorac. Cardiovasc. Surg., 67:3, 1974.

Losay, J., Rosenthal, A., Castaneda, A. R., Bernhard, W. H., and Nades, A. S.: Repair of atrial septal defect primum: Results, course, and prognosis. J. Thorac. Cardiovasc. Surg., 75:248, 1978.

Mair, D. D., and McGoon, D. C.: Surgical correction of atrioventricular canal during the first year of life. Am. J. Cardiol., 40:66, 1977.

McMullan, M. H., McGoon, D. C., Wallace, R. B., Danielson, G. K., and Weidman, W. H.: Surgical treatment of partial atrioventricular canal. Arch. Surg., 107:705, 1973.

McMullan, M. H., Wallace, R. B., Weidman, W. H., and McGoon, D. C.: Surgical treatment of complete atrioventricular canal. Surgery, 6:905, 1972.

Mills, N. D., Ochsner, J. L., and King, T. D.: Correction of Type C complete atrioventricular canal: Surgical considerations. J. Thorac. Cardiovasc. Surg., 71:20, 1976.

Muller, W. H.: Surgical treatment of transposition of pulmonary veins. Ann. Surg., 134:683, 1951.

Murphy, J. W., Kerr, A. R., and Kirklin, J. W.: Intracardiac repair for anomalous pulmonary venous connection of right lung to inferior vena cava. Ann. Thorac. Surg., 11:1, 1971.

Neill, C. A.: Postoperative hemolytic anemia in endocardial cushion defects. Circulation, 30:801, 1964.

Parr, G. V. S., Kirklin, J. W., Pacifico, A. D., Blackstone, E. H., and Lauridsen, P.: Cardiac performance in infants after repair of total anomalous pulmonary venous connection. Ann. Thorac. Surg., 17:6, 1974.

Rastelli, G. C., Kirklin, J. W., and Titus, J. L.: Anatomic observations on complete form of persistent common atrioventricular canal with special reference to atrioventricular valves. Mayo Clin. Proc., 41:296, 1966.

Rastelli, G. C., Weidman, W. H., and Kirklin, J. W.: Surgical repair of the partial form of persistent common atrioventricular canal, with special reference to mitral valve incompetence. Circulation, 31:31, 1965.

Rastelli, G. C., Rahimtoola, S. H., Ongley, P. A., and McGoon, D. C.: Common atrium: Anatomy, hemodynamics, and surgery. J. Thorac. Cardiovasc. Surg., 55:834, 1968.

Roe, B. B.: Posterior approach to correction of total anomalous pulmonary venous return. J. Thorac. Cardiovasc. Surg., 59:5, 1970.

Rudolph, A. M.: Congenital Diseases of the Heart. Chicago, Year Book Medical Publishers, Inc., 1974, p. 259.

Schwartz, S. I. (Ed.): Principles of Surgery. 2nd Ed. New York, McGraw-Hill Book Co., 1974.

Sellers, R. D., Ferlic, R. M., Sterns, L. P., and Lillehei, C. W.: Secundum type atrial septal defects: Results with 275 patients. Surgery, 59:155, 1966.

Spencer, F. C., and Bahnson, H. T.: Intracardiac surgery employing hypothermia and coronary perfusion performed on 100 patients. Surgery, 46:987, 1959.

Stansel, H. C., Jr., Talner, N. S., and Deren, M. M.: Surgical treatment of atrial septal defect. Analysis of 150 corrective operations. Am. J. Surg., 121:485, 1971.

Turley, K., Wilson, J. M., and Ebert, P. A.: Atrial repairs of infant complex congenital heart lesions. Emphasis on the first three months of life. Arch. Surg., 115:1335, 1980.

Turley, K., Tucker, W. Y., Ullyot, D. J., and Ebert, P. A.: Total anomalous pulmonary venous connection in infancy: Influence of age and type of lesion. Am. J. Cardiol., 45:92, 1980.

Yalav, E., Brown, A. H., and Braimbridge, M. V.: Surgery for atrial septal defect in patients over 60 years of age. J. Thorac. Cardiovasc. Surg., 62:5, 1971.

Chapter 33

Major Anomalies of Pulmonary and Thoracic Systemic Veins

JOHN W. HAMMON, JR.

HARVEY W. BENDER, JR.

Major anomalies of pulmonary and systemic venous return represent one of the few forms of congenital heart disease in which the valves and ventricles are usually normal, and thus, correction should offer excellent long-term results. Patients with total anomalous pulmonary venous connection (TAPVC) rarely survive beyond the first year of life without operative correction, and patients with anomalous systemic venous connections often become symptomatic in infancy and childhood. Operative correction of these conditions is usually successful, and knowledge of this relatively uncommon but important group of congeni-

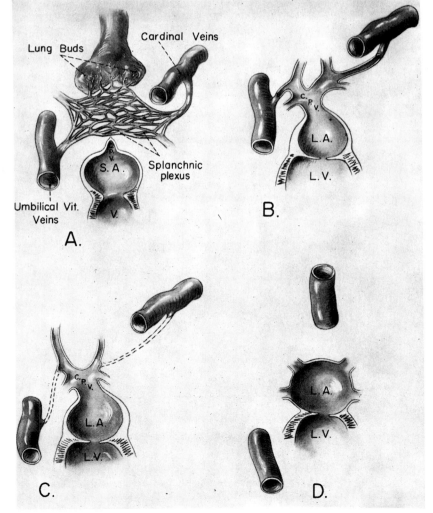

Figure 33–1. Normal development of the pulmonary venous system. *A,* The splanchnic plexus drains the lung buds and shares connections with the cardinal and umbilicovitelline systems. *B,* The common pulmonary vein (C.P.V.) has evaginated from the left atrium (L.A.) and has joined the splanchnic plexus. *C,* As pulmonary venous blood drains to the left heart the primitive connections disappear. *D,* Finally, by differential growth the individual pulmonary veins are incorporated into the left atrium and the common pulmonary vein disappears. (From Lucas, R. V., *et al.:* Congenital causes of pulmonary venous obstruction. Pediatr. Clin. North Am., *10*:781, 1963.)

tal anomalies is essential to insure prompt, accurate diagnosis and therapy. Partial anomalous pulmonary venous connections are considered in the preceding chapter covering atrial septal defect.

EMBRYOLOGY

Pulmonary Venous System

At approximately 3½ weeks' gestation, the lung bud arises from the primitive foregut and becomes surrounded by a plexus of veins that has been called the pulmonary venous plexus (Fig. 33–1A) (Los, 1968). As differentiation proceeds, this venous system has no direct communication with the heart but instead shares the routes of drainage of the splanchnic plexus, i.e., the cardinal and umbilicovitelline systems of veins (Fig. 33–1B). In the normal situation, this pulmonary venous plexus eventually becomes connected to a vessel termed the common pulmonary vein (Neill, 1956), a transient structure that arises from the undivided sinus venosus just to the left of the area in which the atrial septal primum will develop (Fig. 33–1C). Eventually, connections to the systemic venous system are lost, and the common pulmonary vein is incorporated into the developing left atrium (Fig. 33–1D). Abnormal development of the common pulmonary vein provides the embryologic basis for most of the congenital anomalies of the pulmonary veins (Lucas *et al.*, 1962).

If atresia of the common pulmonary vein occurs during the time when systemic communications are present to the cardinal and umbilicovitelline systems, any one or several of these collateral channels can enlarge and provide total anomalous pulmonary venous connection to the systemic venous system (Fig. 33–2). If only the right or left portion of the common pulmonary vein is atretic, partial anomalous venous connection occurs.

Persisting segments of the cardinal veins eventually form the superior vena cava, the innominate vein, the coronary sinus, and the azygos vein. The umbilicovitelline system forms the inferior vena cava, the portal vein, and the ductus venosus. The individual anatomy of the anomalous venous connection is directly related to the early embryologic connection between the pulmonary venous plexus and the particular splanchnic component that persists. Direct anomalous connections to the right atrium are not explained by the aforementioned embryologic accident and are probably best attributed to an abnormality of septation of the two atria, in which the atrial septum forms to the left of the pulmonary veins rather than to the right side of these structures (Shaner, 1961). The systemic venous anatomy and the different systemic veins that can become the site of drainage of pulmonary venous blood in patients with TAPVC are demonstrated in Figure 33–3.

When stenosis of the common pulmonary vein occurs, the result is *cor triatriatum* (Edwards, 1960). In the usual situation, stenosis occurs late, after systemic venous connections have been lost (Fig. 33–4). Occasionally, however, cor triatriatum is associated

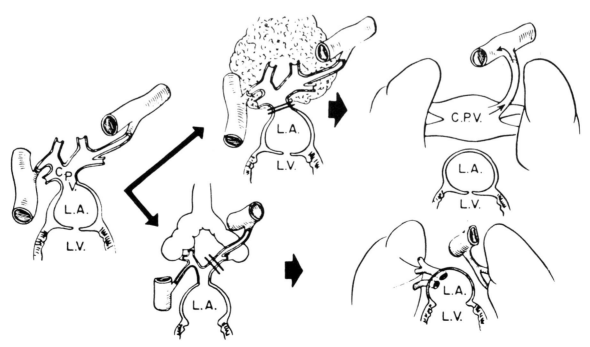

Figure 33–2. The embryologic explanation for anomalous pulmonary venous connections. *Upper,* If atresia of the common pulmonary vein occurs when systemic connections are still present, TAPVC results. *Lower,* Atresia of a branch of the common pulmonary veins results in partial anomalous pulmonary venous connection. (Adapted from Lucas, R. V., and Schmidt, R. E.: *In* Heart Disease in Infants, Children and Adolescents. Edited by A. J. Moss, F. H. Adams, and G. C. Emmanouilides. Baltimore, Williams and Wilkins Co., 1977.)

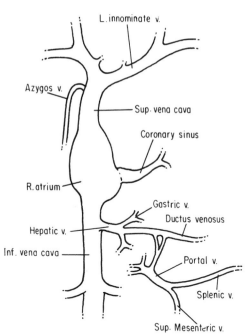

Figure 33–3. The systemic veins that can be the routes of drainage in TAPVC.

with anomalous pulmonary venous connections to systemic veins, suggesting that significant stenosis of the common pulmonary vein is present at a time when systemic venous connections are still present.

Systemic Venous System

The first veins to appear in the embryo are the umbilical and vitelline veins (Fig. 33–5*A*). The cardinal veins are the next to develop (Streeter, 1942). The anterior and posterior cardinal veins unite on each side to form a common cardinal vein. Eventually, the common cardinal, umbilical, and vitelline veins join

the right and left horns of the sinus venosus (Fig. 33–5*B*). By the fourth week of fetal life, the sinus venosus has developed an invagination that separates its left horn from the left atrium and ultimately in which all systemic blood enters the right atrium (Fig. 33–5*C*) (Raghib *et al.*, 1965).

At this stage, the cardinal systemic veins are symmetrical, with the exception of their drainage into the right atrium. During the eighth week of fetal life, the left innominate vein develops, connecting the two anterior cardinal veins. As flow through the left innominate vein increases, the left anterior cardinal vein decreases in size, so that by the sixth fetal month it has become obliterated and the left common cardinal vein remains to drain only the coronary circulation to the right atrium as the coronary sinus (Fig. 33–5*C*). Occasionally, a small portion of the left anterior cardinal vein persists as the oblique ligament or vein of Marshall of the left atrium (Lucas and Schmidt, 1977).

Important abnormalities of the cardinal venous system can be explained on the basis of two developmental aberrations: (1) Failure of obliteration of the left anterior cardinal vein results in persistence of the left superior vena cava. If invagination between the left horn of the sinus venosus has occurred, a coronary sinus is formed, which serves as an outlet for the left superior vena cava. (2) Failure of invagination between the left sinus horn and the left atrium and failure of obliteration of the left anterior cardinal vein result in the left superior vena cava draining directly into the left atrium.

The venous return of the caudal portion of the body continues to drain via the posterior cardinal veins until the sixth week of fetal life. At this point, the inferior vena cava develops in the next two succeeding weeks (McClure and Butler, 1925).

The development of the inferior vena cava depends on the formation of two centrally located systems. The subcardinal system develops ventral and medial to the posterior cardinal veins. The supracar-

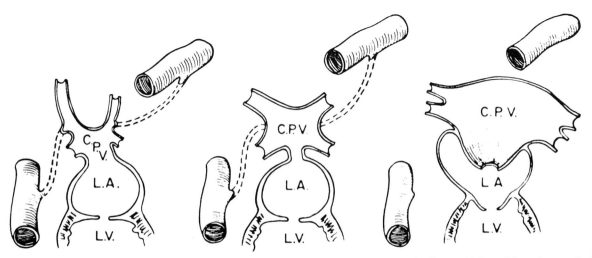

Figure 33–4. When stenosis of the common pulmonary vein occurs, the result is cor triatriatum. (Adapted from Lucas, R. V., and Schmidt, R. E.: *In* Heart Disease in Infants, Children and Adolescents. Edited by A. J. Moss, F. H. Adams, and G. C. Emmanouilides. Baltimore, Williams and Wilkins Co., 1977.)

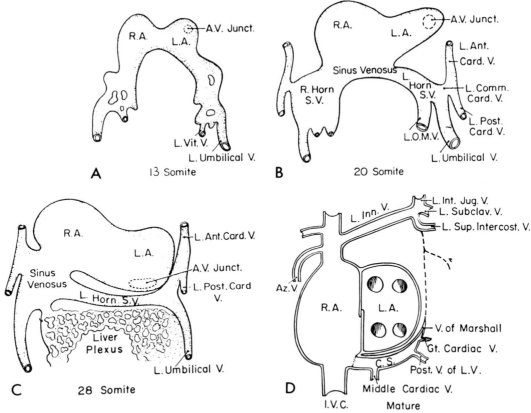

Figure 33–5. Normal embryology of the cardinal venous system. *A,* Bilaterally symmetrical umbilical and vitelline veins drain into the common atrium. Asymmetry begins with the atrioventricular junction to the left. *B,* The cardinal system develops with continuing asymmetrical development of the atrium. *C,* The left and right horns of the sinus venosus are completely separated, and all systemic blood drains to the right atrium. *D,* The left innominate vein (L. Inn. V.) develops, and the left anterior cardinal vein disappears. The left common cardinal vein becomes the coronary sinus (C.S.). (L. Ant. Card. V. = left anterior cardinal vein; L. Post. Card. V. = left posterior cardinal vein; L. Comm. Card. V. = left common cardinal vein; L. Umbilical V. = left umbilical vein; R.A. = right atrium; L.A. = left atrium; L. Int. Jug. V. = left internal jugular vein; L. Subclav. V. = left subclavian vein; L. Sup. Intercost. V. = left superior intercostal vein; V. of Marshall = vein of Marshall; Gt. Cardiac V. = great cardiac vein; Post. V. of L.V. = posterior vein of the left ventricle; Middle Cardiac V. = middle cardiac vein; I.V.C. = inferior vena cava; Az. V. = azygos vein; L. Vit. V. = left vitelline vein; R. Horn S. V. and L. Horn S.V. = right and left horns of the sinus venosus; A.V. Junct. = atrioventricular junction; L.O.M.V. = left omphalomesenteric vein.) (Adapted from Lucas, R. V., and Schmidt, R. E.: *In* Heart Disease in Infants, Children and Adolescents. Edited by A. J. Moss, F. H. Adams, and G. C. Emmanouilides. Baltimore, Williams and Wilkins Co., 1977.)

dinal system forms dorsal and medial to the posterior cardinal veins, and anastomoses develop between the cardinal veins and both systems. The cardinal system atrophies such that no cardinal remnants persist between the iliac veins and the diaphragm. Anastomoses develop between the right and left supra- and subcardinal systems. Flow becomes preferentially directed to the right system, and the left system atrophies; the left supracardinal vein becomes the hemiazygos vein, which joins the right supracardinal (azygos) vein. The right subcardinal vein and hepatic veins join and form the inferior vena cava, which joins the right atrium at the junction of the right common cardinal vein and the atrium.

Failure of connection between the right subcardinal vein and the hepatic vein causes venous blood from the lower half of the body to be directed into the left subcardinal system, resulting in the common anomaly of interruption of the inferior vena cava with azygos continuation. The normal development of the

inferior vena cava and the formation of interrupted inferior vena cava are detailed in Figure 33–6.

Direct *connection* of the inferior vena cava to the left atrium is not well defined embryologically (Meadows *et al.,* 1961). The more common situation in which the inferior vena cava *drains* into the left atrium via an atrial septal defect can be embryologically explained by persistence and overgrowth of the valves of the sinus venosus that usually form the eustachian and thebesian valves. Very rarely, the right valve persists as a membrane that directs all systemic venous blood to the left atrium (Doucette and Knoblich, 1963).

TOTAL ANOMALOUS PULMONARY VENOUS CONNECTION

The term total anomalous pulmonary venous connection (TAPVC) defines the anomaly in which the

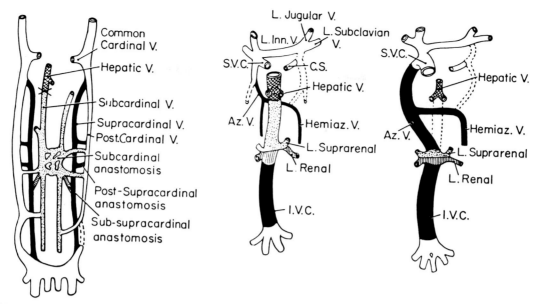

Figure 33–6. Embryology of the inferior vena cava (I.V.C.). *Left,* In early stages of development, blood can reach the heart by way of the posterior cardinal veins (Post. Cardinal V.), supracardinal veins, and the upper portion of the I.V.C. Multiple anastomotic sites exist in the renal area, as demonstrated. *Center,* Normal development of the I.V.C. The I.V.C. is derived, from below upward, from the posterior cardinal system (white), the supracardinal system (black), the renal veins (lined), the subcardinal system (stippled), and the hepatic veins (cross-hatched). The supracardinal veins persist as the hemiazygos and azygos veins. *Right,* Interruption of the I.V.C. with azygos continuation. Absence of the I.V.C. above the renal veins occurs when the right subcardinal vein fails to join with the hepatic vein. The hepatic veins drain directly into the right atrium. All other blood from the lower body drains via the dilated azygos and hemiazygos systems. (From Lucas, R. V., and Schmidt, R. E.: *In* Heart Disease in Infants, Children and Adolescents. Edited by A. J. Moss, F. H. Adams, and G. C. Emmanouilides. Baltimore, Williams and Wilkins Co., 1977.)

pulmonary veins have no direct communication with the left atrium. Instead, they connect to the right atrium or to one of the systemic veins.

Historical Considerations

The first reported case of total anomalous pulmonary venous connection was described in 1798, when Wilson reported a patient in whom the entire pulmonary venous return entered the coronary sinus. Additional reports were uncommon, until 1942, when Brody presented the first authoritative review on the subject with 37 autopsied cases from the literature. In 1957, Darling, Rothney, and Craig added 17 cases and provided a classification of the variants of this anomaly.

The first clinical diagnosis was made by Friedlich and associates in 1950, using cardiac catheterization. In 1951, the first successful operation was reported by Muller, who provided palliation for the patient by anastomosing the left atrial appendage to anomalous veins from the left lung. In 1956, Lewis and coworkers reported the first successful open heart correction of the cardiac type of TAPVC in a 5-year-old patient using hypothermia and inflow occlusion. Cooley and Ochsner (1957) reported the first open heart correction using cardiopulmonary bypass in a patient with a supracardiac anomaly. The first infracardiac anomaly was corrected in 1961 by Sloan, who utilized deep hypothermia, cardiopulmonary bypass, and a period of circulatory arrest (Sloan *et al.*, 1962).

Anatomy

The anatomic prerequisite for TAPVC is an absence of connection between any pulmonary veins and the left atrium. The left atrium has no tributaries and receives all blood by an atrial septal defect. The term total anomalous pulmonary venous *connection* describes this anatomic abnormality and should not be confused with total anomalous pulmonary venous *drainage,* in which the pulmonary veins terminate in the left atrium, but blood passes through an interatrial communication into the right atrium because of atresia of the mitral or aortic valves or a combination of both with total left heart atresia. In 1957, Darling and coworkers described the most frequently used classification of TAPVC. They have divided the anomaly into four subtypes that conveniently describe the anatomic connections of the pulmonary venous to the systemic venous circulation.

Type I — Supracardiac Connection. The anatomic site of anomalous venous connection in this type results in communications to the remnants of the right or left cardinal venous system. The most common form of this anomaly, in which pulmonary venous drainage is to a common pulmonary vein posterior to the left atrium, is demonstrated in Figure 33–7. A left

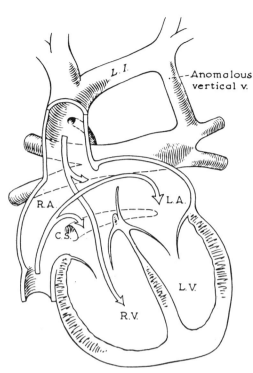

Figure 33–7. A diagrammatic representation of the most common type of supracardiac TAPVC (L.I. = left innominate vein; Anomalous vertical v. = anomalous vertical vein; R.A. = right atrium; L.A. = left atrium; C.S. = coronary sinus; R.V. = right ventricle; L.V. = left ventricle). (Adapted from Eliot, R. S., and Edwards, J. E.: Congenital heart disease. *In* The Heart. Edited by J. W. Hurst and R. B. Logue. New York, McGraw-Hill, 1966.)

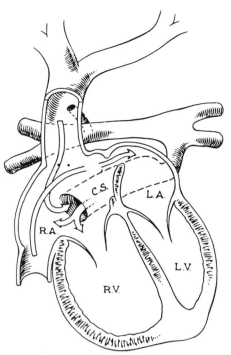

Figure 33–8. The anatomy and blood flow patterns in TAPVC when the pulmonary venous confluence connects to the coronary sinus (C.S.). (Adapted from Eliot, R. S., and Edwards, J. E.: Congenital heart disease. *In* The Heart. Edited by J. W. Hurst and R. B. Logue. New York, McGraw-Hill, 1966.)

vertical vein connects this chamber with the innominate vein, and this vessel usually lies anterior to the left pulmonary artery. When the common pulmonary venous chamber connects with remnants of the right cardinal venous system, the connection may be to the superior vena cava or azygos vein or by an additional right vertical vein draining directly into the innominate vein. Occasionally, pulmonary veins may separately enter the superior vena cava, azygos, and/or innominate vein. This particular type is associated with major cardiac anomalies (Ruttenberg *et al.*, 1964).

Type II — Cardiac Connection. Cardiac connections are divided into two major subtypes. In the most common type, the left and right common pulmonary veins join to form a common venous sinus posterior to the left atrium, which then connects to an enlarged coronary sinus in the atrioventricular groove (Fig. 33–8). In the second major group, the pulmonary veins drain individually or collectively into a sinus in the posterior right atrium (Fig. 33–9).

Type III — Infracardiac Connection. In this group, a common venous chamber posterior to the heart connects to an inferior vein that passes through the diaphragm anterior to the esophagus and then to the portal vein or one of its branches, or with the ductus venosus (Fig. 33–10). Occasionally, the anomalous descending vein passes through an accessory hiatus in the diaphragm and joins one of the systemic

venous channels, most commonly the inferior vena cava or one of its branches.

Type IV — Mixed Connections. In this uncommon group, the pulmonary venous connections are divided such that one lung drains to one of the systemic veins and pulmonary veins from the opposite side usually join one of the cardiac chambers, generally the coronary sinus.

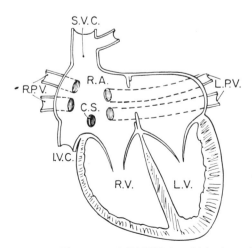

Figure 33–9. The type of TAPVC in which the pulmonary veins directly connect with the right atrium. (Redrawn from Lucas, R. V., and Schmidt, R. E.: *In* Heart Disease in Infants, Children and Adolescents. Edited by A. J. Moss, F. H. Adams, and G. C. Emmanouilides. Baltimore, Williams and Wilkins Co., 1977.)

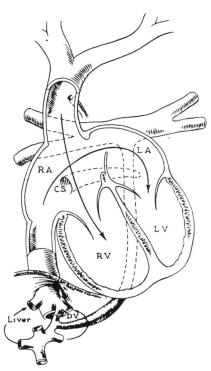

Figure 33–10. The most common type of infracardiac TAPVC in which the anomalous descending vein connects the pulmonary venous confluence with the ductus venosus (D.V.). (Adapted from Eliot, R. S., and Edwards, J. E.: Congenital heart disease. *In* The Heart. Edited by J. W. Hurst and R. B. Logue. New York, McGraw-Hill, 1966.)

Associated Cardiac Defects

An interatrial communication is required for persistence of life beyond the early neonatal period in the patients with TAPVC and is present in nearly all cases. It may vary between a probe-patent foramen ovale to complete absence of the interatrial septum. Patent ductus arteriosus (PDA) is present in 25 to 50 per cent of patients with this defect (Burroughs and Edwards, 1960). In infants with pulmonary venous obstruction, the incidence of PDA is very high and is the physiologic means of decompressing obstructed pulmonary blood flow into the descending thoracic aorta. A particularly high incidence of TAPVC and severe congenital cardiac defects is associated with the asplenia syndrome (Ivemark, 1955).

Incidence

Approximately 1 per cent of infants born with congenital heart disease will have total anomalous pulmonary venous connection (Jensen and Blount, 1971). There is no known genetic predisposition to this lesion; however, males are afflicted nearly twice as often as females. The incidence of the various anatomic types of TAPVC are illustrated in Table 33–1. These data have been gathered from several collected series in the literature. The earlier series represent autopsy reports, and the later series are surgical in nature. It can be seen that supracardiac defects are the most common and make up 50 per cent of those patients affected. The most common supracardiac anomaly is the connection of the pulmonary venous chamber to a left anomalous vertical vein draining to the innominate vein. Type II defects are the second most common, with pulmonary venous connection to the coronary sinus the most prevalent in this group.

Type III and IV defects are the least common, with the incidence of Type III defects being reported more frequently in surgical series, as these infants survive to diagnosis and treatment. Patients with Type IV anomalies are not common in surgical series because most have major intracardiac defects that preclude operative therapy.

Pathophysiology

The factors that influence the pathophysiology of TAPVC include obligatory mixing of pulmonary and systemic blood upstream to or at the right atrium, the presence of obstruction of the anomalous connection, the size of the atrial septal defect, and associated anomalies. The presence or absence of obstruction of the anomalous connection is the most significant factor that influences the patient's clinical condition.

In contrast to patients with atrial septal defects, the mixing of systemic and pulmonary venous blood in TAPVC is obligatory and is not influenced by the compliance of the two ventricles and the end-diastolic pressure in both chambers. In theory, the oxygen saturation should be equal in all four cardiac chambers. This may be altered in patients with small atrial septal defects in which streaming of blood occurs, with the majority of inferior vena caval blood being directed through the patent foramen ovale or small atrial septal defect and with superior vena caval blood entering the right ventricle through the tricuspid valve. If the interatrial communication is large and the anomalous connection is not obstructed, there is adequate flow to the left atrium, and oxygen saturation will be similar in both the right and left heart chambers. In this condition, blood flow through the lungs will be high, and systemic oxygen saturation will be only slightly decreased.

In the patient with unobstructed TAPVC, the entire cardiac output is presented to the right ventricle, and it accepts its maximal end-diastolic volume from the very beginning of life. As the patient grows and performs vigorous exercise, cyanosis increases only when the pulmonary vascular resistance rises and a high pulmonary-systemic flow ratio cannot be maintained. Although not all of these patients develop hyperkinetic pulmonary hypertension, it is clear that the incidence of this complication is higher in patients with TAPVC than in other, high-flow–low-pressure lesions such as atrial septal defect (Gathman and Nadas, 1970; Newfield *et al.*, 1980). Heart failure is more common in patients with hyperkinetic pulmona-

TABLE 33–1. COLLECTED CASES OF TAPVC CLASSIFIED BY TYPE

	BURROUGHS AND EDWARDS (1960)	BONHAM-CARTER ET AL. (1969)	JENSEN AND BLOUNT (1971)	SNELLEN AND BRUINS (1968)	COOLEY ET AL. (1966)	GATHMAN AND NADAS (1971)	BRECKENRIDGE ET AL. (1973)	APPLEBAUM ET AL. (1975)	TURLEY ET AL. (1980)	HAMMON ET AL. (1980)	TOTAL	INCIDENCE (PER CENT)
TYPE I: Supracardiac												
Left anomalous vertical vein	56	34	12	12	28	26	11	21			284	51%
Right superior vena cava	31	9	2	1	7	8	3	2	9	12		
TYPE II: Cardiac												
Coronary sinus	18	18	5	11	12	14	2	3	6	6	156	28%
Right atrium	30	3	6	7	8	3	1	3				
TYPE III: Infracardiac	28	8	2	4	3	16	3	4	6	5	79	14%
TYPE IV: Mixed	16	3	0	3	4	8	1	2	1	2	40	7%
TOTALS	179	75	27	38	62	75	21	35	22	25	559	100%

ry hypertension but is not uncommon in patients with low pulmonary artery pressure and large left-to-right shunts.

The interatrial communication in patients with TAPVC is usually large; however, in a very few patients this communication is small and presents obstruction to flow to the left ventricle. In these patients, a gradient of 3 mm. Hg or greater between the right and left atrium can indicate the presence of an obstructing atrial septal defect (Behrendt et al., 1972). The flow to the left heart and thus the cardiac output can be improved following a balloon atrial septostomy (Miller and Rashkind, 1968).

Anatomic obstruction of the anomalous connection is common in infants and can occur at several sites (Burroughs and Edwards, 1960). In patients with Type I anomalies, the left vertical vein can be constricted as it passes through the pericardial reflection or, rarely, between the left pulmonary artery and left main stem bronchus. In Type III lesions, obstruction most commonly occurs when the ductus venosus closes, if the connection attaches at this level. If the anomalous inferior vein communicates with the portal vein, obstruction is a prerequisite, because pulmonary venous blood must pass through the liver capillary bed before returning to the right heart. Occasionally, anatomic obstruction can occur in infracardiac connections in which the vertical vein passes through the diaphragm and is constricted during tidal ventilation. In Type IV connections, obstruction usually occurs because of inadequate sites of communication between the pulmonary veins and the right heart. Type II connections are rarely obstructed and for this reason present a much more favorable situation for long-term survival.

The pathophysiologic consequences of an obstructed anomalous pulmonary venous connection are pulmonary edema and poor myocardial function. During the first few hours or days of extrauterine life, pulmonary blood flow increases. Pulmonary venous obstruction then causes elevation of pulmonary capillary hydrostatic pressure. When this pressure exceeds the net forces that retain fluid in the vascular space, interstitial pulmonary edema occurs. A vicious cycle then ensues, with interstitial edema causing decreased lung compliance and marked increases in the work of breathing. Ventilation and perfusion are not balanced, and arterial oxygen desaturation results, further compromising the heart's ability to meet the body's oxygen demand. The end result is alveolar flooding and perivascular hemorrhage, resulting in frank pulmonary collapse.

The combination of tachycardia, low coronary perfusion pressure, and cyanosis predisposes the myocardium to subendocardial ischemia. This is especially true in the right ventricle, which, in this condition, usually faces an excessive afterload and will, in most cases, have elevated end-diastolic pressure, which further increases oxygen demand and decreases subendocardial coronary blood flow. The low cardiac output that results promotes anaerobic metabolism, which creates a metabolic acidosis with elevation in plasma lactate. It is because of these related events that infants with obstructed TAPVC rarely survive the first few weeks of life.

Infants born with obstructed connections often retain ductal patency. This serves to decompress the pulmonary artery and help unload the right ventricle. With ductal closure, severe right heart failure and pulmonary and cardiovascular collapse can occur.

Diagnosis

Clinical Manifestations. The severity of the clinical manifestations of TAPVC are directly related to the presence of obstruction of the anomalous connection. With an obstructed connection, the infant usually becomes symptomatic within the first hours or days after birth. Mild to moderate cyanosis is evident, and the respiratory rate is rapid, with evidence of decreased lung compliance, i.e., intercostal retractions, nasal flaring, and sweating. Cardiac output is usually quite low in these infants, as evidenced by decreased pulses and, in some cases, acidosis. In the majority of these infants, the obstruction accompanies infradiaphragmatic connections, but it can be seen with supracardiac or mixed connections. It is uncommon for these infants to present after 3 to 6 months of age because most have expired before this point owing to complications of pulmonary congestion and low cardiac output.

Children with partially obstructed connections or hyperkinetic pulmonary hypertension usually present within the first 1 to 2 years of life. These infants have all the hallmarks of pulmonary hypertension and right ventricular dysfunction, with dyspnea on exertion, poor feeding, lack of weight gain, and cyanosis on crying or exercise. A history of frequent respiratory infections is often evident. On physical examination, the right ventricular impulse is prominent, and a left parasternal flow murmur is usually audible. The second heart sound is widely split and fixed, with a loud pulmonary component. Occasionally, a continuous murmur can be appreciated in the vicinity of the anomalous vertical vein.

Approximately 10 to 20 per cent of infants with TAPVC have no component of obstruction and do not develop pulmonary hypertension. These children can survive into adulthood, although with some restriction. These patients usually have Type I or II anomalous connections. With the exception of slight cyanosis, symptoms and signs are similar to those in patients with ostium secundum atrial septal defects but usually develop sooner. Dyspnea on exertion and fatigue at the end of the day with inability to keep up with their peers are the hallmark symptoms of this type of patient. Cyanosis is usually slight and is not visible to the untrained eye. Respiratory infections may be more common than normal. It is not uncommon for the diagnosis in unobstructed connections to be delayed until the child is seen for a preschool examination. On

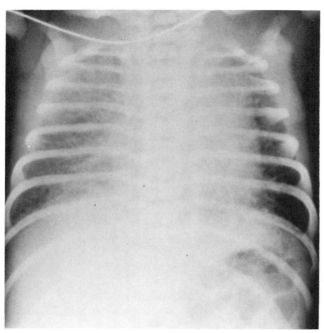

Figure 33–11. The plain chest film in an infant with obstructed TAPVC. Note the fine, reticular lung markings and lack of cardiomegaly.

physical examination, the right ventricle is prominent and hyperactive. The second cardiac sound is split and fixed; however, the pulmonary component is not loud. The parasternal systolic flow murmur is present and is similar to that in patients with atrial septal defects.

Chest Film. In infants with obstructed TAPVC, the heart is frequently not enlarged or is only mildly enlarged. Normally, after a day or two, the typical appearance of pulmonary venous congestion appears on the plain chest film (Fig. 33–11). There is a fine reticular pattern with haziness of the entire lung area. This frequently is the hallmark of the diagnosis and should be considered to be pathognomonic of the condition when seen in the very sick infant. In patients with partially obstructed connections or in those situations in which hyperkinetic pulmonary hypertension is present, the plain chest film shows increased pulmonary vascularity with cardiomegaly due to enlargement of the right atrium and ventricle. In some older children, the mediastinal component of the anomalous connection, the dilated left vertical vein or coronary sinus, may be visualized on the chest film and in this situation can be diagnostic of the condition (Fig. 33–12). In those patients with no pulmonary hypertension, the chest films show an increase in pulmonary vascularity and can show some right atrial and ventricular enlargement. Occasionally, pathognomonic mediastinal silhouettes can be recognized.

Electrocardiogram. The electrocardiogram is least helpful in diagnosing TAPVC. In general, all infants and children with TAPVC have right axis deviation and other electrocardiographic changes indicative of right ventricular hypertrophy. If the condition persists beyond 1 to 2 months, the signs of right atrial enlargement are present, and if this persists for some years, first-degree heart block may be evident, with prolongation of the PR interval.

Echocardiogram. Echocardiographic signs of right ventricular diastolic volume overload predominate in TAPVC. These are increased right ventricular dimension index and paradoxical ventricular septal movement. A highly reliable sign appears to be the finding of an echo-free space posterior to the left atrium representing the pulmonary venous confluence (Paquet and Gutgesell, 1975).

Cardiac Catheterization. As soon as the diagnosis of TAPVC is considered in an infant, cardiac catheterization should be performed. In infants with obstructed connections, oxygen determinations frequently are not as helpful as could be anticipated because of the severe degree of pulmonary vascular obstruction and the degree of shunting, which may not be excessive. Severe pulmonary hypertension is present, usually with a right-to-left ductal shunt. Right ventricular cineangiocardiography may show such a large right-to-left ductal shunt that sluggish and insufficient pulmonary blood flow does not allow the visualization of the pulmonary veins and their drainage. This may be possible only with injection of contrast medium with individual pulmonary arteries or occlusion of the ductus arteriosus with a balloon catheter and injection of contrast material through a proximal port or separate catheter (Fig. 33–13). Left ventricular cineangiocardiography usually reveals a small to normal-sized ventricle and a left atrium that is generally 50 per cent of normal size (Graham and Bender, 1980).

Cardiac catheterization and cineangiocardiography in patients with TAPVC and only mild obstruction or hyperkinetic pulmonary hypertension reveal

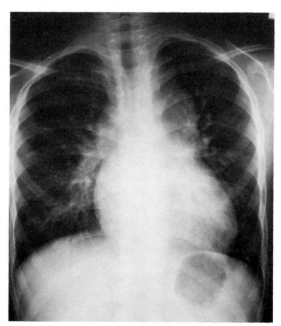

Figure 33–12. A typical chest film in an older child with nonobstructed supracardiac TAPVC. The prominent left upper mediastinal silhouette represents the dilated anomalous left vertical vein.

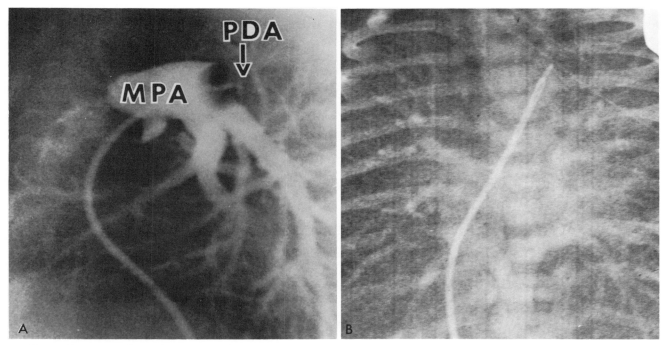

Figure 33–13. *A,* Cineangiocardiogram illustrating occlusion of the ductus arteriosus with a balloon catheter in an infant with infradiaphragmatic TAPVC. *B,* Subsequent contrast injection into the pulmonary artery reveals the pulmonary venous confluence and anomalous descending vertical vein.

findings that are similar to those in infants with pulmonary venous obstruction, except that pulmonary blood flow is usually more than twice the systemic flow and pulmonary capillary wedge pressures and pulmonary vascular resistance are low. Cineangiocardiography reveals a greatly dilated right ventricle, and the anomalous connection can easily be visualized with injection of contrast material into a pulmonary artery. In Type I connections, it is often possible to delineate the connection by passing the catheter through the innominate vein to the anomalous connection, with accurate delineation via an injection of contrast material at this point.

In patients without pulmonary hypertension, the cardiac catheterization findings are similar to those of atrial septal defect, with the exception that systemic oxygen saturations are slightly lower than normal and the anomalous connection is usually visualized without difficulty following injection of contrast material into the pulmonary artery (Fig. 33–14).

Indications for Operation

It is well established now that over 80 per cent of infants born with TAPVC will die before reaching 1 year of age (Burroughs and Edwards, 1980). The one variable that influences longevity is the presence or absence of significant pulmonary venous obstruction (Gathman and Nadas, 1970). Approximately 60 to 75 per cent of infants with TAPVC have obstruction of the anomalous pulmonary venous pathway. Without operation, it is unusual for any of these children to survive past 1 year of age, and most die within the first

3 months after birth (Gathman and Nadas, 1970). Among the remaining 25 to 30 per cent of children with unobstructed TAPVC, hyperkinetic pulmonary hypertension will develop in a significant number at a rate more rapid than in atrial septal defect (Jensen and

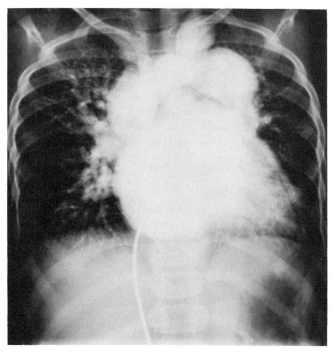

Figure 33–14. Pulmonary angiogram of a child with unobstructed TAPVC. During the venous phase of the study, the greatly dilated anomalous vertical vein connecting to a similarly large left innominate vein is demonstrated.

Blount, 1971). Approximately 50 per cent of these infants die within their first year, and few survive infancy, despite optimal medical management. This leaves only 10 to 20 per cent of all patients with TAPVC who have no pulmonary hypertension. Although heart failure often develops during infancy, most of these patients will survive with proper medical management. The incidence of heart failure or other complications, such as hyperkinetic pulmonary hypertension, then becomes obvious over the succeeding years, for an exceedingly small group reach adolescence and young adulthood without symptoms of any kind.

Because of the poor survival rate of the patient with total anomalous pulmonary venous connection, the diagnosis of TAPVC is in itself the indication for operation. In infants with pulmonary venous obstruction, operation should be performed without delay because of progressive pulmonary insufficiency, low cardiac output, and acidosis that are refractory to any conventional medical therapy. In infants with hyperkinetic pulmonary hypertension, operation can be scheduled at a convenient time but shortly after cardiac catheterization. Children with unobstructed connections should undergo operation within the first 5 years of life, and it is reasonable to repair these connections early so that damage to the distended right cardiac chambers does not occur. In patients with small atrial septal defects and a large pressure gradient between the right and left atrium, balloon atrial septostomy theoretically can be an effective means of increasing cardiac output while these infants are being prepared for operation. In a recent series, this procedure has not been used and is rarely necessary (Hammon et al., 1980).

Operation is contraindicated only in those children in whom irreversible changes of pulmonary vascular obstruction disease have developed. In these patients, intimal hyperplasia and muscular hypertrophy have increased pulmonary vascular resistance to greater than 75 per cent of the systemic level. This situation is very rare in modern medical practice, and contraindication to operation in TAPVC is unusual.

Surgical Treatment

Current practice indicates that cardiopulmonary bypass be used for all operations involving the correction of total anomalous pulmonary venous connection. The defect is best approached through a median sternotomy incision, and the type of perfusion support is dependent upon the age of the patient. In children less than 1 year of age, either surface-induced hypothermia with cardiopulmonary bypass support (Barratt-Boyes, 1973) or cardiopulmonary bypass with profound hypothermia and low-flow perfusion (Turley et al., 1980) is the technique of choice. In small infants and children, the prevention of intraoperative pulmonary venous distention and the construction of an adequate anastomosis are facilitated by circulatory arrest or low-flow perfusion. Cardiopulmonary bypass assists with rapid cooling and rewarming and control of the circulation. The technique for surgically managing infants utilizing profound hypothermia and circulatory arrest has recently been reported (Bender et al., 1979).

Infants are anesthetized with nitrous oxide and halothane, and cutdowns are performed to allow for monitoring of arterial and venous pressures. The infants are then transferred to a hypothermia chamber, where surface cooling to 30°C. is established. Meticulous control of arterial oxygen concentration and acid base balance is essential during this period, because many infants with obstructive TAPVC will have low cardiac output and will require buffering to maintain the pH at normal levels. Acidosis developing during the cooling period can predispose to serious arrhythmias, including ventricular fibrillation, and should be avoided at all cost. The infant is then transferred to the operating table, where a standard median sternotomy incision is made. After heparin is administered, the ascending aorta is cannulated, and the right atrium is cannulated through the right atrial appendage. Cardiopulmonary bypass is initiated, and the infant is further cooled to a nasopharyngeal temperature of 18°C. During this time, ventilation is continued, and the ductus is exposed by careful dissection and ligated. At 18°C., the ascending aorta is clamped and blood drained into the oxygenator. The venous cannula is removed, and the operative repair is performed during a period of circulatory arrest. Following repair, the venous cannula is reinserted, and the patient's blood volume is re-established. Air is carefully vented from the left ventricular apex and ascending aorta, cardiopulmonary bypass is resumed, and the infant is rewarmed to an esophageal temperature of 35° to 37°C. and cardiopulmonary bypass discontinued.

In infants weighing more than 10 kg. or children greater than 1 year of age, standard cardiopulmonary bypass techniques are used. A median sternotomy incision is made and the thymus divided or one lobe resected. After heparinization, the ascending aorta is cannulated, and venous cannulas are placed in the superior and inferior venae cavae after tapes are passed around these structures. Cardiopulmonary bypass is instituted, and moderate hypothermia to 25° to 28°C. is established. The aorta is then cross-clamped, and hyperkalemic cardioplegic solution (10 ml./kg.) is instilled through the aortic root. Topical hypothermic solution is poured over the heart to help reduce the intramyocardial temperature to 15°C. Cardiopulmonary bypass flows are reduced at this time to less than the calculated arterial flow. The repair is then performed and the cardiac chambers closed. The aortic cross-clamp is then removed, and before the heart is defibrillated, air is vented from the apex of the left ventricle and the aorta.

Supracardiac connections can be repaired by dissecting the right atrium and superior vena cava from their pericardial attachments (Fig. 33–15). Using this method, the anastomosis between the left atrium and

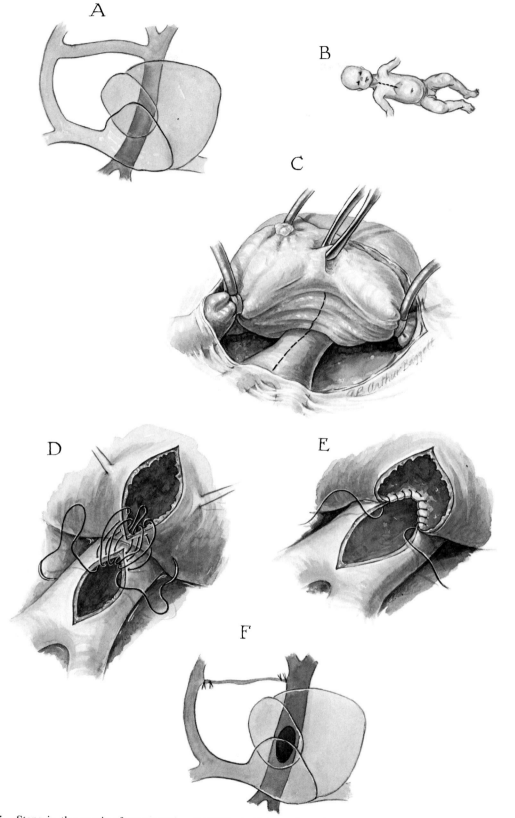

Figure 33–15. Steps in the repair of supracardiac TAPVC. *A*, Schematic anatomy as seen from the surgeon's view. *B*, Median sternotomy incision. *C*, After dissecting pericardial attachments, proposed incisions on the posterior left atrium and pulmonary venous confluence are shown. *D*, Generous incisions are made, and the first few stitches of a double-armed monofilament suture are shown. *E*, After pulling the sutures tight, they should be interrupted in several places to avoid constricting the anastomosis. *F*, The final result. (From Kirklin, J. W.: Surgical treatment for total anomalous pulmonary venous connection in infancy. *In* Heart Disease in Infancy. Edited by B. G. Barratt-Boyes, J. M. Neutze, and E. A. Harris. Baltimore, Williams and Wilkins Co., 1973.)

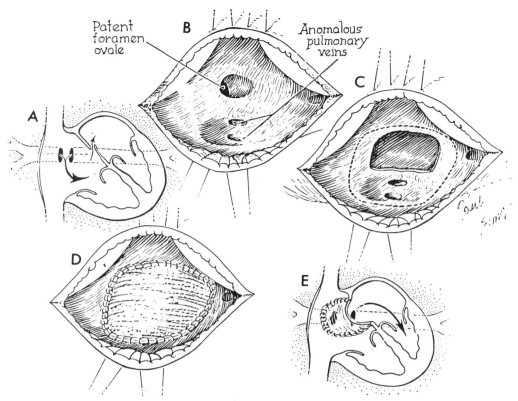

Figure 33–16. Repair of cardiac type of TAPVC in which the pulmonary veins drain directly to the right atrium. *A,* Anatomical representation. *B,* After right atriotomy. *C,* A generous portion of the atrial septum is excised. *D,* A large pericardial patch is used to direct pulmonary venous blood into the left atrium. (From Cooley, D. A., *et al.:* Total anomalous pulmonary venous drainage: Correction with the use of cardiopulmonary bypass in 62 cases. J. Thorac. Cardiovasc. Surg., *51*:88, 1966.)

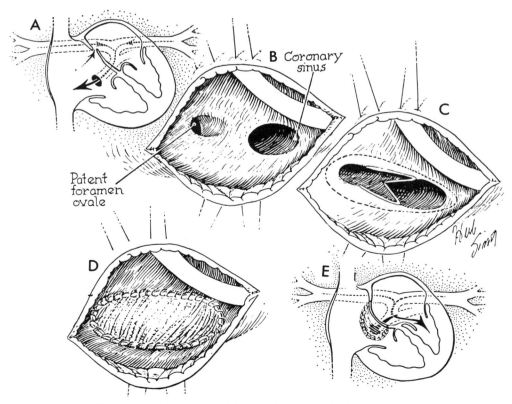

Figure 33–17. Repair of cardiac type of TAPVC in which the pulmonary veins connect with the coronary sinus. *A,* The surgical anatomy. *B,* A view of the dilated coronary sinus ostium after right atriotomy. *C,* The coronary sinus is incised into the left atrial wall and patent foramen ovale. *D,* A large pericardial patch is used to direct coronary sinus blood into the left atrium. *E,* The final result. (From Cooley, D. A., *et al.:* Total anomalous pulmonary venous drainage: Correction with the use of cardiopulmonary bypass in 62 cases. J. Thorac. Cardiovasc. Surg., *51*:88, 1966.)

the posterior venous chamber can be constructed by a combination of lifting the heart upward and completing the anastomosis on the right side of the cavae. Pulmonary veins that have directly entered the right atrium or right superior vena cava are repaired through a right atriotomy (Fig. 33–16). The atrial septal defect is enlarged, and a large pericardial patch is used to form a baffle that directs the pulmonary venous flow through the atrial septal defect. Intracardiac connections that drain into the right atrium via the coronary sinus are repaired in a similar fashion (Fig. 33–17).

It is important in patients with Type II TAPVC draining to the coronary sinus that an oblique right atriotomy be performed so that the crista terminalis is not divided. The coronary sinus is then incised into the foramen ovale or atrial septal defect. The atrial septal defect or foramen ovale is then enlarged, and a pericardial patch is used to direct the coronary sinus blood into the left atrium. Incising the coronary sinus and removing a portion of the atrial septum may injure one or more of the internodal conduction tracts between the sinus and atrioventricular nodes. Preservation of the crista terminalis is usually sufficient to insure sinus rhythm.

For Type III, or intracardiac, connections, the heart is elevated superiorly, and a large anastomosis is created between the posterior venous chamber and the left atrium (Fig. 33–18). In some patients, the posterior venous chamber is not a transverse structure but is an arborized, tree-like structure with the only large point of communication at the confluence of the descending anomalous vein (Kawashima *et al.*, 1977). In such cases, it will be necessary to perform a Y-shaped incision in the anomalous venous chamber and connect this to a similarly shaped incision in the posterior left atrium. If ligating the descending anomalous vein compromises the size of the left atrium, this can easily be left open, as these connections are in all cases obstructed. Mixed (Type IV) TAPVC is repaired using techniques described for the above combination of lesions.

It has been suggested that enlargement of the usually small left atrium may be necessary (Bonham-Carter *et al.*, 1969; Parr *et al.*, 1974). It has been observed on preoperative cineangiography (Graham and Bender, 1980), at operation (Goor *et al.*, 1976), and during the postoperative period (Parr *et al.*, 1974) that left atrial size is small, and reservoir function may be compromised because of poor compliance. Despite these theoretic arguments for using a pericardial patch to enlarge the size of the left atrium, several authors have noted that these maneuvers do not appreciably increase survival (Katz *et al.*, 1978; Hammon *et al.*, 1980). For these reasons, there is no convincing argument that the additional time and the construction of another suture line that may impair internodal conduction are necessary.

Postoperative care may be difficult in patients

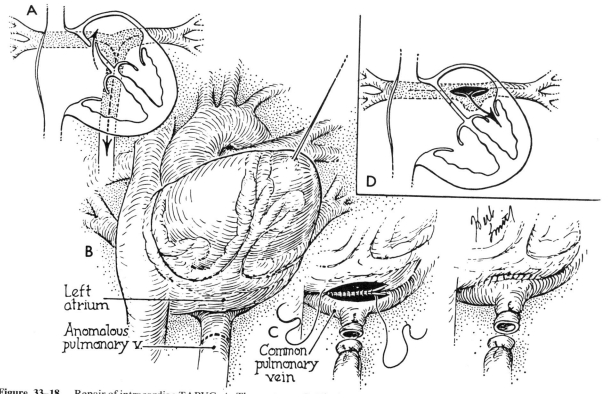

Figure 33–18. Repair of intracardiac TAPVC. *A,* The anatomy. *B,* The heart is deviated superiorly and the anomalous descending vein ligated. *C,* Generous incisions are made in the venous confluence and the left atrium. These are anastomosed with a fine monofilament suture. *D,* The final result after closing the atrial septal defect or patent foramen ovale. (From Cooley, D. A., *et al.:* Total anomalous pulmonary venous drainage: Correction with the use of cardiopulmonary bypass in 62 cases. J. Thorac. Cardiovasc. Surg., *51*:88, 1966.)

with TAPVC, especially in infants. Stiff, wet lungs are difficult to ventilate, and excessive inspiratory pressure serves to further decrease the function of a heart already compromised by pre- and intraoperative ischemia. Positive end-expiratory pressure, when used judiciously, can raise arterial oxygen concentration by better matching ventilation and perfusion and preventing atelectasis. Many infants require the infusion of catecholamines postoperatively. Isoproterenol in low to moderate doses (0.01 to 0.06 mcg./kg./min.) has a positive myocardial inotropic and chronotropic effect and serves to dilate both systemic and pulmonary arteries and thus decrease myocardial oxygen demands. Many infants are quite edematous, and the administration of diuretics encourages the return to normal hydration. In any case, careful attention to the details of blood and fluid replacement, arterial blood gases, and acid-base balance plus maintenance of adequate cardiac output are essential to a successful result.

Results

The results of operations for total anomalous pulmonary venous connection are directly related to the presence of obstruction and thus indirectly related to the type of connection present. Infants with obstructed connections usually present in extremis with very low cardiac output and are at great risk for the development of subendocardial necrosis. They are often very difficult to ventilate because of very poor lung compliance and suffer all the complications of mechanical ventilation that occur in infants with stiff lungs. Cardiac catheterization and operations in this group are usually performed on an emergent basis, and mortality and the rate of complications have been high. In the past few years, the operative mortality in infants has decreased from nearly 50 per cent to less than 30 per cent (Hammon et al., 1980; Turley et al., 1980). With more of these infants surviving to diagnosis and treatment, these results represent a marked improvement in the therapy of this condition. With more prompt diagnosis and therapy, the operative mortality can be expected to improve in these very sick infants.

Operative mortality is even less in patients who are between 3 and 12 months of age (Behrendt et al., 1972). In older children and adults, operative mortality is rare and is probably less than 5 per cent (Gomes et al., 1971). In most of these patients, the operative mortality is related to the presence of increased pulmonary vascular resistance from long-standing left-to-right intracardiac shunts.

Thus, it is the presence of obstruction in the anomalous connection that most significantly affects the patient's survival both with and without operation. In a recent series of infants operated on at Vanderbilt University Hospital between 1970 and 1980, the age of the patient did not directly affect the operative mortality (Hammon et al., 1980). In all surgical series, there have been more deaths in Types I and III TAPVC;

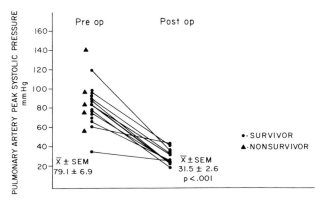

Figure 33–19. Preoperative and postoperative peak pulmonary artery pressures from a group of infants undergoing repair of TAPVC in infancy. Note the marked reduction in postoperative patients. (From Hammon, J. W., et al.: Total anomalous pulmonary venous connection in infancy. J. Thorac. Cardiovasc. Surg., 80:544, 1980.)

however, in these two groups the presence of anatomic obstruction to the anomalous connection is much more prevalent, especially in Type III.

With successful operation, late complications and mortality are rare. In patients with severe pulmonary hypertension and impaired left ventricular function, normal pulmonary artery pressure (Fig. 33–19) and left ventricular function (Fig. 33–20) can be expected with successful operation (Hammon et al., 1980; Mathew et al., 1977). Several reports of postoperative pulmonary venous obstruction due to a hypertrophic lesion in individual pulmonary veins after repair of various types of TAPVC in infancy are now present in the literature (Behrendt et al., 1972; Breckenridge et al., 1973; Whight et al., 1978; Fleming et al., 1979; Turley et al., 1980). Although this complication is rare, it usually results in severe morbidity or the death of the patient. The etiology of this problem is not clear; however, stenosis of individual pulmonary veins has a common embryologic etiology with TAPVC (Lucas et al., 1962), and it may be possible that these infants represent a combination of the two lesions. For older children and adults, late complication is exceedingly

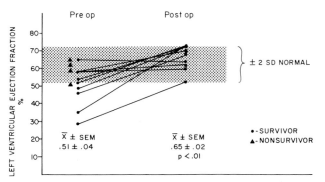

Figure 33–20. Preoperative and postoperative left ventricular ejection fraction calculated from left ventricular volume data obtained at cardiac catheterization. Note the return to normal function in postoperative patients. (From Hammon, J. W., et al.: Total anomalous pulmonary venous connection in infancy. J. Thorac. Cardiovasc. Surg., 80:544, 1980.)

rare and is usually due to an arrhythmia (Gomes *et al.*, 1971).

COR TRIATRIATUM

In *cor triatriatum*, the pulmonary veins enter a chamber superior to the left atrium that then joins the left atrium through a narrow opening. Alternatively, the accessory chamber may be totally separate from the left atrium and have a direct communication with the right atrium or indirectly communicate with the right atrium by way of an anomalous channel.

Historical Considerations

The classic form of cor triatriatum was clearly described in 1868 by Church. Anatomic classifications of cor triatriatum were first given by Loeffler in 1949 and further subdivided by Edwards in 1960. The first successful operation for total correction of cor triatriatum was reported by Vineberg and associates in 1956.

Incidence

Cor triatriatum is an exceedingly unusual anomaly. The frequency of cor triatriatum in all patients with congenital heart disease has been variously reported to be 0.1 to 0.4 per cent (Jegier *et al.*, 1963; Niwayama,

1960). The male-female incidence is approximately equal in most series. Although the etiology is unknown, the currently accepted embryologic explanation is that the accessory atrium is a common pulmonary vein that has failed to become incorporated into the left atrium in a normal fashion (Edwards, 1960).

Anatomy

The large number of subtypes of cor triatriatum demands a somewhat more inclusive classification than that proposed by Loeffler. The following classification is based on contributions of a number of individuals interested in this unusual anomaly (Loeffler, 1949; Edwards, 1960; Niwayama, 1960; Grondin *et al.*, 1964).

Accessory Left Atrial Chamber Receives All Pulmonary Veins and Communicates with the Left Atrium. This is the classic cor triatriatum in which a membranous partition having the shape of a windsock separates the more proximal chamber, which receives the pulmonary veins, from the more distal left atrium, which communicates with the mitral valve (Fig. 33–21A). The windsock-shaped partition is usually directed toward the mitral valve and may have one or more orifices. This anomalous septum contains cardiac muscle fibers and is occasionally calcified. The true left atrium communicates with the left atrial appendage and contains a fossa ovalis. In the majority of patients, there is no communication between the right and left atria; however, occasionally, a patent foramen ovale or

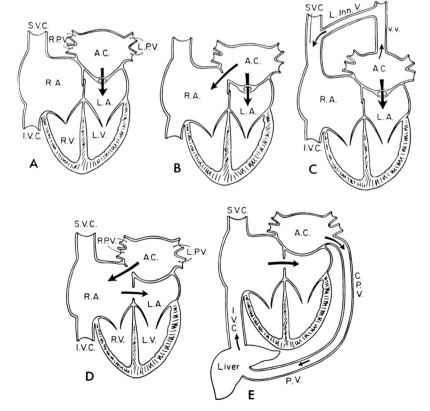

Figure 33–21. Diagrammatic illustration of the various types of cor triatriatum. *A,* Classical cor triatriatum in which the accessory chamber receives the pulmonary veins and communicates with the left atrium. *B,* Classical cor triatriatum in which the accessory chamber communicates both with the left atrium and the right atrium or *C,* the systemic venous circulation via an anomalous venous connection. *D,* Cor triatriatum in which the accessory chamber communicates only with the right atrium or *E,* the systemic venous circulation via an anomalous vein. (Adapted from Lucas, R. V., and Schmidt, R. E.: *In* Heart Disease in Infants, Children and Adolescents. Edited by A. J. Moss, F. H. Adams, and G. C. Emmanouilides. Baltimore, Williams and Wilkins Co., 1977.)

secundum atrial septal defect allows the lower left atrial chamber to communicate with the right atrium (Niwayama, 1960).

In a few patients, the accessory atrial chamber communicates directly with the left atrium through a stenotic opening and with the right atrium directly (Fig. 33–21B) or via an anomalous venous connection (Fig. 33–21C). The anatomy of complete cor triatriatum communicating with the left atrium was recently reported in 20 patients (Marin-Garcia et al., 1975). In 12 of these patients, a classic diaphragm divided the left atrium and contained one or more stenotic orifices. In six patients, the accessory venous chamber was obstructed by either an hourglass configuration or a tubular narrowing that obstructed flow into the normal left atrium. These were invariably associated with very complex associated cardiac lesions. The remaining two patients demonstrated other anomalous connections to the right atrium.

Accessory Atrial Chamber Receives All Pulmonary Veins and Does Not Communicate with the Left Atrium. In this particular anomaly, the diaphragm separating the common venous chamber from the left atrium is complete and prevents the direct flow of pulmonary venous blood to the left atrium. In order for the patient to survive, there is a direct communication from the common pulmonary venous chamber either to the right atrium (Fig. 33–21D) or via an anomalous channel either to the innominate vein or to the portal vein, as in the supracardiac and infracardiac types of total anomalous pulmonary venous connection (Fig. 33–21E).

Pathophysiology

In classic cor triatriatum in which there is no alternative pathway for pulmonary venous blood, the stenotic opening in the membranous partition separating the accessory atrial chamber from the true left atrium results in supravalvular mitral stenosis with all the features of elevated pulmonary venous pressure transmitted to the lungs, causing pulmonary edema. The feature that determines the clinical condition of the patient with this form of cor triatriatum is the size of the opening in the membrane. If the opening is 3 mm. or less in diameter, the symptoms occur in infancy and are similar to those of TAPVC with obstruction. If the opening is larger, the symptoms occur later in infancy, in childhood, or occasionally, later in life.

In other forms of cor triatriatum, the features of unobstructed TAPVC are found, with hyperkinetic pulmonary hypertension and communications of the pulmonary venous system with the right atrium either directly or through an anomalous channel.

Diagnosis

Clinical Manifestations. The majority of patients with cor triatriatum present with symptoms within the first few years of life (Niwayama, 1960). In these patients, signs of pulmonary venous obstruction are always prevalent, with bouts of pulmonary edema, extreme feeding difficulties, and poor weight gain. On physical examination, the predominant features will be moist rales in the lower lung fields associated with a very loud pulmonary second sound compatible with pulmonary hypertension. If there is a communication with the right atrium, there will be a flow murmur at the left sternal border associated with the large left-to-right intracardiac shunt.

In the occasional circumstance in which a patient is discovered with this condition later in life, there will be a history of breathlessness, frequent respiratory infections, and, in some cases, peripheral embolization. As with mitral stenosis, many patients are mistaken to have primary pulmonary disease. The physical examination in these patients will reflect severe pulmonary hypertension, i.e., a loud pulmonary second sound, right ventricular lift, and pulmonary rales. In many patients, the signs of right heart failure will be prominent, with distended peripheral veins and an enlarged liver. The usual cardiac murmur is a soft, blowing, systolic murmur along the left sternal border. In some cases, a diastolic murmur will be heard in the mitral area.

Chest Film. The plain chest film in cor triatriatum usually reflects pulmonary venous obstruction. Fine, diffuse, reticular pulmonary markings fan out from the pulmonary hilus to involve the lower lung fields. In older patients, Kerley's B lines may be present, coupled with prominent venous engorgement of the upper pulmonary vessels. There will also be signs of left atrial enlargement produced by the dilated accessory chamber (Fig. 33–22).

Electrocardiogram. The electrocardiographic findings reflect right ventricular systolic overload. In many cases, there are tall peaked P waves, suggesting right atrial enlargement. Rarely, notched P waves are present, presumably as a consequence of the dilated accessory atrial chamber.

Echocardiogram. The echocardiographic features are variable in cor triatriatum. When the membrane separating the accessory chamber from the true left atrium is thick and prominent, it sometimes can be localized with the echocardiogram. In most cases, however, it is impossible to differentiate the large dilated accessory chamber from TAPVC draining to the coronary sinus or persistent left superior vena cava connecting to the coronary sinus.

Cardiac Catheterization. The hallmark with regard to hemodynamic findings in cor triatriatum is a pressure gradient between the pulmonary capillary wedge pressure and the left atrial pressure. In most cases, oximetry will rule out a left-to-right shunt, and significant pulmonary hypertension is the rule. Selective pulmonary arteriography usually demonstrates cor triatriatum in the venous phase. Pulmonary transit time is prolonged. As the pulmonary veins are opacified, they drain into an accessory left atrial chamber. In most cases, there is a delay between the opacification of this chamber and the visualization of the true

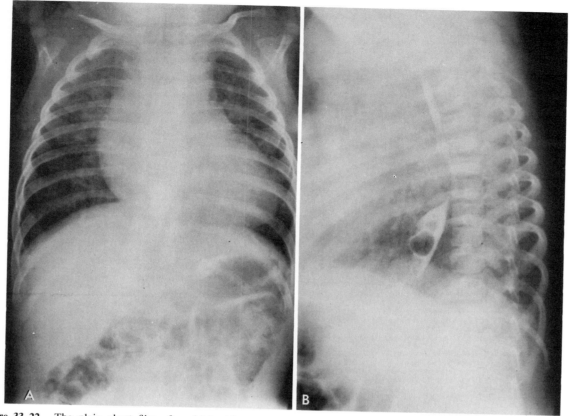

Figure 33–22. The plain chest film of a child with cor triatriatum. *A,* Posteroanterior view demonstrating pulmonary venous engorgement and left atrial enlargement. *B,* Lateral view confirming left atrial enlargement produced by the dilated accessory chamber, which causes posterior displacement of the barium-filled esophagus.

left atrium and left ventricle. With a high-quality study, the interatrial diaphragm can be identified as a linear or windsock-shaped filling defect between the accessory atrial chamber and the true left atrium (Fig.

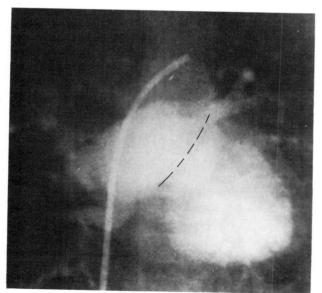

Figure 33–23. Venous phase of the pulmonary angiogram in a child with cor triatriatum. The dotted line indicates the position of the membrane separating the dilated accessory chamber from the left atrium.

33–23). The accessory atrial chamber usually remains opacified for some time and does not contract as does the normal left atrial chamber.

Surgical Treatment

The only successful therapy for cor triatriatum has been surgical. The indications for operation and preoperative preparation are similar to those for patients with TAPVC. Open correction is preferred in all cases. In infants, this is facilitated by hypothermia and circulatory arrest. In most cases, resection of the membrane between the accessory venous chamber and the left atrium can be accomplished through the atrial septum in infants and in older children by an incision into the true left atrium by developing the interatrial groove. If the preoperative diagnosis has suggested TAPVC, exploration of the heart exteriorly will usually demonstrate a dilated pulmonary venous chamber, which can be confused with the operative findings in congenital mitral stenosis. Occasionally, when anomalous connections between the accessory chamber and the systemic venous system are present, the operative findings can be quite confusing, and only a very careful and thorough intra- and extracardiac examination will reveal the true cause of the anomaly, which can then be easily corrected. The number of cases reported in the literature is quite small, and thus, the estimation of the operative mortality is difficult. In general, the very sick infants with pulmonary venous obstruction will have a higher mortality because of their preoperative condition. Mortality should be rare in older children and adults; however, late complications such as arrhythmias will be more common.

MAJOR ANOMALIES OF THE THORACIC SYSTEMIC VENOUS SYSTEM

Recent developments in the diagnosis and treatment of cardiovascular disorders have brought anomalies of the thoracic systemic veins to the attention of the cardiologist and thoracic surgeon alike. The consideration of these diverse anomalies requires a simple and practical system classification. A classification based entirely on anatomy tends to be cumbersome, whereas one based solely on physiology excludes conditions that result in hemodynamic derangement but may provide important information about technical complications that may occur during cardiac catheterization and operation. Therefore, a classification based on embryologic principles provides a more inclusive framework for discussion and for the practical consideration of the defects (Lucas and Schmidt, 1977). This system of classification includes anomalies of the cardinal venous system, anomalies of the inferior vena cava, and anomalies of the valves of the sinus venosus.

Anomalies of the Cardinal Venous System

Anomalies of the cardinal venous system involve aberrations in the development of the right and left superior vena cava and abnormalities of the coronary sinus. These anomalies present problems to the cardiac surgeon during repair of other defects or when the anomaly is associated with the drainage of desaturated blood into the left atrium.

Persistent Left Superior Vena Cava. Persistent left superior vena cava is the most common anomaly of the superior vena caval system. In a series of 4000 unselected autopsies, the prevalence was 0.3 per cent (Geissler and Albert, 1956). The association is much higher in patients with additional cardiac defects, ranging from 2.8 to 4.3 per cent (Loogen and Rippert, 1958). As a rule, persistent left superior vena cava is part of a bilateral superior vena caval system. This is a normal stage in evolutionary development, as well in the growth of the human embryo. Its usual anatomic course begins where it arises from the junction of the left subclavian and the left internal jugular veins. It then descends vertically in front of the aortic arch. A short distance from its origin, it receives the superior left intercostal vein. It then passes in front of the left pulmonary artery and left pulmonary veins or in between these vessels (Winter, 1954). It usually receives a hemiazygos vein and then penetrates the pericardium and crosses the posterior wall of the left atrium obliquely to approach the posterior atrial ven-

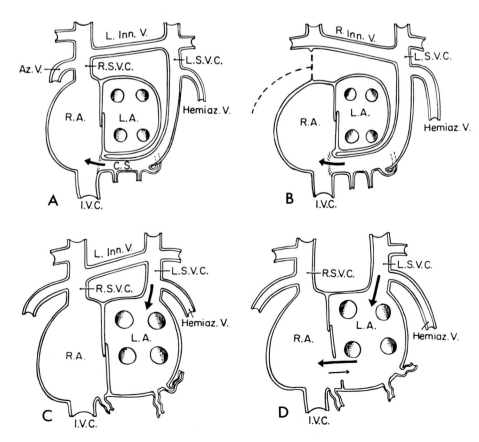

Figure 33–24. Variation of persistent left superior vena cava (L.S.V.C.). *A,* L.S.V.C. drains via the coronary sinus (C.S.) to the right atrium (R.A.). The sizes of the left innominate vein (L. Inn. V.) and L.S.V.C. vary inversely, with the former often being absent. *B,* Uncommonly, the right superior vena cava (R.S.V.C.) is atretic. *C,* The coronary sinus is absent, and the L.S.V.C. drains directly into the left atrium. Simple ligation of the L.S.V.C. is curative. *D,* The coronary sinus is absent, and there is no communication between the two superior venae cavae. A low-lying coronary sinus A.S.D. is present, and treatment requires baffling the L.S.V.C. into the right atrium and closing the A.S.D. (Adapted from Lucas, R. V., and Schmidt. R. E.: *In* Heart Disease in Infants, Children and Adolescents. Edited by A. J. Moss, F. H. Adams, and G. C. Emmanouilides. Baltimore, Williams and Wilkins Co., 1977.)

tricular groove. There it receives the great cardiac vein and becomes the coronary sinus (Fig. 33–24). Rarely, the right superior vena cava may be absent, and thus, the entire venous return from the head and arms enters the coronary sinus (Fig. 33–24). Associated anomalies are very common with persistent left superior vena cava. It is not uncommonly found with sinus venosus atrial septal defect or other congenital syndromes associated with cardiac malposition. Its only clinical importance is that cardiac catheterization is difficult when performed from the left arm. In addition, at the time of open cardiac operations, it is important to recognize the presence of the left superior vena cava so that appropriate cannulation techniques can eliminate the large amount of systemic venous blood that enters the heart through the coronary sinus. It is also very important to recognize the absence of collateral vessels between the left and right superior vena cava or, rarely, the absence of the right superior vena cava, in which case ligation of the persistent left superior vena cava would result in venous engorgement in the head and arms.

Persistent Left Superior Vena Cava Associated with Failure of Coronary Sinus Development (Unroofed Coronary Sinus). In this defect, the left superior vena cava takes its usual course anterior to the aortic arch and the left pulmonary artery. Then, instead of crossing back to the left atrium to enter the coronary sinus, it directly connects to the upper portion of the left atrium between the atrial appendage and the left superior pulmonary veins (Fig. 33–24C).

The physiologic consequences of this defect are almost always overshadowed by other major congenital cardiac malformations. The only contribution this defect makes to the overall hemodynamic findings at cardiac catheterization is a small right-to-left shunt at the atrial level.

This defect is almost invariably associated with other anomalies. In a recent series of eight operated patients, a coronary sinus atrial septal defect was present in all patients (Fig. 33–24D) (Quaegebeur *et al.*, 1979). This anomaly is also associated with primitive-type cyanotic congenital heart defects, such as cor biloculare, anomalies of conotruncal development, and the syndrome of splenic agenesis (Campbell and Deuchar, 1954).

DIAGNOSIS. *Clinical Findings.* In most cases, features of a complex associated defect obscure the clinical effects of left superior vena cava directly connected to the left atrium. When a defect in the atrial septum is associated, the primary manifestations are those found in atrial septal defect. When drainage of the left superior vena cava to the left atrium is an isolated phenomenon, cyanosis is prevalent in early infancy. Although the patient is asymptomatic, clubbing and polycythemia are usual. The heart is normal both on auscultation and on radiographic examination.

Cardiac Catheterization. The precise diagnosis of this defect is possible either by following the course of the cardiac catheter through the left superior vena

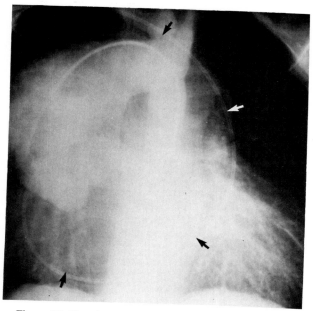

Figure 33–25. A cardiac catheter (arrows) passing from the right arm into a persistent left superior vena cava and into the right atrium in a child with complicated congenital heart disease.

cava or by dye injection in the left arm (Fig. 33–25). These findings in the face of peripheral cyanosis suggest a systemic vein draining anomalously into the left atrium.

Surgical Treatment. The treatment in all cases is surgical. If there are competent bridging veins between the left and right superior vena cava, the surgical treatment is simply ligation of the left superior vena cava and correction of the associated intracardiac defect. If, as in most cases, there are no bridging communications and the coronary sinus septum has not been formed, it is necessary to "roof" the coronary sinus with pericardium or a portion of the left atrium so that the left superior vena cava now drains to the right atrium (Fig. 33–26). Complications are usually related to the magnitude of operation for associated anomalies and not to the operative therapy for this uncommon situation.

Anomalies of the Inferior Vena Cava

Significant anomalies of the inferior vena cava are those that shunt unsaturated blood into the left atrium and that can complicate cardiac catheterization and cardiac operations for congenital heart disease. These anomalies are intrahepatic interruption of the inferior vena cava with azygos continuation, and anomalous drainage of the inferior vena cava into the left atrium.

Interrupted Inferior Vena Cava. Interruption of the inferior vena cava with azygos continuation is much more prevalent in patients with congenital heart disease, particularly those with the polysplenia syndrome and with cardiac malpositions (Anderson and Varco, 1961). When it is present as an isolated anoma-

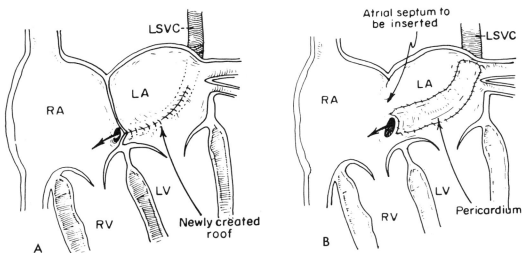

Figure 33–26. Repair (or roofing) of an unroofed coronary sinus associated with a persistent left superior vena cava (LSVC). *A,* The repair is made by bringing together the posterior left atrial wall to form a channel such that the LSVC communicates with the right atrium. *B,* The same repair is accomplished in a patient with a common atrium using pericardium. (From Quaegebeur, J., *et al.:* Surgical experience with unroofed coronary sinus. Ann. Thorac. Surg., *27*:418, 1979.)

ly, it is associated with a normal longevity and no physiologic abnormalities. Problems arise when it occurs with other congenital anomalies requiring surgical correction. During operations for congenital heart disease, ligation of the large azygos vein can result in a fatality and must be recognized (Effler *et al.,* 1951). The anomaly also leads to difficulties in cannulation for cardiopulmonary bypass, and details of this technical problem have been described elsewhere (Bosher, 1959).

Anomalous Drainage of the Inferior Vena Cava into the Left Atrium. In those cases in which the inferior vena cava shunts blood directly into the left atrium, a distinction must be made between connection of the inferior vena cava to the left atrium with intact atrial septum and cases in which a low atrial septal defect allows drainage of inferior vena caval blood into the left atrium. Direct connection of the inferior vena cava to the left atrium is extremely uncommon, and the embryology is obscure. The clinical features in these

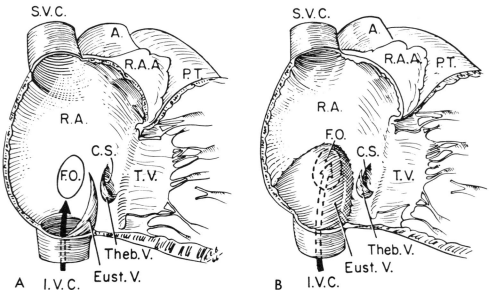

Figure 33–27. Persistence of the valves of the sinus venosus. *A,* Normal persistence of the valves of the sinus venosus results in the eustachian valve (Eust. V.) and the thebesian valve (Theb. V.). *B,* Abnormal persistence of the eustachian valve has resulted in a membrane that completely diverts inferior vena cava (I.V.C.) blood into the left atrium via the foramen ovale (F.O.). In similar fashion, the ostium of the coronary sinus (C.S.), the superior vena cava (S.V.C.) orifice, or all three may be isolated from the true right atrium by abnormal persistence of the valves of the sinus venosus. (R.A.A. = right atrial appendage; T.V. = tricuspid valve; P.T. = pulmonary trunk; A. = aorta.) (From Lucas, R. V., and Schmidt, R. E.: *In* Heart Disease in Infants, Children and Adolescents. Edited by A. J. Moss, F. H. Adams, and G. C. Emmanouilides. Baltimore, Williams and Wilkins Co., 1977.)

cases are comparable to those of left superior vena cava connections to the left atrium (Gardner and Cole, 1955). In these patients, the risk of systemic embolization is present, and surgical therapy should be undertaken. The placement of an interatrial baffle to provide for normal systemic venous drainage is curative (Black *et al.*, 1964). In some cases, persistence of the valves of the sinus venosus can direct inferior vena caval blood into the left atrium by an atrial septal defect or patent foramen ovale (Fig. 33–27) (Doucette and Knoblich, 1963). Treatment is effected simply by incising the persistent valvular tissue and closing the interatrial communication. In some patients with an atrial septal defect, a large eustachian valve may be mistaken for the lower margin of the atrial septal defect. Great care must be taken to close the atrial defect itself, since closure of the atrial septum onto the eustachian valve may then divert inferior vena caval blood into the left atrium (Mustard *et al.*, 1964).

SELECTED REFERENCES

Bender, H. W., Fisher, R. D., Walker, W. E., and Graham, T. P.: Reparative cardiac surgery in infants and small children: Five years experience with profound hypothermia and circulatory arrest. Ann. Surg., *190*:437, 1979.

A recent summary of the results of operations on a large series (128) of infants and children using hypothermia and circulatory arrest. The surgical techniques are detailed and the results illustrated.

Darling, R. C., Rothney, W. B., and Craig, J. M.: Total pulmonary venous drainage into the right side of the heart. Lab. Invest., *6*:44, 1957.

The first publication to carefully characterize the types of TAPVC. Beautifully illustrated description of the pathologic anatomy.

Hammon, J. W., Bender, H. W., Graham, T. P., Boucek, R. J., Smith, C. W., and Erath, H. G.: Total anomalous pulmonary venous connection in infancy. J. Thorac. Cardiovasc. Surg., *80*:544, 1980.

A recent series of operated patients with TAPVC emphasizing pre- and postoperative hemodynamic and ventricular function studies. This article points out that operative survivors will have normal hemodynamic and ventricular function.

Ivemark, B. I.: Implications of agenesis of the spleen on the pathogenesis of conotruncus anomalies in childhood: An analysis of the heart malformations in the splenic agenesis syndrome with fourteen new cases. Acta Paediatr. Scand. (Suppl.), *104*:1, 1955.

One of the best descriptions of the pathologic anatomy, diagnosis, and surgical treatment of this uncommon anomaly.

Katz, N. M., Kirklin, J. W., and Pacifico, A. D.: Concepts and practices in surgery for total anomalous pulmonary venous connection. Ann. Thorac. Surg., *25*:479, 1978.

An excellent review article that discusses many of the controversial features in the diagnosis and management of TAPVC.

Lucas, R. V., and Schmidt, R. E.: Anomalous venous connection, pulmonary and systemic. *In* Heart Disease in Infants, Children and Adolescents. Edited by A. J. Moss, F. H. Adams, and G. C. Emmanouilides. Baltimore, Williams and Wilkins, 1977, pp. 437–470.

A carefully detailed explanation of the embryology of anomalies of pulmonary venous connection to the heart. Well illustrated and easily understandable.

Neill, C. A.: Development of the pulmonary veins: With reference to the embryology of anomalies of pulmonary venous return. Pediatrics, *18*:880, 1956.

A landmark embryologic study that outlines the development of the pulmonary venous system and provides an embryologic explanation for anomalous pulmonary venous connections.

Sloan, H., MacKenzie, J., Morris, J. D., Sterns, S., and Sigmann, J.: Open-heart surgery in infancy. J. Thorac. Cardiovasc. Surg., *44*:459, 1962.

A description of the first successful repair of Type III TAPVC in an infant. This introduced the concept of deep hypothermia induced by surface cooling and cardiopulmonary bypass so that a period of circulatory arrest could be utilized for operative repair.

REFERENCES

Anderson, R. C., and Varco, R. L.: Cor triatriatum: Successful diagnosis and surgical correction in a 3-year-old girl. Am. J. Cardiol., *7*:436, 1961.

Appelbaum, A., Kirklin, J. W., Pacifico, A. D., *et al.*: The surgical treatment of total anomalous pulmonary venous connection. Isr. J. Med. Sci., *11*:89, 1975.

Barratt-Boyes, B. G.: Primary definitive intracardiac operations in infants; total anomalous pulmonary venous connection. *In* Advances in Cardiovascular Surgery. Edited by J. W. Kirklin. New York, Grune and Stratton, 1973, pp. 127–140.

Behrendt, D. M., Aberdeen, E., Waterson, D. J., and Bonham-Carter, R. E.: Total anomalous pulmonary venous drainage in infants. Circulation, *46*:347, 1972.

Bender, H. W., Fisher, R. D., Walker, W. E., and Graham, T. P.: Reparative cardiac surgery in infants and small children: Five years experience with profound hypothermia and circulatory arrest. Ann. Surg., *190*:437, 1979.

Black, H., Smith, G. T., and Goodale, W. T.: Anomalous inferior vena cava draining into the left atrium associated with intact interatrial septum and multiple pulmonary arteriovenous fistulae. Circulation, *29*:258, 1964.

Bonham-Carter, R. E., Capriles, M., and Noe, Y.: Total anomalous pulmonary venous drainage: A clinical and anatomical study of 75 children. Br. Heart J., *31*:45, 1969.

Bosher, L. H.: Problems in extracorporeal circulation relating to venous cannulation and drainage. Ann. Surg., *149*:652, 1959.

Breckenridge, I. M., de Leval, M., Stark, J., and Waterston, D. J.: Correction of total anomalous pulmonary venous drainage in infancy. J. Thorac. Cardiovasc. Surg., *66*:447, 1973.

Brody, H.: Drainage of the pulmonary veins into the right side of the heart. Arch. Pathol., *33*:22, 1942.

Burroughs, J. T., and Edwards, J. E.: Total anomalous pulmonary venous connection. Am. Heart J., *59*:913, 1960.

Campbell, M., and Deuchar, D. C.: The left-sided superior vena cava. Br. Heart J., *16*:423, 1954.

Church, W. S.: Congenital malformation of the heart: Abnormal septum in left auricle. Trans. Pathol. Soc. (Lond.), *19*:188, 1868.

Cooley, D. A., and Ochsner, A.: Correction of total anomalous pulmonary venous drainage. Surgery, *42*:1014, 1957.

Cooley, D. A., Hallman, G. L., and Leachman, R. D.: Total anomalous pulmonary venous drainage: Correction with the use of cardiopulmonary bypass in 62 cases. J. Thorac. Cardiovasc. Surg., *51*:88, 1966.

Darling, R. C., Rothney, W. B., and Craig, J. M.: Total pulmonary venous drainage into the right side of the heart. Lab. Invest., *6*:44, 1957.

Doucette, J., and Knoblich, R.: Persistent right valve of the sinus venosus. Arch. Pathol., *75*:105, 1963.

Edwards, J. E.: Malformations of the thoracic veins. *In* Pathology of the Heart. 2nd Ed. Edited by S. E. Gould. Springfield, Illinois, Charles C Thomas, 1960, p. 484.

Effler, D. B., Greer, A. E., and Sifers, E. C.: Anomaly of the vena cava inferior. Report of fatality after ligation. J.A.M.A., *146*:1321, 1951.

Eliot, R. S., and Edwards, J. E.: Congenital heart disease. *In* The Heart. Edited by J. W. Hurst and R. B. Logue. New York, McGraw-Hill, 1966, pp. 587–620.

Fleming, W. H., Clark, E. B., Dooley, K. J., Hofschire, P. J., Ruckman, R. N., Hopeman, A. R., Sarafian, L., and Mooring, P. K.: Late complications following surgical repair of total anomalous pulmonary venous return below the diaphragm. Ann. Thorac. Surg., *27*:435, 1979.

Friedlich, A., Bing, R. J., and Blount, S. G.: Physiological studies in congenital heart disease: IX. Circulatory dynamics in the anomalies of venous return to the heart, including pulmonary arteriovenous fistula. Am. Heart J., *86*:20, 1950.

Gardner, D. L., and Cole, L.: Long survival with inferior vena cava draining into left atrium. Br. Heart J., *17*:93, 1955.

Gathman, G. H., and Nadas, A. S.: Total anomalous pulmonary venous connection: Clinical and physiologic observations of 75 pediatric patients. Circulation, *42*:143, 1970.

Geissler, W., and Albert, M.: Persistierende linke obere Hohlvene und Mitralstenose. A. Gesamte Inn. Med., *11*:865, 1956.

Gomes, M. M. R., Feldt, R. H., McGoon, D. C., and Danielson, G. K: Long-term results following correction of total anomalous pulmonary venous connection. J. Thorac. Cardiovasc. Surg., *61*:253, 1971.

Goor, D. A., Yellin, A., Frand, M., Smolinsky, A., and Neufeld, H.: The operative problem of small left atrium in total anomalous pulmonary venous connection: Report of 5 patients. Ann. Thorac. Surg., *22*:254, 1976.

Graham, T. P., and Bender, H. W.: Preoperative diagnosis and management of infants with critical congenital heart disease. Ann. Thorac. Surg., *29*:272, 1980.

Grondin, C., Leonard, A. S., Anderson, R. C., Amplatz, K. A., Edwards, J. E., and Varco, R. L.: Cor triatriatum: A diagnostic surgical enigma. J. Thorac. Cardiovasc. Surg., *48*:527, 1964.

Hammon, J. W., Bender, H. W., Graham, T. P., Boucek, R. J., Smith C. W., and Erath, H. G.: Total anomalous pulmonary venous connection in infancy. J. Thorac. Cardiovasc. Surg., *80*:544, 1980.

Ivemark, B. I.: Implications of agenesis of the spleen on the pathogenesis of conotruncus anomalies in childhood: An analysis of the heart malformations in the splenic agenesis syndrome with fourteen new cases. Acta Paediatr. Scand. (Suppl.), *104*:1, 1955.

Jegier, W., Gibbons, J. E., and Wiglesworth, F. W.: Cor triatriatum: Clinical, hemodynamic, and pathologic studies: Surgical correction in early life. Pediatrics, *31*:255, 1963.

Jensen, J. B., and Blount, S. G.: Total anomalous pulmonary venous return: A review and report of the oldest surviving patient. Am. Heart J., *82*:387, 1971.

Katz, N. M., Kirklin, J. W., and Pacifico, A. D.: Concepts and practices in surgery for total anomalous pulmonary venous connection. Ann. Thorac. Surg., *25*:479, 1978.

Kawashima, Y., Matsuda, H., Hakano, S., Miyamoto, K., Fujino, M., Kozuka, T., and Manabe, H.: Tree-shaped pulmonary veins in infracardiac total anomalous pulmonary venous drainage. Ann. Thorac. Surg., *23*:436, 1977.

Kirklin, J. W.: Surgical treatment for total anomalous pulmonary venous connection in infancy. *In* Heart Disease in Infancy. Edited by B. G. Barratt-Boyes, J. M. Neutz, and E. A. Harris. Baltimore, Williams and Wilkins, 1973, pp. 89–100.

Lewis, J., Varco, R. L., Taufic, M., and Niazi, S. A.: Direct vision repair of triatrial heart and total anomalous pulmonary venous drainage. Surg. Gynecol. Obstet., *102*:713, 1956.

Loeffler, E.: Unusual malformation of the left atrium: Pulmonary sinus. Arch. Pathol., *48*:371, 1949.

Loogen, F., and Rippert, R.: Anomalien der grossen Korper und Lungenvenen. Z. Kreislaufforsch., *47*:677, 1958.

Los, J. A.: Embryology. *In* Pediatric Cardiology. Edited by H. Watson. St. Louis, C. V. Mosby Co., 1968.

Lucas, R. V., and Schmidt, R. E.: Anomalous venous connection, pulmonary and systemic. *In* Heart Disease in Infants, Children and Adolescents. Edited by A. J. Moss, F. H. Adams, and G.

C. Emmanouilides. Baltimore, Williams and Wilkins, 1977, pp. 437–470.

Lucas, R. V., Woolfrey, B. F., Anderson, R. C., Lester, R. G., and Edwards, J. E.: Atresia of the common pulmonary vein. Pediatrics, *29*:729, 1962.

Marin-Garcia, J., Tandon, R., Lucas, R. V., Jr., and Edwards, J. E.: Cor triatriatum: Study of 20 cases. Am. J. Cardiol., *35*:59, 1975.

Mathew, R., Thilenius, O. G., Replogle, R. L., and Arcilla, R. A.: Cardiac function in total anomalous pulmonary venous return before and after surgery. Circulation, *55*:361, 1977.

McClure, C. F. W., and Butler, E. G.: The development of the vena cava inferior in man. Am. J. Anat., *35*:331, 1925.

Meadows, W. R., Bergstrand, I., and Sharp, J. T.: Isolated anomalous connection of a great vein to the left atrium. Circulation, *24*:669, 1961.

Miller, W. W., and Rashkind, W. J.: Palliative treatment of total anomalous pulmonary venous drainage by balloon atrial septostomy. Lancet, *2*:387, 1968.

Muller, W. H.: The surgical treatment of transposition of the pulmonary veins. Ann. Surg., *134*:683, 1951.

Mustard, W. T., Firor, W. B., and Kidd, L.: Diversion of the venae cavae into the left atrium during closure of atrial septal defects. J. Thorac. Cardiovasc. Surg., *47*:317, 1964.

Neill, C. A.: Development of the pulmonary veins: With reference to the embryology of anomalies of pulmonary venous return. Pediatrics, *18*:880, 1956.

Newfield, E. A., Wilson, A., Paul, M. H., and Reisch, J. S.: Pulmonary vascular disease in total anomalous venous drainage. Circulation, *61*:103, 1980.

Niwayama, G.: Cor triatriatum. Am. Heart J., *59*:291, 1960.

Paquet, M., and Gutgesell, H.: Echocardiographic features of total anomalous pulmonary venous connection. Circulation, *51*:599, 1975.

Parr, G. V. S., Kirklin, J. W., Pacifico, A. D., Blackstone, E. H., and Lauridsen, P.: Cardiac performance in infants after repair of TAPVC. Ann. Thorac. Surg., *17*:561, 1974.

Quaegebeur, J., Kirklin, J. W., Pacifico, A. D., and Bargeron, L. M.: Surgical experience with unroofed coronary sinus. Ann. Thorac. Surg., *27*:418, 1979.

Raghib, G., Ruttenberg, H. D., Anderson, R. C., Amplatz, K., Adams, P., and Edwards, J. E.: Termination of left superior vena cava in left atrium, atrial septal defect, and absence of coronary sinus. Circulation, *31*:906, 1965.

Ruttenberg, H. D., Neufeld, H. N., Lucas, R. V., Carey, L. S., Adams, P., Anderson, R. D., and Edwards, J. E.: Syndrome of congenital cardiac disease with asplenia: Distinction from other forms of congenital cardiac disease. Am. J. Cardiol., *13*:387, 1964.

Shaner, R. F.: The development of the bronchial veins with special reference to anomalies of the pulmonary veins. Anat. Rec., *140*:159, 1961.

Sloan, H., MacKenzie, J., Morris, J. D., Stern, S., and Sigmann, J.: Open-heart surgery in infancy. J. Thorac. Cardiovasc. Surg., *44*:459, 1962.

Snellen, H. A., and Bruins, C.: Anomalies of venous return. *In* Pediatric Cardiology. Edited by H. Watson. St. Louis, C. V. Mosby Co., 1968.

Streeter, G. L.: Developmental horizons in human embryos. Description of age group XI, 13 to 20 somites, and age group XII, 21 to 20 somites. Carnegie Inst. Contrib. Embryol., *30* (197):211, 1942.

Turley, K., Tucker, W. Y., Ullyot, D. J., and Ebert, P. A.: Total anomalous pulmonary venous connection in infancy: Influence of age and type of lesion. Am. J. Cardiol., *45*:92, 1980.

Vineberg, A., and Gialloreto, O.: Report of a successful operation for stenosis of common pulmonary vein (cor triatriatum). Can. Med. Assoc. J., *74*:719, 1956.

Whight, C. M., Barratt-Boyes, B. G., Calder, A. L., Neutze, J. M., and Brandt, P. W. T.: Total anomalous pulmonary venous connection. J. Thorac. Cardiovasc. Surg., *75*:52, 1978.

Wilson, J.: On a very unusual formation of the human heart. Phil. Trans. (Lond.), *88*:332, 1798.

Winter, F. S.: Persistent left superior vena cava: Survey of world literature and report of thirty additional cases. Angiology, *5*:90, 1954.

Chapter 34

Atrioventricular Canal

Dwight C. McGoon

Francisco J. Puga

Gordon K. Danielson

The various congenital deformities of the atrioventricular canal are usually designated by the inclusive term "persistent common atrioventricular (A-V) canal defect" (Feldt, 1976). The common A-V canal is not an entity recognized in the normal, fully developed human heart but is encountered only in the embryo. It consists of that slightly narrowed zone between the one atrium and the one ventricle when the embryo is in its early tubular stage of development, and it serves as a broad area of connection and communication between the primitive atrium and the primitive ventricle.

During the course of embryonic development, the ventricular septum ascends from the apex and the atrial septum descends from the cephalad atrial wall, thus dividing the heart into right and left halves. As these septa converge at the A-V junction or canal, "cushions" of endothelium form on the anterior and posterior margins of the canal. The progressive enlargement of these cushions contributes to separation of the common A-V canal into right and left A-V orifices and to development of their respective valves. Defective development in this area may result in incomplete septation of the A-V canal and deformity of one or both A-V valves. The underlying embryonic abnormality appears to be failure of normal fusion of the major atrioventricular endocardial cushions. The development of the central cardiac septum and the adjacent portions of the atrioventricular valves is apparently dependent on the normal development of the endocardial cushions.

CLASSIFICATION

When embryonic development of the area of the common A-V canal is abnormal, the resulting malformation is subject to several variations, depending on the extent of involvement of the atrial and ventricular septa as well as of the mitral and tricuspid valves. Concepts about classification of the various congenital cardiac defects have slowly evolved, and for the surgeon, a surgically oriented classification is preferable. Thus, for the surgeon, the first distinction is

whether a given anomaly includes a fully displayed A-V canal septal defect in the center of the heart involving the ostium primum area of the atrial septum as well as the adjacent basal area of the ventricular septum, or, alternatively, whether the anomaly includes some lesser extent of septal defect or none at all and is therefore an incompletely displayed A-V canal septal defect. The classification developed in Table 34–1 is based on this distinction. The table lists each of the 15 theoretically possible types of anomalies according to which combination of the four potential defects in embryogenesis of the A-V canal has occurred. Note that both the ostium primum (O) and basal ventricular (V) septal defects are present in each type of fully displayed form, whereas they are never associated in the same heart in any incompletely displayed form.

TABLE 34–1. THEORETICALLY POSSIBLE FORMS OF A-V CANAL DEFECT

I. Fully displayed A-V canal septal defect (both ostium primum [O] and ventricular [V] septal defects are present)
   1. OVMT
   2. OVM
   3. OVT
   4. OV

II. Incompletely displayed A-V canal septal defect (O and V are not present together)
  A. Septal defect present
    1. VMT
    2. OMT
    3. VM
    4. VT
    5. OM
    6. OT
    7. V
    8. O
  B. No septal defect present
    1. MT
    2. M
    3. T

O = ostium primum atrial septal defect
V = basal (inlet) ventricular septal defect
M = typical mitral defect (cleft of anterior leaflet)
T = typical tricuspid defect (cleft or partial absence of septal leaflet)

Incompletely Displayed Forms

Incompletely displayed forms of the anomaly may result in isolated cleft formation in the anterior (aortic) leaflet of the mitral valve (M), isolated inlet ventricular septal defect (V), isolated atrial septal defect of the ostium primum type (O), or combined inlet ventricular septal defect and cleft mitral valve (VM), and so on. These forms of incompletely displayed A-V canal septal defect should best be classified with mitral valve deformities, atrial septal defects, or ventricular septal defects, whichever best pertains, and can be found in those respective chapters: therefore, they are not a subject of further discussion in this chapter. Thus, emphasis is given to the tenet that to be classified as a fully displayed A-V canal defect, an anomaly must include a central septal defect that involves both the ostium primum area of the atrial septum and the basal portion of the ventricular septum. This concept of a central septal defect involving both atrial and ventricular septa must be emphasized for clear appreciation of the anatomic and surgical aspects of this anomaly.

Fully Displayed Forms

It has been helpful from the surgical point of view to separate the fully displayed A-V canal deformities into three types—partial, intermediate, and complete. **_Partial A-V Canal_** (Fig. 34–1*A*). This is the type of deformity in which there is a centrally located septal

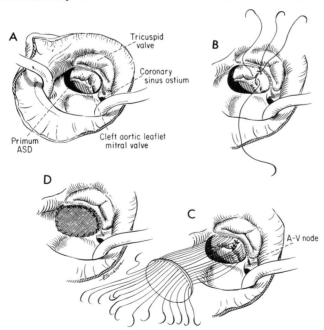

Figure 34–1. Partial A-V Canal. *A*, Surgical exposure, optimized by long atriotomy in the trabecular wall from the apex of the appendage to near the inferior caval orifice, and wide mobilization of venous cannulae. *B*, Beginning closure of the cleft in the anterior (aortic) mitral leaflet. *C*, Sutures placed between the patch and the junction of the mitral and tricuspid valves as initial stage of closure of the ostium primum atrial septal defect (see also Fig. 34–3*A* and *B*). *D*, Repair completed. (Reproduced with permission from Danielson, G. K.: Endocardial cushion defects. *In* Pediatric Surgery, 3rd Ed. Edited by M. M. Ravitch, *et al.* Copyright © 1979 by Year Book Medical Publishers, Inc., Chicago.)

defect with both involvement of the ostium primum area of the atrial septum and a deficiency ("scooping out") in the base of the ventricular septum. The distinctive feature of the partial A-V canal is that the valvular leaflet tissue positioned superadjacent to the ventricular septum has become fused continuously to the underlying crest of the ventricular septum. Although there is a deficiency, or "scooping out," of the base of the ventricular septum in partial A-V canal, the fusion of the valvular leaflets to the crest of this deficient septum prevents a direct interventricular communication deep to the leaflets. This absence of direct interventricular communication is the hallmark of the partial A-V canal anomaly. In addition, there is nearly always a cleft in the anterior (aortic) leaflet of the mitral valve, and furthermore, the majority of hearts (85 per cent) show an incomplete development of the septal leaflet of the tricuspid valve, particularly in its anterior portion. Usually, the cleft in the anterior leaflet of the mitral valve does not extend across the crest of the ventricular septum, i.e., the anterior and posterior portions of the anterior (aortic) mitral leaflet are fused to each other along the crest of the ventricular septum. In turn, this in effect provides a complete circle to the mitral anulus and to the tricuspid anulus, thus dividing the "complete" canal into separated mitral and tricuspid orifices.

The discerning reader of Table 34–1 might object that the theoretical variations of A-V canal defect consisting of OMT, OM, or O are, in fact, defects that should be dealt with in this chapter, since they amount to an ostium primum atrial septal defect, with or without valvular involvement. However, it must be emphasized that a theoretically possible anomaly consisting of an isolated ostium primum defect (i.e., without an associated deficiency, or "scooping out," of the base of the ventricular septum) is *not* representative of a partial A-V canal defect as typically encountered. In fact, deficiency of the basal (inlet) portion of the ventricular septum is a constant component of the typical partial A-V canal defect. As corroboration of this, it is to be noted that the outflow tract of the left ventricle has the appearance of being elongated because of the ventricular septal deficiency into the "goose-neck" deformity typical of partial A-V canal (Rastelli *et al.*, 1967; Baron, 1968; Blieden *et al.*, 1974). Furthermore, the issue of deficiency at the base of the ventricular septum has relevance to the surgeon, particularly if valvular replacement is required, as will be discussed later.

Intermediate A-V Canal. Intermediate A-V canal is the rarest of the three types of fully displayed A-V canal. Unfortunately, this categorization designates widely varying features by various authors (Bharati *et al.*, 1980 a,b). In our usage, it is characterized by two features, one of which it holds in common with the partial form of A-V canal, and one it holds in common with the complete form. In the intermediate form, distinct mitral and tricuspid valvular orifices have been formed as a result of embryonic fusion between the anterior and posterior common leaflets of the common A-V valve at their centers, just as in partial A-V canal.

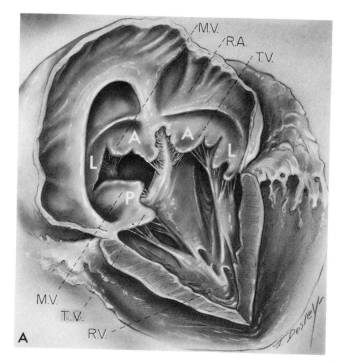

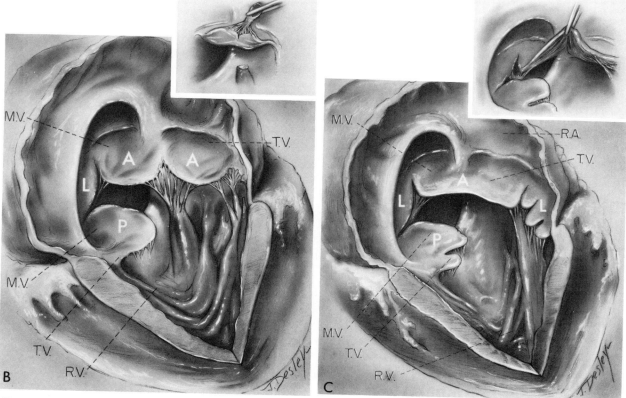

Figure 34–2. The three types of complete atrioventricular canal. *A*, Type A. Anterior common leaflet (A) divided and attached to the crest of the ventricular septum (M.V. = mitral valve; R. A. = right atrium; T. V. = tricuspid valve; P = posterior common leaflet; L = Lateral leaflet; R.V. = right ventricle). *B*, Type B. Anterior common leaflet partially divided, with chordae from the central area of the leaflet attached to a single abnormal papillary muscle arising from the right ventricle. *C*, Type C. Anterior common leaflet is undivided and is not attached to the ventricular septum. The insets in *B* and *C* show the extent of the interventricular communication deep to the common anterior leaflet. Note that the ventricular septum below the valvular attachment approximates the position of the anterior rim of the atrial septal defect above the leaflet. Thus, the surgical incision to be made in the common anterior leaflet (see surgical technique) will be made to this area at the base of the common anterior leaflet. (From Rastelli, G. C., Kirklin, J. W., and Titus, J. L.: Anatomic observations on complete form of persistent common atrioventricular canal with special reference to atrioventricular valves. Mayo Clin. Proc., *41*:296, 1966.)

However, in contrast to partial A-V canal, this centrally connected leaflet tissue does not fully fuse with the underlying crest of the ventricular septum. As a result, a space bordered superiorly by the leaflets and inferiorly by the crest of the ventricular septum allows a direct interventricular communication, just as in the complete form of A-V canal. Thus, this condition is truly intermediate between the partial and complete forms. Other authors have used a more liberal definition for the intermediate designation, so as to include hearts exhibiting any of various atypical features encountered in the three basic types (partial, intermediate, and complete) of fully displayed A-V canal.

Complete A-V Canal (Fig. 34–2). This type of fully displayed A-V canal is characterized by failure of the common A-V valvular orifice to partition into separate mitral and tricuspid orifices, i.e., the anterior and posterior common leaflets of the common A-V valvular orifice are not fused to each other centrally to form two separate orifices. Furthermore, the anterior and posterior common leaflets are not fused with the crest of the underlying ventricular septum; thus, in complete A-V canal, there *is* direct interventricular communication.

These three defined types of fully displayed A-V canal septal defects may be correlated with the extent of involvement of the four possible components of the anomalies, as shown in Table 34–1. As noted previously, all three types involve a central septal defect comprising both an ostium primum atrial septal defect (O) and a deficiency or defect, or "scooping out," of the basilar ventricular septum (V). The complete A-V canal defect always, by definition, has involvement of all four components, i.e., OVMT. However, for the intermediate and partial types of A-V canal, clefts or deformity of either the anterior leaflet of the mitral valve (M) or the septal leaflet of the tricuspid valve (T), or both, may be involved, or these leaflets could, rarely, be fully and normally developed. Thus, intermediate and partial types of A-V canal could be of any one of the four patterns of fully displayed A-V canal septal defect (i.e., OVMT, OVM, OVT, or OV) (Table 34–1). (These abbreviations are used here only as symbols and certainly not as a system of classification apart from the anatomic features for which the symbols stand.)

Subtypes of Complete A-V Canal. A subclassification of complete A-V canal anomalies into three types according to the configuration of the anterior common leaflet of the common A-V valve was established by Rastelli and associates (1966). In Type A (Fig. 34–2A), the anterior common leaflet has a naturally occurring division along the plane separating its mitral and tricuspid components; there are also chordal attachments from the margins of this division to the crest of the underlying ventricular septum. Some 80 per cent of patients with complete atrioventricular canal belong to this group. In Type B (Fig. 34–2B), the anterior common leaflet is partially divided but is not attached by chordae directly to the crest of the underlying ventricular septum; instead, the edges

of the division of the anterior common leaflet are attached by chordae to an abnormal papillary muscle that arises in the right ventricle near the apical portion of the ventricular septum. This is a rare form of complete atrioventricular canal. In Type C (Fig. 34–2C), the anterior common leaflet is undivided and appears as a single continuous leaflet that floats freely over the crest of the underlying ventricular septum, to which it is not attached. The chordal attachments of the leaflet at its right and left margins are to papillary muscles on the free wall of the right and left ventricles. Associated anomalies are common in this type of complete A-V canal; for example, if pulmonary stenosis is associated with atrioventricular canal, it is almost always Type C.

No consistent relationship exists between the configurations of the anterior and posterior common leaflets. The attachment of the posterior common leaflet to the underlying ventricular septum can vary from sparse chordae to an imperforate "frenulum-like" membrane, and the division or notching between mitral and tricuspid portions also is variable. Thus, although the structure of the posterior common leaflet does not enter into the scheme for subclassification of complete A-V canal into Types A, B, and C, it is well, in describing individual hearts, to identify the characteristics of this leaflet, especially the extent of its fusion to the underlying crest of the ventricular septum.

For the sake of completeness, it should be noted that more recently some workers have been persuaded by their studies to modify the aforementioned subtyping of complete A-V canal in various ways (Piccoli *et al.*, 1979; Carpentier, 1978). In our surgical experience, however, the basic classification described above has correlated well with the selection of the best technique of repair, although, of course, the surgeon must be alert to the individual and intermediate variations that are common in biology, and especially in congenital anomalies.

The location of the atrioventricular conduction system in A-V canal defects is important to the surgeon. In all types, whether complete, intermediate, or partial, there is slight posterior displacement of the atrioventricular node compared with its normal relationship to the ostium of the coronary sinus (see Figs. 34–1, 34–3, and 34–6). There is also posterior displacement of the common bundle of His, the course of which is usually intimately related to the posterior rim of the "scooped out" basal portion of the ventricular septum, and hence, it is located at the posteroinferior rim of the septal defect.

ANATOMIC TERMINOLOGY

Anterior and Posterior. In these descriptions of the anatomic and surgical features of these anomalies, it may be helpful to be aware of the ambiguity of the terms "anterior" and "posterior" as they relate to the common leaflets and to the respective portions of the ventricular and atrial septa. It is to be remembered that in the normal heart, the septa are not in a true sagittal plane but are obliquely oriented, the anterior margins being leftward and the posterior margins being rightward. Furthermore, at operation, when the atrium is opened and the anterior lip of the atriotomy is retracted leftward, the heart becomes rotated counterclockwise on its longitudinal axis, as seen from above. Thus, the anterior margins of the septa become situated even more to the left. Indeed, the crest of the ventricular septum, as viewed by the surgeon, appears to be more in the coronal plane than in the sagittal plane, so that which is called anterior becomes more strictly leftward, and vice versa.

Anterior or Posterior Common Leaflet. There is only one A-V valve in complete A-V canal. Anteriorly and posteriorly in such a valve are leaflets common to both the left ventricular and right ventricular inlet orifices. These anterior and posterior common leaflets consist on the leftward side of tissue that would normally have been incorporated into the anterior leaflet (or aortic leaflet in some schemes of terminology) of the mitral valve, and on the rightward side of tissue that would have been incorporated into the septal leaflet of the tricuspid valve. Since in complete A-V canal this normal differentiation into mitral and tricuspid valves does not occur, the leaflet tissue anteriorly and posteriorly remains part of the "common" A-V valve, and hence, they are common leaflets. The terminology can be confusingly complex unless carefully noted, especially when speaking of the anterior leaflet of the mitral valve. Note in Figure 34–2 that the rudimentary components of the normal mitral valve are present, consisting of the lateral (L) leaflet (which would be called the posterior or mural leaflet of the normal mitral valve) and the leftward portion of the anterior common leaflet plus the leftward portion of the posterior common leaflet, which normally would have fused to form the anterior (aortic or septal) leaflet of the mitral valve.

Cleft, Division, or Incision. For precision of terminology, clear distinction between the definitions of these three words should be noted. *Cleft* refers to the separation that partially persists between the two components of the anterior leaflet of the mitral valve, i.e., a separation between the component originating from the anterior common leaflet and that originating from the posterior common leaflet; the term cleft is thus usually used in reference to the partial A-V canal. A tricuspid counterpart of this cleft seldom exists. *Division* of the anterior common leaflet is found in Type A complete A-V canal and refers to the naturally occurring separation, or division, between the mitral and tricuspid components of the common anterior leaflet. Some workers prefer to call this "division" a "commissure." As will be described under operative technique (see Figs. 34–5 and 34–6), it is often necessary for the surgeon to make an *incision* in the anterior or posterior common leaflet in order to expose the underlying crest of the ventricular septum and to place a septal patch between the incised edges of the leaflet,

especially in the Type C variety. Thus, "division" refers to a natural separation between the mitral and tricuspid components of the common leaflet, and "incision" refers to a surgically created separation between the components.

Ventricular Septal Defect and Interventricular Communication. Even the term "ventricular septal defect" is a potential source of confusion when speaking of A-V canal defects, since, as was discussed previously, *all* of the fully displayed forms of A-V canal have a deficiency or defect in the base of the ventricular septum. Therefore, it is *not* appropriate, strictly speaking, to state that a ventricular septal defect is not present in partial A-V canal but is present in complete A-V canal, since a defect is present in both forms. Rather, it *is* appropriate to state that a ventricular septal defect is present in both the partial and complete forms, but an *interventricular communication* is not present in the partial form but is present in the complete A-V canal.

CLINICAL FEATURES

The partial form of A-V canal was much more commonly encountered in earlier surgical experience than was the complete form. This probably was an exaggeration of the true relative frequencies of the partial and complete forms owing to a greater mortality during infancy for babies born with a complete A-V canal. Now that operative intervention has become the appropriate management for infants seriously ill from congenital heart disease, the complete form has become the more commonly encountered at several centers.

The symptoms of A-V canal defect are primarily related to the presence of increased pulmonary blood flow resulting from the septal defect and to the presence of mitral regurgitation resulting from mitral deformity. About two thirds of patients with partial A-V canal are asymptomatic at the time of operation, and only one sixth of patients who are operated on have had severe symptoms, which include dyspnea, fatigue, and frank congestive heart failure. Two thirds of patients with complete A-V canal have developed such symptoms of heart failure, most often during infancy.

On physical examination, a systolic ejection murmur is noted at the pulmonic area owing to increased flow across the pulmonic valve. In addition, a diastolic flow murmur across the tricuspid valve can be heard in many patients. Furthermore, a holosystolic apical murmur is often present but is of variable intensity, depending on the degree of associated mitral regurgitation.

The vectorcardiogram is helpful in confirming the diagnosis, since a counterclockwise frontal loop is almost always present (Toscano-Barbosa *et al.*, 1956); however, such a configuration may, of course, exist in other forms of congenital heart disease. Cardiac catheterization and angiography document the presence and magnitude of intracardiac shunting, help define the degree of mitral regurgitation, and show the classic "goose-neck" configuration of the left ventricular outflow tract. Patients with the partial form of A-V canal are much less likely to develop pulmonary hypertension or pulmonary vascular obstructive disease at an early age, whereas in the complete form, pulmonary hypertension and progressive pulmonary vascular disease are common in childhood and even infancy. The echocardiographic display of these lesions (Bloom *et al.*, 1979), particularly in the two-dimensional mode, is highly useful in distinguishing between the complete and partial forms as well as in defining the anatomic details of the subgroups that are not commonly revealed by angiocardiography alone.

INDICATIONS FOR OPERATION

The guidelines for selecting patients for correction of the atrioventricular canal anomaly are similar to those for patients having any of the various types of congenital anomalies resulting in increased pulmonary blood flow (Berger *et al.*, 1978). Specifically, correction is indicated at any age, even early infancy, when congestive heart failure or significant disability persists despite medical supportive measures.

For the asymptomatic infant with partial A-V canal and absence of significant pulmonary hypertension, postponement of correction until an arbitrary age of approximately 4 years is customary. Operation then seems indicated on the basis of a relatively low anticipated hospital mortality rate for the elective correction of partial A-V canal (approximately 2 per cent) and on the basis that progressive disability and cardiac failure are common during the second decade of life. However, if correction were not accomplished electively at this time, operation would still be indicated later in life, even at such time as clinical disability might impose more compelling reasons for the patient to accept operation. For the patient with a partial A-V canal, the occurrence of progressive pulmonary vascular obstructive disease as a contraindication to operation is uncommon.

Most infants with the complete form of A-V canal will already have significant or even severe pulmonary hypertension, as well as congestive heart failure poorly responsive to medical treatment. Surgical intervention is indicated for these patients. Some controversy remains as to whether palliative banding of the pulmonary artery or corrective operation is the better approach (Epstein *et al.*, 1979; Kirklin and Blackstone, 1979). For surgical teams skilled and experienced in the repair of A-V canal defects and in cardiac surgery for infants, corrective rather than palliative operation seems preferable for two chief reasons. First, the overall risk for early banding of the pulmonary artery and later correction is probably increased over that for correction in infancy. Second, banding of the pulmonary artery does not palliate the hemodynamic effects of mitral regurgitation, and in many instances, this may be an important factor contributing to the presence of congestive heart failure. For the child with complete A-V canal and marked elevation of pulmonary arterial pressure who escapes significant disability and congestive heart failure in infancy, we believe corrective operation is nevertheless indicated electively during the second year of life. If operation were delayed further, pulmonary vascular obstructive disease might continue to progress even after repair at an older age (Newfeld *et al.*, 1977).

OPERATIVE TECHNIQUE

Operation for both the partial and complete types of A-V canal is performed through a median sternotomy and utilizes hypothermic total cardiopulmonary bypass. The ascending aorta is cannulated, and both caval lines are passed through the right atrial appendage so that they can be widely mobilized by the atriotomy to provide optimal intra-atrial exposure. Standard techniques of whole-body perfusion are maintained, including use of a slotted needle air vent in the ascending aorta. Some surgeons have found circulatory arrest during profound hypothermia to be beneficial during repair on very small infants, but the role of this modality is not yet firmly defined. In the past, myocardial protection has been afforded by intermittent aortic cross-clamping for periods of approximately 15 minutes each, with that portion of the suturing that is done in the vicinity of the bundle of His being performed at a time when the heart was actively beating. More recently, cardioplegic arrest has been employed for myocardial protection, since confidence had been gained in the ability to avoid heart block even in the nonbeating heart by precise placement of sutures and since it has been assumed that myocardial protection is greater by this means. Some have questioned whether cardioplegia is well tolerated in the infant. The total time of extracorporeal circulation has averaged about 65 minutes for correction of the partial type of the defect and 100 minutes for the complete type.

Partial Atrioventricular Canal

Repair of the partial type of A-V canal has two principal objectives, namely, the careful approximation and alignment of the edges of the cleft in the mitral valve and closure of the atrial septal defect with a patch (Fig. 34–1). The aim is to close the cleft in such a way as to optimize the competence of the mitral valve. Distortion of the leaflet can best be avoided by suturing the cleft in an alignment that is estimated to be the same as that which had occurred prior to operation during systolic closure of the valve. Fortunately, thickened ridges are typically present along the edges of the cleft, which are of identical length, probably as a result of closure of these edges against each other during systole throughout life. It has been learned not only that accurate approximation of these ridges provides optimal alignment of the valve, but also that the ridges themselves provide strength for the suture line. One or two simple sutures are first placed to approximate the cleft near the mitral ring, and then the thickened edges of the cleft at their farthest margin (closest to the free edge of the leaflet) are approximated, after which the intervening sutures are placed. If incompetence has been minimal or absent preoperatively and if accurate orientation and alignment of the edges of the cleft do not seem possible, it may be best to abandon suturing of the cleft and leave the mitral valve as it was. We have not found that mitral stenosis results from accurate repair of the mitral cleft. It has not been our practice to transect chordae of the mitral valve, including those attached to the ventricular septum, nor have we found it useful to add tissue to the mitral leaflet in the form of a patch of pericardium or synthetic material. Preoperative mitral regurgitation may have been caused by incomplete closure of the cleft in the mitral valve during systole, especially at the base of the valve, in which case the repair of the cleft is effective in reducing or obliterating mitral regurgitation, or the regurgitation could have been caused by a deficiency of leaflet length from base to free edge, in which case the resulting regurgitation through the central portion of the valve during systole is not significantly affected by simple repair of the cleft. In some such hearts, mitral anuloplasty may be effective in reducing the degree of mitral regurgitation. Competency of the valve is tested by distending the ventricle with liquid so that refinements of the repair can then be effected as indicated. Almost never is it so clearly obvious that mitral repair will be unsuccessful that replacement of the mitral valve should be done at the time of the primary repair.

The interatrial communication is closed by a patch of pericardium or prosthetic material. The patch is attached to the junction of the mitral and tricuspid valves along the crest of the ventricular septum using interrupted sutures, which are all placed before the patch is lowered into position (see Fig. 34–1). As this suturing continues toward the posterior (rightward) end of the crest of the ventricular septum, care must be taken to avoid injury to the bundle of His. This is done by placing the interrupted sutures superficially and closely together and by deviating the suture line as far to the left as possible, even onto the base of the mitral valve leaflet (Fig. 34–3). The difficulty of suturing in the region of the posterior A-V valve anulus is heightened by poor delineation of the true line of separation between the right and left atria along the posterior margin of the defect; orientation in this area is facilitated by exerting traction on a suture placed for that purpose in the atrial septal rim of the ostium primum defect. This creates a small ridge that demarcates the right atrium from the left atrium. Sutures anchoring the patch should be placed on the left atrial side of that ridge until the suture line reaches

the clearly defined septal rim of the ostium primum defect (Fig. 34–3). Finally, the cephalad margin of the patch can then be attached to the rim of the atrial septal defect with continuous sutures.

Intermediate Atrioventricular Canal

So few intermediate types of A-V canal have been encountered or reported that techniques for repair have not become standardized. However, the principles of repair are to leave the mitral and tricuspid valves intact, as for repair of the partial A-V canal (repairing the mitral cleft if appropriate), and to place two septal patches, one to close the interventricular communication and one for the interatrial communication. The two patches are separated from each other along their adjacent edges by the midline fused tricuspid and mitral leaflet tissue but are sutured to each other by stitches passing through this leaflet substance.

Complete Atrioventricular Canal

The first step in the repair of complete A-V canal is a careful and deliberate identification of its anatomic characteristics. After the anatomy of the anterior and posterior common leaflets has been carefully determined and the extent of the underlying interventricular communication has been defined, the next step in the repair is approximation of the mitral components of the anterior and posterior common leaflets so as to constitute an anterior (or aortic) leaflet of the mitral valve (Fig. 34–4A). Again, the objective is to avoid distortion of the mitral leaflet tissue as much as possible and to reconstruct the valve in the alignment that it would assume during systole in the preoperative state. This alignment can often be determined best by floating the leaflets into their closed position by instillation of saline under pressure into the left ventricular cavity. Often, thickened ridges along the cleft of the mitral valve, as encountered in the partial form of the defect, are not present in the complete form, which further tends to obscure the appropriate alignment of the mitral valve in the complete form. Sufficient time must be devoted to this step in the reconstruction, even to the necessity, on many occasions, of placing and replacing sutures reconstructing the mitral leaflet in a trial-and-error manner. As was noted for repair of partial A-V canal, valve replacement at the initial operation is rarely justified.

The second step in the repair is to expose the entire length of the crest of the ventricular septal rim of the interventricular communication. In the Type A form of complete A-V canal, the natural division in the anterior common leaflet has already resulted in such exposure of the majority of the underlying ventricular crest (Fig. 34–4). Even when the division in the anterior common leaflet seems to deviate rightward near the anterior anulus, it is found that the

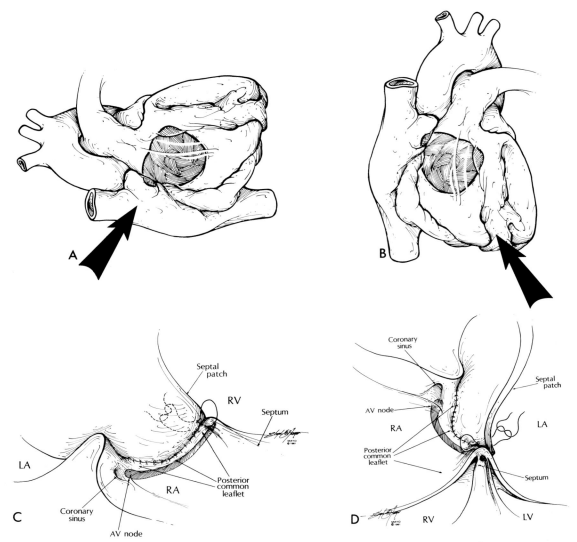

Figure 34–3. Detail of the positioning and suturing of the septal patch posteroinferiorly (posterocaudally) in partial A-V canal. Drawings *A* and *B* provide orientation for the points of view for drawings *C* and *D*, respectively. The viewpoint shown in *A* and *C* is that of the surgeon at the operating table, whereas the viewpoint in *B* and *D* is, surgically speaking, a hypothetical one, as though the viewer were positioned anteroapically within the right ventricle. The central structure shown in *A* and *B* is for the purpose of designating the position within the heart of the septal defect typical of the A-V canal anomaly. In *C* and *D*, the dark structure running along the crest of the ventricular septum, commencing at the A-V node, is the bundle of His; its branches are not illustrated except in *D*, where a part of the left bundle branch complex is seen in the cross-section of the ventricular septum. It should be stressed that views *C* and *D* illustrate only the posterior aspect of the anomaly, the remainder of the heart having been "cut away" by the artist in (1) a transverse plane just superior to the level of the coronary sinus orifice, this "cut" slicing through the posterior atrial wall and septum, and (2) in a coronal plane located toward the posterior part of the ventricular septum, the latter "cut" slicing through the posterior common leaflet and through the septal patch.

To describe the principles for attachment of the patch in partial A-V canal in this critical posteroinferior area, attention is first directed to the anterior aspect of the illustration (anterior is toward the right in both *C* and *D*). The patch is attached anteriorly to the line of junction of the mitral and tricuspid components of the posterior common leaflet, which is fused to the underlying crest of the ventricular septum. However, as the suturing progresses posteriorly, the line of attachment of the patch is deviated to the left, onto the base of the mitral component of the leaflet; still further posteriorly after crossing the mitral anulus, the patch attachment remains leftward, away from the conduction tissue, and to the left of the rim of the atrial septal defect. Thus, the widest possible separation is provided between the suture line and the A-V node and penetrating portions of the conduction bundle. In our experience with many operations in which suturing in this area was accomplished with the heart beating, transient heart block was never encountered during suturing anterior to middle arrow in the diagrams designating the posterior common leaflet, either in partial or complete A-V canal. Thus, the illustrated line of attachment posterior to the middle arrow is accomplished by closely spaced, superficially placed sutures. As mentioned in the text, all sutures illustrated had been placed prior to lowering the patch into position, thus allowing optimal exposure for suture placement.

underlying septum typically deviates similarly, thus facilitating identification of the septal crest. However, in the Type C variant, it is necessary to incise the anterior common leaflet along a line estimated to demarcate the tricuspid from the mitral components of the anterior common leaflet (Fig. 34–5A,B). The ideal line of demarcation may be difficult to identify, and in instances of doubt, it is our preference to err on the side of placing the incision more to the tricuspid aspect than to the mitral aspect of the anterior common leaflet. In this way, one is more likely to preserve adequate leaflet area for mitral function. However, it must be anticipated that in performing the next step in the operation, a septal patch will be placed that must be attached both to the crest of the ventricular septum and to the rim of the atrial septal defect and that must lie between the tricuspid and mitral components of the common leaflet. Therefore, the location of the anular end of the incision in the common leaflet is largely established by the position of the underlying ventricular septum where it joins the anulus of the A-V valve. (This consideration would seem to contradict the suggestion of others to incise the common leaflet in a place remote from that of the underlying ventricular septum.) Thus, since the anular end of the incision to be placed in a common leaflet is at a fixed point, as described, any freedom in placement of the leaflet incision must be exercised along the free edge of the leaflet; usually, the proper site along the free edge for this incision is defined by the line of convergence of chordae from the papillary muscle of the left ventricle with those from the papillary muscle of the right ventricle.

In those instances in the Type A deformity in which the division of the anterior leaflet is incomplete and in most instances of the Type B deformity (Pacifico and Kirklin, 1973), it is necessary to extend the division in the anterior common leaflet by incising the remaining intact bridging portion of the leaflet all the way to the anulus of the atrioventricular valve. A similar incision in the posterior common leaflet is nearly always required, but this incision in the posterior common leaflet extends from the free margin of that leaflet only to the posterior limit of the underlying interventricular communication. Often, this interventricular communication does not reach the true anulus of the atrioventricular valve since there is a variable length of fibrous fusion of the base of the posterior common leaflet to the crest of the ventricular septum in many instances (Figs. 34–4B and 34–6A,B). The latter is a favorable situation, in that it provides a buffer area of intact fibrous septum that protects the conduction bundle from the suture line.

The next step is to close the cardiac septum with a patch of knitted synthetic material. The size of the patch is best estimated by measuring the distance from the atrial septal rim to the ventricular septal rim of the defect with a segment of string and then marking this distance on the patch. Similarly, the distance from the anterior to the posterior aspect of the anulus

of the atrioventricular canal, that is, the anteroposterior dimension of the septal defect, is measured and marked off on the patch. Usually, the two dimensions are approximately equal, and the patch assumes a circular configuration. The edge of the patch that will be approximated to the crest of the ventricular septum is then attached with a row of interrupted sutures, all of which are placed prior to lowering the patch into position (Figs. 34–4C and 34–5C). We prefer to use simple interrupted sutures that pass into the right aspect of the ventricular septum adjacent to its crest. Strong bites can be taken in the anterior two thirds of this suture line adjacent to the right bundle branch, but more posteriorly, the sutures are placed progressively more superficially and more closely together in order to avoid encirclement of the nonbranching and penetrating portions of the conduction tissue.

In the situation described previously in which the posterior limit of the interventricular communication is sealed off by a membrane between the ventricular septum and the overlying leaflet, the incision in the posterior common leaflet will have been extended posteriorly only to the limit of the interventricular communication (Fig. 34–6A,B). From this point on, in a posterosuperior direction, the patch is sutured to the atrial surface of the posterior common leaflet, then to the posterior atrial wall as far leftward as possible, and finally to the atrial septum (Fig. 34–6A,B) in a manner exactly the same as in repair of the partial A-V canal described earlier (see Fig. 34–3C,D).

In the case of hearts in which the interventricular communication (or perforating communication) extends all the way to the posterior valvular anulus (which is to say that the posterior common leaflet is not fused at all to the underlying crest of the ventricular septum [Fig. 34–6C–F]), there is legitimate difference of opinion as to the preferred technique for placement of the patch so as to achieve the least risk of heart block. One choice (Fig. 34–6E,F) would be to extend the incision in the posterior common leaflet along the anulus well to the right of the plane of the ventricular septum, so that the patch would then cross the anulus well to the right of the junction of the anulus and the ventricular septum and, hence, entirely to the right of the conduction tissue, with the option of attaching the patch so that the coronary sinus opens either into the right or left atrium (Thiene et al., 1981). Alternatively, we have most commonly preferred to extend the incision in the posterior common leaflet in such hearts directly to the junction of the ventricular septum and the A-V valvular anulus, with the intent of placing sutures for the patch superficially and closely together in this area (Fig. 34–6C,D).

The next step involves the anchoring of the incised edges of the mitral and tricuspid components of the anterior and posterior common leaflets to their respective left and right sides of the prosthetic septal patch. This is accomplished by a single row of interrupted mattress sutures (Figs. 34–4D and 34–5D). This attachment of the mitral and tricuspid leaflets should

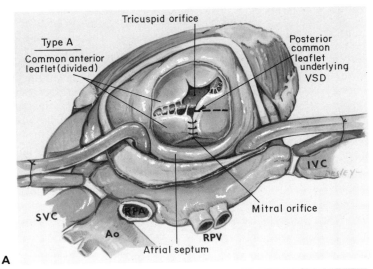

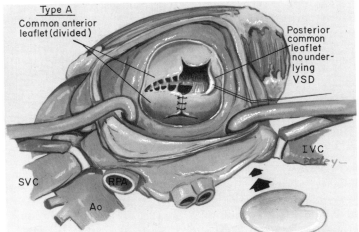

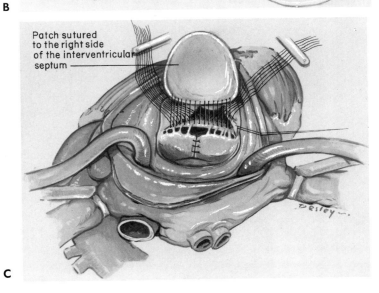

Figure 34–4. Repair of Type A complete A-V canal. *A,* The anterior mitral leaflet has been constructed by approximating the edges of the mitral portions of the anterior and posterior common leaflets. The line for incision of the posterior common leaflet is identified by the dotted line. *B,* In this case, most of the posterior common leaflet is fused to the crest of the ventricular septum. Thus, there is no need to incise the posterior common leaflet, and the appropriately shaped patch (bottom right) can be attached to the atrial surface of the posterior common leaflet. *C,* The prosthetic patch is sewn to the right aspect of the ventricular septum with interrupted sutures (see Fig. 34–6 for further detail).

Illustration continued on opposite page

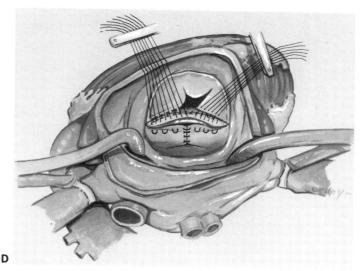

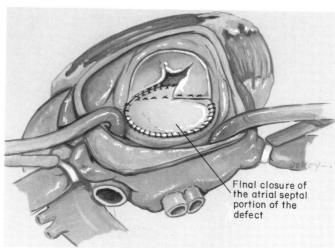

Figure 34–4 *Continued.* *D,* The reconstructed anterior leaflet of the mitral valve is attached to the prosthetic patch with interrupted nonabsorbable mattress sutures in the same plane as the anulus of the A-V valve. Note also in this instance, where the posterior common leaflet was incised, that both edges of this incision (tricuspid and mitral) are attached to the respective surface of the patch. Many surgeons prefer the use of pledgets in these mattress sutures. *E,* The repair is completed by continuous suture approximation to the rim of the atrial septal defect. (SVC = superior vena cava; IVC = inferior vena cava; Ao = aorta; RPA = right pulmonary artery; VSD = ventricular septal defect; RPV = right pulmonary vein.) (From McMullan, M. H., *et al.:* Surgical treatment of complete atrioventricular canal. Surgery, *72:*905, 1972.)

Final closure of the atrial septal portion of the defect

be at a level on the patch that is estimated to correspond to the ideal plane of the orifice of the mitral and tricuspid valves. This ideal level is considered to be along the line to which the leaflet would reach during systole when its retaining chordae would become fully stretched and is also found to be in the same plane as the anulus of the common A-V valve. It should be pointed out that for the Type A deformity, we have considered it appropriate to attach the mitral but not the corresponding tricuspid edge of the naturally divided anterior common leaflet to the patch (Fig. 34–4D). This is because this portion of the tricuspid valve corresponds to the anterior leaflet of the normally developed tricuspid valve, and the base of the anterior tricuspid leaflet does not normally attach to the septum. There is thus a complete deficiency of the anterior portion of the septal leaflet of the tricuspid valve in the Type A deformity (which corresponds, as noted, to the usual situation in partial A-V canal). Fortunately, tricuspid regurgitation does not typically occur postoperatively, despite this deficiency of the septal tricuspid leaflet. In Type C de-

formity, the incised edges of both the tricuspid and mitral components of both the anterior and posterior common leaflets are attached to the patch (Fig. 34–5D). Interest has been rekindled in the use of two patches for the repair of complete A-V canal defects (Carpentier, 1978), and late results of operation by this method are awaited.

The final step of the repair is the attachment of the cephalad edge of the septal patch to the rim of the atrial septal defect, usually with a continuous suture (Figs. 34–4*E* and 34–5*E*).

After completion of the repair in both the partial and complete forms, the right atriotomy is closed, air is evacuated from the heart, continuous aspiration is applied to a slotted needle vent in the ascending aorta, and extracorporeal circulation is gradually discontinued. Atrial and arterial pressures are continuously monitored during this period and throughout the first postoperative day.

The postoperative care of these patients is not different from that of other patients undergoing repair of other forms of complex congenital cardiac defects.

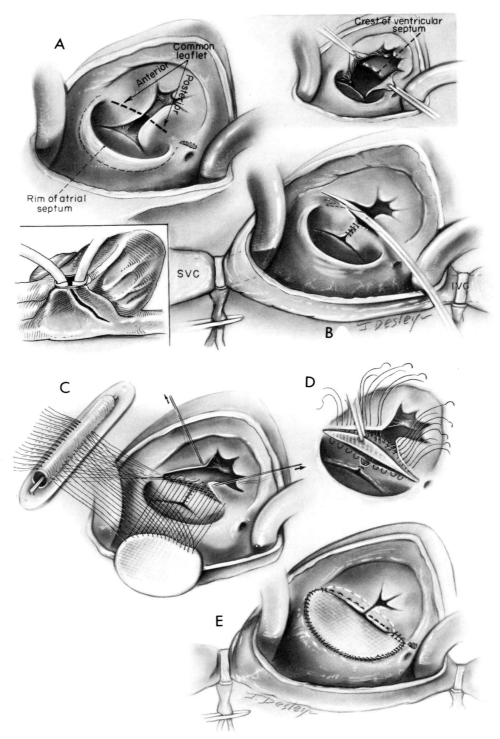

Figure 34–5.   Surgical repair of Type C complete A-V canal. *A*, Heavy broken line indicates line of incision of the common atrioventricular leaflets. *B*, Incisions being accomplished. *C–E*, The remainder of the repair is similar to that illustrated in Figure 34–4, except (as seen in *D* and *E*) both the tricuspid and mitral edges of the incised anterior common leaflet are sutured to the respective sides of the patch. (From Rastelli, G. C., Ongley, P. A., and McGoon, D. C.: Surgical repair of complete atrioventricular canal with anterior common leaflet undivided and unattached to ventricular septum. Mayo Clin. Proc., *44*:335, 1969.)

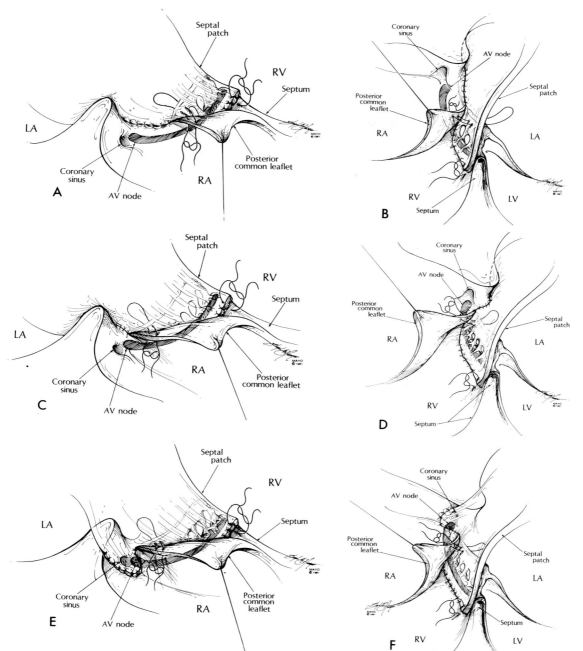

Figure 34–6. Detail for anchoring septal patch posteroinferiorly in complete A-V canal, and for reconstructing posterior common leaflet. The view for *A, C,* and *E* corresponds to orientation described for Figure 34–3*A,* and that for *B, D,* and *F* corresponds to orientation described for Figure 3*B.* Illustrated in *A* and *B* is the repair used for hearts in which the basilar (or anular) portion of the posterior common leaflet is fused to the underlying ventricular septum by a sheet of fibrous tissue; *C* and *D,* and *E* and *F* show alternatives for repair where no such fusion has occurred. In both situations, the posterior common leaflet has been incised beginning at its free margin (at the estimated point of junction of its tricuspid and mitral portions) to the posterior limit of any interventricular communication deep to the valve. In *A* and *B,* the incision extends only part way to the anulus, and in *C, D, E,* and *F,* it extends essentially to the anulus. In *A* and *B,* the septal patch is attached to the right surface of the ventricular septal crest where the leaflet has been incised, but continuing posteriorly the suture line then passes along the edge of the fibrous tissue fusing leaflet to septum until it reaches the apex of the incision in the leaflet. The suturing posteriorly from this point proceeds exactly as for partial A-V canal, as described in Figure 34–3. Remember that in reality all the sutures illustrated have been placed prior to lowering the patch into position, as in Figures 34–4*C* and 34–5*C.*

In *C* and *D,* which is our usual technique, the incision in the posterior common leaflet extends posteriorly to the junction of atrium, ventricular septum, and anulus; the patch is again attached along the right surface of the ventricular septal crest, and the sutures become ever more superficial and more closely spaced as work proceeds posteriorly. The suture at the apex of the leaflet incision (not illustrated) grasps only leaflet tissue near the anulus but does not penetrate the anulus;. the suture line remains superficial as it crosses right to left to reach the left surface of the rim of the atrial septum, as in Figure 34–3.

An alternative method, preferred by some, is shown in *E* and *F,* in which the patch is placed entirely to the right of the conduction tissue; the incision in the posterior common leaflet is extended along the anulus to the right of the level of the coronary sinus ostium; the suture line for the patch passes even further inferiorly on the right ventricular surface of the ventricular septum to reach the apex of the incision in the leaflet; the patch is then attached entirely to the right atrial side of the coronary-sinus ostium. An alternative variant would be to attach the patch along the inferior lip of the ostium, allowing the coronary sinus to drain to the right atrium.

The postoperative course is typically uncomplicated, but when a complication occurs, it is most commonly an arrhythmia of the supraventricular type or reduced cardiac output, which may be exacerbated by the presence of residual mitral regurgitation. Fortunately, the incidence of heart block has been negligible with utilization of the intraoperative precautions noted previously (McMullan et al., 1972, 1973).

The difficult surgical treatment of A-V canal defect associated with anomalies such as tetralogy of Fallot and other conotruncal malformations has received increasing attention and has been increasingly successful (Sridaromont et al., 1975; Bastos et al., 1978; Thiene et al., 1979; Pacifico et al., 1980; Bharati et al., 1980a,b; Villani et al., 1980; Arciniegas et al., 1981).

Mitral Valve Replacement

When it is decided that mitral valve replacement is required, whether at the initial (very rarely) or subsequent operation or whether for the partial or the complete form of A-V canal, an important anatomic feature bears re-emphasis: A deficiency of the basilar portion of the ventricular septum exists in both partial and complete A-V canal lesions, and the patch that is placed to close the septal defect has a ventricular septal portion as well as an atrial septal portion. Or, stated differently, the plane of the mitral anulus lies at a level that does not follow the crest of the ventricular septum; rather it crosses the patch used to close the septal defect at a level centrally on the patch, which is about 1 or 2 cm. cephalad (or atrialward) from the crest of the "scooped-out" portion of the ventricular septum. Thus, the mitral valve prosthesis must be attached in a special way, i.e., along the true plane of the mitral anulus. The prosthesis should be secured to the mural aspect of the mitral anulus as always, but on the septal aspect, the line of attachment leaves the edge of the resected natural valve and follows an imaginary line on the left surface of the septal patch corresponding to the extended true plane of the mitral orifice. In other words, the mitral prosthesis is attached to the septal patch at the junction of its ventricular and atrial portions. There is a threat that if the prosthesis is attached too high on the septal patch, it may face into the left ventricular outflow tract too severely, thus bringing to critical degree the natural confinement of the left ventricular outflow tract present in A-V canal (Piccoli et al., 1982). This could also result in poppet malfunction.

This principle for attachment of the mitral prosthesis holds the additional advantage that the suturing avoids injury to the bundle of His, which courses along the ventricular septal crest and to which the prosthesis would otherwise be attached. The only area in which the bundle of His might be vulnerable, using this technique, is at the junction of the posterior anulus and the septal patch, so that suturing in this small area should be done superficially.

RESULT OF OPERATION

Throughout the entire experience with repair of partial A-V canal, the mortality rate has been at a satisfactory level of about 5 per cent or less. It has not increased with the more frequent recent application of the operation for the occasional infant who develops congestive heart failure in the early months of life. Similarly, repair of partial A-V canal in 52 adults ranging in age up to 75 years and with an average age of 37 years was accomplished at a 6 per cent risk (Hynes et al., 1981). The incidence of late deaths, usually related to arrhythmias or the necessity for mitral valve replacement, is a small fraction of 1 per cent per year (McMullan et al., 1973). The great majority of surviving patients with native valves are completely free of disability; about one-fourth have mild symptoms on strenuous exertion.

The result of operation for complete A-V canal was totally unsatisfactory (McGoon et al., 1959) prior to the development of the current techniques of repair as described previously. After the implementation of these techniques, the in-hospital mortality rate dropped precipitously from more than 60 per cent to approximately 10 per cent (McMullan et al., 1972). However, in our modern experience, in which an ever-increasing proportion of patients operated on are in the infant age group, the mortality rate has increased slightly. In view of the grave prognosis for infants who develop congestive heart failure with complete A-V canal, even a mortality rate of 20 per cent is attractive, although in need of significant improvement (Mair and McGoon, 1977; Mills et al., 1976; McCabe et al., 1977; Culpepper et al., 1978; Berger et al., 1978).

Unquestionably, a key factor relating to the early and late results of repair of atrioventricular canal deformities, whether partial or complete, is the degree of residual mitral valve regurgitation. The results of intraoperative double-sampling dye dilution studies indicate that essentially complete absence of mitral regurgitation is achieved in approximately 50 per cent of the patients; almost all of the remainder have mild to moderate regurgitation at the completion of operation. Although valve replacement at the initial operation might seem attractive for those patients with persistence of moderate mitral regurgitation after repair of their native valve, this is believed to be unwise in most instances because of the inherent limitations of valve replacement. These limitations include an inability of the replacement valve to grow with the patient, the presence of a gradient across a small replacement valve, the need for anticoagulant therapy if a prosthetic valve is employed, and uncertain durability of all prostheses and especially tissue valves. Therefore, it seems preferable to accept both postoperative mitral regurgitation and the necessity of reoperating at some time in the future when mitral valve replacement can no longer be postponed than to replace the mitral valve at the initial operation. The overall incidence of reoperation for severe residual mitral regurgitation has been well under 1 per cent per year, but it appears to be higher after repair during infancy, probably being related to the more severe valvular deformity in the infant group.

SELECTED REFERENCES

Berger, T. J., Blackstone, E. H., Kirklin, J. W., Bargeron, L..M., Jr., Hazelrig, J. B., and Turner, M. E., Jr.: Survival and probability of cure without and with operation in complete atrioventricular canal. Ann. Thorac. Surg., 27:104, 1979.

These workers analyze comparative data for nonsurgically and surgically treated patients with complete atrioventricular canal showing that only 54 per cent of patients who did not undergo operation survived to 6 months of age and 15 per cent to 24 months of age. Although the risk of correction was high in the early months of life, it fell to 17 per cent by the age of 12 months. Among those surviving operation, the 5-year survival rate was excellent (91 per cent).

Carpentier, A.: Surgical anatomy and management of the mitral component of atrioventricular canal defects. *In* Paediatric Cardiology 1977. Edited by R. H. Anderson and E. A. Shinebourne. Edinburgh, Churchill Livingstone, 1978, p. 477.

This author has studied extensively and innovatively the surgical anatomy of atrioventricular canal defects. He espouses a three-leaflet functional concept for the mitral valve and describes techniques for the extensive mobilization of the leaflets and their support structures plus anular plication. Furthermore, for complete malformations, he recommends reconstruction of the septum utilizing two separate patches, one ventricular and the other atrial.

Piccoli, G. P., Wilkinson, J. L., Macartney, F. J., Gerlis, L. M., and Anderson, R. H.: Morphology and classification of complete atrioventricular defects. Br. Heart J., 42:633, 1979.

This is a new look at the anatomy and classification of the complete form of the anomaly resulting from a study of 70 necropsied hearts in the hope of improving on the Rastelli classification. The subdivisions again depended on the morphology of the valve leaflets, but these authors identified five leaflets distinguished by their commissural pattern and support mechanisms. Some innovative surgical implications are discussed.

Thiene, G., Wenink, A. C. G., Frescura, C., Wilkinson, J. L., Gallucci, V., Ho, S. Y., Mazzucco, A., and Anderson, R. H.: The surgical anatomy and pathology of the conduction tissues in atrioventricular defects. J. Thorac. Cardiovasc. Surg., 82:928, 1981.

These authors examined 16 hearts of patients with atrioventricular defects in detail, describing their findings from the surgeon's viewpoint. Ten hearts had complete defects and six had partial ones, with the disposition of the conduction tissue being the same in both groups. The anatomy of the triangle of Koch was found to be distorted, and the authors defined a "nodal triangle" lying between the coronary sinus ostium and the anulus that contained the A-V node. Techniques to avoid injury to the node and bundle were suggested.

REFERENCES

Arciniegas, E., Hakimi, M., Farooki, Z. Q., and Green, E. W.: Results of total correction of tetralogy of Fallot with complete atrioventricular canal. J. Thorac. Cardiovasc. Surg., 81:768, 1981.

Baron, M. G.: Endocardial cushion defects. Radiol. Clin. North Am., 6:343, 1968.

Bastos, P., de Leval, M., Macartney, F., and Stark, J.: Correction of type C atrioventricular canal associated with tetralogy of Fallot. Thorax, 33:646, 1978.

Berger, T. J., Blackstone, E. H., Kirklin, J. W., Bargeron, L. M., Jr., Hazelrig, J. B., and Turner, M. E., Jr.: Survival and probability of cure without and with operation in complete atrioventricular canal. Ann. Thorac. Surg., 27:104, 1979.

Berger, T. J., Kirklin, J. W., Blackstone, E. H., *et al.*: Primary repair of complete atrioventricular canal in patients less than 2 years old. Am. J. Cardiol., 41:906, 1978.

Bharati, S., Kirklin, J. W., McAllister, H. A., Jr., and Lev, M.: The surgical anatomy of common atrioventricular orifice associated with tetralogy of Fallot, double outlet right ventricle and complete regular transposition. Circulation, 61:1142, 1980a.

Bharati, S., Lev, M., McAllister, H. A., Jr., and Kirklin, J. W.: Surgical anatomy of the atrioventricular valve in the intermediate type of common atrioventricular orifice. J. Thorac. Cardiovasc. Surg., 79:884, 1980b.

Blieden, L. C., Randall, P. A., Castaneda, A. R., Lucas, R. V., Jr., and Edwards, J. E.: The "goose neck" of the endocardial cushion defect: anatomic basis. Chest, 65:13, 1974.

Bloom, K. R., Freedom, R. M., Williams, C. M., Trusler, G. A., and Rowe, R. D.: Echocardiographic recognition of atrioventricular valve stenosis associated with endocardial cushion defect: Pathologic and surgical correlates. Am. J. Cardiol., 44:1326, 1979.

Carpentier, A.: Surgical anatomy and management of the mitral component of atrioventricular canal defects. *In* Pediatric Cardiology 1977, Edited by R. H. Anderson and E. A. Shinebourne. Edinburgh, Churchill Livingstone, 1978, p. 477.

Culpepper, W., Kolff, J., Chung-Yuan, L., *et al.*: Complete common atrioventricular canal in infancy — surgical repair and postoperative hemodynamics. Circulation, 58:550, 1978.

Epstein, M. L., Moller, J. H., Amplatz, K., and Nicoloff, D. M.: Pulmonary banding in infants with complete atrioventricular canal. J. Thorac. Cardiovasc. Surg., 78:28, 1979.

Feldt, R. H.: Atrioventricular Canal Defects. Philadelphia, W. B. Saunders Company, 1976.

Hagler, D. J., Tajik, A. J., Seward, J. B., Mair, D. D., and Ritter, D. G.: Real-time wide-angle sector echocardiography: Atrioventricular canal defects. Circulation, 59:140, 1979.

Hynes, J. K., Tajik, A. J., Seward, J. B., Fuster, V., Ritter, D. G., Brandenburg, R. O., Puga, F. J., Danielson, G. K., and McGoon, D. C.: Partial atrioventricular canal defect in adults. Am. J. Cardiol., 47:466, 1981.

Kirklin, J. W., and Blackstone, E. H.: Management of the infant with complete atrioventricular canal. J. Thorac. Cardiovasc. Surg., 78:32, 1979.

Mair, D. D., and McGoon, D. C.: Surgical correction of atrioventricular canal during the first year of life. Am. J. Cardiol., 40:66, 1977.

McCabe, J. C., Engle, M. A., Gay, W. A., *et al.*: Surgical treatment of endocardial cushion defects. Am. J. Cardiol., 39:72, 1977.

McGoon, D. C., DuShane, J. W., and Kirklin, J. W.: The surgical treatment of endocardial cushion defects. Surgery, 46:185, 1959.

McMullan, M. H., McGoon, D. C., Wallace, R. B., Danielson, G. K., and Weidman, W. H.: Surgical treatment of partial atrioventricular canal. Arch. Surg., 107:705, 1973.

McMullan, M. H., Wallace, R. B., Weidman, W. H., and McGoon, D. C.: Surgical treatment of complete atrioventricular canal. Surgery, 72:905, 1972.

Mills, N. L., Ochsner, J. L., King, T. D., *et al.*: Correction of type C complete atrioventricular canal: Surgical considerations. J. Thorac. Cardiovasc. Surg., 71:20, 1976.

Newfeld, E. A., Sher, M., and Paul, M. H.: Pulmonary vascular disease in complete atrioventricular canal defect. Am. J. Cardiol., 39:721, 1977.

Pacifico, A. D., and Kirklin, J. W.: Surgical repair of complete atrioventricular canal with anterior common leaflet attached to an anomalous right ventricular papillary muscle. J. Thorac. Cardiovasc. Surg., 65:727, 1973.

Pacifico, A. D., Kirklin, J. W., and Bargeron, L. M., Jr.: Repair of complete atrioventricular canal associated with tetralogy of Fallot or double outlet right ventricle: Report of 10 patients. Ann. Thorac. Surg., 29:351, 1980.

Piccoli, G. P., Ho, S. Y., Wilkinson, J. L., Macartney, E. J., Gerlis, L. M., and Anderson, R. H.: Left-sided obstructive lesions in atrioventricular septal defects: an anatomical study. J. Thorac. Cardiovasc. Surg., 83:453, 1982.

Piccoli, G. P., Wilkinson, J. L., Macartney, F. J., Gerlis, L. M., and Anderson, R. H.: Morphology and classification of complete atrioventricular defects. Br. Heart J., 42:633, 1979.

Rastelli, G. C., Kirklin, J. W., and Kincaid, O. W.: Angiocardiography of persistent common atrioventricular canal. Mayo Clin. Proc., 42:200, 1967.

Rastelli, G. C., Kirklin, J. W., and Titus, J. L.: Anatomic observations on complete form of persistent common atrioventricular canal with special reference to atrioventricular valves. Mayo Clin. Proc., 41:296, 1966.

Rastelli, G. C., Ongley, P. A., Kirklin, J. W., and McGoon, D. C.: Surgical repair of the complete form of persistent common atrioventricular canal. J. Thorac. Cardiovasc. Surg., 55:299, 1968.

Rastelli, G. C., Ongley, P. A., and McGoon, D. C.: Surgical repair of complete atrioventricular canal with anterior common leaflet undivided and unattached to ventricular septum. Mayo Clin. Proc., 44:335, 1969.

Sridaromont, S., Feldt, R. H., Ritter, D. G., Davis, D. G., McGoon, D. C., and Edwards, J. E.: Double-outlet right ventricle associated with persistent common atrioventricular canal. Circulation, 52:933, 1975.

Thiene, G., Frescura, C., Di Donato, R., and Gallucci, R.: Complete atrioventricular canal associated with conotruncal malformations: Anatomical observations in 13 specimens. Eur. J. Cardiol., 9:199, 1979.

Thiene, G., Wenink, A. C. G., Frescura, C., Wilkinson, J. L., Gallucci, V., Ho, S. Y., Mazzucco, A., and Anderson, R. H.: The surgical anatomy and pathology of the conduction tissues in atrioventricular defects. J. Thorac. Cardiovasc. Surg., 82:928, 1981.

Toscano-Barbosa, E., Brandenburg, R. O., and Burchell, H. B: Electrocardiographic studies of cases with intracardiac malformations of the atrioventricular canal. Mayo Clin. Proc., 31:513, 1956.

Villani, M., Locatelli, G., Tiraboschi, R., Alfieri, O., and Parenzan, L.: Complete atrioventricular canal associated with tetralogy of Fallot. Scand. J. Thorac. Cardiovasc. Surg., 14:51, 1980.

Chapter 35

Surgical Treatment of Ventricular Septal Defect

JOHN W. KIRKLIN

ALBERT D. PACIFICO

JAMES K. KIRKLIN

LIONEL M. BARGERON, JR.

HISTORICAL NOTES

In 1954, Lillehei, Varco, and colleagues at the University of Minnesota in Minneapolis began to repair ventricular septal defects (VSDs) using controlled cross-circulation with an adult human being as the oxygenator (Lillehei et al., 1955). Five of the eight patients were in their first year of life, and three of the five survived, a tribute to the surgeons' skill, the lack of cardiac ischemia (the aorta was not crossclamped, and the perfection of their human oxygenator. The dramatic weight gain of the surgically cured infants with large VSD was documented. Three patients, one aged 4 and two aged 5 years, also survived, one with multiple VSDs.

In 1956, we reported 20 patients with large VSDs who had undergone intracardiac repair with a mechanical pump-oxygenator at the Mayo Clinic, beginning in March 1955 (DuShane et al., 1956). Normothermic flow rates of 70 ml./kg./min. (about 2.1 L/min./M.²) were used as well as an intracardiac sucker system to return blood to the machine. The duration of cardiopulmonary bypass ranged from 10 to 45 minutes. Indicator-dilution curves were recorded in the operating room before and after repair. Four (20 per cent) of the 20 patients died in the hospital.

Lillehei showed the feasibility of an atrial approach to VSDs in 1957 (Stirling et al., 1957). The technique of profound hypothermia and total circulatory arrest, with rewarming by a pump-oxygenator, was applied successfully to infants with VSD by Okamoto and colleagues (1969). Sloan and colleagues reported on the feasibility of primary repair of VSD in infants (Sigmann et al., 1967), as had we (Kirklin et al., 1961). Commencing in 1969, Barratt-Boyes demonstrated that routine primary repair of VSD in sick, small infants was superior to pulmonary artery banding (Barratt-Boyes et al., 1976).

MORPHOLOGY

Location. VSDs can occur anywhere in the ventricular septum (Fig. 35–1). For purposes of surgical approach, a VSD is conveniently related to (1) the anteroseptal commissure of the tricuspid valve, (2) the subpulmonary infundibulum, (3) the region beneath the septal cusp of the tricuspid valve, (4) the trabecular (muscular) portion of the septum, and (5) combinations of the above.

Most commonly, VSDs are in the region of the anteroseptal commissure of the tricuspid valve. When they are up against the anulus of the valve, they are termed *perimembranous* (Soto et al., 1980). VSDs may be a little anterior to this, with a narrow bar of muscle between the defect and the tricuspid anulus. Strictly speaking, these are muscular VSDs.

The VSD may be beneath the septal leaflet of the tricuspid valve. Most of these are, in fact, perimembranous defects that extend particularly far inferiorly, and they extend up to the tricuspid anulus. A few defects in this region are muscular, not perimembranous, and are a little more anteriorly located and have a bar of muscle between themselves and the tricuspid anulus.

About 10 per cent of VSDs are subpulmonary in position. Most of these are immediately beneath the pulmonary *and* aortic valves, and have been called subarterial by Anderson and colleagues (Soto et al., 1980). A few are in the infundibular septum and are completely surrounded by muscle.

Single or multiple muscular defects may occur in the trabecular portion of the ventricular septum. When they are multiple, they are usually located up and down the anterior portion of the septum.

Size. VSDs are infinitely variable in size, and their division into groups is arbitrary. Furthermore, the sizing of VSDs before operation can be a difficult matter. This is especially true when the VSD is associated with another lesion such as coarctation or pulmonary stenosis. The most reliable way of sizing the defect is its measurement on properly profiled cineangiograms, relating this to the length of the septum or correcting the value for the magnification of the cineangiogram.

Large VSDs are approximately the size of the aortic orifice or larger. *Small* VSDs are of insufficient

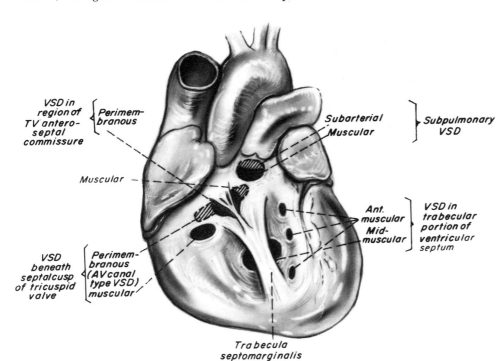

Figure 35–1. Schematic representation of some of the common locations of isolated ventricular septal defects (see text).

size to raise right ventricular systolic pressure, and the pulmonary-systemic flow ratio (Q_P/Q_S) is not increased above 1.75. A third category, *moderate-sized* VSDs, can be useful. Although still "restrictive," these defects are of sufficient size to raise the right ventricular systolic pressure to approximately half the left ventricular pressure and the Q_P/Q_S to 3.5.

Multiple small defects may together behave as a large defect.

ASSOCIATED LESIONS IN "PRIMARY" VSD

Nearly half of the patients undergoing surgical treatment for "primary" VSD have an associated lesion (Blackstone *et al.*, 1976; Barratt-Boyes *et al.*, 1976). A *moderate- or large-sized patent ductus arteriosus* is present in about 6 per cent of the patients of all ages, but in infants in heart failure, about 25 per cent have an associated significant ductus (Barratt-Boyes *et al.*, 1976). A VSD occurs in combination with *severe coarctation* in about 12 per cent of patients. However, this combination is also much more common among infants with large VSD coming to operation when less than 3 months old.

Congenital *valvar or subvalvar aortic stenosis* occurs in about 4 per cent of patients requiring operation for VSD. Subvalvar stenosis is more common (Lauer *et al.*, 1960) and may also occur in association with VSD and infundibular pulmonary stenosis. It may also develop after pulmonary artery banding (Freed *et al.*, 1973). This subvalvar stenosis is of two types. One is in the form of a discrete fibromuscular bar that lies inferior (caudad or upstream) to the VSD. The other is distal (downstream) to the VSD and often

consists of a displacement of infundibular septal muscle into the left ventricular outflow tract. This latter type is often associated with aortic arch anomalies (Dirksen *et al.*, 1978; Moulaert *et al.*, 1976; Van Praagh *et al.*, 1971). Significant *congenital mitral valve disease* occurs in about 2 per cent of patients. One or

TABLE 35–1. ASSOCIATED CONDITIONS OF MINOR ANATOMIC OR FUNCTIONAL SIGNIFICANCE IN 138 PATIENTS WITH LARGE "PRIMARY" VSD AND WITHOUT ASSOCIATED CONDITIONS OF MAJOR ANATOMIC OR FUNCTIONAL SIGNIFICANCE AT UAB (1967–1976)‡

CONDITION	NUMBER AND % OF PATIENTS*
None	73 (53%)
Mild or moderate pulmonary stenosis	27 (20%)
Atrial septal defect†	24 (17%)
Persistent left superior vena cava	12 (9%)
Dextroposition of the aorta	7 (5%)
Aneurysm of membranous septum	2 (1%)
Mild or moderate coarctation of aorta	2 (1%)
Vascular ring	1 (0.7%)
Tricuspid incompetence, mild	2 (1%)
Mitral incompetence, mild	–
Pulmonary valve incompetence	1 (0.7%)
Hepatic veins entering right atrium directly	1 (0.7%)
Anomalous right ventricular muscle band without pulmonary stenosis	1 (0.7%)

*Sum of percentages is > 100%, since some patients had more than one minor associated condition.

†Exclusive of simple patent foramen ovale.

‡Modified from Blackstone, E. H., *et al.*: Optimal age and results in repair of large ventricular septal defects. J. Thorac. Cardiovasc. Surg., 72:661, 1976.

the other pulmonary artery may be absent or severely stenotic. Severe peripheral pulmonary artery stenoses rarely occur. Severe positional cardiac anomalies, such as isolated dextrocardia or situs inversus totalis, exist uncommonly in patients with simple VSD.

A number of minor anomalies may also be present in patients coming to operation for VSD (Table 35–1). In small infants, a large atrial septal defect coexisting with a large VSD may be a significant lesion (Barratt-Boyes et al., 1976).

PULMONARY VASCULAR DISEASE

The classic description of the pathology of hypertensive pulmonary vascular disease is that of Heath and Edwards (1958). They defined Grade 1 changes as being characterized by medial hypertrophy without intimal proliferation; Grade 2 by medial hypertrophy with cellular intimal reaction; Grade 3 by intimal fibrosis as well as medial hypertrophy, and possibly with early generalized vascular dilation; Grade 4 by generalized vascular dilation, an area of vascular occlusion by intimal fibrosis, and plexiform lesions; Grade 5 by other "dilation lesions" such as cavernous and angiomatoid lesions; and Grade 6 by, in addition, necrotizing arteritis.

The pulmonary resistance in patients with a large VSD (and those with a large patent ductus arteriosus) has been positively correlated with the histologic severity of the hypertensive pulmonary vascular disease by Heath and colleagues (1958). However, we have re-analyzed their data and find that the "confidence bands" are rather wide around the probability of severe pulmonary vascular disease as predicted from the pulmonary resistance. This is not unexpected, as the Heath-Edwards classification is based on the most severe lesion seen, regardless of its frequency. Furthermore, as pointed out by Wagenvoort (Wagenvoort et al., 1961; Wagenvoort and Wagenvoort, 1970) and by Yamaki and Tezuka (1976), the grading should include an assessment of the number of vessels affected. Moreover, the calculation of pulmonary vascular resistance is open to many errors.

A somewhat different view of hypertensive pulmonary vascular disease in infants with large VSD has been provided by Reid and colleagues (Hislop et al., 1975). Others had pointed out earlier that intimal proliferation (and thus Heath-Edwards changes of Grade 2 or greater) rarely develops in infants with large VSD until 1 or 2 years of age (Wagenvoort et al., 1961), and yet, infants occasionally do have severely elevated pulmonary resistance. Reid and associates found that infants dying at 3 to 6 months of age with large VSD and high pulmonary vascular resistance (> 8 units $\cdot$ M.^{2}) with intermittent right-to-left shunting have marked medial hypertrophy affecting both large and small pulmonary arteries, including those less than 200 μm. in diameter (Hislop et al., 1975). The usual number of intra-acinar vessels was present. In contrast, they found that infants (3 to 10 months old) with large VSD, dying with a history of large pulmonary blood flow and congestive heart failure and normal or slightly elevated pulmonary vascular resistance, have medial hypertrophy affecting mainly arteries with diameters larger than 200 μm. The intra-acinar vessels were fewer than usual.

The histologic reversibility of pulmonary vascular disease after closure of the VSD has not been documented. The favorable results in infants may be from an increase in the number of arterioles and capillaries as growth proceeds. Presumably, pulmonary vascular disease of Heath-Edwards Grade 3 or greater severity is not reversible.

PATHOPHYSIOLOGY

Determinants of Size and Direction of Shunt. The magnitude and direction of the shunt across a ventricular septal defect depend on the size of the defect and the pressure gradient across it during the various phases of the cardiac cycle. We have observed these relations with biplane cineangiocardiograms in a large number of patients. Jarmakani and colleagues (1968) and Levin and associates (1968) have studied them with special techniques.

When the VSD is small, it offers considerable resistance to flow, and slight variations in the size of the defect are accompanied by large variations in the rate of flow (or shunting). Across small defects, only a large pressure difference, such as occurs during mid and late systole, results in significant flow. When the defect is large, it offers little resistance to flow, and small pressure differences between the left and right ventricle result in shunting. The pressure relations during the entire cardiac cycle must therefore be considered in patients with large defects.

The pressure relations late in systole seem largely related to the output resistance to left and right ventricular ejection. The determinants of those during diastole and early systole are more complex. They include the relative compliance of the two ventricles and the relative pressures in the two atria. Asynchronous systole of the two ventricles relates to the pressure relations in the early portion of systole and diastole.

The size of the VSD itself may vary during various phases of the cardiac cycle. Also, an apparently large VSD may be partially closed during ventricular systole by a flap of muscle or tissue. It is possible that defects in the muscular septum are considerably smaller during systole than during diastole or when viewed at operation or autopsy.

Sequelae of Left-to-Right Shunting. When a left-to-right shunt is present at ventricular level, pulmonary blood flow is increased above normal and systemic blood flow. Consequently, flow through the left atrium and the mitral valve orifice is similarly increased, and greater work is performed by both the left and the right ventricles. The left atrium is enlarged to a degree corresponding to the magnitude of increase in pulmonary blood flow, and a diastolic murmur may be heard over the apex of the heart, reflecting the increase in the blood flow across the mitral valve. Left atrial pressure becomes elevated relative both to normal and to right atrial pressure, as the result of a natural adaptive process related to the Starling-Frank mechanism. The left ventricle is larger than normal, and the right ventricle is dilated.

The elevated left atrial (and pulmonary venous) pressure causes many infants with VSD to have an increased amount of interstitial fluid in the lungs. As a result, they tend to have repeated pulmonary infections. The lungs are relatively noncompliant, and the work of breathing is increased. This increases energy expenditure, which, along with the relatively low systemic blood flow, causes such infants to have striking growth failure. These sequelae are well reflected in the physical findings, chest roentgenograms, and electrocardiograms of patients with VSD and large pulmonary blood flow (DuShane and Kirklin, 1960).

When pulmonary resistance rises in patients with large VSD as a result of the development of pulmonary vascular disease, pulmonary blood flow is reduced, left atrial pressure lessens, and the sequelae of left-to-right shunting lessen. The infant or child seems to improve: as pulmonary infections subside, the work of breathing decreases, and growth improves. Unfortunately, further increases in pulmonary vascular resistance slowly occur, and the classic Eisenmenger complex results. In such patients with severe pulmonary hypertension and bidirectional shunting of equal magnitude in the two directions, the left ventricle is not enlarged and the right ventricle is hypertrophied, but its volume is not increased.

NATURAL HISTORY

Spontaneous Closure. Ventricular septal defects have a tendency to close spontaneously, and this fact is relevant to decisions about operation (Collins *et al.,* 1972). Spontaneous closure can be complete by 1 year of age, or the defect may have only narrowed by then, with complete closure taking considerably longer. The phenomenon of spontaneous closure or narrowing of VSDs explains the infrequency with which large VSDs are encountered in adults. An inverse relationship exists between the probability of eventual spontaneous closure and the age at which the patient is observed (Hoffman and Rudolph, 1965; Keith *et al.,* 1971; Blackstone *et al.,* 1976) (Fig. 35–2). This is highly relevant to clinical decisions about individual patients. According to these data, about 80 per cent of individuals seen at 1 month of age with large VSDs experience eventual spontaneous closure, as do about 60 per cent of those seen at 3 months of age, about 50 per cent of those seen at 6 months of age, and 25 per cent of those seen at 12 months of age.

Pulmonary Vascular Disease. A large ventricular septal defect predisposes the patient to the development of an increased pulmonary vascular resistance from hypertensive pulmonary vascular disease, which tends to worsen as the individual gets older (Auld *et*

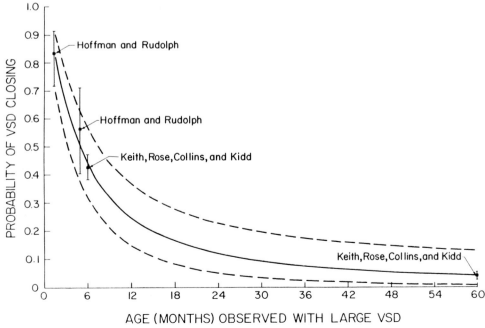

Figure 35–2. Probability of eventual spontaneous closure of a large VSD according to the age at which the patient is observed. The *dotted lines* enclose the 70 per cent confidence limits around the solid probability line. The specific ratios, with the 70 per cent confidence limits, reported by Hoffman and Rudolph (1966) and Keith and associates (1971) are shown centered upon the mean or assumed ages of patients in their reports. (p < 0.0001.) (From Blackstone, E. H., *et al,*: Optimal age and results in repair of large ventricular septal defects, J. Thorac. Cardiovasc. Surg., *72*:661, 1976.)

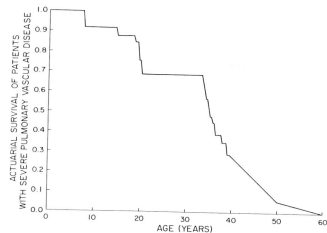

Figure 35–3. Actuarial survival of patients with large VSD who had proven elevation of pulmonary vascular resistance to a level that made them inoperable (≥10 units m²) demonstrated at cardiac catheterization done at various ages. Note that fatalities begin to occur in the second decade of life, that about one half of the patients are dead by age 35, and that a few survive until 50 years of age. (Modified from Clarkson, P. M., et al.: Prognosis for patients with ventricular septal defect and severe pulmonary vascular obstructive disease. Circulation, *38*:129, 1968.)

al., 1963; Lucas et al., 1961). Thus, the proportion of patients with large VSD who have a severely elevated pulmonary vascular resistance is directly related to the age of the patient. Patients with severe pulmonary vascular disease are usually dead by 40 years of age (Fig. 35–3).

The statement that some infants less than 2 years of age with large VSD have severely elevated pulmonary vascular resistance is doubted by some, but its occurrence is well documented (Barratt-Boyes et al., 1976). It is, however, quite uncommon. It occurs in some infants because they do not undergo the usual fall in pulmonary vascular resistance a few weeks to a few months after birth. Others do undergo this but later, in the first 2 years of life, develop a rapid increase in pulmonary vascular resistance (Hoffman and Rudolph, 1966). Some infants with large VSD have normal or mildly elevated resistance, retain this through the first decade of life, and then, if their VSD is still large, develop more severe changes as the years pass (Keith et al., 1971; Kirklin et al., 1963).

Bacterial Endocarditis. This is rare, occurring at a rate of about 0.3 per cent per year in individuals with VSD (Corone et al., 1977; Campbell, 1971; Shah et al., 1966). Often, a pulmonary process is the presenting feature, presumably developing from emboli secondary to right-sided bacterial vegetations. Prognosis with treatment is excellent.

Premature Death. Past experience and reports in the literature indicate that without surgical treatment some infants (about 9 per cent of those with large VSD) die of their disease in the first year of life (Keith et al., 1971; Ash, 1964). Death may result from congestive heart failure, which may devleop very early but usually occurs at about 2 to 3 months of age,

presumably because at about this time the left-to-right shunt becomes larger as the medial hypertrophy present in the small pulmonary arteries at birth regresses. Death also may result from recurrent pulmonary infections secondary to pulmonary edema from the high pulmonary venous pressure. Death is most apt to occur in those infants with large VSD who have associated conditions of major anatomic or functional significance, such as patent ductus arteriosus, coarctation of the aorta, or a large atrial septal defect (Barratt-Boyes et al., 1976).

After the age of 1 year, few if any patients die because of their ventricular septal defect until the second decade of life. By then, most patients whose VSDs have remained large have developed pulmonary vascular disease and in subsequent years die from complications of Eisenmenger complex (Clarkson et al., 1968) (Fig. 35–3). These include hemoptysis, polycythemia, cerebral abscess or infarction, and right heart failure.

Patients with *small* VSDs do not develop pulmonary vascular disease and are unlikely to die prematurely. Their only real risk is bacterial endocarditis, the incidence of which is low (estimated to occur once in 500 patient years [Shah et al., 1966]). It is generally well treated by antibiotics.

Symptoms. Patients with small VSDs rarely have symptoms related to the defect. Patients with large VSDs may have symptoms of intractable heart failure in the first few months of life, with poor peripheral pulses, inability to feed, sweating, and chronic pulmonary edema. About one half of the patients coming to operation in the first 2 years of life do so because of this (Table 35–2) (Barratt-Boyes et al., 1976). During early life, rapid and labored respiration and recurrent pulmonary infections may occur secondary to high pulmonary venous pressure and chronic pulmonary edema. At any time in the first year of life, lobes of the lung may become chronically hyperinflated because of pressure of the large and tense pulmonary arteries on the bronchi, preventing complete escape

Table 35–2. INDICATIONS FOR REPAIR OF VENTRICULAR SEPTAL DEFECT IN PATIENTS OPERATED ON IN THE FIRST 2 YEARS OF LIFE*

INDICATION FOR VSD REPAIR	NO.	% OF TOTAL	AGE IN MONTHS AVERAGE (RANGE)
Intractable congestive heart failure	30	53%	2.9 (1 to 7)
Recurrent respiratory infections	3	5%	8 (6 to 9)
Controlled congestive heart failure and failure to thrive	17	30%	11.4 (4 to 21)
Increased pulmonary vascular resistance	7	12%	14.6 (10 to 19)

*Modified from Barratt-Boyes, B. G., et al.: Repair of ventricular septal defect in the first two years of life using profound hypothermia–circulatory arrest techniques. Ann. Surg., *184*:376, 1976.

of air during expiration (Oh *et al.*, 1978). As a result of all this, many babies with large VSDs are small and physically underdeveloped. It is these symptomatic patients who fail to respond well to medical management who are at particular risk of dying in the first year of life. Some babies who survive through the first year of life with large VSD have controlled heart failure and failure to thrive in the second year of life as well.

Children and young adults with large VSDs are usually symptomatic and tend to be small both in height and weight. As pulmonary vascular disease develops, symptoms may regress.

Development of Aortic Incompetence. A small proportion of patients (probably about 5 per cent in Caucasians and black races) develop aortic valve incompetence as a complication of VSD. The incompetence is not present at birth but develops during the first decade of life. It gradually worsens, so that by the end of the second decade, it is usually severe. As the incompetence increases, the shunt often decreases, owing to occlusion of the VSD by the prolapsed aortic cusp.

Development of Infundibular Pulmonary Stenosis. A small proportion (perhaps 5 to 10 per cent) of patients with large VSD and large left-to-right shunt in infancy develop infundibular pulmonary stenosis (Keith *et al.*, 1971; Gasul *et al.*, 1957; Hoffman and Rudolph, 1970). The mild and moderate infundibular pulmonary stenoses in those patients operated on for "primary" VSD (see Table 35–1) as well as the more important stenoses probably develop in this way. The stenosis may become severe enough to produce shunt reversal and cyanosis, and the condition then can properly be termed tetralogy of Fallot. Somerville's data (1970) indicate that this transformation occurs in about 6 per cent of infants with isolated VSD. Those who undergo the transformation probably are born with some anterior displacement of the infundibular septum and its extensions.

DIAGNOSIS

Examination

The infant with a large ventricular septal defect and increased pulmonary blood flow presents a particular and highly characteristic clinical picture. Tachypnea with marked subcostal retraction, severe growth failure, and lack of subcutaneous tissue are evident. A waxen complexion and evidence of profuse sweating such as hair that is damp or matted from recently dried perspiration may be noted. The external jugular venous pulses are usually quite prominent when the infant is supine and often even when he is held erect. A bulging precordium is a common finding. On palpation, a rapid, overactive heart is apparent. A thrill is maximal in the third to fifth intercostal spaces on the left. The loud pansystolic murmur is also maximal in the third to fifth intercostal spaces on the

left. A short mid-diastolic murmur is usually appreciated at the apex, giving the entire cardiac cycle a gallop quality. The second sound at the base is usually loud and may be slightly split. The liver and spleen are usually enlarged, and the peripheral pulses are rapid and thready. Such infants are obviously in heart failure, and many are actually in shock.

In older patients with large VSDs, a protruding sternum, or so-called pigeon breast deformity, is found rather frequently. Presumably, this is due to the large right ventricle pushing the sternum anteriorly during the period of growth. A systolic thrill over the left precordium is often present. The characteristic murmur of VSD is a pansystolic harsh murmur heard in the second, third, and maximally in the fourth left interspace in the midclavicular line (Leatham and Segal, 1962). In patients with a large pulmonary blood flow, there may be a superimposed systolic ejection murmur originating in the area of the pulmonary valve. Characteristically, an early diastolic filling murmur is heard at the apex, indicating a large flow across the mitral valve. The first heart sound at the base is normal; the second sound at the base is abnormally split, owing both to shortened left ventricular ejection time and to prolonged right ventricular ejection time. The splitting is accentuated in inspiration.

These classic physical findings are altered by the size of the ventricular septal defect and the magnitude of the pulmonary vascular resistance. Patients with small VSDs and small left-to-right shunts have only a systolic murmur. The heart is not hyperactive, and on palpation, there is no enlargement of the left ventricle and no right ventricular lift. Not only do patients with large VSD, mild elevation of pulmonary vascular resistance, and large pulmonary blood flow have the characteristic systolic murmur, but in addition, the heart is hyperactive, the left ventricle is enlarged on palpation, there is a right ventricular lift, there is an apical diastolic rumble, and the second sound at the base is moderately accentuated. In patients with a large VSD and high pulmonary vascular resistance, and consequently with a net left-to-right shunt that is small or with shunts that are bidirectional and of about equal magnitude in the two directions, the heart is quiet on examination. There is no evidence on palpation of left ventricular enlargement, but the right ventricular lift is prominent. The systolic murmur is soft and short, or may be nearly absent. There is no apical diastolic rumble. The second sound at the base is markedly accentuated. Those patients in whom the pulmonary vascular resistance has become higher than systemic resistance are, of course, cyanotic.

Chest Roentgenogram

The chest roentgenogram in a patient with a ventricular septal defect reflects the pathophysiology. Patients with small VSDs and small left-to-right shunts usually have normal chest roentgenograms; those with large VSDs, mild elevation of pulmonary vascular

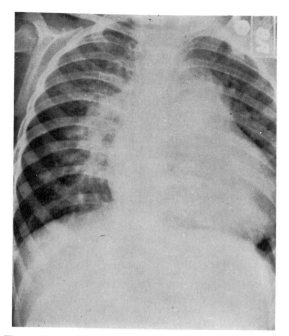

Figure 35–4. Chest roentgenogram of a child with a large VSD, large pulmonary blood flow, and pulmonary hypertension, but only mild elevation of pulmonary vascular resistance. This is reflected in the evidence of left and right ventricular enlargement, enlargement of the main pulmonary artery, and marked increase in pulmonary blood flow.

resistance, and large left-to-right shunts have characteristic chest roentgenograms (Fig. 35–4). In the latter, pulmonary arteries, both centrally and peripherally, are large, indicating large pulmonary blood flow. There may be evidence of some enlargement of the left atrium; the left ventricle is abnormally large; and the right ventricle appears dilated. When one sees *marked* enlargement of the left atrium in a patient suspected of having a ventricular septal defect, the coexistence of significant mitral valvular incompetence should be suspected.

When the patient has a large VSD and severe elevation of pulmonary vascular resistance, the appearance of the chest roentgenogram is quite different. The peripheral pulmonary arteries are normal in size, and there is no evidence of increased pulmonary blood flow. The main pulmonary artery is often markedly enlarged. There is no evidence of left atrial or left ventricular enlargement. The right ventricle may appear somewhat enlarged, but often the cardiac silhouette, other than the large pulmonary artery, is essentially normal (Fig. 35–5).

Electrocardiogram

If the defect is large and the pulmonary vascular resistance only mildly elevated, there is evidence of overload of both ventricles. The R wave from the right precordial leads is tall, and when right ventricular peak pressure is similar to left ventricular peak pres-

sure it is notched on the upstroke. The left precordial leads in this situation have the pattern of ventricular overload previously described although here there may also be a deeper S wave. As long as evidence of left ventricular enlargement exists in these leads, the patient probably has a pulmonary-systemic flow greater than about 1.8 and a pulmonary-systemic resistance less than about 0.6 and is operable. Absence of this pattern by itself is not clear evidence of a higher resistance ratio and inoperability.

Cardiac Catheterization and Cineangiography

Although clinical findings and the chest roentgenogram usually allow estimation of the pulmonary blood flow and Q_P/Q_S and two-dimensional echocardiography can often visualize a large VSD and eliminate the possibility of A-V canal and left ventricular outflow tract obstruction, cardiac catheterization is indicated in patients being considered for operation. A major purpose of this special study is the accurate localization of the defect and the identification of multiple defects and other major associated cardiac anomalies.

INDICATIONS FOR OPERATION

When *infants* with *large VSDs* have severe intractable heart failure or intractable, severe respiratory symptoms at any time during the first 3 months

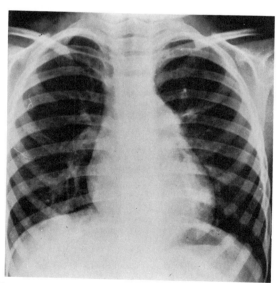

Figure 35–5. This chest roentgenogram is in contrast to that shown in Figure 35–4. The heart is not enlarged overall. The main pulmonary artery is enlarged; there is no evidence of increased pulmonary blood flow. This patient has a large ventricular septal defect, pulmonary hypertension, severe elevation of pulmonary vascular resistance, and pulmonary blood flow that is less than systemic blood flow. The condition is inoperable. (From DuShane, J. W., and Kirklin, J. W.: Selection for surgery of patients with ventricular septal defect and pulmonary hypertension. Circulation, *21*:13, 1960.)

of life, prompt primary repair is indicated. Operation is not advised *electively* in the first 3 months of life, in the hope that spontaneous closure or narrowing of the defect may occur.

When severe symptoms, significant growth failure, or rising pulmonary vascular resistance is present in infants 3 months of age or older, prompt primary repair is advised.

When an infant reaches *6 months* of age with a single, *large ventricular septal defect*, he is rarely truly thriving. The probability of cure by spontaneous closure of the VSD has decreased significantly (see Fig. 35–2). If the pulmonary vascular resistance is high (e.g., about 8 units · M.² or greater), repair is advisable without undue delay, since delay lessens the infant's chances of "surgical cure." If the infant's pulmonary vascular resistance is low (e.g., 10 units · M.²) and stays low and his clinical condition reasonably good, operation can be deferred until about 12 months of age, although the risks of repair are not demonstrably less than at 6 months of age. It should not be delayed after this time.

Patients with *large VSDs* who are first *seen after infancy* must be considered primarily on the basis of the *extent of their pulmonary vascular disease* (Kirklin and DuShane, 1963). When the pulmonary vascular resistance is greater than 10 units · M.², in which circumstance the ratio of pulmonary to systemic blood flow (Q_P/Q_S) is usually less than 1.5 (with the patient at rest and breathing air), and when the clinical data are also consistent with this hemodynamic state (the systolic murmur is soft or absent; no apical diastolic flow murmur is present; the lung fields on roentgenogram are not plethoric; the left ventricle is normal or near-normal in size; and the ECG shows at least moderate right ventricular hypertrophy), operation is not advisable. Closure of the defect under these circumstances precludes right-to-left shunting during exercise; consequently, exercise capacity and life expectancy are not as good with the defect closed as with it open. When pulmonary vascular resistance is elevated but within the "operable range" (5 to 10 units · M.²), operation is generally advisable, with the knowledge that the long-term results may be compromised by persisting and possibly increasing pulmonary vascular disease. However, some patients with resistance values in this range at rest have rather fixed pulmonary vascular resistance, which does not fall during stress. Therefore, in patients with borderline operability who are old enough to cooperate, measurement of pulmonary and systemic blood flow and resistances during moderate exercise is helpful; even if Q_P/Q_S is 1.5 or 1.8 at rest, if it becomes 1.0 or less during moderate exercise (from systemic peripheral vasodilation and increased systemic blood flow, and a fixed and high pulmonary vascular resistance preventing increased pulmonary blood flow), operation is not indicated. The simple finding of a significant fall in arterial oxygen saturation during exercise (from right-to-left shunting across the VSD for the reasons described) is suggestive of inoperability. The response of the pulmonary vascular resistance to inhalation of high oxygen mixtures is not useful in determining operability in borderline situations.

A considerable number of children have a *moderate-sized VSD*, which is not sufficient to raise pulmonary artery pressure above 40 to 50 mm. Hg systolic and which will not result in subsequent elevation of pulmonary vascular resistance and yet produces a Q_P/Q_S of up to 3, moderate cardiomegaly, and significant pulmonary plethora. There are usually few if any symptoms. Such patients should be kept under observation for about 5 years in the hope that there will be spontaneous reduction in the size of the VSD. If there is no change on subsequent recatheterization, closure is indicated.

It is not advised that young patients with *small VSDs* undergo repair, since they are suffering no significant ill effects and the defect will probably close.

Subpulmonary defects are a special situation. Even though apparently small, they should not be left untreated beyond 5 years of age, because aortic incompetence may develop, and they should be repaired promptly at an earlier age if an aortic diastolic murmur develops.

SURGICAL TREATMENT

Ventricular septal defects are usually repaired through the right atrium but, occasionally, are repaired through the right ventricle, and very occasionally through the pulmonary artery or left ventricle.

We generally perform the operations with hypothermic (about 24°C.) cardiopulmonary bypass. The traditional two venous cannulae are used, but in infants, exposure is best when the venae cavae are cannulated directly with special small metal venous cannulae. After opening the right atrium, a small sump sucker is introduced into the left atrium via the foramen ovale. With this, plus cold cardioplegic myocardial protection, exposure and working conditions are superb. When the patient is a very small baby (weighing less than 3 kg.), we usually elect to use a single venous cannula, cooling to 20°C., and total circulatory arrest during the repair. The period of total circulatory arrest should always be less than 45 minutes for this operation, and we consider this quite safe. We recognize that others have obtained excellent results using total circulatory arrest for all infants less than 2 years of age (Barratt-Boyes *et al.*, 1976; Rein *et al.*, 1977).

Before commencing cardiopulmonary bypass, the possible presence of anomalies of pulmonary or systemic venous return is determined. It should be known from preoperative study whether the ductus arteriosus is open or closed. This is a very important matter, for an open ductus during total circulatory arrest and open cardiotomy allows air to enter the aorta and later to go to the brain, and during cardiopulmonary bypass, it increases intracardiac return and overdistends the pulmonary circulation. When a patent ductus is present or suspected, it is ligated from the anterior approach.

Perimembranous VSD. Either a right atrial or a right ventricular approach is satisfactory for this repair, but we prefer a right atrial approach in nearly all cases. The atrium is opened obliquely, and the exposure is arranged during perfusion cooling (Fig. 35–6). The cold cardioplegic solution is then injected into the aortic root. All VSDs are repaired with a patch. The relationship of the bundle of His to the posterior and inferior margin of the defect must be clearly understood in order to accomplish a safe repair.

When a right ventricular approach is used, a transverse incision is made. The repair is basically the same.

Subpulmonary VSD. Subarterial VSDs and muscular defects in the subpulmonary infundibulum are approached through a transverse incision in the infundibulum. These defects are usually large enough to require a patch for closure.

Atrioventricular Canal Type of VSD. This defect is most easily repaired through the right atrium, although it may be done through the right ventricle. Since the defect is beneath the septal leaflet of the tricuspid valve, care must be taken to prevent tricuspid dysfunction postoperatively by avoiding damage to the leaflet or its chordae and by tailoring the patch so that it is not too bulky beneath the septal leaflet. One method of avoiding damage and improving exposure is to temporarily detach the base of the septal leaflet and a portion of the anterior leaflet of the tricuspid valve and retract the leaflets anteriorly. These defects are nearly always repaired with a patch.

Muscular VSD. We select a right-sided approach for repair of muscular VSDs whenever possible. Often, these can be closed through the right atrium. At times, for multiple anterior VSDs, a vertical right ventriculotomy is made near the septum. The defects are closed by mattress sutures placed over felt pledgets (Breckenridge et al., 1972). Left ventriculotomy gives excellent exposure (Aaron and Lower, 1975; Singh et al., 1977), but we prefer not to use it routinely in infants because it has been associated with left ventricular dysfunction early and late postoperatively in some of our small patients. In older patients, avoidance of left ventriculotomy seems to be less important.

The rare "Swiss-cheese" septum usually requires a left ventricular approach. An associated perimembranous defect should be repaired through the right atrium, because its repair from the left ventricular side increases the risk of heart block.

POSTOPERATIVE CARE

Most infants convalesce normally after VSD repair, and special treatment usually is not required. Generally, the patients are extubated within 24 hours of operation and recover rapidly.

In the unusual circumstance of low cardiac output after operation, in addition to the usual supportive treatment (Kirklin and Kirklin, 1981), consideration should be given to the possibility of an overlooked or incompletely closed VSD. This is especially to be considered if the left atrial pressure is considerably higher than the right. If recovery from the low output state does not occur within a few hours and in the absence of secure information from an indicator-dilution study that a residual shunt is not present, urgent recatheterization and possible reoperation are indicated.

If complete atrioventricular dissociation was present for a time after cardiopulmonary bypass, but sinus rhythm reappeared, a demand pacemaker attached to ventricular wires should be in place for a week postoperatively, since, rarely, the A-V dissociation recurs temporarily in the early postoperative period.

RESULTS OF SURGICAL TREATMENT

Early Results of Primary Repair

Hospital mortality rates for repair of VSD now approach 0 per cent in most centers properly prepared for this type of work, even in very small infants (Rizzoli et al., 1980; Rein et al., 1977; Barratt-Boyes et al., 1976; Lincoln et al., 1977). However, in earlier times, deaths did occur, and a number of incremental risk factors could be identified. The current very low hospital mortality rates are the result of the neutralization of most of these risk factors by scientific progress and by minimization of human error.

Type of VSD. The location of the *single large VSD* is not an incremental risk factor with regard to early or late results of repair. In the past, *multiple VSDs* have been an important incremental risk factor (Blackstone et al., 1976; Kirklin et al., 1980). Our more recent experience indicates that it is only a weak one (Rizzoli et al., 1980) (Table 35–3). This improvement is in part related to the general improvements in infant intracardiac surgery, but is also related in a major way to a now higher proportion of patients with complete or nearly complete repair and little or no residual shunting. This can be attributed primarily to better preoperative cineangiographic identification of the presence, size, and location of the multiple VSDs.

Age at Repair. We have had no deaths at the University of Alabama at Birmingham among patients operated on at age 24 months or older for repair of isolated large VSD in the last decade, and thus, for a long time, the risk of operation under these circumstances has approached 0 per cent.

The incremental risk of young age was clearly apparent in our early experience, as it was in many centers (Binet et al. 1970; Ching et al., 1971; Cooley et al., 1962; Johnson et al., 1974). However, a steady decrease in hospital mortality has occurred with time, affecting infants particularly. As a result, the previously apparent incremental risk of young age has been

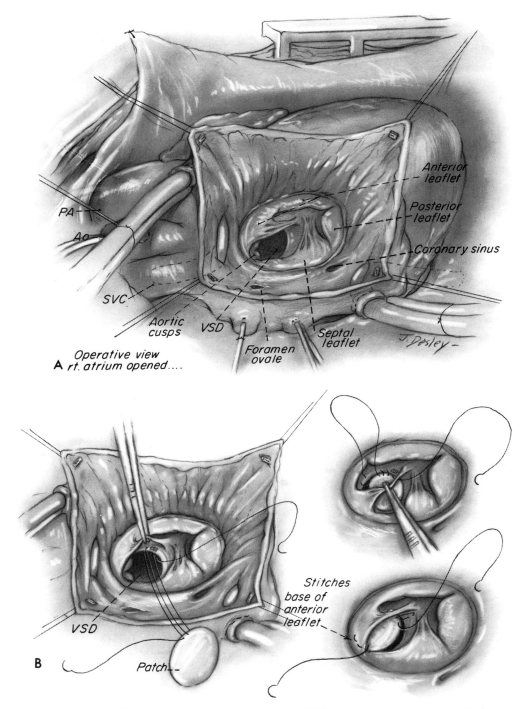

Figure 35–6. *A*, Right atrial incision and exposure of perimembranous VSD in the region of the tricuspid anteroseptal commissure. Stay sutures have been placed in order to somewhat evert the atrial wall. Note that initially the superior edge of this typical perimembranous defect is not visible. The A-V node is in the muscular portion of the atrioventricular septum, just on the atrial side of the commissure between the tricuspid septal and anterior leaflets. The His bundle thus penetrates at the posterior angle of the VSD, where it is vulnerable to injury.

B, The repair of the perimembranous VSD. This is begun by placing a mattress suture of 4-0 Prolene with a small pledget at the 12 o'clock position in the defect as viewed by the surgeon through the tricuspid valve. A piece of knitted Dacron velour is trimmed to be slightly larger than the approximate size of the defect, and one arm of the suture is passed through the Dacron patch, back through the septum, and again through the patch. Either now or after placing several more stitches, the sutures are snugged up as the patch is lowered into place. The suture line between the cephalad rim of the defect and the patch is continued. The traction on the suture exposes the next areas to be stitched and provides good visibility. When the junction of the superior muscular rim (ventriculo-infundibular fold) and tricuspid anulus has been reached, the suture is passed through the base of the contiguous portion of the tricuspid valve (usually the anterior leaflet) from the ventricular to the atrial side, then back from the atrial to the ventricular side of the valve and through the patch. After passing the stitch back through the leaflet, the suture is tagged.

Illustration continued on opposite page

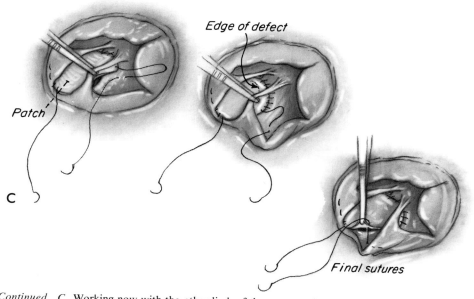

Figure 35–6. *Continued C,* Working now with the other limb of the suture, stitches are taken between the ventricular septum and the patch along the caudad side of the defect. These stitches are placed 3 to 5 mm. away from the edge of the defect *in order to avoid the area most probably occupied by the bundle of His* and more posteriorly 5 to 7 mm. back from the edge.

neutralized in more recent experiences (Barratt-Boyes *et al.,* 1976; Rein *et al.,* 1977; Rizzoli *et al.,* 1980) (Table 35–4 and Fig. 35–7). This has resulted in part from scientific progress, with improved preoperative diagnostic accuracy, improved surgical and support techniques, and improved myocardial preservation. It has also resulted in part from a demonstrated decrease in the fatal human surgical and management errors as institutions have increased their experience and expertise with infant intracardiac surgery.

Pulmonary Artery Pressure and Pulmonary Vascular Resistance. At present, these are not determinants of hospital mortality, although they do affect late results

(Blackstone *et al.,* 1976). This is different from our earlier Mayo Clinic experiences (Cartmill *et al.,* 1966), probably because the upper limit of acceptable (''operable'') pulmonary vascular resistance is better understood and management has improved.

Major Associated Lesions. The frequency of major associated lesions, particularly in symptomatic infants with large VSDs, has already been stressed. These do have, even currently, an incremental risk effect on hospital mortality. At the University of Alabama at Birmingham, among 312 patients operated on for VSD from 1967 to 1979, 16 hospital deaths (*6.3 per cent*; confidence limits (CL) 4.7 to 8.3 per cent)

TABLE 35–3. HOSPITAL MORTALITY IN 29 PATIENTS UNDERGOING PRIMARY REPAIR OF MULTIPLE VSDs WITHOUT MAJOR ASSOCIATED LESIONS AT UAB (1967–1979)*

AGE (MONTHS)	TOTAL				1974–1979‡			
	No.	*Hospital Deaths*			*No.*	*Hospital Deaths*		
		No.	%	70% CL		No.	%	70% CL
< 3	1	0	0%	0%–85%				
≥ 3 < 6	4	2	50%	18%–82%	1	0	0%	0%–85%
≥ 6 < 12	5	1	20%	3%–53%	2	0	0%	0%–61%
≥ 12 < 24	7	3	43%	20%–68%	3	0	0%	0%–47%
≥ 24 < 48	5	3	60%	29%–86%	4	1	25%	3%–63%
≥ 48	7	0	0%	0%–24%	1	0	0%	0%–85%
					3	0	0%	0%–47%
Total	29	9	31%	21%–42%	14	1	7%	1%–22%
	(15	8	53%	37%–69%)†				

p for table (n = 29) = 0.22

*From Rizzoli, G., *et al.:* Incremental risk factors in hospital mortality after repair of ventricular septal defect. J. Thorac. Cardiovasc. Surg., *80*:494, 1980.

‡Numbers in parentheses are for the period from 1967 to 1974.

‡Note the markedly lowered mortality in this period.

TABLE 35–4. EFFECT OF AGE ON HOSPITAL MORTALITY IN 166 PATIENTS UNDERGOING PRIMARY REPAIR OF SINGLE LARGE VSD WITHOUT MAJOR ASSOCIATED LESIONS AT UAB (1967–1979)*

AGE (MONTHS)	TOTAL		Hospital Deaths			1974–1979		Hospital Deaths		
	No.	%	No.	%	70% CL	No.	%	No.	%	70% CL
< 3	14	8.4%	2	14%	5%–31%	11	11.7%	1‡	9%	1%–28%
≥ 3 < 6	12	7.2%	0	0%	0%–15%	10	10.6%	0	0%	0%–17%
≥ 6 < 12	23	13.9%	3	13%	6%–25%	14	14.9%	0	0%	0%–13%
≥ 12 < 24	21	12.7%	1	5%	1%–15%	11	11.7%	0	0%	0%–16%
≥ 24 < 48	27	16.3%	0	0%	0%–7%	15	16.0%	0	0%	0%–12%
≥ 48	69	41.6%	0	0%	0%–3%	33	35.1%	0	0%	0%–6%
Total	166		6	3.6%	2.1%–5.8%	94		1	1.1%	0.1%–3.6%
	(72		5	6.9%	3.9%–11.5)†					

p for table (n = 166) = 0.01

*From Rizzoli, G., *et al.:* Incremental risk factors in hospital mortality after repair of ventricular septal defect. J. Thorac. Cardiovasc. Surg., *80*:494, 1980.

‡Numbers in parentheses are for the period from 1967 to 1974.

‡1.2-month-old baby, preoperative seizures, admitted and to surgery intubated and ventilated. Died on third postoperative day with acute cardiac failure.

occurred among 254 patients with single or multiple VSDs but no major associated lesion, whereas 14 (*24 per cent*; CL 18 to 31 per cent) occurred among 58 patients with major associated lesions (p < 0.0001) (Rizzoli *et al.*, 1980). Additional technical and scientific progress will probably improve this situation.

Surgical Approach. The surgical approach for repair of the VSD (through the right atrium, through the right ventricle, or through both) has not been a determinant of hospital mortality after repair of single VSDs (Table 35–5). Neither has it been after the repair of muscular or multiple VSDs through a left ventriculotomy, an experience also reported by surgeons at the Boston Children's Hospital (Kirklin *et al.*, 1980). However, we remain concerned about the long-term functional results of left ventriculotomy in infants.

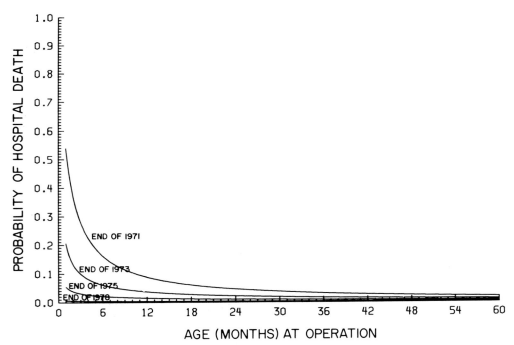

Figure 35–7. Probability of hospital death at UAB after repair of single large VSD in patients without major associated cardiac anomalies. Note that in 1971 and 1973 the risk was considerably increased in very young patients. By 1979, not only was the risk of hospital death less than 1 per cent, but an incremental risk in patients of young age was no longer apparent. (From Rizzoli, G., *et al.*: Incremental risk factors in hospital mortality after repair of ventricular septal defect. J. Thorac. Cardiovasc. Surg., *80*:494, 1980.)

TABLE 35–5. EFFECT OF SURGICAL APPROACH ON HOSPITAL MORTALITY IN 166 PATIENTS UNDERGOING PRIMARY REPAIR OF SINGLE LARGE VSDs WITHOUT MAJOR ASSOCIATED LESIONS AT UAB (1967–1979)*

| | TOTAL | | | | 1974–1979 | | | |
| | | Hospital Deaths | | | | Hospital Deaths | | |
SURGICAL APPROACH	No.	No.	%	70% CL	No.	No.	%	70% CL
Rt Atrium	105	2	1.9%	0.6%–4.5%	65	1	1.5%	0.2%–5.1%
RA → RV	4	0	0%	0%–38%	2	0	0%	0%–61%
RV	57	4	7%	4%–12%	27	0	0%	0%–7%
Total	166	6	3.6%	2.1%–5.8%	94	1	1.1%	0.1%–3.6%

p for table (n = 166) = 0.23
RA = right atrium; RV = right ventricle
*From Rizzoli, G., et al.: Incremental risk factors in hospital mortality after repair of ventricular septal defect. J. Thorac. Cardiovasc. Surg., 80:494, 1980.

Late Results

Repair of VSD in the first year or two of life is curative for most patients, resulting in full functional activity and normal or near-normal life expectancy.

Improved Physical Development. This is a prominent feature of the late postoperative course following repair of large ventricular septal defects in infants (Rein et al., 1977). Lillehei and colleagues first showed an impressive increase in weight after VSD repair in 1955. There is a less impressive increase in length and in head circumference (Clarkson et al., 1973). This improved physical development is usually associated with complete relief of symptoms. We have also reported increase in weight postoperatively in children in whom a large VSD had been repaired later in the first decade of life (Cartmill et al., 1966).

Permanent Heart Block (complete atrioventricular dissociation with independent atrial activity not conducted to the ventricles). This is uncommon with present techniques. For example, heart block was present at death or hospital dismissal in 1.5 per cent (CL — 0.5 to 3 per cent) of patients with large VSDs without associated lesions of major anatomic or functional significance in the UAB experience between 1967 and 1976 (Blackstone et al., 1976). The two patients were both unusual, one having multiple muscular defects and one being a patient with Down's syndrome and a large perimembranous defect. In our earlier report from the Mayo Clinic, no such instance occurred among the 146 patients with large VSD operated on between 1962 and 1966.

Cardiac Function. Cardiac function late postoperatively is essentially normal when repair is done in the first 2 years of life by modern techniques through the right atrium or right ventricle. Graham and colleagues found left ventricular end-diastolic volume, left ventricular systolic output, left ventricular mass, and left ventricular ejection fraction all to be normal about a year after operation in a group of such patients (Cordell et al., 1976). Others have found persisting abnormalities of left ventricular size and function after

repair of large VSDs at an older age, although all patients were asymptomatic (Jarmakani et al., 1971, 1972). This information lends support to the idea that, in general, patients with large VSDs should be operated on before they are 2 years old.

Residual Shunting. Postoperative left-to-right shunts of such magnitude as to indicate reoperation are uncommon when proper techniques are used. One of 138 patients (0.7 per cent; CL — 0.1 to 2 per cent) operated on at UAB for repair of large VSD has required reoperation (and this was for overlooked multiple muscular defects) (Blackstone et al., 1976). A report from Castaneda's group (Rein et al., 1977) states that only one patient out of 48 hospital survivors (2 per cent, CL — 0 to 7 per cent) required reoperation for residual VSD.

Premature Late Deaths. Late death occurs rarely (<2.5 per cent of patients) when pulmonary vascular resistance is low preoperatively. Presumably, these deaths are from arrhythmias, either ventricular fibrillation or the sudden late development of heart block.

Patients with a high pulmonary vascular resistance preoperatively have a tendency for this to progress and cause premature death; this becomes of some magnitude (± 25 per cent dying within 5 years of operation) when the resistance preoperatively is greater than 10 units · M.²

Pulmonary Hypertension. In general, the younger the child at the time of repair, the better his chances of having an essentially normal pulmonary artery pressure 5 years later, and thus, presumably, for the rest of his life (Barratt-Boyes et al., 1976; DuShane and Kirklin, 1973; Hoffman and Rudolph, 1966; Castaneda et al., 1971; Lillehei et al., 1968; Maron et al., 1973; Sigmann et al., 1977; Yacoub et al., 1978). The lower the pulmonary vascular resistance or the pulmonary artery pressure at the time of repair, the better the patient's chances of having normal pulmonary artery pressure postoperatively.

Severe pulmonary hypertension postoperatively can worsen with the passage of time (Friedli et al., 1974) and cause premature late death, usually within

3 to 10 years of operation (DuShane and Kirklin, 1973; Friedli *et al.*, 1974, Hallidie-Smith *et al.*, 1969). However, some patients with pulmonary hypertension and elevated pulmonary vascular resistance late postoperatively have neither progression nor regression of their disease for as long as 20 years, although with some limitation in exercise tolerance (Hallidie-Smith *et al.*, 1975; DuShane and Kirklin, 1973). Their life expectancy, however, is probably not normal.

SPECIAL SITUATIONS

VSD plus Coarctation of the Aorta. Although there has been controversy as to the management of young infants in congestive heart failure because of this combination, most centers, including our own, now practice prompt repair of the coarctation by the subclavian flap method (Bergdahl *et al.*, 1982), *without* concomitant pulmonary artery banding. If the baby remains ventilator-dependent for 72 hours, the VSD is closed then. Usually, this is not the case, and prompt improvement occurs after repair of the coarctation. The VSD may then require repair 3 to 12 months later. Often, however, spontaneous reduction in size and eventual closure occur.

VSD plus Patent Ductus Arteriosus. When a young infant with severe congestive heart failure has a large VSD and a patent ductus arteriosus of any size, operation is advisable, and both are repaired at operation, through a median sternotomy incision.

When the VSD is moderate-sized or small and the patent ductus arteriosus is large and the infant is in the first few months of life, the ductus arteriosus is closed by way of a simple operation through a left thoracotomy incision. The VSD will usually narrow and close spontaneously.

SELECTED REFERENCES

Barratt-Boyes, B. G., Neutze, J. M., Clarkson, P. M., Shardey, G. C., and Brandt, P. W. T.: Repair of ventricular septal defect in the first two years of life using profound hypothermia—circulatory arrest techniques. Ann. Surg., *184*:376, 1976.

This classic paper describes the results of primary repair of VSD in 57 patients less than 2 years of age, with many of the patients being less than 6 months old. Hospital mortality was 4 per cent in the patients without associated coarctation — a remarkable achievement. The late postoperative results are excellent. The method of profound hypothermia and total circulatory arrest and these superb results have had an important and worldwide impact on cardiac surgery.

Hoffman, J. I. E., and Rudolph, A. M.: The natural history of ventricular septal defects in infancy. Am. J. Cardiol., *16*:634, 1965.

This classic paper reports data on 62 infants with ventricular septal defect who were first catheterized under 1 year of age and were followed for 1 to 5 years thereafter. Forty were recatheterized. Fifty per cent of the infants had congestive heart failure. Spontaneous closure of the ventricular septal defect took place in 36 per cent of the patients, and in an additional 28 per cent, marked decrease in the size of the defect took place. In this series, complete spontaneous closure occurred between 7 and 12 months of age. Sixteen per cent of the group studied did not do well. Five had severe and unrelenting congestive heart failure. One baby had a high pulmonary vascular resistance from birth that never regressed. Four babies had low pulmonary vascular resistance when first catheterized at less than 1 year of age, with significant rises of resistance to pathologic levels when recatheterized subsequently. These data form a rational basis for surgical patient management programs.

Lillehei, C. W., Cohen, M., Warden, H. E., Ziegler, N. R., and Varco, R. L.: The results of direct vision closure of ventricular septal defects in eight patients by means of controlled cross circulation. Surg. Gynecol. Obstet., *101*:446, 1955.

This classic article, reporting the first successful closures of ventricular septal defects, still makes superb and informative reading. Although cross-circulation is no longer used, it obviously was a superb support system for these small patients.

Rein, J. G., Freed, M. D., Norwood, W. I., and Castaneda, A. R.: Early and late results of closure of ventricular septal defect in infancy. Ann. Thorac. Surg., *24*:19, 1977.

The superb results obtained by Castaneda and colleagues in the operation of primary repair of VSD in the first year of life in 50 infants are reported here. The Kyoto-Barratt-Boyes technique of profound hypothermia and total circulatory arrest was used. Hospital mortality was 6 per cent, no late death occurred, and the late functional status was excellent. This paper gave strong supportive evidence for the excellence of the results that can be obtained from primary repair of VSD, even in very young infants.

Rizzoli, G., Blackstone, E. H., Kirklin, J. W., Pacifico, A. D., and Bargeron, L. M., Jr.: Incremental risk factors in hospital mortality after repair of ventricular septal defect. J. Thorac. Cardiovasc. Surg., *80*:494, 1980.

This paper describes the incremental risk (degree of difficulty, if you will) of numerous factors in 312 patients undergoing repair of VSD from 1967 to 1979. More importantly, it describes how these incremental risk factors have gradually been neutralized by scientific advances and minimization of human errors. Thus, in the era beginning in 1978, the hospital mortality of repair of single large ventricular septal defects is less than 1 per cent, no matter how young the patient (neutralization of the previous incremental risk of young age), and is about 5 per cent for multiple ventricular septal defects, again without an incremental risk of young age. Major associated cardiac anomalies or procedures (large patent ductus arteriosus, simultaneous repair of coarctation or interrupted arch, and important mitral valve abnormalities) still increase risk.

Soto, B., Becker, A. E., Moulaert, A. J., Lie, J. T., and Anderson, A. H.: Classification of ventricular septal defects. Br. Heart J., *43*:332, 1980.

Many anatomic studies of VSD have been reported through the years, but this one by Anderson and colleagues has been particularly helpful to surgeons. It is their work, described in this paper, that forms the basis for the description of morphology used in this chapter. The ventricular septum is divided into a membranous and muscular portion, and the latter into an inlet, trabecular, and infundibular (outlet) portion. This paper introduces the advisable phrase *perimembranous VSD* for those in the region of the membranous septum, right up against the tricuspid anulus. It also clarifies the fact that so-called atrioventricular canal *type* of VSD is really a perimembranous one, extending particularly beneath the septal tricuspid leaflet. Beautiful anatomic and cineangiographic plates clarify the description.

REFERENCES

Aaron, B. L., and Lower, R. R.: Muscular ventricular septal defect repair made easy. Ann. Thorac. Surg., *19*:568, 1975.

Ash, R.: Natural history of ventricular septal defects in childhood lesions with predominant arteriovenous shunts. J. Pediatr., 64:45, 1964.

Auld, P. A. M., Johnson, A. L., Gibbons, J. E., and McGregor, M.: Changes in pulmonary vascular resistance in infants and children with intracardiac left-to-right shunts. Circulation, 27:257, 1963.

Barratt-Boyes, B. G., Neutze, J. M., Clarkson, P. M., Shardey, G. C., and Brandt, P. W. T.: Repair of ventricular septal defect in the first two years of life using profound hypothermia—circulatory arrest techniques. Ann. Surg., 184:376, 1976.

Bergdahl, L. A. L., Blackstone, E. H., Kirklin, J. W., Pacifico, A. D., and Bargeron, L. M., Jr.: Determinants of early success in repair of aortic coarctation in infants. J. Thorac. Cardiovasc. Surg., 83:736, 1982.

Binet, J. P., Conso, J. F., Langlois, J., Pottemann, M., Cloup, M., Thibert, M., and Lucet, P.: Fermeture de certaines communications interventriculaires congénitales basses par le ventricule gauche. Arch. Mal. Coeur, 63:1345, 1970.

Blackstone, E. H., Kirklin, J. W., Bradley, E. L., DuShane, J. W., and Appelbaum, A.: Optimal age and results in repair of large ventricular septal defects. J. Thorac. Cardiovasc. Surg., 72:661, 1976.

Breckenridge, I. M., Stark, J., Waterston, D. J., and Bonham-Carter, R. E.: Multiple ventricular septal defects. Ann. Thorac. Surg., 13:128, 1972.

Campbell, M.: Natural history of ventricular septal defect. Br. Heart J., 33:246, 1971.

Cartmill, T. B., DuShane, J. W., McGoon, D. C., and Kirklin, J. W.: Results of repair of ventricular septal defect. J. Thorac. Cardiovasc. Surg., 52:486, 1966.

Castaneda, A. R., Zamora, R., Nicoloff, D. M., Moller, J. H., Hunt, C. E., and Lucas, R. V.: High-pressure, high-resistance ventricular septal defect. Surgical results of closure through right atrium. Ann. Thorac. Surg., 12:29, 1971.

Ching, E., DuShane, J. W., McGoon, D. C., and Danielson, G. K.: Total correction of ventricular septal defect in infancy using extracorporeal circulation: Surgical considerations and results of operation. Ann. Thorac. Surg., 12:1, 1971.

Clarkson, P. M.: Growth following corrective cardiac operation in early infancy. In Heart Disease in Infancy. Diagnosis and Surgical Treatment. Edited by B. G. Barratt-Boyes, J. M. Neutze, and E. A. Harris. London, Churchill Livingstone, 1973, p. 75.

Clarkson, P. M., Frye, R. L., DuShane, J. W., Burchell, H. B., Wood, E. H., and Weidman, W. H.: Prognosis for patients with ventricular septal defect and severe pulmonary vascular obstructive disease. Circulation, 38:129, 1968.

Collins, G., Calder, L., Rose, V., Kidd, L., and Keith, J.: Ventricular septal defect: Clinical and hemodynamic changes in the first five years of life. Am. Heart J., 84:695, 1972.

Cooley, D. A., Garrett, H. E., and Howard, H. S.: The surgical treatment of ventricular septal defect: An analysis of 300 consecutive surgical cases. Prog. Cardiovasc. Dis., 4:312, 1962.

Cordell, D., Graham, T. P., Jr., Atwood, G. F., Boerth, R. C., Boucek, R. J., and Bender, H. W.: Left heart volume characteristics following ventricular septal defect closure in infancy. Circulation, 54:294, 1976.

Corone, P., Doyan, F., Gaudeau, S., Guerin, F., Vernant, P., Ducam, H., Rumeau-Rouquette, C., and Gaudeul, P.: Natural history of ventricular septal defect. A study involving 790 cases. Circulation, 55:908, 1977.

Dirksen, T., Moulaert, A. J., Buis-Liem, T. N., and Brom, A. G.: Ventricular septal defect associated with left ventricular outflow tract obstruction below the defect. J. Thorac. Cardiovasc. Surg., 75:688, 1978.

DuShane, J. W., and Kirklin, J. W.: Late results of the repair of ventricular septal defect on pulmonary vascular disease. In Advances in Cardiovascular Surgery. Edited by J. W. Kirklin. New York, Grune and Stratton, 1973, p. 9.

DuShane, J. W., and Kirklin, J. W.: Selection for surgery of patients with ventricular septal defect and pulmonary hypertension. Circulation, 21:13, 1960.

DuShane, J. W., Kirklin, J. W., Patrick, R. T., Donald, D. E., Terry, H. R., Jr., Burchell, H. B., and Wood, E. H.: Ventric-

ular septal defects with pulmonary hypertension: Surgical treatment by means of a mechanical pump-oxygenator. J.A.M.A., 160:950, 1956.

Freed, M. D., Rosenthal, A., Plauth, W. H., Jr., and Nadas, A. S.: Development of subaortic stenosis after pulmonary artery banding. Circulation, 47, 48(Suppl. III):7, 1973.

Friedli, B., Kidd, B. S. L., Mustard, W. T., and Keith, J. D.: Ventricular septal defect with increased pulmonary vascular resistance. Late results of surgical closure. Am. J. Cardiol., 33:403, 1974.

Gasul, B. M., Dillon, R. F., Vrla, V., and Hait, G.: Ventricular septal defects. Their natural transformation into those with infundibular stenosis or into the cyanotic or non-cyanotic type of tetralogy of Fallot. J.A.M.A., 164:847, 1957.

Hallidie-Smith, K. A., Edwards, R. E., Wilson, R., and Zeidifard, E.: Long-term cardiorespiratory assessment after surgical closure of ventricular septal defect in childhood. (Abstract.) Proc. Br. Cardiac Soc., 37:553, 1975.

Hallidie-Smith, K. A., Hollman, A., Cleland, W. P., Bentall, H. H., and Goodwin, J. F.: Effects of surgical closure of ventricular septal defects upon pulmonary vascular disease. Br. Heart J., 31:246, 1969.

Heath, D., and Edwards, J. E.: The pathology of hypertensive pulmonary vascular disease. A description of six grades of structural changes in the pulmonary arteries with special reference to congenital cardiac septal defects. Circulation, 18:533, 1958.

Heath, D., Helmholtz, H. F., Jr., Burchell, H. B., DuShane, J. W., Kirklin, J. W., and Edwards, J. E.: Relation between structural changes in the small pulmonary arteries and the immediate reversibility of pulmonary hypertension following closure of ventricular and atrial septal defects. Circulation, 18:1167, 1958.

Hislop, A., Haworth, S. G., Shinebourne, E. A., and Reid, L.: Quantitative structural analysis of pulmonary vessels in isolated ventricular septal defect in infancy. Br. Heart. J., 37:1014, 1975.

Hoffman, J. I. E.: Diagnosis and treatment of pulmonary vascular disease. Birth Defects (original article series), 8:9, 1972.

Hoffman, J. I. E., and Rudolph, A. M.: The natural history of ventricular septal defects in infancy. Am. J. Cardiol., 16:634, 1965.

Hoffman, J. I. E., and Rudolph, A. M.: Increasing pulmonary vascular resistance during infancy in association with ventricular septal defect. Pediatrics, 38:220, 1966.

Hoffman, J. I. E., and Rudolph, A. M.: The natural history of isolated ventricular septal defect, with special references to selection of patients for surgery. In Advances in Pediatrics. Edited by I. Schulman. Chicago: Year Book Medical Publishers, Inc., 1970, p. 57.

Jarmakani, M. M., Edwards, S. B., Spach, M. S., Canent, R. V., Jr., Capp, M. P., Hagan, M. J., Barr, R. C., and Jain, V.: Left ventricular pressure volume characteristics in congenital heart disease. Circulation, 37:879, 1968.

Jarmakani, J. M., Graham, T. P., Jr., and Canent, R. V., Jr.: Left ventricular contractile state in children with successfully corrected ventricular septal defect. Circulation, 45, 46(Suppl. I):102, 1972.

Jarmakani, J. M. M., Graham, T. P., Jr., Canent, R. V., and Capp, M. P.: The effect of corrective surgery on left heart volume and mass in children with ventricular septal defect. Am. J. Cardiol., 27:254, 1971.

Johnson, D. C., Cartmill, T. B., Celermajer, J. M., Hawker, R. E., Stuckey, D. S., Bowdler, J. D., and Overton, J.: Intracardiac repair of large ventricular septal defect in the first year of life. Med. J. Aust., 2:193, 1974.

Keith, J. D., Rose, V., Collins, G., and Kidd, B. S. L.: Ventricular septal defect: Incidence, morbidity, and mortality in various age groups. Br. Heart J., 33(Suppl.):81, 1971.

Kirklin, J. K., and Kirklin, J. W.: Management of the cardiovascular subsystem after cardiac surgery. Ann. Thorac. Surg., 32:311, 1981.

Kirklin, J. K., Castaneda, A. R., Keane, J. F., Fellows, K. E., and Norwood, W. I.: Surgical management of multiple ventricular septal defects. J. Thorac. Cardiovasc. Surg., 80:485, 1980.

Kirklin, J. W., and DuShane, J. W.: Repair of ventricular septal defect in infancy. Pediatrics, 27:961, 1961.

Kirklin, J. W., and DuShane, J. W.: Indications for repair of ventricular septal defects. Am. J. Cardiol., 12:79, 1963.

Lauer, R. M., DuShane, J. W., and Edwards, J. E.: Obstruction of left ventricular outlet in association with ventricular septal defect. Circulation, 22:110, 1960.

Leatham, A., and Segal, B.: Auscultatory and phonocardiographic signs of ventricular septal defect with left-to-right shunt. Circulation, 25:318, 1962.

Levin, A. R., Boineau, J. P., Spach, M. S., Canent, R. V., Jr., Capp, M. P., and Anderson, P. A. W.: Ventricular pressure flow-dynamics in tetralogy of Fallot. Circulation, 34:4, 1966.

Lillehei, C. W., Anderson, R. C., Eliot, R. S., Wany, Y., and Ferlic, R. M.: Pre- and postoperative cardiac catheterization in 200 patients undergoing closure of ventricular septal defects. Surgery, 63:69, 1968.

Lillehei, C. W., Cohen, M., Warden, H. E., Ziegler, N. R., and Varco, R. L.: The results of direct vision closure of ventricular septal defects in eight patients by means of controlled cross circulation. Surg. Gynecol. Obstet., 101:446, 1955.

Lincoln, C., Jamieson, S., Joseph, M., Shinebourne, E., and Anderson, R. H.: Transatrial repair of ventricular septal defects with reference to their anatomic classification. J. Thorac. Cardiovasc. Surg., 74:183, 1977.

Lucas, R. V., Jr., Adams, P., Jr., Anderson, R. C., Meyne, N. G., Lillehei, C. W., and Varco, R. L.: The natural history of isolated ventricular septal defect. A serial physiologic study. Circulation, 24:1372, 1961.

Maron, B. J., Redwood, D. R., Hirschfeld, J. W., Jr., Goldstein, R. E., Morrow, A. G., and Epstein, S. E.: Postoperative assessment of patients with ventricular septal defect and pulmonary hypertension: Response to intense upright exercise. Circulation, 48:864, 1973.

Moulaert, A. J., Bruins, C. G., and Oppenheimer-Dekker, A.: Anomalies of the aortic arch and ventricular septal defects. Circulation, 53:1011, 1976.

Oh, K. S., Park, S. C., Galvis, A. G., Young, L. W., Neches, W. H., and Zuberbuhler, J. R.: Pulmonary hyperinflation in ventricular septal defect. J. Thorac. Cardiovasc. Surg., 76:706, 1978.

Okamoto, Y.: Clinical studies for open heart surgery in infants with profound hypothermia. Arch. Jpn. Chir., 38:188, 1969.

Rein, J. G., Freed, M. D., Norwood, W. I., and Castaneda, A. R.: Early and late results of closure of ventricular septal defect in infancy. Ann. Thorac. Surg., 24:19, 1977.

Rizzoli, G., Blackstone, E. H., Kirklin, J. W., Pacifico, A. D., and Bargeron, L. M., Jr.: Incremental risk factors in hospital mortality after repair of ventricular septal defect. J. Thorac. Cardiovasc. Surg., 80:494, 1980.

Shah, P., Singh, W. S. A., Rose, V., and Keith, J. D.: Incidence of bacterial endocarditis in ventricular septal defects. Circulation, 34:127, 1966.

Sigmann, J. M., Stern, A. M., and Sloan, H. E.: Early surgical correction of large ventricular septal defects. Pediatrics, 39:4, 1967.

Sigmann, J. M., Perry, B. L., Behrendt, D. M., Stern, A. M., Kirsch, M. M., and Sloan, H. E.: Ventricular septal defect: Results after repair in infancy. Am. J. Cardiol., 39:66, 1977.

Singh, A. K., deLeval, M. R., and Stark, J.: Left ventriculotomy for closure of muscular ventricular septal defects. Ann. Surg., 186:577, 1977.

Somerville, J.: Personal communication, 1970.

Soto, B., Becker, A. E., Moulaert, A. J., Lie, J. T., and Anderson, A. H.: Classification of ventricular septal defects. Br. Heart J., 43:332, 1980.

Stirling, G. R., Stanley, P. H., and Lillehei, C. W.: Effect of cardiac bypass and ventriculotomy upon right ventricular function. Surg. Forum, 8:433, 1957.

Van Praagh, R., Bernhard, W. F., Rosenthal, A., Parisi, L. F., and Fyler, D. C.: Interrupted aortic arch: Surgical treatment. Am. J. Cardiol., 27:200, 1971.

Wagenvoort, C. A., and Wagenvoort, N.: Primary pulmonary hypertension. A pathological study of the lung vessels in 156 clinically diagnosed cases. Circulation, 42:1163, 1970.

Wagenvoort, C. A., Neufeld, H. N., DuShane, J. W., and Edwards, J. E.: The pulmonary arterial tree in ventricular septal defect. A quantitative study of anatomic features in fetuses, infants, and children. Circulation, 23:740, 1961.

Yacoub, M. H., Radley-Smith, R., and deGasperis, C.: Primary repair of large ventricular septal defects in the first year of life. G. Ital. Cardiol., 8:827, 1978.

Yamaki, S., and Tezuka, F.: Quantitative analysis of pulmonary vascular disease in complete transposition of the great arteries. Circulation, 54:805, 1976.

Chapter 36

Tetralogy of Fallot

DAVID C. SABISTON, JR.

One of the most common of the more serious congenital malformations of the heart is the tetralogy of Fallot. In most instances, the condition is associated with cyanosis. The clinical manifestations of this defect are generally rather characteristic, and with cardiac catheterization and angiocardiography, a definite diagnosis can almost always be made with certainty. Since nearly all patients with this condition require surgical correction, it is fortunate that the operative procedures are now well established with excellent clinical results and a low surgical mortality.

HISTORICAL ASPECTS

Although Stensen deserves credit for the first description in 1672 of what is now termed the tetralogy of Fallot, nevertheless it is Etienne-Louis Arthur Fallot (1888) of Marseille, France, whose name is characteristically attached to this congenital cardiac disorder. There were others prior to Fallot who described the malformation, including Sandifort (1777), John Hunter (1784), William Hunter (1784), Farre (1814), Gintrac (1824), Hope (1839), and Peacock (1866). Most of these descriptions were case reports of comical curiosities. However, in his description of the disorder, Fallot was the first to describe accurately the clinical and complete pathologic manifestations of this deformity. He emphasized that with a knowledge of the clinical manifestations, the malformation could be diagnosed accurately during life.

In the original description of this congenital anomaly, Fallot stated, "This malformation consists of a true anatomopathological type represented by the following tetralogy: (1) stenosis of the pulmonary artery; (2) interventricular communication; (3) deviation of the origin of the aorta to the right; (4) hypertrophy, almost always concentric, of the right ventricle. Failure of obliteration of the foramen ovale may occasionally be added in a wholly accessory manner." Fallot reported 55 patients with congenital heart disease, of whom most had the tetralogy malformation. In retrospect, it is remarkable that such a large number of patients could have been reported by a single author in that early day of the recognition of cardiac abnormalities.

Despite the fact that accurate clinical diagnosis could often be established after these contributions by Fallot, nevertheless, many years passed before definitive treatment of the condition became available. In 1944, Blalock operated on a severely ill infant with tetralogy of Fallot who weighed only 4.5 kg. The child was severely cyanotic and had had multiple episodes of unconsciousness due to marked hypoxemia. A systemic-pulmonary anastomosis was achieved by joining the subclavian artery to the pulmonary artery, and the child was greatly benefited. Several months later, Blalock and Taussig (1945) reported this patient together with two others, and a new era had been opened in the field of cardiac surgery. The first open correction of the tetralogy was performed by Scott in 1954 using circulatory arrest with hypothermia. The following year, Lillehei and associates (1955) described open correction using cardiopulmonary bypass, and since that time, many advances have been made in the correction of this malformation and with increasingly improved survival rates.

ANATOMY

It is apparent from the choice of the term *tetralogy* that Fallot originally considered the malformation to comprise four major defects: infundibular pulmonary stenosis, ventricular septal defect, dextroposition of the aorta, and hypertrophy of the right ventricle. It is now recognized by most authorities that the two most important features of tetralogy of Fallot are (1) the right ventricular outflow tract obstruction, which is nearly always infundibular in location, although valvular stenosis may also be present in some 20 per cent of patients, and (2) the ventricular septal defect. The overriding aorta is directly related to the ventricular septal defect and the right ventricular hypertrophy is more appropriately regarded as a secondary phenomenon due to the ventricular response. There is a wide variation in the spectrum of the severity of the anatomic malformations in the tetralogy of Fallot (Johns *et al.*, 1953). The wide differences in the severity of these components have led some to urge discontinuance of the term "tetralogy of Fallot." Nevertheless, from both diagnostic and therapeutic point of view, the term continues to have usefulness. A working definition of the tetralogy includes the basic principle that it is a congenital cardiac malformation with a ventricular septal defect, the size of which approximates the aortic orifice, and with pulmonary stenosis of such a degree that approximately equal pressures result in both ventricles. There are varying degrees of dextroposition of the aorta, and the degree and nature of the infundibular pulmonary stenosis may be quite variable. Several types of infundibular chambers have been described, depending mostly on the size of the chamber (Brock, 1952; Brock and Campbell, 1950). The infundibular chamber may be quite small when the outflow tract obstruction is near the pulmonary valve. At the opposite extreme, the muscular obstruction in the outflow tract may be quite proximally situated, resulting in a large infundibular chamber sometimes called a "third ventricle." Moreover, *stenosis* of the pulmonary valve is common, occurring in as many as one third of patients with tetralogy of Fallot in addition to infundibular stenosis. Rarely, the stenosis is confined solely to the pulmonary valve without the presence of infundibular obstruction.

From a physiologic point of view, the majority of patients with tetralogy of Fallot exhibit a high resistance to right ventricular emptying owing to pulmonary stenosis. The predominant shunt is from right to left, with flow across the ventricular defect into the aorta producing cyanosis and an elevation of the hematocrit. When the pulmonary stenosis is less severe, bidirectional shunting may occur. In some patients, the infundibular stenosis is minimal and the predominant shunt is from left to right, producing what is termed "the pink tetralogy." Although such patients may not appear cyanotic, they often have oxygen desaturation in the systemic arterial blood.

Occasionally, no communication exists between the right ventricle and the pulmonary artery. In these patients, the outflow tract of the right ventricle or the pulmonary valve is *atretic*. The pulmonary valve ring and the main pulmonary artery are often quite small, although the left and right branches may be of significant size. Such infants exhibit severe symptoms and usually require operation early in life. It has also been recognized that some patients with a previous systemic-pulmonary anastomosis may experience a progression of the outflow tract obstruction in the right ventricle. Thus, the infundibular stenosis or valvular stenosis may become more severe and can become total, representing an *acquired* lesion. In this event, life is maintained solely by a previous systemic-pulmonary shunt with additional help from collateral bronchial arterial circulation (Sabiston *et al.*, 1964).

DIAGNOSIS

Clinical Manifestations

The clinical manifestations are dependent on the severity of the anatomic malformation. Infants with pulmonary atresia manifest distress shortly after birth and usually succumb unless operation is performed. Cyanosis is common, especially with crying, but in most infants is not present at *birth,* probably because of a persistent ductus arteriosus. As the child grows older, dyspnea on exertion usually follows, and the characteristic position of *squatting* is assumed by the great majority of these patients to relieve fatigue. Moreover, this position has diagnostic significance and is highly characteristic of the tetralogy of Fallot. It usually produces an increase in systemic arterial oxygen saturation.

Although some patients with pulmonary atresia present desperate problems in infancy, there are rare instances of a reasonably normal life span. One interesting example of this is that of the American composer, Gilbert, who lived to the age of 60 with tetralogy of Fallot and led a relatively productive life without therapy (White and Sprague, 1929). Such a history is obviously rare. Statistics show that the natural history for the entire group of patients with tetralogy of Fallot indicates that half reach the age of 7, one-fifth reach the age of 14, and not more than one-tenth survive to the age of 21 in the absence of operative intervention (Campbell and Deuchar, 1953).

Physical Examination

The patient may appear to be smaller than expected for the age, and cyanosis of the lips and nail beds is usually apparent. The fingers and toes usually show clubbing (hypertrophic pulmonary osteoarthropathy). On palpation of the chest, a thrill is usually present anteriorly. A harsh systolic murmur is audible over the pulmonary area and along the left sternal border. Absence of a murmur in a patient suspected of having the tetralogy is suggestive of pulmonary atresia.

Roentgenograms

In the early stages, the chest film may be normal, but the chest film in the tetralogy of Fallot usually shows diminished vascularity in the lungs and absence of prominence of the pulmonary artery. The shadow of the great vessels in the superior mediastinum is narrow, owing to the diminished caliber of the pulmonary artery. If cyanosis and dyspnea are quite prominent, the pulmonary vascular markings are usually markedly diminished. Later, the classic boot-shaped heart (*coeur en sabot*) may develop, and it is recognized as a hallmark of the tetralogy of Fallot (Fig. 36–1). Diminution or absence of pulsations in the pulmonary arteries can be demonstrated by fluoroscopy. Right ventricular enlargement is present and is best demonstrated in the left anterior oblique position. The barium swallow provides evidence of the side on which the aortic arch descends. This is of considerable importance, since approximately one fourth of the patients with tetralogy of Fallot have a *right* aortic arch. In fact, the presence of a right aortic arch with cyanosis is strong evidence that the malformation is indeed tetralogy of Fallot.

Blood Studies

The hemoglobin, hematocrit, and erythrocyte count are usually elevated. The magnitude of the increase is generally proportional to the cyanosis, with hematocrit values varying from normal to as high as 90 per cent, the majority being between 50 and 70 per cent. Similarly, the oxygen saturation in the systemic arterial blood is variable, usually between 65 and 70 per cent. However, in severe forms of the malformation, the arterial oxygen saturation during exercise may fall to as low as 25 per cent. A bleeding tendency is present in some patients with the tetralogy of Fallot, especially those in whom cyanosis is marked. The usual finding is a diminution in a variety of the factors responsible for blood coagulation, but none of the factors are reduced to critical levels. The platelet count and total blood fibrinogen are frequently slightly diminished, and clot retraction is sometimes poor and associated with prolonged prothrombin and coagulation times. Despite the defects in the clotting mechanism in some patients, the changes are usually insufficient to explain the hemorrhagic tendency noted at the time of operation (Hartmann, 1952; Porter and Silver, 1968).

Electrocardiogram

The electrocardiogram usually shows right ventricular hypertrophy, usually apparent in the standard leads and most consistently found in the unipolar leads. The more commonly encountered findings include tall and peaked T waves, reversal of the RS ratio, and a normal PR interval and QRS duration. If right ventricular hypertrophy is absent, a diagnosis of tetralogy of Fallot should be seriously questioned. *Echocardiography* using ultrasound techniques has

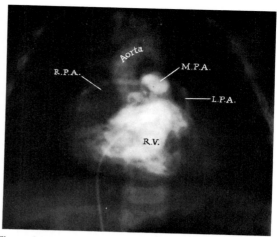

Figure 36–2. Angiocardiogram of an infant with tetralogy of Fallot in whom the pulmonary arteries are very small. In an infant with pulmonary arteries of this size, consideration should be given to the performance of a systemic-pulmonary shunt as the primary procedure rather than an open correction.

also been used in the diagnosis of tetralogy of Fallot and has concentrated on the appearance of the ventricular septal defect (VSD) and evidence of hypertrophy and debilitation (Morris *et al.*, 1975).

Angiocardiogram

The angiocardiogram is of great importance in establishing the diagnosis. Moreover, it demonstrates objectively the magnitude of pulmonary stenosis and the size of the pulmonary arteries (Fig. 36–2). The ventricular septal defect and overriding of the aorta are also shown (Fig. 36–3). An atrial septal defect may also be present. Rarely, only one pulmonary artery is present, and in nearly all patients with a single artery, it is the left one that is absent.

Cardiac Catheterization

Considerable data are provided by cardiac catheterization. The presence of equal pressures in both ventricles distinguishes the condition from isolated valvular pulmonary stenosis, in which the pressure in the right ventricle may be considerably greater than that in the left ventricle. Tracings also establish the level of right ventricular outflow tract obstruction and the presence of valvular stenosis.

INDICATIONS FOR OPERATION

Most patients with tetralogy of Fallot are candidates for surgical correction. When feasible, it is preferable to perform a corrective procedure *electively* before school age, generally when the patient is 3 to 5 years old (Dobell *et al.*, 1968). However, severe symptoms may become manifest much earlier, includ-

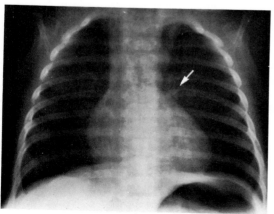

Figure 36–1. Chest film of an infant with tetralogy of Fallot. Note the diminished vascular markings in the lungs and the reduced prominence of the pulmonary artery shadow.

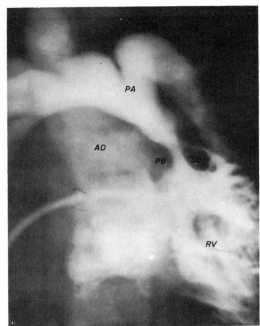

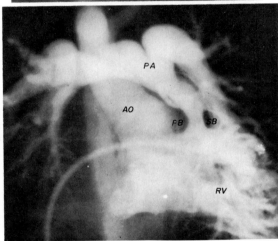

Figure 36–3. Obstruction in the region of the infundibulum. *A,* Frame made in systole. *B,* Frame made in diastole. The negative shadows of the hypertrophied parietal (PB) and septal (SB) bands are particularly well demonstrated. The pulmonary valve appears domed, and at operation was bicuspid, but not stenotic. The aorta (AO) is opacified by this right ventricular injection, and its diameter is three times that of the pulmonary artery. The underdevelopment of the infundibulum of the right ventricle, a basic characteristic of the tetralogy of Fallot, is apparent in this angiocardiogram. (RV = right ventricle; PA = pulmonary artery.) (From Kirklin, J. W., and Karp, R. B.: The Tetralogy of Fallot from a Surgical Viewpoint. Philadelphia, W. B. Saunders Company, 1970.)

ing during the first several days of life, and an operative procedure may be necessary as a lifesaving measure. Some prefer to perform corrective procedures using extracorporeal circulation at almost any age (Calder *et al.,* 1979; Daily *et al.,* 1978; Kirklin *et al.,* 1979); others believe a systemic-to-pulmonary anastomosis is somewhat safer and generally employ a Blalock-Taussig anastomosis as a preliminary proce-

dure (Chopra *et al.,* 1976; Neches *et al.,* 1975; Wood *et al.,* 1973). Those who prefer open correction at any time emphasize that it prevents the necessity for a second operation and that the current results are sufficiently good to support this judgment. One group currently believes that surgery should be performed in all patients with tetralogy of Fallot, irrespective of age or weight, except for those with an anterior descending coronary artery arising from the right coronary artery or those who have associated congenital pulmonary atresia (Castaneda *et al.,* 1977). Those who prefer an initial shunt in infancy emphasize that the overall mortality is lower than if the mortality of the later corrective operation is included. In addition, these observers are concerned about whether or not the small heart in infancy will remain corrected as growth continues, feeling perhaps that outflow tract obstruction of the right ventricle may occur. One group (Arciniegas *et al.,* 1980) considers the Blalock-Taussig shunt to be the shunt of choice in all symptomatic infants and small children with tetralogy of Fallot and that the two-stage surgical approach compares favorably with primary total correction, particularly in infants under 1 year of age. Although controversy continues concerning the preferential operation during *infancy,* there has been a general trend toward open correction (Tucker *et al.,* 1979). If the cardiac malformation is quite severe or if the infant is quite small, anastomotic procedures may be preferable. Such a procedure should be of the Blalock-Taussig type, as the aortic–to–pulmonary artery procedure (Potts and Waterston) is beset with additional Hazards in the long-term postoperative period (Daily *et al.,* 1978; Ebert, 1979).

SURGICAL TECHNIQUES

The most frequently performed *shunt* operation is a systemic-pulmonary anastomosis (Blalock, 1948; Blalock and Taussig, 1945). This procedure has its maximal usefulness in the severely ill infant in whom operation must be performed at an early age, and it is becoming unusual to employ this procedure in patients older than 1 year of age. The goal of the procedure is to produce an increase in blood flow to the lungs. Evidence has been presented that enlargement of the right and left pulmonary arteries is produced by a systemic-pulmonary anastomosis in these patients (Gale *et al.,* 1979). Earlier, an alternate technique was sometimes employed, anastomosis between the left pulmonary artery and the descending aorta (Potts' operation) (Potts *et al.,* 1946). This procedure is rarely used today, since the anastomosis usually enlarges with time and produces an excessive shunt, with pulmonary hypertension and often aneurysmal formation at the site of the anastomosis (Fig. 36–4) (Ross *et al.,* 1958; Stephens, 1967). Moreover, a Potts' anastomosis is more difficult to close at the time of subsequent correction. Another alternate technique is

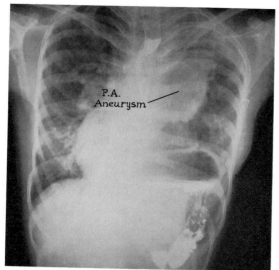

Figure 36–4. Chest film of a patient with previous descending aorta–pulmonary artery anastomosis (Potts'). A large aneurysm is present at the site of the anastomosis. Note the marked vascularity of the lung fields. The aortic and pulmonary pressures were equal, and the patient was markedly cyanotic with a high hematocrit. Open correction is not advisable in this situation.

that of an ascending aorta–to–right pulmonary artery anastomosis (Waterston, 1962), but this procedure has become less often used, owing, among other reasons, to the fact that kinking and stenosis may ensue at the anastomotic site and make subsequent open correction difficult (Gay and Ebert, 1973).

In performance of a *subclavian-pulmonary anastomosis (Blalock-Taussig operation),* the incision is generally made on the side opposite that on which the aorta descends (Fig. 36–5). In the majority of patients, the incision is made on the right side, since the aorta most often descends on the left. When the aorta descends on the right (20 to 25 per cent of patients), the incision is made on the left. Ideally, the subclavian branch of the innominate artery is used for the anastomosis because the angle produced at its origin from its parent vessel is better than that formed when the subclavian artery is used, as shown in Figures 36–6, 36–7, and 36–8 (Sabiston and Blalock, 1959). The latter arises directly from the aorta and is apt to kink at its origin when deflected inferiorly for anastomosis to the pulmonary artery (Fig. 36–9). Experimental studies have shown that approximately three fourths of the blood passing through a subclavian-pulmonary

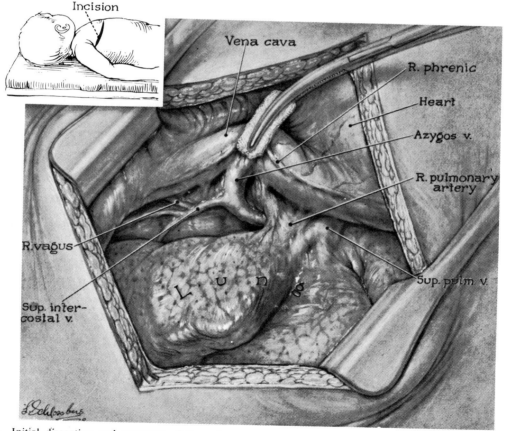

Figure 36–5. Initial dissection and exposure of the pulmonary artery for construction of a right subclavian-pulmonary artery anastomosis. The insert at the top shows the position of the patient on the operating table. The entry into the pleural cavity is through the second intercostal space. (From Blalock, A.: Surgical procedures employed and anatomical variations encountered in the treatment of congenital pulmonic stenosis. Surg. Gynecol. Obstet., 87:385, 1948.)

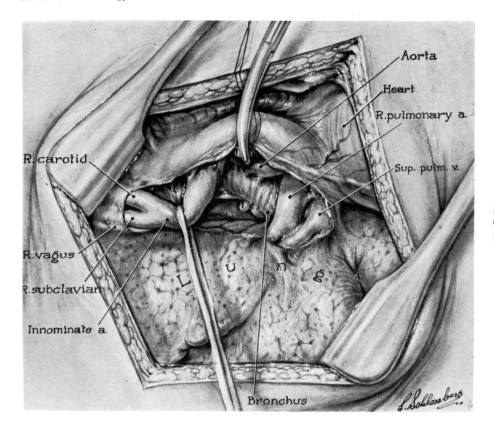

Figure 36–6. Dissection of the innominate artery and its branches. (From Blalock, A.: Surg. Gynecol. Obstet., *87*:385, 1948.)

shunt is directed to the lung on the side of the anastomosis (Fort *et al.,* 1965).

Detailed attention must be given in performing the Blalock shunt, especially in the construction of the anastomosis. Every effort must be made to prevent constriction of the anastomosis, and meticulous technique is essential (Fig. 36–10). In infants, it is preferable to use interrupted sutures.

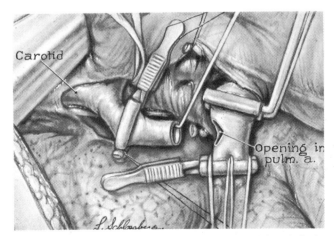

Figure 36–7. Completion of dissection of the right subclavian artery and pulmonary artery with the division of the subclavian artery and arteriotomy made in the pulmonary artery. Note the favorable angle of the right subclavian artery as it originates from the innominate artery. (From Blalock, A.: Surg. Gynecol. Obstet., *87*:385, 1948.)

Other congenital anomalies are encountered frequently with the tetralogy of Fallot. For example, a right aortic arch is quite common, and a single pulmonary artery is occasionally seen. A retroesophageal subclavian artery occurs in approximately 5 per cent of patients and may involve either the right or the left vessel. It is quite *rare* for the retroesophageal subclavian vessels to cause dysphagia. In fact, it is usually not necessary to alter the retroesophageal relationship of the vessel in order to perform a proper anastomosis. A persistent left superior vena cava occurs with about the same incidence (Nagao *et al.,* 1967). Peripheral pulmonary arterial stenosis of the main artery or of branches has also been described (Gregoratos *et al.,* 1965). Although a second subclavian-pulmonary anastomosis has been performed in the past for return of symptoms (Haller, 1958), the appropriate decision today in almost every instance is open correction if a second operation is required.

Anastomosis of the superior vena cava to the right pulmonary artery (Glenn operation) was once advocated in the treatment of tetralogy of Fallot (Bakulev and Kolesnikov, 1959; Glenn and Patino, 1954). In this procedure, the systemic venous blood from the superior vena cava passes directly into the pulmonary circulation, thus bypassing the right heart. Although the procedure has produced good results with respect to symptoms in some patients, more difficulty is experienced in the subsequent total correction. It is rarely employed today in the treatment

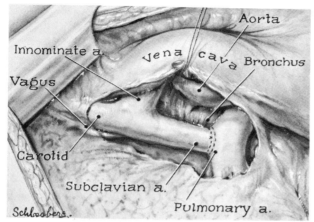

Figure 36–8. Completed anastomosis. Note that the caliber of the subclavian artery at its origin from the innominate artery is circular. When the anastomosis is performed between the subclavian branch of the aorta and the pulmonary artery, there is usually a kink (oval shape) of the left subclavian artery at its origin, thus diminishing the blood flow through the anastomosis. (From Blalock, A.: Surg. Gynecol. Obstet., *87*:385, 1948.)

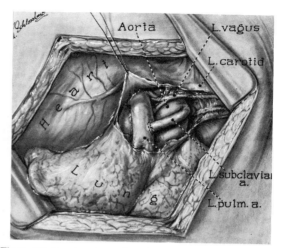

Figure 36–9. Anastomosis of the left subclavian artery as it arises from the aorta to the left pulmonary artery. Note that the angle of the left subclavian is less favorable than that of the subclavian branch of the innominate artery. (From Blalock, A.: Surg. Gynecol. Obstet., *87*:385, 1948.)

of the tetralogy of Fallot. A method for subsequent correction of the ventricular septal defect and relief of the right ventricular outflow obstruction following a superior vena cava–to–right pulmonary artery anastomosis has been described (Claxton and Sabiston, 1969) (Fig. 36–11).

Open Correction

Open correction is the ideal operation for treatment of the tetralogy of Fallot and is accomplished with extracorporeal circulation. Through a median sternotomy, the pericardium is opened. Major

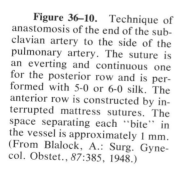

Figure 36–10. Technique of anastomosis of the end of the subclavian artery to the side of the pulmonary artery. The suture is an everting and continuous one for the posterior row and is performed with 5-0 or 6-0 silk. The anterior row is constructed by interrupted mattress sutures. The space separating each "bite" in the vessel is approximately 1 mm. (From Blalock, A.: Surg. Gynecol. Obstet., *87*:385, 1948.)

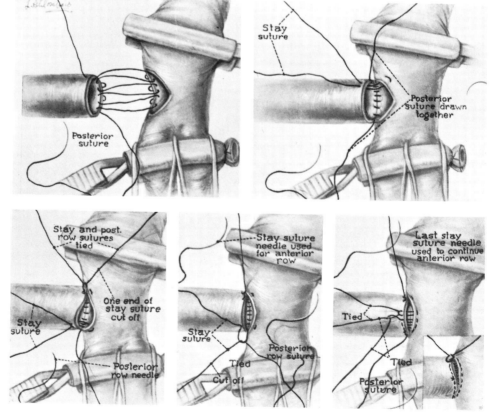

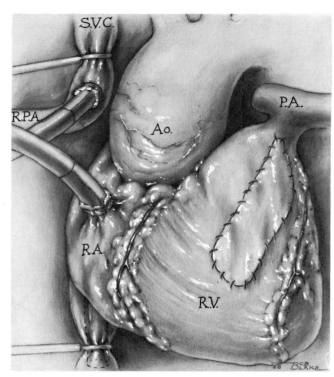

Figure 36–11. Illustration of technique of open correction following a previous superior vena cava-to-right pulmonary artery anastomosis (end-to-end). Note the placement of the superior and inferior vena caval catheters. The interventricular septal defect has been corrected with a Teflon felt prosthesis. A patch graft is inserted in the outflow tract of the right ventricle. The disproportion in size of the aorta and pulmonary artery is evident. At the end of the procedure, the pressure was 25/4 mm. Hg in the right ventricle and 18/5 mm. Hg in the pulmonary artery.

branches of the right coronary artery may pass across the outflow tract to supply the left ventricle; occasionally, the anterior descending coronary artery arises from the right coronary artery and should be avoided (Fig. 36–12). Significant coronary arterial anomalies occur in approximately 5 per cent of these patients (Fellows *et al.*, 1975). Repair of a divided anomalous anterior descending coronary artery has been described (Shaffer *et al.*, 1979). A careful estimate is made of the size of the main pulmonary artery as well as the possible presence of valvular stenosis. The inferior and superior venae cavae are dissected in preparation for insertion of venous cannulas into the right atrium. The left heart is vented through a catheter passed either through the right superior pulmonary vein, through the left atrial appendage, or through the left ventricular apex. The corrective procedure is preferentially performed with use of potassium cardioplegia and topical hypothermia with saline at 4° C. The potassium cardioplegic solution is administered through the aortic root after the ascending aorta has been clamped. Sufficient potassium is perfused into the coronary circulation to place the heart in complete diastolic arrest, and additional injections into the aortic root are made at 15- and 20-minute

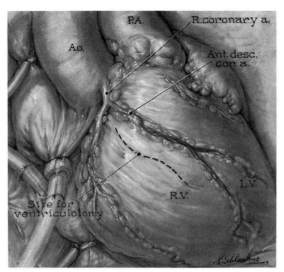

Figure 36–12. Illustration of the anterior descending coronary artery arising from the right coronary artery.

intervals. A transverse or longitudinal ventriculotomy is then made in the outflow tract of the right ventricle (Figs. 36–13 and 36–14*A*). The repair of the ventricular septal defect (VSD) and infundibular stenosis can also be done through an atriotomy (Edmunds *et al.*, 1976). If valvular pulmonary stenosis is present, it is relieved by commissural incisions. The infundibular stenosis is carefully resected, with removal of all obstructing muscle (Fig. 36–14*B*). The ventricular septal defect is then identified. It is usually large and requires a plastic prosthesis for closure (Fig. 36–14*C,D*). It is important to be quite careful in the placement of sutures for the VSD patch, since heart block may otherwise occur.

Following closure of the VSD, the right ventricle

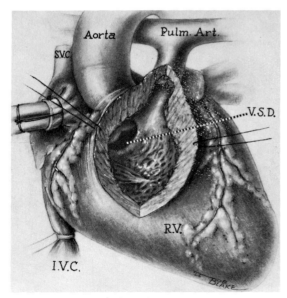

Figure 36–13. Illustration of typical ventricular septal defect in the tetralogy of Fallot. Note the difference in the size of the aorta and the pulmonary artery. The aortic valve is easily seen through the defect.

Figure 36–14. Steps in the total correction of the tetralogy of Fallot. *A,* Note the infundibular chamber and the normal distribution of coronary vessels. The superior and inferior venae cavae are separately cannulated. The left atrium is decompressed by a catheter in the left atrial appendage. The arterial cannula is placed through a purse-string suture in the ascending aorta. The procedure is performed using potassium cardioplegia, with the solution introduced by a small cannula placed proximal to the aortic occlusion clamp. *B,* Marked infundibular stenosis is present in the outflow tract of the right ventricle. The pulmonary valve is normal. The interventricular defect is of the standard type. Through the defect, the cusps of the aortic valve are easily visualized. The aorta is temporarily occluded to prevent reflux of blood that would obscure the operative field in the region of the ventricular septal defect. *C,* The placement of the initial suture in the ventricular septal defect border. Intermittent aortic occlusion is employed. *D,* Completion of placement of a ventricular prosthesis.

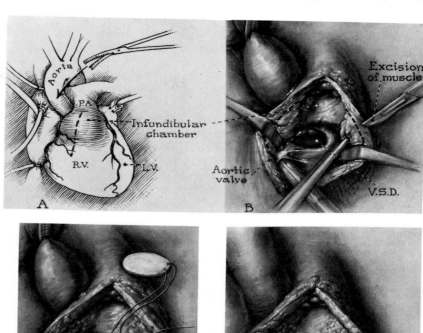

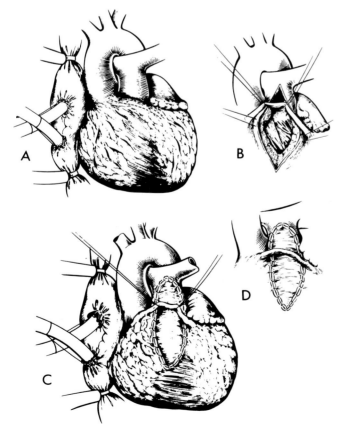

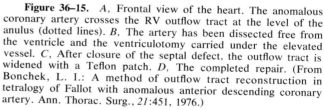

Figure 36–15. *A,* Frontal view of the heart. The anomalous coronary artery crosses the RV outflow tract at the level of the anulus (dotted lines). *B,* The artery has been dissected free from the ventricle and the ventriculotomy carried under the elevated vessel. *C,* After closure of the septal defect, the outflow tract is widened with a Teflon patch. *D,* The completed repair. (From Bonchek, L. I.: A method of outflow tract reconstruction in tetralogy of Fallot with anomalous anterior descending coronary artery. Ann. Thorac. Surg., *21*:451, 1976.)

may be closed primarily or may require a patch. The patch should preferably be of plastic material (woven Dacron) since the pericardial outflow patches have been associated with a significant percentage of right ventricular aneurysm formation (Seybold-Epting *et al.*, 1977). When feasible, primary closure is desirable, but if a primary closure produces excessive obstruction, right ventricular hypertension and a low cardiac output syndrome ensue. A technique has also been described in older children with the anterior descending coronary artery arising from the right coronary artery, in which the artery is dissected and the outflow patch is placed *beneath* the coronary artery and extended across the coronary valve onto the pulmonary artery (Fig. 36–15) (Bonchek, 1976). If the pulmonary artery or the valvular anulus is small, it may be necessary to extend the patch across the valve ring to the proximal portion of the pulmonary artery (Fig. 36–16). This produces pulmonary insufficiency, but it may be unavoidable and is apt to cause few problems. Residual right ventricular pulmonary artery gradients above 50 mm. Hg can be tolerated, although if this level is to be exceeded, judicious assessment of the situation is required. One group has recommended the role of preoperative prediction from cineangiograms of postrepair right ventricular pressure and provides a formula for this determination (Blackstone *et al.*, 1979). The body temperature is then rewarmed and a normal coronary circulation allowed to resume after removal of the aortic clamp. After the procedure has been completed and cardiopulmonary bypass discontinued, a dye dilution curve should be obtained to be certain that there is not any residual shunt present. If the dye curve shows a shunt, the heart should be reopened and the defect found and appropriately

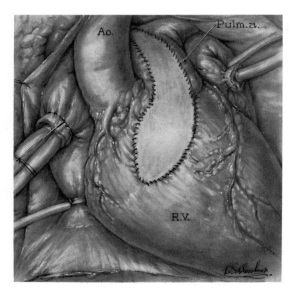

Figure 36–16. In this patient with atresia of the pulmonary valve ring, a large plastic prosthesis was required from the bifurcation of the pulmonary artery in order to decompress the right ventricle adequately. (From Sabiston, D. C., Jr.: *In* Gibbon's Surgery of the Chest. 2nd Ed. Edited by D. C. Sabiston, Jr. and F. C. Spencer. Philadelphia, W. B. Saunders Company, 1969.)

closed. The operation for correction is more difficult in patients with a previous left pulmonary artery–to–descending aortic anastomosis (Potts' operation), and the technique is shown in Figure 36–17.

RESULTS

The tetralogy of Fallot is now being corrected with an ever-diminishing mortality. The results with open correction during the recent past have been impressive. The mortality rate in most series is 5 per cent or less (Daily *et al.*, 1978; Kirklin *et al.*, 1979), particularly in patients older than 1 year. In the majority of patients, the clinical and physiologic status is greatly improved, and good to excellent results have been reported in up to 90 per cent (Malm *et al.*, 1966). Although patients with the more severe anatomic malformations respond less well, even these lesions are now yielding to correction with improved results (Allison *et al.*, 1963; Hallidie-Smith *et al.*, 1967; Theye and Kirklin, 1963). Following open correction, the chest film usually shows slight enlargement of the heart, and murmurs of pulmonary insufficiency may be present. In early experience with the technique of open correction, left-to-right shunts through a ventricular septal defect or reopening of the defect occurred with some frequency, but this is now uncommon.

POSTOPERATIVE MANAGEMENT

Many variables must be followed postoperatively. *Pulmonary function* is maintained by the use of an endotracheal tube and respirator until the patient's cardiac and respiratory status is stable, maintaining relatively normal values for the arterial Po_2, Pco_2, pH. The percentage of oxygen in the inspired air is maintained between 40 and 50 per cent, with attempts made not to exceed 60 per cent to prevent oxygen toxicity. Maintenance of an adequate *cardiac output* is also of crucial importance. It is appropriate to obtain determinations of cardiac output when indicated. In general, the cardiac output can be increased by raising the ventricular end-diastolic pressure, as accomplished by administration of blood or fluids. The atrial pressure can be increased should this be necessary. However, if evidence of *low* cardiac output persists, a search should be conducted for other primary causes. *Cardiac tamponade* is a recognized cause of the low output syndrome and may be present. If tamponade is not present, efforts should be made to improve the contractility of the myocardium and can be accomplished by the use of digitalis if the situation is not acute and with inotropic agents such as isoproterenol if the clinical manifestations are more serious. The use of dopamine is often quite helpful in maintaining adequate arterial pressure. Hypertension may develop, and the judicious use of intravenous nitroprusside may be used for control. Maintenance of *renal* function is of critical importance, and the ure-

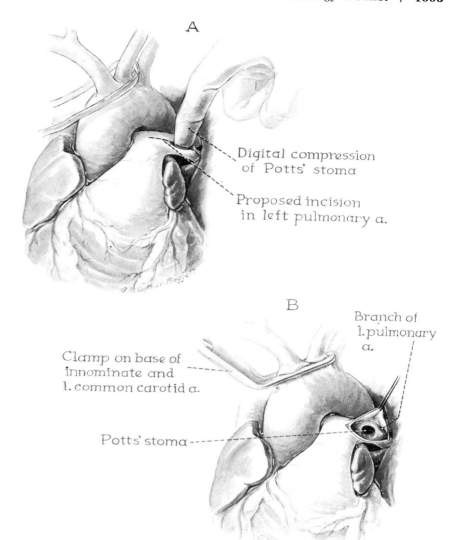

A

Digital compression
of Potts' stoma

Proposed incision
in left pulmonary a.

B

Branch of
l. pulmonary
a.

Clamp on base of
innominate and
l. common carotid a.

Potts' stoma

Figure 36–17. For closure of Potts' anastomosis, the head vessels are clamped at their origin, circulatory arrest is established, and the stoma is visualized through an incision in the left pulmonary artery. (From Kirklin, J. W., and Karp, R. B.: The Tetralogy of Fallot from a Surgical Viewpoint. Philadelphia, W. B. Saunders Company, 1970.)

thral catheter is left in place with a desired output of at least 20 ml. per hour. A study of factors that predispose to renal dysfunction following total correction of tetralogy of Fallot has shown that a combination of a severe form of tetralogy of Fallot and a large left ventricle increases the susceptibility to a low cardiac output syndrome and postoperative renal insufficiency (Tanaka *et al.,* 1980). It is generally necessary to limit fluid intake, especially during the first 24 hours following operation. This is due to the tendency toward development of fluid retention in patients after repair of tetralogy of Fallot. On the first day, approximately 500 ml. of water per square meter of body surface should be administered. After the second postoperative day, the patient is allowed fluids by mouth but is placed on a low-sodium diet (500 mg. daily). Following this, fluid intake may be regulated in accordance with total body weight, which should be obtained on accurate and reliable scales. Furosemide (Lasix) is quite helpful in controlling retained fluid and should be used as indicated. To prevent infection,

especially when prosthetic materials have been used, antibiotics are given routinely. Arrhythmias, especially atrioventricular dissociation, can be a serious postoperative complication. Temporary pacemaker wires are generally inserted into the myocardium and are allowed to remain for several days in the event that they may be needed. If a dissociation pattern occurs in the postoperative period, pacing may be easily instituted. If atrial fibrillation develops, rapid digitalization is indicated.

The hemodynamic results after intracardiac repair of the tetralogy of Fallot have been assessed in several series. Surgical repair of infants under deep hypothermia has been compared hemodynamically with correction by conventional cardiopulmonary bypass, with the finding that the results are equal or better with deep hypothermia (Murphy *et al.,* 1980). In a companion study, left ventricular dysfunction as determined after an afterload stress was found to be present postoperatively for those patients who had open correction at an older age but not in patients who underwent repair during infancy. This raises the possibility that early definitive repair may help to preserve postoperative left ventricular function (Borow et al., 1980). In another study, a group of patients with surgical correction of tetralogy who survived to adulthood were evaluated for their current state as adolescents and adults. Among 233 studied, it was concluded that clinical assessment alone is nonpredictive of the hemodynamic result and that cardiac catheterization should be performed in all patients for objective follow-up. The combination of persistent elevation of right ventricular systolic pressure above 60 mm. Hg and ventricular premature depolarizations placed the patient at risk of sudden death. However, 80 per cent of the patients led a normal life without impairment of intellect, exercise tolerance, or fertility (Garson et al., 1979).

With regard to the incidence of sudden death following correction of the tetralogy, in a study of 243 patients evaluated with special emphasis on postoperative conduction disturbances, sudden death occurred in seven patients, with an average follow-up of 12 years (range—6.5 to 16.5 years). Among these patients, four deaths were in those with right bundle branch block, and three of these four patients had premature ventricular contractions for more than 1 month postoperatively. Premature ventricular contractions were documented in 10 of the 158 patients with right bundle branch block, and sudden death occurred in three. Three of the 10 patients with trifascicular block pattern died suddenly, but no deaths occurred in 24 patients with bifascicular block pattern. The authors of this study concluded that the risk of sudden death in patients with right bundle branch block and premature ventricular contractions following tetralogy repair is high and warrants consideration of suppressive therapy (Quattlebaum et al., 1976). With the advances in detection and surgical treatment of recurrent sustained ventricular tachycardia, a new approach to the therapy of these problems has arisen. Ventricular tachyarrhythmias are estimated to occur in from 0.3 to 3 per cent of patients following complete repair and have not appeared to be related to the hemodynamic success of the repair. A report in patients experiencing from 30 to 150 documented episodes of sustained ventricular tachycardia with failure of pharmacologic and pacing regimens indicated that the source of the arrhythmia was localized to the right ventriculotomy scar by electrophysiologic mapping (Harken et al., 1980). The scar was surgically excised, and ventricular tachycardia was not inducible following operation and has not recurred in the 6 and 18 months, respectively, following surgical excision of the scar in these patients.

Of increasing significance are those patients with tetralogy of Fallot who also have major additional congenital cardiac anomalies. One of the more interesting associations is that with complete atrioventricular canal. Several studies have emphasized the fact that total correction of this combination consists of closure of the VSD as well as of the atrial septal defect (ASD) and reconstruction of the AV valve with relief of right ventricular outflow tract obstruction (Arciniegas et al., 1981). A double-outlet right ventricle has also been reported with successful correction (Pacifico et al., 1980). In addition, patients with tetralogy of Fallot and associated aortic insufficiency (Matsuda et al., 1980), with aorticopulmonary window (Castaneda and Kirklin, 1977), with anomalous origin of the left coronary artery from the pulmonary artery (Akasaka et al., 1981), and with diverticulum of the right ventricle (Magrassi et al., 1980) have undergone successful repair.

It is now possible to correct the tetralogy with extracorporeal circulation in patients with sickle cell anemia, including those with G-6-PD deficiency. Intracardiac procedures can be performed safely on these patients if certain guidelines are observed, especially the avoidance of hypoxia, hypothermia, acidosis, and dehydration. The patient should be prepared for operation with transfusion of normal red cells (Szentpetery et al., 1976).

PULMONARY STENOSIS WITH INTACT VENTRICULAR SEPTUM

Stenosis of the pulmonary valve with intact ventricular septum is one of the most favorable congenital cardiac lesions from the point of view of treatment. The symptoms are generally less pronounced than with the tetralogy of Fallot, although there are numerous examples of infants with extremely severe pulmonary stenosis producing congestive heart failure. Some infants require immediate valvotomy as an emergency procedure, but in the majority, the symptoms develop more slowly. In approximately three fourths of this group, the foramen ovale is patent, and with development of increased pressure in the right atrium, blood is shunted to the left atrium and cyanosis is produced. Clubbing of the fingers may appear later. The pulmonary valvular commissures are fused into a dome-shaped structure with a small central lumen. A jet of blood that is forced through the aperture under great pressure from the right ventricle into the pulmonary artery creates turbulence and a prominent thrill. Poststenotic dilatation of the main pulmonary artery ensues. In rare instances, *infundibular* stenosis may be associated with valvular stenosis and an intact ventricular septum. Moreover, frank atrial septal defects are also encountered, the latter combination being termed the *trilogy of Fallot*. The clinical findings are dependent on the severity of the valvular pulmonary stenosis and the patency of the foramen ovale (Engle and Taussig, 1950). Exertional dyspnea is the most common complaint, and cyanosis is usually present in those patients with a patent foramen ovale or an atrial septal defect. A harsh systolic murmur and thrill are present over the pulmonary area; the thrill can be palpated in the suprasternal notch. The pulmonary second sound is characteristically weak or absent. The chest film is often typical, demonstrating

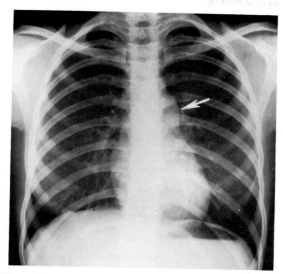

Figure 36–18. Chest film of a patient with isolated valvular pulmonary stenosis, demonstrating typical appearance of dilatation of the pulmonary artery. (From Sabiston, D. C., Jr.: *In* Gibbon's Surgery of the Chest. 2nd Ed. Edited by D. C. Sabiston, Jr. and F. C. Spencer. Philadelphia, W. B. Saunders Company, 1969.)

prominence of the pulmonary artery due to poststenotic dilatation (Fig. 36–18). The angiocardiogram is also helpful in demonstrating the classic dome-shaped pulmonary valve with small aperture and poststenotic dilatation, or an atrial septal defect and infundibular stenosis combined with valvular stenosis. Cardiac catheterization demonstrates a gradient between the right ventricle and the pulmonary artery *without* evidence of a shunt at the ventricular level. In severe forms, the pressure gradient between the pulmonary artery and the right ventricle may exceed 200 mm. Hg.

Pulmonary atresia with an intact ventricular septum represents a very serious condition in infancy. Although this is not a common lesion, it usually demands urgent therapy quite early in life. Infants with the combination of pulmonary atresia and an intact ventricular septum usually present within 24 to 48 hours of birth with dyspnea, tachypnea, and progressive cyanosis. A patent ductus arteriosus is usually present, as well as a right ventricular heave and murmurs of tricuspid insufficiency. Those in whom symptoms are not as prominent until several weeks or several months later usually have a widely patent ductus arteriosus. Arrhythmias, probably the result of right ventricular hypertension and right atrial dilatation, may be present. Cardiomegaly is demonstrated on the chest film together with diminished pulmonary vascular markings. The electrocardiogram usually shows a normal axis with left ventricular predominance in the precordial leads. The size of the right ventricular cavity can be assessed by echocardiography; the diagnosis together with details of anatomic and physiologic changes is best determined by cardiac catheterization and angiocardiography. Factors of considerable importance in planning therapy in these

infants include the size of the main pulmonary artery and the right and left branches, the size and characteristics of the right ventricular cavity, and the presence and relative size of a patent ductus arteriosus (Fig. 36–19) (Moulton *et al.*, 1979). In addition, ultrasound is helpful in determining the presence of a patent ductus arteriosus, its size and relationship in a comparison with the size of the left atrium and the aorta, and also retrograde flow into the descending thoracic aorta.

Treatment

Pulmonary valvotomy was introduced by Brock (1948) and consisted of transventricular valvotomy. A valvulotome was passed through the wall of the right ventricle into the pulmonary artery to open the stenotic valve. Later, an improved valvulotome was designed for transventricular use (Potts *et al.*, 1950). It is now agreed that open repair of the valvular stenosis under direct vision produces the best results (Blount *et al.*, 1954). The use of extracorporeal circulation permits simultaneous correction of coexisting atrial septal defects and of infundibular stenosis when present (McGoon and Kirklin, 1958). Thus, the open approach to the correction of pulmonary valvular stenosis is most often indicated (Fig. 36–20).

Most infants with the combination of pulmonary atresia and intact ventricular septum become critically

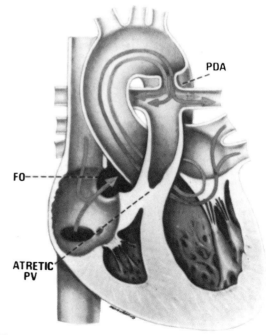

Figure 36–19. Pulmonary atresia with intact ventricular septum demonstrating hypoplastic right ventricle, shunting via a patent foramen ovale, and ductus-dependent pulmonary blood supply (PDA = patent ductus arteriosus; FO = foramen ovale; PV = pulmonary valve). (From Moulton, A. M., Bowman, F. O., Jr., Edie, R. N., Hayes, C. J., Ellis, K., Gersony, W. M., and Malm, J. R.: J. Thorac. Cardiovasc. Surg., 78:527, 1979.)

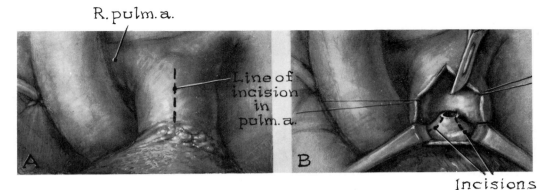

Figure 36-20. Illustration of open correction of pulmonary valvular stenosis employing extracorporeal circulation. An incision is made in the main pulmonary artery, exposing the dome-shaped pulmonary valve. Radial incisions are made in each of the fused commissures, with complete opening of the valve. (From Sabiston, D. C., Jr.: In Gibbon's Surgery of the Chest. 2nd Ed. Edited by D. C. Sabiston, Jr. and F. C. Spencer. Philadelphia, W. B. Saunders Company, 1969.)

ill quite early in life and demand urgent therapy. In most, a patent ductus arteriosus is responsible for maintenance of life, and the infusion of prostaglandin E can be helpful in preventing ductal closure and the associated severe hypoxia and acidosis that would otherwise follow. Although closed valvotomy (Brock), systemic pulmonary shunt (Blalock, Potts, or Waterston), and combination procedures have been used, at present the preferred management appears to be combined valvotomy and shunt. Closed valvotomy can be performed, although in some instances an open procedure using extracorporeal circulation with insertion of an outflow prosthetic patch is preferable (Moulton *et al.*, 1979).

Valvotomy by open correction of pulmonary valvular stenosis yields excellent results, and recurrence of the condition is rare. Moreover, the compensatory infundibular hypertrophy that frequently accompanies the valvular stenosis usually regresses with time. Although the gradient between the right ventricle and the pulmonary artery may not be totally abolished immediately after operation, regression of the secondary hypertrophy of the right ventricular outflow tract occurs, and repeat catheterization later shows a marked reduction in the gradient (Engle *et al.*, 1958).

Isolated infundibular stenosis of the right ventricle may also occur as a congenital anomaly. The symptoms are quite similar to those of valvular stenosis, although the murmur may be located somewhat lower in the precordium. The angiocardiogram demonstrates the lesion wth precision, and cardiac catheterization demonstrates two gradients: (1) between the pulmonary artery and (2) between the infundibulum and the right ventricle. Management of these cases is resection of the infundibular stenosis in the open heart employing extracorporeal circulation. The results are excellent.

SELECTED REFERENCES

Arciniegas, E., Farooki, Z. Q., Hakimi, M., and Green, E. W.: Results of two-stage surgical treatment of tetralogy of Fallot. J. Thorac. Cardiovasc. Surg., 79:876, 1980.

This group reports 109 consecutive patients undergoing palliative shunt as the initial management for symptomatic tetralogy of Fallot. The total early shunt mortality, including the Blalock-Taussig as well as Waterston shunts, was 2.7 per cent. The mean patient age at the time of total repair was 4.8 years, and the second-stage corrective operation had a mortality of 1.6 per cent. They consider the Blalock-Taussig shunt to be the shunt of choice in all symptomatic infants and small children with tetralogy of Fallot and emphasize that the two-stage surgical approach compares favorably with primary total correction, particularly in infants under 1 year of age.

Blalock, A., and Taussig, H. G.: The surgical treatment of malformations of the heart in which there is pulmonary stenosis or pulmonary atresia. J.A.M.A., 128:189, 1945.

In this paper, Dr. Blalock's first three operations for creation of a systemic-pulmonary anastomosis are reported. The first patient, a 15-month-old infant with severe cyanosis, had a history of multiple episodes of loss of consciousness. An anastomosis of the left subclavian artery to the left pulmonary artery was made, and the clinical improvement was striking. Two additional patients with successful results are also described. It is of interest that Dr. Blalock refers to earlier experimental work in which subclavian-pulmonary anastomoses were performed in the dog in an effort to produce pulmonary hypertension. Although these experiments did not succeed in producing an elevated pulmonary arterial pressure, the operation was subsequently used for an entirely different purpose. This procedure was the first of many additional cardiac surgical advances.

Castaneda, A. R., Freed, M. D., Williams, R. G., and Norwood, W. I.: Repair of tetralogy of Fallot in infancy. Early and late results. J. Thorac. Cardiovasc. Surg., 74:372, 1977.

These authors report a series of 41 consecutive infants operated on with primary correction of the tetralogy of Fallot with deep hypothermia and circulatory arrest. The infants ranged in age from 12 days to 1 year, with a mean age of 5.7 months. The authors conclude that the hospital mortality and early and late results justify continued evaluation of primary repair of tetralogy of Fallot in symptomatic infants, regardless of weight or age. The contraindications that they cite to reparative operation in symptomatic infants with the tetralogy are an anterior descending coronary artery arising from the right coronary artery or associated congenital pulmonary atresia.

Chopra, P. S., Levy, J. M., Dacumos, G. C., Jr., Berkoff, H. A., Loring, L. L., and Kahn, D. R.: The Blalock-Taussig operation—the procedure of choice in the hypoxic infant with tetralogy of Fallot. Ann. Thorac. Surg., 22:235, 1976.

These authors advocate systemic-pulmonary anastomosis (Blalock-Taussig operation) as the ideal procedure in the infant. It is their belief that a better long-term result is obtained using a preliminary shunt followed by open correction than by performing the definitive procedure with extracorporeal circulation as the initial operation.

Daily, P. O., Stinson, E. B., Griepp, R. B., and Shumway, N. E.: Tetralogy of Fallot. Choice of surgical procedure. J. Thorac. Cardiovasc. Surg., 75:338, 1978.

The authors review the use of total correction of the tetralogy versus anastomotic procedures in early childhood. From their data, they conclude that the operative mortality for total correction of tetralogy of Fallot after the age of 4 is less than that in infancy, and if surgical therapy is required in the first 24 months of life, total correction is preferred over palliative shunting with later total correction. Moreover, their data indicate that the Blalock-Taussig procedure is definitely preferred to palliative shunts of the Waterston or Potts type. The primary indication for a shunt procedure is the presence of severe hypoplasia of the right and left pulmonary arteries in infancy.

Kirklin, J. W., and Karp, R. B.: Tetralogy of Fallot from a Surgical Viewpoint. Philadelphia, W. B. Saunders Company, 1970.

This is a superb monograph with excellent presentations of the anatomy, natural history, hemodynamics, clinical features, and diagnosis of tetralogy of Fallot. The techniques of palliative and open corrective surgery are superbly described and illustrated. A detailed account of the results is provided and ranks among the best in the world literature. The monograph is highly recommended for a complete analysis of the entire subject.

Lillehei, C. W., Cohen, M., Warden, H. E., Read, R. C., Aust, J. B., DeWall, R. A., and Varco, R.: Vision intracardiac surgical correction of the tetralogy of Fallot, pentalogy of Fallot, and pulmonary atresia defects. Ann. Surg., 142:418, 1955.

In this paper, the original descriptions for surgical correction of the tetralogy of Fallot are provided. The paper is a classic one in the development of surgical techniques for complete correction of this malformation.

Moulton, A. L., Bowman, F. O., Jr., Edie, R. N., Hayes, C. J., Ellis, K., Gersony, W. M., and Malm, J. R.: Pulmonary atresia with intact ventricular septum. Sixteen-year experience. J. Thorac. Cardiovasc. Surg., 78:527, 1979.

This is a review of 30 patients with pulmonary atresia and intact ventricular septum treated by a variety of surgical approaches over a 16-year period. The authors conclude that in the majority of patients, the preferred operation is combined pulmonary valvotomy (or outflow patch) together with a systemic-pulmonary shunt. This approach has yielded the best long-term results thus far.

Sabiston, D. C., Jr.: Role of the Blalock-Taussig operation in the hypoxic infant with tetralogy of Fallot. (Editorial.) Ann. Thorac. Surg., 22:303, 1976.

In this editorial, the use of an initial systemic-pulmonary shunt procedure is contrasted with total correction of the tetralogy of Fallot in infancy. The reasoning advanced by the advocates of each of these methods is discussed in detail.

Sabiston, D. C., Jr., Cornell, W. P., Criley, J. M., Neill, C. A., Ross, R. S., and Bahnson, H. T.: The diagnosis and surgical correction of total obstruction of the right ventricle: An acquired condition developing after systemic artery–pulmonary artery anastomosis for tetralogy of Fallot. J. Thorac. Cardiovasc. Surg., 48:577, 1964.

In this paper, the most severe of the forms of tetralogy of Fallot, those with complete obliteration of the outflow tract of the right ventricle and its communication with the pulmonary artery, are described together with the details of operative corrections and results. It is interesting that in these patients who have no communication between the right ventricle and pulmonary artery and who, following correction, have total pulmonary insufficiency, the subsequent course is generally surprisingly good. In other words, pulmonary valvular insufficiency can be well tolerated.

Taussig, H. B.: Tetralogy of Fallot: Early history and late results. Neuhauser Lecture. Am. J. Roentgenol., 133:423, 1979.

This is a classic and updated reference written by a distinguished pediatric cardiologist. She summarizes the early and late results of the Blalock-Taussig operation in a large series of patients. In addition, an excellent historical review of the subject is included.

Tucker, W. Y., Turley, K., Ullyot, D. J., and Ebert, P. A.: Management of symptomatic tetralogy of Fallot in the first year of life. J. Thorac. Cardiovasc. Surg., 78:494, 1979.

A series of patients is presented in whom correction of symptomatic tetralogy of Fallot in the first year was recommended with excellent results.

REFERENCES

Akasaka, T., Itoh, K., Ohkawa, Y., Nakayama, S., Miyamoto, H., Nishi, T., Satoh, H., and Takarada, M.: Surgical treatment of anomalous origin of the left coronary artery from the pulmonary artery associated with tetralogy of Fallot. Ann. Thorac. Surg., 31:469, 1981.

Allison, P. R., Gunning, A. J., Hamill, J., and Mody, S. M.: Fallot's tetralogy. A postoperative study. Circulation, 28:525, 1963.

Arciniegas, E., Farooki, Z. Q., Hakimi, M., and Green, E. W.: Results of two-stage surgical treatment of tetralogy of Fallot. J. Thorac. Cardiovasc. Surg., 79:876, 1980.

Arciniegas, E., Hakimi, M., Farooki, Z. Q., and Green, E. W.: Results of total correction of tetralogy of Fallot with complete atrioventricular canal. J. Thorac. Cardiovasc. Surg., 81:768, 1981.

Bakulev, A. N., and Kolesnikov, S. A.: Anastomosis of the superior vena cava and pulmonary artery in the surgical treatment of certain congenital defects of the heart. J. Thorac. Surg., 37:693, 1959.

Blackstone, E. H., Kirklin, J. W., Bertranou, E. G., Labrosse, C. J., Soto, B., and Bargeron, L. M., Jr.: Preoperative prediction from cineangiograms of postrepair right ventricular pressure in tetralogy of Fallot. J. Thorac. Cardiovasc. Surg., 78:542, 1979.

Blalock, A.: Surgical procedures employed and anatomical variations encountered in the treatment of congenital pulmonic stenosis. Surg. Gynecol. Obstet., 87:385, 1948.

Blalock, A., and Taussig, H. B.: The surgical treatment of malformations of the heart in which there is pulmonary stenosis or pulmonary atresia. J.A.M.A., 128:189, 1945.

Blount, S. G., Jr., McCord, M. C., Mueller, H., and Swan, H.: Isolated valvular pulmonic stenosis; clinical and physiologic response to open valvuloplasty. Circulation, 10:161, 1954.

Bonchek, L. I.: A method of outflow tract reconstruction in tetralogy of Fallot with anomalous anterior descending coronary artery. Ann. Thorac. Surg., 21:451, 1976.

Borow, K. M., Green, L. H., Castaneda, A. R., and Keane, J. F.: Left ventricular function after repair of tetralogy of Fallot and its relationship to age at surgery. Circulation, 61:1150, 1980.

Brock, R. C.: Pulmonary valvulotomy for the relief of congenital pulmonary stenosis; report of 3 cases. Br. Med. J., 1:1121, 1948.

Brock, R. C.: Congenital pulmonary stenosis. Am. J. Med., 12:706, 1952.

Brock, R. C., and Campbell, M.: Infundibular resection or dilatation for infundibular stenosis. Br. Heart J., 12:403, 1950.

Calder, A. L., Barratt-Boyes, B. G., Brandt, P. W. T., and Neutze, J. M.: Postoperative evaluation of patients with tetralogy of Fallot repaired in infancy. Including criteria for use of outflow patching and radiologic assessment of pulmonary regurgitation. J. Thorac. Cardiovasc. Surg., 77:704, 1979.

Campbell, M., and Deuchar, D. C.: Results of the Blalock-Taussig operation in 200 cases of morbus caeruleus. Br. Med. J., 1:349, 1953.

Castaneda, A. R., and Kirklin, J. W.: Tetralogy of Fallot with aorticopulmonary window. Report of two surgical cases. J. Thorac. Cardiovasc. Surg., 74:467, 1977.

Castaneda, A. R., Freed, M. D., Williams, R. G., and Norwood, W. I.: Repair of tetralogy of Fallot in infancy. Early and late results. J. Thorac. Cardiovasc. Surg., 74:372, 1977.

Chopra, P. S., Levy, J. M., Dacumos, G. C., Jr., Berkoff, H. A., Loring, L. L., and Kahn, D. R.: The Blalock-Taussig operation—the procedure of choice in the hypoxic infant with tetralogy of Fallot. Ann. Thorac. Surg., 22:235, 1976.

Claxton, C. P., Jr., and Sabiston, D. C., Jr.: Correction of tetralogy of Fallot following superior vena cava to pulmonary artery shunt. J. Thorac. Cardiovasc. Surg., 57:475, 1969.

Daily, P. O., Stinson, E. B., Griepp, R. B., and Shumway, N. E.: Tetralogy of Fallot. Choice of surgical procedure. J. Thorac. Cardiovasc. Surg., 75:338, 1978.

Dobell, A. R. C., Charrette, E. P., and Chughtai, M. S.: Correction of tetralogy in the young child. J. Thorac. Cardiovasc. Surg., 55:70, 1968.

Ebert, P. A.: Ascending aorta–right pulmonary artery anastomosis. (Editorial.) J. Thorac. Cardiovasc. Surg., 77:478, 1979.

Edmunds, L. H., Jr., Saxena, N. C., Friedman, S., Rashkind, W. J., and Dodd, P. F.: Transatrial resection of the obstructed right ventricular infundibulum. Circulation, 54:117, 1976.

Engle, M. A., and Taussig, H. B.: Valvular pulmonic stenosis with intact ventricular septum and patent foramen ovale: Report of illustrative cases and analysis of clinical syndrome. Circulation, 2:481, 1950.

Engle, M. A., Holswade, G. R., Goldberg, H. P., Lukas, D. S., and Glenn, F.: Regression after open valvotomy of infundibular stenosis accompanying severe valvular pulmonic stenosis. Circulation, 17:862, 1958.

Fallot, E.-L. A.: Contribution à l'anatomie pathologique de la maladie bleue (cyanose cardiaque). Marseille Med., 25:77, 138, 207, 270, 341, 403, 1888.

Farre, J. R.: Pathological Researches. Essay I. On Malformations of the Human Heart: Illustrated by Numerous Cases, and Preceded by Some Observations on the Method of Improving the Diagnostic Part of Medicine. London, Longmans, Green and Co., 1814.

Fellows, K. E., Freed, M. D., Keane, J. F., Van Praagh, R., Bernhard, W. F., and Castaneda, A. C.: Results of routine preoperative coronary angiography in tetralogy of Fallot. Circulation, 51:561, 1975.

Fort, L., III, Morrow, A. G., Pierce, G. E., Saigusa, M., and McLaughlin, J. S.: The distribution of pulmonary blood flow after subclavian-pulmonary anastomosis. An experimental study. J. Thorac. Cardiovasc. Surg., 50:671, 1965.

Gale, A. W., Arciniegas, E., Green, E. W., Blackstone, E. H., and Kirklin, J. W.: Growth of the pulmonary anulus and pulmonary arteries after the Blalock-Taussig shunt. J. Thorac. Cardiovasc. Surg., 77:459, 1979.

Garson, A., Jr., Nihill, M. R., McNamara, D. G., and Cooley, D. A.: Status of the adult and adolescent after repair of tetralogy of Fallot. Circulation, 59:1232, 1979.

Gay, W. A., Jr., and Ebert, P. A.: Aorta–to–right pulmonary artery anastomosis causing obstruction of the right pulmonary artery. Ann. Thorac. Surg., 16:402, 1973.

Gintrac, E.: Observations et Recherches sur la Cyanose, ou Maladie Bleue. Paris, J. Pinard, 1824.

Glenn, W. W. L., and Patino, J. F.: Circulatory bypass of the right heart. I. Preliminary observation on direct delivery of vena caval blood into pulmonary arterial circulation. Azygos vein–pulmonary artery shunt. Yale J. Biol. Med., 27:147, 1954.

Gregoratos, G., Jones, R. C., and Jahnke, E. J., Jr.: Unilateral peripheral pulmonic stenosis complicating tetralogy of Fallot. J. Thorac. Cardiovasc. Surg., 50:202, 1965.

Haller, J. A., Jr.: Second shunting operations for pulmonary stenosis with cyanosis following failure of original systemic-pulmonary anastomoses. Surgery, 44:919, 1958.

Hallidie-Smith, K. A., Dulake, M., Wong, M., Oakley, C. M., and Goodwin, J. F.: Ventricular structure and function after radical correction of the tetralogy of Fallot. Br. Heart J., 29:533, 1967.

Harken, A. H., Horowitz, L. N., and Josephson, M. E.: Surgical correction of recurrent sustained ventricular tachycardia following complete repair of tetralogy of Fallot. J. Thorac. Cardiovasc. Surg., 80:779, 1980.

Hartmann, R. C.: Hemorrhagic disorder occurring in patients with cyanotic congenital heart disease. Bull. Johns Hopkins Hosp., 91:49, 1952.

Hope, J.: A Treatise on the Diseases of the Heart and Great Vessels, and on the Affections Which May be Mistaken for Them. London, J. Churchill & Sons, 1839.

Hunter, J.: Medical Observations and Inquiries by a Society of Physicians of London. London, 1757–1784.

Hunter, W.: Three cases of malformation of the heart. Case II. Medical Observations and Inquiries by a Society of Physicians in London, 6:291, 1784.

Johns, T. N. P., Williams, G. R., and Blalock, A.: The anatomy of pulmonary stenosis and atresia with comments on surgical therapy. Surgery, 33:161, 1953.

Kirklin, J. W., and Karp, R. B.: The Tetralogy of Fallot from a Surgical Viewpoint. Philadelphia, W. B. Saunders Company, 1970.

Kirklin, J. W., Blackstone, E. H., Pacifico, A. D., Brown, R. N., and Bargeron, L. M., Jr.: Routine primary repair vs. two-stage repair of tetralogy of Fallot. Circulation, 60:373, 1979.

Lillehei, C. W., Cohen, M., Warden, H. E., Read, R. C., Aust, J. B., DeWall, R. A., and Varco, R. L.: Vision intracardiac surgical correction of the tetralogy of Fallot, pentalogy of Fallot, and pulmonary atresia defects. Ann. Surg., 142:418, 1955.

Magrassi, P., Chartrand, C., Guerin, R., Kratz, C., and Stanley, P.: True diverticulum of the right ventricle: Two cases associated with tetralogy of Fallot. Ann. Thorac. Surg., 29:357, 1980.

Malm, J. R., Blumenthal, S., Bowman, F. O., Jr., Ellis, K., Jameson, A. G., Jesse, M. J., and Yeoh, C. B.: Factors that modify hemodynamic results in total correction of tetralogy of Fallot. J. Thorac. Cardiovasc. Surg., 52:502, 1966.

Matsuda, H., Ihara, K., Mori, T., Kitamura, S., and Kawashima, Y.: Tetralogy of Fallot associated with aortic insufficiency. Ann. Thorac. Surg., 29:529, 1980.

McGoon, D. C., and Kirklin, J. W.: Pulmonic stenosis with intact ventricular septum. Treatment utilizing extracorporeal circulation. Circulation, 17:180, 1958.

Morris, D. C., Felner, J. M., Schlant, R. C., and Franch, R. H.: Echocardiographic diagnosis of tetralogy of Fallot. Am. J. Cardiol., 36:908, 1975.

Moulton, A. L., Bowman, F. O., Jr., Edie, R. N., Hayes, C. J., Ellis, K., Gersony, W. M., and Malm, J. R.: Pulmonary atresia with intact ventricular septum. Sixteen-year experience. J. Thorac. Cardiovasc. Surg., 78:527, 1979.

Murphy, J. D., Freed, M. D., Keane, J. F., Norwood, W. I., Castaneda, A. R., and Nadas, A. S.: Hemodynamic results after intracardiac repair of tetralogy of Fallot by deep hypothermia and cardiopulmonary bypass. Circulation, 62 (Suppl. 1):168, 1980.

Nagao, G. I., Daoud, G. I., McAdams, A. J., Schwartz, D. C., and Kaplan, S.: Cardiovascular anomalies associated with tetralogy of Fallot. Am. J. Cardiol., 20:206, 1967.

Neches, W. H., Naifeh, J. G., Parks, S. C., Lenox, C. C., Zuberbuhler, J. R., Siewers, R. D., Pontius, R. G., and Bahnson, H. T.: Systemic-pulmonary artery anastomoses in infancy. J. Thorac. Cardiovasc. Surg., 70:921, 1975.

Pacifico, A. D., Kirklin, J. W., and Bargeron, L. M., Jr.: Repair of complete atrioventricular canal associated with tetralogy of Fallot or double-outlet right ventricle: Report of 10 patients. Ann. Thorac. Surg., 29:351, 1980.

Peacock, T. B.: On Malformations of the Human Heart etc., with Original Cases and Illustrations. 2nd Ed. London, J. Churchill & Sons, 1866.

Porter, J. M., and Silver, D.: Alterations in fibrinolysis and coagulation associated with cardiopulmonary bypass. J. Thorac. Cardiovasc. Surg., 56:869, 1968.

Potts, W. J., Smith, S., and Gibson, S.: Anastomosis of the aorta to a pulmonary artery for certain types of congenital heart disease. J.A.M.A., 132:629, 1946.

Potts, W. J., Gibson, S., Riker, W. L., and Leninger, C. R.: Congenital pulmonary stenosis with intact ventricular septum. J.A.M.A., *144*:8, 1950.

Quattlebaum, T. G., Varghese, P. J., Neill, C. A., and Donahoo, J. S.: Sudden death among postoperative patients with tetralogy of Fallot. A follow-up study of 243 patients for an average of twelve years. Circulation, *54*:289, 1976.

Ross, R. S., Taussig, H. B., and Evans, M. H.: Late hemodynamic complications of anastomotic surgery for treatment of the tetralogy of Fallot. Circulation, *18*:553, 1958.

Sabiston, D. C., Jr.: Role of the Blalock-Taussig operation in the hypoxic infant with tetralogy of Fallot. (Editorial.) Ann. Thorac. Surg., *22*:303, 1976.

Sabiston, D. C., Jr., and Blalock, A.: The tetralogy of Fallot, tricuspid atresia, transposition of the great vessels and associated disorders. *In* Encyclopedia of Thoracic Surgery. Vol. 2. Edited by E. Derra. Heidelberg, Springer-Verlag, 1959.

Sabiston, D. C., Jr., Cornell, W. P., Criley, J. M., Neill, C. A., Ross, R. S., and Bahnson, H. T.: The diagnosis and surgical correction of total obstruction of the right ventricle: An acquired condition developing after systemic artery–pulmonary artery anastomosis for tetralogy of Fallot. J. Thorac. Cardiovasc. Surg., *48*:577, 1964.

Sandifort, E.: Observationes Anatomico-Pathologicae. Lugdunum Batavorum, P.v.d. Eyk et D. Vygh, 1777, Chapter 1, Figure 1.

Scott, H. W., Collins, H. A., and Foster, J. H.: Hypothermia as an adjuvant in cardiovascular surgery. Experimental and clinical observations. Am. Surg., *20*:799, 1954.

Seybold-Epting, W., Chiariello, L., Hallman, G. L., and Cooley, D. A.: Aneurysm of pericardial right ventricular outflow tract patches. Ann. Thorac. Surg., *24*:237, 1977.

Shaffer, C. W., Berman, W., Jr., and Waldhausen, J. A.: Repair of divided anomalous anterior descending artery in tetralogy of Fallot. Ann. Thorac. Surg., *27*:250, 1979.

Stensen, H. (Nicholaus Steno). *In* Bartholin, T.: Acta Medica et Philosophica Hafnienca, 1671–72, Vol. 1, p. 302. Reprinted in Stenosis, N.: Opera Philosophica. Copenhagen, Vilhelm Maar, 1910, Vol. 2, pp. 49–53.

Stephens, H. B.: Aneurysm of the pulmonary artery following a Potts' shunt operation. J. Thorac. Cardiovasc. Surg., *53*:642, 1967.

Szentpetery, S., Robertson, L., and Lower, R. R.: Complete repair of tetralogy associated with sickle cell anemia and G-6-PD deficiency. J. Thorac. Cardiovasc. Surg., *72*:276, 1976.

Tanaka, J., Yasui, H., Nakano, E., Sese, A., Matsui, K., Takeda, Y., and Tokunaga, K.: Predisposing factors of renal dysfunction following total correction of tetralogy of Fallot in the adult. J. Thorac. Cardiovasc. Surg., *80*:135, 1980.

Taussig, H. B.: Tetralogy of Fallot: Early history and late results. Neuhauser Lecture. Am. J. Roentgenol., *133*:423, 1979.

Theye, R. A., and Kirklin, J. W.: Physiologic studies early after repair of tetralogy of Fallot. Circulation, *28*:42, 1963.

Tucker, W. Y., Turley, K., Ullyot, D. J., and Ebert, P. A.: Management of symptomatic tetralogy of Fallot in the first year of life. J. Thorac. Cardiovasc. Surg., *78*:494, 1979.

Waterston, D. J.: Treatment of Fallot's tetralogy in children under 1 year of age. Rozhl. Chir., *41*:181, 1962.

White, P. D., and Sprague, H. B.: The tetralogy of Fallot. Report of a case in a noted musician who lived to his sixtieth year. J.A.M.A., *92*:787, 1929.

Wood, W. C., McCue, C. M., and Lower, R. R.: Blalock-Taussig shunts in the infant. Ann. Thorac. Surg., *16*:454, 1973.

Chapter 37

Truncus Arteriosus

DWIGHT C. MCGOON

Persistent truncus arteriosus is a congenital cardiac deformity of the outflow tracts of the right and left ventricles characterized by the presence of a single outflow valve and a single artery (the truncus) originating from the heart; this truncus sequentially gives origin to the coronary arteries and the pulmonary artery or arteries and then continues as the ascending aorta (Fig. 37–1). The pulmonary artery or arteries typically arise from the left posterolateral aspect of the truncus just downstream from the truncal valve and the coronary ostia. A ventricular septal defect is nearly always present. Typically, this defect lies immediately upstream from the truncal valve, thus replacing the infundibular septum, and usually, it does not extend to the tricuspid anulus (Marcelletti et al., 1977; Crupi et al., 1977).

The preceding definition has undergone periodic revision since the condition was first described by Buchanan in 1864. This current definition excludes closely related anomalies such as pulmonary atresia, in which the pulmonary artery does not take origin from an ascending aortic "truncus" (however, in pulmonary atresia, a coronary artery–to–pulmonary artery fistula may be a source of pulmonary blood flow [Krongrad et al., 1972]). The definition also excludes atresia of the aortic valve, in which a diminutive ascending aorta is present that transports flow from the ductus to the coronary arteries. Similarly, this definition denies the existence of a subclass of truncus arteriosus (Type IV of Collett and Edwards [1949]) in which pulmonary arteries are absent; rather, such a condition is better described as pulmonary atresia totalis. Even the distinction between Types I, II, and

III of Collett and Edwards is highly imprecise. Indeed, the very occurrence of truly lateral origins (Type III) rather than somewhat posterolateral origins of the right and left pulmonary arteries from the truncus is legitimately questioned. Since there is almost never significant distance between the lumen of the truncus and the origin of the right pulmonary artery, a precise distinction seems not to exist between Type I truncus (in which the pulmonary arteries branch from a common pulmonary trunk) and Type II (in which the right and left pulmonary arteries arise closely together from the dorsal wall of the truncus arteriosus). Furthermore, the unfortunate term "pseudotruncus" should be abandoned in favor of the more descriptive designation of a condition characterized by pulmonary atresia and patent ductus arteriosus.

The various anatomic variations encountered in a consecutive series of 92 corrective operations for truncus arteriosus are shown in Table 37–1 (Marcelletti et al., 1977). Probably since these data are derived from a group of 92 patients who were selected by virtue of having survived without severe pulmonary vascular obstructive disease until operation (ages 14 months to 21 years; median 7.3 years), they indicate a higher incidence of patients with protective lesions such as hypoplastic or stenotic pulmonary arteries and a lower incidence of patients with truncal valvular incompetence, absence of one pulmonary artery, or complex associated cardiac anomalies than would be true of unselected newborns having truncus arteriosus. At any rate, the Marcelletti report (1977) showed that about three fourths of patients had the Type I anomaly, two-thirds had a tricuspid truncal

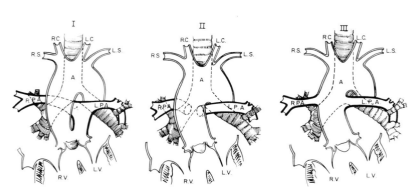

Figure 37–1. These are, from left to right, the classically described variants of truncus arteriosus, Type I, II, and III, respectively. Their features have been exaggerated by the artist for purposes of illustration, but in clinical practice, many patients are encountered in the border zone between Types I and II, and truly lateral origin of the left and right pulmonary arteries from the truncus rarely, if ever, occurs.

TABLE 37-1. ANATOMIC VARIATIONS OF TRUNCUS ARTERIOSUS (92 PATIENTS)*

FEATURES	PER CENT
Type	
I	73
II	27
Truncal valve	
Bicuspid	11
Tricuspid	67
Quadricuspid	9
Pentacuspid	1
Undetermined	2
Truncal valve regurgitation	
Competent	45
Incompetent	55
Mild	(30)
Mild to severe	(25)
Ventricular septal defect	
Infundibular septum	100
Extending to tricuspid anulus	20
Aortic arch	
Left	69
Right	31
Pulmonary arteries	
Normal size and number	50
Bilateral hypoplasia	3
Right hypoplasia	4
Bilateral banding	14
Right stenosis (some banded)	15
Left stenosis (some banded)	3
Right absent	2
Left absent	7
Left from ductus	1
Associated cardiac defects	
Atrial septal defect	9
Anomalous pulmonary veins	2
Patent ductus	5
Interrupted aortic arch	3

*From Marcelletti, C., et al.: Early and late results of surgical repair of truncus arteriosus. Circulation, 55:636, 1977.

TABLE 37-2. NATURAL HISTORY OF TRUNCUS ARTERIOSUS*

AGE (YEARS)	NO. OF PATIENTS	RP (UNITS M.²)†	STATUS
<2	10	4.2	All dead (two lived >2 years)
2–7	8	10.5	All alive except one (died 11 years later)
>7	5	21.8	Three dead (Rp >20 units · M.²) Two alive (Rp <20 units · M.²)

*From Marcelletti, C., et al.: The natural history of truncus arteriosus. Circulation, 54:108, 1976.

†Rp = average pulmonary resistance in Wood units. Data available for only two of 10 in the youngest age group, six of eight in the intermediate age group, and all five in the oldest group.

semilunar valve, over half had some truncal valve incompetence, nearly one-third had a right-sided aortic arch, only one-half had right and left normal-sized (not hypoplastic or stenotic) pulmonary arteries, and one-fifth had associated cardiac anomalies.

Morphogenetically, truncus arteriosus is thus a defect in septation between the outflow tracts of the two ventricles, explainable embryologically by lack of development of the conotruncal ridges that normally form the conotruncal septum and divide the outflow valve into two semilunar valves. The hemodynamic consequence of the malformation is the establishment of a wide intercommunication between the systemic and pulmonary circulations. Since this communication is downstream as well as upstream to the semilunar valve, direct shunting of blood at systemic pressure from the higher- to the lower-resistance circulatory bed can continue throughout the entire duration of the cardiac cycle. This feature may account for an apparent acceleration of the development of pulmonary vascular obstructive disease in this condition.

Persistent truncus arteriosus accounts for only about 2 per cent of all congenital cardiac anomalies. It occurs slightly more frequently in males than in females.

NATURAL HISTORY

The prognosis for patients with truncus arteriosus is generally poor. The median age at death, reported in autopsy series, varies from a few weeks to 6 months (Fontana and Edwards, 1962; Van Praagh and Van Praagh, 1965; Bharati et al., 1974). Congestive heart failure secondary to a large pulmonary blood flow, with or without associated truncal valve regurgitation, is the major cause of death in early infancy. As is true for most congenital anomalies, adequate studies of the natural history of truncus arteriosus had not been conducted prior to the possibility of interfering with the natural history by surgical intervention. In the only available late follow-up study of nonoperated patients, Marcelletti and associates (1976) retrospectively identified 23 patients whose conditions were diagnosed during the 10 years before the availability of correction (1967). Their ages ranged from 8 days to 16 years (Table 37–2), and follow-up ranged from 8 to 18 years. All of the 10 patients whose conditions were diagnosed before 2 years of age had died of congestive heart failure resulting from huge blood flow through the relatively low-resistance pulmonary bed; only two survived beyond 2 years of age, and they died 8.5 and 12 years later, respectively. All but one of the patients surviving infancy whose condition was first diagnosed between the ages of 2 and 7 years had survived to the date of follow-up; apparently, in these patients, just enough elevation of pulmonary resistance had developed to protect them from excessive pulmonary blood flow and its consequences. Patients first seen when they were more than 7 years old showed pronounced elevation of pulmonary resistance, and three of five had died suddenly, presumably of arrhythmia. This study clearly confirms the early lethality of this condition and supports the evidence that operation, either palliative or corrective, should best be considered during infancy for most patients.

DIAGNOSIS

Patients born with truncus arteriosus are typically recognized as having congenital heart disease while they are still infants. During the very first few weeks of life, there may be little evidence of cardiac disease, since persistence of the normal prenatal elevation of pulmonary arteriolar resistance protects the baby from excessive pulmonary blood flow and cardiac overload. Despite the presence of the defect, however, pulmonary resistance eventually tends to decrease in most patients, accompanied by progressively increasing pulmonary blood flow, increasing cardiac workload, and a tendency toward congestive heart failure, as manifested by tachypnea, tachycardia, excessive sweating, and poor feeding. In infants born with severe deformity of the truncal valve resulting in major truncal valvular incompetence, the congestive heart failure may appear during the early neonatal period and may be more fulminant. Should stenosis at the origin of one or both pulmonary arteries or diffuse hypoplasia of the arteries be present, congestive heart failure may not develop, and indeed, in such instances, cyanosis may be the primary manifestation. In those fortunate patients who survive infancy, perhaps because of an enhanced ability to constrict their pulmonary arterioles and thus better control the excessive pulmonary blood flow, cyanosis develops and usually increases progressively during the subsequent 5 to 10 years as pulmonary blood flow becomes suboptimal owing to relentless increase in pulmonary vascular obstructive disease, which ultimately results in death.

The physical findings in truncus arteriosus are related to the anatomic and hemodynamic features of the individual patient. Because the shunt can occur throughout the cardiac cycle, as mentioned previously, diastolic systemic blood pressure falls, increasing the pulse pressure and causing the peripheral pulses to be accentuated or bounding in character. The heart is typically overactive, with the left precordium bulging to accommodate the enlarged heart, and there may be a systolic thrill along the left sternal border. Forceful opening of the truncal valve often causes a loud ejection click, but peculiarly, the closing of the valve (second heart sound) is not always single but may be split, perhaps owing to asynchronous approximation of the semilunar valve cusps. The large pulmonary blood flow may cause a ventricular filling sound (apical third heart sound). For the same reason, an apical mid-diastolic rumbling murmur is often present. A continuous murmur is not typical and, if present, usually is suggestive of an associated pulmonary arterial stenosis. A decrescendo diastolic murmur indicates the presence of truncal valve incompetence. The typical findings of congestive heart failure may be present, such as tachypnea, crepitant rales, hepatomegaly, and neck vein distention.

The electrocardiogram is not distinctive but usually shows combined ventricular hypertrophy and may show left atrial enlargement. The roentgenogram of the chest may provide some specific clues in addition to the typical cardiomegaly and increased pulmonary vascular markings. A right-sided aortic arch in the absence of cyanosis is highly suggestive of the diagnosis of truncus arteriosus, as is the presence of an abnormally high silhouette of the left pulmonary artery.

The two-dimensional echocardiogram is particularly useful in identifying the specific anatomic features of truncus arteriosus (Hagler et al., 1980), including the ventricular septal defect, the presence of a single semilunar valve, a single larger-than-normal arterial trunk, and the origins of the pulmonary arteries, as well as in defining left atrial size as an estimate of the volume of pulmonary blood flow.

Cardiac catheterization and angiocardiography provide precise anatomic and hemodynamic documentation. Detailed right and left heart catheterization studies are designed to provide information as to the pulmonary and systemic blood flows and resistances, identification of pressure gradients within the heart or great arteries, localization of the site of shunting, and the exclusion of other significant associated anomalies. Similarly, angiocardiography should define the specific features of the anomaly and especially demonstrate the origins, sizes, and distribution of the pulmonary arteries. The competence of the truncal valve should be assessed, although this may be unusually difficult because adequate filling of the truncal root with dye may not be possible owing to the preferential run-off of blood into the pulmonary circulation.

The differential diagnosis of truncus arteriosus requires consideration of many other anomalies, particularly those with conotruncal abnormalities. Prominent on the list of similar anomalies should be pulmonary atresia with large patent ductus arteriosus, aorticopulmonary window, double-outlet right ventricle, and even transposition of the great arteries with ventricular septal defect.

TREATMENT

Aside from supportive treatment for associated congestive heart failure, as well as prophylaxis against infective endocarditis, significant intervention in the unfavorable natural history of truncus arteriosus requires operative intervention. Such intervention may be either palliative or corrective.

Pulmonary Arterial Banding

Muller and Dammann (1952) first proposed that the pulmonary arteries could be narrowed so as to reduce pulmonary blood flow and relieve congestive heart failure in patients with large left-to-right shunts between the ventricles or between the great arteries. This procedure seemed particularly applicable before the availability of more corrective-type repair and even since that time has gained frequent application in the management of the infant with truncus arteriosus in congestive heart failure. Although the pulmonary arteries could be reached through a lateral thoracotomy, experience has led to the preference for median sternotomy as the better approach. Since the attempt to band the pulmonary artery proximal to its bifurcation has often resulted in excessive narrowing of one pulmonary arterial branch and inadequate narrowing of the opposite branch, now separate bands are preferably applied at the origin of each pulmonary artery, and the bands are anchored to the vessel to prevent distal migration (Parker *et al.*, 1975).

Palliation is successfully achieved in some infants as a result of banding the pulmonary arteries, but the mortality risk of the operation itself varies between 33 and 100 per cent, according to a review by Poirier and colleagues (1975). At least some of these surviving infants achieve adequate short-term palliation, as demonstrated by Ciaravella and associates (1979), who reported that among 120 of their patients with truncus arteriosus who underwent corrective operation, 41 (34 per cent) had survived previous banding of the pulmonary artery or arteries. Despite the increased technical complexity involved in corrective operation in such patients, these workers noted a lower early mortality rate (17 per cent) for patients who had previously undergone pulmonary arterial banding than for those who had not (32 per cent).

Corrective Operation

Successful corrective operation for truncus arteriosus was accomplished by two groups who were working independently — McGoon and associates (1968) and Weldon and Cameron (1968). Corrective operation involves the use of an extracardiac conduit. The development of this operation followed the successful use of such extracardiac conduits for other conditions (Klinner and Zenker, 1965; Rastelli *et al.*, 1965; Ross and Somerville, 1966; Behrendt *et al.*, 1974).

Technique. The operation is performed through a median sternotomy. Extracorporeal circulation is instituted, usually by cannulation of the external iliac or femoral artery, but in some instances, direct cannulation of the distal ascending aorta is feasible. The left ventricle is vented via either the atrium or the left ventricular apex. During the early moments of perfusion, as body temperature is being lowered quickly to 25°C., a danger exists that the central circulation and ventricles will become overdistended with blood owing to the large communication between the systemic and pulmonary circulations. For this reason, it is preferable to obstruct flow to the pulmonary arteries by clamping the pulmonary artery or its branches. This maneuver also facilitates the injection of cardioplegic solution into the truncal root, since otherwise much of the solution would find its way into the lungs rather than the coronary arteries. Similarly, the presence of significant truncal valve insufficiency might complicate myocardial perfusion with cold cardioplegic solution; in such instances, it is preferable to open the truncus along the anticipated line of excision

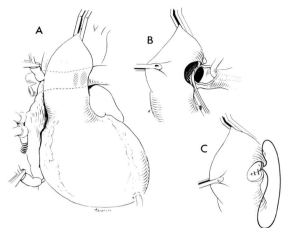

Figure 37–2. First step of surgical repair. *A*, Cardiopulmonary bypass instituted and ascending aorta clamped. *B*, Excision of pulmonary arteries from truncus. *C*, The defect in the truncus (aorta) is being repaired. (From Wallace, R. B., Rastelli, G. C., Ongley, P. A., Titus, J. L., and McGoon, D. C.: Complete repair of truncus arteriosus defects. J. Thorac. Cardiovasc. Surg., 57:95, 1969.)

of the pulmonary arteries from the truncus and, through this orifice, cannulate the coronary arteries individually and perfuse them with cardioplegic solution. The basic steps of the operative repair are three: (1) separation of the pulmonary artery (or arteries) from the truncus and closure of the resulting truncal defect; (2) right ventriculotomy and patch closure of the ventricular septal defect; and (3) establishment of continuity between the right ventricle and the pulmonary artery or arteries.

The pulmonary arteries are separated from the truncus as a single confluence in a Type II truncus arteriosus (Fig. 37–2). It is advisable to leave intact as much proximal length of the truncal (aortic) root as possible so that excision of the pulmonary arteries will not injure the orifice of the left coronary artery and so that distortion of the aortic root will not induce or increase incompetence of the truncal (aortic) valve. It is essential to identify and probe both pulmonary arteries, since the potential exists for misidentification of the left pulmonary artery as the main pulmonary artery, so that, inadvertently, the right pulmonary artery may remain attached to the truncus. After excision of the pulmonary arteries, the resulting defect in the truncus is precisely closed with a continuous, nonabsorbable everting mattress suture that is reinforced with a continuous over-and-over suture.

Experience has demonstrated that a simple longitudinal incision into the most downstream portion of the right ventricle is preferable to circular or oval excision of the free wall (Fig. 37–3*A*). Care is taken to avoid injury to the coronary arteries (Anderson *et al.*, 1978). The ventriculotomy may be carried superiorly nearly to the anulus of the truncal valve. Usually, it is preferable to undermine the ventriculotomy by excising endocardial myocardium from around the ventriculotomy. The ventricular septal defect is usu-

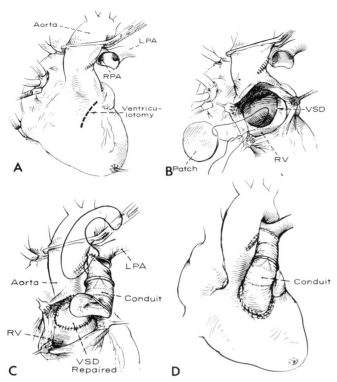

Figure 37–3. Completion of surgical repair (see text).

ally readily accessible since it involves the infundibular septum and often does not reach posteriorly to involve the membranous septum. The patch of synthetic material for closure of the ventricular septal defect is fashioned to an ample size (Fig. 37–3B,C). The patch is attached by continuous or interrupted sutures to the crest of the ventricular septum caudally and to the remaining margins of the ventricular septal defect; its cephalad margin is usually anchored to the epicardium and myocardium at the superior end of the ventriculotomy.

An extracardiac conduit is selected (Fig. 37–3C) that is as large as possible, not only to avoid an immediate gradient across the conduit but also to delay development of a gradient as a result of growth of the patient or peel formation on the inner aspect of the conduit, or both (Agarwal et al., 1981). It seems essential that the conduit contain a valve, since pulmonary arterial pressure is usually elevated to some degree postoperatively as a result of pre-existing elevation of pulmonary resistance. The length of the conduit may be easily estimated by measuring the distance from the caudal end of the ventriculotomy to the orifice of the pulmonary arteries, using a malleable wire. The conduit is trimmed in such a way that its valve lies just proximal to the distal anastomosis with the pulmonary arteries. Attention should be given to the avoidance of compression of a coronary artery (the left) by the rigid portion of the valvular support mechanism of the conduit. The pulmonary artery–to–conduit anastomosis should be accomplished unusually carefully with closely placed continuous

sutures, since the aforementioned elevation in pulmonary arterial pressure after repair poses an increased potential for bleeding along the suture line and since the anastomosis is somewhat inaccessible for placement of additional interrupted sutures at bleeding points later on. The ventricular anastomosis can be accomplished after release of the aortic clamp, during rewarming of the patient and while the heart is beating. The proximal conduit is cut on a wide oblique angle in order to minimize any tendency for contraction and stenosis at that level (Fig. 37–3D).

Several manufacturers supply valved conduits ranging from 12 to 30 mm. in diameter and containing glutaraldehyde-preserved tissue valves of porcine aortic or bovine pericardial origin. The earlier use of homograft aortas with integral aortic valves, sterilized and preserved by high-voltage radiation and freezing, respectively, has been abandoned because of the rapid tendency for calcification of such conduits (Moodie et al., 1976); others who have used fresh preserved homograft conduits remain enthusiastic about their use (Shabbo et al., 1980).

The presence of truncal valve insufficiency, even though mild, complicates the procedure and requires specific attention. If the incompetence is mild, especially in the infant, the valve probably can be left unrepaired; in that case, the chief attention required is that the ventricle not be allowed to overdistend with blood after release of the aortic clamp and before myocardial tone and myocardial contraction resume. Such overdistention of the left ventricle may not be relieved entirely simply by withdrawing blood through the vent in the left ventricle, but, in addition, intermittent manual emptying of the ventricle may be indicated. In instances in which the truncal valve insufficiency is more severe and especially in the older child, the resulting increased postoperative workload on the left ventricle may prevent a satisfactory result; therefore, the operation may need to be extended to allow replacement of the truncal valve (de Leval et al., 1974). Dramatically excellent long-term results can be achieved by such radical correction.

Interrupted aortic arch may coexist with truncus arteriosus, the interruption usually occurring between the left common carotid artery and the left subclavian artery. Repair of this associated anomaly can be accomplished by excising the pulmonary arteries from the posterior aspect of the truncus and repairing the truncus (aorta) in such a way that the ductus arteriosus continues to function as the aortic arch (Gomes and McGoon, 1971). Such a repair was required in three of the 92 truncus repairs encountered by Marcelletti and associates (1977).

Reconstruction of right ventricular outflow continuity is also technically complicated by previously placed pulmonary arterial bands, particularly if hypoplasia of one or both of the proximal pulmonary arteries results. The repair can be accomplished by extending the pulmonary arteriotomy laterally along each pulmonary artery until a satisfactory lumen is reached (Parker et al., 1975); then, a long anastomosis is made to this extended arteriotomy by "fishmouthing" the distal end of the conduit. Alternatively, especially in the presence of extended hypoplasia of the proximal pulmonary artery or arteries, a side-arm graft or a "T" graft to the distal normal pulmonary artery or arteries may be required. As noted previously, this extended technical requirement has not increased the hospital mortality rate, perhaps because pulmonary arteriolar protection was provided by the prior banding.

Results of Corrective Operation. Since corrective operation was first successfully accomplished only in 1967 and since truncus arteriosus is a relatively rare anomaly, usually resulting in death during infancy, relatively few reports of extensive experience with repair of truncus arteriosus are available in the literature. Even in reports that are available, the patients included undoubtedly represent a distortion of the true presentation of the anomaly in the general population, since in the larger series relatively few infants and rather large proportions of patients who have successfully survived earlier banding operations are included. Furthermore, most authors record their experience with repair of truncus arteriosus as part of a comprehensive experience in the use of extracardiac conduits for various anomalies. However, in general, the results of the various reports in the literature are comparable.

The largest review of results of surgical repair for truncus arteriosus as a discrete entity was provided by Marcelletti and colleagues (1977), who reviewed 92 patients. An expansion of this clinical experience to 120 patients has been reported as a part of a comprehensive review of extracardiac conduits by the same group (Ciaravella *et al.*, 1979; McGoon *et al.*, 1982).

In the discrete analysis of repair of truncus arteriosus (Marcelletti *et al.*, 1977), 23 of the 92 patients died within 30 days of operation (25 per cent). The postoperative complications and causes of early death are detailed in Table 37–3. No statistically significant relationship was found between the risk of early mortality and the sex of the patient, the anatomic type of truncus arteriosus, the presence of abnormalities in the pulmonary arterial tree, the presence of truncal valve regurgitation, the presence of associated cardiovascular anomalies, previous operation for palliation or exploration, or even the duration of extracorporeal circulation. However, a positive correlation was found between the age of the patient at the time of surgical repair and the early mortality, the risk being 83 per cent in patients less than 2 years of age and 21 per cent in patients more than 2 years of age (p<0.01) (Table 37–4). Most patients who were less than 2 years of age at operation were encountered in the earlier portion of this experience, and thus, the higher mortality for infants may be partially explained on this basis.

With the passage of time and increased experience and improved selection of patients, a reduction in risk of operation was noted during the evolution of

TABLE 37–3. POSTOPERATIVE COMPLICATIONS AND CAUSES OF EARLY SURGICAL DEATH IN CORRECTION OF TRUNCUS ARTERIOSUS (92 PATIENTS)*

	NO. OF PATIENTS
COMPLICATION	
Low output syndrome	23
Arrhythmia	17
Respiratory insufficiency (tracheostomy required in 15)	35†
Febrile course without identified infection	10‡
Bleeding required reoperation	5
Injury to central nervous system	2
Coagulation deficit with thrombocytopenia	1
Postcardiotomy syndrome	1
Gastrointestinal bleeding	1
Paralysis of left hemidiaphragm	1
Wound infection	1
CAUSES OF DEATH	
Low cardiac output	10§
Cardiac arrest before perfusion (anesthetic)	2
Respiratory insufficiency	4
Arrhythmia (ventricular tachycardia or fibrillation)	3
Hemorrhage	2
Heart block	1
Cardiac arrest	1

*From Marcelletti, C., *et al.*: Early and late results of surgical repair of truncus arteriosus. Circulation, 55:636, 1977.

†Defined as requiring endotracheal intubation 72 hours or more postoperatively.

‡Eight of these patients had received a Dacron conduit containing a porcine valve.

§Includes four patients unable to be discontinued from bypass.

the reported experience (Table 37–5). Thus, the risk of hospital mortality in the 33 more recent patients who had received a valved Dacron conduit was only 9 per cent, whereas the risk in the earlier group had been 34 per cent.

The latest status of these patients, now expanded to 120, is provided in the report by McGoon and colleagues (1982). The late survival of patients dismissed from the hospital after repair of truncus arteriosus was 95 per cent at 1 year, 83 per cent at 5 years, and 75 per cent at 10 years (Fig. 37–4). Of the patients dismissed from the hospital after repair of truncus arteriosus, and at a mean of 65 months later, 53 per cent were considered to have a good result, 25 per

TABLE 37–4. AGE AT TIME OF OPERATION AND SURGICAL RISK (92 PATIENTS WITH TRUNCUS ARTERIOSUS)*

AGE (YEARS)	NO. OF PATIENTS	HOSPITAL DEATHS	
		No.	%
<2	6	5	83†
2–4	20	5	25
5–12	52	10	19 } 21% (18/86)†
>12	14	3	21
Total	92	23	25

*From Marcelletti, C., *et al.*: Early and late results of surgical repair of truncus arteriosus. Circulation, 55:636, 1977.

†Significantly different (p < 0.01).

TABLE 37–5. YEAR OF OPERATION AND RELATIONSHIP TO SURGICAL RISK (92 PATIENTS WITH TRUNCUS ARTERIOSUS)*

PERIOD	NO. OF PATIENTS	HOSPITAL DEATHS	
		No.	%
1967–1972 (Jan.–Oct.)	59†	20	34‡
1967	2	0	0
1968	7	2	29
1969	15	5	33
1970	7	1	14
1971	15	7	47
1972 (Jan.–Oct.)	13	5	38
1972 (Nov.–Dec.)–1975	33	3	9‡
1972 (Nov.–Dec.)	1	0	0
1973	9	2	22
1974	20	1	5
1975	3	0	0

*From Marcelletti, C., *el al.*: Early and late results of surgical repair of truncus arteriosus. Circulation, *55*:636, 1977.

†Patients in the 1967 to 1972 group received an aortic homograft; patients in the 1972 to 1975 group received a Dacron conduit containing a porcine valve. One patient operated on at the end of 1972 received a Dacron conduit.

‡Significantly different (p<0.01).

cent fair, and 2 per cent poor; 19 per cent had died during the late follow-up period. The probability of reoperation (primarily required because of an increasing gradient across the extracardiac conduit) was 1 per cent at 1 year, 10 per cent at 5 years, and 35 per cent at 10 years (Fig. 37–5). However, the great majority of these reoperations were in patients who had received an aortic homograft conduit rather than a Dacron conduit containing a porcine valve; for patients surviving 5 years postoperatively, the likelihood of reoperation was 28 per cent for those having an aortic homograft conduit and only 6 per cent for those with the Hancock conduit.

Of particular interest with respect to late survival was the striking influence of age, in that late mortality was virtually absent among the youngest age group (infancy through 4 years of age) (Fig. 37–6).

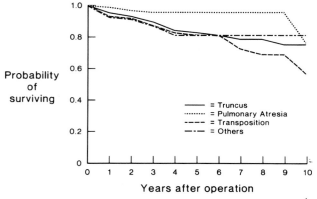

Figure 37–4. Graph showing late survival of patients who received an extracardiac conduit and survived the perioperative period. (From McGoon, D. C., Danielson, G. K., Puga, F. J., Ritter, D. G., Mair, D. D., and Ilstrup, D. M.: Late results after extracardiac conduit repair for congenital cardiac defects. Am. J. Cardiol., *49*:1741, 1982.

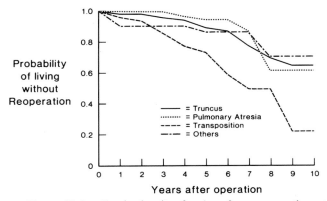

Figure 37–5. Graph showing freedom from reoperation at various postoperative intervals among patients surviving insertion of an extracardiac conduit. (From McGoon, D. C., Danielson, G. K., Puga, F. J., Ritter, D. G., Mair, D. D., and Ilstrup, D. M.: Late results after extracardiac conduit repair for congenital cardiac defects. Am. J. Cardiol., *49*:1741, 1982.)

INDICATIONS AND TIMING FOR OPERATION

Corrective operation is the definitive management for all patients with truncus arteriosus, and therefore, operation is indicated universally, except in the presence of compelling contraindications. The overwhelmingly predominant contraindication for corrective operation of truncus arteriosus is associated severe pulmonary vascular obstructive disease. Studies that have focused on the effect of the level of pulmonary arteriolar resistance on survival (Mair *et al.*, 1974; Marcelletti *et al.*, 1977) have demonstrated that patients with truncus arteriosus who have two pulmonary arteries and a pulmonary arteriolar resistance of greater than 8 units·M.² are at significantly higher early and late risk than are patients with resistances below that level. Of the initial 70 patients with truncus arteriosus who underwent correction in the study by Mair and associates (1974), 42 had pulmonary arteri-

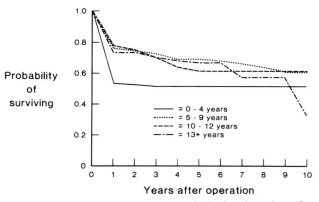

Figure 37–6. Graph showing survival after insertion of an extracardiac conduit, including early deaths, with respect to age grouping. This graph is of all patients receiving an extracardiac conduit, including patients with truncus arteriosus, but the results reflect appropriately the influence of age on late survival after truncus repair. (From McGoon, D. C., Danielson, G. K., Puga, F. J., Ritter, D. G., Mair, D. D., and Ilstrup, D. M.: Late results after extracardiac conduit repair for congenital cardiac defects. Am. J. Cardiol., *49*:1741, 1982.)

olar resistances of less than 8 units · M.², there were six operative deaths (14 per cent) and no late deaths secondary to advancing pulmonary hypertension. However, among the remaining 28 patients with pulmonary arteriolar resistances higher than 8 units · M.², there were 11 hospital deaths (39 per cent), and among the 17 patients surviving operation, there were five late deaths due to progression of pulmonary vascular obstruction disease with resulting right heart failure. Such findings strongly contraindicate corrective operation for patients whose pulmonary arteriolar resistance is greater than 8 units · M.². An exception to this policy exists for the child less than 2 years of age, since evidence suggests that such young patients can, during subsequent growth, develop new alveoli supplied by new undamaged vascular components.

Different criteria of operability are applied to patients with unilateral absence of a pulmonary artery. Since flow is directed to one lung instead of two in such patients, the degree of pulmonary arteriolar changes related to a given level of estimated pulmonary arteriolar resistance would be only half as severe as would be the case if two lungs were being perfused (Mair *et al.*, 1977). Thus, patients with a single pulmonary artery who have pulmonary arteriolar resistances up to 16 units · M.² may still be considered potential surgical candidates. Unfortunately, even though these theoretic projections have proved to be useful in predicting the early mortality after operation in this subset of patients having a single pulmonary artery, pulmonary vascular obstructive disease tends to progress postoperatively more often than it does in patients who have two pulmonary arteries. This observation seems explainable on the basis that the entire cardiac output must still pass through only one lung postoperatively; therefore, the rate of flow through each functioning arteriole would remain approximately doubled, thus producing a potential stimulus for the progression of pulmonary vascular changes.

Everything that is known about the natural history of truncus arteriosus indicates that if surgical correction is to have its greatest influence on the salvage of patients with this congenital anomaly, the ability to intervene surgically with relative safety while patients are still in their infancy must be developed. Unfortunately, with one exception, recent reports (Appelbaum *et al.*, 1976; Norwood *et al.*, 1977; Stark *et al.*, 1978; Locatelli *et al.*, 1980; Parenzan *et al.*, 1980) have shown early plus short-term mortality rates ranging from 46 to 80 per cent for patients younger than 1 or 2 years of age.

The exceptional experience is that of Ebert (Stanger *et al.*, 1977; Ebert, 1981), who reported an 11 per cent mortality rate for repair of truncus arteriosus in 56 infants less than 6 months of age. Twenty-two of Ebert's 56 patients had already required reoperation for replacement of the conduit from 1 to 3 years postoperatively, but without mortality. Although no information as to criteria for selection of patients for operation was provided, this record of achievement

will serve as a challenge to maintain and to emulate. Since even the aforementioned higher mortality rates are almost certainly a significant improvement over the natural history of the condition, and possibly an improvement over the staged approach of early banding and later correction, ample support exists for following a protocol of early corrective operation for patients born with truncus arteriosus.

SELECTED REFERENCES

Marcelletti, C., McGoon, D. C., Danielson, G. K., Wallace, R. B., and Mair, D. D.: Early and late results of surgical repair of truncus arteriosus. Circulation, *55*:636, 1977.

Ninety-two patients had corrective operations for truncus arteriosus between 1967 and 1975. Twenty-three patients died during the first 30 days after operation. No significant differences in risks were found among the many parameters studied, although higher levels of pulmonary resistance appeared to result in greater risk. Ninety-seven per cent of the survivors were asymptomatic or mildly symptomatic. The late result was suggestively less satisfactory in patients with significant preoperative truncal valve regurgitation. The current operative mortality of 9 per cent, as well as the late results, indicated a high degree of success for repair of truncus arteriosus.

Stanger, P., Robinson, S. J., Engle, M. A., and Ebert, P. A.: "Corrective" surgery for truncus arteriosus in the first year of life. (Abstract.) Am. J. Cardiol., *39*:293, 1977.

Management of truncus arteriosus during the first year of life has been a dilemma because of the high mortality of medical management, palliative banding, and previous attempts at complete correction. Eleven infants less than 1 year of age with either Type I or II truncus underwent surgical correction. Three were less than 3 months of age, five between 3 and 6 months, and three between 7 and 12 months. There was one death in the group. In all 11 patients, the ratio of pulmonary to systemic mean pressure was 1 or nearly 1 before operation, and in 10 patients, the ratio decreased to 0.4 or less after separation of the circulations. The one death occurred in an infant whose pulmonary artery pressures were higher than aortic pressure after separation of the circulations. Four patients underwent postoperative catheterizations, and a normal pulmonary vascular resistance was found in each. The low operative mortality in this age group suggests that corrective operation is an acceptable method of intervention to control failure and reduce the likelihood of developing pulmonary vascular disease, even though reoperation for enlargement of the conduit may be required.

REFERENCES

Agarwal, K. C., Edwards, W. D., Feldt, R. H., Danielson, G. K., Puga, F. J., and McGoon, D. C.: Clinicopathological correlates of obstructed right-sided porcine-valved extracardiac conduits. J. Thorac. Cardiovasc. Surg., *81*:591, 1981.

Anderson, K. R., McGoon, D. C., and Lie, J. T.: Surgical significance of the coronary arterial anatomy in truncus arteriosus communis. Am. J. Cardiol., *41*:76, 1978.

Appelbaum, A., Bargeron, L. M., Jr., Pacifico, A. D., and Kirklin, J. W.: Surgical treatment of truncus arteriosus, with emphasis on infants and small children. J. Thorac. Cardiovasc. Surg., *71*:436, 1976.

Behrendt, D. M., Kirsh, M. M., Stern, A., Sigmann, J., Perry, B., and Sloan, H.: The surgical therapy for pulmonary artery–right ventricular discontinuity. Ann. Thorac. Surg., *18*:122, 1974.

Bharati, S., McAllister, H. A., Jr., Rosenquist, G. C., Miller, R. A., Tatooles, C. J., and Lev, M.: The surgical anatomy of truncus arteriosus communis. J. Thorac. Cardiovasc. Surg., *67*:501, 1974.

Buchanan, A.: Malformation of heart: Undivided truncus arteriosus; heart otherwise double. Trans. Pathol. Soc. Lond., *15*:89, 1864.

Ciaravella, J. M., Jr., McGoon, D. C., Danielson, G. K., Wallace, R. B., Mair, D. D., and Ilstrup, D. M.: Experience with the extracardiac conduit. J. Thorac. Cardiovasc. Surg., *78*:920, 1979.

Collett, R. W., and Edwards, J. E.: Persistent truncus arteriosus: A classification according to anatomic types. Surg. Clin. North Am., 1949, p. 1245.

Crupi, G., Macartney, F. J., and Anderson, R. H.: Persistent truncus arteriosus: A study of 66 autopsy cases with special reference to definition and morphogenesis. Am. J. Cardiol., *40*:569, 1977.

de Leval, M. R., McGoon, D. C., Wallace, R. B., Danielson, G. K., and Mair, D. D.: Management of truncal valvular regurgitation. Ann. Surg., *180*:427, 1974.

Ebert, P. A.: Truncus arteriosus. *In* Congenital Heart Disease in the First Three Months of Life, Medical and Surgical Aspects. Edited by L. Parenzan, G. Crupi, and G. Graham. Bologna, Pàtron Editore, 1981, p. 439.

Fontana, R. S., and Edwards, J. E.: Congenital Cardiac Disease: A Review of 357 Cases Studied Pathologically. Philadelphia, W. B. Saunders Company, 1962, p. 95.

Gomes, M. M. R., and McGoon, D. C.: Truncus arteriosus with interruption of the aortic arch. Report of a case successfully repaired. Mayo Clin. Proc., *46*:40, 1971.

Hagler, D. J., Tajik, A. J., Seward, J. B., Mair, D. D., and Ritter, D. G.: Wide-angle two-dimensional echocardiographic profiles of conotruncal abnormalities. Mayo Clin. Proc., *55*:73, 1980.

Klinner, W., and Zenker, R.: Experience with correction of Fallot's tetralogy in 178 cases. Surgery, *57*:353, 1965.

Krongrad, E., Ritter, D. G., Hawe, A., Kincaid, O. W., and McGoon, D. C.: Pulmonary atresia or severe stenosis and coronary artery–to–pulmonary artery fistula. Circulation, *46*:1005, 1972.

Locatelli, G., Alfieri, O., Villani, M., Crupi, G., and Parenzan, L.: Traitement chirurgical du truncus arteriosus dans la première année de la vie. (Surgical treatment of truncus arteriosus in the first year of life.) Chir. Pédiatr., *21*:89, 1980.

Mair, D. D., Ritter, D. G., Danielson, G. K., Wallace, R. B., and McGoon, D. C.: Truncus arteriosus with unilateral absence of a pulmonary artery: Criteria for operability and surgical results. Circulation, *55*:641, 1977.

Mair, D. D., Ritter, D. G., Davis, G. D., Wallace, R. B., Danielson, G. K., and McGoon, D. C.: Selection of patients with truncus arteriosus for surgical correction: Anatomic and hemodynamic considerations. Circulation, *49*:144, 1974.

Marcelletti, C., McGoon, D. C., and Mair, D. D.: The natural history of truncus arteriosus. Circulation, *54*:108, 1976.

Marcelletti, C., McGoon, D. C., Danielson, G. K., Wallace, R. B., and Mair, D. D.: Early and late results of surgical repair of truncus arteriosus. Circulation, *55*:636, 1977.

McGoon, D. C., Rastelli, G. C., and Ongley, P. A.: An operation for the correction of truncus arteriosus. J.A.M.A., *205*:69, 1968.

McGoon, D. C., Danielson, G. K., Puga, F. J., Ritter, D. G., Mair, D. D., and Ilstrup, D. M.: Late results after extracardiac conduit repair for congenital cardiac defects. Am. J. Cardiol., *49*:1741, 1982.

Moodie, D. S., Mair, D. D., Fulton, R. E., Wallace, R. B., Danielson, G. K., and McGoon, D. C.: Aortic homograft obstruction. J. Thorac. Cardiovasc. Surg., *72*:553, 1976.

Muller, W. H., Jr., and Dammann, J. F., Jr.: The treatment of certain congenital malformations of the heart by the creation of pulmonic stenosis to reduce pulmonary hypertension and excessive pulmonary blood flow: A preliminary report. Surg. Gynecol. Obstet., *95*:213, 1952.

Norwood, W. I., Freed, M. D., Rocchini, A. P., Bernhard, W. F., and Castaneda, A. R.: Experience with valved conduits for repair of congenital cardiac lesions. Ann. Thorac. Surg., *24*:223, 1977.

Parenzan, L., Crupi, G., Alfieri, O., Bianchi, T., Vanini, V., Locatelli, G., Tirboschi, R., DiBenedetto, G., Villani, M., Annecchino, F. P., and Ferrazzi, P.: Surgical repair of persistent truncus arteriosus in infancy. Thorac. Cardiovasc. Surg., *28*:18, 1980.

Parker, R. K., McGoon, D. C., Danielson, G. K., Wallace, R. B., and Mair, D. D.: Repair of truncus arteriosus in patients with prior banding of the pulmonary artery. Surgery, *78*:761, 1975.

Poirier, R. A., Berman, M. A., and Stansel, H. C., Jr.: Current status of the surgical treatment of truncus arteriosus. J. Thorac. Cardiovasc. Surg., *69*:169, 1975.

Rastelli, G. C., Ongley, P. A., Davis, G. D., and Kirklin, J. W.: Surgical repair for pulmonary valve atresia with coronary-pulmonary artery fistula: Report of case. Mayo Clin. Proc., *40*:521, 1965.

Ross, D. N., and Somerville, J.: Correction of pulmonary atresia with a homograft aortic valve. Lancet, *2*:1446, 1966.

Shabbo, F. P., Wain, W. H., and Ross, D. N.: Right ventricular outflow reconstruction with aortic homograft conduit: Analysis of the long-term results. Thorac. Cardiovasc. Surg., *28*:21, 1980.

Stanger, P., Robinson, S. J., Engle, M. A., and Ebert, P. A.: "Corrective" surgery for truncus arteriosus in the first year of life. (Abstract.) Am. J. Cardiol., *39*:293, 1977.

Stark, J., Gandhi, D., de Leval, M., Macartney, F., and Taylor, J. F. N.: Surgical treatment of persistent truncus arteriosus in the first year of life. Br. Heart. J., *40*:1280, 1978.

Van Praagh, R., and Van Praagh, S.: The anatomy of common aorticopulmonary trunk (truncus arteriosus communis) and its embryologic implications: A study of 57 necropsy cases. Am. J. Cardiol., *16*:406, 1965.

Wallace, R. B., Rastelli, G. C., Ongley, P. A., Titus, J. L., and McGoon, D. C.: Complete repair of truncus arteriosus defects. J. Thorac. Cardiovasc. Surg., *57*:95, 1969.

Weldon, C. S., and Cameron, J. L.: Correction of persistent truncus arteriosus. J. Cardiovasc. Surg., *9*:463, 1968.

Chapter 38

Congenital Aortic Stenosis

GRADY L. HALLMAN
DENTON A. COOLEY

ANATOMY

Aortic stenosis may occur in one or more of three anatomic sites: supravalvar, valvar, or subvalvar. The most common form of obstruction occurs at the level of the aortic valve. Fusion of cusps restricts the effective orifice and may offer resistance to ejection by the left ventricle and result in hypertrophy, dilatation, and eventual failure of this chamber. Several anatomic forms of aortic stenosis have been described (Ellis and Kirklin, 1962). In our experience, the most common type is one in which the valve is functionally bicuspid (Fig. 38–1). The left and right coronary cusps are fused and are separated by a vestigial commissure represented by a raphe extending centrally from the anulus for varying distances. These two cusps function as a single leaflet and are separated from the noncoronary cusp by a long, fused commissure with a small central or eccentric opening.

Subvalvar aortic stenosis is next in frequency. This may be due to a fibrous diaphragm located a few millimeters below the aortic valve or to a diffuse, fibromuscular "tunnel" beneath the aortic leaflets. A third type of subaortic stenosis is called hypertrophic obstructive cardiomyopathy (also known as idiopathic hypertrophic subaortic stenosis) (Braunwald et al., 1960). In this lesion, outflow obstruction is due to hypertrophy of the interventricular septum and systolic anterior motion of the mitral valve and/or chor-

dae. This motion brings these structures into apposition with the septum and further narrows the left ventricular outflow tract (Henry et al., 1975).

The least common form of left ventricular outflow obstruction occurs in the supravalvar area. The aorta is constricted just above the coronary ostia in a manner somewhat similar to that seen in coarctation of the aorta. Indeed, this anomaly may be considered a coarctation of the ascending aorta. Valve leaflets may be normal or thickened. Intimal hypertrophy is often present in the surrounding aorta and may extend distally into the brachiocephalic vessels or proximally and involve the ostia of the coronary arteries.

HISTORY

According to a review of early literature by Kumpe and Bean (1948), stenosis of the aortic valve was described by Boneti in 1700 and by Morgagni in 1769. Brock (1954) was the first to report successful results in the relief of aortic stenosis by closed transventricular valvotomy. The use of hypothermia to permit open valvotomy under direct vision was reported by Swan and Kortz (1956) and by Lewis and associates (1956). Lillehei and colleagues (1958) utilized temporary cardiopulmonary bypass for aortic valvotomy, and the pump-oxygenator has been universally adopted as the best means of support for such procedures.

Williams and coworkers (1961) were the first to describe the characteristic facies and mental retardation in patients with supravalvar aortic stenosis. McGoon and associates (1961) and Starr and colleagues (1961) reported successful surgical correction of this variant of aortic stenosis.

Surgical treatment of muscular subaortic stenosis was first described by Brock (1957). A comprehensive review of this lesion was provided by Braunwald and coworkers (1960). This form of aortic stenosis is discussed in this chapter, but uncertainty exists about whether to classify it as a congenital or an acquired lesion. Surgical techniques used in patients with this condition include transventricular instrumental dilatation (Brock, 1959), transaortic myotomy (Morrow and Brockenbrough, 1961), excision of subaortic mus-

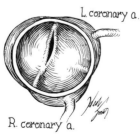

Figure 38–1. Drawing indicating anatomy of common type of aortic valve stenosis. Valve is functionally bicuspid. Left and right coronary cusps are fused and are separated by a vestigial commissure represented by a raphe extending centrally from the anulus. Left and right coronary cusps function as a single leaflet and are separated from noncoronary cusp by a long, fused commissure with a small opening.

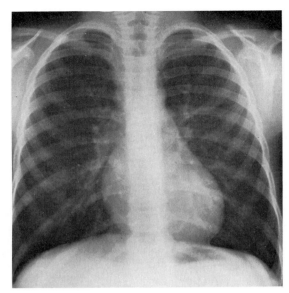

Figure 38–2. Posteroanterior roentgenogram of the chest in a 7-year-old male with aortic valve stenosis showing normal size and configuration of the heart. Gradient across valve was 90 mm. Hg. (From Hallman, G. L., and Cooley, D. A.: Surgical Treatment of Congenital Heart Disease. 2nd Ed. Philadelphia, Lea and Febiger, 1975.)

cle through the left atrium (Lillehei and Levy, 1963) or the left ventricle (Kirklin and Ellis, 1961), and removal of muscle from the right side of the ventricular septum (Harken, 1961; Cooley et al., 1967).

DIAGNOSIS

Aortic stenosis can usually be identified on clinical grounds, but cardiac catheterization should be done to confirm the diagnosis and to quantitate the severity of the obstruction. Patients with mild aortic stenosis may be asymptomatic. Severe aortic stenosis can result in heart failure during the first few days or weeks of life and may be fatal. Syncope may be present in childhood or later, and sudden death may occur during exertion.

An ejection systolic murmur, frequently accompanied by a thrill, is the characteristic auscultatory finding in patients with valvar aortic stenosis. The findings on roentgenography of the chest may vary from a normal cardiac silhouette in patients with mild aortic stenosis to advanced stages of cardiac enlargement, left atrial dilatation, and pulmonary edema (Figs. 38–2 and 38–3). Electrocardiographic findings are variable but usually include left ventricular hypertrophy and possibly strain.

Cardiac catheterization is done to measure the gradient across the outflow tract of the left ventricle, so that the severity of obstruction can be assessed. The level in the left ventricular outflow tract at which pressure change occurs may localize the site of obstruction, but precise identification of the type of aortic stenosis usually requires selective angiocardiog-

raphy with contrast material injected into the left ventricle. A catheter may be passed into this chamber retrograde across the aortic valve or antegrade via the transseptal route.

INDICATIONS FOR OPERATION

Young infants with heart failure who respond poorly to medical therapy should be operated on. Older infants and adults with syncope or cardiac failure should be treated surgically after completion of diagnostic studies. In patients with valvar aortic stenosis and minimal or no symptoms, operation is recommended if the gradient is 70 mm. Hg or greater or if progressive left ventricular hypertrophy is present.

SURGICAL TECHNIQUE

All forms of aortic stenosis require cardiopulmonary bypass for successful treatment (Hallman and Cooley, 1975). We utilize a median sternotomy with the patient in the supine position. Perfusion is conducted at normothermia, using disposable plastic bubble oxygenators (Cooley et al., 1962, 1965). In infants weighing less than 20 pounds, the extracorporeal circuit is primed with heparinized blood. Five per cent dextrose in distilled water is used in patients weighing more than 20 pounds. A sump suction cannula is placed in the left atrium via the right superior pulmonary vein. The coronary arteries are not perfused. The technique used for the relief of left ventricular outflow obstruction depends on the site of stenosis.

Supra-aortic Stenosis. The ascending aorta is thickened, and an indentation or a constriction may be noted 1 cm. or so above the anulus. Coronary arteries are usually dilated, and the aortic valve is normal. After the institution of cardiopulmonary bypass, the ascending aorta is clamped just proximal to the innominate artery. A vertical incision is made in the right anterolateral aspect of the aorta, beginning above the constricted area and extending across it into the noncoronary sinus of Valsalva (Fig. 38–4). If a cleavage plane exists at the site of constriction, an endarterectomy is done. In some cases, it may be necessary to extend the endarterectomy distally to the innominate artery. The valve and subaortic area are examined carefully, because multiple sites of obstruction may be present. An elliptical patch of woven Dacron is sutured into the incision in the ascending aorta to widen the previously constricted area. Wider patches must be used in those patients in whom an endarterectomy is not possible. In some patients, the aortotomy may be closed by primary suture. If the aortic constriction is sharply localized, excision and primary anastomosis may be possible as in coarctation of the aorta.

Valvar Stenosis. The ascending aorta is usually dilated, and a thrill can be felt. A transverse incision is made about 1 to 2 cm. above the anulus. The valve

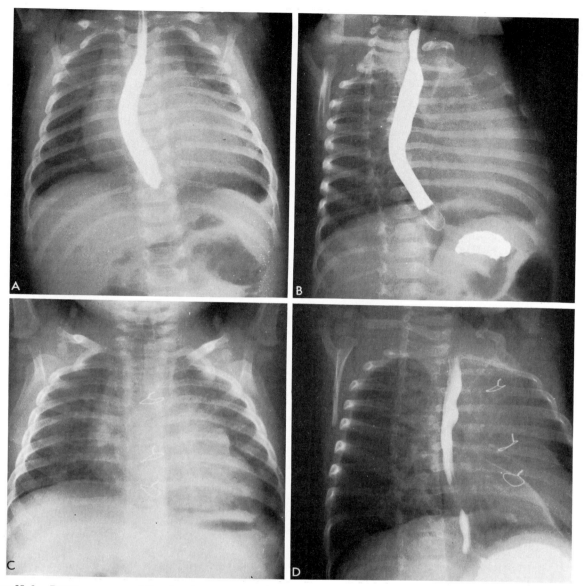

Figure 38–3. Roentgenograms of the chest in an 8-week-old male with aortic valve stenosis. *A,* Posteroanterior view shows marked cardiac enlargement with normal pulmonary arterial markings. *B,* Right anterior oblique view shows considerable displacement of barium-filled esophagus by dilated left atrium. *C,* Posteroanterior roentgenogram of the chest 4 months after valvotomy shows decrease in the size of the heart. *D,* Right anterior oblique view 4 months after operation indicates that the left atrium is no longer dilated. (From Hallman, G. L., and Cooley, D. A.: Surgical Treatment of Congenital Heart Disease. 2nd Ed. Philadelphia, Lea and Febiger, 1975.)

is usually deformed in the manner described earlier in the section on anatomy. An incision is made along the fused commissure between the combined left and right coronary cusps on one side and the noncoronary cusp on the other side. These incisions should stop about 1 or 2 mm. short of the anulus in order to avoid unhinging leaflets and producing aortic insufficiency. The rudimentary commissure between the right and left coronary cusps is not incised, since aortic valvar incompetence may result. The basic technique of valvotomy is the same for other forms of valvar incompetence stenosis (Fig. 38–4). Two incisions are made through fused commissures, creating a bicuspid valve. Rarely, it may be possible to form a tricuspid valve. After examining the subaortic area for evi-

dence of disease, the ascending aorta is closed with continuous suture.

In some adults with congenital aortic stenosis, fibrosis and calcification may make valvotomy and reconstruction impossible. Excision and replacement with a prosthesis constitute the treatment of choice in these patients (Cooley *et al.,* 1965).

Subaortic Stenosis. If subaortic stenosis is due to a fibrous membrane, a transverse incision is made in the proximal ascending aorta (Fig. 38–4). Valve leaflets, which are usually normal, are gently retracted. The membrane is excised with a scalpel blade, avoiding injury to the ventricular septum anteriorly and to the right, and to the mitral valve posteriorly and to the left.

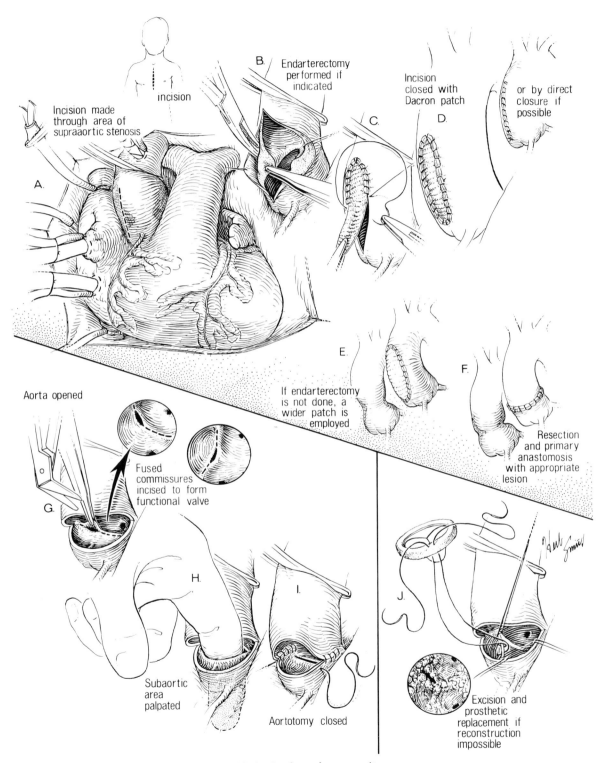

incision

B. Endarterectomy performed if indicated

Incision made through area of supraaortic stenosis

A.

C.

Incision closed with Dacron patch

D. or by direct closure if possible

E. If endarterectomy is not done, a wider patch is employed

F. Resection and primary anastomosis with appropriate lesion

Aorta opened

G. Fused commissures incised to form functional valve

H. Subaortic area palpated

I. Aortotomy closed

J. Excision and prosthetic replacement if reconstruction impossible

Figure 38–4 *See legend on opposite page*

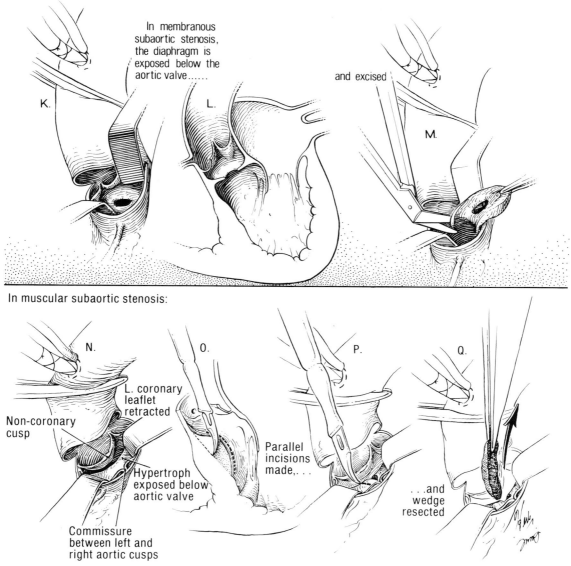

Figure 38–4. Drawings indicating techniques of operation in patients with various types of aortic stenosis. *Inset,* Median sternotomy. *A,* Cannulation done, cardiopulmonary bypass begun, and ascending aorta clamped. In patients with supra-aortic stenosis, a vertical incision is made through constricted area to right of midline extending toward noncoronary sinus of Valsalva (dotted line). *B,* Endarterectomy is performed if cleavage plane exists between inner coats of aorta at constriction. *C* and *D,* Incision is closed with Dacron patch and continuous suture. Direct closure may be utilized if technically feasible. *E,* Larger Dacron patch is used if endarterectomy is not done. *F,* If constriction is well localized, circumferential excision and primary end-to-end aortic anastomosis may be done. *G,* In patients with valvar stenosis, the aorta is incised transversely. Site of commissural incisions depends on anatomic features present. In one type of stenosis shown here, fused commissure between left and right coronary cusps and between left and noncoronary cusps are cut to within 1 to 2 mm. of the anulus. Bicuspid valve results. Also shown is valve in which fused commissures between right and noncoronary cusps and between left and noncoronary cusps are cut. Resulting bicuspid valve has fused left and right cusps on one side and noncoronary cusps on the other. *K,* In patients with membranous subaortic stenosis, a low transverse aortotomy is made and valve leaflets retracted. *L,* Stenosis is caused by a fibrous diaphragm below the valve. *M,* Membrane is excised using scissors or scalpel. *N,* Drawing shows anatomy of idiopathic hypertrophic subaortic stenosis. Leaflets are retracted revealing hypertrophy anteriorly. *O* and *P,* Parallel incisions made at commissure between right and left coronary cusps extending from apex to valve. *Q,* Intervening wedge of muscle excised. See text for discussion of mitral valve replacement. (From Hallman, G. L., and Cooley, D. A.: Surgical Treatment of Congenital Heart Disease. 2nd Ed. Philadelphia, Lea and Febiger, 1975.)

In patients with idiopathic hypertrophic subaortic stenosis, we use a modification of the operative technique originally described by Morrow and Brockenbrough (1961) (Fig. 38–4). The aorta is opened with a low transverse incision, and the aortic leaflets are gently retracted. Coronary arteries are not perfused. The hypertrophied septum is cut vertically at a point beneath the commissure between the right and left coronary cusps. This incision is made with a curved tonsil-type blade and extends from a point near the apex to the area just under the aortic valve. A parallel incision is made about a centimeter to the right of this, and a strip of muscle is excised. Care must be taken not to cut through the septum.

Abnormality of the anterior leaflet of the mitral valve may contribute to outflow obstruction in patients with idiopathic hypertrophic subaortic stenosis. If gross mitral regurgitation is present, selected patients may benefit from replacement of the mitral valve with a prosthesis (Shumacker, 1965; Cooley et al., 1973).

COMPLICATIONS

Hemorrhage may occur from the incision in the aorta. Unusual or persistent drainage of blood from thoracostomy tubes and the appearance of cardiac tamponade or hemothorax are indications for immediate reoperation. Heart failure may be present in infants and is usually a continuation of the process that led to operation. Response to medical therapy is usually satisfactory if valvotomy is adequate. Aortic regurgitation may be noted especially if fused commissures are cut completely to the anulus. There is little cause for concern as long as the diastolic pressure is 60 mm. Hg or greater. Aortic regurgitation has rarely been a problem in the early postoperative period. Small infants seem to tolerate mild insufficiency better than they tolerate stenosis. Heart block may occur during operations for subaortic stenosis. If heart block or A-V dissociation is present, myocardial wires should be implanted in the right ventricle and brought out through the skin. A satisfactory rate can be maintained with an external pacemaker. If a sinus rhythm does not return within 2 weeks, a permanent pacemaker should be implanted before the patient is discharged from the hospital.

SELECTED REFERENCES

Campbell, M.: The natural history of congenital aortic stenosis. Br. Heart J., 30:514, 1968.

The author studied 87 patients and reviewed the literature. One-fifth had subvalvar stenosis. The risk of sudden death is at least 0.4 per cent per annum in the first three decades and twice this in those seen in the hospital.

Cohen, L. S., Friedman, W. F., and Braunwald, E.: Natural history of mild congenital aortic stenosis elucidated by serial hemodynamic studies. Am. J. Cardiol., 30:1, 1972.

The authors studied 15 initially asymptomatic children first seen at an average age of 8.5 years and again at an average age of 15.1 years. They concluded that congenital aortic stenosis may be a progressive disorder, even early in life, in a significant percentage of patients presenting initially with mild obstruction.

Dobell, A. R. C., Bloss, R. S., Gibbons, J. E., and Collins, G. F.: Congenital valvular aortic stenosis: Surgical management and long-term results. J. Thorac. Cardiovasc. Surg., 81:916, 1981.

Case histories of 50 consecutive infants and children with congenital aortic valve stenosis are reviewed. All had valvotomy over a 16-year period. Seven patients died (14 per cent), six of whom were infants. Eight- to 16-year follow-up of the first 25 survivors revealed one late death, four "good" results, five aortic valve replacements, and three secondary valvotomies. Ten patients have recurrent aortic stenosis, and two have moderate aortic insufficiency. The authors emphasize that aortic valvotomy is a palliative operation, and about a third of the children operated on required a second operation within 10 years.

El-Said, G., Galioto, F. M., Mullins, C. E., and McNamara, D. G.: Natural hemodynamic history of congenital aortic stenosis in childhood. Am. J. Cardiol., 30:6, 1972.

In a series of 37 patients, 28 had valvar stenosis. Repeat catheterization demonstrated that in the majority of patients the anomaly increased in severity.

Glew, R. H., Varghese, P. J., Krovetz, L. J., Dorst, J. P., and Rowe, R. D.: Sudden death in congenital aortic stenosis: A review of eight cases with evaluation of premonitory clinical features. Am. Heart J., 78:615, 1969.

The authors describe eight cases of sudden death during a 20-year period at the Pediatric Clinic of Johns Hopkins Hospital, Baltimore. They state that death may be sudden but should not be entirely unexpected because of warning symptoms. They concluded that even mild cases of congenital aortic stenosis may progress and require careful follow-up.

Konno, S., Imai, Y., Nakajima, M., and Tatsuno, K.: A new method for prosthetic valve replacement in congenital aortic stenosis associated with hypoplasia of the aortic valve ring. J. Cardiovasc. Surg., 70:909, 1975.

Many patients with congenital aortic stenosis have a small anulus, making valve replacement difficult should this be necessary after an initial valvotomy. The authors describe a new technique for enlarging the anulus by making an incision through it into the septum and outflow tract of the right ventricle. Patches are inserted to widen the anulus and close the incisions. Thus, a larger prosthesis can be used.

Kugler, J. D., Campbell, E., Vargo, T. A., McNamara, D. G., Hallman, G. L., and Cooley, D. A.: Results of aortic valvotomy in infants with isolated aortic valvular stenosis. J. Thorac. Cardiovasc. Surg., 78:553, 1979.

Thirty-nine infants less than a year of age underwent valvotomy over a 21-year period for isolated aortic valve stenosis. The average age at operation was 10.7 weeks. The mortality rate was 33 per cent (13 patients). Eleven of these early deaths occurred in the 21 infants less than 2 months of age. Follow-up (mean — 7.2 years) of the 26 survivors revealed that 34 had aortic insufficiency clinically, but the only repeat aortic valve operation necessary in the 26 was an aortic valve replacement performed at 17 years of age in a patient with severe aortic insufficiency.

Lindesmith, G. G., Fyler, D. C., Meyer, B. W., and Jones, J. C.: Congenital valvular aortic stenosis: An evaluation of surgical experience. Ann. Thorac. Surg., 3:406, 1967.

Forty-two patients less than 25 years of age were operated on for valvar stenosis. The authors describe the current operative technique of open-heart surgery and mild hypothermia. They emphasize the use of limited commissurotomy to avoid aortic insufficiency.

McGoon, D. C., Geha, A. S., Scofield, E. L., and DuShane, J. S.: Surgical treatment of congenital aortic stenosis. Dis. Chest, 55:388, 1969.

The authors present a series of 169 patients less than 25 years old and state that aortic valvotomy is primarily a palliative procedure. This operation produced adequate relief of gradient in only 56 per cent of patients and left a severe gradient in 20 per cent. Operative mortality was low, and there were no deaths in seven infants.

Mody, M. R., Nadas, A. S., and Bernhard, W. F.: Aortic stenosis in infants. N. Engl. J. Med., 276:832, 1967.

The 24 infants in this report were all those seen at the Children's Hospital Medical Center, Boston, between 1958 and 1966 with a diagnosis of aortic stenosis. The authors recommend surgical treatment for all infants with severe aortic stenosis leading to congestive heart failure. Seventeen infants were operated on. Operative mortality was reduced by using inflow occlusion under hyperbaric conditions.

Mulder, D. G., Katz, R. D., Moss, A. J., and Hurwitz, R. A.: The surgical treatment of congenital aortic stenosis. J. Thorac. Cardiovasc. Surg., 55:786, 1968.

In a series of 45 children, 21 had valvular stenosis. Cardiopulmonary bypass and hypothermia at 30° C. were used and incisions were made to form a bicuspid valve. The authors describe their disappointment with surgical treatment of congenital aortic stenosis because of the limitations imposed by anatomy, i.e., inability to cut far enough to relieve completely the stenosis for fear of causing aortic regurgitation.

REFERENCES

Braunwald, E. A., Morrow, A. G., Cornell, W. P., Aygen, M. M., and Hilbish, T. F.: Idiopathic hypertrophic muscular stenosis: Clinical, hemodynamic, and angiographic manifestations. Am. J. Med., 29:924, 1960.

Brock, R. C.: Valvotomy for aortic stenosis. Br. Heart J., 16:471, 1954.

Brock, R. C.: Functional obstruction of the left ventricle: Acquired aortic subvalvular stenosis. Guy's Hosp. Rep., 126:221, 1957.

Brock, R. C.: Aortic subvalvular stenosis: Surgical treatment. Guy's Hosp. Rep., 108:144, 1959.

Cooley, D. A., Beall, A. C., Jr., and Grondin, P.: Open-heart operations with disposable oxygenators, 5 per cent dextrose prime, and normothermia. Surgery, 52:713, 1962.

Cooley, D. A., Beall, A. C., Jr., and Hallman, G. L.: Open-heart surgery using disposable plastic oxygenators, 5 per cent dextrose for priming and maintenance of normothermia: Ex-perience with 1162 operations. Ann. Chir. Thorac. Cardio-vasc., 4:233, 1965.

Cooley, D. A., Leachman, R. D., and Wukasch, D. C.: Diffuse muscular subaortic stenosis: Surgical treatment. Am. J. Car-diol., 31:1, 1973.

Cooley, D. A., Beall, A. C., Jr., Hallman, G. L., and Bricker, D. L.: Obstructive lesions of the left ventricular outflow tract. Circulation, 31:612, 1965.

Cooley, D. A., Bloodwell, R. D., Hallman, G. L., LaSorte, A. F., Leachman, R. D., and Chapman, D. W.: Surgical treatment of muscular subaortic stenosis: Results from septectomy in twenty-six patients. Circulation, 35, 36(Suppl. I):124, 1967.

Ellis, F. H., and Kirklin, J. W.: Congenital valvular aortic stenosis: Anatomic findings and surgical technique. J. Thorac. Cardio-vasc. Surg., 43:199, 1962.

Hallman, G. L., and Cooley, D. A.: Surgical Treatment of Congen-ital Heart Disease. 2nd Ed. Philadelphia, Lea and Febiger, 1975.

Harken, D. E.: Cited by Morrow, A. G., and Brockenbrough, E. C. (1961).

Henry, W. L., Clark, C. E., Griffith, J. M., and Epstein, S. E.: Mechanism of left ventricular outflow obstruction in patients with obstructive asymmetrical septal hypertrophy (idiopathic hypertrophic subaortic stenosis). Am. J. Cardiol., 35:362, 1975.

Kirklin, J. W., and Ellis, F. H.: Surgical relief of diffuse subvalvular aortic stenosis. Circulation, 24:739, 1961.

Kumpe, C. W., and Bean, W. B.: Aortic stenosis: A study of the clinical and pathologic aspects of 107 proved cases. Medicine, 27:739, 1948.

Lewis, F. J., Shumway, N. E., Niazi, S. A., and Benjamin, R. B: Aortic valvulotomy under direct vision during hypothermia. J. Thorac. Surg., 32:481, 1956.

Lillehei, C. W., and Levy, M. J.: Transatrial exposure for correc-tion of subaortic stenosis. J.A.M.A., 186:8, 1963.

Lillehei, C. W., Gott, V. L., DeWall, R. A., and Varco, R. L.: Surgical treatment of stenotic or regurgitant lesions of the mitral and aortic valves by direct vision utilizing a pump oxygenator. J. Thorac. Surg., 35:154, 1958.

McGoon, D. C., Mankin, H. T., Vlad, P., and Kirklin, J. W.: The surgical treatment of supravalvular aortic stenosis. J. Thorac. Cardiovasc. Surg., 41:125, 1961.

Morrow, A. G., and Brockenbrough, E. C.: Surgical treatment of idiopathic hypertrophic subaortic stenosis. Technic and hemo-dynamic results of subaortic ventriculomyotomy. Ann. Surg., 154:181, 1961.

Shumacker, H. B.: New operative approach in the management of hypertrophic subaortic stenosis. J. Thorac. Cardiovasc. Surg., 49:497, 1965.

Starr, A., Dotter, C., and Griswold, H.: Supravalvular aortic stenosis: Diagnosis and treatment. J. Thorac. Cardiovasc. Surg., 41:134, 1961.

Swan, H., and Kortz, A. B.: Direct vision trans-aortic approach to the aortic valve during hypothermia. Experimental observa-tions and report of successful clinical case. Ann. Surg., 144:205, 1956.

Williams, J. C. P., Barratt-Boyes, B. G., and Lowe, J. B.: Supra-valvular aortic stenosis. Circulation, 24:1131, 1961.

Chapter 39

Congenital Mitral Stenosis

JAMES W. KILMAN

Congenital mitral stenosis is a rare cardiac lesion, almost always associated with other congenital abnormalities of the heart and great vessels (Ferencz et al., 1954). In patients with severe obstruction of the deformed mitral valve, the prognosis without operation is almost hopeless, and the infants die of right heart failure. An analysis of published reports indicates that one fifth of the children with congenital mitral stenosis die in the first month of life, and one half of them die within 1 year. Only one fifth survive to 3 years of age or longer. Surgery offers the opportunity of relief of the obstruction and survival of the infant or child. Since the development of obstructive pulmonary vascular disease probably occurs in the first year of life, there is some evidence that surgery should be done prior to the first birthday for the infant with this type of obstruction (Ruckman and Van Praagh, 1979).

There is some confusion concerning the nomenclature of congenital mitral stenosis, and all of the following terms may be used: stenosis, common narrowing or stricture, incomplete or defective development of valvular tissue, atresia, imperforate mitral valve, and mitral valve arcade. The lesions most commonly associated with congenital mitral stenosis have been patent ductus arteriosus, aortic stenosis, coarctation of the aorta, abnormalities of the cusps of the aortic valve, and, rarely, ventricular or atrial septal defects. Isolated congenital mitral stenosis does occur, but it is less frequent than the simultaneous occurrence with one of the aforementioned anomalies (Lassrich and Keck, 1967).

Surgery for congenital mitral stenosis was not attempted until after the popularization of the closed mitral valvulotomy by Bailey and Harken. The first successful closed mitral commissurotomy for congenital mitral stenosis was done by Manheimer and associates in 1952. The first successful mitral valve replacement in an infant with congenital mitral stenosis was done by Young and Robinson in 1964. In 1971, in a 20-year review of the literature, Humblet and colleagues found reports of 50 patients who had undergone surgery for congenital mitral stenosis. In 42 of these patients, a closed or open mitral commissurotomy was done, with a mortality rate of 50 per cent. Eight infants had had replacement of their mitral valves by either a Starr-Edwards valve prosthesis or a disc-type valve prosthesis. In a study in 1976 by Carpentier and coworkers in which information was pooled from surgical teams

in Italy, France, and the Netherlands, the treatment of all congenital malformations of the mitral valve was reviewed. The surgical approach to these lesions was innovative, and most procedures were of a reparative nature but did not include a large group of small infants. With the use of the newer modes of echocardiography, specifically two-dimensional echocardiography, earlier diagnosis in infancy can be made and these patients could be taken to surgery prior to the development of obstructive pulmonary vascular disease. With the use of profound hypothermia, infant bypass is safe and better results should be obtained in this very difficult, rare lesion. Congenital mitral stenosis is an anomaly that is difficult to manage. In a large group of patients treated at the Boston Children's Hospital, the 18-year survival rate of all patients treated both medically and surgically was only 18 per cent (Collins-Nakai et al., 1977).

EMBRYOLOGY

Congenital mitral stenosis represents the failure of normal embryologic formation of the left-sided atrioventricular valve (Titus, 1969). In many cases, congenital mitral valve defects are combined with more than one fenestration, and since fenestration anomalies are associated with failure of formation of the atrioventricular valve, it can be assumed that congenital mitral stenosis is a canal defect (Edwards, 1971). In some infants with congenital mitral stenosis, the fact that the electrocardiographic pattern is the same as that of persistent atrioventricular canal tends to corroborate the theory, first proposed by Bower in 1953, that congenital mitral stenosis represents a type of persistent atrioventricular canal (Barcia et al., 1962). The associated defects found with congenital mitral stenosis occur at about the same time in fetal development or are formed from the bulbus cordis at about the same time as the mitral valve is being formed from the endocardial cushions (Liberthson et al., 1971).

PATHOLOGY

Edwards (1971) has supported the theory that congenital mitral stenosis is embryologic in ·nature and not an acquired state secondary to some other condition such as endocardial fibroelastosis. Basic congenital mitral stenosis is a type of cushion defect, and it occurs with arrested fetal development of the left heart. Changes in the right heart (e.g., atrial hypertrophy and right ventricular hypertrophy) are probably secondary to the left heart obstruction, and it is very possible that persistence of the patent ductus arteriosus in some patients may be the result of elevated pulmonary pressure caused by obstruction at the mitral valve level. A review of the pathologic findings at autopsy of patients with congenital mitral stenosis showed cardiac enlargement chiefly of both the right and left atrium and the right ventricle. Left ventricular hypertrophy or dilatation is present in most cases as well as some sclerosis of the left atrial endocardium, suggesting acquired endocardial fibroelastosis. It is thought that the left ventricular hypertrophy is due to the fact that the majority of these children have associated patent ductus arteriosus, aortic stenosis, coarctation of the aorta, or a ventricular septal defect that results in enlargement of the left side of the heart. The pulmonary artery is usually dilated, and the aorta is of normal or small size. The mitral valve is markedly deformed and may have more than one fenestration. The chordae tendineae are shortened and thick. The papillary muscles are hypertrophic and fibrotic. Mitral orifices usually measure no more than a few millimeters in diameter. The mitral valve may be one of three types: (1) a funnel-shaped, elongated cone type of congenital stenosis, (2) the ballooning type of valve with short chordae tendineae and hypertrophic papillary muscles obstructing the anulus of the mitral valve, and (3) the so-called "parachute type" of valve in which all of the chordae tendineae of both malformed leaflets are connected to a single large papillary muscle (see Fig. 39–4).

Histologic examination of the mitral valve shows endocardial sclerosis and fibrosis with no evidence of rheumatic fever. Histologic study of the lungs reveals the phenomenon seen in obstructive pulmonary venous disease, namely, medial thickening of the pulmonary veins, medial hypertrophy of the muscular arteries, and engorgement of the capillaries and the presence of obstructed lymphatics. Endocardial fibroelastosis has been reported in more than half of the studies reviewed at autopsy. This appears to be a phenomenon related to the duration and severity of the obstructive lesions, especially in those patients with aortic stenosis or coarctation. Surface changes resembling endocardial fibroelastosis of the left atrium with long-standing mitral stenosis in adults does occur, and the severity of these lesions seems to be related to the severity and duration of the obstructing lesion. Davachi and associates (1979) have done an anatomic analysis of 55 autopsy cases of mitral valvular disease in infancy. This beautiful study defines obstruction of the mitral valve: (1) the leaflets, (2) the chordae tendineae, (3) the commissures, and (4) the papillary muscles. In the study of anatomic material by Edwards and his group (1971), the "parachute" mitral valve seemed to be the most common type of mitral stenosis found at autopsy. A single occurrence of combined congenital and pulmonic mitral stenosis has been reported by Roberts and colleagues (1962). A congenital stenosis of the left atrioventricular canal located above the posterior mitral leaflet and involving the middle portion of the anterior mitral leaflet has been also reported (Chung et al., 1974). In this malformation, a membrane or shelf-like structure with one of the two orifices is located close to the mitral valve and obstructs flow from the left atrium. Location of the foramen ovale and the left atrial appendage above the membrane differentiates this anomaly from cor triatriatum. Duplication of the mitral valve may occur, and the accessory valve leaflets must be removed, as they may be obstructive.

In 1979, Ruckman and Van Praagh reviewed 49 autopsy cases of mitral obstructive lesions with considerations of diagnosis and surgical implications. They divided mitral stenosis into four anatomic types. Type I was shortened or obliterated chordae tendineae and in this series of specimens represented 49 per cent of the cases (24 of 49). Type II was the hypoplastic valve, hypoplastic valve ring, or combinations of the two. These anomalies were usually associated with the severe left heart syndromes in infancy and represented 41 per cent of their cases (20 of 49). Type III consisted of the supramitral ring, and this may or may not be present with some involvement of the mitral valve, chordae tendineae, or papillary muscle mechanisms. This anomaly represented 12 per cent of their specimens (6 of 49). Type IV was the "parachute" mitral valve, which constituted 8 per cent of their specimens (4 of 49). This group of patients had a 96 per cent incidence of associated congenital malformations, a 47 per cent incidence of hypoplastic aortic isthmus, and a 29 per cent incidence of aortic valve stenosis. There was a 29 per cent incidence of aortic atresia, and coarctation of the aorta was present in 27 per cent of the cases.

Congenital mitral stenosis may accompany the complete atrioventricular canal malformation in some patients, and early surgical repair is probably contraindicated in these patients. Echocardiographic demonstration of this combined lesion may contraindicate surgical repair in infancy (Bloom et al., 1979). Supravalvular ring is commonly associated with congenital mitral stenosis and can usually be treated at the same time as the valve (Chung et al., 1974). An anomalous coronary artery has been reported to lie within this ridge by one author and should be avoided at any surgical procedure (Huhta et al., 1981).

CLINICAL DIAGNOSIS

An infant or child with congenital mitral stenosis usually has a heart murmur that is discovered early in life. Symptoms of pulmonary congestion occur in three fourths of the patients prior to 1 year of age and in about one third of the patients before 1 month of age. Those patients with other congenital heart lesions in addition to congenital mitral stenosis have earlier symptoms. Approximately 50 per cent of the patients die within 6 months of the onset of symptoms, and very few have survived beyond 2 years of age without operation. Patients with associated lesions usually are identified early as candidates for surgical intervention because of the effects of the associated lesions. These patients have congestive failure, and this is associated with frequent respiratory infections in 50 per cent of the patients (Khoury *et al.*, 1969). Differential cyanosis can be difficult in those patients with a patent ductus arteriosus and a right-to-left shunt at the ductus level. Cyanosis can also occur in those patients with a right-to-left shunt at the ventricular level.

The examination of the cardiovascular system reveals cardiomegaly in virtually all of the patients, and most of these infants and children have precordial bulges. A mitral "opening snap" is rarely heard, probably because of lack of mobility of the malformed valves. The most common murmur heard is the long, apical diastolic, rumbling murmur, which in some cases has a rough crescendo systolic component. Systolic murmurs are usually associated with the other cardiovascular defects such as aortic stenosis, patent ductus, ventricular septal defect, and coarctation of the aorta that occur along with congenital mitral stenosis.

The electrocardiogram reveals definite or border-

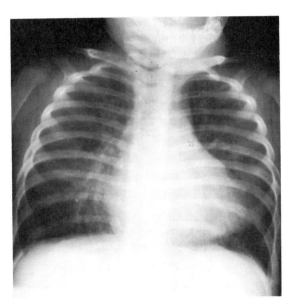

Figure 39–2. Plain chest film of a child with congenital mitral stenosis. Left atrial enlargement can easily be seen as a double density with some elevation of the left main stem bronchus. There is evidence of passive congestion of the lungs.

line right atrial overload in almost 90 per cent of the children with congenital mitral stenosis. The incidence of left atrial hypertrophy, as detected by electrocardiography, is almost 90 per cent. Right ventricular overload is almost always present. Left ventricular overload is a rare finding in isolated congenital mitral stenosis but is almost always present in those patients with associated aortic stenosis, coarctation, patent ductus, and ventricular septal defect (Fig. 39–1).

The plain chest film reveals that the shape of the heart in patients with congenital mitral stenosis is similar to that seen in adults with acquired mitral stenosis. There is a straight left heart border, except in those patients examined in early infancy. Almost all patients have radiologic evidence of left atrial enlargement, either on plain films or with barium swallow. The radiologic findings of passive congestion of the lungs are present in all symptomatic patients (Figs. 39–2 and 39–3). Some older children show the radiologic findings of severe pulmonary venous obstruction, including the obstructed lymphatic lines of Kerley.

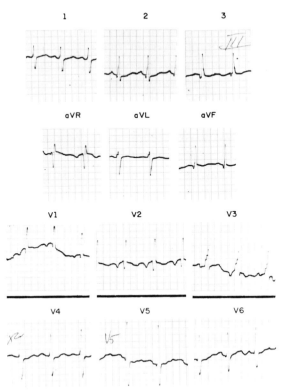

Figure 39–1. Electrocardiogram of a child with coarctation of the aorta and congenital mitral stenosis. The coarctation has been repaired and the child presents at 18 months of age for surgical therapy of his congenital mitral stenosis. The EKG shows evidence of left atrial enlargement and right ventricular hypertrophy. There is a suggestion of left ventricular hypertrophy. The rhythm is sinus.

Echocardiography

The earliest use of echocardiography was in the diagnosis of mitral stenosis in adults. M-mode echocardiography is quite specific for the diagnosis of left ventricular inflow obstruction, but it has been difficult to differentiate at what level the obstruction occurs with this simple form of echocardiography. The development of two-dimensional echocardiography has allowed the demonstration of congenital valvular anomalies in infants and children and may clearly define the distinct types of anatomic obstruction, owing to its ability to define spatial display of obstruc-

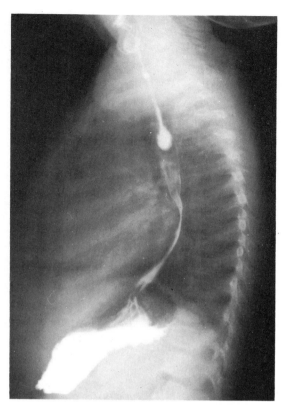

Figure 39–3. The lateral chest film of a cardiac series of the child in Figure 39–2. Left atrial enlargement can easily be identified as an indication of the barium column within the esophagus.

tive lesions (Snider *et al.*, 1980). In a review of the clinical uses of two-dimensional echocardiography in 1980, Cottler demonstrated accurate determinations of mitral valve area anomalies with two-dimensional echocardiography and thought that these could be well correlated with the findings at surgery, even in infants and small children, and that they could also be correlated with the cardiac catheterization data. They did demonstrate that the type of anomaly present could not be determined with plain two-dimensional echocardiography. Shunt lesions and valvular obstructive lesions were clearly defined by echocardiography, and a suggestion was made to use M-mode cardiography and perhaps contrast M-mode cardiography in defining the level of obstruction in these lesions (Williams *et al.*, 1978).

The very small infants with severe stenosis of the mitral valve tended to have a greater decrease in the rate of early diastolic closure and exhibited abnormal motion of the posterior mitral leaflet (Driscoll *et al.*, 1978). In general, the advent of echocardiography and, most recently, the use of two-dimensional echocardiography with current contrast enhancement have made the diagnosis of obstructive mitral lesions by noninvasive means easier in infants and children. The use of this diagnostic modality will allow some decisions to be made as to surgical procedures that might be indicated in these very small infants, as well as the degree of safety of these procedures, if the level of obstruction can be defined.

Cardiac Catheterization

Cardiac catheterization reveals elevated pulmonary arterial wedge pressure and pulmonary hypertension. More than 50 per cent of patients with congenital mitral stenosis have elevated pulmonary vascular resistance. This is particularly common in older children, indicating that repair should be undertaken early in life.

Conventional angiocardiography reveals enlargement of the right atrium, right ventricle, and pulmonary artery in all patients. The pulmonary circulation is delayed, and as a rule, the left atrium is large, although early in infancy it may be small. The mitral valve anulus is usually smaller than normal, and the valve frequently has a funnel-shaped appearance. There is decreased flow from the lungs, indicating obstruction at the mitral valve level. In isolated congenital mitral stenosis, the left ventricular chamber is usually of normal size or smaller, but with other lesions contributing to distal left-sided obstruction, the left ventricle is enlarged. The aorta tends to be small in all cases.

With the use of better angiographic techniques, there is some evidence that there is a classic appearance to the left ventricular angiogram with biplane views of this structure. There are characteristic filling defects of the left ventricular cavity in "mitral valve arcade" or "hammock" valve. This "thumb printing" is very characteristic of the disorganized papillary muscle structures within the left ventricle. There is characteristic appearance of the "parachute" valve on the lateral left ventricular view, which shows a single filling defect in the lower half of the posterior medial wall. The papillary muscle type of obstruction demonstrates filling defects and a severe rigidity of the posterior mural leaflet (Carpentier *et al.*, 1976).

Differential Diagnosis

The differential diagnosis of congenital mitral stenosis includes other anomalies that produce a high pulmonary venous pressure because of pulmonary venous obstruction or secondary to left ventricular failure or defects with a large left or right shunt with pulmonary hypertension. Clinical findings similar to those in congenital mitral stenosis may be encountered in such anomalies as cor triatriatum, a stenotic ring of the left atrium, stenosis or atresia at the entrance of pulmonary veins into the left atrium, left atrial myxoma, and some cases of total anomalous venous return, especially the infradiaphragmatic type. Endocardial fibroelastosis with mitral insufficiency may mimic congenital mitral stenosis because of the left ventricular failure and the enlarged left atrium (Van der Horst and Hastreiter, 1967).

The diastolic murmur is the *sine qua non* of congenital mitral stenosis. The "opening snap" of adult mitral stenosis is not usually present, but some differentiation can be related to the presence or absence of the diastolic murmur. In cor triatriatum, the murmur is more of a continuous type, and there is only slight cardiomegaly. Left atrial enlargment may be present in cases of cor triatriatum, but usually, differentiation from congenital mitral stenosis can be made by means of angiocardiography. Infradiaphragmatic total anomalous venous return may be easily confused with congenital mitral stenosis, but children with this defect generally present at a very early age, are much more ill, and are cyanotic in the neonatal period. The heart is not enlarged, and there is no left atrial enlargement. In the supradiaphragmatic type of anomalous venous return, the symptoms are less severe than those of congenital mitral stenosis, and although the patient may have some degree of cardiomegaly, the classic "figure-of-eight" or "snowman-type" heart is usually diagnostic. Angiocardiography will easily differentiate the supracardiac type of total anomalous venous return from congenital mitral stenosis.

Stenosis of the entrance of pulmonary veins into the left atrium can be confused with congenital mitral stenosis, but good angiocardiography will differentiate the two conditions. The left atrium is almost always of normal size in stenosis of the pulmonary veins.

Left atrial myxoma is very rare in infants and small children, but the presence of a changing murmur or peripheral emboli would be suggestive and indicate the need for angiocardiography.

There is a great debate about whether endocardial fibroelastosis, which does occur in congenital mitral stenosis, is a secondary endocardial change or a primary cause of mitral constriction. Endocardial fibroelastosis usually causes mitral insufficiency, which may be confused with congenital mitral stenosis, but usually, the apical diastolic murmur is absent and there is predominant left ventricular hypertrophy on the electrocardiogram. Angiocardiography will differentiate congenital mitral stenosis from the heart involved with endocardial fibroelastosis and mitral insufficiency.

Children in whom coarctation of the aorta or aortic stenosis is present usually have earlier symptoms than those with congenital mitral stenosis. The presence of the apical diastolic murmur favors congenital mitral stenosis, but again, angiocardiography and cardiac catheterization will easily differentiate the two entities. Supravalvular ring of the left atrium is a difficult diagnosis to establish even by angiocardiography. Two-dimensional echocardiography may well differentiate the level of obstruction even in small infants. This noninvasive technique will indicate further study by angiography for the small symptomatic infant and perhaps can lead to earlier therapy if a surgical procedure is indicated. Good cardiac catheterization and angiocardiography are required for differential diagnosis, and once these studies are done, surgical approach can be undertaken. The typical angiocardiographic finding of congenital mitral stenosis is that of delayed emptying of an enlarged left atrium. This finding in the incapacitated symptomatic child requires surgical exploration.

BASIC SURGICAL ANATOMY

The classification of congenital mitral stenosis into three different anatomic types of deformed valves is a useful guide in choosing different forms of surgical therapy (Fig. 39–4). The valves can usually be classified into one of three anatomic types, depending on the level of obstruction of the valve: Type I — obstruction at the leaflet level; Type II — obstruction at the chordae tendineae level; and Type III — obstruction at the papillary muscle level. The Type I valve, which appears to be the most common type presenting with symptoms in infancy, is usually an elongated cone with fusion of the cusps in their anatomic commissures to form a pinpoint opening deep in the ventricular cavity. This valve probably will respond to commissurotomy, but there will be residual mitral

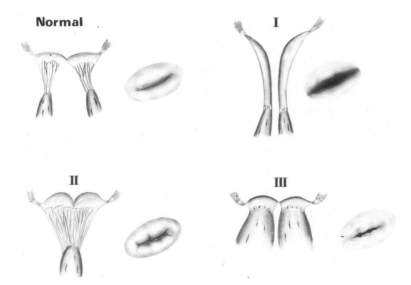

Figure 39–4. The surgical anatomy of the location of the obstruction in congenital mitral stenosis is very important. The normal mitral valve is made up of three components: (1) the valve leaflets; (2) the chordae tendineae; and (3) the papillary muscles. Type I congenital mitral stenosis is the most common in infancy, and the main obstruction is at the leaflet level owing to its elongated cone shape. Type II congenital mitral stenosis is the "parachute mitral valve" type in which the chordae tendineae insert into a single papillary muscle and the obstruction is at the chordae tendineae level. In Type III congenital mitral stenosis, there are short chordae tendineae attached to very hypertrophied papillary muscles. The obstruction is therefore at the papillary muscle level.

insufficiency. This is probably the type of valve that responded well to "blind" commissurotomy in the past. The Type II valve is the classic "parachute mitral valve" with all chordae tendineae inserted into a single papillary muscle (Glancy *et al.*, 1971; Prado *et al.*, 1965; Schachner *et al.*, 1975). Davachi and associates (1971) have reported success in removal of some chordae tendineae to enhance flow through the valve in an infant. The Type III valve is that in which the obstruction is due to large papillary muscles attached to short, fused chordae tendineae. This type of valve must be replaced with a prosthesis.

SURGICAL MANAGEMENT

Vigorous medical management would ideally allow the child with congenital mitral stenosis to grow to a size at which surgery could be undertaken electively, but unfortunately, medical therapy is often ineffective. Surgical intervention may well prove to be lifesaving, although in most cases, the relief will be only partial. The closed procedures that were done early in the history of heart surgery for congenital mitral stenosis resulted in some mitral insufficiency but did permit survival in a few cases. Open mitral commissurotomy using total cardiopulmonary bypass with profound hypothermia has been successful in infants at an early age, but in some cases, especially those of Type II and Type III congenital mitral stenosis with obstruction at the chordae tendineae of papillary muscle level, excision of the valve and replacement with a prosthesis are required. Infants less than 1 year of age with obstructive valvular lesions still have a high surgical risk, but with the use of profound hypothermia and cardioplegic solutions, surgical approach to the obstructive mitral lesions is quite possible. Many infants and children have had a successful prosthetic replacement of the mitral valve for this anomaly, and several authors have reported re-replacement at a later age of these valves replaced in infancy (Bloodwell *et al.*, 1969; Carpentier *et al.*, 1976; Castaneda *et al.*, 1969; Collins-Nakai *et al.*, 1977; Geha *et al.*, 1979). Mitral commissurotomy may relieve the obstructive problem but usually results in mitral insufficiency, and a valve replacement may be indicated at a later point. Carpentier and associates (1976) have devised innovative approaches to mitral obstructive lesions avoiding valve replacement if at all possible and employing reconstruction with the Carpentier valve ring.

Surgical Approach

The surgical approach to congenital mitral stenosis is dependent on the age of the child, the anatomic type of congenital mitral stenosis, and the presence of other associated congenital defects. Accompanying patent ductus arteriosus, coarctation of the aorta, or aortic stenosis causes severe congestive failure earlier in the clinical course than does isolated congenital mitral stenosis. If possible, the diagnosis should be made prior to 1 year of age, and if the type of mitral obstruction can be delineated, the conditions that are amenable to surgery in this age group would be best relieved prior to 1 year of age because of the development of obstructive pulmonary vascular disease. The best approach in the child with associated lesions is to relieve the most distal obstruction first, usually with a closed procedure, and then to proceed to an open heart procedure through a sternal splitting incision using profound hypothermia and cardioplegic solution for cardiac protection. If at the time of the open procedure a conservative operative procedure can be done in order to preserve the mitral valve and relieve the obstruction, this should be undertaken. If the child will tolerate the relief of the distal obstruction and a delay in time, then perhaps a delay in the correction of the obstructing mitral lesion, particularly if it is the type that will require mitral valve replacement, should be made until the child is big enough for a small prosthetic valve to be used. In the review of the literature of 69 cases of congenital mitral stenosis, patent ductus was associated in 36 of the cases, coarctation in 23, and aortic stenosis in 21 (Humblet *et al.*, 1971). Eight had ventricular septal defects, and nine had atrial septal defects (Dahlback *et al.*, 1968). The remainder of the defects mainly concerned malformations of the tricuspid valve or the aortic valve or hypoplasia of the left side of the heart. In 16 of the cases, relief of the associated defect was provided before surgery for the congenital mitral stenosis. The overall frequency of associated significant cardiovascular abnormalities in one series was 74 per cent (28 of 38 patients). These findings were equally distributed among patients with mild and severe mitral obstructions (Collins-Nakai *et al.*, 1977).

The approach to the congenital mitral stenotic valve should be by open cardiopulmonary bypass, and the choice between profound hypothermia and mild hypothermia depends on the preference of the operating surgical team. The left atrium is usually large enough to allow a direct approach through the left atrium, and the mitral valve can be well visualized from this approach (Fig. 39–4). The decision to do an open mitral commissurotomy or replacement of the stenotic valve will depend on many factors; among them, of course, is the size of the patient, the anatomy of the mitral valve, and the type of congenital mitral stenosis that is being dealt with. The ideal candidate for a commissurotomy is the patient with a cone-shaped stenosis of the mitral valve with anatomic commissures. Once the valve is opened, and provided there is no obstructing musculature below the valve, these patients appear to do well, even if there is residual mitral insufficiency. If there is obstructing musculature below the mitral leaflet, resection and replacement with a prosthesis will probably be necessary, although in a recent series of patients reviewed by Carpentier and colleagues (1976), it was possible to do innovative types of relief of obstruction in the

TABLE 39-1. CONGENITAL MITRAL STENOSIS*

PATIENT	YEAR	AGE	SEX	ASSOCIATED LESIONS	DIASTOLIC MURMUR	CYANOSIS	PULMONARY ARTERY PRESSURE	ENLARGED LEFT ATRIUM	ANATOMIC TYPE VALVE	SURGERY	RESULTS
1. E.F.	1959	14	M	—	+	−	90/50	+	I	Open valvulotomy	Alive with significant mitral insufficiency
2. S.A.	1961	3	M	Coarctation	+	+	72/26	+	?	Resection of coarctation and closed valvulotomy	Alive with mild mitral stenosis
3. T.W.	1961	10	M	—	+	−	54/32	+	III	Open valvulotomy	Expired—pulmonary hypertension
4. D.O.	1962	4	F	Coarctation and patent ductus arteriosus	+	−	60/28	+	?	Resection of coarctation and ligation of patent ductus arteriosus with closed valvulotomy	Alive with mild mitral insufficiency
5. K.K.	1966	1½	M	Coarctation	+	+	110/40	+	?	Resection of coarctation and closed valvulotomy	Expired—pulmonary hypertension
6. L.M.	1969	2 mo.	F	Coarctation and patent ductus arteriosus	+	+	65/19	−	I	Resection of coarctation and ligation of patent ductus arteriosus	Expired—mitral stenosis not recognized
7. D.S.	1969	3	F	Coarctation	+	−	57/25	+	I	Resection of coarctation, year later open commissurotomy	Alive with significant mitral insufficiency
8. D.D.	1971	1½	M	Coarctation	+	−	60/70	+	I	Resection of coarctation, 3 months later open commissurotomy	Alive with mild mitral insufficiency
9. T.L.	1974	8 mo.	M	Ventricular septal defect	+	+	55/45	+	III	Closure of ventricular septal defect and valve replacement	Expired—pulmonary hypertension
10. C.C.	1976	12 mo.	M	Coarctation	+	−	85/60	+	I	Open valvulotomy	Alive with mitral insufficiency
11. V.C.	1979	2	M	Coarctation and patent ductus arteriosus	+	−	60/40	+	I	Open valvulotomy	Alive with mitral insufficiency
12. T.M.	1980	11	F	Coarctation	+	+	80/50	+	III	Valve replacement	Alive and well

*Study done at the Columbus Children's Hospital of the Ohio State University College of Medicine.

chordae tendineae and in the papillary musculature below the mitral valve, sculpturing these in such a way as to allow the obstruction to be surgically relieved. This approach was made through an opening, usually through the posterior leaflet of the mitral valve, and then a repair was made using the Carpentier ring prosthesis if there was any residual insufficiency caused by the sculpturing of the mitral valve. Division of the obstructed chordae in the "parachute mitral valve" may create a functional valve, but most often, these children require valve replacement later in childhood or as adults (Vlad, 1971; Schachner, 1975). The youngest child reported to have had mitral valve replacement was 10 months old (Castaneda *et al.*, 1969). It is obvious that when a mitral valve is replaced at this age, it will almost certainly require re-replacement at a later date. The selection of the valve for replacement will depend on many factors, guided by the anatomic size of the mitral ring and the volume of the left ventricular cavity. A low-profile valve may be the most desirable, but ball-type prostheses have been used in small infants with success. One must carefully weigh the desirable aspects of a xenograft prosthetic valve in children, since there have been reports of early deterioration and degeneration due to fibrocalcific changes in these valves when used in young children (Geha *et al.*, 1979; Kutsche *et al.*, 1979). If any operative procedure is required at a very early age in these infants, perhaps a bypass type of conduit might be used, as described by Laks and associates in 1980. In this procedure, a valve-bearing conduit was used from the left atrium to the distal left ventricle to bypass the mitral valve with an obstructive or tiny mitral ring in which a prosthesis would not fit. This procedure might have some application in the very small infant with significant obstructive pulmonary vascular disease in order to relieve that obstruction, and then, obviously, a further surgical procedure would be required at a later date.

RESULTS

Closed mitral valvulotomy for congenital mitral stenosis in 42 patients resulted in a mortality rate of 50 per cent. This was done by the finger-fracture technique or with a mechanical dilator. The open technique using cardiopulmonary bypass has better results, according to reports by Gotsman and associates (1973), Khalil and coworkers (1975), and Collins-Nakai and colleagues (1977). Good results with prosthetic valve replacement in small infants and children have been reported in many instances in the literature.

At the Columbus Children's Hospital of The Ohio State University College of Medicine, 12 children have had operative procedures for congenital mitral stenosis (Table 39–1). Eight have survived the operative procedure, for an overall mortality rate of 44 per cent. Eleven of the 12 had accompanying congenital defects. Nine had coarctation of the aorta, and three had significant patent ductus arteriosus in addition to coarctation. One patient had a ventricular septal defect repaired at the time of valve replacement. In three patients, blind, instrumental, closed valvulotomies were done at the time of coarctation repair and there were two survivors; all of these were done prior to 1969. Of the seven children who had open valvulotomy, five survived. Prosthetic replacement has been done in one patient with survival. In one patient, the diagnosis was missed at the time of catheterization; therefore, no attempt at valvulotomy was undertaken at the time of coarctation repair.

The approach that seems reasonable at this time is to correct the accompanying lesion at the first procedure and then to treat congenital mitral stenosis by an open procedure at the time of the correction of the distal obstructing lesion, using total cardiopulmonary bypass, profound hypothermia, and cardioplegic solution if the child's clinical course indicates such an approach. If the child is doing well, the distal obstructing lesion, such as coarctation, should be relieved, and a delay should be made in order to allow the child's heart to reach a size that would accept a prosthesis if this is indicated. Using the newer diagnostic techniques such as two-dimensional echocardiography, a clearer definition of the level of obstruction of the mitral stenotic lesion may be possible. If the level of obstruction is Type I, or valvular in nature, then an early open procedure might be indicated in order to prevent the development of chronic pulmonary obstructive vascular disease. If the obstruction is at the muscle level in the heart, then an attempt should be made at management with medical means until the child is of a size to accept a prosthetic valve at the time of surgical correction of the problem. There has been one recent success with a bypass conduit in a tiny infant with obstruction at the mitral valve level, and this may be a feasible approach to delay the development of pulmonary vascular obstructive disease if this procedure could be done prior to 1 year of age.

SELECTED REFERENCES

Bloom, K. R., Freedom, R. M., Williams, C. M., Trusler, G. A., and Rowe, R. D.: Echocardiographic recognition of atrioventricular and valve stenosis associated with endocardial cushion defect: Pathologic and surgical correlates. Am. J. Cardiol., *44*:1326, 1979.

A high incidence of associated mitral stenosis and endocardial cushion defect should make one cautious of surgery in these patients. Surgery may be contraindicated for infants with this combination of defects, and therefore, echocardiography is of great importance as a diagnostic tool.

Carpentier, A., Branchini, B., Cour, J. C., Asfaou, E., Villani, M., Parenzan, L., Brom, G., *et al.*: Congenital malformations of mitral valve in children: Pathology and surgical treatment. J. Thorac. Cardiovasc. Surg., *72*:854, 1976.

A study of all cases of congenital anomalies of the mitral valve treated by a combined experience in France, Italy, and the Netherlands. This group of surgeons prefer valve restructuring for the congenital mitral lesions if at all possible, and their results support this. Seven patients with pure mitral stenosis were cared for; six had repair, and only one replacement was needed — for a patient with a parachute mitral valve. A direct repair of a hammock valve ("mitral valve arcade") was done using a Carpentier ring in the repair.

Collins-Nakai, R. L., Rosenthal, A., Castaneda, A. R., Bernhard, W. F., and Nadas, A. S.: Congenital mitral stenosis — a review of 20 years' experience. Circulation, 56:1039, 1977.

A summary of the clinical course of 38 patients with congenital mitral stenosis. Significant cardiovascular abnormalities were present in 74 per cent (28 of 38) of the patients. Diagnosis is difficult, and echocardiography offers the ability to define anatomy but is not reliable for determining the severity of the disease. Pulmonary vascular obstructive disease develops during early childhood, as defined by histologic examination of the lung. The 18-year survival rate in all patients (medical and surgical) is 18 per cent.

Davachi, F., Moller, J. H., and Edwards, J. E.: Diseases of the mitral valve in infancy: An anatomic analysis of 55 cases. Circulation, 43:565, 1971.

This is an excellent review of the anatomy of congenital diseases of the mitral valve of all types, including stenosis and insufficiency. The basic interpretation of the type of obstruction that can occur in congenital mitral stenosis is carefully defined and presented. The article has excellent photographs of the various mitral valve anomalies.

Humblet, L., Stainier, I., Joris, J., Collignon, P., Kulbertus, H., and Delvigne, J.: La sténose mitrale congénitale, Acta Cardiol., 26:500, 1971.

This article is in French. It is a superb review of the literature concerning congenital mitral stenosis during 20 years. Support of the concept that the congenital mitral stenotic valve is really a canal defect is carefully documented. A good chart concerning concurrent defects is presented.

Kutsche, L. M., Oyer, P., Shumway, N., and Baum, D.: An important complication of Hancock mitral valve replacement in children. Circulation, 60(Suppl. I):98, 1979.

Fibrocalcific recurrent mitral stenosis of a heterograft valve in children. This is a significant factor in the determination of the type of valve for use in children.

Ruckman, R. N., and Van Praagh, R.: Anatomic types of congenital mitral stenosis: Report of 49 autopsy cases with consideration of diagnosis and surgical implications. Am. J. Cardiol., 42:592, 1979.

Excellent autopsy review of congenital mitral stenosis. Divides mitral stenosis into four anatomic types: Type I — shortened or obliterated chordae tendineae — 49 per cent (24 of 49); Type II— hypoplastic valve, hypoplastic valve ring, or combinations; usually associated with left heart syndrome — 41 per cent (20 of 49); Type III — supramitral ring — 12 per cent (6 of 49); and Type IV— parachute mitral valve — 8 per cent (4 of 49). This group of patients had a 96 per cent incidence of associated malformations, a 47 per cent incidence of endocardial fibroelastosis or sclerosis, a 37 per cent incidence of hypoplastic aortic isthmus, a 29 per cent incidence of aortic atresia and coarctation of the aorta in 27 per cent of cases.

Snider, A. R., Roge, C. L., Schiller, N. B., and Silverman, N. H.: Congenital left ventricular inflow obstruction evaluated by two-dimensional echocardiography. Circulation, 61:848, 1980.

M-mode echocardiography is valuable for the diagnosis of left ventricular inflow obstruction but does not differentiate the distinct types of obstruction. Two-dimensional echocardiographic demonstration of congenital mitral valve anomalies clearly defines the distinct types owing to its spatial anatomic display capability.

Titus, J. L.: Congenital malformations of the mitral and aortic valves and related structures. Dis. Chest, 55:358, 1969.

The normal embryology of the mitral and aortic valves is carefully presented, and the basic embryology of congenital mitral valve stenosis is carefully developed. This article includes excellent pictures and is a very important basic discussion of the embryology of the mitral valve.

Van der Horst, R. L., and Hastreiter, A. R.: Congenital mitral stenosis. Am. J. Cardiol., 20:773, 1967.

This article is a review of the literature and of the pathologic material available at their particular institution. It reveals excellent clinical correlation of catheterization findings with autopsy findings and operative results.

REFERENCES

Barcia, A., Titus, J. L., Swan, H. J. C., Ongley, P. A., and Calene, J. G.: Congenital mitral stenosis: A case studied by selective angiocardiography and necropsy. Proc. Mayo Clin., 37:632, 1962.

Bloodwell, R. D., Hallman, G. L., McNamara, D. G., and Cooley, D. A.: Cardiac valve replacement for congenital mitral valvular disease in children. J. Pediatr. Surg., 4:9, 1969.

Bloom, K. R., Freedom, R. M., Williams, C. M., Trusler, G. A., and Rowe, R. D.: Echocardiographic recognition of atrioventricular and valve stenosis associated with endocardial cushion defect: Pathologic and surgical correlates. Am. J. Cardiol., 44:1326, 1979.

Carpentier, A., Branchini, B., Cour, J. C., Asfaou, E., Villani, M., Parenzan, L., Brom, G., et al.: Congenital malformations of the mitral valve in children: Pathology and surgical treatment. J. Thorac. Cardiovasc. Surg., 72:854, 1976.

Castaneda, A. R., Anderson, R. C., and Edwards, J. E.: Congenital mitral stenosis resulting from anomalous arcade and obstructing papillary muscles: Report of correction by use of ball valve prosthesis. Am. J. Cardiol., 24:237, 1969.

Chung, K. J., Manning, J. A., Lipchik, E. O., Gramiak, R., and Mahoney, E. B.: Isolated supravalvular stenosing ring of left atrium: Diagnosis before operation and successful surgical treatment. Chest, 65:25, 1974.

Collins-Nakai, R. L., Rosenthal, A., Castaneda, A. R., Bernhard, W. F., and Nadas, A. S.: Congenital mitral stenosis — a review of 20 years' experience. Circulation, 56:1039, 1977.

Dahlback, O., Kugelberg, J., and Schuller, H.: Congenital mitral stenosis. Scand. J. Thorac. Cardiovasc. Surg., 2:209, 1968.

Davachi, F., Moller, J. H., and Edwards, J. E.: Diseases of the mitral valve in infancy: An anatomic analysis of 55 cases. Circulation, 43:565, 1971.

Driscoll, D. J., Gutgesell, H. P., and McNamara, D. G.: Echocardiographic features of congenital mitral stenosis. Am. J. Cardiol., 42:259, 1978.

Edwards, J. E.: Straddling and displaced atrioventricular orifices and valves. Circulation, 43:613, 1971.

Ferencz, C., Johnson, A. L., and Wiglesworth, F. W.: Congenital mitral stenosis. Circulation, 9:161, 1954.

Geha, A. S., Laks, H., Stanser, H. C., Cornhill, J. F., Kilman, J. W., Buckley, M. J., and Roberts, W. C.: Late failure of porcine valve heterografts in children. J. Thorac. Cardiovasc. Surg., 78:351, 1979.

Glancy, D. L., Chang, M. Y., Corney, E. R., and Roberts, W. C.: Parachute mitral valve. Further observations and associated lesions. Am. J. Cardiol., 27:309, 1971.

Gotsman, M. S., Van der Horst, B. T., le Roux, B., and Williams, M. A.: Mitral valvulotomy in childhood. Thorax, 28:453, 1973.

Huhta, J. C., Edwards, W. D., and Danielson, G. K.: Supravalvular mitral ridge containing the dominant left circumflex coronary artery. J. Thorac. Cardiovasc. Surg., 81:577, 1981.

Humblet, L., Stainier, I., Joris, J., Collignon, P., Kulbertus, H., and Delvigne, J.: La sténose mitrale congénitale. Acta Cardiol., 26:500, 1971.

Khalil, K. G., Shapiro, I., and Kilman, J. W.: Congenital mitral stenosis. J. Thorac. Cardiovasc. Surg., 70:40, 1975.

Khoury, G., Hawes, C. R., and Grow, B.: Coarctation of the aorta with obstructive anomalies of the mitral valve and left ventricle. J. Pediatr., 76:652, 1969.

Kotler, M. N., Mintz, G. S., Segal, B. L., and Parry, W. R.: Clinical uses of two-dimensional echocardiography. Am. J. Cardiol., 45:1061, 1980.

Kutsche, L. M., Oyer, P., Shumway, N., and Baum, D.: An important complication of Hancock mitral valve replacement in children. Circulation, 60 (Suppl. I): 98, 1979.

Laks, H., Hellenbrand, W. E., Kleinman, C., and Talner, N.: Left atrial–left ventricular conduit for relief of congenital mitral stenosis in infancy. J. Thorac. Cardiovasc. Surg., 80:782, 1980.

Lassrich, A., and Keck, E. W.: The congenital isolated mitral stenosis. Ann. Radiol., 10:523, 1967.

Liberthson, R. R., Paul, M. N., Muster, A. J., Arcilla, R. A., Eckner, F. A. O., and Lev, M.: Straddling and displaced atrioventricular orifices and valves with primitive ventricles. Circulation, 43:213, 1971.

Mannheimer, R., Bengtsson, E., and Winberg, J.: Pure congenital mitral stenosis due to fibro-elastosis. Cardiologia, 21:574, 1952.

Pappas, G., Grover, F. L., Sarche, M. A., and Blount, S. G.: Congenital mitral stenosis treated by aortic homograft valve replacement. J. Thorac. Cardiovasc. Surg., 62:51, 1971.

Prado, S., Levy, M., and Varco, R. L.: Successful re-replacement of parachute mitral valve in a child. Circulation, 32:130, 1965.

Roberts, W. C., Goldblatt, A., Mason, D. T., and Morrow, A. G.: Combined congenital pulmonic and mitral stenosis. N. Engl. J. Med., 267:1298, 1962.

Ruckman, R. N., and Van Praagh, R.: Anatomic types of congenital mitral stenosis: Report of 49 autopsy cases with consideration of diagnosis and surgical implications. Am. J. Cardiol., 42:592, 1979.

Schachner, A., Varsano, I., and Levy, M. J.: The parachute mitral valve complex: Case report and review of literature. J. Thorac. Cardiovasc. Surg., 70:451, 1975.

Schwarze, E. W., and Bernhard, A.: The pathological anatomy of surgically reconstructable or prosthetically correctable congenital valvular malformations of the mitral region. Virchows Arch. (Pathol. Anat.), 367:149, 1975.

Shem-Tov, A., Yahini, J. H., Deutsch, V., Katznelson, D., and Neufeld, H.: Congenital mitral stenosis. Cardiologia, 54:65, 1969.

Singh, S. P., Gotsman, M. S., Abrams, L. D., Astley, R., Parsons, C. G., and Roberts, K. D.: Congenital mitral stenosis. Br. Heart J., 29:83, 1967.

Snider, A. R., Roge, C. L., Schiller, N. B., and Silverman, N. H.: Congenital left ventricular inflow obstruction evaluated by two-dimensional echocardiography. Circulation, 61:848, 1980.

Titus, J. L.: Congenital malformations of the mitral and aortic valves and related structures. Dis. Chest, 55:358, 1969.

Van der Horst, R. L., and Hastreiter, A. R.: Congenital mitral stenosis. Am. J. Cardiol., 20:773, 1967.

Vlad, P.: Mitral valve anomalies in children. Circulation, 43:465, 1971.

Williams, R. G., and Lacorte, M. A.: Echocardiographic evaluation of valvular and shunt lesions in children. Prog. Cardiovasc. Dis., 20:432, 1978.

Young, D., and Robinson, G.: Successful valve replacement in an infant with congenital mitral stenosis. N. Engl. J. Med., 270:660, 1964.

Chapter 40

Transposition of the Great Arteries

I   THE MUSTARD PROCEDURE

GEORGE A. TRUSLER

ROBERT M. FREEDOM

Transposition of the great arteries (TGA) is a severe cardiac malformation in which the aorta arises from the right ventricle and the pulmonary artery arises from the left ventricle in the patient with atrioventricular concordance. The physiologic effects are acute, with cyanosis and distress usually obvious soon after birth. Survival depends on mixing of blood between pulmonary and systemic circulations, chiefly through a patent foramen ovale, and with the assistance of a patent ductus arteriosus and sometimes a coexistent ventricular septal defect. Untreated, many infants die in the first week of life, and most are dead by one year of age. Survival is extended by procedures that increase mixing, mainly by enlarging the atrioseptal communication.

Although TGA was considered for many years to be lethal and uncorrectable, methods of repair were developed gradually through the work of many individuals. Once these techniques were widely available, there was a great upsurge in interest, study, and knowledge of TGA in both its simple and complex forms.

HISTORY

In 1797, Matthew Baillie first described the pathologic anatomy of TGA. The first palliative operation, an ingenious closed technique for creating an atrial septal defect (ASD), was done by Blalock and Hanlon in 1948. Lillehei and Varco (1953) attempted to transfer the inferior vena cava to the left atrium and the right pulmonary veins to the right atrium. In 1956, Baffes described a palliative procedure, which was in fact a partial repair, that consisted of suturing the right pulmonary veins to the right atrium and connecting the inferior vena cava to the left atrium with a graft. For some years, this procedure provided effective palliation for many children.

The first attempts at repair of TGA were directed toward the great arteries. In 1954, Mustard and associates described a technique for switching the arteries plus one coronary artery. They were unsuccessful, as were Bailey and coworkers (1954), Bjork and Bouckaert (1954), Kay and Cross (1955), Senning (1959),

Idriss and colleagues (1961), and Baffes and associates (1961). It was not until 1975 that the first successful arterial repair was reported by Jatene and coworkers (1975, 1976). This encouraged other surgeons to attempt this operation, but the mortality rate was high. It is only in the last few years that the risk of arterial repair has improved, owing to better patient selection and management.

A technique for complete repair by rearranging venous inflow at the atrial level was first suggested by Albert (1955), who later attempted an intra-arterial repair with a patch of plastic material. Subsequent trials by Merindino and colleagues (1957), Kay and Cross (1957), Creech and coworkers (1958), and Wilson and associates (1962) using various materials were all unsuccessful. The first successful intra-atrial repair was described by Senning in 1959 with a clever but complicated procedure involving flaps of atrial wall and septum. Kirklin and colleagues (1961) employed Senning's technique with success, but the mortality rate was high. In 1961, Barnard and coworkers performed a successful intra-atrial repair using a large crimped tube of Teflon to connect the pulmonary veins to the tricuspid valve. In 1963, Mustard applied Albert's principle, using a patch or baffle of pericardium to partition the atria and redirect venous inflow to match the transposed arteries. This operation was not only relatively simple but reproducible and safe; its success stimulated an immediate and widespread awakening of interest in the repair of TGA.

Other historical highlights include the development of the Rastelli procedure in 1969 for TGA with ventricular septal defect (VSD) and pulmonary stenosis (PS) and of intraventricular repair by McGoon in 1972 for those patients with very large and suitably positioned VSDs.

PATHOLOGIC ANATOMY

Definition

Transposition of the great arteries refers to that condition in which the aorta originates from the morphologically right ventricle and the pulmonary artery is supported by the morphologically left ventricle. When so-called complete transposition of the great arteries is present, the atrioventricular connections are concordant. That is, the morphologically right atrium connects with the morphologically right ventricle, and the left atrium connects with the morphologically left ventricle. This definition of "transposition" excludes the concept of spatial relationships between the two great arteries because they are so variable and, by utilizing a "connections" approach, is independent of infundibular anatomy.

Anatomy

Complete TGA can occur in hearts exhibiting dextrocardia or mesocardia, but our experience indicates that in more than 95 per cent of patients, levocardia is evident. Similarly, more than 95 per cent of patients with complete transposition exhibit visceroatrial situs solitus, with only a few patients demonstrating visceroatrial situs inversus. We have identified a few patients with isomeric left atria, but with the right-sided atrium receiving the entire systemic venous return and the left-sided atrium receiving the pulmonary venous connections. In this situation, the presence of normal or noninverted ventricles and discordant ventriculoarterial connections will result in the physiology of complete TGA. Among most patients with complete TGA and visceroatrial situs solitus, the ventricular relationship is normal. That is, the ventricular relationship is that of a noninverted pattern—the so-called d-loop or "right-hand" pattern. In this pattern, the inlet–apical trabecular–outlet axis of the morphologically right ventricle is from right to left, with the outlet or infundibular component of the right ventricle to the left of the inlet zone. With very rare exception, the presence of concordant atrioventricular connections implies a d-ventricular loop. Hearts with so-called superoinferior ventricles or crossed atrioventricular connections can exhibit discordant ventriculoarterial connections (Freedom et al., 1978). About 70 per cent of patients with complete TGA will have an intact ventricular septum, absence of left ventricular outflow tract obstruction (LVOTO), a small and inadequate interatrial communication, and a small patent ductus arteriosus (PDA).

Major Anomalies Associated with Transposition

The most common associated anomalies among patients with complete TGA include VSD and/or LVOTO (Rowe et al., 1981). VSDs can occur in any portion of the ventricular septum and may occur as a single defect or may be multiple. Using a tripartite schema of the ventricular septum, as advocated by Soto and associates (1980), the septum can be viewed as having an inlet component, an apical trabecular component, and an infundibular or subarterial component. In the majority of patients, the VSD will involve either the infundibular septum or the perimembranous septum (Oppenheimer-Dekker, 1978). As might be anticipated, a defect of one zone may be confluent with that of another zone. The infundibular (or subarterial) VSD can result from an isolated defect or deficiency of the infundibular septum (analogous to the so-called isolated supracristal VSD in the otherwise normal heart), or it can result from a malalignment between the infundibular septum (that portion of interventricular septum separating the aorta from the pulmonary artery) and the trabecula septomarginalis. When a malalignment defect is present, the infundibular septum is almost always deviated posteriorly, encroaching on the left ventricular outflow tract and resulting in a muscular subpulmonary stenosis. Anterosuperior deviation of the infundibular septum is infrequently identified in these patients. Such deviation will encroach on the right ventricular subaortic outflow tract and may be seen in the patient with complete TGA, VSD, and an obstructive anomaly of the aortic arch. The complete form of atrioventricular defect can rarely occur in the patient with complete TGA, but it is more frequently identified in the patient with isomeric right or left atria and thus an ambiguous atrioventricular connection. Distinctly uncommon as well is the isolated defect of the inlet component of the ventricular septum. Such a defect can be accompanied by straddling of the tricuspid valve.

It is difficult to consider the morphologic basis of LVOTO without first considering the basic patterns of infundibular anatomy among patients with complete TGA. About 95 per cent of patients will have a subaortic infundibulum; thus, the aortic valve is separated from the tricuspid valve, whereas the pulmonary and mitral valves are in fibrous continuity. About 4 per cent of patients will have bilateral muscular infundibula with neither semilunar valve in fibrous continuity with the atrioventricular valve. A very rare patient will have bilaterally deficient infundibula, with both semilunar valves in continuity with the atrioventricular valves (Van Praagh et al., 1980).

Left ventricular outflow tract obstruction can result from one or more pathologic mechanisms (Jimenez and Martinez, 1974; Shrivastava, et al., 1976; Idriss et al., 1977; Van Gils, 1978; Van Gils et al., 1978; Aziz et al., 1979; Sansa et al., 1979). These include (1) posterior malalignment of the infundibular septum; (2) fibrous subpulmonary membrane; (3) accessory tissue tags, often pedunculated and mobile, originating from an atrioventricular valve and contiguous structures; (4) a muscular or tunnel form of subpulmonary obstruction; (5) aneurysm of the membranous or perimembranous interventricular septum; (6) straddling atrioventricular valve tissue; (7) pulmonary valve stenosis; (8) maladherent anterior leaflet of the mitral valve; (9) dynamic subvalvular obstruction due to posterior systolic bulging of the ventricular septum; or (10) combinations of the above. The most common mechanism results from the leftward and posterior deviation of a malaligned infundibular septum (Van Gils *et al.*, 1978). This is consistent with the observation that most of the patients with LVOTO complicating complete TGA have an associated VSD.

The spatial relationships between the great arteries at semilunar valve level in hearts exhibiting atrioventricular concordance and ventriculoarterial discordance are quite variable, and, at least in part, the relative positions of the great arteries are predicated on the infundibular anatomy. By far, the most common relationship is location of the aorta to the right of and anterior to the pulmonary valve, but side-by-side, left-anterior, right-anterior, and left-posterior relationships have all been described. Thus, "transposition" should *not* be defined in terms of the relative position of the great arteries, but rather should be viewed in terms of the ventriculoarterial connection.

Less Common Anomalies Associated with Transposition

Left juxtaposition of the right atrial appendage (Rosenquist *et al.*, 1974) has been identified in about 1 to 2 per cent of our patients with complete transposition. These patients have had dextrocardia or mesocardia and often an unusual spatial ventricular relationship. Almost any anomaly of the atrioventricular valve can complicate complete transposition (Layman and Edwards, 1967). Straddling of the tricuspid valve can be identified in some patients. It is particularly important to rule out an abnormality of the right atrioventricular junction in the patient with right ventricular hypoplasia (Riemenschneider *et al.*, 1968). Structural anomalies of the mitral valve are not uncommon in patients with complete transposition (Rosenquist *et al.*, 1975), but fortunately, functional disturbances seem less frequent. Thus, although mitral stenosis or straddling of the anterior leaflet of the mitral valve has been recorded, such instances are uncommon. Perhaps tricuspid atresia is more common than mitral atresia.

Obstructive anomalies of the aortic arch, including coarctation, atresia, and complete interruption of the aortic arch, have been identified in about 6 per cent of our patients. Although severe coarctation can be found when the ventricular septum is intact and when the right ventricle is of normal size, such aortic arch anomalies are more frequently identified when a VSD is present or when the morphologically right ventricle is underdeveloped. Finally, aortic valve atresia can rarely complicate the condition of the patient with complete TGA with an intact ventricular septum (McGarry *et al.*, 1980).

Laterality of the Aortic Arch

A left aortic arch is found in about 90 to 92 per cent of patients with complete TGA. In 8 to 10 per cent, the aortic arch is right-sided. The lowest frequency of right aortic arch (about 4 per cent) is found in patients with an intact ventricular septum, and the highest incidence (about 16 per cent) is seen among those with VSD and left ventricular outflow tract stenosis (Mathew *et al.*, 1974).

The Coronary Arteries

Knowledge of the aortic origin of the coronary arteries and their epicardial distribution is necessary for the operative management of some forms of transposition. The epicardial distribution must be defined prior to interposition of a right ventricular–pulmonary artery conduit. Because the anterior descending coronary artery can cross the right ventricular outflow tract, this distribution may prevent or make difficult interposition of a right ventricular conduit in the young or small patient. Since 1975, when Jatene and colleagues successfully performed an anatomic repair with coronary artery reimplantation, there has been a resurgence of interest in the anatomy and variations of the coronary artery origin in these patients (see the third section of this chapter on anatomic correction of transposition).

Wall Thickness of Ventricular Chambers in Transposition

Bano-Rodrigo and colleagues (1980) have examined the wall thickness of ventricular chambers in TGA. The surgical implications of these findings with regard to the arterial switch are obvious. Among their patients with TGA and an intact ventricular septum, a significant decrease in the left ventricular–right ventricular ratio was found after the neonatal period, and after 8 months of age the thickness of the left ventricular wall in this group was under the 95 per cent confidence limits for normality. For patients with an associated large VSD, the same was true after 18 months of age. In view of their findings, these authors could not recommend anatomic correction after 8 months of age for the patients with an intact ventricular septum, or after 18 months of age for the patient with a large VSD. A similar study was recently published by Huhta and colleagues (1982).

The Pulmonary Arteries

Among patients with complete TGA and an intact ventricular septum, the main and branch pulmonary arteries are usually dilated when compared with normal ones, especially after the newborn period. Furthermore, after the newborn period, one can recognize asymmetric distribution of the pulmonary blood flow between the right and left lungs (Muster *et al.*, 1976). The inclination or geometry of the left ventricular outflow tract favors blood flow from the main pulmonary artery to the right pulmonary artery. This maldistribution of flow may be increased when there is LVOTO or when there are anatomic stenoses in the left pulmonary artery. The disparity in perfusion between the two lungs may be progressive.

Patients with associated VSD and left ventricular outflow tract stenosis can exhibit all of the anomalies of pulmonary arteries anticipated in patients with Fallot's tetralogy (see Chapter 36). Among the patients with pulmonary atresia and VSD (but posterior pulmonary artery), it will be necessary to define the site(s) of origin of the pulmonary arteries (i.e., single ductus; ascending aorta; aortopulmonary collaterals; bilateral homologous ducts when the right and left pulmonary arteries are not confluent; and so on).

PATHOPHYSIOLOGY

The neonate with complete TGA, an intact ventricular septum, a small ASD and a closing PDA can be viewed as having two parallel circulations: a systemic circulation and a pulmonary circulation. Survival in this group of patients for even a short time is predicated on affording adequate mixing between the two parallel circulations. The presence of a large VSD or a large PDA affords some mixing between the two circulations. Thus, intense cyanosis is less common, and frequently, these patients are only mildly to moderately cyanotic. Yet, in this group, congestive heart failure may be very conspicuous and unresponsive to anticongestive therapy.

The patient with associated VSD and LVOTO has a natural history similar to that of the patient with Fallot's tetralogy. An increasing severity of LVOTO will result in inadequate pulmonary blood flow, and for this reason, hypoxia and polycythemia may become progressive. When the pulmonary arteries are not in continuity with the heart, pulmonary blood flow may be entirely duct-dependent, or, depending on the site of origin of the pulmonary arteries, the patient may have reasonable saturation in the aorta.

CLINICAL MANIFESTATIONS

Two thirds of patients with complete transposition are males (Fyler, 1980). Although 9 per cent of patients with complete transposition included in the New England Regional Infant Cardiac Program had extracardiac congenital anomalies, the majority of these anomalies were minor. In reviewing 140 clinical and autopsy cases of complete transposition, Landtman and colleagues (1975) found extracardiac malformations in 39 patients, which were thought to be responsible for the death of 22 of these patients. Low birth weight is not a consistent feature.

The clinical manifestations will, of course, depend on the presence or absence of associated cardiovascular anomalies. Because the majority of patients with complete transposition will have inadequate circulatory mixing, these patients will inevitably present in the newborn period. The most striking physical sign

of TGA is persistent cyanosis unresponsive to an increased oxygen concentration (Shannon et al., 1972; Tooley and Stanger, 1972; Goldman et al., 1973; Jones et al., 1976). Cyanosis, usually progressive, may be intense, especially when the neonate is also relatively polycythemic. It may be less intense, or even equivocal, in the patient with good circulatory mixing. When ductal patency is responsible for only equivocal cyanosis, the reprieve may be transient, and ductal closure may lead to rapid clinical deterioration (Rowe et al., 1981). Differential cyanosis with relatively pink lower extremities and deeper cyanosis of the upper extremities may be found in the patient with associated severe thoracic coarctation or interruption of the aortic arch. After cyanosis, the next most conspicuous finding in these patients is congestive heart failure, with tachycardia, tachypnea, dyspnea, and an enlarged liver. It would be distinctly uncommon for the patient with severe LVOTO to have signs of heart failure. Conversely, the patient with a large VSD or ductus arteriosus or severe obstructive anomaly of the aortic arch may present in severe cardiorespiratory distress, with relatively mild to moderate hypoxia and cyanosis. The profoundly acidotic infant may present in extremis.

The heart is usually overactive, with a prominent left parasternal lift. The heart sounds are usually loud and crisp. The second sound is single. When the ventricular septum is intact, there may be no murmur, or a soft systolic ejection murmur may be audible along the left sternal border. A soft pansystolic murmur may indicate the presence of a small or moderate VSD. It is uncommon to appreciate a typical "machinery" murmur of a PDA in the immediate newborn period. The caliber and timing of the femoral pulses may indicate an obstructive anomaly of the aortic arch.

LABORATORY FINDINGS

Radiologic Features. The typical radiographic appearance of TGA is that of an enlarged heart with the appearance of an egg on its side (Fig. 40–1). Pulmonary plethora may be conspicuous, and beyond the first 1 or 2 months of life, a disparity in pulmonary perfusion may be apparent, with the right lung being more plethoric than the left. Characteristically, the cardiac pedicle is narrow (Kurlander et al., 1968; Nogrady and Dunbar, 1969; Guerin et al., 1970; Moes, 1975; Tonkin et al., 1976). Although these features can be seen in the first few days of life, there are numerous exceptions to the classic appearance. Indeed, Counahan and colleagues (1973) suggested that 10 per cent of plain chest radiographs obtained from infants less than 1 month of age with complete TGA were interpreted as normal.

Electrocardiography. Most patients exhibit normal sinus rhythm or a sinus tachycardia. About 2 per cent exhibit the so-called coronary sinus rhythm, with a negative P wave in leads 2, 3 and aVf, and a normal

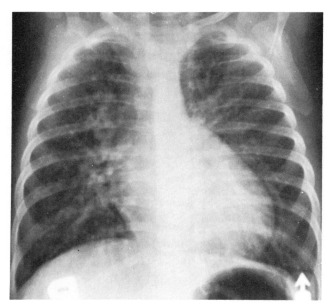

Figure 40–1. Chest radiograph of a youngster with complete transposition of the great arteries. The cardiac pedicle is narrow, and the configuration is "egg-shaped." Pulmonary plethora is conspicuous. (Courtesy of C.A.F. Moes, M.D., Department of Radiology, The Hospital for Sick Children, Toronto.)

P-R interval. The mean QRS axis congregates around +100° to +120°, although some patients exhibit profound right-axis deviation of +150° to +240°. It is distinctly uncommon to identify left-axis deviation in patients with uncomplicated TGA.

There is not a clear-cut relationship between the pattern of ventricular hypertrophy and the presence or absence of a VSD and/or LVOTO. Most patients, especially hypoxic neonates, show a pattern of right ventricular hypertrophy or dominance, and our data indicate that left ventricular hypertrophy or combined ventricular hypertrophy is uncommonly observed in the neonate. Even in the patient with severe LVOTO with or without a VSD, it is unusual for the electrocardiogram to demonstrate severe left ventricular hypertrophy.

ST-T wave changes are not uncommon and may reflect some degree of myocardial ischemia, especially in the severely hypoxic and acidotic neonate.

Echocardiography. Both M-mode and two-dimensional echocardiographic examinations have had a major impact on the noninvasive diagnosis of complete TGA. Using the two-dimensional technique, the demonstration of the abnormal spatial relationship between the aorta and the pulmonary artery (when compared with the normal relationship) and their respective origins from the discordant ventricle can be done in a matter of only a few minutes (Houston *et al.*, 1978; Bierman and Williams, 1979b). But what is the relevance of the echocardiographic examination to the surgeon?

Once the diagnosis of complete transposition has been unequivocally confirmed, two-dimensional echocardiographic techniques should allow (1) visualiza-

tion of the atrial septum and the adequacy of balloon atrial septostomy; (2) longitudinal assessment of ventricular contractility and wall motion; (3) assessment of the atrioventricular junction in the patient with complex transposition; (4) the recognition of the type of LVOTO when left ventricular angiography is unsatisfactory (Aziz *et al.*, 1978, 1979); (5) imaging of the ventricular septum and quantitation of the number and type of VSD; and (6) imaging of the aortic isthmus and juxtaductal or juxtaligamental level with regard to the question of coarctation.

Following the Mustard operation, echocardiographic techniques allow visualization of the baffle and serial assessment of right ventricular function. The use of microcavitation facilitates recognition of baffle leaks in the postoperative period or residual shunting at the ventricular level.

Angiocardiography. There is currently an extensive literature devoted to the angiocardiography of patients with complete TGA (Barcia *et al.*, 1967; Deutsch *et al.*, 1970; Fisher *et al.*, 1970; Silove and Taylor, 1973; Freedom *et al.*, 1974, 1983; Paul, 1977; Sansa *et al.*, 1979).

Selective right ventriculography is usually performed in frontal and lateral projections, and currently most institutions will perform selective angiocardiograms in the biplane mode. Frontal and lateral right ventriculograms are most frequently performed and will demonstrate the discordant ventriculoarterial connection, the subaortic infundibulum, the size and function (when using cine technique) of the right ventricle, and the presence or absence of tricuspid regurgitation, and when the ventricular septum is intact (or when only a small VSD is present), the status of the aortic isthmus, ductus arteriosus, and the presence or absence of a juxtaductal coarctation or other obstructive anomaly of the aortic arch (Figs. 40–2 and 40–3). When a significant VSD is present, opacification of the main and left pulmonary arteries may obscure the aortic isthmus. Thus, selective aortography may be necessary to more fully define the caliber of the aortic isthmus and to exclude obstructive anomalies of the aortic arch (Fig. 40–4). Furthermore, the origin of the coronary arteries is best visualized by aortography filmed in the biplane mode.

Selective biplane left ventriculography is best filmed using axial cineangiography. Such projections, as initially advocated by Bargeron and colleagues (1977) and Elliott and associates (1977), will elongate the left ventricular outflow tract. This has two immediate advantages. First, it allows precise definition of the left ventricular outflow tract, without the "shoulder" of the left ventricle compromising the immediate subpulmonary area (Fig. 40–5). Second, the left long axial oblique projection should profile the majority of the VSD involving the infundibular or perimembranous septum. When a more posteriorly positioned VSD is suspected, it would be advantageous to utilize the hepatoclavicular four-chamber projection. This more adequately profiles the inlet and posterior aspects of the ventricular septum.

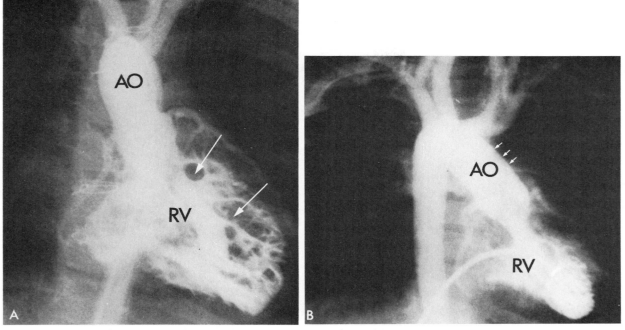

Figure 40–2. Complete transposition of the great arteries. *A*, Frontal right ventriculogram with opacification of aorta (AO). The right ventricle (RV) is heavily trabeculated (white arrows). The ascending aorta is in the usual position. *B*, In this patient with complete transposition, the aorta is relatively levo-positioned and the ascending aorta (white arrows) forms the left border of the cardiac silhouette.

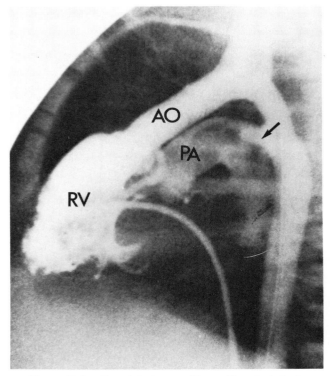

Figure 40–3. Complete transposition with patent ductus arteriosus. Lateral right ventriculogram demonstrates an anteriorly positioned, discordantly connected aorta (AO). The larger and posteriorly positioned pulmonary artery (PA) is opacified via a moderate-sized patent ductus arteriosus (arrow). (RV = ventricle.)

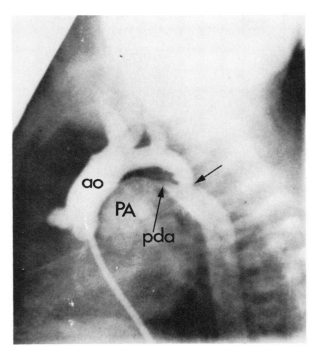

Figure 40–4. Coarctation of the aorta (arrow on right) complicating complete transposition of the great arteries. This aortogram demonstrates a relatively small ascending aorta (ao), a small aortic isthmus, and a discrete coarctation of aorta with a posterior shelf. The small patent ductus arteriosus (pda) opacifies the pulmonary artery (PA).

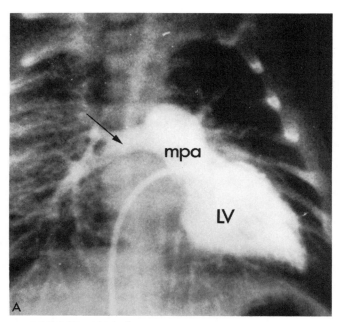

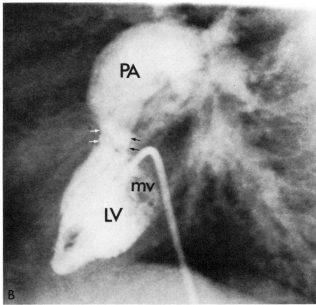

profiled using this projection, but the exact degree of obliquity must be individualized for every patient (Figs. 40–6 to 40–8).

Selective atrial angiography (right or left) may be necessary to define the presence or absence of a straddling atrioventricular connection. We advocate such atrial angiography in those patients with the superointerior ventricular relationship or the appearance of crossed atrioventricular connections, both conditions in which a straddling atrioventricular valve might be encountered. Atrial angiography may be useful in evaluating the atrioventricular junction when the concordant ventricle is underdeveloped. Furthermore, when mesocardia or dextrocardia is present, a selective right atrial angiogram will exclude left juxtaposition of the right atrial appendage, a condition that makes the Blalock-Hanlon atrial septectomy or intra-atrial repair more difficult, especially in the very young and small patient (Rosenquist *et al.,* 1975; Urban *et al.,* 1976).

Figure 40–5. Left ventriculogram in a patient with complete transposition of the great arteries and an intact ventricular septum. *A,* Frontal left ventriculogram opacifies the discordantly connected pulmonary artery (mpa). There is preferential flow into the right pulmonary artery (arrow) because of the inclination of the left ventricular outflow tract. (LV = left ventricle.) *B,* An intact ventricular septum and absence of left ventricular outflow tract obstruction (between white and black arrows) (mv = mitral valve).

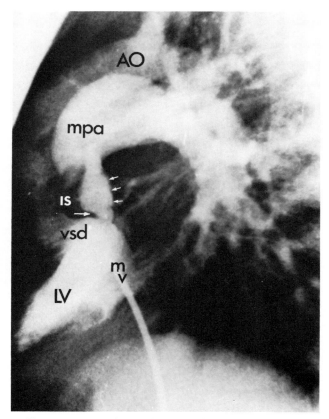

Figure 40–6. Left ventricular outflow tract obstruction at several sites in a child with complete transposition of the great arteries and malalignment type of ventricular septal defect. This long axial oblique left ventriculogram shows that the pulmonary artery (mpa) is supported by the left ventricle (LV). The infundibular septum (IS) is deviated posteriorly (solitary white arrow) and is seen superior to the large ventricular septal defect (vsd). The subpulmonary infundibulum is an elongated muscular structure (small white arrows), and because it is well developed but poorly expanded, there is discontinuity between the pulmonary valve and the anterior leaflet of the mitral valve (mv). (AO = aorta.)

As mentioned earlier, there is considerable heterogeneity among these anatomic causes of LVOTO. The left long axial oblique projection is ideal to demonstrate posterior malalignment of the infundibular septum and the resulting VSD. The presence of associated pulmonary valve stenosis, fibrous diaphragm, fibromuscular tunnel form of subpulmonary stenosis, and accessory tissue tags is also usually best

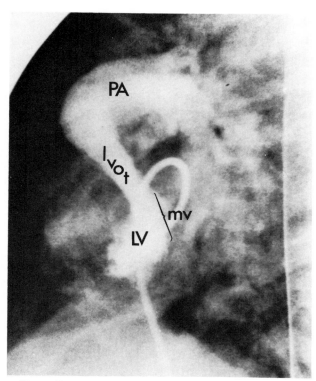

Figure 40–7. Muscular tunnel form of subpulmonary stenosis in a patient with complete transposition of the great arteries and multiple small ventricular septal defects. This lateral left ventriculogram demonstrates the markedly elongated left ventricular outflow tract (lvot). The main pulmonary trunk (PA) is of good caliber. Clearly, the mitral valve (mv) is not in continuity with the pulmonary valve. (LV = left ventricle.)

NATURAL HISTORY OF THE PATIENT WITH COMPLETE TRANSPOSITION OF THE GREAT ARTERIES

Prior to the introduction of balloon atrial septostomy by Rashkind and Miller in 1966, the natural history for these patients was quite clear: 90 per cent of patients with TGA would *not* survive to their first birthday, and nearly half of all these patients would die by 1 month of age (Liebman *et al.*, 1969). Although nonoperative atrial septostomy has irrevocably altered the natural history, a substantial number of patients with transposition will still die before reaching their first birthday. Data compiled from the New England Infant Cardiac Program (Fyler, 1980) reveal a crude first-year mortality rate of 39 per cent for patients with complete transposition. In reviewing 112 consecutive neonates with complete transposition seen at the Texas Children's Hospital from 1967 to 1977, Gutgesell and colleagues (1979) found that the first month of life was the period of greatest risk, with an 8 per cent mortality rate. Between the balloon atrial septostomy and baffle repair, 14 of 103 patients at risk either died or sustained a cerebrovascular accident. The mortality rate at baffle repair in their series was 14 per cent, with three late postoperative deaths. Their

actuarial analysis suggested that approximately 50 per cent of newborns with transposition of the great arteries will survive for 5 years with excellent function and that an additional 15 to 20 per cent will survive with one or more medical handicaps.

Plauth and associates (1968) reviewed serial hemodynamic studies among a cohort of patients with complete TGA. Like the patient with a small VSD and an otherwise normal heart, the small VSD in the patient with complete transposition can undergo spontaneous diminution in size or spontaneous closure. Diminution in size may be accompanied by so-called aneurysmal transformation. Because the aneurysm protrudes into the left ventricular outflow tract, this may result in subpulmonary stenosis (Vidne *et al.*, 1976). We would assume that the spontaneous closure rate of a small VSD in the patient with complete transposition is about the same as that in the individual with an otherwise normal heart.

LVOTO can develop or may worsen with time in the patient with an associated VSD or in the patient with an intact ventricular septum. Our own data indicate that the development of LVOTO in the individual with an intact ventricular septum is in the range

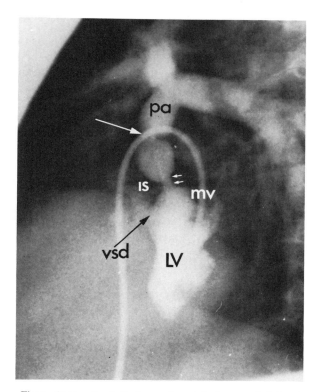

Figure 40–8. A relatively small ventricular septal defect (vsd) and severe subpulmonary obstruction are demonstrated by this long axial oblique left ventriculogram performed via the mitral valve (mv). The ventricular septal defect is inferior to the posteriorly malaligned infundibular septum (IS). There is concentric stenosis (two small white arrows) of the left ventricular outflow tract. The severely stenotic pulmonary valve (long white arrow) is partially obscured by the catheter. The muscular subpulmonary infundibulum prevents pulmonary valve–mitral valve fibrous continuity. (LV = left ventricle.)

of 2 to 3 per cent and is somewhat higher in the patient with an associated VSD. Tonkin and coworkers (1980) have provided beautiful angiographic verification of developing LVOTO in patients with complete transposition and an intact ventricular septum.

Pulmonary vascular obstructive disease is distinctly uncommon within the first few years of life in the patient with complete TGA and an intact ventricular septum. Nonetheless, Lakier and colleagues (1975) and Newfeld and associates (1974) have described early onset of pulmonary vascular obstruction in a small number of patients. Far more common is the development of pulmonary vascular arteriopathy in those patients with an associated large VSD or large PDA (Newfeld *et al.*, 1974; Waldman *et al.*, 1977). Although it is difficult and unwise to generalize, many patients with complete transposition and an unrestrictive VSD or ductus arteriosus may develop severe pulmonary vascular obstruction by 1 year of age (Yamaki and Tezuka, 1976).

MEDICAL TREATMENT

The initial medical therapy of the severely hypoxic neonate should be directed toward (1) correction of metabolic acidosis, (2) treatment of congestive heart failure with parenteral digoxin and diuretics, (3) maintenance of normothermia, (4) treatment of hypoglycemia, and (5) provision of adequate ventilation for the profoundly distressed infant. Echocardiographic examination should then be performed as expeditiously as possible, and the neonate should be transferred to the cardiac catheterization laboratory. If the clinical and echocardiographic features of complete transposition are unequivocal in the critically ill neonate, we perform balloon atrial septostomy prior to hemodynamic and angiocardiographic investigations. Balloon atrial septostomy should be performed with the largest balloon catheter that can be safely introduced. This can be done via a saphenofemoral venous cutdown, by the percutaneous approach, via the umbilical vein. We perform the septostomy maneuver a number of times until no further resistance is met at the atrial septum. When hemodynamic recordings are obtained prior to balloon atrial septostomy, we routinely record a withdrawal pressure tracing from the left to the right atrium following balloon septostomy, as well as obtaining arterial Po_2 and saturation data before and after the procedure.

In some neonates, the clinical and echocardiographic features may not be entirely consistent with complete transposition. When this situation is encountered, complete hemodynamic data are obtained, and indicator dilution curves are obtained by injection of indocyanine green dye initially in the right atrium with withdrawal from the aorta, and then by injection in the left atrium, again sampling in the aorta, which will provide the correct diagnosis (Gingell *et al.*, 1979). We prefer to use dye dilution techniques to confirm the diagnosis in the acidotic infant, because contrast material may hasten clinical deterioration. Again, once the unequivocal diagnosis of complete transposition has been made, balloon atrial septostomy is then indicated. Finally, complete hemodynamic and angiocardiographic investigations should be performed. The use of flow-directed catheters will facilitate entry into all the cardiac chambers, and usually both great arteries can be entered (Kelly *et al.*, 1971). When possible, it is desirable to position an umbilical artery catheter proximal to the origin of the ductus arteriosus. This will allow efficient blood-gas analysis and may expedite the catheter study. Unless the left ventricular pressure is half systemic or less, we routinely attempt to record the pulmonary artery pressure.

There is not unanimity as to the definition of an adequate response to balloon atrial septostomy (the pertinent literature is summarized in Rowe *et al.*, 1981). Some neonates will remain hypoxic, despite what would seem to be an adequate balloon atrial septostomy. The adequacy of the balloon atrial septostomy can be viewed in terms of abolishing the interatrial pressure gradient and visualization of the atrial septum following septostomy to quantitate the adequacy of the tear (Korns *et al.*, 1972; Clark *et al.*, 1977; Bierman and Williams, 1979a).

We have tried two maneuvers to facilitate atrial mixing in neonates in whom we would have anticipated a better response to balloon atrial septostomy. If congestive heart failure is not a feature, hypertransfusion with 5.0 to 10 ml./kg. of whole blood, by increasing atrial filling, may afford a substantial improvement in arterial oxygen saturation. Or, when we are convinced of an adequate tear of the atrial septum, the administration of an E-type prostaglandin may improve systemic oxygenation (Benson *et al.*, 1979; Driscoll *et al.*, 1979; Lang *et al.*, 1979; Henry *et al.*, 1981). The action of the E-type prostaglandin is to maintain patency of the ductus arteriosus (Coceani and Olley, 1973; Olley *et al.*, 1978). The increase in pulmonary venous blood to the left atrium facilitated by the prostaglandin may alter the compliance of the left atrium; if an adequate interatrial communication is present, increased mixing may result. We would certainly urge caution in the use of prostaglandins when the interatrial communication is marginal (Benson *et al.*, 1979). When the interatrial defect is restrictive, E-type prostaglandins, by increasing pulmonary blood flow, may actually precipitate or worsen congestive heart failure. Despite an "adequate" balloon atrial septostomy, hypertransfusion, and the administration of an E-type prostaglandin, some babies, fortunately few, will remain severely hypoxic. Such babies may appear reasonably comfortable, despite an arterial Po_2 of 20 to 25 mm. Hg, and one might be tempted into complacency. Yet it is this type of patient who is prone to a hypoxic cerebrovascular accident. For this reason, if a neonate maintains an arterial Po_2 consistently below 30 mm. Hg, we advocate a Blalock-Hanlon atrial septectomy. In other institutions, a second balloon atrial septostomy might be performed or an early intra-atrial baffle or Senning repair may be done.

The medical management of the neonate with an associated small or moderate VSD is the same as that for the patient with an intact ventricular septum.

The patient with a large VSD and/or a large PDA poses a somewhat different problem, and our views about the surgical therapy of these groups of patients are changing. Congestive heart failure rather than hypoxia may be the more conspicuous sign, and, indeed, some of these babies will have arterial oxygen saturations of from 80 to 85 per cent. Nonetheless, we strongly urge that all patients with complete transposition (no matter what the associated lesion) undergo balloon atrial septostomy. Even a large ductus can close, and babies in whom this occurs can become acutely hypoxic. Furthermore, if a clinically "malignant" ductus requires surgical ligation, the magnitude of interatrial mixing will become very important. At present, the timing and type of surgery reserved for the patient with TGA, a large VSD or a large PDA, and systemic levels of left ventricular hypertension are undergoing review. The surgical options for the baby with a large VSD and pulmonary artery hypertension include (1) intra-atrial repair and VSD closure, (2) pulmonary artery banding, followed by the Mustard repair, VSD closure and debanding, or debanding with anatomic repair, or (3) primary anatomic repair. Because most patients with a nonrestrictive VSD develop pulmonary vascular obstruction, some form of surgical intervention will certainly be necessary within the first year of life. Other patients with intractable congestive heart failure and severe growth retardation may require surgical intervention within the first few weeks or months of life. Similarly, for the patient with transposition, an intact ventricular septum, and pulmonary artery (and left ventricular) hypertension secondary to a large ductus arteriosus, the surgical options include early duct ligation followed by Mustard repair or surgery within 3 months to 1 year of life with duct ligation and Mustard repair or duct ligation and anatomic repair.

SURGICAL TREATMENT

Palliative Procedures

The basic principle of all palliation is to improve mixing between the pulmonary and systemic circulations by creating or enlarging an ASD. Enlargement of an ASD by means of the Rashkind balloon atrial septostomy (Rashkind and Miller, 1966) is employed universally at the time of initial cardiac catheterization in almost all infants with TGA.

Before the development of balloon atrial septostomy, some form of surgical atrial septectomy was an essential component in the management of infants with TGA and an intact ventricular septum. Although closed techniques using various ingenious instruments or open excision of the septum with inflow caval

occlusion were often effective, the resultant ASD was relatively small and the palliation sometimes barely adequate. The original operation by Blalock and Hanlon (1950) creates a large ASD and remains the surgical procedure of choice for palliation (Fig. 40–9). The technique is demanding, but if it is done carefully, the results are excellent. Cooley reported that 23 to 28 children operated on from 1958 to 1960 have survived (Ochsner et al., 1961). In 20 cases treated by Spencer (1973) only one death occurred. Since 1968, at the Hospital for Sick Children in Toronto, there have been 8 deaths in 112 Blalock-Hanlon operations performed. Conduction disturbances may occur (Hamilton et al., 1968), and it is important to leave part of the atrial septum to preserve the artery to the sinoatrial (SA) node and internodal pathways (Trusler et al., 1980).

Over the past decade, improved operative techniques and better perioperative management have reduced the mortality of TGA repair. The elective age for repair has been lowered, and many surgeons now recommend primary repair at an early age whenever the protection afforded by balloon atrial septostomy is no longer adequate. Others continue to recommend surgical septectomy for most infants who require surgery in the first 2 to 3 months of life on the basis that repair at this age carries a slightly higher operative risk and the chance of postoperative complications is greater. The choice rests with the surgeon, who must consider his experience with both the Blalock-Hanlon operation and the repair.

Infants with TGA and a large VSD require treatment before they are 6 months old to prevent pulmonary vascular disease and often earlier to relieve congestive heart failure. Balloon atrial septostomy soon after birth helps by eliminating left atrial hypertension and improving oxygen saturation. At one time, pulmonary artery banding was the mainstay of palliation for these infants (Trusler and Mustard, 1968). Now early repair, either intra-atrial or arterial, is preferred. Occasionally, in very small or very ill infants or when there is some complicating feature such as a muscular VSD or a hypoplastic ventricle, pulmonary artery banding rather than repair is advisable. In such cases, in order to apply an adequate band, there must be a satisfactory ASD. If there is not, a Blalock-Hanlon septectomy should be done with the banding. Both procedures can be performed through a right anterolateral thoracotomy. Edwards and associates (1964) described a modification of the Blalock-Hanlon operation in which the atrial septum is not resected but is sutured to the posterior wall of the left atrium medial to the right pulmonary venous orifices. This produces obligatory mixing of the right pulmonary venous return in the right atrium and appears to provide better palliation than the Blalock-Hanlon procedure when associated with pulmonary artery banding.

Infants with TGA plus a VSD and LVOTO often require palliation before they are old enough for repair. When the VSD is large and the LVOTO is a

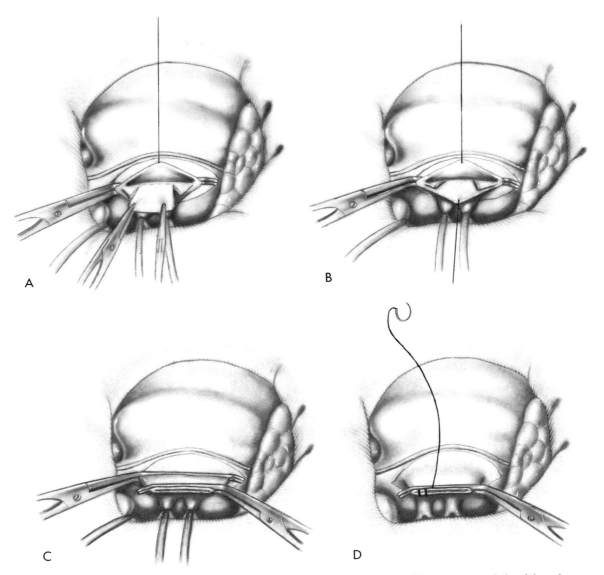

Figure 40–9. Approach by a right lateral thoracotomy through the fifth interspace with snares around the right pulmonary artery and the upper and lower right pulmonary veins, and a partial occlusion clamp with one jaw posterior to the pulmonary veins and the other anterior, so that a portion of the right and left atria has been included. The pericardium has been opened posterior to the right phrenic nerve, and the right and left atria have been opened by an incision parallel to the atrial septum. The atrial septum has been incised with scissors, the free edges have been grasped with hemostats, and an extra portion of atrial septum has been withdrawn from the heart while the partial occlusion clamp was gently released (*A*). The mobilized flap of atrial septum is then cut through its pedicle (*B*), and a smaller partial-occlusion clamp is applied to the free edges of the incision in the left and right atria and lies anterior to the right pulmonary veins (*C*). The larger occlusion clamp is then released, as are the snares on the pulmonary veins and the pulmonary artery. The incision in the atria can then be closed at leisure (*D*). (From Aberdeen E.: Blalock-Hanlon operation and Rashkind procedure. *In* Rob, C., and Smith, R.: Operative Surgery. 2nd Ed. London, Butterworth, 1968, Vol, 2, pp. 193–199.)

type that cannot be relieved directly, the best treatment is a Rastelli operation, but this procedure should not be done until some time after the child's fifth birthday. Prior to that time, if palliation is required, a shunt is done, preferably a Blalock-Taussig anastomosis, which is the easiest shunt to close at repair and is associated with the fewest complications. In the series of Stark and coworkers (1971), 54 of 58 children who had Blalock-Taussig shunts between 1953 and 1968 survived. From 1960 to 1980, at the Hospital for Sick Children in Toronto, 54 Blalock-

Taussig shunts were done in children with TGA, with one death.

Other shunts have been used, but most have serious disadvantages. In patients more than 6 months of age, the Glenn operation (Glenn, 1958) is effective and safe, but it is much more difficult to take down later and should not be used. The Potts anastomosis is the easiest shunt to construct in a small infant but causes serious stenosis and scarring of the pulmonary artery in many infants. It should be used only in exceptional circumstances. Similarly, the Waterston anastomosis, although easier to take down than a Potts anastomosis, often causes severe pulmonary artery narrowing. The problem cases are small infants who weigh less than 3 kg. Blalock-Taussig anastomoses are not only difficult to construct in infants at this early age but are unreliable and often, depending on the size of the subclavian artery, provide meager and short-lived palliation. An alternative described by de Leval and associates (1981), which consists of using a prosthesis from the subclavian artery to the pulmonary artery, has shown some promise.

In infants with TGA and LVOTO without a VSD, creation of a large ASD usually provides adequate palliation until repair can be accomplished. If the LVOTO is severe and in a form that cannot be relieved by a direct attack, it may be advisable to provide palliation for the child for some years with a Blalock-Taussig shunt as well as the Blalock-Hanlon septectomy. Patients who have undergone such palliative procedures may be at risk for the early onset of pulmonary vascular obstructive disease.

Surgical Repair

A variety of repair procedures are now available, and the choice is generally dictated by the anatomy. Arterial repair is usually used for TGA with a VSD and is considered separately. The Rastelli procedure is used for TGA with a VSD and LVOTO and intraventricular repair is employed for exceptional patients with very large VSDs. There are two primary operations for intra-atrial repair: the Senning operation and the Mustard operation. The Senning operation is dealt with in another section of this chapter, as is the arterial switch procedure. A description of the Mustard procedure follows.

The Mustard Procedure

Through a median sternotomy, the anterior aspect of the pericardial sac is cleared for a width of 5 to 6 cm. and superiorly to the great arteries, where the thymus is reflected. The pericardium is incised close to the diaphragm and a relatively rectangular patch of pericardium is taken for use as the intra-atrial baffle. The patch is hollowed or made concave on both sides to create a waist that is 2.5 to 3.0 cm. wide. Both ends are rounded for adequate caval channels. The inferior vena caval end is slightly larger (5 cm.) and more rounded to allow flexibility of choice in the position of the suture line. In a child weighing 10 kg., the main dimensions are 4 cm. by 7 cm. In a 5-kg. infant, the dimensions are 0.5 cm. less on all sides. The long side of the patch is taken some distance from but approximately parallel to the right phrenic nerve. It extends from the diaphragm below to the most prominent point on the ascending aorta above. Once this margin is cut (Fig. 40–10), its measured length serves as a tentative guide for the length of the other borders. This is particularly useful in older children who are outside the usual size range at operation.

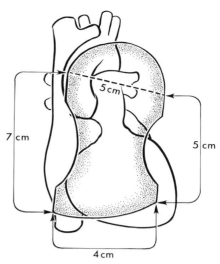

Figure 40–10. Artist's depiction of the pericardial patch (stippled area) for the intra-atrial baffle. Basic dimensions are 7 × 4 cm. for a 10-kg. child, 0.5 cm. less for a 5-kg. child. The slightly convex superior vena cava portion is taken along the diaphragm. The long border is on the right atrium, extending up to the ascending aorta. The other two borders are basically 5 cm. long, but the superior border is fully rounded to allow flexibility in choosing the suture line position around the inferior vena cava.

At present, most patients with TGA undergo intracardiac repair in the first year of life, with deep hypothermia and circulatory arrest. Older children weighing more than 10 kg. undergo repair with cardiopulmonary bypass and moderate hypothermia. Low-flow bypass and aortic cross-clamping are useful adjuncts to improve exposure for short periods of time.

In infants, cannulas are inserted into the ascending aorta and right atrial appendage after the pericardial baffle is prepared. Moderate cooling is allowed during the early part of the operation. Once the cannulas are in place, the child is placed on bypass and core-cooled until the rectal temperature is 16° to 18°C. At this point, the esophageal temperature is usually about 10° to 12°C. During cooling, tourniquets are placed around the cavae and the aorta, the in and out lines for the cold pericardial bath are positioned, and the cardioplegia line is filled and inserted in the ascending aorta.

When cooling is done on bypass, the esophageal and blood temperatures are close. The rectal temperature falls more slowly and is likely to be a safer guide to brain temperature. When the rectal temperature reaches 16° to 18°C., the pump is stopped and the aortic line and the aorta are clamped. The caval tourniquets are snugged, the venous cannula is removed, and the right atrium is opened with a longitudinal incision well away from the SA node (Fig. 40–11). Cold (4°C.) potassium is injected into the aortic root (300 ml./M.² of surface area) to induce cardioplegia. The pericardial bath (4°C.) is also started, dripping onto a gauze square covering the right ventricle.

After cardioplegia is obtained, the interior of the

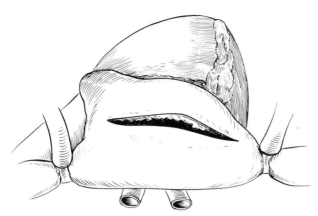

Figure 40–11. With circulatory arrest and the venous cannula removed, the caval tourniquets are tightened and a longitudinal incision is made in the right atrium.

right atrium is examined (Fig. 40–12). If there is a VSD or LVOTO, it should be examined and the pulmonary venous orifices, left atrial appendage, and mitral valve identified. The remaining atrial septum is partly excised. The first cut is made from the superior border of the ASD up to the middle of the superior vena caval (SVC) orifice. The ridge of septum to the left of this cut is preserved, for it often contains the artery to the SA node and may act as a conduction pathway between the SA node and the AV node. The atrial septum to the right of this cut is excised completely. This excision is extended to include any septal remnant near the inferior vena cava (IVC). The coronary sinus is cut back into the left atrium for a distance of approximately 1.5 cm., and any residual septum between the IVC and the coronary sinus is excised. The raw cut margins left by excising septum are oversewn with a 5-0 suture material, taking relatively small bites to avoid a purse-string effect (Fig. 40–13).

The intra-atrial baffle is now sutured into the common atrium using a double-armed continuous 3-0 braided synthetic suture (Fig. 40–14). The midpoint of the long side of the baffle is sutured and tied to the anterior margin of the internal orifices of the left pulmonary veins. From here, the continuous suture

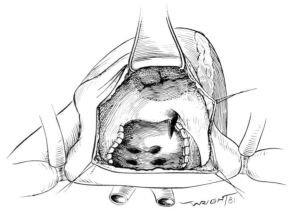

Figure 40–13. The first cut is made from the superior border of the ASD up to the middle of the superior vena caval orifice. The ridge of septum to the left of this cut is preserved, for it often contains the artery to the SA node and may act as a conduction pathway between the SA node and the AV node. The atrial septum to the right of this cut is excised completely. This excision is extended to include any septal remnant near the inferior vena cava. The coronary sinus is cut back into the left atrium for a distance of approximately 1.5 cm., and any residual septum between the inferior vena cava and the coronary sinus is excised. The raw cut margins left by the excision of septum are oversewn with 5-0 suture material taking relatively small bites to avoid a purse-string effect.

line passes around the orifice of the left superior pulmonary vein to reach the posterior wall of the left atrium, crosses that wall, curving inferiorly for a short distance to create a larger SVC channel, and then passes between the right superior pulmonary vein and the SVC orifice. The first corner of the baffle (i.e., one end of the long border) should reach the lateral wall of the right atrium. The short SVC border of the baffle is then sutured around the internal orifice of the SVC, and the second corner of the baffle reaches part of the way across the roof of the right atrium between the SVC and the residual ridge of atrial septum. Initially, on this border, relatively large bites of baffle

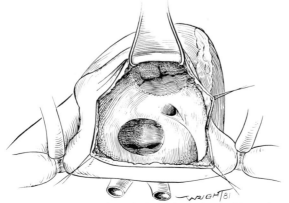

Figure 40–12. Interior of the right atrium with moderately large ASD.

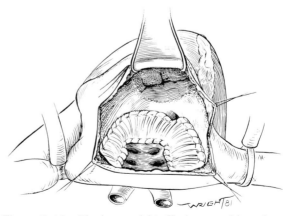

Figure 40–14. The intra-atrial baffle is sutured into the common atrial chamber with a double-armed continuous 3-0 braided synthetic suture. The inferior vena caval tourniquet is loosened to improve exposure for choice of suture line position. At the coronary sinus, which has been cut back, the suture line runs 5 to 8 mm. to the left of the original coronary sinus orifice.

and small bites of SVC orifice are taken to increase ballooning of the channel and to avoid flattening of the baffle across the SVC orifice. The SA node, which is located about 1 cm. away from this orifice, should be carefully avoided. This suture line continues onto the third border of the baffle, which, like the first, is slightly concave. Part of this border is sutured to the roof of the right atrium and then to the residual atrial septum near the tricuspid valve, stopping at the middle of the septum.

The second end of the original 3-0 suture is now used to suture the rest of the long border of the baffle around the internal orifice of the left inferior pulmonary vein and across the posterior wall of the left atrium to the right atrium. In crossing, the suture line curves up slightly to enlarge the IVC channel, but it should not be too close to the previous superior suture line or future baffle contraction may obstruct the left pulmonary veins. The corner of the baffle between the long border and the fully curved IVC border reaches the lateral wall of the right atrium between the right inferior pulmonary vein and the IVC, in a position that will allow ample flow through both pulmonary and caval venous channels.

At this point, if there is a circulatory arrest, it is expedient to remove the IVC tourniquet. With suction in the IVC, the anatomy can be seen easily and an appropriate path for the baffle suture line selected. If the eustachian valve is well formed and sturdy, the baffle may be sutured to it directly. If it is not, either the base of the eustachian valve or some ridge nearby on the right atrial wall will serve. The last corner of the baffle, marking the end of the IVC border, should reach a point approximately midway along the ridge that extends from the eustachian valve to the coronary sinus. The final border of the baffle is then sutured to this ridge. At the coronary sinus, the suture line runs down one cut edge of coronary sinus for 5 to 8 mm., across the sinus 5 to 8 mm. from its orifice, and then back up to the other cut edge and along the atrial septum for a short distance to meet the first suture and complete the baffle. Before tying the suture, the left side of the heart is gently filled with saline to reduce the amount of trapped air. Once finished, the baffle is inspected briefly, and then the right atrial incision is closed.

The venous cannula is reinserted into the right atrium, and the infant is placed back on bypass for rewarming. The cardioplegia line is removed from the aortic root, but the suture is left loose to allow bleeding and evacuation of air. The tip of the venous cannula is gently inserted through the tricuspid valve for a few seconds to remove any major amount of air from the right ventricle. Reinserting the venous cannula into the right atrial appendage is simple and convenient. Since this is now the pulmonary venous atrium, there is some reduction in venous return to the pump for 2 to 3 minutes. Gentle cardiac massage and ventilating the lungs move blood from the systemic venous side through the lungs to the cannula. Once the heart starts to beat spontaneously, the venous return becomes stable. During rewarming, two atrial and two ventricular temporary pacemaker wires are inserted for postoperative support and monitoring.

Variations in Surgical Repair

When there is left juxtaposition of the right atrial appendage, the right appendage remains on the systemic venous side after repair. The new pulmonary venous atrium is smaller than usual and should, in most cases, be enlarged with a patch of pericardium. Mesocardia or dextrocardia with situs solitus makes access to the right atrium difficult from an anterior approach. A right lateral thoracotomy may provide better exposure.

Moderate to large VSDs are closed from the right atrium through the tricuspid valve. Very small VSDs are left untouched, not only to save time, but also to avoid the danger of creating right bundle branch block. LVOTO is approached through the pulmonary artery and valve. When repair of a VSD or LVOTO is necessary in conjunction with a Mustard procedure, the time required may exceed the limits of safety for a single period of circulatory arrest. To avoid excessive ischemia, part of the repair is performed on bypass by switching to two acutely curved cannulas that are inserted into the cavae through the open atriotomy.

In patients in whom pulmonary vascular disease has progressed to a severe level, improvement can still be obtained by doing a Mustard operation but leaving the VSD open (Lindesmith et al., 1972). Occasionally, severe pulmonary vascular disease develops in children with TGA and an intact ventricular septum. Palliation can be provided for these children by doing a Mustard operation and creating an apical ventricular septal defect (Byrne et al., 1978).

Occasionally, infants with TGA and an intact ventricular septum have a severe form of LVOTO that cannot be relieved by operation. It is best to provide palliation for the infant with a Blalock-Taussig shunt with or without a Blalock-Hanlon operation until he is older. When intra-atrial repair is done, the LVOTO should be relieved as completely as possible by direct means, and, if necessary, the balance of the obstruction can be bypassed using a valved conduit between the left ventricle and the pulmonary artery (Crupi et al., 1979).

If there is a very large and high VSD, an option is the intraventricular repair described originally by McGoon (1972) and reported more recently by Pitlick and associates (1981). The VSD is exposed through a right ventriculotomy, and a large curved patch directs blood from the left ventricle across the VSD to the aorta while leaving a channel for right ventricular blood to cross the VSD and reach the pulmonary artery (Fig. 40–15).

Rastelli (1969) devised a repair for children with a substantial VSD and LVOTO (Fig. 40–16). The VSD is closed with a patch that extends to include the aortic root, thus diverting flow from the left

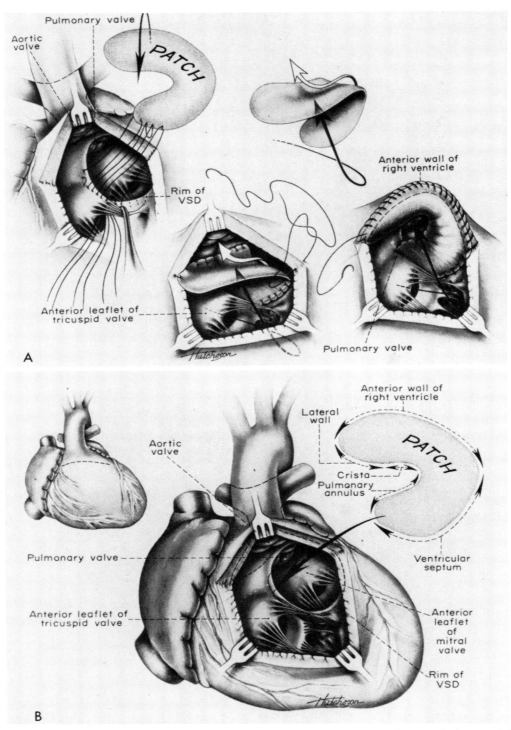

Figure 40–15. *A,* Anatomy of transposition of the great arteries associated with large basilar ventricular septal defect. Line and sites of attachment of knitted Teflon patch and its preferred shape are shown. *B, left,* Initial attachment of patch is the same as for any posterior high ventricular septal defect. *Middle and right,* Subsequent steps in attachment of patch. (From McGoon, D.C.: Intraventricular repair of transposition of the great arteries. J. Thorac. Cardiovasc. Surg., *64*:430, 1972.)

ventricle to the aorta. The pulmonary artery channel is closed, either within the ventricle or through the VSD or by closing the pulmonary artery from without. The ventricular incision is then joined to the distal pulmonary artery with a valved conduit, either a homograft aorta with an aortic valve or one of the commercially available Dacron tubes with porcine valves. This repair is particularly appropriate in cases in which the LVOTO cannot be relieved surgically. It requires a VSD that is the same size as the aortic root or at least one that can be enlarged to that size.

Arterial repair has always seemed a major surgical

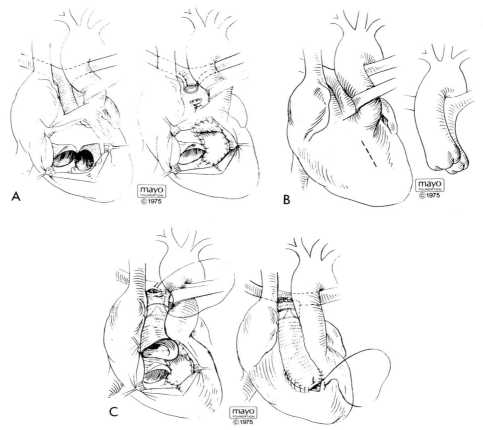

Figure 40–16. *A*, A longitudinal right ventriculotomy is made from the midportion of the anterior right ventricular wall to the base of the heart toward the site of the distal anastomosis. *B*, If the ventricular septal defect is smaller than the diameter of the aorta or if the defect is obscured by a muscle bar or chordal attachments, it is enlarged by resecting the septum in the shaded area. A tunnel is constructed from the ventricular septal defect to the aorta by means of a knitted Teflon patch. The cephalad end of the patch is anchored to the cephalad end of the ventriculomyotomy. The main pulmonary artery is divided, and the proximal end is ligated and oversewn. The distal pulmonary artery is incised to increase the size for anastomosis. *C*, Continuity between the right ventricle and the pulmonary artery is restored with a Dacron graft containing a glutaraldehyde-preserved porcine valve. (From Marcelletti, C, *et al.*: The Rastelli operation for transposition of the great arteries. Early and late results. J. Thorac. Cardiovasc. Surg., *72*:427, 1976.)

tour de force. Not only are the arteries divided and switched, but the coronary arteries must also be transferred to the new aorta. Since the first successful arterial repair by Jatene in 1975, this operation has been attempted widely, but usually with high mortality. It seems best suited to patients with TGA with a normal left ventricular outflow tract, low pulmonary vascular resistance, and a left ventricle that is able to generate systemic pressures. Thus, the most suitable children are those with TGA and a VSD in the first 6 months of life before pulmonary vascular resistance increases. In this particular group of children, the results of intra-atrial repair are poorest, with relatively high early and late mortality and a high incidence of late problems. Arterial repair should especially be considered if the right ventricle contracts poorly.

Recently, the mortality of arterial repair has been reduced to a relatively low and acceptable level (Yacoub *et al.*, 1980; Freedom *et al.*, 1981; Williams *et al.*, 1981). Furthermore, Yacoub has performed arterial repair successfully in children with TGA and an intact ventricular septum by doing preliminary pulmonary artery banding to prepare the left ventricle.

Several months later, when the left ventricular pressure is at or close to a systemic level, the pulmonary artery is debanded and the great arteries are switched. It will be some time before the usefulness of this two-stage procedure can be properly assessed. Intra-atrial repair now carries a low operative mortality, and the main problem is the incidence of late complication and the question of late right ventricular function. It remains to be seen whether Yacoub's early results can be achieved by other surgeons and what the late results of this two-stage arterial repair are.

Results

Early Mortality. The overall early and late results at the Hospital for Sick Children are shown in Table 40–1 by this simple classification of patients into four groups and by comparing the first decade with the years from 1974 to 1980. In the total group of 349 patients, there were 45 early hospital deaths. The early mortality (within 30 days of operation) has gradually decreased for all types of transposition. The results of the Mustard procedure alone are evident in

TABLE 40–1. RESULTS OF THE MUSTARD OPERATION FOR TRANSPOSITION OF THE GREAT ARTERIES AT THE HOSPITAL FOR SICK CHILDREN, TORONTO

| | MAY 1963–DEC. 1973 | | | JAN. 1974–DEC. 1980 | | |
	Number	Early Death	Late Death	Number	Early Death	Late Death
With intact ventricular septum	108	11	15	119	2	6
With VSD	35	14	5	32	7	3
VSD + LVOTO	13	6	3	18	0	5
IVS + LVOTO	9	3	1	17	2	1
Total	163	34	24	186	11	15

the 225 infants and children with TGA and an intact ventricular septum in whom the early mortality rate decreased from 11 per cent in the first group to 1.7 per cent in the last 119 patients. Mortality is highest in those with a VSD.

The results reflect changing patterns of treatment. For instance, in TGA with a VSD, mortality was high at first because most children were operated on at an older age, when they had pulmonary hypertension. Mortality was reduced by preliminary palliation with pulmonary artery banding and surgical septostomy and was decreased further when primary repair in the first 6 months of life became routine. Now some children in this group have an arterial repair.

Similarly, the mortality for children with transposition with a VSD and LVOTO changed when selected patients were treated by the Rastelli procedure. The only patients now treated with intra-atrial repair are those with a relatively small VSD and an obstruction that can be relieved surgically. In this group, there has been no early mortality recently, but obviously, these patients are highly selected.

The most common causes of early mortality in the whole series were low output myocardial failure (23 patients), pulmonary vascular disease (10 pa-

tients), and dysrhythmias (4 patients). Pulmonary vascular disease is now largely avoided, but myocardial failure remains the chief cause of death, particularly in complex cases. Other causes were bleeding (2 patients), other cardiac malformation (3 patients), and miscellaneous causes (3 patients).

Many authors have reported excellent results with the Mustard repair recently, some with low or zero mortality in uncomplicated TGA (Table 40–2). Mortality is higher in complicated cases (Tables 40–3 and 40–4).

Late Mortality. From May 1963 to December 31, 1980 in our series, there were 304 early survivors, among whom there were 39 late deaths. These occurred in all types of transposition, but more commonly in those with a VSD or a VSD and LVOTO.

Cardiac failure is the most common cause of death (14 patients). This is likely related in part to the conduction of the operation and has been reduced in recent years by improved myocardial protection, using lower temperatures, cardioplegia, shorter periods of myocardial ischemia, and local myocardial cooling. Inexplicable instances of failure still occur, and perhaps myocardial damage can result from mild low output cardiac failure or even dysrhythmias postoperatively.

Dysrhythmia caused death in 10 patients and was the possible cause in another two who died suddenly. Pulmonary venous obstruction was responsible for death in five patients but rarely occurs now. Pulmonary vascular disease caused three late deaths early in the series. Other isolated causes of death were

TABLE 40–2. RESULTS OF THE MUSTARD OPERATION FOR SIMPLE TGA WITH AN INTACT VENTRICULAR SEPTUM (IN CHILDREN OF ALL AGES)

AUTHORS (YEAR OF REPORT)	NO. OF PATIENTS	HOSPITAL DEATHS	MORTALITY RATE
Clarkson *et al.* (1972)	45	7	15.5%
Danielson *et al.* (1971)	25	3	12%
Ebert *et al.* (1974)	54	3	5.5%
Kilman *et al.* (1973)	15 (or 16)	0	0%
Lindesmith *et al.* (1972)	31	2	6%
Parr *et al.* (1974)	24	3	12.5%
Shumway *et al.* (1975)	32	2	6%
Sorland *et al.* (1976)	32	3	9%
Subramanian and Wagner (1973)	34	3	9%
Waldhausen *et al.* (1971)	18	0	0%
Oelert *et al.* (1977)	60	0	0%
Arciniegas *et al.* (1981)	82	4	4.8%
Stark *et al.* (1980)	307	27	9%

TABLE 40–3. TGA AND VSD: THE MUSTARD OPERATION AND VSD CLOSURE (IN PATIENTS OF ALL AGES)

AUTHORS (YEAR OF REPORT)	NO. OF PATIENTS	HOSPITAL DEATHS	MORTALITY RATE
Danielson *et al.* (1971)	29	16	55%
Ebert *et al.* (1974)	13	1	8%
Kilman *et al.* (1973)	6	1	16.6%
Mori *et al.* (1976)	23	9	39%
Arciniegas *et al.* (1981)	23	6	26%
Stark *et al.* (1980)	95	25	26%

TABLE 40–4. TGA, VSD, AND LVOTO: THE MUSTARD OPERATION AND VSD CLOSURE AND OUTFLOW TRACT CORRECTION (IN PATIENTS OF ALL AGES)

AUTHORS (YEAR OF REPORT)	NO. OF PATIENTS	HOSPITAL DEATHS	MORTALITY RATE
Chiarello et al. (1975)	17	10	59%
Danielson et al. (1971)	14	5	36%
Ebert et al. (1974)	14	2	14%
Idriss et al. (1974)	8	0	0%
Arciniegas et al. (1981)	7	2	28.5%
Stark et al. (1980)	33	7	21%

baffle detachment, congenital respiratory problems, pulmonary venous thrombosis, septicemia, and inferior vena caval obstruction.

The quality of life in the surviving children is really quite good. Levy and associates (1978) and Takahashi and colleagues (1977) found that infants and children grew at a more normal rate after TGA repair, and they considered this an indication for early repair. Stark and coworkers (1980) noted that many of their patients achieved a normal working capacity, but as a group, there was a statistically significant reduction in exercise tolerance when compared with that of healthy children. They did not find a significant difference between the group of patients who underwent repair in infancy and those who did so later.

Complications

Many of the complications of intra-atrial repair for TGA are identical to those following any major cardiac repair. Postoperative bleeding, hemothorax, and cardiac tamponade may occur, particularly if there are pericardial adhesions from a previous palliative procedure, but can be prevented by meticulous hemostasis and maintenance of blood coagulability with appropriate blood clotting factors. Low output cardiac failure may occur after repair, especially in complicated cases, causing early death or residual impairment of right ventricular contractility. It is likely that this is due to inadequate myocardial protection and can be prevented by avoiding prolonged myocardial ischemia. Air embolism, a constant danger, is rarely a problem if appropriate preventive measures are taken.

Phrenic nerve paralysis occurs occasionally, probably from dissection of the large pericardial patch. The nerve injury may be related to local mechanical trauma or cautery, particularly above, at the great vessel level, where the space between the two phrenic nerves is narrower; alternatively, strong traction on pericardial stay sutures near a phrenic nerve may cause injury.

Dysrhythmia. Dysrhythmia is a relatively common and potentially serious complication following the Mustard operation owing to the wide excision of the atrial septum and the long atrial suture line. It is generally accepted now that most dysrhythmias are due to interference with function of the SA node either directly or from injury to the SA node artery (El-Said et al., 1976; Edwards et al., 1978; Gillette et al., 1980). Preservation of the node and its artery is an important principle of any operation. The significance of obliterating or excising the pathways of impulse transmission from the SA node to the AV node is less clear, but it is likely that preservation of at least one pathway for internodal conduction is important.

There was a relatively high incidence of dysrhythmias in the early series, and some dysrhythmias were responsible for both early and late deaths, including a number of sudden, unexpected deaths, which likely were due to this cause. Temporary atrial and ventricular pacemaker wires are inserted routinely at operation and are monitored carefully for the first few days after operation. In one follow-up study of 102 surviving children in Toronto, only 66 children were still in sinus rhythm 1 year or more following repair. Thirty-one had junctional rhythm, and five had atrial flutter, atrial fibrillation, or complete heart block (Trusler et al., 1977). Major dysrhythmias were more common in children who had had a VSD repair in addition to the Mustard procedure. A few with bradyarrhythmias required pacemakers.

In recent years, with knowledge of the problem and attention to detail, the incidence of dysrhythmias is much lower, and most children remain in sinus rhythm. Over the 7-year period from 1974 to 1980, 91 per cent of the children with isolated transposition who had a Mustard operation in Toronto were in sinus rhythm when discharged from the hospital. Eighty-six per cent were still in sinus rhythm at their last visit, but 8 per cent of these showed some evidence of sinus node dysfunction. In other series, there is a similar low incidence of dysrhythmias (Lewis et al., 1977; Clarkson et al., 1976; Southall et al., 1980; Turley and Ebert, 1978). However, it has been shown that the true incidence of abnormal rhythm can be identified only by exercise studies and 24-hour monitoring (Rakowski et al., 1979; Southall et al., 1980).

Baffle Complications. Many complications are related to changes in the atrial partition, and it is useful to consider what happens to it following operation. Mohri and associates (1970) found that the partition, regardless of material used, is soon covered by a layer of fibrin that subsequently fibroses, forming a neoendocardium, which, with the underlying graft material, gradually contracts to about 50 per cent of its original area. The neoendocardium that formed over Dacron was thicker than that which formed over pericardium. They concluded that adequate atrial volume would be maintained by growth of normal atrial wall.

Our observations at reoperation and necropsy indicate that baffle shrinkage is limited or restricted by tension. When the pericardium partially encircles a venous orifice, the appropriate channel is maintained if the sutures are secure. If several sutures pull out, the pericardium will contract between the points of fixation, partly obstructing the venous channel and creating a leak between the atrial chambers. When using pericardium, a relatively large patch can be utilized, and the final shape will be determined by relative pressures and flow within the two atria as well as by the security and position of the suture line. Soon after insertion, the mobile pericardium, covered by fibrin, may adhere to itself or to other raw areas, so that a very redundant baffle should be avoided and raw areas of atrial wall should be oversewn.

Synthetic materials do not shape as easily as pericardium; therefore, the patch must be tailored precisely to avoid ridges or narrow channels. Excessive shrinkage or an error in the line of suture is more critical, especially in infants, in whom all the venous orifices and channels are smaller and there is less margin for error. This does not mean that synthetic materials should not be used, but it does seem that pericardium is safer for repairs in infants.

The most common late complication is a leak around the baffle. By December 31, 1980, 131 of 304 early survivors had had one or more cardiac catheterizations following the Mustard repair. Thirty-four of these children were found to have leaks. Fortunately, 27 were small and only seven were significant (five with a left-to-right shunt over 1.5:1, and two with a right-to-left shunt). The leaks were easily repaired, but when they were associated with caval obstruction, it was necessary to patch the baffle to relieve the associated venous obstruction.

Superior vena caval obstruction may cause symptoms and signs of increased SVC pressure soon after operation, although many cases are asymptomatic and only identified at late cardiac catheterization. Occasionally, there is persistent bilateral pleural effusion or chylothorax. The obstruction usually occurs where the new SVC channel crosses the plane of the atrial septum and may be due to a residual ridge of atrial septum or flattening of the baffle (Figs. 40–17 and 40–18). If several sutures pull out, the baffle may contract across the caval orifice, causing obstruction. In our series, there was a 4 per cent incidence of SVC obstruction. Recently, this incidence has increased owing to a change in the technique of atrial septal excision, and more children have mild to moderate SVC narrowing due to the residual ridge of atrial septum between the superior vena cava and the tricuspid valve. This is now avoided by using a slightly larger baffle in this area. The total number of patients in whom this occurred is 19 among 304 early survivors, a known incidence of 6 per cent. However, only three (1 per cent overall) required repair, two in association with baffle leaks. Many authors, including Hagler and coworkers (1978) and Arciniegas and colleagues (1981), described an increased incidence of SVC obstruction when Dacron was used for the baffle material (Doty et al., 1975; Shumway et al., 1975; Egloff et al., 1978). Stark and associates (1974) and Wyse and coworkers (1979) find the jugular flow profile recording

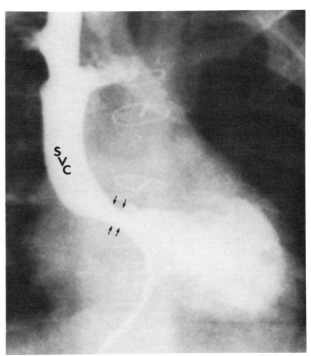

Figure 40–17. Mild narrowing of (arrows) the superior limb of the baffle following the Mustard operation (SVC = superior vena cava).

to be the most effective way to screen for SVC obstruction.

Inferior vena caval obstruction is uncommon but can occur at the plane of the atrial septum or by the coronary sinus from a tight baffle or at the IVC orifice if several sutures pull out. Severe obstruction is associated with increased IVC pressure, causing hepatomegaly and ascites or even a low output state. Inferior vena caval obstruction was identified in five of our 304 early survivors. In one child, it was associated with a baffle leak and required repair. In another child, it was identified at autopsy. The other three children are asymptomatic with partial obstruction that has not been repaired. Stark and colleagues (1974) described an increased incidence of IVC obstruction when Dacron was used as a baffle material in infants.

Pulmonary venous obstruction is a less common but more serious complication, causing five of the late deaths. There were nine cases in the 304 early survivors, an incidence of 3 per cent. In five of the nine cases, all four pulmonary veins were involved. The obstruction occurred where the new pulmonary venous channel crossed the plane of the atrial septum just anterior to the entrance of the right pulmonary veins and seemed to be caused by progressive adherence and fibrous stenosis between the baffle and the adjacent right lateral atrial wall. It appears to occur more often if the raw cut margin of the atrial septum is not oversewn and there is a large redundant baffle that can make contact with the wall of the atrium. If diagnosed early, it can be treated successfully by patching both the baffle and the atrial wall between

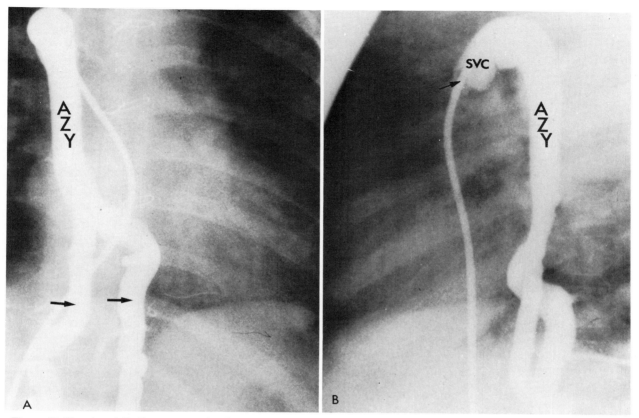

Figure 40–18. *A* and *B*, Severe stenosis of the superior limb of the baffle following the Mustard operation. This asymptomatic patient was found to have paravertebral densities that proved to be venous in origin (Castellino *et al.*, 1968; Polansky and Culham, 1980). Although the superior vena cava (SVC) could be probed from the venous route, most of the superior vena caval blood passed via large azygos (AZY) and hemiazygos collaterals (arrows) and through the inferior limb of the baffle.

the two right pulmonary veins. With delayed diagnosis, there is rapid progression of severe pulmonary vascular disease. A higher incidence has been noted in several series, and it seems more common in infants and when Dacron is used (Driscoll *et al.*, 1977; Doty *et al.*, 1975; Oelert *et al.*, 1977; Hagler *et al.*, 1978).

An uncommon variant is isolated obstruction of the left pulmonary venous channel, which appears to result from excessive contraction of the baffle when the upper and lower suture lines between the right and left pulmonary veins are brought too close together on the posterior wall of the left atrium. Affected children may present with chronic left pulmonary edema and pleural effusion. On angiocardiography, there is marked reduction in pulmonary blood flow into the left lung. Repair requires patching of both the posterior left atrial wall and the baffle itself at the site of obstruction.

Other Complications. Some degree of LVOTO appears to be common in children with TGA (Idriss *et al.*, 1977; Vidne *et al.*, 1976; Gomes *et al.*, 1980; Stark *et al.*, 1976). A pressure gradient of 10 mm. Hg or greater across the left ventricular outflow tract was identified in 36 children in our series. Most cases were minor and due to bulging of the muscular septum into the outflow tract. Only 14 patients had gradients over 25 mm. Hg. Although some of these patients repre-

sented residual obstruction incompletely relieved by operation, the majority were children who were considered to have uncomplicated TGA. Fortunately, none have required operative intervention as yet.

Other complications that have been identified include small persistent VSDs. Most of these are small defects that were recognized originally but not treated because they were of no physiologic significance. Pulmonary vascular disease and mitral incompetence have developed in a few children with isolated TGA.

Of greater significance is the recognition of some diminution of right ventricular contractility on angiocardiography. In our patients, this is a subjective assessment by the radiologist and was recognized in 55 (42 per cent) of children at follow-up cardiac catheterization. Many also have a degree of tricuspid valve incompetence (Tynan *et al.*, 1972), and occasionally, the incompetence occurs alone. The incidence is higher in the complicated forms of transposition in which there is repair of a VSD. A reduction of right ventricular contractility was noted in 31 of 90 children (34 per cent) with uncomplicated transposition and 14 of 24 children (58 per cent) who also had a VSD repair. The incidence of accompanying tricuspid incompetence was higher in the latter group, suggesting that VSD repair may lead to tricuspid incompetence.

Right ventricular dysfunction following intra-atrial repair of TGA has been described. Graham and associates (1975a) and Jarmakani and Canent (1974) found that the right ventricular end-diastolic volume was increased and right ventricular ejection fraction was decreased, evidence of poor right ventricular function both before and after repair. These findings were verified by Hagler and coworkers (1979), Alpert and colleagues (1979), and Shirotani (1980).

It is likely that some of these problems originate at operation, and the right ventricle in transposition is more susceptible to ischemic damage than the left ventricle in a normal heart. If this is so, every effort should be made to protect the myocardium during repair. Low output cardiac failure postoperatively may have a deleterious effect on the myocardium and should be avoided if possible. Some cases of poor right ventricular contractility, however, occur in children who appear to have had a good operation and a good postoperative course, and there is concern about the long-term fate of the right ventricle in transposition. Fortunately, close to two thirds of the children have apparently normal right ventricular contractility at follow-up catheterization.

In the largest group of patients, those with uncomplicated TGA and an intact ventricular septum, the operative risk is now low (1.7 per cent) and the subsequent survival is very satisfactory. There is every indication that the incidence of early and late mortality and complications will continue to decrease in years to come. At the same time, the results of other forms of repair continue to improve, and a frequent reappraisal will be needed to determine the optimal treatment for each child.

SELECTED REFERENCES

Alpert, B. S., Bloom, K. R., Olley, P. M., Trusler, G. A., Williams, C. M., and Rowe, R. D.: Echocardiographic evaluation of right ventricular function in complete transposition of the great arteries: Angiographic correlates. Am. J. Cardiol., *44*:270, 1979.

This group assessed the right ventricular function in patients with complete transposition of the great arteries using M-mode echocardiographic techniques. Their data suggested that right ventricular function can be predicted reliably by echocardiography. Although right ventricular function was depressed in some patients, the data from the Hospital for Sick Children in Toronto suggested that most patients with poor right ventricular function had associated anatomic malformations and had undergone prolonged cardiopulmonary bypass with postoperative right bundle branch block and tricuspid regurgitation. The data from this institution were not as bleak as those suggested by Hagler and his group.

Gillette, P. C., Kugler, J. D., Garson, A., Jr., Gutgesell, H. P., Duff, D. F., and McNamara, D. G.: Mechanism of cardiac arrhythmias after the Mustard operation for transposition of the great arteries. Am. J. Cardiol., *45*:1225, 1980.

In this publication, intracardiac electrophysiologic studies were performed in 52 children after the Mustard operation. Sinus nodal automaticity was abnormal in over half of the children. The members of this group from Houston were among the first to point out the relationship between damage to the sinus node and arrhythmias,

one of the most common complications seen after the Mustard operation. This study further supports this belief.

Hagler, D. J., Ritter, D. G., Mair, D. D., Tajik, A. J., Seward, J. B., Fulton, R. E., and Ritman, E. L.: Right and left ventricular function after the Mustard procedure in transposition of the great arteries. Am. J. Cardiol., *44*:276, 1979.

The Mayo Clinic has assessed right and left ventricular function using video-densito-metric determination of ejection fraction and ventricular volume data, and for the right ventricle, ventricular volumes were obtained by computerized videoanalysis utilizing Simpson's rule. Their data suggested that after the Mustard operation, right ventricular function is severely decreased, with relatively preserved left ventricular function. This group is so concerned about diminished right ventricular function in patients having undergone the Mustard operation that they feel that the left ventricle should be utilized whenever possible as a systemic ventricle in correction of complete transposition of the great arteries.

Stark, J., Weller, P., Leanage, R., Cunningham, K., de Leval, M., Macartney, F., and Taylor, J. F. N.: Later results of surgical treatment of transposition of the great arteries. Adv. Cardiol., *27*:254, 1980.

This is a comprehensive review of the late results following repair of TGA by the group at Great Ormond Street in London who have the greatest experience with transposition repair. Early results reported in the literature are reviewed. There is a discussion of the incidence and cause of arrhythmias and the effect of different surgical techniques. The late functional results are described in detail. Although many patients achieved a normal working capacity, the overall exercise performance of asymptomatic patients 6 to 13 years after the Mustard operation was somewhat diminished compared with that of a group of normal children.

REFERENCES

Aberdeen, E.: Blalock-Hanlon operation and Rashkind procedure. *In* Rob, C., and Smith, R.: Operative Surgery. 2nd Ed. London, Butterworth, 1968, Vol. 2, pp. 193–199.

Albert, H. M.: Surgical correction of transposition of the great vessels. Surg. Forum, *5*:74, 1954.

Alpert, B. S., Bloom, K. R., Olley, P. M., Trusler, G. A., Williams, C. M., and Rowe, R. D.: Echocardiographic evaluation of right ventricular function in complete transposition of the great arteries: Angiographic correlates. Am. J. Cardiol., *44*:270, 1979.

Arciniegas, E., Farooki, A. Q., Hakimi, M., Perry, B. L., and Green, E. W.: Results of the Mustard operation for dextro-transposition of the great arteries. J. Thorac. Cardiovasc. Surg., *81*:580, 1981.

Aziz, R. U., Paul, M. H., and Muster, A. J.: Echocardiographic assessment of left ventricular outflow tract in d-transposition of the great arteries. Am. J. Cardiol., *41*:543, 1978.

Aziz, R. U., Paul, M. H., Idriss, F. S., Wilson, A. D., and Muster, A. J.: Clinical manifestations of dynamic left ventricular outflow tract stenosis in infants with d-transposition of the great arteries with intact ventricular septum. Am. J. Cardiol., *44*:290, 1979.

Baffes, T. G.: A new method for surgical correction of transposition of the aorta and pulmonary artery. Surg. Gynecol. Obstet., *102*:227, 1956.

Baffes, T. G., Ketola, F. H., and Tatooles, C. J.: Transfer of coronary ostia by "triangulation" in transposition of the great vessels and anomalous coronary arteries: A preliminary report. Dis. Chest, *39*:648, 1961.

Bailey, C. P., Cookson, B. A., Downing, D. F., and Neptune, W. B.: Cardiac surgery under hypothermia. J. Thorac. Surg., *27*:73, 1954.

Baillie, M.: The Morbid Anatomy of Some of the Important Parts of the Human Body. London, Johnson and Nicol, 1797, p. 38.

Bano-Rodrigo, A., Quero-Jimenez, M., Moreno-Granado, F., and Gamallo-Amat, C.: Wall thickness of ventricular chamber in transposition of the great arteries. Surgical implications. J. Thorac. Cardiovasc. Surg., 79:592, 1980.

Barcia, A., Kincaid, O. W., Davis, G. D., Kirklin, J. W., and Ongley, P. A.: Transposition of the great arteries. An angiocardiographic study. Am. J. Roentgenol., 100:249, 1967.

Bargeron, L. M., Jr., Elliott, L. P., Soto, B., Bream, P. R., and Curry, G. C.: Axial cineangiography in congenital heart disease. Section I. Concept, technical and anatomical considerations. Circulation, 56:1075, 1977.

Barnard, C. N., Schrire, V., and Beck, W.: Complete transposition of the great vessels: A successful complete correction. J. Thorac. Cardiovasc. Surg., 43:768, 1962.

Benson, L. N., Olley, P. M., Patel, R. G., Coceani, F., and Rowe, R. D.: Role of prostaglandin E1 infusion in the management of transposition of the great arteries. Am. J. Cardiol., 44:691, 1979.

Bierman, F. Z., and Williams, R. G.: Subxiphoid two-dimensional imaging of the interatrial septum in infants and neonates with congenital heart disease. Circulation, 60:80, 1979a.

Bierman, F. Z., and Williams, R. G.: Prospective diagnosis of d-transposition of the great arteries in neonates by subxiphoid two-dimensional echocardiography. Circulation, 60:1496, 1979b.

Bjork, V. O., and Bouckaert, L.: Complete transposition of the aorta and the pulmonary artery: An experimental study of the surgical possibilities for its treatment. J. Thorac. Surg., 28:632, 1954.

Blalock, A., and Hanlon, C. R.: The surgical treatment of complete transposition of the aorta and the pulmonary artery. Surg. Gynecol. Obstet., 90:1, 1950.

Byrne, J., Clarke, D., Taylor, J. F. N., Macartney, F., de Leval, M., and Stark, J.: Treatment of patients with transposition of great arteries and pulmonary vascular obstructive disease. Br. Heart J., 40:221, 1978.

Castellino, R. A., Blank, N., and Adams, D. F.: Dilated azygos and hemiazygos veins presenting as paravertebral intrathoracic masses. N. Engl. J. Med., 278:1087, 1968.

Chiarello, L., Agosti, J., Vlad, P., and Subramanian, S.: Management of left ventricular outflow tract obstruction in complex transposition. A critical review of our experience. Circulation, 51(Suppl. 2):169, 1975.

Clark, E. B., Sweeny, L. J., and Rosenquist, G. C.: Atrial defect size after Blalock-Hanlon atrioseptectomy. Am. J. Cardiol., 40:405, 1977.

Clarkson, P. M., Barratt-Boyes, B. G., and Neutze, J. M.: Late dysrhythmias and disturbances of conduction following Mustard operation for complete transposition of the great arteries. Circulation, 53:519, 1976.

Clarkson, P. M., Barratt-Boyes, B. G., Neutze, J. M., and Lowe, J. B.: Results over a ten year period of palliation followed by corrective surgery for complete transposition of the great arteries. Circulation, 45:1251, 1972.

Coceani, F., and Olley, P. M.: The response of the ductus arteriosus in prostaglandins. Can. J. Physiol. Pharmacol., 51:220, 1973.

Counahan, R., Simon, G., and Joseph, M.: The plain chest radiograph in d-transposition of the great arteries in the first month of life. Pediatr. Radiol., 1:217, 1973.

Creech, O., Jr., Mahaffey, D. E., Sayegh, S. F., and Sailors, E. L.: Complete transposition of the great vessels: A technique for intracardiac correction. Surgery, 43:349, 1958.

Crupi, G., Anderson, R. H., Ho, S. Y., and Lincoln, C.: Complete transposition of the great arteries with intact ventricular septum and left ventricular outflow tract obstruction. J. Thorac. Cardiovasc. Surg., 78:730, 1979.

Danielson, G. K., Mair, D. D., Ongley, P. A., Wallace, R. B., and McGoon, D. C.: Repair of transposition of the great arteries by transposition of the venous return. J. Thorac. Cardiovasc. Surg., 61:96, 1971.

de Leval, M. R., McKay, R., Jones, M., Stark, J., and Macartney, F. J.: Modified Blalock-Taussig shunt. J. Thorac. Cardiovasc. Surg., 81:112, 1981.

Deutsch, V., Shem-Tov, A., Yahini, J. H., and Neufeld, H. N.: Cardioangiographic evaluation of the relationship between atrioventricular and semilunar valves: Its diagnostic importance in congenital heart disease. Am. J. Roentgenol., 110:474, 1970.

Doty, D. B., Lauer, R. M., and Ehrenhaft, J. L.: Congenital cardiac anomalies: One stage repair in infancy. Ann. Thorac. Surg., 20:316, 1975.

Driscoll, D. J., Kugler, J. D., Nihill, M. R., and McNamara, D. G.: The use of prostaglandin E1 in a critically ill infant with transposition of the great arteries. J. Pediatr., 95:259, 1979.

Driscoll, D. J., Nihill, M. R., Vargo, T. A., Mullins, C. E., and McNamara, D. G.: Late development of pulmonary venous obstruction following Mustard's operation using a Dacron baffle. Circulation, 55:484, 1977.

Ebert, P. A., Gay, W. A., Jr., and Engle, M. A.: Correction of transposition of the great arteries: Relationship of the coronary sinus and postoperative arrhythmias. Ann. Surg., 180:433, 1974.

Edwards, W. D., and Edwards, J. E.: Pathology of the sinus node in d-transposition following the Mustard operation. J. Thorac. Cardiovasc. Surg., 75:213, 1978.

Edwards, W. S., Bargeron, L. M., Jr., and Lyons, C.: Reposition of right pulmonary veins in transposition of great vessels. J.A.M.A., 188:522, 1964.

Egloff, L. P., Freed, M. D., MacDonald, D., Norwood, W. I., and Castaneda, A. R.: Early and late results with the Mustard operation in infancy. Ann. Thorac. Surg., 26:474, 1978.

Elliott, L. P., Bargeron, L. M., Jr., Bream, P. R., Soto, B., and Curry, G. D.: Axial cineangiography in congenital heart disease. Section II. Specific lesions. Circulation, 56:1084, 1977.

El-Said, G. M., Gillette, P. C., Cooley, D. A., Mullins, C. E., and McNamara, D. G.: Protection of the sinus node in Mustard's operation. Circulation, 53:788, 1976.

Fisher, E. H. R., Muster, A. J., Lev, M., and Paul, M. H.: Angiocardiographic and anatomic findings in transposition of the great arteries with left ventricular outflow tract gradients. Am. J. Cardiol., 25:95, 1970.

Freedom, R. M., Culham, J. A. G., and Moes, C. A. F.: The Angiocardiography of Congenital Heart Disease. New York, Macmillan, 1983.

Freedom, R. M., Culham, J. A. G., and Rowe, R. D.: The criss-cross and supero-inferior ventricular heart: An angiocardiographic study. Am. J. Cardiol., 42:620, 1978.

Freedom, R. M., Harrington, D. P., and White, R. I., Jr.: The differential diagnosis of levo-transposed or malposed aorta: An angiocardiographic study. Circulation, 50:1040, 1974.

Freedom, R. M., Culham, J. A. G., Olley, P. M., Rowe, R. D., Williams, W. G., and Trusler, G. A.: Anatomic correction of transposition of the great arteries: Preoperative and postoperative cardiac catheterization with angiocardiography in 5 patients. Circulation, 63:905, 1981.

Fyler, D. C.: Report of the New England Regional Infant Cardiac Program. Pediatrics, 65(Suppl.):422, 1980.

Gillette, P. C., Kugler, J. D., Garson, A., Jr., Gutgesell, H. P., Duff, D. F., and McNamara, D. G.: Mechanisms of cardiac arrhythmias after the Mustard operation for transposition of the great arteries. Am. J. Cardiol., 45:1225, 1980.

Gingell, R. L., Freedom, R. M., Hawker, R. E., Krovetz, L. J., and Rowe, R. D.: Indicator dilution curves in the diagnosis of d-transposition of the great arteries in infancy. Cathet. Cardiovasc. Diagn., 5:119, 1979.

Glenn, W. W. L.: Circulatory bypass of the right side of the heart: IV. Shunt between superior vena cava and distal right pulmonary artery—report of clinical appearance. N. Engl. J. Med., 259:117, 1958.

Goldman, H. E., Maralit, A., Sun, S., and Lanzkowsky, P.: Neonatal cyanosis and arterial oxygen saturation. J. Pediatr., 82:319, 1973.

Gomes, A. S., Nath, P. H., Singh, A., Lucas, R. V., Amplatz, K., Nicoloff, D. M., and Edwards, J. E.: Accessory flaplike tissue causing ventricular outflow obstruction. J. Thorac. Cardiovasc. Surg., 80:211, 1980.

Graham, T. P., Jr., Atwood, G. F., Boucek, R. J., Boerth, R. C., and Bender, H. W., Jr.: Abnormalities of right ventricular function following Mustard's operation for transposition of the great arteries. Circulation, 52:678, 1975a.

Graham, T. P., Jr., Atwood, G. F., Boucek, R. J., Jr., Boerth, R.

C., and Nelson, J. H.: Right heart volume characteristics in transposition of the great arteries. Circulation, 51:881, 1975b.

Guerin, R., Soto, B., Karp, R. B., Kirklin, J. W., and Barcia, A.: Transposition of the great arteries. Determination of the position of the great arteries in conventional chest roentgenograms. Am. J. Roentgenol., 110:747, 1970.

Gutgesell, H. P., Garson, A., and McNamara, D. G.: Prognosis for the newborn with transposition of the great arteries. Am. J. Cardiol., 44:96, 1979.

Hagler, D. J., Ritter, D. G., Mair, D. D., Davis, G. D., and McGoon, D. C.: Clinical angiographic and hemodynamic assessment of late results after Mustard operation. Circulation, 57:1214, 1978.

Hagler, D. J., Ritter, D. G., Mair, D. D., Tajik, A. J., Seward, J. B., Fulton, R. E., and Ritman, E. L.: Right and left ventricular function after the Mustard procedure in transposition of the great arteries. Am. J. Cardiol., 44:276, 1979.

Hamilton, S. D., Bartley, T. D., Miller, R. H., Schiebler, G. L., and Marriott, H. J. L.: Disturbances in atrial rhythm and conduction following the surgical creation of an atrial septal defect by the Blalock-Hanlon technique. Circulation, 38:73, 1968.

Henry, C. G., Goldring, D., Hartman, A. F., Weldon, C. S., and Strauss, A. W.: Treatment of d-transposition of the great arteries. Management of hypoxemia after balloon atrial septostomy. Am. J. Cardiol., 47:299, 1981.

Houston, A. B., Gregory, N. L., and Coleman, E. N.: Echocardiographic identification of aorta and main pulmonary artery in complete transposition. Br. Heart J., 40:377, 1978.

Huhta, J. C., Edwards, W. D., Feldt, R. H., and Puga, F. J.: Left ventricular wall thickness in complete transposition of the great arteries. J. Thorac. Cardiovasc. Surg., 84:97, 1982.

Hvass, U.: Coronary arteries in d-transposition. A necropsy study of reimplantation. Br. Heart J., 39:1234, 1977.

Idriss, F. S., Aubert, J., Paul, M., Nikaidoh, H., Lev, M., and Newfeld, E. A.: Transposition of the great vessels with ventricular septal defect: Surgical and anatomic considerations. J. Thorac. Cardiovasc. Surg., 68:732, 1974.

Idriss, F. S., DeLeon, S. Y., Nikaidoh, H., Muster, A. J., Paul, M. A., Newfeld, E. A., and Albers, W.: Resection of left ventricular outflow obstruction in d-transposition of the great arteries. J. Thorac. Cardiovasc. Surg., 74:343, 1977.

Idriss, F. S., Goldstein, I. R., Grana, L., French, D., and Potts, W. J.: A new technique for complete correction of transposition of the great vessels: An experimental study with a preliminary clinical report. Circulation, 24:5, 1961.

Jarmakani, J. M. M., and Canent, R. V., Jr.: Preoperative and postoperative right ventricular function in children with transposition of the great vessels. Circulation, 49(Suppl. 2):39, 1974.

Jatene, A. D., Fontes, V. F., Paulista, P. P., Sousa, L. C. B., Neger, F., Galantier, M., and Sousa, J. E. M. R.: Successful anatomic correction of transposition of the great vessels. A preliminary report. Arq. Bras. Cardiol., 28:461, 1975.

Jatene, A. D., Fontes, V. F., Paulista, P. P., Sousa, L. C. B., Neger, F., Galantier, M., and Sousa, J. E. M. R.: Anatomic correction of transposition of the great vessels. J. Thorac. Cardiovasc. Surg., 72:364, 1976.

Jiminez, M. Q., and Martinez, V. P.: Uncommon conal pathology in complete dextro-transposition of the great arteries with ventricular septal defect. Chest, 66:411, 1974.

Jones, R. W. A., Baumer, J. H., Joseph, M. C., and Shinebourne, E. A.: Arterial oxygen tension and response to oxygen breathing in differential diagnosis of congenital heart disease in infancy. Arch. Dis. Child., 51:667, 1976.

Kay, E. B., and Cross, F. S.: Surgical treatment of transposition of the great vessels. Surgery, 38:712, 1955.

Kay, E. B., and Cross, F. S.: Transposition of the great vessels corrected by means of atrial transposition. Surgery, 41:938, 1957.

Kelly, D. T., Krovetz, L. J., and Rowe, R. D.: Double-lumen flotation catheter for use in complex congenital cardiac anomalies. Circulation, 44:910, 1971.

Kilman, J. W., Williams, T. E., Jr., Kakos, G. S., Craenen, J., and Hosier, D. M.: Surgical correction of the transposition complex in infancy. J. Thorac. Cardiovasc. Surg., 66:387, 1973.

Kirklin, J. W., Devloo, R. A., and Weidman, W. H.: Open intracardiac repair for transposition of the great vessels: 11 cases. Surgery, 50:58, 1961.

Korns, M. E., Garabedian, H. A., and Lauer, R. M.: Anatomic limitation of balloon atrial septostomy. Hum. Pathol., 3:345, 1972.

Kurlander, G. J., Petry, E. L., and Girod, D. A.: Plain film diagnosis of congenital heart disease in the newborn period. Am. J. Roentgenol., 103:66, 1968.

Lakier, J. B., Stanger, P., Heymann, M. A., Hoffman, J. I., and Rudolph, A. M.: Early onset of pulmonary vascular obstruction in patients with aortopulmonary transposition and intact ventricular septum. Circulation, 51:875, 1975.

Landtman, B., Louhimo, I., Rapola, J., and Tuuteri, L.: Causes of death in transposition of the great arteries. A clinical and autopsy study of 140 cases. Acta Paediatr. Scand., 64:785, 1975.

Lang, P., Freed, M. D., Bierman, F. Z., Norwood, W. I., Jr., and Nadas, A. S.: Use of prostaglandin E1 in infants with d-transposition of the great arteries and intact ventricular septum. Am. J. Cardiol., 44:76, 1979.

Layman, T. E., and Edwards, J. E.: Anomalies of the cardiac valves associated with complete transposition of the great vessels. Am. J. Cardiol., 19:247, 1967.

Levy, R. J., Rosenthal, A., Castaneda, A. R., and Nadas, A. S.: Growth after surgical repair of simple d-transposition of the great arteries. Ann. Thorac. Surg., 25:225, 1978.

Lewis, A. B., Lindesmith, G. G., Takahashi, M., Stanton, R. E., Tucker, B. L., Stiles, Q. R., and Meyer, B. W.: Cardiac rhythm following the Mustard procedure for transposition of the great vessels. J. Thorac. Cardiovasc. Surg., 73:919, 1977.

Liebman, J., Cullum, L., and Belloc, N. B.: Natural history of transposition of the great arteries. Anatomy and birth and death characteristics. Circulation, 40:237, 1969.

Lillehei, C. W., and Varco, R. L.: Certain physiologic, pathologic and surgical features of complete transposition of the great vessels. Surgery, 34:376, 1953.

Lindesmith, G. G., Stiles, Q. R., Tucker, B. L., Gallaher, M. E., Stanton, R. E., and Meyer, B. W.: The Mustard operation as a palliative procedure. J. Thorac. Cardiovasc. Surg., 63:75, 1972.

Marcelletti, C., Mair, D. D., McGoon, D. C., Wallace, R. B., and Danielson, G. K.: The Rastelli operation for transposition of the great arteries. Early and late results. J. Thorac. Cardiovasc. Surg., 72:427, 1976.

Mathew, R., Rosenthal, A., and Fellows, K.: The significance of the right aortic arch in d-transposition of the great arteries. Am. Heart J., 87:314, 1974.

McGarry, K. M., Taylor, J. F. N., and Macartney, F. J.: Aortic atresia occurring with complete transposition of great arteries. Br. Heart J., 44:711, 1980.

McGoon, D. C.: Intraventricular repair of transposition of the great arteries. J. Thorac. Cardiovasc. Surg., 64:430, 1972.

Merendino, K. A., Jesseph, J. E., Herron, P. W., Thomas, G. I., and Vetto, R. R.: Interatrial venous transposition—a one stage intracardiac operation for the conversion of complete transposition of the aorta and pulmonary artery to corrected transposition: Theory and clinical experience. Surgery, 42:898, 1957.

Moes, C. A. F.: Analysis of the chest in the neonate with congenital heart disease. Radiol. Clin. North Am., 13:251, 1975.

Mohri, H., Barnes, R. W., Rittenhouse, E. A., Reichenbach, D. D., Dillard, D. H., and Merendino, K. A.: Fate of autologous pericardium and Dacron fabric used as substitutes for total atrial septum in growing animals. J. Thorac. Cardiovasc. Surg., 59:501, 1970.

Mori, A., Ando, F., Setsuie, N., Yamaguchi, K., Oku, H., Kanzaki, Y., Kawai, J., Shirtoni, H., Makino, S., and Yokoyama, T.: Operative indication for corrective surgery in cases of complete transposition of the great arteries associated with large ventricular septal defect. J. Thorac. Cardiovasc. Surg., 71:750, 1976.

Mustard, W. T.: Successful two-stage correction of transposition of the great vessels. Surgery, 55:469, 1964.

Mustard, W. T., Chute, A. L., Keith, J. D., Sirek, A., Rowe, R. D., and Vlad, P.: A surgical approach to transposition of the great vessels with extracorporeal circuit. Surgery, 36:39, 1954.

Muster, A. J., Paul, M. H., Van Grondelle, A., and Conway, J. J.: Asymmetric distribution of the pulmonary blood flow between the right and left lungs in d-transposition of the great arteries. Am. J. Cardiol., 38:352, 1976.

Newfeld, E. A., Paul, M. H., Muster, A. J., and Idriss, F. S.: Pulmonary vascular disease in complete transposition of the great arteries. A study of 200 patients. Am. J. Cardiol., 34:75, 1974.

Newfeld, E. A., Paul, M. H., Muster, A. J., and Idriss, F. S.: Pulmonary vascular disease in transposition of the great vessels and intact ventricular septum. Circulation, 59:525, 1979.

Nogrady, M. B., and Dunbar, J. S.: Complete transposition of the great vessels. Re-evaluation of the so-called "typical configuration" on plain films of the chest. J. Can. Assoc. Radiol., 20:124, 1969.

Ochsner, J. L., Cooley, D. A., Harris, L. C., and McNamara, D. G.: Treatment of complete transposition of the great vessels with the Blalock-Hanlon operation. Circulation, 24:51, 1961.

Oelert, H., Laprell, H., Piepenbrock, S., Luhmer, I., Kallfelz, H. C., and Borst, H. G.: Emergency and non-emergency intra-atrial correction for transposition of the great arteries in 43 infants: Indications, details for the operative technique and results. Thoraxchirurgie, 25:305, 1977.

Olley, P. M., Coceani, F., and Rowe, R. D.: Role of prostaglandin E1 and E2 in the management of neonatal heart disease. Adv. Prostaglandin Thromboxane Res., 4:345, 1978.

Oppenheimer-Dekker, A.: Interventricular communications in transposition of the great arteries. In Embryology and Teratology of the Heart. Edited by L. H. S. Van Mierop, A. Oppenheimer-Dekker, and C. L. D. Bruins. Leiden, Leiden University Press, 1978, p. 136.

Parr, G. V. S., Blackstone, E. H., Kirklin, J. W., Pacifico, A. D., and Lauridsen, P.: Cardiac performance early after interatrial transposition of venous return in infants and small children. Circulation, 49(Suppl. 2):2, 1974.

Paul, M. H.: D-transposition of the great arteries. In Heart Disease in Infants, Children and Adolescents. Edited by A. J. Moss, F. H. Adams, and G. S. Emmanoulides. Baltimore, Williams and Wilkins Co., 1977, p. 301.

Pitlick, P., French, J., Guthaner, D., Shumway, N., and Baum, D.: Results of intraventricular baffle procedure for ventricular septal defect and double outlet right ventricle or d-transposition of the great arteries. Am. J. Cardiol., 47:307, 1981.

Plauth, W. H., Jr., Nadas, A. S., Bernhard, W. F., and Gross, R. E.: Transposition of the great arteries: Clinical and physiological observations on 74 patients treated by palliative surgery. Circulation, 37:316, 1968.

Polansky, S. M., and Culham, J. A. G.: Paraspinal densities developing after repair of transposition of the great arteries. Am. J. Roentgenol., 134:394, 1980.

Rakowski, H., Drobac, M., Bonet, J. F., Benson, L., McLaughlin, P. R., Olley, P. M., Rowe, R. D., and Morch, J. E.: Long term follow-up of Mustard's operation. Circulation, 59,60 (Suppl. 2):111, 1979.

Rashkind, W. J., and Miller, W. W.: Creation of an atrial septal defect without thoracotomy: A palliative approach to complete transposition of the great arteries. J.A.M.A., 196:991, 1966.

Rastelli, G. C.: A new approach to "anatomic" repair of transposition of the great vessels. Mayo Clin. Proc., 44:1, 1969.

Rastelli, G. C., McGoon, D. C., and Wallace, R. B.: Anatomic correction of transposition of the great arteries with ventricular septal defect and subpulmonary stenosis. J. Thorac. Cardiovasc. Surg., 58:545, 1969.

Riemenschneider, T. A., Vincent, W. R., Ruttenberg, H. D., and Desilets, D. T.: Transposition of the great vessels with hypoplasia of the right ventricle. Circulation, 38:386, 1968.

Rosenquist, G. C., Stark, J., and Taylor, J. F. N.: Anatomical relationships in transposition of the great arteries. Juxtaposition of the atrial appendage. Ann. Thorac. Surg., 18:456, 1974.

Rosenquist, G. C., Stark, J., and Taylor, J. F. N.: Congenital mitral valve disease in transposition of the great arteries. Circulation, 51:731, 1975.

Rowe, R. D., Freedom, R. M., Mehrizi, A., and Bloom, K. R.: The neonate with congenital heart disease. Major Probl. Clin. Pediatr., 5:3, 1981.

Rowlatt, U. F.: Coronary artery distribution in complete transposition. J.A.M.A., 179:109, 1972.

Sansa, M., Tonkin, I. L., Bargeron, L. M., Jr., and Elliott, L. P.: Left ventricular outflow tract obstruction in transposition of the great arteries: An angiographic study of 74 cases. Am. J. Cardiol., 44:88, 1979.

Senning, Å.: Surgical correction of transposition of the great vessels. Surgery, 45:966, 1959.

Shaher, R. M., and Puddu, G. C.: Coronary arterial anatomy in complete transposition of the great vessels. Am. J. Cardiol., 17:355, 1966.

Shannon, D. C., Lusser, M., Goldblatt, A., and Bunnell, J. B.: The cyanotic infant—heart disease or lung disease? N. Engl. J. Med., 287:951, 1972.

Shirotani, H.: Results over a two-year period in complete transposition of the great arteries after Mustard's procedure. Jpn. Circ. J., 44:916, 1980.

Shrivastava, S., Tadavarthy, S. M., Fukuda, T., and Edwards, J. E.: Anatomic causes of pulmonary stenosis in complete transposition. Circulation, 54:154, 1976.

Shumway, N. E., Griepp, R. B., and Stinson, E. B.: Surgical management of transposition of the great arteries. Am. J. Surg., 130:233, 1975.

Silove, E. D., and Taylor, J. F. N.: Angiographic anatomical features of subvalvular left ventricular outflow obstruction in transposition of the great arteries. The possible role of the anterior mitral valve leaflet. Pediatr. Radiol., 1:87, 1973.

Sorland, S. J., Tjonneland, S., and Hall, K. V.: Transposition of the great arteries. Early results of Mustard's operation in paediatric patients. Br. Heart J., 38:584, 1976.

Soto, B., Becker, A. E., Moulaert, A. J., Lie, J. T., and Anderson, R. H.: Classification of ventricular septal defects. Br. Heart J., 43:332, 1980.

Southall, D. P., Keeton, B. R., Leanage, R., Lam, L., Joseph, M. C., Anderson, R. H., Lincoln, C. R., and Shinebourne, E. A.: Cardiac rhythm and conduction before and after Mustard's operation for complete transposition of the great arteries. Br. Heart J., 43:21, 1980.

Spencer, F. C.: Monitoring techniques during palliative operations for transposition of the great vessels. In Heart Disease in Infancy: Diagnosis and Surgical Treatment. Edited by B. G. Barratt-Boyes, J. M. Neutze, and E. A. Harris. Baltimore, Williams and Wilkins Co., 1973, p. 261.

Stark, J., de Leval, M. R., and Taylor, J. F. N.: Mustard operation and creation of ventricular septal defect in two patients with transposition of the great arteries, intact ventricular septum and pulmonary vascular disease. Am. J. Cardiol., 38:524, 1976.

Stark, J., Hucin, B., Aberdeen, E., and Waterston, D. J.: Cardiac surgery in the first year of life: Experience with 1049 operations. Surgery, 69:483, 1971.

Stark, J., Silove, E. D., Taylor, J. F. N., and Graham, G. R. L.: Obstruction to systemic venous return following the Mustard operation for transposition of the great arteries. J. Thorac. Cardiovasc. Surg., 68:742, 1974.

Stark, J., Weller, P., Leanage, R., Cunningham, K., de Leval, M., Macartney, F. J., and Taylor, J. F. N.: Late results of surgical treatment of transposition of the great arteries. Adv. Cardiol., 27:254, 1980.

Subramanian, S., and Wagner, H.: Correction of transposition of the great arteries in infants under surface-induced deep hypothermia. Ann. Thorac. Surg., 16:391, 1973.

Takahashi, M., Lindesmith, G. G., Lewis, A. B., Stiles, Q. R., Stanton, R. E., Meyer, B. W., and Lurie, P. R.: Long term results of the Mustard procedure. Circulation, 56(Suppl. 2):85, 1977.

Tonkin, I. L., Kelley, M. J., Bream, P. R., and Elliott, L. P.: The frontal chest film as a method of suspecting transposition complexes. Circulation, 53:1016, 1976.

Tonkin, I. L., Sansa, M., Elliott, L. P., and Bargeron, L. M., Jr.: Recognition of developing left ventricular outflow tract obstruction in complete transposition of the great arteries. Radiology, 134:53, 1980.

Tooley, W. H., and Stanger, P.: The blue baby—circulation or ventilation or both? N. Engl. J. Med., 287:983, 1972.

Trusler, G. A., and Mustard, W. T.: Selection of palliative procedure in transposition of the great vessels. Ann. Thorac. Surg., 5:528, 1968.

Trusler, G. A., Mulholland, H. C., and Takeuchi, Y.: Long term results of intra-atrial repair of transposition of the great arteries. In The Second Henry Ford Hospital International Symposium on Cardiac Surgery. Edited by J. C. Davila. New York, 1977, p. 368.

Trusler, G. A., Williams, W. G., Izukawa, T., and Olley, P. M.: Current results with the Mustard operation in isolated transposition of the great arteries. J. Thorac. Cardiovasc. Surg., 80:381, 1980.

Turley, K., and Ebert, P. A.: Total correction of transposition of the great arteries. Conduction disturbances in infants younger than three months of age. J. Thorac. Cardiovasc. Surg., 76:312, 1978.

Tynan, M., Aberdeen, E., and Stark, J.: Tricuspid incompetence after the Mustard operation for transposition of the great arteries. Circulation, 45(Suppl. 1):111, 1972.

Urban, A. E., Stark, J., and Waterston, D. J.: Mustard's operation for transposition of the great arteries complicated by juxtaposition of the atrial appendages. Ann. Thorac. Surg., 21:304, 1976.

Van Gils, F. A. W.: Left ventricular outflow tract obstruction in transposition with interventricular communication: Anatomical aspects. In Embryology and Teratology of the Heart. Edited by L. H. S. Van Mierop, A. Oppenheimer-Dekker, and C. L. D. Bruins, Leiden, Leiden University Press, 1978, p. 160.

Van Gils, F. A. W., Moulaert, A. J., Oppenheimer-Dekker, A., and Wenink, A. C. G.: Transposition of the great arteries with ventricular septal defect and pulmonary stenosis. Br. Heart J., 40:494, 1978.

Van Praagh, R., Layton, W. M., and Van Praagh, S.: The morphogenesis of normal and abnormal relationship between the great arteries and the ventricle: Pathologic and experimental data.

In Etiology and Morphogenesis of Congenital Heart Disease. Edited by R. Van Praagh and A. Takao. Mt. Kisco, New York, Futura Publishing Co., 1980, p. 271.

Vidne, B. A., Subramanian, S., and Wagner, H. R.: Aneurysm of the membranous ventricular septum in transposition of the great arteries. Circulation, 53(1):157, 1976.

Waldhausen, J. A., Pierce, W. S., Park, C. D., Rashkind, W. J., and Friedman, S.: Physiologic correction of transposition of the great arteries: Indications for and results of operation in 32 patients. Circulation, 43:738, 1971.

Waldman, J. D., Paul, M. H., Newfeld, E. A., Muster, A. J., and Idriss, F. S.: Transposition of the great arteries with intact ventricular septum and patent ductus arteriosus. Am. J. Cardiol., 39:232, 1977.

Williams, W. G., Freedom, R. M., Culham, G., Duncan, W. J., Olley, P. M., Rowe, R. D., and Trusler, G. A.: Early experience with arterial repair of transposition, Ann. Thorac. Surg., 32:8, 1981.

Wilson, H. E., Nafrawi, A. G., Cardozo, R. H., and Aguillon, A.: Rational approach to surgery for complete transposition of the great vessels. Ann. Surg., 155:258, 1962.

Wyse, R. K. H., Hawroth, S. G., Taylor, J. F. N., and Macartney, F. J.: Obstruction of superior vena caval pathway after Mustard's repair. Reliable diagnosis by transcutaneous Doppler ultrasound. Br. Heart J., 42:162, 1979.

Yacoub, M., Bernhard, A., Lange, P., Radley-Smith, R., Keck, E., Stephan, E., and Heintzen, P.: Clinical and hemodynamic results of the two-stage anatomic correction of simple transposition of the great arteries. Circulation, 62(Suppl. 1):190, 1980.

Yamaki, S., and Tezuka, F. L.: Quantitative analysis of pulmonary vascular disease in complete transposition of the great arteries. Circulation, 54:805, 1976.

II   THE SENNING PROCEDURE

Åke Senning

The logical approach to correct a d-transposition of the great arteries (d-TGA) is a redirection of the bloodstream on the ventricular level if there is a large VSD present or to switch the great arteries, including the coronary arteries. The prerequisites are that the anatomic situation is favorable and that the left ventricle is prepared to assume the load of the systemic circulation. Several such operations were performed but without success, until 1975, when Jatene performed such an arterial switch (Jatene et al., 1975, 1976). Yet, the first successful hemodynamic correction of a d-TGA in 1958 (Senning, 1958, 1959) was based on a redirection of inflow to the heart on the atrial level. Albert (1955) had already suggested such a method, but his technique was impractical.

Today, the advances in diagnostic methods, operative techniques, and postoperative care allow us to operate on children at a very early age and to choose between hemodynamic corrective procedures that switch either the inflow or the outflow of the heart. When a correction is made at the atrial level, the function of the reconstructed atrial chambers should

be normal or near normal. These chambers must function as conduits without obstruction to the systemic or pulmonary venous inflow and have a good reservoir capacity, and perhaps most important, the pumping function must be optimal. In addition, the chambers should be able to grow with the child's increasing cardiac output. The surgical procedure should not disturb the atrial or ventricular conduction system in order to avoid different forms of arrhythmias. A final important condition is that the tricuspid valve and the right ventricle must be able to chronically assume the load of the systemic circulation.

Long-term follow-up is needed to verify if these conditions are fulfilled. The first patient operated on in 1958 at the age of 10 years lived a normal life of 18 years, playing football as a teenager, completing an education as a mechanic, marrying, and having a healthy daughter. In 1976, he developed a tricuspid valve endocarditis with several systemic emboli from the ulcerated, finally insufficient tricuspid valve and died with Staphylococcus aureus sepsis.

The tactics of the surgical treatment of TGA have

changed during the last 5 to 10 years. Earlier, a preliminary palliative operation, a Blalock-Hanlon septectomy, was performed to achieve good mixing at the atrial level. In addition, pulmonary flow was altered. If low, pulmonary flow was increased by a systemic artery–to–pulmonary artery shunt; if it was too high, a banding of the pulmonary artery and closure of the patent ductus arteriosus were performed. Today, a Rashkind balloon septostomy is done in conjunction with the initial diagnostic cardiac catheterization. If the resultant oxygen saturation of the arterial blood is sufficient and the pulmonary vascular resistance is within normal limits, a definitive operation can be postponed until the patient is approximately 6 months old. On the other hand, if the arterial saturation remains low after the Rashkind septostomy, the risk of cerebral damage as well as myocardial necrosis is high, and therefore, a corrective procedure should not be delayed.

TECHNIQUE

A right thoracotomy can be used, but a standard median sternotomy is preferred. The surgical correction is performed with extracorporeal circulation combined with hypothermia of 17° to 22°C. At this temperature, it is questionable if cardioplegia has any advantage compared with periods of cross-clamping of the aorta. One venous cannula is placed in the superior vena cava (SVC) about 15 mm. cranial to the junction with the right atrium. The inferior cannula is placed just below the right auricle in the inferior vena cava (IVC). The flow is adjusted according to the temperature level.

In infants, especially those less than 3 months of age, it is preferable to do the correction of a simple TGA with extracorporeal circulation combined with deep hypothermia and circulatory arrest. In this situation, only one cannula is introduced through the right atrial appendage, and the child is rapidly cooled to about 20°C. If the perfusate is pre-cooled to approximately 5°C., the heart usually stops within 2 minutes. After the aorta is cross-clamped and the extracorporeal circulation stopped, the venous system is drained and the caval veins are occluded. When the last atrial suture has been placed, the venous cannula is reintroduced through the right atrial appendage in the anterior part of the newly constructed pulmonary venous atrium. The extracorporeal circulation is started again, and the circulation is filled with blood and the infant rewarmed to 34° to 35°C. To achieve a sufficient flow, it is usually not necessary to have a cannula in the systemic venous atrium. All air must be carefully emptied before the heart is allowed to beat. Frequently, a short period of electrically induced ventricular fibrillation is of benefit in preventing air embolism.

The correction is started with an incision in the right atrium in front of and parallel to the caval veins that is extended into the atrial appendage (Fig. 40–19). Another incision is made as long as possible in the

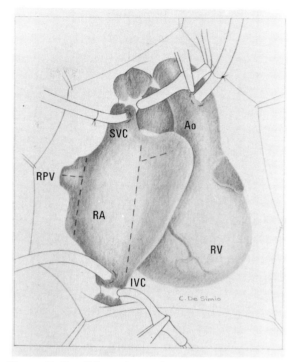

Figure 40–19. Schematic drawing of the atrial incisions. One incision is parallel to and in front of the caval veins. The upper part of the incision is extended into the atrial appendage. After dissection into the interatrial groove, an incision is made as far as possible into the left atrium. The superior pulmonary vein is incised to the insertion of the pericardium. (Ao = aorta; RV = right ventricle; IVC = inferior vena cava; SVC = superior vena cava; RA = right atrium; RPV = right pulmonary vein.)

interatrial groove into the left atrium. Vertical to this incision, the superior right pulmonary vein is split to the pericardial insertion. The atrial septum is now incised to form a flap as large as possible, fixed posteriorly between the caval veins (Fig. 40–20). In the anterior upper corner, it is important to leave some tissue to avoid disturbing the arterial circulation of the sinus node and to spare the anterior conducting tissue from the sinus node to the AV node. The anterior conduction pathway goes anterior to the coronary sinus and the posterior pathway passes posterior to the coronary sinus. Therefore, the coronary sinus is unroofed to increase the atrial septal defect. The middle pathway is cut when forming the flap. Since the posterior conduction pathway passes in the posterior atrial wall bridge between the caval veins, this tissue must be treated with utmost care and any trauma avoided. The lower incision in the septum is extended along the insertion in the bottom of the left atrium.

The first step is to separate the left pulmonary venous blood flow from the mitral valve area. With double-armed 4-0 silk suture material, the apex of the flap is fixed in front of the atrial orifices of the left pulmonary veins (silk is used because it will disintegrate) (Fig. 40–21). With one suture line, the upper edge of the flap is sutured to the posterior wall of the

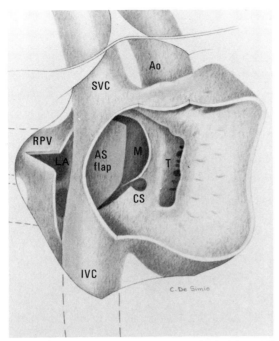

Figure 40–20. Demonstration of the atrial incisions. The left atrium (LA) is opened, and the right pulmonary vein (RPV) is incised. Between the superior vena cava (SVC) and the inferior vena cava (IVC), the right atrium is incised, and the incision is extended into the appendage. The atrial septum is incised leaving a flap (AS flap) fixed posteriorly. The coronary sinus (CS) is also incised. The tricuspid valve (T) is visible. (M = mitral valve.)

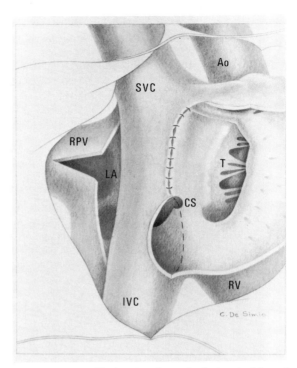

Figure 40–22. This drawing shows the first part of the suturing of the anterior edge of the posterior part of the right atrial wall to the septal remnant. It will continue inside the coronary sinus and down to the IVC.

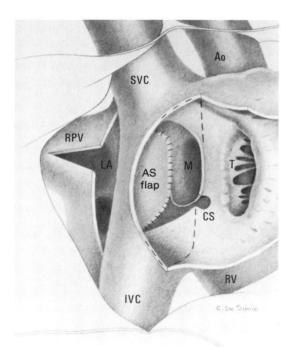

Figure 40–21. The first step of the suturing. The atrioseptal flap (AS flap) has been sutured in front of the left pulmonary veins and behind the left atrial appendage. The tricuspid valve (T) as well as the mitral valve (M) is seen. In the next step, the anterior edge of the posterior part of the right atrial wall will be sutured to the anterior part of the septal defect, and the dotted lines will be sutured to each other.

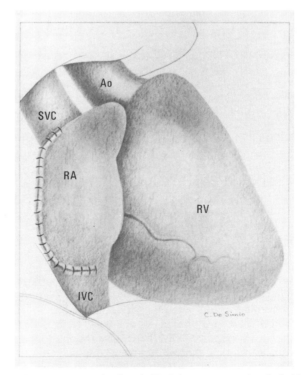

Figure 40–23. The first half of the reconstruction is finished. Now the posterior edge of the anterior part of the right atrial wall will be sutured around the caval veins along the dotted lines and to the left atrial wall.

left atrium. With the other suture line, the edge below the pulmonary veins is sutured first to the atrial wall behind the atrial appendage, and then the suture line is continued along the left atrial wall to the end of the incision, using part of the incised coronary sinus. With a nerve hook or a similar instrument, the suture line is probed for leaks, thus diverting all left pulmonary venous blood flow behind the atrial septal flap to the right.

The next step is to divert the systemic venous blood from the systemic circulation to the mitral valve and left ventricle (Fig. 40–22). The edge of the posterior part of the incised right atrial wall is sutured in front to the atrial septal remnant. The suturing is continued cranially to the posterior right atrial wall. The lower part is continued through the inside of the coronary sinus orifice (Fig. 40–23) (to avoid damage to the AV node) and to the right atrial wall, down to the bottom of the incision or to the eustachian valve, if the tissue is good. The snares around the caval veins are now loosened, and the atrial chamber is allowed to fill with systemic blood to ensure that the suture lines do not leak.

The final step is to direct the pulmonary venous blood to the tricuspid valve area (Fig. 40–24). Therefore, the edge of the anterior part of the incised right atrial wall is sutured around the caval veins and to the incised left atrium. The suturing is started in the upper part of the incision at the base of the caval vein, and the incised atrial appendage is stretched posteriorly and sutured above the SA node to the lowest part of the superior caval vein, avoiding the

sinus node. This suturing is continued over to the incised left atrium. In most cases, it may be advantageous to place a separate short suture to approximate the upper portion of the incised left atrium to the superior vena caval wall. The lower part of the edge of the anterior wall is sutured around the caval vein and in the direction of the incised left atrium. It is important to stretch the caval wall during the suturing to avoid an obstruction of the inflow. As the atrial appendix has been incised, there is plenty of tissue to suture the posterior edge of the anterior part of the right atrial wall around the caval veins and to the incised left atrium and the superior pulmonary vein. Before the suturing is finished, a drainage cannula for air is inserted through the pulmonary venous chamber into the right ventricle.

When this last suture line is started, rewarming of the patient begins and if the ventricle starts to beat, electric ventricular fibrillation is induced to avoid air embolism. This is continued until the suture line is finished and the heart is carefully emptied of air. A small incision is also made in the uppermost part of the aorta to allow any air remaining in the chambers to leave the circulation when the heart resumes beating.

A VSD of perimembranous type complicating TGA can usually be closed through the tricuspid valve. Iatrogenic tricuspid insufficiency is deleterious; therefore, utmost care must be taken not to disturb papillary muscle function or the attachments of the muscles and the chordae tendineae to the septal and anterior cusps of the tricuspid valve. Only in rare cases does a right ventricular outflow ventriculotomy have to be done to close defects in the subpulmonary parts of the conus. For multiple trabecular septal defects, a left ventriculotomy is preferred.

Depending on the relationship of the great vessels to each other, the transpulmonary correction of left ventricular outflow tract obstruction (LVOTO) (stenosis) can be performed either posterior to or to the left of the aorta. The pulmonary artery is separated from the aorta and incised longitudinally down to the valve. If necessary, a valvular commissurotomy is performed. A muscular stenosis can be resected through the valve, although Oelert (1981) suggests a resection through the mitral valve. When the myocardium is flaccid, the anterior cusp of the mitral valve is retracted, allowing a resection of the obstructing myocardium. A resection of a subvalvular fibrotic stenosis can be done only through the pulmonary artery when it is important to liberate the anterior surface of the mitral valve from fibrotic tissue.

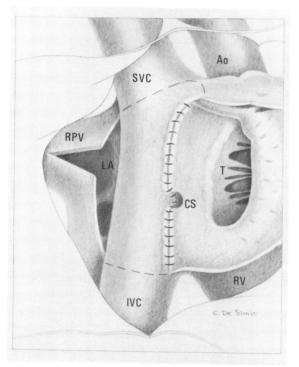

Figure 40–24. The reconstruction is now finished. The upper suture line is cranial to the sinus node location.

RESULTS

In most instances, the hospital mortality rate for children 6 months of age or older who undergo the Senning procedure is now around 5 per cent, but in several series, the reported mortality rate has been even lower (Parenzan *et al.*, 1977).

Previously, when the operation was performed in children less than 3 months old, the mortality rate was high, but recently, Chalant (1981), Ebert (1981), and others have shown that even in this age group, mortality rate can be kept extremely low, even lower than the combined mortality rates from a palliative operation, waiting time, and the final correction. It is therefore preferable to operate on the child as soon as possible.

Small ventricular septal defects in infants can be left alone, since they will usually close spontaneously. If, on the other hand, a VSD is large, closure of the defect is necessary. In these patients, the mortality rate still remains high, mainly because of the pathologic changes of the pulmonary vessels.

Late mortality after correction of a simple TGA or of a TGA combined with pulmonary stenosis has been low in our experience. In a group of 16 patients in whom a VSD had been corrected, there were three late deaths, two from increasing pulmonary vascular resistance in spite of a good VSD closure and one from an AV block. Two other patients had a correction at the atrial level, and the VSD was left open because of high pulmonary resistance. Both of these patients died 1½ to 2 years postoperatively. Lindesmith and associates (1975) reported good results after palliative flow redirection at the atrial level, leaving the VSD open. Several of their patients have survived for many years.

There has been only one reoperation in our series, including patients followed up to 19 years, in contrast to many series in which the Mustard operation was performed. Oelert (1981), for example, had to reoperate on 34 of 221 patients.

During a 10- to 19-year follow-up of our 51 patients, the atrial chambers created by the operation were studied, especially concerning their function as conduits, reservoirs, and pumps, as well as with regard to arrhythmias following the surgical interventions.

With regard to the function of the atrial chambers as a conduit, none of the patients operated on according to the original Senning method has had any stenosis of the pulmonary venous return, and there has been no obstruction to the IVC flow. Postoperative evaluation revealed no significant pressure gradients indicative of obstruction to systemic or pulmonary venous flow. In one patient, a minimal gradient of 3 mm. Hg between the superior caval vein and the systemic venous atrium was found. Likewise, no visual evidence of obstruction was found by postoperative angiograms (Fig. 40–25).

Concerning the reservoir function, in the early postoperative period the systemic venous atrium is a little smaller than normal, but it enlarges with growth and increased flow. In addition, early postoperatively an edematous swelling of the atrial walls can cause some hindrance to the flow, but this disappears after

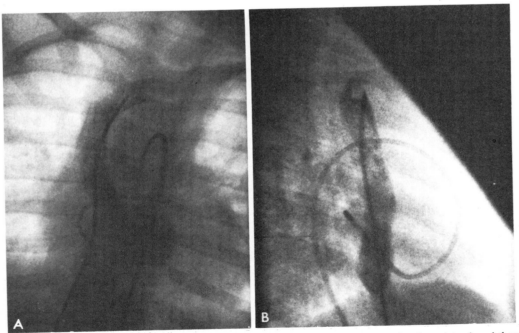

Figure 40–25. Postoperative angiograms. *A*, Anteroposterior projection. A venous catheter has been introduced through the inferior vena cava. A small injection of contrast medium indicates that the superior vena cava and inferior vena cava clearly have wide entrances into the systemic atrium. The catheter is straight between the caval veins, indicating that the atrial chamber has adapted itself to the flow. A retrograde arterial catheter passes from the aorta to the anatomic right ventricle and through the tricuspid valve into the posterior part of the pulmonary venous atrium. Note the large distance between the systemic venous catheter and the pulmonary venous atrium catheter, indicating the wide connection between the pulmonary veins and the anterior part of the pulmonary venous atrium. *B*, Lateral view. There is no obstruction of the superior vena cava and good filling of the systemic venous atrium. Note also here the large distance between the posterior wall of the systemic atrium and the catheter in the pulmonary venous atrium, indicating no obstruction to the pulmonary venous return.

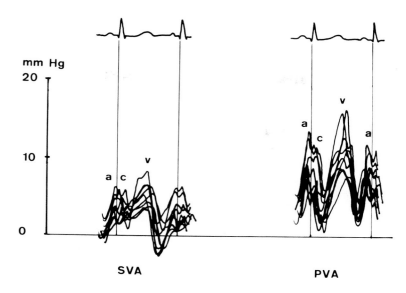

20 pts with sinus rhythm

	a	c	v	m
SVA	3.7 ± 2.0	4.8 ± 2.0	6.1 ± 1.8	2.8 ± 1.2 mm Hg
PVA	7.2 ± 2.0	6.3 ± 2.4	8.7 ± 2.4	4.8 ± 1.7 mm Hg

Figure 40–26. Atrial pressure curves in TGA after the Senning operation. The pulmonary venous atrium (PVA), in general, has a good-sized a wave, which is higher than the c wave but smaller than the v wave. The ratio a/v (0.83 ± 0.16) is comparable to that of a normal left atrium. The systemic venous atrium (SVA) shows dominant v and c waves. Atrial function, particularly that of the more important PVA, seems to be less impaired after the Senning operation than after the Mustard procedure.

a few days. The concave inflow from the caval veins to the systemic atrium also seems to disappear with the growth of the child.

As only living contracting tissue has been used to construct the new atrial chambers, practically normal contractions can be expected. Postoperative angiograms have shown large differences in volume between diastole and systole for both atrial chambers. The active contractions of the atrial chambers can also be demonstrated with the pressure curves, as shown in Figure 40–26. There are practically normal atrial contraction waves in the more important pulmonary venous atrial chamber. The slight deviation from normal in the systemic atrial pressure curves can be explained by the slightly insufficient volume of this chamber. Since the pressure curves in the pulmonary venous atrium were recorded in the posterior part of this chamber near the left pulmonary vein, they excluded any obstruction of the pulmonary venous return. The pressure waves also show a normal function of the tricuspid valve and exclude any significant tricuspid insufficiency. The normal atrial pressure also confirms the ability of the right ventricle to handle the systemic load. In our 51 patients followed for 10 to 19 years, there have been no clinical signs of tricuspid valve insufficiency. However, in a later series, two patients with ventricular septal defects showed tricuspid valve insufficiency; one instance occurred after the repair of the VSD, and the other

was pre-existing and was corrected with an anulorraphy according to DeVega's technique. None of the patients have shown impairment of right ventricular function.

A common complication after the Senning operation as well as after the Mustard operation is a disturbance of the normal rhythm. Of 41 patients followed for 4 to 66 months after a Senning correction, 33 were in a stable sinus rhythm, four had an intermittent nodal rhythm, and two had a constant nodal rhythm. One patient had a flutter with a 2:1 block, and another patient finally had AV block (Table 40–5). Impairment of the sinus node function now occurs less frequently, as we have learned to avoid damaging the sinus node blood supply by not going too high in

TABLE 40–5. HEMODYNAMIC CORRECTION OF TGA — FOLLOW-UP 4 TO 66 MONTHS (MEAN 21 MONTHS)

RHYTHM	NUMBER OF PATIENTS	
Sinus	33	A-V block
SR nodal	4	I – II 8
Nodal	2	
Atrial flutter + 2:1 block	1	
A-V block	1	
Total	41	

the septum while making the atrial septal flap. Additional care is taken to avoid the anterior and posterior conduction pathways. Nodal rhythm or tachyarrhythmias or bradyarrhythmias are relatively rare today. Complete AV block is usually seen only after correction of cases complicated by a VSD.

Suture line leaks can be avoided by careful intraoperative inspection. In our series, leaks of 20 to 30 per cent have been found in four of 51 patients; one patient underwent reoperation. A preoperative redistribution of the blood flow through the lungs is seen in some patients but was not seen as a postoperative complication. The redistribution of the pulmonary flow with underperfusion of the left lung is in some cases explained by anatomic conditions but in other cases can be explained by an obstruction of the left pulmonary veins after correction. This was not observed in this series.

As reported in the literature, in a certain percentage of the patients, correction of TGA is complicated by impairment of cerebral function. In a few patients, this has been due to complications during the surgical correction, but most are pre-existing. In some instances, it may be congenital, but probably most cases are due to cerebral hypoxia before correction. It is also possible that the right ventricular myocardial insufficiency (Trusler *et al.*, 1980) is a consequence not only of the anatomic architecture of the ventricle or insufficient intraoperative myocardial protein, but also of the preoperative myocardial hypoxia.

Therefore, it seems important to correct TGA as early as possible, that is, before cerebral and myocardial impairment occurs and before progressive pulmonary vascular changes become irreversible. Although our perfusion and surgical techniques have been developed to a point that allows us to perform correction of TGA in the first days of an infant's life, it will be another two decades before we will have the long-term follow-up data to know which is the best technique for correction of TGA.

REFERENCES

Albert, H. M.: Surgical correction of transposition of the great vessels. Surg. Forum, *5*:74, 1954.

Chalant, C. H.: Communication at the XV World Congress of the International Cardiovascular Society, Athens, 1981.

Ebert, P. A.: Personal communication, 1981.

Jatene, A. D., Fontes, V. F., Paulista, P. P., Sousa, L. C. B., Neger, F., Galantier, M., and Sousa, J. E. M. R.: Successful anatomic correction of transposition of the great vessels. A preliminary report. Arq. Bras. Cardiol., *28*:461, 1975.

Jatene, A. D., Fontes. V, F., Paulista, P. P., Sousa, L. C. B., Neger, F., Galantier. M., and Sousa, J. E. M. R.: Anatomic correction of transposition of the great vessels. J. Thorac. Cardiovasc. Surg., *72*:364, 1976.

Lindesmith, G. G., Stanton, R. E., Lurie, P. R., Takahashi, M., Tucker, B. L., Stiles, Q. R., and Meyer, B. W.: An assessment of Mustard's operation as a palliative procedure for transposition of the great arteries. Ann. Thorac. Surg., *19*:514, 1975.

Oelert, H.: Communication at the XV World Congress of the International Cardiovascular Society, Athens, 1981.

Parenzan, L., Locatelli, G., Alfieri, O., Villani, M., and Invernizzi, G.: The Senning operation for transposition of the great arteries. J. Thorac. Cardiovasc. Surg., *76*:305, 1977.

Senning, Å.: Transposition av aorta och arteria pulmonalis. Opuscula Medica, nr, 2, 1958.

Senning, Å.: Surgical correction of transposition of the great vessels. Surgery, *45*:966, 1959.

Trusler, G. A., Williams, W. G., Izukawa, T., and Olley, P. M.: Current results with the Mustard operation in isolated transposition of the great arteries. J. Thorac. Cardiovasc. Surg., *80*:381, 1981.

III   ANATOMIC CORRECTION OF TRANSPOSITION OF THE GREAT ARTERIES AT THE ARTERIAL LEVEL

Magdi Yacoub

As the basic abnormality in complete transposition of the great arteries (TGA) is the abnormal connections between the ventricles and great arteries, the most direct and obvious way of treating this anomaly is anatomic correction at the arterial level. It is not surprising, therefore, that this approach was used in some of the earliest attempts at surgical correction of this anomaly (Mustard *et al.*, 1954; Bailey *et al.*, 1954; Kay and Cross, 1955). However, for a variety of reasons, it was abandoned in favor of atrial repair by the Mustard or Senning operation until the early 1970s, when the concept of arterial repair was revived and applied successfully.

HISTORICAL ASPECTS

The first attempt at anatomic correction was performed by Mustard in Toronto, who in 1954 described a technique for "re-transposition of the great vessels," which was tried in seven patients, using monkey lung as an oxygenator (Mustard *et al.*, 1954). The technique included transfer of the left coronary artery in continuity with the distal aorta. In the same year, Bjork and Boukaert (1954), working in Sweden, described an experimental technique for "switch over anastomosis" of the great arteries, leaving the coronary arteries to be supplied by the pulmonary ventricle. This technique involved the use of segments of aortic homografts as permanent shunts between the great arteries, followed by interruption of the aorta and pulmonary arteries between the shunts. Around the same time, several clinical attempts at switching the great arteries without coronary transfer were made utilizing hypothermia (Bailey *et al.*, 1954), temporary plastic shunts (Cross *et al.*, 1954), or sequential anastomosis (Kay and Cross, 1955). None of these patients survived.

In 1959, Åke Senning, working at the Karolinska Institute in Stockholm, reported the use of a technique that involved disinsertion of the pulmonary valve from the left ventricular outflow tract and closure of the gap so created, followed by insertion of an intraventricular baffle to direct blood from the left ventricle through a ventricular septal defect to the aorta. The mobilized pulmonary valve and artery were then anastomosed directly to the right ventricular outflow tract. The technique was tried in three children, with no survivors. This report represents the first attempt at restoring normal connections between both coronary arteries and the left ventricle.

In 1961, Idriss and associates described another technique for retransposition of the great arteries with coronary transfer. This consisted of mobilization of a complete ring of ascending aorta carrying the two coronary orifices. The ring was then rotated and sutured in place to form a segment of the pulmonary artery. The three children who underwent this operation could not be weaned off cardiopulmonary bypass. Although this is an ingenious technique, the rotation of the aortic disc through an angle of 180 degrees could produce severe torsion and narrowing of the proximal coronary arteries.

Experimental techniques for coronary transfer were described by Anagnostopoulos and colleagues from Chicago (Anagnostopoulos, 1973; Anagnostopoulos *et al.*, 1973). In 1972, I developed and used a technique similar to the one currently used. This technique was initially tried in three children with simple transposition and low preoperative left ventricular pressure operated on between November 1972 and March 1975. Although the initial left ventricular function was good, all of the children died during the early postoperative period owing to progressive left ventricular failure This technique was later applied successfully in September 1975 (Yacoub *et al.*, 1976). Earlier in the same year, Adib Jatene, working independently in Sao Paolo, successfully relocated the great arteries with coronary transfer in a patient who had a large ventricular septal defect (Jatene *et al.*, 1975). This child was the first survivor of the arterial switch operation, and the results of the procedure in this instance emphasized the importance of the development of the left ventricle for the success of this operation. Following that, several children with complex TGA underwent successful correction (Ross *et al.*, 1976; Kreutzer *et al.*, 1976). In 1976, a two-stage operation for anatomic correction of simple TGA was developed and applied (Yacoub *et al.*, 1977). Several

modifications and refinements have since been described (Yacoub, 1977; Le Compte *et al.*, 1981).

An alternative technique to avoid mobilization of the coronary ostia was reported by Aubert and co-workers (1978). To date, the results of four series have been reported (Yacoub, 1979; Williams *et al.*, 1981; Le Compte *et al,*, 1981; Jatene *et al.*, 1982).

A different concept for correction of TGA at the arterial level was suggested by Paul Damus in 1975 while he was completing his residency. This operation consists of end-to-side anastomosis of the transected pulmonary artery to the ascending aorta, followed by insertion of a valved conduit from the right ventricle to the distal pulmonary artery. This technique was also suggested by Kaye (1975) and Stansel (1977), and later successfully performed by Danielson and associates (1978) and Damus and colleagues (1982).

In 1978, Bex and coworkers suggested and applied mobilization of the aortic root with the proximal coronary arteries, followed by direct anastomosis to the pulmonary root after excision of the pulmonary valve (Bex *et al.*, 1980). The distal pulmonary artery is then anastomosed directly to the right ventricular outflow duct without insertion of a valve.

PREOPERATIVE EVALUATION

Prior to anatomic correction, it is essential to define accurately the anatomy and function of the atrioventricular valves, the interventricular septum, the coronary arteries, the left ventricular outflow tract, the pulmonary arterial tree, and the left ventricle.

Atrioventricular Valves. Anatomic abnormalities of the atrioventricular (AV) valves in TGA are relatively rare (Layman and Edwards, 1967; Elliott *et al.*, 1963; Shaher, 1973; Rosenquist *et al.*, 1975; Huhta *et al.*, 1982). The majority of these abnormalities, such as cleft mitral valve or abnormal attachment of tricuspid valve chordae, have little functional significance and do not interfere with the technique or results of anatomic correction. Severe mitral valve abnormalities such as parachute mitral valve (Shone *et al.*, 1963) must be excluded. The presence of a straddling AV valve (Bharati *et al.*, 1979), best defined by two-dimensional echocardiography (Seward *et al.*, 1978) and angiography, is not a contraindication to anatomic correction, except when associated with a hypoplastic ventricular chamber. Tricuspid regurgitation with or without impaired right ventricular function is an indication for anatomic correction rather than atrial repair.

Interventricular Septum. The presence, number, and location of ventricular septal defects should be defined by careful examination and by scrutinizing the appropriate angiographic projections of the ventricular septum. This is of particular importance because ventricular septal defects in TGA could have unusual locations (Lev *et al.*, 1961; Idriss *et al.*, 1974) and therefore may be missed or prolong the time of myocardial ischemia and cardiopulmonary bypass.

Left Ventricular Outflow Tract. Varying degrees

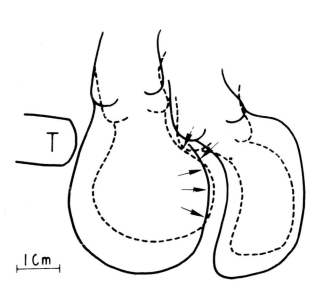

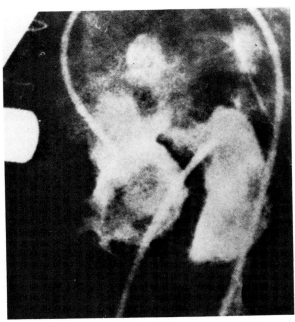

Figure 40–27. Simultaneous right and left ventricular angiocardiogram showing bulging of the right ventricle into the left ventricular outflow tract. (From Park, S.C., *et al.*: Echocardiographic and hemodynamic correlation in transposition of the great arteries. Circulation, *57*:291, 1978.)

of left ventricular outflow tract obstruction (LVOTO) are common in TGA and are usually due to functional subpulmonary stenosis produced by abnormal bulging of the interventricular septum to the left (Tynan, 1972; Vidne *et al.*, 1976; Park *et al.*, 1978; Aziz *et al.*, 1979) (Fig. 40–27). This can be aggravated by secondary deposition of subendocardial fibroelastic tissue, which simulates a shelf or membrane (Fig. 40–28), or by protrusion of tricuspid valve tissue through a ventricular septal defect (Ashby, 1881; Riemenschneider *et al.*, 1969). Fixed or tunnel subpulmonary stenosis is less common and is usually associated with pulmonary valve stenosis (Shaher *et al.*, 1967; Shrivastava *et al.*, 1976; Sansa *et al.*, 1979).

The presence of LVOTO is suspected from the

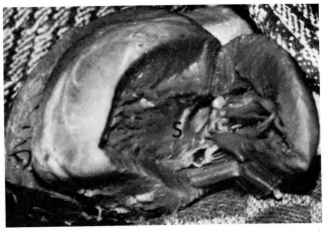

Figure 40–28. Heart showing "shelf" (S) caused by deposition of subendocardial fibroelastic tissue in the left ventricular outflow tract.

presence of a pulmonary ejection murmur associated with electrocardiographic and vectorcardiographic evidence of left ventricular hypertrophy and lack of severe pulmonary plethora observed on a plain film. The diagnosis is confirmed and the anatomic type determined by M-mode and two-dimensional echocardiography as well as biplane angiography.

In the presence of a normal pulmonary valve, functional subpulmonary stenosis with or without an additional fibromuscular ridge is not a contraindication to anatomic correction and usually does not require surgical resection, as it disappears immediately after restoration of the normal pressure relationship between the two ventricles. Similarly, obstruction due to prolapse of the tricuspid valve through a ventricular septal defect (VSD) can be easily corrected at the time of repair.

In contrast, long tunnel obstruction or any degree of pulmonary valve stenosis constitutes a contraindication to the arterial switch operation.

Coronary Anatomy. Because anatomic correction of TGA involves transfer of the coronary ostia from the aorta to the pulmonary artery, it is essential to be familiar with the different modes of origin, course, and early branching of the coronary arteries in TGA. Despite the existence of many variations of coronary anatomy (Shaher and Puddu, 1966; Elliott *et al.*, 1966), the vast majority of patients have one of three types, which have been designated Types A, D, and E (Yacoub and Radley-Smith, 1978). In Type A, the right and left coronary arteries arise from the center of the right posterior aortic sinus and the left posterior aortic sinus respectively (Fig. 40–29). The left coronary artery divides soon after its origin into anterior descending and circumflex branches, which are dis-

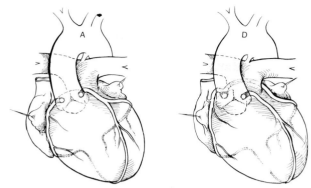

Figure 40–29. The origin, course, and branching pattern of the coronary arteries in Type A (*left*) and Type D (*right*) anatomies.

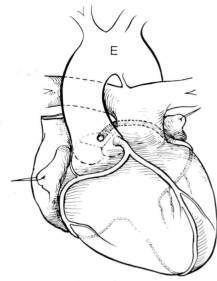

Figure 40–30. The origin, course, and branching pattern of the coronary arteries in Type E anatomy.

tributed in a manner similar to that present in a normal heart. The right coronary artery passes backwards and to the right for a very short distance before curving forward toward the atrioventricular groove between the right atrial appendage and the right ventricle.

Types B and C are extremely rare and differ from Type A only in the location of the coronary ostia. In Type B, they are located very close to each other on either side of the posterior aortic commissure. In Type C, a single coronary orifice is located on either side of the posterior commissure.

Type D, which is present in approximately 14 per cent of patients, differs from Type A in the mode of branching and course of the proximal coronary arteries. Almost immediately after its origin, the right coronary artery gives origin to the circumflex branch, which curves around the right lateral and posterior aspects of the root of the pulmonary artery to reach the atrioventricular groove between the left atrial appendage and the left ventricle (Fig. 40–29). The left coronary artery courses to the top of the anterior interventricular groove and continues as the left anterior descending artery.

Type E is present in approximately 10 per cent of patients, in whom the great arteries are situated side by side. In this type of coronary anatomy, the right coronary artery arises from the left anterior aortic sinus, gives origin to the left anterior descending branch, and crosses in front of the right ventricular outflow tract to reach the right atrioventricular groove (Fig. 40–30). The circumflex artery arises separately from the posterior aortic sinus and passes behind the root of the pulmonary artery in a manner similar to that found in Type D anatomy to reach the left atrioventricular groove.

The particular type of coronary anatomy can usually be diagnosed preoperatively from the available angiogram. This exercise is important to familiarize the surgeon and investigator with different types of coronary anatomy but is not of crucial importance for individual patients, since all types are amenable to transfer and can be readily identified at the time of operation.

Pulmonary Flow and Vascular Resistance. The choice of procedure for anatomic correction of both simple and complex TGA may be influenced by the levels of pulmonary flow and pulmonary vascular resistance. In simple TGA, pulmonary flow can be predicted from heart size and the degree of pulmonary plethora, as observed from a standard chest radiograph. More accurate information can be obtained at cardiac catheterization from the formula:

$$\text{Total pulmonary flow} = \frac{\text{Oxygen consumption}}{\substack{\text{Pulmonary venous} \\ \text{oxygen content} - \\ \text{pulmonary arterial} \\ \text{oxygen content}}}$$

or from angiographic left ventricular volume measurements using the formula:

$$\text{Pulmonary flow} = (\text{LVEDV} - \text{LVESV}) \times \text{HR}$$

where LVEDV = left ventricular end-diastolic volume; LVESV = left ventricular end-systolic volume; and HR = heart rate.

In patients with simple TGA and low pulmonary artery pressure, banding of the pulmonary artery without additional shunt (to prepare the left ventricle for anatomic correction) is only well tolerated in patients with a high pulmonary flow. In the remaining patients, who have a relatively reduced pulmonary flow, an additional systemic–to–pulmonary artery shunt is required (Yacoub *et al.,* 1980).

In patients with TGA and a large VSD, the presence of a pulmonary vascular resistance equal to or more than 12 units constitutes a contraindication to closure of the VSD at the time of anatomic repair. In these patients, pulmonary vascular disease is usually severe and irreversible and, therefore, may produce early or late severe, fatal right ventricular failure if the VSD is closed. In contrast, excellent palliation is obtained if the VSD is left open at the time of anatomic correction.

The Left Ventricle. For the success of anatomic correction, it is essential for the left ventricle to support the systemic circulation immediately after operation. This poses no problems in patients with additional defects that maintain a high peak systolic pressure in the left ventricle, or PLVP (within 20 mm. Hg of that in the systemic circulation). Such defects include large ventricular septal defects, a patent ductus arteriosus, an aortopulmonary window, or subpulmonary stenosis. The most reliable guide to the state of the left ventricle is the level of PLVP. Additional helpful guides include conventional electrocardiography, vectorcardiography, systolic time intervals, and measurements of posterior wall thickness and left ventricular muscle mass using M-mode echocardiography or angiography. The reliability of these methods in assessing the suitability of the left ventricle for supporting the systemic circulation will be discussed in the following section dealing with preparation of the left ventricle.

PROCEDURE FOR ANATOMIC CORRECTION OF TGA AT THE ARTERIAL LEVEL

Preparation of the Left Ventricle

Although the shape and fiber orientation of the right and left ventricles appear to be genetically determined, the ventricular volume, wall thickness, and muscle mass represent functional adaptation to the hemodynamic load to which each ventricle is subjected both before and after birth. This view is supported by the fact that at birth the right and left ventricles are nearly equal in weight and wall thickness (Scammon, 1927; Keen, 1955). This observation was first made in 1628 by William Harvey, who stated that in the embryo "there is not such a difference between the two ventricles, but as in a double nut they are nearly equal in all respects." A similar relationship has been reported in the newborn pig (Booth *et al.,* 1966), rabbit (Gluck *et al.,* 1964), and dog (Latimer, 1965). Two studies, however, have shown that in the newborn human heart the left ventricular wall is slightly thicker than the right (De La Cruz *et al.,* 1960; Smith *et al.,* 1982). In TGA with an intact interventricular septum, the relationship between right and left ventricular wall thickness and muscle mass at birth is similar to that found in the normal heart at that age (Bano-Rodrigo *et al.,* 1980; Smith *et al.,* 1982).

The normal drop in pulmonary artery pressure after birth results in fall of PLVP in TGA and progressive regression or failure of the left ventricle to grow. These changes are analogous to those observed in the right ventricle of a normal heart after birth, which represents an actual decrease in size previously attained (Keen, 1955; Averill *et al.,* 1963; Recavarren and Arias-Stella, 1964) or failure to grow (Emery and Mithal, 1961). The drop in pulmonary artery pressure in simple TGA occurs largely during the first 4 weeks

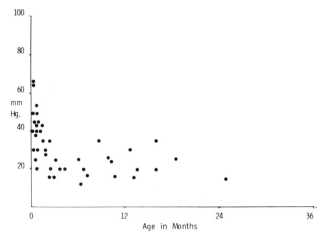

Figure 40–31. The relationship between peak pulmonary artery pressure and age at catheterization in simple TGA.

of life (Tynan, 1972) (Fig. 40–31). By the end of this period, most patients have a PLVP equal to or less than 65 per cent of that in the systemic circulation (Fig. 40–32). The temporal relationship between the drop in PLVP and diminution in the left ventricular wall thickness to render the left ventricle incapable of supporting the systemic circulation is not known, but probably represents a short period of time.

One-stage anatomic correction of simple TGA at a very young age (during the first 2 to 3 weeks of life) is feasible (Ebert, 1981) but has not been widely tried because of the increased risks of prolonged cardiopulmonary bypass at this age as well as the elevated pulmonary vascular resistance normally present during this period. Furthermore, many children are referred for surgical correction at an age when the left ventricle is already too thin to support the systemic circulation. The postnatal fall in pulmonary vascular resistance in simple TGA leads to acceleration of flow in the pulmonary circuit, resulting in a large pulmonary flow compared with that in the systemic circulation in most patients (Graham *et al.,* 1970; Plauth *et*

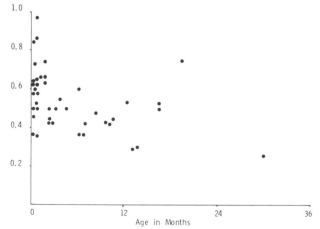

Figure 40–32. Relation of peak left ventricular–to–right ventricular pressure ratio with age in simple TGA.

al., 1970; Tynan, 1972). This imposes a diastolic overload on the left ventricle, which results in adaptive increase in left ventricular cavity volume. This increase in volume has been documented in both clinical studies (Graham et al., 1970; Plauth et al., 1970) and pathologic studies (Lev et al., 1969). Although the calculated left ventricular muscle mass measured by echocardiography or angiography is increased in these patients owing to the increased cavity volume, left ventricular wall thickness is too low to support the systemic circulation.

Because of these considerations, a technique for redeveloping the left ventricle has been introduced and regularly applied since 1976 (Yacoub et al., 1977; Yacoub et al., 1980; Bernhard et al., 1981). This technique consists of banding of the pulmonary artery with or without the addition of a systemic–to–pulmonary artery shunt. A shunt is usually necessary in patients with a relatively low total pulmonary flow, as indicated by a cardiothoracic ratio of 0.54 or less; the need for a shunt is also determined by the degree of pulmonary plethora, as judged from the chest radiograph, and the calculated pulmonary flow measured by oximetry and/or from angiographic left ventricular volume measurements, This first-stage operation is usually performed using a right lateral thoracotomy through the fourth intercostal space. A limited incision œ the pericardium is performed in front of the phrenic nerve and a nylon band is used to constrict the main pulmonary artery 2 to 3 mm. below the lower border of the right pulmonary artery (Fig. 40–33). Dissection between the aorta and the pulmonary artery is limited to avoid migration of the band. The exact position of the band should be as far as possible from the top of the pulmonary valve commissures without encroaching on the pulmonary arterial bifurcation (Fig. 40–34). The band is tightened progressively to achieve the highest peak systolic pressure in the proximal pulmonary artery while maintaining a pulsatile pressure in the distal segment (Fig.

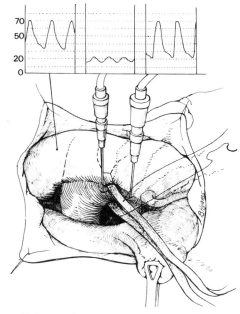

Figure 40–34. Pulmonary artery band tightened to obtain a peak proximal artery pressure at the systemic level while maintaining pulsatile distal flow. The band is positioned away from both the pulmonary valve and the bifurcation.

40–34) and a drop in arterial oxygen saturation of not more than 10 per cent. If this cannot be achieved, a modified Blalock-Hanlon procedure is performed in patients with a gradient between the left and right atria. In addition, a systemic–to–pulmonary artery shunt, consisting of a 4-mm. Gore-Tex tube from the root of the subclavian artery to the pulmonary artery is utilized (Fig. 40–35). In our experience, larger shunts tended to produce severe pulmonary congestion and edema in these patients.

Immediately following banding, the peak systolic pressure in the left ventricle and proximal pulmonary artery rises to near systemic pressure in all patients

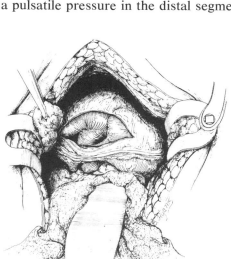

Figure 40–33. Technique for banding of the main pulmonary artery through a limited incision of the pericardium in front of the phrenic nerve.

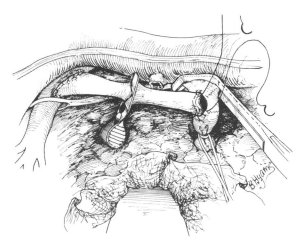

Figure 40–35. Additional Gor-Tex shunt from the right subclavian artery to the right pulmonary artery in patients with inadequate pulmonary flow.

INTRA - OPERATIVE PRESSURES IN T.G.A. WITH INTACT SEPTUM

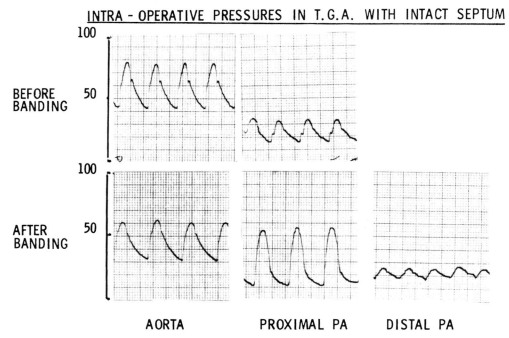

BEFORE BANDING

AFTER BANDING

AORTA   PROXIMAL PA   DISTAL PA

Figure 40–36. Pressures in the aorta and the proximal and distal pulmonary artery before and after banding.

(Fig. 40–36), regardless of the age of the patient at the time of operation or the preoperative PLVP. Because the preoperative PLVP is higher in patients operated on during the first few weeks of life, the change in pressure produced by banding is smaller. In spite of the fact that the postbanding PLVP is similar to that in the systemic ventricle, myocardial oxygen demand is significantly lower than that required to sustain the systemic circulation. This is due to the fact that following banding, the shape of the left ventricular pressure tracing is different from that of a systemic ventricle in that the peak systolic pressure is not sustained (Fig. 40–37), and therefore, the systolic time tension index, which is one of the main determinants of myocardial oxygen consumption (Sarnoff *et al.*, 1958), is lower. In addition, following banding, the presence of a large interatrial communication prevents excessive rise of the left ventricular end-diastolic pressure. Furthermore, whereas a temporary drop in left ventricular systolic output can be of critical importance after anatomic correction, it can be well tolerated after the first-stage operation, particularly in patients with an additional shunt.

The increase in left ventricular muscle mass following the first-stage operation is probably similar to that accompanying normal growth, particularly when performed early in life. Although normal myocardial growth includes a limited degree of hyperplasia at a very young age, resulting in actual increase in the number of myocardial cells (Overy and Priest, 1966; Zhinkin and Andreeva, 1963), the main process of postnatal growth is achieved by hypertrophy or increase in the size of the myocardial cells (Enesco and Leblond, 1962). For many years, it had been assumed that, beyond critical upper size limits, the growth of myocardial muscle cells by hypertrophy exceeded that

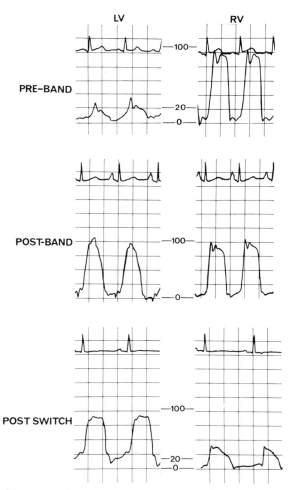

LV   RV

PRE–BAND

POST–BAND

POST SWITCH

Figure 40–37. Left and right ventricular pressure curves before and after banding and after anatomic correction.

ANATOMICAL CORRECTION OF SIMPLE TRANSPOSITION OF THE GREAT ARTERIES

AGE AT BANDING   1 DAY - 44 MONTHS (MEAN 10.5)
AGE AT CORRECTION   4.5 - 47 MONTHS (MEAN 14.3)
INTERVAL BETWEEN OPERATIONS   5 WEEKS - 11 MONTHS (MEAN 4.9)

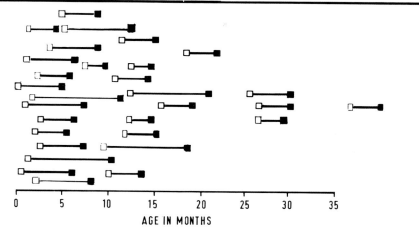

AGE IN MONTHS

Figure 40–38. Age at operation and interval between banding and anatomic correction.

of their accompanying blood vessels (Shipley *et al.*, 1937; Wearn, 1941). Now, however, evidence has indicated that vascularization does keep pace with hypertrophy of heart muscles (Linzbach, 1956; Tepperman and Pearlman, 1961; Kerr *et al.*, 1968).

The first-stage operation should ideally be performed during the first 2 to 3 months of life to allow for continued growth of the left ventricular myocardium, to prevent fragmentation of the elastica of the pulmonary arterial wall, and to allow anatomic correction within the first 6 to 9 months. This policy would also reduce the incidence of cerebral complications (Keck *et al.*, 1981) and pulmonary vascular disease, which is progressive in patients with uncorrected TGA (Viles *et al.*, 1969; Newfeld *et al.*, 1974). However, it is to be noted that successful two-stage correction can be accomplished in patients undergoing the first-stage operation at ages of up to 3½ years (Fig. 40–38).

The development of adequate left ventricular "hypertrophy" to support systemic circulation depends on the level of PLVP attained after banding and the period of time during which the left ventricle has been subjected to such a pressure (Yacoub *et al.*, in press). When the postbanding PLVP is within 10 mm. Hg of that in the systemic circulation, anatomic correction can be safely performed 2 to 3 months after the first-stage operation. In contrast, if the postbanding PLVP is 65 mm. Hg or below (about two thirds that in the systemic circulation), an interval of 6 to 9 months between the two stages appears to be necessary if severe postoperative left ventricular failure is to be avoided (Yacoub *et al.*, in press). During the waiting period between the two operations, several noninvasive tests can be of some value in determining the

state of the left ventricle. The development of an R wave of 4 mm. or more in V5 or V6 of a conventional 12-lead electrocardiogram is a useful guide; however, because of the marked preponderance of the electrical forces from the right ventricle in TGA, the electrocardiogram has been found to be a poor predictor of the state of the left ventricle (Khoury *et al.*, 1966; Mair *et al.*, 1970). Frank vectorcardiography is a more sensitive test (Khoury *et al.*, 1967; Mair *et al.*, 1970; Restieaux *et al.*, 1972). In our experience, the development of counterclockwise initial QRS forces in the horizontal plane has been found to be a reliable indicator of the development of an adequate left ventricle for anatomic correction. Changes in systolic time intervals, such as the ratio of left ventricular pre-ejection period to ejection time, are poor predictors of the state of the left ventricle after the first-stage operation (Yacoub *et al.*, in press).

Technical Considerations

Although the technique of anatomic correction of TGA at the arterial level is now fairly well standardized, there are still several variations in some of the technical details. In addition, several modifications have recently been introduced either on theoretical grounds or to prevent recently recognized complications. Critical evaluation of the medium-term and late results may necessitate further modifications. The current technique consists of several stages, which include division of the great arteries, coronary transfer, bridging the gap between the proximal aorta and the distal pulmonary artery, and anastomosis of the distal aorta to the proximal pulmonary artery.

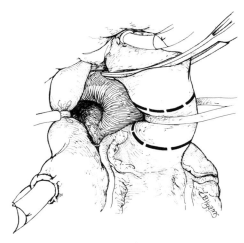

Figure 40–39. Position of the aortic incision. The lower level is utilized if a dural tube is to be used, and the upper level is utilized if direct anastomosis is to be used.

Transection of the Great Arteries

The initial part of the operation consists of opening the pulmonary artery 3 mm. above the top of the commissures of the pulmonary valve, or just below the level of the band if prior banding has been performed. The pulmonary valve is scrutinized. Any significant abnormality is regarded as a contraindication to this type of operation, as this valve will function as an aortic valve postoperatively. The level of division of the aorta depends on the particular technique to be used for bridging the gap between the proximal aorta and the distal pulmonary artery (Fig. 40–39). If a dural tube is to be used, the aorta is incised 3 mm. above the top of the sinuses of Valsalva. This preserves a relatively long segment of ascending aorta below the aortic clamp to prevent compression of the anastomosis between the dural tube and the distal pulmonary artery. In contrast, if the Le Compte-Hazan method (Le Compte *et al.*, 1981) of threading the aortic arch behind the pulmonary arterial bifurcation is to be used, the aortic incision is made at a higher level (15 mm. above the aortic sinuses) (Fig. 40–39). This prevents arching of the ascending aorta forward and possible stretching of the main branches of the pulmonary artery that straddle the ascending aorta.

Coronary Transfer

Coronary transfer constitutes one of the most crucial parts of the operation. The technique used should avoid tension, torsion, or kinking of the main coronary arteries, avoid injury to the proximal branches, and allow for growth of the origins of the coronary arteries from the aorta. To achieve these objectives, the following principles should be observed:

1. The angle of rotation of the coronary ostia in the horizontal plane should not be more than 90 degrees.

2. The level of the anastomoses should correspond to the site of origin from the anterior vessels in the vertical plane. As the aortic valve and sinuses in TGA are higher (more cephalad) than the pulmonary valve, it is usually necessary to anastomose the coronary ostia at a point above the level of the pulmonary valve sinuses.

3. The spatial relationship between the mobilized aortic discs surrounding the coronary ostia and the proximal coronary arteries should be maintained, as any rotation of the discs during anastomoses may produce torsion of the proximal coronary arteries.

4. Kinking or injury of an early branch should be avoided. This can be achieved by identifying these branches and performing minimal mobilization of the coronary arteries.

5. Apposition between the proximal coronary artery and the future aortic wall should be avoided, because postoperative distention of the aorta during exercise or periods of hypertension may result in stretching of the coronary artery and sudden myocardial ischemia, as is known to happen in patients with abnormal origin of the left coronary artery from the anterior sinus (Mustafa *et al.*, 1981).

The technique commonly used for most patients who have Type A, D, or E coronary anatomy consists of mobilization of the coronary ostia with a surrounding disc of aortic wall (Fig. 40–40). The size of the disc should be as large as possible to prevent kinking of the proximal coronary artery or one of its branches and to allow for future growth. The site of anastomosis to the pulmonary artery can be chosen before transecting the great arteries or after anastomosing the distal aorta to the proximal pulmonary artery and releasing the aortic clamp. At the chosen site, a generous disc of pulmonary arterial wall is excised to compensate for the tendency of the new aortic root to enlarge. Although the anastomosis between the aortic discs and the pulmonary artery is generally performed at a level higher than the top of the sinuses of the pulmonary valve, care should be taken not to distort the components of this valve, because this may result in postoperative aortic regurgitation.

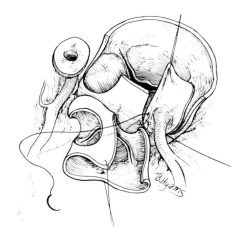

Figure 40–40. Method of transfer of Type A, D, and E coronary arteries.

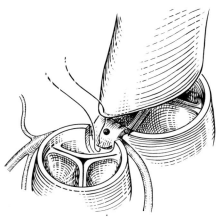

Figure 40–41. Technique for dealing with Type B .and C anatomy without rotation of the coronary ostium. (From Yacoub, M. H., and Radley-Smith, R.: Anatomy of the coronary arteries in transposition of the great arteries and methods for their transfer in anatomical correction. Thorax, *33*:418, 1978.)

In patients with Type B or C coronary anatomy, in whom the coronary ostium (or ostia) is facing almost directly forward, rotation of the disc would involve an angle of 180 degrees, with resultant severe torsion of the proximal coronary arteries. For these patients, another technique, which requires minimal or no rotation of the disc, has been devised (Yacoub and Radley-Smith, 1978) (Fig. 40–41). A similar but not

identical principle has been described by Aubert and associates (1977) for "transfer" of all varieties of coronary anatomy. This technique involves creating a circular communication between the two great arteries just above the coronary ostia, then placing a prosthetic patch inside the aorta to direct blood from the pulmonary artery through the newly created communication to the coronary ostia (Fig. 40–42). This technique has the advantage of not mobilizing the coronary arteries at all but suffers the theoretical disadvantage of creating a small "aneurysmal" recess with a relatively small entrance, two small outlets, and prosthetic material forming part of its wall. In theory, the flow pattern inside such a recess and the nature of its wall may interfere with coronary flow and could predispose to embolization. The occurrence as well as the importance of these possible complications, however, has not as yet been documented.

Another technique that avoids any manipulations near the coronary arteries is that described by Damus (1975), Kaye (1975), and Stansel (1977). The technique entails end-to-side anastomosis of the transected proximal pulmonary artery to the ascending aorta and restoration of continuity between the right ventricle and the distal pulmonary artery using a valved conduit (Fig. 40–43). In spite of the obvious advantages of this technique, it has several theoretical disadvantages, including the use of a foreign valve and conduit, the creation of a defect in the right ventricular wall,

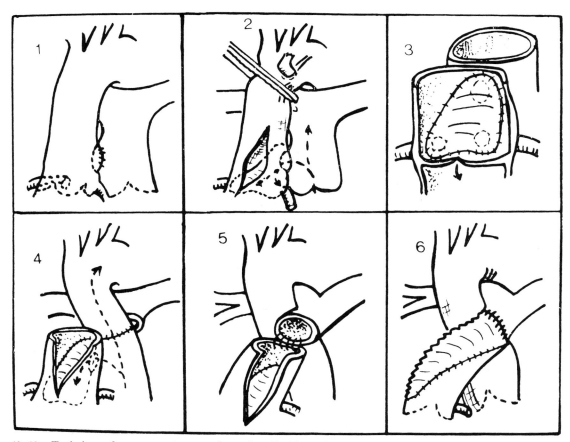

Figure 40–42. Technique of coronary artery transfer as described by Aubert and associates. (From Aubert, J., *et al.*: Transposition of the great arteries. New technique for anatomical correction, Br. Heart J., *40*:204, 1978.)

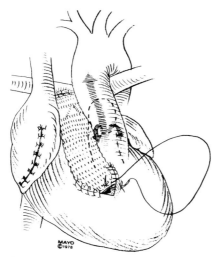

Figure 40–43. Technique for "correction" without relocation of the coronary arteries entailing the use of a valve conduit to restore continuity between the right ventricle and the distal pulmonary arteries. (From Danielson, G. K., *et al.*: Great-vessel switch operation without coronary relocation for transposition of the great arteries. Mayo Clin. Proc., *53*:675, 1978.)

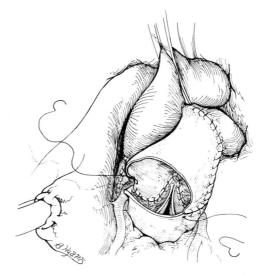

Figure 40–44. Proximal anastomosis of the dural tube with refashioning of the end of the tube to fill defects in the aorta left by the coronary arteries.

and the possibility of formation of clot owing to stagnation of blood in the aortic root. In addition, if pressure rises in the right ventricle postoperatively because of narrowing of the conduit, the aortic valve might open, resulting in cyanosis or even systemic embolism. Further experience is required to establish the balance between the obvious advantages and possible disadvantages of this technique.

Bridging the Gap Between the Proximal and Distal Pulmonary Artery

Direct anastomosis of these two structures can be achieved in a small number of patients, particularly those with side-by-side relationship of the great arteries. In the majority of patients, however, attempts at performing direct anastomosis produce stretching of the pulmonary artery with subsequent stenosis or, more seriously, pressure on one of the coronary arteries. To bridge the gap between these structures, two techniques may be used. The first entails the use of a large tube made of homologous dura mater measuring 2.5 cm. in diameter. This tube should be placed to the left of the newly reconstructed ascending aorta. Placing the tube on the right side may predispose to late supravalvular pulmonary stenosis (Yacoub *et al.*, 1982c). The proximal end of the tube is anastomosed to the proximal aorta after releasing the aortic clamp to enable trimming of the tube to the exact length without any redundancy or tension that might compress the proximal coronary arteries. The defects in the root of the aorta created by mobilization of the discs bearing the coronary ostia can be repaired by refashioning the end of the dural tube to fill these gaps (Fig. 40–44).

An alternative method for bridging the gap between the proximal aorta and the distal pulmonary

artery has been described by Le Compte and associates (1981). This technique entails wide mobilization of the distal pulmonary artery and its two branches as far as possible into the pulmonary hila. The ascending aorta is then threaded behind the pulmonary arterial bifurcation. This enables direct anastomosis of the proximal aorta to the distal pulmonary artery without interposition of foreign material (Fig. 40–45).

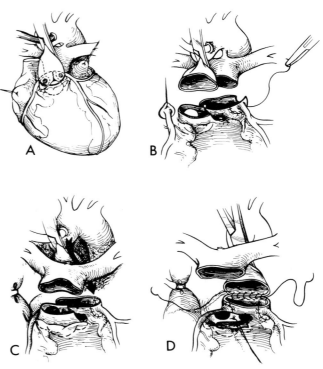

Figure 40–45. Method devised by Le Compte and associates (1981) for direct anastomosis of the proximal aorta and the distal pulmonary artery, entailing mobilization of the distal pulmonary artery and threading of the aorta behind the pulmonary artery bifurcation.

Anastomosis of the Proximal Pulmonary Artery to the Distal Aorta

Although the distal aorta is usually smaller than the proximal pulmonary artery, the two structures can usually be easily matched by cutting the distal aorta obliquely. In performing this anastomosis, special care is needed to avoid any torsion of the root of the pulmonary artery, which may distort the origins of the coronary arteries or interfere with the function of the future aortic valve.

The use of interrupted sutures for part of this anastomosis is preferred. However, repeat catheterization in 30 patients 1 to 5 years after operation (Yacoub *et al.*, 1982a) showed normal growth of this anastomosis in all patients, including those in whom interrupted sutures were not used.

POSTOPERATIVE MANAGEMENT

Following operation, varying degrees of temporary left ventricular failure may occur. For this reason, routine monitoring of left atrial pressure and the use of inotropic support and afterload reduction for several days are recommended. In addition, intensive antifailure treatment with diuretics for 2 to 4 months is usually required.

FOLLOW-UP AND EVALUATION

Although anatomic correction of TGA is intellectually appealing and is probably the only operation that offers hope for cure of this anomaly, it has several potential problems, including (1) a relatively high initial mortality; (2) the ability of the left ventricle to take the load of the circulation immediately after operation and to continue to function normally for life; (3) the ability of the aortic, coronary, and pul-

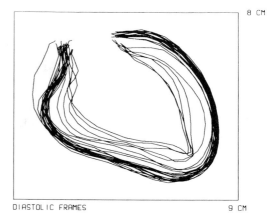

DIASTOLIC FRAMES

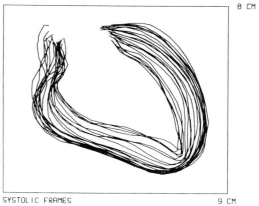

SYSTOLIC FRAMES

Figure 40–47. Frame-by-frame computer analysis of left ventricular contraction and relaxation pattern obtained from angiography after anatomic correction. (From Yacoub, M.H., *et al.*: Clinical and haemodynamic results of the two-stage anatomic correction of simple transposition of the great arteries. Circulation, *62*(Suppl. 1):190, 1980.)

monary anastomoses to grow normally; (4) bridging the gap between the proximal aorta and the distal pulmonary artery; and (5) the ability of the new aortic root and valve to grow normally without progressive dilatation and regurgitation.

The role of this operation in the management of patients with TGA depends on accurate definition of the relative importance of these potential problems. Recent experience has shown that the initial high mortality (learning curve) has dropped to levels comparable to those obtained by inflow correction (Fig. 40–46). In addition, following anatomic correction, there has been no incidence of sudden death. Studies of ventricular function and shape for periods of up to 5 years have shown that following a period of temporary failure, the left ventricle continues to function normally with a normal ejection fraction and end-diastolic pressure and pattern of contraction and relaxation (Fig. 40–47) (Lange *et al.*, 1981; Yacoub *et al.*, 1982b). Left ventricular shape, however, appears to be more globular, and left ventricular end-diastolic volume is relatively increased in the majority of patients (Yacoub *et al.*, 1982b).

Sequential postoperative angiographic and echocardiographic studies have shown that the aortic,

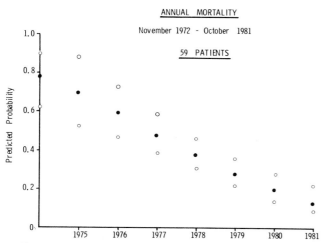

Figure 40–46. Predicted annual mortality rate of patients who have undergone anatomic correction of transposition of the great arteries. (From Yacoub, M. H., *et al.*: Supravalvar pulmonary stenosis after anatomic correction of transposition of the great arteries: Causes and prevention. Circulation, *66*:I–193, 1982.)

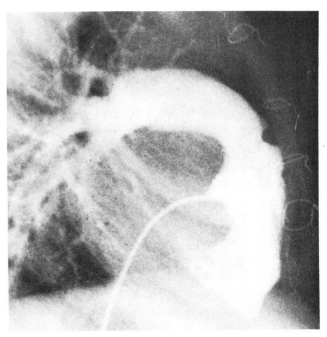

Figure 40–48. Right ventricular angiogram in the lateral projection 13 months after anatomic correction. The pulmonary artery was reconstructed with a dura mater conduit placed to the left of the aorta, with a normal pulmonary valve and ring and good distal pulmonary arteries without any narrowing.

coronary, and pulmonary anastomoses continue to grow normally in all patients (Figs. 40–48 and 40–49) (Yacoub *et al.,* 1982a). However, when nonvalved conduits used for bridging the gap between the proximal aorta and the distal pulmonary artery were placed on the right side of the aorta, about 20 per cent of the

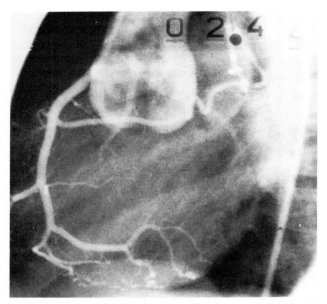

Figure 40–49. Aortogram 18 months after correction showing slight discrepancy between the size of the aortic root and the ascending aorta, but no narrowing in the area of the anastomosis. The coronary arteries appear normal with no narrowing or kinking,

patients developed supravalvular pulmonary stenosis. This appears to be a preventable complication (Yacoub *et al.,* 1982c). Postoperative aortograms have shown discrepancy between the size of the aortic root and the ascending aorta in most patients (Fig. 40–48) and trivial aortic regurgitation in approximately 20 per cent. In patients undergoing more than one reinvestigation postoperatively, no progression of these changes was noted. Longer periods of follow-up are required to accurately define the importance of these possible complications; however, the available evidence suggests that anatomic correction should play a major role in the management of TGA.

SELECTED REFERENCES

Bernhard, A., Yacoub, M., Regensburger, D., Sievers, H. H., Smith, R. R., Stephan, E., Lange, P. E., Keck, E. W., and Heintzen, P. H.: Further experience with the two-stage anatomic correction of simple transposition of the great arteries. Thorac. Cardiovasc. Surg., 29:138, 1981.

This article describes 25 patients with simple transposition of the great arteries, ranging in age from 4 months to 4 years, who underwent a two-stage anatomic correction. The first stage consisted of banding of the pulmonary artery to redevelop the left ventricle, including a Blalock-Taussig anastomosis in four patients. Among the 33 patients undergoing first-stage correction, there were three deaths (9 per cent). The interval between the first and second stages varied from 5 weeks to 9 months. After the first-stage operation, the peak systolic left ventricular pressure rose from an average of 34 to 80 mm. Hg without significant change in end-diastolic pressure. Following anatomic correction, there were five early deaths (20 per cent), four of which were due to left heart failure. The coronary arteries, with different types of origin, could be reimplanted to the posterior vessels without kinking, tension, or torsion in all cases. After anatomic correction of the great arteries, recatheterization in 11 patients showed normal left ventricular pressure at rest in all except two, and these patients were catheterized early after correction.

Jatene, A. D., Fontes, V. F., Sousa, L. C. B., Paulista, P. P., Neto, C. A., and Sousa, J. E. M. R.: Anatomic correction of transposition of the great arteries. J. Thorac. Cardiovasc. Surg., *83*:20, 1982.

In this paper, 33 patients undergoing anatomic correction of transposition of the great arteries since 1975, when the senior author reported his first experience, are reviewed. Fourteen patients were under the age of 6 months, and 23 were under the age of 1 year. In all but one patient, the left ventricular pressure was at a systemic level. A VSD was present in 29 patients, a patent ductus arteriosus in nine, and only one patient had absence of a PDA and VSD. The entire hospital mortality rate was 51.5 per cent, although among the last 12 consecutive patients there were only two deaths (16.6 per cent). In retrospect, the operation in 10 patients was considered inadequate, in nine of these because of an exceedingly high pulmonary vascular resistance and in one because of a hypoplastic left ventricle, with each of these patients dying. The remaining 23 patients, all with a VSD, had an adequate left ventricle, as indicated by left ventricular pressure at physiologic levels. Fourteen of these patients had low pulmonary vascular resistance, without any significant pulmonary outflow tract stenosis. There were five deaths (35.7 per cent) postoperatively. Follow-up studies up to 51 months revealed a clinical course considered very satisfactory. The lower mortality and successful clinical recovery of the patients operated on more recently support the usefulness of this technique in properly selected patients.

Williams, W. G., Freedom, R. M., Culham, G., Duncan, W. J., Olley, P. M., Rowe, R. D., and Trusler, G. A.: Early experience with arterial repair of transposition. Ann. Thorac. Surg., 32:8, 1981.

The authors of this article emphasize that major anomalies associated with isolated complete transposition of the great arteries (TGA) may produce systemic pressure in the left ventricle without fixed stenosis of the left ventricular outflow tract. In this situation, arterial repair may be particularly advantageous. Eight patients, aged 10 days to 15 years, had arterial repair of TGA. Major associated anomalies included patent ductus arteriosus, bulging interventricular septum, VSD, tricuspid atresia, and the Taussig-Bing type of double-outlet right ventricle. There were two operative deaths related to acute left ventricular failure. The survivors underwent postoperative echocardiographic, hemodynamic, and angiographic assessment, and all were in sinus rhythm and well 6 months to 2 years postoperatively.

REFERENCES

Anagnostopoulos, C. E.: A proposed new technique for correction of transposition of the great arteries. Ann. Thorac. Surg., 15:565, 1973.

Anagnostopoulos, C. E., Athanasuleas, C. L., and Arcilla, R.: Towards a rational operation for transposition of the great arteries. Ann. Thorac. Surg., 16:458, 1973.

Ashby, H.: A case of transposition of the aorta and pulmonary artery in a child of 7 months. J. Anat. Physiol., 16:90, 1881.

Aubert, J., Pannetier, A., Couvelly, J. P., Unal, D., Rounault, F., and Delarue, A.: Transposition of the great arteries. New technique for anatomical correction. Br. Heart J., 40:204, 1978.

Averill, K. H., Wagner, W. W., and Vogel, J. H. K.: Correlation of right ventricular pressure with right ventricular weight. Am. Heart J., 66:632, 1963.

Aziz, K. U., Paul, M. H., Idriss, F. S., Wilson, A. D., and Muster, A. J.: Clinical manifestations of dynamic left ventricular outflow tract stenosis in infants with d-transposition of the great arteries with intact ventricular septum. Am. J. Cardiol., 44:290, 1979.

Bailey, C. P., Cookson, B. A., Downing, D. F., and Neptune, W. B.: Cardiac surgery under hypothermia. J. Thorac. Surg., 27:73, 1954.

Bano-Rodrigo, A., Quero-Jimenez, M., Moreno-Granado, F., and Gamallo-Amat, C.: Wall thickness of ventricular chambers in transposition of the great arteries, surgical implications. J. Thorac. Cardiovasc. Surg., 79:592, 1980.

Bernhard, A., Yacoub, M. H., Regensburger, D., Sievers, H. H., Radley-Smith, R., Stephan, E., Lange, P. E., Keck, E. W., and Heintzen, P. H.: Further experience with the two-stage anatomic correction of simple transposition of the great arteries. Thorac. Cardiovasc. Surg., 29:138, 1981.

Bex, J. P., Le Compte, Y., Baillot, F., and Hazan, E.: Anatomical correction of transposition of the great arteries. Ann. Thorac. Surg., 29:86, 1980.

Bharati, S., Molthan, M. E., Veasey, L. G., and Lev, M.: Conduction system in two cases of sudden death two years after the Mustard procedure. J. Thorac. Cardiovasc. Surg., 77:101, 1979.

Bjork, V. O., and Bouckaert, L.: Complete transposition of the aorta and pulmonary artery. An experimental study of the surgical possibilities for its treatment. J. Thorac. Cardiovasc. Surg., 28:632, 1954.

Booth, N. H., Hastings, S. G., Hopwood, M., and Maaske, C. A.: Postnatal changes in the cardiac ventricles of the pig. Proc. Soc. Exp. Biol. Med., 122:186, 1966.

Cross, F., Kay, E. B., and Jones, R. D.: A simple shunting technique for surgery of the aorta and pulmonary valves and proximal great vessels. An experimental study. J. Thorac. Cardiovasc. Surg., 28:229, 1954.

Damus, P. S.: Letter to the Editor. Ann. Thorac. Surg., 20:724, 1975.

Damus, P. S., Thomson, N. B., and McLoughlin, T. G.: Arterial repair without coronary relocation for complete transposition of the great vessels with ventricular septal defect. J. Thorac. Cardiovasc. Surg., 83:316, 1982.

Danielson, G. K., Tabry, I. F., Mair, D. D., and Fulton, R. E.: Great-vessel switch operation without coronary relocation for transposition of the great arteries. Mayo Clin. Proc., 53:675, 1978.

De La Cruz, M. V., Anselmi, G., Romero, A., and Monroy, G.: A qualitative and quantitative study of the ventricles and great vessels of normal children. Am. Heart J., 60:675, 1960.

Ebert, P. A.: Discussion of Williams, W. G., Freedom, R. M., Culham, G., Duncan, W. J., Olley, P. M., Rowe, R. D., and Trusler, G. A.: Ann. Thorac. Surg., 32:8, 1981.

Elliott, L. P., Neufeld, H. N., Anderson, R. C., Adams, P., Jr., and Edwards, J. E.: Complete transposition of the great vessels. An anatomic study of sixty cases. Circulation, 27:1105, 1963.

Elliott, L. P., Amplatz, K., and Edwards, J. E.: Coronary arterial patterns in complete transposition complexes. Anatomic and angiographic studies. Am. J. Cardiol., 17:362, 1966.

Emery, J. L., and Mithal, A.: Weights of cardiac ventricles at and after birth. Br. Heart J., 23:313, 1961.

Enesco, M., and Leblond, C. P.: Increase in cell number as a factor in the growth of the organs and tissues of the young male rat. J. Embryol. Exp. Morphol., 10:530, 1962.

Gluck, L., Talner, N. S., Gardner, T. H., and Kulovich, M. V.: RNA concentrations in the ventricles of full term and premature rabbits following birth. Nature, 202:770, 1964.

Graham, T. R., Jr., Barnett, W. L., Jarmakani, M. M., Canent, R. V., Jr., and Capp, M. P.: Left heart volume and mass quantification in children with left ventricular pressure overload. Circulation, 41:203, 1970.

Harvey, W.: An anatomical disquisition on the motion of the heart and blood in animals (1628). Translated from the Latin by Willis, R., 1847. In Everyman's Library. Edited by E. A. Parkyn. London, J. M. Dent, 1906, p. 98.

Huhta, J. C., Edwards, W. D., Danielson, G. K., and Feldt, R. H.: Abnormalities of the tricuspid valve in complete transposition of the great arteries with ventricular septal defect. J. Thorac. Cardiovasc. Surg., 83:569, 1982.

Idriss, F. S., Goldstein, I. R., Grana, L., French, D., and Potts, W. J.: A new technique for complete correction of transposition of the great vessels. Circulation, 24:5, 1961.

Idriss, F. S., Aubert, J., Paul, M., Nikaidoh, H., Lev, M., and Newfeld, E. A.: Transposition of the great vessels with ventricular septal defect. Surgical and anatomic considerations. J. Thorac. Cardiovasc. Surg., 68:732, 1974.

Jatene, A. D., Fontes, V. F., Paulista, P. P., Sousa, L. C. B., Neger, F., Galantier, M., and Sousa, J. E. M. R.: Successful anatomic correction of transposition of the great vessels. A preliminary report. Arq. Bras. Cardiol., 28:461, 1975.

Jatene, A. D., Fontes, V. F., Sousa, L. C. B., Paulista, P. P., Neto, C. A., and Sousa, J. E. M. R.: Anatomic correction of transposition of the great arteries. J. Thorac. Cardiovasc. Surg., 83:20, 1982.

Kay, E. B., and Cross, F. S.: Surgical treatment of transposition of the great vessels. Surgery, 39:712, 1955.

Kaye, M. P.: Anatomic correction of transposition of the great arteries. Mayo Clin. Proc., 50:638, 1975.

Keck, E. W., Kimm, E., Grävinghoff, L., Sieg, K., Lagenstein, I., and Kühne, D.: Neurologische Veränderungen und cerebrale Läsionen bei Kindern mit Transposition des grossen Arterien (TGA). Monatsschr. Kinderheilkd., 129:45, 1981.

Keen, E. N.: The postnatal development of the human cardiac ventricles. J. Anat., 89:484, 1955.

Kerr, A., Jr., Bommer, W. J., and Pilato, S.: Letter: Coronary artery enlargement in experimental cardiac hypertrophy. Am. Heart J., 75:144, 1968.

Khoury, G. H., Shaher, R. M., and Fowler, R. S.: The vectorcardiogram in complete transposition of the great arteries. Analysis of 50 cases. Circulation, 35:178, 1967.

Khoury, G. H., Shaher, R. M., Fowler, R. S., and Keith, J. D.: Preoperative and postoperative electrocardiogram in complete transposition of the great vessels. Am. Heart J., 72:199, 1966.

Kreutzer, G., Neirotti, R., Galindez, E., Coronel, A. R., and Kreutzer, E.: Anatomic correction of transposition of the great arteries. J. Thorac. Cardiovasc. Surg., 73:538, 1977.

Lange, P. E., Onnasch, D. G. W., Stephen, E., Wessel, A., Radley-Smith, R., Yacoub, M. H., Regensburger, D., Bernhard, A., and Heintzen, P. H.: Two-stage anatomic correction of complete transposition of the great arteries. Ventricular volumes and muscle mass. Herz, 6:336, 1981.

Latimer, H. B.: The weight and thickness of the two ventricular walls in the newborn dog heart. Anat. Rec., 152:225, 1965.

Layman, P. E., and Edwards, J. E.: Anomalies of the cardiac valves associated with complete transposition of the great vessels. Am. J. Cardiol., 19:247, 1967.

Le Compte, Y., Zannini, L., Hazan, E., Jarreau, M. M., Bex, J. P., Tu, T. V., and Neveux, J. Y.: Anatomic correction of transposition of the great arteries. A new technique without use of prosthetic conduit. J. Thorac. Cardiovasc. Surg., 82:629, 1981.

Lev, M., Alcalde, V. M., and Baffes, T. G.: Pathologic anatomy of complete transposition of the arterial trunks. Pediatrics, 28:293, 1961.

Lev, M., Rimoldi, H. J. A., Paiva, R., and Arcilla, R. A.: The quantitative anatomy of simple complete transposition. Am. J. Cardiol., 23:409, 1969.

Linzbach, A. J.: Über das Langenwachstum der Herzmuskelfasern und ihrer Kerne in Beziehung zur Herzdilatation. Arch. Pathol. Anat. Histol., 328:165, 1956.

Mair, D. D., Macartney, F. J., Weidenman, W. H., Rutter, D. G., Ongley, P. A., and Smith, R. E.: The vectorcardiogram in complete transposition of the great arteries. Correlation with anatomic and hemodynamic findings and calculated left ventricular mass. J. Electrocardiol., 3:217, 1970.

Mustafa, I., Gula, G., Radley-Smith, R., Durrer, D., and Yacoub, M.: Anomalous origin of the left coronary artery from the anterior aortic sinus: A potential cause of sudden death. Anatomic characterization and surgical treatment. J. Thorac. Cardiovasc. Surg., 82:297, 1981.

Mustard, W. T., Chute, A. L., Keith, J. D., Srek, A., Rowe, R. D., and Vlad, P.: A surgical approach to transposition of the great vessels with extracorporeal circuit. Surgery, 3:39, 1954.

Newfeld, E. A., Paul, M. H., Muster, A. J., and Idriss, F. S.: Pulmonary vascular disease in complete transposition of the great arteries. A study of 200 patients. Am. J. Cardiol., 34:75, 1974.

Overy, H. R., and Priest, R. A.: Mitotic cell division in postnatal cardiac growth. Lab. Invest., 15:1100, 1966.

Park, S. C., Neches, W. H., Zuberbuhler, J. R., Mathews, R. A., Lenox, C. C., and Fricker, F. J.: Echocardiographic and hemodynamic correlation in transposition of the great arteries. Circulation, 57:291, 1978.

Plauth, W. H., Jr., Nadas, A. S., Bernhard, W. F., and Fyler, D. C.: Changing hemodynamics in patients with transposition of the great arteries. Circulation, 42:131, 1970.

Recavarren, S., and Arias-Stella, J.: Growth and development of the ventricular myocardium from birth to adult life. Br. Heart J., 26:187, 1964.

Restieaux, N. J., Ellison, R. C., Albers, W. H., and Nadas, A. S.: The Frank electrocardiogram in complete transposition of the great arteries. Its use in assessment of left ventricular pressure. Am. Heart J., 83:219, 1972.

Riemenschneider, T. A., Goldberg, S. J., Ruttenberg, H. D., and Gyepes, M. T.: Subpulmonic obstruction in complete (d) transposition produced by redundant tricuspid tissue. Circulation, 39:603, 1969.

Rosenquist, G. C., Stark, J., and Taylor, J. F. N.: Congenital mitral valve disease in TGA. Circulation, 51:731, 1975.

Ross, D., Rickards, A., and Somerville, J.: Transposition of the great arteries: Logical anatomical arterial correction. Br. Med. J., 1:1109, 1976.

Sansa, M., Tonkin, I. L., Bargeron, L. M., and Elliott, L. P.: Left ventricular outflow tract obstruction in transposition of the great arteries: An angiographic study of 74 cases. Am. J. Cardiol., 44:88, 1979.

Sarnoff, S. T., Braunwald, E., Welch, G. H., Case, R. B., Stainsby, W. N., and Macruz, R.: Hemodynamic determinants of oxygen. Consumption of the heart with special reference to tension-time index. Am. J. Physiol., 192:148, 1958.

Scammon, R. E.: Studies on the growth and structure of the infant thorax. Radiology, 9:89, 1927.

Senning, Å.: Surgical correction of transposition of the great vessels. Surgery, 45:966, 1959.

Seward, J. S., Tajik, A. J., Hagler, D. J., and Mair, D. D.: Straddling atrioventricular valve. Diagnostic two-dimensional echocardiographic features. (Abstract.) Am. J. Cardiol., 41:354, 1978.

Shaher, R. M.: Cardiac pathology. In Complete Transposition of the Great Arteries. New York, Academic Press, 1973, p. 128.

Shaher, R. M., and Puddu, G. C.: Coronary arterial anatomy in complete transposition of the great vessels. Am. J. Cardiol., 17:355, 1966.

Shaher, R. M., Puddu, G. C., Khoury, G., Moes, C. A. F., and Mustard, W. T.: Complete transposition of the great vessels with anatomic obstruction of the outflow tract of the left ventricle. Surgical implications of anatomic findings. Am. J. Cardiol., 19:658, 1967.

Shipley, R. A., Shipley, L. J., and Wearn, J. T.: The capillary supply in normal and hypertrophied hearts of rabbits. J. Exp. Med., 65:29, 1937.

Shone, J. D, Sellers, R. D., Anderson, R. C., Adams, P., Jr., Lillihei, C. W., and Edwards, J. E.: The developmental complex of parachute mitral valve, supravalvular ring of left atrium, subaortic stenosis and coarctation of the aorta. Am. J. Cardiol., 11:714, 1963.

Shrivastava, S., Tadavarthy, S. M., Fukuda, T., and Edwards, J. E.: Anatomic causes of pulmonary stenosis in complete transposition. Circulation, 54:154, 1976.

Smith, A., Wilkinson, J. L., Arnold, R., Dickinson, D. F., and Anderson, R. H.: Growth and development of ventricular walls in complete transposition of the great arteries with intact septum (simple transposition). Am. J. Cardiol., 49:362, 1982.

Stansel, H. C., Jr.: A new operation for d-loop transposition of the great vessels. Ann. Thorac. Surg., 19:565, 1977.

Tepperman, J., and Pearlman, D.: Effects of exercise and anaemia on coronary arteries of small animals as revealed by the corrosion-cast technique. Circ. Res., 9:576, 1961.

Tynan, M.: Transposition of the great arteries. Changes in circulation after birth. Circulation, 46:809, 1972.

Tynan, M., Carr, I., Graham, G., and Bonham-Carter, R. E.: Subvalvar pulmonary obstruction complicating the postoperative course of balloon atrial septostomy in transposition of the great arteries. Circulation, 39(Suppl. 1):223, 1969.

Vidne, B. A., Subramanian, S., and Wagner, H. R.: Aneurysm of the membranous ventricular septum in transposition of the great arteries. Circulation, 53:157, 1976.

Viles, P. H., Ongley, P. A., and Titus, J. L.: The spectrum of pulmonary vascular disease in transposition of the great arteries. Circulation, 40:31, 1969.

Wearn, J. T.: Alterations in the heart accompanying growth and hypertrophy. Bull. Johns Hopkins Hosp., 68:363, 1941.

Williams, W. G., Freedom, R. M., Culham, G., Duncan, W. J., Olley, P. M., Rowe, R. D., and Trusler, G. A.: Early experience with arterial repair of transposition. Ann. Thorac. Surg., 32:8, 1981.

Yacoub, M. H.: Anatomical correction of transposition of the great arteries. In Operative Surgery. 3rd Ed. Edited by J. W. Jackson. London, Butterworth, 1977, p. 136.

Yacoub, M. H.: The case for anatomic correction of transposition of the great arteries. J. Thorac. Cardiovasc. Surg., 78:3, 1979.

Yacoub, M. H., and Radley-Smith, R.: Anatomy of the coronary arteries in transposition of the great arteries and methods for their transfer in anatomical correction. Thorax, 33:418, 1978.

Yacoub, M. H., Radley-Smith, R., and Hilton, C.: Anatomical correction of complete transposition of the great arteries and ventricular septal defect in infancy. Br. Med. J., 1:1111, 1976.

Yacoub, M. H., Radley-Smith, R., and MacLaurin, R.: Two-stage operation for anatomical correction of transposition of the great arteries with intact interventricular septum. Lancet, *1*:1275, 1977.

Yacoub, M. H., Bernhard, A., Lange, P., Radley-Smith, R., Keck, E., Stephan, E., and Heintzen, P.: Clinical and hemodynamic results of the two-stage anatomic correction of simple transposition of the great arteries. Circulation, *62*(Suppl. 1):190, 1980.

Yacoub, M. H., Bernhard, A., Lange, P., and Radley-Smith, R.: Fate of aortic, pulmonary and coronary anastomoses after anatomical correction of transposition of the great arteries. (Abstract.) Br. Heart J., *4* :194, 1982a.

Yacoub, M. H., Arensman, F. W., Lange, P., Bernhard, A., Heintzen, P., and Radley-Smith, R.: Left ventricular shape and function one year or more after anatomic correction of transposition of the great arteries. (Abstract.) Am. J. Cardiol., *49*:986, 1982b.

Yacoub, M. H., Bernhard, A., Radley-Smith, R., Lange, P., Sievers, H., and Heintzen, P.: Supravalvar pulmonary stenosis after anatomic correction of transposition of the great arteries: Causes and prevention. Circulation, *66*(Suppl. 1):193, 1982c.

Yacoub, M. H., Arensman, F. W., Bernhard, A., Heintzen, P., Lange, P., and Radley-Smith, R.: Preparation of the left ventricle for anatomical correction of transposition of the great arteries. Ped. Cardiol., in press.

Zhinkin, L. N., and Andreeva, L. F.: DNA synthesis and nuclear reproduction during embryonic development and regeneration of muscle tissue. J. Embryol. Exp. Morphol., *11*:353, 1963.

Chapter 41

Pulmonary Atresia with Intact Ventricular Septum

JAMES R. MALM
KATHLEEN W. MCNICHOLAS

INTRODUCTION AND ANATOMY

Pulmonary atresia with intact ventricular septum is an uncommon congenital cardiac anomaly associated with a high infant mortality. One third of the patients with this lesion are dead by the second week of life, and 50 per cent die within 1 month without surgical intervention. Longer survival depends on patency of the ductus arteriosus, and only rare survival has been reported beyond childhood (Keith *et al.*, 1978). This lesion was first described by Hunter in 1783 (Hunter, 1869), but the clinical significance was not appreciated until 1951 (Novelo *et al.*, 1951). Pulmonary atresia with intact ventricular septum occurs in less than 1 per cent of the total group of congenital malformations in most series, although Subramanian and associates (1972) and Parisi-Buckley and colleagues (1975) noted such an occurrence in 3 per cent of cases. This anomaly was described by Edwards and coworkers in 1965 as complete obstruction of the pulmonary valve associated with a patent tricuspid valve and two distinct ventricles. The pulmonary valve is most frequently a diaphragm composed of three thickened, fused leaflets, and the anulus is often hypoplastic. The pulmonary arteries are confluent and normal in size as a result of flow through the patent ductus arteriosus. The main pulmonary artery is usually present to the level of the atretic pulmonary valve, and only a small segment of this atretic valve is in contact with the right ventricular cavity. There is hypertrophy of the muscle bundles related to the pulmonary cusp, leading to narrowing of the right ventricular infundibulum. The infundibulum is short and separated from the right ventricle by a muscle mass. There is marked endocardial thickening with speckling secondary to fibroelastosis.

The lesion has been classified into two ventricular types by Greenwold and associates (1956). Group I is defined as having a small or minuscule right ventricle, whereas Group II has an anatomically larger or normal right ventricle. This classification is too rigid, however. There is, rather, a spectrum of right ventricular mass and diastolic volume. The tricuspid valve leaflets and orifice vary from normal to dysplastic valve leaflets with a stenotic anulus. Some degree of tricuspid valve insufficiency is always present.

The right atrium is always enlarged, and with massive tricuspid regurgitation, it may reach aneurysmal proportions. Embryonic intramyocardial spaces may be kept open by the elevated right ventricular pressures, with resulting sinusoids that may communicate with coronary arteries and contribute to a right-sided circular shunt. A patent foramen ovale and ductus arteriosus are essential for survival. The fea-

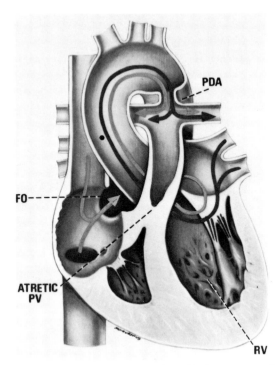

Figure 41–1. Schematic illustration of pulmonary atresia with intact ventricular septum showing the following anatomic features: (1) A thick-walled right ventricle (RV) with a small cavity. (2) Pulmonary valve atresia (PV) with a normal size pulmonary artery. (3) A patent foramen ovale (FO), and patent ductus arteriosus (PDA). (From Moulton, A. L., *et al* : Pulmonary atresia with intact ventricular septum: A sixteen year experience. J. Thorac. Cardiovasc. Surg., *78*:527, 1979.)

tures of pulmonary atresia with intact ventricular septum are illustrated in Figure 41–1.

CLINICAL FINDINGS

Infants with pulmonary atresia and intact ventricular septum present characteristically with extreme cyanosis shortly after birth, often with a Pa_{O_2} as low as 19 to 24 torr. This is secondary to a large obligatory right-to-left shunt at the atrial level, which occurs secondary to the right ventricular outflow tract obstruction, and to inadequate pulmonary blood flow through the patent ductus arteriosus, which frequently closes during the first weeks of life. Patients may have dyspnea and tachypnea and signs of right-sided congestive heart failure secondary to tricuspid insufficiency. Hepatomegaly is present with right heart failure. Frequently, no murmur is audible, but a soft systolic murmur of tricuspid regurgitation may be heard in addition to a continuous murmur of patent ductus arteriosus. The electrocardiogram is either normal or shows right axis deviation in the frontal plane. Progressive changes occur with degrees of right axis deviation, signs of right atrial overload, and right ventricular hypertrophy. The chest roentgenogram may be normal in patients with normal-sized or small right ventricles, but marked cardiomegaly, particularly to the right, is seen with right ventricular enlargement. Pulmonary vascular markings may be decreased or normal in the presence of a patent ductus arteriosus. The chest roentgenogram may suggest tricuspid atresia or tetralogy of Fallot, but the presence of cardiomegaly with rapidly increasing heart size soon after birth favors the diagnosis of pulmonary atresia. In the majority of patients the echocardiogram shows a small right ventricle with a thick wall. Tricuspid valve motion is frequently impaired. The pulmonary root is small and often difficult to visualize. Aortic–to–mitral valve continuity is seen, as is a normal left atrium and left ventricle.

DIAGNOSIS

Cardiac catheterization soon after birth is crucial for the establishment of a definitive diagnosis and plan of management. A right atrial angiogram shows an obligatory right-to-left shunt, but it does not reliably define right ventricular anatomy or the source of pulmonary blood flow. Selective right ventricular angiography (Fig. 41–2) demonstrates the size of the right ventricular chamber and allows for measurement of right ventricular pressure in an estimate of the degree of tricuspid regurgitation. Left ventricular angiography (Fig. 41–3) shows the pulmonary artery filling retrograde through a patent ductus arteriosus and demonstrates the level of atresia. Simultaneous visualization of the right coronary artery and left ventricle (Fig. 41–4) is useful in estimating the size of the right ventricle compared with the opacified left

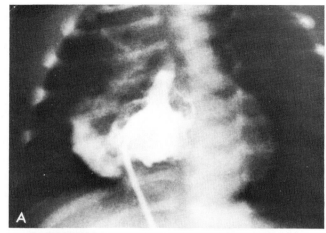
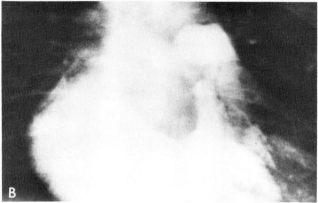

Figure 41–2. *A,* Anteroposterior right ventricular angiogram shows a small trabeculated right ventricular chamber with complete obstruction at the level of the pulmonary valve. *B,* This right ventricular angiogram demonstrates tricuspid regurgitation resulting in marked right atrial enlargement. (From Bowman, F. O., Jr., *et al.*: Pulmonary atresia with intact ventricular septum. J. Thorac. Cardiovasc. Surg., *61*:85, 1971.)

ventricle. Ideally, both right ventricular and left ventricular angiograms should be obtained, but either is sufficient for the diagnosis, as the clinical status of the patient limits the study.

SURGICAL MANAGEMENT

Most infants with pulmonary atresia and intact ventricular septum are critically ill with extreme cyanosis in the first hours of life when the ductus arteriosus constricts. These patients need urgent operative intervention. Recent introduction of prostaglandin E_1 infusion (Elliot *et al.*, 1975; Heymann and Rudolph, 1977; Olley *et al.,* 1976, Rudolph *et al.,* 1975) has been useful in maintaining duct patency and in delaying the onset of severe hypoxemia and resultant acidosis. Catheterization and operation may then be performed under more stable conditions. Formalin infiltration of the ductus has also been suggested by Rudolph and associates (1975) to maintain pulmonary blood flow.

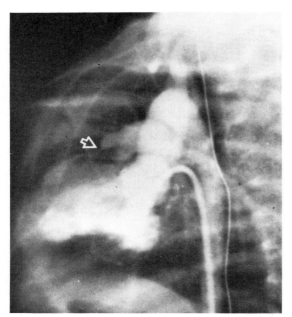

Figure 41–3. A lateral left ventricular angiogram shows a normal-sized left ventricle with intact ventricular septum and a normal-sized main pulmonary artery filling from a patent ductus arteriosus to the level of the atretic pulmonary valve (arrow). (From Ellis, K., et al.: Pulmonary atresia with intact ventricular septum: New developments in diagnosis and treatment. Am. J. Roentgenol., *116*:501, 1972.)

An occasional patient with a large right ventricle will improve following pulmonary valvotomy. The pulmonary valvotomy has, however, been unreliable in providing pulmonary blood flow adequate for survival. The initial increase in Po_2 following valvotomy is usually followed by gradual fall in saturation, low cardiac output, and death. However, pulmonary valvotomy is important in decompressing the hypertensive right ventricle, for right ventricular pressure, in part, may lead to myocardial fibrosis and papillary muscle infarct. This decompression may also delay progressive tricuspid regurgitation and allow growth of a small right ventricle into a large functioning chamber in preparation for total correction.

A systemic–to–pulmonary artery shunt as a single procedure results in prompt improvement in arterial saturation, but again, the early (Bowman *et al.*, 1971) and late (Miller *et al.*, 1969) mortality is high.

Shunt or valvotomy alone is not satisfactory as an initial procedure for patients with pulmonary atresia and intact ventricular septum. Successful palliation depends on an increase in pulmonary blood flow and adequate decompression in the right ventricle. Simultaneous valvotomy and shunt best fulfill the criteria for successful initial surgical intervention. The operative technique of shunt and valvotomy has been described by Bowman. Preoperative preparation includes correction of acidosis. Intubation and mechanical ventilatory support may be needed. Prostaglandin E_1 infusion through a central line is used, and anesthesia is induced by inhalation technique followed by

a combination of inhalation agents and muscle relaxants. The patient is positioned for the combined procedure of valvotomy and shunt. A right anterior thoracotomy of the fourth intercostal space is performed with transsternal extension as necessary. Pulmonary valvotomy may be performed through a transventricular approach using small calibrated valvulotomes that accommodate the small size of the right ventricle and small pulmonary anulus. An excision valvotomy is performed through the two anterior cusps of the pulmonary valve with a specifically designed valvulotome. The pulmonary outflow tract is then calibrated. Initial clinical improvement following valvotomy is seen with an increase in Pa_{O_2}, and the right ventricular color becomes pink. This allows time for the shunt to be performed in an unhurried fashion and sustains the infant during the performance of a Waterston or Blalock-Taussig shunt when a pulmonary artery is occluded. Increased pulmonary blood flow and right ventricular decompression are thus achieved. Pulmonary valvotomy also allows for the increased pulmonary blood flow if ductal closure occurs.

The ascending aorta–to–right pulmonary artery anastomosis has been performed most frequently. Accurate size and placement posteriorly on the aorta are necessary to prevent kinking of the anastomosis and distortion. Anastomosis in infants should not exceed 3 mm. A larger anastomosis may lead to pulmonary overcirculation with pulmonary edema,

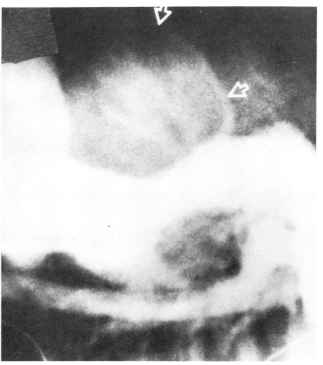

Figure 41–4. This lateral left ventriculogram demonstrates the course of the right coronary artery (arrows) and is useful in estimating the right ventricular size.

and a smaller anastomosis frequently results in adequate palliation. On occasion, if the ductus is large and pulmonary blood flow is excessive after the combined procedure, an interruption of the patent ductus arteriosus may be necessary. The advantages of the Waterston anastomosis was felt to be ease of construction, effective palliation, and ease of closure at the time of correction. These goals have not been universally achieved, and complications secondary to the Waterston shunt have been reported by our group and several others. Because of this, alternative shunts have been attempted with increasing success. The use of microsurgical techniques allows for the performance of a Blalock-Taussig anastomosis even in the neonate. This shunt may be performed through an anterior thoracotomy or through the usual posterolateral approach. Retrograde pulmonary valvotomy through a full left thoracotomy followed by placement of a 5 mm. Gore-Tex shunt from the subclavian artery to the left pulmonary artery has been successful in achieving good initial palliation. Prostaglandin E_1 infusion may be continued following this procedure for the first 2 to 3 days, if necessary.

Close follow-up of patients surviving the initial valvotomy and shunt is imperative. Repeat catheterization at 6 to 12 months of age is indicated to confirm the adequacy of valvotomy and to assess right ventricular development and function. A second valvotomy, either open or closed, is necessary in some patients to improve right ventricular decompression.

RESULTS OF PALLIATIVE SURGERY

Prior to 1967, there were only three reported cases of survival in patients operated on for pulmonary atresia and intact ventricular septum. Our present surgical management has evolved from an experience with 30 patients, 26 of whom were less than 3 days of age, treated at Babies' Hospital of the Columbia-Presbyterian Medical Center between 1960 and 1978. Transventricular valvotomy was performed in six patients with no survivors and resulted in unpredictable and inadequate pulmonary blood flow. Six other patients underwent the shunt procedure alone. There were three early survivors. The shunt provided adequate pulmonary blood flow, but in follow-up, there was failure of right ventricular development and significant progressive tricuspid regurgitation. There was a high incidence of late sudden death in this group, possibly related to arrhythmias. There were no long-term survivors.

The initial approach must not only increase pulmonary blood flow and relieve hypoxia by shunt, but also decompress the right ventricle and allow for growth. The present approach is that of combined shunt and pulmonary valvotomy. Seventeen patients underwent this procedure, and 14 survived the neonatal period with significant palliation. Eight have undergone correction, with five long-term survivors.

TOTAL CORRECTION

The goals of correction are relief of right ventricular obstruction and closure of the atrial septal defect. Shunt closure is also necessary.

The atrial septal defect is closed to insure adequate preload for the right ventricle in the postoperative period. The problem of right ventricular reconstruction is more difficult and is a good case for construction of a pulmonary valve at the right ventricular outflow tract with a patch or a conduit. A vertical right ventriculotomy is extended across the atretic pulmonary valve. The pulmonary valve is excised, and thick, fibrous muscle of the right ventricular outflow tract is resected. The outflow tract patch is used to reconstruct the anulus, and the valve is incorporated to avoid pulmonary insufficiency in these patients with varying degrees of tricuspid regurgitation. The right ventricular outflow tract was enlarged with a unicusp aortic homograft in the first five cases and with Hancock conduits in the more recent cases (Fig. 41–5). There were two operative deaths and one late death. The late death occurred in the patient with pre-existing pulmonary vascular obstructive disease. The five long-term survivors are all active.

Total correction is feasible in initial palliation in patients with pulmonary atresia and intact ventricular

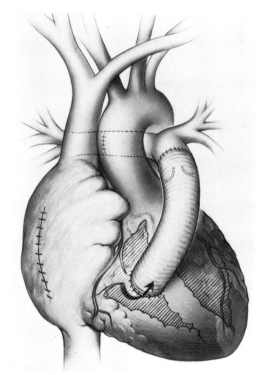

Figure 41–5. This schematic illustration shows the completed correction for pulmonary atresia with intact ventricular septum. It illustrates closure of the foramen ovale, closure of the Waterston shunt through the aortotomy, and placement of a valved conduit between the right ventricle and the pulmonary artery. (From Moulton, A. L., *et al.*: Pulmonary atresia with intact ventricular septum: A sixteen year experience. J. Thorac. Cardiovasc. Surg., *78*:527, 1979.)

septum, and treatment is undertaken with this goal in mind. Extreme tricuspid valve hypoplasia may be the only limiting factor.

REFERENCES

Bowman, F. O., Jr., Hancock, W. D., and Malm, J. R.: A valve-containing Dacron prosthesis. Arch. Surg., *107*:724, 1973.

Bowman, F. O., Jr., Malm, J. R., Hayes, C. J., Gersony, W., and Ellis, K.: Pulmonary atresia with intact ventricular septum. J. Thorac. Cardiovasc. Surg., *61*:85, 1971.

Edwards, J. E., Carey, L. S., Neufeld, H. N., and Lester, R. G.: Congenital Heart Disease. Vol. II. Philadelphia, W. B. Saunders Company, 1965, pp. 575—578.

Elliot, R. B., Starling, M. P., and Neutze, J. M.: Medical manipulation of the ductus arteriosus. Lancet, *1*:140, 1975.

Ellis, K., Casarella, W. J., Hayes, C. J., Gersony, W., Bowman, F. O., Jr., and Malm, J. R.: Pulmonary atresia with intact ventricular septum: Report of 50 cases. Pediatrics, *47*:370, 1971.

Ellis, K., Casarella, W. J., Hayes, C. J., Gersony, W., Bowman, F. O., Jr., and Malm, J. R.: Pulmonary atresia with intact ventricular septum: New developments in diagnosis and treatment. Am. J. Roentgenol., *116*:501, 1972.

Grant, R. T.: Unusual anomaly of coronary vessels in malformed heart of a child. Heart, *13*:273, 1926.

Greenwold, W. E., DuShane, J. W., Burchell, H. B., Brewer, A., and Edwards, J. E.: Congenital pulmonary atresia with intact ventricular septum. Two anatomic types. (Abstract.) Circulation, *14*:945, 1956.

Heymann, M. A., and Rudolph, A. M.: Ductus arteriosus dilatation by prostaglandin E1 in infants with pulmonary atresia. Pediatrics, *59*:325, 1977.

Hunter, J.: Observations and Enquiries, 6:291, 1973. Cited in Peacock, T. B.: Malformations of the heart; atresia of the orifice of the pulmonary artery; aorta communicating with both ventricles. Trans. Pathol. Soc. Lond., *20*:61, 1869.

Keith, J. D., Rowe, R. D., and Vlad, P.: Heart Disease in Infancy and Childhood, 3rd Ed. New York, Macmillan, 1978.

Lauer, R. M., Fink, H. P., Petry, E. L., Dunn, M. I., and Diehl, A. M.: Angiographic demonstration of intra-myocardial sinusoids in pulmonary valve atresia with intact ventricular septum and hypoplastic right ventricle. N. Engl. J. Med., *271*:68, 1964.

Marchand, P.: The use of the cusp-bearing homograft patch to the outflow tract in pulmonary atresia in Fallot's tetralogy and pulmonary valve stenosis. Thorax, *22*:497, 1967.

Miller, W. W., Beligere, N., Waldhausen, J. A., Chatten, J., and Rashkind, W. J.: Congenital pulmonary atresia with intact ventricular septum. Am. J. Cardiol., *23*:128, 1969.

Moller, J. H., Girod, D., Amplatz, K., and Jarco, R. L.: Pulmonary valvotomy in pulmonary atresia with hypoplastic right ventricle. Surgery, *68*:630, 1970.

Moulton, A. L., Bowman, F. O., Jr., Edie, R. N., Hayes, C. J., Ellis, K., Gersony, W. and Malm, J. R.: Pulmonary atresia with intact ventricular septum: A sixteen year experience. J. Thorac. Cardiovasc. Surg., *78*:527, 1979.

Murphy, D. A., Murphy, D. R., Gibbons, J. E., and Dobell, A. R. C.: Surgical treatment of pulmonary atresia with intraventricular septum. J. Thorac. Cardiovasc. Surg., *62*:213, 1971.

Novelo, S., Chait, L. O., Zapata-Diaz, J., and Valasquez, T.: Atresia pulmonary estenosis tricuspidea sin co minicaciones interventricular. Arch. Inst. Cardiol. Mex., *21*:325, 1951.

Olley, P. M., Cocean, F., and Bodach, E.: E-type prostaglandin: A new emergency therapy for certain cyanotic congenital heart malformations. Circulation, *53*:728, 1976.

Parisi-Buckley, L., Dooley, K. J., and Fyler, D. C.: Pulmonary atresia and intact ventricular septum in New England. (Abstract.) Circulation, *11*(51–52):225, 1975.

Rao, P. S., Liebman, J., and Borkget, G.: Right ventricular growth in a case of pulmonary stenosis with intact ventricular septum and hypoplastic right ventricle. Circulation, *53*:389, 1976.

Rudolph, A. M., Heymann, M. A., Fishman, N., and Lankier, J. B.: Formalin infiltration of the ductus arteriosus. A method for palliation of infants with selected congenital cardiac lesions. N. Engl. J. Med., *292*:1263, 1975.

Shams, A., Fowler, R. J., Trusler, G. A., Keith, J. D., and Mustard, W. T.: Pulmonary atresia with intact ventricular septum: Report of 50 cases. Pediatrics, *47*:370, 1971.

Subramanian, S., Wagner, H., Teshai, G., and Menon, C. A.: Pulmonary atresia with intact ventricular septum. Ann. Clin. Inf., *13*:225, 1972.

Chapter 42

Univentricular Heart

Aart Brutel de la Rivière

James R. Malm

In 1824, Holmes described a heart with one ventricle. In 1936, Abbott reported 27 instances of single ventricle alone and with associated defects in a total of 1000 congenital heart malformations. Since that time, the pathologic anatomy of hearts with one ventricle has been studied by many authors, resulting in various views of the entity itself as well as its embryology and classification. Van Praagh and associates (1964, 1965, 1972), Lev and coworkers (1969), and Anderson's group (1974, 1976, 1978) have made major contributions to the understanding of the anatomy of single ventricle. A clinical diagnosis has become possible with the use of biplane cineangiocardiography and two-dimensional echocardiography, and in selected cases, palliation or surgical correction has been performed.

Anderson's terminology is practical for surgeons and has therefore been used throughout this chapter.* A univentricular heart (UVH) is defined by the commitment of the atrioventricular (AV) valves to only one chamber in the ventricular mass. A rudimentary chamber (being either an outlet chamber or a trabecular pouch) is usually present. If this chamber gives rise to (more than half) a great artery, it is termed an outlet chamber; otherwise, it is termed a trabecular pouch. Common ventricle is defined by the absence or rudimentary presence (as a posterior rim) of the interventricular septum, with both right and left ventricular sinus myocardium present, and this form may be considered as a huge ventricular septal defect.

EMBRYOLOGY, ANATOMY, AND CLASSIFICATION

Three variations of UVH exist (Fig. 42–1). The most common form is UVH of left ventricular (LV) type, in which the ventricle has a trabecular component of left ventricular morphology, associated with a rudimentary chamber of right ventricular (RV) type. Less common is UVH of RV type, associated with a rudimentary chamber of LV type. Finally, there has been defined a UVH of indeterminate morphology, without rudimentary chamber. The incidence of UVH of LV type has been reported to be about 63 to 80 per cent of all cases of single ventricle, whereas UVH or RV type was found to be present in about 5 per cent. Ventricular arterial discordance (transposition of the great arteries [TGA]) was found in 76 to 90 per cent of the hearts, with rather equal distribution of cases in which the aorta was anterior and to the right

---

*Exclusive of tricuspid and mitral atresia.

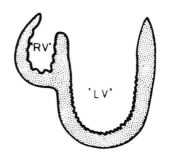

a) UVH of Left Ventricular Type with Rud. Chamber of RV Type   b) UVH of Right Ventricular Type with Rud. Chamber of LV Type   c) UVH of Indeterminate Type without Rudimentary Chamber

Figure 42–1. The ventricular morphologies of univentricular hearts. *Note:* Rudimentary chambers may be right-sided or left-sided in either left ventricular or right ventricular varieties of univentricular heart. (LV = chamber of left ventricular morphology; RV = chamber of right ventricular morphology; Indet. = chamber of indeterminate morphology.)

of the pulmonary artery and anterior and to the left of the pulmonary artery. Common ventricle (i.e., the absence of the ventricular septum in an otherwise "normal" heart) is now considered a large ventricular septal defect (VSD).

Single ventricle and *l*-transposition of the great arteries may be associated with a number of varieties of intestinal malrotation, most commonly with the asplenia syndrome. Asplenia includes abdominal situs ambiguus and bilateral right bronchi, which will facilitate the diagnosis on routine chest film. Details of the embryology and anatomy of these defects can be read in the selected references.

Several aspects of the surgical anatomy of UVH deserve special attention: (1) the conduction tissue, (2) subarterial stenosis, (3) AV valves, and (4) coronary arteries.

1. *The conduction tissue.* In UVH of LV type with outlet chamber and discordant ventriculoarterial connection, (i.e., transposed great arteries), the regular posterior AV node is rudimentary (Fig. 42–2). An anterolateral (right-sided) accessory AV node adjacent to the AV ring is present, from which the penetrating bundle descends onto the right rim of the trabecular septum at the outlet foramen. The relationship of the bundle and the posterior great artery (taking origin from the main chamber) is dependent on the position of the rudimentary chamber. A left-sided rudimentary chamber (again, in situs solitus of the atria) will be

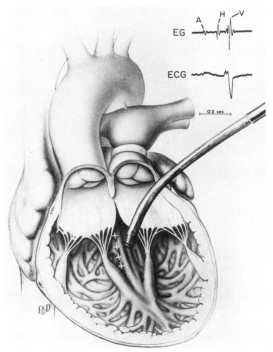

Figure 42–3. An illustration of the intraventricular location of the bundle of His (+ +) in one patient with common ventricle. The electrical probe used for recording the operative electrogram (EG) is seen. Note on the EG the characteristic His (H) spike between the atrial (A) and ventricular (V) recordings. (From Edie, R. N., Ellis, K., Gersony, W. M., Krongrad, E., Bowman, F. O., and Malm, J. R.: Surgical repair of single ventricle. J. Thorac. Cardiovasc. Surg., 66:350, 1973.)

associated with a long bundle in close proximity to the ostium of the posterior great artery (the pulmonary artery) (Fig. 42–2), whereas in the case of a right-sided rudimentary chamber, the bundle will stay remote from the posteriorly located pulmonary artery, in fact remaining on top of the trabecula septomarginalis and therefore not being related to the pulmonary artery.

In common ventricle, the conduction tissue has an anatomy analogous to that of the conduction tissue in VSD, i.e., the AV node is situated posteriorly and medially at the right AV valve orifice near the posterior ridge. The penetrating bundle runs at the posterior rim, i.e., at the rim of the rudimentary interventricular septum (Fig. 42–3).

Detailed descriptions of the localization of the conduction tissue in the following other types of UVH have been reported: UVH of LV type without outlet chamber (Wilkinson *et al.*, 1976), UVH of RV type with right-sided outlet chamber (Essed *et al.*, 1980), and UVH of RV type with left-sided outlet chamber (Wilkinson *et al.*, 1979).

2. *Subarterial stenosis* (Fig. 42–4). Obstruction at the arterial outlet, either from the main chamber or from the rudimentary chamber, may be valvular or subvalvular. The obstruction can be present at birth or may be acquired during life. The obstruction can also form at the site of the bulboventricular foramen. There is some suggestive evidence that banding of the

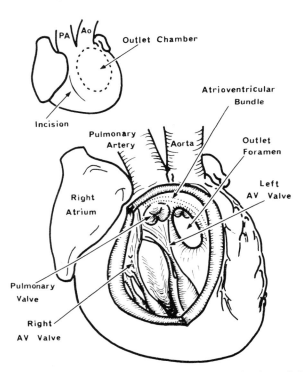

Figure 42–2. Drawing illustrating the surgeon's view of the conducting tissue in univentricular heart of left ventricular type with double inlet and left-sided rudimentary chamber. (From Anderson, R. H., Arnold, R., Thapar, M. K., Jones, R. S., and Hamilton, D. I.: Cardiac specialized tissues in hearts with an apparently single ventricular chamber (double inlet left ventricle). Am. J. Cardiol., *33*:95, 1975. By kind permission of Martinus Nyhoff, The Hague.)

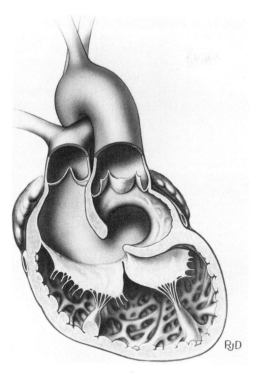

Figure 42–4. An illustration of the univentricular heart with LV morphology and left-sided subaortic outflow chamber with *l*-transposition of the great vessels. A single anatomical left ventricle is seen into which enter two separate AV valves. The rudimentary right ventricular infundibulum is in an inverted position and leads to a narrow aortic outflow tract. (From Edie, R. N., Ellis, K., Gersoney, W. M., Krongrad, E., Bowman, F. O., and Malm, J. R.: Surgical repair of single ventricle. J. Thorac. Cardiovasc. Surg., 66:350, 1973.)

pulmonary artery may accelerate the development of subaortic stenosis if the anatomy is favorable to its formation.

The presence of a restrictive bulboventricular foramen has been shown to be an incremental risk factor in open repair of UVH. In UVH of LV type with rudimentary chamber, the outlet foramen was found to be restrictive in 33 per cent of cases with ventriculoarterial discordance, resulting in obstruction to aortic flow, and in 70 per cent of cases with ventriculoarterial concordance, resulting in obstruction to pulmonary flow. In one series, pulmonic stenosis was found in 83 of 145 cases of common ventricle.

Occasionally, there is obstruction to both pulmonary and aortic flow.

3. *AV valves.* AV valve anomalies such as parachute deformities, clefts, valve stenoses, common papillary attachments, and common AV valves occur with a relatively high incidence. They are of surgical significance; therefore, not only should preoperative analysis with echocardiography (especially two-dimensional and contrast M-mode) and cineangiocardiography be undertaken to establish valve anatomy and function, but also sufficient time should be taken at operation for a complete evaluation of both AV valve apparatuses.

A special problem is presented by *straddling of AV valves*. In UVH, an overriding anulus is present when one AV valve ring is committed to both the ventricle and the rudimentary chamber; this is also called *anular straddling*. A straddling valve is defined as that condition in which either AV valve tensor apparatus enters both the ventricle and the rudimentary chamber with papillary and chordal attachments in both; this is also termed *peripheral straddling*. Peripheral straddling will preclude the insertion of a new interventricular septum, unless an AV valve prosthesis is used. Detachment of the straddling papillary muscles and/or chordae will usually result in severe AV valve insufficiency. Therefore, in patients with straddling AV valve, a septation procedure is undesirable; a modified Fontan procedure is indicated.

Finally, it should be mentioned that AV valve regurgitation may develop, mostly after the first decade. This may be due to congenitally abnormal valve leaflets and/or tensor apparatus, but more commonly, it is due to ventricular dilatation. This may be particularly prominent if an effective systemic–to–pulmonary artery shunt has been created resulting in volume overloading of the ventricle. Most probably, AV valve dysfunction is, apart from pulmonary vascular disease, the major precipitating cause of heart failure in adult life in the natural history of the disease.

4. *Coronary arteries.* In the absence of an interventricular septum, the presence of a proper anterior descending coronary artery is unlikely. The terms right and left delimiting coronary arteries have been introduced, referring to those vessels that demarcate the outlet chamber in UVH of LV type. Keeton and associates (1979b) studied the coronary anatomy in 26 UVHs, 24 of which were of LV type with outlet chamber. Right and left delimiting coronary arteries outlined the outlet chamber in 16 (76 per cent). In 95 per cent of the hearts, large delimiting parallel branches of the right coronary artery crossed over the anterior wall of the heart. Especially since all hearts studied had marked hypertrophy with a poorly developed collateral circulation and little cross-circulation between the main coronary arterial systems, ischemic injury to the myocardium at the time of surgery had occurred frequently. It should be mentioned that apparently normal coronary anatomy has also been described in UVH of LV type. Therefore, during repair, the coronary anatomy should be determined intraoperatively.

NATURAL HISTORY

The incidence of single ventricle is approximately 3 per cent of all congenital cardiac malformations, with a male predominance of 2.5 to 1. In the first year of life, single ventricle constitutes up to 10 per cent of symptomatic cyanotic heart disease. Until recently, all diagnoses were made at autopsy, and in Abbott's series (1936), death occurred in a range from infancy to 37 years, with a mean of 7¾ years. Since that time, one fifth of all reported patients have survived to adult life, with the mortality rate in the first year of life being 47 per cent.

The Mayo Clinic reported 122 patients with the diagnosis of common (single) ventricle who have been followed for a period of 6 months to 15 years (mean 9 years), after the diagnosis has been made at the age of 7 days to 38 years (mean 9.4 years). It was found that 44 patients had died from congestive heart failure, dysrhythmias, or sudden unexplained death. Seventy-eight patients were alive (age 9 months to 40 years), of whom 62 were cyanotic and had diminished exercise tolerance. A positive or negative correlation with the presence or absence of an outlet chamber or obstruction to pulmonary blood flow could not be established. The oldest patient reported with one ventricle was 69 years old; he died from congestive heart failure and atrial fibrillation, having mild pulmonary stenosis. Our own experience suggests that survival will depend on adequate resistance to pulmonary blood flow proximal to the pulmonary vascular bed. Longevity is most often associated with a flow-limiting degree of pulmonary stenosis.

PATHOPHYSIOLOGY, CLINICAL PRESENTATION, AND DIAGNOSIS

Univentricular heart and common ventricle are admixture types of lesions with clinical features dependent on the relative amount of systemic and pulmonary blood flow. Although it has been shown that preferential streaming in the ventricle may contribute to favorable (i.e., physiologic) blood flow, the major determinant of the hemodynamic presentation is the presence of obstruction to pulmonary blood flow and its degree. Patients presenting without obstruction to pulmonary blood flow demonstrate clinical features typical of a large left-to-right shunt with congestive heart failure. Their natural clinical course is determined by the development of pulmonary vascular disease.

If severe obstruction to pulmonary blood flow exists, patients are markedly cyanotic; lesser degrees of pulmonary stenosis are associated with arterial desaturation compatible with normal life.

Additional lesions (e.g., patent ductus arteriosus) will contribute to the pathophysiology and clinical presentation according to their nature. Physical findings are not pathognomonic and depend largely on the associated anomalies (e.g., pulmonic stenosis). The chest film is not specific, with pulmonary vascular markings dependent on pulmonary blood flow—oligemic lung fields and a small heart in patients with severe obstruction to pulmonary blood flow and plethoric lung fields with cardiomegaly in patients with pulmonary overcirculation. The determination of the cardiac position (e.g., dextrocardia) is of prime importance, and the atrial situs can be predicted. The EKG is not diagnostic in UVH because of wide variations in the precordial lead patterns.

Echocardiography is of great value in establishing the diagnosis. Special criteria have been described with reference to the AV valves, the absence of the interventricular septum with apposition of the "septal" leaflets of the AV valves, the presence (or absence) of an outlet chamber, and echocardiographic continuity between the posterior great artery and the AV valves. Echocardiographic contrast studies have proved most useful, particularly to show a common AV valve. Two-dimensional echocardiography has proved to be superior for an accurate diagnosis of UVH. The most diagnostic view in this technique is the apical four-chamber view. Echocardiography gives an indication of ventricular performance, provides cardiac dimensions, and allows the diagnosis of straddling AV valve. Although some echocardiographic studies have shown normal ventricular performance, Gibson and colleagues (1979) showed abnormal ventricular contraction patterns in UVH using cineangiographic data.

Cardiac catheterization and cineangiocardiography will provide the definitive diagnosis. Pressure tracings will reveal outflow tract obstruction and its degree, and oximetry data will show shunting. Flows as well as resistances should be calculated in order to make proper decisions regarding operation. Cineangiocardiography will show the anatomic and functional state of the major cardiac segments (Fig. 42–5).

To classify and manage UVH, the following features should be identified: AV valve anatomy and function, ventricular morphology, and the presence of a rudimentary chamber and the ventriculoarterial connection.

It has been shown that ejection fraction, independent from pulmonary stenosis, is depressed in single ventricle. Ventricular function and ventricular volume can be measured. Finally, the presence and nature of additional congenital cardiac malformation can be determined. The differentiation between UVH and common ventricle is important in view of surgical treatment.

The most reliable sign to differentiate between UVH and common ventricle is the presence of a posterior rim between morphologic left and right ventricular trabecular portions. Echocardiography will be most helpful, but, again, cineangiocardiography will provide the definitive diagnosis.

TREATMENT

Surgical treatment is usually required at some time for patients with UVH. Patients with a naturally occurring obstruction to pulmonary blood flow will require treatment when pulmonary blood flow is limited. When a severe, marked decrease in arterial desaturation occurs, a systemic–to–pulmonary artery shunt is indicated. The shunt procedure of choice is the Blalock-Taussig anastomosis, using either the native subclavian artery or a Gore-Tex prosthetic graft (connecting the subclavian artery to the pulmonary artery). It is possible to increase pulmonary blood flow by a transvalvular pulmonary valvotomy (Brock

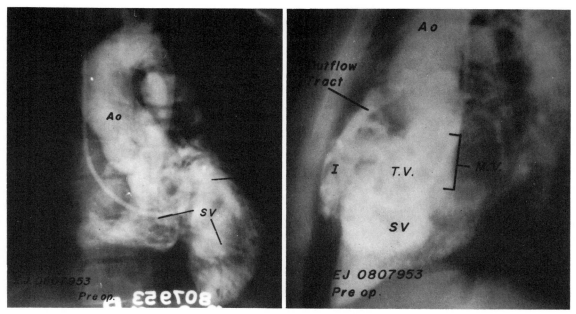

Figure 42–5. Preoperative antero-posterior and lateral angiocardiograms in a single ventricle of right ventricular morphology with normal relationships of the great vessels. The catheter is through the tricuspid valve (T.V.) with the injection into a large, poorly defined single left ventricle (SV), which gives origin to both the aorta (Ao) and the narrow pulmonary outflow tract. The lateral view shows both the mitral (MV) and tricuspid (T.V.) valves entering the single ventricle with an anterior infundibulum (I) leading to the pulmonary outflow tract. (From Edie, R. N., Ellis, K., Gersony, W. M., Krongrad, E., Bowman, F. O., and Malm, J. R.: Surgical repair of single ventricle. J. Thorac. Cardiovasc. Surg., *66*:350, 1973.)

procedure) in selected cases. A purely infundibular obstruction can be relieved by the insertion of a palliative outflow tract patch (with or without the aid of cardiopulmonary bypass). In older patients, a Glenn shunt (connecting the superior vena cava to the right pulmonary artery) can be performed; its advantage over a Blalock-Taussig or Waterston shunt is the absence of volume loading (overloading) of the ventricle with subsequent ventricular dilatation and AV valve dysfunction. A Glenn shunt conditions the heart favorably for a Fontan-type procedure. If pulmonary blood flow is adequate with normal pressure in the pulmonary artery, no treatment is necessary.

Patients with systemic pressure in the pulmonary artery will develop pulmonary vascular obstructive disease without surgery. Banding of the pulmonary artery should be performed at an early age, preferably during the first 6 months of life. The banding should be sufficient to reduce systolic pressure in the pulmonary artery distal to the band to 30 to 35 per cent of systemic arterial pressure.

If proper palliation or an adequate degree of pulmonary stenosis has allowed the patient to grow to the age of 4 to 8 years, two options exist for definitive repair of univentricular heart: ventricular septation, which consists of the insertion of a prosthetic interventricular septum to divide the ventricle and thereby make it into a physiologic biventricular pump, or a modified Fontan procedure, by which a univentricular pumping heart is established. Elevated resistance in the pulmonary vascular bed is a contraindication to both types of repair.

Ventricular Septation (Fig. 42–6)

Replacement of the excised ventricular septum by a prosthetic patch has been shown to allow long-

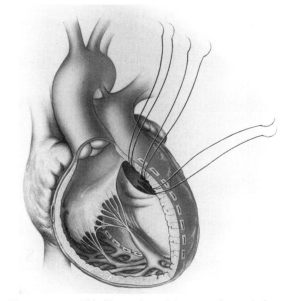

Figure 42–6. This illustration of the operative technique used for reconstruction of the ventricular septum demonstrates the large prosthesis separating the two AV valve mechanisms. The anterior sutures have been inserted from the outside of the heart through the entire wall thickness. (From Edie, R. N., Ellis, K., Gersony, W. M., Krongrad, E., Bowman, F. O., and Malm, J. R.: Surgical repair of single ventricle. J. Thorac. Cardiovasc. Surg., *66*:350, 1973.)

term survival in dogs. Although the animal model is more similar to the common ventricle, the results obtained have been used to advocate septation for univentricular heart. Attention will be focused upon UVH of LV type with ventriculoarterial discordance (*l*-transposition of the great arteries).

Median sternotomy, or in young females, a horizontal submammary skin incision, is performed before the median sternal split. Cardiopulmonary bypass using hemodilution with hypothermia (18° to 24°C., which will allow short periods of total circulatory arrest if needed) is employed, combined with low arterial flow, one period of aortic cross-clamping, and myocardial preservation using cold potassium cardioplegia. Ventricular decompression via the right superior pulmonary vein or foramen ovale is established. Septation can be done through the atrium or using a ventriculotomy. The main advantage of the former is preservation of myocardial muscle; its disadvantage is the poor exposure for mapping the conducting tissue, as well as frequent inadequate exposure in general.

A longitudinal ventriculotomy is made either in the plane of the anticipated attachment of the prosthetic patch, carefully avoiding the coronary arteries, or as a left-sided apical incision between the papillary muscles. The bundle of His can be localized using a probe in 50 per cent of patients, and its course can be anticipated by published anatomic studies. It is obvious that mapping should be done before cardioplegia has been induced, since the cessation of all electrical activity after administration of the cardioplegic solution will prevent electrophysiologic studies.

A restrictive bulboventricular outlet foramen should be enlarged before septation, carefully avoiding the conduction tissue. The septal patch, for which a rather heavy noncompliant material (such as knitted Teflon) should be used, is shaped according to the anatomy. Insertion starts at the posterior aspect of the ventricle, between the AV valves. Obviously, a common AV valve will preclude the insertion of an interventricular septum unless a right-sided AV valve prosthesis is also inserted. Common atrium, which accompanies common AV valve, will require atrial septation. Although the presence of a noncontractile interatrial prosthetic septum will impede atrial contraction after a modified Fontan procedure, that operation has also been used in patients with common AV valve.

Interrupted mattress sutures are used in the heavily trabecular areas; some of them are taken to the outside of the heart to prevent leaking. Papillary muscles are assigned to the appropriate ventricles; the patch is carefully sutured between them.

At the level of the semilunar valves, two options exist: the patch can be inserted between the semilunar valves, or both arterial outlets can be allowed to remain to the left side of the patch, creating a double-outlet left ventricle. The former, especially in patients with *l*-transposition of the great arteries, implies suturing in the danger area between the semilunar valves with a high risk of inducing complete heart block. In the latter, re-establishment of right ventricular pulmonary arterial continuity is necessary using an external conduit. The use of a conduit is required when pulmonary stenosis is present, since reconstruction of the pulmonary outflow tract is extremely hazardous, if at all possible, owing to its posterior localization.

Both ventricles are made of equal size. Too large a patch will tend to cause obstruction to the new right ventricular outflow tract, and too narrow a patch will impair diastolic filling of both ventricles as a result of approximation of the anterior and posterior ventricular wall.

Apart from septation of the ventricle, additional abnormalities should be corrected and palliative shunts closed. Temporary pacing wires on the right atrium and the right ventricle are left in place. Complete heart block occurs in about 50 per cent of the patients; hence, permanent pacing wires are implanted in all cases. The postoperative complications include low cardiac output and rhythm disturbances. Besides the usual causes after open heart surgery, low cardiac output may be the result of excessive systolic bulging of the interventricular patch into the right ventricle. This can be easily detected using M-mode echocardiography. The use of intraoperative echocardiography will detect this complication early. The most common arrhythmias are supraventricular and junctional tachyarrhythmias; they should be treated medically and/or by use of atrial pacing. Complete heart block requires the insertion of a permanent pacemaker, by reference, the AV sequential type.

Modified Fontan Procedure

The modified Fontan procedure requires special venous cannulation techniques. In order to minimize surgical trauma to the right atrium, both venae cavae are directly cannulated using right-angled Rygg cannulas. The right atrium is opened at the level of the right atrial appendage by a limited incision, which later will be used to attach the valved conduit between the right side of the heart and the pulmonary artery. After the intracardiac anatomy has been determined, the right AV valve orifice is closed using a pericardial patch. The patch is sutured in such a way as to avoid the conduction tissue; therefore, it is attached to the atrial wall at some distance from the AV valve ring. The coronary sinus can be left draining into the ventricle beneath the patch or, by suturing the patch inside the coronary sinus, carefully away from the posterior AV node, can be left draining into the right atrium, thereby obtaining complete physiologic venous return.

The conduit between the right atrium and the pulmonary artery, which should be closed off by division and oversuturing, may be valved or non-valved. Obviously, again, all other anomalies should be corrected and palliative shunts closed. Special problems such as arterial stenosis are managed by more specific techniques (Doty *et al.*, 1981).

If, coming off bypass, the patient's right atrial

pressure is greater than 35 mm. Hg, a superior vena cava–to–right pulmonary artery anastomosis (Glenn shunt) can be performed to unload the right atrium. A chest tube is left in place to drain pleural effusions, which usually accompany Fontan procedures. Postoperatively, early extubation will promote pulmonary blood flow, as will optimal positioning of the patient (semi-Fowler position). Maintenance of an adequate cardiac output usually will require high systemic venous filling pressure and inotropic support. The use of drugs that lower pulmonary and systemic vascular resistance, such as sodium nitroprusside, is often helpful.

Treatment of common ventricle follows a course analogous to surgical therapy for VSD, although primary repair in infancy carries a higher risk. Palliation is usually accomplished by banding. Since AV valve anatomy and arterial outlet are normal and the conduction tissue has a location similar to that in VSD, ventricular septation is the procedure of choice. Patch closure of the defect can be performed, carefully avoiding the bundle at the posterior ridge of the rudimentary interventricular septum. If normal (ventriculoarterial concordant) relationship of the great arteries is present (in atrioventricular concordance), physiologic blood flow is obtained by just septating the ventricle, leaving the arterial outlets to their respective ventricles. However, if ventriculoarterial discordance (i.e., transposition) is present, various options exist: a venous rerouting procedure at the atrial level (Mustard or Senning operation) can be done; a valved external conduit can be used, closing the pulmonary valve; a spiral interventricular patch can be inserted, resulting in adequate interventricular rerouting; or an arterial switch procedure could be added to septation in order to achieve physiologic blood flow.

RESULTS

Palliative surgical treatment in UVH carries a substantial hospital mortality, mostly related to the age of the patient and the complexity of the lesion. The hospital mortality rate in patients with UVH and elevated pressure in the pulmonary artery who require banding has been reported to be 10 to 25 per cent. The hospital mortality rate in patients with decreased pulmonary blood flow requiring shunt procedures has been reported to range from 0 to 33 per cent. The Blalock-Taussig anastomosis has a lower mortality

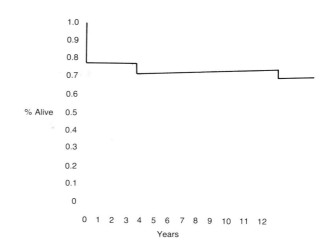

Figure 42–7. Actuarial survival after palliation of univentricular heart.

rate (6.2 to 11 per cent) than the Waterston shunt (33 to 40 per cent). However, these results should be interpreted in view of the difference in age between patients receiving Waterston shunts (mostly neonates) and those receiving Blalock-Taussig anastomoses (mostly infants). Some patients may require multiple palliative procedures.

Late mortality is limited, and actuarial survival curves show a nearly horizontally shaped curve after a few years' follow-up, the first part of the curve being greatly influenced by hospital mortality (Fig. 42–7). In a series of 84 patients with common (single) ventricle, 70 per cent were alive 10 years after diagnosis followed by palliative treatment. Recently, a survey has been published concerning palliative treatment of single ventricle during the first year of life. The overall mortality rate was 47 per cent; it was 41 per cent for the surgically treated patients and 58 per cent for the medically treated patients. (Report of the New England Regional Infant Cardiac Program, 1980).

Experience with total correction is limited (Table 42–1). Ventricular septation has a reported hospital mortality rate of 50 per cent. Hospital mortality has been related to ventricular size, a restrictive outlet foramen, age, and complete heart block after operation.

Long-term results are influenced by various factors, such as myocardial infarction (i.e., the extent of myocardial injury during operation), the presence of residual pathology (such as ventricular shunts and arterial obstruction), sometimes necessitating reoperation, the occurrence of "new" pathology (such as

TABLE 42–1. RESULTS OF VENTRICULAR SEPTATION FOR UVH*

	NO. OF PATIENTS	HOSPITAL MORTALITY	LATE MORTALITY	CUMULATIVE MORTALITY	70% CV OF CUM. MORTALITY
Mayo Clinic	45	24	8	32 (72%)	
UAB	16	7	—	7 (44%)	29–60
CPMC	10	7	—	7 (70%)	

UAB = University of Alabama at Birmingham.
CPMC = Columbia Presbyterian Medical Center, New York, N. Y.
*From Danielson, G. K.: Modified Fontan procedure. *In* Congenital Heart Surgery: Current Techniques and Controversies. Edited by A. L. Moulton. Pasadena, California, Appleton Davies, Inc., 1983 (in press).

TABLE 42–2. RESULTS OF MODIFIED FONTAN PROCEDURE FOR UVH (MAYO CLINIC)*

	NO. OF PATIENTS	MORTALITY	% MORTALITY
1974–March 1979	14	4	29
Apr. 1971–Feb, 1981	52	13	25
Total	66	17	26

*From Danielson, G. K.: Modified Fontan procedure. *In* Congenital Heart Surgery: Current Techniques and Controversies. Edited by A. L. Moulton. Pasadena, California, Appleton Davies, Inc., 1983, (in press).

AV valve dysfunction, rhythm disturbances, valve degeneration, and conduit obstruction), and the presence of surgically induced complete heart block (i.e., pacemaker dependency).

Follow-up studies have shown that if normal sinus rhythm is present, myocardial function is unimpaired, and there is no residual intracardiac pathology, long-term survival is possible after septation with good cardiac performance and functional class. Whether long-term results of septations performed recently with low hospital mortality will attain superior results with regard to improved long-term survival remains to be established, but the prospect is good.

Hospital mortality for the modified Fontan operation is much less than that for septation. In one series (Table 42–2), the hospital mortality rate is 25 per cent. In addition, the incidence of complications such as complete heart block is less with the modified Fontan procedure. However, follow-up is shorter, and the long-term results of operations that leave the patients without a right ventricle still remain to be elucidated.

Surgical treatment of common ventricle is by septation. The results of the limited experience reported are good. Hospital mortality is low, and long-term results are excellent. Recent functional follow-up studies after septation of common ventricle showed a near-normal ejection fraction with the use of a straight interventricular patch and a slightly depressed ventricular function after the insertion of a spiral patch (to obtain physiologic flow in the presence of transposed great vessels).

PROPOSED SURGICAL TREATMENT

Patients with univentricular heart will usually require surgical treatment, most often in the first months of life. The indications for palliative surgery are clearly defined: Elevated pressure in the pulmonary artery will necessitate banding of that vessel, whereas decreased pulmonary blood flow causing hypoxic symptoms will require the creation of a systemic–to–pulmonary artery shunt.

When the patient has reached the age of 4 to 8 years, two options exist for total surgical correction: ventricular septation and a modified Fontan procedure. Both operations can only be performed safely in the presence of low pulmonary vascular resistance (Fig. 42–8). In selected cases (UVH of LV type with two AV valves; *l*-transposition of the great arteries

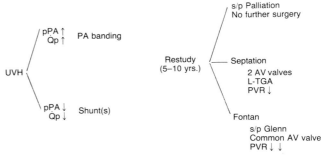

Figure 42–8. Proposed surgical treatment for univentricular heart.

and no major additional abnormalities, such as subaortic obstruction), we tend to favor ventricular septation in view of the recent good hospital results and good long-term survival reported with this type of repair. Adequate ventricular size seems of paramount importance, so that the newly created right and left ventricles are of normal or greater than normal size (both naturally occurring and after previous pulmonary artery banding). A modified Fontan procedure is the correction of choice when a single AV valve is present. The surgical management of univentricular heart is evolving, and the final chapter has not been written.

SELECTED REFERENCES

Anderson, R. H., and Shinebourne, E. A. (Eds.): Pediatric Cardiology, 1977. Edinburgh, Churchill Livingstone, 1978, pp. 305–406.

In various chapters, morphology, angiography, hemodynamics, and surgery are all covered by different authors. An excellent review of Anderson's terminology is presented, as well as detailed descriptions of the conduction tissue, especially outlined for surgeons.

Elliott, L. P., Bream, P. R., and Gessner, I. H.: Single and common ventricle. *In* Heart Disease in Infants, Children and Adolescents. 2nd Ed. Edited by A. J. Moss, F. H. Adams and C. Emmanouilides. Baltimore, Williams and Wilkins Co., 1977, p. 387.

This chapter is a good review of the clinical and diagnostic aspects of the entire subject. The pathologic anatomy and clinical features are emphasized with detailed description of electrocardiographic, roentgenographic, and angiocardiographic findings.

Van Praagh, R., Plett, J. A., and Van Praagh, S.: Single ventricle. Herz, *4*(2) 113, 1972.

This article contains an excellent review of the pathology, embryology, terminology, and classification of single ventricle. It has an exhaustive bibliography consisting of 126 references. This particular volume is completely devoted to univentricular heart (pages 78 to 266).

REFERENCES

Abbott, M. E.: Atlas of Congenital Heart Disease. New York, American Heart Association, 1936.
Anderson, R. H., and Shinebourne, E. A. (Eds.): Paediatric Cardiology, 1977. Edinburgh, Churchill Livingstone, 1978, pp. 305–406.
Anderson, R. H., Arnold, R., Thapar, M. K., Jones, R. S., and Hamilton, D. I.: Cardiac specialized tissues in hearts with an

apparently single ventricular chamber (double inlet left ventricle). Am. J. Cardiol., 33:95, 1974.

Anderson, R. H., Becker, A. E., Wilkinson, J. L., and Gerlis, L. M.: Morphogenesis of univentricular hearts. Br. Heart J., 38:558, 1976.

Anderson, R. H., Shinebourne, E. A., Becker, A. E., Macartney, F. J., Quero-Jimenez, M., Tynan, M. J., Arnold, R., Smith, A., and Wilkinson, J. L.: Tricuspid atresia. J. Thorac. Cardiovasc. Surg., 74:325, 1977 (with a reply by Bharati, S., and Lev, M., p. 328).

Beardshaw, J. A., Gibson, D. G., Pearson, M. C., Lipton, M. K., and Anderson, R. H.: Echo cardiographic diagrams of primitive ventricle with two AV valves. Br. Heart J., 39:266, 1977.

Bharati, S., and Lev, M.: Course of conductive tissue in single ventricle with l-loop and transposition of the great arteries. Circulation, 57:723, 1975.

Doty, D. B., Marin, W. J., and Lauer, R. M.: Single ventricle with aortic outflow obstruction. J. Thorac. Cardiovasc. Surg., 81:636, 1981.

Doty, D. B., Schrieken, R. M., and Lauer, R. M.: Septation of univentricular heart: Transatrial approach. J. Thorac. Cardiovasc. Surg., 78:423, 1979.

Edie, R. N., Ellis, K., Gersony, W. M., Krongrad, E., Bowman, F. O., and Malm, J. R.: Surgical repair of single ventricles. J. Thorac. Cardiovasc. Surg., 66:350, 1973.

Elliott, L. P., Bream, P. R., and Gessner, I. H.: Single and common ventricle. In Heart Disease in Infants, Children and Adolescents. 2nd Ed. Edited by A. J. Moss, F. H. Adams, and C. Emmanouilides. Baltimore, Williams and Wilkins Co., 1977, p. 387.

Elliott, L. P., Bargeron, L. M., Soto, B., and Bream, P. R.: Axial cineangiography in congenital heart disease. Radiol. Clin. North Am., 18:515, 1980.

Essed, C. E., Ho, S. Y., Hunter, S., and Anderson, R. H.: Atrioventricular conducting system in univentricular heart of right ventricular type with right-sided rudimentary chamber. Thorax, 35:123, 1980.

Feldt, R. H., Mair, D. D., Danielson, G. K., Wallace, R. B., and McGoon, D. C.: Current status of the septation procedure for univentricular heart, J. Thorac. Cardiovasc. Surg., 82:93, 1981.

Freedom, R. M., Sondheimer, H., Dische, R., and Rowe, R. D.: Development of "subaortic" stenosis after pulmonary artery banding for common ventricle. Am. J. Cardiol., 39:78, 1977.

Gale, A. G., Danielson, G. K., McGoon, D. C., and Mair, D. D.: Modified Fontan operation for univentricular heart and complicated congenital anomalies. J. Thorac. Cardiovasc. Surg., 78:831, 1979.

Gibson, D. G., Traill, T. A., and Brow, D. J.: Abnormal ventricular function in patients with univentricular heart. Herz, 4:226, 1979.

Hallerman, F. J., Davis, G. D., Ritter, D. G., and Kincaid, O. K.: Roentgenographic patterns of common ventricle. Radiology, 87:409, 1966.

Holmes, W. F.: Case of malformation of the heart. Trans. Med. Clin. Soc. Edinburgh, 4:252, 1824 (reprinted in Abbott, M. E.: Montreal Med. J., 30:522, 1901).

Kaiser, G. A., Waldo, A. L., Beach, P. M., Bowman, F. O., Hoffman, B. F., and Malm, J. R.: Specialized cardiac conduction system: Improved electrophysiologic identification techniques at surgery. Arch. Surg., 101:673, 1970.

Keeton, B. R., Macartney, F. J., Hunter, S., Mortera, C., Rees, P., Shinebourne, E. A., Tynan, M. J., Wilkinson, J. L., and Anderson, R. H.: Univentricular heart of RV type with double or common inlet. Circulation, 59:403, 1979a.

Keeton, B. R., Lie, J. L., McGoon, D. C., Danielson, G. K., Ritter, D. G., and Wallace, R. B.: Anatomy of coronary arteries in univentricular hearts and its surgical implications. Am. J. Cardiol., 43:569, 1979b.

Kitamura, S., Kawashima, Y., Shimazaki, Y., Mori, T., Nakano, S., Beppu, S., and Kozuka, T.: Characteristics of ventricular function in single ventricle. Circulation, 60:849, 1979.

Lev, M., Liberthson, R. R., Kirckpatrick, J. K., Eckner, F. A. O., and Arcilla, R. A.: Simple (primitive) ventricle. Circulation, 39:577, 1969.

Liberthson, R. R., Paul, M. H., Muster, A. J., Arcilla, R. A., Echner, F. A. O., and Lev, M.: Straddling and displaced AV

orifices and valves with primitive ventricle. Circulation, 53:213, 1976.

Macartney, F. J., Partridge, J. B, Scott, O., and Deverall, P. B.: Common or single ventricle. Circulation, 53:543, 1976.

McGoon, D. C., Danielson, G. K., Ritter, D. G., Wallace, R. B., Maloney, J. D., and Marcelletti, C.: Correction of univentricular hearts having two AV valves. J. Thorac. Cardiovasc. Surg., 74:148, 1977.

McKay, R., Pacifico, A. D., Blackstone, E. H., Kirklin, J. W., and Bargeron, L. M.: Septation of univentricular heart with left anterior subaortic outlet chamber. J. Thorac. Cardiovasc. Surg., 84:77, 1982.

Milo, S., Ho, S. Y., Macartney, F. J., Wilkinson, J. L., Becker, A. E., Wenink, A. C. G., Gittenberger-de Groot, A. C., and Anderson, R. H.: Straddling and overriding atrioventricular valves: Morphology and classification. Am. J. Cardiol., 44:1122, 1979.

Moodie, D. S., Tajik, A. J., and Ritter, D. G.: The natural history of common (single) ventricle. (Abstract.) Am. J. Cardiol., 39:311, 1977.

Moodie, D. S., Tajik, A. J., Ritter, D. G., and O'Falla, W. M.: Long term follow-up of patients with common (single) ventricle after palliative surgery. (Abstract.) Am. J. Cardiol., 41:390, 1978.

Quero-Jimenez, M., Perez-Martinez, V., Sarrion-Guzman, M., Rodriguez-Alonso, M., and Perez-Diaz, L.: Altérations des valves auriculo-ventriculaires dans les ventricules uniques et anomalies similaires. Arch. Mal. Coeur, 68:323, 1975.

Report of the New England Regional Infant Cardiac Program. Pediatrics, 65:377, 1980.

Sakakibara, S., Tominaga, S., Imai, Y., Vehara, K., and Matsumuro, M.: Successful total correction of common ventricle. Chest, 61:192, 1972.

Schatz, J., Fenoglio, J., and Krongard, E.: Electrophysiologic histologic correlation of the cardiac specialized conduction system in two cases of single ventricle and levo transposition of the great arteries. Am. Heart J., 96:235, 1978.

Seki, S., and McGoon, D. C.: Surgical technique for replacement of the interventricular septum. J. Thorac. Cardiovasc. Surg., 62:919, 1971.

Seward, J. B., Tajik, A. J., and Hagler, D. J.: 2D echocardiographic features of univentricular heart. In Pediatric Echocardiography – Cross Sectional, M Mode and Doppler. Edited by N. R. Lundstrom. Amsterdam, Elsevier North Holland Biomedical Press, 1981, p. 129.

Seward, J. B., Tajik, A. J., Hagler, D. J., and Ritter, D. G.: Contrast echocardiography in single or common ventricle. Circulation, 55:513, 1977.

Shimazaki, Y., Kawashima, Y., Mori, T., Matsudo, H., Kitamora, S., and Yokota, K.: Ventricular function of single ventricle after ventricular septation. Circulation, 61:653, 1980a.

Shimazaki, Y., Kawashima, Y., Mori, T., Kitamora, S., Marsudo, H., and Yokota, K.: Ventricular volume characteristics of single ventricle before corrective surgery. Am. J. Cardiol., 45:806, 1980b.

Shinebourne, E. A., Lau, K. C., Calcaterra, G., and Anderson, R. H.: UVH of RV type: Clinical, angiographic and electrocardiographic features. Am. J. Cardiol., 46:439, 1980.

Somerville, J., Becu, L., and Ross, D. N.: Common ventricle with acquired subaortic obstruction. Am. J. Cardiol., 34:206, 1974.

Van Praagh, R., Ongley, P. A., and Swan, H. J. C.: Anatomic types of single or common ventricle in man. Am. J. Cardiol., 13:307, 1964.

Van Praagh, R., Plett, J. A., and Van Praagh, S.: Single ventricle. Herz, 4(2):113, 1972.

Van Praagh, R., Van Praagh, S., Vlad, P., and Keith, J. D.: Diagnosis of the anatomic types of single or common ventricle. Am. J. Cardiol., 15:345, 1965.

Wenink, A. G. C.: Conducting tissue in primitive ventricle with outlet chamber. J. Thorac. Cardiovasc. Surg., 75:747, 1978.

Wilkinson, J. L., Anderson, R. H., Arnold, R., et al.: The conducting tissues in primitive ventricular hearts without an outlet chamber. Circulation, 53:930, 1976.

Wilkinson, J. L., Dickerson, D., Smith, A., and Anderson, R. H.: Conducting tissue in univentricular heart of right ventricular type with double or common inlet. J. Thorac. Cardiovasc. Surg., 77:691, 1979.

Chapter 43

Tricuspid Atresia

ROBERT M. SADE

HISTORICAL NOTE

Although tricuspid atresia was clearly described by Kreysig in 1817, no surgical relief for the symptoms of this malformation was possible until Taussig suggested and Blalock performed a subclavian–to–pulmonary artery anastomosis for tricuspid atresia in 1945. The next year, Potts and associates (1946) performed a descending aorta–to–left pulmonary artery anastomosis. Waterston introduced the ascending aorta–to–right pulmonary artery anastomosis in 1962.

Enlargement of a restrictive interatrial septal communication by closed atrial septectomy was introduced by Blalock and Hanlon in 1950. Rashkind and Miller introduced balloon atrioseptostomy 16 years later (1966). Accomplished at cardiac catheterization, it may be used as an initial procedure to enlarge the interatrial communication.

The small group of patients with tricuspid atresia, transposition of the great arteries, large ventricular septal defect, and no pulmonary stenosis (Type IIc) (see Fig. 43–1) usually responds well to pulmonary artery banding, which was first done by Muller in 1952 (Muller and Dammann, 1952).

The development of a corrective operation for tricuspid atresia depended on a fundamental conceptual change: recognition that pulmonary vascular resistance is normally so low that a pumping ventricle is not necessary to maintain adequate pulmonary circulation (Sade and Castaneda, 1975). The right ventricle was successfully bypassed experimentally by Carlon and colleagues (1951), Warden and coworkers (1954), and others subsequently. Clinical application of this principle was undertaken by Glenn (1958) when he did the first cavopulmonary anastomosis in man. Based on the foundation laid by these workers, Fontan performed the first successful correction of tricuspid atresia on April 25, 1968, utilizing a right atrium–to–pulmonary artery aortic allograft and a pulmonary valve allograft in the inferior vena cava (Fontan *et al.*, 1971). Several modifications of Fontan's operation have been described since his initial report in 1971.

INTRODUCTION

Tricuspid atresia is a congenital malformation of the heart characterized by absence of direct communication between the right atrium and the right ventricle. Three additional anomalies are nearly always associated with tricuspid atresia: (1) interatrial septal communication; (2) enlargement of the mitral valve and the left ventricle, and (3) underdevelopment of the right ventricle.

The lesion is uncommon but is not rare. In the total series of congenital cardiac malformations at Children's Hospital Medical Center, the incidence is 1.1 per cent (Nadas and Fyler, 1972). In the autopsy series reported by Keith and coworkers (1979), the incidence was higher — 3.1 per cent. It is the third most common anomaly producing cyanosis, after tetralogy of Fallot and transposition of the great arteries, representing 2.5 per cent of all infants with heart disease hospitalized or dying during the first year of life (Rosenthal, 1980).

ANATOMY

Van Praagh and associates (1971) have classified tricuspid atresia into three anatomic types: (1) muscular, (2) fibrous (membranous), and (3) Ebstein's malformation with no opening through the abnormal tricuspid valve. In the muscular form, the usual type (84 per cent), a central fibrotic umbilication is present in the region where the tricuspid valve would be expected. Microscopically, muscle bundles radiate from the central dimple. The membranous type (8 per cent) is always associated with juxtaposition of the atrial appendages. This form transilluminates well; microscopically, it is composed of fibrous tissue. In the Ebstein's type of atresia (8 per cent), the atrialized right ventricle forms a blind pouch beneath the right atrium, and there is no opening in the tricuspid valve. These types of tricuspid atresia appear to constitute a spectrum that may be related to developmental arrests at different stages during the formation of the tricuspid valve from the developing right ventricle. In 1973 Van

Praagh identified another very rare anatomic type, in which an atrioventricular valve leaflet of a total atrioventricular canal malformation completely closes the entrance to the right ventricle. We have also observed such a case during successful surgical correction.

The right atrium is invariably enlarged, with a thickened muscular wall; the left atrium is frequently affected in the same way. The interatrial communication is usually a patent foramen ovale but may be a true defect in the atrial septum. There is occasionally complete absence of the atrial septum.

The mitral valve is large and normally located; it occasionally comprises more than two leaflets. The left ventricle is always enlarged, with hypertrophic walls. The hypertrophy can sometimes reach extreme proportions.

The right ventricle is hypoplastic, especially its inflow portion. The exception to this is the Ebstein's type of atresia, in which the atrialized right ventricle serves as the right ventricular inflow tract. If pulmonary atresia is present, the right ventricle may be undetectable by gross examination.

CLASSIFICATION ACCORDING TO ASSOCIATED LESIONS

Kühne (1906) was the first to recognize that either normally related or transposed great arteries may occur in patients with tricuspid atresia. Edwards and Burchell (1949) classified tricuspid atresia in terms of the associated anomalies: transposition, obstruction to pulmonary blood flow, and size of ventricular septal

Figure 43–1. Classification of tricuspid atresia according to associated lesions. *Ia,* The pulmonary atresia can be valvar, or the main artery itself can be atretic. The right ventricular cavity is either slit-like or entirely absent on gross inspection. The ductus arteriosus is often patent but usually inadequate in size. *Ib,* This is the most common type of tricuspid atresia. The VSD is small, and the right ventricle is diminutive. The pulmonary anulus is narrow and the leaflets are usually thickened and bicuspid. The pulmonary artery is hypoplastic from its origin to its intrapulmonary branches. The ductus arteriosus is patent in about one fourth of these patients. *Ic,* There is a medium-sized VSD with normal or large pulmonary valve and main pulmonary artery. *IIa,* The VSD is large, and the right ventricular wall is thicker than it is in Type I. There is pulmonary atresia and the aorta arises from the right ventricle. The ductus arteriosus is often patent but usually inadequate in size. *IIb,* The VSD is large and high, extending to the semilunar valves. The aorta is occasionally overriding. The pulmonary stenosis can be valvar, subpulmonary, or both. *IIc,* The VSD is usually large; the pulmonary artery can be two to four times the diameter of the aorta. Systemic blood flow is frequently reduced owing to right ventricular infundibular stenosis, small VSD, aortic coarctation, aortic atresia, or relative hypoplasia of the aorta. Aortic coarctation or hypoplasia is commonly associated with this type. *III,* Tricuspid atresia in *l*-transposition with *d*-bulboventricular loop is very rare; it has been described in association with both subpulmonary and subaortic stenosis. Two patients have been described with *l*-transposition and *l*-bulboventricular loop with atresia of the left atrioventricular valve (tricuspid atresia); both had obstruction of the pulmonary outflow tract. Modified from Keith, J. D., Rowe, R. D., and Vlad, P.: Heart Disease in Infancy and Childhood. New York, Macmillan Co., 1967.

TRICUSPID ATRESIA WITH NORMALLY RELATED GREAT ARTERIES

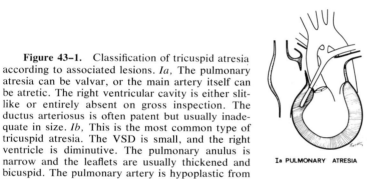

Ia PULMONARY ATRESIA

Ib PULMONARY HYPOPLASIA, SMALL VENTRICULAR SEPTAL DEFECT

Ic NO PULMONARY HYPOPLASIA, LARGE VENTRICULAR SEPTAL DEFECT

TRICUSPID ATRESIA WITH *d*-TRANSPOSITION

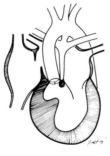
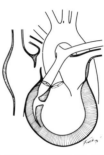
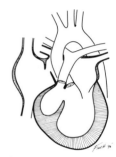

IIa PULMONARY ATRESIA

IIb PULMONARY STENOSIS

IIc LARGE PULMONARY ARTERY

TRICUSPID ATRESIA WITH *l*-TRANSPOSITION

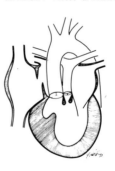
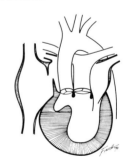
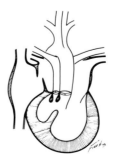

III SUBPULMONARY OR SUBAORTIC STENOSIS

defect (VSD). This classification was later expanded by Keith and associates (1979) and by Paul (1968) to include a small group of patients with *l*-transposition of the great arteries. It is illustrated in Figure 43–1: Type I is tricuspid atresia without transposition; Type II is tricuspid atresia with *d*-transposition; and Type III is tricuspid atresia with *l*-transposition. Each of these major divisions is further subdivided according to other associated anomalies. Rao's recent classification (1980) retains the same Types I and II but subdivides Type III into several malpositions and adds Type IV, persistent truncus arteriosus.

PATHOPHYSIOLOGY

Certain hemodynamic features are shared by all patients with tricuspid atresia: (1) The entire systemic venous return must traverse the atrial septum; therefore, if the atrial septal defect is small, the systemic venous pressure is high and can produce the clinical picture of right heart failure. (2) All the return from both the systemic veins and the pulmonary veins is mixed in the left atrium; this admixture leads to systemic arterial desaturation. (3) The right ventricle is small, so that the burden of the workload for both circulations falls on the left ventricle.

There are two distinct physiologic variants associated with different anatomic types. One group has reduced pulmonary blood flow and includes Types Ia, Ib, IIa, and IIb, representing 71 per cent of patients with tricuspid atresia (Keith *et al.*, 1979). Because of the relatively low pulmonary flow, a small volume of saturated blood is available for mixing in the left atrium; therefore, these patients usually have moderate to severe clinical cyanosis. The small pulmonary flow also results in a proportionately reduced volume load on the left ventricle, so that left heart failure is minimal or absent.

A different physiologic pattern is associated with Types Ic and IIc, in which there is no obstruction to pulmonary blood flow. Because of the increased volume of pulmonary flow, these patients have only mild to moderate desaturation and clinically may have no cyanosis. Both groups may present with congestive heart failure, often mild in Type Ic, but usually severe in Type IIc. The prognosis is quite different in these two groups. Because of the severe pulmonary plethora, congestive heart failure, and high incidence of associated coarctation or hypoplasia of the aorta, patients with type IIc tricuspid atresia are likely to die before they are 2 or 3 months old (Marcano *et al.*, 1969); those who do not die often develop pulmonary vascular obstructive disease (Dick *et al.*, 1975). Patients without transposition (Type Ic), on the other hand, frequently develop progressive cyanosis with a decrease in pulmonary blood flow and a decrease in heart size, possibly due to a closing VSD (Gallaher and Fyler, 1967; Marcano *et al.*, 1969). These patients are, in effect, converted to Type Ib: most will require shunt surgery.

A few patients with transposition and increased pulmonary flow (Types IIc and III) have obstruction to systemic arterial flow because of either subaortic infundibular stenosis or a small VSD. Obstruction to systemic blood flow can be progressive, owing to a closing VSD, and can require operative intervention (Neches *et al.*, 1973).

CLINICAL FEATURES

The most constant clinical finding in tricuspid atresia is cyanosis (Nadas and Fyler, 1972). The occurrence of cyanotic spells, manifested by dyspnea, cyanosis, and occasionally syncope, is a grave sign, since it usually indicates a decreasing pulmonary blood flow due to an inadequate ventricular septal defect or a closing ductus arteriosus. Squatting occurs rarely, but clubbing is constantly present in patients over the age of 2 years. Dyspnea may be a striking clinical feature; it appears to be directly related to the degree of hypoxia. Signs of systemic venous congestion, including hepatomegaly, pulsation of jugular veins and of the liver, and peripheral edema, may be associated either with a small atrial septal communication or with congestive heart failure. When increased pulmonary blood flow is present, signs of pulmonary congestion or pulmonary edema may appear.

About three fourths of patients with diminished pulmonary blood flow have a systolic murmur (Robicsek *et al.*, 1956). In patients with increased pulmonary blood flow, there is always a relatively loud systolic murmur along the left sternal border or at the apex; a mid-diastolic rumble is occasionally heard. The murmur of a patent ductus arteriosus suggests the presence of pulmonary atresia but may also be heard in Type Ib tricuspid atresia.

On the electrocardiogram, left axis deviation is found in almost 90 per cent of patients; its presence in a cyanotic child should raise a strong suspicion of tricuspid atresia. Right axis deviation occurs with transposition of the great arteries with a large pulmonary artery (Type IIc). Left ventricular hypertrophy is almost always present and can progress with age (Fig. 43–2). The P wave may show right atrial hypertrophy, left atrial hypertrophy, or combined atrial hypertrophy. P-tricuspidale (notched P wave with a taller initial peak) is sometimes seen.

The appearance of the chest roentgenograms (Fig. 43–3) is extremely variable (Wittenborg *et al.*, 1951). In most patients, the heart size is either normal or only slightly increased. Cardiomegaly may become quite marked, however, when pulmonary blood flow is large. The cardiac silhouette is usually not helpful. A characteristic configuration of the heart in tricuspid atresia 'has been described: a flattened right heart border, an abnormally rounded left border, an elevated apex, and a concave pulmonary artery segment. However, the cardiac configuration may resemble the "coeur-en-sabot" that is seen in tetralogy of Fallot or the "egg-shaped heart" with a narrow vascular pedicle that is typical of transposition of the great arteries.

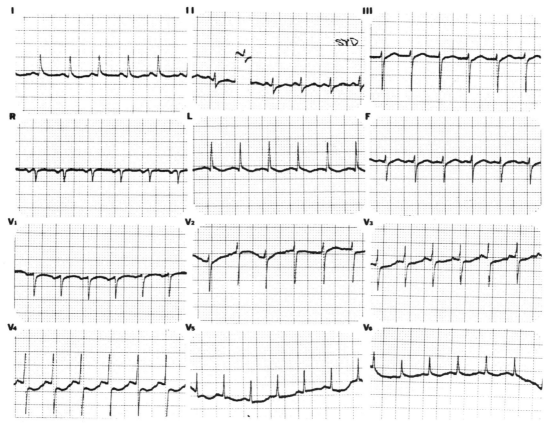

Figure 43–2. Electrocardiogram of a newborn with tricuspid atresia. Diagnostic features are left axis deviation, left ventricular hypertrophy, and almost complete absence of right ventricular forces.

The pulmonary vascular markings are usually reduced. Older patients sometimes have evidence of extensive pulmonary collateral circulation. Radiographic patterns of normal flow can be seen, especially in Types Ic and IIb. Pulmonary plethora can be seen in a number of circumstances: transposition of the great arteries with a large pulmonary artery, normally related great arteries with a large ventricular septal defect, pulmonary atresia with a large patent ductus arteriosus, and postoperatively in patients who have

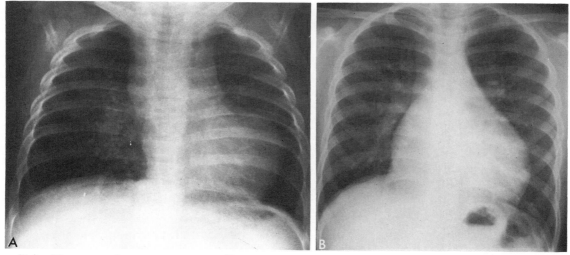

Figure 43–3. These two chest roentgenograms illustrate the extremely wide variation in appearance of tricuspid atresia. *A,* Tetralogy-like appearance. This patient has decreased pulmonary blood flow, a "coeur-en-sabot" configuration of the left heart border with elevated apex and concave pulmonary artery segment, and no evidence of right atrial enlargement. *B,* Transposition-like appearance. In contrast to the patient in *A,* this patient has increased pulmonary blood flow, a rounded left heart border, enlarged right atrial shadow, and narrow great vessels shadow. There is no diagnostic or consistent plain chest film finding in tricuspid atresia.

had systemic–to–pulmonary artery shunts (Keith *et al.*, 1979). A right aortic arch is seen in 8 per cent of patients.

CARDIAC CATHETERIZATION AND ANGIOCARDIOGRAPHY

Angiocardiography is diagnostic for tricuspid atresia (Cooley *et al.*, 1950). There is a typical sequence of appearance of contrast material in the cardiac chambers after a venous or right atrial injection: The contrast material appears in the left atrium, the left ventricle, and, finally, the great arteries. This sequence is not pathognomonic since it can also be seen in such lesions as pulmonary atresia with intact ventricular septum and tricuspid stenosis. Also typical

of tricuspid atresia is the so-called "right ventricular window," which is a triangular area within the heart shadow that fails to fill with contrast medium early in the ventricular phase. The triangular defect has its base on the diaphragm; its sides are formed by the right atrium and inferior vena cava on the right and by the left ventricle on the left (Fig. 43–4). This shadow is due to the absence of the inflow portion of the right ventricle. The triangle sometimes opacifies late in the injection owing to filling of a small right ventricle through the VSD.

Angiography also gives information about the size of the cardiac chambers and the relations of the great arteries. The size and location of the VSD and of the great arteries are sometimes best delineated by selective injection of the left ventricle, especially in the left anterior oblique or lateral projections.

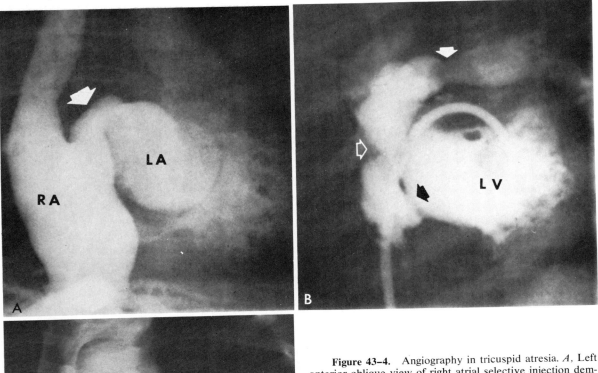

Figure 43–4. Angiography in tricuspid atresia. *A,* Left anterior oblique view of right atrial selective injection demonstrates flow of contrast material directly into the left atrium through septal communication (arrow), and no flow into the right ventricle. *B,* Left anterior oblique view of left ventricular selective injection demonstrates three levels of obstruction to pulmonary blood flow: small ventricular septal defect (black arrow), obstructive infundibulum (open arrow), and pulmonary anular stenosis (white arrow). *C,* Late frame from anteroposterior projection of right atrial angiogram shows filling of the cardiac chambers and great vessels. The radiolucent triangular "right ventricular window" diagnostic of tricuspid atresia is clearly seen (arrow). It represents the atretic inflow portion of the right ventricle. The triangle is based on the diaphragm, bordered on the right by the right atrium and on the left by the left ventricle. (LA = left atrium; LV = left ventricle; RA = right atrium.)

Cardiac catheterization data are characteristic. The right ventricle cannot be entered through the tricuspid valve. There is a very prominent A wave in the right atrium, a right-to-left shunt at the atrial level, and often a pressure gradient across the atrial septum. The magnitude of the gradient depends on the size of the atrial septal defect and on the left atrial pressure: The gradient is large when there is a small atrial septal defect or decreased pulmonary blood flow; conversely, the gradient is small when there is a large atrial septal defect or increased pulmonary blood flow. Identical oxygen saturations are found in the left atrium, left ventricle, right ventricle, and great arteries. The systemic arterial oxygen saturation is directly related to the magnitude of pulmonary blood flow.

NATURAL HISTORY

The natural history of tricuspid atresia indicates a tendency toward early death (Keith et al., 1979). Only half of these patients are alive at the age of 6 months, and only a third survive for 1 year. By 10 years, 90 per cent are dead.

The prognosis correlates closely with pulmonary blood flow. Children with extremely high pulmonary blood flow (Type IIc) or extremely low pulmonary blood flow (Types Ia and IIa) usually die before the age of 3 months. The longest survivors are those with the most nearly normal pulmonary flow: the average survival of patients with Type Ib is 11 months, that of those with Type Ic is 8 years, and that of those with Type IIb is over 7 years (Keith et al., 1979). The oldest survivors are patients with Type IIc; the oldest on record was 56 years.

A poor prognosis is foretold by the early onset of cyanosis, absence of a significant murmur, and a roentgenographic pattern of either markedly increased or markedly decreased pulmonary blood flow. A good prognosis is associated with the converse findings: late onset of cyanosis, a loud systolic murmur, and normal vascular markings on the chest roentgenogram.

PALLIATIVE TREATMENT

Three clinically important physiologic abnormalities associated with tricuspid atresia can be surgically palliated: (1) Cyanosis can be improved by systemic–to–pulmonary artery shunt procedures. (2) Right heart failure due to inadequate atrial septal communication can be relieved by atrial septostomy or septectomy. (3) Increased pulmonary blood flow can be decreased by pulmonary artery banding.

Increasing Pulmonary Blood Flow

The most common indication for palliation in tricuspid atresia is the presence of symptomatic cyanosis, which is seen in patients with decreased pulmonary blood flow (Types Ia, Ib, IIa, and IIb). The objective of operation is to increase the delivery of desaturated blood to the pulmonary capillary bed. The systemic arterial blood is markedly desaturated in these children; therefore, a systemic artery–to–pulmonary artery shunt can provide the desired increase in pulmonary flow, as can a systemic vein–to–pulmonary artery anastomosis. Each type of shunt has distinctive advantages and disadvantages, related to both technical and physiologic considerations.

The first palliative operation for cyanotic congenital heart disease was performed by Blalock on November 19, 1944 (Blalock and Taussig, 1945): a subclavian–to–pulmonary artery shunt in a patient with tetralogy of Fallot. Within a few months, he performed the same operation in a patient with tricuspid atresia, the first palliation for that disease (Taussig et al., 1973). The anastomosis is ideally performed on the side on which the subclavian artery arises from the innominate artery, that is, on the side opposite the aortic arch. There had been a high incidence of shunt failure with use of the subclavian artery arising from the aortic arch (Taussig et al., 1971), until Laks and Castaneda (1975) described subclavian arterioplasty, which has markedly improved the results of ipsilateral shunts. The major advantage of the Blalock-Taussig anastomosis is that the shunt is seldom excessive: The size of the anastomosis is limited by the cross-sectional diameter of the subclavian artery, and the flow is further limited by resistance along the length of the subclavian artery segment. Of 33 patients with tricuspid atresia who survived Blalock-Taussig shunts at Great Ormond Street, only three had mild congestive heart failure and one had moderate congestive heart failure. None required reoperation (Deverall et al., 1969). The main disadvantage of this shunt is the small size of the subclavian artery in small infants. This problem is demonstrated by the Great Ormond Street series: The mortality rate after Blalock-Taussig anastomosis in patients under the age of 6 months was 63 per cent, and in those over the age of 6 months, it was 3 per cent. Much better results have been achieved in infants in some recent series.

The year after Blalock and Taussig introduced their anastomosis, Potts and coworkers (1946) described their clinical results with a descending aorta–to–left pulmonary artery anastomosis. Its advantages include relative ease of construction and low incidence of thrombosis, even in very small infants. However, too large a shunt results in congestive heart failure, which may be severe enough to require reoperation and a narrowing procedure; such failure can occur early if a large anastomosis is made at surgery, or late if the anastomosis grows disproportionately (Cole et al., 1971; Hallman et al., 1968; Paul et al., 1969). In children with large flow who survive congestive heart failure, pulmonary artery hypertension due to pulmonary vascular obstructive disease may complicate the late clinical picture (von Bernuth et al., 1971). An additional technical problem posed by the

Potts shunt is the difficulty attending its obliteration at the time of definitive repair in patients with correctable lesions. The possibility of correction now weighs against the use of the Potts shunt in patients with tricuspid atresia.

In 1962, Waterston introduced the ascending aorta–to–right pulmonary artery shunt, performed intrapericardially. Like the Potts operation, the Waterston shunt can be done relatively easily in small infants, even those with a small pulmonary artery. However, it is not as difficult to close at the time of definitive operation as the Potts anastomosis; in most cases, the aorta can be cross-clamped and opened, and the anastomosis can be closed by suture or patch (Sade *et al.*, 1977). It shares a major disadvantage with the Potts shunt, however, in that there is a relatively high incidence of congestive heart failure, sometimes requiring reoperation to narrow the anastomosis (Edmunds *et al.*, 1971; Somerville *et al.*, 1969). Kinking at the anastomosis can cause obstruction of the right pulmonary artery; this requires reconstruction of the pulmonary artery at the time of corrective surgery. The incidence of this complication varies widely in different series (Ashcraft, 1973; Gay and Ebert, 1973).

Ascending aorta–to–main pulmonary artery anastomosis has also been performed successfully in tricuspid atresia (Arguero *et al.*, 1969) and was first described by Davidson (1955) (Fig. 43–5). The advantages of this anastomosis are similar to those of the Waterston shunt; in addition, there is almost no ten-

sion on the suture line, kinking of the pulmonary artery is unlikely to occur, blood flow through the pulmonary artery is not interrupted during the operation, and the anastomosis can be closed through the pulmonary artery at the time of corrective surgery. The distribution of blood flow through the shunt may be more symmetric than after other, more peripheral shunts.

The introduction of the polytetrafluoroethylene tube graft has made possible construction of a prosthetic conduit from a systemic artery to a pulmonary artery with a good probability of continued patency. Long-term experience with this technique is not available as yet, but in the medium term, the graft remains patent in 80 per cent of the patients. McKay and associates (1980) and Donahoo and coworkers (1980) have suggested constructing the graft from side of subclavian artery to side of pulmonary artery (Fig. 43–6). A large graft (5 mm.) can then be used even in the newborn, since flow through the graft is limited by the diameter of the subclavian artery. We have used this technique in 17 children, with three shunt failures (17 per cent) and no instance of congestive heart failure.

The wall of the ductus arteriosus may be infiltrated with formaldehyde in the newborn to maintain patency for palliation of cyanotic congenital heart disease (Hatem *et al.*, 1980). Because palliation with this technique is measured only in months, we believe it is not appropriate for palliation of tricuspid atresia.

The diversion of vena caval blood directly into

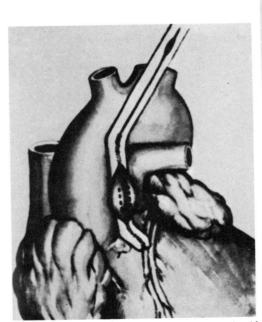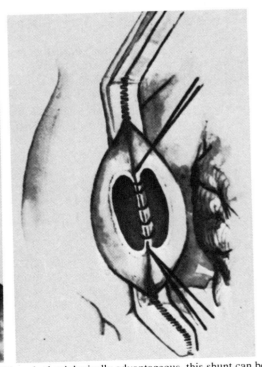

Figure 43–5. Main pulmonary artery–to–aorta anastomosis. Although physiologically advantageous, this shunt can be used in only a limited number of tricuspid atresia patients because of the frequently small size or posterior location of pulmonary artery. (From Arguero, R., *et al.*: Surgical production of aorticopulmonary window in congenital heart disease with ischemic lung. J. Thorac. Cardiovasc. Surg., 57:786, 1969.)

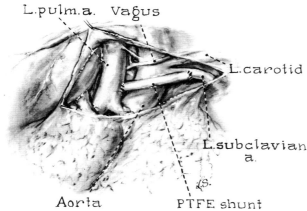

L.pulm.a. Vagus

L.carotid

L.subclavian a.

Aorta   PTFE shunt

Figure 43–6. Modified Blalock-Taussig anastomosis. In newborn infants, a length of large (5-mm.) Gore-Tex graft may be interposed between the subclavian artery and the pulmonary artery. Shunt flow is limited by the diameter of the subclavian artery. (PTFE = polytetrafluorethylene). (From Donahoo, J. S., Gardner, T. J., Zahka, K., and Kidd, B. S. L.: Systemic-Pulmonary shunts in neonates and infants using microporous expanded polytetrafluoroethylene: Immediate and late results. Ann. Thorac. Surg., *3* :146, 1980.)

the pulmonary arterial tree was first suggested as a means of treating cyanotic congenital heart disease and was proved to be feasible experimentally by Carlon and coworkers in 1951. Further observations were made by Glenn and Patino (1954) (see Fig. 43–5). These early studies and their own experimental observations led Robicsek and associates (1958, 1969) to cite the following advantages of cavopulmonary anastomosis over arterial anastomoses: (1) The operation is technically easy to perform. (2) Pure venous blood is supplied to the right lung, and pulmonary blood flow is adequate despite only slightly higher systemic venous pressure than normal. (3) Ventilation and oxygen exchange on the side of the shunt are almost the same as in the contralateral lung. (4) The bypass places no extra workload on the heart. (5) The blood pressure in the pulmonary arterial tree is not increased and thus does not lead to the pulmonary hypertension that is sometimes seen after systemic artery shunts. (6) Endarteritis is less likely to occur with a venous than with an arterial shunt.

Since the initial clinical reports in the United States by Glenn (1958) and in the Soviet Union by Bakulev and Kolesnikov (1959), a large clinical experience with the cavopulmonary anastomosis has demonstrated two major problems associated with it: the early development of the superior vena cava syndrome and late deterioration of function of the shunt. The superior vena caval syndrome, consisting of venous distention and edema of the upper half of the body, can develop in about 20 per cent of patients with tricuspid atresia who have a cavopulmonary shunt (Mathur and Glenn, 1973; Trusler *et al.*, 1971). This incidence can be markedly reduced if the superior vena cava pressure is kept below 30 cm. of water by incomplete ligation of the cavoatrial junction (Saki-

yalak *et al.*, 1971) or by delayed ligation of the azygos vein (Edwards and Bargeron, 1968). Because of the likelihood of obstruction, a cavopulmonary shunt should not be done when the pulmonary artery is less than the diameter of the superior vena cava (Edwards and Bargeron, 1968; Glenn *et al.*, 1968; Trusler *et al.*, 1971). In his collected series of 255 patients with tricuspid atresia who had cavopulmonary shunts, Glenn found that the mortality rate in patients under 1 month of age was 95 per cent, in those between 1 and 6 months old, it was 46 per cent; and in those over 6 months old, it was 18 per cent (Glenn *et al.*, 1966). The very high mortality during infancy has been attributed to the high pulmonary vascular resistance at that age and to the small size of the pulmonary artery. Edwards and Bargeron (1968) reported a series of 23 cavopulmonary shunts using vigorous fluid replacement and delayed ligation of the azygos vein, with only two deaths, both of which occurred in infants under the age of 1 month. There were eight infants under 3 months old, and three between 3 and 6 months of age.

The second major problem with cavopulmonary anastomosis has been late clinical deterioration. Increasing cyanosis with rising hematocrit and hemoglobin may appear at 1 to 5 years after cavopulmonary shunt (Martin *et al.*, 1970; Robicsek *et al.*, 1969; Sakiyalak *et al.*, 1971), although in some series this has been a rare problem (Edwards, 1971). Deterioration can be associated with obstruction to blood flow to the left lung due to infundibular hypertrophy (Gabriele, 1970), progressive closure of the ventricular septal defect, or increasing pulmonary valvar obstruction (Glenn *et al.*, 1968). It might also be due to imbalance of ventilation and perfusion of the right lung, as caval flow is displaced to the lower lobe by increasing bronchial collateral flow to the upper and middle lobes (Mathur and Glenn, 1973). However, increasing cyanosis is more frequently associated with decreasing blood flow through the right lung. The nature of the declining shunt flow has been the subject of considerable interest. Early in the experience with cavopulmonary shunts, there was concern that the development of collateral circulation between the superior and inferior vena cava might deprive the right lung of some of its flow. Extensive collaterals sometimes develop (Mathur and Glenn, 1973) and have been cited as a major cause of late clinical deterioration in one series (Laks *et al.*, 1977). Long-term follow-up has revealed, however, that 80 to 85 per cent of the superior vena cava flow may continue to pass through the right pulmonary artery, both experimentally (Calabrese *et al.*, 1968) and clinically (Glenn *et al.*, 1970). A left superior vena cava can "steal" blood flow from the right lung; the flow can be improved by ligation (Sakiyalak *et al.*, 1971) or banding (Oparil *et al.*, 1972) of the anomalous vessel. The decreasing shunt flow could be related to high pulmonary vascular resistance caused by increasing viscosity of blood due to rising hematocrit (Mathur and Glenn, 1973). It is probably not due to thromboemboli

(Boruchow *et al.*, 1970). The increasing pulmonary vascular resistance is associated with a progressive decrease in perfusion of the upper and middle lobes of the right lung (Boruchow *et al.*, 1970; Trusler *et al.*, 1971).

Whatever the reasons for the late deterioration after cavopulmonary shunt, additional surgery to improve oxygenation is necessary in many patients (Sachs *et al.*, 1968; Sakiyalak *et al.*, 1971), usually between the ages of 8 and 12 years (Glenn and Fenn, 1972). These additional operations can be a systemic artery–to–left pulmonary artery shunt, ligation of collateral venous connections, correction of the cardiac defect (Mathur and Glenn, 1973), or construction of a right axillary arteriovenous fistula (Glenn and Fenn, 1972). The number of patients requiring such additional surgery can be high (11 of 17 patients in one series [Pennington *et al.*, 1981]) or low (only three of 52 survivors in another series [Rosenthal, 1980]). In Glenn's series (Mathur and Glenn, 1973), only 22 of 56 long-term survivors of cavopulmonary shunt (39 per cent) had adequate arterial saturations with cavopulmonary shunt alone. When pulmonary arteriovenous fistulas develop after cavopulmonary anastomosis, some patients may benefit by reconstruction of the cavoatrial junction and ligation of the right pulmonary artery (Van Den Bogaert-Van Heesvelde, *et al.*, 1978).

Because the cavopulmonary anastomosis is mutilating and normal anatomy is difficult to reconstruct, the presence of a correctable congenital heart lesion is generally considered to be a contraindication to its use. Tricuspid atresia is now a correctable lesion (Fontan and Baudet, 1971). Although the original clinical correction employed the construction of a cavopulmonary shunt, this procedure is probably not necessary (Kreutzer *et al.*, 1973); indeed, it may be disadvantageous because it deprives the right lung of a pulsatile blood flow (Furuse *et al.*, 1972). For these reasons, in addition to the problems already discussed, we no longer use the cavopulmonary shunt in the treatment of tricuspid atresia, despite its proven safety.

Trusler and Williams (1978) reviewed the Toronto experience with palliative operation for 148 children with tricuspid atresia. The Potts anastomosis was used in 52 patients, the Blalock-Taussig in 46, the Glenn in 22, and others in 28. The mortality rate after the initial operation in patients under 6 months of age was 47 per cent; in those over 6 months of age, it was 14 per cent. The patients who survived their first operation had an 84 per cent chance of living at least 10 years and 72 per cent chance of living for 15 years (Fig. 43–7). Thus, after the first operation, the overall initial mortality rate was 30 per cent, that at 10 years postoperatively was 41 per cent, and that at 15 years postoperatively was 49 per cent. These figures are similar to those from the series at Children's Hospital in Boston (Dick *et al.*, 1975) and at the Johns Hopkins Hospital (Taussig *et al.*, 1973).

An alternative to systemic–to–pulmonary artery anastomosis to increase pulmonary blood flow was suggested by Brock (1964): reconstructing the right ventricular outflow tract. Annecchino and associates (1980) reported five patients who had a previous shunt that was failing and did not satisfy the criteria for corrective operation. Their patients underwent enlargement of a restrictive VSD and infundibuloplasty or pulmonary valvotomy. All survived, and four had significant clinical improvement. Besides improving

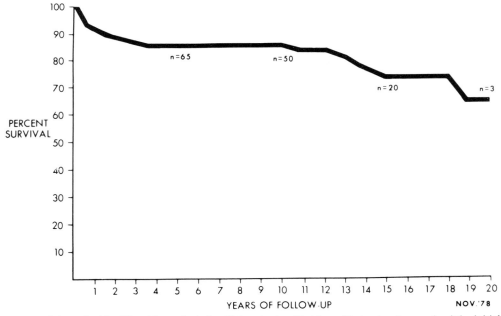

Figure 43–7. Actuarial survival by life-table analysis for 104 patients with tricuspid atresia who survived the initial shunt operation. (From Trusler, G. A., and Williams, W. G.: Long-term results of shunt procedures for tricuspid atresia. Ann. Thorac. Surg., *29*:312, 1978.)

pulmonary blood flow, this technique may provide a suitable stimulus for symmetric growth of hypoplastic pulmonary arteries, allowing later completion of corrective operation by closure of the VSD and connection of the right atrium to the right ventricle.

We now use palliative operations for two subgroups of patients with tricuspid atresia: those who are physiologically unsuited for corrective operation, and patients under 2 to 3 years of age. All others undergo corrective operation. Within the limitations noted above, we believe that any systemic–to–pulmonary artery anastomosis that can be performed safely by the surgeon is suitable palliation. Our own preference is either a Blalock-Taussig shunt or, in newborns, a prosthetic shunt of 5-mm. polytetrafluoroethylene from the side of the subclavian artery arising from the aortic arch to the side of the ipsilateral pulmonary artery. When the initial shunt fails, we do a corrective operation if possible; if it is not possible, we perform a Blalock-Taussig shunt on the opposite side or reconstruct the right ventricular outflow tract.

Enlargement of Atrial Septal Communications

The interatrial communication is a patent foramen ovale in two thirds of the patients with tricuspid atresia and a defect of the atrial septum in the remaining third (Keith et al., 1979). The communication is probably inadequate if there are pulsatile neck veins and a pulsatile liver, the EKG shows tall P waves, a large right atrium is seen on the chest roentgenogram (Keith et al., 1979), and there is a significant pressure difference between the two atria (> 5 mm. Hg) (Nadas and Fyler, 1972). In such a situation, it is necessary to enlarge the interatrial communication. Since it can be difficult to judge the adequacy of the interatrial communication, some recommend that every newborn with tricuspid atresia have a balloon septostomy at the time of initial catheterization (Deverall et al., 1969; Pujatti et al., 1967; Rashkind and Miller, 1966; Rashkind et al., 1969; Singh et al., 1968). Balloon septostomy has been used successfully in a 21-month-old child with tricuspid atresia (Lenox and Zuberbuhler, 1970).

Surgical creation of an atrial septal defect by a closed technique was first described by Blalock and Hanlon (1950); their method remains the most widely used of several available. Open atrial septectomy performed under inflow occlusion has been used in tricuspid atresia (Hallman et al., 1968; Lindesmith et al., 1966). Other closed techniques of enlarging the atrial septum have also been described (Fonkalsrud and Linde, 1971; Rastan and Koncz, 1971). Surgical septectomy is rarely necessary in tricuspid atresia.

Pulmonary Artery Banding

Patients with tricuspid atresia associated with transposition of the great arteries and a large ventricular septal defect (Type IIc) usually have pulmonary artery hypertension and excessive pulmonary blood flow associated with severe congestive heart failure. The clinical course can be complicated by respiratory infections, severe limitation of activity, and failure to thrive. These patients usually die by 2 months of age.

Longer survival can be achieved and symptoms effectively relieved by constriction of the pulmonary artery with a band, as originally suggested by Muller and Dammann (1952). This procedure increases resistance to flow from the right ventricle to the pulmonary artery, consequently reducing pulmonary blood flow. The resulting reduction in the left-to-right shunt improves congestive heart failure and protects the pulmonary arterioles against the development of pulmonary vascular obstructive disease.

Almost all infants with tricuspid atresia who require pulmonary banding have Type IIc, which constitutes only 18 per cent of patients with tricuspid atresia (Keith et al., 1979). There has been no single large experience with banding for this lesion, but combining several small series from the literature (Glenn et al., 1968; Hallman et al., 1968; Idriss et al., 1968; Neches et al., 1973; Ochsner et al., 1962; Rashkind et al., 1969) with our own cases produces a total of 20 patients with tricuspid atresia who had pulmonary artery banding, six of whom died (30 per cent). Of those who survived operation, almost all had marked improvement of symptoms.

Although patients without transposition with a large VSD (Type Ic) often have increased pulmonary flow, they usually respond to medical management and rarely require pulmonary artery banding; only one child without transposition who required banding has been reported (Tingelstad et al., 1971), and we have seen two in our series. These patients often develop decreasing flow with increasing cyanosis, owing to closing VSD, and later require a palliative shunt (Gallaher and Fyler, 1967; Marcano et al., 1969).

CORRECTIVE OPERATION

Surgical correction of tricuspid atresia was made possible by an important conceptual change, the realization that a ventricle is not necessary to maintain an adequate pulmonary circulation (Sade and Castaneda, 1975). The development of corrective operations was stimulated in part by the availability of valve-bearing conduits for cardiovascular reconstruction.

Experimental Background

Experimental bypass of a semilunar valve was first performed by Carrel in 1910, when he temporarily bypassed the aortic valve by placing a vein graft between the left ventricle and the descending aorta. Rodbard and Wagner (1949) bypassed the pulmonary valve by anastomosing the right atrial appendage to the main pulmonary artery distal to a ligature on the pulmonary artery (Fig 43–8a). Right ventricular bypass was not complete in their animals because of

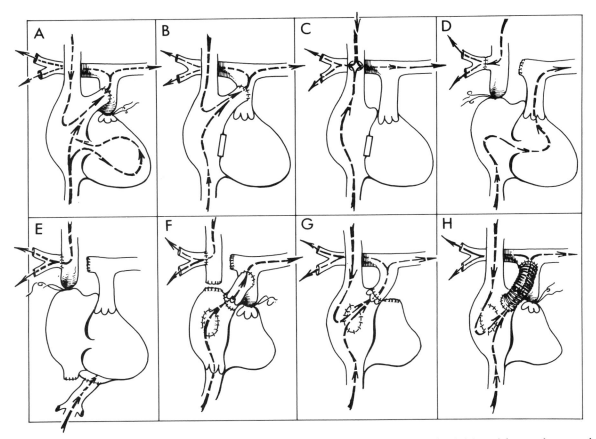

Figure 43–8. Successive steps in the development of right ventricular bypass. *a,* Anastomosis of right atrial appendage to pulmonary artery (Rodbard and Wagner, 1949). *b,* Anastomosis of right atrial appendage to pulmonary artery with ligation of tricuspid valve (Warden *et al.,* 1954). *c,* Anastomosis of side of vena cava to side of right pulmonary artery (Haller *et al.,* 1966). *d,* Anastomosis of side of vena cava to end of distal right pulmonary artery with ligation of cavo-atrial junction (Carlon *et al.,* 1951). *e,* Same as *d* but with inferior vena cava divided and connected to left atrium (Robicsek *et al.,* 1966). *f,* Fontan's original operation (Fontan *et al.,* 1971). (See text.) *g,* One of Kreutzer's modifications of Fontan's procedure, simply closing atrial septal defect and connecting pulmonary anulus directly to right atrial appendage (Kreutzer *et al.,* 1973). *h,* Same as *g* but using prosthetic graft from right atrium to pulmonary artery (Henry *et al.,* 1974). (From Sade, R. M., and Castaneda, A. R.: The dispensable right ventricle. Surgery, 77:624, 1975.)

functional tricuspid regurgitation, but survival was achieved.

The first use of a valve-bearing conduit to bypass the pulmonary valve was by Donovan (1950), who used preserved valve-containing femoral and jugular allografts to conduct blood from the right ventricle to the left pulmonary artery distal to a ligature. He later used allograft veins to bypass the pulmonary valve completely, from the right ventricle to the proximally ligated main pulmonary artery (Donovan *et al.,* 1951).

The use of aortic allografts in clinical surgery was introduced by Gross and associates in 1949 for the treatment of coarctation of the aorta. An aortic allograft with an intact, functional valve was first used clinically for reconstruction of the pulmonary artery by Ross and Somerville (1966); such grafts were popularized by the Mayo Clinic group (McGoon *et al.,* 1973). Pulmonary artery reconstruction with a valve-bearing conduit has also been accomplished with a Dacron tube containing either an allograft valve (Kouchoukos *et al.,* 1971) or a preserved xenograft valve (Bowman *et al.,* 1973).

Warden and coworkers (1954) did the classic experiments proving the right ventricle to be unnec-

essary (Fig. 43–8*b*). They succeeded in bypassing the right ventricle and pulmonary valve by a staged ligation of the tricuspid valve and anastomosis of the right atrial appendage to the main pulmonary artery. They had several long-term survivors. Haller and colleagues (1966) also succeeded in completely bypassing the right ventricle; they ligated the tricuspid valve and did a side-to-side anastomosis between the superior vena cava and the right pulmonary artery (Fig 43–8*c*). It should be pointed out that both Warden and Haller's groups had long-term survivors among their animals despite the fact that there was no valve at all in the right heart circuit. Just-Viera and associates (1971, 1973) bypassed the right ventricle by closing the tricuspid valve and placing a pulmonary artery valve-bearing allograft between the right atrium and the pulmonary artery. In a similar preparation, Puga and McGoon (1973) showed an acute rise in cavoatrial pressures and a fall in cardiac output after right ventricular bypass in dogs.

Robicsek and coworkers (1956) were able to bypass the entire right heart with a multistage operation that diverted the inferior caval return into the left atrium and the superior caval return into the right lung

(Fig. 43–8*e*). This procedure was well tolerated by some animals, in one for over 4 years (Robicsek *et al.*, 1966), thus proving that exclusion of both the right atrium and the right ventricle from the circulation is compatible with long-term survival.

Recent experimental work has defined more clearly cardiopulmonary hemodynamics after right heart bypass in dogs with open chest (Matsuda *et al.*, 1981; Sade and Dearing, 1981; Shemin *et al.*, 1979). In these preparations, the tricuspid valve or pulmonary artery was closed and the right atrium was connected with the pulmonary artery by a valve-bearing conduit. In one model, a parallel conduit was placed without a valve (Shemin *et al.*, 1979) (Fig. 43–9). By measuring intracardiac flows and pressures under a variety of conditions, the investigators were able to reach several conclusions. A pulmonary valve after right heart bypass probably is not necessary, since pulmonary blood flow was not different whether a valve was present or not. The right atrium is not an effective pump immediately after right heart bypass, and the atrial rhythm is not an important determinant of cardiac output. Manipulation of ventilation characteristics did not change mean pulmonary blood flow, although phasic flow could be altered (Shemin *et al.*, 1979).

The most important determinants of pulmonary blood flow in dogs after right heart bypass are right

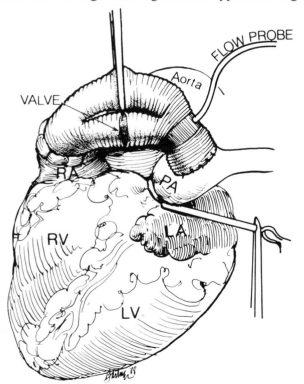

Figure 43–9. Experimental evaluation of right heart function after right ventricular bypass. Pulmonary blood flow was not changed by the presence or absence of a valve in the pulmonary artery. (From Shemin, R. J., Merrill, W. H., Pfeifer, J. S., Conkle, D. M., and Morrow, A. G.: Evaluation of right atrial–pulmonary artery conduits for tricuspid atresia. Experimental Study. J. Thorac. Cardiovasc. Surg., 77:685, 1979.)

atrial pressure, left atrial pressure, and pulmonary arterial resistance. Increasing right atrial pressure is directly and nearly linearly related to pulmonary blood flow (Matsuda *et al.*, 1981; Shemin *et al.*, 1979), mostly owing to declining resistance as pulmonary vessels are distended (Sade and Dearing, 1981). Since flow varies directly wih pressure difference across the capillary bed (Sade *et al.*, 1981), it is not surprising that lowering left atrial pressure results in rising pulmonary blood flow. This has been achieved with inotropic agents (Shemin *et al.*, 1979) and with left heart bypass (Sade and Dearing, 1981). Left ventricular function is a major determinant of cardiac output after right heart bypass (Sade and Dearing, 1981). Pulmonary vascular resistance can be manipulated with vasodilators and by controlling PCO_2 and pH. Reduction of resistance increases cardiac output by increasing pulmonary blood flow (Sade and Dearing, 1981).

Clinical Correction

The earliest clinical attempts to bypass the right ventricle were those of Hurwitt and coworkers (1955) and Shumacker (1955). They both connected the right atrial appendage to the pulmonary artery; Hurwitt and colleagues' patient died at operation; Shumacker's died a few hours after the operation. In 1962, Harrison described an infant who had a Glenn operation at the age of 15 months, anastomosis of the right atrial appendage to pulmonary artery at the age of 37 months, and closure of his atrial septal defect at the age of 44 months. This patient did well immediately after the third and final stage, with blood pressure in the normal range and caval pressure not markedly elevated, but died later with anuria.

Fontan and coworkers were the first to apply successfully the concept of right atrium–to–pulmonary artery bypass for clinical correction of tricuspid atresia (Fontan and Baudet, 1971; Fontan *et al.*, 1971). They originally thought it necessary to insert two allograft valves into the right heart circuit: one at the junction of the inferior vena cava with the right atrium to avoid splanchnic pooling and massive ascites, which had also been observed by others (Noland *et al.*, 1958; Robicsek *et al.*, 1956), and the other in the atrium–to–pulmonary artery conduit. In their original technique, the right pulmonary artery was transected, a superior vena cava–to–pulmonary artery anastomosis constructed, a valved aortic allograft inserted between the right atrial appendage and the proximal end of the right pulmonary artery, a pulmonary allograft valve placed at the inferior vena caval orifice, and atrial septal defect closed (Fig. 43–8*F*). Thus, inferior vena caval blood flowed into the right atrium and was then pumped through the valve-bearing conduit into the proximal stump of the right pulmonary artery and into the left lung. A small enough allograft was not available for one of their three patients, so they used only an inferior vena caval valve in that patient, suturing the proximal stump of the right pulmonary artery directly to the right atrium. The patient had a good clinical result.

Many modifications of Fontan's original operation have been successful. Division of the right pulmonary artery with anastomosis to the vena cava and the right atrium was shown to be unnecessary by Ross and Somerville in 1973. They placed an aortic allograft valve in the inferior vena cava and an allograft conduit from the right atrium to the main pulmonary artery. In the same year, Kreutzer and coworkers (1973) not only omitted cavopulmonary anastomosis, but also did not use a valve in the inferior vena cava; they simply closed the atrial septal communication and connected the right atrium to the pulmonary artery with an aortic allograft. A similar operation was described using a Dacron graft with a porcine valve from the atrium to the pulmonary artery (Henry *et al.*, 1974) (Fig. 43–8*H*). Kreutzer and associates (1973) corrected tricuspid atresia using no prosthetic material by disinserting the pulmonary anulus with its valve from the ventricle and connecting it to the right atrial appendage (Fig. 43–8*G*). Several surgeons have reported successful operations in which no valves were included in the pulmonary circuit by directly anastomosing the right atrial appendage to the pulmonary artery.

Other approaches to correction have been used under special anatomic circumstances. In patients who have normally related great arteries with right ventricular outflow chamber, pulmonary anulus, and pulmonary valve of adequate size, it is possible to connect the right atrium directly to the right ventricle, either by prosthetic conduit, with or without a valve, or by direct anastomosis of the right atrial appendage to the right ventricle (Fig. 43–10) (Bjork *et al.*, 1979; Bowman

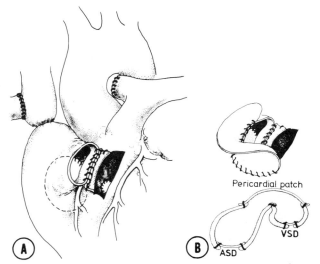

Figure 43–10. Anastomosis of the right atrial appendage to the right ventricular outflow tract. The cavopulmonary shunt shown here is not required. A pericardial patch is not always needed. The right atrial appendage may also be connected directly to the pulmonary artery with good result. (From Bjork, V. O., Olin, C. L., Bjarke, B. B., and Thoren, C. A.: Right atrial–right ventricular anastomosis for correction of tricuspid atresia. J. Thorac. Cardiovasc. Surg., *77*:452, 1979.)

et al., 1978; Fontan *et al.*, 1978; Henry *et al.*, 1974; Laks *et al.*, 1980; Murray *et al.*, 1977). This procedure has the advantage of allowing some potential for growth of the right ventricle, while using the patient's own pulmonary valve in situ. There has been one report of reconstruction of a right ventricular chamber using a sheet of Dacron containing a porcine valve (Gago *et al.*, 1976). A patient with tricuspid atresia, transposition of the great arteries, and previous pulmonary artery band underwent correction by arterial switch with coronary reimplantation and connection of the right atrium to the right ventricle with a valve-bearing conduit (Freedom *et al.*, 1980).

Results of Correction

Early in the experience with right ventricular bypass, the hospital mortality rate was high, up to 50 per cent (Tatooles *et al.*, 1976). Survival rates in recent series have been considerably better. For example, four of the first eight children (50 per cent) corrected by Fontan died. He then performed correction in 21 consecutive patients without a death (Fontan *et al.*, 1978). At the Mayo Clinic, three of the first seven patients undergoing right ventriclar bypass died (43 per cent), but only one of their next 22 patients died (4 per cent) (Gale *et al.*, 1980). Much of this improvement was due to better selection of patients for the procedure, avoiding those with high pulmonary vascular resistance (for example, small pulmonary arteries or obstructive pulmonary arterial disease) or high left atrial pressure (for example, left ventricular failure or mitral valve disease).

The hemodynamic results documented by follow-up cardiac catheterization have been satisfactory, although several abnormalities have been found (Hellenbrand *et al.*, 1981; Shachar *et al.*, 1981). At rest, right atrial pressure is usually in the range of 14 to 17 mm. Hg, with little or no pressure difference between right atrium and the pulmonary artery. The cardiac index is usually 2 to 3 L./min./M.² During exercise, right atrial pressure rises by 8 to 12 mm. Hg and pressure differences between the right atrium and the right ventricle appear in some cases. The cardiac index rises to 4 to 5 L./min./M.²; this increase is due mostly to rise in heart rate, since stroke volume changes little. Pulmonary arterial oxygen saturation falls from 68 to 32 per cent. The aortic oxygen saturation is usually good, in the range 87 to 97 per cent, but some residual right-to-left shunt through the atrial septum or across the pulmonary capillary bed is often detected. It should be pointed out that the patients with the best hemodynamic results may have a right atrial pressure less than 10 mm. Hg, no pressure difference between the atrium and the pulmonary artery, a cardiac index over 3 L./min./M.² at rest, and nearly normal responses to exercise.

Clinically, most patients do well postoperatively, despite hemodynamic abnormalities. Almost all have mild or moderate pleural effusion and ascites postoperatively, usually clearing within a week. They are rarely chronic problems. Although the cardiac rhythm is usually sinus, many patients have been reported with junctional rhythm and even heart block with little apparent deleterious effect. After a decade of follow-up, Fontan and associates (1978) reported only one patient who developed atrial fibrillation, which was successfully cardioverted to sinus rhythm. Obstruction of blood flow from the vena cava to the pulmonary artery may occur at several different levels: narrowing of anastomosis, residual pulmonary valve stenosis, prosthetic valve calcification, and fibrosis or thrombosis of the prosthetic conduit (Behrendt and Rosenthal, 1980). These complications have been reported in only a few patients, but they are expected to increase in incidence with the passage of time.

After repair, residual left-to-right shunts may remain because of incomplete closure of pre-existing shunt, residual ventricular septal defect, or extensive aortopulmonary collateral vessels. These seldom present a major problem. Liver dysfunction due to systemic venous hypertension may also be a long-term problem (Behrendt and Rosenthal, 1980).

Unresolved Questions about Right Ventricular Bypass

How Many Valves Are Necessary in the Right Heart? Fontan initially believed that valves in the inferior cavoatrial orifice and in the pulmonary artery were necessary (Fontan and Baudet, 1971). He used only an inferior cavoatrial valve in one of his original patients, however, and many patients have been reported since then in whom only one valve was used in the pulmonary position, either prosthetic or autogenous. Experimental data from the work of Rodbard and Wagner (1949), Warden and associates (1954), Haller and coworkers (1966), Shemin and colleagues (1979), and Sade and Dearing (1981) suggest that no valve is needed. Clinically, no valve has been used in many reported patients, with good results. Doty and associates (1981) described several methods of achieving direct anastomosis of the right atrium to the pulmonary artery, leaving no valves in the right heart. Of eight patients undergoing this procedure in their series, only one died.

Several workers have observed identical pressure curves in the venae cavae, right atrium, and pulmonary artery in patients who have only a pulmonary valve in place, and they have concluded that no valve is necessary. Hellenbrand and associates (1981) have documented antegrade flow throughout the cardiac cycle in six of seven patients late after right heart bypass, suggesting lack of function of the pulmonary valve. Yacoub (1978), however, has presented theoretical arguments and clinical follow-up data that suggest that inflow valves for both venae cavae and the pulmonary artery markedly improve the hemodynamic results of right heart bypass. In his patients with three right heart valves, the A wave was lower

in the venae cavae than it was in the right atrium and the pulmonary artery diastolic pressure was higher than that of the right atrium. Serial chest films showed reduction of heart size to within normal limits for three patients with caval valves, whereas the heart size increased in four patients without additional valves. The number of patients reported by Yacoub was small, and the postoperative hemodynamic data were not complete, but his analysis strongly suggested that two inflow valves in combination with a pulmonary valve may make an important hemodynamic difference late postoperatively.

Is It Useful to Include the Right Ventricle in the Repair? Many surgeons have demonstrated that the right ventricular outflow tract can be used in the correction of tricuspid atresia with normally related great arteries, thereby retaining the patient's own pulmonary valve. (Bjork et al., 1979; Bowman et al., 1978; Fontan et al., 1978; Henry et al., 1974; Laks et al., 1980; Murray et al., 1977). The right ventricular chamber seems likely to be too hypoplastic to serve as an effective pumping chamber, even with moderate growth. Nevertheless, Bowman and coworkers (1978) have reported nine patients who underwent repair with a valve-bearing conduit between the right atrium and the hypoplastic right ventricle, eight of whom survived. In the five recatheterized patients, the morphology of the atrial and pulmonary artery pressure curves was said to be normal, although the right atrial pressure and the right ventricular end-diastolic pressure were elevated. All right ventricles were said to have increased in size compared with the preoperative study. Each patient had angiographic evidence of contraction of the right ventricle. Bjork and associates (1979) anastomosed the right atrium directly to the right ventricle and reported growth of the right ventricle with reasonable function in one patient but no function in another. The value of using the hypoplastic right ventricle in the right heart circuit is not yet clear.

What is the Long-Term Incidence of Arrhythmias, and What is Their Effect on Cardiac Function? There have been several reports of junctional rhythm, atrial tachycardia, and complete heart block after right heart bypass. In most instances, there was little apparent effect on cardiac function, although a few patients developed a low output state that responded to cardioversion to sinus rhythm. The incidence of late arrhythmias has remained low, even after follow-up of more than a decade; nevertheless, much longer follow-up will be necessary before the true incidence and consequences of arrhythmias in these patients with hypertrophied and hypertensive right atria become apparent.

What Are the Proper Criteria for Selection of Suitable Candidates for Right Heart Bypass? The most detailed description of selection criteria is that of the Bordeaux group (Choussat et al., 1978). They recommend operation only for patients older than 4 and younger than 15 years of age, with a weight of at least 13 kg., normal cardiac rhythm, a normal or large right atrium, and normal caval drainage. The pulmonary arterial mean pressure must be less than 15 mm. Hg, the resistance less than 4 units · M.², and the pulmonary arteries of normal size, with a pulmonary artery–aorta diameter ratio of 0.75 or more. The left ventricular ejection fraction must be higher than 0.60. The mitral valve must be normal, with no incompetence. Selecting patients by these criteria, Fontan and associates (1978) have had excellent results.

The criteria, however, may be overly restrictive. In the Mayo Clinic series (Furuse *et al.*, 1972), 18 patients did not satisfy the criteria, and 14 survived (78 per cent). Several of their patients had more than one contraindication to operation. For example, a 33-year-old man had a mean pulmonary artery pressure of 34 mm. Hg, a resistance of 6.1 units · M.², and severe mitral insufficiency. Mitral valve replacement was done simultaneously with right ventricular bypass, and he did well postoperatively. A 2-year-old patient with increased pulmonary blood flow, a pulmonary arterial pressure of 39 mm. Hg, and a resistance of 2.7 units · M.² also did well. Five of their six patients with left ventricular end-diastolic pressure above normal (16 to 23 mm. Hg) survived operation, four with a good late result. Age was a factor in mortality, since only one of 18 patients (6 per cent) in the ideal age range of between 4 and 15 years died at operation, whereas three of 11 patients (28 per cent) outside that age range died. We have reported a patient with only one pulmonary artery, which was of good size, who did well postoperatively (Sade *et al.*, 1980).

The criteria we now use for operability are physiologic ones. We prefer to do a palliative operation, usually a Blalock-Taussig shunt, in infants under the age of 2 to 3 years. Total pulmonary vascular resistance must be low: arteriolar resistance less than 4 units · M. and adequate size of at least one pulmonary artery by the criteria of Pacifico and coworkers (1977). The left ventricular end-diastolic pressure should be 15 mm. Hg or less, or if it is higher, there must be a correctable cause of the higher pressure, such as mitral stenosis or insufficiency. As demonstrated by Gale and associates (1980), the use of less strict criteria for operability than Fontan's may result in a higher operative mortality rate but will offer corrective operation, with its potential for marked improvement in clinical status and perhaps longevity, to a much larger group of patients than could otherwise be helped. We emphasize, however, that longer follow-up and additional physiologic data are needed to clarify the best choice of operation for individual patients.

SELECTED REFERENCES

Fontan, F., Choussat, A., Brown, A. G., Chauve, A., Deville, C., and Castro-Cels, A.: Repair of tricuspid atresia — surgical considerations and results. *In* Paediatric Cardiology, 1977. Edited by R. H. Anderson and E. A. Shinebourne. Edinburgh, Churchill Livingstone, 1978, pp. 567–580.

Fontan and his coworkers have a large series of patients undergoing corrective operations for tricuspid atresia. This chapter summarizes their experience with their first 40 cases over nearly a 10-year period. Their overall hospital mortality rate was 17.5 per cent, with a late mortality rate of 7.5 per cent. Of their last 31 patients, however, only two died (6.5 per cent). These excellent recent results were due mostly to selection of patients for operation based on anatomic and physiologic criteria outlined in the paper.

Gale, A. W., Danielson, G. K., McGoon, D. C., Wallace, R. B., and Mair, D. D.: Fontan procedure for tricuspid atresia. Circulation, *62*:91, 1980.

The Mayo Clinic series of patients undergoing correction for tricuspid atresia included 29 patients, of whom four died (13.8 per cent). As in Fontan's series, recent results have been much better, with only one death in the most recent 22 consecutive patients (4.5 per cent). Many of their patients did not meet the criteria of operability enumerated by Fontan, but 14 of these 18 patients survived (78 per cent). This paper contains a useful discussion of the anatomy and physiology required preoperatively to permit corrective operation.

Rao, P. S.: A unified classification for tricuspid atresia. Am. Heart J., *99*:799, 1980.

The anatomic classification of tricuspid atresia has been the subject of much discussion. This paper summarizes previous attempts at classification and proposes a unified classification that includes aspects of several previous systems, yet is similar to the original classification of Edwards and Burchell that has been, in modified form, more commonly used than any other.

Sade, R. M., and Castaneda, A. R.: The dispensable right ventricle. Surgery, *77*:624, 1975.

The development of the concept of right ventricular bypass, based on the realization that a ventricle is not required in the pulmonary circuit, is discussed. Unanswered questions are raised regarding the ultimate clinical course in patients who undergo right ventricular bypass: the importance of cardiac rhythm late postoperatively, the number of valves required for correction, and the possible effects of artificial ventilation on pulmonary blood flow after right heart bypass.

Trusler, G. A., and Williams, W. G.: Long-term results of shunt procedures for tricuspid atresia. Ann. Thorac. Surg., *29*:312, 1978.

The experience at the Hospital for Sick Children in Toronto with shunt procedures for tricuspid atresia is summarized. In children under 6 months of age, the hospital mortality rate was 47 per cent, and in those over 6 months, it was 14 per cent. About half of the survivors required a second operation an average of 5.3 years after the first procedure, and 15 per cent of those children required a third operation an average of 4.3 years after the second procedure. The authors' preference is for a Blalock-Taussig shunt in older children and a Potts shunt in early infancy. Whenever possible, a Fontan operation should be the second procedure.

REFERENCES

Annecchino, F. P., Fontan, F., Chauve, A., and Quaegebeur, J.: Palliative reconstruction of the right ventricular outflow tract in tricuspid atresa: A report of 5 patients. Ann. Thorac. Surg., *29*:317, 1980.

Arguero, R., Perez-Alvarez, J. J., Franco-Vazquez, S., Perez-Trevino, C., and Jimenez-Martinez, M.: Surgical production of aorticopulmonary window in congenital heart diease with ischemic lungs. J. Thorac. Cardiovasc. Surg., *57*:786, 1969.

Ashcraft, K. W.: Discussion of Gay and Ebert, 1973.

Bakulev, A. N., and Kolesnikov, S. A.: Anastomosis of superior vena cava and pulmonary artery in the surgical treatment of certain congenital defects of the heart. J. Thorac. Surg., 37:693, 1959.

Behrendt, D. M., and Rosenthal, A.: Cardiovascular status after repair by Fontan procedure. Ann. Thorac. Surg., 29:322, 1980.

Bjork, V. O., Olin, C. L., Bjarke, B. B., and Thoren, C. A.: Right atrial–right ventricular anastomosis for correction of tricuspid atresia. J. Thorac. Cardiovasc. Surg., 77:452, 1979.

Blalock, A., and Hanlon, C. R.: The surgical treatment of transposition of the aorta and the pulmonary artery. Surg. Gynecol. Obstet., 90:1, 1950.

Blalock, A. and Taussig, H. B.: The surgical treatment of malformations of the heart in which there is pulmonary stenosis or pulmonary atresia. J.A.M.A., 128:189, 1945.

Boruchow, I. B., Swenson, E. W., Elliott, L. P., and Wheat, M. W.: Study of the mechanisms of shunt failure after superior vena cava–right pulmonary artery anastomosis. J. Thorac. Cardiovasc. Surg., 60:531, 1970.

Bowman, F. O., Hancock, W. D., and Malm, J. R.: A valve-containing Dacron prosthesis: Its use in restoring pulmonary artery–right ventricular continuity. Arch. Surg., 107:724, 1973.

Bowman, F. O., Jr., Malm, J. R., Hayes, C. J., and Gersony, W. M.: Physiological approach to surgery for tricuspid atresia. Circulation, 58(Suppl. 1), 83, 1978.

Brock, R. E.: Tricuspid atresia: A step toward corrective treatment. J. Thorac. Cardiovasc. Surg., 47:17, 1964.

Calabrese, C. T., Carrington, C. B., Hurley, R. A., Jr., Rojas, R. H., and Glenn, W. W. L.: Circulatory by-pass of the right side of the heart. J. Surg. Res., 8:593, 1968.

Carlon, C. A., Mondini, P. G., and DeMarchi, R.: Surgical treatment of some cardiovascular diseases (a new vascular anastomosis). J. Int. Coll. Surg., 16:1, 1951.

Carrel, A.: On the experimental surgery of the thoracic aorta and the heart. Ann. Surg., 52:83, 1910.

Choussat, A., Fontan, F., Besse, P., Vallot, F., Chauve, A., and Bricaud, H.: Selection criteria for Fontan's procedure. In Paediatric Cardiology, 1977. Edited by R. H. Anderson and E. A. Shinebourne. Edinburgh, Churchill Livingstone, 1978, pp. 559–566.

Clarkson, S., Sade, R. M., and Hohn, A.: Clinical and hemodynamic results of extracardiac conduit reconstruction of the pulmonary artery. Clin. Cardiol., 3:42, 1980.

Cole, R. B., Muster, A. J., Fixler, D. E., and Paul, M. H.: Long-term results of aortopulmonary anastomosis for tetralogy of Fallot. Morbidity and mortality. 1946–1969. Circulation, 43:263, 1971.

Cooley, R. N., Sloan, R. D., Hanlon, C. R., and Bahnson, H. T.: Angiocardiography in congenital heart disease of cyanotic type. II. Observations on tricuspid stenosis or atresia with hypoplasia of the right ventricle. Radiology, 54:848, 1950.

Coronel, A. R., Pedrini, M., Anania, R., and Parente, A. G.: Hemodynamics of tricuspid atresia corrected with a surgical technique. Rev. Argent. Cardiol., 41:382, 1973.

Davidson, J. S.: Anastomosis between the ascending aorta and the main pulmonary artery in the tetralogy of Fallot. Thorax, 10:348, 1955.

Deverall, P. B., Lincoln, J. C. R., Aberdeen, E., Bonham-Carter, R. E., and Waterston, D. J.: Surgical management of tricuspid atresia. Thorax, 24:239, 1969.

Dick, M., Fyler, D. C., and Nadas, A. S.: Tricuspid atresia: Clinical course in 101 patients. Am. J. Cardiol., 36:327, 1975.

Donahoo, J. S., Gardner, T. J., Zahka, K., and Kidd, B. S. L.: Systemic-pulmonary shunts in neonates and infants using microporous expanded polytetrafluoroethylene: Immediate and late results. Ann. Thorac. Surg., 30:146, 1980.

Donovan, T. J.: The experimental use of homologous vein grafts to circumvent the pulmonic valves. Surg. Gynecol. Obstet., 90:204, 1950.

Donovan, T. J., Hufnagel, C. A., and Eastcott, H. H. G.: Permanent ligation of the left main pulmonary artery. Surg. Forum, 2:229, 1951.

Doty, D. B., Marvin, W. J., Jr., and Lauer, R. M.: Modified Fontan procedure. Methods to achieve direct anastomosis of right atrium to pulmonary artery. J. Thorac. Cardiovasc. Surg., 81:470, 1981.

Edmunds, L. H., Jr., Fishman, N. H., Heymann, M. A., and Rudolph, A. M.: Anastomoses between aorta and right pulmonary artery (Waterston) in neonates. N. Engl. J. Med., 284:464, 1971.

Edwards, J. E., and Burchell, H. B.: Congenital tricuspid atresia: A classification. Med. Clin. North Am., 33:1177, 1949.

Edwards, W. S.: Discussion of Sakiyalak et al., 1971.

Edwards, W. S., and Bargeron, L. M.: The superiority of the Glenn operation for tricuspid atresia in infancy and childhood. J. Thorac. Cardiovasc. Surg., 55:60, 1968.

Fonkalsrud, E. W., and Linde, L.: Experience with atrial septectomy for transposition of the great vessels using a biconical punch. Surg. Forum, 22:158, 1971.

Fontan, F., and Baudet, E.: Surgical repair of tricuspid atresia. Thorax, 26:240, 1971.

Fontan, F., Choussat, A., Brown, A. G., Chauve, A., Deville, C., and Castro-Cels, A.: Repair of tricuspid atresia — surgical considerations and results. In Paediatric Cardiology, 1977. Edited by R. H. Anderson and E. A. Shinebourne. Edinburgh, Churchill Livingstone, 1978, pp. 567–580.

Fontan, F., Mournicot, F. B., Baudet, E., Simmoneau, J., Gordo, J., and Gouffrant, P.: "Correction" de l'atrésie tricuspidienne. Rapport de deux cas "corriges" par l'autilisation d'un technique chirurgical nouvelle. Ann. Chir. Thorac. Cardiovasc., 10:39, 1971.

Freedom, R. M., Williams, W. G., Fowler, R. S., Trusler, G. A., and Rowe, R. D.: Tricuspid atresia, transposition of the great arteries, and banded pulmonary artery. Repair by arterial switch, coronary artery reimplantation, and right atrioventricular valved conduit. J. Thorac. Cardiovasc. Surg., 80:621, 1980.

Furse, A., Brawley, R. K., and Gott, V. L.: Pulsatile cavo-pulmonary artery shunt. J. Thorac. Cardiovasc. Surg., 63:495, 1972.

Gabriele, O. F.: Progressive obstruction of pulmonary blood flow in tricuspid atresia. J. Thorac. Cardiovasc. Surg., 59:447, 1970.

Gago, O., Salles, C. A., Stern, A. M., Spooner, E., Brandt, R. L., and Morris, J. D.: A different approach for the total correction of tricuspid atresia. J. Thorac. Cardiovasc. Surg., 72:209, 1976.

Gale, A. W., Danielson, G. K., McGoon, D. C., Wallace, R. B., and Mair, D. D.: Fontan procedure for tricuspid atresia. Circulation, 62:91, 1980.

Gallaher, M. E., and Fyler, D. C.: Observations on changing hemodynamics in tricuspid atresia without associated transposition of the great vessels. Circulation, 35:381, 1967.

Gamboa, R., Gersony, W. M., and Nadas, A. S.: The electrocardiogram in tricuspid atresia and pulmonary atresia with intact ventricular septum. Circulation, 34:24, 1966.

Gay, W. A., Jr., and Ebert, P. A.: Aorta–to–right pulmonary artery anastomosis causing obstruction of the right pulmonary artery. Management during correction of tetralogy of Fallot. Ann. Thorac. Surg., 16:402, 1973.

Glenn, W. W. L.: Circulatory bypass of the right side of the heart. IV. Shunt between superior vena cava and distal right pulmonary artery — report of a clinical application. N. Engl. J. Med., 259:117, 1958.

Glenn, W. W. L., and Fenn, J. E.: Axillary arteriovenous fistula, a means of supplementing blood flow through a cava-pulmonary artery shunt. Circulation, 46:1013, 1972.

Glenn, W. W. L., and Patino, J. F.: Circulatory bypass of the right heart. I. Preliminary observations on the direct delivery of vena caval blood into the pulmonary arterial circulation. Azygos vein–pulmonary artery shunt. Yale J. Biol. Med., 27:147, 1954.

Glenn, W. W. L., Browne, M., and Whittemore, R.: Circulatory bypass of the right side of the heart. Cava-pulmonary artery shunt — indications and results: Report of a collected series of 537 cases. In The Heart and Circulation in the Newborn and Infant. Edited by D. E. Cassels. New York, Grune and Stratton, 1966, p. 345.

Glenn, W. W. L., Gardner, T. H., Jr., Talner, N. S., Stansel, H. C. Jr., and Matano, I.: Rational approach to the surgical management of tricuspid atresia. Circulation, 37(Suppl. 2):62, 1968.

Glenn, W. W. L., Spencer, R. P., Deren, M. M., and Tanae, H.: Functional changes in pulmonary circulation following cava-pulmonary artery shunt. Circulation, 42(Suppl. 3):157, 1970.

Gross, R. E., Bill, A. H., Jr., and Peirce, E. C., II: Methods for preservation and transplantation of arterial grafts. Surg. Gynecol. Obstet., 88:689, 1949.

Haller, J. A., Adkins, J. C., Worthington, M.,and Rauenhorst, J.: Experimental studies on permanent bypass of the right heart. Surgery, 59:1128, 1966.

Hallman, G. L., Stasney, C. R., and Cooley, D. A.: Surgical treatment of tricuspid atresia. J. Cardiovasc. Surg., 9:154, 1968.

Harrison, R.: Discussion of Bopp, R. K., Larsen, P. B., Caddell, J. L., Patrick, J. R., Hipona, F. A., and Glenn, W. W. L.: Surgical considerations for treatment of congenital tricuspid atresia and stenosis: With particular reference to vena cava–pulmonary artery anastomosis. J. Thorac. Cardiovasc. Surg., 43:97, 1962.

Hatem, J., Sade, R. M., Upshur, J. K., and Hohn, A. R.: Maintaining patency of the ductus arteriosus for palliation of cyanotic congenital cardiac malformations. Ann. Surg., 192:124, 1980.

Hellenbrand, W. E., Laks, H., Kleinman, C. S., and Talner, N. S.: Hemodynamic evaluation of the Fontan procedure at rest and with exercise. Am. J. Cardiol., 47:432, 1981.

Henry, J. N., Devloo, R. A. E., Ritter, D. G., Mair, D. D., Davis, G. D., and Danielson, G. K.: Tricuspid atresia. Successful surgical "correction" in two patients using porcine xenograft valves. Mayo Clin. Proc., 49:803, 1974.

Hurwitt, E. S., Young, D., and Escher, D. J. W.: The rationale of anastomosis of the right auricular appendage to the pulmonary artery in the treatment of tricuspid atresia. J. Thorac. Surg., 30:503, 1955.

Idriss, F. S., Riker, W. L., and Paul, M. H.: Banding of the pulmonary artery: A palliative surgical procedure. J. Pediatr. Surg., 3:465, 1968.

Jennings, R. B., Jr., Crisler, C., Johnson, D. H., and Brickman, R. D.: Tricuspid atresia with dextrotransposition, dextrocardia, and mitral insufficiency: Successful circulatory correction. Ann. Thorac. Surg., 29:369, 1980.

Just-Viera, J. O., Rive-Mora, E., Altieri, P. I., and Girod, C. E.: Tricuspid atresia and the hypoplastic right ventricular complex: Complete correction for long-term survival. Surg. Forum, 22:165, 1971.

Just-Viera, J. O., Rive-Mora, E., Rodriquez, O. L., Altieri, P. I., and Girod, C. E.: Atriopulmonary shunt. Ann. Thorac. Surg., 15:41, 1973.

Keith, J. D., Rowe, R. D., and Vlad, P.: Heart Disease in Infancy and Childhood. 3rd Ed. New York, Macmillan Company, 1979.

Kouchoukos, N. T., Barcia, A., Bargeron, L. M., and Kirklin, J. W.: Surgical treatment of congenital pulmonary atresia with ventricular septal defect. J. Thorac. Cardiovasc. Surg., 61:70, 1971.

Kreutzer, G., Galindez, E., Bono, H., dePalma, D., and Laura, J. P.: An operation for the correction of tricuspid atresia. J. Thorac. Cardiovasc. Surg., 66:613, 1973.

Kreysig, F. L.: Krankenheiten des Herzens. Vol. 3. Berlin, Maurer, 1817.

Kühne, M.: Über zwei Fälle kongenitaler Atresie des Ostium venosum dextrum. Jahresb. Kinderh., 63:225, 1906.

Laks, H., and Castaneda, A. R.: Subclavian arterioplasty for the ipsilateral Blalock-Taussig shunt. Ann. Thorac. Surg., 19:319, 1975.

Laks, H., Mudd, J. G., Standeven, J. W., Fagan, L., and Willman, V. L.: Long-term effect of the superior vena cava–pulmonary artery anastomosis on pulmonary blood flow. J. Thorac. Cardiovasc. Surg., 74:253, 1977.

Laks, H., Williams, W. G., Hellenbrand, W. E., Freedom, R. M., Talner, N. S., Rowe, R. D., and Trusler, G. A.: Results of right atrial to right ventricular and right atrial to pulmonary

artery conduits for complex congenital heart disease. Ann. Surg., 192:382, 1980.

Lenox, C. C., and Zuberbuhler, J. R.: Balloon septostomy in tricuspid atresia after infancy. Am. J. Cardiol., 25:723, 1970.

Lindesmith, G. G., Gallaher, M. E., Durnin, R. E., Meyer, B. W., and Jones, J. C.: Cardiac surgery in the first month of life. Ann. Thorac. Surg., 2:250, 1966.

Litwin, S. B., Plauth, W. H., Jr., Jones, J. E., and Bernhard, W. F.: Appraisal of surgical atrial septectomy for transposition of the great arteries. Circulation, 43(Suppl. 1):7, 1971.

McGoon, D. C., Wallace, R. B., and Danielson, G. K.: The Rastelli operation — its indications and results. J. Thorac. Cardiovasc. Surg., 65:65, 1973.

Mahoney, E. B.: Discussion of Brock, 1964.

Marcano, B. A., Riemenschneider, T. A., Ruttenberg, H. D., Goldberg, S. J., and Gyepes, M.: Tricuspid atresia with increased pulmonary blood flow. Analysis of 13 cases. Circulation, 40:399, 1969.

Martin, S. P., Anabtawi, I. N., Selmonosky, C. A., Folger, G. M., Ellison, L. T., and Ellison, R. G.: Long-term follow-up after superior vena cava–right pulmonary artery anastomosis. Ann. Thorac. Surg., 9:339, 1970.

Mathur, M., and Glenn, W. W. L.: Long-term evaluation of cava-pulmonary artery anastomosis. Surgery, 74:899, 1973.

Matsuda, H., Kawashima, Y., Takano, H., Miyamoto, K., and Mori, T.: Experimental evaluation of atrial function in right atrium–pulmonary artery conduit operation for tricuspid atresia. J. Thorac. Cardiovasc. Surg., 81:762, 1981.

McGoon, D. C., Wallace, R. B., and Danielson, G. K.: The Rastelli operation — its indications and results. J. Thorac. Cardiovasc. Surg., 65:65, 1973.

McKay, R., de Leval, M. R., Rees, P., Taylor, J. F. N., Macartney, F. J., and Stark, J.: Postoperative angiographic assessment of modified Blalock-Taussig shunts using expanded polytetrafluoroethylene (Gore-Tex). Ann. Thorac. Surg., 30:137, 1980.

Miller, R. A., Pahlajani, D., Serratto, M., and Tatooles, C.: Clinical studies after Fontan's operation for tricuspid atresia. Am. J. Cardiol., 33:157, 1974.

Muller, W. H., Jr., and Dammann, J. F., Jr.: The treatment of certain congenital malformations of the heart by the creation of pulmonary stenosis to reduce pulmonary hypertension and excessive pulmonary blood flow. Surg. Gynecol. Obstet., 95:213, 1952.

Murray, G. F., Herrington, R. T., and Delany, D. J.: Tricuspid atresia: Corrective operation without a bioprosthetic valve. Ann. Thorac. Surg., 23:209, 1977.

Nadas, A. S., and Fyler, D. C.: Pediatric Cardiology. 3rd Ed. Philadelphia, W. B. Saunders Company, 1972.

Neches, W. H., Park, S. C., Lenox, C. C., Zuberbuhler, J. R., and Bahnson, H. T.: Tricuspid atresia with transposition of the great arteries and closing ventricular septal defect. Successful palliation by banding of the pulmonary artery and creation of an aorticopulmonary window. J. Thorac. Cardiovasc. Surg., 65:538, 1973.

Nuland, S. B., Glenn, W. W. L., and Guilfoil, P. H.: Circulatory by-pass of the right heart. III. Some observations on long-term survivors. Surgery, 43:184, 1958.

Ochsner, J. L., Cooley, D. A., McNamara, D. G., and Kline, A.: Surgical treatment of cardiovascular anomalies in 300 infants younger than one year of age. J. Thorac. Cardiovasc. Surg., 43:182, 1962.

Oparil, S., Greenblatt, A., and Hendren, W. H.: Left-superior-vena-cava steal syndrome. N. Engl. J. Med., 286:303, 1972.

Pacifico, A. D., Kirklin, J. W., and Blackstone, E. H.: Surgical management of pulmonary stenosis in tetralogy of Fallot. J. Thorac. Cardiovasc. Surg., 74:382, 1977.

Paul, M. H.: Tricuspid atresia. In Pediatric Cardiology. Edited by H. Watson. St. Louis, C. V. Mosby Co., 1968, p. 451.

Paul, M. H., Greenwood, R. D., Cole, R. B., and Muster, A. J.: Aortic-pulmonary anastomosis for tricuspid atresia. 1946–1968. Presented at American Heart Association, Dallas, Nov. 14, 1969.

Pennington, D. G., Nouri, S., Ho, J., Secker-Walker, R., Patel, B., Sivakoff, M., and Willman, V. L.: Glenn shunt: Long-term results and current role in congenital heart operations. Ann. Thorac. Surg., *31*:532, 1981.

Potts, W. J., Smith, S., and Gibson, S.: Anastomosis of the aorta to a pulmonary artery. J.A.M.A., *132*:627, 1946.

Puga, F. J., and McGoon, D. C.: Exclusion of the right ventricle from the circulation: Hemodynamic observations. Surgery, *73*:607, 1973.

Pujatti, G., Lise, M., and Morea, M.: Septal and arterial shunts in tricuspid atresia. Lancet, *2*:1311, 1967.

Rao, P. S.: A unified classification for tricuspid atresia. Am. Heart J., *99*:799, 1980.

Rashkind, W. J., and Miller, W. W.: Creation of an atrial septal defect without thoracotomy. A palliative approach to complete transposition of the great arteries. J.A.M.A., *196*:991, 1966.

Rashkind, W., Waldhausen, J., Miller, W., and Friedman, S.: Palliative treatment in tricuspid atresia. Combined balloon atrioseptostomy and surgical alteration of pulmonary blood flow. J. Thorac. Cardiovasc. Surg., *57*:812, 1969.

Rastan, H., and Koncz, G.: A new method of closed atrioseptectomy for palliative treatment of complete transposition of the great vessels. J. Thorac. Cardiovasc. Surg., *61*:705, 1971.

Robicsek, F., Temesvari, A., and Kadar, R. L.: A new method for the treatment of congenital heart disease associated with impaired pulmonary circulaton. Acta Med. Scand., *154*:151, 1956.

Robicsek, F., Sanger, P. W., Gollucci, V., and Daugherty, H. K.: Long-term circulatory exclusion of the right heart. Surgery, *59*:431, 1966.

Robicsek, F., Magistro, R., Foti, E., Robicsek, L., and Sanger, P. W.: Vena cava–pulmonary artery anastomosis for vascularization of the lung. J. Thorac. Surg., *35*:440, 1958.

Robicsek, F., Sanger, P. W., Moore, M., Daugherty, H. K., Robicsek, L. K., and Bagby, E.: Observations following four years of complete circulatory exclusion of the right heart. Ann. Thorac. Surg., *8*:530, 1969.

Rodbard, S., and Wagner, D.: By-passing the right ventricle. Proc. Soc. Exp. Biol. Med., *71*:69, 1949.

Rosenthal, A.: Current status of treatment for tricuspid atresia. Introduction to symposium. Ann. Thorac. Surg., *29*:304, 1980.

Ross, D. N., and Somerville, J.: Correction of pulmonary atresia with a homograft aortic valve. Lancet, *2*:1446, 1966.

Ross, D. N., and Somerville, J.: Surgical correction of tricuspid atresia. Lancet, *1*:845, 1973.

Sachs, B. F., Pontius, R. G., and Zuberbuhler, J. R.: The clinical use of the superior vena cava–pulmonary artery shunt: A report of 20 cases. J. Pediatr. Surg., *3*:364, 1968.

Sade, R. M.: Orthoterminal correction of congenital cardiovascular defects. Ann. Thorac. Surg., *19*:105, 1975.

Sade, R. M., and Castaneda, A. R.: The dispensable right ventricle. Surgery, *77*:624, 1975.

Sade, R. M., and Dearing, J. P.: Augmentation of pulmonary blood flow after right ventricular bypass. J. Thorac. Cardiovasc. Surg., *81*:928, 1981.

Sade, R. M., Riopel, D. A., and Taylor, A. B.: Orthoterminally corrective operation in the presence of severe hypoplasia of a pulmonary artery. J. Thorac. Cardiovasc. Surg., *80*:424, 1980.

Sade, R. M., Lubbe, J. J. D., Simpser, M. D., and Strieder, D. J.: Mechanical ventilation as a pump for the pulmonary circulation. Eur. Surg. Res., *13*:414, 1981.

Sade, R. M., Sloss, L., Treves, S., Bernhard, W. F., and Castaneda, A. R.: Repair of tetralogy of Fallot after aortopulmonary anastomosis. Ann. Thorac. Surg., *23*:32, 1977.

Sakiyalak, P., Ankeney, J. L., Liebman, J., and DeMeules, J.: Results of superior vena cava–to–pulmonary artery shunt in the treatment of cyanotic congenital heart disease. Ann. Thorac. Surg., *12*:514, 1971.

Serratto, M., Miller, R. A., Tatooles, C., and Ardekani, R.: Hemodynamic evaluation of Fontan operation in tricuspid atresia. Circulation, *54*(Suppl. 3):99, 1976.

Shachar, G. B., Fuhrman, B. P., Wang, Y., Lucas, R. V., and

Lock, J. E.: Rest and exercise hemodynamics after Fontan procedure. Am. J. Cardiol., *47*:432, 1981.

Sharratt, G. P., Johnson, A. M., and Monro, J. L: Persistence and effects of sinus rhythm after Fontan procedure for tricuspid atresia. Br. Heart J., *42*:74, 1979.

Shemin, R. J., Merrill, W. H., Pfeifer, J. S., Conkle, D. M., and Morrow, A. G.: Evaluation of right atrial–pulmonary artery conduits for tricuspid atresia. Experimental study. J. Thorac. Cardiovasc. Surg., *77*:685, 1979.

Shumacker, H. B.: Discussion of Hurwitt *et al.*, 1955.

Singh, S. P., Astley, R., and Parsons, C. G.: Haemodynamic effects of balloon septostomy in tricuspid atresia. Br. Med. J., *1*:225, 1968.

Somerville, J., Yacoub, M., Ross, D. N., and Ross, K.: Aorta to right pulmonary artery anastomosis (Waterston's operation) for cyanotic heart disease. Circulation, *39*:593, 1969.

Stanford, W., Armstrong, R. G., Cline, R. E., and King, T. D.: Right atrium–pulmonary artery allograft for correction of tricuspid atresia. J. Thorac. Cardiovasc. Surg., *66*:105, 1973.

Tatooles, C. J., Ardekani, R. G., Miller, R. A., and Seratto, M.: Results following physiological repair for tricuspid atresia. Ann. Thorac. Surg., *22*:578, 1976.

Taussig, H. B., Crocetti, A., Eshaghpour, E., Keinonen, R., Yap, K. N., Bachman, D., Momberger, N., and Kirk, H.: Long-time observation on the Blalock-Taussig operation. I. Results of first operation. Johns Hopkins Med. J., *129*:243, 1971.

Taussig, H. B., Keinonen, R., Momberger, H., and Kirk, H.: Long-time observatons on the Blalock-Taussig operation. IV. Tricuspid atresia. Johns Hopkins Med. J., *132*:135, 1973.

Tingelstad, J. B., Lower, R. R., Howell, T. R., and Eldredge, W. J.: Pulmonary artery banding in tricuspid atresia without transposed great arteries. Am. J. Dis. Child., *121*:434, 1971.

Trusler, G. A., and Williams, W. G.: Long-term results of shunt procedures for tricuspid atresia. Ann. Thorac. Surg., *29*:312, 1978.

Trusler, G. A., MacGregor, D., and Mustard, W. T.: Cavopulmonary anastomosis for cyanotic congenital heart disease. J. Thorac. Cardiovasc. Surg., *62*:803, 1971.

Van Den Bogaert-Van Heesvelde, A. M., Derom, F., Kunnen, M., Van Egmond, H., and Devloo-Blancquaert, A.: Surgery for arteriovenous fistulas and dilated vessels in the right lung after the Glenn procedure. J. Thorac. Cardiovasc. Surg., *76*:195, 1978.

Van Praagh, R.: Discussion of Vlad P: Pulmonary atresia with intact ventricular septum. *In* Heart Disease in Infancy: Diagnosis and Surgical Treatment. Edited by B. G. Barratt-Boyes, J. Neutze, and E. A. Harris. Baltimore, Williams and Wilkins, 1973, pp. 246.

Van Praagh R., Ando, M., and Dungan, W. T.: Anatomic types of tricuspid atresia: Clinical and developmental implications. Circulation, *44*(Suppl. 2):115, 1971.

von Bernuth, G., Ritter, D. G., Frye, R. L., Weidman, W. H., Davis, G. D., and McGoon, D. C.: Evaluation of patients with tetralogy of Fallot and Potts anastomosis. Am. J. Cardiol., *27*:259, 1971.

Warden, H. E., DeWall, R. A., and Varco, R. L.: Use of the right auricle as a pump for the pulmonary circuit. Surg. Forum, *5*:16, 1954.

Waterston, D. J.: The treatment of Fallot's tetralogy in children under one year of age. Rozhl. Chir., *41*:181, 1962 (in Czech).

Wittenborg, M. H., Neuhauser, E. B. D., and Sprunt, W. H.: Roentgenographic findings in congenital tricuspid atresia with hypoplasia of the right ventricle. Am. J. Roentgenol., *66*:712, 1951.

Yacoub, M. H.: Fontan's operation — are caval valves necessary? *In* Paediatric Cardiology, 1977. Edited by R. H. Anderson and E. A Shinebourne. Edinburgh, Churchill Livingstone, 1978, pp. 581–588.

Chapter 44

Ebstein's Anomaly

GORDON K. DANIELSON

PATHOLOGIC ANATOMY

The anomalous development of the tricuspid valve described by Wilhelm Ebstein in 1866 (Mann and Lie, 1979) is characterized by a deformity of the valve in which there is a downward displacement of the posterior and septal leaflets in a spiral fashion below the true anulus (Fig. 44–1) (Anderson *et al.*, 1979; Zuberbuhler *et al.*, 1979). The displaced leaflets are hypoplastic, thickened, and often adherent to the wall of the right ventricle. Their displacement leaves a portion of the ventricle above the valve as an integral part of the right atrium; this is referred to as the "atrialized ventricle."

The anterior leaflet of the tricuspid valve in Ebstein's anomaly is typically larger than normal and has been described as "sail-like." It may be fenestrated, and variable portions of the free edge may be attached to the right ventricular endocardium. The chordae tendineae and papillary muscles of the tricuspid valve are anomalous and abnormally positioned. The malformed tricuspid valve is usually incompetent, but it may occasionally be stenotic or, rarely, imperforate.

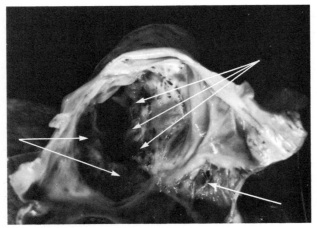

Figure 44–1. Ebstein's malformation in a 9-day-old infant, view from right atrium. The single arrow indicates a patent foramen ovale. The anterior leaflet is enlarged and hooded (double arrow). The posterior and septal leaflets are dysplastic and displaced in a spiral fashion toward the apex of the right ventricle (triple arrow).

The atrialized ventricle is characteristically thinned and dilated, but careful observation shows that the entire wall of the right ventricle, both proximal and distal to the abnormal insertion of the tricuspid leaflets, including the infundibulum, is also dilated. Dilatation of the right ventricular wall is associated not only with thinning of the wall, but also with an absolute decrease in the number of myocardial fibers (Anderson and Lie, 1979). The atrioventricular node is located at the apex of the triangle of Koch, and the conduction system is normally situated. Atrial septal defect and other associated anomalies are common (Watson, 1974).

In those congenital cardiac anomalies in which there is atrioventricular discordance with ventriculoarterial discordance (corrected transposition), Ebstein's anomaly of the left atrioventricular valve is a common finding. The nature of the displacement of the septal and posterior leaflets in left-sided Ebstein's anomaly is similar to that in the right-sided form, but the anterior leaflet is smaller and anatomically quite different (Anderson *et al.*, 1978). Other differences relate to the functional portion of the morphologically right ventricle, which is rarely dilated, and the atrialized portion of the ventricle, which has less thinning of the wall. The atrioventricular conduction tissue in corrected transposition is right-sided and anterior, at a distance from the left-sided tricuspid valve (Anderson *et al.*, 1974). Thus, insertion of a prosthetic valve in the anatomic position has less risk of producing complete heart block in left-sided Ebstein's anomaly than in the right-sided form.

PATHOLOGIC PHYSIOLOGY

The functional impairment of the right ventricle and the incompetence of the deformed tricuspid valve retard forward flow of blood through the right heart. Moreover, during contraction of the atrium, the atrialized portion of the right ventricle is in diastole and balloons out (if very thin) or acts as a passive reservoir, decreasing the volume to be ejected; during ventricular systole, it contracts, creating a pressure wave that impedes venous filling of the right atrium, which is in the diastolic phase. In most cases, the atrial septum is deficient owing to patency or fenestration of the foramen ovale; sometimes, there is a distinct secundum atrial septal defect. The movement of blood through the septal opening is predominantly from right to left but occasionally may be from left to right. The overall effect of these structural abnormalities on the right atrium is to produce gross dilatation, which may reach enormous proportions, even in infancy. This dilatation leads to further incompetence of the tricuspid valve and further widening of the interatrial communication.

CLINICAL FEATURES

Ebstein's anomaly is a rare cardiac anomaly, accounting for less than 1 per cent of all congenital heart disease. It involves both sexes equally. Although a few patients reach advanced age, life expectancy for most is limited. The most common causes of death are congestive heart failure, hypoxia, and cardiac arrhythmias. When the diagnosis of Ebstein's anomaly is made in infancy, the prognosis is worse; one third to one half of these patients will die before 2 years of age (Kumar *et al.*, 1971; Giuliani *et al.*, 1979).

Because there is a broad spectrum of pathologic changes in Ebstein's anomaly, the hemodynamic alterations are variable. Symptoms are related to the severity of the incompetence of the tricuspid valve, the presence or absence of an associated atrial septal defect, the impairment of right ventricular function, and the presence of associated cardiac anomalies.

In the early neonatal period, any tricuspid incompetence is accentuated by the normally occurring elevated pulmonary arteriolar resistance, and infants with Ebstein's anomaly may develop severe congestive heart failure. Because the foramen ovale is patent in early infancy, severe tricuspid incompetence, with its resultant elevation of right atrial pressure, will produce a right-to-left atrial-level shunt, and such infants may be deeply cyanotic. If the infant survives this critical period, the degree of cyanosis and the symptoms will often diminish as the fetal pulmonary hypertension regresses.

In older patients, the predominant symptoms are fatigability, dyspnea on exertion, and cyanosis. Less frequently, peripheral edema and palpitations in the form of paroxysmal atrial arrhythmias and premature ventricular beats are encountered.

In an experience with 67 patients who had a mean follow-up of 12 years, Giuliani and associates (1979) found that 39 per cent remained in functional Class I or II and 61 per cent progressed at some time into Class III or IV. Death occurred in 21 per cent of the patients, and these were characterized by one or more of the following features: (1) they were in functional Class III or IV; (2) the cardiothoracic ratio was greater than 0.65; (3) they had cyanosis or an arterial oxygen saturation of less than 90 per cent; and (4) they were infants when the diagnosis was made.

The physical signs are variable. Heart sounds are usually soft, and there is often a multiplicity of sounds and murmurs, all originating from the right heart. A systolic murmur of tricuspid regurgitation is heard along the left sternal border. There may be diastolic and presystolic murmurs of low intensity that are due to anatomic or functional tricuspid stenosis. These murmurs characteristically become louder with inspiration. There is wide splitting of both the first and the second heart sounds. Atrial and ventricular filling sounds are relatively common and contribute to the cadence quality that is so often found in patients with Ebstein's anomaly. There may be summation of these gallop sounds due to prolongation of atrioventricular conduction.

The arterial and jugular venous pulse forms are usually normal. A large V wave can sometimes be seen in the jugular venous pulse, but usually this is not prominent. The liver may be palpably enlarged, but it is almost never pulsatile.

DIAGNOSTIC CRITERIA

Electrocardiography. The electrocardiogram is usually abnormal, but it is not diagnostic. Typically, there is complete or incomplete right bundle branch block and right axis deviation. The P waves are large, and the R waves in leads V_1 to V_4 are small. Often, the P-R interval is prolonged and the QRS complex slurred. Arrhythmias are common. Ventricular pre-excitation (Wolff-Parkinson-White syndrome) is seen in some cases and is almost always of the right ventricular free-wall type.

Roentgenography. The cardiac silhouette may vary from near-normal to the typical configuration, which consists of a globular-shaped heart with a narrow waist similar to that seen with pericardial effusion. This appearance is produced by enlargement of the right atrium and displacement of the right ventricular outflow tract outward and upward. Vascularity of the pulmonary fields is either normal or decreased.

Cardiac Catheterization. The right atrial pressure is usually moderately elevated, and the pulse contour most often shows a dominant V wave with a steep Y descent. However, in patients with a markedly dilated right atrium, the atrial pressure pulse may be normal despite the presence of severe tricuspid incompetence. Right ventricular pressure is most often normal, although the end-diastolic pressure may be elevated. One method of establishing the diagnosis is by intracardiac electrocardiography: On pull-back of the catheter from the right ventricle, the intracardiac electrocardiogram demonstrates continued right ventricular electrical potentials after the pressure pulse has changed from a ventricular to an atrial contour. In some patients with very severe tricuspid incompetence, however, the pressure pulses in the right atrium and right ventricle may be of very similar contour, thus making interpretation of the intracardiac electrocardiogram difficult. Pulmonary artery pressure is normal or decreased. In patients with an associated atrial septal defect and right-to-left shunt, oximetry will demonstrate systemic arterial desaturation, and intracardiac dye dilution curves from the venae cavae will confirm the shunt.

Angiography. Injection of contrast medium into the right atrium demonstrates enlargement of this chamber and normal position of the tricuspid anulus. There may be an indentation on the inferior wall of the right ventricle some distance to the left of the tricuspid anulus, which represents the site of origin of the displaced leaflets of the tricuspid valve. The leaflets sometimes appear as radiolucent lines laterally and superiorly within the body of the right ventricle. Contrast medium often moves back and forth between the right atrium and the right ventricle, and right-to-left shunting at atrial level may be found in the presence of an atrial septal defect or a patent foramen ovale. Flow through the right heart and lungs is slow.

Echocardiography. The M-mode echocardiogram is abnormal; the most reliable single criterion is the relationship of mitral valve closure to tricuspid valve closure (Giuliani *et al.,* 1979). Two-dimensional echocardiography has greatly improved the ability to make the diagnosis of Ebstein's anomaly without catheterization. This allows accurate evaluation of the anatomic relationships of the tricuspid leaflets to the right heart, the size of the right atrium, including the atrialized portion of the right ventricle, and the size and function of the right ventricle. When two-dimensional echocardiography is combined with the use of peripheral venous injections of indocyanine dye, the presence of a right-to-left shunt at atrial level can be detected and semi-quantitations of tricuspid regurgitation can be made by viewing reflux into the inferior vena cava and the hepatic veins during systole.

SURGICAL CONSIDERATIONS

Medical management has little to offer patients with Ebstein's anomaly, except for management of fluid retention and treatment of some arrhythmias. The prognosis is poorest in those who have congestive heart failure, marked cyanosis, associated cardiac anomalies, extreme cardiomegaly (cardiothoracic ratio >0.65), and diagnosis in infancy (Kumar *et al.,* 1971; Giuliani *et al.,* 1979). Serious cardiac arrhythmias may develop without associated congestive failure or hypoxemia. Those patients who have survived infancy generally do well for a number of years; as long as they are only mildly symptomatic, medical management alone is advised. Operative correction is generally postponed until deterioration is evident. However, since all patients with Ebstein's anomaly will sooner or later show progressive deterioration, all will ultimately become candidates for surgical correction.

Surgical attempts to treat Ebstein's anomaly began in the 1950s with the establishment of systemic-to-pulmonary artery shunts for relief of cyanosis, but results were uniformly poor. A superior vena cava-to-pulmonary artery shunt was then proposed as a more physiologic means of improving oxygenation, but this approach has proved to be of limited usefulness. In a collected series of 36 cases of cava–pulmonary artery shunts performed for Ebstein's anomaly, 17 patients survived operation and 14 were benefited by the procedure (Glenn *et al.,* 1966). In 1954, Wright and coworkers made a direct attack on a patent foramen ovale that was associated with Ebstein's anomaly; although the patient survived and was improved, a residual shunt was demonstrated at atrial level.

An operation for total correction of the hemodynamic abnormalities of Ebstein's anomaly was reported in 1958 by Hunter and Lillehei (Lillehei *et al.,* 1967). Their method included repositioning the displaced posterior and septal leaflets, excluding the atrialized ventricular chamber, and closing the atrial septal defect when one was present. Two of their patients sustained complete heart block, and none survived.

Hardy and coworkers revived and modified the Hunter-Lillehei operation in 1964. They placed interrupted sutures close together on the spiral line of the displaced posterior and septal cusp bases and wider apart at the anulus. The tying of the sutures created multiple tucks in the leaflets, narrowed the tricuspid orifice, and pulled the displaced leaflets back toward the tricuspid anulus. The technique was employed in six patients; four are late survivors, one having complete heart block (Hardy and Roe, 1969). Although some good results have subsequently been reported with this procedure, it has not been generally effective in establishing a competent valve in the moderate and severe forms of Ebstein's anomaly. With suture placement in the septum as originally shown, heart block may occur. Moreover, it is not possible to transpose the septal leaflet and medial portions of the posterior leaflet to the tricuspid anulus, because the ventricular septum cannot be plicated in the same way as the free wall of the right ventricle. Finally, direct approximation of the displaced leaflet to the tricuspid anulus along the free wall does not obliterate the atrialized ventricle, which protrudes below the heart as an aneurysmal sac and, in spite of efforts to the contrary, usually remains in communication with the right ventricle.

Prosthetic replacement of the deformed tricuspid valve was accomplished successfully by Barnard and Schrire in 1963. In their technique, the sutures for anchoring the prosthesis were deviated cephalad to the coronary sinus and atrioventricular node to avoid injuring the node and the conduction bundle. With the sutures thus placed, blood from the coronary sinus drained directly into the right ventricle. The atrialized portion of the ventricle was not obliterated.

In 1967, Lillehei and colleagues reported tricuspid valve replacement with a Starr-Edwards ball valve in five patients with Ebstein's anomaly. In two patients, the prosthetic valve was sutured to the true anulus, causing complete atrioventricular dissociation; one of

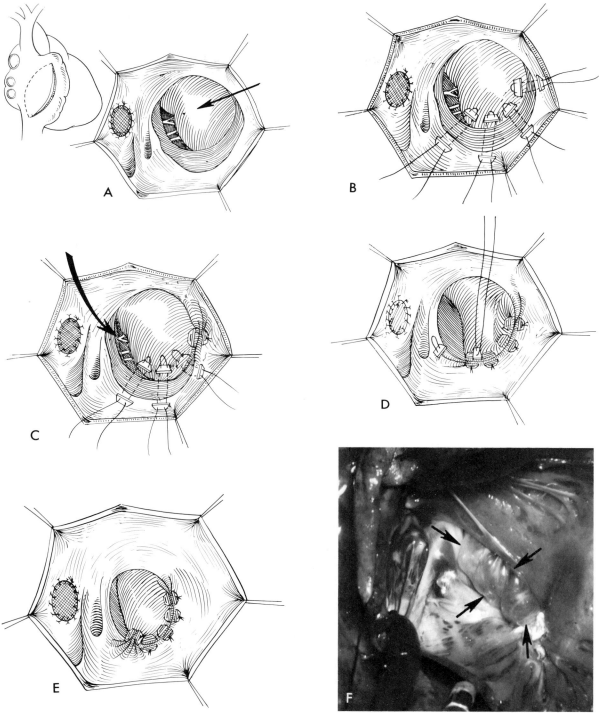

Figure 44–2. Diagram of repair. *A, Left,* The right atrium is incised from the atrial appendage to the inferior vena cava. Redundant portion of the right atrium is excised (dotted line) so that the final size of the right atrium is normal. *Right,* Atrial septal defect is closed with a patch. The large anterior leaflet is indicated by arrow. The posterior leaflet is displaced down from the anulus. The septal leaflet is hypoplastic and is not seen in this view. *B,* Mattress sutures passed through pledgets of Teflon felt are used to pull the tricuspid anulus and tricuspid valve together. Sutures are placed in the atrialized portion of the right ventricle, as shown, so that when they are subsequently tied, the atrialized ventricle is plicated and the aneurysmal cavity is obliterated. *C,* Sutures are tied down sequentially. Hypoplastic, markedly displaced septal leaflet is now visible (arrow). *D,* Posterior anuloplasty is performed to narrow the diameter of the tricuspid anulus. Coronary sinus marks posteroleftward extent of the anuloplasty, which is terminated there to avoid injury to the conduction bundle. Occasionally, one or two additional mattress sutures are required to obliterate the posterior aspect of the anuloplasty repair in order to render the valve totally competent. At this time, tricuspid anulus will admit two or more fingers. *E,* Completed repair, which allows anterior leaflet to function as a monocusp valve. *F,* Operative photograph of completed repair. Large anterior leaflet forms competent monocusp valve (arrows). (From Danielson, G. K., Maloney, J. D., and Devloo, R. A. E.: Surgical repair of Ebstein's anomaly. Mayo Clin. Proc., *54*:185, 1979.)

the two died. In the remaining three patients, attachment of the prosthesis according to the Barnard-Schrire technique avoided heart block.

Other operations include atrioventricular plication combined with tricuspid valve replacement (Timmis et al., 1967) and replacement of the tricuspid valve with a tissue valve combined with obliteration of the atrialized portion of the right ventricle and closure of the atrial septal defect (Ross and Somerville, 1970).

Prosthetic valve replacement, although it remains the most popular method for repair of Ebstein's anomaly, has given less than ideal results for some patients. Valve replacement in the tricuspid area is associated with a higher frequency of valve malfunction and thrombotic complications than is replacement of the other cardiac valves. Tissue valves do not have the thromboembolic complications of mechanical valves, but they do have a limited life expectancy, particularly in infants and children. In our experience, the failure-free rate of porcine heterograft valves in children is only 58.5 per cent at 5 years (Williams et al., 1982).

Since 1972, we have employed a repair that consists of plication of the free wall of the atrialized portion of the right ventricle, posterior tricuspid anuloplasty, and right atrial reduction (Danielson et al., 1979). The repair is based on the construction of a monocusp valve by the use of the anterior leaflet of the tricuspid valve, which, as noted earlier, is usually enlarged in this anomaly (Fig. 44–2). Repair is preferred to valve replacement whenever it is feasible because it avoids the problems of prosthetic valve dysfunction, anticoagulation, and, in children, the need for replacement of the prosthesis because of growth.

Our operative management of patients with Ebstein's malformation consists of (1) electrophysiologic mapping for localization of accessory conduction pathways in those patients having ventricular pre-excitation, (2) patch closure of the atrial septal defect or patent foramen ovale, (3) plication of the atrialized portion of the right ventricle, (4) plastic repair of the tricuspid valve, when feasible, or valve replacement with a bioprosthesis, (5) correction of associated anomalies, such as relief of pulmonary stenosis or division of accessory conduction pathways, and (6) excision of redundant right atrial wall.

The ventricular plication sutures are placed so as to avoid the posterior descending coronary artery and obvious large branches of the right coronary artery. When all plication sutures have been tied, the anterior and posterior aspects of the right ventricle are inspected to be certain that no injury has occurred to the major coronary arteries.

At the completion of the procedure, the tricuspid valve is tested by injecting saline under pressure into the right ventricle with a bulb syringe and large catheter. Finally, after venous decannulation, an exploring finger is introduced into the right atrium for direct palpation of the tricuspid valve in the beating heart. Temporary pacemaker wires are attached to the right atrium and the right ventricle for postoperative monitoring of rhythm and for pacing in selected cases.

Modification of the procedure is necessary in a few patients. In those instances in which the tricuspid valve is only moderately displaced from the anulus but in which the leaflets are adherent to the ventricular endocardium, the plicating sutures are extended across the leaflet down toward the apex of the right ventricle to the same level that would be appropriate if the leaflets had been displaced to the level of their adherence to the ventricular wall. This modification has given results as good as those in cases in which there is no adherence of the displaced leaflet to the right ventricle.

Because repair is based on the presence of an enlarged anterior leaflet, significant abnormalities of the leaflet may compromise the result. For most patients with fenestrations or perforations of the anterior leaflet, the defects can be satisfactorily repaired with fine continuous sutures. If more significant abnormalities are present, such as attachment of the free edge of the leaflet to the ventricular wall, this plastic repair will not be applicable, and prosthetic valve replacement will be required.

SURGICAL RESULTS

Thirty-four consecutive patients underwent repair of Ebstein's anomaly by this plastic repair between April 1972 and November 1981. The ages ranged from 11 months to 52 years. In three patients with Wolff-Parkinson-White syndrome and right free-wall accessory conduction pathways, the pathways were successfully interrupted. There were no instances of permanent complete heart block.

Three hospital deaths occurred (8.8 per cent), two caused by sudden ventricular fibrillation in patients who were otherwise doing well, but who had massive cardiomegaly. The third patient was an infant who had an associated hypoplastic right ventricular outflow tract. Two late deaths have occurred, both in patients who had significant preoperative ventricular arrhythmias. There have been no early or late deaths in the last 17 patients who underwent repair. During this same time interval, eight patients underwent other types of repair, with no early or late deaths (Table 44–1).

TABLE 44–1. REPAIR OF EBSTEIN'S ANOMALY APRIL 1972 TO NOVEMBER 1981

OPERATION	NUMBER OF PATIENTS	OPERATIVE MORTALITY No.	%
Plastic repair	34	3	8.8
Valve replacement with ventricular plication	6	0	0
Modified Fontan procedure*	2	0	0
Total	42	3	7.1

*Both patients had prior Glenn anastomoses.

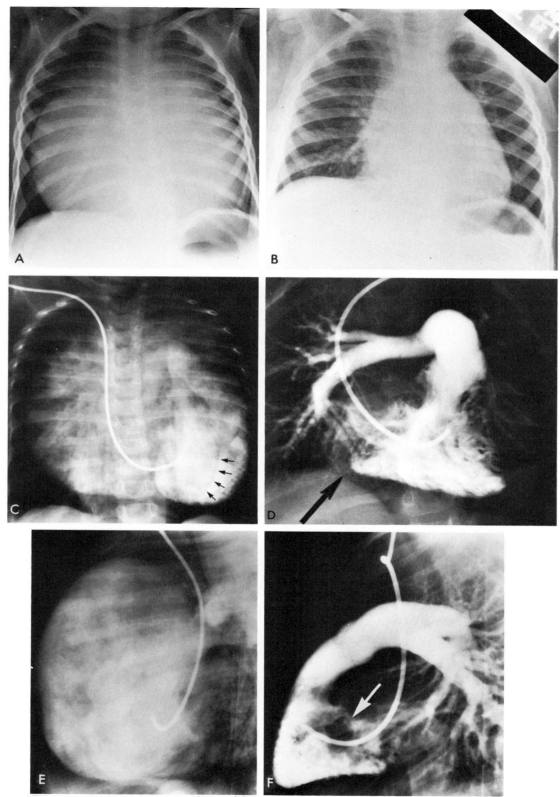

Figure 44–3. Two-year-old girl with Ebstein's anomaly and history of pneumonia, cardiorespiratory arrest, and failure to thrive. Chest roentgenograms: *A*, Preoperative (cardiothoracic ratio – 0.9). *B*, Thirteen days postoperatively (cardiothoracic ratio – 0.55). Right ventricular angiogram, anteroposterior view: *C*, Preoperative. The contrast medium refluxes through the tricuspid valve to fill the entire cardiac silhouette. A radiolucent line within the cavity of the ventricle shows the location of the displaced tricuspid leaflets (arrows). *D*, Postoperative. There is rapid transit of contrast medium from the right ventricle to the pulmonary arteries with only a trace of tricuspid insufficiency. The arrow indicates the new plane of the tricuspid valve. Right ventricular angiogram, lateral view: *E*, Preoperative. *F*, Postoperative. The tricuspid valve is competent. Arrow points to filling defect created by the anterior leaflet. This patient is now 10 years old. She is asymptomatic, is taking no cardiac medications, and is an "A" student. (From Danielson, G. K., Maloney, J. D., and Devloo, R. A. E.: Surgical repair of Ebstein's anomaly. Mayo Clin. Proc., *54*:185, 1979.)

Long-term follow-up in the first 22 survivors, who were all in New York Heart Association functional Class III or IV preoperatively, showed that all but four had improved to Class I or II. Postoperative reduction in heart size was often dramatic (Fig. 44–3*B*). The cardiothoracic ratio decreased in all patients who had a preoperative ratio greater than 0.5. Postoperative cardiac catheterizations have shown satisfactory tricuspid valve function (Fig. 44–3 *D, F*). Analysis by two-dimensional echocardiography revealed significant reduction in the atrialized portion of the right ventricle, reduced right atrial size, and good function of the reconstructed tricuspid valve. Injections of indocyanine green dye in the venae cavae confirmed absence of residual right-to-left shunting. These results compare very favorably with the natural history of patients having Ebstein's anomaly who are in functional Class III or IV (Giuliani *et al.*, 1979).

SELECTED REFERENCES

Kumar, A. E., Fyler, D. C., Miettinen, O. S., and Nadas, A. S.: Ebstein's anomaly: Clinical profile and natural history. Am. J. Cardiol., *28*:84, 1971.

The clinical features, cardiac catheterization data, and natural history of 55 patients with Ebstein's anomaly are described. This review gives a good perspective of the clinical aspects of this anomaly, but current indications for operation and techniques for repair are not discussed.

Special Review of Ebstein's anomaly. Mayo Clin. Proc., *54*:163, 1979.

This monograph describes the historical, clinical, morphologic, and surgical aspects of Ebstein's anomaly. The clinical features and natural history of 67 consecutive patients with Ebstein's anomaly who were followed a mean of 12 years are described. This monograph gives a good overview of the current knowledge of Ebstein's anomaly.

REFERENCES

Anderson, K. R., and Lie, J. T.: The right ventricular myocardium in Ebstein's anomaly. A morphometric histopathologic study. Mayo Clin. Proc., *54*:181, 1979.

Anderson, K. R., Danielson, G. K., McGoon, D. C., and Lie, O. T.: Ebstein's anomaly of the left-sided tricuspid valve: Pathological anatomy of the valvular malformation. Circulation, *58*:87, 1978.

Anderson, R. H., Becker, A. E., Arnold, R., and Wilkinson, J. L.: The conducting tissues in congenitally corrected transposition. Circulation, *50*:911, 1974.

Anderson, K. R., Zuberbuhler, J. R., Anderson, R. H., Becker, A. E., and Lie, J. T.: Morphologic spectrum of Ebstein's anomaly of the heart: A review. Mayo Clin. Proc., *54*:174, 1979.

Barnard, C. N., and Schrire, V.: Surgical correction of Ebstein's malformation with prosthetic tricuspid valve. Surgery, *54*:302, 1963.

Danielson, G. K., Maloney, J. D., and Devloo, R. A. E.: Surgical repair of Ebstein's anomaly. Mayo Clin. Proc., *54*:185, 1979.

Ebstein, W.: Über einen sehr seltenen Fall von Insufficienz der Valvula Tricuspidalis, Bedingt durch eine angeborene hochgradige Missbildung derselben. Arch. Anat. Physiol., 1866, pp. 238–254.

Giuliani, E. R., Fuster, V., Brandenburg, R. O., and Mair, D. D.: The clinical features and natural history of Ebstein's anomaly of the tricuspid valve. Mayo Clin. Proc., *54*:163, 1979.

Glenn, W. W. L., Browne, M., and Whittemore, R.: Circulatory bypass of the right side of the heart: Cava–pulmonary artery shunt — indications and results (report of a collected series of 537 cases). *In* The Heart and Circulation in the Newborn and Infant. Edited by D. E. Cassels. New York, Grune and Stratton, 1966, pp. 345–357.

Hardy, K. L., and Roe, B. B.: Ebstein's anomaly. Further experience with definitive repair. J. Thorac. Cardiovasc. Surg., *58*:553, 1969.

Hardy, K. L., May, I. A., Webster, C. A., et al.: Ebstein's anomaly: a functional concept and successful definitive repair. J. Thorac. Cardiovasc. Surg., *48*:927, 974, 1964.

Hunter, S. W., and Lillehei, C. W.: Ebstein's malformation of the tricuspid valve: Study of a case, together with suggestions of a new form of surgical therapy. Dis. Chest, *33*:297, 1958.

Kumar, A. E., Fyler, D. C., Miettinen, O. S., and Nadas, A. S.: Ebstein's anomaly: Clinical profile and natural history. Am. J. Cardiol., *28*:84, 1971.

Lillehei, C. W., Kalke, B. R., and Carlson, R. G.: Evolution of corrective surgery for Ebstein's anomaly. Circulation, *35*, *36*(Suppl. 1):111, 1967.

Mann, R. J., and Lie, J. T.: The life story of Wilhelm Ebstein (1836–1912) and his almost overlooked description of a congenital heart disease. Mayo Clin. Proc., *54*:197, 1979.

Ross, D., and Somerville, J.: Surgical correction of Ebstein's anomaly. Lancet, *2*:280, 1970.

Special review of Ebstein's anomaly. Mayo Clin. Proc., *54*:163, 1979.

Timmis, H. H., Hardy, J. D., and Watson, D. G.: The surgical management of Ebstein's anomaly. The combined use of tricuspid valve replacement, atrioventricular plication and atrioplasty. J. Thorac. Cardiovasc. Surg., *53*:385, 1967.

Watson, H.: Natural history of Ebstein's anomaly of tricuspid valve in childhood and adolescence: An international co-operative study of 505 cases. Br. Heart J., *36*:417, 1974.

Williams, D. B., Danielson, G. K., McGoon, D. C., Puga, F. J., Mair, D. D., and Edwards, W. D.: Porcine heterograft valve replacement in children. J. Thorac. Cardiovasc. Surg., *84*:446, 1982.

Wright, J. L., Burchell, H. B., Kirklin, J. W., et al.: Symposium on physiologic, clinical and surgical interdependence in study and treatment of congenital heart disease; congenital displacement of tricuspid valve (Ebstein's malformation); report of case with closure of associated foramen ovale for correction of right-to-left shunt. Proc. Staff Meet. Mayo Clin., *29*:278, 1954.

Zuberbuhler, J. R., Allwork, S. P., and Anderson, R. H.: The spectrum of Ebstein's anomaly of the tricuspid valve. J. Thorac. Cardiovasc. Surg., *77*:202, 1979.

Chapter 45

Acquired Disease of the Tricuspid Valve

Siavosh Khonsari

Albert Starr

HISTORICAL NOTES

Surgery for acquired disease of the tricuspid valve entered a new era in February 1963 (Starr *et al.*, 1964) when the first triple valve replacement was successfully performed in a desperately ill patient at the Oregon Health Sciences University. Since then, numerous ingenious prostheses and reconstructive techniques have evolved and important contributions have been made toward a better understanding of the functional anatomy of the right ventricle and tricuspid valve.

Kay and associates (1965) recommended bicuspidization of the tricuspid valve for tricuspid insufficiency by exclusion of the anulus of the posterior leaflet, and Boyd and colleagues (1974) reported a technique of measured tricuspid anuloplasty nearly a decade later. Carpentier and associates (1971) revolutionized the management of tricuspid valve disease by emphasizing that the septal segment of the tricuspid anulus does not participate in the anular dilatation process and by introducing a nondeformable prosthetic ring for their technique of anular remodeling.

DeVega reported a simple and ingenious method of semicircular anuloplasty in 1972. Duran and co-workers (1975) recommended a flexible atrioventricular ring to be used in tricuspid anuloplasty. Since then, Carpentier introduced a semicircular flexible open ring (Deloche *et al.*, 1975; Hanania *et al.*, 1975; Carpentier and Relland, 1979), and Puig Massana introduced an adjustable anuloplasty ring (Shiley, Inc., 1981).

Many other notable contributions have been made by investigators in the field, but the work of Wooler and Danielson (as cited by West and Weldon, 1978), and Bex (Hecart *et al.*, 1980) is of particular merit.

SURGICAL AND FUNCTIONAL ANATOMY OF THE TRICUSPID VALVE

The tricuspid valve guards the right ventricular orifice. It consists of a septal leaflet and a large anterior and a smaller posterior leaflet, which are attached to and blend with the tricuspid ring. Small accessory leaflets are occasionally present in the angle between the major leaflets. These valve leaflets are folds of endocardium that are strengthened by fibrous tissue. The right ventricular cavity is tubular and triangular in configuration in contrast to that of the left ventricle, which is conical. It is bounded by concave anterior and posterior walls and a convex septal wall. There are at least three groups of papillary muscles that stem from the inner aspect of the right ventricular cavity. Chordae tendineae, which are nonelastic cords of tissue, diverge from papillary muscles and become anchored to the edges as well as the ventricular aspects of the leaflets of the tricuspid valve. The chordae of each papillary muscle control the contiguous margins of two cusps. Hence, chordae pass from a large anterior papillary muscle to the anterior and posterior leaflets; from a posterior papillary muscle, often represented by two or more components, chordae become anchored to the posterior and septal leaflets; and finally, from a variable group of small septal papillary muscles, chordae fan out to become fastened to the anterior and septal leaflets of the tricuspid valve. A chord of the specialized tissue associated with the conducting mechanism, the moderator band, stems from the septum, crosses the cavity of the right ventricle, and gives origin to the anterior papillary muscle. The A-V node lies in the atrial septum superior to the septal leaflets just anterior to the opening of the coronary sinus (Fig. 45–1).

The atrioventricular bundle or bundle of His extends from the A-V node, adjacent to the septal leaflet of the tricuspid valve, through the fibrous skeleton of the heart to the membraneous part of the ventricular septum. It is about 2 mm. thick and pale and consists of bundles of fine muscular fibers. There is normally no muscular continuity between the atria and the ventricle except through the conducting tissue of the A-V node and the A-V bundle, but aberrations may exist that can give rise to rhythm disturbances.

In ventricular systole, the contraction of the free wall and the papillary muscle pulls the tricuspid valve ring downward toward the apex, and an effective right ventricular ejection is generated by the free wall moving toward the convex septal wall (Fig. 45–2). The fibrous ring prevents the orifice from stretching,

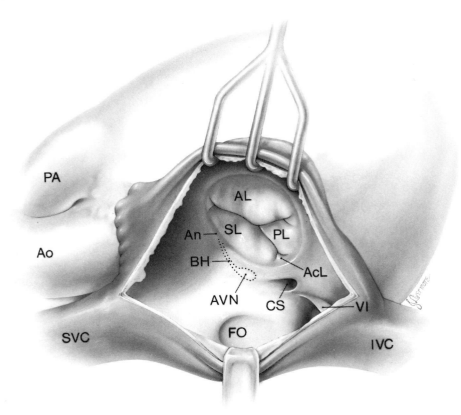

Figure 45–1. Surgical anatomy of right atrium (SVC = superior vena cava; IVC = inferior vena cava; Ao = aorta; PA = pulmonary artery; VI = valve of inferior vena cava (eustachian); CS = coronary sinus; AVN = atrial ventricular node; BH = bundle of His; AL = anterior leaflet of tricuspid valve; PL = posterior leaflet of tricuspid valve; SL = septal leaflet of tricuspid valve; AcL = accessory leaflet of tricuspid valve; AN = anulus of tricuspid valve; FO = fossa ovalis).

which may render the valve incompetent. The right ventricle is capable of ejecting a large volume of blood into a normally low-pressure pulmonary system. This is based on the shape of the chamber, which allows considerable increase in stroke volume at a small cost in wall tension and, hence, in O_2 requirement. When it becomes conical or globular, the right ventricle is put at a tremendous disadvantage and any increase in end-diastolic volume will have a profound deleterious effect on wall tension, and hence, O_2 requirements are greatly increased. When pulmonary arterial pressure rises rapidly, as in acute pulmonary embolism, right ventricular ejection becomes hampered, with catastrophic results. During ventricular contraction, the septal wall bulges inward, giving the right ventricle a flattened cavity (Fig. 45–2), but the role of the interventricular septum and right ventricular function (Armour *et al.*, 1970) is not well defined as evidenced by cineangiography. In the laboratory, however, it has been shown that septal walls can function effectively when the right ventricular free wall becomes destroyed (Zaus and Kearns, 1952).

ETIOLOGY

Rheumatic fever (Chopra and Tandon, 1977) is the most common cause of organic tricuspid valve disease. However, it usually attacks the mitral and aortic valve with such vigor that there has been some doubt in the past on an anatomic basis concerning the clinical importance of tricuspid involvement. With

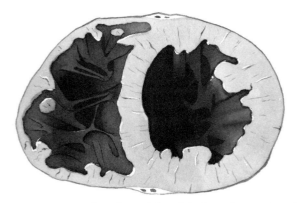
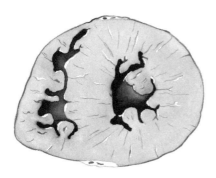

Figure 45–2. Cross-section of ventricles of the heart in systole and diastole. The septal wall bulges inward, giving the right ventricle a flattened cavity during systole.

rare exceptions, organic tricuspid valve disease is associated with mitral valve disease and, in the majority of patients, with aortic valve disease as well.

Tricuspid valve dysfunction is sometimes, but rarely, due to atrial myxoma (Suri *et al.*, 1978), blunt trauma (Stephenson *et al.*, 1979), pericardial disease (Dillon, 1977), perforation of a leaflet by a rigid transvenous electrode (Gould *et al.*, 1974; Lee *et al.*, 1977), metastatic tumor (Fortt and Mackay, 1978; Thomas *et al.*, 1977), chronic use of methysergide (Mason *et al.*, 1977; Barrillon and Baragan, 1978), or aneurysm of the ventricular septum (Eshaghpour *et al.*, 1978). It may also occasionally be a manifestation of carcinoid syndrome (Hendel *et al.*, 1980; Honey and Paneth, 1975), caused by subendothelial plaque-like thickening of valve leaflets (Ferrans and Roberts, 1976).

Commonly, both stenosis and insufficiency coexist in organic tricuspid valve disease, and pure tricuspid stenosis is rarely seen. Tricuspid insufficiency is by far the more common, and in addition to having an organic cause, it can result from anular dilatation and right heart failure.

Tricuspid incompetence as a result of right ventricular infarction (Collings and Daly, 1977; McAllister *et al.*, 1976) is an uncommon entity, but it is being reported with increasing frequency in recent years. Endocarditis of the tricuspid valve (Roberts and Buchbinder, 1972) can occasionally be seen as an isolated condition or as a part of the general picture of infective endocarditis. Of great concern is the recent emergence of a specific bacterial endocarditis in narcotic addicts (Arbulu *et al.*, 1973).

PATHOPHYSIOLOGY

The pathologic changes in rheumatic tricuspid valve disease are easily recognized and, although less extensive than in rheumatic mitral valve disease, involve the same elements of fibrous thickening of the leaflet, thickening and shortening of the chordae tendineae, and fusion of the commissures (Chopra and Tandon, 1977). Calcification is rarely extensive (Fig. 45–3). Patients with functional tricuspid regurgitation do not have these changes, and their condition is classified as reversible if tricuspid regurgitation, which was palpable prior to bypass, has disappeared completely on palpation following bypass. The condition of patients in the functional group is classified as irreversible on the basis of the following criteria: (1) prebypass palpation reveals significant tricuspid regurgitation with no evidence of scarring or fusion of the commissures; (2) inspection of the valve at operation or at reoperation confirms the absence of significant scarring, chordal thickening, or commissural fusion; and (3) considerable regurgitation persists after bypass is discontinued.

These patients are viewed as having ventricular valvular disproportion based on long-standing right ventricular hypertrophy and dilatation. On palpation, the leaflets may be pulled down into the right ventricle. The anulus is usually dilated but may be of normal size. Inspection of the decompressed heart reveals an essentially normal valve, except that there may be slight thickening of the leaflets that gives it a whitish discoloration. Inspection of these valves reveals very slight leaflet and chordal thickening that does not appear to be related to rheumatic fever and may result from turbulence injury due to long-standing functional regurgitation. The classification of tricuspid valve disease into organic, reversible functional, and irreversible functional types has important therapeutic and prognostic significance. There are some patients, however, who appear to have greatly reduced tricuspid regurgitation after mitral correction, indicating a partially reversible lesion, but who subsequently develop recurrent severe regurgitation as blood volume is

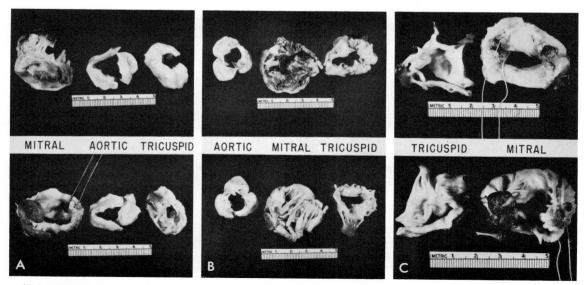

Figure 45–3. Typical resected pathologic specimens. In each instance, there was complete destruction of the mitral valve and organic disease of the tricuspid valve. *A,* Tricuspid stenosis. *B,* Mixed lesion. *C,* Pure tricuspid regurgitation.

restored in the postoperative period. Such patients may require prophylactic reparative surgery.

DIAGNOSIS, PREOPERATIVE ASSESSMENT, AND MANAGEMENT

The clinical picture in patients with tricuspid valve disease is dominated by the signs and symptoms of long-standing mitral and aortic disease. Indeed, early in our experience, significant tricuspid valve disease was unsuspected preoperatively in one third of our patients who subsequently required repair or replacement of the valve. More commonly, murmurs of tricuspid regurgitation or stenosis are easily detected, together with peripheral findings of edema, hepatosplenomegaly, ascites, and abnormal venous pulsations.

Right atrial dilatation may displace a tricuspid valve many centimeters to the left of the sternum. In such cases, the pansystolic murmur of tricuspid regurgitation may be mistakenly considered to be of mitral origin. An opening tricuspid snap is unusual in tricuspid stenosis, but when present, it is diagnostic. Two thirds of the patients have chronic atrial fibrillation, and a sinus rhythm may be present in many with sufficiently severe tricuspid valve disease to warrant operation.

Jaundice is uncommon. Abnormal liver functions occur in most patients, and about 25 per cent of the patients who require tricuspid valve surgery have depression of prothrombin function as well. Cardiac cachexia is common and correlates well with the characteristic preoperative hemodynamic findings or marked reduction of cardiac output and wide arterial venous oxygen difference at rest. Mean right atrial pressure is frequently but not always elevated.

Tricuspid stenosis causes an increase in right atrial pressure, and a diastolic pressure gradient of only 2 mm. Hg between the right atrium and the right ventricle is suggestive. A pressure gradient greater than 5 mm. Hg may precipitate gross right heart failure, manifested by peripheral edema, jugular venous distention, and ascites (Braunwald, 1980). Characteristically, the right atrial and right ventricular end-diastolic pressures are elevated in tricuspid insufficiency. The right atrial wave increasingly resembles a right ventricular wave as the degree of tricuspid incompetence increases (Grossman, 1980).

Indicator dilution techniques (Sinclair-Smith, 1974; Hoffman and Rowe, 1959) and determination of blood flow patterns (Wexler et al., 1968; Kalmanson et al., 1974; Nichols et al., 1977; Pepine et al., 1978) in the vena cava are more sophisticated tools in assessing tricuspid insufficiency. Right ventriculography using a Bourassa catheter from the inferior vena cava and indicator injected into the right ventricle and sampled in the right atrium and femoral arteries have been used to determine the severity of regurgitation (Grondin et al., 1975; Lingamneni et al., 1979; Pepine et al., 1979).

In the investigations of patients with clinical evidence of tricuspid valve disease, right ventricular systolic pressure less than 40 mm. Hg usually suggests organic tricuspid valvular disease. However, right ventricular pressure greater than 60 mm. Hg suggests tricuspid insufficiency due to right ventricular failure and dilatation. Unfortunately, it is not possible to quantify right ventricular function in terms of end-diastolic volume and systolic volume ejection fraction with sufficient precision at this time. Echocardiography and nuclear techniques are currently under evaluation and may play an important role in the very near future (Johnson et al., 1979; Berger et al., 1979; Berger and Matthay, 1981; Winzelberg et al., 1981).

Supravalvular aortography is of special value in detecting subclinical but anatomically significant aortic valve disease. In some instances, left ventriculography may provide useful information concerning myocardial contractility and severity and anatomic basis of concomitant mitral valve disease.

Coronary arteriography is very useful in patients over 40 years of age. In some patients, the need for valvular surgery is sufficiently clear from clinical and simple laboratory data, so that operation is undertaken without extensive cardiac studies and a complete assessment of mitral, aortic, and tricuspid valve function is made at the time of operation.

The duration of preoperative hospitalization may vary from a few days to a few months for patients with tricuspid valve disease. Most patients, even those with far advanced disease, reach a point of diminishing return after a few weeks of hospitalization, but some with very severe hepatic dysfunction and marked cachexia may profit from prolonged bed rest. Peritoneal dialysis and intensive diuretic treatment are occasionally indicated. For most patients, however, intensive preoperative measures are best avoided, and major reliance should be placed on the correction of the valvular disease at operation to produce postoperative improvement in cardiac function. Supplemental potassium is given preoperatively, and digitalis is withheld for a few days prior to operation. Vitamin K is given preoperatively to patients with hepatic dysfunction.

TRICUSPID VALVE ENDOCARDITIS

Tricuspid valve endocarditis is no longer a rare entity and is seen with increasing frequency in narcotic addicts. At least 25 per cent of heroin addicts with infective endocarditis have tricuspid valve involvement (Banks et al., 1973; Dreyer and Fields, 1973; Menda and Gorbach, 1973). Congenital heart malformations and occasionally an infected permanent transvenous pacemaker electrode can give rise to endocarditis. Staphylococci are the causative organisms in the majority of the patients (Roberts and Buchbinder, 1972; Menda and Gorbach, 1973; Robin et al., 1974), but the incidence of endocarditis due to mixed infections (Simberkott et al., 1974), particularly Pseudo-

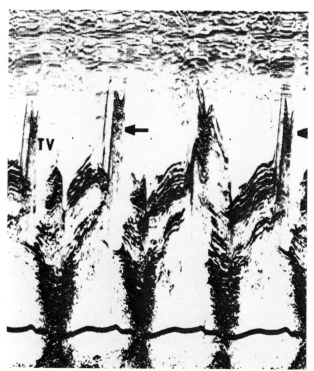

Figure 45-4. Echocardiogram of a patient with an infective endocarditis of the tricuspid valve. Arrow points to shaggy echoes reflecting vegetations on the valve leaflets. (Courtesy of Dr. M. Sheikh.)

monas, has been increasing (Rosenblatt et al., 1973; Carruthers and Kanovechayant, 1973; Cherubin et al., 1968; Conway, 1969). The triad of pyrexia, multiple lung lesions, and narcotic addiction should raise the suspicion of right-sided endocarditis. Fever and multiple septic pulmonary emboli that may progress to form lung abscesses with a murmur of tricuspid insufficiency are the most prominent features of tricuspid valve endocarditis. The chest roentgenogram may reveal multiple peripheral densities due to these septic emboli. Shaggy echoes suggestive of bacterial endocarditis vegetation affecting the tricuspid valve can be detected on echocardiography (Fig. 45-4). These findings are more clearly delineated in the presence of an enlarged right ventricle, which may be the outcome of long-standing tricuspid insufficiency and pulmonary hypertension (Sheikh et al., 1979; Dillon et al., 1973; Roy et al., 1976; Wann et al., 1976; Andy et al., 1977).

Antibiotic therapy alone can eradicate staphylococcal endocarditis. When infection is due to drug-resistant organisms or when suprainfection develops, surgical intervention with removal of the septic focus becomes mandatory. Rarely, it may be possible to shave off the localized vegetation from the valve leaflet (Chandraratna et al., 1978; Khonsari and Starr, 1980), but complete excision of the tricuspid valve can assure complete eradication of infectious vegetations. Valve replacement in the presence of active endocarditis has not been uniformly successful in the past, and a two-stage approach to tricuspid valve replacement has therefore been advocated (Arneborn et al., 1977; Arbulu et al., 1972, 1973).

Removal of the tricuspid valve necessarily results in the right atrium and right ventricle becoming a single chamber. The hemodynamic consequence may not be revealed in the immediate postoperative period, partly because of the otherwise healthy nature of the myocardium, in these patients, but right heart failure will ensue in due course (Robin et al., 1975).

Our approach to tricuspid valve endocarditis that has not responded to antibiotic therapy is to recommend excision and removal of the tricuspid valve. Valve replacement is indicated approximately 3 months after all evidence of residual infection has disappeared. Drug addicts, in addition, should be completely free of their habit before being subjected to further valve surgery in order to lessen the risk of subsequent prosthetic endocarditis. This can be difficult to establish with certainty, and there is inherent risk in valve replacement in these patients owing to the high incidence of recurrent drug addiction.

OPERATIVE TECHNIQUE

Median sternotomy is the preferred approach for acquired valvular heart disease because it allows complete exploration of the mitral, aortic, and tricuspid valves. In severely ill patients, the safety of the supine position and the decreased interference with the ventilation provide additional advantages to this approach. Changes in pulmonary artery or systemic pressures, cardiac output, and circulatory volume influence the degree of tricuspid regurgitation. However, digital palpation of the tricuspid valve prior to bypass remains an essential feature of the operative procedure. Both venae cavae are cannulated via the right atrial appendage, with arterial inflow by direct cannulation of the ascending aorta through a simple purse-string suture (Fig. 45-5a). A disposable bubble oxygenator is primed with 5 per cent dextrose and water, Ringer's lactate solution, and 10 per cent mannitol (Harlan et al., 1980). The caval tapes are tightened in order to establish total cardiopulmonary bypass. The aorta is cross-clamped just prior to the infusion of cold (4°C.) cardioplegic solution (Harlan et al., 1980). When aortic valve surgery is contemplated or when there is mild aortic insufficiency, the infusion is done through hand-held cannulas into each coronary artery ostium; in the absence of aortic valve disease, the cardioplegic solution is infused through a large-bore needle into the aortic root. The cold solution traversing the coronary circulation reaches the right atrial cavity through the coronary sinus and is discarded into a waste suctioning system through an opening in the right atrium.

A needle thermistor introduced into the interventricular septum provides continuous monitoring of myocardial temperature, which is kept between 10° and 14°C. by reinfusion of cardioplegic solution every

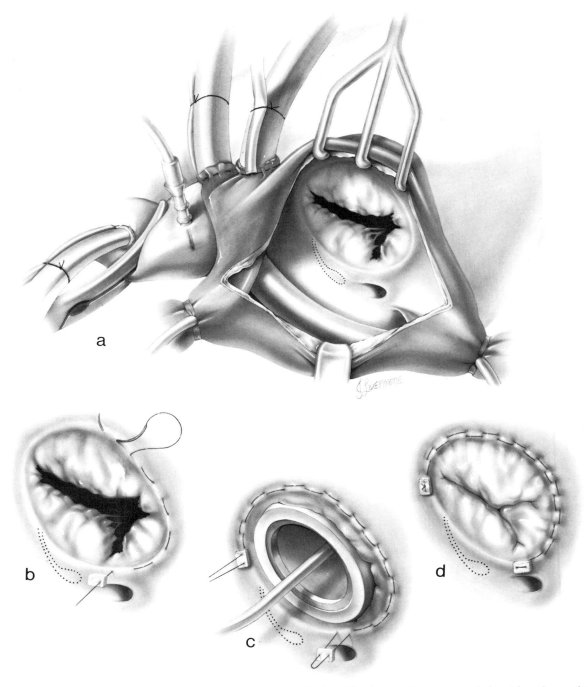

Figure 45–5. DeVega's technique of anuloplasty. *a,* Exposure of tricuspid valve; aortic root cannulation; bicaval cannulation via right atrial appendage with IVC cannula lying in the posterior gutter of right atrium; aortic needle air vent also used for infusion of cardioplegic solution. *b,* Deep bites are taken into the tricuspid anulus using 2-0 Prolene suture material. *c,* A second row of similar sutures traverses the same routes as in *b* and is then tied around a Starr-Edwards mitral prosthesis of desired size. Pledgets of Teflon are used at both ends of the suture for a buttressing effect. *d,* The completed anuloplasty.

30 to 40 minutes or as deemed necessary. For added protection, the heart is bathed in 4°C. Physiosol solution, and the anterior surface of the right ventricle is protected from the heat of the operating room light with an ice-cold soaked sponge.

The left atrium is opened behind the interatrial groove, either for a left-sided vent during the course of aortic valve surgery or for exposure of the mitral valve. The aortic valve is repaired or replaced after the mitral surgery has been completed. The tricuspid procedure is left as the last step in the multiple-valve procedure. Usually, the Foley catheter, placed through the mitral prosthesis and brought out through the left atriotomy, is left in place until the tricuspid operation is completed.

The right atrium is explored when there is either preoperative hemodynamic diagnosis of tricuspid valvular disease or a prior history of tricuspid insufficiency. The suggestion of some abnormality on digital palpation of the tricuspid valve prior to bypass is another equally important indication for opening the right atrium.

In organic valve disease, the morphology is distorted and is characterized by severe leaflet deficiency associated with stenosis of the commissures. A reparative procedure is always attempted in these patients, but valve replacement may have to be performed.

Reversible functional disease is characterized by the disappearance of regurgitation following a satisfactory repair of associated valvular disease. The regurgitation is usually due to right ventricular damage with increased pulmonary vascular resistance, giving rise to right ventricular dilatation and stretching of the tricuspid anulus.

Irreversible functional tricuspid insufficiency is the outcome of chronic right ventricular damage with permanent increase in right ventricular volume and loss of the bellows shape. Following satisfactory relief of associated valvular disease, the regurgitant jet will remain and may even progress, resulting in increased postoperative mortality and morbidity.

The controversy regarding the management of functional tricuspid insufficiency reflects the inadequacy of precisely distinguishing the two stages of the same disease process. Both the DeVega and Carpentier techniques of tricuspid anuloplasty are satisfactory and do not incorporate the margin of the septal leaflet that is usually minimally involved in functional dilatation (Carpentier et al., 1971).

The DeVega Anuloplasty

DeVega's anuloplasty (Rabago et al., 1980) is an effective method in the management of reversible functional tricuspid insufficiency. We recommend this technique even in patients in whom the only indication may be prior history of tricuspid insufficiency. Because of its simplicity, little additional time is required, and it can be performed with the initial mitral valve surgery.

The right atrium is opened in a longitudinal direction, and the tricuspid valve is inspected. A double-armed needle suture, usually 2-0 Prolene, is started on the septal ring just before the anterior septal commissure. It is then extended forward by taking (every 5 to 6 mm.) deep bites into the endocardium and the fibrous ring of the posterior septal commissure, posterior leaflet, anteroposterior commissure, anterior leaflet, anterior septal commissure, and about 4 to 5 mm. of septal ring. The second needle of the suture traverses the same route in the same fashion. At each end of the suture, a small pledget of Teflon

is used for a buttressing effect, and the suture is then tied securely around a 28- or 30-mm. Starr-Edwards mitral prosthesis obturator to ensure an anuloplasty of predictable size (Fig. 45–5).

Carpentier Ring Anuloplasty (Carpentier et al., 1974; Carpentier and Relland, 1979)

Criticism of the efficacy of DeVega's semicircular anuloplasty has alluded to the inability to concentrate the plication at the commissures, where dilatation is predominant. At times, infolding of the leaflets as a consequence of anular plication may interfere with the normal function of the valve. Carpentier's current prosthesis is a flexible semicircle with a large opening at the septal leaflet (Fig. 45–6). It conforms to the normal shape of the tricuspid valve. The sizes vary according to the length of the septal fibrous ring. Mattress sutures of 3-0 Dacron are placed in the fibrous anulus, excluding that of septal leaflet, and then brought out through the prosthetic ring at shorter intervals in order to reduce the size of the anulus. They are then individually tied in place (Fig. 45–7). The Carpentier prosthesis is useful in valvular reconstruction. It restores the valvular ring to its normal configuration when severe anular dilatation or mixed disease is present.

Once the decision is made to repair a tricuspid valve for pure regurgitation based on the findings at operation, the plan must go to completion. When the decompressed heart is opened, the tricuspid valve may look completely competent. The features of ventricular valvular disproportion are missed in the decompressed heart, and the slight thickening of the subvalvular mechanism is not easily detected from the atrial view.

This aggressive approach to tricuspid valve disease, either by replacement or by Carpentier ring anuloplasty, is supported by the results in 50 patients undergoing mitral valve replacement early in our experience in whom tricuspid valve disease was either not treated or treated inadequately. Twelve patients

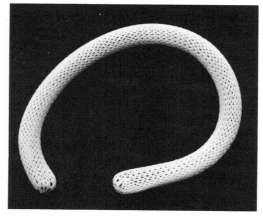

Figure 45–6. Carpentier-Edwards anuloplasty ring (Model 4500).

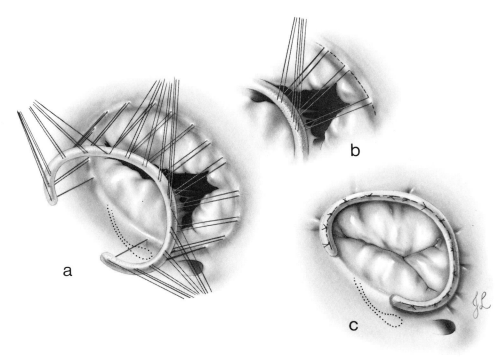

Figure 45–7. Technique of Carpentier ring anuloplasty. *a*, Deep mattress sutures of 3-0 Dacron are placed in the fibrous anulus, excluding the septal segment, and are then brought out at shorter intervals through the ring. *b*, Wider bites are taken at the commissural anulus in order to reduce the size of as well as remodel the anulus of tricuspid valve. *c*, The semicircular prosthesis tied in position, thus restoring a normal configuration to the valvular ring.

required a second-stage tricuspid valve replacement, and three required further reparative surgery as a result of recurrent symptoms.

Tricuspid Commissurotomy

In patients with pure or predominant tricuspid stenosis, direct-vision commissurotomy may be attempted, but at times, division of the fused chordae tendineae may become necessary. Because separation of all the fused commissures may produce tricuspid regurgitation, commissurotomy is limited to one or two commissures (Fig. 45–8). The use of the Carpentier ring in association with commissurotomy has been in those patients with reasonable leaflet pliability and surface area. The technique of closed tricuspid commissurotomy as attempted in the past in conjunction with closed mitral commissurotomy is likely to injure the tricuspid valve and has been discarded as definitive treatment for tricuspid stenosis. However, in the patient with very tight tricuspid stenosis, temporary improvement may be achieved prior to bypass by increasing the tricuspid orifice by mild digital pressure at the time of palpation.

Tricuspid Valve Replacement

When the severity of valvular distortion prevents a satisfactory reconstructive procedure, valve replacement is performed. Resection of the tricuspid valve is started by incising the attached margin of the anterior and posterior leaflets and dividing the papillary muscles deep in the right ventricle. The mobilized valve

may now be inverted into the right atrium, and under visual control from both the atrial and ventricular sides, the septal leaflet is resected. A broad zone of attached margin of septal leaflet and its chordal support are left in place. Size 3-0 Teflon-impregnated

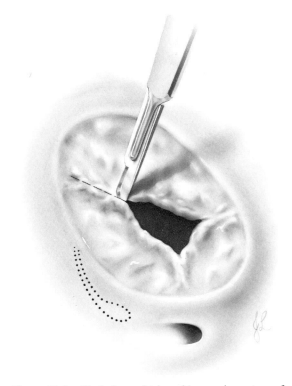

Figure 45–8. Technique of tricuspid commissurotomy for tricuspid stenosis. Commissurotomy is limited to one or two commissures. The anteroseptal commissure is "rarely" incised.

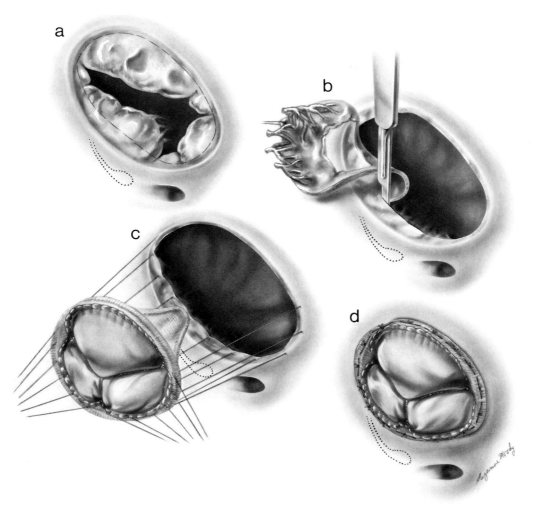

Figure 45–9. Technique of tricuspid valve replacement. *a,* Diseased tricuspid valve. Dotted line shows line of valvular resection. *b,* The diseased tricuspid valve is resected leaving a broad zone of the septal leaflet with its supporting chordal attachment intact. *c,* Deep mattress sutures of 3-0 Dacron are passed through the anulus and through the septal leaflet tissue to avoid heart block. If the structures are friable or delicate, horizontal pledgeted sutures are preferred. *d,* The bioprosthesis sewn in place.

Dacron sutures are passed through the anulus, except in the region of the septal leaflet. In this area, sutures are placed only through leaflet tissue and its supporting structure to avoid heart block. The sutures are then passed through the cloth margin of the prosthesis exactly as in mitral valve replacement. The prosthesis is slipped down into its bed, and the sutures are tied and cut (Fig. 45–9). Care is taken to avoid injury to the right ventricular endocardium by pressing the prosthesis into the decompressed ventricle. As in mitral valve replacement, the size selection is based not only on the diameter of the atrioventricular ring but also on the size of the right ventricular cavity. No problems have been encountered in narrowing the anulus by placing sutures close together in the prosthesis. However, serious injury to the septum may occur if too large a prosthesis is selected.

Following closure of the right heart, the patient is tilted with the right side up so that the air may be removed from the left heart via the partially closed left atrial incision. A needle vent is placed in the ascending aorta, and the heart is defibrillated. The Foley catheter is removed from the mitral prosthesis, and the bleeding residual left atrial incision is closed. Prolonged mechanical ventilatory assistance is required in about 75 per cent of these patients with far-advanced disease. This is done with a nasotracheal tube, with care being taken to avoid pressure necrosis of the nares. Tracheostomy is rarely indicated.

RESULTS OF TRICUSPID VALVE REPLACEMENT

From 1963 to 1980, we have implanted 136 tricuspid valves either as an initial operation or as a re-replacement of a previous prosthesis in 121 patients. Fifty-five patients had triple-valve replacement; 58 patients had mitral and tricuspid valve replacement; seven had isolated tricuspid replacement; and one patient had aortic and tricuspid replacement. Except for patients with Ebstein's disease, infective endocarditis, or prosthetic valve malfunction, no tricuspid valve has been replaced in our institution since 1973.

The operative mortality rate was 21 per cent (25 of 118) for primary operations and 6 per cent (1 of 18) for re-replacement. The overall operative mortality rate was 19 per cent (26 of 136). Consideration must be given to the early time frame of operation in this series and the high percentage of replacements done for functional regurgitation with end-stage right ventricular disease. Thus, there was a significant difference between the operative risk for organic tricuspid valve disease (13 per cent) and that for functional tricuspid valve disease (32 per cent). It is of interest that during the time frame involved in this review, the addition of tricuspid valve replacement as an independent variable to other variables associated with multivalvular procedures did not significantly alter the operative risk.

All patients with tricuspid valve replacement for acquired heart disease have received anticoagulant therapy because the tricuspid valve surgery was associated with replacement of other valves. When tricuspid valve replacement was performed for an isolated lesion, as in Ebstein's disease, anticoagulation has not proved necessary.

Caged Ball Prostheses. In describing the results obtained with replacement of the tricuspid valve, emphasis will be placed on the 95 patients in this series with acquired multiple valvular disease in whom the tricuspid valve was replaced with a caged ball valve prosthesis (Fig. 45–10), since this group constitutes the largest number of patients. The most recent ball valve was implanted in our institution in 1973. The overall operative mortality rate in the caged ball valve series was 23 per cent (22 of 97). The operative mortality rate was 18 per cent (12 to 67) for organic disease, 40 per cent (10 of 25) for functional irreversible disease, and 0 per cent (0 of 5) for re-replacement of a previous prosthesis. There were 56 Silastic ball valves and 41 metal ball valves in this series. Of the 75 patients who survived the ball valve operation, 41 died from 1 to 17 years postoperatively; eight have had valves removed and re-replaced from 1 to 15 years postoperatively; and 26 are presently alive with

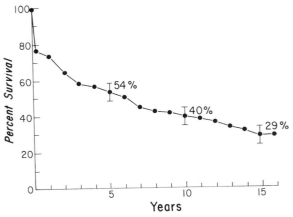

Figure 45–11. Actuarial survival curve following tricuspid valve replacement with caged-ball prosthesis.

caged ball valves in place. Twenty-one patients are alive more than 10 years after operation, and six patients are alive more than 15 years after operation. The longest surviving patient is now in her eighteenth postoperative year and is enjoying a satisfactory life-style. Causes of late death have been thrombotic occlusion of the tricuspid valve, arrhythmia, congestive failure due to myocardial fibrosis, infection, myocardial infarction, cerebrovascular accident, pneumonia, and drug idiosyncrasy. Of note is the absence of any clinical evidence of pulmonary embolism. The 5-, 10-, and 15-year survival rates, including operative mortality, are 54 ± 5 per cent, 40 ± 5 per cent, and 29 ± 6 per cent, respectively (Fig. 45–11).

There have been 12 patients with thrombotic stenosis in the caged ball valve series, occurring from 1 to 15 years postoperatively: In five patients, it was fatal; seven patients underwent successful re-replacement. The thrombosis-free rates at 5, 10, and 15 years are 87 ± 4 per cent, 82 ± 5 per cent, and 72 ± 9 per cent, respectively (Fig. 45–12). The pathology at autopsy or reoperation was similar in all patients with thrombosed ball valve prostheses. The cage was found

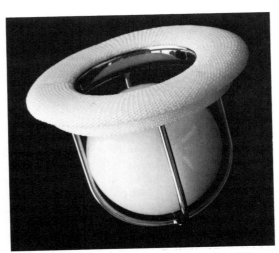

Figure 45–10. Silastic ball valve (Model 6120).

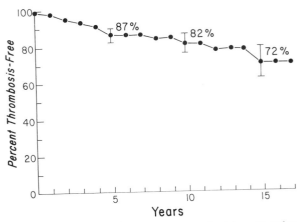

Figure 45–12. Thrombosis-free curve for tricuspid valve replacement with caged ball prosthesis.

to be partially embedded in the right ventricular endocardium, and thrombus was primarily on the ventricular side of the valve. A review of patients with fatal thrombosis revealed that symptoms are gradual in onset and should allow successful reoperation in the majority of cases.

The experience with tricuspid valve replacement at the Mayo Clinic (Sanfelippo et al., 1971) included 154 patients whose valves were replaced with a Starr-Edwards ball valve prostheses. Despite an operative mortality rate of 28 per cent, 70 per cent of the surviving patients were alive after 3 years, and 93 per cent of these patients were functionally improved. Experience with tricuspid valve replacement at the University of Alabama Medical Center (Kouchoukos and Stephenson, 1976) included 87 patients, with an operative mortality rate of 22 per cent during a 7.5-year period. The prostheses used were 33 Starr-Edwards Silastic ball valves, 25 Starr-Edwards metallic ball valves, nine Braunwald-Cutter ball valves, 16 Bjork-Shiley tilting disc valves, and four porcine xenografts. No death was due to malfunction of the prostheses, and the incidence of thromboembolism was only 4 per cent among the surviving patients. Myocardial dysfunction accounted for over 75 per cent of late deaths. Bjork (Péterffy et al., 1978) reported his experience of 66 patients whose tricuspid valves were replaced with Bjork-Shiley prostheses, with an operative mortality rate of 21 per cent. Three of the surviving patients (14 per cent) developed thrombosis of the tricuspid valve, which had to be excised and re-replaced. Acute catastrophic accidents are major drawbacks associated with tilting disc valves (Azpitarte et al., 1975; Bourdillon and Sharratt, 1976). Other reports from Glasgow (Baxter et al., 1975) and Edmondton (Jugdutt et al., 1977) relate similar experiences.

At the National Heart, Lung and Blood Institute in Bethesda, Maryland, clinical and hemodynamic results were compared in patients who underwent triple-valve replacement with mechanical and xenograft prostheses. Mechanical valves were selected during the period from 1966 to 1972, and xenografts were chosen from 1972 to 1975. The authors concluded that xenografts compared favorably with mechanical valves, although their 6-year experience included two different time frames (Rhodes et al., 1977). Dura mater (Zerbini and Puig, 1979) valves and pericardial valves (Becker et al., 1981) are currently under evaluation and may have an important place, especially in patients with a small right ventricular cavity. However, degenerative and calcific changes in the tissue valves (Lamberti et al., 1979; Sade et al., 1979; Allen et al., 1982) continue to be of concern.

A review of our own experience does not allow a firm conviction concerning the ideal prosthesis for tricuspid valve replacement, because our experience with the xenograft is small. Our experience with the disc valves reveals a higher thrombosis rate than with ball valves. If those patients with functional irreversible tricuspid regurgitation, a condition for which

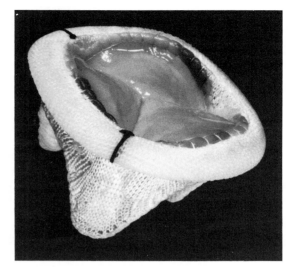

Figure 45–13. Carpentier-Edwards improved bioprosthesis (Model 6625).

tricuspid valve replacement is currently contraindicated, are excluded, our results with the ball valve are acceptable. The question is one of balancing the risk of reoperation for thrombosis with a Silastic ball valve against the risk of reoperation for valve failure with the xenograft. Since the long-term durability of the xenograft in the tricuspid position is not known at this time, a decision based on quantitative results is not possible. However, the low profile of the xenograft and the possibility of at least 10 years of adequate function for the majority of patients would lead us to select this prosthesis as the valve of choice for tricuspid valve replacement at present (Fig. 45–13). However, when the right ventricular cavity is large and the patient is young with a reasonable life expectancy, and mechanical prostheses that require anticoagulation have been implanted at other valve sites, the Silastic ball valve (Fig. 45–12) may provide a more suitable replacement. We look forward to future reports of long-term results for comparison in order to better define the relative merits of alternative devices for replacement of the tricuspid valve.

RESULTS OF CONSERVATIVE SURGERY

Recent reports on the long-term follow-up of patients who have undergone tricuspid valve anuloplasty have all been impressive. The Carpentier, DeVega, Duran, and other techniques have all proved to be satisfactory in clinics all over the world. A collaborative report from the Montreal Heart Institute and from Madrid (Grondin et al., 1975) has confirmed the efficacy of both the Carpentier ring and DeVega technique of anuloplasty, with 77 per cent of the patients having had a good result. Most patients who had residual tricuspid insufficiency had, in fact, incomplete repair of a left-sided lesion. Duran and associates (1980) reported their vast experience with

368 patients who required tricuspid valve surgery during a 5-year period from 1974 to 1979. Of 350 patients who underwent tricuspid valve anuloplasty, the Duran flexible ring was used in 306, the Carpentier ring in 31, the DeVega technique of anuloplasty in 13, isolated commissurotomy in nine, and valve replacement in nine, with an overall hospital mortality rate of 8.4 per cent. Detailed comparison of preoperative and postoperative parameters such as functional class, tricuspid gradient, tricuspid insufficiency, and right ventricular volume revealed a significant improvement in the absence of poor right ventricular myocardium, increased pulmonary hypertension, and residual lesions of the left heart. Thus, at the end stages of acquired valvular heart disease, especially in patients with massive long-standing cardiomegaly, a point is reached beyond which valvular replacement or anuloplasty is ineffective in restoring cardiac function. Although residual pulmonary vascular disease may be responsible for this in a few patients, the primary problem appears to be myocardial, which may be manifested as myocardial fibrosis on microscopic examination. In others, the cause of persistent cardiomegaly is obscure. It is now apparent that conservative corrective operation for acquired valvular heart disease should be attempted early in the course of the disease, thus preventing the possbiility of irreversible myocardial damage.

SELECTED REFERENCES

Chopra, P., and Tandon, H. D.: Pathology of chronic rheumatic heart disease with particular reference to tricuspid valve involvement. Acta Cardiol., 32:423, 1977.

A detailed study of pathologic changes in chronic and acute rheumatic heart disease in 144 autopsied cases forms the basis of this report. The incidence of tricuspid valve involvement was 46 per cent, and its association with severe pulmonary vascular changes, particularly in the juvenile age group, was noteworthy.

Duran, C. M., Pomar, J. L., Colman, T., et al.: Is tricuspid valve repair necessary? J. Thorac. Cardiovasc. Surg., 80:849, 1980.

This is an excellent review of 150 patients who were studied by full catheterization and biventricular angiography both preoperatively and postoperatively to delineate the indication for tricuspid valve surgery and to evaluate the efficacy of tricuspid valve remodeling. The authors conclude that early satisfactory repair of the left-sided lesions is most important to prevent the development of functional tricuspid insufficiency. Seventy-eight patients had organic tricuspid disease, and 72 patients had functional tricuspid disease. Anuloplasty was performed in 115 patients and commissurotomy in 46 patients, and the tricuspid valve was left alone in the remaining patients. When pulmonary vascular resistance can be predicted to fall after adequate repair of associated valvular disease, functional tricuspid insufficiency may be surgically ignored. Tricuspid anuloplasty is indicated in all patients with organic disease and in those with irreversible functional tricuspid insufficiency.

Grondin, P., Meere, C., Limet, R., et al.: Carpentier's annulus and DeVega's annuloplasty: The end of the tricuspid challenge. J. Thorac. Cardiovasc. Surg., 70:852, 1975.

This is a combined study from Montreal and Madrid on the efficacy of Carpentier and DeVega techniques of tricuspid valve remodeling. Cardiac catheterization and biventricular angiography were carried out on all patients 6 to 38 months postoperatively. Both procedures proved to be satisfactory, and any residual tricuspid insufficiency was attributed to inadequate repair of the left-sided heart lesions.

Kay, J. H., Mendez, A. M., and Zubiate, P.: A further look at tricuspid annuloplasty. Ann. Thorac. Surg., 22:498, 1976.

This report reviews the experience with the bicuspidization technique of anuloplasty of the tricuspid valve, as described by Kay, in 96 patients. The operative mortality was 10 per cent and the actuarial curve showed a 64 per cent survival rate at 12 years.

Pepine, C. J., Nichols, W. W., and Selby, J. H.: Diagnostic tests for tricuspid insufficiency: How good? (Editorial.) Cathet. Cardiovasc. Diagn., 5:1, 1979.

This editorial reviews in some depth the current techniques and methods for the evaluation of tricuspid insufficiency.

Robin, E., Thomas, N. W., Arbulu, A., et al.: Hemodynamic consequences of total removal of the tricuspid valve without prosthetic replacement. Am. J. Cardiol., 35:481, 1975.

Hemodynamic data before and after tricuspid valvulectomy without prosthetic replacement in 10 heroin addicts with infective endocarditis did not offer a differentiating factor in anticipation of the late development of right heart failure. Three patients developed right heart failure within 19 months postoperatively and required valve replacement. The remaining patients were asymptomatic but did develop a rise in right atrial mean pressure.

Sanfelippo, P. M., Giuliani, E. R., Danielson, G. K., et al.: Tricuspid valve prosthetic replacement. Early and late results with the Starr-Edwards prosthesis. J. Thorac. Cardiovasc. Surg., 71:441, 1975.

This is a valuable review of 154 patients with Starr-Edwards ball valve replacement of the tricuspid valve at the Mayo Clinic. Tricuspid valve replacement with mitral valve replacement had a 70 per cent 3-year survival rate, with 94 per cent of the surviving patients showing functional improvement. Triple valve replacement had a 50 per cent 3-year survival rate, with 93 per cent of the surviving patients showing functional improvement.

REFERENCES

Allen, D. J., Highison, G. J., Didio, L. J. A., et al.: Evidence of remodeling in dura mater cardiac valves. J. Thorac. Cardiovasc. Surg., 84:267, 1982.

Andy, J. J., Skeikh, M. I., Ali, N., et al.: Echocardiographic observations in opiate addicts with active infective endocarditis. Am. J. Cardiol, 40:17, 1977.

Arbulu, A., Thomas, N. W., and Wilson, R.: Valvulectomy without prosthetic replacement. J. Thorac. Cardiovasc. Surg., 64:102, 1972.

Arbulu, A., Kafi, A., Thomas, N. W., et al.: Right-sided bacterial endocarditis. Ann. Thorac. Surg., 16:136, 1973.

Armour, J. A., Page, J. B., and Randall, W. C.: Interrelationship of architecture and function of right ventricle. Am. J. Physiol., 218:174, 1970.

Arneborn, P., Bjork, V. O., Rodriguez, L., et al.: Two-stage replacement of tricuspid valve in active endocarditis. Br. Heart J., 39:1276, 1977.

Azpitarte, J., DeVega, N. G., Santalla, A., et al. Thrombotic obstruction of Bjork-Shiley tricuspid valve prosthesis. Report of three cases reoperated with success. Acta Cardiol., 30:419, 1975.

Banks, T., Fletcher, R., and Ali, N.: Infective endocarditis in heroin addicts. Am. J. Med., 55:444, 1973.

Barrillon, A., and Baragan, J.: Methysergide and tricuspid valve lesions. Circulation, 58:578, 1978.

Baxter, R. H., Bain, W. H., Rankin, R. J., et al.: Tricuspid valve replacement: A five-year appraisal. Thorax, 30:158, 1975.

Becker, R. M., Sandor, L., Tindel, M., *et al.*: Medium-term follow-up of the Ionescu-Shiley heterograft valve. Ann. Thorac. Surg., *32*:120, 1981.

Berger, H. J., and Matthay, R.: Radionuclide right ventricular ejection fraction. (Editorial.) Chest, *79*:497, 1981.

Berger, H. J., Johnstone, D. E., Sands, J. M., *et al.*: Response of right ventricular ejection fraction to upright bicycle exercise in coronary artery disease. Circulation, *60*:1292, 1979.

Bourdillon, P. D., and Sharratt, G. P.: Malfunction of Bjork-Shiley valve prosthesis in tricuspid position. Br. Heart J., *38*:1149, 1976.

Boyd, A. D., Engelman, R. M, Isom, O. W., Reed, G. E., and Spencer, F. C.: Tricuspid annuloplasty. Five and one-half years' experience with 78 patients. J. Thorac. Cardiovasc. Surg., *68*:344, 1974.

Braunwald, E. (Ed.): Heart Disease: A Textbook of Cardiovascular Medicine. Philadelphia, W. B. Saunders Company, 1980.

Carpentier, A., and Relland, J.: Carpentier rings and tricuspid insufficiency. Ann. Thorac. Surg., *27*:96, 1979.

Carpentier, A., Deloche, A., Dauptain, J., *et al.*: A new reconstructive operation for correction of mitral and tricuspid insufficiency. J. Thorac. Cardiovasc. Surg., *61*:1, 1971.

Carpentier, A., Deloche, A., Hanania, G., *et al.*: Surgical management of acquired tricuspid valve disease. J. Thorac. Cardiovasc. Surg., *67*:53, 1974.

Carruthers, M. M., and Kanovechayant, R.: *Pseudomonas aeruginosa* endocarditis. Report of a case, with review of the literature. Am. J. Med., *55*:811, 1973.

Chandraratna, P. A. N., Reagan, R. B., Imaizumi, T., *et al.*: Infective endocarditis cured by resection of a tricuspid valve vegetation. Ann. Intern. Med., *89*:517, 1978.

Cherubin, C. E., Baden, M., Kavaler, F., *et al.*: Infective endocarditis in heroin addicts. Ann. Intern. Med., *69*:1091, 1968.

Chopra, P., and Tandon, H. D.: Pathology of chronic rheumatic heart disease with particular reference to tricuspid valve involvement. Acta Cardiol., *32*:423, 1977.

Collings, R., and Daly, J. J.: Tricuspid incompetence complicating acute myocardial infarction. Postgrad. Med. J., *53*:51, 1977.

Conway, N.: Endocarditis in heroin addicts. Br. Heart J., *31*:543, 1969.

Deloche, A., Carpentier, A., Hanania, G., *et al.*: Annuloplastie reconstitutive tricuspidienne (résultats cliniques sur 250 patients). Coeur, numéro spécial:673, 1975.

DeVega, N. G.: La anuloplastia selectiva, regulable y permanente. Rev. Esp. Cardiol., *25*:555, 1972.

Dillon, J. C.: Tricuspid stenosis secondary to pericardial disease. (Editorial.) Chest, *71*:690, 1977.

Dillon, J. C., Feigenbaum, H., Konecke, L. L., *et al.*: Echocardiographic manifestations of valvular vegetations. Am. Heart J., *86*:698, 1973.

Dreyer, N. P., and Fields, B. N.: Heroin associated infective endocarditis. Ann. Intern. Med., *78*:699, 1973.

Duran, C. M., Pomar, J. L., Colman, T., *et al.*: Is tricuspid valve repair necessary? J. Thorac. Cardiovasc. Surg., *80*:849, 1980.

Duran, C. M., Cucchiara, G., Ubago, J. L., and Pomar, J. L.: A new flexible ring for atrioventricular annuloplasty. Proceedings of the Annual Meeting of the Society of Thoracic and Cardiovascular Surgeons of Great Britain and Ireland, Glasgow, Scotland, September 26, 1975.

Eshaghpour, E., Kawai, N., and Linhart, J. W.: Tricuspid insufficiency associated with aneurysm of the ventricular septum. Pediatrics, *61*:586, 1978.

Ferrans, V. J., and Roberts, W. C.: The carcinoid endocardial plaque. Hum. Pathol., *7*:387, 1976.

Fortt, R. W., Mackay, A. D.: A solitary cardiac metastasis involving the tricuspid valve ring. Pathol. Res. Pract., *162*:420, 1978.

Gould, L., Reddy, C. V., Yacoub, U., *et al.*: Perforation of the tricuspid valve by a transvenous pacemaker. J.A.M.A., *230*:86, 1974.

Grondin, P., Meere, C., Limet, R., *et al.*: Carpentier's annulus and DeVega's annuloplasty: The end of the tricuspid challenge. J. Thorac. Cardiovasc. Surg., *70*:852, 1975.

Grossman, W. (Ed.): Cardiac Catheterization and Angiography. 2nd Ed. Philadelphia, Lea and Febiger, 1980.

Hanania, G., Sellier, P., Deloche, A., *et al.*: Résultats à moyen terme de l'annuloplastie tricuspide reconstitutive de Carpentier. Arch. Mal. Coeur, *67*:875, 1975.

Harlan, B. J., Starr, A., and Harwin, F. M.: Manual of Cardiac Surgery. Vol. I. New York, Springer-Verlag, 1980.

Hecart, J., Blaise, C., Bex, J. P., *et al.*: Technique for tricuspid annuloplasty with a flexible linear reducer. J. Thorac. Cardiovasc. Surg., *79*:689, 1980.

Hendel, N., Leckie, B., and Richards, J.: Carcinoid heart disease: Eight-year survival following tricuspid valve replacement and pulmonary valvotomy. Ann. Thorac. Surg., *30*:391, 1980.

Hoffman, J. I. E., and Rowe, G. G.: Some factors affecting indicator dilution curves in the presence and absence of valvular incompetence. J. Clin. Invest., *38*:138, 1959.

Honey, M., and Paneth, M.: Carcinoid heart disease: Successful tricuspid valve replacement. Thorax, *30*:464, 1975.

Johnson, L. L., McCarthy, D. M., Sciacca, R. R., *et al.*: Right ventricular ejection fraction during exercise in patients with coronary artery disease. Circulation, *60*:1284, 1979.

Jugdutt, B. I., Fraser, R. S., Lee, S. J., *et al.*: Long-term survival after tricuspid valve replacement. Results with seven different prostheses. J. Thorac. Cardiovasc. Surg., *74*:20, 1977.

Kalmanson, D., Veyrat, C., Chiche, P., *et al.*: Non-invasive diagnosis of right heart disease and of left to right shunts using directional Doppler ultrasound. *In* Cardiovascular Applications of Ultrasound. Edited by R. S. Reneman. New York, American Elsevier, 1974, p. 361.

Kay, J. H., Maselli-Campagna, G., and Tsuji, H. K.: Surgical treatment of tricuspid insufficiency. Ann. Surg., *162*:53, 1965.

Kay, J. H., Mendez, A. M., and Zubiate, P.: A further look at tricuspid annuloplasty. Ann. Thorac. Surg., *22*:498, 1976.

Khonsari, S., and Starr, A.: Unpublished data, 1980.

Kouchoukos, N. T., and Stephenson, L. W.: Indications for and results of tricuspid valve replacement: Clinical application of current techniques and treatment in cardiology. Adv. Cardiol., *17*:199, 1976.

Lamberti, J. J., Wainer, B. H., Fisher, K. A., *et al.*: Calcific stenosis of the porcine heterograft. Ann. Thorac. Surg., *28*:28, 1979.

Lee, M. E., Chaux, A., and Matlogg, J. M.: Avulsion of a tricuspid valve leaflet during traction on an infected, entrapped endocardial pacemaker electrode. The role of electrode design. J. Thorac. Cardiovasc. Surg., *74*:433, 1977.

Lingamneni, R., Cha, S. D., Maranhao, V., *et al.*: Tricuspid regurgitation: Clinical and angiographic assessment. Cathet. Cardiovasc. Diagn., *5*:7, 1979.

Mason, J. W., Billingham, M. E., and Friedman, J. P.: Methysergide induced heart disease, a case of multivalvular and myocardial fibrosis. Circulation, *56*:889, 1977.

McAllister, R. G., Jr., Friesinger, G. C, and Sinclair-Smith, B. C.: Tricuspid regurgitation following inferior myocardial infarction. Arch. Intern. Med., *136*:95, 1976.

Menda, K. B., and Gorbach, S. L.: Favorable experience with bacterial endocarditis in heroin addicts. Ann. Intern. Med., *78*:25, 1973.

Nichols, W. W., Conti, C. R., Pepine, C. J., *et al.*: Instantaneous force velocity length relations in the intact human heart. Am. J. Cardiol., *40*:754, 1977.

Pepine, C. J., Nichols, W. W., and Conti, C. R.: Aortic input impedance. Circulation, *58*:460, 1978.

Pepine, C. J., Nichols, W. W., and Selby, J. H.: Diagnostic tests for tricuspid insufficiency: How good? (Editorial.) Cathet. Cardiovasc. Diagn., *5*:1, 1979.

Péterffy, A., Henze, A., Jonasson, R., *et al.*: Clinical evaluation of the Bjork-Shiley tilting disc valve in the tricuspid position. Early and late results in 10 isolated and 51 combined cases. Scand. J. Thorac. Cardiovasc. Surg., *12*:179, 1978.

Rabago, G., DeVega, N. G., Castillon, L., *et al.*: The new DeVega technique in tricuspid annuloplasty (results in 150 patients). J. Cardiovasc. Surg., *21*:231, 1980.

Rhodes, G. R., McIntosh, C. L., Redwood, D. R., *et al.*: Clinical and hemodynamic results following triple valve replacement: Mechanical vs. porcine xenograft prostheses. Circulation, *56*:122, 1977.

Roberts, W. C., and Buchbinder, N. A.: Right-sided valvular infective endocarditis. A clinicopathologic study of twelve necropsy patients. Am. J. Med., *53*:7, 1972.

Robin, E., Belamaric, J., Thoms, N. W., *et al.*: Consequences to total tricuspid valvulectomy without prosthetic replacement in treatment of Pseudomonas endocarditis. J. Thorac. Cardiovasc. Surg., *68*:461, 1974.

Robin, E., Thomas, N. W., Arbulu, A., *et al.*: Hemodynamic consequences of total removal of the tricuspid valve without prosthetic replacement. Am. J. Cardiol., *35*:481, 1975.

Rosenblatt, J. E., Dahlgren, J. G., Fishbach, R. S., *et al.*: Gram-negative bacterial endocarditis in narcotic addicts. Calif. Med., *55*:811, 1973.

Roy, P., Tajik, A. J., Giuliani, E. R., *et al.*: Spectrum of echocardiographic findings in bacterial endocarditis. Circulation, *53*:474, 1976.

Sade, R. M., Greene, W. B., and Kurtz, S. M.: Structural changes in a porcine heterograft. Am. J. Cardiol., *44*:761, 1979.

Sanfelippo, P. M., Giuliani, E. R., Danielson, G. K., *et al.*: Tricuspid valve prosthetic replacement. Early and late results with the Starr-Edwards prosthesis. J. Thorac. Cardiovasc. Surg., *71*:441, 1976.

Sheikh, M. U., Ali, N., Covarrubias, E., *et al.*: Right-sided infective endocarditis: An echocardiographic study. Am. J. Med., *66*:283, 1979.

Shiley, Inc., Irving, California: Personal Communication, 1981.

Simberkott, M. S., Isom, W., Smithivas, T., *et al.*: Two-stage tricuspid valve replacement for mixed bacterial endocarditis. Arch. Intern. Med., *133*:212, 1974.

Sinclair-Smith, B. C.: Measurement of valvular insufficiency. *In*

Dye Curves: The Theory and Practice of Indicator Dilution. Edited by D. A. Bloomfield. Baltimore, University Park Press, 1974.

Starr, A., McCord, C. W., Wood, J., *et al.*: Surgery for multiple valve disease. Ann. Surg., *160*:596, 1964.

Stephenson, L. W., MacVaugh, H., 3rd, and Kastor, J. A.: Tricuspid valvular incompetence and rupture of the ventricular septum caused by nonpenetrating trauma. J. Thorac. Cardiovasc. Surg., *77*:768, 1979.

Suri, R. K., Pattankar, V. L., Smith, H., *et al.*: Myxoma of the tricuspid valve. Aust. N.Z. J. Surg., *48*:429, 1978.

Thomas, J. H., Panoussopoulos, D. G., Jewell, W. R., *et al.*: Tricuspid stenosis secondary to metastatic melanoma. Cancer, *39*:1732, 1977.

Wann, L. S., Dillon, J. C., Weyman, A. E., *et al.*: Echocardiography in bacterial endocarditis. N. Engl. J. Med., *295*:135, 1976.

West, N. W., and Weldon, C. S.: Reconstructive valve surgery. Ann. Thorac. Surg., *25*:167, 1978.

Wexler, L., Bergel, D. K., Gabe, I. T., *et al.*: Velocity of blood flow in normal vena cava. Circ. Res., *23*:349, 1968.

Winzelberg, G. G., Boucher, C. A., Pohost, G. M., *et al.*: Right ventricular function in aortic and mitral valve disease. Chest, *79*:520, 1981.

Zaus, E. A., and Kearns, W. M., Jr.: Massive infarction of the right ventricle and atrium. Circulation, *6*:593, 1952.

Zerbini, E. J., and Puig, L. B.: The dura mater allograft valve. *In* Tissue Heart Valves, Edited by M. I. Ionescu. London, Butterworth and Co., Ltd., 1979.

Chapter 46

Acquired Disease of the Mitral Valve

FRANK C. SPENCER

HISTORICAL DATA

In 1923, after detailed pathologic studies of diseased mitral valves, Cutler and Levine made a bold effort to perform mitral valvulotomy for mitral stenosis but, unfortunately, reasoned erroneously that resection of part of the stenosed valve was necessary. The first patient survived, but the next several died from insufficiency, so that the procedure was abandoned. In England, a digital commissurotomy was also performed in 1925 by Souttar on one patient, but for obscure reasons, no further patients were operated on. It is curious that the field then remained static for over 20 years, until Harken and associates (1948) and Bailey (1949) independently demonstrated the feasibility and value of digital commissurotomy. This was a dramatic advance, for mitral stenosis was inevitably a fatal disease, from either recurrent heart failure or cerebral emboli. Impressive results were quickly obtained in hundreds of patients, resulting in widespread adoption of the procedure throughout the world.

Because of the limitations of the extent to which the stenosed valve could be opened by digital commissurotomy, the stenosis recurred in as many as 50 per cent of the patients within 4 to 5 years. In the following decade, a mitral valve dilator was developed in England by Tubbs (Logan and Turner, 1959). This permitted a more extensive commissurotomy, although mitral insufficiency resulted in a significant percentage of patients.

Open heart surgery had become feasible by this time, with the first successful operation by Gibbon in 1953, and the independent landmark achievements by Lillehei and Kirklin in 1955. Hence, there was increasing interest in the performance of commissurotomy by an open technique. Initially, the complications of cardiopulmonary bypass made the closed digital commissurotomy a safer procedure, but with improvements in cardiopulmonary bypass, an open valvulotomy with cardiopulmonary bypass has been adopted by virtually all groups in the past decade. Only in areas where a heart lung machine is not available is digital commissurotomy still performed with any frequency.

With mitral insufficiency, none of the ingenious closed techniques attempted before 1955 proved durable. With cardiopulmonary bypass (1955), different forms of anuloplasty were tried in many patients, with good results in a few, but a distressingly high failure rate. An intensive search in many cardiac laboratories was quickly initiated to develop a prosthetic mitral valve. The landmark accomplishment of Starr and Edwards (a mechanical engineer) in 1961, the development of their ball valve prosthesis, launched the modern era of prosthetic valve replacement. They correctly reasoned from the previous work of Hufnagel, who implanted a ball valve in the descending aorta of patients with aortic insufficiency without the use of a heart lung machine, that a ball valve prosthesis could be successfully implanted. Hence, at this time, successful valve replacement became possible for the first time. In the subsequent 20 years, numerous prosthetic valves have been evaluated.

For the past 20 years, anuloplasty has been performed in a minority of patients, usually children with pliable leaflets. In recent years, as will be detailed in this chapter, the outstanding work of Carpentier in Paris has demonstrated that mitral valve reconstruction may be performed much more frequently than it has been in the past.

The ideal type of prosthetic valve is still being determined. The original ball valve, after problems with the manufacture of the Silastic ball were corrected in 1966, remains in use and is the prosthesis of choice in some centers. The other most popularly used mechanical valve is the Bjork disc valve, introduced in the late 1960s and used in over 200,000 patients (Bjork, 1979). All metallic prostheses require permanent anticoagulation and carry the lifelong threat of hemorrhage from anticoagulants as well as thromboembolism.

Different types of tissue valves have also been investigated during the past 20 years, including fascia lata valves, homograft valves, and heterograft valves. All tissue valves ultimately failed from fibrosis with stenosis or insufficiency until the glutaraldehyde-preserved porcine valve appeared, developed primarily by Carpentier in Paris and Hancock in the United States. In the past 5 years, it has become the valve of choice for prosthetic replacement in many centers, although its durability beyond 8 or 9 years is of serious concern. At least 5 per cent of valves have failed between 6 and 8 years after insertion. Ionescu, in Leeds, England, began investigating valves constructed of bovine pericardium preserved in glutaraldehyde in the late 1960s and has periodically reported experiences since that time. His data are described in more detail later in this chapter.

An unanswerable question at present is whether patients should have a metal valve, which requires permanent anticoagulation but has known durability, or a porcine valve, which rarely requires anticoagulation but whose durability at 8 to 10 years is as yet unknown. With this uncertainty, the type of valve inserted has varied widely among different centers. For the past 4 years at New York University, the porcine valve has been inserted in over 90 per cent of patients undergoing mitral valve replacement. Experiences with over 700 patients were reported by Isom and colleagues (1980).

MITRAL STENOSIS

Etiology and Pathology

Rheumatic fever is the only known cause of mitral stenosis, although a definite clinical history can be obtained in only about 50 per cent of patients. For unknown reasons, women are affected much more frequently than men. With the widespread effective prophylaxis of rheumatic fever in children for the past decades, the frequency of mitral stenosis has decreased markedly in this country, although in many areas of the world with limited health facilities, such as India and South Africa, mitral stenosis of advanced degree is commonly seen in childhood. Congenital mitral stenosis is very rare. Fewer than 150 cases were found in the review by Tsuji and associates in 1967.

Although the rheumatic inflammatory process is a pancarditis involving the endocardium, myocardium, and pericardium, permanent injury is almost always limited to the cardiac valve. Rheumatic myocarditis is apparently seldom of permanent harm, although there is a puzzling, unexplained variation in cardiac reserve among patients following mitral replacement that could conceivably be due to injury from a previous myocarditis.

Rheumatic valvulitis produces at least three distinct pathologic changes, with the degree varying widely among different patients: fusion of the valve leaflets along the commissures; fibrosis of the leaflets with stiffening, retraction, and ultimate calcification; and fusion and shortening of the chordae tendineae. The more extensive changes are usually seen in patients with recurrent attacks of rheumatic fever.

Fusion of the valve leaflets is the most common result of rheumatic inflammation, as the endocardium ulcerates where the two leaflets normally oppose in systole. If commissural fusion alone is present, excellent results can be obtained by commissurotomy. However, if the valve leaflets have become fibrotic, contracted, and calcified, restoration of pliable valve leaflets is impossible and prosthetic replacement is necessary. An intermediate form of injury exists in which the underlying chordae tendineae are fibrotic and shortened. Often, by surgically separating these fused and divided chordae, perhaps combined with a form of anuloplasty if insufficiency is present, valve replacement can be avoided, although the long-term

course of these diseased valves is as yet uncertain. A large number, however, have functioned satisfactorily for more than 5 years.

The pathologic changes in mitral stenosis progress slowly, evolving over decades. Symptoms may not appear for several years after an initial attack of rheumatic fever. For a long time, it was thought that heart failure in a child was due to a recurrence of rheumatic fever. However, recurrent episodes of rheumatic fever can produce gross valvular destruction and calcification even by 10 to 12 years of age. With modern pediatric therapy in this country, this is very rare.

In most patients, the process appears in adults from fusion and gradual fibrosis and stiffening of the valve. It is a remarkable biologic phenomenon to see patients in the fifth, sixth, or seventh decade with valvular stenosis, who surely had rheumatic fever as a child. In the ensuing three to four decades, the progressive stiffening and fibrosis of the valve probably resulted from turbulent flow of blood. This concept, presenting a picture similar to that seen with congenital aortic stenosis, was suggested by Selzer and Cohen in 1972.

Pathophysiology

Although the cross-sectional area of the normal mitral valve is between 4 and 6 cm.^{2}, varying with body size, significant hemodynamic changes do not appear until the cross-sectional area is reduced to less than 2.0 to 2.5 cm.^{2}. Patients with this mild degree of mitral stenosis may have classic physical findings but become symptomatic only with extreme exertion (Class I). With more severe reduction in cross-sectional area to between 1 and 2 cm.^{2}, symptoms appear more readily with lesser degrees of exertion (Class II). A patient with a mitral valve opening as small as 1 cm.^{2} is usually symptomatic at rest (Class III). An opening near 0.5 cm.^{2} is said to be about the smallest size compatible with life (Class IV).

The dominant physiologic change with mitral stenosis is a chronic increase in mean left atrial pressure above the normal limit of 10 to 12 mm. Hg. Many of the symptoms of mitral stenosis can be interpreted as resulting from this chronic elevation in left atrial pressure. The restriction to flow of blood into the left ventricle from the mitral stenosis also causes a reduction in cardiac output and, in some patients (discussed subsequently), an increase in pulmonary vascular resistance. In addition, the chronic elevation in left atrial pressure leads to the sequential changes of left atrial hypertrophy, atrial fibrillation, and, eventually, development of mural thrombi and systemic embolism.

The degree of increase in left atrial pressure above the normal limit of 10 to 12 mm. Hg varies with three factors: the severity of the mitral stenosis, the cardiac output, and the cardiac rate, which determines the duration of diastolic filling of the left ventricle. Accordingly, any measurement of left atrial pressure must be related to the cardiac output. The most precise physiologic measurement, of course, is the cross-sectional area of the valve, calculated from the pressure gradient across the stenotic valve in combination with the cardiac output. Elevation in atrial pressure to levels of 15 to 20 mm. Hg is commonly found at catheterization in patients with moderately severe stenosis. If mean left atrial pressure exceeds 30 mm. Hg above the oncotic pressure of plasma, transudation of fluid into the pulmonary interstitial tissues occurs. Pulmonary edema may or may not develop, depending on the transport capacity of the pulmonary lymphatic circulation.

Hence, the dominant symptoms of mitral stenosis are those of pulmonary congestion, such as cough, hemoptysis, orthopnea, paroxysmal nocturnal dyspnea, and pulmonary edema.

Because mitral stenosis restricts the flow of blood into the left ventricle, this chamber is often small, appearing underdeveloped. For this reason, patients with mitral stenosis may be treated medically for many years, using different measures to limit exercise activities and to avoid the accumulation of fluid in the lungs.

The decrease in cardiac output from restriction of flow through the stenotic orifice leads to fatigue, weakness, and the muscular wasting typically seen with cardiac cachexia. Any attempt by the patient to increase cardiac output with exercise results in severe dyspnea. The patient quickly learns to avoid such exertion. The widely recognized classic symptom of mitral stenosis, therefore, is "dyspnea on exertion." Patients with severe mitral stenosis may live for many years with a sedentary, semi-invalid type of existence.

The left atrial hypertension often produces pulmonary vasoconstriction and an increase in pulmonary vascular resistance. Hypertrophy of the intima and media of the pulmonary arterioles may be found on histologic studies of the lung, but permanent organic obstruction probably results principally from pulmonary emboli and thrombosis. There is great variation among individual patients in the degree of increase in pulmonary vascular resistance; probably over 50 per cent of patients never develop any significant increase, whereas others may develop an increase in resistance four to five times greater than normal, with pulmonary artery systolic pressures as great as 100 to 140 mm. Hg. Fortunately, in the great majority, the increase in vascular resistance subsides markedly after operation, in sharp contrast to the grim picture in congenital heart disease, in which elevated pulmonary vascular resistance often is an irreversible disease. A corollary to this fortunate fact is that pulmonary hypertension from mitral stenosis in adults, although it increases the operative risk, is never per se a contraindication to operation. Associated hypertrophy of the right ventricle, however, makes it necessary to protect the right ventricle as well as the left ventricle while the aorta is occluded at operation.

Eventually, as mentioned earlier, atrial fibrillation develops from hypertrophy of the smooth muscle of the left atrial wall. Cardiac output decreases 10 to 15 per cent when this occurs, but the most serious complication is the development of thrombi from stasis in the left atrium. Rarely, huge thrombi, 5 to 10 cm. in diameter, develop and virtually fill the left atrial cavity. Systemic emboli, especially to the brain, are a constant threat, constituting a major indication for early operation, because the likelihood of systemic embolism can never be predicted. Emboli after successful commissurotomy, with closure of the atrial appendage, are fortunately rare, even though atrial fibrillation persists (Fig. 46–1).

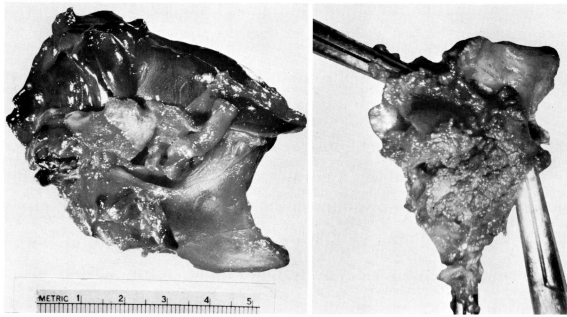

Figure 46–1. Massive left atrial thrombi removed from two different patients during cardiopulmonary bypass. The thrombi virtually filled the left atrial cavity and would obviously have led to catastrophic results if closed digital commissurotomy had been attempted.

Diagnostic Considerations

As mentioned previously, the characteristic symptom of mitral stenosis is dyspnea on exertion. Often, this is the only symptom, except for general weakness and fatigability. The severity of mitral stenosis correlates to some degree with the degree of exertion required to produce dyspnea. As the symptoms of mitral stenosis primarily result from pulmonary congestion, the type of symptom varies with the effect of gravity on body fluids. Hence, with a patient in the supine position, dyspnea is called orthopnea. In addition, at night, there may be paroxysmal nocturnal dyspnea or even pulmonary edema. Fortunately, hemoptysis, an alarming symptom, is rarely of great magnitude. Occasionally, it is severe enough to require urgent mitral commissurotomy to prevent death from asphyxia.

When right heart failure develops, the familiar findings of chronic congestive failure with hepatomegaly, engorged veins, and peripheral edema gradually appear. With right heart failure, the presence of either pulmonary hypertension or tricuspid insufficiency, or both, should be investigated. Right heart failure may develop primarily or with either or both of the aforementioned conditions.

On physical examination, patients with chronic mitral stenosis are often thin and frail with diffuse muscular atrophy, a reflection of long-standing restriction of cardiac output. These chronic metabolic abnormalities, often reflected by anergy to skin tests and a negative nitrogen balance, decrease the overall tolerance to operation and increase the susceptibility to infection.

If right heart failure has developed, engorged cervical veins, hepatomegaly, and peripheral edema are evident. Rubor or cyanosis of the lips, cheeks, and fingers is distinctive in some, a manifestation of increased oxygen extraction from the slow rate of blood flow through the peripheral capillaries because of the low cardiac output. The pulse is decreased in volume and often irregular from atrial fibrillation. On examination of the chest, basilar inspiratory rales are frequently heard.

An important point to emphasize is that the heart size is usually normal, with an apical impulse of normal or decreased intensity. This occurs, of course, because the left ventricle is small. Finding a forceful apical impulse immediately suggests that additional valvular disease, such as mitral insufficiency or aortic valvular disease, has produced hypertrophy of the left ventricle. If pulmonary hypertension has produced hypertrophy of the right ventricle, a forceful systolic impulse may be palpable in the left parasternal area.

The three characteristic auscultatory findings of mitral stenosis, termed "the auscultatory triad," include an apical diastolic rumble, an increased first sound, and an opening snap. These are sufficiently characteristic to establish the diagnosis with an accuracy approaching 100 per cent on physical examination alone. The apical diastolic rumble, produced by blood flowing through the stenotic orifice, may be sharply localized to an area at the apex no larger than 1 inch in diameter. The intensity varies, usually Grade II or III, but in some patients, it is loud enough to produce a palpable thrill. However, the intensity of the murmur does not correlate with the severity of the stenosis. Actually, in some far-advanced cases with a calcified immobile valve, so-called "silent" mitral stenosis is present, with no murmur detectable even by phonocardiography.

The increased first sound, probably resulting from thickening of the mitral leaflets, is one of the earliest findings. The opening snap can be identified on careful examination in most patients but is absent with rigid, immobile leaflets. A short apical systolic murmur occurs frequently and is of little significance, but a loud pansystolic murmur, transmitted to the axilla, usually indicates mitral insufficiency. Associated tricuspid insufficiency may produce a systolic murmur near the apex, but usually, the murmur is loudest near the xiphoid process and characteristically varies with inspiration.

Several abnormalities are seen on the chest roentgenogram. The earliest change is enlargement of the left atrium, typically seen on the posteroanterior roentgenogram with a double contour visible behind the right atrial shadow (Fig. 46-2A). The earliest enlargement of the left atrium can be determined by the lateral roentgenogram exposed during a barium swallow, showing concave indentation of the middle third of the esophagus (Fig. 46-2B). However, with the simplicity and precision of echocardiography, this test is now seldom performed.

The overall cardiac size is often normal, but the enlargement of the left atrium and pulmonary artery obliterates the normal concavity between the aorta and the left ventricle, producing a "straight" left heart border. Calcification of the mitral valve, very extensive in an occasional patient, can be readily detected on fluoroscopy. In the lung fields, different signs of pulmonary congestion may be recognized. These include distention of the pulmonary arteries and veins, engorgement of pulmonary lymphatics, and pleural effusion. Engorged pulmonary lymphatics, often termed "Kerley's lines," are seen with severe mitral stenosis and can be recognized as distinct horizontal linear opacities in the lower lung fields.

The electrocardiogram is an inaccurate guide to assessment of the severity of the mitral stenosis and may be completely normal, even in patients with severe disease. An increased amplitude of the P wave from hypertrophy of the left atrium is the earliest change, but the changes are not consistent enough to be of clinical value. Signs of right ventricular hypertrophy appear if there is an increase in pulmonary vascular resistance. If left ventricular hypertrophy is seen on the electrocardiogram, some disease other than isolated mitral stenosis, such as mitral insufficiency or aortic valvular disease, is probably present.

In recent years, echocardiography has become a valuable noninvasive technique for evaluating changes with mitral stenosis, measuring the cross-sectional area of the valve as well as the size of the left atrium

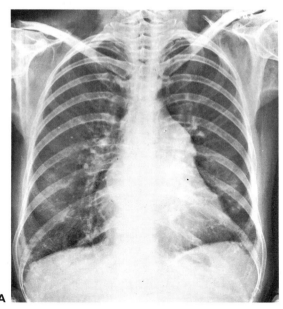 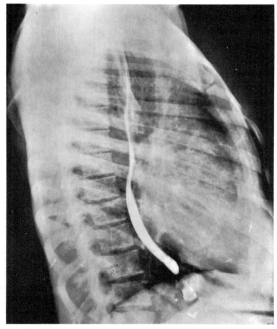

Figure 46–2. *A*, Chest roentgenogram of a patient with mitral stenosis showing a heart of normal size. The prominent pulmonary artery along the left cardiac border is characteristic of this condition. The enlarged left atrium can be seen as a double density behind the shadow normally formed by the right atrium. *B*, Lateral roentgenogram of the same patient showing enlargement of the left atrium producing a concave displacement of the barium-filled esophagus.

and the left ventricle. This is discussed in detail in the section on mitral insufficiency later in the chapter.

Cardiac catheterization and angiography are unnecessary to establish the diagnosis of mitral stenosis but should be done routinely to evaluate associated diseases, such as pulmonary hypertension, mitral insufficiency, coronary disease, or aortic disease. This information, of course, is of particular value in estimating the risk of operation, the likelihood of benefit, and the likelihood of prosthetic valve replacement being required. For example, if significant mitral insufficiency is present with severe calcification, prosthetic replacement will surely be necessary. The significant points that can be determined from catheterization include not only the presence of mitral stenosis and insufficiency, but also the presence of aortic stenosis and insufficiency; the nature of left ventricular function, reflected by left ventricular enddiastolic pressure, ejection fraction, and cardiac index; the presence of pulmonary hypertension; and the presence of coronary artery disease or calcification in the mitral valve or other areas.

Tricuspid stenosis or insufficiency may be difficult to detect on cardiac catheterization. Hence, an important routine is to always palpate the tricuspid valve at the time of operation by insertion of a finger through the right atrial appendage before the venous cannula is inserted.

Operative Treatment

Indications for Operation

In general, I feel strongly that any patient with significant mitral stenosis should be operated on, unless concomitant disease creates a serious operative risk (Spencer, 1978). This is an opinion held by a minority and not shared by many cardiologists because patients with few symptoms may be managed medically for many years. However, during this time, there is the ever-present risk of cerebral embolism and the inevitable, slowly progressive changes of fibrosis and ultimate calcification in the diseased valve because of turbulent flow of blood through the stenotic orifice. The risk of early operation is very small, less than 1 per cent, with a likelihood of greater than 90 per cent that a commissurotomy can be done, which will provide almost complete protection from arterial embolism and may also avoid ultimate valve replacement if the valve leaflets become fibrotic and calcified. The latter possibility, of course, will probably always remain a hypothesis, because it is almost impossible to subject it to meaningful scientific analysis.

Although it occurs infrequently, a grim clinical experience is seeing a patient for the first time who was asymptomatic until a massive cerebral embolus produced massive hemiplegia with aphasia and permanent neurologic deficit. Rarely, a patient has such a cerebral embolism without even being aware of the presence of heart disease.

At the other extreme, it should be emphasized that patients rarely have such far-advanced disease that operation cannot be performed. Even in terminal patients with isolated mitral disease, operative risk with modern supportive techniques seldom exceeds 15 to 20 per cent. Long-term results in patients operated on in a terminal state are not nearly as good as those in patients operated on earlier: The 5-year survival rate in Class IV patients is 50 to 60 per cent, as compared with 90 to 95 per cent in Class II patients, but remarkable improvement can be obtained. This is true even in the presence of severe pulmonary hypertension, with the pulmonary systolic pressure exceeding 120 mm. Hg. Such excellent results have become fairly common with the present technique of hypothermic potassium cardioplegia with cold blood. Therefore, as stated earlier, unless there is advanced disease in other organ systems, such as severe emphysema, cerebral atrophy, or irreversible renal disease, operation can virtually always be performed for mitral valve disease.

Some near-terminal patients require operation as an emergency procedure. In such instances, a remarkable diffuse hyperemic "flush" appears throughout the body after operation, resembling the hyperemic response when an ischemic extremity is revascularized. This apparently is due to the increase in cardiac output to tissues that have been chronically anoxic from the low cardiac output.

The risk of operation in Class IV patients can be greatly decreased by intensive therapy with bed rest, digitalis, and diuretics for several days or weeks before operation. An extremely important concept to understand is that the duration of effective preoperative therapy varies widely; hence, a fixed schedule cannot be planned. Preoperative therapy should be continued as long as there is continuing improvement, usually manifested by resolution of peripheral edema. Some patients gradually improve for 2 to 3 weeks or longer, ultimately reaching a plateau, at which time operation should be performed. The most remarkable example seen in our center in the past decade was a patient operated on several years ago who lost *80 pounds* of edema fluid during intensive diuretic therapy and bed rest over a period of 2 months in the hospital. Her subsequent convalescence following mitral valve replacement was strikingly uneventful: The patient left the hospital in good condition in less than 2 weeks and remained well in the subsequent 2 or 3 years of follow-up.

The metabolic changes that improve with bed rest and diuretic therapy are not fully understood but include changes in protein metabolism, probably an increase in resistance to infection, and an improvement in blood coagulation because of decrease in chronic passive congestion of the liver.

A useful warning sign that operation may be required promptly is a gradual rise in blood urea nitrogen or creatinine, indicating that cardiac output is no longer able to maintain adequate renal function. Progressive failure of renal function is one of the earliest and most significant objective signs that cardiac function will decrease to a lethal degree unless operation is performed.

In the 2 to 3 days immediately preceding operation, both digitalis and diuretic therapy are decreased. Apparently, the myocardium is more sensitive to digitalis immediately following operation, probably because of operative trauma. This can be more precisely determined in many patients by measurement of serum digoxin levels.

Open Versus Closed Commissurotomy

In an earlier edition of this text, closed digital commissurotomy, with the heart-lung machine on a standby basis, was recommended. With the astonishing safety of open heart procedures, such an approach has been considered obsolete for several years. I have not personally performed a closed digital commissurotomy in almost 10 years. Although good results have been reported by several groups with closed digital commissurotomy, I consider the procedure obsolete, subjecting the patient to the unreasonable hazard of cerebral embolism and also often resulting in an inferior commissurotomy as compared with that which can be obtained by an open technique. Probably the only indication for a closed commissurotomy is the unavailability of a heart-lung machine, either because of emergency circumstances or because of geographic factors that exist in many parts of the world.

With open commissurotomy, the risk of cardiopulmonary bypass per se is less than 1 per cent; the risk of cerebral embolism is virtually 0 per cent; mitral insufficiency can often be precisely evaluated and treated; and a more effective commissurotomy can be performed by separating fused chordae tendineae as well as fused commissures. As early as 1974, Mullin and associates reported experiences from New York University with open commissurotomy in 100 consecutive patients operated on between 1966 and 1973, with no operative deaths among the 94 patients with valvular disease alone. In a report in 1981, the New York University series was brought up to date in a report by Gross and coworkers describing 202 patients undergoing commissurotomy between 1967 and 1978, with a follow-up that was 98 per cent complete. The operative mortality rate was 1.7 per cent, and the long-term mortality rate was 2.5 per cent. Postoperative emboli occurred in 3 per cent of the patients, often in association with failure to obliterate the left atrial appendage. Five years following operation, 87 per cent of the patients who had no residual valve dysfunction were completely free of any complications.

Similar results were reported by Halseth and colleagues in 1980 in a review of 222 patients operated on over a period of 10 years, ending in December 1978. Quite impressive is the fact that during this time, mitral valve replacement was necessary in only 11 per cent of the patients operated on. There were only three deaths (1.5 per cent operative risk), and two of these occurred in patients operated on on an emergency basis. Seven per cent of the 191 patients surviving commissurotomy required mitral valve replacement between 2 and 92 months after operation, usually for mitral insufficiency. The 10-year survival rate for the 197 patients was 81 per cent.

In addition, in 1977, Housman and associates reported late results following open commissurotomy in 100 patients. They had used open commissurotomy exclusively for 15 years. In the 100 operations, there was only one operative death, from pancreatitis, and one late death, from cancer. The actuarially projected survival rate at 10 years was 97 per cent. Sixteen patients required reoperation on the mitral valve because of functional deterioration.

The *concept* of radical open valvuloplasty is not to simply open the valve enough to correct stenosis, but to open the valve as widely as possible without producing significant insufficiency. With the techniques to be described subsequently for correcting insufficiency produced at operation, this can be done more boldly than in the past, with the knowledge that any insufficiency that is produced can be corrected. The objective is not only to eliminate the diastolic gradient but also to minimize the turbulent flow of blood across the diseased mitral orifice. Although a mitral valve opening of 2 cm.² may have little or no gradient across it at rest, the orifice is still much smaller than the normal size of 4 to 6 cm.².

In the decade that followed the widespread adoption of digital commissurotomy around 1950, excellent short-term results were reported. As late as 1961, however, mitral stenosis had recurred within 5 years in 20 to 50 per cent of patients. The gradients following digital commissurotomy were usually not reported at that time. It seems probable that residual stenosis, with a valve opening of about 2.5 cm.² and turbulent flow of blood, led to progressive fibrosis and calcification of the valve leaflets that required repeat operation within 5 to 10 years.

Whether better long-term results can be obtained by radical open commissurotomy will take decades to determine, but at present, over the past 8 years, reoperation for recurring stenosis has been necessary only in a few patients in whom a small residual gradient was left at the initial operation. It seems probable that stenosis recurs primarily in valves that were not opened widely at the initial operation. The late development of mitral insufficiency, occurring unpredictably in some patients between 5 and 10 years after mitral commissurotomy, is probably due to the turbulent flow of blood across the diseased orifice, a hypothesis proposed by Selzer and Cohen in 1972.

Technique of Open Commissurotomy

Our concepts about and technique for open mitral commissurotomy were described Mullin and associates in 1974. A median sternotomy incision is regularly used. The tricuspid valve is always palpated with a finger introduced through an opening in the right atrial appendage to determine if any insufficiency or stenosis is present. If there is any uncertainty about tricuspid insufficiency, the thickness of the right atrial wall is a useful guide, because a thin atrial wall indicates that any tricuspid insufficiency present is of recent origin and probably clinically insignificant.

The bypass technique is a standard one, with sufficient heparinization to produce an activated clotting time above 400 seconds usually at least 4 mg./kg., and with cannulation of the ascending aorta for aortic return and cannulation of the venae cavae with two cannulas for venous return. The oxygenator is a membrane oxygenator primed with a balanced crystalloid solution, 40 ml./kg of patient weight, adding sufficient blood to fill the oxygenator, if necessary. The flow rate is about 25 liters per square meter per minute. Perfusion is usually performed near a temperature of 25°C. Blood is added to the pump if the hematocrit decreases below 20 per cent.

Once bypass has been established and the temperature has been lowered to 25°C, the aorta is occluded and the heart is arrested by infusing 1200 to 1400 ml. of cold blood (10° to 12°C.) containing potassium, 35 mEq. per liter, with sufficient THAM added to adjust the pH to near 7.60. The blood is collected from the pump-oxygenator in a reservoir, and the potassium and THAM are added. This technique of cardioplegia was modified from that developed at UCLA by Buckberg, Maloney, and associates, differing principally in the fact that calcium concentration is not decreased.

Once the heart has been arrested and blood infused, it is important to check the temperature in different areas of the heart with a needle thermistor and to pour iced electrolyte solution (4°C.) over the heart until the myocardial temperature is below 15°C. This is a modification of the original Shumway technique. After the temperature has been lowered, the heart is wrapped in a sponge, and cold fluid is continually dripped into the sponge, about 1 liter every 5 to 10 minutes, removing the fluid from the operative field through a sump introduced through a stab wound and placed at the bottom of the pericardial cavity. Careful adjustment of the drape around the heart, the fluid infusion line, and the sump tube permit the heart to be kept bathed in cold fluid without having the cold fluid enter the atriotomy incision. This is particularly important in patients with pulmonary hypertension and hypertrophy of the right ventricle. Almost certainly in the past, problems with right heart failure in such patients were due to inadequate protection of the hypertrophied right ventricle, which, because of its anatomic position, is readily exposed to rewarming by lights in the operating room and other factors. With careful draping, as described, both ventricles are completely covered, and their temperature will often decrease to temperature between 8° and 12°C. during the period of aortic occlusion. Every 30 minutes, 400 to 500 ml. of cold blood is reinfused and additional cold fluid is poured over the heart to be certain that the temperature remains below 15°C. The perfusate in the pump is maintained at a temperature between 25° and 30°C. Without the topical hypothermia, the heart will gradually rewarm because of the aorta lying posteriorly, the diaphragm inferiorly, and the operating room lights above.

Many techniques of cardioplegia are currently used in different centers throughout the world, with no definitive data showing that one is superior. Techniques of cardioplegia have been a leading subject of investigation in our laboratories for the past few years. Three significant reports from these experimental

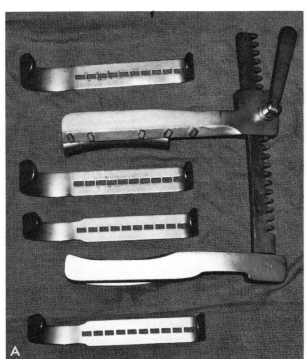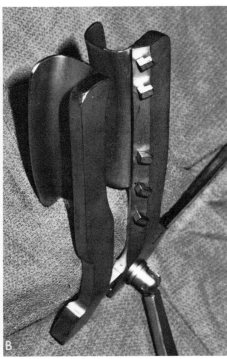

Figure 46–3. *A,* The sternal retractor developed by Carpentier in Paris with a variety of blades that can be attached to facilitate exposure of the mitral valve, greatly enhancing techniques of reconstruction. The instrument is very useful, with five different areas on the blades where the retractors can be attached with different degrees of tension. Adequate exposure is, of course, essential for complex techniques of reconstruction, even more so than for simple prosthetic replacement. *B,* Side view of the same instrument.

studies are those by Cunningham and associates (1979), Srungaram and coworkers (1981), and Catinella and colleagues (1981).

Once the heart has been arrested and cooled, the left atrium is opened with a long incision in the interatrial groove, extending the atriotomy beneath and over to the left of both the superior and inferior venae cavae. A special malleable retractor developed by Carpentier (Fig. 46–3) has been especially valuable for providing adequate exposure, because its unique design permits multiple adjustments of the different blades. The crucial consideration is to adjust the tips of the retractor blades to apply traction to the atrial wall about 2 cm. superior to the mitral anulus, exposing the mitral ring nicely. Deeper insertion of the retractor will actually obscure the operative field.

Initially, the atrial cavity is carefully examined for thrombi, especially inside the atrial appendage (see Fig. 46–1). For more than 8 years, the atrial appendage has been excluded from the left atrium by closing the orifice of the appendage with a continuous suture of 3-0 Prolene. This suture is carefully placed in a horizontal direction, barely beneath the endocardium, so that the shaft of the needle is faintly visible beneath the endocardium. This direction of needle insertion parallels the course of the circumflex coronary artery and has been found to be uniformly safe. It is surprising that this method has not been more widely adopted; this is principally due to the persisting myth that closure of the atrial appendage is dangerous. Our data from the past 8 years amply refute this statement

and support the policy that routine closure should always be done unless anatomic factors obscure the atrial appendage, which occurs in probably no more than 1 to 2 per cent of patients. Unless the appendage is closed, the patient remains at risk after operation from emboli developing within the fibrillating appendage.

Nearly a decade ago, we became alerted to the grave possibility of emboli arising from the atrial appendage, rather than from the prosthetic valve, by having an unfortunate experience with four patients who sustained a cerebral embolus a few weeks to a few months after open mitral commissurotomy. In one of these patients, a devastating embolus occurred 6 weeks after an uneventful recovery from commissurotomy when the cardiac rhythm abruptly changed from atrial fibrillation to a sinus rhythm. It seems highly probable that a thrombus in a fibrillating appendage was expelled when the atrium began to contract. This potential mechanism has been visualized in at least five patients, who, at the time of operation, were found to have 3- to 5-mm. fragments of thrombus lying "free" in the cavity of the atrial appendage. Why the thrombi were not fused to the endocardium is unclear, but the frightful possibility was clear that such emboli would be quickly expelled from the appendage if atrial contractions returned with a sinus rhythm.

Following closure of the appendage, the mitral valve is exposed by what is termed the "triple right angle" technique. A heavy suture is inserted in each

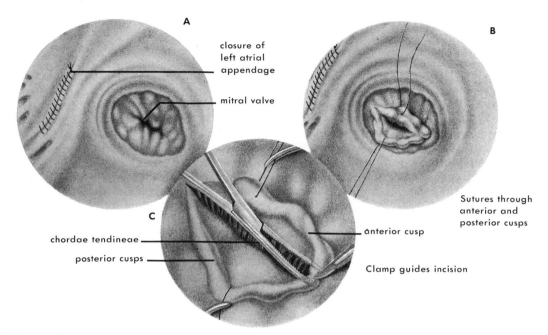

Figure 46–4. *A*, Closure of left atrial appendage. *B*, Exposure of mitral valve with horizontal traction on sutures. *C*, Third right-angle clamp guides incision.

leaflet, which in turn is grasped with a right-angle clamp to apply "horizontal" traction to the leaflet, as opposed to simple vertical traction (Fig. 46–4). Application of horizontal traction stretches the leaflets and facilitates identification of the commissures. Several landmarks identify a commissure, such as the typical depressed area where the leaflets are fused, the thickened tissue, the difference in color from adjacent leaflets, and the method of attachment of the underlying chordae. There is wide variation, however, among patients. In many patients, fused commissures are immediately obvious; in other patients, the exact site of commissural fusion has to be determined cautiously because landmarks have been obscured by the inflammatory process.

Once the commissure has been identified, the third right-angle clamp is introduced beneath the fused commissure between the chordae, and the blades are separated enough to stretch the fused commissure.

The commissure is then cautiously incised with a knife, 2 to 3 mm. at a time, being certain that the separated margins are each attached to chordae tendineae. This is obviously a crucial part of the operative technique to avoid mitral insufficiency.

Occasionally, landmarks are grossly distorted, with fusion of the leaflets directly to underlying papillary muscles from shortening or obliteration of chordae tendineae. Where to start the incision in such instances is uncertain. The incision may be begun initially by stabbing through the fused commissure with a small blade (No. 15, about 3 cm. wide) beyond the site of fusion with the papillary muscle, making the stab wound where the commissure is clearly visible. The stab wound may be separated slightly with forceps, after which the incision may be cautiously extended to the free margin of the mitral orifice, incising the underlying papillary muscle for 5 to 10 mm. (Fig. 46–5).

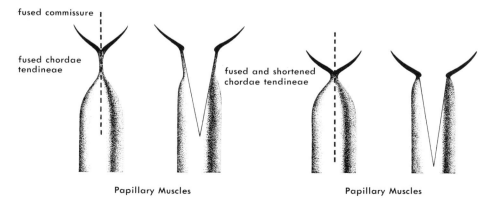

Figure 46–5. *A*, Separation of fused chordae tendineae with incision into papillary muscle. *B*, Deeper incision into papillary muscle when valve leaflets are fused to underlying papillary muscle.

Needless to say, this technique is a delicate one, requiring a dry operative field with excellent exposure and careful identification of all structures before any incision is made. Incorrect division of chordae tendineae resulting in production of a flail leaflet almost mandates prosthetic replacement.

In all operations, both commissures are opened as widely as possible, stopping a few millimeters from the valve anulus where the valve tissue becomes thin. This is a normal anatomic change, for the normal mitral commissure stops a few millimeters from the valve anulus.

Following completion of the commissurotomy, leaflet mobility is assessed. Restricted motion may be improved by further division of fused chordae. In a few patients, cautious debridement of calcium from the leaflets with rongeurs and a bone curette is feasible, but perforation of the leaflet is a serious hazard. Usually, with extensive calcification, prosthetic replacement is necessary.

The importance of performing more than a simple commissurotomy is evident from a review of the operative records, which indicate that in more than 30 per cent of patients, more than a simple commissurotomy is needed, usually separation of underlying fused chordae and splitting of papillary muscles. A similar observation was recorded more than a decade ago by Roe and associates (1971).

Once the valvuloplasty has been completed, the presence of any mitral insufficiency is assessed by selective induction of aortic insufficiency with a technique specifically designed for that purpose. A small plastic cannula (10 French) with multiple side perforations over an area of 6 to 7 cm. is introduced into the ascending aorta through a stab wound made 4 to 5 cm. above the aortic ring. The catheter is then manipulated across the aortic valve into the left ventricle, usually while the aorta is temporarily occluded to permit collapse of the aortic valve leaflets. Care must be taken during these maneuvers to avoid inadvertently introducing air into the aorta.

With the catheter in its final position, some of the perforations remain in the aorta, whereas the distal ones are in the outflow tract of the left ventricle (Fig. 46–6). When the aortic clamp is released and intra-aortic air is removed, blood refluxes into the ventricle, ballooning the aortic leaflet of the mitral valve and seating it firmly against the mural leaflet. Focal areas of regurgitation can be readily identified and corrected, usually with one or two sutures. If the insufficiency is in the central portion of the mitral orifice, anuloplasty can be performed. Previously, patients have been treated with the anuloplasty described by Reed in 1973. The Carpentier ring anuloplasty is probably a superior method, distributing tension more properly, but it has not been used sufficiently with such patients as yet. Its use for mitral insufficiency is described later in this chapter.

The selective catheter method of assessing regurgitation before closing the left atrium has now been used for more than 8 years and has constituted a valuable addition to mitral valvuloplasty, permitting a bolder approach than previously seemed feasible. For some years, the reliability of the method was routinely checked by subsequent digital palpation of the mitral valve with the heart beating and systolic pressure near the preoperative level and with bypass either slowed or stopped. Because insufficiency was not found by the digital palpation approach, this additional palpation was abandoned several years ago as being superfluous.

The report by Halseth and associates in 1980 describes their method of inducing insufficiency by distortion of the aortic anulus, a technique described by Sterling Edwards long ago. We have utilized this technique somewhat but find the catheter technique

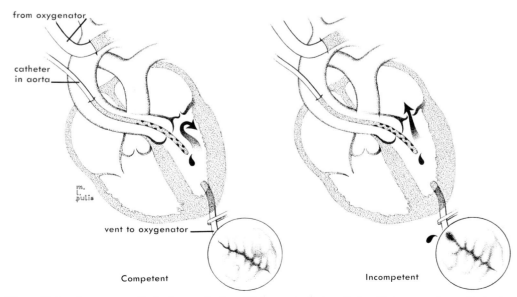

from oxygenator

catheter in aorta

m. l. pulis

vent to oxygenator

Competent

Incompetent

Figure 46–6. Assessment of mitral regurgitation utilizing controlled aortic insufficiency to close mitral valve.

more precise and more effective than either the Halseth method or retrograde injection of fluid either through a left ventricular vent or directly through the mitral orifice.

Following completion of valvuloplasty and closure of the atriotomy incision, fibrillation is induced while the aortic clamp is removed and air is removed from the aorta, left atrium, and left ventricle. This requires a variety of maneuvers, because removal of air from the heart is one of the most difficult and important steps in the operative procedure.

Before the aortic clamp is released, the venous cannulas are constricted to permit distention of the right ventricle with blood, after which compression of the right ventricle will force blood retrograde from the coronary sinus through the right coronary artery and into the aorta, covering the coronary ostia with blood. Otherwise, a small bolus of air may be trapped within the proximal right coronary artery. A stab wound is then made in the superior portion of the aorta and the aortic clamp is released, slowing the perfusion rate to about 500 ml. per minute and permitting all air to be removed from the aorta before full flow is resumed. When this has been accomplished, with the heart fibrillating, air is then removed from the left atrium by vigorously ventilating the lungs, with the atriotomy suture line held open with forceps.

For years, a left ventricular vent was employed to remove air from the left ventricle, but the left ventricle is small in many patients with mitral stenosis. A transatrial vent is now usually employed, using the vent developed by the Sarns Corporation, which is introduced across the mitral valve and fixed in position with a suture so that the tip is near the apex of the left ventricle. Gentle suction on this catheter is usually adequate for removing air, although it does not seem as reliable as the left ventricular vent.

Finally, once all air apparently has been removed, but with the heart still fibrillating, the aorta is compressed about 90 per cent with a vascular clamp, leaving the only patent segment of the aorta near the undersurface of the aortic arch. The heart is then defibrillated, permitting the left ventricle to expel through the stab wound in the ascending aorta for 2 to 3 minutes. The coronary arteries are perfused during this time by blood coming through the aorta in the small area not compressed by the clamp, so that the heart will contract vigorously and expel air against the aortic clamp. After 2 or 3 minutes, the aortic clamp can be removed, and the incision in the aorta is sutured. As a final precaution, a small catheter is left in the aorta and gentle suction is applied until bypass is terminated.

Removal of air from the heart is so difficult and unpredictable that the safest procedure is to assume "some" air is always trapped in some area in the heart and to employ safety precautions accordingly. This is the purpose of continuous gentle suction on the ascending aorta until bypass is stopped. One example of the myriad causes of air embolism is the simple fact that a foramen ovale may constitute a source of fatal air embolism if certain circumstances exist. These require that one of the cannulas in the atrium be inadequately secured with a purse-string suture, usually from tearing of the purse-string suture. Inadvertent excessive removal of blood from the patient into the oxygenator may partly collapse the right atrium and permit air to enter the right atrium. If the heart is vigorously beating, this air may be transmitted through a foramen ovale into the left atrium and into the aorta.

Another tragic example occurred when vigorous ventilation resulted in rupture of a bleb in the lung, with air passing from a bronchus into a pulmonary vein. Undoubtedly, there are other rare mechanisms by which air can be trapped in the left heart or pulmonary vascular bed, all of which lead to the conclusion that air cannot be simply removed but requires a variety of maneuvers and a number of safety precautions that initially might seem superfluous.

Following bypass, when normal cardiac contractility and blood pressure have returned, the correction of the mitral stenosis is confirmed by measuring left atrial and ventricular end-diastolic pressures, demonstrating that no gradient remains. The presence of any gradient, even one as small as 4 mm., indicates residual stenosis. In a few such patients in whom this small gradient has been left, usually because of calcifications in a commissure, recurrent stenosis has developed within 2 to 4 years. Hence, it may be best in such patients to perform prosthetic replacement rather than to leave the diseased valve.

Obviously, if reconstruction of the mitral valve cannot be done, prosthetic replacement is necessary. The most common abnormality requiring replacement is dense calcification, especially across the commissures, or rigidity of the leaflets that converts the entire valve into a rigid, fixed structure. Such valves may have an opening greater than 1 cm., even though on catheterization severe mitral stenosis was demonstrated, indicating that the principal obstruction was rigidity of the leaflets rather than a narrow orifice. Usually, if both insufficiency and stenosis are present, valve replacement is necessary, although Carpentier has successfully employed reconstruction with his ring technique in a series of patients with impressive results. The techniques of prosthetic valve replacement are described in the following section.

Prosthetic Replacement of the Mitral Valve

At New York University, the Starr-Edwards cloth-covered steel ball prosthesis (Fig. 46–7) was used almost exclusively for over a decade. Experiences with 1375 such prostheses in the aortic and mitral position were reported by Isom and associates in 1977. Although functional results were excellent, widespread dissatisfaction gradually increased with long-term complications from cloth wear and hemolysis. The prosthesis was gradually abandoned, and its manufacture by the Starr-Edwards Company stopped.

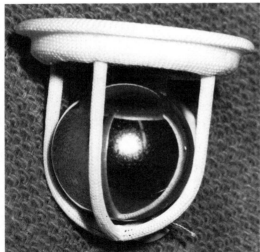

Figure 46–7. The Starr-Edwards cloth-covered steel ball prosthesis used at New York University for over a decade in over 1500 patients. The prosthesis was ultimately abandoned because of cloth wear, but it gave excellent results for many years. A bare-strut prosthesis is currently the prosthetic valve of choice if a ball valve prosthesis is employed, using the Silastic ball, originally developed by Starr around 1965.

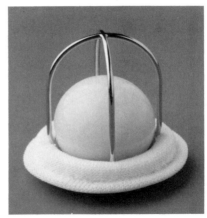

Figure 46–8. The mitral bare-strut Starr-Edwards Silastic ball valve currently in use. This was developed in 1965–1966, and is still widely used.

The Starr-Edwards prosthesis now used by several groups is the bare-strut prosthesis (Fig. 46–8).

Around 1976 and 1977, the porcine prosthesis (Hancock and Carpentier-Edwards) (Fig. 46–9) was adopted by us for the majority of patients, as sufficient data had become available to indicate that its function was good for at least 5 years. Subsequently, it has been used for prosthetic replacement in over 90 per cent of patients, with the Bjork tilting disc valve being employed in the remainder (Fig. 46–10).

The type of prosthesis used should vary with the individual patient, depending on his age, personal circumstances, and personal preferences. The metallic prostheses, such as the disc valve and the ball valve, have the advantage of seemingly unlimited durability but the disadvantage of the necessity for permanent anticoagulation, with the hazards of bleeding and a greater risk of thromboembolism than from porcine prostheses. Hence, with porcine prostheses, the hazards of neurologic injury are decreased for two reasons: There is less risk of cerebral hemorrhage and less risk of cerebral embolism. Among the few patients having emboli, a permanent neurologic deficit has been very rare, suggesting that most emboli are small and probably due to platelets, rather than fibrin.

However, there is uncertainty about the durability of porcine prostheses. At this time, sufficient data have accumulated to indicate that 90 to 95 per cent of prostheses function well for at least 8 years, but there is a definite increased frequency of deterioration after 6 or 7 years. Because only a few patients were operated on more than 10 years ago, there are insignificant 10-year follow-up data at present. An important but unanswerable question with porcine prostheses is whether deterioration is inevitable at some unpredictable date, or whether durability may be altered by methods of preservation or by handling of the valve at operation, such as the method of fixation in glutaraldehyde, washing of the prosthesis at the time of operation, and the avoidance of trauma at operation (e.g., drying of the leaflets).

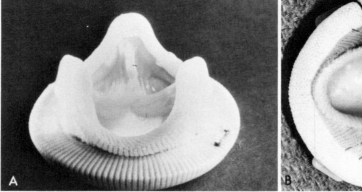
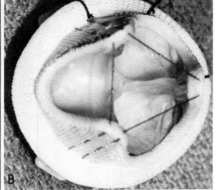

Figure 46–9. *A,* The Hancock porcine prosthesis. *B,* The Carpentier-Edwards porcine prosthesis. These are two of the most popular porcine prostheses currently in use. A comparison of the two prostheses at New York University, described in the text, found little difference in their performance over a short period of observation, averaging between 2 and 3 years.

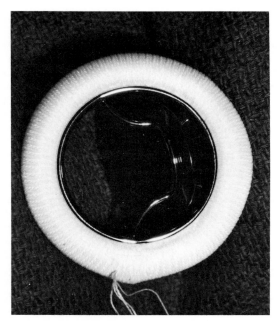

Figure 46–10. The Bjork tilting-disc prosthesis, an excellent low-profile prosthetic valve, and the valve of choice in many institutions.

In 1980, Isom and associates reported our 4 years of experience at New York University (1976 through 1979), during which 714 porcine valves were inserted, 303 Hancock prostheses and 411 Carpentier-Edwards prostheses. The series was analyzed to see if there was any discernible difference between the two types of valve. The prostheses differ slightly in their methods of preparation: The Hancock valve is prepared with a Dacron sewing ring and the Carpentier-Edwards valve is prepared with a Teflon sewing ring. The stent is made of plastic in the Hancock valve, with wire in the Carpentier-Edwards. The Hancock prosthesis is sterilized in a 0.2 per cent concentration of glutaraldehyde, although the exact method is patented and secret. The Carpentier-Edwards technique is well-publicized, consisting of 0.5 per cent glutaraldehyde and a final rinse in dilute formaldehyde. Although precise details are not known, the cloth in the Carpentier-Edwards valve seems to be significantly more porous than that in the Hancock valve, permitting better tissue ingrowth and less hazard of loose attachment of fibrin that might detach and embolize.

The series of 714 patients was consecutive, with the porcine prosthesis being employed in about 90 per cent of the patients operated on. As virtually no patients were considered inoperable, the series includes a large number of seriously ill patients. Eighty-five were classified as Class III or Class IV; 30 per cent required multiple cardiac procedures (as compared with 10 per cent in most reports from other groups); and about 25 per cent had a concomitant coronary bypass. There were 327 aortic valve replacements, with a 6.4 per cent mortality rate; 186 mitral valve replacements, with an 8.1 per cent mortality rate; and 201 multiple valve replacements, with a 17

per cent mortality rate. The follow-up was 98 per cent complete, with a mean follow-up of 24 months.

There were 71 operative deaths, 41 of which were cardiac in origin, due to low output, infarction, or arrhythmias that could presumably be prevented with the techniques of myocardial preservation now available. Seventeen deaths occurred from infection. There were only five deaths from neurologic injuries, less than 1 per cent of the total group. The frequency of deaths from arrythmias, 15 per cent of the group, indicates the importance of careful monitoring both during hospitalization and during the next 3 to 5 years.

The 4-year survival rate after discharge from the hospital, calculated by actuarial methods, was near 90 per cent for both types of prosthesis and was also similar for either aortic or mitral valve replacement. Substantial improvement occurred in 85 to 90 per cent of patients, supporting the policy of operating on all patients, regardless of the severity of congestive failure. This policy is also supported by the fact that only seven late deaths occurred from congestive heart failure, about 1 per cent of the total number of patients discharged from the hospital.

Thirty patients died after leaving the hospital. In about half of these, death was sudden, either from an arrhythmia or from unknown causes, probably an unrecognized arrhythmia. This high frequency of sudden death after discharge further emphasizes the importance of frequent long-term monitoring. Only three deaths occurred from myocardial infarction, perhaps a result of the concomitant bypass grafting in 25 per cent of the group. There were only two deaths from cerebral embolism, both in patients with Hancock prostheses in the mitral position who were receiving anticoagulants. Three patients died from complications of anticoagulation, supporting the policy of not continuing warfarin for more than 3 months after operation. Because patients are under the care of their private physicians after discharge from our institution, we recommend that anticoagulants be stopped 3 months after operation, as noted previously. Two of the three deaths mentioned occurred in patients who were maintained on anticoagulants, with death occurring about a year later. Our general policy with anticoagulation is to give warfarin in a conservative amount, keeping the prothrombin time no higher than 20 seconds, for about 3 months after operation. After this time, warfarin is stopped, and an antiplatelet drug, usually aspirin, is given for about 2 years.

Malfunction of the prosthetic valve occurred in nine patients, equally divided between the Hancock and the Carpentier-Edwards groups. This appeared between 2 and 44 months after operation. The early instances of malfunction almost surely represent some mechanical defect, either operative trauma or a defect in the valve manufacturing process or possibly in the pig from which the valve was taken. There were no instances of severe calcification or thrombosis. The calculated rate of malfunction was 0.7 per cent per patient year, but this figure is of little significance because of the short follow-up.

Endocarditis remains a constant hazard, well documented by all reports with long-term studies of prosthetic valves. The calculated frequency was about 1.7 per cent per patient year. There were a total of 20 cases of endocarditis, 15 of which occurred on the aortic valve. Fortunately, there were no deaths from endocarditis; 12 patients recovered with antibiotic therapy, and eight required reoperation. This fortunate absence of any deaths supports our policy of aggressive treatment of endocarditis, operating within 4 or 5 days if the patient does not promptly respond to appropriate antibiotic therapy. There were no instances of recurrent infection.

Very liberal criteria were used to diagnosis thromboembolism, with all dizzy spells and similar episodes considered as possibly representing tiny platelet emboli. Undoubtedly, a number of unexplained neurologic syndromes were erroneously attributed to emboli, because the total frequency is considerably higher than that recorded in other reports. The frequency rate was 5.1 per cent per patient year with the Hancock valve and 2.4 per cent per patient year for the Carpentier-Edwards valve. The difference was not statistically significant. Supporting the point that the use of these criteria probably resulted in the inclusion of a number of episodes that were not embolic in nature is that the frequency of residual neurologic defects was very small, 0.7 per cent in the Hancock series and 0.2 per cent in the Carpentier-Edwards series.

The aortic series was particularly encouraging, for only one patient of the entire group of more than 300 who underwent aortic valve replacements had a significant neurologic defect.

With the mitral series, there were slightly more problems. A total of 22 embolic episodes occurred, 16 in the Hancock series and six in the Carpentier-Edwards series. Among this group of 22 patients, two died and four had residual neurologic defects. Both of the deaths from emboli occurred in patients receiving warfarin.

Experiences at Stanford University with 1407 patients receiving Hancock porcine prostheses between 1971 and 1979 were reported by Oyer and colleagues in 1980. Of these patients, 179 have been followed for more than 5 years and 67 for more than 6 years. Twenty-one aortic prosthetic valves and 23 mitral valves had failed. The probability of freedom from primary tissue failure in adults was 99 per cent at 5 years in patients with aortic prostheses, and 95 per cent in patients with mitral prostheses at 6 years.

In 1980, Magilligan and associates described experiences at the Henry Ford Hospital in Detroit with 490 patients operated on between 1971 and 1979. Twenty-three valves had been subsequently removed because of degeneration. Valve survival without degeneration was 99 per cent at 4 years, 96 per cent at 5 years, 91 per cent at 6 years, and 84 per cent at 7 years.

Experiences at the University of Alabama in Birmingham with 425 patients operated on between 1973 and 1978 were described by Williams and co-workers in 1980. This series differs from the two reported in the previous paragraphs in that the Bjork metal prosthesis was used in the majority of the patients. Hence, the Alabama series is a selected one. The actuarial survival rate with porcine prostheses at 36 months was almost 88 per cent for patients with aortic prostheses and was 80 per cent for those with mitral prostheses. Degeneration of the prosthesis had been recognized in nine of the 425 patients.

In 1981, Jamieson and colleagues reported experiences with thromboembolism in 465 patients from the University of British Columbia in Vancouver. Emboli occurred soon after operation in six patients and at a later date in 18. Among the 18 late embolic episodes, five were fatal and three resulted in permanent sequelae. The calculated frequency of embolism was 1.3 per cent per 100 patient years for aortic prostheses and 3.3 per cent per 100 patient years for mitral prostheses. Atrial fibrillation was present in the majority of patients who had late embolic episodes.

Emboli have been noted more frequently in the first 3 months after operation and also in patients with atrial fibrillation. For this reason, as mentioned previously, we have employed conservative anticoagulation with warfarin for about 3 months, keeping the prothrombin time near 20 seconds. Warfarin is usually stopped at that time, and antiplatelet therapy, generally aspirin, is employed for at least 2 years.

The necessity for permanent anticoagulation for patients remaining in atrial fibrillation is uncertain because of the variation in the frequency with which the atrial appendage is routinely closed at operation among different centers. At New York University, where this is routinely done, the vast majority of patients with chronic atrial fibrillation have not received permanent anticoagulation.

It is already clear from several reports that porcine prostheses are unsatisfactory in children because of the development of rapid calcification with stenosis. This surprising finding is probably related to the more rapid metabolism of calcium in the growing child.

In 1979, Geha and associates reported experiences with porcine valves in 25 children between 17 months and 16 years of age, with a mean follow-up of 33 months. Severe degeneration had already occurred in five children (20 per cent of the group) with sufficient stenosis to require reoperation between 18 and 45 months after the initial operation.

Similar experiences were reported in 1979 by Kutsche and coworkers at Stanford. These included nine children between 2 and 15 years of age. Six were well, but three required reoperation for calcific stenosis between 3 and 5 years after the initial operation, representing one third of the total group.

Naturally, with children, prosthetic replacement should be avoided if at all possible because of the strong probability of the necessity for replacement as the child becomes an adult. Experiences with 92 children undergoing aortic or mitral valve replacement at the Sick Children's Hospital in Toronto between

1963 and 1980 were reported by Williams and associates in 1981. The mortality rate with mitral valve replacement was 32 per cent, and the actuarial survival rate at 5 years after operation was only 50 per cent. Major complications occurred frequently, following both aortic and mitral valve replacement.

A different type of tissue prosthesis is the pericardial xenograft, developed by Ionescu in Leeds, England, and used clinically since 1971. The xenograft is constructed as a three-cusp valve on a Dacron-covered titanium frame. Subsequently, the pericardium is stabilized with 0.5 per cent glutaraldehyde and sterilized and stored in 4 per cent buffered formaldehyde. Since 1976, the pericardial xenograft valve has been manufactured by the Shiley Laboratories in California. An early report was given by Tandon and associates in 1978, comparing experiences over a period of 6 years (1971 to 1977) with Bjork prostheses in 42 patients, Braunwald-Cutter prostheses in 52 patients, and the pericardial xenograft in 126 patients. The actuarial survival rate with the pericardial prosthesis 7 years following insertion was 89 ± 9 per cent. The frequency of thromboembolism was 1.5 episodes per 100 patient years.

Subsequently, at the meeting of the International Surgical Society in San Francisco in September 1979, Ionescu reported the following data: He had operated on 535 patients, with 100 valves functioning for more than 5 years and a few for as long as 9 years. Interestingly enough, he stated that he had not had any prosthetic valve failures after 5 years, a curious experience, contrary to that of others with tissue valves. The rate of endocarditis was low, ranging from 0.5 per cent per 100 patient years for aortic prostheses to 0.9 per cent per 100 patient years for mitral prostheses. Valve dysfunction was calculated as 0.8 per cent per 100 patient years.

Almost all emboli occurred in the first few weeks after operation, rarely after the first year. Emboli had a frequency of 0.9 per cent per 100 patient years with mitral prostheses and of 0.4 per cent with aortic prostheses. Some patients had had four serial catheterizations during the 5 years following operation, without any changes being found. The valve had not been used in anyone under 15 years of age.

Cooley adopted the Ionescu prosthesis for almost routine use in July 1978 and reported in 1981 in a discussion of a report by Becker and associates that he had used the valve in almost 1400 patients in the aortic and mitral positions, with a frequency of embolism near 1 per cent patient year in the short follow-up available.

More recently, Zerbini (1981) in São Paulo, Brazil, has begun employing the pericardial xenograft valve extensively. Previously, Zerbini had implanted a dura mater valve, preserved in glycerol, in almost 2000 patients over a period of more than 10 years. The dura mater valve has been virtually abandoned in the aortic position because of a distressingly high frequency of stiffening of the valve with rupture of a cusp between 9 and 11 years after operation.

Metallic Prostheses. The longest follow-up data available for any type of valve prosthesis, of course, are with the Starr-Edwards ball valve prosthesis, introduced by Starr in 1961. This landmark achievement not only demonstrated that a prosthetic valve could function in man, but also opened the door for numerous clinical investigations of different types of valve prostheses in the next 20 years. Hence, all new prostheses should be compared with the Starr-Edwards ball valve prosthesis, as it has the best long-term data available.

Reporting from Starr's group in 1981, Teply and coworkers described total experiences with 2135 Starr-Edwards ball valve prostheses over a period of 20 years, 34 per cent of which were mitral valve replacements. The 15-year survival rate for mitral valve replacement was 47 per cent. For unknown reasons, the frequency of emboli decreased sharply after 1973, even though there was no known change in design of the prosthesis or operative technique. Before 1973, only 69 per cent of patients were free of emboli 5 years after operation, but after 1973, 95 per cent were free of emboli. This fortunate event is as yet unexplained, especially as the valve prosthesis used (a Silastic ball with bare struts – Model 6120) had not been modified since 1966. It is hoped that other experiences will confirm this significant improvement in the rate of embolism.

In a panel discussion on valve prostheses at the annual meeting of the American College of Cardiology in March 1981, of which I was the moderator, Pluth reported a large series from the Mayo Clinic of mitral replacements with the Model 6120 Starr-Edwards valve. The survival rate at 8 years was 73 per cent, at 10 years 63 per cent. All patients were maintained on warfarin, with the addition of an antiplatelet agent in some. The frequency of thromboembolism was impressively low, 0.4 per cent per 100 patient years.

In 1979, Bjork and Henze described their experiences with insertion of 1800 Bjork-Shiley valves over a period of 10 years. Subsequent experiences were mentioned by Bjork in a discussion of the paper by Cheung and associates in 1981. The 5-year survival rate after aortic valve replacement was 82 per cent; it was 66 per cent after mitral valve replacement. The frequency of embolism was 0.7 per cent per year after aortic valve replacement and 4.2 per cent per year after mitral valve replacement. The frequency of obstruction by thrombosis was 0.3 per cent per year for aortic valve replacement and 1.3 per cent per year for mitral valve replacement.

In 1981, Karp and coworkers reported experiences with 643 patients operated on at the University of Alabama in Birmingham, with a mean follow-up of 38 months. Valve thrombosis occurred in 15 patients and caused 13 deaths. The survival rate at 4 years was between 83 and 86 per cent. Thromboembolism, occurred in 65 patients, 36 of whom had aortic prostheses.

One of the newer prostheses being evaluated is the St. Jude prosthesis, a type of disc valve with a wider orifice. Experiences with 88 patients operated on since 1978 were described by Chaux and colleagues in 1981. Early results have been encouraging. However, with any new prosthesis, at least 5 years of evaluation are required before a decision can be made about its effectiveness.

A sobering report in this regard appeared by Bowen and associates in 1980, describing long-term results with 80 patients undergoing mitral valve replacement with the Kay-Shiley plastic disc prosthesis between 1966 and 1972. Long-term follow-up found thromboembolism in 64 per cent of the patients and a 5-year survival rate of only 49 per cent. With these dismal results, the prosthesis was abandoned, and 18 of the 26 survivors underwent elective reoperation for replacement of the prosthesis. The principal problem was deterioration of the plastic disc.

Technique of Operation. The initial approach for mitral valve replacement is identical to that described earlier for open mitral commissurotomy. The tricuspid valve is routinely palpated at the time of insertion of the venous cannulas. Hypothermic potassium cardioplegia, described in detail in the section on mitral commissurotomy, has greatly increased the safety of mitral valve replacement. In patients without coronary disease, periods of aortic occlusion as long as 2 or 3 hours are surprisingly well tolerated. The actual limit of safe occlusion is uncertain, but it is probably between 3 and 4 hours. Much shorter times, 45 to 60 minutes, are adequate in the majority of patients, but the fact that the aorta can be safely occluded for over 3 hours clearly indicates that adequate time is present to correct any pathologic abnormality found at operation.

The treatment of tricuspid disease is described in Chapter 45. At New York University, our approach has remained unchanged for more than 8 years: We employ the conservative anuloplasty that obliterates the posterior leaflet of the tricuspid valve, described by Boyd and associates in 1974. The anuloplasty is a simple one, outlining a length of 8 cm. along the circumference of the tricuspid valve, starting at the coronary sinus and progressing medially. The anulus in excess of 8 cm. is then identified by marking sutures and plicated with mattress sutures of Dacron but-

tressed with Dacron pledgets. This has been uniformly successful in a large number of patients in whom organic disease of the valve leaflets was not present. With organic disease, which is fortunately rare, a porcine prosthesis is implanted, preserving the septal leaflet of the tricuspid valve to avoid heart block.

For removal of the mitral valve, the Carpentier type of retractor provides excellent exposure (see Fig. 46–3). After obliteration of the atrial appendage with sutures, the location of the anulus at the site of the anterolateral commissure is marked with a suture. The valve is then removed, dividing the leaflets 3 to 4 mm. from the anulus. Preservation of this small rim of leaflet tissue is quite important. A potentially hazardous technical problem exists when calcium extends from the leaflet tissue into the anulus. In such instances, the calcium must be cut with heavy scissors or rongeurs, carefully identifying the ventricular wall beforehand so that excision is not extended into the anulus itself. A usually hazardous problem exists when calcium infiltrates the ventricular wall below the valve. Special rongeurs have been designed for this purpose (Culliford *et al.,* 1979) (Fig. 46–11). Appropriate precautions are also taken to avoid loss of tissue or calcium fragments that could cause emboli. The chordae tendineae are divided near their junction with the papillary muscles.

A fortunately rare, but usually lethal, complication of mitral valve replacement is rupture of the left ventricle. This can occur from at least three causes. The most frequently recognized cause is partial avulsion of the mitral anulus from the underlying ventricular muscle from application of excessive traction during removal of the valve or insertion of the prosthesis (Zacharias *et al.,* 1975). This can almost always be prevented by avoiding excessive traction during all parts of the operation and also by inserting the sutures along the mural leaflet into the *anulus,* rather than into the underlying ventricular muscle.

A second type of left ventricular rupture results when a prosthesis is inserted that is too large for the ventricular cavity. The likelihood of this complication is probably greater with the use of potassium cardioplegia because the arrested heart is relaxed in diastole. Hence, a prosthesis that appears appropriate in

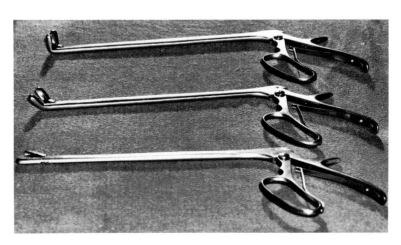

Figure 46–11. Rongeurs developed especially for the difficult, often lethal, problem of removal of calcium from the left ventricular wall in patients with calcific mitral stenosis. The condition is rare, with calcium infiltrating both the valve and the wall of the left ventricle for 3 to 5 cm. These instruments were developed in conjunction with the Pilling Corporation in Philadelphia.

the arrested heart may be too large when the heart begins to contract. In most patients the 29- or 31-mm. prosthesis of the Carpentier-Edwards type can be inserted satisfactorily, depending on body size. An important routine check at operation, however, is to examine the relationship between the posterior post of the prosthesis and the adjacent ventricular wall, being certain that the post is at least 3 to 4 mm. from the ventricular wall and not lying against the ventricular endocardium.

In 1974, Treasure and colleagues analyzed these two types of left ventricular rupture. Subsequently, in 1978, Nuñez and coworkers reported from Spain the death of two patients from strut perforation and stated that this complication occurred in a series of 322 patients with mitral valve replacement. They also noted that such a rupture had been previously reported in only three patients.

The third type of ventricular rupture is the most puzzling, occurring as a transverse rupture between the anulus of the mural leaflet and the papillary muscles. In 1978, Miller and associates reported two patients dying from a transverse rupture of the ventricle following insertion of a Bjork prosthesis. One patient died 2 weeks after operation with refractory heart failure and was found to have a pseudoaneurysm at the site of a transverse ventricular rupture between the mitral valve anulus and the base of the papillary muscles. In the other patient, exsanguination occurred in the recovery room from a 4.5-cm. transverse tear.

In detailed analyses of previous reports of this catastrophe, Cobbs and colleagues at Emory University (1977) and Treasure and associates (1974) concluded that three types of ventricular rupture could occur: one at the atrioventricular groove, one near the base of the papillary muscle, probably representing perforation by a post of the prosthesis, and one in the mid-portion of the ventricle. The most plausible explanation for the third variety, the most lethal, was advanced by Cobbs and coworkers (1977). Transverse rupture results from changes in tensile forces in the left ventricle after excision of the chordae of the mural leaflet. In a series of 14 patients, Miller and associates (1979) adopted a technique of partial or complete preservation of the posterior leaflet with the attached chordae, referring to the concept originally suggested by Lillehei and colleagues in 1964.

The largest experience with this problem was reported in a second report by Cobbs and associates in 1980, describing experiences with seven patients. A subsequent change in operative technique resulted in the disappearance of this problem to date. Their hypothesis was that strong contraction of the left ventricle following removal of the chordae attached to the mural leaflet could rupture the posterior ventricular wall. Preventing forceful contraction of the left ventricle for at least 20 to 30 minutes after unclamping the aorta, during which the effects of potassium on the left ventricular muscle should be greatly diminished, seems to have prevented this deadly complication. Another approach, without adequate data at present, is to preserve some of the chordae attached

to the mural leaflet of the mitral valve when possible. This was suggested by Miller and associates (1979) and also, for a different reason, by Lillehei and coworkers (1964).

The final solution to this deadly, though infrequent, problem is not yet clear. It is particularly prone to occur in older patients of small stature, usually in those over 60 years of age and weighing less than 130 pounds.

Following removal of the mitral valve, the size of the prosthesis is selected with a plastic sizer, noting the relationship of the posts to the ventricular cavity as well as to the aortic outflow tract. The prosthesis is inserted with 12 to 16 mattress sutures of 0 Dacron, all buttressed with Dacron pledgets, a technique employed routinely for the past decade (Isom et al., 1972). As mentioned earlier, in the area of the mural leaflet, it is important to insert the sutures in the anulus rather than in the ventricular muscle. In the area of the aortic leaflet, where no true anulus is present, insertion of sutures in the residual leaflet tissue avoids the circumflex coronary artery, which lies beyond the zone of the anulus. The routine use of Dacron pledgets on all mattress sutures has virtually eliminated the postoperative problem of paravalvular leakage for the past decade.

When the prosthesis is lowered into position, one of the many maneuvers to avoid tension during operation is to tie the sutures gently, applying only enough tension to create a visible dimple on the surface of the cloth of the prosthesis. Greater force during tying of the sutures may inadvertently avulse the anulus from the underlying ventricular muscle.

Until the past two years, a left ventricular vent was used routinely in the majority of patients, but since then, a transatrial catheter has been used more frequently. Air embolism with mitral valve replacement can occur from many causes, as described in the section on open mitral commissurotomy. A standardized technique for air removal should be employed in all patients because of the many mechanisms by which air emboli can occur. These techniques were described in the preceding section on mitral commissurotomy.

In 10 to 15 per cent of patients, depending on patient preference, the presence of a small left ventricular cavity, or the presence of massive calcification, the Bjork-Shiley disc prosthesis has been used. This is inserted with mattress sutures with the pledgets placed above the anulus, rotating the disc so that the downward portion of the disc is opposite the aortic outflow tract. It is very important to be certain that the disc can be rotated freely before it is inserted, because subsequent checking of the motion of the disc after insertion may reveal protruding tissue that can interfere with disc motion. Rotation of the disc at this time, with appropriate precaution to avoid tearing the sutures anchoring the prosthesis, can prevent this problem.

Following operation, the mediastinal soft tissues are closed superiorly to cover the aorta, leaving the remaining pericardium open. Care is taken to avoid entering either pleural cavity. The mediastinum is drained with a sump tube in the pericardial cavity and a chest tube in the mediastinum.

Technique of Closed Commissurotomy

As noted earlier, I have not performed this operation in almost 10 years, considering it an inferior operation, indicated only in the rare instance when an open heart procedure cannot be safely performed. It is described here for this purpose.

The two main hazards with digital commissurotomy are hemorrhage from laceration of the left atrium and cerebral embolism from thrombi in the left atrium or calcific fragments dislodged from the mitral valve.

A left posterolateral thoracotomy in the fourth intercostal space, with the patient turned slightly beyond a true lateral position, approximately 110 degrees rather than 90 degrees, is best. The increased rotation facilitates exposure of the posterior aspect of the left atrium.

The pericardium is incised anterior to the phrenic nerve, and stay sutures are inserted for traction on the pericardial edges. The atrial appendage is then examined. An appendage containing an organized thrombus often has a rubbery consistency, very different from the soft, compressible feel of a normal appendage. A fibrotic, contracted appendage usually indicates chronic fibrotic organization of a thrombus over a long period of time.

A heavy purse-string suture is placed around the base of the appendage and secured with a snare that can be tightened around the finger to minimize the loss of blood. An important adjunct with the operation is to have the anesthesiologist identify both carotid pulses at the start of the operation, so that intermittent digital occlusion for 30 to 60 seconds can be performed during all intracardiac manipulations. With this technique, cerebral embolism is fortunately rare.

When the atrial appendage is incised, a jet of blood is allowed to flush from the opening momentarily to dislodge any free-floating thrombi. Rarely, a thrombus as large as 1 to 2 cm. in diameter is expelled. Subsequently, the index finger is introduced, cautiously watching for undue resistance or laceration. If a tear begins, the finger should be withdrawn promptly and the atrial incision extended superiorly toward the left pulmonary vein. Lacerations in this area can be readily controlled, whereas those extending toward the circumflex coronary artery or beneath the pulmonary artery can produce lethal hemorrhage.

Once the index finger has been introduced into the atrium, the degree of stenosis, insufficiency, and valvular calcification is noted. If friable calcific granules are felt along the margins of the valve, there is a great risk of cerebral embolization. Hence, temporary occlusion of the carotid vessels is of particular importance, if it is necessary to proceed with the procedure. If possible, the procedure should be terminated and an open commissurotomy performed.

In the absence of a dangerous degree of calcification, commissurotomy is performed by pressure with the index finger on the two commissures, opening each commissure gradually and noting any mitral insufficiency that results after each manipulation. A variety of digital maneuvers, varying with individual patients, is necessary to open a densely fused commissure.

Usually repeated efforts are necessary to open a fused commissure, gradually weakening and tearing the rigid scar tissue that initially may be quite resistant. A mechanical transventricular dilator can be used, which applies more mechanical force than is possible with the finger. However, insufficiency can readily result, and therefore, use of the dilator is no longer recommended. It is better to terminate the procedure and perform an open commissurotomy later.

Under ideal circumstances, unless mitral insufficiency appears, both commissures should be opened to within a few millimeters of the mitral anulus. Subsequently, after removal of the finger from the atrium, any gradient remaining across the mitral valve can be measured by needle puncture of the left atrium and left ventricle. It is hoped that the end-diastolic gradient will have been abolished.

With adequate precautions, the risk of operation is surprisingly small, 1 to 2 per cent. As discussed earlier, the main objections are the inability to open the valve properly if fused chordae are present and the inability to correct any insufficiency produced at operation.

Postoperative Considerations

Following Open Commissurotomy. In most patients, the postoperative course is so uncomplicated that they can be discharged within 8 to 10 days and gradually resume normal activities in the next 8 to 12 weeks.

Prophylactic antibiotics, started before operation and given in large amounts during the procedure, should be selected according to the prevailing bacterial flora found in wound infections in the hospital. These vary from year to year, so that appropriate adjustment of the antibiotic program is necessary. Our current program is to give cefamandole (Mandol) in a dosage of 2 gm. before operation, 2 gm. at the start of bypass, and an additional 2 gm. repeated in the operating room after 4 hours if necessary. Following operation, it is continued in a dosage of 2 gm. every 6 hours for 48 to 72 hours, until intracardiac catheters and central lines have been removed.

Arrhythmias are common, especially atrial fibrillation, even though a sinus rhythm may have been present beforehand. Attempts to convert fibrillation to a sinus rhythm, usually by cardioversion, are often unsuccessful in the early postoperative course, when cardiac irritability is marked, but may be successful at a later date. A pleural effusion, even though the pleural cavity was not entered, often requires one or two thoracenteses in the first few days after operation.

A pericardiotomy syndrome is a frequent complication, occurring to some extent in about 10 to 15 per cent of patients. The clinical manifestations vary. Although the syndrome has been recognized for over 25 years, the etiology remains obscure. It is usually manifested by a low-grade fever, a white blood cell count of less than 10,000 cells per cubic millimeter, a pericardial or pleural effusion, and often a pericardial friction rub. Therapy with steroids is almost always effective, starting with prednisone, 50 to 60 mg. per day, and gradually decreasing the amount over 4 to 5 days. If symptoms recur, prednisone may be necessary in smaller doses for some period of time, even for 4 to 6 weeks in unusual refractory cases.

An echocardiogram is a valuable method for following the degree of pericardial effusion present. In some instances, a dramatic decrease in the size of the effusion can be seen with intense diuretic therapy, decreasing the patient's weight 5 or more pounds below that before operation.

As mentioned earlier, results are excellent in the majority of patients, but evaluation by the patient's physician should be done at periodic intervals indefinitely because of the hazard of arrhythmias or recurrent mitral disease, usually mitral insufficiency developing from fibrosis caused by turbulent flow of blood across the diseased mitral orifice.

Following Prosthetic Replacement of the Mitral Valve. Following bypass, left atrial pressure is measured while blood is gradually infused, noting the response of the arterial pressure to the increase in blood volume and elevation of left atrial pressure. Cardiac output is usually determined by thermodilution from a previously placed Swan-Ganz catheter in the pulmonary artery. A cardiac index above 2 liters per minute usually indicates a satisfactory postoperative course. If cardiac output is not measured, a small catheter can be left in the pulmonary artery and the oxygen tension of the mixed venous blood periodically measured, a technique developed by Boyd and associates (1959) at Johns Hopkins more than 20 years ago and used almost routinely since that time. If a Swan-Ganz catheter is not used, left atrial pressure should be monitored with a small plastic catheter left in the left atrium. With a Swan-Ganz catheter, the left atrial pressure may be estimated from the pulmonary artery diastolic pressure, noting the relationship between pulmonary artery diastolic pressure and left atrial pressure at the time of operation. Alternately, the wedge pressure can be measured, although this carries the rare but dangerous hazard of rupture of the pulmonary artery.

Pacemaker wires are routinely left in the right ventricle and right atrium for several days. Intracardiac catheters are usually removed 24 to 48 hours after operation.

The low cardiac output syndrome has virtually disappeared from clinical practice since the introduction of effective myocardial preservation with potassium cardioplegia. The preferred technique was described earlier in the chapter. We consider the use of topical hypothermia an important adjunct to potassium cardioplegia, especially in patients with hypertrophy of the right ventricle from pulmonary hypertension and carefully wrap the heart with a large sponge soaked with cold fluid, so that the myocardial temperature remains lower than 15°C. throughout the operation. With this technique, significant problems with decreased cardiac output are rare. If a cardiac index of 2 liters per minute is not present for any reason and does not respond to appropriate elevation of left atrial pressure by infusion of fluid, an inotropic agent, usually dobutamine, 500 μg./min., is administered for 24 to 48 hours. If peripheral vascular resistance is increased, it can be decreased to normal levels by infusion of nitroprusside or nitroglycerin.

A cardiac rate between 80 and 90 beats per minute is preferable. The pacemaker wires are invaluable for maintaining the proper rate, and atrioventricular pacing is preferred if atrial fibrillation is not present. Otherwise, ventricular pacing can be used until the spontaneous rhythm is satisfactory.

Cardiac arrhythmias occur frequently, so that constant monitoring for several days is essential. With premature contractions, different antiarrhythmic drugs may be necessary, including propranolol (Inderal), procainamide (Pronestyl), quinidine, or other agents. Digoxin is given cautiously, with monitoring of the serum level as well as the blood potassium concentration.

Prophylactic antibiotics are given in a manner similar to that described previously following open mitral commissurotomy.

If for any reason antibiotics are given for more than 3 or 4 days, nystatin (Mycostatin), 500,000 units every 8 hours, is given by mouth. The routine use of Mycostatin with antibiotics for several days has virtually eliminated superimposed infection with a yeast organism, which was seen in several patients a few years ago.

Anticoagulant therapy is begun 3 or 4 days after operation with sodium warfarin (Coumadin), elevating the prothrombin time to near 20 seconds. A greater degree of anticoagulation, with the prothrombin time about twice normal levels, was found to be unnecessary several years ago. Hemorrhage occurred more often with the higher degree of anticoagulation, and a lesser degree of anticoagulation has been equally effective in preventing thromboembolism.

With porcine prostheses, anticoagulation is usually stopped after 3 months. However, patients are then under the management of their referring cardiologists, some of whom prefer to continue anticoagulation if atrial fibrillation is present. As mentioned earlier, if the atrial appendage has been obliterated, we have not found long-term anticoagulation necessary, despite continued atrial fibrillation.

When Coumadin therapy is stopped 3 months after operation, antiplatelet therapy, usually with acetylsalicylic acid, 0.3 to 0.6 gm. per day, is recommended for at least 2 years to lessen the hazard of platelet emboli. The efficacy of the antiplatelet therapy has not been completely proved, but available data are supportive.

Patients are usually discharged from the hospital in less than 2 weeks and resume normal activities over the next 2 to 3 months. A restriction in sodium intake may be necessary for a few months, checking the weight daily and using diuretics as necessary. Three to 6 months may be required to obtain full benefit from operation, especially in patients with advanced failure preoperatively.

If a Bjork metallic prosthesis has been inserted, anticoagulation with sodium warfarin is continued permanently, keeping the prothrombin time near 20 seconds.

Long-term Management of Patients with a Prosthetic Mitral Valve. An important principle to emphasize is that any patient with a prosthetic valve requires lifelong periodic surveillance by his physician, similar to a patient with diabetes. Complications that may occur include thromboembolism, endocarditis, malfunction of the prosthesis, arrhythmias, and cardiac failure.

THROMBOEMBOLISM. Fortunately, with porcine prostheses, thromboembolism is rare. As mentioned earlier, warfarin is normally stopped 3 months after operation but restarted if thromboemboli occur. In the rare instance in which a patient has recurrent thromboembolic problems despite the combination of warfarin and an antiplatelet drug, a mechanical problem with the prosthesis requiring reoperating should be seriously considered. The frequency of thromboembolism in the group of 714 patients having a porcine prosthesis inserted at New York University between 1976 and 1979 was described earlier (Isom *et al.,* 1980).

ENDOCARDITIS. Any patient with a prosthetic valve has a permanent susceptibility to bacterial endocarditis during periods of transient bacteremia. Representative episodes would be a dental extraction or cystoscopic procedures. This is similar to the well-known susceptibility of patients with valvular disease from rheumatic fever. Hence, it is of great importance that appropriate antibiotic therapy be given for a short period of time before and after such elective surgical procedures. This is effective in many patients, but others may develop endocarditis from unknown causes.

In the New York University series of 714 porcine prostheses inserted before 1980, endocarditis occurred 20 times, with a mean follow-up of 24 months, a frequency of 1.7 per cent per patient year. Fortunately, in 12 of the 20 patients, prompt institution of antibiotic therapy cured the problem, obviating the need for reoperation. The other eight patients were successfully operated on, so that there were no fatalities from endocarditis. A most important principle with endocarditis, however, is that if a patient remains septic after 3 or 4 days of treatment with the appropriate antibiotic, operation should be done promptly. Continued antibiotic therapy is often not only ineffective, but also hazardous because of erosion of the valve anulus with formation of para-anular abscesses as well as cerebral emboli from bacterial vegetation.

Fortunately, the risk of reoperation is small, and with the use of appropriate antibiotics, recurrent endocarditis is surprisingly rare.

PROSTHESIS MALFUNCTION. With the porcine prosthesis, malfunction is rare in the first 4 to 5 years after operation. A systolic murmur may be audible, probably from turbulent flow of blood around a strut in the outflow tract. Paravalvular leakage has virtually disappeared over the past decade with the routine use of pledgeted mattress sutures. Hemolysis, previously seen in some patients with the steel ball prosthesis, is not a problem.

If any question exists about either stenosis or insufficiency, investigation should be done promptly with echocardiography and cardiac catheterization.

In the New York University series reported by Isom and associates in 1980, malfunction of the prosthetic valve (aortic or mitral) required reoperation in nine of 632 patients within 2 to 44 months. Insufficiency was the usual problem. No instances of calcification or thrombosis were seen. Some of the early failures were possibly due to methods of valve preservation, operative trauma, or unknown factors, because several occurred too soon to represent heterograft degeneration.

ARRHYTHMIAS. In the 5 to 10 years following insertion of a prosthetic valve, some patients may die suddenly without known cause. Sudden death, with or without known arrhythmias, caused nearly 50 per cent of the 30 late deaths occurring in the New York University porcine valve series of 632 patients (Isom *et al.,* 1980). Frequently, a postmortem examination is not done. When a postmortem examination is performed, often the only finding is seemingly insignficant scattered areas of myocardial fibrosis. In such patients, it seems probable that an arrhythmia was the cause of death. How commonly this occurs is unknown, but with the increasing ability to detect and treat arrhythmias, periodic monitoring of patients with any arrhythmias should be done, including 24-hour Holter monitoring. As the death rate in the first 5 years after operation is significantly greater in the Class IV patients, this group should be monitored with particular care.

In the Seattle series reported by Cobb and colleagues (1980) of a 10-year experience with cardiac resuscitation for sudden death occurring outside the hospital, averaging about 300 cases of ventricular fibrillation a year in recent years, over 50 per cent of the patients resuscitated had no signs of myocardial necrosis whatsoever (CPK-MB enzymes), even though the majority had coronary disease.

CARDIAC FAILURE. The degree of improvement following mitral valve replacement varies widely and cannot be predicted with certainty from individual patients. This is well reflected in the wide variation in the 5-year survival rate, depending on the degree of cardiac failure beforehand. The 5-year survival rate following valve replacement in patients in Class II or III is usually between 85 and 90 per cent, but it is as low as 55 to 60 per cent in patients with advanced failure (Class IV). As this has been observed by different groups with various prostheses, the difference in late mortality is probably due to pre-existing myocardial injury and not to either operative trauma or the type of prosthesis employed. These data clearly support the need for early operation once significant cardiac disability appears, because with advanced failure, some degree of irreversible myocardial injury has probably already occurred.

When cardiac failure appears months or years after mitral valve replacement, several possibilities should be evaluated.These include paravalvular leak, the development of additional valvular disease, such as aortic or tricuspid disease, or deterioration of the prosthetic valve, such as stenosis or insufficiency with porcine prostheses. These possibilities should be promptly evaluated by cardiac catheterization.

At catherization, the distinction can be readily made between cardiac failure from prosthetic malfunction and primary left ventricular failure, manifested by an elevated end-diastolic pressure. It is hoped that the sad clinical picture of patients with advanced left ventricular failure 2 to 3 years following mitral valve replacement will decrease and disappear in the future with the combination of present operative techniques that minimize injury to the heart and the earlier performance of operation on patients before irreversible injury has developed.

PROGNOSIS. Long-term results with porcine prostheses and Bjork prostheses were mentioned earlier in the section concerning mitral valve replacement and the choice of prosthesis. The longest follow-up data are with the ball valve prosthesis, as this was the first successful prosthesis, developed by Starr more than 20 years ago and summarized in the 1981 report by Teply and associates.

MITRAL INSUFFICIENCY

Etiology and Pathology

Although mitral stenosis is almost always due to rheumatic fever, mitral insufficiency can result from several causes. Four different types of structural injuries to the mitral valve may produce insufficiency. These include leaflet retraction from fibrosis and calcification; dilatation of the anulus abnormalities of the chordae tendineae, including rupture, elongation, or shortening; and papillary muscle dysfunction. The presence of each of these injuries must be assessed when reconstructive operations, rather than prosthetic valve replacement, are undertaken.

Rheumatic fever is probably the most common cause of mitral insufficiency, although the frequency is gradually decreasing, and a definite rheumatic history often cannot be obtained. The dominant changes from rheumatic fever are the inflammatory changes in the valve leaflets. These include fibrosis and contraction, shortening and fusion of the chordae tendineae, and, eventually, calcification of the leaflets and the anulus (Fig. 46–12).

Why the rheumatic process produces mitral insufficiency in one patient and mitral stenosis in another is unknown and is probably fortuitous. Often, both stenosis and insufficiency are present.

Dilatation of the mitral anulus varies with different disorders, but is probably uniformly present with ruptured chordae tendineae and prolapse. Hence, reconstructive procedures should uniformly include an anuloplasty to correct the deformity of the anulus. Carpentier in Paris has been the leading contributor to innovative techniques of anuloplasty for the past

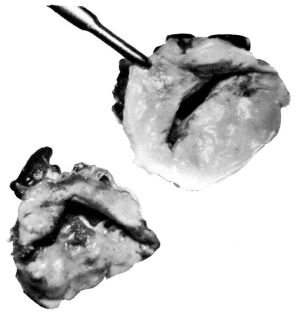
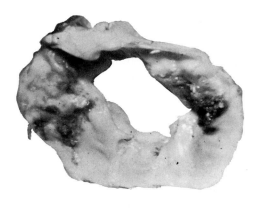

Figure 46–12. Mitral valves removed from three different patients, illustrating the fibrosis and calcification commonly encountered in patients with mitral insufficiency. An effort is made to remove the mitral valve intact to avoid fragmentation and possible displacement of calcium fragments into the left ventricle when the valve is removed.

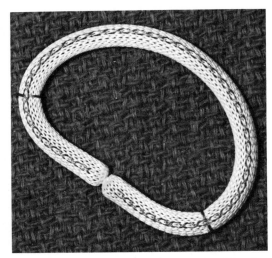

Figure 46–13. The prosthetic ring developed by Carpentier and used for mitral valve reconstruction. The ring is incomplete, facilitating its insertion and function.

several years, developing a special ring for this purpose (Fig. 46–13).

Probably the second most common cause of mitral insufficiency is prolapse of the mitral valve, a congenital abnormality varying widely in its severity but surprisingly common in its milder forms. It has been estimated to occur to a slight degree in nearly 5 per cent of the normal female population. Fortunately, in the majority of patients, it is of minor physiologic significance, but it is seen more frequently with increasing age, probably because turbulent flow of blood over a period of decades produces fibrosis and calcification of the leaflets. Before widespread recognition of the frequency of mitral valve prolapse, such patients were erroneously assumed to have had rheumatic fever, although a clinical history could not be obtained.

Unusual causes of mitral insufficiency include ruptured chordae tendineae; bacterial endocarditis; primary dilatation of the anulus, as with rheumatoid arthritis; and papillary muscle dysfunction from either coronary artery disease or a myopathy, especially asymmetric septal hypertrophy with associated obstruction in the aortic outflow tract (idiopathic hypertrophic subaortic stenosis [IHSS]).

Rupture of chordae tendineae is a clinical condition of particular significance. The basic cause is unknown but is probably some defect in the collagen of the mitral valve. It is of particular clinical importance because reconstructive techniques can often be used, with an excellent prognosis. It can occur from endocarditis or other inflammatory processes, but in the majority of patients, it appears without any known cause. It can be suspected when mitral insufficiency develops acutely without any previous symptoms of heart disease and can be diagnosed readily by echocardiography and angiography.

Papillary muscle dysfunction is typically seen with far-advanced coronary artery disease, as the papillary muscles readily become ischemic with cor-

onary insufficiency. Focal papillary muscle dysfunction may follow myocardial infarction, either from fibrosis or from rupture of the muscle.

Pathophysiology

The basic physiologic burden with mitral insufficiency is reflux of part of the stroke volume of the contracting left ventricle into the left atrium, reducing systemic blood flow and elevating left atrial pressure. Left atrial pressure tracings will accordingly reveal a systolic spike as high as 30 to 40 mm. Hg, occasionally as high as 70 to 80 mm. Hg, followed by an abrupt decline in diastole. At the end of diastole, pressure may remain slightly elevated, with a 5 to 10 mm. Hg gradient across the mitral valve, even though no organic stenosis is present, the gradient representing a "flow gradient" resulting from increased flow of blood during diastole. The mean left atrial pressure is usually between 15 and 20 mm. Hg; in some patients, it is normal.

Pulmonary vascular resistance is increased less often than in patients with mitral stenosis, probably because left atrial pressure is elevated only intermittently. Similarly, left atrial thrombi and systemic emboli occur less frequently than with mitral stenosis because of the absence of stasis in the left atrium. Left ventricular function may be adequate for surprisingly long periods of time, despite massive mitral regurgitation. This is indicated both by the absence of symptoms and by a left ventricular end-diastolic pressure less than 12 mm. Hg. Once left ventricular failure occurs, however, the course progressively worsens, usually at a fairly rapid rate.

The blood regurgitating into the left atrium with each systolic contraction leads to progressive enlargement of the left atrium, often to gigantic proportions. A grotesque cardiac shadow may result in which the left atrial contour extends almost to the right chest wall, some of the largest degrees of left atrial enlargement encountered in clinical medicine. The degree of left atrial enlargement, however, does not correspond to the degree of mitral insufficiency. Why the degree of dilatation varies so much is unknown, but it probably reflects an inherent variation in distensibility of left atrial muscle.

Diagnostic Considerations

In patients with mild mitral insufficiency, an apical systolic murmur is present without any disability. Such patients may remain well for many years, with the left ventricle adapting adequately to the increased workload. An increased susceptibility to bacterial endocarditis is the only hazard. The characteristic adaptation of the left ventricle is dilatation, increasing stroke volume by increasing the diastolic fiber length of the ventricular muscle. Hence, the principal question in evaluating the severity of mitral insufficiency is the degree of left ventricular enlargement present.

As insufficiency progresses, the most common symptoms are weakness, fatigability, and palpitations, with some dyspnea on exertion. These reflect a decreased cardiac output as well as left atrial hypertension. Gradually, symptoms of pulmonary congestion become more prominent, as described in the section on mitral stenosis. If right heart failure appears, hepatic enlargement and peripheral edema develop with a rapidly worsening course, even more rapid than that with mitral stenosis.

On physical examination, the two characteristic findings are the apical systolic murmur and the forceful apical impulse with cardiac enlargement. The apical murmur is harsh and blowing in quality, transmitted to the axilla. Usually, it is Grade II or III in intensity, although there is wide variation. The severity of the insufficiency does not correlate with the intensity of the murmur, but the pansystolic characteristic does. With mild mitral insufficiency, the systolic murmur does not extend completely through systole, whereas with severe insufficiency, it occupies all of systole. A diastolic murmur may also be heard because of the increased volume of blood flowing across the mitral valve. However, in contrast to mitral stenosis, there is neither an opening snap nor an increased first sound.

The most important clinical finding on physical examination is the forceful apical impulse, reflecting the degree of enlargement of the left ventricle. This finding contrasts sharply with the normal or decreased apical impulse with mitral stenosis, in which the work requirements of the left ventricle are decreased rather than increased.

The characteristic change on the chest roentgenogram is enlargement of the left atrium and the left ventricle (Fig. 46–14). Precise determination of the degree of enlargement of the left ventricle is the single most valuable measurement for determining prognosis

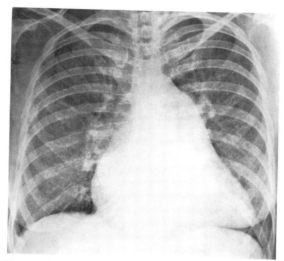

Figure 46–14. Chest roentgenogram of a patient with mitral insufficiency. The distinctive features include an enlarged cardiac shadow with a prominent pulmonary artery. The shadow of the left atrium is visible in the right border of the cardiac shadow behind the shadow of the right atrium. The pulmonary vascular markings are prominent.

and therapy. As long as left ventricular size is normal, a nonoperative approach is satisfactory. With progressive degrees of enlargement of the left ventricle, however, operation should be undertaken before irreversible injury occurs. A leading area of clinical investigation is to determine by echocardiography and other noninvasive techniques which abnormality of left ventricular function has the most accurate prognostic value for indicating when operation should be done.

Changes in the pulmonary vasculature, similar to those described for mitral stenosis, may be present. Calcification of the mitral valve occurs less frequently but is of considerable surgical importance. Extensive calcification almost always indicates that replacement, rather than reconstruction, will be necessary.

The electrocardiogram is not a precise guide. Signs of left ventricular hypertrophy are prominent in about half of the patients, whereas in other patients, right ventricular hypertrophy is more evident because of increased pulmonary vascular resistance. Atrial fibrillation is common. In some patients with extensive insufficiency, the electrocardiogram is nearly normal.

Echocardiography is highly sensitive and specific in the diagnosis of mitral stenosis. Two-dimensional echocardiography can quantitate the lesion, determining the cross-sectional area even more precisely than data obtained by cardiac catheterization. Following mitral commissurotomy, serial echocardiography permits periodic evaluation of the patient for any signs of recurring stenosis.

With mitral insufficiency, echocardiography is not diagnostic but is valuable for defining the degree to which ventricular function is impaired. Different abnormalities that cause mitral insufficiency can be recognized. For example, the impaired contraction of segments of the ventricular wall with coronary artery disease can be defined, which, in turn, usually result from infarction or from papillary muscle ischemia. Prolapse of the mitral valve can readily be detected. Active endocarditis may be recognized by visualizing vegetations on the mitral leaflets. With idiopathic hypertrophic subaortic stenosis (IHSS), the echocardiogram is highly sensitive and specific.

A separate important aspect of echocardiography in the evaluation of the patient with mitral insufficiency is its role in determining serial changes in left ventricular function. Increasing data indicate that patients should be operated on because of progressive deterioration of ventricular function, not because of disabling symptoms. The echocardiogram can measure the internal volume of the ventricle in both systole and end-diastole, and from these measurements, calculation of the stroke volume and the ejection fraction is possible. The left ventricular wall thickness as well as the left ventricular wall systolic thickness can be measured, a normal muscle increasing its thickness in systole by 30 per cent or more. The mean circumferential fiber shortening velocity can also be measured, probably the best precise measurement at present for left ventricular contractility.

The ability to make these determinations represents a great advance in noninvasive diagnostic techniques and will undoubtedly become increasingly important in the future management of patients. At present, for example, the end-systolic volume in the patient with aortic insufficiency seems to be the best prognostic indicator of ventricular function and the most reliable guide of indicating when operation should be performed.*

After evaluation by echocardiography, mitral insufficiency is best evaluated by catheterization and angiography. Injection of radiopaque material into the left ventricle, usually by retrograde insertion of a catheter across the aortic valve, can visually demonstrate the degree of regurgitation. The degree of elevation of left atrial pressure will vary with the degree of heart failure present, usually with the mean left atrial pressure between 15 and 20 mm. Hg. Cardiac failure is also reflected by a decrease in ejection fraction from the normal range of 0.65 to 0.70.

Operative Treatment

In contrast to mitral stenosis, in which early operation is indicated because commissurotomy may be performed with a low operative risk, operation is usually considered for mitral insufficiency only when disability has progressed to a significant degree or there is progressive cardiac enlargement with other signs of hemodynamic deterioration. In at least 80 to 90 per cent of patients, prosthetic valve replacement has been necessary. Because of the permanent hazards with prosthetic valves, discussed in the preceding sections, a more conservative approach to operation is indicated than with mitral stenosis. However, current data clearly indicate that better long-term results are obtained when operation is performed before irreversible ventricular injury has occurred.

Operative techniques for prosthetic replacement have been described previously. In the following section, the technique of anuloplasty and repair of ruptured chordae tendineae will be briefly discussed. Thus far, these have been applied only to a small percentage of patients with mitral insufficiency, but with recently developed techniques, it is probable that this percentage can be significantly increased in the future.

Mitral Valve Anuloplasty

An anuloplasty may be successful in patients with isolated insufficiency, usually with dilatation of the mitral anulus and absence of calcification of the leaflets. The procedure has been intermittently described for more than two decades. Enthusiasm for anuloplasty has varied widely among different cardiac cen-

ters, with only a few significant long-term results being reported. At New York University, anuloplasty has been used for more than 15 years, as described by Reed in 1973. These experiences have been primarily with children and young adults.

Published techniques of anuloplasty have varied. Kay and Egerton (1963) employed sutures primarily along the anulus of the mural leaflet, usually at the posteromedial commissure. Reed (1973), by contrast, performed asymmetric anuloplasty at both commissures, selectively narrowing the mural leaflet to a greater degree, with the goal of uniformly reducing the mitral valve to a cross-sectional area of between 3.0 and 3.5 cm.^{2}.

In 1980, Reed and associates reported 17 years' experience with 196 patients who had undergone mitral anuloplasty. This series represented 35 per cent of all of those operated on for mitral disease during that time. Anuloplasty was performed on 115 patients, and commissurotomy and anuloplasty on another 81 patients. The operative mortality rate was low, 4.5 per cent, and the later mortality rate was 8.7 per cent. Only six episodes of embolism occurred in the entire series over this period of 17 years. Eight per cent of the patients have required subsequent operation. These experiences indicate that anuloplasty is a durable and effective operation in a certain type of patient, especially younger patients without extensive calcification of the valve leaflets.

Similarly, Kay and colleagues (1980) reported operating on 61 patients with mitral insufficiency secondary to coronary disease between 1970 and 1978, performing a different type of anulopasty in which most of the mural leaflet was obliterated by sutures at each commissure. Ruptured chordae tendineae were treated by suturing the flail leaflet to the underlying papillary muscle, after which the anulus of the mural leaflet was obliterated, as described. There were five hospital deaths among the 61 patients, most of the deaths occurring in patients with an ejection fraction less than 0.40.

The principal uncertainty thus far with anuloplasty has been its durability as well as its applicability to different patients.

For the past several years, Carpentier in Paris has employed a prosthetic ring that he developed to more effectively distribute tension in narrowing and remolding the deformed mitral anulus. His experiences include several hundred patients and suggest that anuloplasty may be applied much more widely than it has been in the past. This is particularly true because the techniques of shortening chordae tendineae and excising segments of valve leaflets with ruptured chordae seem to be reliable. Long-term hemodynamic data, however, are not yet available.

With ruptured chordae tendineae, different techniques of reconstruction have been employed in selected cases for more than 20 years, including an ingenious suggestion by McGoon in 1960, and a variety of techniques periodically reported by Kay and associates (Kay and Egerton, 1963; Kay et al., 1980).

---

*The information about echocardiography was provided through the generosity of Dr. Itzhak Kronzon, Associate Professor of Clinical Medicine and Director of the Echocardiography Laboratories at New York University.

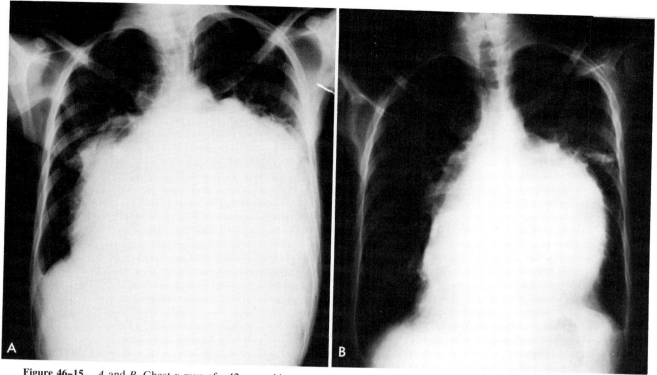

Figure 46–15. *A* and *B*, Chest x-rays of a 42-year-old woman with long-standing mitral regurgitation who was operated on in August 1981. The preoperative film (*A*) shows the massive cardiac enlargement, found at operation to consist primarily of a gigantic left atrium with a tiny left ventricle. The postoperative film (*B*) was taken in September 1981, 6 weeks after operation. The Carpentier ring used for the anuloplasty can be faintly seen through the cardiac silhouette. Tricuspid anuloplasty was also done. At operation, the patient had rheumatic mitral insufficiency with fusion of the mural leaflet to the wall of the left ventricle. There were no ruptured chordae. The fused leaflets were mobilized, dividing secondary chordae, after which a Carpentier ring was inserted. The dramatic improvement well supports the role of anuloplasty in selected patients.

With the experiences of Carpentier, it may be that the majority of patients with rupture of the chordae tendineae involving the mural leaflet can be treated by simply excising the flail leaflet, approximating the leaflets and the anulus with interrupted sutures, and inserting an appropriate Carpentier ring to restore the deformed anulus to its normal size and shape. An additional elongated chordae may be treated at the same time. A final decision about the reliability of this approach can be made only when significant 5- and 10-year follow-up data become available.

Following a visit by one of the faculty at New York University to Paris to study techniques with Carpentier in 1981, his techniques have been employed in a variety of patients at New York University with excellent short-term results to date (Fig. 46–15). Carpentier has periodically reported extensive experiences over the past 10 years. In 1976, he and his associates reported experiences with 47 children between 4 months and 12 years of age, describing a wide variety of pathologic abnormalities, including both stenosis and insufficiency. Valve reconstruction was possible in 38 of the patients, and valve replacement was necessary in nine. Some insufficiency remained in the majority of patients, but it was fortunate that valve replacement at that time had not become necessary, with the obvious advantage that if valve re-

placement ultimately became necessary, it could be done when the patients reached adulthood.

In 1978, Carpentier and colleagues reported experiences with 213 operations for prolapse of the mitral valve performed between 1969 and 1977. These included 109 patients with ruptured chordae tendineae treated by quadrangular resection of the prolapsed leaflet and 103 patients with elongated chordae tendineae treated by shortening of the elongated chordae. A Carpentier ring was used in the majority of patients to restore the deformed anulus to normal size and shape. Only six reoperations were necessary, and only one patient had a late thromboembolic complication. Actuarial curve analysis demonstrated a 91 per cent survival rate at 8 years. These impressive results strongly suggest that techniques of reconstruction can be much more widely applied for patients with abnormalities of the chordae tendineae than has been done in the past. Others, however, have not yet reported similar experiences.

In a discussion of this report, Liddle, of Salt Lake City, reported that the late Dr. Ray Rumel had performed reconstructive procedures in 71 patients between 1961 and 1975, with good results in the majority. Objective hemodynamic data were not given.

More recently, Carpentier and coworkers (1980) reported their 10 years of experience with 551 patients operated on from 1969 to 1978. The operative mortality rate was 4 per cent in patients with isolated mitral disease, with a late mortality rate of 7 per cent. The actuarial survival curve at 9 years was 85 per cent. Only 37 patients, 11 per cent of the group, required reoperation for residual incompetence. In addition, only 12 patients of the entire group (2 per cent) had had thromboembolic problems.

Precise data defining the degree of remaining incompetence are not available for the majority of these patients, because postoperative angiograms were performed in only 52 patients. The clinical results, however, are certainly superior to those following prosthetic valve replacement.

Hence, the data from Carpentier, Reed, and Kay and associates, all of whom have performed some form of anuloplasty for more than a decade with durable results, indicate clearly that anuloplasty may be employed in selected patients much more frequently than it has been in the past. The recent dramatic improvements in myocardial preservation should facilitate techniques of reconstruction, as a complex reconstruction requires a longer period of myocardial ischemia than insertion of a prosthetic valve.

SELECTED REFERENCES

Bjork, V. O., and Henze, A.: Ten years' experience with the Bjork-Shiley tilting disc valve. J. Thorac. Cardiovasc. Surg., 78:331, 1979.

A major development with prosthetic valves was the tilting disc valve, popularized by Bjork over 10 years ago. His decade of experience with over 1800 patients is summarized in this report, quoted in detail in this chapter.

Boyd, A. D., Engelman, R. H., Isom, O. W., Reed, G. E., and Spencer, F. C.: Tricuspid annuloplasty. J. Thorac. Cardiovasc. Surg., 68:344, 1974.

Many types of tricuspid valve reconstruction have been described in recent years. It remains a curiosity to me why the technique of simple posterior leaflet anuloplasty has not been utilized more widely. As described initially in this report 9 years ago, it is simple and reliable and has been used at New York University for over a decade with satisfactory results, unless advanced organic disease of the tricuspid valve requires valvular replacement.

Carpentier, A., Chauvaud, S., Fabiani, J. N., Deloche, A., Relland, J., Lessana, A., D'Allaines, C., Blondeau, P., Piwnica, A., and Dubost, C.: Reconstructive surgery of mitral valve incompetence—Ten-year appraisal. J. Thorac. Cardiovasc. Surg., 79:338, 1980.

A major development of the recent years has been the elaboration of techniques of mitral valve reconstruction, as opposed to prosthetic valve replacement. Many contributions have been made by the group led by Carpentier in Paris. Experiences with 551 patients are summarized in this report. The prosthetic ring, developed by Carpentier, has been a major contribution.

Carpentier, A., Relland, J., Deloche, A., Fabiani, J. N., D'Allaines, C., Blondeau, P., Piwnica, A., Chauvaud, S., and Dubost, C.: Conservative management of the prolapsed mitral valve. Ann. Thorac. Surg., 26:294, 1978.

This remarkable paper describes the repair of prolapsed mitral valves in 213 patients between 1969 and 1977, 109 of whom

had ruptured chordae as well. For uncertain reasons, Carpentier's methods of reconstruction have not become popular in this country, although they have been enthusiastically adopted at New York University in the past year. Probably a simple lack of familiarity with this technique is the principal reason, although only time and meaningful data will provide the ultimate answer.

Cobbs, B. W., Jr., Hatcher, C. R., Jr., Craver, J. M., Jones, E. L., and Sewell, C. W.: Transverse midventricular disruption after mitral valve replacement. Am. Heart J., 99:33, 1980.

An infrequent but lethal complication of mitral valve replacement is rupture of the posterior wall of the left ventricle. This can occur in at least three areas, as described in detail in this chapter. The most bizarre is a transverse rupture of the muscle of the posterior ventricular wall, between the mitral anulus above and the stumps of the papillary muscles below. This paper is the most extensive report in the English literature of this unusual complication, which is perhaps a result of removal of the posterior papillary muscle in elderly people with small left ventricles.

Gross, R. I., Cunningham, J. N., Jr., Snively, S. L., Catinella, F. P., Nathan, I. M., Adams, P. X., and Spencer, F. C.: Long-term results of open radical mitral commissurotomy: Ten-year follow-up study of 202 patients. Am. J. Cardiol., 47:821, 1981.

With the increasingly good results with prosthetic valves, the value of mitral commissurotomy, as opposed to valve replacement, has been periodically questioned. This long-term follow-up conclusively demonstrates that commissurotomy is far superior to valve replacement if the gradient can be corrected without producing significant insufficiency.

Isom, O. W., Culliford, A. T., Colvin, S. B., Adams, P. X., Cunningham, J. N., Jr., Trehan, N., Leist, A., Cordone, R., Shemin, R. J., Glassman, E., and Spencer, F. C.: Porcine valves: Is there a difference? Presented at the American Heart Association, Miami, November 1980.

This paper summarizes experiences with over 700 patients undergoing replacement with a porcine prosthesis at New York University, where porcine valves have been used in about 90 per cent of valvular replacements for the past 3 to 4 years. Emboli causing permanent neurologic defects have been very rare, which is the reason for the strong preference for the porcine prosthesis, as well as the freedom from anticoagulants. The principal question is the durability of the prosthesis, as data currently being reported indicate that degeneration is far more common after 7 or 8 years following operation. Whether all such prostheses will ultimately require replacement is the major question, presently unanswerable.

Miller, D. W., Jr., Johnson, D. D., and Ivey, T. D.: Does preservation of the posterior chordae tendineae enhance survival during mitral valve replacement? Ann. Thorac. Surg., 28:22, 1979.

The transverse ventricular rupture after the mitral valve replacement, described in the previously cited report by Cobbs and associates, may be avoided by preservation of the chordae to the anulus of the mural leaflet of the mitral valve. This report, although certainly not conclusive, describes preliminary experiences with this technique, a concept suggested by Lillehei in the early 1960s for a different reason.

Oyer, P. E., Miller, D. C., Stinson, E. B., Retiz, B. A., Moreno-Cabral, R. J., and Shumway, N. E.: Clinical durability of the Hancock porcine bioprosthetic valve. J. Thorac. Cardiovasc. Surg., 80:824, 1980.

This report is one of the most extensive in the surgical literature about experiences with porcine prostheses, describing operations upon 1407 patients between 1971 and 1979.

Teply, J. F., Grunkemeier, G. L., Sutherland, H. D., Lambert, L. E., Johnson, V. A., and Starr, A.: The ultimate prognosis after valve replacement: An assessment at twenty years. Ann. Thorac. Surg., *32*:111, 1981.

The year 1981 marked the passage of 20 years since the introduction of the caged ball prosthesis by Albert Starr, the first successful prosthetic valve to be regularly used. This paper summarizes the authors' 20-year experience with 2135 patients.

REFERENCES

Bailey, C. P.: The surgical treatment of mitral stenosis (mitral commissurotomy). Dis. Chest, *15*:377, 1949.

Becker, R. M., Sandor, L., Tindel, M., and Frater, R. W. M.: Medium-term follow-up of the Ionescu-Shiley heterograft valve. Ann. Thorac. Surg., *32*:120, 1981.

Bjork, V. O., and Henze, A.: Ten years' experience with the Bjork-Shiley tilting disc valve. J. Thorac. Cardiovasc. Surg. *78*:331, 1979.

Bowen, T. E., Zajtchuk, R., Brott, W. H., and deCastro, C. M.: Isolated mitral valve replacement with the Kay-Shiley prosthesis. Long-term follow-up and recommendations. J. Thorac. Cardiovasc. Surg., *80*:45, 1980.

Boyd, A. D., Tremblay, R. E., Spencer, F. C., and Bahnson, H. T.: Estimation of cardiac output soon after intracardiac surgery with cardiopulmonary bypass. Ann. Surg., *150*:613, 1959.

Boyd, A. D., Engelman, R. H., Isom, O. W., Reed, G. E., and Spencer, F. C.: Tricuspid annuloplasty. J. Thorac. Cardiovasc. Surg., *68*:344, 1974.

Carpentier, A., Branchini, B., Cour, J. C., Asfaou, E., Villani, M., Deloche, A., Relland, J., D'Allaines, C., Blondeau, P., Piwnica, A., Parenzan, L., and Brom, G.: Congenital malformations of the mitral valve in children. Pathology and surgical treatment. J. Thorac. Cardiovasc. Surg., *72*:854, 1976.

Carpentier, A., Chauvaud, S., Fabiani, J. N., Deloche, A., Relland, J., Lessana, A., D'Allaines, C., Blondeau, P., Piwnica, A., and Dubost, C.: Reconstructive surgery of mitral valve incompetence—Ten-year appraisal. J. Thorac. Cardiovasc. Surg., *79*:338, 1980.

Carpentier, A., Relland, J., Deloche, A., Fabiani, J. N., D'Allaines, C., Blondeau, P., Piwnica, A., Chauvaud, S., and Dubost, C.: Conservative management of the prolapsed mitral valve. Ann. Thorac. Surg., *26*:294, 1978.

Catinella, F. P., Cunningham, J. N., Jr., Srungaram, R. K., Knopp, E. A., Paone, G., Adams, P. X., and Spencer, F. C.: Comparison of myocardial protection offered by three different techniques of blood potassium cardioplegia administration. Arch. Surg., *116*:1509, 1981.

Chaux, A., Gray, R. J., Matloff, J. M., Feldman, H., and Sustaita, H.: An appreciation of the new St. Jude valvular prosthesis. J. Thorac. Cardiovasc. Surg., *81*:202, 1981.

Cheung, D., Flemma, R. J., Mullen, D. C., Lepley, D., Anderson, A. J., and Weirauch, E.: Ten-year follow-up in aortic valve replacement using the Bjork-Shiley prosthesis. Ann. Thorac. Surg., *32*:138, 1981.

Cobb, L. A., Werner, J. A., and Trobaugh, G. B.: Sudden cardiac death. I. A decade's experience with out-of-hospital resuscitation. Mod. Concepts Cardiovasc. Dis., *49*:31, 1980.

Cobbs, B. W., Jr., Hatcher, C. R., Jr., Craver, J. M., and Jones, E. L.: Transverse midventricular disruption after mitral valve replacement. Circulation. *56*(Suppl. 3):111, 1977.

Cobbs, B. W., Jr., Hatcher, C. R., Jr., Craver, J. M., Jones, E. L., and Sewell, C. W.: Transverse midventricular disruption after mitral valve replacement. Am. Heart J., *99*:33, 1980.

Culliford, A. T., Boyd, A. D., and Spencer, F. C.: A special rongeur for removal of extensively calcified mitral valves. Ann. Thorac. Surg., *28*:605, 1979.

Cunningham, J. N., Jr., Adams, P. X., Knopp, E., Baumann, G., Snively, S., Gross, R. I., Nathan, I., and Spencer, F. C.: Preservation of ATP, ultrastructure, and ventricular function following aortic cross-clamping and reperfusion—clinical use of blood potassium cardioplegia. J. Thorac. Cardiovasc. Surg., *78*:708, 1979.

Cutler, E. C., and Levine, S. A.: Cardiotomy and valvulotomy for mitral stenosis. Boston Med. Surg. J., *188*:1023, 1923.

Geha, A. S., Laks, H., Stansel, H. C., Jr., Cornhill, J. F., Kilman, J. W., Buckley, M. J., and Roberts, W. C.: Late failure of porcine valve heterografts in children. J. Thorac. Cardiovasc. Surg., *78*:351, 1979.

Gross, R. I., Cunningham, J. N., Jr., Snively, S. L., Catinella, F. P., Nathan, I. M., Adams, P. X., and Spencer, F. C.: Long-term results of open radical mitral commissurotomy: Ten-year follow-up study of 202 patients. Am. J. Cardiol., *47*:821, 1981.

Halseth, W. L., Elliott, D. P., Walker, E. L., and Smith, E. A.: Open mitral commissurotoy: A modern re-evaluation. J. Thorac. Cardiovasc. Surg., *80*:842, 1980.

Harken, D. E., Ellis, L. B., Ware, P. F., and Norman, L. R.: The surgical treatment of mitral stenosis. N. Engl. J. Med., *239*:801, 1948.

Housman, L. B., Bonchek, L., Lambert, L., Grunkemeier, G., and Starr, A.: Prognosis of patients after mitral commissurotomy. Actuarial analysis of late results in 100 patients. J. Thorac. Cardiovasc. Surg., *73*:742, 1977.

Isom, O. W., Williams, C. O., Falk, E. A., Glassman, E., and Spencer, F. C.: Long-term evaluation of cloth-covered metallic ball prostheses. J. Thorac. Cardiovasc. Surg., *64*:354, 1972.

Isom, O. W., Spencer, F. C., Glassman, E., Teiko, P., Boyd, A. D., Cunningham, J. N., Jr., and Reed, G. E.: Long-term results in 1375 patients undergoing valve replacement with the Starr-Edwards cloth-covered steel ball prosthesis. Ann. Surg., *186*:310, 1977.

Isom, O. W., Culliford, A. T., Colvin, S. B., Adams, P. X., Cunningham, J. N., Jr., Trehan, N., Leist, A., Cordone, R., Shemin, R. J., Glassman, E., and Spencer, F. C.: Porcine valves: Is there a difference? Presented at the American Heart Association, Miami, November 1980.

Jamieson, W. R. E., Janusz, M. T., Miyagishima, R. T., Munro, A. I., Tutassura, H., Gerein, A. N., Burr, L. H., and Allen, P.: Embolic complication of porcine heterograft cardiac valves. J. Thorac. Cardiovasc. Surg., *81*:626, 1981.

Karp, R. B., Cyrus, R. J., Blackstone, E. H., Kirklin, J. W., Kouchoukos, N. T., and Pacifico, A. D.: The Björk-Shiley valve. Intermediate-term follow-up. J. Thorac. Cardiovasc. Surg., *81*:602, 1981.

Kay, J. H., and Egerton, W. S.: The repair of mitral insufficiency associated with ruptured chordae tendineae. Ann Surg., *157*:351, 1963.

Kay, J. H., Zubiate, P., Mendez, M. A., Vanstrom, N., Yokoyama, T., and Gharavi, M. A.: Surgical treatment of mitral insufficiency secondary to coronary disease. J. Thorac. Cardiovasc. Surg, *79*:12, 1980.

Kronzon, I.: Personal communication, 1981.

Kutsche, L. M., Oyer, P., Shumway, N., and Baum, D.: An important complication of Hancock mitral valve replacement in children. Circulation, *60*(Suppl. 1):1, 1979.

Lillehei, C. W., Levy, M. J., and Bonnabeau, R. C.: Mitral valve replacement with preservation of papillary muscles and chordae tendineae. J. Thorac. Cardiovasc. Surg. *47*:532, 1964.

Logan, A., and Turner, R.: Surgical treatment of mitral stenosis with particular reference to the transventricular approach with a mechanical dilator. Lancet, *2*:874, 1959.

Magilligan, D. J., Jr., Lewis, J. W., Jr., Jara, F. M., Lee, M. W., Alam, M., Riddle, J. M., and Stein, P. D.: Spontaneous degeneration of porcine bioprosthetic valves. Ann. Thorac. Surg., *30*:259, 1980.

McGoon, D. C.: Repair of mitral insufficiency due to ruptured chordae tendineae. J. Thorac. Surg., *39*:357, 1960.

Miller, D. W., Jr., Johnson, D. D., and Ivey, T. D.: Does preservation of the posterior chordae tendineae enhance survival during mitral valve replacement? Ann. Thorac. Surg., *28*:22, 1979.

Mullin, M. J., Engelman, R. M., Isom, O. W., Boyd, A. D., Glassman, E., and Spencer, F. C.: Experience with open mitral commissurotomy in 100 consecutive patients. Surgery, *76*:974, 1974.

Nuñez, L., Gil-Aguado, M., Cerron, M., and Celemin, P.: Delayed rupture of the left ventricle after mitral valve replacement with bioprosthesis. Ann. Thorac. Surg., *27*:465, 1979.

Oyer, P. E., Miller, D. C., Stinson, E. B., Reitz, B. A., Moreno-Cabral, R. J., and Shumway, N. E.: Clinical durability of the Hancock porcine bioprosthetic valve. J. Thorac. Cardiovasc. Surg., *80*:824, 1980.

Pluth, J. R.: The case for the Starr-Edwards valve. Presented at the American College of Cardiology, San Francisco, March 1981.

Reed, G. E.: Repair of mitral regurgitation. Am. J. Cardiol. *31*:494, 1973.

Reed, G. E., Pooley, R. W., and Moggio, R. A.: Durability of measured mitral annuloplasty. Seventeen-year study. J. Thorac. Cardiovasc. Surg., *79*:321, 1980.

Roe, B. B., Edmunds, H., Jr., Fishman, N. H., and Hutchinson, J. C.: Open mitral commissurotomy. Ann. Thorac. Surg., *12*:483, 1971.

Selzer, A., and Cohen, K. E.: Natural history of mitral stenosis: A review. Circulation, *45*:878, 1972.

Spencer, F. C.: A plea for early, open mitral commissurotomy. Am. Heart J., *95*:668, 1978.

Srungaram, R. K., Cunningham, J. N., Jr., Catinella, F. P., Knopp, E. A., Nathan, I. M., and Spencer, F. C.: Blood versus crystalloid cardioplegia. Which is superior for prolonged aortic cross-clamping? Surg. Forum, *32*:288, 1981.

Starr, A., and Edwards, M. L.: Mitral replacement: Clinical experience with a ball valve prosthesis. Ann. Surg., *154*:726, 1961.

Tandon, A. P., Sengupta, S. M., Lukacs, L., and Ionescu, M. I.: Long-term clinical and hemodynamic evaluation of the Ionescu-Shiley pericardial xenograft and the Braunwald-Cutter and Björk-Shiley prosthesis in the mitral position. J. Thorac. Cardiovasc. Surg., *76*:763, 1978.

Teply, J. F., Grunkemeier, G. L., Sutherland, H. D., Lambert, L. E., Johnson, V. A., and Starr, A.: The ultimate prognosis after valve replacement: An assessment at twenty years. Ann. Thorac. Surg., *32*:111, 1981.

Treasure, R. L., Rainer, W. G., Strevey, T. E., et al.: Intraoperative left ventricular rupture associated with mitral valve replacement. Chest, *66*:511, 1974.

Tsuji, H. K., Shapiro, M., Redington, J. V., and Kay, J. H.: Congenital mitral stenosis. Report of two cases and a review of the literature. J. Thorac. Cardiovasc. Surg., *53*:850, 1967.

Williams, J. B., Karp, R. B., Kirklin, J. W., Kouchoukos, N. T., Pacifico, A. D., Zorn, G. L., Jr., Blackstone, E. H., Brown, R. N., Piantadosi, S., and Bradley, E. L.: Considerations in selection and management of patients undergoing valve replacement with glutaraldehyde-fixed porcine bioprostheses. Ann. Thorac. Surg., *30*:247, 1980.

Williams, W. G., Pollock, J. C., Geiss, D. M., Trusler, G. A., and Fowler, R. S.: Experience with aortic and mitral valve replacement in children. J. Thorac. Cardiovasc. Surg., *81*:326, 1981.

Zacharias, A., Grones, L. K., Cheanvechai, C., Loop, F. D., and Effler, D. B.: Rupture of the posterior wall of the left ventricle following mitral valve replacement. J. Thorac. Cardiovasc. Surg., *69*:259, 1975.

Zerbini, E. J.: Personal communication, 1981.

Chapter 47

Complications from Cardiac Prostheses

I INFECTION, THROMBOSIS, AND EMBOLI ASSOCIATED WITH INTRACARDIAC PROSTHESES

ELLIS L. JONES

STEPHEN W. SCHWARZMANN

WILLIAM A. CHECK

CHARLES R. HATCHER, JR.

INFECTION OF INTRACARDIAC DEVICES

As experience with infectious complications of prosthetic valve surgery has accumulated, it has become increasingly evident that a useful purpose is served by classifying infective prosthetic valve endocarditis (PVE) according to the time infection occurs after surgical insertion of the valve. Infection occurring within the first 60 days after surgery is generally due to organisms acquired during or shortly after surgery, whereas infection occurring 2 months or longer after surgery shares a pathogenesis with endocarditis occurring on native heart valves. This classification also seems to relate to the relative morbidity and mortality of the infection and to the organism(s) causing the infection. Reports of the incidence of early prosthetic valve endocarditis range between 0 and 7 per cent, with an average of 1 per cent, and the mortality rate ranges between 56 and 88 per cent, with an average of 72 per cent. The incidence of late PVE obviously relates to the duration of follow-up of the patient. At 6 months, the incidence of PVE averages 1.2 per cent, but in at least one study (Clarkson and Barratt-Boyes, 1970), this increased to 2.2 per cent by 5 years after surgery. The mortality rate from late PVE has been reported to be between 31 and 66 per cent, with an average of 45 per cent. In both the early and late groups, mortality seems to be lowest with streptococcal infection and highest in nonstreptococcal infections (staphylococci, gram-negative bacteria, and fungi). The fact that streptococcal infection occurs most commonly in late PVE may explain in part the lower mortality from late PVE. Obviously, other factors, such as a recent postoperative state with incomplete healing of the surgical field and tissue trauma, also prejudice the outcome of early PVE.

Early Prosthetic Valve Endocarditis

It is generally thought that the organisms responsible for early PVE are acquired either during surgery or in the early postoperative period. In a study designed to identify potential sources of contamination (Kluge *et al.*, 1974), it was found that the air in the operating room contained several organisms, most commonly staphylococci and diphtheroids, and that the greatest microbial density occurred immediately above the operative field. Cultures taken from the operative site, i.e., the repaired area of myocardium or the prosthesis, were more often positive than not, especially when tested just before closure. Again, diphtheroids and staphylococci were the most commonly isolated organisms. Donor blood bags and the pump reservoir following bypass were other less common sources of bacterial contamination, the former being particularly likely to harbor gram-negative rods and yeasts as well as more common skin contaminants. In the postoperative period, opportunities for infection of the freshly operated tissues include transient bacteremia complicating wound infections, pneumonia, emergency reoperation, urinary tract infections, and especially contaminated intravascular catheters. In one study, 50 per cent of intravascular catheter tips yielded a variety of gram-positive and gram-negative organisms and fungi when routinely cultured immediately after removal. These infected catheters can then become a source of bacteremia, with potential secondary seeding of microorganisms on the newly inserted prosthetic heart valve. Measures such as removal of intravascular lines at the earliest possible time and frequent flushing of the lines seem to reduce the incidence of contamination, whereas manipulation without flushing seems to increase the likelihood of contamination.

The placement of a prosthetic valve in the setting of active native heart valve endocarditis could be considered to predispose the patient to subsequent early infection of the implanted prosthetic valve. Surprisingly, however, this complication has not been a major factor, occurring at a rate of approximately 4 per cent, although the operative mortality rate when active infection is present is reported to be 20 to 30 per cent. There appears to be no major difference in the risk of PVE between the use of a mechanical valve or heterograft tissue valve in this situation.

Late Prosthetic Valve Endocarditis

Late PVE may be acquired intraoperatively or postoperatively and simply reflect a long incubation period, perhaps induced by the use of prophylactic antibiotics. In this situation, prophylactic antibiotics may have served only to suppress growth of bacteria introduced intraoperatively or perioperatively, thereby delaying the clinical manifestations of the infection. This is supported by data in one study that revealed a high incidence of valve infection due to staphylococci, diphtheroids, and gram-negative organ-

isms in the first 18 months after surgery, following which streptococci accounted for 37 per cent of all infections. This change in microbiologic etiology and the less acute clinical course in patients with delayed PVE suggest that the sources of the infection are much the same as in native heart valve infection. These sources would include transient bacteremias from genitourinary tract surgery, dental manipulation or extraction, primary skin infection, or upper respiratory tract infections (Karchmer et al., 1978). It follows that patients who have prosthetic heart valves require very aggressive antibiotic prophylaxis when submitted to procedures known to predispose to endocarditis.

Epidemiology and Pathology

The results of a study involving 51 patients who developed PVE out of a group of 2184 patients who received either heterograft tissue or mechanical heart valves pointed out several other features that further characterize the epidemiology of this disease (Rossiter et al., 1978). As mentioned previously, there appeared to be no major difference in the risk of developing PVE between the use of heterograft tissue valves and mechanical valves. In contrast to another study in which no early PVE was seen on heterograft tissue valves in the aortic position (Magilligan et al., 1977), this study of Rossiter and associates showed a significantly higher incidence of early PVE in heterograft tissue valves when compared with mechanical valves

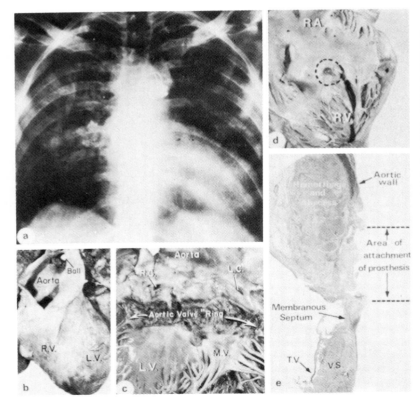

Figure 47–1. *Staphylococcus epidermidis* prosthetic aortic valve endocarditis in a 48-year-old man. He had been well for 11 months following insertion of the Starr-Edwards prosthesis when, 1 month before death and 6 weeks after dental extraction, shaking chills appeared and blood cultures were positive for *Staphylococcus epidermididis*. Despite intensive antibiotic therapy, signs of aortic regurgitation appeared, and minutes before death he complained of "feeling funny." *a*, Chest roentgenogram immediately post mortem revealed that the prosthesis had dislodged and migrated to the aortic arch. *b*, Anterior view of the heart and opened ascending aorta. The detached prosthesis ball is visible, lodged in the transverse aorta. (L.V. = left ventricle; R.V. = right ventricle.) *c*, Opened aorta, aortic valve "ring," and left ventricle showing a totally necrotic aortic anulus. (M.V. = anterior mitral leaflet; R.C. = ostium of right coronary artery; L.C. = ostium of left coronary artery.) *d*, Opened right atrium (R.A.), tricuspid valve, and right ventricle (R.V.) showing a ring abscess (circle) that had extended from the aortic prosthetic anulus. *e*, Photomicrograph through the aortic valve "ring" showing a large ring abscess and the necrotic aortic anulus material, which extended through the membranous ventricular septum into the right atrium. (Hematoxylin and eosin stain; original magnification × 2.) (T.V. = tricuspid valve leaflet; V.S. = ventricular septum.) (From Arnett, E. N., and Roberts, W. C.: Active infective endocarditis: A clinicopathologic analysis of 137 necropsy patients. Curr. Probl. Cardiol., *1*:2, 1976.)

in the aortic position. It was, however, pointed out that concomitant aortocoronary bypass grafting was performed considerably more commonly in the tissue valve group, resulting in increased operative time and the added risk of contamination by the saphenous vein graft. On the other hand, once infection was established, heterograft tissue valves appeared to be more easily sterilized. This impression was supported by the pathologic findings on recovered specimens that infection of heterograft valves was often limited to the valve leaflets, whereas ring infection was nearly always present in the case of mechanical valves. Obviously, a ring abscess, whether associated with a heterograft valve or a mechanical valve, renders antibiotic sterilization virtually impossible. Another highly statistically significant finding that is universally reported is the much greater risk of developing PVE at the aortic site as opposed to the mitral site. This is opposite to the situation in native valve endocarditis.

The pathologic focus of PVE is most often found at the valve seat. Abscess formation and destruction of tissue are the hallmarks and frequently involve the entire circumference of the valve seat. With prosthetic aortic valves, the process may progress to dehiscence, with resulting paravalvular leaks and formation of mycotic aneurysms bordering the prosthetic valve seat (Fig. 47–1). Extension of the ring infection to adjacent cardiac structures and the aorta is common and may produce fistula and disturbances of atrioventricular conduction (Fig. 47–2). Clinically, these changes may be translated into new regurgitant murmurs and the appearance of varying degrees of heart block. The appearance of left bundle branch block does not seem to indicate inflammatory invasion of the conduction system as reliably as does the presence of AV block.

In contrast to the situation in aortic prosthetic valve endocarditis, infection of a mitral prosthesis more commonly results in obstruction than regurgitation. This may occur as a result of immobilization of the disc or ball, in which case regurgitation may also occur, or by fusion of the growths over the atrial surface of the valve, which causes obstruction of the inflow site (Fig. 47–3). The development of obstruction by valve immobilization can often be recognized by changes in valve sounds and fluoroscopic evaluation of ball motion. Obstruction occurring solely from infectious growth interfering with transmitral flow without interference of valve motion may appear simply as pulmonary congestion associated with evidence of pulmonary venous hypertension. In this situation, obstruction can be confirmed by measurement of a significant transmural gradient. Case reports of patients with rapidly fatal disease due to significant obstruction of left ventricular flow with minimal evidence of valvular dysfunction have been reported, and these symptoms must always be acted on rapidly in the situation of possible prosthetic mitral valve endocarditis (McAllister *et al.*, 1974). In addition to producing anular infection and abscess formation with its resulting complications, endocarditis involving heterograft valves may be limited to the valve cusps (Fig.

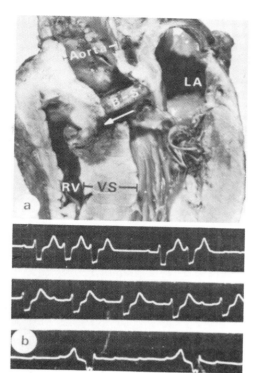

Figure 47–2. *Staphylococcus epidermidis* prosthetic aortic valve endocarditis in a 51-year-old man. His stenotic bicuspid aortic valve had been replaced with a Bjork-Shiley prosthesis 83 days before death. Fever was present in the early postoperative period, and shortly before death, complete heart block and signs of congestive heart failure appeared. *a*, Longitudinal section of the heart with the anterior portion removed. The Bjork-Shiley (B-S) prosthesis is partially detached, and the ring abscess (arrow) has burrowed through the ventricular septum (VS) into the right ventricle (RV). (LA = left atrium.) (From Arnett, E. N., and Roberts, W. C.: Active infective endocarditis: A clinicopathologic analysis of 137 necropsy patients. Curr. Prob. Cardiol., *1*:2, 1976.)

47–4). This results in either total destruction of the cusp(s) or vegetations that stiffen and obstruct the valve, making its replacement mandatory even if the infection has been eradicated.

Diagnosis and Microbiology

The diagnosis of PVE is generally accepted (1) if there are at least two positive blood cultures for the same organism in a patient with a compatible clinical syndrome and no other potential source for the bacteremia, or (2) if histopathologic evidence of endocarditis is found in a surgical or autopsy specimen. A compatible clinical syndrome may include fever, developed splenomegaly, or evidence of peripheral emboli. In most series, fever is the most common clinical finding and is reported in 95 per cent of patients with early and late PVE. When it occurs, a new regurgitant murmur and septic shock are usually seen in early PVE, whereas manifestations of peripheral emboli and splenomegaly are more commonly seen in late PVE.

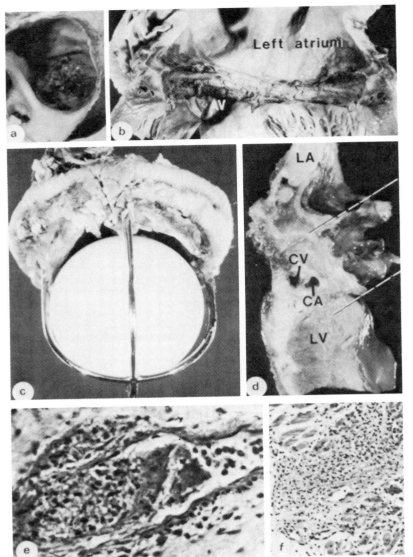

Figure 47–3. *Staphylococcus aureus* prosthetic mitral valve endocarditis in a 47-year-old man who had the onset of symptoms of infective endocarditis 4 months after valve replacement. He had done well during the first 3 months following operation but developed symptoms of infection following grafting of a cutaneous ulcer. Signs of prosthetic dysfunction were never detected clinically. *a,* Prosthetic mitral orifice obstructed by vegetative material, as viewed from the left atrium. *b,* Opened left atrium, mitral anulus, and left ventricle after removal of the mitral prosthesis. The entire anulus is necrotic. (AV = aortic valve.) *c,* Mitral prosthesis showing infected thrombus at its base. *d,* Longitudinal section through left atrium (LA), mitral anulus, and left ventricle (LV). The former site of attachment of the prosthesis is designated by the dashed lines. The infective process burrowed through the wall of the heart and caused pericarditis. (CA = coronary artery; CV = coronary vein in the right atrioventricular sulcus.) (From Arnett, E. N., and Roberts, W. C.: Active infective endocarditis: A clinicopathologic analysis of 137 necropsy patients. Curr. Prob. Cardiol., *1*:2, 1976.)

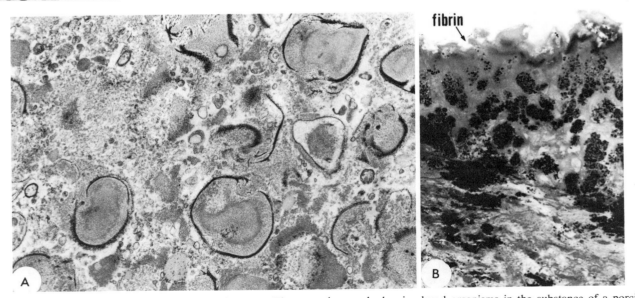

Figure 47–4. Infection of porcine bioprostheses. *a,* Electron micrograph showing lysed organisms in the substance of a porcine valve removed from a patient who developed signs of prosthetic stenosis and regurgitation and who had blood cultures positive for *Staphylococcus* (× 30,000). *b,* Clusters of gram-positive organisms in a fibrin meshwork on the surface of the valve leaflet shown in *a,* with invasion of the underlying valve tissue (toluidine blue stain, × 600). (Courtesy of Victor J. Ferrans, M.D., Ph.D.)

This difference probably relates to the duration of endocarditis before the diagnosis is made.

The differential diagnosis of early PVE may be especially difficult in the early postoperative period when complications of sternal wound infection, pneumonia, septic phlebitis, or urinary tract infections have occurred. It may be difficult to discern whether positive blood cultures at this time are indicative of infection on the prosthetic heart valve. It has been reported that PVE was not usually the source of a sustained bacteremia due to gram-negative rods occurring less than 25 days after surgery with obvious potential sites of origin in the absence of any changes in heart murmurs (Sande *et al.,* 1972). However, multiple positive blood cultures involving gram-positive organisms occurring after the twenty-fifth postoperative day were likely to originate from the heart, especially if accompanied by new or changing heart murmurs. Unfortunately, exceptions to this clinical dictum exist, particularly as it relates to bacteremia with gram-negative rods in the early postoperative setting. Thus, one cannot confidently dismiss the diagnosis of PVE in this situation. The initiation of treatment for PVE is therefore often employed in an effort to avoid its dismal prognosis.

The less acute course of late PVE may often be diagnosed as influenza or some other nonspecific cause of fever and weakness. In any event, the diagnosis must first be considered and then usually confirmed by blood culture. In one study, at least one of five blood samples was positive in 91 per cent of patients, the very first culture being positive in 87 per cent, and all blood cultures were positive in 73 per cent of patients (Masur and Johnson, 1980). Antibiotic administration within a 2-week period before blood cultures are obtained reduces positive cultures only modestly and is therefore still very useful. In the case of fungal PVE, blood cultures are much less reliable, and diagnosis is sometimes made by examination of peripheral emboli or histologic examination of the resected valve. When confronted with a negative blood culture in a patient with strong clinical features of PVE, the physician should either initiate empiric antibiotic therapy or, preferably, perform cardiac exploration. This procedure will both confirm the diagnosis and allow replacement of the infected valve.

Other diagnostic aids have included assessment of prosthetic valve stability by cinefluoroscopy and angiography. The former test generally requires a previous study for comparison, although a single study showing valve rocking greater than 7 to 10 degrees is considered abnormal. Angiography may also be employed to assess secure attachment of the valve to the valve seat or to identify the presence of a myocardial abscess or fistula.

The presence of growths on both native and prosthetic heart valves has been demonstrated by two-dimensional echocardiography. As opposed to M-mode echocardiography, which provides a relatively poor spatial impression of vegetations, the two-dimensional technique shows size, shape, attachment, and

TABLE 47–1. MICROBIOLOGY OF PROSTHETIC VALVE ENDOCARDITIS

ORGANISM	INCIDENCE IN EARLY ENDOCARDITIS (%)	INCIDENCE IN LATE ENDOCARDITIS (%)
Staphylococcus epidermidis	27.2	23.9
Staphylococcus aureus	18.6	12.7
Streptococci	6.2	38.5
Diphtheroids	8	4
Gram-negative (aerobic) organisms	21.5	12.8
Other bacteria	7.2	3.4
Fungi	11.3	4.7

motion of vegetations. Unfortunately, this diagnostic aid is most likely to be helpful in a more advanced infection, at which point salvageability is at its lowest.

The microbiology of prosthetic valve endocarditis is reasonably consistent among several series of patients reported in the literature. Approximate proportions of the various organisms in early and late PVE are listed in Table 47–1. Staphylococcal species make up the greatest proportion of cases in early PVE, and streptococcal species, including *Streptococcus viridans,* Enterococcus, *S. pneumoniae,* and others make up the largest group in late PVE. The fungal agents are most commonly Candida followed by Aspergillus. These appear much more frequently in early PVE. As can be seen, organisms that make up normal skin flora and are so commonly considered nonpathogens (i.e., *Staphylococcus epidermidis* and diphtheroids) are very prominent in both early and late PVE, and attempts at antibiotic prophylaxis should be made for these organisms in addition to those for *Staphylococcus aureus.* No correlation between specific microorganisms and the type of prosthetic valve involved has been demonstrated.

Diphtheroids may pose a particularly difficult problem, both in their isolation from blood specimens and in establishing *in vitro* sensitivity testing. These organisms, which belong to the genus Corynebacterium and form part of the normal skin flora, are generally unclassified, except for *C. diphtheriae.* They often grow very slowly and require 3 to 14 days of incubation before recognition can be made. Growth is best accomplished in brain-heart infusion (BHI) broth supplemented by 5 per cent rabbit serum. Because of their very slow growth, usual methods of antibiotic sensitivity testing are often ineffective, and the use of rabbit serum–supplemented BHI broth is useful for determination of broth dilution minimal inhibitory concentrations (MICs). By and large, diphtheroids are susceptible to gentamicin, amikacin, streptomycin, erythromycin, tetracycline, and vancomycin. A newly identified species of Corynebacterium, designated by the Special Bacteriology Section of the Centers for Disease Control as group JK, has recently been recognized as an important cause of serious and fatal diphtheroid infection in several clinical settings, including PVE. This organism is generally more antibiotic-resistant than other diphtheroid species, and only vancomycin has been shown to have reliable activity against it (Murray *et al.*, 1980).

Management

The therapeutic options available in the treatment of PVE include antibiotic therapy with or without replacement of the infected prosthetic valve. The decision as to which approach should be taken in a given situation can be made by reviewing factors associated with mortality. Those elements that significantly relate to increased mortality include early onset, nonstreptococcal etiology, paravalvular leak, heart failure, presence of multiple systemic emboli, and relapse of bacteremia after medical therapy. Generally, then, medical therapy alone is reserved for patients who have late onset of PVE due to a streptococcal organism and in whom there is no evidence of a paravalvular leak, congestive heart failure, or multiple systemic emboli. Under these circumstances, the mortality rate is approximately 35 per cent. When medical therapy alone is applied to patients in other categories, the mortality rate increases markedly: In medically treated early-onset PVE, the mortality rate is 78 per cent. When PVE, either early or late, is complicated by a paravalvular leak or congestive heart failure, the mortality rate is 80 to 100 per cent.

The contrast of this dismal prognosis with the success that has been enjoyed in the treatment of native valve bacterial and fungal endocarditis by means of prompt valve replacement suggested application of this modality to these high-risk PVE patients. A comparison of the outcome of valve replacement plus antibiotic therapy versus antibiotic therapy alone for PVE at three medical centers demonstrated statistically significant benefit in some patient categories. The overall mortality rates in antibiotic-treated groups and valve replacement groups were 60 per cent and 23 per cent, respectively. When examined relative to early or late onset PVE, the results were somewhat different. In early PVE, the mortality rate in the group receiving antibiotic therapy only was 80 per cent, compared with 60 per cent in the group receiving antibiotic therapy plus valve replacement. In late PVE, the mortality rates were 42 per cent and 12 per cent, respectively. Valve replacement in addition to antibiotic therapy is recommended for all patients who have early PVE and in those with late PVE who have any of the following conditions: infection by a non-streptococcal organism, paravalvular leak, congestive heart failure, systemic emboli, or recurrence of medically treated infection. In addition to providing a better operative risk, early surgical intervention should achieve several desirable objectives, including the prevention of extension of infection into vital or inaccessible myocardial tissue and reduction of the risk of systemic embolism and congestive heart failure (Saffle *et al.*, 1977). The replacement of an infected prosthetic valve, however, may entail significant tech-

nical difficulties and in some situations may be impossible. The occurrence of a grossly necrotic anulus at the time of reoperation poses major difficulties in the placement of a new valve, both in seating the prosthesis and in burrowing the sewing ring of the prosthesis into the necrotic anulus (Fig. 47–5). Despite these obstacles, valve replacement in this setting does appear to be helpful in some cases.

The initial choice of an antibiotic regimen depends on identification of the organism and results of *in vitro* susceptibility tests modified by serum bactericidal assays. Bactericidal antibiotics are generally required because of barriers to host defense mechanisms presented by the prosthesis and infectious growth. Serum bactericidal levels of 1:8 or greater are generally associated with a favorable outcome, although not in the setting of high-risk PVE.

Antibiotics are preferably administered by the intravenous route on an intermittent schedule. Bactericidal levels should be obtained 2 to 3 days after antibiotics are begun, and blood samples should be taken at a time estimated to represent the peak antibiotic blood level, i.e., 30 to 60 minutes after administration. The selection and dose of antibiotic according to organism are listed in Table 47–2. Disc sensitivity testing for *Staphylococcus epidermidis* is frequently unreliable when compared with more stringent methods of susceptibility testing, and serum bactericidal assays should always be done to ensure efficacy. Testing with inocula of 10^5 to 10^8 organisms in a broth assay has been recommended. Once desired bactericidal antibiotic levels are achieved, they should be maintained for 6 to 8 weeks. Blood cultures should be obtained daily for the first few days to demonstrate efficacy and then once weekly for the duration of antibiotic therapy and once weekly for a month after antibiotics have been discontinued to confirm microbiologic cure. If relapse of infection occurs, replacement of the valve and another course of bactericidal antibiotics should be instituted.

THROMBOEMBOLISM OF PROSTHETIC CARDIAC VALVES

When successful replacement of diseased aortic and mitral heart valves began in the early 1960s, it became clear that a substantial number of recipients suffered complications from emboli that formed on the valve surfaces. Occasionally, the valve surfaces themselves became occluded by slowly developing thrombi. These problems seemed to be due to both the inherent thrombogenicity of the materials used and abnormalities in blood flow through the valves due to the presence of a centrally occluding ball. In the last two decades, the problem of thromboembolic complications has been approached by altering materials used, changing valve design, and using systemic anticoagulation. The most recent valves, made from porcine xenografts or bovine pericardium, offer to many patients improved cardiac function with a

Figure 47–5. *Staphylococcus epidermidis* endocarditis originally involving a Bjork-Shiley aortic valve prosthesis, which was excised and replaced with a Magovern prosthesis 28 days before death in a 69-year-old man. Fever and signs of aortic regurgitation appeared 7 months following aortic valve replacement with the Bjork-Shiley prosthesis. After replacement with the Magovern prosthesis, a murmur of aortic regurgitation reappeared. At necropsy, the sewing ring of the aortic wall, probably producing prosthetic aortic stenosis. *a*, Longitudinal section of the heart through the aortic anulus with the Magovern prosthesis in place, and *b*, after removal of the prosthesis. The frame of the prosthesis has

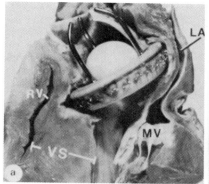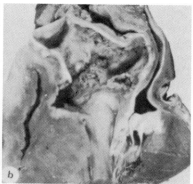

burrowed deeply into the necrotic anulus. (VS = ventricular septum; RV = right ventricular cavity; MV = mitral valve; LA = left atrium.) (From Arnett, E. N., and Roberts, W. C.: Active infective endocarditis: A clinicopathologic analysis of 137 necropsy patients. Curr. Prob. Cardiol., *1*:2, 1976.)

TABLE 47–2. RECOMMENDED ANTIBIOTIC THERAPY FOR PROSTHETIC VALVE ENDOCARDITIS IN AVERAGE-SIZED ADULTS WITH NORMAL RENAL FUNCTION

ORGANISM	ANTIBIOTIC	TOTAL DAILY DOSE	FREQUENCY
Streptococci	Penicillin G +	20 million units	q 4 h IV
	Gentamicin or	3–5 mg./kg.	q 8 h IV
	Vancomycin +	2 gm./day	q 6 h IV
	Gentamicin	3–5 mg./kg.	q 8 h IV
Staphylococcus aureus *Staphylococcus epidermidis*	± Nafcillin Rifampin†	12 gm. 120 mg.	q 4 h IV q 12 h PO
Methicillin-resistant staphylococci	± Vancomycin Rifampin†	2 gm./day 1200 mg.	q 6 h IV q 12 h PO
Diphtheroids penicillin-sensitive	Penicillin G +	20 million units	q 4 h IV
	Gentamicin	3–5 mg./kg.	q 8 h IV
JK strain—penicillin-resistant (strain)	Vancomycin	2 gm.	q 6 h IV
Aerobic gram-negative bacilli*	Carbenicillin or	30 gm.	q 4 h IV
	Ticarcillin or	18 gm.	q 4 h IV
	Cefamandole +	8–12 gm.	q 4–6 h IV
	Gentamicin	3–5 mg./kg.	q 8 h IV
Fungal: Candida	Amphotericin B +	0.5–1.0 mg./kg.	qd IV
	5-Fluorocytosine	150 mg./kg.	q 6 h PO
Aspergillus	Amphotericin B	0.5–1.0 mg./kg.	qd IV
Etiologic agent unknown	Vancomycin +	1 gm./day	q 6 h IV
	Gentamicin +	3–5 mg./kg.	q 8 h IV
	Penicillin G	20 million units	q 4 h IV

*Aerobic gram-negative bacilli will show variable antibiotic sensitivity, and selection must be made appropriately.

†May be added if serum bactericidal levels are inadequate on a single drug. Gentamicin can also be tested for presence of synergy when added to the beta-lactam antibiotic if the above is not effective.

greatly reduced clotting risk and freedom from anticoagulant drugs. Not all surgeons, however, are willing to use them in all patients. Several good reviews of the issues involved are available (Bonchek, 1981; Lefrak and Starr, 1979; Murphy and Kloster, 1979).

Incidence of Thromboembolic Complications with Mechanical Prosthetic Valves

The first type of valve used, the caged ball valve, proved highly thrombogenic. The initiation of long-term systemic anticoagulation with warfarin or its derivatives greatly reduced the incidence of these complications. It has been estimated that only 20 per cent of patients receiving the early Starr-Edwards caged ball valves would be free of emboli at 10 years without anticoagulation. Introduction of anticoagulant use reduced the rate of these complications to approximately 5 per cent in the aortic position and 7 per cent in the mitral position per year. With recent changes in the selection of patients, these rates may be even lower.

In 1967, the addition of a cloth covering over the cage struts, with inclusion of metal tracks for the ball to move in, apparently reduced the thrombogenicity of this type of valve. The 10-year embolus-free survival rate without anticoagulants was raised to about 50 per cent. With anticoagulants thromboembolic incidents occurred in about 2 per cent of replaced aortic valves per year and in 3 to 5 per cent of mitral valves per year. Unfortunately, the cloth covering tends to wear, and the metal ball moving in a metal track creates a noise that is quite audible to most patients (Fig. 47–6).

The design of the tilting disc valves, such as the Bjork-Shiley valve (introduced in 1969) and the Lillehei-Kaster valve, was supposed to allow more central blood flow than the caged ball design. It was hoped that reduced turbulence would decrease fibrin and thrombin deposition around the valve and reduce thromboembolic complications. Unfortunately, flow through tilting disc valves has been found to be less than ideal, with such phenomena as eddy currents around the minor orifice creating the potential for platelet and thrombin accumulation. As a result, these valves appear to be no less thrombogenic than the caged ball valves, and patients receiving them still require lifelong anticoagulation. In one comparative study (Dale et al., 1980), deaths from thromboembolism occurred at a rate of 1.5 to 2 per cent over a 5-year period with either the caged ball or tilting disc valves in the presence of continuous anticoagulation. With tilting disc valves, nonfatal thromboembolic complications occur in various series at about 1 to 3 per cent in the aortic position and 3 to 5 per cent per year in the mitral position (Borst et al., 1979), a rate similar to that found with caged ball prostheses. An additional problem with tilting disc valves is the occurrence of "sudden" thrombosis, the formation of a

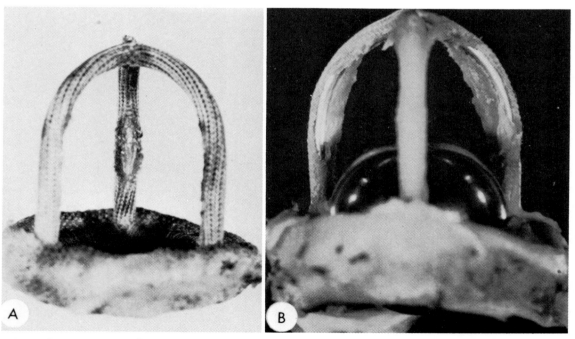

Figure 47–6. Starr-Edwards aortic prostheses from two patients; each shows cloth wear. *a*, Model 2300, size 8A prosthesis removed at operation 16 months after insertion. Focal wearing of the cloth was observed on the inner aspects of each of the three struts (the inner portion of only one strut is seen here). The cloth of the struts is nearly free of tissue ingrowth. *b*, Severe through-and-through wearing of the cloth exposing the metallic struts in this size 10A, Model 2310 prosthesis implanted for 25 months in a 47-year-old man who died suddenly and unexpectedly shortly after the onset of chest pain. Fibrin-platelet thrombus also is present on the struts. (From Winter, T. Q., Reis, R. L., Glancy, D. L., Roberts, W. C., Epstein, S. W., and Morrow, A. G.: Current status of the Starr-Edwards cloth-covered prosthetic cardiac valves. Circulation, *45, 46*(Suppl. 1): 14, 1972.)

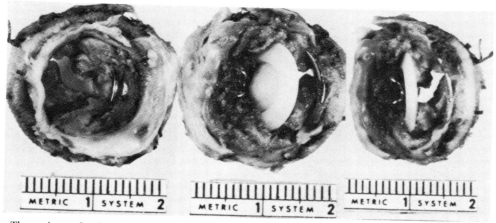

Figure 47–7. Three views of a thrombosed (noninfected) Bjork-Shiley aortic valve prosthesis. This prosthesis had been in place for 270 days, and the patient had not been receiving warfarin sodium. *Left,* View from ventricular side. *Center,* View from aortic side showing immobilization of the Delrin disc. *Right,* View from aortic side showing orifice in its maximal dimension. Severe prosthetic obstruction was present. (From Roberts, W. C., and Hammer, W. J.: Cardiac pathology after valve replacement with a tilting disc prosthesis [Bjork-Shiley type]. Am. J. Cardiol., *37:*1024, 1976.)

thrombus on the valve itself (Fig. 47–7). This causes rapid loss of function and, in the absence of prompt reoperation, can result in very high mortality. Bjork and Henze (1977) have reported that sudden thrombosis in the absence of anticoagulation strikes at the rate of about 3 per cent per year. Even with anticoagulation, up to 1 per cent of patients with a tilting disc valve in the mitral position may experience this complication.

In 1977, the St. Jude bileaflet valve was introduced. This device is designed to produce even more central flow. Early reports cited a very low incidence of thromboembolism, but the rate appears to be rising with an increase in the number of valves inserted and the time of observation (Cohn, 1981). Two cases of valve thrombus have been reported. Evaluation of this device will have to await further results.

Tissue Valves

Although anticoagulation was largely successful in reducing thromboembolic complications with mechanical prosthetic valves, the drugs themselves caused problems. "Serious" or "major" bleeding (requiring transfusion or hospitalization) occurs at the rate of 1 to 3 per cent each year with anticoagulation medication. To avoid this problem, several investigators attempted to use valves made of cardiac tissue.

One approach was to use human cadaver valves, rendered sterile with antibiotics and quick-frozen. Although these valves appear to be very effective in trained hands, they are difficult to obtain, and appropriate sizes are not always available.

In 1969, Carpentier and associates reported what has been a much more practical and effective prosthetic tissue valve, an aortic valve taken from a pig heart, treated with glutaraldehyde to cross-link collagen fibers, and mounted on a support. Both the Carpentier-Edwards and the Hancock porcine xeno-

graft have been widely used, and this type of valve prosthesis is now the first choice of many surgeons in most patients. The device has very low thrombogenicity, perhaps because of its nearly central flow and the reduced use of "unnatural" materials. Even without anticoagulation, porcine xenografts have a thromboembolic rate of only 1 to 3 per cent per year in the aortic position and 2 to 4 per cent per year in the mitral position (Jamieson *et al.,* 1981). In one recent publication (Cohn *et al.,* 1981), the actuarial embolus-free survival rate at 8 years with Hancock valves was 97 per cent for patients with aortic valve replacement, 82 per cent for those with prosthetic mitral valves, and 72 per cent when multiple valve replacement was done. Most patients were not taking anticoagulant medication.

Use of porcine heterograft tissue valves greatly reduces, but does not completely eliminate, the need for anticoagulants. Because of a high incidence of thrombi early after surgery, anticoagulant drugs have been recommended for the first 6 to 8 weeks after insertion of the valve in the mitral position.

In addition, experience has demonstrated that certain cardiac conditions predispose to clotting problems. These include atrial fibrillation, enlarged left atrium, and low output syndrome (Fig. 47–8). (In these situations, it may well be the disease itself, rather than the prosthetic valve, that induces the thromboembolic incidents.) For instance, in the series reported by Cohn and colleagues (1981) the 8-year embolus-free survival rate was approximately 95 per cent for patients in sinus rhythm, but only 70 per cent for those in atrial fibrillation. Therefore, recipients having any of these three conditons (which frequently occur together) are put on long-term systemic anticoagulation. One additional indication for anticoagulation cited by some authors is a history of emboli or the finding of thrombus during surgery. Overall, Cohn and colleagues (1981) reported that 27 per cent of their tissue valve recipients were receiving anticoagulation for one or more of these indications.

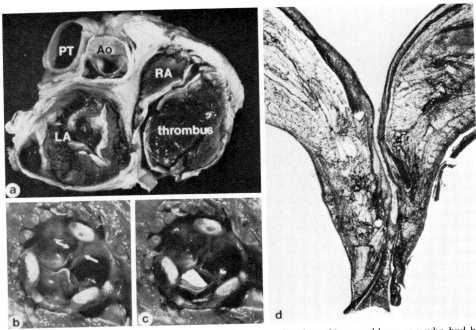

Figure 47–8. Stenosis of porcine bioprosthesis implanted 32 days earlier in a 61-year-old woman who had had rheumatic mitral stenosis and tricuspid regurgitation. The patient sustained an air embolus intraoperatively and remained comatose with severe low cardiac output after operation. *a,* At necropsy, both the right atrium (RA) and the left atrium (LA) were filled with organizing thrombi. (Ao = aortic root; PT = pulmonary trunk. *b,* View of the 31-mm. porcine bioprosthesis in the tricuspid position from the ventricular aspect as seen in systole. Thrombus is present in two of the three cusp sinuses, and there is fusion of the commissure between these leaflets (arrows). *c,* Bioprosthesis in simulated ventricular diastole. The fusion of two leaflets permits opening of only the one mobile leaflet, with resulting valve stenosis. *d,* Section through fused leaflets at level of arrows in *b,* showing adherence of the leaflets by fibrin thrombus. (Phosphotungstic acid–hematoxylin stain, × 16, reduced by 24 per cent.) (From Spray, T. L., and Roberts, W. C.: Structural changes in porcine xenografts used as substitute cardiac valves. Am. J. Cardiol., *40*:319, 1977.)

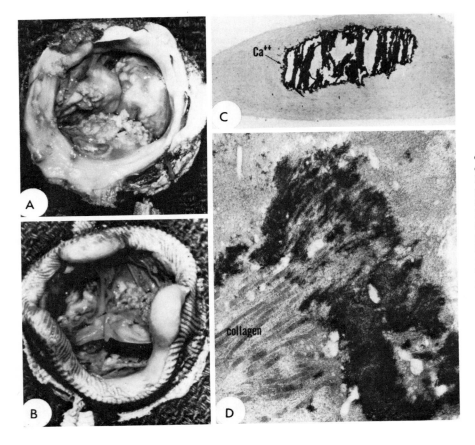

Figure 47–9. Calcification of porcine bioprostheses. *a* and *b,* Nodular calcific deposits in the leaflets of a mitral Hancock porcine valve implanted for 4 years in a 12-year-old male. Reoperation was required for prosthetic stenosis. *c,* Histologic section of one leaflet from a similar valve showing nodular calcific deposits (Ca++) in the substance of the valve leaflet. (VonKossa stain. × 40.) *d,* Electron micrograph showing calcium deposition associated with the collagen bundles in the valve leaflet (× 47,000).

Since many recipients of porcine xenograft tissue valves do not need to take anticoagulants, these valves would seen to be ideal for those patients who will have the grafts the longest—children and young adults. Unfortunately, increasing experience with bioprostheses in this population has shown that the failure rate with porcine tissue valves is much higher in younger persons. In one series of children receiving Hancock valves for reconstruction of the right ventricular outflow tract, it was projected that the failure rate would be 30 per cent at 6 years (Bissett et al., 1981). In another group of patients between the ages of 1 and 20 years, eight of the 25 Hancock valve recipients who survived for more than 20 months after surgery required valve replacement (Sanders et al., 1980). Another group calculated a failure rate of almost 10 per cent per year in a group of patients less than 15 years of age having aortic or mitral valve replacement with porcine tissue valves (Oyer et al., 1980). Since removed xenograft valves have been found to be heavily calcified and a high rate of xenograft failure is also seen in persons on renal dialysis, it has been postulated that failure may be closely related to hyperactive calcium metabolism

(Fig. 47–9). The increased failure rate appears to extend to age 30, and Magilligan and colleagues (1980) have even claimed an increased risk in patients as old as 35 years.

In older persons, the Hancock xenograft valve has a very low rate of primary failure, about 1 per cent per year. Studies of tissue valves recovered at autopsy suggest the possibility of increased failure over the longer term (Ferrans et al., 1978) (Figs. 47–10 and 47–11), and a few authors have found a noticeable acceleration of the failure rate between 5 and 6 years after insertion (Lakier et al., 1980; Casarotto et al., 1979; Oyer et al., 1980), but more extensive observation will be necessary to settle this question.

The Ionescu-Shiley xenograft tissue valve, composed of bovine pericardial tissue fixed with glutaraldehyde and mounted on a metal support, has been less widely used. In one large series, Ott and colleagues (1980) at the Texas Heart Institute became dissatisfied with hemodynamic performance of the Hancock valve and inserted Ionescu-Shiley valves in 326 patients during 1978 and 1979. Follow-up of these patients has been short, averaging 6 months. No

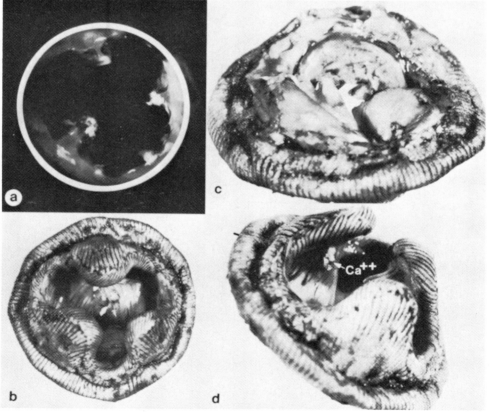

Figure 47–10. Tissue degeneration and calcification in a 75-month-old porcine bioprosthesis that had been in the mitral position. *a,* Roentgenogram of the removed bioprosthesis showing focal calcific deposits in the leaflets. *b,* View of the bioprosthesis from the ventricular aspect showing bowing-in of all three struts. *c,* View of the bioprosthesis from the atrial aspect showing tears and fraying of two of the three leaflets and prolapse of the leaflets toward the atrial side of the valve. The resulting regurgitation required reoperation and replacement of the bioprosthesis with a fresh prosthesis. *d,* Side view showing nodular calcific deposits (Ca^{++}) at the commissural attachment of two leaflets. (From Spray, T. L., and Roberts, W. C.: Structural changes in porcine xenografts used as substitute cardiac valves. Am. J. Cardiol., *40:*319, 1977.)

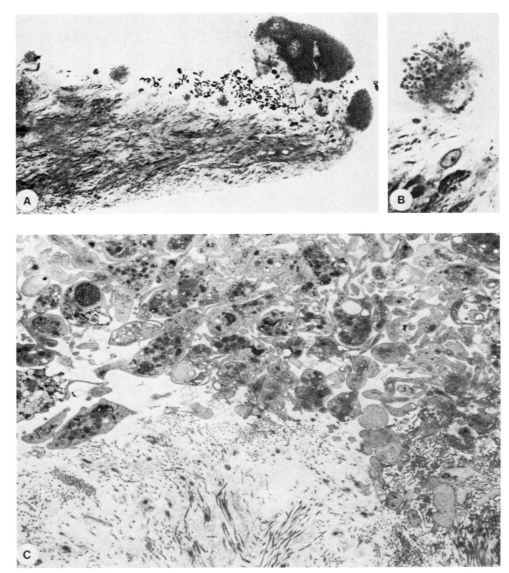

Figure 47–11. Light (*A* and *B*) and electron (*C*) micrographs of aggregates of platelets in a valve. *A,* Section through the area adjacent to a tear (the edge of which is seen at far right) in the leaflet. Collagen in this area is greatly disrupted, and layers of valve connective tissue are not recognizable. The outflow surface (top) is covered with red blood cells and with several aggregates of platelets. (Alkaline toluidine blue stain, × 250). *B,* Aggregate of platelets (shown at upper left in *A*) is connected to the surface of the valve by a narrow pedicle (× 750). *C,* Base of a platelet aggregate similar to that shown in *B*. The platelets are in direct contact with severely disrupted collagen in the valve surface; they are well preserved and contain abundant glycogen. (× 13,000.) (From Ferrans, V. J., Spray, T. L., Billingham, M. E., and Roberts, W. C.: Structural changes in glutaraldehyde-treated porcine heterografts used as substitute cardiac valves. Am. J. Cardiol., *41*:1159, 1978.)

emboli have occurred in patients with aortic valve bioprostheses, despite the lack of anticoagulation. One nonfatal femoral artery thromboembolism occurred in a patient with a replaced mitral valve, even though she was taking anticoagulants. The patient was in atrial fibrillation. The overall time-related incidence of thromboembolic complications to date among these recipients has been 0.7 per cent per year. Using the same indications as Cohn and colleagues (1981), the Houston surgeons have found it necessary to maintain 42 per cent of their 287 surviving patients on long-term anticoagulation. Hemodynamic performance of the Ionescu-Shiley valve was judged ''excellent.''

Anticoagulation

The basis for systemic long-term anticoagulation is warfarin or a derivative. In one study, the rate of emboli in patients receiving cloth-covered Starr-Edwards valves with no anticoagulation was 4 per cent per year (Moggio *et al.,* 1978). A similar group of patients treated concurrently with Coumadin sustained only about one embolus per 100 patients per year. The same study demonstrated the possible effectiveness of aspirin used alone, since the embolic rate with this drug was 2.6 per cent per year. However, in this situation, most use both drugs in combination. Among a group of high-risk patients receiving caged ball valves for aortic replacement, emboli occurred at the rate of 9 per cent per year when the patients were taking warfarin (Dale *et al.*, 1977). When the same patients were subsequently treated with the addition of aspirin, the rate of emboli dropped to 2 per cent per year. (It should be noted that aspirin had to be stopped in one third of these patients, mostly because of bleeding problems.) In a study done in the reverse order (Brott *et al.*, 1981), 50 patients receiving dipyridamole (Persantine) and aspirin sustained thromboembolic events at the rate of almost 9 per cent per year. The addition of warfarin reduced this incidence to 1 per cent.

Steele and colleagues (1979) showed that *in vitro* measurement of platelet survival time correlated strongly with a reduction in embolic events in patients taking aspirin. In this study, patients having decreased platelet survival time after valve replacement received antiplatelet drugs in addition to warfarin. Over the next 4 years, there were no emboli among the 59 patients whose platelet survival time increased on aspirin therapy, whereas one third of the patients whose platelet survival time remained subnormal despite aspirin administration had emboli. These findings suggest that the effect of aspirin in reducing emboli is due to its antiplatelet action. They also show that effective antiplatelet therapy can be monitored by this *in vitro* test.

Dipyridamole may be less effective than aspirin in these situations, although the evidence is far from conclusive. Dipyridamole was given to a group of patients who received tilting disc valves in Great Britain (Thomsen and Alstrup, 1979). Over the next few years, these patients sustained a 22 per cent incidence of thromboembolism. A similar group of patients concurrently operated on for valve replacement but receiving warfarin experienced only a 7 per cent incidence of thromboembolism over the same period.

Interruption of warfarin for short periods in patients undergoing noncardiac surgery has been found to carry a minimal risk of thromboembolic complications (Katholi *et al.*, 1978; Tinker and Tarhan, 1978). Heparin may be given soon after surgery to restore anticoagulation. Heparin can also be substituted for warfarin in women with prosthetic valves who become pregnant, but more recently, the need for valve replacement in a woman of child-bearing age is seen as a strong indication for insertion of a tissue valve.

Diagnosis and Treatment of Valve Thrombosis

Clinically, the presence of thrombus formation on a valve can often be detected by the appearance of pulmonary edema associated with the disappearance of valve clicks, especially in cases of sudden valve thrombosis. Systolic murmurs may appear. Echocardiography may show an alteration in disc motion, especially if a baseline study is available. With tissue valves, serial echocardiography can reveal progressive thickening of the cusps. Magilligan and associates (1980) have reported that cusp thickening greater than 3 mm. is highly correlated with tissue valve dysfunction. Phonocardiography is a valuable tool and can detect a decrease in ejection time with aortic valves and a prolonged diastolic rumble with thrombosed mitral valves. In a recent innovation, computer-assisted real-time sound spectrum analysis allowed detection of three out of seven cerebral emboli and all four valve thrombi among 127 patients with disc valves (Kagawa *et al.*, 1980). Two-dimensional echocardiography has also been reported to be very accurate (Martin *et al.*, 1980). Among 40 patients with suspected Hancock valve dysfunction, this technique correctly diagnosed seven patients with normal valves; 18 of 19 with suspected endocarditis (12 positive, 6 negative); six cases of suspected recent cerebrovascular accident (three with a valvular mass as a source of the embolus); and eight cases of abnormal left ventricular function causing congestive heart failure. The overall accuracy was 97 per cent, compared with 67 per cent with one-dimensional echocardiography in the same patients. The two-dimensional modality is more difficult to use, the authors warn, and the settings must be adjusted accurately, because the sewing ring and stents produce stronger echoes than the valve leaflets.

The most common treatment for thrombosed or failed valves is reoperation and replacement. Recently, thromboembolic problems have been successfully resolved by replacing mechanical valves with tissue valves. In one series, this strategy resulted in a 90 per cent operative survival rate and 50 per cent 10-year survival rate (Shemin *et al.*, 1979).

An intitial report from Europe using fibrinolysis to treat valve thromboembolism was moderately encouraging (Witchitz *et al.*, 1980). Of 13 episodes treated with intravenous streptokinase or urokinase for 1 to 4 days, complete regression resulted in eight. Some of these patients had later thromboembolic episodes, however, and required reoperation. This technique may find a place in the treatment of the acute episode so that the patient can undergo reoperation in a nonemergency state.

Acknowledgment

Appreciation is expressed to Dr. Thomas L. Spray for preparing the illustrations for this section.

REFERENCES

Arnett, E. N., and Roberts, W. C.: Active infective indocarditis: A clinicopathologic analysis of 137 necropsy patients. Curr. Probl. Cardiol., *1*:2, 1976.
Bissett, G. S., III, Schwartz, S. C., Benzing, G., III, Helmsworth, J., Schrieber, J. T., and Kaplan, S.: Late results of reconstruction of the right ventricular outflow tract with porcine heterografts in children. Ann. Thorac. Surg., *31*:437, 1981.

Bjork, V. O., and Henze, A.: Isolated mitral valve replacement with the Bjork-Shiley tilting disc prosthesis. Scand. J. Thorac. Cardiovasc. Surg., *11*:181, 1977.

Bonchek, L. I.: Current status of cardiac valve replacement: Selection of a prosthesis and indications for operation. Am. Heart J., *101*:96, 1981.

Borst, H. G., Papagiannakis, N., Beddermann, C., and Oelert, H.: Cardiac valve replacement. Problems solved and unsolved. Thorac. Cardiovasc. Surg., *27*:76, 1979.

Brott, W. H., Zajchuck, R., Bowen, T. E., Davia, J., and Green, D. C.: Dipyridamole-aspirin as thromboembolic prophylaxis in patients with aortic valve prosthesis. J. Thorac. Cardiovasc. Surg., *81*:632, 1981.

Carpentier, A., Lemaigre, G., Robert, L., Carpentier, S., and Dubost, C.: Biological factors affecting long-term results of valvular heterografts. J. Thorac. Cardiovasc. Surg., *48*:467, 1969.

Casarotto, D., Bortolotti, U., Thiene, G., Gallucci, V., and Cévese, P. G.: Long-term results (from 5 to 7 years) with the Hancock S-G-P bioprosthesis. J. Cardiovasc. Surg., *20*:399, 1979.

Clarkson, P. M., and Barratt-Boyes, B. G.: Bacterial endocarditis following homograft replacement of the aortic valve. Circulation, *42*:987, 1970.

Cohn, L. H.: Valve replacement in children. Ann. Thorac. Surg., *31*:491, 1981.

Cohn, L. H., Mudge, G. H., Pratter, F., and Collins, J. J., Jr.: Five- to eight-year follow-up of patients undergoing porcine heart-valve replacement. N. Engl. J. Med., *304*:258, 1981.

Dale, J., Levang, O., and Enge, I.: Long-term results after aortic valve replacement with four different prostheses. Am. Heart J., *99*:155, 1980.

Dale, J., Myhre, E., Storstein, O., Stormorken, H., and Efskind, L.: Prevention of arterial thromboembolism with acetylsalicylic acid. A controlled clinical trial in patients with aortic ball valves. Am. Heart J., *94*:101, 1977.

Ferrans, V. J., Spray, T. L., Billingham, M. E., and Roberts, W. C.: Structural changes in glutaraldehyde-treated porcine heterografts used as substitute cardiac valves. Am. J. Cardiol., *41*:1159, 1978.

Jamieson, W. R., Janusz, M. T., Miyagishima, R. T., Munro, A. I., Tutassura, H., Gerein, A. N., Burr, L. H., and Allen, P.: Embolic complications of procine heterograft cardiac valves. J. Thorac. Cardiovasc. Surg., *81*:626, 1981.

Kagawa, Y., Sato, N., Nitta, S., Hongo, T., Tanaka, M., Mohri, H., and Horiuchi, T.: Real-time spectroanalysis for diagnosis of malfunctioning prosthetic valves. J. Thorac. Cardiovasc. Surg., *79*:671, 1980.

Karchmer, A. W., Dismukes, W. E., Buckley, M. J., and Austen, W. G.: Late prosthetic valve endocarditis. Am. J. Med., *64*:199, 1978.

Katholi, R. E., Nolan, S. P., and McGuire, L. B.: The management of anticoagulation during noncardiac operations in patients with prosthetic heart valves. A prospective study. Am. Heart J., *96*:163, 1978.

Kluge, R. M., Calia, F. M., McLaughlin, J. S., and Hornick, R. B.: Source of contamination in open heart surgery. J.A.M.A., *230*:1415, 1974.

Lakier, J. B., Khaja, F., Magilligan, D. J., Jr., and Goldstein, S.: Porcine xenograft valves. Long-term (60–89 month) follow-up. Circulation, *62*:313, 1980.

Lefrak, E. A., and Starr, A.: Current heart valve prostheses. Am. Fam. Physician, *20*:93, 1979.

Magilligan, D. J., Jr., Quinn, E. L., and Davila, J. C.: Bacteremia, endocarditis and the Hancock valve. Ann. Thorac. Surg., *24*:508, 1977.

Magilligan, D. J., Jr., Lewis, J. W., Jr., Jara, F. M., Lee, M. W., Alan, M., Riddle, J. M., and Stein, P. D.: Spontaneous degeneration of porcine bioprosthetic valves. Ann. Thorac. Surg., *30*:259, 1980.

Martin, R. P., French, J. W., and Popp, R. L.: Clinical utility of two-dimensional echocardiography in patients with bioprosthetic valves. Adv. Cardiol., *27*:294, 1980.

Masur, H., and Johnson, W. D., Jr.: Prosthetic valve endocarditis. J. Thorac. Cardiovasc. Surg., *80*:31, 1980.

McAllister, R. G., Jr., Samet, J., Mazzoleni, A., and Dillon, M. L.: Endocarditis on prosthetic mitral valves. Chest, *66*:682, 1974.

Moggio, R. A., Hammond, G. L., Stansel, H. C., Jr., and Glenn, W. W.: Incidence of emboli with cloth-covered Starr-Edwards valve without anticoagulation and with varying forms of anticoagulation. Analysis of 183 patients followed for 3½ years. J. Thorac. Cardiovasc. Surg., *75*:296, 1978.

Murphy, E. S., and Kloster, F. E.: Late results of valve replacement surgery. II. Complications of prosthetic heart valves. Mod. Concepts Cardiovasc. Dis., *48*:59, 1979.

Murray, B. E., Karchmer, A. W., Moellering, R. C., Jr.: Diphtheroid prosthetic valve endocarditis. Am. J. Med., *69*:838, 1980.

Ott, D. A., Coelho, A. T., Cooley, D. A., and Reul, G. J., Jr.: Ionescu-Shiley pericardial xenograft valve: Hemodynamic evaluation and early clinical follow-up of 326 patients. Cardiovasc. Dis. Bull. Texas Heart Inst., *7*:137, 1980.

Oyer, P. E., Miller, D. C., Stinson, E. B., Reitz, B. A., Moreno-Cabral, R. J., and Shumway, N. E.: Clinical durability of the (Hancock) porcine bioprosthesis valve. J. Thorac. Cardiovasc. Surg., *80*:824, 1980.

Roberts, W. C., and Hammer, W. J.: Cardiac pathology after valve replacement with a tilting disc prosthesis (Bjork-Shirley type). Am. J. Cardiol., *37*:1024, 1976.

Rossiter, S. J., Stinson, E. B., Oyer, P. E., Miller, D. C., Schapira, J. N., Martin, R. P., and Shumway, N. E.: Prosthetic valve endocarditis. J. Thorac. Cardiovasc. Surg., *76*:795, 1978.

Saffle, J. R., Gardner, P., Schoenbaum, S. C., and Wild, W.: Prosthetic valve endocarditis. The case for prompt valve replacement. J. Thorac. Cardiovasc. Surg., *73*:416, 1977.

Sande, M. A., Johnson, W. D., Hook, E. W., *et al.*: Sustained bacteremia in patients with prosthetic cardiac valves. N. Engl. J. Med., *286*:1067, 1972.

Sanders, S. P., Levy, R. J., Freed, M. D., Norwood, W. I., and Castaneda, A. R.: Use of Hancock porcine xenografts in children and adolescents. Am. J. Cardiol., *46*:429, 1980.

Shemin, R. J., Guadiana, V. A., Conkle, D. M., and Morrow, A. G.: Prosthetic aortic valves. Indications for and results of reoperation. Arch. Surg., *114*:63, 1979.

Spray, T. L., and Roberts, W. C.: Structural changes in porcine xenografts used as substitute cardiac valves. Am. J. Cardiol., *40*:319, 1977.

Steele, P., Rainwater, J., and Vogel, R.: Platelet suppressant therapy in patients with prosthetic cardiac valves. Relationship of clinical effectiveness to alteration of platelet survival time. Circulation, *60*:910, 1979.

Thomsen, P. B., and Alstrup, P.: Thromboembolism in patients without anticoagulants after aortic valve replacement with the Lillehei-Kaster disc valve. Thorac. Cardiovasc. Surg., *27*:313, 1979.

Tinker, J. H., and Tarhan, S.: Discontinuing anticoagulant therapy in surgical patients with cardiac valve prostheses. J.A.M.A., *239*:738, 1978.

Winter, T. Q., Reis, R. L., Glancy, D. L., Roberts, W. C., Epstein, S. W., and Morrow, A. G.: Current status of the Starr-Edwards cloth-covered prosthetic cardiac valves. Circulation, *45*, *46*(Suppl. 1):14, 1972.

Witchitz, S., Veyrat, C., Moisson, P., Scheinman, N., and Rozenstajn, L.: Fibrinolytic treatment of thrombus on prosthetic heart valves. Br. Heart J., *44*:545, 1980.

II. THROMBOEMBOLIC COMPLICATIONS OF CARDIAC AND VASCULAR PROSTHESES

FRED H. KOHANNA

EDWIN W. SALZMAN

Thromboembolism is a major cause of morbidity and death following implantation of prosthetic devices within the circulation or passage of blood through extracorporeal circuits and is a potential hazard in all applications in which the blood contacts artificial surfaces. The tendency of the blood to solidify into a gel when exposed to surfaces other than the normal lining of blood vessels was pointed out by William Hewson in the eighteenth century. A century later, Lord Joseph Lister observed that blood clotted more rapidly in a latex rubber tube than in a tube lined with paraffin. More recent workers have considered the physical and chemical characteristics of surfaces with respect to their interaction with the blood. Detailed reviews of the subject are available (Forbes and Prentice, 1978; Berger and Salzman, 1974).

Activation of the intrinsic coagulation pathway occurs whenever blood contacts a damaged vessel wall or artificial surface (Fig. 47–12). Factor XII is activated, leading to thrombin generation and formation of a fibrin network. In addition, activated factor XII can initiate the kinin-forming pathway, leading to the production of bradykinin and activation of the intrinsic fibrinolytic system.

Activated platelets contribute to the coagulation cascade by exhibiting a critical membrane property called platelet factor 3, by virtue of which clotting factors Xa and Va and Ca^{++} reversibly bind to the platelet membrane and facilitate conversion of prothrombin to thrombin. Thrombin, in turn, exerts potent stimulatory effects on platelets, which can also be activated by contact with surfaces other than normal endothelium (Fig. 47–13). The key plasma protein, von Willebrand's factor, is essential for platelet adhesion. After adhesion of individual platelets, additional platelets are recruited in the form of aggregates, and there may be secretion of platelet contents, including serotonin and adenine nucleotides (e.g., ADP). ADP and thromboxane A_2, a product of platelet arachidonic acid metabolism, are chiefly responsible for platelet aggregation and secretion. The substances released by adherent platelets together with thrombin influence other platelets to aggregate and fully cover the endothelial defect or foreign surface.

The relative composition of a thrombus, either plasma fibrin clot or cellular platelet aggregate, is dictated largely by local blood flow conditions. In areas of sluggish blood flow, where fluid shear stress is low or where recirculating eddies permit long residence times of blood elements near prosthetic surfaces, activation of clotting factors leads to a local build-up in concentration of procoagulants and ultimately to the formation of a plasma clot. Thus, the "red thrombus" or "stasis thrombus" is a clot composed of red cells entrapped in fibrin strands. It predominates in peripheral veins, behind stenotic cardiac valves, around the sewing rings of prosthetic heart valves, and in extracorporeal reservoirs. In regions where blood flow is brisk and fluid shear stress is greater, as in peripheral arteries, the "white thrombus" or "platelet thrombus" is more common. The white thrombus is characteristic of arteries, of the tubing and cannulas of artificial circulatory systems, and of the cages or struts of prosthetic heart valves that jut out into the bloodstream.

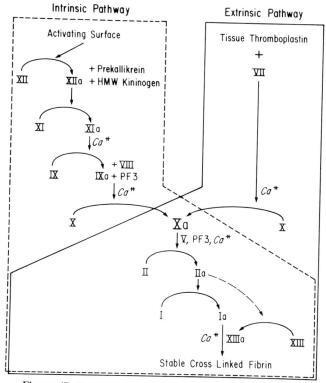

Figure 47–12. Intrinsic and extrinsic coagulation pathways demonstrating their convergence at Xa (a = activated; PF3 = platelet factor 3; Ca^{++} = calcium; II = prothrombin; IIa = thrombin; I = fibrinogen; Ia = fibrin monomer; HMW kininogen = high–molecular-weight kininogen). (Modified with permission from Brozovic, M., and Mibashan, R. S.: Disorders of hemostasis in surgery. *In* Recent Advances in Surgery. 9th Ed. Edited by S. F. Taylor. London, Churchill Livingstone, 1977.)

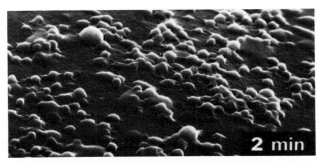

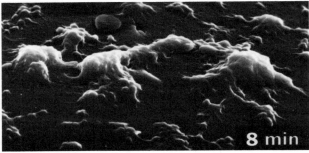

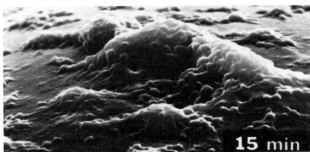

Figure 47–13. Scanning electron micrograph of platelet-rich plasma exposed to a polymethyl acrylate surface for varying periods of time. At 2 minutes, platelets adhere. Progressive aggregation is seen at 8 and 15 minutes. (From Salzman, E. W., Lindon, J., Brier, D., *et al.*: Surface-induced platelet adhesion, aggregation, and release. Ann. N.Y. Acad. Sci., *283*:114, 1977.)

Thrombosis induced by artificial surfaces may be manifested in several ways:

1. Gross thrombus may form in an artificial intravascular device as a deposit on the surface facing the blood. Thrombosis on prosthetic heart valves can impair movement of the ball, disc, or leaflet. In conduits such as arterial grafts, obliteration of the lumen may result.

2. Bits of the thrombus or all of it may break free and embolize downstream, sometimes leaving little trace behind. In patients with nontissue prosthetic mitral and/or aortic valves, peripheral arterial embolism is the leading source of morbidity. With porcine tissue valves, peripheral embolization shares roughly equal importance with other valve complications such as degeneration, calcification, and infection.

3. Repeated generation of microscopic platelet aggregates and cellular debris may result from interaction of blood with artificial surfaces. This can occur with prosthetic arterial graft segments or cardiac valvular prostheses and especially with extracorporeal circulation (ECC) (Dutton *et al.*, 1974).

4. Even when gross or microscopic thromboembolism is not demonstrable, accelerated consumption of hemostatic elements such as platelets and fibrinogen can be found (Harker and Slichter, 1972). Shortened platelet survival has been reported in patients with A-V shunts for hemodialysis, vascular grafts, and artificial heart valves. In the last group, Weily and associates (1974) found a significant correlation between short platelet survival and prior history of or subsequent risk for thromboembolism. Davies and coworkers (1980) showed a rise in fibrinopeptide A (FPA) and thromboxane B_2 levels in patients undergoing ECC for coronary bypass or valve replacement. FPA was elevated prior to ECC, indicating stimulation of coagulation even prior to exposure to the extracorporeal circuit, probably as a result of the contact of blood with intravascular cannulas.

5. Activation of the hemostatic mechanism can lead to profound systemic effects. Contact activation of Factor XII (intrinsic pathway) leads to production of kinins, which mediate blood vessel dilatation, vascular permeability, leukocyte migration, and pain production. Platelet activation with release of platelet constituents (e.g., serotonin) may be responsible for phenomena such as bronchoconstriction with pulmonary embolism (Rosoff *et al.*, 1971) or cerebral vasoconstriction with subarachnoid hemorrhage (Zervas *et al.*, 1973).

6. Exposure of blood to foreign surfaces can have deleterious effects on the function of platelets and other hemostatic elements. This is particularly true with extracorporeal circulation, where air bubbles oxidize as well as oxygenate and lead to denaturation of plasma proteins and alterations of lipids. Platelets, too, are profoundly affected and demonstrate a qualitative defect that may be secondary to partial release of intracellular secretory granules (Beurling-Harbury and Galvan, 1978).

PROSTHETIC HEART VALVES

The fundamental considerations of surface chemistry that governs interactions of blood with artificial materials are largely unknown. The present-day utility of artificial circulatory devices depends less on the availability of bland thromboresistant surfaces than on skillful design aimed to insure favorable flow patterns and on antithrombotic drugs used to retard the response of the blood to foreign surface contact.

In the early days of cardiac valve replacement, the frequency of thromboembolic complications approached 50 per cent if oral anticoagulants were not used (Duvoisin *et al.*, 1967). Subsequent changes in design and materials and increasing use of tissue valves have reduced thromboembolic complications considerably. Table 47–3 categorizes prosthetic valves according to flow type and materials.

Thrombi that develop on prosthetic heart valves are complicated structures. In the neighborhood of the sewing ring at the base of a valve, where disturbed lines of flow with vortices and recirculating eddies

TABLE 47–3. CHARACTERISTICS OF THE MAJOR TYPES OF PROSTHETIC CARDIAC VALVES

VALVE	FLOW	MATERIAL	WARFARIN USUALLY REQUIRED	HEMOLYSIS	COMMENTS
Caged Ball Valve	Peripheral	*Ball:* Metal or silicon *Base and struts:* Metal *Cloth covering:* Polypropylene, Dacron, knitted Teflon	Yes	+	Recent "track" model reduces cloth wear
Caged Disc Valve	Peripheral	*Disc:* Teflon, pyrolytic carbon *Base and struts:* Metal *Cloth covering:* Teflon, Dacron	Yes	+	Pyrolytic carbon disc is more durable and may be less thrombogenic
Tilting Disc Valve	Central	*Disc:* Delrin, Teflon, pyrolytic carbon *Base and struts:* Metal *Cloth covering:* Polypropylene, Dacron, knitted Teflon	Yes	±	Convex-concave disc decreases stagnation of blood behind the pivot points between the disc and valve ring; disc no longer overlaps valve ring, thereby decreasing hemolysis
Tissue Valve	Central	*Valve:* Pericardium, fascia lata, dura mater, porcine valve, cadaver homograft valve *Stent:* Polypropylene or metal *Cloth covering of stent:* Dacron, Teflon	No	−	Anticoagulation may be advisable for patients in atrial fibrillation receiving mitral valves

lead to a long residence time for blood constituents, a red fibrin clot is the rule. On the cage or struts of the valve, out in the fluid stream where flow rates are brisk and the surfaces are constantly washed in rapidly moving blood, a white platelet thrombus is more typical. The composite nature of the thrombus probably accounts for the limited ability of long-term treatment with oral anticoagulants to completely prevent thromboembolic complications of prosthetic valves (Cohn, 1977). Thromboembolic rates are higher when more than one valve is implanted, reflecting the cumulative risk of each additional prosthetic valve, but have shown steady improvement over the years with innovations such as cloth covering and the use of tissue valves. Prosthetic valves whose fixed parts are totally covered by cloth may acquire an adherent layer of thrombus that under ideal circumstances is well tolerated by the blood and serves as a compatible coating (Braunwald *et al.*, 1972). The thrombus layer is initially thin and delicate; its propagation into the orifice of the valve is limited by flow. Eventually, the thrombus is invaded by well-vascularized fibrous tissue growing up from the base of the valve. When an endothelial coat develops, it appears to lessen the frequency of embolic complications (Isom *et al.*, 1973). Starr and colleagues (1976) reported an embolus-free rate at 6 years of 66 per cent and 85 per cent, respectively, for mitral valve replacement (MVR) with non–cloth-covered and cloth-covered caged ball prostheses in patients who were anticoagulated with warfarin. In a similar analysis of isolated aortic valve replacement (AVR), 75 per cent of the patients with non–cloth-covered valves and 91 per cent of the patients with cloth-covered valves were embolus-free at 6 years (Starr *et al.*, 1977). These rates are in general agreement with those of other

published series (Forman *et al.*, 1978; Salomon *et al.*, 1977; Rubin *et al.*, 1977; MacManus *et al.*, 1978).

Other valve designs such as the tilting disc and caged disc have slightly fewer thromboembolic complications than their caged ball counterparts but still require anticoagulation (Bjork and Henze, 1979; Rubin *et al.*, 1977). Karp and associates (1981) evaluated a large group of patients surviving aortic and/or mitral valve replacement with a tilting disc valve. All patients were anticoagulated with warfarin. At 4 years, 85 per cent of the MVR group and 88 per cent of the AVR group were free of thromboembolic complications, but of concern was an overall incidence of gross valve thrombosis of 13 per cent for MVR and 3 per cent for AVR. Thrombotic obstruction is a life-threatening complication, which, although not unique to tilting disc valves, is more common with them. Inadequate anticoagulation or outright cessation of warfarin has been shown to raise the incidence of thrombotic obstruction (Bjork and Henze, 1979).

Tissue valves such as the glutaraldehyde-preserved porcine valve ("bioprostheses") have proved to be less thrombogenic and in many instances can be used without long-term anticoagulation (Cohn *et al.*, 1979). It is not clear whether this relative thromboresistance derives from their natural surface, which is biologic but abnormal, not being covered with living endothelium or from their favorable fluid mechanical configuration, with soft flexible leaflets opening at the center.

Cohn and associates (1981) reported that at 96 months, patients with bioprostheses in the mitral or aortic position were 82 per cent and 97 per cent free of emboli, respectively. Most of their patients were not anticoagulated, but a handful of the AVR patients and about a third of the MVR patients did receive warfarin. In other studies of porcine valves, similar thromboembolic rates were noted, although the use of anticoagulation varied widely (Cohn et al., 1976; Davila et al., 1978; Oyer et al., 1979). A number of studies have emphasized the higher incidence of thromboemboli in patients with atrial fibrillation undergoing valve replacement. (Hetzer et al., 1978; Jamieson et al., 1977; Williams et al., 1980; Cohn et al., 1981). In the latter series, the probability of freedom from emboli at 96 months after mitral, aortic, and double valve replacement with bioprostheses was approximately 98 per cent for patients with normal sinus rhythm and 75 per cent for patients with atrial fibrillation. Use of anticoagulants after MVR with a porcine valve in patients with atrial fibrillation is controversial. Several studies have shown no significant benefit of warfarin in these patients (Stinson et al., 1977). Hetzer and coworkers (1978) demonstrated a protective effect of aspirin in a group of patients with atrial fibrillation who had undergone porcine MVR.

The risk of thromboembolism must, of course, be balanced against the risk of anticoagulants (Forfar, 1979), and absolute guidelines for their use with tissue valves cannot yet be delineated.

EXTRACORPOREAL CIRCULATION

Extracorporeal circulation of the blood for cardiopulmonary bypass (CPB) or for long-term respiratory assistance invariably results in damage to platelets and red cells, denaturation of plasma proteins, and activation of the coagulation mechanism. Bachman and colleagues (1975) noted a 4 per cent incidence of postoperative bleeding in a large series of patients undergoing CPB. Half of these patients had surgically correctable bleeding, 25 per cent had a predominant coagulopathy, and 25 per cent had a major acquired platelet defect. The enormous artificial surface of the heart-lung machine coupled with areas of stagnation and eddy currents offers ample opportunity for blood-surface interaction. Recirculation of extravasated blood from cardiotomy suction aggravates the problem by introducing partially activated blood, which may also contain procoagulant tissue juices, fat, and bone fragments (Wisch et al., 1973).

Consumptive coagulopathies can occur if anticoagulation with heparin is inadequate, leading to fibrin production and fibrinogen depletion. Heparin may be administered according to several arbitrary formulas (Nyman et al., 1974), but the reliability of these methods for achieving optimal anticoagulation is open to question (O'Brien et al., 1981). Alternatively, tests such as the protamine titration test or activated coagulation time can be used to guide heparin dosage (Jobes et al., 1981). Heparin must be neutralized with protamine to insure adequate surgical hemostasis prior to closure of the chest (Gans and Castaneda, 1967). Recommendations for protamine dosage vary (Nyman et al., 1974); 1 mg. per 100 units of heparin activity is a reasonable dose. Protamine in excess of heparin can exert an anticoagulant effect (Hougie, 1958); however, this tends to be overrated, as three times the neutralizing dose of protamine must be given to yield a major anticoagulant effect (Perkins et al., 1956; Ellison et al., 1971).

Free heparin may reappear in the circulation up to 18 hours after initially adequate neutralization with protamine. This phenomenon, known as heparin rebound, may be secondary to splitting of heparin-protamine complexes, more rapid metabolism of protamine than of heparin, or sequestering of heparin in the microcirculation or extravascular spaces preventing neutralization with the initial protamine dose. A recent report by Pifarre and associates (1981) suggested that use of the automated protamine titration test in the early postoperative period was beneficial in decreasing blood loss secondary to unneutralized heparin.

Thrombocytopenia occurs within minutes of contact of the blood with the extracorporeal circuit (Gralnick and Fischer, 1971). This fall in platelet number is accounted for by hemodilution, adherence to foreign surfaces, sequestration in spleen, liver, and lungs (deLeval et al., 1975), formation and filtration of microaggregates (Dutton et al., 1974), and destruction in the cardiotomy suction system (Edmunds et al., 1978). The problem of circulating platelet aggregates and particulate matter during extracorporeal circulation has led to the development of micropore filters to remove them (Pastoriza-Pinol et al., 1979). Such emboli are responsible for postoperative dysfunction of many viscera, including the brain, kidneys, and lungs (Ashmore et al., 1972; Byrick and Noble, 1978).

Platelet *function* also is profoundly affected by extracorporeal circulation. Platelets may undergo partial "release" of intracellular granules, resulting in an acquired storage pool deficiency (Beurling-Harbury and Galvan, 1978). Platelets recently released from bone marrow stores are more metabolically active and may be more likely to react with foreign surfaces (Karpatkin, 1969), which could leave a circulating population of platelets with reduced capacity for adhesion and aggregation (Hirsh et al., 1968).

Despite the inherent procoagulant effects of ECC, disseminated intravascular coagulation (DIC) is a rare complication (Umlas, 1976). Fibrinolysis occurs in parallel with intravascular fibrin production and with DIC may be so brisk as to deplete stores of fibrinogen and other clotting factors. Fibrinogen-fibrin degradation products (FDP) are formed, which themselves are anticoagulants and help prevent further thrombosis. Attempts to limit fibrinolysis pharmacologically with agents such as epsilon-aminocaproic acid (EACA) in the face of ongoing fibrin formation can lead to catastrophic thrombotic complications (Gans, 1966). Fibrinolysis *rarely* occurs as an isolated hemostatic derangement after CPB but rather is an appropriate response to intravascular coagulation.

Extracorporeal circulation with membrane oxygenators appears to produce less hematologic derangement than bubble-type oxygenators, inciting less hemolysis, platelet loss, and protein denaturation (Mortensen, 1977; Clark *et al.*, 1979). Postoperative dysfunction of vital organs such as the brain, lungs, and kidneys secondary to particulate emboli (Allardyce *et al.*, 1966; Hill *et al.*, 1969) is reduced by in-line micropore filters (Patterson and Twichell, 1971; Solis and Gibbs, 1972) and appears to be lessened by membrane oxygenators (Byrick and Noble, 1978). Nevertheless, attempts to provide long-term respiratory support using extracorporeal circulation have been frustrated by marked thrombocytopenia and serious bleeding complications (Bloom *et al.*, 1974).

ARTIFICIAL VENTRICLE

Development of a total artificial heart or left ventricular assist device would have obvious clinical usefulness, including (1) support of intraoperative or postinfarction heart failure; (2) temporary support while awaiting cardiac transplantation; and (3) definitive treatment of end-stage heart disease when all other modalities fail. In addition to problems of pump design and energy supply, the artificial heart offers a large thrombogenic surface to the blood. Early designs utilizing sacs of Silastic with Dacron-fibril intimas resulted in severe hemolysis and consumption of hemostatic elements (Stanley and Kolff, 1973). With advances in design and development of less thrombogenic materials, the goal of a total artificial heart or a left ventricular assist device is closer to being reached. Kolff and associates (1979) implanted a flexible diaphragm heart with a smooth polyurethane surface in calves and noted normal platelet counts and plasma hemoglobin levels. Some activation of the coagulation system did occur, and platelet survival was half of normal. Fuqua and colleagues (1981) reported the use of an abdominally implanted left ventricular assist device that employs a polyurethane pumping diaphragm and woven Dacron inlet and outlet conduits containing glutaraldehyde-preserved porcine xenograft valves. These surfaces underwent accretion of thrombus, which was apparently kept in check by ongoing fibrinolytic activity. A left ventricular assist device was successfully used for 94 hours to support a patient who sustained an intraoperative myocardial infarction and cardiac failure following coronary bypass surgery (Berger *et al.*, 1979).

A challenge for the future is to design a total artificial heart or left ventricular assist device with flow characteristics and blood compatibility that will permit long-term application in man.

INTRA-AORTIC BALLOON CARDIAC ASSISTANCE

Intra-aortic balloon pumping has become a standard form of circulatory assistance for cardiogenic shock due to acute infarction or cardiac dysfunction after open heart surgery. In recent years, its use has been extended to patients with unstable angina or life-threatening arrhythmias and to support of preoperative patients with severe left ventricular failure. High fluid shear rates in the thoracic aorta coupled with streamlined design of the balloon and use of thromboresistant materials (i.e., polyurethane) have kept the rate of thromboembolic complications low.

The most common complication with this device is compromise of the circulation to the legs. Arterial insufficiency usually requires balloon removal and thrombectomy. Patients who are dependent on intra-aortic balloon pumping may benefit from cross-femoral grafts. Alpert and colleagues (1976) reported a 36 per cent incidence of serious vascular complications following femoral artery cannulation for intra-aortic balloon pumping. Most of these required operative intervention, which usually prevented limb loss, but a 54 per cent mortality rate in this group underscores the serious nature of such complications. Late ischemic complications can also occur secondary to stenosis or occlusion at the site of a previous arteriotomy (Kozloff *et al.*, 1980). Doppler monitoring of the lower extremity while the intra-aortic balloon pump catheter is in place permits early detection and correction of vascular compromise.

Other vascular complications with this device include intimal injury, aortoiliac dissection, perforation, and insertion site bleeding. Thrombocytopenia is virtually universal with intra-aortic balloon pumping; however, the effects of CPB and multisystem failure are difficult to sort out. The fall in platelet count is usually modest, and a bleeding diathesis from intra-aortic balloon pumping alone is rare (Subramanian *et al.*, 1980).

Antithrombotic drugs such as heparin, dextran, and aspirin have been employed to prevent consumption of hemostatic elements during balloon assistance, but their efficacy is questionable (DeLaria *et al.*, 1972; Bregman, 1974).

The percutaneous intra-aortic balloon pump catheter obviates the need for a prosthetic graft anastomosed end to side to the femoral artery for balloon insertion. Lower thromboembolic rates have been reported in several small series (Subramanian *et al.*, 1980; Bregman and Casarella, 1980).

VASCULAR PROSTHESES

Replacement of peripheral arteries and veins has been successfully performed for three decades despite the unavailability of truly nonthrombogenic materials for construction of vascular prostheses. Most graft materials in clinical use today rely on deposition of a lining layer of adherent thrombus in order to create a relatively bland, thromboresistant surface. Large grafts, such as those to the aortoiliac vessels, have high patency rates because the neointimal thrombus does not significantly encroach upon the lumen. High flow rates minimize layering of the thrombus, which, if progressive, would eventually compromise the internal diameter of the graft. Prosthetic grafts to small vessels such as the tibial and coronary arteries have

TABLE 47–4. CHARACTERISTICS OF MATERIALS USED FOR FABRICATION OF PROSTHETIC VASCULAR GRAFTS

MATERIAL	CONSTRUCTION	POROSITY	PRE-CLOTTING REQUIRED	NEOINTIMAL FORMATION	PLATELET ADHESION TO GRAFT
Dacron	Woven	Microporous	Optional	Yes	+
	Knitted (internal velour, external velour, or double velour)	Macroporous	Yes	Yes	+
Teflon	Expanded reinforced	Microporous	No	Yes	+
Human umbilical vein	Glutaraldehyde-stabilized (reinforced with Dacron mesh)	Nonporous	No	No	+
Autologous saphenous vein	Reversed because of valves	Nonporous	No	No (true endothelium preserved or regenerated)	− (+ if endothelium is injured)

had limited success. Even larger grafts have shown a disappointing frequency of thrombotic occlusion if the prosthetic graft is subjected to repeated bending as it crosses a joint or if it is employed in the venous tree rather than in arteries.

Several materials, which vary in thrombogenicity and mechanical properties, have been used for fabrication of prosthetic vascular grafts (Table 47–4).

Dacron grafts, either woven or knitted, rely on early deposition of plasma proteins, platelets, and fibrin to render their internal surfaces relatively thromboresistant. Within months, a neointimal lining of fibroblasts, smooth muscle cells, collagen, and elastin develops, although this lining is incomplete, and patches covered only by fibrin can be found (Fig. 47–14). True endothelium grows in from the ends of the graft for 1 to 2 cm. (Sauvage *et al.*, 1974), but in humans, endothelium in other more central areas of the graft is rare (Sauvage *et al.*, 1975). In other species, endothelial recovering tends to be more nearly complete. Neointimal formation is facilitated by ingrowth of fibroblasts from the outside of the graft through its interstices. Factors such as wall thickness, porosity, and filamentous projections on the surface of the graft (i.e., velour) profoundly affect this ingrowth. Thrombotic occlusion of prostheses as a result of fracture of the neointima remains a hazard long after implantation.

Autogenous saphenous vein is a nearly ideal vessel substitute, constrained only by its limited size. It functions as a living tissue with considerable tensile strength and the inherent thromboresistance of its endothelial lining. Care must be taken in the harvesting of the vein to prevent spasm or overdistention leading to endothelial sloughing and exposure of subendothelial elements with subsequent platelet adhesion (Baumann *et al.*, 1981).

Grafts made of expanded microporous polytetrafluorethylene (PTFE) have shown promising results in a variety of smaller vessel applications (Rosenthal *et al.*, 1979; Gupta and Veith, 1980). Like Dacron, these grafts rely on neointimal formation, but because of

their low porosity, they do not require preclotting. Campbell and associates (1975) in a study in dogs found that the major determinant for tissue ingrowth, neointimization, and patency using 4-mm. PTFE grafts was pore size. Wall thickness and PTFE density were relatively less important. Human umbilical vein grafts stabilized with glutaraldehyde and reinforced with

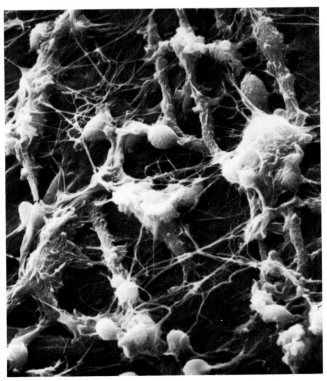

Figure 47–14. Scanning electron micrograph of the blood-contacting surface of a Dacron graft after implantation for 2 years. Adherence of platelets and fibrin on a "glistening pseudo neo-intima" is demonstrated. (From Baier, R. E., and Abbott, W. M.: Comparative biophysical properties of the flow surfaces of contemporary vascular grafts. *In* Graft Materials in Vascular Surgery. Edited by H. Dardick, Miami, Florida. Symposia Specialists, 1978.)

Dacron mesh have shown promise when saphenous vein is unavailable. Processing renders the graft non-antigenic, and its nonporous structure prevents ingrowth of neointimal cells. After initial remodeling *in vivo*, the internal elastic membrane is retained and serves as the interface with the blood and is apparently thromboresistant. Amorphous material is commonly found to line the graft when it is harvested after several months.

Bonding heparin to existing prosthetic materials is another approach to lessening thrombogenicity. Donahoo and colleagues (1977) reported a 10-year experience (25 patients) with heparin-bonded polyvinyl shunts for intraoperative bypass of the thoracic aorta. There were no thrombotic complications of the shunt. Heparin can be bonded to other polymers as well and may even be affixed to glutaraldehyde-preserved human umbilical vein. The efficacy of such grafts is yet to be established.

Oral anticoagulants have failed to alter long-term patency of vascular grafts, and the use of antiplatelet drugs is controversial. Harker and associates (1977) observed shortened platelet survival after placement of prosthetic arterial grafts in baboons. Dipyridamole or dipyridamole plus aspirin improved platelet survival; however, aspirin alone did not. Blakely and Pogoriler (1977) found no improvement in patency using sulfinpyrazone in patients undergoing aortoiliac or femoropopliteal grafts followed up to 3 years. Oblath and coworkers (1978) noted that platelet adhesion and subsequent neointimal fibrous hyperplasia were decreased in dogs receiving aspirin and dipyridamole following femoral artery bypass with Dacron or PTFE grafts. Since platelets play a key role in thrombotic occlusion of grafts, antiplatelet therapy

may be a promising modality for improving graft patency, but further investigation is necessary.

VENA CAVAL INTERRUPTION

Interruption of the inferior vena cava may be necessary to prevent pulmonary emboli when systemic anticoagulation is contraindicated or has been ineffective. Transabdominal operations to ligate or partially occlude the inferior vena cava are associated with an operative mortality rate of about 10 to 15 per cent (Bernstein, 1978). Risk of subsequent fatal pulmonary emboli persists, presumably from large collateral veins or from the infrarenal inferior vena cava if the interruption is performed too low. The cumulative death rate from recurrent emboli following various transabdominal interruption procedures is about 2 per cent (DeWeese, 1980). Other complications associated with these techniques include nonfatal pulmonary emboli (7.3 per cent), postoperative occlusion of the inferior vena cava (at least 30 per cent), chronic leg edema, recurrent phlebitis, and venous stasis ulceration (Bernstein, 1978; DeWeese, 1980). Development of transvenously inserted devices for inferior vena caval interruption has reduced the morbidity and mortality for this procedure. Three devices are currently in use: the Kim-Ray Greenfield filter (KGF), the Mobin-Uddin umbrella (MUU), and the Hunter-Sessions balloon (HSB). Table 47–5 lists the complications of each device. The HSB totally occludes the inferior vena cava in all cases. The KGF and MUU filter caval blood and are only totally occluding if subsequently clogged with large emboli or an in situ thrombus. Anticoagulation with heparin, if not con-

TABLE 47–5. COMPLICATIONS OF DEVICES USED FOR TRANSVENOUS INTERRUPTION OF THE INFERIOR VENA CAVA

DEVICE	INSERTION COMPLICATIONS	DISPLACEMENT AFTER INSERTION	FILTER INJURY TO IVC OR ADJACENT STRUCTURE	FATE OF MATERIALS AFTER IMPLANTATION	RECURRENT PULMONARY EMBOLI	LATE PATENCY
Kim-Ray Greenfield Filter	Air embolus; cardiac arrhythmia; vein too small; misplacement; dislodgement of IVC thrombus	No proximal displacement; may displace distally into right iliac vein, leaving left iliac vein unprotected	Pericaval bleeding secondary to struts	No change	0–3%	90%
Mobin-Uddin Umbrella	Same as with KGF	1% incidence; causes include: 1. Umbrella too small 2. Filter occlusion with clot, causing caval distention 3. Dislodgement during cardiopulmonary resuscitation	1. Pericaval bleeding secondary to umbrella struts 2. Penetration of struts into ureter or duodenum	No change (one reported case of umbrella breakage)	3–12%	30%
Hunter-Sessions Balloon	Same as with KGF	Rare	None	Balloon deflates over 1 year and is entrapped in scar	Late results unavailable	0%

traindicated, may be a useful adjunct to maintain patency of the inferior vena cava and lessen the incidence of recurrent pulmonary emboli and post-phlebitic venous stasis. Heparin bonding to the MUU is intended to improve inferior vena caval patency rates but awaits clinical validation.

VASCULAR CATHETERS

Thrombotic occlusion of vessels that contain catheters for intravenous infusion is frequent and may occur even after the catheter has been removed (McNeill, 1981). Thrombosis is influenced by duration of infusion and type of fluid infused, presence of bacteria, and the size and composition of the catheter (Fonkalsrud, 1968). Catheters that are less irritating to the endothelium and less inherently thrombogenic will improve patency and lower the incidence of phlebitis. Anticoagulants may also be beneficial in reducing thromboses secondary to vascular cannulation. Bedford and Ashford (1979) reported that aspirin reduced the incidence of postcannulation radial artery occlusion in both men and women.

Thrombus formation on angiographic catheters with subsequent embolization is a major hazard of radiographic procedure (Moore et al., 1970). Thromboembolic complications are particularly troublesome in examinations of the intracranial and coronary circulation, where the target organs are intolerant of embolic occlusion and where interference with flow is easily recognized.

Development of a sleeve of thrombus on an indewelling angiographic catheter has been demonstrated by "pull-out angiography" and "washout thrombectomy" in as many as 95 per cent of angiocardiographic procedures performed by percutaneous puncture of the femoral artery using polyethylene and polyurethane catheters (Eldh and Jacobsson, 1974). As the catheter is removed, the sleeve of thrombus may be stripped off and passed to the lower extremities or may be advanced into the proximal circulation if the catheter is replaced by a guide wire.

Testing of thromboresistant catheters in dogs using techniques such as fibrinopeptide A measurement (Casarella and Wilner, 1977) and ^{111}In labeling of platelets (Lipton et al., 1980) should lead to improved materials and catheter design.

Systemic heparin is an important adjunct to the clinical use of angiographic catheters. Wallace and associates (1972) found that systemic heparinization significantly decreased thromboembolic complications during angiography. Dextran has also been reported to be beneficial (Jacobsson, 1968). Aspirin, on the other hand, did not reduce the incidence of brachial artery occlusion following cardiac catheterization (Hynes et al., 1973). Heparin prior to angiographic catheter insertion, later neutralized with protamine after catheter removal, seems to be a reasonable adjunct for patients in whom anticoagulation is not contraindicated. Heparin-bonded angiographic catheters currently undergoing testing may soon obviate the need for systemic anticoagulation.

ANTITHROMBOTIC DRUGS

Pharmacologic agents that interfere with hemostatic processes may reduce the thrombotic tendency that complicates exposure of the blood to artificial surfaces. The drugs available include heparin and coumarin compounds, which interfere with fibrin formation, and a large number of agents that alter platelet activity. Heparin is a strongly anionic sulfated polysaccharide, which must be given parenterally. Heparin binds to and activates antithrombin III, a natural inhibitor of several serine protease coagulation factors, including thrombin and Factors XIIa, XIa, IXa, and Xa. Cleavage by thrombin of fibrinopeptide A and B from fibrinogen is prevented, thereby shutting down fibrin production. Unfortunately, heparin does not have an inhibitory effect on platelets. In fact, heparin has been shown to promote platelet aggregation in whole blood in vitro (Kohanna et al., 1981). Silane and collagues (1981) demonstrated circulating platelet aggregates in rabbits shortly after heparin administration. Numerous reports of early thrombocytopenia and arterial thrombosis after institution of heparin therapy suggest that this phenomenon also occurs in humans (Towne et al., 1979).

Extracorporeal circulation for cardiopulmonary bypass and partial cardiac bypass for circulatory or respiratory assistance require anticoagulation with heparin to prevent the formation of fibrin in the extracorporeal circuit. In cases of partial bypass, such as extracorporeal hemodialysis, regional heparinization of the extracorporeal circuit without anticoagulation of the patient is possible (Maher et al., 1963). Heparin is added to the blood as it leaves the patient and is neutralized with an appropriate amount of protamine at the inflow end of the extracorporeal circuit. In practice, achievement of an exact balance between heparin and protamine is difficult, and regional heparinization often results in a degree of anticoagulation of the patient. Regional use of heparin has even been successfully employed with the intracorporeal artificial heart (Murashita et al., 1978). An alternative system for hemodialysis is to utilize "fractional heparinization," in which a modest degree of interference with coagulation is achieved through the use of small doses of heparin. Natural defenses against thrombosis, including fibrinolysis and restoration of depleted clotting factors through natural synthesis, are depended on to support the patient's hemostatic processes (Kjellstrand and Buselmeier, 1972).

For long-term anticoagulation of patients bearing vascular or valvular prostheses, "oral anticoagulants" (e.g., warfarin) are preferred to heparin because of the ease of their administration compared with that of heparin, which must be given by parenteral injection, relatively simple regulation of dosage, and freedom from side effects peculiar to heparin, such as osteoporosis and alopecia. Warfarin inhibits the synthesis of vitamin K–dependent Factors VII, IX, X, and prothrombin. Clinical response varies, depending on vitamin K stores, albumin binding, and hepatic degradation. Warfarin is essential in patients with nontissue cardiac valvular prostheses. In these patients, thromboembolic complications can be held to below 5 per cent using this agent. High-risk patients such as those with atrial fibrillation or mural thrombus who receive tissue valves (i.e., porcine xenografts) may also require anticoagulation with warfarin. The use of oral anticoagulants in patients who have undergone arterial reconstruction with vascular prostheses has not been shown to be beneficial. Late patency rates are not improved by anticoagulation, nor is the ultimate progression of arteriosclerosis affected. The principal value of oral anticoagulants in such patients appears to be to prevent venous thromboembolism in the early postoperative period.

Bleeding during the administration of warfarin is dose-related. Patients should therefore be monitored with a clotting test such as the prothrombin time. A patient who bleeds despite proper anticoagulation should be suspected of harboring an underlying lesion, such as an ulcer, neoplasm, or A-V malformation.

Drugs that alter platelet function have also been shown to have an antithrombotic effect. These drugs function by a variety of mechanisms (Fig. 47–15). Aspirin in small doses inhibits platelet synthesis of prostaglandins by irreversibly blocking the enzyme cyclo-oxygenase. Platelet secretion and aggregation are impaired. Other nonsteroidal anti-inflammatory agents block the same platelet synthetic pathway that aspirin does, but their effect is reversible and dose-related. Dipyridamole raises platelet cyclic AMP levels by inhibiting the phosphodiesterase enzyme, which normally degrades cyclic AMP. Increased intracellular cyclic AMP inhibits platelet adhesion and aggregation. A combination of aspirin and warfarin is more effective than warfarin alone in patients with prosthetic

valves (Sullivan *et al.*, 1968), although the shortened platelet survival in patients with prosthetic heart valves is not corrected to normal by administration of aspirin (Harker and Slichter, 1970).

Sulfinpyrazone, a drug originally introduced as a uricosuric agent, is an inhibitor of platelet prostaglandin synthesis, although its precise mechanism of action is not understood. It has been found to reduce the thrombotic occlusion rate of arteriovenous shunts employed for hemodialysis (Kaegi *et al.*, 1974) and to correct shortened platelet survival in patients with prosthetic heart valves (Weily and Genton, 1970).

Low–molecular-weight dextran impairs platelet adhesion and aggregation by coating the platelet membrane, interacting with plasma proteins necessary for coagulation, and interfering with fibrin polymerization. The effect is dose-related and with higher–molecular-weight dextran is more pronounced. Dextran has been used to protect platelets during cardiopulmonary bypass (Long *et al.*, 1961) and may be helpful in preventing thromboembolic complications during intra-aortic balloon pumping.

In general, the use of an antiplatelet agent in combination with an anticoagulant such as heparin or warfarin predisposes to bleeding and is extremely hazardous. Although dipyridamole has been used to lessen platelet loss during cardiopulmonary bypass (Nuutinen *et al.*, 1977), similar use of dextran (Smith *et al.*, 1964) and aspirin (Torosian *et al.*, 1978) has led to unacceptable bleeding.

Prostaglandin E_1 (PGE$_1$) and prostacyclin (PGI$_2$) are promising new antiplatelet agents with reversible short-lived antiplatelet effects. PGE$_1$ and PGI$_2$ both raise intracellular levels of cyclic AMP, thereby inhibiting platelet adhesion and aggregation. Cardiopulmonary bypass utilizing PGE$_1$ preserved platelet number and function without undue bleeding in monkeys (Addonizio *et al.*, 1978). Regional infusion of PGI$_2$ in sheep undergoing extracorporeal membrane oxygenation successfully preserved platelet function and protection against thrombocytopenia (Coppe *et al.*, 1979). Hemodialysis or cardiopulmonary bypass may even be possible using PGI$_2$ without any heparin whatsoever (Woods *et al.*, 1978). Use of prostaglandins for extracorporeal circulation in humans must await further clinical investigation but holds considerable promise for the future.

NONTHROMBOGENIC MATERIALS

Normal endothelium possesses a metabolic armamentarium capable of plasminogen activation and prostacyclin synthesis that actively impedes thrombosis. Artifical surfaces, on the other hand, must rely on inherent physicochemical properties that render them relatively blood-compatible. Prosthetic devices are less than perfect in this regard, owing much of their *in vivo* success to the cleansing effects of blood flow, limited surface area, antithrombotic drugs, and deposition of neointimal thrombus (Salzman, 1975).

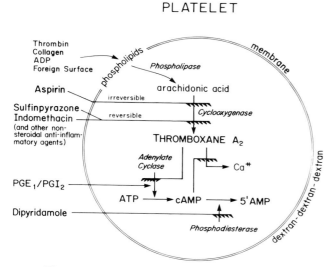

Figure 47–15. Site of action of antiplatelet drugs.

The properties of a surface that dictate its reactivity toward the blood are not entirely understood. Proteins are adsorbed by foreign surfaces within seconds after contact with blood. These proteins appear to mediate subsequent interactions with platelets and formation of thrombus. The importance of these early protein-surface interactions is illustrated by the fact that a material coated with albumin will be relatively thromboresistant, whereas the same material coated with fibrinogen will foster platelet reactivity (Lyman et al., 1974; Zucker and Vroman, 1969).

Surface charge was thought to play an important part in blood compatibility after early reports that electrodes placed across a blood vessel in an animal caused thrombosis at the positive pole (Sawyer and Pate, 1953). Much effort has been expended to produce materials bearing a fixed negative charge at their surface, the goal being to achieve a surface that would electrostatically repel negatively charged blood elements such as plasma proteins and platelets. Unfortunately, surface charge is an average value that results from summation of a mosaic of molecular charges arrayed at a surface, and it has proved of limited value for prediction of the behavior of an artificial material in contact with blood.

Surface wettability as an expression of surface-free energy is also cited as an important characteristic of artificial surfaces. Wettable surfaces have traditionally been thought to promote thrombosis (Neubauer and Lampert, 1930). More recent evidence suggests that hydrophobic (nonwettable) surfaces may actually be more thrombogenic than more hydrophilic surfaces (Merrill et al., 1981). Other properties that may influence thrombogenicity include surface roughness, capacity for electrostatic (ionic) interaction, chain flexibility in polymers, and a host of contaminants, such as waxes, plasticizers, and mold-release agents.

One strategy for improving blood compatibility has been to bind heparin to a polymer surface. This would seem at first to be a paradoxic approach, since heparin dissolved in blood does nothing to impede platelet adhesion or other platelet reactions, except those mediated by thrombin. In fact, heparin induces platelet aggregation in platelet-rich plasma and whole blood in vitro and "sensitizes" the platelets to subsequent stimulation with ADP, epinephrine, or collagen. Why then does binding heparin to various polymers render them less thrombogenic? First, heparin bonded to a surface electrostatically or ionically may leach from the material, creating a thin layer of anticoagulated blood in contact with the surface. Second, heparin that does remain bound to the material may participate in formation of heparin-antithrombin complexes, which have been shown in vitro to "passivate" artificial surfaces (Salzman et al., 1981). Improved techniques for binding heparin to artificial surfaces as well as use of heparin "fractions" selected for high antithrombin III affinity and low platelet reactivity may lead to materials with better blood compatibility in the future.

The development of thromboresistant surfaces is a subject of active investigation in many laboratories because of their potential practical applications, and additional developments in this fast-moving field can be anticipated.

SELECTED REFERENCES

Forbes, C. D., and Prentice, C. R. M.: Thrombus formation and artificial surfaces. Br. Med. Bull., 34:201, 1978.

This article is a comprehensive review of the interaction of blood with artificial surfaces in a variety of clinical settings.

Kohanna, F., and Salzman, E. W.: Surgical bleeding and hemostasis. In Basic Surgery. Edited by H. Polk et al. New York, Appleton-Century-Crofts, 1983.

This a basic review of congenital and acquired bleeding disorders and their significance in surgical patients. Discussions of the common tests of coagulation and the approach to the bleeding patient are included.

Salzman, E. W., Silane, M., and Lindon, J.: Thromboresistance of heparin-coated surfaces. In Chemistry and Biology of Heparin. Edited by R. L. Lunderblad et al. New York, Elsevier North-Holland, Inc., 1981, p. 435.

This is an up-to-date review of heparin-bonded artificial surfaces.

Shattil, S. J., and Bennett, J. S.: Platelets and their membranes in hemostasis: Physiology and pathophysiology. Ann. Intern. Med., 94:108, 1981.

This article presents an authoritative review of platelet physiology, including its role in the coagulation cascade.

Sobel, M., and Salzman, E. W.: Hemorrhagic and thrombotic complications after cardiac surgery. In Thoracic and Cardiovascular Surgery. 4th Ed. Edited by A. Baue and A. Geha. New York, Appleton-Century-Crofts, 1983.

This is an extensive review of hematologic abnormalities following cardiopulmonary bypass.

REFERENCES

Addonizio, V. P., Strauss, J. F., Macarak, E. J., et al.: Preservation of platelet number and function with prostaglandin E during total cardiopulmonary bypass in rhesus monkeys. Surgery, 83:619, 1978.

Allardyce, D. B., Yoshida, S. H., and Ashmore, P. G.: The importance of microembolism in the pathogenesis of organ dysfunction caused by prolonged use of the pump oxygenator. J. Thorac. Cardiovasc. Surg., 52:706, 1966.

Alpert, J., Ezhuthachan, K. B., Gielchinsky, I., et al.: Vascular complications of intraaortic balloon pumping. Arch. Surg., 111:1990, 1976.

Ashmore, P. G., Swank, R. L., Gallery, R., et al.: Effect of Dacron wool filtration on the microembolic phenomenon in extracorporal circulation. J. Thorac. Cardiovasc. Surg., 63:240, 1972.

Bachman, F., McKenna, R., Cole, E. R., et al.: Hemostatic mechanism after open-heart surgery. I. Studies on plasma coagulation factors and fibrinolysis in 512 patients after extracorporeal circulation. J. Thorac. Cardiovasc. Surg., 70:76, 1975.

Baumann, F. G., Catinella, F. P., Cunningham, J. N., Jr., et al.: Vein contraction and smooth muscle cell extensions as causes of endothelial sloughing during graft preparation. (Abstract.) Thromb. Haemost., 46:222, 1981.

Bedford, R. F., and Ashford, T. P.: Aspirin pretreatment prevents post-cannulation radial-artery thrombosis. Anesthesiology, *51*:176, 1979.

Berger, R. L., Merin, G., Carr, J., et al.: Successful use of a left ventricular assist device in cardiogenic shock from massive postoperative myocardial infarction. J. Thorac. Cardiovasc. Surg., *78*:626, 1979.

Berger, S., and Salzman, E. W.: Thromboembolic complications of prosthetic devices. Prog. Hemostasis Thromb., *2*:273, 1974.

Bernstein, E. F.: The role of inferior vena cava interruption in the management of venous thromboembolism. World J. Surg., *2*:61, 1978.

Beurling-Harbury, C., and Galvan, C. A.: Acquired decrease in platelet secretory ADP associated with increased post-operative bleeding in post-cardiopulmonary bypass patients with severe valvular heart disease. Blood, *52*:13, 1978.

Bjork, V. O., and Henze, A.: Ten years experience with the Bjork-Shiley tilting disc valve. J. Thorac. Cardiovasc. Surg., *78*:331, 1979.

Blakely, J. A., and Pogoriler, G.: A prospective trial of sulfinpyrazone after peripheral vascular surgery. Thromb. Haemostasis, *38*:238, 1977.

Bloom, S., Zapol, W., Wonders, T., et al.: Platelet destruction during 24 hour membrane lung perfusion. Trans. Am. Soc. Artif. Intern. Organs, *20*:29, 1974.

Braunwald, N. S., O'Rourke, R., and Paterson, K.: Postoperative clinical and hemodynamic evaluation of a new fabric covered ball-valve prosthesis. Circulation, *45*(Suppl. 2):92, 1972.

Bregman, D.: Management of patients undergoing intraaortic balloon pumping. Heart and Lung, *3*:916, 1974.

Bregman, D., and Casarella, W. J.: Percutaneous intraaortic balloon pumping: Initial clinical experience. Ann. Thorac. Surg., *29*:153, 1980.

Byrick, R. J., and Noble, W. H.: Postperfusion lung syndrome. J. Thorac. Cardiovasc. Surg., *76*:685, 1978.

Campbell, C. D., Goldfarb, D., and Roe, R.: A small arterial substitute: Expanded microporous polytetrafluoroethylene: Patency versus porosity. Ann. Surg., *182*:138, 1975.

Casarella, W. J., and Wilner, G. D.: Guide wire thrombogenicity measured by fibrinopeptide A radioimmunoassay. Am. J. Roentgenol., *128*:363, 1977.

Clark, R. E., Beauchamp, R. A., Magrath, R. A., et al.: Comparison of bubble and membrane oxygenators in short and long perfusions. J. Thorac. Cardiovasc. Surg., *78*:655, 1979.

Cohn, L. H.: Evolution and present state of cardiac valve substitutes: Which should I use? Durability of mechanical and biologic prostheses for aortic valve replacement. *In* Henry Ford Hospital International Symposium for Cardiac Surgery. Edited by J. C. Davila. New York, Appleton-Century-Crofts, 1977, pp. 380–388.

Cohn, L. H., Sanders, J. H., Jr., and Collins, J. J.: Aortic valve replacement with the Hancock porcine xenograft. Ann. Thorac. Surg., *22*:221, 1976.

Cohn, L. H., Mudge, G. H., Pratter, F., et al.: Five- to eight-year follow-up of patients undergoing porcine heart-valve replacement. N. Engl. J. Med., *304*:258, 1981.

Cohn, L. H., Koster, J. K., Mee, R. B. B., et al.: Long-term follow-up of the Hancock bioprosthesis heart valve: A 6-year review. Circulation, *60*:(Suppl. 1):87, 1979.

Coppe, D., Wonders, T., Snider, M., et al.: Preservation of platelet number and function during extracorporeal membrane oxygenation by regional infusion of prostacyclin. *In* Prostacyclin. Edited by J. R. Vane. New York, Raven Press, 1979, p. 371.

Davies, G. C., Sobel, M., and Salzman, E. W.: Elevated plasma fibrinopeptide A and thromboxane B_2 levels during cardiopulmonary bypass. Circulation, *61*:808, 1980.

Davilla, J. C., Magilligan, D. J., and Lewis, J. W.: Is the Hancock porcine valve the best cardiac valve substitute today? Ann. Thorac. Surg., *26*:303, 1978.

DeLaria, G. A., Nyilas, E., and Bernstein, E. F.: Intraaortic balloon pumping without heparin. Trans. Am. Soc. Artif. Intern. Organs, *18*:501, 1972.

de Leval, M., Hill, J. D., Mielke, C. H., et al.: Blood platelets and extracorporeal circulation: Kinetic studies on dogs on cardi-

opulmonary bypass. J. Thorac. Cardiovasc. Surg., *69*:144, 1975.

DeWeese, M. S.: Complications of caval ligation and transabdominal partial interruption of the vena cava. *In* Vascular Surgery. Edited by V. M. Bernhard, and J. B. Towne. New York, Grune and Stratton, 1980, p. 311.

Donahoo, J. S., Brawley, R. K., and Gott, V. L.: The heparin-coated vascular shunt for thoracic aortic and great vessel procedures: A ten-year experience. Ann. Thorac. Surg., *23*:509, 1977.

Dutton, R. C., Edmunds, L. H., Hutchinson, J. C., et al.: Platelet aggregate emboli produced in patients during cardiopulmonary bypass with membrane and bubble oxygenators and blood filters. J. Thorac. Cardiovasc. Surg., *67*:258, 1974.

Duvoisin, G. E., Brandenburg, R. O. and McGoon, D. C.: Factors affecting thromboembolism associated with prosthetic heart valves. Circulation, *35*:(Suppl. 1):70, 1967.

Edmunds, L. H., Saxena, N. C., Hillyer, P., et al.: Relationship between platelet count and cardiotomy suction return. Ann. Thorac. Surg., *25*:306, 1978.

Eldh, P., and Jacobsson, B.: Heparinized vascular catheters: A clinical trial. Radiology, *111*:289, 1974.

Ellison, N., Ominsky, A. J., and Wollman, H.: Is protamine a clinically important anticoagulant? A negative answer. Anesthesiology, *35*:621, 1971.

Fonkalsrud, E. W.: The effect of pH in glucose infusions on development of thrombophlebitis. J. Surg. Res., *8*:539, 1968.

Forbes, C. D., and Prentice, C. R. M.: Thrombus formation and artificial surfaces. Br. Med. Bull., *34*:201, 1978.

Forfar, J. C.: A 7-year analysis of hemorrhage in patients on long-term anticoagulation treatment. Br. Heart J., *42*:128, 1979.

Forman, R., Beck, W., and Barnard, C. N.: Results after initial valve replacement with cloth-covered Starr-Edwards prostheses. Br. Heart. J., *40*:612, 1978.

Fuqua, J. M., Jr., Igo, S. R., Hibbs, C. W., et al.: Development and evaluation of electrically activated abdominal left ventricular assist systems for long-term use. J. Thorac. Cardiovasc. Surg., *81*:718, 1981.

Gans, H.: Thrombogenic properties of epsilon-aminocaproic acid. Ann. Surg., *163*:175, 1966.

Gans, H., and Castaneda, A. R.: Problems in hemostasis during open-heart surgery. VIII. Changes in fibrinogen concentration during and after cardiopulmonary bypass with particular reference to the effect of heparin in neutralization of fibrinogen. Ann. Surg., *165*:551, 1967.

Gralnick, H. R., and Fischer, R. D.: The hemostatic response to open-heart operations. J. Thorac. Cardiovasc. Surg., *61*:909, 1971.

Gupta, S. K., and Veith, F. J.: Three year experience with expanded polytetrafluoroethylene arterial grafts for limb salvage. Am. J. Surg., *140*:214, 1980.

Harker, L. A., and Slichter, S. J.: Platelet and fibrinogen consumption in man. N. Engl. J. Med., *287*:999, 1972.

Harker, L. A., and Slichter, S. J.: Studies of platelet and fibrinogen kinetics in patients with prosthetic heart valves. N. Engl. J. Med., *283*:1302, 1970.

Harker, L. A., Slichter, S. J., and Sauvage, L. R.: Platelet consumption by arterial prostheses: The effects of endothelialization and pharmacologic inhibition of platelet function. Ann. Surg., *186*:594, 1977.

Hetzer, R., Hill, J. D., and Kerth, W. J.: Thromboembolic complications after mitral valve replacement with Hancock xenograft. J. Thorac. Cardiovasc. Surg., *75*:651, 1978.

Hill, J. D., Aguiler, M. J., Baranco, A., et al.: Neuropathological manifestations of cardiac surgery. Ann. Thorac. Surg., *7*:409, 1969.

Hirsh, J., Glynn, M. F., and Mustard, J. F.: The effect of platelet age on platelet adherence to collagen. J. Clin. Invest., *47*:466, 1968.

Hougie, C.: Practical considerations in the control of bleeding associated with extracorporeal circulation. Proc. Soc. Exp. Biol. Med., *98*:130, 1958.

Hynes, K. J., Gau, G. T., Rutherford, B. D., et al.: Effect of aspirin in brachial artery occlusion following brachial arteriotomy for coronary arteriography. Circulation, *47*:544, 1973.

Isom, O. W., Williams, D., Falk, E. A., et al.: Evaluation of anticoagulant therapy in cloth-covered prosthetic valves. Circulation, 48(Suppl. 3):48, 1973.

Jacobsson, B.: Use of dextran in prophylaxis against thromboembolic complications in arterial catheterization. Acta Chir. Scand. (Suppl.), 387:103, 1968.

Jamieson, W. R. E., Munro, A. I., and Allen, P.: Study of porcine xenograft replacement without long-term anticoagulants. (Abstract.) Ann. R. Coll. Phys. Surg. Can., 10:36, 1977.

Jobes, D. R., Schwartz, A. J., Ellison, N., et al: Monitoring heparin anticoagulation and its neutralization. Ann. Thorac. Surg., 31:161, 1981.

Kaegi, A., Pineo, G. F., Shimize, A., et al.: Arteriovenous-shunt thrombosis. Prevention by sulfinpyrazone. N. Engl. J. Med., 290:304, 1974.

Karp, R. B., Cyrus, R. J., Blackstone, E. H., et al.: The Bjork-Shiley valve: Intermediate-term follow-up. J. Thorac. Cardiovasc. Surg., 81:602, 1981.

Karpatkin, S.: Heterogenicity of human platelets. I. Metabolic and kinetic evidence suggestive of young and old platelets. J. Clin. Invest., 48:1073, 1969.

Kjellstrand, C. M., and Buselmeier, T. J.: A simple method for anticoagulation during pre- and post-operative hemodialysis, avoiding rebound phenomenon. Surgery, 72:630, 1972.

Kohanna, F., and Salzman, E. W.: Surgical bleeding and hemostasis. In Basic Surgery. Edited by H. Polk et al. New York, Appleton-Century-Crofts, 1983.

Kohanna, F., Ransil, B., Smith, M. S., et al.: Sex difference in heparin induced platelet aggregation in whole blood. (Abstract.) Thromb. Haemost., 46:378, 1981.

Kolff, W. J., Hershgold, E. J., Hadfield, C., et al.: The improving hematologic picture in long-term surviving calves with total artificial hearts. Artif. Organs, 3:97, 1979.

Kozloff, L., Rich, N. M., Brott, W. H., et al: Vascular trauma secondary to diagnostic and therapeutic procedures: Cardiopulmonary bypass and intra-aortic balloon assist. Am. J. Surg., 140:302, 1980.

Lipton, M. J., Doherty, P. W., Goodwin, D. A., et al.: Evaluation of catheter thrombogenicity in vivo with indium-labelled platelets. Radiology, 135:191, 1980.

Long, D. M., Jr., Sanchez, L., Varco, R. L., et al.: The use of low molecular weight dextran and serum albumin as plasma expanders in extracorporeal circulation. Surgery, 50:12, 1961.

Lyman, D. J., Metcalf, L. C., Albo, D., Jr., et al.: The effect of chemical structure and surface properties of synthetic polymers on the coagulation of blood. III. In-vivo adsorption of proteins onto polymer surfaces. Trans. Am. Soc. Artif. Intern. Organs, 20:474, 1974.

Macmanus, Q., Grunkemeier, G., Thomas, D., et al.: The Starr-Edwards Model 6000 valve. Circulation, 56:623, 1977.

Maher, J. F., Lapierre, L., Schreiner, G. E., et al.: Regional heparinization for hemodialysis. N. Engl. J. Med., 268:451, 1963.

McNeill, R.: Internal jugular vein thrombosis. Head Neck Surg., 3:247, 1981.

Merrill, E. W., Salzman, E. W., Sa da Costa, V., et al.: Molecular factors in blood polymer interactions: Hydrophobic, hydrophilic, hydrogen bonding and aromatic. AIChE Symposium, 1981.

Moore, C. H., Wolma, F. J., Brown, R. W., et al.: Complications of cardiovascular radiology. A review of 1204 cases. Am. J. Surg., 120:591, 1970.

Mortensen, J. D.: Evaluation of tests for blood damage produced by oxygenators. Trans. Am. Soc. Artif. Intern. Organs, 23:747, 1977.

Murashita, J., Nakagaki, M., and Taguchi, K.: On the local heparinization of the artificial heart pump. Blood Vessels, 9:224, 1978.

Neubauer, O., and Lampert, H. A.: A new blood transfusion apparatus. Munch. Med. Wochenschr., 77:582, 1930.

Nuutinen, L. S., Pihlajaniemi, R., Soavela, E., et al.: The effect of dipyridamole on the thrombocyte count and bleeding tendency in open-heart surgery. J. Thorac. Cardiovasc. Surg., 74:295, 1977.

Nyman, D., Thurnherr, N., and Duckert, F.: Heparin dosage in extracorporeal circulation and its neutralization. Thromb. Diath. Haemorrh., 33:102, 1974.

Oblath, R. W., Buckley, F. O., Jr., Green, R. M., et al.: Prevention of platelet aggregation and adherence to prosthetic vascular grafts by aspirin and dipyridamole. Surgery, 84:37, 1978.

O'Brien, P. F., Savidge, G. F., and Williams, B.: Heparin and antithrombin III levels during cardiopulmonary bypass surgery — a pilot study. (Abstract.) Thromb. Haemost., 46:214, 1981.

Oyer, P. E., Stinson, E. B., Reitz, B. A., et al.: Long-term evaluation of porcine xenograft bioprosthesis. J. Thorac. Cardiovasc. Surg., 78:343, 1979.

Pastoriza-Pinol, J. V., McMillan, J., Smith, B. F., et al.: An analysis of micro-embolic particles originating in the extracorporeal circuit before bypass. J. Extracorporeal Technol., 11:221, 1979.

Patterson, R. H., Jr., and Twichell, J. B.: Disposable filter for microemboli. Use in cardiopulmonary bypass and massive transfusion. J.A.M.A., 215:76, 1971.

Perkins, H. A., Osborn, J. J., Hurt, R., et al.: Neutralization of heparin in vivo with protamine; a simple method of estimating the required dose. J. Lab. Clin. Med., 48:223, 1956.

Pifarre, R., Babka, R., Sullivan, H. J., et al.: Management of postoperative heparin rebound following cardiopulmonary bypass. J. Thorac. Cardiovasc. Surg., 81:378, 1981.

Reimers, J. J., Kinlough-Rathbone, R. L., Cazenave, J. P., et al.: In vitro and in vivo functions of thrombin-treated platelets. Thromb. Haemostasis, 35:151, 1976.

Rosenthal, D., Deterling, R. A., Jr., O'Donnell, T. F., et al.: Interposition grafting with expanded polytetrafluoroethylene for portal hypertension. Surgery 148:387, 1979.

Rosoff, C. B., Salzman, E. W., Gurewich, V., et al.: Reduction of platelet serotonin and the response to pulmonary emboli. Surgery, 70:12, 1971.

Rubin, J. W., Moore, V. H., Hillson, R. F., et al.: Thirteen year experience with aortic valve replacement. Am. J. Cardiol., 40:345, 1977.

Salomon, N. W., Stinson, E. B., Griepp, R. B., et al.: Mitral valve replacement: Long-term evaluation of prosthesis-related mortality and morbidity. Circulation, 56(Suppl. 3):94, 1977.

Salzman, E. W.: Platelets, drugs and prosthetic surfaces. In Platelets, Drugs and Thrombosis. Edited by J. Hirsh. Basel, S. Karger, 1975, p. 226.

Salzman, E. W., Lindon, J., Brier, D., et al.: Surface-induced platelet adhesion, aggregation, and release. Ann. N.Y. Acad. Sci., 283:114, 1977.

Salzman, E. W., Silane, M., Lindon, J., et al.: Thromboresistance of heparin-coated surfaces. In Chemistry and Biology of Heparin. Edited by R. L. Lunderblad, et al. New York, Elsevier North-Holland Inc., 1981, p. 435.

Sauvage, L. R., Berger, K., Wood, S. J., et al.: Interspecies healing of porous arterial prostheses: Observations, 1960–1974. Arch. Surg., 109:698, 1974.

Sauvage, L. R., Berger, K., Beilin, L., et al.: Presence of endothelium in an axillary-femoral graft of knitted Dacron with an external velour surface. Ann. Surg., 182:749, 1975.

Sawyer, P. N., and Pate, J. W.: Bioelectric phenomena as an etiologic factor in intra-vascular thrombosis. Am. J. Physiol., 175:103, 1953.

Shattil, S. J., and Bennett, J. S.: Platelets and their membranes in hemostasis: Physiology and pathophysiology. Ann. Intern. Med., 94:108, 1981.

Silane, M., Lindon, J. N., Ransil, B. J., et al.: Platelet aggregation induced in vivo by heparin and heparin fractions. Thromb. Haemost., 46:194, 1981.

Smith, B., Omeri, M. A., Melrose, D. G., et al.: Blood loss after cardiopulmonary bypass. Lancet, 2:273, 1964.

Sobel, M., and Salzman, E. W.: Hemorrhagic and thrombotic complications after cardiac surgery. In Thoracic and Cardiovascular Surgery. 4th Ed. Edited by A. Bane and A. Geha. New York, Appleton-Century-Crofts, 1982.

Solis, R. T., and Gibbs, M. B.: Filtration of the microaggregates in stored blood. Transfusion, 12:245, 1972.

Stanley, T. H., and Kolff, W. J.: Effects of smooth vs. Dacron-lined Silastic artificial hearts on RBC destruction, blood proteins, and peripheral embolization. Surg. Forum, 24:171, 1973.

Starr, A., Grunkemeier, G. L., Lambert, L. E., et al.: Aortic valve replacement: A ten-year follow-up of non-cloth-covered vs. cloth-covered caged-ball prostheses. Circulation, 56(Suppl. 2):133, 1977.

Starr, A., Grunkemeier, G., Lambert, L., et al.: Mitral valve replacement. A ten-year follow-up of non-cloth-covered vs. cloth-covered caged-ball prostheses. Circulation, 54(Suppl. 3):47, 1976.

Stinson, E. B., Griepp, R. B., Oyer, P. E., et al.: Long-term experience with porcine aortic valve xenografts. J. Thorac. Cardiovasc. Surg. 73:54, 1977.

Subramanian, V. A., Goldstein, J. E., Sos, T. A., et al.: Preliminary clinical experience with percutaneous intraaortic balloon pumping. Circulation, 62(Suppl. 1):123, 1980.

Sullivan, J. M., Harken, D. E., and Gorlin, R.: Pharmacologic control of thromboembolic complications of cardiac valve replacement. N. Engl. J. Med., 279:576, 1968.

Torosian, M., Michelson, E. L., Morganroth, J., et al.: Aspirin- and Coumadin-related bleeding after coronary artery bypass graft surgery. Ann. Intern. Med., 89:325, 1978.

Towne, J. B., Bernhard, V. M., Hussey, C., et al.: White clot syndrome. Arch. Surg., 114:372, 1979.

Umlas, J.: Fibrinolysis and disseminated intravascular coagulation in open-heart surgery. Transfusion, 16:460, 1976.

Wallace, S., Medellin, H., DeJongh, D., et al.: Systemic heparinization for angiography. Am. J. Roentgenol. Radium Ther. Nucl. Med., 116:204, 1972.

Weily, H. S., and Genton, E.: Altered platelet function in patients with prosthetic mitral valves. Effects of sulfinpyrazone therapy. Circulation, 42:967, 1970.

Weily, H. S., Steele, P. P., Davies, H., et al.: Platelet survival in patients with substitute heart valves. N. Engl. J. Med., 290:534, 1974.

Williams, J. B., Karp, R. B., Kirklin, J. W., et al.: Considerations in selection and management of patients undergoing valve replacement with glutaraldehyde-fixed porcine bioprostheses. Ann. Thorac. Surg., 30:247, 1980.

Wisch, N., Litwak, R. S., Luckban, S. B., et al.: Hematologic complications of open-heart surgery. Am. J. Cardiol., 31:282, 1973.

Woods, H. F., Ash, G., Weston, M. J., et al.: Prostacyclin can replace heparin in haemodialysis in dogs. Lancet, 2:1075, 1978.

Zervas, N. T., Kuwayama, A., Rosoff, C. B., et al.: Cerebral arterial spasm. Arch. Neurol., 28:400, 1973.

Zucker, M. B., and Vroman, L. Platelet adhesion induced by Fibrogen absorbed onto glass. Proc. Soc. Exp. Biol. Med., 131:318, 1969.

Chapter 48

Acquired Disease of the Aortic Valve

IVAN K. CROSBY

WILLIAM H. MULLER, JR.

Surgery for acquired heart disease was first performed in 1896, when Rehn successfully repaired a stab wound of the heart (Rehn, 1897). In 1914, Tuffier reported six experimental aortic and pulmonary valvulotomies and described the first attempt to correct human aortic stenosis by digital dilatation of the aortic valve through the aortic wall. Thereafter, with the exception of chronic constrictive pericarditis, the efforts of cardiac surgery were directed largely to the management of cardiac wounds and a few pioneering efforts in procedures for mitral stenosis (Cutler and Beck, 1929).

During World War II, a number of successful cardiac procedures were performed to repair cardiac injuries and remove intracardiac foreign bodies. Since then, cardiac surgery and the management of acquired diseases of the aortic valve have progressed rapidly. In 1952, Bailey and associates devised an operation for the relief of aortic stenosis, using transventricular dilatation with a mechanical dilator to separate the fused valvular commissures. The following year, Hufnagel and Harvey (1953) inserted a plastic ball valve in the descending aorta, thereby reducing aortic regurgitation by approximately 75 per cent.

The development of the pump-oxygenator by Gibbon and associates in 1954 opened a new vista in the management of aortic valvular disease. This permitted accurate valvulotomy and removal of calcium deposits for the treatment of aortic stenosis, as well as reconstructive procedures for the treatment of aortic insufficiency. It soon became apparent, however, that simple debridement and valvulotomy were inadequate for the management of many patients with aortic valvular stenosis, and many valves were not suitable for commissurotomy alone; further relief of severe stenosis was achieved by excision of the most severely diseased leaflet and replacement with a prosthetic leaflet. Bahnson and colleagues (1960), Harken and coworkers (1960), McGoon (1961), and Lillehei and associates (1961) reported successful partial prosthetic replacements of the aortic valve; however, results of partial valvular replacement were still suboptimal in many cases, and in the latter part of 1958, Lillehei and Muller both replaced the entire aortic valve with a prosthesis (Lillehei et al., 1961; Muller et al., 1961).

Starr's original ball valve prosthesis, developed in 1960, was a significant advance in aortic valvular replacement surgery (Starr et al., 1963), but all of the early mechanical or tissue valve substitutes have been abandoned or have undergone multiple modifications because of structural failure or embolic complications. Some mechanical prostheses have withstood 12 to 16 years of clinical experience in terms of function and durability, and with better techniques of tissue valve preparation and preservation, encouraging results of valve replacement with heterograft valve substitutes have been experienced over the last 7 to 10 years. Thus, with better valve substitutes currently available and superior techniques for myocardial protection being used almost universally, the morbidity and mortality associated with aortic valve replacement have been progressively reduced.

ANATOMY AND FUNCTION OF THE AORTIC VALVE

The aortic valve, situated at the junction of the left ventricular outflow tract in the ascending aorta, consists of three pocket-like cusps, or leaflets: the right and left coronary cusps and the posterior or noncoronary cusp. Each cusp forms a truncated parabola (Nolan and Muller, 1981). Between the cusps themselves and the aortic wall lie three cavities, the sinuses of Valsalva, whose distal limits extend to the uppermost attachment of the commissures. The coronary arteries arise in the upper third of those sinuses formed by the right and left coronary cusps. Analysis of normal and abnormal cardiac cycles in the animal laboratory demonstrated that when the ventricular pressure equalled the aortic pressure, in the normal expansile aortic root, the commissures expand 10 per cent and the valve opens with a stellate orifice before the onset of forward flow and without a rise in aortic pressure (Thubrikar et al., 1979, 1980).

With the beginning of ejection, all three cusps rapidly retract to form a triangular orifice. Eddy currents within the sinuses of Valsalva cause a slow wave-like motion of the free edge and billowing of the base of each cusp, thus preventing occlusion of the coronary ostia and maintaining a posture that allows slight reversal of flow to result in immediate closure without regurgitation (Nolan and Muller, 1981).

Diastolic blood flow, which accounts for 80 per cent of the total coronary blood flow, is enhanced by increased aortic pressure and decreased intramural pressure of the ventricles. When left ventricular pressure exceeds aortic pressure, however, systolic left ventricular ejection occurs; diastolic blood flow is retarded by increased right atrial and intraventricular pressures. The forward pressure gradient ceases during the first half of systole; forward flow is maintained thereafter by a mass-acceleration effect. Closure of the normal aortic valve is accompanied by reversal of the flow, rather than by reversal of the pressure gradient.

During aortic valvular replacement, as the leaflets are excised, one can see the anterior leaflet of the mitral valve extending up to the aortic anulus. The ventricular septum appears in the area of the comissure between the right and noncoronary cusps, and below the noncoronary cusp.

ETIOLOGY OF AORTIC VALVULAR DISEASE

Rheumatic Valvular Aortic Stenosis

Rheumatic fever, characterized by pancarditis and specific involvement of the heart valves, begins with inflammation and swelling of the aortic anulus, extending throughout the cusps and causing valvulitis (Friedberg, 1966). The cusps become thickened by edema, capillary vascularization, and cellular infiltration (predominantly lymphocytes and occasionally polymorphonuclear leukocytes). Verrucae, which may be present when the disease is active, consist of wartlike vegetations of hyaline eosinophilic material, resulting from swollen, degenerated collagen and disintegrated cells near the valvular surface.

The inflammatory exudate produces thickening and deformity of the valve and commissural fusion between the adjacent cusps (Friedberg, 1966). Adherence usually begins at the less mobile portion of the cusps where they are attached to the aortic wall. The cusps become thickened and fixed into position and ultimately fuse to form a solid ring, resulting in a small triangular or irregular aperture in the center of the valve and leading to stenosis as well as insufficiency (Fig. 48–1A). Significant symptoms appear clinically only when the normal valvular area of 3 cm.^{2} is reduced to 0.5 cm.^{2} or less (Friedberg, 1966). Occasionally, inordinate fusion of the right and left cusps creates an apparent bicuspid valve, resembling a congenitally bicuspid valve. Calcification is usually more pronounced in the anterior cusps (Friedberg, 1966).

Rheumatic aortic stenosis may be associated with disease of the mitral or tricuspid valve. Severe mitral stenosis may reduce the systolic pressure gradient across the aortic valve, partially masking evidence of aortic stenosis.

Subacute Bacterial Endocarditis

Subacute or acute bacterial endocarditis involving the aortic valve usually causes aortic regurgitation and may occur in patients who have had rheumatic valvulitis (Friedberg, 1966) or who have a predominantly abnormal aortic valve (e.g., a bicuspid valve), in perennial drug-abuse patients, and even in some patients with normal aortic valvular architecture (Silber and Katz, 1975).

Valvular vegetations develop and, if large enough, may prevent accurate apposition of the cusps and closure of the aortic orifice. Frequently, the bacterial process erodes the valvular substance, producing either an aneurysm or perforation of the cusp, thereby creating or intensifying valvular insufficiency (Silber and Katz, 1975).

Nontraumatic rupture of an aortic valve is usually due to bacterial endocarditis but occurs rarely with syphilitic aortitis or in rheumatic or atheromatous valves. Perforation of a leaflet in bacterial endocarditis causes a change in the character of the diastolic murmur (Fig. 48–2A). Progressive congestive heart

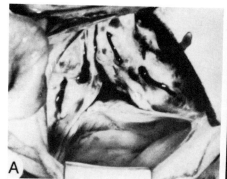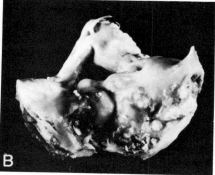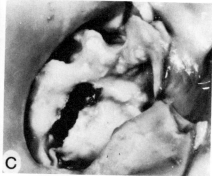

Figure 48–1. *A,* Fusion of all three commissures secondary to rheumatic valvulitis results in a central triangular orifice. The exposure of this valve at surgery reveals the calcific degeneration of the cusps. *B,* The valvular leaflets are calcified, and the sinus areas are filled with calcific aggregations that extend to involve adjacent aortic root structures. This valve is typical of idiopathic calcific aortic stenosis. *C,* The excessive calcific degeneration in this functionally bicuspid valve extends to involve the supravalvular and infravalvular structures. The normally pliable aortic valve has been transformed into an immobile bony shelf with an eccentric fixed orifice.

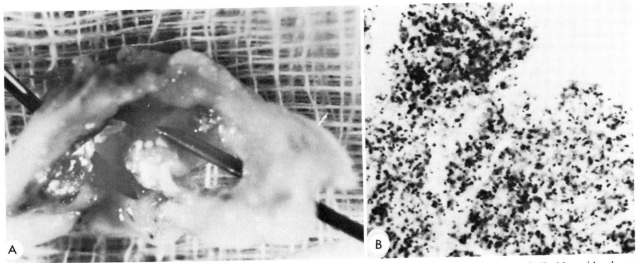

Figure 48–2. *A,* Probes are inserted through two large perforations in the noncoronary leaflet of a congenitally bicuspid valve with severe aortic regurgitation; the vegetations of bacterial endocarditis on the valve are obvious. *B,* A high-powered photomicrograph of a valve excised at operation in a patient after a long course of antibiotics shows multiple gram-positive cocci present within the substance of the valve.

failure secondary to aortic regurgitation is a common cause of death in this disease; however, valvular destruction resulting in precipitous heart failure is the most common cause of death today (Manhas *et al.,* 1970; Crosby *et al.,* 1973; Silber and Katz, 1975). Emboli from vegetations, mycotic aneurysms, and septicemia also account for some deaths.

Two-dimensional echocardiography can describe the movement of all aortic cusps, can measure any vegetations present on the valve, and can indicate whether the aortic valve anulus is normal or involved with abscess formation.

Until recently, a 6-week course of antibiotics was believed to be imperative prior to valvular replacement (Friedberg, 1966). During this interval, some patients died from intractable heart failure. Currently, a more aggressive short course of antibiotics prior to surgery has yielded improved overall results in the treatment of bacterial endocarditis (Crosby *et al.,* 1973; Silber and Katz, 1975). Even when the patient is afebrile and has had an appropriate course of antibiotics, organisms may be seen within the substance of the excised valve on microscopic examination (Fig. 48–2*B*); thus, prolongation of antibiotic therapy for 6 weeks is indicated, especially for organisms relatively resistant to medications (Silber and Katz, 1975).

Syphilis

Syphilitic valvular disease, infrequently seen in the United States today despite the increase in venereal disease generally, begins in the aorta around the vasa vasorum (Friedberg, 1966). Initially, a perivascular cellular infiltration compromises the nutrient vessels, destroying the muscular and elastic layers of the tunica media as well as roughening the intima. Valvular dysfunction occurs when the process affects

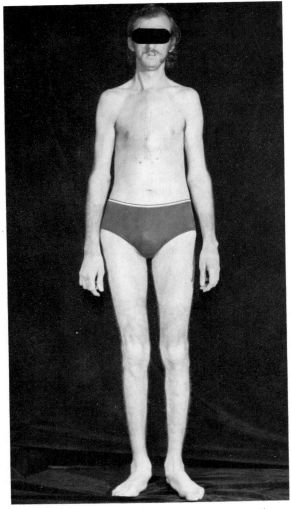

Figure 48–3. All the classic stigmata of Marfan's disease are present in this 6-foot, 7-inch man who presented with acute total aortic dissection.

the aortic root, resulting in dilatation of the valvular ring and widening of the commissures (Friedberg, 1966). The cusps may be everted, retracted, stiffened, and shortened, and the most common result is aortic insufficiency. Since the coronary ostia are narrowed, coronary insufficiency occurs in many of these patients (Friedberg, 1966; Silber and Katz, 1975). A review of 258 autopsy reports of aortic regurgitation indicated that syphilis accounts for less than 5 per cent of such cases (Barondess and Sande, 1969).

Traumatic Aortic Valvular Disease

Aortic valvular regurgitation, the most common traumatic valvular lesion, occurs infrequently (Friedberg, 1966). Although the aortic valve is injured more often than any other cardiac valve, the only types of injury causing aortic regurgitation, other than penetrating wounds, are those produced by unusually strenuous effort or direct trauma, such as a heavy blow to the chest wall or a fall from a tree (Levine *et al.*, 1962; Friedberg, 1966). Injury presumably occurs when the ventricles are in early diastole and the aortic

valve is under maximal tension; usually, a single cusp is torn from its commissural attachment. Traumatic regurgitation may also be caused by a penetrating wound to the heart. Such cases usually involve a linear opening in the cusp. Occasionally, more than one cusp may be affected. Although the ruptured valve or aorta usually has some pre-existing disease such as syphilis or bacterial endocarditis, the normal aortic valve may also rupture (Friedberg, 1966).

Clinically, traumatic aortic regurgitation is characterized by a sudden onset of chest pain, a musical diastolic murmur, signs of free aortic regurgitation, and progressive intractable heart failure.

Marfan's Syndrome

This heritable disorder is characterized by myxoid degeneration of the medial layer of the aorta, which contains stellate cells surrounded by basophilic ground substance in the loose myxomatous stroma (Muller *et al.*, 1960; Friedberg, 1966). The classic features include a tall, slim physique; elongated arms and legs; long, tapering fingers; hyperextensibility of the joints;

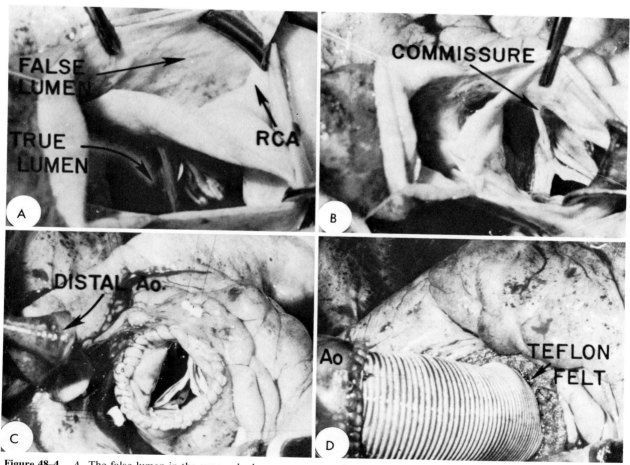

Figure 48–4. *A,* The false lumen in the supravalvular area causes prolapse of the valvular suspensory apparatus, resulting in aortic valvular regurgitation (RCA = right coronary artery). *B,* Resuspension of the commissure reveals a normal trileaflet aortic valve. *C,* A continuous 5-0 suture coapts the two layers of the proximal aorta, and pledgeted sutures at the commissures resuspend the aortic valve (Distal Ao. = distal aorta). *D,* A layer of Teflon felt externally is included in the proximal suture line and adds strength to the prosthetic graft insertion. (Ao. = distal aorta).

pectus deformity of the thorax; subluxation of the lens of the eye with a predisposition to ultimate blindness; a high arched palate (Silber and Katz, 1975); as well as such cardiovascular anomalies as aortic regurgitation and ascending aortic aneurysm, with a peculiar predisposition to aortic dissection (Friedberg, 1966). If all these classic stigmata are present, the condition is called Marfan's syndrome (Fig. 48–3); when aortic insufficiency and ascending aortic aneurysm occur, with cystic medial necrosis and none of the other classic stigmata, the condition is termed the "forme fruste" or incomplete form of Marfan's syndrome (Golden and Lakin, 1959). Cystic medial necrosis per se is not pathognomonic of Marfan's syndrome; rather, it is a degenerative change in the aortic wall and can occur in otherwise normal individuals more than 40 years of age (Friedberg, 1966).

Two manifestations of Marfan's syndrome are (1) progressive aneurysmal dilatation of the ascending aorta secondary to cystic medial necrosis, resulting in gradual anular dilatation and secondary valvular regurgitation, and (2) dissecting aneurysm or hematoma of the ascending aorta, frequently resulting in acute aortic regurgitation (Friedberg, 1966).

Initial corrective procedures involved the creation of a bicuspid valve by excision of the noncoronary leaflet (Muller *et al.*, 1960) and replacement of the ascending aorta with a woven prosthetic graft. If dissection is present but the aortic valve is not involved, prosthetic replacement of the aorta at the site of the intimal tear, converting the distal double lumen to a single lumen, will suffice (Fig. 48–4). However, if regurgitation is secondary to retrograde extension of the dissection and/or valvular disease, then both the valve and the ascending aorta must be replaced (Bentall and DeBono, 1968; Edwards and Kerr, 1970). Earlier attempts at this combined replacement entailed the usual subcoronary insertion of the prosthetic valve and attachment of the ascending aorta prosthetic graft to a rim of aortic wall 2 cm. above the valvular anulus, so that the coronary ostia were left undisturbed (Symbas *et al.*, 1970). This left a remnant of diseased aortic wall that could undergo progressive dilatation and eventually cause death. Currently, a more aggressive approach entails a suturing of the tubular prosthetic graft directly to the prosthetic valvular rims before the prosthetic valve is inserted in the normal subcoronary position. Two windows in this tubular graft are sutured to the right and left coronary ostia (Figs. 48–5 and 48–6). By this technique, the proximal aorta is totally replaced from the valvular anulus to a point

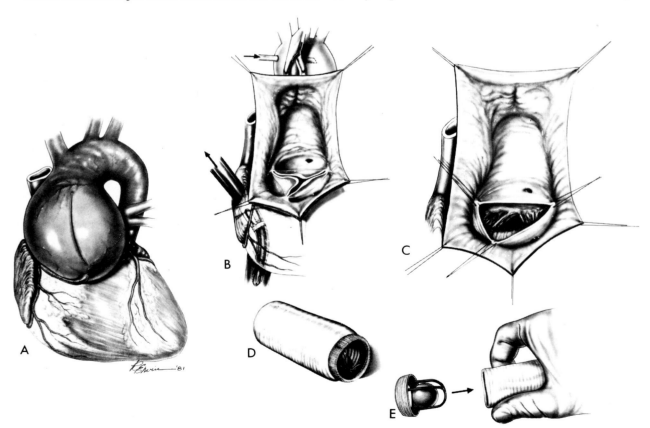

Figure 48–5. *A,* The pulmonary artery and the superior vena cava are obscured by the aneurysm of the ascending aorta. *B,* With the patient on cardiopulmonary bypass and the aneurysm opened, the anular dilatation that prevents coaptation of the valvular leaflets is obvious. In some patients, organic valvular disease (thickening and shrinkage of the leaflets) can be an additive cause of valvular regurgitation. *C,* With the valve excised, the traction sutures through the commissures reveal the true size of the dilated anulus and display the subvalvular anatomy. *D,* A composite valve–tubular graft prosthesis utilizing the Bjork-Shiley tilting disc valve simplifies the surgical procedure. *E,* Some surgeons prefer to manufacture their own composite prosthesis by sewing a Starr-Edwards Model 1260 valve to a tubular graft.

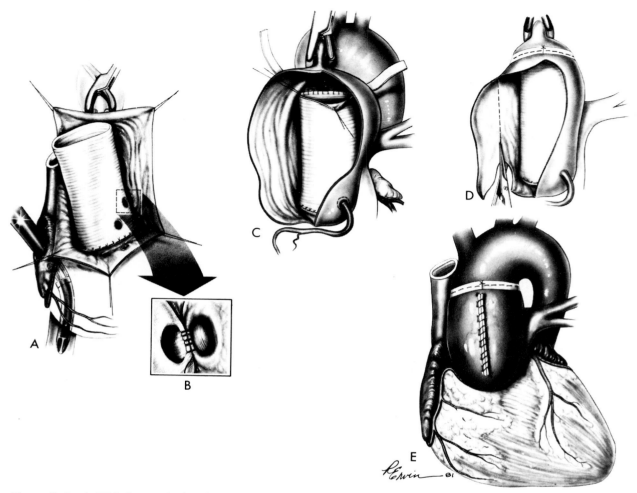

Figure 48–6. *A,* With the prosthetic valve secured in the subcoronary position, two windows are created by electrocautery in the tubular prosthesis for anastomosis to the coronary ostia. *B,* A continuous suture technique utilizing 4-0 or 5-0 monofilament suture material provides excellent hemostasis in anastomosing the coronary ostium to the window in the tubular prosthesis. *C,* The distal end of the tubular graft is anastomosed to the distal aorta from inside the aneurysm. Strips of Teflon felt externally, especially in cases of acute aortic dissection, add strength and hemostasis to this anastomosis. *D,* With all anastomoses completed, the redundant wall of the aneurysm is trimmed and wrapped around the composite prosthesis externally. The excellence of the hemostasis in the aortic root area and of both coronary ostial anastomoses should be checked prior to sewing the aneurysm wall over the composite prosthesis. *E,* With the reconstruction completed, the reduction in bulk of the ascending aorta can be dramatic and allows visualization of the pulmonary artery and the superior vena cava.

just proximal to the origin of the innominate artery (Bentall and DeBono, 1968; Edwards and Kerr, 1970; Crosby *et al.,* 1973).

Calcific Aortic Valvular Disease

Congenital Aortic Valvular Disease. In adult life, congenital anomalies of the aortic valve usually become calcified and often produce acquired stenosis. A bicuspid valve, the most common congenital valvular anomaly, may have no initial dysfunction or may be associated with aortic regurgitation. The incidence and degree of calcification of the congenitally anomalous valve increase with age; calcification is present therefore in a large majority of these patients by the age of 20 years and in virtually all by the age of 30 years (Friedberg, 1966). Of 162 patients over the age of 15 years dying of aortic stenosis, Roberts (1973)

found that 52 per cent had congenital valvular deformities.

Congenital aortic stenosis may occur with other cardiac lesions, particularly patent ductus arteriosus and coarctation of the aorta (Friedberg, 1966). The pathologic configuration of a congenitally deformed valve may also be obscured by subsequent calcific degenerative changes, atheromatous superimposition, or secondary bacterial endocarditis. In severely diseased valves, it may be difficult to distinguish between a congenitally bicuspid valve and one that is bicuspid secondary to rheumatic inflammation with leaflet fusion (see Fig. 48–1*C*); however, in the latter case, characteristic pathologic rheumatic stigmata sometimes may be found. Calcific aortic stenosis has been described following bacterial endocarditis (Friedberg, 1966; Silber and Katz, 1975).

The congenitally stenotic aortic valve treated by valvulotomy in infancy or childhood usually becomes calcified in later life (Friedberg, 1966) and often requires replacement.

Idiopathic Calcific Valvular Aortic Stenosis. Although rheumatic fever has been presumed to cause calcific aortic stenosis in the majority of patients, there is doubt as to the frequency of this relationship in patients over 50 years of age (Friedberg, 1966). It seems probable that in many instances, calcific aortic stenosis is secondary to aging, degeneration, and atherosclerosis. It appears unlikely that rheumatic valvular disease would first produce a cardiac murmur after middle age, unless the patient has a definite history of rheumatic fever in adult life (Friedberg, 1966).

Calcification may involve structures adjacent to aortic cusps and the sinuses of Valsalva (see Fig. 48–1*B*) and may extend by way of the intervalvular fibrosis, like the extension of luetic aortitis, to involve the anterior leaflet of the mitral valve, the bundle of His in the interventricular septum, or, occasionally, the mitral anulus (Friedberg, 1966) (see Fig. 48–1*C*). Other, less frequent complications include coronary atherosclerosis and myocardial infarction. Therefore, the diagnostic work-up of patients with aortic stenosis should include two-dimensional echocardiographic visualization of the aortic and mitral valves, left heart catheterization, left ventricular function studies (either ventriculography or gated blood pool scan), and, in patients over 30 years of age, coronary arteriography (Triestman and El-Said, 1975).

PATHOPHYSIOLOGY OF AORTIC STENOSIS

Hemodynamic Alterations

Left heart catheterization in valvular aortic stenosis reveals on catheter pull-back a gradient between the systolic pressure in the left ventricle and that in the ascending aorta. This gradient varies, depending on the degree of stenosis, but in patients with severe aortic stenosis, the gradient may range from 90 to 180 mm. Hg. When no regurgitation is present, elevation of the ventricular end-diastolic pressure is often an early sign of left ventricular failure (Friedberg, 1966); indeed, when left ventricular failure is established, the gradient across the valve may fall, as the myocardial contractility is no longer able to maintain the high interventricular pressure. In patients with both systolic and diastolic aortic murmurs, left heart catheterization may demonstrate a significant gradient across the aortic valve, and a root aortogram will illustrate the degree of insufficiency; this is termed a mixed lesion. Simultaneous monitoring of the left ventricular and aortic pressures demonstrates the gradient across the aortic valve (Fig. 48–7).

Pathologic Changes

Classically, there is enormous concentric hypertrophy of the left ventricular muscle, without significant dilatation of the ventricular chamber. The heart itself may be greatly enlarged, and when cardiac failure occurs, dilatation of the left ventricular chamber develops, as well as dilatation and hypertrophy of the right atrium and right ventricle. A "jet" lesion, produced by blood streaming through the stenotic orifice and striking the aortic wall, may result in local thickening and fibrosis in the ascending aorta (Friedberg, 1966). In long-standing severe aortic stenosis, significant poststenotic dilatation of the proximal ascending aorta usually occurs (Friedberg, 1966).

Clinical Features

The patient with moderate or moderately severe aortic stenosis may be entirely asymptomatic. However, dizziness is a significant symptom of advanced stenosis, and syncope may even lead to sudden death (Friedberg, 1966; Silber and Katz, 1975). Many patients present with nocturnal dyspnea or pulmonary edema as a manifestation of their left ventricular failure. Severe angina pectoris in the presence of a normal coronary arterial circulation has also been documented (Friedberg, 1966); however, concomitant coronary artery disease may be partly responsible for the angina. Complete heart block, bundle branch block, or intraventricular conduction delay frequently is associated with calcific aortic stenosis and may be related to extension of calcification from the aortic valve onto the fibrous septum (Friedberg, 1966).

PATHOPHYSIOLOGY OF AORTIC REGURGITATION

Hemodynamic Alterations

The size of the regurgitant orifice and the amount of pressure between the ascending aorta and the left ventricle in early diastole are directly proportional to the dynamic effects of aortic regurgitation (Silber and Katz, 1975). The magnitude of the reflux into the left ventricle can be estimated by clinical assessment of

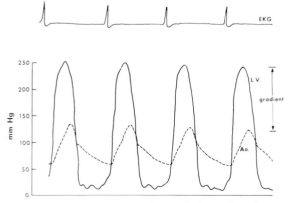

Figure 48–7. Simultaneous left ventricular and aortic pressure tracings reveal a peak-to-peak gradient of 110 mm. Hg across the stenotic aortic valve.

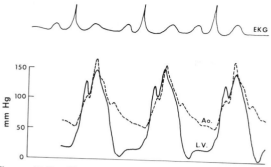

Figure 48–8. Simultaneous left ventricular and aortic pressures fail to demonstrate any gradient across the aortic valve, but the aortic diastolic pressure is approaching the left ventricular end-diastolic pressure in this patient with aortic regurgitation.

the intensity of the regurgitant murmur, the degree of left ventricular thrust, and the roentgenographic size of the left ventricle. Cineangiographic assessment affords an estimation of the regurgitant volume into the left ventricle when dye is injected under pressure into the ascending aorta (Friedberg, 1966). Left heart catheterization with simultaneous pressure recordings in the left ventricle and the ascending aorta (Fig. 48–8) will reveal no gradient across the aortic valve in pure valvular regurgitation, but the diastolic pressure in the ascending aorta will be collapsing and may approximate the left ventricular end-diastolic pressure. Left heart catheterization may reveal a normal left ventricular end-diastolic pressure in patients with compensated regurgitation. However, elevation above 25 mm. Hg is usually present in patients with cardiac failure (Friedberg, 1966).

Pathology

If there is dilatation of the valvular anulus, the leaflets are frequently pliable, thick, and without microscopic evidence of gross disease; in the absence of anular dilatation, there may be perforation, fenestration, thickening, or shrinking of the leaflets or prolapse of a floppy leaflet, preventing adequate central coaptation (Fig. 48–9A). Especially in cases of rheumatic valvulitis, commissural fusion and calcification may be present (Silber and Katz, 1975). The increased stroke volume and workload in aortic regurgitation cause progressive dilatation and hypertrophy of the left ventricle (the so-called ox heart or cor bovinum). The chest roentgenogram reveals a left ventricular contour indicative of gross enlargement (Fig. 48–9B). In long-standing regurgitation, the coronary arteries often appear larger than normal and are usually free of disease.

Clinical Features

Aortic regurgitation is characterized by a prolonged history of minor symptoms, followed by an abrupt onset of congestive heart failure. Precordial chest pain is uncommon in the early stages. Physical examination usually reveals a hyperkinetic circulatory state, accompanied by a left ventricular lift on palpation of the precordium, and an early decrescendo diastolic murmur that is maximal to the left of the sternum in the second intercostal space. Whereas the chest film shows marked left ventricular dilatation, the electrocardiogram demonstrates a strain pattern secondary to the left ventricular dilatation and hypertrophy. Clinical features of advanced disease include angina pectoris (seen in 50 per cent of patients when the aortic diastolic pressure is less than 50 mm. Hg [Friedberg, 1966]) and left ventricular failure; with progressive disease, the symptoms of left heart failure are combined with, or even overshadowed by, those of right ventricular failure (Friedberg, 1966).

Indications for Surgery

In the absence of complicating features, patients with moderate aortic regurgitation may lead a normal life for years with no change in their symptoms.

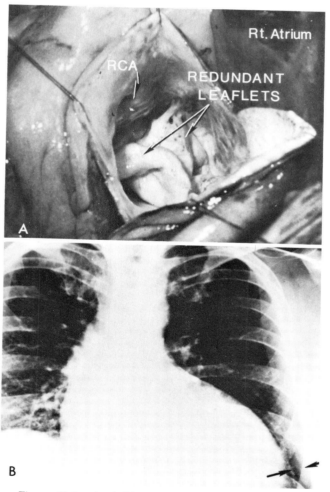

Figure 48–9. *A.* A bicuspid valve with floppy redundant leaflets causes severe aortic regurgitation (Rt. atrium = right atrium; RCA = right coronary artery). *B.* The left ventricular enlargement of the classic "cor bovinum" is so enormous that the ventricular apex almost touches the chest wall laterally (arrows).

Indications for surgery include a progressive increase in cardiac size on serial chest roentgenograms, significant limitation of functional capacity despite digitalis and diuretic therapy, the presence of severe regurgitation (diastolic pressure below 50 mm. Hg) with intolerable angina pectoris, or clinically significant left heart failure or left and right heart failure (Friedberg, 1966). Regurgitation due to bacterial endocarditis or anular dilatation is often progressive, necessitating valvular replacement.

In Segal and associates' study (1956) of 100 cases of severe aortic insufficiency, death occurred an average of 6.5 years after the development of symptoms. After diagnosis, approximately 75 per cent of patients with moderately severe to severe aortic regurgitation will survive for 5 years. Fifty per cent will survive for 10 years. Without surgery, death usually occurs within 5 years after the development of angina and within 2 years after the development of congestive heart failure (Silber and Katz, 1975). Thus, although the need may not be as urgent as in aortic stenosis, surgery should be undertaken before severe or intractable cardiac failure occurs. A decreased cardiac index or a marked increase in left ventricular end-diastolic pressure indicates a poor prognosis for the surgical candidate (Friedberg, 1966).

With the currently lowered mortality rate after aortic valve replacement and with the improvement in valvular substitutes, surgery should be considered for the young person with a normal-sized heart who is unable to perform physically demanding work.

PREOPERATIVE EVALUATION

Patients with symptomatic aortic stenosis, aortic regurgitation, or mixed aortic valvular lesions require critical assessment of their cardiovascular, pulmonary, neurologic, and renal functions prior to surgery. Pulmonary and renal function studies, cardiac roentgenograms, electrocardiograms, and two-dimensional echocardiography are performed routinely prior to cardiac catheterization. Patients considered for valvular replacement should also have coronary arteriography performed at the time of cardiac catheterization. Smoking should be discontinued before surgery, as it predisposes the patients to postoperative atelectasis; abrupt cessation for a few days preoperatively diminishes the circulating carbaminohemoglobin, thus increasing the oxygen-carrying capacity for the critical postoperative period. Carious teeth should be removed prior to valve replacement to prevent bacteriologic seeding of the prosthesis at subsequent dental procedures.

Preoperative physical and respiratory therapy, bathing with a bacteriostatic soap, and prophylactic antibiotics are important considerations. Stabilization of cardiac medications and cessation of digitalis and diuretic therapy 24 to 36 hours prior to surgery are recommended. Antiarrhythmic drugs usually may be discontinued, but coronary artery dilating medications may be continued up to the time of operation. Blood coagulation studies routinely screen any detectable coagulopathy. Psychologic preparation of the patient and his family by interviews with members of the surgical team, nurse practitioners, anesthesiologists, and intensive care unit nursing personnel helps the patient develop a positive attitude toward the operation.

If an ascending aortic aneurysm is suspected, aortography for computed tomography should be performed to delineate the extent of the pathology.

SURGICAL TECHNIQUE

Anesthetic Technique

Modern cardiac anesthetic techniques entail monitoring of the filling pressures of the heart and the cardiac output prior to the induction of anesthesia and during the period of cannulation for bypass. The blood pressure can be stabilized pharmacologically, the left ventricular workload can be reduced by unloading agents, and any electrocardiographic changes suggestive of ischemia can be treated with intraoperative nitroglycerin. This results in a safer induction of anesthesia for the patient, with significantly fewer hypotensive or arrhythmic crises in patients with aortic valvular pathology alone or that associated with advanced coronary occlusive disease. These aggressive anesthetic measures have been efficacious in patients with critically compromised cardiac function.

Cannulation for Extracorporeal Circulation

Refinement of the technology of extracorporeal circulation has led to an overall diminution in mortality and morbidity for patients undergoing open heart surgery in general. For aortic valvular replacement, a right atrial venous return line, in conjunction with an ascending aortic perfusion cannula and a left ventricular vent inserted through the right superior pulmonary vein, constitutes standard cannulation for extracorporeal circulation. The transatrial ventricular vent causes no damage to the hypertrophied left ventricular muscle, obviating occasional troublesome ventricular bleeding and preventable technical problems, as well as avoiding myocardial irritability secondary to manipulation of the hypertrophied left ventricle. Partial occlusion of the venous return after insertion of the prosthetic valve, with the heart beating and the apex of the heart elevated, allows air to be flushed through the left atrium and left ventricle and out of the transatrial ventricular vent.

Myocardial Protection During Cardiopulmonary Bypass

The concentrically hypertrophied, stiff-walled, small-chambered left ventricle associated with critical aortic stenosis requires special attention in terms of myocardial protection techniques during aortic valve replacement. On the other hand, the physical enormity of the 1000-gram "cor bovinum" typical of aortic regurgitation, by its very largeness, also requires careful myocardial protection. Historically, perfusion of one or both coronary arteries by means of rigid or soft cannulas and packing the heart in saline slush have led to more refined techniques of myocardial protection (Friedberg, 1966; Kay et al., 1961; Nolan and Muller, 1981); moderate core hypothermia to 30°C. was usually utilized in conjunction with these techniques. Enthusiasm for ischemic arrest at normothermia was prevalent in many centers in the early 1970s, but because of the obvious deficiencies of this technique, protection of the myocardium by profound hypothermia resulted in safer valve replacement (Mulder et al., 1976).

Cold (4° to 8°C.) cardioplegic myocardial protection is used almost universally at present (Buckberg, 1979; Ebert, 1978; Scott et al., 1978), as this technique allows immediate postbypass restoration of left ventricular function almost to the prebypass level, with only minor changes in left ventricular compliance (Cunningham et al., 1979; Follette et al., 1978). Whether blood or crystalloid cardioplegia is utilized is probably less important; what is of the utmost importance is the monitoring of the degree of myocardial cooling and of the electrical activity of the arrested heart. A thermistor probe inserted in the interventricular septum is a simple means of monitoring the degree of myocardial protection. Cardioplegic solution should be infused until the myocardial temperature is reduced to between 5° and 15°C. (Ebert, 1978, Buckberg, 1979). The use of iced saline at 4°C. in the pericardial well (Landymore et al., 1981) and systemic hypothermia to 20° to 25°C. allow rapid and controlled cooling of the myocardium and extend the safe period for uninterrupted aortic cross-clamping up to 90 minutes or more (Cunningham et al., 1979). This allows the more complicated valvular operations (e.g., multiple valve surgery, valve replacement with multiple coronary revascularization, or anulus enlargement procedures) to be performed with a greater degree of safety.

Valvular Excision and Insertion of a Prosthesis

When the valve is calcified, excision and debridement of the aortic anulus must be done as carefully as possible. The use of a pituitary rongeur to remove calcium from the sinus provides better delineation of the base of the cusp, allowing one to leave a short fibrous rim of 1 to 2 mm. of cusp tissue (Fig. 48–10A,B). When the calcification extends onto the anterior leaflet of the mitral valve or onto the ventricular septum, minimal debridement of these areas should be undertaken to prevent such technical complications as heart block or perforation of the mitral leaflet. Fragments of the calcified valve should be

prevented from falling into either the coronary orifices or the left ventricular chamber.

The various suture techniques utilized to secure the valvular prosthesis in the subcoronary position (Fig. 48–10C,D) include simple, figure-of-eight, or pledgeted mattress sutures. The sutures should not simply encompass the thickened remnant of the diseased cusp but should take a partial bite through the media of the aortic wall.

Concomitant Coronary Revascularization

When the patient undergoing aortic valve replacement has severe coronary occlusive disease, monitoring the interventricular septal temperature is helpful to ensure the adequacy of the myocardial protection. Infusion of cold cardioplegic solution directly into the coronary ostia may be inadequate or ineffective in achieving distal myocardial protection because of the severe proximal coronary occlusions; in this situation, once the heart is arrested, the anterior descending aorta should be immediately revascularized so that additional cardioplegic solution can be infused through the graft to afford greater myocardial protection. Sequential grafting and infusion of cardioplegic solution through the other occluded vessels should be performed prior to the valve replacement. With the prosthesis inserted, the aorta closed, air evacuated from the heart, and the cross-clamp released, the patient can be rewarmed while the vein grafts are anastomosed to the ascending aorta using a partial occlusion clamp.

If the patient is hemodynamically stable, some surgeons prefer to perform the proximal graft anastomoses to the ascending aorta prior to the commencement of cardiopulmonary bypass. Then, with the heart arrested and cooled by cardioplegic infusion, the distal coronary anastomoses are made to the occluded vessels serially, and cardioplegic solution is infused through the proximal graft anastomoses via a cannula. After the valve insertion and closure of the aorta, the oxygen debt is repaid more promptly through the functioning bypass grafts.

POSTOPERATIVE MANAGEMENT

Careful preoperative assessment of all pathology and meticulous intraoperative correction of the pathologic cardiovascular problems utilizing improved myocardial protection techniques have been effective in lowering the morbidity of aortic valve replacement surgery. However, sophisticated around-the-clock postoperative management is an important factor in achieving these better results. The hemodynamic parameters that are monitored in the operating room are continuously analyzed for the first 24 hours postoperatively to optimize cardiac output. Patients with hypertrophy of the left ventricle are particularly susceptible to ventricular arrhythmia; in the early post-

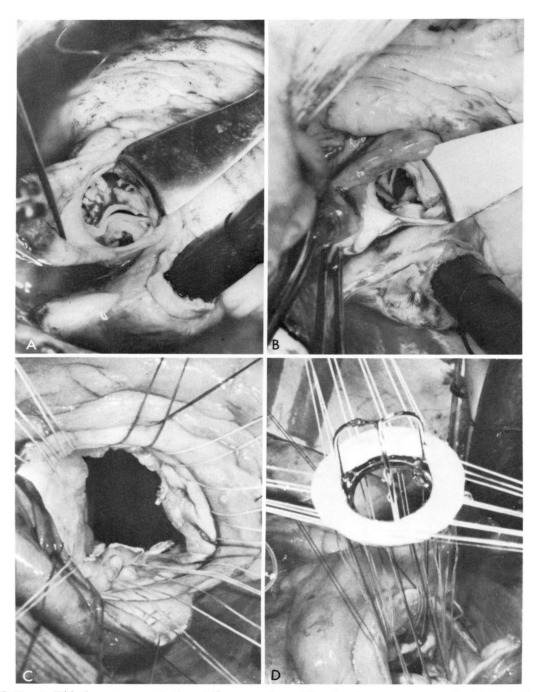

Figure 48–10. *A,* With the aorta opened, the calcific aggregations obliterating the sinus areas can be debrided using a pituitary rongeur. *B,* The valve is then excised in preparation for insertion of the prosthesis. *C,* Interrupted pledgeted mattress sutures are simple and effective for secure fixation of the prosthesis. *D,* After the interrupted sutures have been passed through the sewing ring of the prosthesis, the valve is carefully secured in the subcoronary position.

operative stage, any evidence of ventricular ectopy should be treated aggressively by infusion of antiarrhythmic agents and occasionally by "overdrive" atrial pacing.

Pulmonary Support

Pulmonary support by controlled ventilation and oxygenation, particularly if muscle relaxants used during the anesthesia are not neutralized, is essential until the patient can breathe spontaneously. The increased oxygenation helps prevent hypoxia due to inadequate tidal exchange until respiratory and cardiovascular dynamics are stable. To ensure synchronous respiration, some surgeons administer narcotics as a respiratory depressant; others prefer to neutralize the muscle relaxants and have the patient breathe oxygen-enriched air through a face mask as soon as possible after the operation. Whichever technique is used, a thorough understanding and smooth cooperation among the surgical team, respiratory therapists, and anesthesiologists are essential for cohesive management of the patient's postoperative respiratory status. Intra-arterial blood-gas determinations are mandatory, and a blood-gas analyzer in or near the intensive care unit is desirable, if not essential. Patients should not be returned to their rooms until pulmonary support has been discontinued. Rarely, patients who do not respond neurologically after surgery because of a central nervous system injury may require prolonged nasotracheal intubation with a tissue-compatible, nonirritant Silastic tube, along with assisted ventilatory support for several days. This method of ventilatory maintenance has almost eliminated the need for tracheostomy, although the latter technique is still necessary on occasion.

Renal Support

After the anesthetic is administered, a urinary catheter is inserted, and the volumes of urine produced before, during, and after cardiopulmonary bypass are monitored. Postoperative assessment of urine output is equally important. Blood or hemoglobin in the urine secondary to excessive hemolysis usually clears spontaneously; this process is aided by the intravenous administration of mannitol or a diuretic. A steady fall in the postoperative urine output may be the first sign of low cardiac output, and measures to ensure continued urine production should be started. Severe renal failure after extracorporeal circulation is unusual today. Adequate perfusion during operation and monitoring of the blood urea nitrogen, serum creatinine, urine and blood osmolality, and daily urine output, together with the careful control of nephrotoxic medications, have made postoperative

hemodialysis or peritoneal dialysis rarely necessary. However, patients with postoperative left ventricular failure requiring heavy inotropic support may have renal failure secondary to low cardiac output, or drug-induced renal arterial vasoconstriction.

Neurologic Status

The probability of air embolism is usually evident when the ascending aorta is unclamped by the evacuation of an excessive amount of air from the aorta or the left ventricular vent after the heart resumes contraction. If the patient has generalized obtundation or hemiparesis postoperatively, intracerebral edema should be suspected and treated prior to the onset of any seizure disorders. The administration of high doses of dexamethasone (Decadron) intravenously and antiarrhythmics, together with prolonged ventilatory support, is used to manage air embolism.

MECHANICAL VALVULAR PROSTHESES

Mechanical aortic valvular substitutes can be either the caged ball type or the tilting disc prosthesis (Fig. 48–11) (Chaux et al., 1981; Hehrlein et al., 1980a). However, all mechanical substitutes require long-term anticoagulant therapy (Stein et al., 1976; Semb et al., 1980; Nicoloff and Emery, 1979; Macmanus et al., 1980). It is well known that, annually, approximately 1.4 to 3 per cent of patients on anticoagulants will have some minor or major hemorrhagic complications, for example, hematuria, gastrointestinal hemorrhage, or intracerebral hemorrhage (Macmanus et al., 1980). This frustrating need for permanent anticoagulation and the risks thereof have caused repeated waves of enthusiasm for tissue valvular substitutes, which do not require long-term anticoagula-

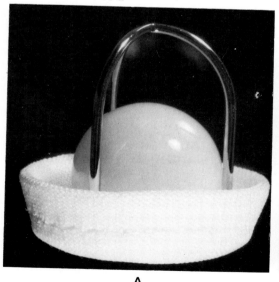
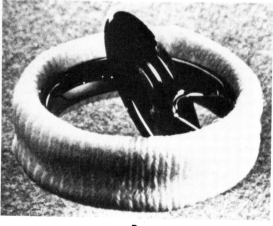

A **B**

Figure 48–11. *A,* The Model 1260 Starr-Edwards prosthesis with the barium-impregnated Silastic poppet has enjoyed widespread clinical use since 1968. *B,* The Bjork-Shiley low-profile tilting disc prosthesis has a low incidence of thromboembolic problems and is particularly suitable for insertion in the small aortic root.

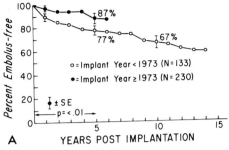

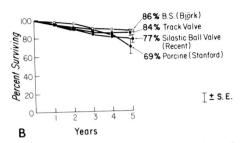

Embolus-free curves for the Model 1200/60 aortic valve.

Actuarial survival for operative survivors with several current aortic prostheses.

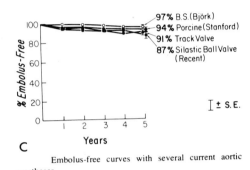

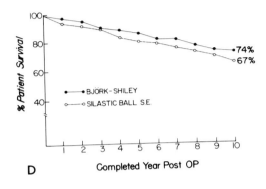

Embolus-free curves with several current aortic prostheses.

Figure 48–12. *A*, Embolus-free curves for the Model 1200/60 aortic valve. *B*, Actuarial survival for operative survivors with several current aortic prostheses. *C*, Embolus-free curves with several current aortic prostheses. *D*, The long-term survival of operative survivors with the Starr-Edwards Model 1200/60 prosthesis compared with that of those with the Bjork-Shiley tilting disc prosthesis.

tion (Barratt-Boyes *et al.*, 1969; Pipkin *et al.*, 1976). Abrupt cessation of anticoagulant therapy in patients with mechanical aortic valves undergoing unrelated surgical procedures may be accompanied by rebound coagulopathy (Macmanus *et al.*, 1980; Robicsek and Harbold, 1976), which can result in the obstruction of the coronary orifices, embolic complications, or sudden death.

The true incidence of postoperative thromboembolic complications in patients with mechanical valves is difficult to ascertain. However, it appears that the permanent maintenance of anticoagulation and the greater availability of laboratory facilities to control the anticoagulation have resulted in a lower thromboembolic rate and have improved survival rates generally for patients undergoing aortic valve replacements with mechanical valves in the last 5 to 8 years (Macmanus *et al.*, 1980) (Fig. 48–12*A*). Historically, the incidence of thromboembolic complications in a 6-year follow-up of patients with the caged ball prosthesis has diminished from the 37 per cent seen with the Series 1000 Starr-Edwards valve in 1961, to 30 per cent for the series 1200/60 (see Fig. 48–10*A*) inserted prior to 1973 (5 per cent per patient year), to 20.4 per cent with the Model 1260 implanted between 1973 and 1979 (3.4 per cent per patient year), to 2.2 per cent per patient year for the composite-strut Starr-Edwards valve (Macmanus *et al.*, 1980). The overall incidence of thromboembolic complications with the low-profile disc valves (Fig. 48–12*C*) is quite similar, although

there is a small but worrisome incidence of sudden and catastrophic valve thrombosis. Macmanus and associates (1980) compared actuarial patient survival and thromboembolic rates reported by Bjork for his patients with the Bjork-Shiley valve, Stanford University's experience with xenograft prostheses, and Starr's own series with caged ball prostheses; they found that there was no statistically significant difference at the 5-year level (Fig. 48–12*B*,*C*).

Hemolysis, seen more frequently after mitral valve replacement, can occur after aortic valvular replacement (Magilligan *et al.*, 1980a) and may be a complication of paraprosthetic regurgitation. Especially in aortic roots that have been the site of subacute bacterial endocarditis or severe calcific degeneration, paraprosthetic regurgitation predisposing to infection as well as hemolysis is a small (2.6 per cent) but worrisome complication (Nicoloff and Emery, 1979; Arrigoni *et al.*, 1973; Callaghan and Singh, 1968), which may lead to recurrent septic emboli, severe regurgitation, generalized sepsis, and even death. Replacement of the infected prosthesis must therefore be considered (Sandza *et al.*, 1977).

TISSUE VALVULAR SUBSTITUTES

Tissue valvular substitutes currently include homograft aortic valves, porcine aortic valves mounted on flexible supporting stents, and biologic prosthetic valves constructed from such homograft or heterograft tissues as dura mater or pericardium.

Homograft Aortic Valves

Although some surgeons, including Ross and Yacoub (1969), Barratt-Boyes and associates (1967, 1969), and Angell and colleagues (1972), have achieved good long-term survival rates in selected patients undergoing aortic valve replacement with fresh homograft valves, and although the longitudinal results compare most favorably with the best survival curves for patients receiving prosthetic valves (Thompson *et al.*, 1979), homograft aortic valves currently have a very limited use in the United States. The freedom from anticoagulation and good long-term survival rates reported in patients undergoing homograft aortic valve replacement are offset by the very limited availability of these valves. The difficulty in procuring fresh homograft valves has thus greatly diminished their use in this country.

Porcine Xenograft Aortic Valves

Perhaps the most commonly used tissue valvular substitute is the porcine aortic valve cured in glutaraldehyde (Fig. 48–13). Long-term follow-up studies by Cohn and associates (1981), Oyer and coworkers (1979, 1980), Magilligan and colleagues (1980a), and Jamieson and associates (1980) show actuarial patient survival and embolus-free survival rates comparable to those with the Bjork or the Starr-Edwards prostheses (Macmanus *et al.*, 1980) (see Fig. 48–11*B*, *C*). Freedom from the hemorrhagic complications of anticoagulation is a decided advantage for patients with the porcine xenograft prosthesis. This advantage is offset by the questionable durability of these prostheses at 10- and 15-year levels (Riddle *et al.*, 1981; Magilligan *et al.*, 1980a, 1980b; Pipkin *et al.*, 1976). The calcific degeneration seen in children with porcine bioprostheses has rendered their use in patients under the age of 30 years inappropriate (Curcio *et al.*, 1981; Williams *et al.*, 1981). Similarly, patients with deranged calcium metabolism should not receive

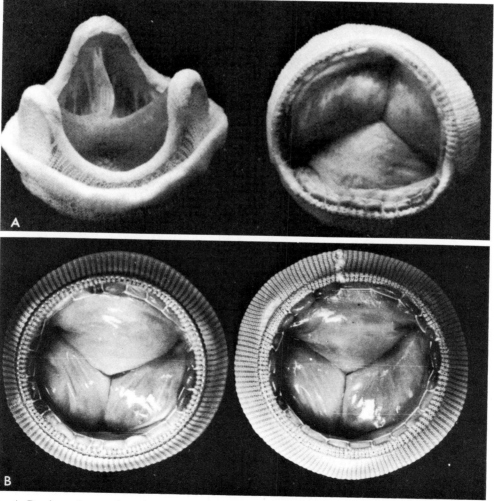

Figure 48–13. *A*, Porcine valves such as the Carpentier-Edwards are particularly appropriate in the noncompliant or elderly patient in whom the size of the valvular anulus is 25 mm. or more. *B*, The Hancock standard valve with the muscular bar in one leaflet (right) is compared with the modified orifice valve with a greater effective orifice area in the same size prosthesis (left).

this bioprosthesis as an aortic valvular substitute. From Oyer and associates' studies (1979, 1980), 5 per cent of the survivors at the 7-year postoperative level had bioprosthesis failure requiring reoperation. It is likely that this percentage will increase with additional years of follow-up, and many patients with porcine bioprostheses may require valve re-replacement 10 to 20 years postoperatively. When the porcine valve does fail, it is usually a gradually progressive problem, which is certainly superior to the often sudden and catastrophic valve failure (valve thrombosis, poppet migration, or jamming of the poppet in the open position [Macmanus et al., 1980]) found with artificial valves. The use of the porcine bioprosthesis is particularly appropriate in the elderly patient population in whom long-term survival is less likely for obvious physiologic reasons. Similarly, it is the prosthesis of choice in all patients for whom anticoagulation is dangerous or inappropriate.

BIOLOGIC PROSTHETIC VALVES

Other forms of biologic valves currently in use include the pericardial xenograft of Ionescu (Ott et al., 1980; Tandon et al., 1980) and the dura mater valve (Zerbini, 1975). Although these prostheses have optimal hemodynamic features and the early clinical results seem excellent, the long-term durability of these biologic valves is unknown (Nuno-Conceicao et al., 1975).

THE CHOICE OF PROSTHESIS

Since the inception of aortic valve replacement, the mortality rate for these patients has been progressively reduced by improvement in cardiovascular anesthesia, better intraoperative myocardial protection, and superior postoperative care. With the current reduction in hospital mortality, emphasis is now placed on the long-term survival of patients and the long-term function of aortic valvular prostheses. Before recommending a particular valvular substitute for an individual patient, the physician must take into account the individual patient's age and occupation, the availability of medical care, the patient's compliance with medical supervision, and the presence of such associated medical problems as peptic ulcer disease, hypertension, and/or bleeding diathesis. From Figure 48–12B,C, no statistical difference in terms of actuarial survival or embolus-free survival can be seen between the Bjork-Shiley valve, the Starr-Edwards Model 1260 valve, the composite-strut valve, and the Hancock porcine xenograft valve. Thus, the selection of the valvular substitute to be used in an individual patient should take into account the aforementioned variables, the size of the aortic anulus, and the patient's own attitude concerning the long-term durability of the prosthesis and the attendant possibility of reoperation, versus the inconvenience and risk of

anticoagulation associated with a mechanical prosthesis.

RESULTS OF AORTIC VALVULAR REPLACEMENT

Survival after aortic valvular replacement appears related to a variety of factors, including the age of the patient (Copeland et al., 1977b), the extent of the cardiac disease, the presence of concomitant disease at the time of cardiac surgery, the expertise of the intraoperative and postoperative management of the patient, and the effectiveness of the valvular prosthesis. In elective patients with a normal cardiothoracic ratio and no evidence of significant coronary artery disease, the hospital mortality rate for aortic valvular replacement is less than 2 per cent (DeBoer and Midell, 1974). However, because of advanced age of the patient, severe cardiomegaly, left ventricular dysfunction, advanced coronary artery disease (Duvoisin and McGoon, 1969), and/or active endocarditis (Wilcox et al., 1977), the mortality rate ranges from 2 to 12 per cent in many centers (Copeland et al., 1977a; Macmanus et al., 1980). One significant preoperative prognostic sign is the size of the cardiac silhouette (Braun et al., 1973) on roentgenogram (Fig. 48–14). If the cardiothoracic ratio is more than 0.61, the 6-month survival rate is 78 per cent, whereas if this ratio is less than 0.61, the 6-month survival rate is between 93 and 96 per cent (Braun et al., 1973).

Factors predisposing to late mortality include severe preoperative functional disability (New York Heart Association Class III or IV), gross cardiomegaly, preoperative congestive cardiac failure, associated advanced coronary artery occlusive disease, pulmonary emboli, and preoperative bacterial endocarditis (Duvoisin and McGoon, 1969). There is an annual postoperative attrition rate of approximately 4 per cent related to arrhythmia, thromboembolic complications, coronary occlusive disease, and congestive heart failure (Macmanus et al., 1980). The 10-year actuarial survival rate (see Fig. 48–12D) for operative survivors ranges from 67 to 74 per cent (Macmanus et al., 1980; Bjork and Henze, 1979). After successful aortic valve replacement, most patients will have a gratifying improvement in exercise tolerance and a modest reduction in cardiac size (Fig. 48–14), will return full time to their preoperative occupations (DeBoer and Midell, 1974), and will be able to participate in desirable recreational activities. Still somewhat controversial is the concept of coronary revascularization at the time of aortic valve replacement. Although it seems logical to combine revascularization with valve replacement in the quest for improved long-term survival and a lower incidence of coronary artery disease complications postoperatively, some authors feel that there is an incremental risk in hospital mortality when revascularization is added to valve replacement, and for this reason, they believe concomitant revascularization is inappropriate

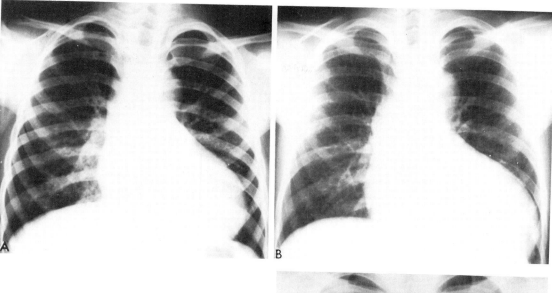

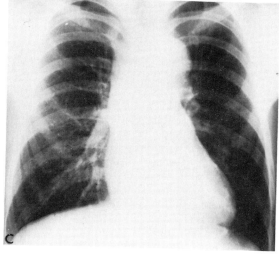

Figure 48–14. The preoperative left ventricular dilatation and hypertrophy *(A)* seemed to increase in the immediate postoperative period *(B),* but 6 months after surgery *(C),* there has been a progressive reduction in the size of the left ventricle on the chest roentgenogram.

(Bonow *et al.,* 1981; Friedberg, 1966). However, with improved myocardial protection allowing more complicated cardiac reconstruction to be performed more safely, Kirklin and Kouchoukos (1981) and many others believe that incremental risk with combined revascularization and valve replacement increases primarily with age, and many centers revascularize 10 to 30 per cent of all patients undergoing aortic valve replacement (Macmanus *et al.,* 1980; Callard *et al.,* 1976).

THE SMALL AORTIC ANULUS

In a certain percentage of patients undergoing aortic valve replacement, it will be obvious after the valve has been excised and the anulus inspected that the anulus is too small to accept an adequate-sized caged ball prosthesis or porcine bioprosthesis. Porcine or mechanical caged ball prostheses with a diameter of less than 23 mm. have unacceptable gradients across the valve with exercise (Hatcher, 1981). In these situations, some surgeons will insert a tilting

disc prosthesis (such as a Bjork-Shiley or a St. Jude Medical valve) where orifice–to–sewing ring diameter ratio is greater (Aberg and Holmgren, 1981; Bjork *et al.,* 1973; Nicoloff and Emery, 1979). However, especially in an adult with a large body surface area, a 21-mm. Bjork-Shiley or similar valve will still result in a significant valvular gradient with exercise, and alternative measures must be taken. There are five possible reconstructive procedures that can be done to offset the problem of the small aortic root:

1. A technique described by Nicks and associates in 1970, by Blank and coworkers in 1976, and by Pupello and colleagues in 1978 entails an incision through the mid-portion of the noncoronary cusp across the anulus down into the upper part of the anterior leaflet of the mitral valve (Fig. 48–15*I*). This V-shaped incision is then patched and results in an approximately 3-mm. increase in the diameter of the aortic root (Mori *et al.,* 1981), allowing insertion of a larger tilting disc prosthesis or utilization of a porcine bioprosthesis (Fig. 48–16*I*).

2. A technique described by Manouguian and associates (1979a) consists of a more radical incision

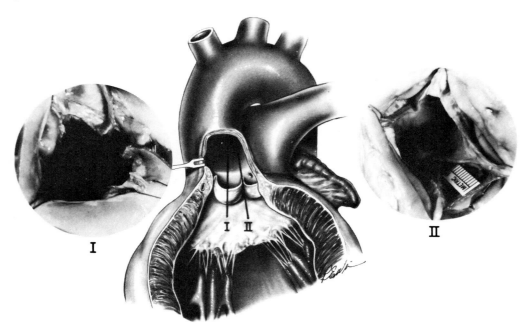

Figure 48–15. The artist's impression depicts the possible sites for division of the aortic valvular anulus. *I,* From the surgeon's perspective, the anulus is incised through the mid-portion of the noncoronary cusp. *II,* An incision through the commissure between the left and noncoronary cusps can be extended down onto the anterior leaflet of the mitral valve from 10 to 15 mm., allowing a slightly more radical enlargement of the aortic anulus.

down the commissure between the left and the noncoronary cusps and deeply into the anterior leaflet of the mitral valve (Fig. 48–15*II*). This allows a greater enlargement of the aortic root (10- to 25-mm. increase in anular circumference) than is possible with the technique of Nicks, Blank, Pupello and associates. An adequate-sized prosthesis can easily be inserted, and a patch is utilized to bridge the defect in the anulus (Fig. 48–16*II*).

3. Especially in children with hypoplastic left ventricular outflow tracts, a Konno (1975) procedure can be performed (Fig. 48–17). The aortotomy is extended inferiorly across the anulus and divides the interventricular septum. The incision is then extended to cut across the right ventricular outflow tract as well, resulting in the creation of a large ventricular septal defect. A two-layered patch is used to bridge the defect in the septum, allowing an adult-sized prosthesis to be sewn in this greatly expanded aortic valve anulus. The second layer of the patch is used to repair the right ventricular outflow tract. This is a more aggressive root enlargement procedure and is more suitable for use in children, in whom the enlargement of the root to accommodate an adult-sized prosthesis will eliminate the need for repeated valve replacement as the child grows.

4. When the aortic anulus is hypoplastic and has been operated on several times previously for congenital valvular aortic stenosis and is thus deemed unreconstructable, a valved conduit can be inserted in the left ventricular apex and joined to the abdominal or thoracic aorta, thus creating a double-outlet left ventricle (Norman *et al.,* 1976).

5. When the left ventricular outflow tract is quite small (or when the subcoronary area has been destroyed by bacterial endocarditis and is thus unsuitable for the subcoronary fixation of a valvular prosthesis) and when there is poststenotic dilatation of the aorta, consideration should be given to implanting a larger-sized prosthetic valve more distally in the aorta. The native coronary ostia would be oversewn and saphenous vein grafts attached from the aorta distal to the valvular prosthesis to both the right and the left coronary system (Reitz *et al.,* 1981). This would ensure that coronary perfusion would be maximum in the diastolic phase of the cardiac cycle.

Although the problem of the moderately small aortic anulus can be circumvented by utilizing a tilting disc prosthesis in most cases, some type of formal anulus enlargement will be necessary in from 1 to 5 per cent of the patients undergoing aortic valve replacement.

IDIOPATHIC HYPERTROPHIC SUBAORTIC STENOSIS

Idiopathic hypertrophic subaortic stenosis (IHSS), which has gained increasing attention in recent years, is a muscular obstruction of the left ventricular outflow tract generally characterized by marked hypertrophy of the left ventricle, particularly the interventricular septum. During systole, the hypertrophied outflow tract muscle often narrows sufficiently to obstruct left ventricular ejection.

There are two configurations of hypertrophied myocardium: (1) nonsymmetric hypertrophy (Braunwald *et al.,* 1964; Henry *et al.,* 1973), particularly

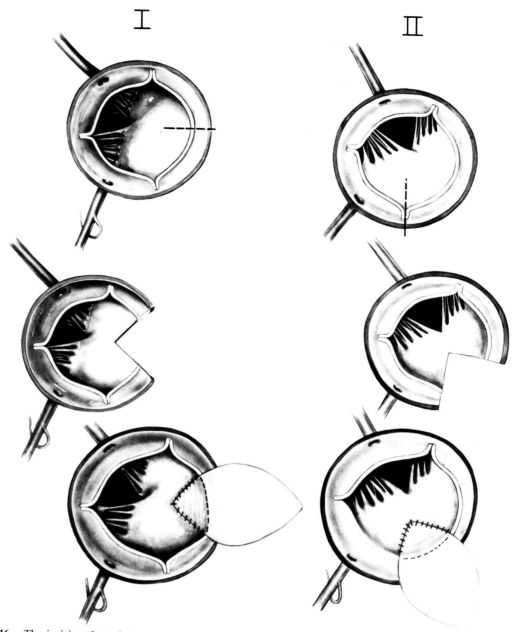

Figure 48–16. The incision through the aortic valve anulus, either in the mid-portion of the noncoronary cusp (*I*) or through the commissure between the noncoronary and left cusps (*II*), is extended into the anterior leaflet of the mitral valve. A prosthetic patch is inserted with considerable enlargement of the circumference of the valve anulus.

involving the interventricular septum and outflow tract area (Cohen *et al.,* 1964), but also with marked enlargement of the papillary muscles and trabeculae carneae; and (2) diffuse concentric hypertrophy of the entire left ventricle. Enlargement of the papillary muscles, thickening of the anterior leaflet of the mitral valve, and functional deformity of the mitral valvular anulus frequently combine to cause mitral regurgitation (Cooley *et al.,* 1973). Septal hypertrophy can be so great as to encroach upon the right ventricular cavity; on bimanual palpation, it can feel as though a golf ball is lodged in the interventricular septum.

Microscopic examination reveals a bizarre arrangement of the left ventricular muscle bundles. Individual muscle fibers are often greatly thickened, tend to be shorter than normal, and sometimes are separated by clefts in which endothelium-lined channels between the muscle bundles may open into the ventricular cavities. Electron-microscopic examination shows an increase in the size and number of nerve fibrils, elastic tissue, and mitochondria, and the myofibril bands are fragmented into short pieces. Cooley and associates (1973) found a striking resemblance between these abnormal IHSS fibers and the

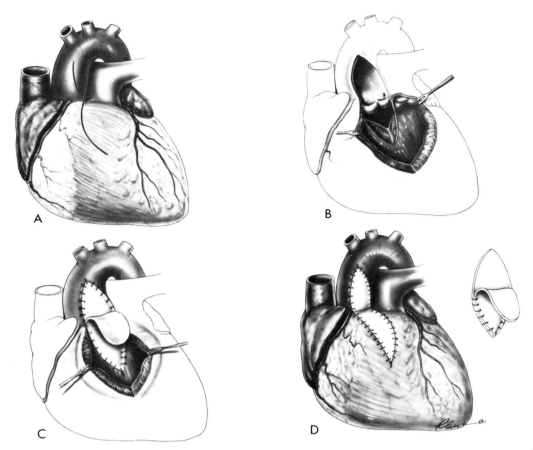

Figure 48–17. *A,* The Konno procedure incorporates an incision from the aorta anteriorly down into the right ventricular outflow tract. *B,* The valve anulus is radically enlarged by cutting deeply into the interventricular septum. *C,* A two-layered patch increases the circumference of the valve anulus, allowing insertion of an adult-sized disc prosthesis. *D,* The second layer of the patch enlarges the right ventricular outflow tract.

normal sinoatrial nodal cells and atrial muscle and speculated that IHSS may represent a developmental anomaly consisting of displacement of atrial muscle or an abnormal proliferation of cardiac sympathetic nerves.

Clinical Features

Braunwald and colleagues (1964), in a series of 64 patients with IHSS, found that the overall male-to-female distribution was 2 to 1, although patients with the familial form of the disease were distributed equally between the two sexes (Cohen *et al.,* 1964). Ages of the patients ranged from 6 to 56 years, with an average of 25.7 years.

The disease was usually manifested clinically as a heart murmur, progressing into symptoms of dyspnea, angina, dizziness, and syncope. Fourteen of the 48 symptomatic patients had clear evidence of cardiac decompensation. Physical examination revealed an enlarged heart with a left ventricular lift. A systolic thrill was present in 50 per cent of the patients, and a fourth heart sound was usually heard in patients in sinus rhythm. An ejection systolic murmur was most prominent along the left sternal border or at the apex.

Electrocardiography showed that normal sinus rhythm was usually present, and obstruction of the left ventricular outflow tract tended to be more severe in those patients whose electrocardiograms showed delta waves. There was a relationship between the abnormally deep and broad Q waves related to gross septal hypertrophy and the familial form of IHSS. On chest roentgenography, half of the patients showed an increased cardiothoracic ratio, and all had enlarged left ventricles (Braunwald *et al.,* 1964; Cohen *et al.,* 1964). Mitral regurgitation was present in nearly half of the

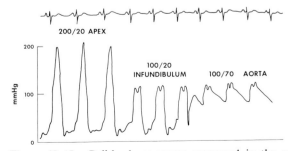

Figure 48–18. Pull-back pressures measured in the apex, infundibulum, and ascending aorta reveal a gradient from the apex to the infundibular area of the left ventricle, but no gradient across the aortic valve in IHSS.

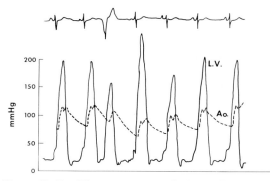

Figure 48–19. The postextrasystolic beat when pressures in the aorta and left ventricle are monitored simultaneously shows an increased gradient for that beat with a gradual reduction of the gradient over the next several beats.

patients in the older age group, and they tended to be more symptomatic.

Critical hemodynamic studies are necessary to document IHSS, and simultaneous measurements of the left ventricular and aortic pressures demonstrate the pressure gradient across the outflow tract (Figs. 48–18 and 48–19). This gradient varies from one patient to another, and in individual patients from the resting state to the institution of certain physical and pharmacologic maneuvers. In the basal state, the peak systolic left ventricular outflow pressure gradient exceeded 100 mm. Hg in 14 patients and ranged between 50 and 100 mm. Hg in 15 patients in Braunwald and associates' series (1964). The other 14 patients did not exhibit significant gradients in the basal resting state. This gradient is significantly increased by digitalis therapy, isoproterenol infusion, amyl nitrate inhalation, nitroglycerin administered sublingually, the Valsalva maneuver, and exercise. Hemorrhagic shock causes a reflex positive inotropic effect, resulting in an increased gradient; beta-receptive blockage specif-

ically reduces the gradient across the left ventricular outflow tract; and propranolol is important in the management of this condition. Elevation of the legs, hypervolemia, and aortic cross-clamping during surgery all help to lower the gradient (Braunwald *et al.*, 1964).

In recent years, echocardiography has been increasingly helpful in diagnosing IHSS and documenting its prevalence in asymptomatic members of the same family (Clark *et al.*, 1973; Henry *et al.*, 1973; Tajik and Giuliani, 1974). This completely noninvasive technique delineates clearly the asymmetric septal hypertrophy and the dynamics of the mitral valve (Fig. 48–20). This thickness of the ventricular septum is compared with that of the posterior left ventricular free wall at the level of the tips of the papillary muscles; a ratio of greater than 1.3 to 1.0 is considered diagnostic of IHSS (Henry *et al.*, 1973; Tajik and Giuliani, 1974).

The anterior leaflet of the mitral valve normally moves in a posterior direction in systole for coaptation with the posterior leaflet; in IHSS, however, it moves anteriorly in systole as it takes part in obstructing the outflow. Other abnormalities of mitral valve motion seen on the echocardiogram include diastolic apposition against the ventricular septum and decreased diastolic closure rate (Fig. 48–20) (Clark *et al.*, 1973; Henry *et al.*, 1973; Tajik and Giuliani, 1974).

Treatment

Approximately two of every three patients respond satisfactorily to propranolol therapy and require no surgical intervention. In the remaining patients, however, a variety of surgical approaches for resection of the hypertrophied septum in the outflow tract have been employed. Morrow (1969), Kittle and as-

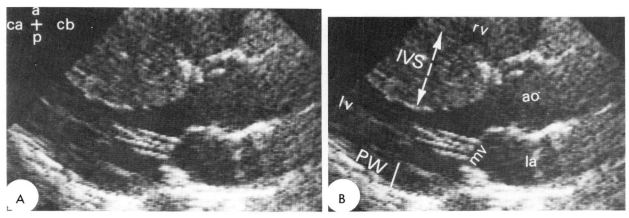

Figure 48–20. A stop-frame image of a patient with marked echocardiographic findings of IHSS. These images are obtained from a parasternal transducer position and are oriented like a left lateral view of the heart. The orientation is marked in the upper left corner of *A*, which is an unlabeled photograph. *B* is the identical image labeled. The interventricular septum (IVS) can be seen approximately 2½ times the size of the left ventricular posterior wall (PW). This septum measured 3.5 cm. in comparison to the posterior wall, which measured 1 cm. The mitral valvular structures (mv) are easily visualized. This patient was on extremely high doses of Inderal and therefore did not have any prominent systolic anterior motion. (a = anterior; ao = aortic root; ca = cardiac apex; cb = cardiac base; la = left atrium; lv = left ventricle; p = posterior; rv = right ventricle.) (Courtesy of Randolph P. Martin, M.D., Department of Internal Medicine, University of Virginia Medical Center.)

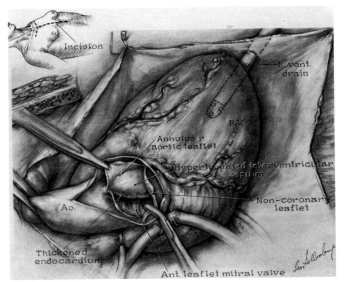

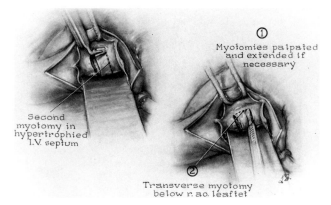

Figure 48–21. General operative exposure utilized in the treatment of hypertrophic subaortic stenosis. After institution of cardiopulmonary bypass, the patient is cooled at 30°C., the aorta occluded, and the left ventricle drained through the apex. A vertical incision is made in the ascending aorta and extended down into the noncoronary sinus of Valsalva. The normal aortic valve is retracted, and the ridge or bulge of the hypertrophic muscle in the interventricular septum can be seen beneath the base of the right coronary leaflet. Opposite it is the anterior leaflet of the mitral valve, which is also thickened and opaque. The heart is allowed to go into flaccid arrest; the right coronary leaflet is then retracted, and much of the septum can be rotated anteriorly into the operative field. On the most prominent aspect of the hypertrophied septum, the endocardium is always seen to be thickened and "heaped up" into a transverse ridge of fibrous tissue. This endocardial scarring is the site at which the septum is contacted by the mitral leaflet during systole.

Figure 48–23. A second myotomy is made in the same manner, parallel to the first and about 1 cm. to the right, or clockwise, from the initial one. Both incisions are then palpated and deepened by digital pressure if necessary. At the most prominent part of the septum, the incision should be about 1.5 cm. in depth. With a conventional knife, a transverse incision is then made at the base of the right coronary leaflet, connecting proximal portions of the two myotomies.

sociates (1964), and Dong and coworkers (1962) have resected the obstructing muscle adequately using a supravalvular aortotomy alone; Kirklin and Ellis (1961) used a combined approach through the aorta and a small counterincision in the left ventricular wall to achieve symptomatic improvement in 9 of 13 surviving patients. The best-documented approach, Morrow's ventriculomyotomy and myomectomy (Figs. 48–21 to 48–26), seems to have yielded the most consistent results (Dong *et al.*, 1962; Kay *et al.*, 1961; Kirklin and Ellis, 1961; Kittle *et al.*, 1964; Morrow *et*

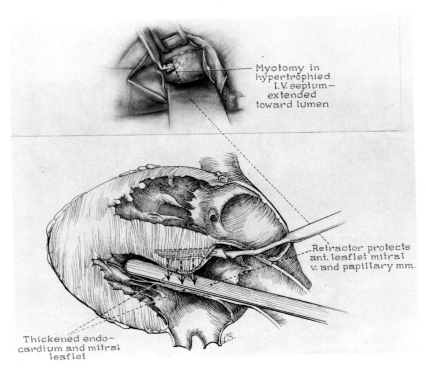

Figure 48–22. From an assortment of flat ribbon retractors, one is selected that will pass freely but snugly through the aortic anulus. The retractor is passed to the apex of the heart, displacing and protecting the anterior mitral leaflet and papillary muscles behind it. The tip of a No. 10 knife blade, attached to an angled handle, is passed into the septum just below the base of the right coronary leaflet at a point 2 or 3 mm. to the right of the commissure between the left and right coronary leaflets. The blade is inserted through the septum toward the apex for a distance of about 4 cm. and is then withdrawn as its cutting edge incises the septum with a sawing motion directed toward the ventricular lumen and the retractor.

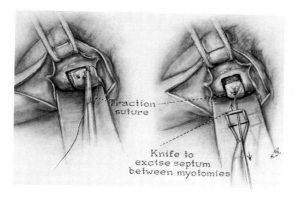

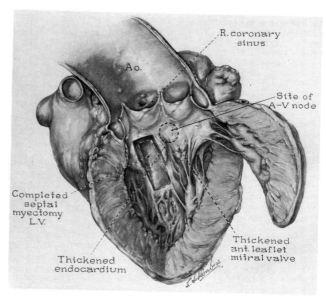

Figure 48–24. A traction suture is placed in the bar of muscle that has been isolated, and the bar is then freed from the septum for a variable distance by incision of its attachment under direct vision. The resection is usually not possible deep within the ventricle, and the suture is then passed through the opening of a special knife, the blade of which is 1 cm. in length.

Figure 48–26. The appearance of the resected area of the septum and its relation to the aortic valve leaflets are shown semidiagrammatically. Also illustrated is the area of the conduction tissue, which must be avoided in performing the procedure.

al., 1975; Pearse, 1964). Cooley and colleagues (1973) have advocated mitral valvular replacement alone. In 9 patients treated in this way, the pressure gradients, which had ranged from 50 to 135 mm. Hg preoperatively, were reduced to 0 to 15 mm. Hg postoperatively. The excised mitral valve appeared thickened and fibrotic, but there was no evidence of previous inflammation or calcification.

Although surgical management clearly relieves the obstruction, it does not influence the underlying cardiomyopathy; therefore, operative treatment is best reserved for patients with disabling symptoms who have not responded to medical management and for patients with severe resting obstruction. Complete postoperative heart block has a significant influence on mortality. Preoperative mitral regurgitation often disappears after a ventriculomyotomy and myomectomy. Surgery also often reduces preoperative elevation of the left ventricular end-diastolic pressure and relieves symptoms (McGoon, 1961).

SELECTED REFERENCES

Bjork, V. O., and Henze, A.: Ten years' experience with the Bjork-Shiley tilting disk valve. J. Thorac. Cardiovasc. Surg., 78:331, 1979.

Bjork shares some of the developmental steps taken in designing and improving his tilting disc prosthesis since 1968. An encouraging aspect of this paper is the excellent 10-year actuarial survival rate of 74 per cent for operative survivors with the Bjork-Shiley prosthesis. There is a clear need for permanent anticoagulation with this prosthesis, and although the thromboembolic complications are no greater than with other types of valvular substitutes, there is a small but disappointing incidence (0.2 per cent per year) of acute valve thrombosis. Several minor technical points related to the insertion of the prosthesis are important for the reader.

Braun, L. O., Kincaid, O. W., and McGoon, D. C.: Prognosis of aortic valve replacement in relation to preoperative heart size. J. Thorac. Cardiovasc. Surg., 65: 381, 1973.

This article examines the relationship between preoperative heart size and early and late results after aortic valve replacement in 548 patients. A preoperative cardiothoracic ratio above 0.57 is associated with a significantly higher mortality rate in both the early and late postoperative periods; the differences increase progressively as the follow-up period lengthens.

Buckberg, F. D.: A proposed "solution" to the cardioplegic controversy. J. Thorac. Cardiovasc. Surg., 77:803, 1979.

The author, a pre-eminent authority in the field of myocardial protection, explains the pathophysiology of ischemic and reperfusion injuries, the principles of myocardial energy supply and demand that must underlie the composition of any cardioplegic solution, and the means of developing a strategy for delivering and maintaining a properly designed solution to all myocardial regions. The reader can easily understand the physiologic requirements of a cardioplegic solution and can appreciate that, during aortic clamping, all hearts receive flow from noncoronary collateral sources that washes away all cardioplegic solutions and diminishes the salutary effect of "ideal" solutions. The reader of this article

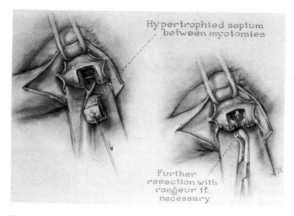

Figure 48–25. As traction is made on the suture, the rectangular knife is pushed toward the apex, freeing the remainder of the muscle bar from the septum. The bar of muscle can usually be excised intact, but sometimes it breaks or fragments. In this case, the resection is completed with a special angled rongeur.

has a better understanding of the deleterious effects of ischemic and reperfusion injury and is stimulated to review his current cardioplegic technique in the interests of superior myocardial protection.

Kirklin, J. W., and Kouchoukos, N. T.: Aortic valve replacement without myocardial revascularization. (Editorial.) Circulation, 63:252, 1981.

In their characteristically precise way, Kirklin and Kouchoukos scientifically analyze what is known and what is unknown about aortic valve replacement with and without concomitant myocardial revascularization. The experience from January 1975 to July 1979 with 489 patients undergoing simple aortic valve replacement demonstrated a 2 per cent hospital mortality rate. Of 251 patients who had aortic valve replacement plus revascularization, the mortality rate was 3.6 per cent (the p value of 0.21 shows no statistical difference in terms of hospital mortality). Obvious improvements in myocardial protection and superior intraoperative technique allow revascularization to be included in patients undergoing aortic valve replacement without a significant increment of risk. Kirklin and Kouchoukos stress that the limited follow-up data in terms of patient survival do not prove that concomitant revascularization results in superior long-term survival in patients undergoing aortic valve replacement (although they do it almost routinely).

Konno, S., Imai, Y., Iida, Y., Nakajima, M., and Tatsuno, K.: A new method for prosthetic valve replacement in congenital aortic stenosis associated with hypoplasia of the aortic valve ring. J. Thorac. Cardiovasc. Surg., 70:909, 1975.

The authors illustrate clearly the clinical applications of a well-designed laboratory experiment carried out in 1969 in dogs. In the hypoplastic aortic valve ring, simple valvulotomy is ineffective in increasing the valvular orifice area significantly. An incision in the supravalvular aorta anteriorly is extended inferiorly into the right ventricular outflow tract and divides the aortic valve anulus by aggressively incising the interventricular septum between both coronary orifices. A large two-layered patch bridges the defect in the septum and allows the insertion of an adult-sized prosthesis. One layer of the patch increases the diameter of the aortic outflow tract, and the other layer increases the pulmonary outflow area.

Macmanus, Q., Grunkemeier, G. L., Lambert, L. E., Teply, J. F., Harlan, B. J., and Starr, A.: Year of operation as a risk factor in the late results of valve replacement. J. Thorac. Cardiovasc. Surg., 80:834, 1980.

Macmanus, Starr, and associates identify many of the variables that result in improved quality of life with fewer postoperative problems for patients undergoing aortic valve replacement in the past few years, compared with patients operated on a decade ago. They show good evidence that there is currently a significant reduction in postoperative thromboembolic complications for patients with the Model 1200/60 aortic prosthesis. They compare the actuarial survival and the embolus-free survival rates of patients who underwent porcine xenograft aortic valve replacement at Stanford University, Bjork-Shiley replacement at the Karolinska Institute in Stockholm, and caged ball aortic valve replacement in Oregon. In this analysis, there is no statistically significant superiority of one prosthesis over the others. The authors emphasize that mechanical prostheses all require anticoagulation; the risk of anticoagulation should be weighed against the questioned durability of the porcine prosthesis in deciding which valvular substitute should be used for an individual patient.

Magilligan, D. J., Jr., Lewis, J. W., Jr., Jara, F. M., Lee, M. W., Alam, M., Riddle, J. M., and Stein, P. D.: Spontaneous degeneration of porcine bioprosthetic valves. Ann. Thorac. Surg., 30:259, 1980.

From a data base of 560 porcine bioprosthetic valves in 490 patients from 1971 to 1979, valuable information concerning the durability of the porcine xenograft is presented. The bioprosthetic valve survival rate without degeneration was 98.9 per cent at 4 years, 96.4 per

cent at 5 years, 90.8 per cent at 6 years, 84.2 per cent at 7 years. There was no difference in valve degeneration observed with regard to sex, valve position, or whether the valves were rinsed in antibiotics prior to implantation. Patients younger than 35 years old had an increase in valve degeneration compared with those more than 35 years old. When the porcine xenograft valve does fail, it is a gradual failure, which is detectable by echocardiography and phonocardiography. The ubiquitous enthusiasm for the porcine xenograft is tempered by the rather sobering durability statistics presented by Magilligan and coworkers.

Pupello, D. F., Blank, R. H., Bessone, L. N., Harrison, E., and Sbar, S.: Surgical management of the small aortic annulus: Hemodynamic evaluation. Chest, 74:163, 1978.

In a series of 253 patients undergoing aortic valve replacement, 9 per cent (22 patients) required anulus enlargement. This large, pioneering series in anulus enlargement utilized an extension of the aortotomy across the mid-portion of the noncoronary cusp down into the base of the anterior leaflet of the mitral valve. There were no deaths in the 22 patients, and 12 underwent postoperative catheterization 1 to 10 months later. The routine use of the porcine xenograft valve in larger sizes resulted in a gratifying reduction in the transvalvular gradient, an increase in cardiac output, and an increase in the aortic valve orifice area.

REFERENCES

Aberg, B., and Holmgren, A.: Haemodynamic evaluation of the convex-concave Bjork-Shiley prosthesis in patients with narrow aortic annulus. Scand. J. Thorac. Cardiovasc. Surg., 15:117, 1981.

American Edwards Laboratories: Carpentier-Edwards Bioprostheses. Pub. #106189-1. Santa Ana, California, February 1980.

Angell, W. W., Shumway, N. E., and Cosek, J. C.: A five-year study of viable aortic valve homografts. J. Thorac. Cardiovasc. Surg., 64:329, 1972.

Arrigoni, M. G., Danielson, G. K., Mankin, H. T., and Pluth, J. R.: Aortic valve replacement with cloth covered composite-seat Starr-Edwards prostheses: A review of thirty-two months clinical experience. J. Thorac. Cardiovasc. Surg., 65:376, 1973.

Bahnson, H. T., Spencer, F. C., Busse, E. F. G., and Davis, F. W., Jr.: Cusp replacement in coronary artery perfusion in open operations on the aortic valve. Ann. Surg., 152:494, 1960.

Bailey, C. P., Ramirez, H. P., and Larselere, H. B.: Surgical treatment of aortic stenosis. J.A.M.A., 150:1647, 1952.

Barondess, J. A., and Sande, M.: Some changing aspects of aortic regurgitation. Arch. Intern. Med., 124:600, 1969.

Barratt-Boyes, B. G.: Homograft replacement for aortic valve disease. Mod. Concepts Cardiovasc. Dis., 36:1, 1967.

Barratt-Boyes, B. G., Roche, A. H. G., Brandt, P. W. T., Smith, J. C., and Lowe, J. B.: Aortic valve replacement—a long-term follow-up in an initial series of 101 patients. Circulation, 40:763, 1969.

Bentall, H., and DeBono, A.: A technique for complete replacement of the ascending aorta. Thorax, 23:338, 1968.

Bjork, V. O.: The improved Bjork-Shiley tilting disc valve prosthesis. Scand. J. Thorac. Cardiovasc. Surg., 12:81, 1978.

Bjork, V. O., and Henze, A.: Ten years' experience with the Bjork-Shiley tilting disc valve. J. Thorac. Cardiovasc. Surg., 78:331, 1979.

Bjork, V. O., Henze, A., Holmgren, A., and Szamosi, A.: Evaluation of the 21 mm. Bjork-Shiley tilting disc valve in patients with narrow aortic roots. Scand. J. Thorac. Cardiovasc. Surg., 7:203, 1973.

Blank, R. H., Pupello, D. F., Bessone, L. N., Harrison, E. E., and Sbar, S.: Method of managing the small aortic annulus during valve replacement. Ann. Thorac. Surg., 22:356, 1976.

Bonow, R. O., Kent, K. M., Rosing, D. R., Lipson, L. C., Borer, J. S., McIntosh, C. L., Morrow, A. G., and Epstein, S. E.: Aortic valve replacement without myocardial revascularization in patients with combined aortic valvular and coronary artery disease. Circulation, 63:243, 1981.

Braun, L. O., Kincaid, O. W., and McGoon, D. C.: Prognosis of aortic valve replacement in relation to preoperative heart size. J. Thorac. Cardiovasc. Surg., 65:381, 1973.

Braunwald, E., Lambrew, C. T., Rockoff, S. D., Ross, J., Jr., and Morrow, A. G.: Idiopathic hypertrophic subaortic stenosis. Circulation, 30(Suppl. 4):1, 1964.

Brott, W. H., Zajtchuk, R., Bowen, T. E., Davia, J., and Green, D. C.: Dipyridamole-aspirin as thromboembolic prophylaxis in patients with aortic valve prosthesis: Prospective study with the Model 2320 Starr-Edwards prosthesis. J. Thorac. Cardiovasc. Surg., 81:632, 1981.

Buckberg, G. D.: A proposed "solution" to the cardioplegic controversy. J. Thorac. Cardiovasc. Surg., 77:803, 1979.

Callaghan, J. C., and Singh, S.: The follow-up of 80 consecutive valve replacements. Ann. Thorac. Surg., 6:40, 1968.

Callard, G. M., Flege, J. B., Jr., and Todd, J. C.: Combined valvular and coronary artery surgery. Ann. Thorac. Surg., 22:338, 1976.

Chapman, D. W., Beazley, H. L., Peterson, P. K., Webb, J. A., and Cooley, D. A.: Annulo-aortic ectasia with cystic medial necrosis. Am. J. Cardiol., 16:679, 1965.

Chaux, A., Gray, R. J., Matloff, J. M., Feldman, H., and Sustaita, H.: An appreciation of the new St. Jude valvular prosthesis. J. Thorac. Cardiovasc. Surg., 81:202, 1981.

Clark, C. E., Henry, W. L., and Epstein, S. E.: Familial prevalence and genetic transmission of idiopathic hypertrophic subaortic stenosis. N. Engl. J. Med., 289:709, 1973.

Cohen, J., Effat, H., Goodwin, J. F., Oakley, C. M., and Steiner, R. E.: Hypertrophic obstructive cardiomyopathy. Br. Heart J., 26:16, 1964.

Cohn, L. H., and Collins, J. J., Jr.: Local cardiac hypothermia for myocardial protection. Ann. Thorac. Surg., 17:135, 1974.

Cohn, L. H., Mudge, G. H., Pratter, F., and Collins, J. J., Jr.: Five- to eight-year follow-up of patients undergoing porcine heart-valve replacement. N. Engl. J. Med., 304:258, 1981.

Cooley, D. A., Leachman, R. D., and Wukasch, D. C.: Diffuse muscular subaortic stenosis: Surgical treatment. Am. J. Cardiol., 31:1, 1973.

Copeland, J. G., Griepp, R. B., Stinson, E. B., and Shumway, N. E.: Long-term follow-up after isolated aortic valve replacement. J. Thorac. Cardiovasc. Surg., 74:875, 1977a.

Copeland, J. G., Griepp, R. B., Stinson, E. B., et al.: Isolated aortic valve replacement in patients older than 65 years. J.A.M.A., 237:1578, 1977b.

Crawford, F. A., Sethi, G. K., Scott, S. M., and Takaro, T.: Systemic emboli due to cloth wear in a Starr-Edwards Model 2320 aortic prosthesis. Ann. Thorac. Surg., 16:614, 1973.

Crosby, I. K., Ashcraft, W. C., and Reed, W. A.: Surgery of the proximal aorta in Marfan's syndrome. J. Thorac. Cardiovasc. Surg., 66:75, 1973.

Cunningham, J. N., Abbas, J. S., Adams, P. X., Nathan, I., Klugman, I., and Spencer, F. C.: Constant-pressure aortic root perfusion versus cardioplegia and hypothermia: Comparison of methods of myocardial protection. J. Thorac. Cardiovasc. Surg., 77:496, 1979.

Curcio, C. A., Commerford, P. J., Rose, A. G., Stevens, J. E., and Barnard, M. S.: Calcification of glutaraldehyde-preserved porcine xenografts in young patients. J. Thorac. Cardiovasc. Surg., 81:621, 1981.

Cutler, E. C., and Beck, C. S.: The present status of the surgical procedures in chronic valvular disease of the heart. Arch. Surg., 18:403, 1929.

DeBoer, A., and Midell, A. I.: Isolated aortic valve replacement: Analysis of factors influencing survival after replacement with the Starr-Edwards prosthesis. Ann. Thorac. Surg., 17:360, 1974.

Dong, E., Jr., Hurley, E. J., Hancock, E. W., Stofer, R. C., and Shumway, N. E.: Surgical treatment of aortic stenosis. Surgery, 52:720, 1962.

Duvoisin, G. E., and McGoon, D. C.: Aortic valve replacement with a ball-valve prosthesis. Arch. Surg., 99:684, 1969.

Ebert, P. A.: Aspects of myocardial protection. (Editorial.) Ann. Thorac. Surg., 26:495, 1978.

Edwards, W. S., and Kerr, A. R.: A safer technique for replacement of the entire ascending aorta and aortic valve. J. Thorac. Cardiovasc. Surg., 59:837, 1970.

Edwards Laboratories, Santa Ana, California: Clinical report: Starr-Edwards cardiac valve prostheses, 1973.

Ferlic, R. M., Goott, B., Edwards, J. E., and Lillehei, C. W.: Aortic valvular insufficiency associated with cystic medial necrosis. Ann. Surg., 165:1, 1967.

Follette, D. M., Mulder, D. G., Maloney, J. V., Jr., and Buckberg, G. D.: Advantages of blood cardioplegia over continuous coronary perfusion or intermittent ischemia: Experimental and clinical study. J. Thorac. Cardiovasc. Surg., 76:604, 1978.

Friedberg, C. K.: Diseases of the Heart. 3rd Ed. Philadelphia, W. B. Saunders Company, 1966.

Gibbon, J. H.: Application of a mechanical heart and lung apparatus to cardiac surgery. Minn. Med., 37:171, 1954.

Golden, R. L., and Lakin, H.: The forme fruste in Marfan's syndrome. N. Engl. J. Med., 260:797, 1959.

Grunkemeier, G. L., Macmanus, Q., Thomas, D. R., Luber, J. M., Lambert, L. E., Suen, Y.-F., and Starr, A.: The use of time-interrelated covariates to predict survival following aortic valve replacement. Ann. Thorac. Surg., 30:240, 1980.

Hancock Laboratories, Inc. (Vascor Labs) Anaheim, California: Durability assessment of the Hancock porcine bioprosthesis: A multicenter retrospective analysis of patients operated on prior to 1975. April 1980.

Harken, D. E., Sorof, H. S., Taylor, W. J., Lefemine, A. A., Gupta, S. K., and Lunzer, S.: Partial and complete prostheses in aortic insufficiency. J. Thorac. Cardiovasc. Surg., 40:744, 1960.

Hatcher, C. R., Jr.: Aortic valve replacement: The problem of the small aortic annulus. Editorial from the Division of Thoracic and Cardiovascular Surgery, Emory University School of Medicine, Atlanta, Georgia, 1981.

Hehrlein, F. W., Gottwik, M., Fraedrich, G., and Mulch, J.: First clinical experience with a new all-pyrolytic carbon bileaflet heart valve prosthesis. J. Thorac. Cardiovasc. Surg., 79:632, 1980a.

Henrlein, F. W., Gottwik, M., Mulch, J., Walter, P., and Fraedrich, G.: Heart valve replacement with the new all-pyrolytic bileaflet St. Jude Medical prosthesis. J. Cardiovasc. Surg., 21:395, 1980b.

Henry, W. L., Clark, C. E., and Epstein, S. E.: Asymmetric septal hypertrophy: Echocardiographic identification of the pathognomonic anatomic abnormality of IHSS. Circulation, 47:225, 1973.

Herr, R. H., Starr, A., Pierie, W. R., Wood, J. A., and Bigelow, J. C.: Aortic valve replacement: A review of six years' experience with the ball valve prosthesis. Ann. Thorac. Surg., 6:199, 1968.

Hufnagel, C. A., and Harvey, W. P.: The surgical correction of aortic regurgitation: Preliminary report. Bull. Georgetown U. Med. Ctr., 6:60, 1953.

Jamieson, W. R. E., Janusz, M. T., Miyagishima, R. T., Munro, A. I., Tutassura, H., Gerein, A. N., Burr, L. H., and Allen, P.: Embolic complications of porcine heterograft cardiac valves. J. Thorac. Cardiovasc. Surg., 81:626, 1981.

Jamieson, W. R. E., Janusz, M. T., Munro, A. I., Miyagishima, R. T., Tutassura, H., Gerein, A. N., Burr, L. H., and Allen, P.: Early clinical experience with the Carpentier-Edwards porcine heterograft cardiac valve. Can. J. Surg., 23:132, 1980.

Kalil, R. K., Azambuja, P. C., Bertoletti, V. E., Lucchese, F. A., Prates, P. R., and Nesralla, I. A.: Surgical treatment of annuloaortic ectasia with composite grafts including homologous dura mater valves. Ann. Thorac. Surg., 26:142, 1978.

Karp, R. B., Cyrus, R. J., Blackstone, E. H., Kirklin, J. W., Kouchoukos, N. T., and Pacifico, A. D.: The Bjork-Shiley valve: Intermediate-term follow-up. J. Thorac. Cardiovasc. Surg., 81:602, 1981.

Kay, E. B., Nogueira, C., Suzuki, A., Postigo, J., and Mendelsohn, D.: Myocardial protection during aortic valvular surgery. Ann. Surg., 154(Suppl.):159, 1961.

Kihlgren, M., and Dubiel, W. T.: Rehabilitation after aortic valve replacement with autologous fascia lata: A sociomedical study. Ann. Thorac. Surg., 24:346, 1977.

Kirklin, J. W.: The replacement of cardiac valves. (Editorial.) N. Engl. J. Med., *304*:291, 1981.

Kirklin, J. W., and Ellis, F. H.: Surgical relief of diffuse subvalvular aortic stenosis. Circulation, 25:739, 1961.

Kirklin, J. W., and Kouchoukos, N. T.: Aortic valve replacement without myocardial revascularization. (Editorial.) Circulation, *63*:252, 1981.

Kittle, C. F., Reed, W. A., and Crockett, J. E.: Infundibulectomy for subaortic hypertrophic stenosis. Circulation, 29 (Suppl.):119, 1964.

Konno, S., Imai, Y., Iida, Y., Nakajima, M., and Tatsuno, K.: A new method for prosthetic valve replacement in congenital aortic stenosis associated with hypoplasia of the aortic valve ring. J. Thorac. Cardiovasc. Surg., 70:909, 1975.

Landymore, R. W., Tice, D., Trehan, N., and Spencer, F. C.: Does topical hypothermia prevent sublethal intraoperative injury during coronary artery bypass surgery? Presented at the Annual Meeting of the American Association for Thoracic Surgery, Washington, D. C., May 13, 1981.

Lawrence, R. S., Mena, I., Jengo, J. A., Walkinshaw, M. D., and Nelson, R. J.: Noninvasive evaluation of late left ventricular function after aortic valve replacement. J. Thorac. Cardiovasc. Surg., 79:504, 1980.

Lee, G., Grehl, T. M., Joye, J. A., Kaku, R. F., Harter, W., DeMaria, A. N., and Mason, D. T.: Hemodynamic assessment of the new aortic Carpentier-Edwards bioprosthesis. Cathet. Cardiovasc. Diagn., 4:373, 1978.

Levine, R. J., Roberts, W. C., and Morrow, A. G.: Traumatic aortic regurgitation. Am. J. Cardiol., 10:752, 1962.

Lillehei, C. W., Barnard, C. N., Long, D. M., et al.: Aortic valve reconstruction and replacement by total valve prostheses. In Prosthetic Heart Valves for Cardiac Surgery. Edited by K. A. Merendino. Springfield, Illinois, Charles C Thomas, 1961, pp. 527–575.

Macmanus, Q., Grunkemeier, G. L., Lambert, L. E., Teply, J. F., Harlan, B. J., and Starr, A.: Year of operation as a risk factor in the late results of valve replacement. J. Thorac. Cardiovasc. Surg., 80:834, 1980.

Magilligan, D. J., Jr., Fisher, E., and Alam, M.: Hemolytic anemia with porcine xenograft aortic and mitral valves. J. Thorac. Cardiovasc. Surg., 79:628, 1980a.

Magilligan, D. J., Jr., Lewis, J. W., Jr., Jara, F. M., Lee, M. W., Alam, M., Riddle, J. M., and Stein, P. D.: Spontaneous degeneration of porcine bioprosthetic valves. Ann. Thorac. Surg., 30:259, 1980b.

Manhas, D. R., Hessel, E. A., Winterscheid, L. C., Dillard, H., and Merendino, K. A.: Open heart surgery in infective endocarditis. Circulation, 41:841, 1970.

Manouguian, S., and Seybold-Epting, W.: Patch enlargement of the aortic valve ring by extending the aortic incision into the anterior mitral leaflet. J. Thorac. Cardiovasc. Surg., 78:402, 1979a.

Manouguian, S., Abu-Aishah, N., and Neitzel, J.: Patch enlargement of the aortic and mitral valve rings with aortic and mitral double valve replacement. J. Thorac. Cardiovasc. Surg., 78:394, 1979b.

McGoon, D. C.: Prosthetic reconstruction of the aortic valve. Staff Meet. Mayo Clin., 36:88, 1961.

Mori, T., Kawashima, Y., Kitamura, S., Nakano, S., Kawachi, K., and Nakata, T.: Results of aortic valve replacement in patients with a narrow aortic annulus: Effects of enlargement of the aortic annulus. Ann. Thorac. Surg., 31:111, 1981.

Morrow, A. G.: Hypertrophic subaortic stenosis: Some physiologic concepts and the role of operative treatment. Arch. Surg., 99:677, 1969.

Morrow, A. G., Reitz, B. A., Epstein, S. E., Henry, W. L., Conkle, D. M., Itscoitz, S. B., and Redwood, D. R.: Operative treatment in hypertrophic subaortic stenosis: Techniques and the results of pre- and postoperative assessment in 83 patients. Circulation, 52:88, 1975.

Mulder, D. G., Olinger, G. N., McConnell, D. H., Maloney, J. V., Jr., and Buckberg, G. D.: Myocardial protection during aortic valve replacement. Ann. Thorac. Surg., 21:123, 1976.

Muller, W. H., Jr., and Littlefield, J. B.: Kinetics and clinical application of a prosthetic aortic valve. Surg., Gynec. Obstet., *117*:330, 1963.

Muller, W. H., Jr., Dammann, J. F., Jr., and Warren, W. D.: Surgical correction of cardiovascular deformities in Marfan's syndrome. Ann. Surg., *152*:506, 1960.

Muller, W. H., Jr., Littlefield, J. B., and Dammann, J. F.: Subcoronary prosthetic replacement of the aortic valve. In Prosthetic Heart Valves for Cardiac Surgery. Edited by K. A. Merendino. Springfield, Illinois, Charles C Thomas, 1961, pp. 493–526.

Najafi, H., Ostermiller, W. E., Jr., Javid, H., Dye, W. S., Hunter, J. A., and Julian, O. C.: Narrow aortic root complicating aortic valve replacement. Arch. Surg., *99*:690, 1969.

Nicks, R., Cartmill, T., and Bernstein, L.: Hypoplasia of the aortic root: The problem of aortic root replacement. Thorax, *25*:339, 1970.

Nicoloff, D. M., and Emery, R. W.: Current status of the St. Jude cardiac valve prosthesis. Contemp. Surg., *15*, 1979.

Nolan, S. P., and Muller, W. H., Jr.: Acquired disorders of the aortic valve. In Davis-Christopher Textbook of Surgery. 12th Ed. Edited by D. C. Sabiston, Jr. Philadelphia, W. B. Saunders, 1981, pp. 2356–2363.

Norman, J. C., Cooley, D. A., Hallman, G. L., and Nihill, M. R.: Left ventricular apical-abdominal aortic conduits for left ventricular outflow tract obstructions: Clinical results in nine patients with a special composite prosthesis. Circulation, 54 (Suppl.):100, 1976.

Nuno-Conceicao, A., Puig, L. B., Verginelli, G., Iryia, K., Bittencourt, D., and Zerbini, E. J.: Homologous dura mater cardiac valves: Structural aspects of eight implanted valves. J. Thorac. Cardiovasc. Surg., 70:499, 1975.

Ott, D. A., Coelho, A. T., Cooley, D. A., and Reul, G. J., Jr.: Ionescu-Shiley pericardial xenograft valve: Hemodynamic evaluation and early clinical follow-up of 326 patients. Cardiovasc. Dis., 7:137, 1980.

Oyer, P. E., Miller, D. C., Stinson, E. B., Reitz, B. A., Morena-Cabral, R. J., and Shumway, N. E.: Clinical durability of the Hancock porcine bioprosthetic valve. J. Thorac. Cardiovasc. Surg., 80:824, 1980.

Oyer, P. E., Stinson, E. B., Reitz, B. A., Miller, D. C., Rossiter, S. J., and Shumway, N. E.: Long-term evaluation of the porcine xenograft bioprosthesis. J. Thorac. Cardiovasc. Surg., 78:343, 1979.

Pearse, A. G. E.: The histochemistry and electronmicroscopy of obstructive cardiomyopathy. Ciba Foundation Symposium on Cardiomyopathies. Boston, Little, Brown and Co., 1964.

Pently, G., Morton, M., and Rahimtoola, S. H.: Effects of successful, uncomplicated valve replacement on ventricular hypertrophy, volume, and performance in aortic stenosis and in aortic incompetence. J. Thorac. Cardiovasc. Surg., 75:383, 1978.

Pipkin, R. D., Buch, W. S., and Fogarty, T. J.: Evaluation of aortic valve replacement with a porcine xenograft without long-term anticoagulation. J. Thorac. Cardiovasc. Surg., 71:179, 1976.

Pupello, D. F., Blank, R. H., Bessone, L. N., Harrison, E., and Sbar, S.: Surgical management of the small aortic annulus: Hemodynamic evaluation. Chest, 74:163, 1978.

Rehn, L.: Ueber Penetrirende Herzwunden und Herznaht. Arch. Klin. Chir., 55:315, 1897.

Reitz, B. A., Stinson, E. B., Watson, D. C., Baumgartner, W. A., and Jamieson, S. W.: Translocation of the aortic valve for prosthetic valve endocarditis. J. Thorac. Cardiovasc. Surg., 81:212, 1981.

Riddle, J. M., Magilligan, D. J., and Stein, P. D.: Surface morphology of degenerated porcine bioprosthetic valves four to seven years following implantation. J. Thorac. Cardiovasc. Surg., 81:279, 1981.

Roberts, W. C.: Valvular, subvalvular, and supravalvular aortic stenosis: Morphologic features. Cardiovasc. Clin., 5:97, 1973.

Robicsek, F., and Harbold, N. B., Jr.: Management of the patient with a prosthetic heart valve. Ann. Thorac. Surg., 22:389, 1976.

Robinson, M. J., and Ruedy, J.: Sequela of bacterial endocarditis. Am. J. Med., *32*:922, 1962.

Ross, D., and Yacoub, M. H.: Homograft replacement of the aortic valve: A critical review. Prog. Cardiovasc. Dis., *11*:275, 1969.

Rothkopf, M., Davidson, T., Lipscomb, K., Narahara, K., Hillis, L. D., Willerson, J. T., Estrera, A., Platt, M., and Mills, L.: Hemodynamic evaluation of the Carpentier-Edwards bioprosthesis in the aortic position. Am. J. Cardiol., *44*:209, 1979.

Sandza, J. G., Jr., Clark, R. E., Ferguson, T. B., Connors, J. P., and Weldon, C. S.: Replacement of prosthetic heart valves: A fifteen-year experience. J. Thorac. Cardiovasc. Surg., *74*:864, 1977.

Scott, W. C., Shemin, R. J., Gaudiani, V. A., and Conkle, D. M.: Limits of myocardial protection with potassium cardioplegia. Ann. Thorac. Surg., *26*:507, 1978.

Segal, J., Harvey, W. P., and Hufnagel, C.: A clinical study of one hundred cases of severe aortic insufficiency. Am. J. Med., *21*:200, 1956.

Semb, B. K. H., Nitter-Hauge, S., and Hall, K. V.: The Hall-Kaster disc valve prosthesis: Clinical and hemodynamic observations in patients undergoing aortic valve replacement. J. Cardiovasc. Surg., *21*:387, 1980.

Silber, E. N., and Katz, L. N.: Heart Disease. New York, Macmillan Co., 1975.

Starr, A., Edwards, M. L., McCord, C. W., and Griswold, H. E.: Aortic replacement: Clinical experience with a semirigid ball-valve prosthesis. Circulation, *27*:779, 1963.

Starr, A., Bonchek, L. I., Anderson, R. P., Wood, J. A., and Chapman, R. D.: Late complications of aortic valve replacement with cloth-covered, composite-seat prostheses. Ann. Thorac. Surg., *19*:289, 1975.

Stein, D. W., Rahimtoola, S. H., Kloster, F. E., Selden, R., and Starr, A.: Thrombotic phenomena with nonanticoagulated, composite-strut aortic prostheses. J. Thorac. Cardiovasc. Surg., *71*:680, 1976.

Symbas, P. N., Baldwin, B. J., Silverman, M. E., and Galambos, J. T.: Marfan's syndrome with aneurysm of ascending aorta and aortic regurgitation. Am. J. Cardiol., *25*:483, 1970.

Syracuse, D. C., Bowman, F. O., Jr., and Malm, J. R.: Prosthetic valve reoperations: Factors influencing early and late survival. J. Thorac. Cardiovasc. Surg., *77*:346, 1979.

Tajik, A. J., and Giuliani, E. R.: Echocardiographic observations in idiopathic hypertrophic subaortic stenosis. Mayo Clin. Proc., *49*:89, 1974.

Tandon, A. P., Whitaker, W., and Ionescu, M. I.: Multiple valve replacement with pericardial xenograft: Clinical and hemodynamic study. Br. Heart J., *44*:534, 1980.

Thompson, R., Ahmed, M., Seabra-Gomes, R., Ilsley, C., Rickards, A., Towers, M., and Yacoub, M.: Influence of preoperative left ventricular function on results of homograft replacement of the aortic valve for aortic regurgitation. J. Thorac. Cardiovasc. Surg., *77*:411, 1979.

Thubrikar, M., Bosher, L. P., and Nolan, S. P.: The mechanism of opening of the aortic valve. J. Thorac. Cardiovasc. Surg., *77*:863, 1979.

Thubrikar, M., Nolan, S. P., Bosher, L. P., and Deck, J. D.: The cyclic changes and structure of the base of the aortic valve. Am. Heart J., *99*:217, 1980.

Triestman, B., and El-Said, G.: Valvular aortic stenosis and coronary artery disease. Cardiovasc. Dis., *2*:193, 1975.

Tuffier, T.: Étude expérimentale sur la chirurgie des valves de coeur. Bull. Acad. Méd. Paris, *71*:293, 1914.

Walker, D. K., Scotten, L. N., Modi, V. J., and Brownlee, R. T.: *In vitro* assessment of mitral valve prostheses. J. Thorac. Cardiovasc. Surg., *79*:680, 1980.

Wallace, R. B., Londe, S. P., and Titus, J. L.: Aortic valve replacement with preserved aortic valve homografts. J. Thorac. Cardiovasc. Surg., *67*:44, 1974.

Wilcox, B. R., Murray, G. F., and Starek, P. J. K.: The long-term outlook for valve replacement in active endocarditis. J. Thorac. Cardiovasc. Surg., *74*:860, 1977.

Williams, J. B., Karp, R. B., Kirklin, J. W., Kouchoukos, N. T., Pacifico, A. D., Zorn, G. L., Jr., Blackstone, E. H., Brown, R. N., Piantadosi, S., and Bradley, E. L.: Considerations in selection and management of patients undergoing valve replacement with glutaraldehyde-fixed porcine bioprostheses. Ann. Thorac. Surg., *30*:247, 1980.

Williams, W. G., Pollock, J. C., Geiss, D. M., Trusler, G. A., and Fowler, R. S.: Experience with aortic and mitral valve replacement in children. J. Thorac. Cardiovasc. Surg., *81*:326, 1981.

Wortham, D. C., Tri, T. B., and Bowen, T. E.: Hemodynamic evaluation of the St. Jude Medical valve prosthesis in the small aortic annulus. J. Thorac. Cardiovasc. Surg., *81*:615, 1981.

Zerbini, E. J.: Results of replacement of cardiac valves by homologous dura mater valves. (Abstract.) J.A.M.A., *233*:1433, 1975.

Chapter 49

Cardiac Pacemakers and Cardiac Conduction System Abnormalities

G. Frank O. Tyers

HISTORY

The invention early in the eighteenth century of timing mechanisms accurate enough for counting of the human pulse, combined with careful clinical and pathologic observations, allowed the potentially detrimental effects of cardiac arrhythmias to be recognized over 150 years ago (Schechter, 1979; Sutton *et al.*, 1980a; Thalen, 1979). In 1761, Morgagni described the combination of bradycardia and seizures but believed that the neurologic problem was primary and the arrhythmia secondary. In 1827, based on postmortem findings, Robert Adams suggested that the combination of bradycardia and syncope was probably of cardiac rather than cerebral origin. Although Adams' findings were not accepted by many authorities of the time, William Stokes supported his concept in 1846 based on his own experience and a review of the literature. The first recordings of complete heart block using a sphygmograph were made by Galaban in 1875, and the syndrome of bradycardia and syncopal attacks was called Stokes-Adams disease by Huchard in 1890. During the same period, the effects of electric irritation of the heart were reported. Initially, biologic current sources (frog legs, eels) were used and, subsequently, the Leyden jar, with which Von Humboldt was able to control the rate of an isolated heart at will. The first report of resuscitation of a human using surface electrostimulation was in 1774. Transthoracic needle cardiac stimulation was reported by Krimer in 1828 and transvenous atrial stimulation by Floresco in 1905.

The electrophysiologic and technical developments that underlie current cardiac pacing practice occurred thereafter at regular intervals (Schechter, 1979; Sutton *et al.*, 1980a; Thalen, 1979). The importance of proper timing of atrial contraction was noted by Gesell in 1911, and the role of the sinoatrial node as the natural cardiac pacemaker was confirmed by Marmorstein in 1927. An artificial external atrial pacemaker and bipolar leads were designed and used successfully in patients by Hyman, who reported his results in 1932. It is to Hyman that we owe the origin of the designation artificial cardiac pacemaker. An external ventricular pacemaker that was triggered and timed to follow atrial contraction was designed by Butterworth and Poindexter in 1942. In 1949, Bigelow and Callaghan reported their experience with an external pacemaker and transvenous right atrial leads that were used to overcome severe bradycardia in their studies of hypothermia. A most significant advance in the development of cardiac pacing was made by Zoll in 1952, when he undertook external ventricular pacing in patients with complete heart block and syncope (Stokes-Adams syndrome). The high risk of this condition, which was associated with a mortality rate in the range of 50 per cent per year, was recognized. Zoll was able to eliminate Stokes-Adams attacks by applying rhythmic electric stimuli directly to the surface of the chest, although the patients experienced significant discomfort and stimulation of skeletal as well as cardiac muscle. There was little chance of long-term benefit, but with the repeated demonstration of elimination of devastating symptoms with controlled rhythmic electrotherapy, a new era began. Only a year later, Dammann reported the development of an external ventricular pacemaker that automatically turned on only when the patient's heart rate fell below a predetermined level. This was the first "demand" pacemaker. A device of this type was used clinically in 1956 by Leathem and associates, and in the same year, Lillehei and Bakken developed mixed transthoracic pacing for patients with a newly developed condition, postoperative complete heart block. The bare ends of insulated wires were attached to the heart at the time of surgery and brought through the chest wall and skin to be attached to an external pulse generator. This mixed (external pacer, internal leads) approach eliminated much of the discomfort associated with external pacing and for the first time provided the potential for a degree of mobility and long-term survival. However, related both to the risk of thoracotomy and to the frequent flexion-related failure of the electrodes then available, this method of pacing was infrequently applied to patients with complete heart block.

In 1958, Furman made one of the first of his many significant contributions to the field of cardiac pacing. An electrode was passed through the skin and, by way of superficial vein, vena cava, and right atrium, into the apex of the right ventricle and was connected to an external pulse generator. Thus evolved mixed transvenous cardiac pacing, which could be applied to the majority of heart block patients at a reasonable risk. However, many potential problems remained, including infection tracking down the transcutaneous leads, accidental disconnection, and wetting of the external pulse generator.

Subsequently, more than a decade was required to achieve small, relatively reliable, internal (totally implanted) pulse generators and electrodes (Schechter, 1977; Sutton *et al.*, 1980a; Tyers and Brownlee, 1978). An important first step was taken by Senning and Elmqvist in 1958 when they developed a small pacemaker and electrode system powered by a rechargeable nickel-cadmium battery. Although the batteries in this device proved to be short-lived, even with recharging, the first totally implantable cardiac pacing system had been achieved. In that same year, a mixed radiofrequency pacemaker was reported by Mauro and Glenn. This system involved implantation of electrodes and a receiver coil in conjunction with an external power source that transmitted its energy through the intact skin.

Numerous mixed systems not requiring percutaneous leads were developed and used clinically, but the inconvenience of an external power source remained, limiting the patient's ability to bathe and presenting the constant risk of external transmitter dislocation with recurrence of symptoms. However, at the time and for several years thereafter, only these systems allowed for years of continuous cardiac pacing without reoperation.

The course of pacemaker development for the next 20 years was set in 1959 when Chardack and Greatbatch introduced a totally implantable pacemaker system powered by a primary or nonrechargeable mercury-zinc multicell battery, and Hunter and associates introduced an improved bipolar intramyocardial electrode. A marked improvement in the grave morbidity and mortality associated with nonpacemaker therapy of patients with Stokes-Adams syndrome resulted. However, thoracotomy and implantation of a permanent internal pacemaker in elderly patients with complete heart block continued to be associated with significant risk. This was reduced after 1961, when Davidson and associates recommended temporary transvenous pacing prior to implantation of permanent transthoracic electrodes and an internal pacemaker. The following year, 1962, Lagergren and Johansson reported connecting a permanent subcutaneous pacemaker to a lead passed transvenously into the right ventricle, and the same year, permanent internal physiologic pacing was introduced by Keller and associates with the development of an implantable, atrially triggered, ventricular pacemaker, the Cordis Atricor.

In 1963, "programmable pacing" was reported by Kantrowitz and colleagues. Closure of a reed switch by placing a magnet over the pacemaker resulted in change in the pacemaker stimulation rate. That same year, Medtronic, Inc. introduced a permanent pacemaker that was both rate-programmable and output-energy–programmable. Triangular needles were passed through self-sealing ports into potentiometer receptacles. Turning in one direction lowered the parameter, and turning in the other direction increased it. Also in 1963, totally implantable pacing on demand was described by Zacouto, Castellanos, and coworkers, including Berkovits. Two years later, in 1965, Tyers and associates reported the development of a totally implantable, electromechanical, multiprogrammable pacemaker that allowed for the noninvasive selection of 120 different combinations of six parameters, including rate, output, polarity, stimulation site, and a choice of unipolar or bipolar pacing (Tyers *et al.*, 1966). The 2-year durability of mercury-zinc batteries and epoxy and silicone rubber packages that allowed gradual fluid ingress remained major limitations (Tyers and Brownlee, 1976, 1978). Use of nuclear power sources for pacemakers was reported by Piwnica and Laurens in 1969; the Siemens Elema Company investigated the use of lithium power sources as early as 1970, and Telectronics developed a hermetically sealed, primary, mercury-zinc battery–powered pacemaker the same year. A hermetically sealed, rechargeable, mercury-zinc–powered pacemaker with direct telemetry readout of power cell voltage was developed at Pennsylvania State University in 1971. In 1973, in spite of numerous difficulties encountered by previous investigators, a highly reliable, hermetically sealed, nickel-cadmium cell–powered, rechargeable pacemaker was achieved by workers at Johns Hopkins University and introduced commercially by Pacesetter, Inc. Numerous lithium anode cells were investigated and used clinically, but the reliability of the first widely available hermetically sealed lithium-iodine cell–powered pacer, introduced by Cardiac Pacemakers, Inc. in 1972, eventually led to the elimination from serious contention of most other lithium cell configurations as well as rechargeable and nuclear power sources. Reliability and longevity were to become expected characteristics rather than the exception.

Important changes were also taking place in the design and construction of leads and electrodes (Furman *et al.*, 1979; Schechter, 1979; Sutton *et al.*, 1980a; Thalen, 1979; Tyers and Brownlee, 1981). A single transvenous catheter with two spaced electrodes, for atrial sensing and ventricular stimulation, respectively, was described by Battye in 1960. Multistrand wires were in general replaced by a flexible helix (miniature spring), which markedly improved lead durability. Elgiloy, a flex-resistant alloy developed by the Elgin watch company and pioneered for use in pacing by the Cordis Corporation, and platinum-iridium alloy, pioneered by Chardack and Medtronic, Inc., became the materials of choice. Placement of a permanent transvenous electrode in the coronary sinus for atrial pacing was recommended by Moss in 1967, and shortly thereafter, Messenger and associates began to use this route and the Cordis Ectocor for atrially triggered demand atrial pacing. A J-shaped lead for placement in the right atrial appendage was developed by Smyth and associates in 1969, and with the introduction of improved materials, this has proved to be the technique of choice for atrial pacing. Until recently, during manufacture of a lead, the wire conductor was inserted into a relatively thick-walled tube of silicone rubber. This material is relatively porous, thrombogenic, and of low tensile strength. In our long-term studies of rechargeable pacemakers in goats at Pennsylvania State University in the early 1970s, we were experiencing a high incidence of electrode breakage because these very active animals function as an accelerated test. A segmented polyurethane-coated (Biomer) lead was developed and tested extensively in animals and in an accelerated flex tester. This lead proved to be a thousand times more durable than commercially available Elgiloy coil electrodes in silicone tubes. In the last few years, two major manufacturers (Medtronic, Inc. and Intermedics, Inc.) have independently introduced electrodes that incorporate this technology and earlier manufacturing methods. The metallic conductor is placed into segmented polyurethane tubes of markedly improved elasticity and tensile strength relative to silicone rubber. It is possible that these leads will have improved long-term durability. Another major problem with pervenous electrodes has been their tendency to displace from right atrial and/or ventricular cavities. Fixed and remotely activated tines, barbs, and clamps have been developed to minimize early and late postoperative displacement, with varying degrees of success. Currently, transvenous electrode dislodgement occurs very infrequently following implantation by a careful, experienced operator.

The present era of electronic and technical sophistication (Schechter, 1979; Thalen, 1979; Tyers and Brownlee, 1981; Furman, 1973; Mirowski *et al.*, 1980) began in 1969 with the development, by Berkovits and associates, of a pacemaker that sequentially paced the atrium and subsequently the ventricle to preserve the atrial contribution to cardiac function. This device was "demand," in that it sensed in the ventricle, but it did not sense in the atrium. Compared with the earlier "physiologic," atrially triggered, ventricular stimulating pacemaker, which became a simple, fixed-rate ventricular pacemaker when atrial sensing was disrupted, this was an important advance. In 1971, Rogel described an atrially triggered ventricular pacemaker that sensed in the ventricle and was activated either by an atrial rate exceeding the patient's ventricular rate or by ventricular bradycardia. An electromechanically programmable, dual-function (rate and current) pacemaker was introduced clinically by Terry and Tarjan of the Cordis Corporation in 1972. The development and implantation of a pacemaker with an internal diagnostic radiotransmitter (telemetry) of

physiologic and electronic data (pulse rate and cell voltage) were achieved by Brownlee and Tyers in 1974, followed in 1978 by a multiparameter real data transmitter that allowed the physician following the patient to measure internal pacemaker power cell voltage, power cell impedance, electrode and stimulation impedance, refractory interval, and crude hermeticity. Diagnostic telemetry was combined with the first clinical introduction of a totally electronic multiparameter programmable pacemaker, the Intermedics Cyberlith I, in conjunction with the work of Calfee and associates in 1978 and with the first electronic multiprogrammable, unipolar, AV sequential pacer, the Cyberlith IV, in 1980. The first clinical, three-parameter, electromechanically programmable, bipolar, AV sequential clinical pacemaker (the Byrel) had been achieved by Berkovits and associates at Medtronic, Inc. in 1978. That same year, Funke described the automatic pacemaker. This dual-chamber device can on its own "decide" to function as an atrial demand pacemaker, a ventricular demand pacemaker, an atrially triggered ventricular pacemaker, or a dual-chamber atrial and ventricular demand pacemaker, depending on what is most appropriate for the underlying arrhythmia at the time. Clinical evaluation of small devices of this type has begun.

A final area of fairly recent development is implantable cardiac stimulator treatment of tachyarrhythmias (Furman, 1973; Mirowski *et al.*, 1980). Furman and others have worked with patient-activated, radiofrequency, rapid atrial stimulators for arrhythmia termination for several years, and in 1979, the Medtronic team led by Berkovits began the clinical evaluation of an automatically activated, underdrive, atrioventricular sequential (double-demand) pacemaker for re-entry tachyarrhythmias. More recent developments in antiarrhythmia pacing include the ongoing clinical trials of implantable defibrillators (Medrad Intec AID), automatic scanning stimulators with therapy memory functions for delivery of critically timed extra stimuli (Teletronics Autodecremental Pacer), and automatic multiparameter programmable burst and train stimulators with an arrhythmia treatment memory function (Intermedics CyberTach).

As a result of recent electronic developments, many deriving from the space program, change in the field of cardiac stimulation is now occurring so rapidly that refinements that formerly took years are now achieved within months. At no time in the history of cardiac electrostimulation has the future had such propensity to become the past or has the problem of staying abreast of developments and separating gadgetry from necessity been so acute. However, the gains in longevity, reliability, and therapeutic scope have the potential to more than justify the complexity.

PACEMAKER TYPES AND DESCRIPTIVE CODES

The first internal pacemakers developed were asynchronous or fixed-rate devices that sent electric stimuli at regular preselected intervals through an insulated lead wire to the ventricular myocardium. In those patients with only intermittent loss of conduction and/or bradytachyarrhythmias, these devices of necessity competed with the natural cardiac pacemaker whenever the natural rhythm exceeded the rate of the pacemaker. A logical step was to develop pulse generators that sensed normal cardiac activity and turned on only when required for maintenance of a satisfactory heart rate. Two types of on-demand pacers were developed, triggered and inhibited. A ventricular triggered pacemaker responds to ventricular depolarization by firing immediately into the refractory ventricular myocardium. An atrially triggered pacemaker may fire immediately into the refractory atrium or, with a system with leads in both an atrium and a ventricle, it may fire into the ventricle after an appropriate delay to allow for hemodynamic filling. In the past, some triggered devices put out low-amplitude, subthreshold stimuli and were known as tracking pacemakers. Potential disadvantages of same chamber-triggered pacemakers were energy waste and distortion of the electrocardiogram. Potential advantages included confirmation of the exact time of sensing and the substitution of competitive pacing for inappropriate suppression by noncardiac electric signals. In contrast to triggered devices, inhibited pacemakers respond to cardiac electric signals by turning off. Especially during their early phase of development, these devices could also be turned off by numerous other electromagnetic signals, such as those generated by pulsatile theft detection instruments in department stores, gasoline motor ignition systems, and so on. Apart from the energy-saving advantages of inhibiting or turning off a pacemaker when it is not required, competitive delivery of relatively high-energy and, in particular, anodal electric stimuli during ventricular repolarization (T wave) may on occasion induce ventricular fibrillation. It was thought that demand pacemakers would reduce patient risk and last longer, but the sensing circuit draws a small amount of energy, and inhibition by electromagnetic interference with syncope or even death in a pacemaker-dependent patient was an uncommon but real problem. Thus, at least until recently, improved survival with demand pacers versus competitive or fixed-rate pacers had not been demonstrated (Tyers and Brownlee, 1976b). On-demand or sensing pacers have generated problems with terminology as well as electrocardiographic and functional interpretation. Ventricular sensing devices (inhibited or triggered) have also been called ventricular programmed pacers, and similarly, atrial sensing devices have also been called atrially programmed pacers. It became apparent that a widely accepted terminology was required.

To assist with communication and understanding of pacemaker operating types and modes, an Intersociety Commission for Heart Disease Resources recommmended a three-letter identification code in 1974 (Parsonnet *et al.*, 1974). Table 49–1 illustrates the ICHD three-letter code as currently applied. The first

TABLE 49–1. INTERSOCIETY COMMISSION FOR HEART DISEASE RESOURCES (ICHD) PULSE GENERATOR THREE-LETTER IDENTIFICATION CODE

1st Letter (Chamber[s] Paced)	2nd Letter (Chamber[s] Sensed)	3rd Letter (Mode of Response)
V, A, or D	V, A, D, or O	I, T, D, or O

letter may be a V for ventricle, an A for atrium, or D for double (both atrium and ventricle), indicating the chamber or chambers paced. As stimulation came before sensing in the development of pacing, this should help with remembering the order of the code. The second letter indicates the sensed chamber and again it is V, A, D, or O, the last indicating no sensing function. The third letter indicates the mode of response, if any, to sensing, with I indicating inhibited (output blocked by a sensed signal), T indicating triggered (output discharged by a sensed signal), D indicating both triggered and inhibited function, and 0 indicating not applicable. Examples of the different types of pacemakers currently or previously available are presented in Table 49–2. Thus, VOO is the simplest device, pacing in the ventricle, not sensing in either chamber, and thus having no mode of response. At the opposite extreme is DDD, pacing in both chambers, sensing in both chambers, and responding in either an inhibited or triggered fashion as physiologically indicated. A review of the generic descriptions will facilitate understanding the code. Other designations, some still used, are also included and are self-explanatory, with the exception of DDT*I/I. This indicates pacing in both chambers (first D), sensing in both chambers (second D), ventricular triggered pacing in response to atrial sensing (T*), inhibition of atrial pacing by atrial depolarization (first I), and inhibition of ventricular pacing by ventricular depolarization (second I).

As multiprogrammable and antitachycardia pacing has developed, the three-letter code has not allowed accurate description of all pacemaker functions. A five-letter code was more recently presented (Table 49–3) as a preliminary attempt to address these limitations (Parsonnet *et al.*, 1981). Positions 1, 2, and 3 are essentially unchanged, whereas position 4 indicates absence or presence and type of programmable function, and position 5 indicates antitachyarrhythmia function. As will be seen in the section on antiarrhythmia treatment, a large number of therapy types, including implantable defibrillators, automatic burst and train stimulators, and simultaneous dual-chamber pacing, are currently under evaluation, and it is probable that a number of antiarrhythmia modes will be included in a single device in the near future and that the pacemaker will automatically try different modes of electric antiarrhythmia therapy, beginning with the safest. The same device might treat supraventricular arrhythmias with burst pacing and ventricular arrhythmias with automatic defibrillation. Thus, still more

TABLE 49–2. EXAMPLES OF ICHD PULSE GENERATOR TERMINOLOGY CODE

CHAMBER(S) PACED	CHAMBER(S) SENSED	MODE OF RESPONSE	GENERIC DESCRIPTION	PREVIOUSLY USED DESIGNATION
V	O	O	Ventricular pacing, no sensing function	Asynchronous; fixed rate; set rate
V	V	T	Ventricular pacing and sensing, triggered mode	Ventricular triggered; R triggered; R-wave stimulated; noncompetitive triggered; following; R synchronous; demand; standby
V	V	I	Ventricular pacing and sensing, inhibited mode	Ventricular inhibited; R inhibited; R blocking; R suppressed; noncompetitive inhibited; demand; standby
A	O	O	Atrial pacing, no sensing function	Atrial fixed rate; atrial asynchronous
A	A	T	Atrial pacing and sensing, triggered mode	Atrial triggered; P triggered; P stimulated; P synchronous
A	A	I	Atrial pacing and sensing, inhibited mode	Atrial inhibited; P inhibited; P blocking; P suppressed
V	A	T	Ventricular pacing, atrial sensing, triggered mode	Atrial synchronous, atrial synchronized, AV synchronous
V	D	D	Ventricular pacing and sensing, inhibited mode; atrial sensing, triggered mode	VDT*/I ASVIP
D	O	O	Atrioventricular pacing, no sensing function	AV sequential fixed rate (asynchronous)
D	V	I	Atrioventricular pacing, ventricular sensing, inhibited mode	Bifocal sequential demand; AV sequential
D	D	D	Atrioventricular pacing and sensing, the latter with both triggered and inhibited responses	DDT*I/I

detailed codes will be required in the future. One recent approach has been a two-line code, similar to a complex fraction, with atrial activity indicated above the line and ventricular activity indicated below it (Brownlee *et al.*, 1981). P represents pacing, S sensing, I_A inhibition by a sensed atrial event, I_V inhibition by a sensed ventricular event, T_A triggering by a sensed atrial event, and T_V triggering by a sensed ventricular event. Table 49–4 describes the ICHD three-letter modes listed in Table 49–2 in terms of

the new code. Funke's fully automatic pacemaker would be described as $\dfrac{PSI_A\, I_V}{PST_A\, I_V}$. This device paces and senses in both chambers; the atrial output is inhibited by a sensed event in either the atrium or the ventricle, whereas the ventricular output is inhibited by a sensed ventricular event or triggered by an atrial event, if no spontaneous ventricular event occurs during an appropriate A-V delay. Although apparently more complex and less verbal than the ICHD

TABLE 49–3. FIVE-POSITION PACEMAKER CODE (ICHD)

POSITION	I (CHAMBER[S] PACED)	II (CHAMBER[S] SENSED)	III (MODE OF RESPONSE)	IV (PROGRAMMABLE FUNCTIONS)	V (SPECIAL TACHYARRHYTHMIA FUNCTIONS)
Letters Used	V – Ventricle	V – Ventricle	T – Triggered	P – Programmable (rate and/or output)	B – Bursts
	A – Atrium	A – Atrium	I – Inhibited	M – Multiprogrammable	N – Normal rate competition
	D – Double	D – Double	D – Double* 0 – None		S – Scanning
		0 – None	R – Reverse	0 – None	E – External

*Atrially triggered and/or inhibited and ventricularly inhibited.

TABLE 49-4. THE ICHD MODES DESCRIBED IN TERMS OF CHAMBER ACTIVITY

$$VOO = \frac{O}{P} \qquad\qquad VAT = \frac{S}{PT_A}$$

$$VVT = \frac{O}{PST_V} \qquad\qquad VDD = \frac{S}{PSI_VT_A}$$

$$VVI = \frac{O}{PSI_V} \qquad\qquad DOO = \frac{P}{P}$$

$$AOO = \frac{P}{O} \qquad\qquad DVI = \frac{PI_V}{PSI_V}$$

$$AAT = \frac{PST_A}{O} \qquad\qquad DDD = \frac{PSI_VI_A}{PSI_VT_A}$$

$$AAI = \frac{PSI_A}{O}$$

O = No activity; P = pace; S = sense; I_V = inhibited by ventricular activity; I_A = inhibited by atrial activity; T_V = triggered by ventricular activity; T_A = triggered by atrial activity

code, the Brownlee teaching code clearly and accurately describes even the most complex forms of dual-chamber pacing. It could be easily expanded to indicate a variety of antiarrhythmia functions, in the order attempted by the pacemaker, with letters added above the line for atrial arrhythmia treatment modes and below the line for ventricular arrhythmia treatment modes. Programmability will probably not require an indicator in the future, as current levels of miniaturization and reliability indicate that only clinical and economic disadvantages will derive from the use of nonprogrammable pacers (Lopman *et al.*, 1980), which will undoubtedly go the way of the VOO pacer. From this point on, pacemakers will be described in this chapter using the three-letter ICHD code, as it is currently the most widely accepted descriptive means. It is therefore essential that Tables 49–1 and 49–2 be understood before proceeding.

PACEMAKER TECHNOLOGY

Although details of pacemaker power source chemistry and construction, electronic design, lead insulating materials, and electrode surface area may seem unimportant to the physician primarily involved in pacemaker implantation or follow-up, a basic understanding of this information is essential for making wise hardware and follow-up schedule selections. Physicians who continued to use nonhermetically sealed mercury-zinc battery–powered pulse generators to the very end of their availability, because of lack of understanding the newer, longer-lived pulse generators available, did their patients and health care cost effectiveness a disservice. Similarly, those who now believe that most lithium-powered pulse generators will last 10 or more years, without recognizing the critical roles played by physician-controlled variables such as electrode surface area and pulse width, will be lulled into inadequate follow-up procedures. This section will review current knowledge of and the

continuing search for improved power sources, electronics, and leads and the interactions of hardware selection and patterns of use that inevitably determine longevity and reliability.

Power Sources (Tyers and Brownlee, 1978, 1981)

Pacing systems are described as external, mixed, or internal. With external systems, the power source is outside the patient and the electrodes are applied to the integument, as described in the history section of this chapter. With adequate monitoring and grounding, this system remains both simple and potentially useful for transient emergency resuscitation. However, mixed ventricular or atrial pacing should be the primary choice for even temporarily extended emergency pacing. The so-called mixed systems utilize an external power source that is connected to the heart either by a percutaneous transvenous lead—for example, in the coronary care unit for temporary treatment of bradyarrhythmias after myocardial infarction—or by a percutaneous transthoracic lead brought out through the chest wall at the time of cardiac surgery for the temporary treatment of both postoperative bradyarrhythmias and tachyarrhythmias. Both transvenous and transthoracic mixed pacing systems may be used to pace either the atrium or the ventricle, or both chambers sequentially. Historically, mixed systems with external power sources and totally implanted coil and lead systems, utilizing inductive or radiofrequency energy transmission through the intact skin, were utilized for permanent pacing, but only a small number of these systems are still in clinical use. Internal or totally implanted pacing systems, in which the power source, electronics, and electrodes are all totally contained within the body, are currently the systems of choice worldwide, with more than 260,000 implants performed in 1981 (more than 100,000 in North America) and 330,000 implants estimated for 1985 (more than 150,000 in North America).

Power sources for internal pacemakers may be biologic, rechargeable, nuclear, or chemical. A number of biologic systems have been developed that successfully convert the mechanical or chemical energy of the body into electrical energy using piezoelectric crystals, biogalvanic cells, or bioautofuel cells. Although these energy sources are potentially renewable for the lifetime of the recipient, they have yet to be reduced to clinical practicality. Nuclear-powered pacemakers have been implanted in over 3000 patients worldwide. The radioactive power sources used were primarily promethium-147 and plutonium-238. The promethium photoelectric system was discarded, as it is not theoretically superior to the improved chemical power sources now available, but the plutonium thermoelectric system, which converts heat into electricity, is potentially the longest-lived primary (nonrechargeable) power source developed. Nuclear units are infrequently used, however, because of a number of factors, including cost, the similar longevity of newer chemical power sources, legislative restrictions, and continuing questions regarding the risk of years of low-level radiation exposure.

Chemical power cells have been and continue to be the primary power sources for implantable cardiac pacemakers. Chemical cells are described as primary (used once and discarded) or secondary (rechargeable), with the vast majority of pacemaker implants now powered by primary lithium anode chemical cells. To facilitate understanding of the chemical cells now in use and the need for continuing power cell development and improvement, several definitions will be considered. The terms cell and battery are often employed more or less interchangeably. A power *cell* is composed of an anode (e.g., zinc or lithium), a cathode (e.g., mercuric oxide or iodine polymer), and an electrolyte (e.g., sodium hydroxide or lithium iodide). Cells are generally named for the materials used in the anode and cathode, for example, lithium-iodine. They produce electricity as a result of a chemical reaction or a combination of reactions. Cells are referred to as wet, dry, or solid state, depending on the nature of the electrolyte, the chemical substance within the cell that conducts ions and electrons between the anode and the cathode. In a *wet cell* (Dupont/Cordis, SAFT, automobile lead-acid), the electrolyte is liquid. A *dry cell,* such as a standard flashlight battery, has a paste-like conductive electrolyte. *Solid state cells* (lithium-iodine and Mallory lithium) have a dry, crystalline, nonspillable electrolyte between the anode and the cathode. To produce electric current, the anode of a cell ionizes, resulting in the migration of positively charged metallic ions through the electrolyte toward the cathode. Electrons are left behind on the anode, which becomes negatively charged relative to the cathode. When the anode and the cathode are connected by a conductive pathway, as, for example, in a pacemaker electronic circuit, an electric current (flow of electrons) passes from the anode to the cathode. The higher the resistance in the conductor, the slower the flow of electrons and the longer the power cell will last. In a lithium-iodine cell, the migrating, positively charged ions are lithium, and they combine with iodine from the cathode to form a lithium-iodide electrolyte barrier. A *battery* is a group of cells connected either in parallel (anode to anode, cathode to cathode) to increase battery capacity, or in series (anode to cathode) to increase battery voltage (single cell voltage × the number of cells in the battery = battery voltage). The majority of currently available lithium-powered pacemakers contain single power cells, whereas the original mercury-zinc pacemakers were all powered by multiple-cell batteries.

When a voltmeter is placed in the circuit between the anode and the cathode of a cell, the voltage measured is a function of the chemical reactions occurring. The beginning of life voltage of a Mallory mercury-zinc cell is 1.35 volts, compared with 2.8 volts for a lithium-iodine cell. Other voltages for other lithium anode cells used in pacemakers are shown in

TABLE 49–5. TYPES OF LITHIUM CELLS USED IN PACEMAKERS*§

ANODE	CATHODE	CELL VOLTAGE†	MANUFACTURER
Lithium	Iodine polymer	2.8	Catalyst Research Corp. Wilson Greatbatch Ltd. Ener Tech
Lithium	Silver chromate	3.4	SAFT
Lithium	Cupric sulfide	2.1	Cordis/Dupont
Lithium	Thionyl chloride‡	3.6	GTE/ARCO
Lithium	Lead sulfide, lead iodide	1.9	Mallory

*In order of frequency
†Beginning of life
‡More accurately a reactive electrolyte than the cathode
GTE = General Telephone and Electronics
§From Tyers, G. F. O., and Brownlee, R. R.: Power pulse generators, electrodes and longevity. Prog. Cardiovasc. Dis., 23:421, 1981.

Table 49–5. To estimate the potential life of a pacemaker, it is necesary to know not only the power cell voltage but also the cell capacity, which is a function of its size. Standard Mallory mercury-zinc cells were rated at 1 ampere-hour: that is, they could produce a current of 1 ampere for a duration of 1 hour, or 1 milliampere for a duration of 1000 hours. Most pacemakers of that era required approximately a 20-microampere current and were therefore theoretically good for 50,000 hours or 5.7 years. *Ampere-hour capacity* by itself, however, is not a reliable means of estimating the usable energy of a power cell. It must be combined with cell voltage to determine *watt-hour capacity* and with knowledge of other cell variables, including internal resistance and voltage decay with time. Thus, a 1 ampere-hour, 1.3-volt, mercury-zinc cell has a capacity of 1.3 watt-hours (1 ampere-hour × 1.3 volts), whereas a 1.2 ampere-hour, lithium-iodine cell has a capacity of greater than 3 watt-hours (1.2 ampere-hours × 2.8 volts). By dividing the watt-hour capacity of a cell by its weight or volume, its energy density can be determined in terms of watt-hours per gram and watt-hours per cm.^{3}, respectively. Both *volumetric and gravimetric energy densities* are important considerations in pacemaker design, because the higher the ratings, the smaller the resulting pacemaker of equivalent theoretical functional life. However, it is stressed that no single factor can be taken in isolation. The lithium–thionyl chloride cell (see Table 49–5) has significantly better energy density than any other extensively used power cell system, but it is no longer available because of unreliable end-of-life characteristics. Knowledge of the lithium–thionyl chloride cell, however, is not academic, as thousands of highly mobile patients have pacers powered by it.

The *self-discharge rate* of a power cell is a measure of the rate at which it loses energy spontaneously during storage or in addition to the energy being removed by the circuit following pacemaker manufacture. Temperature, humidity, and rate of discharge affect the measurement of the capacity lost to other than useful work. The self-discharge rate of all of the lithium anode power cells has been satisfactory, in the range of 1 per cent or less per year.

A final concept with regard to pacemaker power sources relates to *energy availability*. For example, a rechargeable system may have a relatively low capacity, but if the energy can be renewed repeatedly, a very long-lived pacemaker can be developed. In contrast, if a low-resistance pathway (short circuit) develops within a battery or within the pacemaker circuitry, even a high-capacity cell will run out of energy very quickly. A unique feature of the lithium-iodine system is a gradual increase in resistance within the cell as lithium and iodine combine to form a progressively thickening lithium-iodide electrolyte barrier. Toward the end of life of the power cell, as the cathode is depleted of iodine, its resistance also rises significantly. Although the development of the lithium-iodide barrier plays an important role in the high reliability of this power cell, it also has the potential to limit energy availability. With some early lithium-iodine cells, significant chemical energy remained at a time when they would no longer drive a pacemaker circuit, because high *internal resistance* had reduced current flow to too low a level. Energy and high current availability are important areas of research, because high current drain applications (multichamber and antiarrhythmia pacing), increase the rate of resistance build-up within a standard lithium-iodine cell, and thus have the potential to markedly reduce the functional life of the pacemaker.

Rechargeable chemical cell–powered pacemakers using both hermetically sealed nickel-cadmium and silver-mercury–silver-zinc power sources have proved to be highly reliable after 7 to 8 years of clinical implantation. The Johns Hopkins/Pacesetter nickel-cadmium systems were implanted in approximately 3000 patients but were discontinued by the manufacturer, primarily because of physician and, on occasion, patient resistance to the necessity for weekly recharging. The rechargeable silver-mercury–silver-zinc cell–powered pacemakers developed at the Pennsylvania State University required relatively infrequent recharging and were capable of providing several years of pacing without recharging, but although still functioning in a limited number of patients, like the nuclear and nickel-cadmium systems, they have been supplanted by the development and availability of highly reliable and practical primary chemical power sources.

As primary chemical power cells are the overwhelming preference of the majority of pacemaker manufacturers and implanting physicians, they will be considered in more detail. The vast majority of pacemakers manufactured between 1960 and 1972 were powered by primary mercury-zinc batteries. Design improvements were made by both the Mallory Com-

pany and General Electric, but only occasional units achieved their potential 5- to 7-year longevity. The era of the lithium pacemaker power source began in 1972, when Cardiac Pacemakers, Inc., of St. Paul, Minnesota, introduced the Maxilith. This pacemaker was powered by a single lithium-iodine cell, and it introduced a period of unprecedented pacemaker longevity and reliability. Major advantages over the mercury-zinc battery power sources included increased energy density, lack of gas generation during discharge (versus hydrogen gas generation), lack of pressure build-up during discharge (versus an operating level of 300 p.s.i.), ease of adaptability to hermetic sealing, and generation of a self-healing lithium-iodide barrier between the anode and cathode (versus the tendency for the development of dendritic growth and short circuiting through a mechanical barrier). Subsequently, a number of other lithium anode pacemaker power cells were developed and used clinically, as listed in Table 49–5. A potential disadvantage of the SAFT and Dupont cells versus the lithium-iodine, GTE, and Mallory cells was their reliance on crimped pressure seals rather than metallic welded seals. In addition, all of the more recent lithium anode cells needed internal barriers between the anode and cathode, as with the older mercury-zinc cells. Disadvantages of the GTE and Mallory power sources included volume changes during discharge, which in the case of the Mallory cell required mechanical spring loading and led to a higher premature failure rate than with lithium-iodine cells. A potential advantage of the GTE lithium–thionyl chloride cell over the lithium-iodine cell was its apparently superior energy density, the highest of all the lithium power sources listed in Table 49–5. A final advantage of the lithium-iodine cell, shared by only the Mallory lithium cell, is its solid state nature, with no liquid electrolyte as present in the SAFT, GTE, and Dupont cells.

All of the lithium power sources listed in Table 49–5 have been shown to have markedly improved reliability and durability versus the earlier mercury-zinc systems, but in by far the greatest percentage of current pacemaker implants worldwide a solid state lithium-iodine cell is used, which appears to be the power source of choice at this time. The relative experience with the different lithium anode power cells through June 1979 is shown in Table 49–6. Lithium-iodine cell–powered pacemaker implants now number in the range of 500,000, compared with only modest increases in implants containing other lithium power sources.

The relative reliability of a selection of pacemakers powered by the different cells is shown in Table 49–7. A monthly failure rate of 0.02 per cent indicates that two out of every 10,000 patients being followed are at risk. However, the numbers must be interpreted in relation to the duration of exposure. With a large number of very recent implants, the monthly failure rate may be much lower than that finally achieved prior to power cell depletion, at which

TABLE 49–6. EXPERIENCE WITH LITHIUM ANODE POWER CELLS THROUGH JUNE 1979§

PACEMAKER COMPANY	Thionyl Chloride	Iodine Polymer	Silver Chromate	Lead Sulfide and Iodide	Cupric Sulfide	NO. OF IMPLANTS*
			CELL TYPE BY CATHODE			
ARCO	16	—	—	—	—	16
CPI	—	45	10	—	—	55
Coratomic	—	—	—	3	—	3
Cordis†	—	—	—	—	3-cell—28 2-cell—1	29
Edwards	—	—	6	—	—	6
Intermedics	—	48	—	5	—	53
Medcor	—	2	3	—	—	5
Medtronic‡	—	2-cell—121 1-cell—11	—	—	—	132
Pacesetter	—	5	—	—	—	5
Telectronics	—	27	13	—	—	40
Vitatron	—	5	5	—	—	10
Total	16	264	37	8	29	354

*Nearest thousand
†3-cell Lambda; 2-cell Theta
‡2-cell Xyrel; 1-cell Mirel
§From Tyers, G. F. O., and Brownlee, R. R.: Power pulse generators, electrodes and longevity. Prog. Cardiovasc. Dis., *23*:421, 1981.

time the failure rate will rise sharply. With all of the lithium anode power cell types grouped together, the relative reliability of nuclear, lithium, and mercury-zinc power sources is shown in Figure 49–1. The results with rechargeable units essentially parallel those with nuclear power sources. The recent increase in pacemaker reliability is readily apparent. Electronic, packaging, and electrode improvements have also played a role in the better results with lithium-powered pacers versus mercury-zinc battery–powered pacers. Unfortunately, however, because of wound, electrode, and functional problems relating to

TABLE 49–7. RELATIVE PACEMAKER RELIABILITY WITH DIFFERENT LITHIUM ANODE POWER CELLS†

LITHIUM ANODE CELL TYPE	COMPANY/MODEL	NO. OF IMPLANTS	MAXIMUM EXPOSURE (MONTHS)	MONTHLY FAILURE RATE (PER CENT) 90% CONFIDENCE LEVEL*
Thionyl chloride	ARCO	12,000	57	0.027
Iodine polymer WG 702E	CPI Maxilith	15,265	72	0.030
Iodine polymer WG 752	CIP Minilith	14,247	39	0.016
Silver chromate SAFT Li210	CPI Minilith	10,029	48	0.021
Cupric sulfide 3-cell	Cordis Omnicor Lambda	25,000	35	0.037
Cupric sulfide 3-cell	Cordis Stanicor Lambda	3000	24	0.027
Silver chromate SAFT Li210	Edwards 20/21 series	5000	23	0.018
Iodine polymer CRC 802-23	Intermedics Interlith 223	23,860	39	0.018
Lead sulfide and iodide Mallory LSA 900-6	Intermedics 221	2912	39	0.091

*June 1979
†From Tyers, G. F. O., and Brownlee, R. R.: Power pulse generators, electrodes and longevity. Prog. Cardiovasc. Dis., *23*:421, 1981.

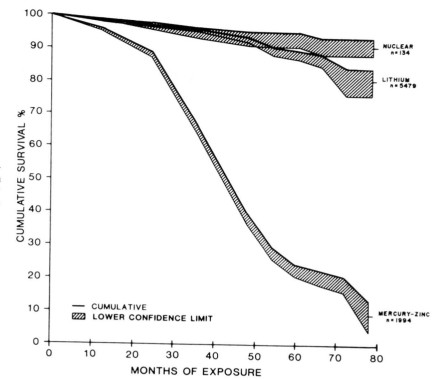

Figure 49–1. Overall pulse generator performance by basic power source types. (From Bilitch, M., Hauser, R. G., Goldman, B. S., *et al.*: Performance of cardiac pacemaker pulse generators, PACE *4*:254, 1981.)

pacing and sensing, clinical results are not quite as good, with approximately 20 per cent of patients having required reoperation by between 4 and 5 years following implantation of a lithium-powered pacemaker.

A major remaining limitation is the potential for a markedly reduced pacemaker life in situations requiring high current drains. Lithium-iodine cell manufacturers are addressing this problem with studies of increased iodine-to-polymer ratios in the cathode and treated, corrugated anodes with increased surface areas to allow more nearly full utilization of the cell's capacity even under high-output conditions. A lithium-bromine cell with double the energy capacity of the original lithium-iodine cells, a voltage of 3.5, and the ability to provide current drains of up to 2 amperes for short durations has been developed (Greatbatch, 1979), and rechargeable and primary plus rechargeable power sources also have potential for use in the development of long-life, high-output, and lifetime pacing systems (Tyers and Brownlee, 1981).

In summary, a variety of significantly improved pacemaker power sources have been developed. With low or moderate current drain requirements, the 5-year pacemaker is a proven entity and a 10-year pacemaker a probability. Many commonly encountered situations can, however, markedly increase energy requirements and shorten pacemaker life to less than 2 years, even with the best available power cells. When patients ask how long a pacemaker will last or specifically for a long-life device, a pat answer will in certain cases lead to false expectations and disappointment. This is especially true since every one of the lithium systems has been associated with an incidence of random or early failure (Welti, 1981b).

Electronics

In addition to improved power sources, important advances have also been made in pacemaker circuit function and reliability (Bowers, 1979). The first pacemakers were assembled using individual or discrete components, including resistors, capacitors, diodes, transistors, reed switches, and coils of wire for induction. Individual components were mounted either on or between printed circuit boards. The original Chardack-Greatbatch VOO pacemaker of 1959 utilized two transistors (Greatbatch, 1979). A subsequent advance was the utilization of "hybrid" circuits. Hybrid technology allows some components — in particular, resistors — to be printed on a thin, wafer-like structure called a substrate, whereas capacitors and semiconductors, including transistors, diodes, and integrated circuits, are attached to the substrate and electrically connected, usually using very tiny wires and microscopic techniques. In contrast to the so-called thick film technique just described, in which components are printed on the surface of the substrate, in thin film techniques all components of the circuit, including semiconductors, resistors, and capacitors, are diffused into a substrate to produce a monolithic silicon chip. Advantages of the single-chip circuit are its small size and the overall reduction in size of the whole pacemaker that it allows. A custom, digital, silicon, large-scale, integrated circuit, as used in virtually all multiprogrammable pacemakers, may include as many as 40,000 transistors on a 4-mm. square wafer. These technologies have made possible the development and use in pacemakers of single-chip, low-current microprocessors, to which have been added various peripheral circuits, including memory circuits and linear or sensing circuits for input/output capability. However, despite increased complexity, many currently available multiprogrammable pacemakers are smaller, lighter, and more reliable than their much simpler predecessors.

Although custom integrated circuit design is reliable, and capable of providing both multiprogrammable and physiologic pacing functions, its capacity for monitoring and data processing is limited, and design changes are time-consuming and expensive. Single-chip microcomputers are now commercially available, although high current drain and software reliability limitations prevent their direct use in pacemaker applications. Future pacemakers will probably utilize low current drain, custom microcomputers, consisting of a central processing unit, a memory unit, and an input/output circuit (Hartlaub, 1981), specifically designed for cardiac pacemaker applications. Pacemakers with electronics of this level of sophistication will be capable of computing the proper response to a variety of physiologic changes, including threshold energy needs, endocardial electrogram size, and cardiac output requirements, as determined by online pH and Po_2 measurements. There will also be the potential for automatic selection of an appropriate therapeutic cascade for a variety of arrhythmias and for design modifications following implantation.

Two areas of long-standing concern in circuit design relate to reed switch reliability and pacemaker rate stability. The components of a reed switch are an elongated, hollow glass bead and two wires. The wires project externally from both ends and into the center of the glass bead, where they extend past each other without touching. When a magnetic field is applied, the wires become opposite magnetic poles and move together, closing the circuit and allowing current flow. The first use of reed switch devices was in programmable pacers, but the most common application is in demand pacemakers. Application of a magnet over the pacemaker bypasses the sensing circuitry by closing the reed switch, causing the pacemaker to function asynchronously. This mechanism is used to confirm pacemaker function and capture during office visits and transtelephonic monitoring in those patients who at test time are exhibiting faster intrinsic rates and suppressing their pacemaker because of normal demand function. In addition, until 1978, all programmable pacemakers utilized reed switches as part of the programming sequence, and some recent units still utilize this mechanism as a lead-in or coupling mechanism for programming. As with any mechanical device, occasional problems (e.g., sticking in the open or the closed position) occur (Tyers *et al.*, 1981). The current levels of pacemaker circuit sophistication already described have relegated the reed switch to noncritical roles within the pacemaker, and devices that utilize a reed switch for protection or activation of programming circuitry are not recommended. The first totally electronic programming system was introduced clinically in the Cyberlith pacemaker in 1978 (Tyers *et al.*, 1981).

A second problem relates to stimulation rate variations. A number of individual and even whole design series of pacemakers have, over the years, exhibited gradual upward or downward rate drift following implantation, which, at the very least, complicated follow-up. In addition, many circuits are temperature-sensitive, so that pacemakers run different rates when measured at room temperature prior to implantation from those measured at body temperature following implantation. There have even been units that ran slightly slower rates during cold winter months. With the availability of multiprogrammable pacing and a wide range of rate selections, gradual wandering of any parameter should be avoided if possible. The availability of quartz-crystal controlled timing circuits, also used clinically in the Intermedics Cyberlith pacemaker in 1978, provides parameter accuracy to one decimal point, allows accurate assessment of each pacemaker prior to implantation, and precludes misdiagnosis of phantom programming when, in reality, rate drift or end of power cell life is the reason for the observed rate change.

The development of demand pacing presented two problems requiring electronic solutions—oversensitivity and self-inhibition. Lack of selectivity of the sensing mechanism in early pacers led to suppression by multiple noncardiac energy sources, including microwave ovens, electric hairdryers, electric drills, and tractor ignition systems, in addition to inhibition by cardiac electric signals (Tyers *et al.*, 1980). The spectral characteristics of the majority of electromagnetic interference signals are quite dissimilar to a cardiac electrogram, and a variety of filters and metallic shields have markedly reduced pacemaker sensitivity to electromagnetic interference. This problem could be essentially eliminated even in the most heavily contaminated electronic environment by including a second detection system on the surface of the pacemaker and electronically subtracting the signals it receives from those received on the endocardiac electrode, leaving only the cardiac electrogram to enter the pacemaker sensing circuitry (Brownlee *et al.*, 1978). Pacemakers that utilize the case as the anodal component of the circuit are potentially more susceptible to electromagnetic interference and are, even with current electronics, on occasion inhibited by motion and skeletal muscle potentials from near the implant, usually from the pectoral muscles.

Another problem with demand pacemakers is self-inhibition or recycling. With a VOO pacer running at a rate of 60 p.p.m., the interval between pacemaker spikes would be 1 second or 1000 milliseconds. (At the more common rate of 72, the interstimulus interval is approximately 830 msec.) If instead of VOO the device was VVI, during the interval between pacemaker spikes, the sensing circuit in the pacemaker would constantly be alert for cardiac electric activity. If the pacemaker detected or sensed an electric signal with the slope and amplitude of a typical QRS complex, it would recycle or reset itself to start a new interstimulus escape interval. Although this need not be the case, the escape interval would probably also be 1000 milliseconds, as in most pacemakers the interval from one pacemaker stimulus to the next is the same as the interval between a sensed beat and the delivery of a pacemaker stimulus. However, following each pacemaker spike, there should be an induced ventricular depolarization, represented on the surface EKG by the QRS complex, and repolarization, represented by the T wave. A functioning sensing circuit would detect these events terminating in the range of 300 msec. after each stimulus and recycle, creating an interspike interval of approximately 1300 msec., or a rate of 46 p.p.m. rather than the selected 60 p.p.m. This led to the development of what is known as the refractory interval. Following each delivered pacemaker stimulus, there is a brief period, averaging somewhat over 300 msec., during which the pacemaker acts as a VOO device and is unable to sense. The refractory interval largely precludes self-recycling, although there are still products with which this has been a not infrequent problem (Welti, 1981a). While reducing the risk of self-inhibition, the refractory interval also makes the pacemaker blind to premature ventricular contractions occurring early after a paced beat, providing at least the potential for pacemaker stimulation during the vulnerable period of ventricular repolarization.

The refractory interval problem and the potential for self-inhibition have been further complicated by the development of dual-chamber pacemakers. With these devices, there is the potential for self-inhibition or triggering of the ventricular output by an atrial stimulus and triggering of the atrial output by a ventricular stimulus. With careful positioning of bipolar electrodes, self-inhibition or crosstalk can be minimized, as in the Medtronic Byrel. Crosstalk is more of a risk with unipolar DVI systems. In the Intermedics Cyberlith DVI unit and the more recently available smaller Pacesetter Programolith and Intermedics Avius AV units, this risk was eliminated by making the ventricular sensing circuit refractory following both the atrial and the ventricular stimuli. Another recent approach is provided by the availability of blanking circuits. These add an additional refractory period that blinds the pacemaker sensing circuit to its own electric stimuli for just a few carefully timed milliseconds. Thus, the atrial spike cannot be sensed by the ventricular lead and vice versa. However, testing will be required to confirm effectiveness, as many self-inhibition and recycling problems relate not to the pacemaker stimulus but to the summation of stimulation afterpotentials and ventricular repolarization. Electronic reduction of afterpotentials is now used in two widely available multiprogrammable pacemakers, the Intermedics Cyberlith and the Medtronic Spectrax.

With DDD devices, self-triggering can result from retrograde conduction of the ventricular artifact up to the bundle of His, where it frequently arrives after the end of the atrial refractory period and induces atrial sensing and atrially triggered ventricular pacing.

This pacemaker-induced or -maintained arrhythmia has been called pacemaker re-entry tachycardia and is functionally similar to the Wolff-Parkinson-White syndrome, with the pacemaker and its atrial and ventricular electrodes providing the accessory AV pathway (Wolff-Parkinson-Funke syndrome?). The presence or absence of retrograde conduction frequently cannot be ascertained prior to pacemaker implantation, and second-generation DDD pacemakers will require greatly expanded refractory and mode programmability to maximize their usefulness and safety. Retrograde VA conduction occurs in 30 to 40 per cent of pacemaker patients at initial electrophysiologic evaluation and may occur intermittently in as many as 90 per cent of pacemaker patients, including some with fixed AV block. As the retrograde pathway may activate the atrium as late as 300 to 400 msec. after ventricular depolarization, a safe DDD unit must have the potential for programming the atrial refractory period to these durations after ventricular pacing or sensing or for programming atrioventricular triggering off (i.e., DDI).

Hermeticity

For the first 10 years following the introduction of completely implantable pacemakers, the electronics and power source were protected by a variety of relatively fluid-impervious materials, in particular epoxy resins and silicone rubber. These materials were fairly well accepted by the body, but moisture gradually intruded into the interior of the pacemaker, with the not infrequent development of short circuits, sudden cessation of pacing, battery explosion, pacemaker runaway (pacing at extremely rapid unphysiologic rates), and ventricular fibrillation. Fluid-related problems were responsible for the massive recalls that terminated the mercury-zinc-epoxy era and generated several of the newer pacemaker manufacturers (Tyers and Brownlee, 1976a; Brownlee and Tyers, 1976). Workers at Telectronics, Inc. played a major role in the commercial introduction of hermetically sealed pacemakers even prior to the lithium era (Wickham and Cartmill, 1971), and the Cordis Corporation and Edwards also produced a limited number of hermetically sealed mercury-zinc battery–powered pacemakers.

Literally, a hermetic enclosure is airtight and fluid-tight. Manufacturers describe hermeticity in terms of a leak rate for an inert gas under standard conditions, an apparent contradiction. However, an "acceptable" helium leak rate of 10^{-8} standard ml. per second at 1 atmosphere involves the passage of less than 1/100 of a ml. per 24 hours, and permeability to fluid is many orders of magnitude lower. Because of the current practice of defining hermeticity in terms of a leak rate, it is probably better to discuss both pacemakers and their contained power cells in terms of sealed metal containers versus containers with

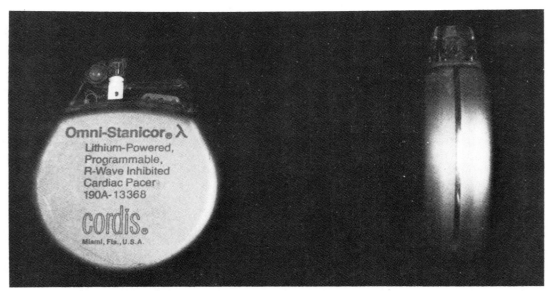

Figure 49–2. A typical round pacer with exposed circumferential weld. (From Tyers, G. F. O., and Brownlee, R. R.: Power pulse generators, electrodes, and longevity. Prog. Cardiovasc. Dis., *23*:421, 1981.)

gasket-type crimp seals or other mechanical nonsolid enclosures. It is probable that sealed metal containers, for both the power cell within and the pacemaker, provide greater protection than gasket-type mechanical seals. As noted previously, a major potential advantage of the lithium-iodine power cell over lithium–silver chromate and lithium–cupric sulfide power sources is availability only in sealed metallic enclosures. Although there may be some question regarding the absolute necessity for a welded enclosure for the internal power source, all current opinion favors a water-impervious encapsulation for the implantable pacemaker device. My preference is for a drawn metallic container with rounded corners into which

the pacemaker electronics and power source are placed, somewhat akin to building a ship in a large-necked bottle. This configuration, widely used by Telectronics, Intermedics, Pacesetter, and Vitatron, allows for the shortest weld, which, in addition, is covered by the epoxy or silicone connector material. Minimization of internal heating of components during welding is also simplified in short peripheral seam designs, and we have calculated that a rounded or oval pacemaker with a peripheral weld or seal (Fig. 49–2) has almost 2 miles of seal at risk for every 10,000 pacemakers implanted versus just over 0.5 mile of seal for rectangular units of our design (Fig. 49–3). The material selected for the external pacemaker

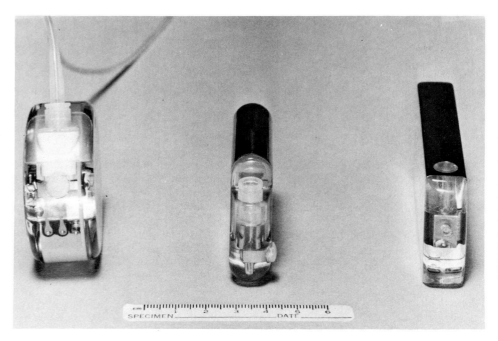

Figure 49–3. *Left,* A multiple mercury-zinc cell, nonhermetic, epoxy-encased pacemaker (Medtronic Xytron). *Center,* A hermetically sealed, thinly epoxy-covered seam, lithium-iodide pacer (Intermedics Interlith). *Right,* A hermetically sealed, deeply epoxy-protected, short seam, rechargeable, silver-mercury silver-zinc pacer. Note that in the unit to the right, the hermetic seal is recessed within the metallic can, so that it is protected by a 2-cm. epoxy cap, which also functions as the connector. (From Tyers, G. F. O., and Brownlee, R. R.: Current status of pacemaker power sources. Ann. Thorac. Surg., *25*:571, 1978.)

enclosure should be compatible with body tissue, noncorrosive, nontoxic, easy to form into a suitably shaped pacemaker package, and easy to seal while retaining a nonreactive internal environment, without undue heating or risk to the internal components. Materials used to date include stainless steel, Haynes alloy, and titanium, with the last very light material being chosen most frequently, in spite of its higher cost.

The final packaging question relates to treatment of the void around the cell and electronic components within the welded external pacemaker enclosure. If the interstices are filled with an inert gas, the pacemaker is light, but failure of the external seal results in more or less immediate wetting of internal components. Filling the unit with silicone rubber or epoxy increases its weight but slows moisture penetration into electronic components, even under gross leak conditions. However, especially in the case of epoxy, contraction during curing will stress components and cause failures. A satisfactory compromise may be achieved by coating internal components with a thin layer of parylene, as this material has proved to be an effective electrolyte barrier.

Leads and Electrodes

When used precisely, lead indicates the insulated wire used to connect the pacemaker to the heart and electrode indicates the uninsulated, electrically active, metal tip in contact with the myocardium. The lead-electrode system serves two equally important functions in a demand pacemaker: carrying the electric stimulus from the pacemaker to the myocardium, and carrying the endocardial electrogram from the myocardium to the pacemaker.

Conductor and electrode materials should be electrochemically inert, nontoxic, resistant to electrolysis, of low resistance, and of high tensile strength and flexibility. A cardiac lead is subjected to 35 to 40 million contractile cycles per year, which combine with respiratory and skeletal muscle movements to produce flexing, torsion, and elongation stresses. Materials used in the lead include platinum-iridium (10 per cent), Elgiloy, MP35N, silver–stainless steel alloy, and nonmetallic conductors, including graphite. Multiple twisted strand construction has been replaced by helical coils and metallic ribbons, a spiral wrapped around a nonconductive flexible core. More recently, multifilar helical-coil electrodes have been introduced where the spiral is formed by multiple, parallel, fine wires rather than a single larger-diameter coiled wire. The larger the diameter of the helix and the smaller the diameter of the wires used to form it, the greater the flexibility and the greater the stress resistance of the resulting lead. The exposed electrode tip is usually formed of Elgiloy or platinum-iridium and may be either porous (metallic or carbon) or solid. Previously, a lead was most commonly insulated in a tube of silicone rubber, but more recently, segmented polyu-

rethane insulating sheaths have been introduced. Their advantages include greater elasticity and tensile strength for reduced lead size and improved durability, and a much smoother surface, which improves handling characteristics during multilead placements and reduces the risk of venous thromboembolism (Williams et al., 1978). Experience with segmented polyurethane–insulated leads, however, is insufficient at this time to recommend them unequivocally over silicone rubber–insulated leads.

Electrodes are of two general types, those passed transvenously to lodge against the endocardium of the right atrium or right ventricle, and those passed transthoracically to be directly attached to the myocardium of any chamber. Transthoracic leads (not epicardial—the epicardium is an insulating layer) are primarily indicated in very small children, after repeated failure of the transvenous approach and at a time when the chest is already open, such as following open heart surgery. Because it requires a more extensive surgical procedure, the direct placement of intramyocardial electrodes is seldom, if ever, indicated primarily, although corkscrew-like, screw-in, sutureless myocardial electrodes have resulted in renewed popularity of this approach. Exit block, that is, late rise of threshold energy requirement above the output of a standard pacemaker, and lead and electrode fractures are more common with the sutureless transthoracic screw-in electrodes than with other approaches (Lawrie et al., 1977). From a surgical-technical view, the Telectronics 030-170 is the best transthoracic myocardial lead. The end of the helical lead coil is exposed to form the electrode, which can be drawn into either the atrial or ventricular myocardium using a suture that projects from one end of the coil and terminates in a swedged, curved needle. Unfortunately, the surface area of this electrode is somewhat large (55 mm.²).

Transvenous leads are currently the systems of choice. They may be described as active or passive. Passive leads have a small flange expansion just proximal to the exposed metallic distal electrode, which is designed to catch beneath trabeculae and reduce the chance of dislodgement, the incidence of which should be less than 5 per cent for any experienced operator (Furman et al., 1981). However, when faced with a large, smooth-walled, ventricular cavity, tricuspid insufficiency, or the need for lead placement in the atrial appendage, the incidence of dislodgement of standard transvenous leads increases. Metallic and plastic tines, barbs, hooks, jaws, arrowheads, balloons, sharpened screws, and dull helices, some remotely activated and retractable, have been designed and provide the implanting surgeon with a wide range of actively adhering electrodes (Fig. 49–4). There is even a transatrial septal, toggle-ended lead that is pulled back against the left side of the interatrial septum and an orthogonol lead with inline ventricular and atrial electrodes, the latter being held against the atrial wall by pressure. My preferences include segmented polyurethane–coated, tined leads (Intermedics and Medtronic); sharp, endocardial, corkscrew-like, screw-in

**REPRESENTATIVE PASSIVE FIXATION TRANSVENOUS
VENTRICULAR LEADS (STATE-OF-THE-ART 1982)**

DISTAL TIP	POLARITY	MANUFACTURER/ MODEL	AVAILABILITY 1982
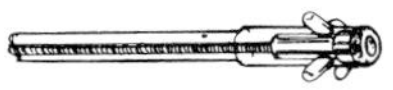	Bipolar Unipolar	Medtronic® 6962 Medtronic® 6961	Yes Yes
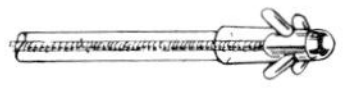	Bipolar Unipolar	Intermedics 476-02 Intermedics 477-02	Yes Yes
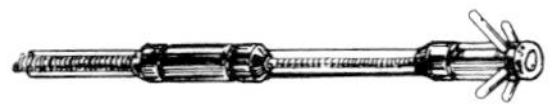	Bipolar Bipolar	Medtronic® 6972 Intermedics 476-03	Yes Yes
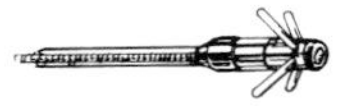	Unipolar Unipolar	Medtronic® 6971 Intermedics 493-01	Yes Yes
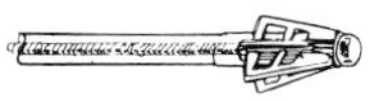	Unipolar	Cordis Fin-Tip	Yes
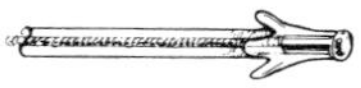	Unipolar	Telectronics Trailing Tine	Yes
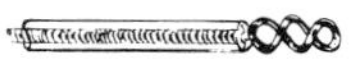	Unipolar	Vitatron Helifix	Yes
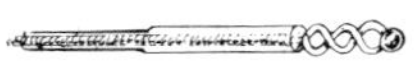	Unipolar	Vitatron Helifix Ball Tip	Yes
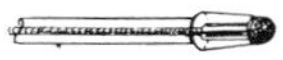	Unipolar Bipolar	CPI14116 Porous CPI14226 Porous	Yes Yes
A 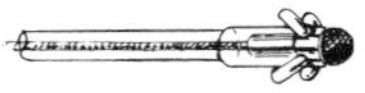	Unipolar Bipolar	CPI4130 Porous Tined CPI4230 Porous Tined	Yes Yes

Figure 49–4. Different types of endocardial unipolar electrode tips with the three upper electrodes showing active fixation devices, including metallic hooks, screws, and tines. From Stokes, K., and Stephenson, N. L.: The implantable cardiac pacing lead—just a simple wire? *In* The Third Decade of Cardiac Pacing. Edited by S. S. Barold and J. Mugica, Mt. Kisco, N.Y., Futura Publishing Co., 1982, 480 pp.

Illustration continued on opposite page

**EXAMPLES OF EARLY ACTIVE FIXATION TRANSVENOUS
VENTRICULAR LEADS**

DISTAL TIP	POLARITY	MANUFACTURER/ MODEL	AVAILABILITY 1982
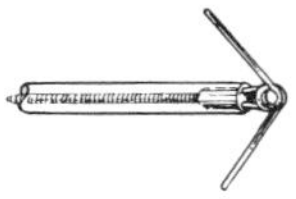	Unipolar	Biotronik IVE-85	Yes
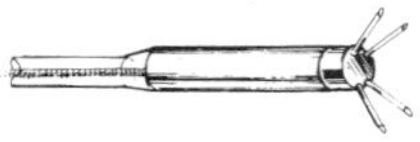	Unipolar	Vitatron MIP2000	Yes
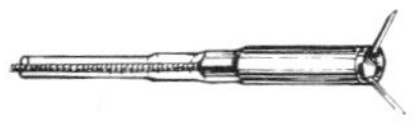	Unipolar	Biotronik IE651	Yes
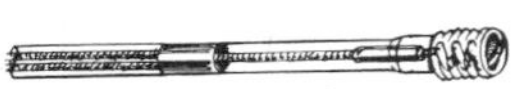	Bipolar	Medtronic® 6954	No
B	Unipolar	Coratomic Endo Loc L-40	No

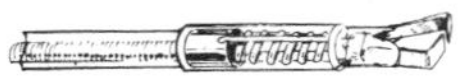

electrodes (Medtronic Bisping); and a pull-activated lead with a distal jaw-like electrode (Coratomic Endo-loc). These electrodes may be placed in either the right atrium or the right ventricle, and even under adverse circumstances the rate of dislodgement is very low. Leads designed primarily for transvenous atrial use differ from ventricular leads in that once the stylet is withdrawn, they assume a distal J shape, which allows them to be hooked up into the atrial appendage. Not all of the active leads are equally effective, and one has been reported to displace more frequently than standard designs (Furman *et al.,* 1979, 1981). In addition, because of their multielement nature, there is the risk of artifact generation and demand pacer

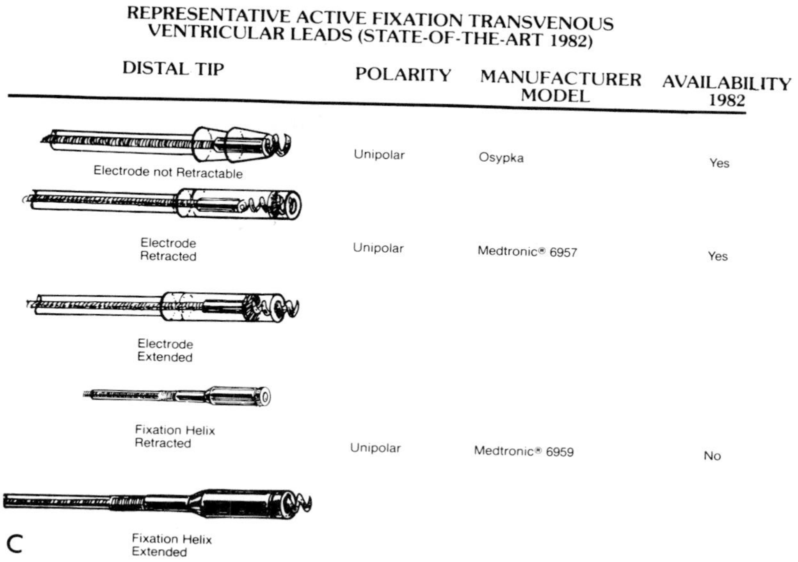

REPRESENTATIVE ACTIVE FIXATION TRANSVENOUS
VENTRICULAR LEADS (STATE-OF-THE-ART 1982)

DISTAL TIP	POLARITY	MANUFACTURER MODEL	AVAILABILITY 1982
Electrode not Retractable	Unipolar	Osypka	Yes
Electrode Retracted	Unipolar	Medtronic® 6957	Yes
Electrode Extended			
Fixation Helix Retracted	Unipolar	Medtronic® 6959	No
Fixation Helix Extended			

Figure 49–4. *Continued*

C

suppression (Brownlee *et al.,* 1980). Especially for physiologic pacing, it is important for the implanter to be familiar with a range of myocardial and transvenous electrodes so that he can respond most appropriately to a variety of clinical situations.

Pacemaker electrode systems are described as bipolar or unipolar. All electrode systems are in reality bipolar; that is, they involve cathodal (negative) and anodal (positive) terminals. By common usage, however, bipolar systems are considered to be those in which both the anodal and cathodal electrodes contact the myocardium, whereas unipolar systems are those in which the case of the pacemaker forms or contains the anode and only the cathodal electrode contacts the heart. Advantages of the unipolar system include a more simple connection, a decreased failure rate for both pacemaker and electrode, decreased voltage and therefore slightly decreased energy requirements, decreased risk of fibrillation, potential for detection of larger sensing signals, and decreased risk of anodal corrosion. Because of the last problem, only noble metal electrodes can be used with bipolar systems. Advantages of bipolar pacing include reduced risk of muscle stimulation, decreased susceptibility to electromagnetic interference, elimination of the potential for pacemaker suppression by myopotentials, decreased risk of crosstalk between atrial and ventricular electrodes and stimuli, and increased sensing selectivity (improved endocardial signal–to–interference ratio for sensing). Thus, although the unipolar systems may present the pacemaker sensing circuit with larger endocardial signals, this advantage may be outweighed by also presenting the sensing circuit with larger spurious or unwanted signals. The issues of greater connector complexity and increased incidence of electrode failure with the bipolar systems may be ameliorated by the recent introduction of coaxial or inline bipolar systems, in which a smaller lead lies within a larger one rather than having two leads of equal size

lying side by side within an insulating sheath. Furthermore, the inner lead is shielded from electromagnetic interference in the coaxial design. However, the coaxial system does necessitate very close apposition of the anodal and cathodal outputs of the pacemaker, providing at least the potential for connector short circuiting, and time will be required to prove the effectiveness of the inline bipolar design.

Cardiac pacing electrodes are involved in an electrochemical hemodynamic-physiologic interface. The rate of myocardial contraction is more rapid and the cardiac output is higher when the ventricle is activated through the Purkinje system (approximately 30 msec.) versus single-site myocardial stimulation (over 100 msec.). Thus, conducted rhythms are almost always preferable to ventricular pacing. Simultaneous stimulation of multiple ventricular sites improves cardiac output, whereas stimulation sites near the left ventricular outflow tract restrict cardiac output (Tyers, 1970). Threshold energy requirements (the smallest product of voltage, current, and pulse width) are dependent on multiple factors. Electrodes with small surface areas are associated with decreased current and, to a lesser degree, voltage requirements at threshold (Tyers *et al.,* 1974) and, as could be ascertained from Ohm's law $\left(R = \dfrac{V}{I} \right)$, are associated with higher stimulation (electrode plus electrode tissue interface) impedances (variable resistances), measured in ohms. Stimulation impedance is also affected by stimulus duration and electrode material (Tyers *et al.,* 1979). "Normal" acute stimulation impedances currently seen clinically vary from as little as 200 ohms with large–surface-area intramyocardial leads (Telectronics 030-170) to over 1000 ohms with 8-mm.^{2} Elgiloy (Cordis) and platinum-iridium (Intermedics) ball-shaped electrodes. Some experimental electrodes with very small surface areas and no metal-to-tissue contact eliminate electrode tip polarization, exhibit stimulation impedances in the range of 2000 to 3000 ohms, and are associated with the lowest recorded threshold energy requirements for pacing. High stimulation impedance in association with small–surface-area, high–current-density electrodes is beneficial, as it markedly reduces pacemaker power cell current drain and prolongs pacemaker life. However, the electrode-tissue interface resistance is several times higher for passage of the endocardial signal from the myocardium into the electrode on its way to the pacemaker than for passage of the stimulus from the pacemaker and electrode to the myocardium. Especially with smaller electrodes, sensing function is directly related to electrode area and adversely affected by small electrode size (Hughes *et al.*, 1976). A compromise between pacing and sensing efficiency seems to be found in the electrode tip surface area range of 12 to 20 mm.^{2}. The rationale behind the development of porous-tipped electrodes is their improved sensing function for a given size, as the interstices increase the sensing area without increasing stimulation energy requirements (MacGregor *et al.*, 1979).

When electrode shape, material, and surface area are held constant, surgically placed intramyocardial electrodes provide lower thresholds than transvenous endocardial electrodes, and left ventricular intramyocardial electrodes provide lower energy requirements than right ventricular intramyocardial electrodes (Tyers *et al.*, 1975). In addition to the well-known effects of electrolyte disturbances, acid-base imbalance also adversely affects threshold energy requirements (Hughes *et al.*, 1975), the usual cause of failure to pace during cardiac resuscitation associated with ventricular arrest.

Lead-Pacemaker Connectors

Although less developmental work has been done on leads and electrodes than on pacemaker power sources and circuitry, the least attention of all has been paid to the lead hub connector receptacle on the pacemaker. The standard Medtronic lead pin is smaller than the standard Cordis pin (both metal and insulation), and to the chagrin of many, they are not interchangeable. The ideal pacemaker connector should be tangential in order to reduce electrode stress, universal in order to simply accept both the Cordis and Medtronic leads without adaptors, simple, and short circuit–proof. Various bayonet and screw-on connectors have been used clinically in the past but were not widely accepted. Whether the recently introduced coaxial bipolar connector will fare better remains to be seen.

Summary

In summary, research over the last decade has centered on the development and testing of more reliable and adaptable low-drain circuitry, the development of methods to reduce energy requirements for pacing (reduced pulse width, small–surface-area electrodes), methods to improve packaging techniques to protect the electronic implant from moisture and other rigors of the biologic environment, and the development and application of longer-lived power sources. However, a large number of pacemaker removals have nothing to do with failure of the pacemaker, and, primarily because of the current state of the electrode and implantation art, approximately 20 per cent of patients still require reoperation between 4 and 5 years following their initial pacemaker implant. Furthermore, with newer multiprogrammable and dual-chamber units, which may require wider pulse widths or higher output voltage, the function of many lithium power sources is doubly jeopardized, both by the high current drain and the more rapid build-up of resistance within the power cell, limiting energy availability. Figure 49–5 illustrates how the physician's choice of pacing rate, pulse width, and electrode surface area can result in a range of from 3 to 9 years between

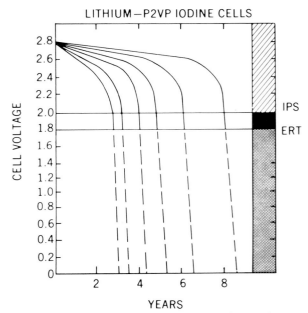

Figure 49–5. The effects of different loads (lead surface areas, pulse widths, pacing rates, etc.) on the duration of pacemaker function provided by a lithium iodine cell are illustrated. The higher the load, the greater the current drain and the shorter the pacemaker life. The interval between the increased patient surveillance point (IPS) and the elective replacement time (ERT) will be longer or shorter, depending on the multiple variables discussed. Although not evident for these voltage curves, the gradual build-up in resistance in a lithium iodine cell with very slow discharge, as in many pacemaker applications, may lead to a situation in which current output is too limited to run a pacemaker circuit but cell voltage has dropped so minimally and gradually that voltage-sensitive end-of-life rate change indication is lacking. Furthermore, if intermittent loss of capture due to falling cell voltage should occur somewhere approaching the knee of the curve, programming to a "high-output" setting could result in a sudden drop in power cell and output voltage and induce precipitous pacemaker failure. (From Tyers, G. F. O., and Brownlee, R. R.: Power pulse generators, electrodes, and longevity. Prog. Cardiovasc. Dis., *23*:421, 1981.)

reoperations for power source replacement. When the variables of dual-chamber pacing are added to potentially increase energy requirements and the variables of very narrow pulse width and low-voltage pacing are added to further reduce energy requirements, the range of functional life for a single pacemaker model may vary from as little as 1.5 years to as long as 15 years. When considered in conjunction with the information on power cell capacity and energy density, a fair degree of skepticism should be generated regarding some very tiny, multiprogrammable, dual-chamber pacemakers now in design and preclinical phases. A very small pacemaker contains a very small battery, and the smaller the battery, the shorter the life of the pacemaker for any given battery design and chemistry. It is thus almost certain that some manufacturers are reinventing the 1-year pacemaker. It is the conscientious and informed physician's duty not to select such a device for his patients.

PROGRAMMABLE PACING

It has been possible to noninvasively change the function of implanted pacemakers since 1962. Although there is some question as to whether these units should be called programmable or externally adjustable, the former is the most commonly used term. The development of programmable pacing was reviewed in the first section of this chapter. Although more than 10 multiprogrammable pacemakers are currently being evaluated clinically, the Intermedics Cyberlith, the Medtronic Spectrax, and the Pacesetter Programalith have been used most frequently, with clinical implants numbering in the range of 31,000, 23,000, and 10,000, respectively, early in 1981. The presently available range of externally adjustable parameters is summarized in Table 49–8, although no single unit includes all of these selections and not all are required with equal frequency. However, as it is never possible in an individual case to accurately predict future requirements, it is virtually certain that the range of available programmable functions will continue to increase.

TABLE 49–8. AVAILABLE RANGE OF PROGRAMMABLE PARAMETERS*

Rate	0 to 150 p.p.m.
Pulse width	0.05 to 2.3 msec.
Voltage	≈ 1 to $\approx 3 \times$ cell voltage
Current	2 to 9 mA.
Sensitivity	0.6 to 8 mV.
Modes	VOO or AOO, VVI or AAI, VVT or AAT, DVI, DOO, VAT, VDD, DDD
Refractory period	200 to 500 msec.
Hysteresis	0 to 600 msec.
Telemetry	On-off

*The recently released DDD pacemakers (see Table 49–9) also have a programmable upper ventricular rate limit on response to rapid intrinsic atrial rates, a range of responses to the upper rate limit (Wenckebach vs. 2:1 block vs. fallback to VVI pacing), and a programmable range of AV intervals up to 250 msec.

Pacemaker programming requires coupling, checking, and information transmission techniques if spurious, unplanned, or so-called "phantom programming" is to be avoided (Tyers et al., 1981). All early programmable pacemakers utilized mechanical methods, including reed-switch closure, percutaneous screwdriver-like needles, magnetic rotational cranks, and reed-switch dithering, for either a portion of or the entire programming technique. Even some recently developed multiprogrammable pacers utilize reed-switch closure and conversion to VOO pacing as part of their coupling mechanism. Dithering techniques, introduced by the Cordis Corporation in 1972, rely on the reed switch not only to couple but also to carry information to the pacemaker. In simplified terms, the pacemaker programming circuit counts the number of rapid sequential closures and openings of the reed switch, and the number indicates the selected setting. For example, 10 rapid closures might indicate a rate of 70, and 15 a rate of 80, whereas a different range of closure rates might indicate a variety of output currents. Although "state of the art" at the time of its introduction, reed-switch dithering was particularly susceptible to phantom programming because of the frequent use of magnets around pacemakers for conversion to VOO for rate change follow-up (Fieldman et al., 1977; Furman, 1980a; Sinnaeve et al., 1980). Reed switches are used in the Spectrax SX and Programalith units only for coupling, but there are still pacemakers available that utilize reed-switch dithering for the entire programming process. They are not recommended. The Cyberlith system entirely eliminates the use of a reed switch during programming (the reed switch limitations were discussed in the preceding section on pacemaker technology), with coupling accomplished by induction and with checking and information transmission accomplished with redundant reciprocal transmission of 80 precisely timed impulses organized in pairs and binary coded data, including special key codes for different models. This type of system eliminates misprogramming even between different models in the same series and largely precludes the potential for phantom programming. It is probable that the next generation of programmable pacemakers from all manufacturers will rely entirely on nonmechanical electron programming techniques.

The potential benefits of being able to change multiple pacemaker stimulation settings noninvasively include the following (Tyers et al., 1981): *Rate* may be increased or decreased to optimize cardiac output and control arrhythmias. An increased stimulation rate often increases cardiac output in patients with fixed stroke volume and poor ventricular function. A decreased stimulation rate is more commonly used to increase cardiac output in patients having sinus rates of between 50 and 70 p.p.m. much of the time, as they will usually have a better cardiac output with sinus rhythm at 60 to 70 p.p.m. than with ventricular pacing at faster rates. Stimulation rate may also be decreased to observe the patient's underlying rhythm and to obtain an undistorted electrocardiogram for diagnostic purposes (e.g., digitalis toxicity, myocardial infarction).

Output energy (pulse width, voltage, and/or current) may be increased to assure capture or decreased to conserve energy and to eliminate stimulation of diaphragmatic or pectoral muscles. Narrow pulse width programming has been conclusively shown to prolong pacemaker life (Furman and Pannizzo, 1981), but programming to a lower voltage or current output may on occasion be more effective in reducing unwanted stimulation of pericardiac structures. A combination of voltage and pulse width programmability is required to accurately determine safe minimal stimulus energy requirements for long-term pacing (Tyers *et al.*, 1981). For example, with doubling the pulse width from 0.1 to 0.2 milliseconds, the effective stimulus energy is doubled, but when increasing the pulse width from 1 to 2 milliseconds, the effective stimulus energy is increased only very slightly. Thus, if several months following pacemaker implantation, capture is just achieved at a pulse width of 0.1 milliseconds, a setting of 0.2 milliseconds provides a large safety margin. If, on the other hand, ventricular capture is obtained with a pulse duration of 1 millisecond, only a marginal capture energy can be provided even with an infinitely wide pulse width, as any duration over 1.5 milliseconds is physiologically almost worthless. The potential for loss of capture is further aggravated, as wider pulse widths put a higher current drain on the battery and lower stimulation voltage. Thus, effective stimulus energy could actually be reduced by programming to an inappropriately wide pulse width. In pacemakers that have both programmable stimulus voltage and pulse width, the voltage should be reduced to one-half nominal, and if capture persists, the pulse width should then be gradually narrowed until capture is lost. At this point, regardless of where it is within the available pulse width range, doubling the voltage will provide a very effective energy safety margin for pacing. For the higher pacing energy requirements that occasionally develop with all electrodes and that are more common with the intramyocardial sutureless screw-in electrodes (Lawrie *et al.*, 1977), increased current or voltage programmability is more effective than pulse width programmability, especially if durations greater than 1.25 milliseconds are required. Wider pulse widths are relatively ineffective because of the shape of strength duration curves, which become relatively flat beyond 1.5 milliseconds.

As with stimulation energy programmability, *sensitivity* to cardiac signals for demand pacing may have to be increased or decreased to maintain optimal pacer function. Sensitivity may be decreased to eliminate oversensing, for example, of T waves and myopotentials, and to minimize susceptibility to electromagnetic interference. Sensitivity may be increased to eliminate undersensing of premature ventricular contractions, poor ventricular signals, and P waves for demand atrial pacing.

Mode may be changed to eliminate otherwise insoluble sensing problems; to eliminate muscle inhi-

bition (VVT); to allow patients to work in difficult occupational settings where there is severe electromagnetic interference (AOO, VOO, AAT, VVT, DOO); to provide for the safe use of electrocautery during subsequent operations (AOO, VOO, DOO); for analysis of sensing effectiveness and timing, particularly in atrial applications (triggered modes); and for energy conservation (AOO, VOO, DOO). Control of difficult oversensing problems by programming to VOO, AOO, or DOO eliminates the risk of the pacer being suppressed, which is especially important in pacemaker-dependent patients (i.e., those with a very slow or no spontaneous ventricular rate of their own). Programming the sensing amplifier out of the circuit in these situations and in patients who essentially never run a rate faster than the pacemaker stimulation rate also saves power-cell current drain, because otherwise the sensing circuit constantly requires energy over and above that needed for stimulation. Programming to a triggered rather than an asynchronous mode will eliminate competitive pacing in the patient who on occasion has a faster spontaneous rhythm than the pacemaker rate setting, although energy consumption will be increased rather than decreased as with inhibited pacing. Temporary programming to the triggered mode also confirms the precise site and timing of sensing, which may otherwise be difficult, especially with AAI pacing.

The *refractory interval* may require lengthening if atrial demand pacing is complicated by recycling on the trailing edge of the ventricular electrogram. Because of the added duration of the PR interval following the pacemaker stimulus prior to ventricular depolarization, ventricular electric events occur much later after an atrial than after a ventricular stimulus. However, with careful design of the sensing circuit and proper patient selection, usual refractory periods should infrequently cause clinical problems. The refractory period may be shortened to allow sensing of the occasional premature ventricular contraction not sensed with a nominal refractory period. Separate (from ventricular) programmable control of the atrial refractory interval in DDD pacemakers is particularly important in view of the frequency of retrograde VA conduction of ventricular events, which, if sensed by the atrial channel, may lead to pacemaker re-entry tachycardia.

High-rate *hysteresis* pacing, in which the pacemaker turns on at a more rapid rate than the nominal stimulation rate of 70, utilized in most standard pacemakers, may occasionally be beneficial to patients with aortic insufficiency or extremely poor ventricular function. Hysteresis pacing, as more commonly used to allow the spontaneous rate to fall below the paced rate, is considered by some to be more physiologic than nonhysteresis pacing, because it allows the pulse rate to slow, as for example, during sleep, without inducing pacing. Hysteresis, in this context, indicates that the pacemaker will not turn on until the spontaneous rate drops relatively low, for example, to 60 p.p.m., but that when activated, the pacemaker will begin to stimulate at the nominal (70 p.p.m.) or programmed rate. However, most of the so-called physiologic indications for hysteresis are better served by AAI, VDD, DVI, DDD, or rate-programmable VVI (VVI, M) pacing. With hysteresis pacing, sinus rhythm is maintained only while the natural rhythm is dropping to the trigger rate, whereas during VVI pacing at a low programmed rate, the patient remains in sinus rhythm whether the spontaneous rate is increasing or decreasing between the trigger rate and the stimulation rate.

A fairly extensive experience with multiprogrammable pacemaking has now accrued, establishing the reliability of the available technology and the ability to reduce the need for reoperation (Tyers et al., 1981; Hauser et al., 1981; Furman, 1981). In my experience, over 75 per cent of patients with multiprogrammable pacemakers benefit from permanent therapeutic programming, not infrequently of multiple parameters. In addition, 43 per cent of patients have required multiple programming of a single parameter, such as rate increase during an acute illness and subsequent reprogramming back to a base rate, or a pulse width increase acutely and subsequent decrease to a very short, energy-conserving pulse duration. Rate, pulse width, and mode were the most frequently programmed therapeutic parameters in over 60, 50, and 30 per cent of patients, respectively. Rate was usually reduced to maximize the patient's time in sinus rhythm but was occasionally increased to improve cardiac output or to suppress ventricular or atrial arrhythmias. Pulse width was usually decreased to extend pacemaker cell life, but in four cases, the primary indication for reducing stimulus energy was diaphragmatic or chest wall stimulation.

During preliminary experience with multiprogrammable pacing, approximately two thirds of patients received multiprogrammable units and one third of patients received nonprogrammable demand pacemakers. Early in the study, one patient with a VVI pacemaker required reoperation for implantation of a high-output unit and had to undergo the cost, risk, inconvenience, and discomfort of a repeat hospitalization. This could have been avoided by the initial implantation of a multiprogrammable pacemaker. More recently, a patient with late loss of capture has had pacing returned nonoperatively by increasing her pacemaker's pulse width. Triggered or asynchronous mode programming was undertaken temporarily to allow use of the electrocautery during unrelated surgical procedures in three patients. One patient, an industrial electrician, was programmed to VOO because of the extremely severe electromagnetic interference in his place of work, and one patient was programmed to DOO from DVI because of symptomatic pacemaker inhibition by myopotentials. Sensitivity programming was seldom required for ventricular pacing, but early in the series, one patient with a VVI unit exhibited clear-cut myopotential inhibition, and the problem was solved by implanting a multiprogrammable unit with variable sensitivities. Again, this

reoperation could have been eliminated by selecting a multiprogrammable pacemaker at the initial procedure. In contrast to ventricular pacing, sensitivity programming has been frequently useful for maintaining demand function during chronic atrial pacing.

Indications for diagnostic or temporary reprogramming have included change to a slow rate (30 p.p.m.) to allow nonpaced assessment of a patient with idiopathic hypertrophic subaortic stenosis during cardiac catheterization and, more commonly, to allow observation of the underlying rhythm in evaluating the level of digitalization or the extent of myocardial ischemia or both. Initially, patient selection for a multiprogrammable pacer was based on the implanting physician's estimate of probability of need for pacemaker parameter adjustment. However, avoidance of a single reoperation more than pays for the modest additional cost of several multiprogrammable pacemakers. As pulse width programmability alone can significantly reduce the incidence of reoperation, and several reports now show early prevention of reoperation using other adjustable parameters, there can be no doubt that multiprogrammable pacemakers will be cost-effective, reducing the need for reoperation in any large series of pacemaker patients (Lopman et al., 1980; Tyers et al., 1981; Billhardt et al., 1981).

In terms of both scope and reliability, several currently available multiprogrammable pacemakers represent advances over the pacing technology of just a few years ago. In the future, the range of programmable options will undoubtedly increase. Multiple physiologic pacing modes will be available in the majority of pacemakers and apart from sensitivity programming for endocardial electrograms of differing magnitudes, slew rate (endocardial electrogram slope responsiveness) and unipolar-to-bipolar programming and vice versa will also be available. Future pacemakers will also have the potential for automatic programming or self-programming to achieve optimal sensitivity and stimulus energy parameters, as well as appropriate antiarrhythmia mode, frequency, and duration settings for treatment of most common, troublesome arrhythmias. Dual-chamber pacemakers will require separate programmable control of the atrial and ventricular outputs, and antiarrhythmia pacemakers will require, in addition, separate adjustability or antiarrhythmic stimulus parameters from 30 joules for defibrillation to two to three times standard for less invasive dysrhythmia termination techniques. Software-based pacemakers allowing noninvasive postimplantation program modifications will assure an optimal range of parameters for selection relative to both new knowledge and changing patient needs.

PHYSIOLOGIC PACING

The designation "physiologic pacing" has been criticized as being trendy and self-serving (Furman, 1980b). This criticism is well taken, as who would want to favor antiphysiologic or nonphysiologic pacing. Even fixed-rate ventricular pacing was more physiologic than spontaneous ventricular rates of 20 to 30 p.p.m. associated with frequent Stokes-Adams attacks. However, as no other phrase seems to better describe attempts to provide patients with the best cardiac function possible, within the limits of current technology, physiologic pacing will probably persist as a generic term, at least for the present.

Physiologic pacing is provided by techniques that maintain an approximation of the normal cardiac electric and contractile sequence, with the atria contracting first, followed by a delay—the AV interval, to allow the ventricles to fill—and, finally, ventricular contraction. When normal atrial rate change responses to increased metabolic requirements are intact, physiologic pacing indicates that ventricular stimulation will be timed to appropriately follow atrial contraction. When atrial rates are inappropriate, truly physiologic pacemakers will sense changes in oxygen demand, temperature, and tissue pH and automatically increase the rate of atrial and ventricular or dual-chamber pacing and adjust the AV delay to maximize cardiac output. The advances described in the section on pacemaker technology have brought us to the point of experimental pacemakers that respond to pH changes, but the advent of truly physiologic dual-chamber units (i.e., those that automatically select optimal rates and AV intervals) is still some time in the future. It is of interest to note, however, that the very first implantable physiologic pacemakers, the Cordis VAT units, did allow for ventricular rate adjustments coincident with spontaneous atrial rate changes.

Atrial synchronous or VAT pacing had been available for 20 years, and AV sequential and atrial pacing for 10 years; yet, in 1980, in only approximately 3 per cent of the more than 100,000 North American implants was an attempt made to preserve atrioventricular synchrony. Prior to 1980, the use of physiologic pacing was even less frequent, with the total number of patients having received dual-chamber, atrial and atrially triggered pacemakers being about 15,000. Reasons for infrequent use of physiologic pacing have included bulky pacemakers and leads, frequent complications, and the potential problems associated with lead positioning and pacing in the atrium. Because the atrium is thin-walled, there is more risk of perforating it during electrode placement and also more risk of significant bleeding following a perforation. Furthermore, historically, there has been much more frequent displacement of atrial leads, and in addition, atrial pacing may be associated with smaller sensing signals and larger threshold energy requirements than ventricular pacing. Is preservation of atrioventricular synchrony worth the associated complexities?

Both atria function as reservoirs to collect blood returning to the heart throughout the cardiac cycle. Even this function is compromised with loss of AV synchrony. One of the most important functions of the atria is to optimize preloading, or filling of the ventricles just prior to each ventricular contraction, the so-called atrial kick. Optimization of left ventricular filling and left ventricular fiber stretch maximizes cardiac output through the Frank-Starling mechanism. Appropriate atrioventricular synchronization also provides pressure protection for the pulmonary circuit. Atrial synchrony minimizes the period during which atrial pressure must be elevated to provide ventricular filling, and thus, with appropriate left atrial timing, there are consistently lower pulmonary venous and wedge pressures. On the other hand, pulmonary venous pressures are highest when there is retrograde ventricular-to-atrial conduction, with an atrial contraction following rather than preceding each ventricular ejection. Thus, proper timing of the atrioventricular conduction system refractory period is important, not only in the suppression of re-entrant arrhythmias but also in optimizing pulmonary diastolic hemodynamics. As might be expected from this, proper atrioventricular sequencing provides more efficient cardiac function, with reduced work per unit of blood pumped and an overall reduction of myocardial oxygen demand. Finally, atrial contraction assists with closure of the atrioventricular valves through both mechanical and electric effects. Rebound waves from rapid flow across the atrioventricular valves following atrial contraction may aid in completing closure. With appropriate AV conduction and rapid, synchronized ventricular contraction, the mitral and tricuspid valvular insufficiency present with ventricular pacing is eliminated. Although it seems obvious that atrial function and atrioventricular synchrony are worth preserving, it is necessary to question the degree of improvement achieved clinically and the severity of the problems, if any, encountered with "nonphysiologic" or ventricular pacing.

That brings us to consideration of what has been called the *pacemaker syndrome* (Erbel, 1979). This entity comprises a multiplicity of adverse sequelae to ventricular pacing, including the induction of congestive heart failure, low cardiac output, and/or syncope. Numerous studies have confirmed that patients with the sick sinus syndrome continue to complain of fatigue, lightheadedness, and angina as frequently after implantation of a ventricular pacemaker as before (Sutton *et al.*, 1980a; El Gamal and Van Gelder, 1981; Crelinsten *et al.*, 1980; Hass and Strait, 1974; Johnson, 1978; Alicandri, 1978; Ogawa *et al.*, 1978). This is in spite of the fact that syncope is usually eliminated. In those patients with preserved retrograde ventricular-to-atrial conduction, ventricular contraction may be uniformly followed by an atrial contraction against the closed atrioventricular valves, with resulting high-pressure Cannon A waves projected back into the pulmonary circuit, syncope, severe pulmonary venous hypertension, and marked loss of exercise tolerance. Under these circumstances, atrial pacing will give a 34 per cent increase in cardiac output compared with ventricular pacing. Numerous acute and chronic clinical studies have confirmed reduced hemodynamics with ventricular pacing versus normal or nearly normal function with atrial or dual-chamber stimulation (Sutton et al., 1980a, 1980b, 1981; Kappenberger et al., 1981; Bognolo et al., 1981). Certainly, patients with complete heart block, loss of AV conduction, and low spontaneous ventricular rates usually feel better with ventricular pacing, although cardiac output measurements remain subnormal. Of special interest with regard to the elderly population with complete heart block and Stokes-Adams disease was a recent study of cerebral blood flow in animals with compromised carotid circulations, comparing the effect of atrial and ventricular stimulation (Hossmann et al., 1981). The subcritical decrease in cerebral blood flow due to vascular occlusion was aggravated by ventricular pacing. Corroborating studies have now been performed in patients, and it would seem that even with complete heart block, atrial or dual-chamber pacing is preferable to ventricular pacing, especially in the elderly population, in whom atherosclerotically narrowed cerebral vessels are common (Miller et al., 1981). The fact that some patients have complete antegrade atrioventricular block but conduct 1:1 retrograde cannot be overlooked, as this allows a patient with complete heart block to develop the full-blown pacemaker syndrome.

Current physiologic pacemaker systems include atrial pacemakers (AOO, AAI, AAT), atrially triggered pacemakers (VAT, VDD), and dual-chamber pacemakers (DVI, DDD) (Sutton et al., 1980a). All physiologic pacemakers potentially require increased sensitivity to cardiac signals because of smaller atrial depolarization waves, increased stimulation energy, and modified frequency and spectral characteristics. Thus, output energy programmability, and sensitivity, and/or refractory period programmability are essential for low-risk, reliable atrial pacing. In addition, optimally, there should be separate output, sensitivity, and refractory period programmability for both the atrial and ventricular circuits of DDD units, as minimal energy requirements should be determined for each lead in order to maximize pacemaker functional life. Refractory period programmability should be included for isolated atrial pacing but will be required infrequently because of the active discharge and blanking circuit technologies already described and the general contraindication to atrial pacing in patients with AV intervals much longer than 200 milliseconds.

Atrial pacing for supraventricular rhythm disorders is appealing because it provides the hemodynamic benefits of AV synchrony in association with natural ventricular activation and treats the underlying rhythm disorder at its site of occurrence with relatively simple and reliable technology, compared with the greater complexities of dual-chamber pacing. Potential problems with atrial pacing versus ventricular pacing include the increased risks of atrial perforation and, historically, increased atrial lead instability. In addition, there is some risk of slower-than-programmed rate stimulation because of atrial output suppression

by the far field effects of the ventricular electrogram. With the three multiprogrammable units discussed in the preceding section, the lead and electronic problems have been largely solved. Potential limitations of atrial pacing versus dual-chamber pacing relate particularly to progression of the supraventricular conduction disorder to complete heart block. This may be due to evolution of the conduction disorder, iatrogenic causes, including drugs such as digitalis, or vagal effects, such as those in the sensitive carotid sinus syndrome, in which atrial rhythm suppression is not infrequently associated with transient heart block. However, in spite of recent recommendations regarding implantation of both atrial and ventricular leads in all patients at the time of the initial procedure, in appropriately selected patients (1:1 AV conduction at a normal interval with rapid atrial pacing) there is a low rate of progression of sick sinus syndrome to complete heart block. In any patient whose atrioventricular conduction system tests normal, atrial pacing is a treatment of choice for symptomatic bradyarrhythmias or tachyarrhythmias.

There are essentially no current indications for VAT pacemakers. These devices were markedly limited by functioning in the VOO mode in response to loss of atrial sensing or with slow atrial rates. They can be mistriggered by premature ventricular contractions sensed by the atrial amplifier, leading to the potential for T-wave pacing. In addition, abrupt decreases in ventricular stimulation rate occurred with high spontaneous atrial rates, leading to presyncopal and syncopal symptoms in patients with intermittent atrial tachycardias. VDD (or ASVIP) devices are less limited, as they do provide ventricular demand pacing in case of atrial sensing failure. Despite the capability of the VAT and VDD devices to provide true ventricular physiologic rate response to normal atrial function, their dependence on atrial sensing, the weakest link in the chain, and the coming availability of satisfactory DDD pacemakers, which automatically include this function when indicated, mean that this type of device will disappear in the near future (Sutton et al., 1980a).

For an increasing number of patients with bradyarrhythmias or tachyarrhythmias, angina, and congestive heart failure, dual-chamber pacing modes, with both the atria and the ventricles stimulated in the appropriate sequence, are the treatment choice. Devices that are now generally available do not offer meaningful programmability of the AV interval between the two stimuli, and for many patients, there is relatively little effect on cardiac output with AV intervals between 150 and 250 msec. However, when the effects of reduced ventricular function, previous myocardial damage, and different rates are introduced, there can be little doubt that in some patients, AV interval optimization will be as important as cardiac rate optimization. Certainly, for antiarrhythmia treatment, as will be covered in the next section, the optimal AV interval is very short, with simultaneous atrial and ventricular stimulation markedly limiting the opportunity for circus or re-entrant rhythms. Both DVI and DDD pacing increase cardiac output and blood pressure, reduce heart size, myocardial ischemia, and pulmonary congestion, and continue to provide physiologic pacing in the face of the unexpected development of junctional rhythm or AV conduction problems (Sutton *et al.*, 1980a). DVI pacing, with sequential stimulation of both chambers but only ventricular sensing and thus the potential for atrial competition, has two potential advantages in the face of atrial tachyarrhythmias. First, rapid triggered ventricular pacing does not ensue, and second, atrial competitive pacing will, in certain cases, result in underdrive termination of the atrial arrhythmia (see the following section on antitachycardia pacing). However, as atrial competition also has the potential to induce arrhythmias, including atrial fibrillation, careful preimplant testing of each patient and the potential for DVI-DDD intermodal programming will be essential. Although atrial fibrillation, like atrial atony, would seem to be an absolute contraindication to physiologic pacing, patients with intermittent atrial fibrillation frequently note a marked reduction in the incidence of their problem following the institution of DVI pacing, and some also note more rapid conversion back to sinus rhythm on those occasions when atrial fibrillation recurs.

The DDD or fully automatic pacemaker combines multiple physiologic pacing modes and the ability to convert from one type of operation to another automatically on a beat-to-beat basis. The usual DDD device stimulates the atria only in response to sinus bradycardia, the atria and the ventricles sequentially in sinus bradycardia with AV block, P wave synchronously during normal atrial rhythms associated with AV block, or neither chamber during normal sinus rhythm with normal AV conduction. To review the DDD designation, the first D indicates that this device has a potential to pace in both the atrium and the ventricle, the second D indicates the potential to sense in both the atrium and ventricle, the third D indicates both triggered and inhibited responses to sensing. The ventricle may be triggered by atrial activity, whereas the atrial output is inhibited by atrial activity and the ventricular output is inhibited by ventricular activity. As with all physiologic pacemakers, DDD devices would be contraindicated in patients with atrial atony and chronic and persistent atrial fibrillation but, in contradistinction to the DVI devices, would also be contraindicated in the face of a number of malignant atrial tachyarrhythmias. DDD devices are being developed and evaluated by all of the pacemaker manufacturers. They are currently undergoing the clinical trial and are not generally available. A number of complications have occurred wih first-generation DDD devices (see footnote, Table 49–9), including rapid ventricular stimulation due to sensing of and triggering from large atrial fibrillation potentials and pacemaker re-entry tachycardias (see previous section on electronics).

In contrast, three DVI pacemakers have been used generally, the American Pacemaker Company (APC) Bifocal 2, the Medtronic Byrel, and the Intermedics Cyberlith IV. Their characteristics are out-

TABLE 49–9. AV SEQUENTIAL PACEMAKER COMPARISONS*

	APC BIFOCAL 2	METRONIC BYREL	INTERMEDICS CYBERLITH IV
Programmable combinations	0	8	3375
Weight (gm.)	130	135	92
Volume (ml.)	59	75	34
Thickness (mm.)	16	18.2	15
Encapsulation	Hermetic	Hermetic	Hermetic
Power source capacity (AH)	SAFT (2.7)	LI (1.4)	LI (3.2)
Projected longevity (years)	5	4	Depends on mode and programming
"Guarantee" (years)	2	2	4
Lead configuration	Bipolar	Bipolar	Unipolar
Lead size	+2	+2	+1
V sensing in AV interval	+	+	−
Postatrial output	V sensing	V sensing	Committed
Potential for self-inhibition	+	+	−
Programming	N.A.	Reed-switch activated, 3-second minimum	80-impulse binomial code; 1/25 second; EMI-insensitive
Modes	0	P × 2	P × 3
P-wave sensitivity	0	0	0
R-wave sensitivity (mv.)	2	2.2	P × 7; 0.6 to 2.8 in VVI + DVI
Pulse width (msec.)	A − 1; V − 0.8	A − 1; V − 0.8	P × 15; 0.15 to 2.29; A + V + all modes
Rate (p.p.m.)	71	P × 5; 63 to 109 in DVI; 70 only in VVI	P × 15; 30 to 120 in all modes
AV delay (msec.)	225	P × 3; 125 to 250	155

P = programmable; A = atrial; V = ventricular; LI = lithium-iodine cell; SAFT = lithium–silver chromate cell; APC = American Pacemaker Co.; EMI = electromagnetic interference; P × 2 = programmable to 2 different settings; P × 3 = programmable to 3 different settings; etc.

*More recently introduced units include the Pacesetter Programalith AV and the Intermedics Avius AV (both substantially smaller DVI pacemakers) and the Cordis Sequicor, Medronic Versatrax, and Telectronics Autima (all first-generation DDD pacemakers with longevity [Sequicor] and/or programmability limitations relative to the problems associated with retrograde conduction and pacemaker-induced tachycardias).

lined in Table 49–9. For comparison, the original epoxy-potted, American Pacemaker Bifocal, SAFT lithium-powered unit weighed 150 gm. and displaced 80 ml. All of the units are hermetically sealed. Projected longevity will be very variable, as previously discussed in the sections on programmability and lead impedance. A major difference between the Intermedics Cyberlith IV and the Medtronic and APC units is the unipolar lead configuration of the Cyberlith, which reduces its size but necessitates that it function as a committed unit. When a ventricular impulse is not sensed after an appropriate duration, all of the units produce an atrial stimulus. The American Pacemaker and Medtronic units then begin to sense and will inhibit the ventricular output if natural ventricular depolarization takes place prior to completion of the pacemakers' AV interval, whereas the atrial output in the Cyberlith is always followed by a ventricular output, thus the committed designation. The committed function can lead to the appearance of apparent ventricular triggered pacing, but this is coincidental. Because of the fixed AV interval of 155 msec. in the Cyberlith, T-wave pacing is very unlikely, despite the committed mode. Sandwich beats, in which the atrial stimulus falls prior to the ventricular depolarization and the ventricular stimulus follows ventricular depolarization, and a phenomenon called pseudo-pseudofusion have been described (Barold et al., 1981). Neither indicates a patient or pacemaker problem. In pseudofusion, a ventricular stimulus falls coincident with a ventricular depolarization but plays no role in ventricular activation, whereas with true fusion, part of the ventricle is captured by a natural depolarization and part by the electric stimulus or an aberrant focus. In pseudo-pseudofusion, the atrial output of a pacemaker may appear to fall on either the QRS or the T wave, but this is spurious, as the stimulus is falling in the atrium, far from the electric events observed on the surface EKG.

The Bifocal DVI unit is not programmable, although four models with different rate and AV delay parameters are available. The Medtronic Byrel has a choice of two modes, DVI or VVI, five rates in DVI only, and a choice of three AV intervals overall, two at a stimulation rate of 70 and two at a stimulation rate of 80 with one overlap. At DVI stimulation rates of 63, 92, and 109 p.p.m., the AV interval is fixed in the Byrel. The Cyberlith has a choice of three modes, DVI, DOO, and VVI. In all modes, there is a choice of seven sensitivities, 15 pulse widths, and 15 rates—all programmable options affecting both the atrial and ventricular outputs (except sensitivity, as, by definition, DVI units do not sense in the atrium).

With the available DVI units, there is little in the way of meaningful AV delay programmability, as the Byrel intervals increase with power-cell depletion and the Cyberlith AV delay is fixed at 155 msec. The VVI mode is important in case of loss of atrial function, as programming to it will result in energy conservation. It also allows for a more accurate assessment of end-of-life characteristics in the Cyberlith. Rate pro-

grammability in the VVI mode is required, as many DVI pacemakers are implanted because of reduced ventricular function, arrhythmias, or angina. The DOO mode in the Cyberlith conserves energy otherwise consumed by sensing functions in those patients with chronic slow ventricular rates, allows the pacemaker to be used for competitive arrhythmia termination, and also makes it totally insensitive to electromagnetic interference and myopotential inhibition, which may otherwise cause symptoms in a small number of patients.

Although there are still limitations, very significant improvements in the available leads and pacemakers now make atrial and AV sequential pacing appropriate considerations for the majority of patients requiring long-term pacing. As illustrated in Figure 49–6, cardiac size frequently returns to normal with atrial or dual-chamber pacing, and it is often possible to achieve chronic atrial pacing at very low stimulus energies, thus ensuring a good potential for prolonged duration of function between pacemaker replacements. With the current state of the art (both medical and technical), atrial pacing deserves far more consideration than it receives. Atrial pacemakers have advantages over dual-chamber pacemakers in terms of simplicity and size, the need for only a single lead, and energy conservation. Yet, whenever natural AV conduction is preserved, atrial pacing provides all of the advantages of dual-chamber pacing, including a 20 per cent increase in cardiac index in 70 per cent of patients; an increase in stroke work index in all patients; a decrease in wedge pressure in all patients; and systemic pressure stabilization and decreased arrhythmias, compared with ventricular pacing in the same patients (Sutton et al., 1980a). From current practice, it appears that dual-chamber pacemakers are indicated in 40 per cent of patients, atrial pacemakers in 15 per cent of patients, and ventricular pacemakers in 45 per cent of patients. It must be recognized that many of the latter are also paced physiologically, because stimulation rate is programmed down to allow the patient to remain in sinus rhythm a great proportion of the time. In the near future, the nonprogrammable ventricular demand pacemaker will have few, if any, indications (Sutton et al., 1980a). With the advent of reliable transvenous atrial leads and improved pacemaker technology, the benefits of systems that restore the normal cardiac sequence should be considered prior to every pacemaker insertion.

ANTITACHYCARDIA PACING

Theories of tachycardia initiation involve the presence of an irritable focus or a re-entrant (circus) loop. (Hart et al., 1978; Wellens et al., 1978; Fisher et al., 1977). The older theory of an irritable focus holds that an area of ischemic or otherwise abnormal conducting tissue begins to fire at a rapid rate, initiating the tachyarrhythmia. The re-entrant loop theory

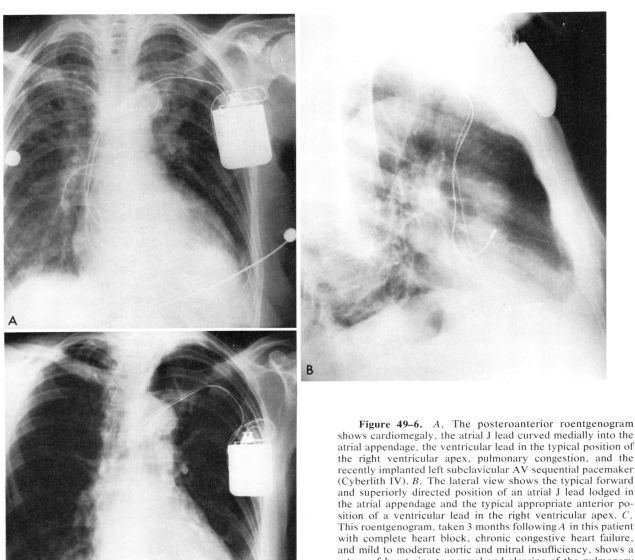

Figure 49–6. *A*, The posteroanterior roentgenogram shows cardiomegaly, the atrial J lead curved medially into the atrial appendage, the ventricular lead in the typical position of the right ventricular apex, pulmonary congestion, and the recently implanted left subclavicular AV sequential pacemaker (Cyberlith IV). *B*, The lateral view shows the typical forward and superiorly directed position of an atrial J lead lodged in the atrial appendage and the typical appropriate anterior position of a ventricular lead in the right ventricular apex. *C*, This roentgenogram, taken 3 months following *A* in this patient with complete heart block, chronic congestive heart failure, and mild to moderate aortic and mitral insufficiency, shows a return of heart size to normal and clearing of the pulmonary congestion. The prepacing cardiac index was only 1.4 L./min./M², but 1 week following the institution of DVI pacing, and again 6 months later, cardiac index was within normal limits, with optimal rate AV sequential pacing, but significantly lower with VVI pacing.

is based on the presence of parallel conducting pathways. If one of the pathways has a slow rate or is unidirectional, any electric activity will have the potential to become self-perpetuating. Reciprocating atrioventricular tachycardias in the Wolff-Parkinson-White syndrome are potentiated by the presence of accessory pathways (usually rapidly conducting) and the His-Purkinje system. Less well-known are dual pathways within an anatomically single AV nodal system, with slow conduction from the atrium to the ventricle but rapid retrograde conduction to restimulate the atrium, as well as the opposite condition, in which there is rapid AV and slow VA conduction. Re-entrant and reciprocating conduction loops probably underlie the majority of symptomatic tachyarrhythmias.

Implantable antitachycardia pacing modalities are outlined in Table 49–10. All of the techniques are at least potentially applicable to both atrial and ventricular arrhythmias. Standard atrial or ventricular *pacing at a nominal rate* will prevent the occurrence of certain tachyarrhythmias that are triggered only when the patient's spontaneous rate falls below 70 p.p.m. (Wellens *et al.*, 1978). *Dual-chamber pacing* (DVI, DOO, DDD) may suppress and/or terminate initiating atrial or ventricular tachycardia re-entrant loops (Dreifus *et al.*, 1975) by ensuring a short interval between atrial and ventricular depolarization and by relieving myocardial ischemia. The latter is accomplished both by increasing cardiac output and decreasing myocardial oxygen demand. The longer the interval between atrial depolarization and the initiation of ventricular

TABLE 49–10. ANTITACHYCARDIA PACING
TECHNIQUES

Single-chamber suppression
Dual-chamber suppression and termination
Overdrive suppression and termination
Underdrive termination
Critically timed single or double stimuli
Entrainment and weaning
Burst pacing
Train pacing
Automatic internal defibrillation

depolarization, the more likely the development of an arrhythmia.

The technique of *overdrive suppression and termination* of either atrial or ventricular arrhythmias is an extension of standard rate pacing suppression (Wellens *et al.*, 1978; Fisher *et al.*, 1977). The faster the pacing rate, the less heart tissue is repolarized, excitable, and capable of generating premature beats or responding to re-entrant stimuli. Overdrive suppression requires chronic rapid rate pacing, which some patients will tolerate for prolonged periods, even at rates in excess of 100 p.p.m. Overdrive pacing is also frequently used temporarily in the postoperative setting for suppression of tachyarrhythmias and conversion of atrial flutter back to sinus rhythm by gradually weaning from rapid rate pacing.

Underdrive termination (Wellens *et al.*, 1978; Fisher *et al.*, 1977) of tachyarrhythmias involves fixed rate stimulation at less than the arrhythmia rate, which occasionally, by chance, produces an appropriately timed stimulus to interrupt the arrhythmia. Competitive underdrive pacing works fairly well in some patients with atrial tachycardias but only occasionally and intermittently in patients with ventricular tachycardias. Its success rate depends on the length of the critical timing period and the rate of underdrive stimulation. It may take a very long time for the appropriately timed stimulus to occur by chance and interrupt the arrhythmia. It is probable that the critical termination period begins at or near to the end of the atrial or ventricular refractory period, depending on the chamber in which the arrhythmia originated.

Critically timed ("programmed") single or double stimuli may be thought of as tuned underdrive termination. Initially, stimuli are delivered sequentially throughout the critical termination period until the precise termination point is found by a more selective trial-and-error method than that available with simple underdrive termination. Once the effective area has been determined, however, through a memory process, the termination stimulus is delivered to precisely the effective point when the pacemaker again recognizes a similar arrhythmia (Fisher *et al.*, 1977; Ward *et al.*, 1980).

Critically timed paired ventricular pacing, although not necessarily effective in terminating ventricular tachycardias, may be used to improve hemodynamics temporarily in patients unresponsive to cardioversion. The second stimulus may slow ventricular rate response and increase systemic blood pressure, but at the risk of inducing ventricular fibrillation. This technique is now used for temporary pacing, but it could be included in a sophisticated implantable device that was also capable of automatically treating ventricular fibrillation. *Paired atrial pacing* can also be used in the temporary treatment of ventricular tachycardias to promote better ventricular filling. The determination of the timing of delivery of critically timed stimuli, called scanning, eliminates the random nature of underdrive pacing for arrhythmia termination.

Train pacing (Fisher *et al.*, 1977) at rates in excess of 1000 p.p.m. provides the ultimate in delivery of a critically timed stimulus because the whole potential termination area is covered, but only a single stimulus, one of the first out of the myocardial refractory period, captures the heart and, it is hoped, terminates the arrhythmia. Train pacing has no more risk of inducing ventricular fibrillation than does a single (functionally equivalent) critically timed stimulus.

Burst pacing is akin to very rapid overdrive termination (Furman, 1973; Fisher *et al.*, 1977; Lister *et al.*, 1973; Waxman *et al.*, 1978). It involves rapid-rate, short-duration, and fixed-rate pacing. This is intended to be a multiple capture technique, with the heart following the pacemaker at a rate usually in the range of 200 p.p.m. and then reverting to a normal rhythm upon sudden cessation of pacing. This, of course, does not always occur, and in some cases, a more gradual weaning from rapid pacing, requiring up to several hours, may be necessary to achieve normal sinus rhythm. No permanent pacemaker yet available involves automatic gradual weaning, but this would be a useful programmable feature. Optimal burst rates and durations may be determined in the electrophysiologic laboratory (Hart *et al.*, 1978; Fisher *et al.*, 1977), but because requirements vary from patient to patient and change with time in the same patient, custom parameter pacers are often only temporarily effective and full programmability is essential. Burst pacing has a high therapeutic index for supraventricular tachycardias but has a lower rate of success and potentially greater risks in the treatment of ventricular tachycardias.

Automatic internal defibrillation, the last technique to be presented, involves the recognition and automatic termination of ventricular fibrillation and certain ventricular tachycardias by the delivery of large energy charges from an implanted device (Mirowski *et al.*, 1980).

A number of implantable devices are available for treatment of recurrent arrhythmias. Atrial and ventricular pacing suppression, overdrive suppression and termination, and underdrive termination may be accomplished with any of the available multiprogrammable pacemakers that include rate and mode programmability for conversion to VOO or AOO pacing. The Medtronic Byrel and ASVIP, the Intermedics Cyberlith IV, the Cordis 208 VAT, the Medtronic Byrel DD, and the American Pacemaker Bifocal 2 are all inherently antiarrhythmia devices because they eliminate the occurrence of prolonged intervals between atrial and ventricular depolarization (Dreifus *et al.*, 1975). In addition, because of its programmability to the DOO mode, the Cyberlith IV can be used for dual-chamber underdrive termination in conjunction with its rate programmability. The Byrel 5992 DD has been called a double-demand AV sequential pacemaker, as it automatically converts from DVI to what might be termed DVO function in response to a detected arrhythmia (Castellanos *et al.*, 1980). The DVI mode is similar to that of the standard Byrel pacemaker (see Table 49–9), with inhibition by spontaneous rates of from 71 to 149 p.p.m. At spontaneous rates of less than 70 p.p.m., the DVI unit differs from the standard Byrel in that the AV interval is fixed at 150 msec. When this device detects five or six consecutive ventricular depolarizations at a rate of 150 p.p.m. or faster, it converts to apparent fixed-rate AV sequential pacing at a rate of 65 p.p.m. with an initial AV interval of 150 msec. and subsequent AV intervals of 70 msec. However, this cannot accurately be described as DOO pacing, because the unit continues to sense in the ventricle, and upon arrhythmia termination, it converts back to its previous DVI function. Although it does not scan and therefore functions randomly, this device has been used successfully for arrhythmia termination. It may function by re-entrant loop blocking (short intervals between atrial and ventricular depolarization) and/or competitive underdrive termination. The ultimate in dual-chamber re-entrant loop blocking would be simultaneous DOO stimulation.

Related single-chamber devices have also been used in clinical trials. Called dual-demand pacemakers (Curry *et al.*, 1979), they are basically VVI or AAI, with automatic conversion to VVO or AAO, respectively, when a tachyarrhythmia is detected. The ventricular or atrial sensing is for monitoring of termination of the arrhythmia, which then results in termination of competitive pacing. Dual-demand pacing is inferior to double-demand pacing for re-entrant tachycardias, since the original dual-demand units involved minimal delay prior to institution of arrhythmia treatment and were more electrode position–sensitive, as the single stimulation site reduces the chance of interrupting a re-entry pathway. The devices have been effective in less than 15 per cent of cases.

The original burst pacemakers were manually activated by radiofrequency signals or by placing a magnet over the pacemaker. When the patient recognized a tachyarrhythmia, treatment was self-initiated and resulted in delivery of a burst of stimuli at a preset rate and number. Second-generation devices would recognize arrhythmias by a rate counting technique and automatically deliver burst pacing for a limited duration. Because different burst rates and durations are effective in different patients, extensive preimplantation electrophysiologic testing was required, but many patients' requirements changed with time, limiting the applicability of nonprogrammable antiarrhythmia devices.

TABLE 49–11. MULTIPROGRAMMABLE SELECTIONS OF THE BURST AND TRAIN PACER (INTERMEDICS CYBERTACH 60 [BIPOLAR MULTIPROGRAMMABLE])

2 modes	AAI or VVI and AAI or VVI plus antitachycardia
7 sensitivities	0.6 to 2.8 mV.
15 pulse widths	0.15 to 2.3 msec.
2 VVI or AAI rates	60 and 80 b.p.m.
2 tachycardia criteria	
8 burst rates	
5 burst durations	
4 telemetry functions	

A recently developed bipolar multiprogrammable burst and train pacemaker (Intermedics CyberTach 60) solves at least some of these problems (Griffin and Mason, 1981). Its programmable features (Table 49–11), in addition to sensitivity, pulse width, and rate, include noninvasive selection of a variety of tachycardia criteria, burst rates, burst durations, and either standard demand atrial or ventricular pacing, depending on lead placement plus standard demand pacing with automatic arrhythmia recognition and termination by burst or train pacing. The tachycardia rate that the physician may choose to activate the burst or train feature of the CyberTach 60 is above 137 p.p.m. or above 180 p.p.m., although special units with different tachycardia recognition criteria can be obtained on request. When the pacemaker detects eight consecutive intervals shorter than the selected rate, it diagnoses a tachycardia. Burst rates of from 180 p.p.m. to train rates of over 1400 p.p.m. may be selected, with rates of between 200 and 300 p.p.m. found to be effective in most patients. The duration of the burst or train pacing can also be noninvasively set from a fraction of a second to over 5 seconds. This pacemaker includes the Cyberlith telemetry follow-up functions of cell voltage, which will be described later, but, in addition, has a memory function that notes if an arrhythmia is treated between patients' visits to the physician, and this information can be determined when the patient returns for follow-up or over the telephone.

Automatic scanning overdrive pacing has been reduced to implantable form by Telectronics, Inc. (1980). Overdrive pacing is initiated at a rate just faster than the tachycardia for a preselected duration. Suppression of the tachycardia leads to demand pacing or automatic pacer suppression if the spontaneous rhythm is fast enough. If, on the other hand, the arrhythmia continues after a preset interval, the overdrive rate is increased slightly. This sequence continues until the arrhythmia converts or until an upper rate limit is reached. Potential advantages of autodecremental pacing include reduced risk of induced atrial or ventricular flutter or fibrillation versus double extra stimuli, underdrive or overdrive pacing, because of the self-selected initial rate. There is an increased potential for arrhythmia termination because progressive acceleration of the overdrive or underdrive rate results in stimulation of different phases of a tachycardia cycle during a shorter period. Optimization of the autodecremental system will require programmable choice of (1) stimulus voltage, width, and amplitude; (2) duration of each therapeutic cycle; (3) maximum rate; (4) decremental duration; (5) both underdrive and overdrive progression; (6) interdecremental interval; and (7) memory.

All of the antiarrhythmia implantable devices require a mechanism for recognition and treatment of lethal arrhythmias. This can potentially be accomplished with the Medrad/Intec AID, an automatic internal defibrillator currently undergoing clinical trials at two centers (Mirowski *et al.*, 1980). The first-generation devices are bulky, 250 gm. and 145 ml., versus 135 gm. and 75 ml. for the Medtronic Byrel. The device is triggered by the absence of isoelectric potentials in cases of ventricular fibrillation or ventricular tachycardia and can deliver up to 100 25- to 30-joule discharges over a maximal period of 3 years. Up to three defibrillation cycles can be delivered in fairly rapid succession. Originally, the device was implanted with the aid of a thoracotomy or a median sternotomy, but currently, recommended techniques include transvenous placement of a high, superior vena caval electrode and subxiphoid placement of a large-area, epicardial electrode. The first defibrillatory shock is delivered 23 seconds after the recognition of ventricular fibrillation. A magnet placed over the unit disables it and allows direct checking of the discharge intensity by an external analogue meter to determine when replacement of the device is indicated. The first automatic defibrillator was implanted on February 4, 1980, and by the summer of 1981, 24 patients had been treated, with over 75 per cent being males and over 75 per cent having coronary artery disease as their primary underlying pathologic condition, although six had cardiomyopathy. All of the patients selected for the implantable defibrillator had two episodes of documented cardiac arrest with poor response to standard therapy. Initially, the unit was designed to treat only ventricular fibrillation, but it will now also recognize most ventricular tachycardias with rates greater than 250 p.p.m. and some with slower rates. Prior to widespread clinical trials, it would seem that the unit would need to be combined with some of the relatively low-energy pacemaker suppression and arrhythmia treatment techniques previously presented in order to, if possible, reduce the need for and frequency of defibrillation. Furthermore, a method of recognizing atrial arrhythmias not responsive to the other techniques already discussed would be valuable.

Candidates for implantable antitachycardia pacemakers should be subject to recurrent symptomatic episodes with poor response to drug therapy (Fisher *et al.*, 1977). Patients with very frequent episodes or who are unable to recognize arrhythmia occurrence or to cope with the responsibility are candidates for automatic devices. Some of the advantages of antitachycardia pacemakers over drug therapy include

patient compliance (the patient does not have to remember to take it) and the rapidity and stability of effect, with minimal side reactions. In addition, the duration from diagnosis to therapy is much shorter, as the work-up for antiarrhythmia drug therapy must, of necessity, include protracted sequential multiagent trials. As recurrent arrhythmias may necessitate prolonged hospitalization, up to several months in some cases, widespread availability of antitachycardia pacing techniques will in all probability reduce the costs of care of these patients who are so very difficult to treat, as well as improve the quality of life by more reliably preventing or treating severe tachyarrhythmias.

Potential disadvantages of implantable antitachycardia treatment devices include the lower success rate and higher complication rate in patients with ventricular versus supraventricular arrhythmias (Griffin and Mason, 1981), the potential for acceleration into more lethal arrhythmias, the testing required prior to implantation, the changing patient requirements for effective termination, and the physician confusion resulting from the availability of multiple treatment modes. With the inclusion of a back-up defibrillator, the risks of acceleration into more lethal arrhythmias would be reduced and effectiveness of treatment of ventricular arrhythmias could be increased. Multiprogrammability will almost entirely eliminate problems with changing patient requirements, especially since scanning techniques, with automatic parameter adjustment, could be adapted to all of the antitachycardia therapeutic modalities. Again, because of changing patient requirements and the potential for availability of multiple antiarrhythmia therapeutic modes within a single device, chronic *in vivo* testing will partially replace extensive and detailed preimplant testing following general availability of these devices. However, criteria for patient selection will require continuing refinement in clinical research centers.

It will be a considerable time before multimodal autoprogramming antiarrhythmia devices with the ability to differentiate between different tachycardia types, to memorize and record the occurrence of all arrhythmias, and to defibrillate when all else fails are available. Current practice would indicate that the majority of patients with supraventricular tachyarrhythmias can be effectively treated by antitachycardia pacing techniques, but that ventricular tachyarrhythmias will be best handled by pharmacologic therapy in over 50 per cent of cases, by direct surgical techniques such as endocardial or aneurysm resection in 10 per cent of cases, and by a combination of antitachycardia pacing and/or drug therapy and surgery in the remainder. With presently available techniques, atrial flutter with rapid ventricular response, atrial fibrillation with rapid ventricular response, ventricular fibrillation and external defibrillator–induced pacer damage are all potentially serious complications of antiarrhythmia pacing. Only multiprogrammable single- and dual-chamber pacing devices are currently generally available, except in research centers, and even these are not specifically approved for antiar-rhythmia therapy. Chronic AV sequential pacing alone has proved effective in the treatment of approximately 40 per cent of patients with paroxysmal supraventricular tachycardias and the tachycardia/bradycardia syndrome of slow inherent rhythm with period escape tachycardias. When combined with drug therapy, effective treatment is achieved in 50 to 60 per cent of patients. Treatment of AV junctional and ventricular tachycardias and prevention of ventricular fibrillation have been achieved with chronic AV sequential pacing (Adinolfi *et al.*, 1981), but the improvements are often partial, and full rate and mode programmability in combination with varying drug therapies is essential to achieve long-term satisfactory results. Often, patients with recurrent ventricular arrhythmias have serious underlying myocardial damage that limits their life expectancy, although certainly there are patients, including those with the mitral prolapse syndrome, in whom no ventricular myocardial abnormality can be detected after death from recurrent ventricular arrhythmias.

Predictions regarding the future use of pacing for tachyarrhythmias vary from inconsequential to equal or greater than that of pacing for bradyarrhythmias. Significant developmental device work remains to be done before the full role of this form of therapy can be assessed.

PATHOPHYSIOLOGY, PATIENT EVALUATION, DIFFERENTIAL DIAGNOSIS, AND INDICATIONS FOR DIFFERENT PACEMAKER MODES

Anatomy and Function of the Cardiac Conduction System

The cardiac conduction system begins at the sinoatrial node, located in the wall of the right atrium near its junction with the superior vena cava. The sinus node is approximately 15 mm. in diameter, and because of its location just beneath the epicardium and its significant connective tissue content, it is susceptible to injury and to pericardial, collagen, and small vessel diseases. The sinus node is organized around a comparatively large central artery, which is probably involved in a biofeedback mechanism through pressure and diameter changes. The node is composed of slender, elongated transitional cells that probably have a conducting function and round P cells that are grouped in clusters. The P cells are probably the site of impulse formation. The heart responds to the most rapidly occurring available stimulus, which normally arises from the sinus node. The location of the node on the most superior portion of the heart provides parallel positioning of the initiation of both hemodynamic and electric events. Normal sinus node rates are between 60 and 100 p.p.m. The sinus node blood supply is from the right coronary artery in just over 50 per cent of cases and from the circumflex coronary artery by one of two routes in the remainder. The impulse produced by the sinus node spreads through the walls of both atria and through three specialized internodal pathways to reach the atrioventricular node.

The atrioventricular node, a small elliptic structure, lies just beneath the right atrial endocardium and just anterior to the ostium of the coronary sinus. It receives its blood supply from the right coronary artery in 90 per cent of cases and from the circumflex artery in 10 per cent of cases. Its intrinsic rate is between 40 and 55 p.p.m., and thus, it is usually suppressed in the presence of normal sinus node function. The atrioventricular node slows conduction to allow for hemodynamic priming of the ventricle. The midportion of the node is capable of completely blocking impulses that are inappropriately rapid.

The bundle of His arises from the distal atrioventricular node and travels in the posteroinferior margin of the membranous septum to the crest of the muscular interventricular septum. It gradually moves from right to left and gives off small right and larger left bundle branches. The blood supply to the His bundle and its branches is similar to that of the AV node. The His bundle is encased in the collagen of the central fibrous body between the mitral and aortic valves, so that a relatively small focal lesion can destroy its function as the only normal electric connection between the atria and ventricles. Abnormal accessory pathways are considered with the Wolff-Parkinson-White syndrome and will not be discussed here. The intrinsic rate of the His bundle and branches ranges between 25 and 40 p.p.m.

The electrical signals of the tissue masses of the sinus node, AV node, and His bundle and branches are too small to register on the surface electrocardiogram, which shows primarily atrial depolarization and ventricular depolarization and repolarization, because these structures have relatively much larger muscle masses and produce comparatively very large electric signals (Resnekov and Lipps, 1972; James, 1979). Following its delay in the AV node, the impulse travels through the His bundle and into its branches and subsequently into the Purkinje system, which rapidly spreads it throughout the ventricular myocardium, resulting in rapid activation and contraction, as are necessary for effective pumping (Tyers, 1967). The majority of the intramyocardial conduction system is vascularized from the left anterior descending coronary artery.

Pathophysiology

All cardiac conditions that cause a sudden diminution in the output of the left ventricle produce episodic cerebral ischemia and the potential for Stokes-Adams seizures. The degrees of cerebral ischemia vary, so that symptoms may be less dramatic than syncope with convulsions, and include dizziness, lightheadedness, brief lapses of consciousness, and fainting without convulsions (Furman, 1977a). The underlying mechanism may be marked bradycardia, asystole, ventricular tachycardia, transient ventricular fibrillation, or a sudden decrease in rate from a relatively well-tolerated tachycardia. During periods when atrioventricular conduction is temporarily or permanently absent and a slow idioventricular rate of 25 to 40 p.p.m. ensues, the cardiac output is reduced and stroke volume is maximal. Thus, increased venous return to the heart, as occurs with exercise, does not result in increased cardiac output, because the heart has been deprived of both rate and stroke volume responses to preload. The arterial venous oxygen difference increases, right ventricular and pulmonary artery pressures are elevated, and because of the maximal stroke volume, left ventricular and systemic arterial pressures are also increased. If sinoatrial function continues, atrial contraction will, on occasion, coincidentally precede ventricular contraction, resulting in a cyclic variation in systemic and pulmonary pressures and cardiac output. Even when slow rates are persistent and syncope does not occur, low cardiac output results in reduced renal and cerebral function, with the BUN and creatinine levels frequently elevated and mentation slowed. A low cardiac output, potential ventricular ischemia, and slow intramyocardial conduction of the idioventricular rhythm provide an ideal substrate for the development of re-entrant loops and ventricular tachycardia or fibrillation.

Etiology of Cardiac Conduction System Dysfunction

An outline of the causes of cardiac conduction system dysfunction is presented in Table 49–12. All

TABLE 49–12. CAUSES OF CARDIAC CONDUCTION SYSTEM DYSFUNCTION

Degenerative:	Cardiac skeletal sclerosis Paget's disease Anular calcification
Traumatic:	Cardiac surgery Projectiles Stab wounds
Vascular, hematologic:	Ischemic heart disease Fibromuscular dysplasia Thrombocytopenic purpura
Metabolic, toxic:	Cardiac drugs Parasiticides Electrolyte disturbances Hypothyroidism Hypothermia Hemochromatosis Amyloidosis
Congenital	
Inflammatory, Myocarditides:	Microorganisms Rheumatic disease Collagen diseases Sarcoidosis
Neoplastic:	Metastases Primary tumor

of the listed conditions may attack any part of the system, interfering with impulse formation in the sinoatrial node or propagation lower down in the conduction system. Degenerative causes of conduction system disruption are by far the most common. The His bundle and branches are particularly susceptible where they pass through the collagen of the central fibrous body. Familial noninflammatory degeneration without marked fibrosis or calcification is called Lenegre's disease; destructive fibrosis of the conductive system usually associated with calcification is known as Lev's disease (James, 1979). Both Paget's disease and the sequelae of rheumatic myovalvulitis are usually associated with calcification. Although gunshot and stab wounds of the heart are increasing in frequency in many centers, the most common traumatic injuries to the heart follow open heart surgery and may be related to hemorrhage, infarction, or suturing or division of the conduction tissue. Aortic valve replacement (the bundle is very superficial in the region of the junction of the right and noncoronary cusps) and operations involving large ventricular septal defects, corrected transposition, or Ebstein's anomaly are associated with the greatest risk.

Of the vascular causes, ischemic heart disease is by far the most common. In the past, it was overemphasized that myocardial infarction infrequently results in permanent complete heart block. Although the percentage of infarction patients developing heart block is small, the very large number of infarctions each year provide at least 5 per cent of patients requiring pacemakers. The sinoatrial node, the AV node, and/or the bundle of His and distal branches may all be compromised by ischemia. Fibromuscular dysplasia has a particular affinity for the AV nodal artery.

Although true of any of the causes of conduction system dysfunction, the metabolic causes in particular may be functional (or temporary) rather than organic. Amyloidosis has an affinity for the sinus node, whereas hemochromatosis is more likely to involve the atrioventricular node. Parasiticides that can produce heart block include the antimalarial drug chloroquine and antimony, which is commonly used in the Orient. Electrolyte disturbances that can result in heart block include both hypokalemia and hyperkalemia as well as hypocalcemia. By far the most common toxic agents causing conduction delays are cardiac drugs, including digitalis, procainamide, quinidine, and the beta-blockers. In the management of angina and arrhythmias, it may be preferable to continue the drug and institute pacemaker therapy rather than discontinue the drug because of bradycardia.

Congenital causes of conduction system dysfunction are associated with other forms of congenital heart disease in 50 per cent of cases and have a tendency to produce the most severe symptoms in infancy and then again in later life, beginning in the teens. Sinus of Valsalva aneurysms may be associated with the late development of heart block. Pacing is required for congenital heart block if the patient is symptomatic or if the duration of the QRS complex is greater than 0.12 seconds (Furman, 1977a). Although most deaths occur in infancy and the majority of children who survive reach adulthood without severe symptoms, sudden death may be the first clinical manifestation of a worsening of the conduction defect at any age. It may be located lower, but the anatomic discontinuity in patients with congenital heart block surviving infancy is usually between the internodal pathways and the AV node, so that a relatively rapid escape rate of about 60 p.p.m. may be present.

Infectious causes of conduction system dysfunction include any condition causing pericarditis, which may affect the sinus node, and viral, bacterial, fungal, spirochetal, protozoan and helminthic myocarditides. Chagas' disease, caused by a protozoan, is the most common indication for pacing in South America. Unlike the other infectious causes of conduction disturbances, the heart block in this condition is rarely temporary. Possibly because of the high collagen content of the sinus node, it is particularly susceptible to collagen diseases, including lupus and scleroderma.

Neoplastic causes of conduction system disturbances are predominantly metastatic and usually occur late in the course of a terminal condition. Primary tumors include fibromas of the central fibrous body, which can compress the node or bundle, and benign congenital polycystic tumors of the atrioventricular node (commonly called mesothelioma of the AV node); both of these can lead to sudden death. A number of patients coming to postmortem examination for unexplained sudden death subsequent to a pacemaker implantation have been determined to have this condition, which, paradoxically, may be less well treated by ventricular pacing than other causes of conduction system dysfunction (James and Galakhov, 1977).

It is apparent that most of the diseases that affect the conduction system of the heart may be multifocal. Causes of abnormality of function of the sinus node may also affect the internodal pathways and the AV node or the bundle of His. The seriousness of sinus node dysfunction is increased when the underlying pathologic condition also prevents emergence of a relatively benign (stable and rapid) escape rhythm further down in the conduction system. The multifocal nature of many of the causes of conduction system dysfunction also explains the limited acceptance of atrial pacing as an isolated modality (Furman, 1977a

Indications by Pacemaker Type and Differential Diagnosis

Conditions that may require pacing by an atrial, dual-chamber, or ventricular device are outlined in Table 49–13. The sick sinus syndrome is recognized in patients with severe persistent or episodic supraventricular bradycardia, sinus arrest for brief or prolonged periods, sinoatrial block not related to drug

TABLE 49–13. CONDITIONS THAT MAY REQUIRE PACING

SUPRAVENTRICULAR OR DUAL-CHAMBER DEVICE
  Sick sinus syndrome
    Sinus bradycardia <60 p.p.m. or sinus arrest
    Slow rate induced escape rhythms
      Tachycardia
      Flutter
      Fibrillation
    ± Sinoatrial block
    ± Conduction system disease
    ± Syncope
  Tachycardias
  Chronotropic incompetence
  Atrial fibrillation with slow ventricular response

VENTRICULAR OR DUAL-CHAMBER DEVICE
  Fixed complete heart block
  Intermittent complete heart block
  Mobitz Type II second-degree block
  Intraventricular conduction defects
  Sensitive carotid sinus syndrome

therapy, episodic alternating tachyarrhythmias with a normal sinus rate or sinus bradycardia between attacks, and slow recovery of sinus function after cardioversion (Furman, 1977a). Chronotropic incompetence is considered to be present in those patients who run an inappropriately slow supraventricular rate in the presence of congestive heart failure and limited stroke volume response, where an adequate cardiac output could be achieved only at a higher rate (Greenburg et al., 1978). Although unusual, atrial fibrillation can be associated with a persistent slow ventricular response and symptoms of cerebral ischemia, indicating the need for the ventricular rate to be increased by pacing (Furman, 1977a).

Fixed complete heart block is an absolute indication for cardiac pacing in the absence of an imminently life-threatening intercurrent illness. As the mortality rate for complete heart block is about 50 per cent per year, only severe senility or terminal cancer would preclude implantation of a pacemaker in most of these patients. Nursing home residents often seem inappropriate candidates for a pacemaker, but their care is made significantly more difficult if they suffer with periodic Stokes-Adams attacks. Heart block, as determined from the surface electrocardiogram, is divided into first, second, and third degrees (Furman, 1977a). First-degree heart block is in fact only a conduction delay and is present if the PR interval is greater than 210 msec. Second-degree heart block is divided into Mobitz Types I and II. In Mobitz Type I or Wenckebach block, the PR interval progressively lengthens, until conduction is transiently blocked. The pathology is usually in the atrioventricular node and is often due to a temporary or reversible cause such as increased vagal tone. In Mobitz Type II second-degree block, the PR interval is constant between occasional random nonconducted impulses. The pathology is usually below the node and is associated with a prolonged HV (His-ventricular) interval during His bundle studies. This condition is likely to proceed to symptomatic complete heart block without warning. In third-degree or complete heart block there is total loss of atrial and ventricular synchrony. The lower the level of the block in the nodal-His-Purkinje system, the wider the QRS complex and the slower the escape rate. Complete heart block can result from injury to or disease of the AV node, the bundle of His, a combination of the left and right bundles, or the right bundle and both fascicles of the left bundle. Bifascicular and trifascicular blocks may have poor prognostic implications in some patients following myocardial infarction, and if the HV interval is longer than 65 msec., the mortality rate can be reduced to less than 33 per cent by the institution of permanent cardiac pacing (Furman, 1977a).

Inclusion of the sensitive carotid sinus syndrome under conditions requiring ventricular or dual-chamber pacing is due to the frequent occurrence of autonomically induced transient heart block in association with sensitive carotid sinus–induced sinus arrest or bradycardia. The differential diagnosis of neurologic dysfunction based on a primary cardiac rhythm disturbance includes epilepsy, transient ischemic or embolic attacks, hypoglycemia, aortic stenosis, intracardiac tumors, and drug toxicity. A careful neurologic, cerebrovascular, and cardiovascular evaluation is frequently indicated, as are metabolic studies and elimination of potential functional or toxic causes of bradycardia.

Patient Evaluation and Clinical Decision Making

Evaluation of a patient for cardiac pacing includes the usual clinical assessment by history and physical examination with a complete CNS and cardiovascular examination. Noninvasive or invasive aortic arch studies to delineate the carotid and vertebral circulation may be required. In patients with intermittent symptoms, the electrocardiogram is frequently normal, and on occasion, Holter ambulatory electrocardiographic recordings may have to be repeated over and over to capture a bradyarrhythmia or tachyarrhythmia. The association of the arrhythmia and the patient's symptoms then has to be confirmed. The clinical evaluation has a confidence level (with regard to making the correct treatment decision) of about 80 per cent. This may be increased 15 per cent by electrophysiologic studies, including His bundle electrograms and sinus node recovery times, with the final 5 per cent provided by instinct. Normal values for sinus node recovery time following rapid pacing are in the range of 525 msec. or less, and certainly, if the recovery time is greater than 3 seconds, the patient requires a pacemaker. However, the sinus node recovery time may be totally normal in a patient with a life-threatening but intermittent bradyarrhythmia or tachyarrhythmia. The surface electrocardiogram exhibits only a portion of cardiac electric activity, with the small mass of the conduction system being completely masked by the atrial and ventricular myocar-

dium. This has led to endocardial His bundle electrogram recordings that require fluoroscopic positioning of a bipolar electrode in contact with both ends of the AV node in the right atrium. His bundle studies provide information regarding passage of impulses from the sinoatrial node through the atrioventricular node. The PR interval of the surface electrocardiogram is divided into AH (atrial-His) and HV (His-ventricular) intervals. A prolonged AH interval indicates a conduction delay from the sinus node through the AV node; a prolonged HV interval indicates a conduction delay distal to the AV node. The normal AH interval is up to 130 msec., whereas a normal HV interval is up to 55 msec.

Sophisticated patient evaluation for physiologic pacing should include whenever possible (1) comparison of natural rhythm with atrial, ventricular, and dual-chamber pacing at a variety of rates, (2) determination of sinus node recovery time with and without anticholinergics, (3) His bundle electrogram recordings with and without carotid massage, and (4) determinations of wedge, pulmonary artery, and systemic arterial pressures and cardiac index with natural rhythm, ventricular pacing, and a pacing technique that preserves atrioventricular synchrony. Atrial electrograms are also required to answer questions regarding adequate sensing signals versus threshold energy requirements. When an electrophysiologic laboratory is not available, an estimate of the effects of physiologic pacing can be obtained from observing the systemic pressure response to random intermittent AV synchrony. Usually, the systemic pressure will increase 20 mm. Hg acutely and may stabilize at even higher levels with chronic pacing. To decide whether the patient needs an atrial or a dual-chamber pacemaker, rapid atrial pacing can be undertaken during implantation. One-to-one ventricular capture with a relatively normal PR interval during atrial pacing at rates of up to 120 p.p.m. indicates only a low risk of progression to complete heart block and the probability that atrial pacing will suffice (Greenburg *et al.*, 1978). A further indication that the patient will benefit from re-establishment of AV synchrony is the electrocardiographic evidence of retrograde ventriculoatrial conduction, which is consistently associated with very poor hemodynamics. When the decision still cannot be made, temporary pacing with the preferred mode can be undertaken to confirm its value in terms of patient response, arrhythmia elimination, and angina threshold.

Permanent and intermittent complete heart block with or without symptoms is an absolute indication for cardiac pacing, but definitive information ends there. There is no test result that absolutely confirms the need or the absence of need for a pacemaker. Demonstration of complete heart block on an electrocardiogram may not infrequently indicate the need for digitalis or beta-blocker dosage reduction, not for a pacemaker, and conversely, both the electrocardiogram and invasive conduction and recovery studies may be entirely normal between intermittent symptomatic attacks of complete heart block. Patients with a syncopal history may undergo several Holter studies during ambulatory monitoring, with no significant conduction or rhythm abnormality detected, only to subsequently suffer a syncopal attack and have complete heart block demonstrated on the emergency room electrocardiogram. This can be quite difficult to explain to the patient and family, especially when it occurs within hours of discharge after a prolonged hospitalization and normal work-up results.

It cannot be overemphasized that the decision to pace or not to pace is primarily based on careful history taking and clinical judgment. The lack of specific tests and the newer physiologic and antiarrhythmia indications for pacing underlie the recent literature (Goldberg, 1981; Friedman, 1981; Preston, 1981; Check, 1980) as well as discussions in lay publications regarding the possibility that too many pacemakers are being implanted. Because of the low risk of pacemaker insertion, the high potential benefit, and the high risk of withholding treatment when needed, the threshold for pacemaker insertion should be in the area of a 15 per cent chance of benefiting the patient (Pauker and Salem, 1981). Certainly, this will lead to a small incidence of nonessential implant procedures, but this is a standard occurrence in quality medical practice. All removed appendices are not inflamed, and all biopsied pulmonary masses do not confirm the presence of carcinoma of the lung. If the indications for pacemaker therapy are too restricted, patients in real need will be denied benefit, with the potential for unnecessary deaths due to the Stokes-Adams syndrome.

In 1970, 75 per cent of patients received their pacemakers for complete heart block, 13 per cent for second-degree heart block, and 12 per cent for other conditions. In 1980, complete heart block accounted for a similar number of implants, but these were only 35 per cent of the total. An additional 35 per cent of units were implanted for the sick sinus syndrome, 10 per cent for the sensitive carotid sinus syndrome, 10 per cent for second-degree heart block, and 10 per cent for tachyarrhythmias and congestive failure. The matching of appropriate pacing modes to the clinical conditions requires some thought (Sutton et al., 1980a). VOO pacing would be indicated for patients with complete antegrade and retrograde AV block, fixed atrial fibrillation or atrial atony, and a very high-risk electromagnetic interference environment. Indications for VVI or VVT pacing would include intermittent antegrade and retrograde AV block, noncomplex spontaneous ventricular rhythm, and atrial fibrillation or atrial atony. Ventricular pacing gives as good a functional result as can be obtained, in approximately 20 per cent of patients requiring pacemakers, those with poor or absent atrial function. AOO pacing would be indicated in patients with fixed sinus or atrial bradycardia and pacemaker dependence, normal AV conduction, and intermittent supraventricular tachycardias responsive to competitive atrial stimulation. Indications for AAI or AAT pacing

would include the sick sinus syndrome with normal AV conduction and slow rate–induced escape tachycardias. Dual-chamber pacing is indicated in most patients with tachybradycardia arrhythmias, angina, and congestive heart failure. DVI pacing is now indicated for supraventricular arrhythmias with AV conduction disturbance, sensitive carotid sinus syndrome, bradycardias during drug therapy with continued need for beta-blockers, parasiticides, or other bradycardia-inducing drugs, atrial and ventricular ectopic rhythms, and re-entry tachyarrhythmias. For both atrial and dual-chamber pacing, a responsive atrium is required. Assuming unlimited availability of a reliable long-lived DDD device, it would be indicated in (1) all patients with atrioventricular block and evidence of sinus node dysfunction, as indicated by a sinus rate of less than 120 p.p.m. with maximal exercise, sinoatrial block on Holter monitoring, or abnormal sinus node recovery time, (2) all patients with sick sinus syndrome who show evidence of His-Purkinje dysfunction, including bifascicular block, prolonged HV interval greater than 55 msec. at atrial rates of 80 to 180 p.p.m., or Mobitz I block at atrial pacing rates greater than or equal to 140 p.p.m., and (3) carotid sinus syndrome with evidence of sinus node dysfunction (Sutton et al., 1980a). DDD pacing will not be applicable to patients with rapid atrial tachyarrhythmias, in whom programming "down" to the DVI mode will be safer.

The place of atrial pacing is still in question. It seems to be the logical approach in patients with supraventricular bradyarrhythmias and a normal atrioventricular conduction system. With careful preoperative and intraoperative evaluation and selection, a relatively low incidence of progression to complete heart block has been noted (Greenburg et al., 1978). However, because of the incidence of associated AV conduction disease, the pathologic overlap (see Table 49–12), the possibility of late development of AV block, and the ineffectiveness of atrial pacing in the presence of atrial fibrillation or flutter, some authorities are still skeptical (Furman, 1977a). Certainly, there should no longer be a "nonthinking," reflex implantation of a VVI pacemaker in every patient who is symptomatic from a bradyarrhythmia, and all implanted units should be multiprogrammable. It is probable that within 5 years only 20 per cent of implants will be ventricular pacemakers, 55 per cent will be automatic dual-chamber devices, and 25 per cent will be either ventricular or dual-chamber devices with a range of antitachycardia therapy modes.

OPERATIVE TECHNIQUES

Pacemaker implantation should always be performed in an operating room provided with a wide range of pacemakers and leads and an image intensifier. Both the transvenous and transthoracic procedures can be performed under local or general anesthesia, although in the majority of transvenous implantations the former is used, and in transthoracic procedures the latter is employed. With current intraoperative support and anesthetic techniques and the use of temporary pacing when needed, there is very little additional risk in performing transvenous implantation under general anesthesia. However, local 1 per cent Xylocaine infiltration is still recommended, because it allows for the performance of better provocative lead dislodgement maneuvers (e.g., coughing, deep breathing) and better assessment of the occurrence of pericardiac stimulation. Although implantation may on occasion have to be performed in an angiographic suite or a cardiac catheterization laboratory, these settings are associated with an increased wound infection rate. Regardless of the planned approach, the whole anterior chest from below the umbilicus to the tip of the chin and from bed to bed, including both axillae, should be disinfected and draped. This allows for conversion from one transvenous technique to another or even to a limited anterior thoracotomy without time-consuming interruption of the procedure for redraping. Even when a general anesthetic is not being used, an anesthesiologist should be involved on a standby basis because of the potential for lifethreatening cardiac dysrhythmias and the occasional need to convert to general anesthesia in the middle of the procedure.

During the implantation of more than 400 pacemakers between 1969 and 1978, alternate patients received prophylactic antibiotics beginning prior to surgery and continuing for 4 days. In addition, all wounds were thoroughly washed with a dilute bacitracin solution prior to closure to remove all loose tissue fragments, and drainage was never used. There were no early or late infections in either group of patients. Subsequently, antibiotic usage was discontinued for 2 years, and during that period, one patient returned 3 months following surgery with a draining sinus over the pacemaker that, when cultured, demonstrated *Staphylococcus epidermidis*. Because of the proven beneficial effects of properly timed prophylactic antibiotic administration with general cardiac and thoracic procedures (Ives *et al.*, 1981; Ronald, 1981), a therapeutic dose of an antistaphylococcal antibiotic is now given to all patients on call to the operating room and for 24 to 48 hours postoperatively. Wound treatment is unchanged. There have been no subsequent infections.

Regardless of the technique of pacemaker placement and the choice of supportive therapy, infection should be very uncommon, but when it occurs, early or late, it is essential to remove all foreign bodies, including the pacemaker and attached electrode, because of the tendency for bacteria to track down the electrode to cause endocarditis or pericarditis. The most common organisms infecting a pacemaker site in addition to *S. epidermidis* are *S. aureus*, streptococci, and *Escherichia coli*. Although there are reports in the literature of patients being placed on cardiopulmonary bypass to remove an entrapped, infected right ventricular lead, tourniquets can be placed around the

superior vena cava proximally and distally through a limited right anterior thoracotomy and the electrode removed with its attached infected material with relatively minimal trauma. Once the foreign body has been removed, the endocarditis almost always responds to antibiotic therapy.

The Pacemaker Pocket

Regardless of the method of lead placement, a site must be chosen for the pacemaker pocket. In general, the pacemaker is placed over the upper chest beneath the junction of the inner and middle thirds of the clavicle on the nondominant side. This is especially important in someone who uses a rifle. However, if the patient plays the violin or is a golfer, the pacemaker should be placed on the dominant side, as otherwise it may interfere with proper positioning of the violin or with the patient's backswing. Pacemaker erosion essentially never occurs (0 in more than 600 implants) if the pocket is made either deep to a muscle layer, usually the pectoralis major, or deep to the premuscular fascia so that the foreign body is covered with the full thickness of the skin and subcutaneous tissue. The pocket is always made long enough (Fig. 49–7) so that it can be closed off from the wound with a continuous absorbable suture layer after the implantation is completed in order to preclude intrusion of either the lead or the pulse generator against the subcutaneous or cutaneous closures. Whether placed from above during transvenous electrode implantation or from below during a limited thoracotomy, positioning of the pacemaker in the prefascial

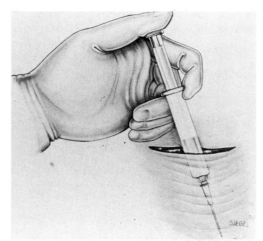

Figure 49–7. Pocket formation. The pocket should be as far medial as comfortable and only slightly larger than the pulse generator, so that the chance of migration (which tends to follow the curvature of the chest wall laterally) and rotation of the pacemaker is minimized. All bleeders must be carefully controlled to avoid postoperative hematoma formation, one cause of late pacemaker extrusion. The dissection plane should be either just superficial to the pectoralis major or beneath the muscle in very thin patients. Planes within the subcutaneous tissue lead to a high incidence of skin devascularization and pulse generator extrusion. (From Parsonnet, V.: Implantation of Transvenous Pacemakers. Tarpon Springs, Florida, Tampa Tracings, 1972.)

plane beneath the breast results in minor augmentation with present pacemaker sizes and a nearly undetectable pulse generator. Even in a baby, generators are now small and thin enough to be placed subpectorally, and there is no longer any need for the elaborate intrathoracic or intra-abdominal deep placement procedures used at one time. In addition, introducer techniques widen the applicability of transvenous electrode placement in children (Whitman *et al.*, 1978). The pocket is formed prior to lead placement, and an electrocautery is used to minimize hematoma formation. The pocket is packed during the remainder of the procedure to further reduce the risk of delayed bleeding.

Reported complications with either transvenous or transthoracic electrode placement are infection, erosion, lead fracture, threshold increases, and extraneous noncardiac stimulation. The mortality rate is slightly higher with the transthoracic approach (2 per cent versus 1 per cent), but there are essentially no lead displacement problems with the transthoracic technique, and stimulation of extraneous sites is more easily controlled (Tyers *et al.*, 1975). A small incidence of transvenously placed electrode dislodgement continues to occur for all operators.

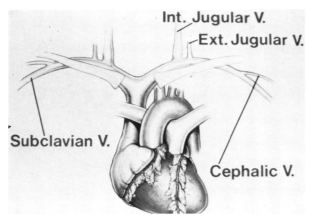

Figure 49–8. Anatomy for preferred venous approaches. Any vein in the neck, chest, or shoulder may be used for a permanent transvenous lead, but it is preferable to expose the vein through the same incision used for making the pocket. In order of preference, acceptable veins are as follows: (1) Cephalic vein, a tributary of the subclavian vein. It lies in the deltopectoral groove and is usually big enough to admit a lead up to 7 or 8 French. In 10 per cent of patients, it is quite delicate and may not be usable. It is occasionally absent. (2) Subclavian vein or tributary. If the cephalic vein cannot be used, it is always possible to expose another tributary of the subclavian or the subclavian vein itself through the same incision by freeing the pectoralis major from its lateral origin from the inferior surface of the clavicle. The subclavian vein is now commonly used as the primary choice for lead insertion with introducer techniques. (3) External jugular vein. This is usually the most prominent visible vein in the neck, although it may be absent in 10 per cent of patients. Because of the necessity of tunneling the electrode over or under the clavicle, with an increased incidence of fracture and erosion, this is a poor choice for permanent pacing. (4) Internal jugular vein. This is also a poor choice, except if there are purulent infections at every other potential site, or if an unusually large electrode is required as for an implantable defibrillator. (From Parsonnet, V.: Implantation of Transvenous Pacemakers. Tarpon Springs, Florida, Tampa Tracings, 1972.)

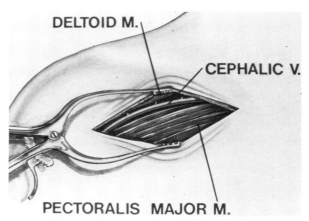

Figure 49–9. Cephalic vein approach. After making the incision below the clavicle, the deltopectoral groove is identified. The cephalic vein is usually found with ease in the fat pad that fills the groove. Division of a few fibers of the pectoralis major from the clavicle will allow dissection of the vein proximally, and if gentle traction is applied, the angle of entrance of the cephalic vein into the subclavian vein can be made more oblique. This facilitates passage of the electrode toward the heart rather than into the axilla. (From Parsonnet, V.: Implantation of Transvenous Pacemakers. Tarpon Springs, Florida, Tampa Tracings, 1972.)

Temporary Electrode Placement

Temporary electrodes should be placed with the same respect for sterility as used during permanent electrode placement. Brachial and subclavian transvenous approaches hasten mobilization, whereas the femoral approach is better for arrhythmia studies. Transthoracic temporary leads are usually placed following cardiac surgery for overdrive pacing of arrhythmias. Because of its detrimental hemodynamic effects, ventricular stimulation alone (versus atrial or AV sequential stimulation) should be avoided whenever the atrium is responsive. Most temporary transthoracic electrodes have a needle swaged on the end of an insulated wire with a small section exposed just proximal to the needle hub to form the electrode. The needle can be passed into either the atrial or ventricular myocardium, drawing the electrode behind it, but bleeding may ensue. A speedy and bloodless technique for atrial electrode placement involves rolling the atrial muscle around the electrode like a bun on a hot dog and clipping the muscle over the electrode with one or two Weck clips or a similar device.

Permanent Transvenous Electrode Placement

Permanent transvenous electrodes are used with over 90 per cent of permanent internal pacemaker implantations. Cephalic, subclavian, jugular, and inferior vena caval routes are used (and are mentioned here in order of preference) (Parsonnet, 1972). The anatomy of the preferred venous approaches to the heart is illustrated in Figure 49–8. The cephalic vein is approached through a small incision over the deltopectoral groove, and the vein is identified by dis-

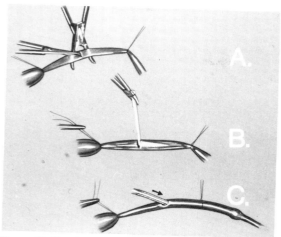

Figure 49–10. Small vein introduction technique. If the vein is large, insertion of an electrode can be performed simply by any standard method. When the vein is small, gentle handling and care will permit insertion of an electrode that at first may seem to be much larger than the vein. The vein is ligated distally, a loose, nonabsorbable suture is placed proximally, and a transverse incision is made one third of the way across the anterior wall of the vessel (*A*). A plastic inserter (present in the lead packages from many manufacturers) is carefully slipped into the opening (*B*). With upward traction on the inserter, which is concave on its inferior surface, the electrode can be passed underneath the inserter, which is not withdrawn until the tip of the electrode has passed medially a centimeter or so. As the electrode is advanced, the proximal ligature is loosened and then tightened to prevent bleeding. Countertraction on the distal ligature is maintained to assist passage into the subclavian vein (*C*). Traction on the distal ligature is easily maintained by pulling it over the self-retaining retractor shown in Figure 49–9 and placing a straight hemostat across it, with the tip of the hemostat underneath the ratchet of the retractor. (From Parsonnet, V.: Implantation of Transvenous Pacemakers. Tarpon Springs, Florida, Tampa Tracings, 1972.)

secting in the fatty and areolar tissue within the groove (Fig. 49–9). (The incision is, for the purpose of the illustration, larger than would usually be made.) Once the vein is identified, it is tied distally and snared proximally, and a small transverse incision is made, into which the electrode is introduced (Fig. 49–10). With a gentle, twisting motion and sometimes with partial withdrawal of the stylet, the electrode can usually be advanced into the superior vena cava in the 90 per cent of patients in whom an adequate cephalic vein is identified. Occasionally, the electrode

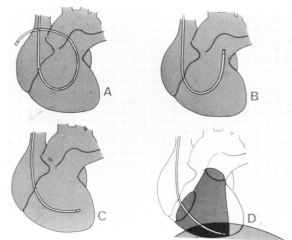

Figure 49–11. Right ventricular lead positioning technique. If the catheter is advanced into the pulmonary artery (*A*), which is easily confirmed by seeing the tip in the lung fields, there can be no question that on slow withdrawal of the electrode tip (*B*), it will fall into the ventricle (*C*), assuming the absence of ventricular septal defects. The shaded area in *D* reflects the approximate shape of the right ventricle. Note that the apex is far lateral and that the electrode usually lies below the dome of the left diaphragm as seen fluoroscopically. (From Parsonnet, V.: Implantation of Transvenous Pacemakers. Tarpon Springs, Florida, Tampa Tracings, 1972.)

will become hung up in a lateral thoracic vein, and the incision will have to be extended up along the vein to identify this point for direct steering of the electrode. At one time, the preferred technique for advancing the electrode from the right atrium into the right ventricle was to form a loop and to pass the loop across the tricuspid valve with the electrode subsequently pulled across backwards, as this avoided entering the coronary sinus and/or middle cardiac vein. However, the current tined electrodes tend to hang up on the tricuspid apparatus with this technique, and the preferred method now is to create a J in the guide wire, once the lead tip is in the right atrium, and steer the lead directly across the tricuspid valve. Position within the right ventricle is confirmed by running the electrode out through the pulmonary valve (Fig. 49–11*A*). Next, the curved guide wire is replaced with a straight wire. The electrode is then gradually withdrawn (Fig. 49–11*B,C*) until it flops down behind

Figure 49–12. Coronary sinus electrode. Incorrect position (unless intended) of the electrode tip in the coronary sinus is shown. On the anteroposterior projection, the electrode position appears a little high. The lateral view, however, will show that the electrode is far posterior, and the cardiogram will confirm the abnormal axis and right bundle branch block, or atrial pacing pattern (From Parsonnet, V.: Implantation of Transvenous Pacemakers. Tarpon Springs, Florida, Tampa Tracings, 1972.)

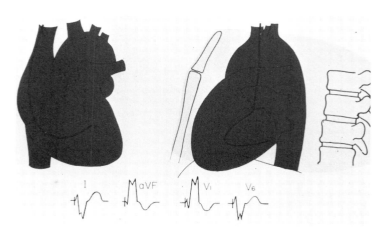

the apex of the left diaphragm, short of the apex of the heart (Fig. 49–11*D*). The guide wire may then be withdrawn a few millimeters, and the lead is gently maneuvered ahead to lodge it beneath the right ventricular trabeculae. Withdrawal of the guide wire is recommended to reduce the risk of perforation of the right ventricular myocardium, which, because of the overlapping structures, is difficult to recognize fluoroscopically. If the coronary sinus is inadvertently entered, the lead position will appear high on the posteroanterior view, as shown on the left in Figure 49–12, and will curve posteriorly rather than anteriorly in the lateral view, as shown on the right in Figure 49–12. If the lead lodges in the middle coronary vein, it will appear slightly lower on the posteroanterior view and almost straight down with a slightly forward distal direction terminally on the lateral view.

Optimal pacemaker pocket and electrode placement are shown in position 2 of Figure 49–13, where the electrode is gently looped and coiled beneath the generator to limit risk of damage at the time of pacemaker replacement. The generator should be placed medially to limit interference with shoulder motion and to reduce the risk of myopotential inhibition of unipolar devices. Position 1 of Figure 49–13 shows an electrode with multiple kinks, which increase the risk of fracture adjacent to the pulse generator.

An introducer technique has recently been popularized for rapid placement of single or multiple leads into the subclavian vein (Parsonett *et al.,* 1980b; Belott, 1981). An incision is made beneath the middle third of the clavicle and extended down to the prepectoral fascia. The pocket is formed first in the usual manner, with adequate administration of local anesthetic (see Fig. 49–7). The patient is positioned with the legs elevated to modestly increase venous pres-

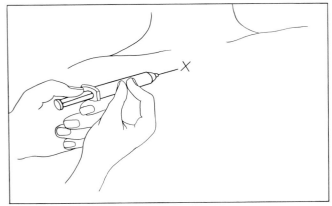

Figure 49–14. Venipuncture for introducer technique. An 18-gauge needle with an attached syringe is used. As soon as the needle tip penetrates the tissue, gentle suction is applied to the syringe. (From Belott, P. H.: A variation on the introducer technique for unlimited access to the subclavian vein. PACE, *4*:43, 1981.)

sure, because of the risk of air embolism. With an index finger marking the suprasternal notch, an 18-gauge needle is directed posteriorly and superiorly, between the clavicle and the first rib, aiming for a position just deep to and above the suprasternal notch. As the needle is advanced, suction is applied to an attached syringe using a one-handed technique. As the subclavian vein is entered, dark blood flows back into the syringe (Fig. 49–14). A guide wire with a J tip is then advanced through the needle under fluoroscopic control (Fig. 49–15), and when it is positioned in the superior vena cava, the needle is withdrawn. A sheath and dilator are then pushed forward over the

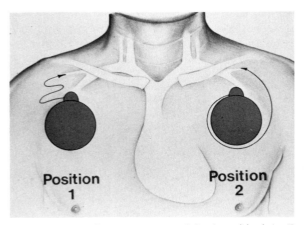

Figure 49–13. Correct pacer and lead positioning. Even though the electrode is placed properly in the heart, it may kink in the axilla and eventually fracture, as made more probable by position 1. The best position is one with a gentle lead curve, preferably behind the pacemaker, where it is not vulnerable to accidental damage during incision for pulse generator replacement and where it does not buckle during shoulder movements (position 2). (From Parsonnet, V.: Implantation of Transvenous Pacemakers. Tarpon Springs, Florida, Tampa Tracings, 1972.)

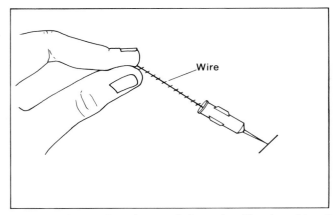

Figure 49–15. Introducer technique. A guide wire with a J tip is gently fed through the needle into the subclavian vein and superior vena cava under fluoroscopic control. Most needles supplied with the introducer kits are approximately 2 inches long, and a much greater portion of the needle usually exits from the wound than shown in the illustration because of the superficial nature of the subclavian vein. Occasionally, especially when there has been previous electrode placement and scarring has occurred in the subclavian vein, it may be necessary to place the needle, guide wire, and introducer into the innominate vein by starting the introduction above the clavicle with the needle directed inferiorly, posteriorly, and medially behind the manubrium. (From Belott, P. H.: A variation on the introducer technique for unlimited access to the subclavian vein. PACE, *4*:43, 1981.)

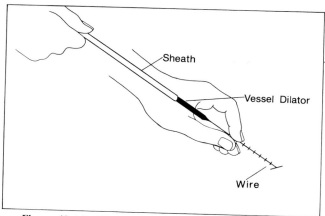

Figure 49–16. Placement of vessel dilator and sheath over the guide wire following removal of the needle. The sheath and dilator are inserted as one unit with quite forcible rotating motion. (From Belott, P. H.: A variation on the introducer technique for unlimited access to the subclavian vein. PACE, *4*:43, 1981.)

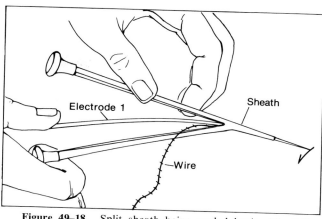

Figure 49–18. Split sheath being peeled back. All of the introducer sheaths are partially split so that they can easily be peeled off the electrode in two halves. (From Belott, P. H.: A variation on the introducer technique for unlimited access to the subclavian vein. PACE, *4*:43, 1981.)

guide wire into the superior vena cava with a rotational motion (Fig. 49–16). The vessel dilator is then removed with or without the guide wire, which may be left in place for subsequent adjacent introducer and lead insertions. Alternately, for dual-chamber pacing, two electrodes can be passed through a single large sheath, or two separate smaller sheaths can be placed through separate subclavian punctures. Bleeding and the risk of air embolism are minimized by holding a fingertip over the sheath, or compressing it, until the electrode, with stylet in place, is ready for insertion (Fig. 49–17).

Once position of the electrode in the superior

vena cava is confirmed by fluoroscopy, the sheath is withdrawn over the electrode, split, and removed (Fig. 49–18). If a dual-chamber procedure is planned, it is my preference to place the second guide wire a centimeter or so away from the first electrode, repeating the subclavian puncture technique, as this limits frictional and braiding interference between the two leads (Fig. 49–19). Ventricular lead placement is then accomplished in the previously described manner. If an atrial J lead has been inserted, pulling the guide wire back an inch or two will allow the electrode end of the lead to form a J, which is then bobbed up and down until it lodges in the right atrial appendage.

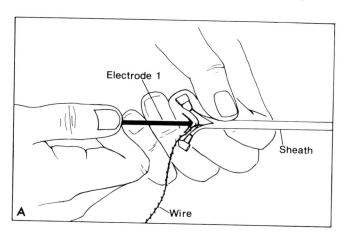

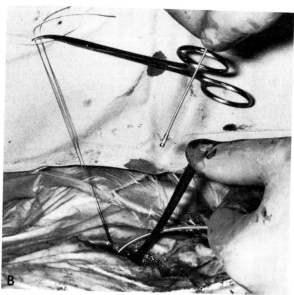

Figure 49–17. Dilator removed and lead ready for advancing. *A,* The electrode is about to be advanced into the sheath, with finger compression of the sheath to prevent bleeding or drawing in of air until the moment the lead is to be advanced. The guide wire is placed within the lead, and pressure is applied to it to prevent kinking of the lead as it is passed through the sheath. In this illustration, the guide wire has been left in place for passage of a subsequent sheath and introducer adjacent to the first lead, although both atrial and ventricular leads may be passed through one large introducer. *B,* An operative photograph shows a different type of sheath (rigid) in place, with bleeding prevented by the operator's thumb, and a ventricular tined lead ready for insertion. This is a two-introducer, dual-lead technique, with approximately a centimeter between the lead entrance sites to avoid friction and twining of the leads, which is especially likely to occur with the rotational motion sometimes required for atrial electrode placement. (*A,* From Belott, P. H.: A variation on the introducer technique for unlimited access to the subclavian vein. PACE, *4*:43, 1981.)

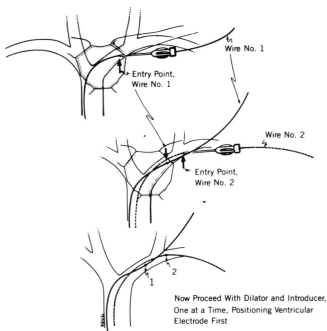

Figure 49–19. Two–entry point dual-lead introducer technique. Method for inserting separate guide wires, introducers, and sheaths with a small distance between the electrode entrance sites. (From Parsonnet V., *et al.:* Transvenous insertion of double set of permanent electrodes; atraumatic technique for atrial synchronous and atrial ventricular sequential pacemakers. J.A.M.A., *243*:62, 1980.)

Secure positioning is rewarded by a characteristic side-to-side bobbing motion of the electrode. Biplane fluoroscopy will confirm the correct anterior position (see Fig. 49–6*B*). If a coronary sinus atrial position is sought, the characteristic motion, rather than from side to side, is back and forth obliquely. If stable positioning of an atrial J lead cannot be obtained, with a J that does not flatten on deep inspiration or become overly redundant on full expiration and with good threshold and sensing signals, the lead of second choice is a Bisping-type, endocardial screw-in electrode, which is placed into the wall of the right atrium. With all of the transvenous techniques, and especially with the newer preferred segmented-polyurethane tined electrodes, very secure multiple ligatures must be placed at the fascial or venous exit site if slipping of the electrode either inward by spring action or outward by traction is to be avoided.

Potential complications of the subclavian puncture technique are air embolism, pneumothorax or hemothorax, and arterial or nerve puncture. If the vein cannot be punctured superficially, the needle should be checked for obstruction and a different angle tried. Serious problems are uncommon. The great advantage is the speed with which multiple leads can be placed in all patients not having superior vena caval obstructions.

If the two preceding techniques fail, part of the lateral portion of the clavicular head of the pectoralis major can be incised and retracted to expose the subclavian vein and its subscapular tributaries for direct lead placement through a purse-string or looping suture. With the preceding three techniques, it is rarely necessary to use an external jugular approach (incision above the clavicle over the lateral border of the sternocleidomastoid muscle), an internal jugular approach (deepening of the aforementioned incision and division of the omohyoid muscle), or an inferior vena caval approach (same incision as for a right lumbar sympathectomy or a vena caval clipping). An exception would be insertion of a very large electrode, as is required with the implantable defibrillator.

Permanent Transthoracic Electrode Placement

Less than 10 per cent of permanent pacemaker implantations are accomplished with electrodes attached directly to the atrial and/or ventricular myocardium. The left ventricle is the first choice for myocardial electrode placement because of decreased threshold energy requirements, increased sensing signals, increased cardiac output compared with right ventricular pacing, and technical safety compared with the thin-walled right ventricle (Tyers *et al.*, 1975). Electrodes should be placed near but not at the apex, because in many patients this area is very thin. Stimulation sites toward the base of the heart should be avoided, because they cause early contraction of the outflow tract and decrease cardiac output.

Chest incisions utilized have included median sternotomy, left parasternal vertical incision, limited right and left anterior fourth or fifth intercostal space thoracotomies, left transaxial thoracotomy, and routine left posterolateral thoracotomy. Nonthoracic approaches have included upper abdominal midline and left subcostal incisions. The midline abdominal incision involves division of the aponeurosis between the rectus muscles, resection of the xiphoid process, and separation of the diaphragm from the chest wall anteriorly and in the midline. This portion of the incision is enlarged and retracted to expose the diaphragmatic surface of the right ventricle. With a left subcostal approach (Bhattacharya *et al.*, 1972), the left rectus is transected and essentially the same approach to the heart is taken, although it may be possible to place the electrodes on the left ventricle. These abdominal incisions provide poor exposure (Fig. 49–20) should bleeding or another complication occur and are not recommended for first consideration. The incision of choice for myocardial lead placement is a limited anterolateral one (Fig. 49–21) or a parasternal one (Fig. 49–22), as either brings the surgeon down on the generally bare anterolateral left ventricular myocardial wall without the necessity of opening the left pleural space (Reed *et al.*, 1969; Garcia and Bengochea, 1972). With a little larger incision, intrapericardial access to the left atrial appendage is provided.

The pericardium is opened well in front of the phrenic nerve, both to avoid injury to the nerve and to facilitate electrode placement in a site that will not later result in phrenic nerve or diaphragmatic stimulation. The intramyocardial, screw-in, sutureless elec-

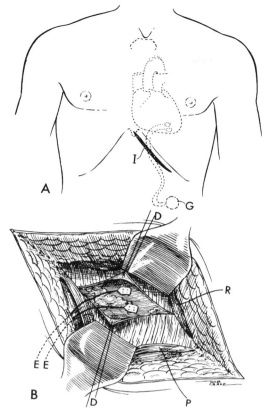

Figure 49–20. Left subcostal approach. *A*, Site of incision (I) for transdiaphragmatic approach (G = pacemaker). *B*, Exposure of undersurface of the right ventricle for intramyocardial pacing. (D = diaphragm; EE = pacing electrodes; P = peritoneum; R = rectus muscle). (From Bhattacharya, S. K., *et al.*: A method of epicardial pacing without thoracotomy: Treatment of heart block in patients with tricuspid valve prosthesis. Chest, *62*:112, 1972.)

trodes, available from several manufacturers, are associated with an increased incidence of electrode fracture and the development of high threshold energy requirements for pacing and are not recommended. The preferred currently available lead for direct intramyocardial placement is the Telectronics 030-170, which utilizes a suture with a swaged needle coming directly out of the bare end of the conducting helical coil. The electrode can be placed at any angle and any depth within either the atrial or the ventricular myocardium to reduce angulation- and contraction-induced trauma. It can be placed through an incision at least as small as required for placement of the screw-in electrode, with greater versatility and with less risk. Once the suture is pulled through the myocardium, a metallic clip is applied to it, completing a very simple procedure. A single fixing suture may be placed through an expansion just proximal to the electrode, if desired. The major disadvantage of this electrode is its large surface area (55 mm.², 200 ohms), which will reduce pacemaker generator life. A final technique involves placement of a posterior left atrial electrode through a mediastinoscope (Lagergren, 1966). This was not very effective previously, but with the advent of dual-chamber pacing, it may deserve reinvestigation using intramyocardial modifications of

the Bisping-type screw-in or Coratomic Endo-loc grasping electrodes.

Should pacemaker replacement be required, it is preferable to open the previous incision, unless the generator has migrated severely. Great care must be taken to avoid injury to the electrode, although with the Cordis lead repair kit a new connector can be securely attached to any of the helical coil electrodes within 1 or 2 minutes. Should the electrode be firmly held in the connector block of a pacemaker to be replaced, it is preferable to drill the back of the block and push the lead out rather than to pull on the lead with excessive force and damage it (O'Neill and Tyers, 1975).

Intraoperative and Postoperative Testing

Complete testing of threshold energy requirements, atrial and ventricular endocardial signals, pacemaker parameters, and physiologic-pacemaker interaction should be performed at every procedure, whether a new implant or a replacement (Calvin, 1978; Kleinert *et al.*, 1979; Parsonnet *et al.*, 1980a; Venkataraman and Bilitch, 1979). High-voltage settings are used to detect diaphragmatic or phrenic nerve stimulation requiring lead repositioning. Deep breathing and coughing procedures are performed to attempt to produce electrode dislodgement, which is preferable to having to return the patient to the operating room for lead repositioning during the early postoperative period. The pulse width and rate at which the threshold tests are performed must always be recorded. Pulse width, in particular, is a determinant of stimulus energy, and without knowing it, current and voltage measurements are meaningless. Similarly, both threshold current and voltage must be recorded to verify stimulation (electrode + electrode tissue interface) impedance (Tyers *et al.*, 1979). With a pulse width of 0.5 msec. (the nominal range of most current pacemakers), a threshold voltage of 0.5 or less should be obtained. The current will, of course, depend on the impedance of the electrode tissue system and, with small–surface-area electrodes (impedances approximating 1000 ohms), will also be 0.5 milliamperes or less, but with electrodes with surface areas in the range of 12 to 20 mm.², with stimulation impedances of about 500 ohms, satisfactory threshold current will be about 1 milliampere. Occasionally, even with multiple repositionings, higher energy requirements cannot be avoided. In addition, most patients go through a period of chronically higher energy requirements for capture over a period of weeks or months following electrode placement before thresholds return to values just greater than those determined acutely. It is believed that these threshold rises are caused by the maturing of scar tissue around the electrode tip. Contamination of the electrode with glove powder should be avoided.

The size of the endocardial signal recorded will depend on whether the electrode is attached to the atrium or the ventricle, on the electrode's surface

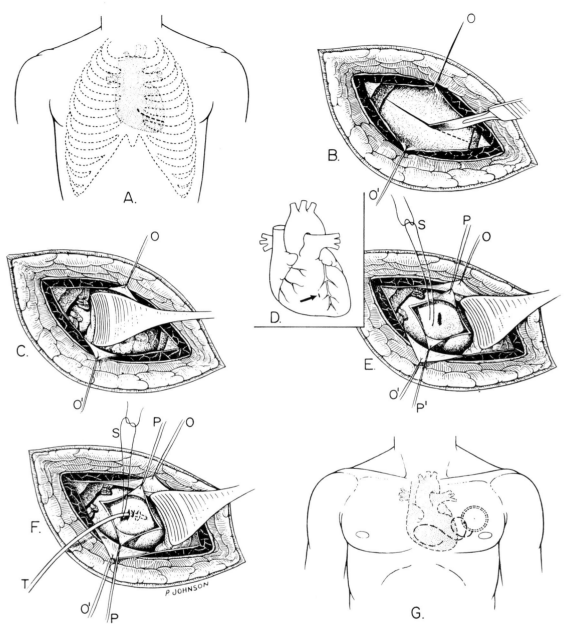

Figure 49–21. Limited thoracotomy approach. *A,* The heavy broken line indicates the site of the skin incision, beginning over the sternum and centered over the lowest costal cartilage that articulates freely with the sternum. *B,* The cartilage has been resected from the sternum to the costochondral junction. The perichondrium is being incised posteriorly. O and O′ are sutures placed in the perichondrium anteriorly. *C,* The internal mammary artery and vein have been ligated and divided. Beginning medially, the propericardial tissue (fat, sometimes pleura) is being reflected laterally in the plane of the fibrous pericardium. *D,* The arrow points to a right ventricular electrode site just to the right side of the left anterior descending coronary artery. A left ventricular site lateral to the anterior descending coronary artery is preferred. *E,* The pericardium (P and P′) has been opened. A heavy suture (S) has been placed in the myocardium just to the right of the entrance point chosen for the electrode. *F,* A standard transvenous lead can be passed into a myocardial tunnel, in a manner similar to performing a Vineburg technique, as shown, or a Telectronics Model 030–170 Intramyocardial Electrode can be drawn into the myocardium with the attached distal suture and swaged on needle, as described in the text. The Telectronics electrode has a small tension-reducing expansion, with two holes for passage of a suture just proximal to the myocardial entrance site. *G,* A large, gentle loop of electrode has been formed within the pericardial space, and the hub of the electrode is drawn out through the intercostal space once or twice removed from the incision. The pulse generator is placed in a prepectoral or subpectoral pocket, which is prepared at the time of performance of the minithoracotomy. (From Reed, G. F., *et al.:* A new technique for pacemaker implantation: Extrapleural, intramyocardial. J. Thorac. Cardiovasc. Surg., *57*:507, 1969.)

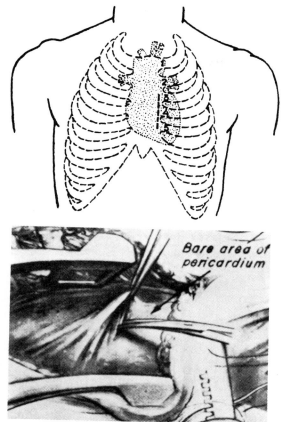

Figure 49–22. Parasternotomy. The heavy broken line indicates the left parasternal incision site over the fourth, fifth, and sixth left costal cartilages, which are divided as close as possible to the sternal junction. The intercostal muscles are divided at the sternal border, and the left internal mammary vessels and adjacent pleura are freed from pericardial adhesions and retracted laterally. It may be necessary in some cases to excise approximately an inch of the cartilages. Finally, the pericardium is opened longitudinally, and the pacemaker electrodes are inserted directly onto the right ventricular wall. This approach does not give good exposure to the more laterally placed left ventricle. (From Garcia, J. B., and Bengochea, J. B.: Extrapleural implantation of epicardial leads under local anesthesia. J. Cardiovasc. Surg., 63:144, 1972.)

that a diagnosis of early or late sensing made from the surface ECG is inappropriate. New intraoperative testing equipment allows the endocardial signal to be run through the pacemaker and into the analyzer, which will determine the safety margin for the particular pacemaker-patient combination being tested (Intermedics CompuPace). Finally, the pacemaker should be completely checked, including rate, interval, pulse width, voltage, current, sensitivity, refractory period, and AV interval, if applicable. Even with complete checking following manufacture, the occasional pacemaker will go out of specification during delivery and storage, and implantation of such a unit should be avoided.

Compared with the knowledge of technical details now required, the operative techniques and intraoperative testing are relatively simple. However, early postoperative technical and equipment-related problems are not unknown. Lead position by posteroanterior and lateral chest radiographs, pacemaker capture and sensing by electrocardiographic monitoring, and pacemaker functional parameters (i.e., pulse width, intervals, power cell voltage, and so on) should be checked as frequently as indicated. P waves to confirm atrial capture are usually best seen on the V1 and V2 leads, and atrial sensing is best confirmed by programming to AAT. Pacemaker procedures, especially pacemaker generator replacement, may be performed on an outpatient basis; however, monitoring for several days may be indicated in pacemaker-dependent patients with new implants.

COMPLICATIONS, MONITORING, AND FOLLOW-UP PROGRAMS FOR PACEMAKER PATIENTS

The patient and the pacemaker system (stimulator and electrode) and their interaction require periodic testing to detect subclinical but potentially serious malfunctions and to follow trends that allow prediction of approaching end of battery life. Reasons for removal of 188 lithium cell–powered pacemakers out of 14,000 being followed are listed in Table 49–14. Transvenous electrode problems have not been significantly increased in patients with corrected transposition, although this would have been expected because of the decreased trabeculation of the embryologic left ventricle. Wound complications can occur, as with any operation, and risk of infection increases with the number of repeated operations at the same site. Infected hardware should always be removed because of the potential for bacteria to track down the lead system to the heart. Perforation or distortion of the tricuspid valve by a transvenous lead can occur, but serious tricuspid regurgitation is rare. Adherence to the chordae or valve leaflets can, however, occasionally lead to severe insufficiency following lead removal. Both the tricuspid and mitral valves (via a patent foramen or septal defect) have been injured. Cardiac perforation by a transvenous lead prob-

area, on polarity, and on circuit design parameters (Kleinert *et al.,* 1979; Parsonnet *et al.,* 1980a; Hughes *et al.,* 1980; Brownlee *et al.,* 1976). Endocardial P-wave equivalents may be 3 millivolts or less, whereas ventricular endocardial electrograms are generally in the range of 5 to 6 millivolts or greater. Apart from the absolute size, the slew rate, or rate of rise of the endocardial signal, is also important, because a tall wave, with a very gradual slope may be more difficult for the sensing amplifier to recognize than a smaller signal with a sharp upstroke. In addition to the slew rate, the overall shape of the electrogram is important, as pacemaker sensing circuits may only recognize signals that are monophasic. Thirty per cent of acute ventricular electrograms are monophasic downward (negative), 58 per cent are biphasic, and 12 per cent are monophasic upward (positive). The surface ECG may be earlier or later than the endocardiogram, so

TABLE 49–14. EXPLANTATION OF LITHIUM CELL–POWERED PACEMAKER SYSTEMS*

REASON FOR REMOVAL	NUMBER REMOVED	PERCENTAGE OF TOTAL REMOVALS
Erratic rate change	10	5.31
Loss of sensing	12	6.38
Loss of sensing and capture	17	9.04
Recall, patient is pacer-controlled	6	3.19
Erosion	18	9.57
Rate decline	19	10.10
Loss of capture	23	12.23
Broken electrode	11	5.85
High pacer rate	3	1.59
No evidence of pacer activity	17	9.04
Component failure	9	4.78
Elective removal	5	2.65
Infection	22	11.70
Unknown	11	5.85
Skeletal muscle twitch	2	1.06
Threshold changes	2	1.06
Rate decline and loss of capture	1	0.53
Total	188	

*From Tyers, G. F. O., and Brownlee, R. R.: Power pulse generators, electrodes and longevity. Prog. Cardiovasc. Dis., *23*: 421, 1981.

ably occurs not uncommonly, but tamponade, hemopericardium, and/or loss of pacing or sensing are very uncommon during either early or late follow-up. Thrombosis and/or fibrosis of veins containing a transvenous electrode occur not uncommonly with silicone rubber insulated electrodes (Williams *et al.*, 1978). The right atrial appendage is a common site for thrombus formation in patients with a low cardiac output and, as with a right ventricular thrombus (most commonly at the apex), may frustrate the achievement of low threshold energy requirements by preventing close apposition of an electrode and the endocardium. Subclavian vein thrombosis, the superior vena caval syndrome, and pulmonary embolism occur but produce clinically recognizable problems very infrequently. Misdiagnosis of a complication, when none has occurred, is now a common problem related to circuit complexities (committed versus noncommitted DVI pacers), natural variations in timing of contractile complex appearance on the surface ECG versus the endocardial electrogram, poor quality of telemetry and ECG monitoring and recording equipment and failure to examine multiple ECG leads, pseudofusion, pseudo-pseudofusion, and loss of sensing due to the pacer functioning normally in the presence of interference (electromagnetic interference, myopotentials).

Pacemaker Follow-up

Better power sources, improved electronics, and hermetic encapsulation now make 10-year pacemakers a probability. Although problems with electromagnetic interference suppression, phantom programming, and fluid entry are much less common than previously, it has been emphasized that this does not imply that pacemaker follow-up is no longer important (Parsonnet, 1977). Random electrode and electronic component malfunctions continue. Premature failure of most current power cells is uncommon but does occur (Welti, 1981b), and all primary power sources will eventually exhaust their energy supplies. Prophylactic replacement at a fixed, supposedly safe interval has been commonly practiced as a safe alternative to regular follow-up, but it is not recommended. Compared with premature replacement of an earlier epoxy-potted mercury-zinc battery–powered pacemaker, which might have cost the patient a few months of operation-free life, too early prophylactic replacement of a lithium- or nuclear-powered generator after a fixed interval may waste years of functional pacemaker life and thousands of dollars for unnecessary hospitalization or, at the other extreme, may be preceded by pacemaker failure in high-output applications. Pacemaker follow-up should maximize patient safety and confidence and reduce health care costs (Furman, 1977b; Pennock *et al.*, 1972). Both aims require more accurate follow-up over long periods with the improved pacemakers now available from all manufacturers.

Patients with pacemakers have generally been followed (1) by regular visits to follow-up physicians' offices or clinics, (2) by pacemaker stimulus variable trends, (3) by transtelephonic monitoring, and (4) by special electronic techniques. Stimulus variables followed include rate, interval, pulse width, and pulse amplitude. The rate of some early pacemakers increased as battery voltage decreased. The upward rate trend signaled the end of pacemaker battery life but occasionally led to dangerously rapid rates—pacemaker runaway. Voltage-dependent circuits were then designed to slow just before end of power-cell life. Stimulus amplitude also decreases as the power cell depletes, and some circuits cause the pulse width to widen as battery energy is used, increasing the rate of voltage decline but providing a secondary indication of approaching end of life. This is an inefficient end-of-life indicator in a multiprogrammable pacemaker. Most mercury-zinc–powered pacemakers of the pre-lithium era still had a few weeks of effective life left when the rate had slowed 5 to 8 p.p.m., for example, from 70 to 65 p.p.m., allowing end-of-life prediction and elective pacemaker replacement in a high percentage of patients by weekly monitoring. However, no standard rate decrease indicator was ever accepted, and apart from unit-to-unit variations in a given manufacturing series, whole pacemaker series have had rate drift upward and downward before end of life (Tyers and Brownlee, 1976a). The introduction of rate-programmable pacemakers plus occasional phantom programming has further reduced the value of rate change for following battery voltage indirectly and predicting end of life (Brownlee *et al.*, 1977; Furman and Fisher, 1977). The interval between pacemaker spikes is also used to express rate; for example, a rate of 60 is equal to a 1000-msec. interval. Rate changes may be followed by the patient and/or the physician (1) by checking the radial pulse; (2) with an

TABLE 49–15. PROPOSED TRANSTELEPHONIC MONITORING SCHEDULES FOR LITHIUM (LI)- AND MERCURY-ZINC (Hg-Zn)–POWERED PACING SYSTEMS†

Power Source	Risk Level*	Every 8 Weeks	Every 4 Weeks	Every 2 Weeks	Weekly
LI	0.5%	Months 3–17	Months 18–23	Month 24	—
Hg-Zn	0.5%	Months 3–6	Months 7–15	Months 16–19	After month 20
LI	1%	Months 3–23	Month 24	—	—
Hg-Zn	1%	Months 3–15	Months 16–19	Months 20–23	After month 24

*Risk level reduces further with increased monitoring frequency. As several lithium systems have shown failure earlier than anticipated (Welti, 1981b), more frequent early monitoring is warranted.

†From Tyers, G. F. O., and Brownlee, R. R.: Power pulse generators, electrodes and longevity. Prog. Cardiovasc. Dis., *23*:421, 1981.

inexpensive transistor radio that ticks in sequence with the pacemaker when placed near to it, or with an electronically similar device with digital readouts for rate, interval, AV interval, and pulse width, (3) with an electrocardiogram that confirms the relationship of the pacer spike to cardiac depolarization, (4) with an oscilloscope that also allows for accurate determination of pulse amplitude within the limitations of varying body impedances, and (5) with an electronic digital or other physiologic pulse detector. Inaccuracies often arise with the first two techniques from observer error and from the frequent occurrence of spontaneous rhythms faster than the preset demand pacemaker rate. Placing a magnet over most demand pacemakers closes a reed switch, disabling the sensing circuit, resulting in asynchronous pacing, which allows stimulation rate to be measured. In spite of the occasional malfunction of reed switches, which has already been discussed, their continued use in this noncritical area is at this time universal.

Follow-up visits to a physician's office or a pacemaker clinic are begun shortly after discharge following pacemaker implantation. The patient should have the wound checked, and depending on the perceived need for interventions such as programming, additional office or pacemaker clinic visits are scheduled at one- to six-month intervals initially, with the potential for less frequent visits as conditions stabilize and transtelephonic monitoring is established. Oscilloscopic stimulus wave-form analysis is best performed at a pacemaker clinic but has limitations (Furman, 1977b).

Transtelephonic monitoring can be performed from as close as the patient's home in the same city or from as far away as any international location with a telephone. The pacer stimulus, the patient's digital pulse, and the electrocardiogram can all be changed into audible signals and transmitted via telephone. The electrocardiographic-based system confirms capture, sensing, and arrhythmias, but only the pulse detection methods that transmit a digital pulse, if present, after each pacemaker spike, can assure that the electric activity is accompanied by adequate tissue flow (Pennock *et al.,* 1972). Recommended follow-up guidelines, depending on implant age and power source type, are shown in Table 49–15 (Tyers and Brownlee, 1981). The 0.5 and 1 per cent levels indicate the risk of unpredicted failure of each patient's pacemaker between follow-up measurements, resulting in

the need for emergency replacement as well as the potential for patient injury and death.

Follow-up techniques that provide additional data have been developed. Edwards Pacemakers Systems had a rate tracking circuit that confirmed sensing function of a demand pacemaker with a subliminal triggered pulse. Vitatron, Siemens, and Medtronic, Inc. provide some units with a physician-activated stepwise output reduction method for measurement of capture threshold, and Pacemaker Diagnostic Clinic of America developed a method of transtelephonic wave-form analysis. However, employing only physiologic rates (1 to 2 hertz—a hertz is a cycle per second) to transmit data severely limits the pacemaker functions that can be noninvasively assessed. Telemetry is a common engineering technique, and a pacemaker telemetry system that employs a simple, high-frequency, AM/FM transmitter within the pacemaker, to send data about the pacemakers's power source, electronics, and hermetic integrity has been developed (Brownlee *et al.,* 1977).

Telemetry covers a variety of techniques employed to remotely monitor the functioning of devices or processes. The best-publicized biotelemetry systems have been employed for long-distance monitoring of the physiologic condition of astronauts during space flight. However, radiotelemetry is not new to the medical or pacemaker field. Remote monitoring of ambulatory electrocardiograms is commonplace in intermediate care, and the stimulation output of all pacemakers generates a radiofrequency signal that can be received transcutaneously on an inexpensive transistor radio to confirm pacemaker output and rate. The development, testing, and refinement of an independent multiparameter data surveillance transmitter for inclusion within all pacemaker implants have been accomplished (Tyers and Brownlee, 1979). With this system, follow-up data can be recorded in the physician's office or in a pacemaker clinic or transmitted by telephone locally or internationally, just as with standard transtelephonic pacemaker follow-up. Initial lithium-powered pacemakers (Intermedics 221-T) transmitted cell voltage and stimulation rate and confirmed hermetic integrity of the encapsulation. In subsequent pacemakers, with implants now numbering several thousand, the additional parameters of electrode impedance, cell impedance, and refractory interval were added (Intermedics 223–04 and Cyberliths). Cell voltage can be determined directly, by

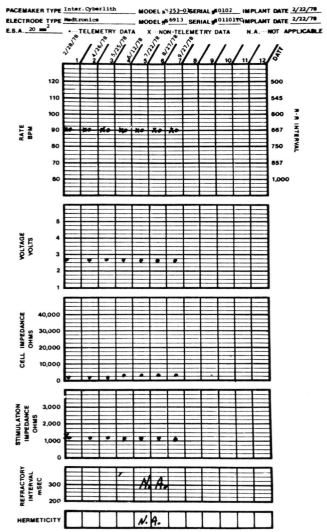

Figure 49–23. Multiparameter telemetry follow-up data illustrating the linear rise in cell impedance, with minimal voltage decline, in a lithium iodine cell-powered pacer. End of life of lithium iodine units is best predicted by sequential monitoring of cell impedance, as currently used by Intermedics, Vitatron, and Pacesetter. (From Tyers, G. F. O., and Brownlee, R. R.: Power pulse generators, electrodes, and longevity. Prog. Cardiovasc. Dis., 23:421, 1981.)

reading a metered device placed near the skin over any of these implanted pacemakers. Impedance determinations require use of an Ohm's law nomogram and are performed without charge through Intermedics Trace-A-Pace, a commercial follow-up service. Multiparameter follow-up data from a typical telemetry pacemaker are shown in Figure 49–23. Nontelemetry rate data from the electrocardiogram and stimulation impedance data determined at the time of implantation are indicated by X's to confirm reliability of the telemetry transmitter.

A digital system for in-office determination of power-cell impedance, electrode impedance, and battery current drain as well as programmed settings was subsequently introduced (all Pacesetter Programalith models). Because of the digital readout of the data,

this system is easier to use for in-office follow-up. However, it does not permit transtelephonic follow-up. More recently, a 15-parameter digital system was introduced (Intermedics Quantum series) and is currently being evaluated. It includes provision for in-office or clinic plus transtelephonic determination of all programmed settings, all pacemaker performance indices, and a variety of follow-up data, including cell voltage. Cell voltage, which is not transmitted by the Programalith series, will again be a very important follow-up parameter with the newer, lower-impedance power cells being developed (see the section on pacemaker technology).

An ideal pacemaker follow-up program should minimize emergency pacemaker replacements, maximize safe pacemaker implant duration, reassure both the patient and physician, and reduce medical care costs. The original follow-up method of prophylactic replacement at an average 80 per cent power source utilization time achieved none of these aims. Second-generation pacemaker follow-up, including regular monitoring of rate change, which was made a function of battery voltage, has also proved to be limited. In a primary mercury-zinc battery–powered pacemaker, with a sudden drop of voltage when one cell failed, rate change was a relatively satisfactory late warning system, although it provided no assessment of remaining capacity until just prior to end of pacemaker life, when only a few weeks of function remained. A further limitation to simple, indirect, rate-change monitoring of cell voltage has arisen with the advent of the lithium-iodine, single-cell power sources now used in the majority of pacemakers. With these cells, there may be no sudden drop in voltage but rather a very gradual decline with a terminal "knee," the slope of which depends on many factors. It has also become increasingly difficult to arbitrarily predict end of life when current drain is related to and modified by not only electronics and design, but also multiple lead factors, including electrode surface area, and m ultiple programmable factors, including mode, rate, and pulse width. In the same unit, the current drain may be higher by a factor of 10 in a pacemaker programmed to the AV sequential mode, a wide pulse width, and a high rate, versus standard rate, asynchronous, narrow pulse width pacing. Further complexities are added by the inclusion of a number of physicians in the follow-up process and the potential for lack of accurate recording of programmed parameters. The relative simplicity of a multiparameter telemetric, follow-up system, which gives accurate information on all programmed parameters, as well as an array of useful pacemaker and physiologic data, is illustrated by the complexity of end-of-life rate change and interval follow-up of one programmable DVI pacer (Table 49–16).

The choice of some of the follow-up parameters requires elaboration. The resistance within presently used lithium cells rises gradually throughout useful life. Initial and end-of-life impedances are known for all lithium-iodine configurations. Noninvasive transmission of power-cell impedance data allows both

TABLE 49–16. TIMING INTERVALS[1] OF MEDTRONIC MODEL 5992 BYREL PULSE GENERATOR

PROGRAM MODE	INITIAL PARAMETERS								RECOMMENDED REPLACEMENT POINT							
	Without Magnet				With Magnet				Without Magnet				With Magnet			
	VA[2]	AV[3]	VV[4]	Rate[5]	VA	AV	VV	Rate	VA	AV	VV	Rate	VA	AV	VV	Rate
VVI	–	–	850	70.6	–	–	765	78.4	–	–	918	65.4	–	–	826	72.6
DVI	700	250	950	63.2	700	155	855	70.2	700	326	1026	58.5	700	223	923	65.0
DVI	700	150	850	70.6	700	65	765	78.4	700	218	918	65.4	700	126	826	72.6
DVI	600	250	850	70.6	600	165	765	78.4	600	318	918	65.4	600	226	826	72.6
DVI	600	150	750	80.0	600	75	675	88.9	600	210	810	70.1	600	129	729	82.3
DVI	500	250	750	80.0	500	175	675	88.9	500	310	810	70.1	500	229	729	82.3
DVI	500	150	650	92.3	500	85	585	102.6	500	202	702	85.5	500	132	632	94.9
DVI	425	125	550	109.1	425	70	495	121.2	425	169	594	101.0	425	110	535	112.0

[1]VA, AV, and VV intervals may vary by tolerances given in the specifications on the first page of manual.*
[2]VA = time measured from ventricular pacing artifact or sensed QRS to atrial pacing artifact.
[3]AV = time measured from atrial pacing artifact to ventricular pacing artifact.
[4]VV = time measured from ventricular pacing artifact or sensed QRS to ventricular pacing artifact.
[5]In DVI modes, programmed rate values apply only when both chambers are stimulated.
*Technical Manual for Model 5992 AV Sequential, Ventricular-Inhibited (DVI), Medtronic, Inc., 1979.

prediction of end of life and also a fairly accurate prediction of remaining capacity at any time during the pacemaker implant. Monitoring of lithium-cell impedance is analogous to the function of a fuel gauge in a motor vehicle (Fig. 49–24). Electrode stimulation impedance may range from as little as 200 ohms to as much as 3000 ohms with the available electrode surface areas and designs that were discussed in the section on pacemaker technology. Knowing the normal range of and previous impedances for a given implant, a dramatic drop in stimulation impedance signals the loss of insulation integrity of the connector or electrode, whereas a dramatic rise indicates fracture of the conductor. For example, the combination of pectoral muscle stimulation and low stimulation impedance immediately following pacemaker implantation confirms either a poor seal at the connector, loss of the set screw covering cap, or a break in the lead insulation. Monitoring of hermetic integrity of the pacemaker capsule is important, because even with current encapsulation technology, random failures may occur. This could lead to a costly and unnecessary recall of all units in a related manufacturing series. A variety of techniques are being assessed for noninvasive follow-up of humidity levels within biologic implants, as knowledge of a stable internal humidity would confirm hermetic integrity. Transmission of the precise duration of the refractory interval for the particular pacemaker implanted allows assessment of the potential causes of oversensing and undersensing.

Follow-up of the first telemetry pacemakers, which transmit signals for cell voltage, pulse rate, and hermetic integrity, continues after 8 years. Reasonable accuracy of all systems has been confirmed. Newer commercial systems (Intermedics 223–04, Cyberlith, and Quantum series and Pacesetter Programalith series) have been implanted in several thousand patients. The slow decline in cell voltage and the progressive rise in cell impedance with time have been confirmed. Electrode impedance transmitted by the telemetry system has ranged from 3000 to 200 ohms, verifying within narrow limits the impedances determined at pacemaker implantation and removal with the varying electrode surface areas and designs used.

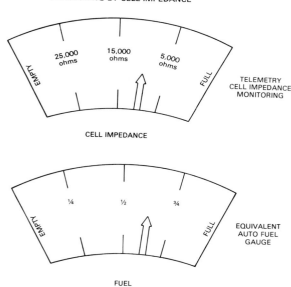

Figure 49–24. Comparision of telemetry monitoring of implanted lithium iodine power cell impedance (above) to a standard auto fuel gauge (below). With cell-impedance monitoring, the physician performing the follow-up examination can determine, within 10 per cent, the relative capacity remaining in the power source at any time during its implantation life. In contrast, rate-change monitoring, with all its limitations, only attempts to indicate end of life by indirectly monitoring battery voltage. (From Tyers, G. F. O., and Brownlee, R. R.: A multiparameter telemetry system for cardiac pacemakers. In Cardiac Pacing, A Concise Guide to Clinical Practice. Edited by P. Varriale and E. A. Naclerio. Philadelphia, Lea and Febiger, 1979, pp. 349–368.)

The Quantum telemetry series allows for the noninvasive determination and follow-up of all programmed settings, as well as the actual values of stimulation rate, interval, pulse width, amplitude, and output current and power cell voltage, current drain, and impedance. Because of changes with time and circuit variations, output parameters are not necessarily the same as those programmed, and the need to be able to determine not only intended settings but actual performance is critical. Most major pacemaker manufacturers are now working on telemetry follow-up systems. Multiparameter, noninvasive, detailed, biologic and electronic assessment is on the threshold of widespread clinical implementation. An optimal system should be capable of interrogation in an office or transtelephonically from anywhere in the world. Electrocardiogram, endocardial electrogram, and blood chemistry values are in the process of being added to implantable transmitters, and online PO_2 determination using platinum electrodes, for true physiologic pacemaker self-adjustment, is now a possibility. A new era of patient monitoring management that is precise, as well as convenient and noninvasive, is within current capacity.

Each previous advance (e.g., improved electrodes, improved power sources, hermetic sealing, transtelephonic follow-up and multiprogrammability) has proved to be cost-effective (Lopman et al., 1980; Tyers et al., 1981; Pennock et al., 1972) both by decreasing rehospitalization, reoperation, and follow-up costs and by markedly reducing the number of implantable pacemakers each patient requires during his lifetime. A less-expensive pacemaker that must be replaced more frequently provides poor-quality care at increased cost, especially as the 50 per cent survival point for pacemaker patients now approaches 8 years. On the other hand, reuse of presently available, high technology, high individual unit cost pacing devices that have been implanted for only a short time would save health care resources with no decrease in the quality of patient care (Zipes, 1981). Telemetry systems allowing noninvasive evaluation of multiple parameters will facilitate pacemaker reuse, especially with direct assessment of remaining power-cell capacity through impedance monitoring. Although implantable devices will continue to entail substantial unit costs, it is probable that physiologic and antiarrhythmia pacing will also reduce overall cost per patient by reducing the need for frequent medical care and hospitalization.

Pacemaker Performance Statistics

A final problem relates to the physician's understanding or misunderstanding of the usual pacemaker performance statistics supplied by the manufacturers to support their reliability claims. Although not always justified, a degree of skepticism is not unreasonable. Each manufacturer's collection of its own data is a situation that is the converse of a double-blind study (Welti, 1980). Commonly used reports include (1)

random failure rate, (2) mean time implanted, (3) mean time between failures, (4) failure rate curves, (5) cumulative survival curves (see Fig. 49–1), and (6) performance index.

Random failure rates are recorded as the percentage of monthly failures. The total number of failures divided by the total number of months all devices have been implanted is multiplied by 100. As an example, if 35,000 pacemakers had been implanted for 632,000 months with 116 failures, the failure rate would be 0.018 per cent per month. The standard set by the Association for Advancement of Medical Instrumentation and for nuclear-powered pacemakers was a failure rate of less than 0.15 per cent per month. As can be seen from Table 49–7, the majority of lithium-powered pacers have been more reliable.

Mean time implanted is obtained by dividing the total number of months that all devices have been implanted by the number of implants; for the preceding example, it would be 18 months. *The mean time between failures,* reported in hours, is calculated by dividing the total number of months that all devices have been implanted by the total number of failures times 730.5, which is the mean number of hours per month. *Failure rate curves* show duration of implantation across the X-axis and number of failures along the Y-axis. This method clearly illustrates which months carry the highest risk of failure and can be useful in assessing patient risk and making management decisions. *Cumulative survival curves* show the percentage of functioning units on the Y-axis versus the months or years implanted on the X-axis. The monthly failure rate is subtracted from 1 to obtain the fraction surviving each month (1 − 0.018 = 0.982), and the monthly survival fractions are multiplied to obtain the cumulative fraction surviving. In addition, life table analysis techniques, which take into account units removed from service for non–failure-related indications, and probability calculations for the percentage of units continuing to function are used. This type of data allows comparison of different series and units if the data base is reliable. The *performance index* is derived from the failure rate curve and the complement of the current monthly failure rate. Any value greater than 0.99 is indicative of a reliable unit (within the limitations of the data). This index is usually used to assist in management of patients with pacemakers involved in an advisory or recall situation.

Apart from some deceptive practices, some of these reporting methods are inherently obscure. Random failure rate and mean time between failures obscure time-dependent failures and thus look very good during early periods following introduction of a new series. For example, if a large number of units have been implanted for less than a year and only a small number have been implanted for more than a year, the random failure rate and the mean time between failures will look very presentable even if all the older units have failed. Similarly, a popular series with a very large number of new implants will produce random failure rate and mean time between failures statistics that are deceptively good. Cumulative survival curves, however, accurately illustrate time-dependent failures, and it behooves the physician selecting pacemakers for implantation to request this additional data. Periodic failure rate charts show the percentage of monthly failures on the Y-axis and months implanted along the X-axis. This type of reporting often produces curves with a somewhat higher failure rate in the first few months as defective units are eliminated, a low intermediate failure rate, and then an increasing monthly failure rate as the units age and begin to fail. No matter how many recent implants are added, the late upward trend and incidence of periodic failures are never obscured as they are in the random failure rate statistics.

Inaccuracies also arise because of the nature of the data base and various manufacturer practices. Most manufacturers collect passive data; that is, they wait for registration cards and subsequent reports of failure. This, of necessity, underreports patient deaths and failures and has on occasion, such as during the massive recalls of mercury-zinc units, approached resistance to receiving information (Tyers and Brownlee, 1976a; McGuire et al., 1981). In contrast, active data–based systems require direct contact with physicians and patients to confirm findings and will usually result in discovery of three times the patient deaths collected by a passive system and a variable increase in unit failures. Furthermore, one manufacturer defines failures as units that are not only out of specification but also result in a clinically recognized problem. This has permitted them to report very low but also meaningless failure statistics. Another manufacturer does not count failed units that are returned unless they were registered for warranty at the time of implant. However, units that fail at the time of implant, as, for example, because of sticking reed switches, are often not registered and so are excluded from the company's reports. Finally, because of a minimum time of from 2 to 3 months required for reporting and recording failures, even with the best intentions all results must be somewhat poorer than advertised. These limitations underline the need for in-depth physician involvement in follow-up of all patients, and several independent comparative sources are now available (Welt, 1981b; Bilitch et al., 1981; Hurzeler et al., 1980).

SELECTED REFERENCES

Sutton, R., Perrins, J., and Citron, P.: Physiological cardiac pacing. PACE, 3:207, 1980.

This excellent paper reviews the history and theory of physiologic cardiac pacing and describes the different pacing modes and their indications. An extensive clinical experience with 176 patients is reviewed, and the markedly improved hemodynamic function accruing from the maintenance of proper atrioventricular sequence is confirmed. The previous limitations of atrial leads and atrial and dual-chambered pacemakers are reviewed, as are the development of and indications for DDD pacemakers.

Thalen, H. J. T., and Meere, C. (Eds.): Fundamentals of Cardiac Pacing. The Hague, Martinus Nijhoff, 1979.

This is an excellent introductory text covering the broad range of pathophysiology of cardiac conduction disorders and the current management of patients requiring pacemaker therapy.

Tyers, G. F. O., and Brownlee, R. R.: Power pulse generators, electrodes and longevity. Prog. Cardiovasc. Dis., 23:421, 1981.

This is a comprehensive review of the development of pacemaker power sources, the relative merits of the different power cells available, and the multiple physician-controlled nonpower source factors, including electrode selection, programmability and dual-chambered modes that affect pacemaker longevity. Applied electronics and power cell chemistry are explained for the physician in nontechnical terms.

Tyers, G. F. O., Williams, E. H., Larrieu, A. J., Jamieson, W. R. E., Calfee, R., and Hardage, M.: Multiprogrammable pacemakers. Can. J. Surg., 24:252, 1981.

The history of the development of, technology of, and indications for multiprogrammable pacemakers are reviewed in detail. The potential benefits of noninvasive alteration and control of rate, output energy, sensitivity, mode, refractory interval, and hysteresis are given, and the most widely used programmable pacemakers are compared. A large clinical experience with follow-up of 164 multiprogrammable pacemakers for up to 3 years is reviewed, with contrasting illustrations of reoperative procedures avoided by the availability of multiprogrammability and the need for reoperations that could have been avoided in patients who, during the same period, did not receive multiprogrammable pacemakers. The need for multiparameter follow-up data, including power cell voltage and power cell impedence, is stressed, and the simplicity and reliability relative to rate change monitoring of complex and multiprogrammable devices are explained.

Varriale, P., and Naclerio, E. A.: Cardiac pacing, A Concise Guide to Clinical Practice. Philadelphia, Lea and Febiger, 1979.

This is an advanced textbook covering the whole range of clinical practice of cardiac pacing in detail. Special interest areas, including pacing in children, pacemaker insertion at the time of cardiac surgery, pacing for refractory arrhythmias, follow-up, and the management of complications, are covered in depth.

REFERENCES

Adinolfi, L., Perticone, F., Curzio, G., and Critelli, G.: Iterative ventricular tachycardia controlled by programmable A-V sequential pacing. PACE, 4:28, 1981.

Alicandri, C.: Three cases of hypotension and syncope with ventricular pacing: Possible role for atrial reflexes. Am. J. Cardiol., 42:132, 1978.

Barold, S. S., Falkoff, M. D., Ong, L. S., and Heinle, R. A.: Apparent VVI (or ?VOO) pacing by AV sequential demand (DVI) pulse generator. PACE, 4:321, 1981.

Belott, P. H.: A variation on the introducer technique for unlimited access to the subclavian vein. PACE, 4:43, 1981.

Bhattacharya, S. K., Sutaria, M., and Braunstein, E. E.: A method of epicardial pacing without thoracotomy: Treatment of heart block in patients with tricuspid valve prosthesis. Chest, 62:112, 1972.

Bilitch, M., Hauser, R. G., Goldman, B. S., Furman, S., and Parsonnet, V.: Performance of cardiac pacemaker pulse generators. PACE, 4:254, 1981.

Billhardt, R. A., Rosenbush, S. W., and Hauser, R. G.: Noninvasive correction of pacing system malfunctions by multiprogrammable pacemakers. Am. J. Cardiol., 47:393, 1981.

Bognolo, D., Vijayanagar, R., Eckstein, P., Cromartie, S., and Janss, B.: Clinical experience with 100 consecutive physiologic pacing systems. PACE, 4:35, 1981.

Bowers, D. L.: Pacemaker technology. In Fundamentals of Cardiac Pacing. Edited by H. J. T. Thalen and C. Meere. The Hague, Martinus Nijhoff, 1979, pp. 181–188.

Brownlee, R. R., and Tyers, G. F. O.: Pacemaker recall. IEEE Spectrum, *13*:32, 1976.

Brownlee, R. R., Hughes, H. C., Jr., and Tyers, G. F. O.: Effects of increasing pacemaker sensing circuit impedance on R wave detection. Surg. Forum, *27*:251, 1976.

Brownlee, R. R., Shimmel, J. B., and Del Marco, C. J.: A new code for pacemaker operating modes. PACE, *4*:396, 1981.

Brownlee, R. R., Hughes, H. C., Jr., Tyers, G. F. O., and Neff, P. H.: Monitoring systems for cardiac pacemakers. Trans. Am. Soc. Artif. Intern. Organs, *23*:65, 1977.

Brownlee, R. R., Tyers, G. F. O., Neff, P. H., and Hughes, H. C., Jr.: New interference sensing demand pacemaker functions. IEEE Trans. Biomed. Eng., *25*:264, 1978.

Brownlee, R. R., Hughes, H. C., Jr., Tyers, G. F. O., Neff, P. H., and Del Marco, C. J.: Cardiac electrodes and electrograms: Some new observations and concerns. PACE, *3*:266, 1980.

Calvin, J. W.: Intraoperative pacemaker electrical testing. Ann. Thorac. Surg., *26*:165, 1978.

Castellanos, A., Waxman, H. L., Moleiro, F., Berkovits, B. V., and Sung, R. J.: Preliminary studies with an implantable multimodal AV pacemaker for reciprocating atrioventricular tachycardias. PACE, *3*:257, 1980.

Check, W. A.: Have pacemakers found their way into too many patients? J.A.M.A., *243*:2371, 1980.

Crelinsten, G. L., Byers, J., and Morin, J.: Permanent pacemaker therapy in the sick sinus syndrome: An evaluation using 24 hour ambulatory ECG monitoring. Can. Cardiovasc. Soc. Prog., *33*:65, 1980.

Curry, P. V. L., Rowland, E., and Krikler, D. M.: Dual-demand pacing for refractory atrioventricular re-entry tachycardia. PACE, *2*:137, 1979.

Dreifus, L. S., Berkovits, B. V., Kimibiris, D., Moghadam, K., Haupt, G., Walinski, P., Thomas, P., and Brockman, S. K.: Use of atrial and bifocal cardiac pacemakers for treating resistant dysrhythmias. Eur. J. Cardiol., *3*:257, 1975.

El Gamal, M. I. H., and Van Gelder, L. M.: Chronic ventricular pacing with ventriculo-atrial conduction versus atrial pacing in three patients with symptomatic sinus bradycardia. PACE, *4*:100, 1981.

Erbel, R.: Pacemaker syndrome. Am. J. Cardiol., *44*:771, 1979.

Fieldman, A., Dobrow, R. J., and Katz, A. M.: Phantom pacemaker programming. Am. J. Cardiol., *39*:306, 1977.

Fisher, J. D., Cohen, H. L., Mehra, R., Altschuler, H., Escher, D. J. W., and Furman, S.: Cardiac pacing and pacemakers. II. Serial electrophysiologic-pharmacologic testing for control of recurrent tachyarrhythmias. Am. Heart J., *93*:658, 1977.

Friedman, H. S.: Are too many permanent pacemakers being implanted? PACE, *4*:232, 1981.

Furman, S.: Therapeutic uses of atrial pacing. Am. Heart J., *86*:835, 1973.

Furman, S.: Cardiac pacing and pacemakers. I. Indications for pacing, bradyarrhythmias. Am. Heart J., *93*:523, 1977a.

Furman, S.: Cardiac pacing and pacemakers. VIII. The pacemaker follow-up clinic. Am. Heart J., *94*:795, 1977b.

Furman, S.: Spurious pacemaker programming. PACE, *3*:517, 1980a.

Furman, S.: Physiologic pacing. PACE, *3*:639, 1980b.

Furman, S.: Pacemaker longevity. PACE, *4*:1, 1981.

Furman, S., and Fisher, J. D.: Cardiac pacing and pacemakers. V. Technical aspects of implantation and equipment. Am. Heart J., *94*:250, 1977.

Furman, S., and Pannizzo, F.: Output programmability and reduction of secondary intervention after pacemaker implantation. J. Thorac. Cardiovasc. Surg., *81*:713, 1981.

Furman, S., Pannizzo, F., and Campo, I.: Comparison of active and passive adhering leads for endocardial pacing. PACE, *2*:417, 1979.

Furman, S., Pannizzo, F., and Campo, I.: Comparison of active and passive leads for endocardial pacing—II. PACE, *4*:78, 1981.

Garcia, J. B., and Bengochea, J. B.: Extrapleural implantation of epicardial leads under local anesthesia. J. Cardiovasc. Surg., *63*:144, 1972.

Goldberg, E.: How does our garden grow. PACE, *4*:230, 1981.

Greatbatch, W.: Energy sources. *In* Fundamentals of Cardiac Pacing. Edited by H. J. T. Thalen and C. Meere. The Hague, Martinus Nijhoff, 1979, pp. 189–210.

Greenburg, P., Castellanet, M., Messenger, J., and Ellestad, M. H.: Coronary sinus pacing. Circulation, *57*:98, 1978.

Griffin, J. C., and Mason, J. W.: Clinical experience with an automatically activated tachycardia terminating pacemaker. PACE, *4*:48, 1981.

Hart, R., Peters, R., Rubinstein, M., Desai, J., O'Young, J., Thomas, A., and Scheinman, M. M.: A review of instrumentation and therapeutic techniques in the diagnosis and management of supraventricular tachycardia. Med. Instrum., *12*:268, 1978.

Hartlaub, J.: The application of microcomputers in implantable pacemakers. Medtronic News, *11*:16, 1981.

Hass, J. M., and Strait, G. B.: Pacemaker induced cardiovascular failure, hemodynamic and angiographic observations. Am. J. Cardiol., *33*:295, 1974.

Hauser, R. G., Klodnycky, M., Stewart, J. A., Staller, B. J., Edwards, L. M., Prabhu, R., Wyndham, C., Belic, N., Wilner, G., Bicoff, J., Davis, A., Smith, C. R., Uret, E. F., and Moran, J. F.: Clinical reliability of programmable pacemakers. PACE, *4*:50, 1981.

Hossmann, V., van den Kerckhoff, W., Matsuoka, Y., and Hossmann, K. A.: The effect of atrial versus ventricular stimulation on cerebral blood flow in cats with one occluded carotid artery. PACE, *4*:14, 1981.

Hughes, H. C., Jr., Brownlee, R. R., and Tyers, G. F. O.: Failure of demand pacing with small surface area electrodes. Circulation, *54*:128, 1976.

Hughes, H. C., Jr., Tyers, G. F. O., and Torman, H. A.: Effects of acid-base imbalance on myocardial pacing thresholds. J. Thorac. Cardiovasc. Surg., *69*:743, 1975.

Hughes, H. C., Jr., Brownlee, R. R., Bertolet, R. D., Neff, P. H., Sluetz, J. E., and Tyers, G. F. O.: The effects of electrode position on the detection of the transvenous cardiac electrogram. PACE, *3*:651, 1980.

Hurzeler, P., Morse, D., Leach, C., Sands, M. J., Pennock, R., and Zinberg, A.: Longevity comparisons among lithium anode power cells for cardiac pacemakers. PACE, *3*:555, 1980.

Ilves, R., Cooper, J. D., Todd, T. R. J., and Pearson, F. G.: Prospective, randomized double-blind study using prophylactic cephalothin for major, elective, general thoracic operations. J. Thorac. Cardiovasc. Surg., *81*:813, 1981.

James, T. N.: Anatomy and pathology of the conduction system of the human heart. *In* Fundamentals of Cardiac Pacing. Edited by H. J. T. Thalen and C. Meere. The Hague, Martinus Nijhoff, 1979, pp. 23–56.

James, T. N., and Galakhov, I.: Fatal electrical instability of the heart associated with benign congenital polycystic tumor of the atrial ventricular node. Circulation, *56*:667, 1977.

Johnson, A. D.: Hemodynamic compromise associated with VA conduction following transvenous pacemaker implantation. Am. J. Med., *65*:75, 1978.

Kappenberger, L., Gloor, H. O., Babotai, I., Steinbrunn, W., and Turina, M.: Benefit of long term physiologic pacing. PACE, *4*:52, 1981.

Kleinert, M., Elmqvist, H., and Strandberg, H.: Spectral properties of atrial and ventricular endocardial signals. PACE, *2*:11, 1979.

Lagergren, H.: Step by step pacemaker procedure lowers risk. Med. World News, *7*:56, 1966.

Lawrie, G. M., Seale, J. P., Morris, G. C., Jr., Howell, J. F., Whisennand, H. H., and DeBakey, M. E.: Results of epicardial pacing by the left subcostal approach. Ann. Thorac. Surg., *28*:561, 1977.

Lister, J. W., Gosselin, A. J., Nathan, D. A., and Barold, S. S.: Rapid atrial stimulation in the treatment of supraventricular tachycardia. Chest, *63*:995, 1973.

Lopman, A., Langer, C. L., Furman, S., and Esher, D. J. W.: A 15 year comparative study of cardiac pacing costs. Am. J. Cardiol., *47*:392, 1980.

MacGregor, D. C., Wilson, G. J., Lixfeld, W. Pilliar, R. M., Bobyn, J. D., Silver, M. D., Smardon, S., and Miller, S. L.: The porous-surfaced electrode, a new concept in pacemaker lead design. J. Thorac. Cardiovas. Surg., *78*:281, 1979.

McGuire, L. B., Breit, R. A., Steinberg, S., and Nolan, S. P.:

Reflections on an epidemic of premature pacemaker failures. PACE, 4:335, 1981.

Miller, M., Fox, S., Jenkins, R., Schwartz, J., and Toonder, F. G.: Non-invasive evaluation of cerebral blood flow during ventricular and AV sequential pacing. Am. J. Cardiol., 47:435, 1981.

Mirowski, M., Reid, P. R., Mower, M. M., Watkins, L., Gott, V. L., Schauble, J. F., Langer, A., Heilman, M. S., Kolenik, S. A., Fischell, R. E., and Weisfeldt, M. L.: Termination of malignant ventricular arrhythmias with an implanted automatic defibrillator in human beings. N. Engl. J. Med., 303:322, 1980.

Ogawa, S., Dreifus, L. S., Shenoy, P. N., Brockman, S. K., and Berkovitz, B.: Hemodynamic consequences of atrioventricular and ventriculo-atrial pacing. PACE, 1:8, 1978.

O'Neill, M. J., and Tyers, G. F. O.: Safe release of impacted pacemaker electrodes. Ann. Thorac. Surg., 19:77, 1975.

Parsonnet, V.: Implantation of transvenous pacemakers. Tarpon Springs, Florida, Tampa Tracings, 1972, pp. 1–21.

Parsonnet, V.: Cardiac pacing and pacemakers. VII. Power sources for implantable pacemakers (Part I). Am. Heart J., 94:517, 1977.

Parsonnet, V., Furman, S., and Smyth, N. P. D.: Implantable cardiac pacemakers: Status report and resource guideline. Am. J. Cardiol., 34:487, 1974.

Parsonnet, V., Furman, S., and Smyth, N. P. D.: A revised code for pacemaker identification. PACE, 4:400, 1981.

Parsonnet, V., Myers, G. H., and Kresh, Y. M.: Characteristics of intracardiac electrograms. II. Atrial endocardial electrograms. PACE, 3:406, 1980a.

Parsonnet, V., Werres, R., Atherley, T., and Littleford, P. O.: Transvenous insertions of double sets of permanent electrodes; atraumatic technique for atrial synchronous and atrial ventricular sequential pacemakers. J.A.M.A. 243:62, 1980b.

Pauker, S. G., and Salem, D. N.: Decision analysis techniques as applied to permanent pacemaker implantation. Presentation at Tufts University School of Medicine, Pacemaker Symposium, June 26, 1981.

Pennock, R. S., Driefus, L. S., Morse, D. P., and Watanabe, Y.: Cardiac pacemaker function. J.A.M.A. 222:1379, 1972.

Preston, T. A.: Pacemaker utilization: The need for information. PACE, 4:235, 1981.

Reed, G. E., Cortes, L. E., Clauss, R. H., and Reppert, E. H.: A new technique for pacemaker implantation: Extrapleural, intra-myocardial. J. Thorac. Cardiovasc. Surg., 57:507, 1969.

Resnekov, L., and Lipp, H.: Pacemaking and acute myocardial infarction. Prog. Cardiovasc. Dis., 14:475, 1972.

Ronald, A. R.: Pros and cons of antimicrobial prophylaxis in surgery. Can. J. Surg., 24:113, 1981.

Schechter, D. C.: Cardiac pacing in perspective. In Cardiac Pacing, A Concise Guide to Clinical Practice. Edited by P. Varriale and E. A. Naclerio. Philadelphia, Lea and Febiger, 1979, pp. 1–12.

Sinnaeve, A., Piret, J., and Stroobandt, R.: Potential causes of spurious programming. PACE, 3:541, 1980.

Stokes, K., and Stephenson, N. L.: The implantable cardiac pacing lead—just a simple wire? In The Third Decade of Cardiac Pacing. Edited by S. S. Barold and J. Mugica. Mt. Kisco, New York, Futura Publishing Co., 1982.

Stopczyk, M. J.: Electrodes, leads and interface problems. In Fundamentals of Cardiac Pacing. Edited by H. J. T. Thalen and C. Meere. The Hague, Martinus Nijhoff, 1979.

Sutton, R., Perrins, J., and Citron, P.: Physiological cardiac pacing. PACE, 3:207, 1980a.

Sutton, R., Perrins, J., Kalebic, B., and Richards, E.: Physiological cardiac pacing in atrio-ventricular block: Acute and long term studies. PACE, 3:388, 1980b.

Sutton, R., Perrins, J., Morley, C., Kalebic, B., Richards, E., and Chan, S. L.: Long term benefits of physiological pacing systems in atrio-ventricular block. PACE, 4:74, 1981.

Telectronics product note 6A. Tachyarrhythmia control pacer, currently undergoing clinical investigation. October, 1980.

Thalen, H. J. T.: History of cardiac pacing. In Fundamentals of Cardiac Pacing. Edited by H. J. T. Thalen and C. Meere, The Hague, Martinus Nijhoff, 1979, pp. 1–22.

Thalen, H. J. T., and Meere, C. (Eds.): Fundamentals of Cardiac Pacing. The Hague, Martinus Nijhoff, 1979.

Tyers, G. F. O.: Maximum cardiac performance after complete heart block. Surg. Forum, 18:132, 1967.

Tyers, G. F. O.: Comparison of effect on cardiac function of single site and simultaneous multiple site ventricular stimulation after AV block. J. Thorac. Cardiovasc. Surg., 59:211, 1970.

Tyers, G. F. O., and Brownlee, R. R.: The non-hermetically sealed pacemaker myth or Navy-Ribicoff 22,000—FDA-Weinberger O. J. Thorac. Cardiovasc. Surg., 71:253, 1976a.

Tyers, G. F. O., and Brownlee, R. R.: The unfulfilled promise of demand pacing. J. Thorac. Cardiovasc. Surg., 72:813, 1976b.

Tyers, G. F. O., and Brownlee, R. R.: Current status of pacemaker power sources. Ann. Thorac. Surg., 25:571, 1978.

Tyers, G. F. O., and Brownlee, R. R.: A multiparameter telemetry system for cardiac pacemakers. In Cardiac Pacing, A Concise Guide to Clinical Practice. Edited by P. Varriale and E. A. Naclerio. Philadelphia, Lea and Febiger, 1979, pp. 349–368.

Tyers, G. F. O., and Brownlee, R. R.: Power pulse generators, electrodes and longevity. Prog. Cardiovasc. Dis., 23:421, 1981.

Tyers, G. F. O., Noto, J. A., and Danielson, G. K.: A new device for nonoperative repair of internal cardiac pacemakers. Arch. Surg., 92:901, 1966.

Tyers, G. F. O., Torman, H. A., and Hughes, H. C., Jr.: Comparative studies of "state of the art" and presently used clinical cardiac pacemaker electrodes. J. Thorac. Cardiovasc. Surg., 67:849, 1974.

Tyers, G. F. O., Hughes, H. C., Jr., Torman, H. A., and Waldhausen, J. A.: The advantages of transthoracic placement of permanent cardiac pacemaker electrodes. J. Thorac. Cardiovasc. Surg., 69:8, 1975.

Tyers, G. F. O., Brownlee, R. R., Hughes, H. C., Jr., Shaffer, C. W., Williams, E. H., and Kao, R. L.: Myocardial stimulation impedance: The effects of electrode, physiological and stimulus variables. Ann. Thorac. Surg., 27:63, 1979.

Tyers, G. F. O., Larrieu, A. J., Nishimura, A., William, E. H., Kurusz, M., and Brownlee, R. R.: Suppression of a demand pacemaker in the presence of redundant transvenous right ventricular leads. PACE, 3:84, 1980.

Tyers, G. F. O., Williams, E. H., Larrieu, A. J., Jamieson, W. R. E., Calfee, R., and Hardage, M.: Multiprogrammable pacemakers. Can. J. Surg., 24:252, 1981.

Varriale, P., and Naclerio, E. A.: Cardiac Pacing, A Concise Guide to Clinical Practice. Philadelphia, Lea and Febiger, 1979.

Venkataraman, K., and Bilitch, M.: Intracardiac electrocardiography during permanent pacemaker implantation: Predictors of cardiac perforation. Am. J. Cardiol., 44:225, 1979.

Ward, D. E., Camm, A. J., Gainsborough, J., and Spurell, R. A. J.: Autodecremental pacing—a microprocessor based modality for the termination of paroxysmal tachyarrhythmias. PACE, 3:178, 1980.

Waxman, M. B., Wald, R. W., Bonet, J. F., MacGregor, D. C., and Goldman, B. S.: Self-conversion of supraventricular tachycardia by rapid atrial pacing. PACE, 1:35, 1978.

Wellens, H. J. J., Bar, F. W., Gorgels, A. P., and Muncharaz, J. F.: Electrical management of arrhythmias with emphasis on the tachycardias. Am. J. Cardiol., 41:1025, 1978.

Welti, J. J.: Pacesetter: With respect to a statistic. PACE, 3:510, 1980.

Welti, J. J.: T-wave recycling of programmable CPI 505 pacemakers. PACE, 4:251, 1981a.

Welti, J. J.: Premature lithium batteries depletion. PACE, 4:349, 1981b.

Whitman, V., Berman, W., Jr., and Tyers, G. F. O.: Pacemakers in young patients. J. Pediatr., 92:722, 1978.

Wickham, G. G., and Cartmill, T. B.: The water vapor permeability of implantable cardiac pacemakers and its effect. Med. J. Aust., 2:138, 1971.

Williams, E. H., Tyers, G. F. O., and Shaffer, C. W.: Symptomatic deep vein thrombosis of the arm associated with permanent transvenous pacing electrodes. Chest, 73:613, 1978.

Zipes, D. P.: Pacing 1980. PACE, 4:182, 1981.

Chapter 50

The Coronary Circulation

I   PHYSIOLOGY OF THE CORONARY CIRCULATION AND INTRAOPERATIVE MYOCARDIAL PROTECTION

J. Scott Rankin
David C. Sabiston, Jr.

During the course of most cardiac operations, it is necessary to temporarily interrupt coronary blood flow for varying periods, and under these circumstances, intraoperative preservation of the heart is of utmost importance. Unlike operations on other organs, the heart must resume full functional activity immediately at the conclusion of the procedure. Prevention of myocardial injury during the ischemic interval, therefore, is critical to the survival of the patient and has been the subject of intense investigation during the past decade. Improvements in myocardial protection resulting from this work have contributed significantly to reductions in mortality and morbidity in most patients undergoing cardiac surgery.

PATHOPHYSIOLOGY OF ISCHEMIC INJURY

From a clinical viewpoint, myocardial protection is not subtle. Whenever a patient enters the operating suite with adequate cardiac pump function, the heart should resume the circulation without difficulty after a technically satisfactory procedure. If myocardial dysfunction is encountered at the conclusion of cardiopulmonary bypass, inadequate myocardial preservation must be considered as a very likely causative factor. The significance of this problem is emphasized by several earlier series (Taber et al., 1967; Henson et al., 1969; Cooley et al., 1972) in which low cardiac output was a major cause of perioperative mortality and morbidity. In several publications, postmortem subendocardial necrosis of the left ventricle was identified as the cause of postoperative low cardiac output (Najafi et al., 1969, 1971). Buckberg and associates (1972a) made the important observation that redistribution of total coronary blood flow away from the subendocardium could occur in the presence of anatomically normal coronary arteries. This finding stimulated the imagination of cardiac surgeons and physiologists, who began to consider the pathophysiology

of myocardial injury in more detail and attempted to develop methods to more effectively protect the heart intraoperatively.

Under basal conditions, average coronary blood flow is approximately 80 ml. per 100 grams of myocardium per minute (Rowe et al., 1959). This value is approximately 10 times that observed for the body as a whole, reflecting the high energy requirements of cardiac muscle. Because oxygen requirements are so high, even short periods of ischemia produce significant derangements in cellular metabolism and abnormalities in myocardial function (Fig. 50–1). The normally beating heart utilizes approximately 10 ml. of oxygen per 100 grams of myocardium each minute. Since 75 per cent of the oxygen is extracted from the arterial blood as it traverses the coronary capillaries, very little additional oxygen is available during periods of increased metabolic demand. Therefore, the added oxygen required by the heart during stress is provided primarily by an increase in coronary blood flow and represents one of the unique characteristics of the coronary circulation.

The heart is the only organ in the body that consistently has a greater arterial blood flow in diastole than in systole (Sabiston and Gregg, 1957; Sabiston, 1974). Through a vascular waterfall effect (Permutt and Riley, 1963), myocardial wall stress increases coronary vascular resistance and limits systolic blood flow to the myocardium. Diastolic coronary flow is mainly determined by aortic perfusion pressure, diastolic wall stress, and coronary vascular resistance. Elevations in diastolic cavitary pressure increase mural stress, especially in the subendocardium, and can redistribute myocardial blood flow, leading to subendocardial ischemia (Bache et al., 1974). During cardiopulmonary bypass, diminished perfusion pressure, ventricular distention, ventricular fibrillation, or atherosclerotic limitations to coronary flow predisposes the vulnerable subendocardium to ischemic injury.

Normal myocardial metabolism is almost totally

1356

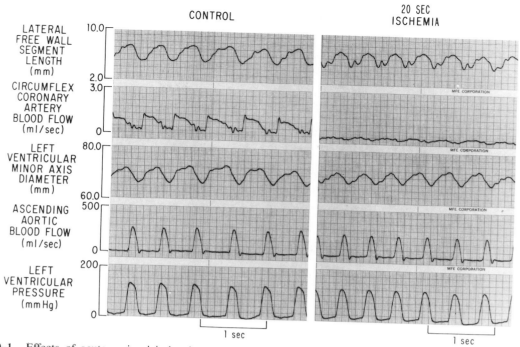

CONTROL

20 SEC ISCHEMIA

LATERAL FREE WALL SEGMENT LENGTH (mm)

CIRCUMFLEX CORONARY ARTERY BLOOD FLOW (ml/sec)

LEFT VENTRICULAR MINOR AXIS DIAMETER (mm)

ASCENDING AORTIC BLOOD FLOW (ml/sec)

LEFT VENTRICULAR PRESSURE (mmHg)

1 sec

1 sec

Figure 50–1. Effects of acute regional ischemia on myocardial function. The circumflex coronary artery was occluded in this conscious dog, and within 10 to 20 seconds, significant regional and global dysfunction was evident. Myocardial dimensions were measured with implanted ultrasonic transducers, flows were measured with electromagnetic flow probes, and pressures were obtained with micromanometers.

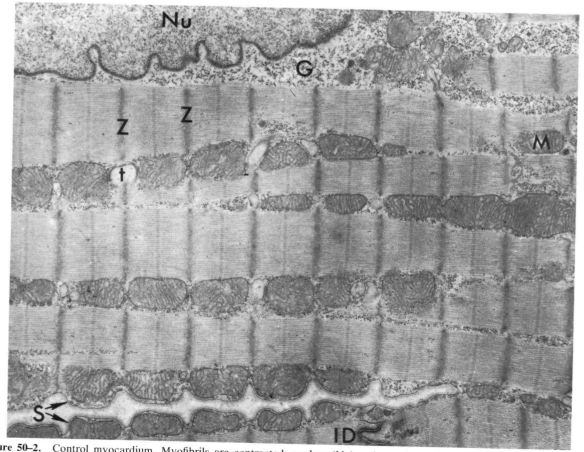

Figure 50–2. Control myocardium. Myofibrils are contracted; nuclear (Nu) and sarcolemmal (S) membranes are scalloped. No I bands are visible adjacent to the Z bands (Z). Mitochondria (M) show tightly packed cristae. Glycogen (G) is abundant in the sarcoplasm. Transverse tubules (t) are at some Z bands. An intercalated disc is at ID. (Osmium fixation; magnification × 8100.) (From Jennings, R. B., and Ganote, C. E.: Structural changes in myocardium during acute ischemia. Circ. Res., *34, 35* (Suppl. 3):156, 1974.)

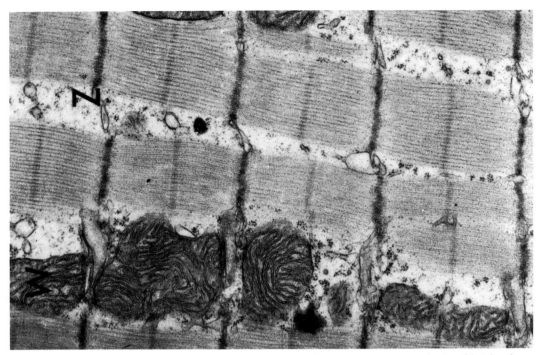

Figure 50–3. Fifteen minutes of ischemia, reversible injury. This sample shows relaxed myofibrils with I bands on either side of the Z band (Z). Little glycogen is present. The mitochondria are similar to those found in nonischemic control left ventricle. (Osmium fixation; magnification × 66,400.) (From Jennings, R. B., and Ganote, C. E.: Structural changes in myocardium during acute ischemia. Circ. Res., *34, 35* (Suppl. 3):156, 1974.)

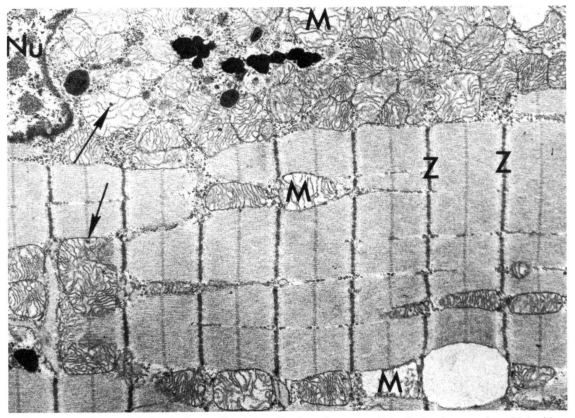

Figure 50–4. Forty minutes of ischemia, irreversible injury. Portion of a myocardial cell showing a nucleus (Nu) with peripherally aggregated chromatin and numerous swollen perinuclear mitochondria (M). Some mitochondria contain tiny amorphous matrix densities. The Z bands (Z) bisect the I bands of the myofibrils. The dark bodies in the perinuclear zone are pigment granules (lysosomes, lipofuchsin) and are structurally intact. (Osmium fixation; magnification × 31,000.) (From Jennings, R. B., and Ganote, C. E.: Structural changes in myocardium during acute ischemia. Circ. Res., *34, 35* (Suppl. 3):156, 1974.)

aerobic, producing 36 moles of adenosine triphosphate (ATP) for each mole of glucose. During global ischemic arrest, ATP stores are replenished primarily by anaerobic metabolism, yielding only 3 moles of ATP per mole of glucose. Because inefficient anaerobic pathways are inadequate to maintain normal energy requirements, cellular injury occurs rapidly after the onset of normothermic ischemia. In addition, accumulation of lactate and acidosis interfere with continued anaerobic energy production and further compound the energy deficit.

Morphologically, early ischemic injury is associated with cellular edema and mitochondrial disruption (Jennings and Ganote, 1974). In the early period of reversible ischemic injury (10 to 15 minutes), primary ultrastructural changes include depletion of glycogen and relaxation of the myofibrils. A normal section of control myocardium magnified 8100 times is shown in Figure 50–2 and may be contrasted with findings after 15 minutes of ischemia, which are shown in Figure 50–3. These changes are reversible. It should be emphasized that at 15 minutes of ischemia, early changes are necessarily uniform, and many cells are identical to those in the control sections, whereas others show characteristic features of glycogen depletion and relaxation. Few cells may show evidence of mitrochondria that appear to be slightly swollen. With increasing periods of ischemia, ultrastructural changes also become more prominent, and distinct irreversible

changes are present at 40 minutes of ischemia (Fig. 50–4). At 60 minutes of ischemia, the myocardium shows the changes present earlier, but in addition, glycogen is virtually absent and the myofibrils are stretched to an even greater extent (Fig. 50–5). The mitochondria are swollen with an enlarged matrix, and the sarcolemma may be lifted off the involved cells and may exhibit tiny defects in the plasma membrane. A striking mitochondrial finding is the appearance of one or more amorphous densities in the matrix space of each mitochondrial profile (Jennings and Ganote, 1974). In later stages, myofibrillar disruption is noted along with development of osmiophilic matrix densities and distortion of Z lines. When severely injured myocardium is reperfused, explosive cellular swelling, deposition of calcium phosphate, and intense contracture are observed, which progress to cell rupture and death. This process can be favorably modified either by reducing the energy demands of the myocardium or by supplying additional oxygen and substrate during the ischemic period. Both of these measures are used clinically to facilitate myocardial protection during induced global ischemia.

GENERAL TECHNIQUES OF PROTECTION

Hypothermia was the first method of myocardial protection to be applied to clinical intracardiac pro-

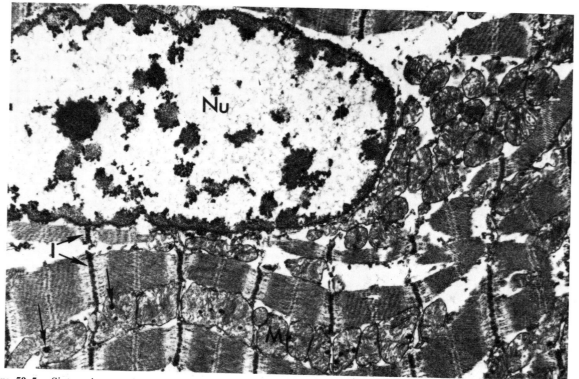

Figure 50–5. Sixty minutes of ischemia, irreversible injury. Note the margination of the chromatin in the nucleus (Nu). The myofibrils are relaxed and have prominent I bands (I); an N band also is present in the I bands. The mitochondria are swollen and contain amorphous matrix densities at the arrows. Little or no glycogen is expected to be present at this time, but this tissue cannot be used to illustrate the fact because the fixative extracts glycogen during processing. (Osmium fixation with uranyl acetate in block; magnification × 16,628.) (From Jennings, R. B., and Ganote, C. E.: Structural changes in myocardium during acute ischemia. Circ. Res., *34, 35* (Suppl. 3):156, 1974.)

cedures (Lewis and Taufic, 1953; Bigelow *et al.*, 1954). When the viability of the brain and myocardium was sustained with moderate systemic hypothermia (30° C.), vena caval inflow was occluded and the heart opened for brief periods. Although this approach provided limited operative time, simple anomalies such as atrial septal defects could be repaired with a high degree of success (Brock and Ross, 1955). After the development of mechanical cardiopulmonary bypass, extracorporeal circulation was combined with profound systemic hypothermia in an effort to improve the protection of body organs during periods of ischemic cardiac arrest (Sealy *et al.*, 1957, 1960; Drew and Anderson, 1959). By lowering the body temperature to 15° C., the circulation could be reduced or stopped for periods of up to 1 hour, providing optimal technical conditions for cardiac surgical procedures. The patient was then rewarmed using the extracorporeal circuit, and the operation was concluded. As time progressed, most surgeons largely abandoned this technique, but interestingly, it has re-emerged in recent years as a highly acceptable method for repair of several categories of cardiovascular disorders (Barratt-Boyes *et al.*, 1971; Crawford and Saleh, 1981).

Chemical arrest of the heart was introduced by Melrose and associates in 1955 (Melrose *et al.*, 1955; Melrose, 1978). After occlusion of the ascending aorta, a 2.5 per cent solution of potassium citrate in blood was injected into the aortic root, achieving a flaccid arrest of the myocardium. The intracardiac repair was then performed with a quiet, motionless operative field. With re-establishment of coronary blood flow and washout of the potassium, normal myocardial contraction resumed. Although a moderate clinical experience with this method was obtained, subsequent reports of direct myocardial injury by the potassium citrate led to abandonment of this practice (Helmsworth *et al.*, 1959; McFarland *et al.*, 1960). As with hypothermia, however, the principle of chemical arrest was to be modified over the next decade and reintroduced into clinical practice in the 1970s.

After the experience with potassium citrate, most surgeons adopted moderate systemic hypothermia and continuous or intermittent coronary perfusion as the routine method of myocardial protection. During aortic valve replacement, the coronary ostia were perfused with blood through indwelling cannulas for as much of the procedure as possible. In other operations, the ascending aorta was occluded intermittently for periods of up to 15 minutes to arrest the heart and improve exposure. Between periods of ischemic arrest, the coronary arteries were perfused for 5 to 10 minutes to allow "payback of oxygen debt" and maintenance of myocardial viability. Although this method reduced operative mortality rates, it soon became evident that myocardial injury occurred in a significant number of patients. Subendocardial necrosis was observed frequently in hypertrophied ventricles, even with relatively short periods of ischemia (Najafi *et al.*, 1971). In addition, problems associated with coronary perfusion cannulas, continued myocar-

dial tone, and coronary venous effluent impaired operative exposure and complicated the technical conduct of the procedure.

An important addition to the technique of intermittent ischemic arrest was topical cardiac hypothermia (Shumway *et al.*, 1959). Reduction of myocardial temperature during the ischemic period slowed metabolic processes and improved tolerance to anoxia. As early as 1964, Shumway and associates achieved excellent results with this method and reported a marked reduction in operative mortality (Hurley *et al.*, 1964). At the beginning of the arrest, irrigation with 4° C. saline was done continuously over the heart and into the pericardium. Myocardial temperatures as low as 15° C. could be obtained with topical cooling alone, although regional myocardial temperature gradients tended to occur and potentially jeopardized vulnerable subendocardial tissue. The addition of topical endocardial cooling provided better transmural myocardial protection, and ischemic periods of over 2 hours were tolerated with good recovery. The principles developed by the Stanford University group are widely accepted today and constitute a major contribution to cardiac surgery.

Although chemical arrest of the heart generally had been abandoned in the early 1960s, Bretschneider (1964) continued to pursue the concept of induced cardioplegia. Using a solution with a low sodium concentration to depolarize the myocardial cells, mannitol to maintain osmolarity, and procaine to stabilize cell membranes, Bretschneider could achieve rapid arrest and preservation of tissue ATP levels for prolonged periods (Bretschneider *et al.*, 1975). Kirsch and associates (1972) developed a similar solution containing magnesium, procaine, and aspartate, which was injected into the ascending aorta as a bolus to arrest the heart. Like Bretschneider, Kirsch believed that elimination of sodium, potassium, and calcium prevented the utilization of ATP for membrane transport and slowed the decay of organic phosphate. Excellent clinical results with both of these solutions were later reported (Søndergaard *et al.*, 1975; Bleese *et al.*, 1978).

Hearse and associates at St. Thomas' Hospital in London took a slightly different approach to chemical cardioplegia. Rather than using an intracellular solution, these investigators developed a predominantly *extracellular formula* based on sodium as the primary cation (Hearse *et al.*, 1976a). Emphasis was placed on making the solution as physiologic as possible. Specific additives were included to arrest the heart and maintain membrane integrity, as will be described in subsequent sections. The extensive validation performed by this group is a model of systematic scientific investigation and constitutes one of the major advances in the area of myocardial preservation. The St. Thomas' solution has been used clinically since 1975 (Braimbridge *et al.*, 1977) and has gained widespread acceptance and application.

In 1973, Gay and Ebert reintroduced the concept of potassium cardioplegia into clinical practice. Using a solution containing 25 mM./liter of potassium chloride, they demonstrated effective protection of isolated dog hearts for up to 1 hour of normothermic ischemia. They hypothesized that direct myocardial injury with the Melrose solution had been caused by the high potassium concentration and hypertonicity. By reducing the potassium level, rapid diastolic arrest could be achieved and the tolerance of ischemia safely prolonged. Clinical experience with the infusion of cold hyperkalemic solutions subsequently has been excellent, and the combination of profound myocardial hypothermia and rapid potassium arrest has emerged as the most widely used method today.

A recent modification, introduced by Buckberg and associates, is the use of cold, hyperkalemic blood to induce and maintain cardiac arrest (Follette et al., 1978a, 1978b). The physiologic nature of blood as well as the improved buffering and oxygen transport capacity makes this technique an attractive option. Blood cardioplegia is rapidly gaining clinical application (Cunningham et al., 1979; Olin et al., 1981), and excellent results have been recently published.

SPECIFIC METHODS OF PROTECTION

Minimizing Operative Injury

Most surgeons would agree that the period of induced ischemia should be kept as short as possible by appropriate planning of the operation. Even with current methods of hypothermic cardioplegia, ischemic tissue injury progresses exponentially with time, thus emphasizing the fact that there is no substitute for an expeditiously performed procedure. With modern surgical technique, however, even the most complicated intracardiac operations can be accomplished within 90 to 120 minutes, a period of ischemia that is well tolerated with appropriate myocardial protection. Care should be taken during the operation to minimize retraction of cardiac structures, since direct damage to the heart may negate even the best method of myocardial preservation. Finally, it is becoming clear that certain commonly employed cardioplegic techniques, such as the use of Ringer's lactate infusion (Hearse et al., 1976b), can cause direct myocardial injury and compromise the beneficial effects of hypothermia and chemical arrest.

During cardiopulmonary bypass, close attention should be given to maintaining adequate coronary perfusion pressure and ensuring satisfactory transmural blood flow distribution. Ventricular distention can limit subendocardial flow and should be prevented by either venting or appropriate perfusion techniques. Ventricular fibrillation creates a continuous myocardial wall stress, which, together with increased oxygen demand, predisposes the heart to subendocardial injury (Buckberg and Hottenrott, 1975). Thus, during the procedure, periods of ventricular fibrillation should be avoided or minimized. Finally, there is no substitute for a well-performed operation. Good my-

ocardial protection combined with complete correction of the physiologic defect should give optimal operative results.

Hypothermia

Hypothermia probably remains the most important component of myocardial preservation during ischemia. The protective effects of hypothermia are related to reduction in heart rate and slowing of basal cellular metabolism (Buckberg et al., 1977). The metabolic effect diminishes energy and ATP consumption during ischemia and reduces the toxic products of metabolism such as carbon dioxide (Fig. 50–6) and hydrogen ions (Flaherty et al., 1979). Because tissue acidosis directly inhibits anaerobic metabolism and may produce ultrastructural damage (Gevers, 1977), inhibition of proton production is one of the most important considerations. In the chemically arrested, nonworking heart, oxygen consumption is reduced directly with hypothermia (Fig. 50–7), such that myocardial oxygen consumption at 10° to 20° C. is less than 5 per cent of the normal value (Chitwood et al., 1979).

Although several investigators have shown a continued beneficial decrement in oxygen consumption at temperatures below 10° C. (Shragge et al., 1978; Rosenfeldt and Arnold, 1980), there is some evidence that hypothermic injury related to cellular swelling and metabolic derangements is more likely at these

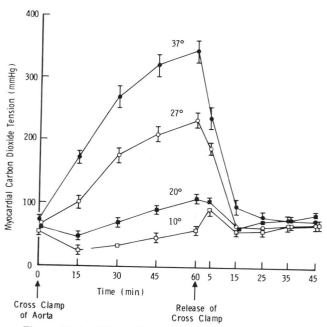

Figure 50–6. Effect of hypothermia on myocardial carbon dioxide tension during ischemic arrest of the isolated cat heart. Myocardial Pco$_2$ was measured with mass spectrometry by a probe positioned at the mid-myocardial level. (From Flaherty, J. T., et al.: Metabolic and functional effects of progressive degrees of hypothermia during global ischemia. Am. J. Physiol., 236:H839, 1979.)

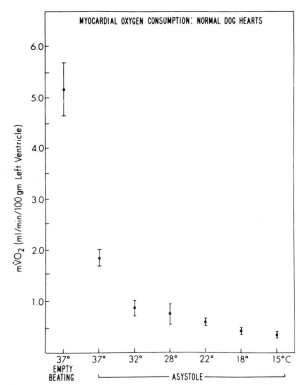

Figure 50–7. Effects of hypothermia on myocardial oxygen consumption in the potassium-arrested dog heart. (From Chitwood, W. R., et al.: The effects of hypothermia on myocardial oxygen consumption and transmural coronary blood flow in the potassium-arrested heart. Ann. Surg., 190:106, 1979.)

temperatures (Tyers et al., 1977a; Flaherty et al., 1979). However, it is extremely difficult to obtain myocardial temperatures below 10° C. in the clinical setting, and the controversies about cold injury are largely superfluous. Clearly, clinically achievable myocardial hypothermia has been shown repeatedly to be quite safe. Myocardial injury has been reported with exposure to intrapericardial ice slush (Speicher et al., 1962), and pathologic changes consistent with subepicardial coagulation necrosis have been observed experimentally. Transient phrenic nerve injury is also occasionally seen with intrapericardial slush, producing mild degrees of ventilatory impairment. Nevertheless, it is likely that in actual practice, the more effective topical hypothermia achieved throughout the procedure with a combination of cold saline and slush offsets the significance of epicardial cold injury.

Myocardial temperature can be most effectively reduced and maintained using combinations of a number of techniques. *External topical cooling* is one important method and is best accomplished by a continuous infusion of 4° C. saline at 50 to 100 ml./min. over the heart and into the pericardial cavity (Shumway et al., 1959; Hurley et al., 1964). Excess fluid is removed by a suction catheter in the inferior aspect of the incision. Placement of a corrugated rubber pad in the posterior pericardium improves the cooling of the posterior cardiac wall and diminishes

heat transmission from the aorta (Rosenfeldt and Watson, 1979; Hearse et al., 1981). The effectiveness of myocardial cooling with the topical method seems to be related to cardiac size. In large hypertrophied ventricles, cooling may be rather slow and reduction in endocardial temperature less uniform. Endocardial cooling can be facilitated by continuous or intermittent *intracavitary infusion* of cold saline either directly into the heart, as in aortic or mitral valve replacement, or through an indwelling catheter (Schachner et al., 1976; Rosenfeldt and Watson, 1979; Hearse et al., 1981).

Initial rapid induction of myocardial hypothermia is best accomplished by infusion of *cold cardioplegic solution* into the aortic root. We usually infuse 1 liter of 4° C. crystalloid solution over a 2- to 4-minute interval to achieve a measured myocardial temperature 12° to 15° C. Occasionally, with markedly hypertrophied ventricles or in the presence of a highly developed noncoronary collateral circulation, 1500 to 2000 ml. are required to produce the desired myocardial hypothermia. Recirculation of the cardioplegic fluid between infusions with a commercially available cannula system* and a roller pump has been helpful in maintaining uniform temperature of the solution.

In the presence of severe proximal coronary stenosis or occlusion, mild impairment in regional cooling can occur because of the obstruction. In this situation, the first bypass graft is usually placed to the involved vessel, and then cardioplegic solution is delivered through the graft. Reinfusion of cardioplegic solution every 20 to 30 minutes is generally performed, and most studies would support periodic reinfusion to replenish the arresting agents, to maintain myocardial hypothermia, and to wash out metabolic wastes (Nelson et al., 1976; Buckberg, 1979). Some surgeons prefer to maintain hypothermia primarily by topical cooling rather than reinfusion. Whatever the individual preference, it is likely that direct coronary infusion of cold cardioplegic solution is the preferred technique for rapid, uniform reduction of myocardial temperature.

Two other techniques are useful for maintaining hypothermia. First, increasing evidence is accumulating about the importance of *individual vena caval cannulation* (Rosenfeldt and Watson, 1979; Hearse et al., 1981). Recent data from our institution (Smith and Cox, 1981) as well as other centers indicate that significant atrial and right ventricular warming is produced by the systemic venous return (Fig. 50–8), which may contribute to postoperative atrioventricular conduction abnormalities and atrial dysrhythmias. These problems can be reduced significantly by using total cardiopulmonary bypass, perhaps combined with topical endocardial cooling (Hearse et al., 1981).

Along with bronchial blood flow and noncoronary collateral circulation, return of the systemic perfusate to the heart is probably the major source of rewarming during hypothermic arrest (Rosenfeldt and Watson, 1979). Therefore, the second technique, *profound sys-*

*DIP, Inc., Walker, Michigan.

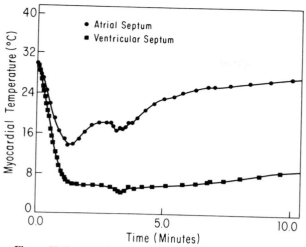

Figure 50–8. Atrial and ventricular temperature curves during cold cardioplegic arrest in a patient undergoing coronary artery bypass grafting. Temperatures were measured with implanted thermistors for 10 minutes after infusion of 800 ml. of 4°C. crystalloid solution into the aortic root. Systemic perfusate temperature was 30°C., and a single venous cannula was used in the right atrial appendage. Note that the atrial septum cooled less and rewarmed faster than the ventricular septum. The second inflection was produced by topical 4°C. saline. (Data reproduced from unpublished work of Drs. Peter K. Smith and James L. Cox.)

temic hypothermia, is highly effective in minimizing rewarming during the period of aortic occlusion (Fig. 50–9) (Conti *et al.*, 1978; Grover *et al.*, 1981). Our practice is to lower systemic perfusate temperature to 20° to 24° C. when the aorta is occluded and to begin rewarming 5 minutes before release of the aortic

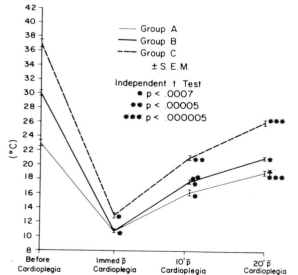

Figure 50–9. Effects of lowering systemic perfusate temperature on myocardial rewarming. Ventricular septal temperature (°C.) was measured after infusion of 4°C. potassium cardioplegic solution into the aortic root. In Group A, systemic perfusate temperature was maintained at 23°C., in Group B at 30°C., and in Group C at 37°C. Lowering systemic perfusate temperature reduced the rate of myocardial rewarming. (From Grover, F. L., *et al.*: Does lower systemic temperature enhance cardioplegic myocardial protection? J. Thorac. Cardiovasc. Surg., *81*:11, 1981.)

clamp. Although used originally in coronary bypass operations, systemic hypothermia to this level during the ischemic period has been extended in our practice to most cardiac procedures.

An additional advantage of this technique is reduction in *total* body oxygen requirement. Below core temperatures of 30° C., systemic flow can be reduced by half, which is effective in decreasing noncoronary collateral blood flow (Hurley *et al.*, 1964; Hearse *et al.*, 1981). Therefore, coronary washout of cardioplegic solution and rewarming by this mechanism can be minimized. One disadvantage of profound hypothermia is that core temperature is lowered progressively with the length of aortic occlusion, and the period of rewarming can be long. However, longer rewarming may have inherent advantages because of a longer obligatory reperfusion of the coronary circulation. Thus, for simple operations such as double coronary bypass or mitral valve replacement with 20- to 35-minute ischemic times, rewarming usually can be accomplished within 15 to 20 minutes. Procedures with longer ischemic times require 30 to 45 minutes for rewarming, which may be beneficial for recovery from longer periods of cardioplegic arrest.

A slower induction of myocardial hypothermia by coronary perfusion with cold blood from the pump-oxygenator without chemical arrest is probably not advisable. During cooling, strong myocardial contraction or fibrillation occurs, which can increase the oxygen demand beyond supply and deplete energy stores in the prearrest period (Hearse *et al.*, 1981; Nordbeck *et al.*, 1974; Archie and Kirklin, 1973). Therefore, it is probably better to arrest the heart suddenly with cold cardioplegic solution from a temperature of around 32° C. in the empty beating state. Finally, it should be emphasized that the full energy-sparing effects of hypothermia are only realized in conjunction with rapid chemical arrest of the myocardium at the onset of ischemia.

Cardioplegic Additives

Rapid diastolic arrest can be achieved with a number of chemical components. Perhaps the most widely used technique at present is potassium arrest. High extracellular potassium reduces the transmembrane potassium gradient, depolarizes the cell, and eliminates the energy cost of maintaining membrane gradients and myocardial work. The concentration of potassium is critical, with 15 to 20 mM./liter achieving optimal results in most studies (Hearse *et al.*, 1975; Tyers, 1975). It should be remembered that *high* concentrations of potassium (such as are present in the Melrose solution) are associated with myocardial contracture and other forms of injury. Conversely, lower concentrations of potassium are less effective in producing immediate arrest. There is evidence that potassium levels in the range of 25 to 30 mM./liter may be necessary with blood cardioplegia (Buckberg, 1979).

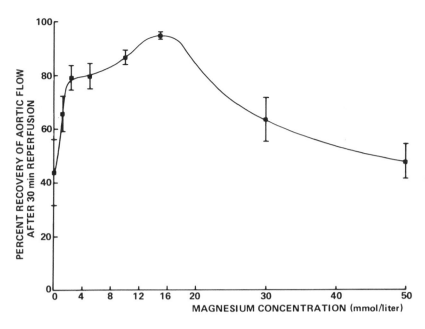

Figure 50–10. Hypothermic dose response curve for magnesium in the ischemic isolated rat heart. After a 2-minute infusion with magnesium concentrations of 0 to 50 mmol./liter, the hearts were subjected to 70 minutes of ischemia at 28°C. Recovery of aortic flow was measured after 20 minutes of reperfusion. (From Hearse, D. J., *et al.*: Myocardial protection during ischemic cardiac arrest. The importance of magnesium in cardioplegic infusates. J. Thorac. Cardiovasc. Surg., *75*:877, 1978.)

Magnesium is a major intracellular cation contained primarily within mitrochondria and myofibrils. On the cell membrane, magnesium competes for calcium receptor sites and delays calcium influx into the cell. It is an important component of high-energy phosphate molecules and a cofactor for cellular enzyme systems. When used to induce arrest, magnesium seems to inhibit excitation-contraction coupling, although it is not a very good arresting agent because of its slow onset of action. Absence of magnesium during ischemia or reperfusion can impair synthesis of ATP. Therefore, it seems preferable to include magnesium in most crystalloid cardioplegic solutions. During the ischemic interval, magnesium concentrations in the range of 15 to 20 mM./liter provide the best protection in isolated rat heart systems (Fig. 50–10) (Hearse *et al*, 1978b). Although there are theoretical problems with isolated rat heart experiments, such as possible species differences with man and the artificial nature of the perfusion technique, these preparations are, in many ways, the most valid for studying pure myocardial drug effects because of the highly controllable nature of the experimental design. Therefore, isolated rat heart data as shown in Figure 50–10 are extremely important and have direct relevance to clinical practice.

Calcium is an essential component of actin-myosin interaction and contributes importantly to the regulation of myocardial contraction (Katz, 1977). Calcium also is required for maintenance of membrane integrity and numerous intracellular functions. Because intracellular calcium deposition plays a significant role in ischemic and reperfusion injury (Shen and Jennings, 1972), extracellular calcium should be carefully regulated during cardioplegic arrest. Reduction in calcium has been shown to diminish the cellular influx associated with ischemic injury and to improve functional recovery (Hearse *et al.*, 1977). Myocardial perfusion with calcium-free solutions can produce cardioplegia by limiting calcium availability for my-

ocardial contraction. In fact, hypocalcemia is a necessary component of the Bretschneider technique (Bretschneider *et al.*, 1975). Minute quantities of calcium, however, are essential for maintenance of cellular integrity. Ischemic arrest of isolated myocardium with calcium-free solutions is associated with severe reperfusion injury upon re-exposure to calcium, probably on the basis of altered membrane permeability and massive cellular influx of calcium (Zimmerman *et al.*, 1967). The magnitude of this "calcium paradox" can be reduced by hypothermia and is influenced to some extent by the severity of the ischemic insult. In the *in vivo* situation, calcium paradox may not be a major factor, because small amounts of calcium are provided to the myocardium through the noncoronary collateral circulation. However, maintaining a minimal concentration of calcium is probably useful in any cardioplegic formulation (Jynge *et al.*, 1977).

The availability of calcium during the ischemic period can be diminished in a number of ways. First, in crystalloid solutions, the concentration of calcium can be reduced to the range of 0.5 to 1.0 mM./liter, which has been shown to be beneficial in numerous studies (Hearse *et al.*, 1981). When blood cardioplegia is used, calcium in the blood can be chelated with small amounts of citrate (Follette *et al.*, 1978a). Cellular calcium influx can be limited by cardioplegic additives such as magnesium and procaine (Hearse *et al.*, 1981). Finally, slow channel calcium-blocking agents are under investigation in a number of centers (Lowe *et al.*, 1977; Robb-Nicholson *et al.*, 1978; Clark *et al.*, 1981). These drugs selectively inhibit the sarcolemmal slow calcium channel and prevent cellular calcium accumulation and degradation of ATP. They can be used to induce and maintain cardiac arrest either singly or in combination with other agents. Although quite effective in preventing ischemic and reperfusion injury, the clinical application of the slow channel blockers may be limited by the prolonged myocardial depression that occurs following reperfu-

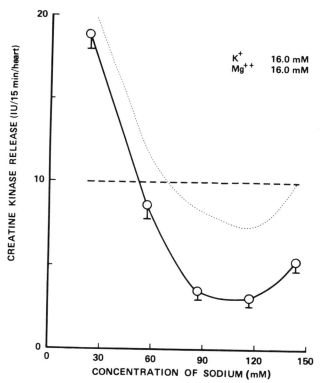

Figure 50–11. Effect of sodium concentration on the patterns of ischemic injury in the isolated rat heart. Protection against 30 minutes of normothermic ischemic arrest was best with sodium concentrations of 100 to 130 mmol./liter. The dotted line indicates enzyme leakage if magnesium and potassium were at their normal levels of 1.2 and 5.9 mmol./liter, respectively. (From Hearse, D. J., et al.: Protection of the Ischemic Myocardium: Cardioplegia. New York, Raven Press, 1981.)

sion. It is also not clear how much additional protection is afforded by these agents beyond that provided by currently utilized crystalloid cardioplegia techniques.

The optimal concentration of sodium to be used in cardioplegic solutions has been a subject of controversy. The formulations of Bretschneider and Kirsch are based on an *intracellular* composition with little or no sodium in the solutions (Kirsch *et al.*, 1972; Bretschneider *et al.*, 1975). Sudden sodium depletion rapidly arrests the heart because of elimination of transmembrane gradients and cell depolarization. However, arrest by sodium depletion favors influx of calcium into the cell, and strict control or elimination of calcium with this technique is essential. Most now favor physiologic *extracellular* sodium concentrations, based on the data from the group at St. Thomas' Hospital and others (Hearse *et al.*, 1981; Tyers *et al.*, 1977b). As with magnesium, one protective effect of sodium is exerted through its control of intracellular calcium movement. Sodium concentrations in the range of 100 to 130 mM./liter are associated with the best protection of isolated myocardium when used in conjunction with hyperkalemic arrest (Fig. 50–11). Extensive clinical experience with extracellular cardioplegic solutions has been very favorable.

Local anesthetic agents have been used for car-

dioplegia for many years. Procaine has received extensive evaluation, especially in Europe, and constitutes a major protective component of the Bretschneider solution (Bretschneider, 1964). These agents induce cardiac arrest by blocking the sodium channel of the sarcolemma and also afford protection by inhibiting the cellular influx of calcium. Inclusion of local anesthetics in cardioplegic solutions may diminish the incidence of ventricular dysrhythmias in the early reperfusion period and thereby improve myocardial oxygen supply/demand ratios and high-energy phosphate levels. When used with hyperkalemic extracellular solutions, procaine or lidocaine concentrations in the range of 0.05 to 1.0 mM./liter have proved most effective in isolated heart studies (Hearse *et al.*, in press).

Buffering

As discussed previously, tissue acidosis during ischemia inhibits anaerobic metabolism and can produce direct myocardial injury. Therefore, maintenance of appropriate pH is important for repletion of ATP and for sustaining low levels of cellular function. Hydrogen ions are produced continuously during the ischemic period, so that a stable source of buffering is required. In most cardioplegic formulations, pH is carefully controlled by the addition of specific buffering systems. The choice of cardioplegic buffers varies, but most clinically tested solutions utilize bicarbonate, phosphate, or TRIS as the major buffering component. Lactate should be avoided because of its poor buffering capacity and because lactate inhibits anaerobic metabolism independent of pH (Tyers *et al.*, 1975; Hearse *et al.*, 1976a).

Available information suggests that cellular function during hypothermia is best maintained with a slightly alkaline pH (Rahn *et al.*, 1975; White, 1981; Becker *et al.*, 1981). Normally, when blood is cooled, pH increases approximately 0.15 per 10° C. of hypothermia (Rosenthal, 1948). Thus, at temperatures below 20° C., cellular pH in excess of 7.70 may be necessary. This concept is further substantiated by the observation that the pH of poikilothermic animals increases to about 7.8 with hypothermia. Although more investigation is needed, recovery of myocardial function has been better when a pH of 7.6 to 7.8 was maintained (Follette *et al.*, 1981). Most investigators currently recommend appropriate composition and buffering of cardioplegic solutions to maintain pH in the alkaline range of normal.

TABLE 50–1. BLOOD CARDIOPLEGIA

CONSTITUENT	CONCENTRATION
Autologous blood	1000 ml.
TRIS buffer (0.3 moles/liter)	50 ml.
CPD solution	20 ml.
Potassium chloride	30 mM./liter
Ionized calcium	0.3 mM./liter

355 mOsm./kg. of H_2O; pH — 7.7; hematocrit — 20%

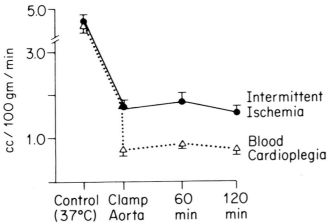

Figure 50–12. Myocardial oxygen consumption during 2 hours of aortic clamping in the dog. Oxygen requirement was lower in the potassium-arrested cold-blood cardioplegia group (dashed line) than in the hearts receiving 20-minute reinfusions of unmodified cold blood. (From Follette, D. M., *et al.*: Advantages of intermittent blood cardioplegia over intermittent ischemia during prolonged hypothermic aortic clamping. Circulation, *58* (Suppl. 1):200, 1978.)

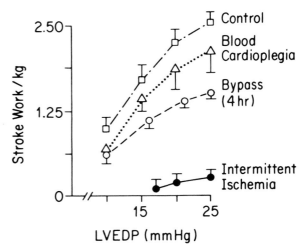

Figure 50–13. Work function after 2 hours of ischemic arrest with potassium cold-blood cardioplegia was minimally depressed from control. Function was severely diminished with unmodified cold-blood reinfusion and moderately depressed after 4 hours of cardiopulmonary bypass without ischemia. (From Follette, D. M., *et al.*: Advantages of intermittent blood cardioplegia over intermittent ischemia during prolonged hypothermic aortic clamping. Circulation, *58* (Suppl. 1):200, 1978.)

Osmolarity

Cellular swelling and myocardial edema consistently accompany ischemic injury (Leaf, 1970). The primary mechanisms responsible seem to be altered cellular energetics and permeability related to the ischemic state (MacKnight and Leaf, 1977; Lee *et al.*, 1980). Thus, one important aspect of minimizing water gain is the efficacy of myocardial protection, with less edema occurring in well-protected hearts. The osmolarity of the perfusate also influences myocardial edema, and hearts perfused with hypotonic solutions rapidly gain water (Foglia *et al.*, 1979). Conversely, hyperosmotic formulations in excess of 400 mOsm./kg. of H_2O produce myocardial dehydration and impair functional recovery (Wildenthal *et al.*, 1969; Hearse *et al.*, 1978a). Although the direct influence of minor degrees of cellular edema on ultimate functional recovery is unclear, most would recommend slightly hyperosmolar cardioplegic solutions at present. The

importance of oncotic agents such as albumin in preventing myocardial edema is controversial and requires further investigation.

Blood Cardioplegia

The concept of using blood as the vehicle for cardioplegic arrest was reintroduced by Buckberg and associates (Follette *et al.*, 1978a, 1978b). Blood is diluted to a hematocrit of 20 per cent with cardioplegic solution such that the final potassium concentration is 25 to 30 mM./liter. TRIS buffer is used to adjust the pH to 7.8, and citrate is added to reduce the ionized calcium to 0.3 mM./liter (Table 50–1). The solution is oxygenated, cooled, and delivered through standard cannulas. Initially, 500 to 750 ml. are administered at 16° to 20° C., and then 250 ml. are reinfused every 20

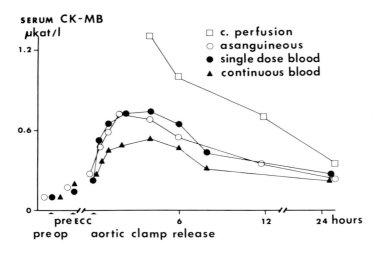

Figure 50–14. Serum CK-MB concentrations after aortic valve replacement with several myocardial protection techniques. Direct coronary perfusion was associated with the greatest myocardial injury and continuous blood cardioplegia with the least myocardial injury. (From Olin, C. L., *et al.*: Myocardial protection during aortic valve replacement: Comparison of different methods by intraoperative coronary sinus blood sampling and postoperative serial serum enzyme determinations. J. Thorac. Cardiovasc. Surg., *82*:837, 1981.)

TABLE 50–2. BRETSCHNEIDER'S CARDIOPLEGIC SOLUTION NUMBER 3

CONSTITUENT	CONCENTRATION
Sodium chloride	12.0 mM./liter
Potassium chloride	10.0 mM./liter
Magnesium chloride	2.0 mM./liter
Procaine chloride	7.4 mM./liter
Mannitol	239.0 mM./liter

320 mOsm./kg. of H_2O; pH — 5.5–7.0

TABLE 50–4. CRAVER'S CARDIOPLEGIC SOLUTION

CONSTITUENT	CONCENTRATION
Sodium chloride	154.0 mM./liter
Potassium chloride	25.0 mM./liter
Sodium bicarbonate	11.0 mM./liter
Dextrose	11.1 mM./liter

391 mOsm./kg. of H_2O; pH —7.5

minutes. Before releasing the aortic clamp, 500 to 750 ml. of 37° C. blood cardioplegic solution are infused to warm and reoxygenate the heart while maintaining arrest (Follette et al., 1981).

When used in this manner, blood cardioplegia has several advantages. Blood is the most physiologic of all solutions. The heart is arrested while being oxygenated, so that ATP is not depleted prior to asystole. Reinfusion of oxygenated blood provides a source of oxygen for continued metabolism and ATP repletion during the period of hypothermic arrest. Although little oxygen is released from hemoglobin during hypothermia, enough is probably dissolved in the plasma to sustain metabolism when reinfusion is performed every 20 minutes. Reinfusing the solution maintains myocardial hypothermia, washes out waste products, and provides metabolic substrate. Initial concerns about rouleaux formation, blood sludging, and inequalities of perfusion have not proved significant; hyperkalemia maintains chemical arrest with its inherently lower metabolic requirements (Fig. 50–12). Formulation of the blood from the oxygenator is simple, and hemodilution is usually not significant, unlike certain asanguineous cardioplegic techniques. The buffering and oncotic characteristics of blood are excellent. Trace metals, cofactors, hormones, or other as yet undefined but important constituents are provided. Finally, reperfusion with alkalotic, hyperkalemic, hypocalcemic blood is facilitated with this system, minimizing fibrillation and reperfusion injury and providing a source of oxygen during the initial rewarming period (Follette et al., 1981).

Clinical experience with blood cardioplegia has been excellent. Follette and associates (1978b) reduced the perioperative myocardial infarction rate from 6.4 per cent with intermittent ischemia to 1.3 per cent with blood cardioplegia. Myocardial function was improved experimentally (Fig. 50–13), and the operative mortality diminished. Similar results have been reported by Culliford and associates (1980), who also noted good preservation of myocardial ultrastructure and ATP. These authors indicated that the "safe" aortic clamping time was extended beyond 2 hours with this technique. Barner and colleagues (1981) confirmed these findings, and recently, Olin and associates (1981) infused blood cardioplegic solution almost continuously at low flow rates during the arrest period. Myocardial enzyme release (Fig. 50–14) and metabolic parameters were improved with continuous blood cardioplegia as compared with coronary perfusion or asanguineous solutions. Thus, blood cardioplegia may offer distinct advantages in certain clinical situations and is apt to be modified and improved in future years.

CARDIOPLEGIC SOLUTIONS

Chemical cardioplegia, as reintroduced by Bretschneider (1964), utilized a low-sodium, calcium-free, procaine solution to achieve rapid diastolic arrest. The constituents of this solution as used clinically by Søndergaard and coworkers (1975) are shown in Table 50–2. The heart was precooled with a liter of 4° C. blood before slow infusion of the solution to achieve diastolic arrest. The relatively high concentration of procaine was the major protective component of this solution. A low-sodium, calcium-free solution, with added potassium, magnesium, and TRIS as the buffer, is used clinically at the University of California, San Francisco, with good results (Roe et al., 1977) (Table 50–3).

Craver's solution (Craver et al., 1978) (Table 50–4) and Tyers' solution (Tyers et al., 1977b) (Table 50–5) are both formulated with extracellular sodium

TABLE 50–3. ROE'S CARDIOPLEGIC SOLUTION

CONSTITUENT	CONCENTRATION
Sodium chloride	27.0 mM./liter
Potassium chloride	20.0 mM./liter
Magnesium chloride	1.5 mM./liter
TRIS buffer	1.0 mM./liter

347 mOsm./kg. of H_2O; pH — 7.6

TABLE 50–5. TYERS' CARDIOPLEGIC SOLUTION

CONSTITUENT	CONCENTRATION
Sodium	138.0 mM./liter
Chloride	98.0 mM./liter
Potassium	25.0 mM./liter
Bicarbonate	20.0 mM./liter
Magnesium	1.5 mM./liter
Calcium	0.5 mM./liter
Acetate	27.0 mM./liter
Gluconate	23.0 mM./liter

275 mOsm./kg. of H_2O; pH — 7.8

TABLE 50–6. BIRMINGHAM SOLUTION

CONSTITUENT	CONCENTRATION
Sodium	100.0 mM./liter
Potassium	30.0 mM./liter
Chloride	84.0 mM./liter
Bicarbonate	28.0 mM./liter
Calcium	0.7 mM./liter
Glucose	27.7 mM./liter
Albumin	50.0 mM./liter
Mannitol	27.5 mM./liter

300–385 mOsm./kg. of H O; pH — 7.5

concentrations and use potassium to arrest the heart. Both have the advantage of being simple modifications of readily available intravenous solutions (normal saline and Normosol pH 7.4, respectively). Tyers' solution also contains magnesium and low concentrations of calcium, which are probably beneficial. Buffering is accomplished with bicarbonate, acetate, and gluconate. We utilize Tyers' solution clinically and have been quite pleased with the results.

Birmingham solution (Table 50–6) is also an extracellular formulation using potassium to achieve arrest (Conti et al., 1978). Bicarbonate is the predominant buffer, and small concentrations of calcium are added to prevent calcium paradox. The solution contains albumin for oncotic purposes, and a large clinical experience with this formulation has been favorable.

The components of St. Thomas' solution are presented in Table 50–7. Every facet of its formulation has been validated in the isolated rat heart (see previous sections), and from a proved physiologic point of view, this may well be the best cardioplegic solution currently available. Concentrations of sodium, potassium, and magnesium are optimal for prolonged chemical protection. It is buffered with bicarbonate, and lidocaine is usually added to improve electrical stability of the heart.

In summary, most currently utilized cold chemical cardioplegic techniques utilize buffered extracellular solutions as a vehicle for hyperkalemic arrest. Most are slightly hyperosmolar and contain small concentrations of calcium. Magnesium, procaine, or lidocaine can be used for additional protection. Oxygen delivery during the ischemic period can be accomplished with blood cardioplegia. Although the exact concentrations of the components are quite variable, these basic concepts are common to most current methods of intraoperative myocardial preservation.

TABLE 50–7. ST. THOMAS' CARDIOPLEGIC SOLUTION

CONSTITUENT	CONCENTRATION
Sodium chloride	110.0 mM./liter
Potassium chloride	16.0 mM./liter
Magnesium chloride	16.0 mM./liter
Calcium chloride	1.2 mM./liter
Sodium bicarbonate	10.0 mM./liter
Lidocaine	1.0 mM./liter

324 mOsm./kg. of H_2O; pH — 7.8

SELECTED REFERENCES

Berne, R. M., and Rubio, R.: Coronary circulation. In Handbook of Physiology. Bethesda, Maryland, American Physiological Society. 1979, Vol. I, pp. 873–952.

A comprehensive review of the physiology of coronary blood flow by two outstanding authorities.

Braunwald, E. (Ed.): Symposium on myocardial metabolism. Proceedings of a symposium held in Ponte Vedra, Florida, November 4–6, 1973. American Heart Association Monograph No. 44. Circ. Res., 34, 35 (Suppl. 3):1, 1974.

This is an outstanding collection of contributions from a number of basic workers in the field of myocardial metabolism with a broad coverage of the entire subject.

Follette, D. M., Fey, K., Mulder, D., Maloney, J. V., and Buckberg, G. D.: Advantages of blood cardioplegia over intermittent ischemia during prolonged hypothermic aortic clamping. Circulation, 58 (Suppl. 1):200, 1978.

This is the original work on blood cardioplegia upon which clinical application has been based.

Gay, W. A., and Ebert, P. A.: Functional, metabolic and morphologic effects of potassium-induced cardioplegia. Surgery, 74:284, 1973.

This paper was responsible for reintroducing potassium cardioplegia into clinical practice. The work is not only a major contribution but also a model of simplicity and innovation.

Gregg, D. E.: The natural history of coronary collateral development. Circ. Res., 35:335, 1974.

This is a classic analysis of the natural history of development of coronary collaterals written by the physiologist who has probably contributed more to the basic understanding of the coronary circulation than any other investigator. This issue of Circulation Research is devoted to a variety of aspects of myocardial metabolism and contains numerous other contributions relative to the coronary circulation.

Hearse, D. J., Braimbridge, M. V., and Jynge, P.: Protection of the Ischemic Myocardium: Cardioplegia. New York, Raven Press, 1981.

This is the definitive work on myocardial preservation, with emphasis on both basic science and practical surgical technique. The world literature on this subject is reviewed and analyzed by the investigators from St. Thomas' Hospital, London.

Sabiston, D. C., Jr.: The coronary circulation. The William F. Rienhoff, Jr. Lecture, Johns Hopkins Med. J., 134:314, 1974.

This is a review of the anatomy, physiology, and pathologic aspects of the coronary circulation. The data presented are based on experimental and clinical findings in the normal and pathologic coronary circulation.

REFERENCES

Archie, J. P., and Kirklin, J. W.: Effect of hypothermic perfusion on myocardial oxygen consumption and coronary resistance. Surg. Forum, 24:186, 1973.
Bache, R. J., Cobb, R. F., and Greenfield, J. C., Jr.: Myocardial blood flow distribution during ischemia-induced coronary vasodilation in the unanesthetized dog. J. Clin. Invest., 54:1462, 1974.
Barner, H. B., Kaiser, G. C., Codd, J. E., Tyras, D. H., Pennington, D. G., Laks, H., and Willman, V. L.: Clinical experience

with cold blood as the vehicle for hypothermic potassium cardioplegia. Ann. Thorac. Surg., 29:224, 1981.

Barratt-Boyes, B. G., Simpson, M., and Neutze, J. M.: Intracardiac surgery in neonates and infants using deep hypothermia, surface cooling, and limited cardiopulmonary bypass. Circulation, 43,44(Suppl. 1):25, 1971.

Becker, H., Vinten-Johansen, J., Buckberg, G. D., Robertson, J. M., Leaf, J. D., Lazar, H. L., and Manganaro, A. J.: Myocardial damage caused by keeping pH 7.40 during systemic deep hypothermia. J. Thorac. Cardiovasc. Surg., 81:810, 1981.

Berne, R. M., and Rubio, R.: Coronary circulation. In Handbook of Physiology. Bethesda, Maryland, American Physiological Society, 1979, Vol. I, pp. 873–952.

Bigelow, W. G., Mustard, W. T., and Evans, J. G.: Some physiologic concepts of hypothermia and their application to cardiac surgery. J. Thorac. Cardiovasc. Surg., 28:463, 1954.

Bleese, N., Doring, V., Kalmar, P., Pokar, H., Polonium, M. J., Steiner, D., and Rodewald, G.: Intraoperative myocardial protection by cardioplegia in hypothermia: Clinical findings. J. Thorac. Cardiovasc. Surg., 75:405, 1978.

Braimbridge, M. V., Chayen, J., Bitensky, L., Hearse, D. J., Jynge, P., and Cankovic-Darracott, S.: Cold cardioplegia or continuous coronary perfusion? Report on preliminary clinical experience as assessed cytochemically. J. Thorac. Cardiovasc. Surg., 74:900, 1977.

Braunwald, E. (Ed.): Symposium on myocardial metabolism. Proceedings of a symposium held in Ponte Vedra, Florida, November 4–6, 1973. American Heart Association Monograph No. 44. Circ. Res., 34,35(Suppl. 3):1, 1974.

Bretschneider, H. J.: Überlebenszeit und Wiederbelebungszeit des Herzens bei Normo-und Hypothermie. Verh. Dtsch. Ges. Kreislaufforsch., 30:11, 1964.

Bretschneider, H. J., Hubner, G., Knoll, D., Lohr, B., Nordbeck, H., and Spieckermann, P. G.: Myocardial resistance and tolerance to ischemia: Physiological and biochemical basis. J. Cardiovasc. Surg., 16:241, 1975.

Brock, R. C., and Ross, D. N.: Hypothermia. III: Clinical application of hypothermic techniques. Guy's Hosp. Rep., 104:99, 1955.

Buckberg, G. D.: A proposed "solution" to the cardioplegic controversy. J. Thorac. Cardiovasc. Surg., 77:803, 1979.

Buckberg, G. D., and Hottenrott, C. E.: Ventricular fibrillation: Its effect on myocardial flow, distribution and performance. Ann. Thorac. Surg., 20:76, 1975.

Buckberg, G. D., Fixler, D. E., Archie, J. P., and Hoffman, J. I. E.: Experimental subendocardial ischemia in dogs with normal coronary arteries. Circ. Res., 30:67, 1972a.

Buckberg, G. D., Towers, B., Paglia, D. E., Mulder, D. G., and Maloney, J. V., Jr.: Subendocardial ischemia after cardiopulmonary bypass. J. Thorac. Cardiovasc. Surg., 64:669, 1972b.

Buckberg, G. D., Brazier, J. R., Nelson, R. H., Goldstein, S. M., McConnell, D. H., and Cooner, N.: Studies on the effects of hypothermia on regional myocardial blood flow and metabolism during cardiopulmonary bypass. I. The adequately perfused beating, fibrillating, and arrested heart. J. Thorac. Cardiovasc. Surg., 73:87, 1977.

Chitwood, W. R., Sink, J. D., Hill, R. C., Wechsler, A. S., and Sabiston, D. C., Jr.: The effects of hypothermia on myocardial oxygen consumption and transmural coronary blood flow in the potassium-arrested heart. Ann. Surg., 190:106, 1979.

Clark, R. E., Christlieb, I. Y., Ferguson, T. B., Weldon, C. S., Marbarger, J. P., Biello, D. R., Roberts, R., Ludbrook, P. A., and Sobel, B. E.: The first American clinical trial of nifedipine in cardioplegia: A report of the first 12 months experience. J. Thorac. Cardiovasc. Surg., 82:848, 1981.

Conti, V. R., Bertranou, E. G., Blackstone, E. H., Kirklin, J. W., and Digerness, S. B.: Cold cardioplegia versus hypothermia for myocardial protection: Randomized clinical study. J. Thorac. Cardiovasc. Surg., 76:577, 1978.

Cooley, D. A., Reul, G. J., and Wukasch, D. C.: Ischemic contracture of the heart: "Stone heart." Am. J. Cardiol., 29:575, 1972.

Craver, J. M., Sams, A. B., and Hatcher, C. R.: Potassium-induced cardioplegia: Additive protection against ischemic myocardial injury during coronary revascularization. J. Thorac. Cardiovasc. Surg., 76:24, 1978.

Crawford, E. S., and Saleh, S. A.: Transverse aortic arch aneurysm: Improved results of treatment employing new modifications of aortic reconstruction and hypothermic cerebral circulatory arrest. Ann. Surg., 194:180, 1981.

Culliford, A. T., Cunningham, J. N., Jr., Adams, P. X., Isom, O. W., and Spencer, F. C.: Clinical experience with potassium cold blood cardioplegia at New York University Medical Center. In Surgery for the Complications of Myocardial Infarction. Edited by J. M. Moran and L. L. Michaelis. New York, Grune and Stratton, 1980, pp. 119–134.

Cunningham, J. N., Jr., Adams, P. X., Knopp, E. A., Baumann, F. G., Snively, S. L., Gross, R. I., Nathan, I. M., and Spencer, F. C.: Preservation of ATP, ultrastructure, and ventricular function after aortic crossclamping and reperfusion: Clinical use of blood potassium cardioplegia. J. Thorac. Cardiovasc. Surg., 78:708, 1979.

Drew, C. E., and Anderson, I. M.: Profound hypothermia in cardiac surgery: Report of 3 cases. Lancet, 1:748, 1959.

Flaherty, J. T., Schaffy, H. V., Goldman, R. A., and Gott, V. L.: Metabolic and functional effects of progressive degrees of hypothermia during global ischemia. Am. J. Physiol., 236:H839, 1979.

Foglia, R. P., Steed, D. L., Follette, D. M., Deland, E., and Buckberg, G. D.: Iatrogenic myocardial edema with potassium cardioplegia. J. Thorac. Cardiovasc. Surg., 78:217, 1979.

Follette, D. M., Fey, K., Mulder, D., Maloney, J. V., and Buckberg, G. D.: Advantages of blood cardioplegia over continuous coronary perfusion or intermittent ischemia: Experimental and clinical study. J. Thorac. Cardiovasc. Surg., 76:604, 1978a.

Follette, D. M., Steed, D. L., Foglia, R., Fey, K., and Buckberg, G. D.: Advantages of intermittent blood cardioplegia over intermittent ischemia during prolonged hypothermic aortic clamping. Circulation, 58(Suppl. 1):200, 1978b.

Follette, D. M., Fey, K., Buckberg, G. D., Helly, J. J., Jr., Steed, D. L., Foglia, R. P., and Maloney, J. V., Jr.: Reducing postischemic damage by temporary modification of reperfusate calcium, potassium, pH, and osmolarity. J. Thorac. Cardiovasc. Surg., 82:221, 1981.

Gay, W. A., and Ebert, P. A.: Functional, metabolic and morphologic effects of potassium-induced cardioplegia. Surgery, 74:284, 1973.

Gevers, W.: Generation of protons by metabolic processes in heart cells. J. Mol. Cell. Cardiol., 9:867, 1977.

Gregg, D. E.: The natural history of coronary collateral development. Circ. Res., 35:335, 1974.

Grover, F. L., Fewel, J. G., Ghidoni, J. J., and Trinkle, J. K.: Does lower systemic temperature enhance cardioplegic myocardial protection? J. Thorac. Cardiovasc. Surg., 81:11, 1981.

Hearse, D. J., Braimbridge, M. V., Jynge, P.: Protection of the Ischemic Myocardium: Cardioplegia. New York, Raven Press, 1981.

Hearse, D. J., Garlick, P. B., and Humphrey, S. M.: Ischemic contracture of the myocardium: Mechanisms and prevention. Am. J. Cardiol., 39:986, 1977.

Hearse, D. J., O'Brien, K., and Braimbridge, M. V.: Protection of the myocardium during ischemic arrest: Dose-response curves for procaine and lignocaine solutions. J. Thorac. Cardiovasc. Surg., in press.

Hearse, D. J., Stewart, D. A., and Braimbridge, M. V.: Hypothermic arrest and potassium arrest, metabolic and myocardial protection during elective cardiac arrest. Circ. Res., 36:481, 1975.

Hearse, D. J., Stewart, D. A., and Braimbridge, M. V.: Cellular protection during myocardial ischemia: The development and characterization of a procedure for the induction of reversible ischemic arrest. Circulation, 54:193, 1976a.

Hearse, D. J., Stewart, D. A., and Braimbridge, M. V.: Myocardial protection during bypass and arrest: A possible hazard with lactate-containing infusates. J. Thorac. Cardiovasc. Surg., 72:880, 1976b.

Hearse, D. J., Stewart, D. A., and Braimbridge, M. V.: Myocardial protection during ischemic cardiac arrest. Possible deleterious effects of glucose and mannitol in coronary infusates. J. Thorac. Cardiovasc. Surg., 76:16, 1978a.

Hearse, D. J., Stewart, D. A., and Braimbridge, M. V.: Myocardial protection during ischemic cardiac arrest. The importance of magnesium in cardioplegic infusates. J. Thorac. Cardiovasc. Surg., 75:877, 1978b.

Helmsworth, J. A., Kaplan, S., Clark, L. C., Jr., McAdams, A. J., Matthews, E. C., and Edwards, F. K.: Myocardial injury associated with asystole induced with potassium citrate. Ann. Surg., 149:200, 1959.

Henson, D. E., Najafi, H., Callaghan, R., Coogan, P., and Julian, O.: Myocardial lesions following open heart surgery. Arch. Pathol., 88:423, 1969.

Hurley, E. J., Lower, R. R., Dong, E., Jr., Pillsbury, R. C., and Shumway, N. E.: Clinical experience with local hypothermia in elective cardiac arrest. J. Thorac. Cardiovasc. Surg., 47:50, 1964.

Jennings, R. B., and Ganote, C. E.: Structural changes in myocardium during acute ischemia. Circ. Res., 34,35(Suppl. 3):156, 1974.

Jynge, P., Hearse, D. J., and Braimbridge, M. V.: Myocardial protection during ischemic cardiac arrest. A possible hazard with calcium-free cardioplegic infusates. J. Thorac. Cardiovasc. Surg., 73:848, 1977.

Katz, A. M.: Physiology of the Heart. New York, Raven Press, 1977.

Kirsch, U., Rodewald, G., and Kalmar, P.: Induced ischemic arrest. J. Thorac. Cardiovasc. Surg., 63:121, 1972.

Leaf, A.: Regulation of intracellular fluid volume and disease. Am. J. Med., 49:291, 1970.

Lee, B. Y., Wilson, G. J., Domnech, R. J., and MacGregor, D. C.: Relative roles of edema versus contracture in the myocardial "no-reflow" phenomenon. J. Surg. Res., 29:50, 1980.

Lewis, F. J., and Taufic, M.: Closure of atrial septal defects with the aid of hypothermia: Experimental accomplishments and the report of one successful case. Surgery, 33:52, 1953.

Lowe, J. E., Kleinman, L. H., Reimer, K. A., Jennings, R. B., and Wechsler, A. S.: Effects of cardioplegia produced by calcium flux inhibition. Surg. Forum, 28:279, 1977.

MacKnight, A. C., and Leaf, A.: Regulation of cellular volume. Physiol. Rev., 57:510, 1977.

McFarland, J. A., Thomas, L. B., Gilbert, J. W., and Morrow, A. G.: Myocardial necrosis following elective cardiac arrest induced with potassium citrate. J. Thorac. Cardiovasc. Surg., 40:200, 1960.

Melrose, D. G.: Elective cardiac arrest: Historical perspective. In Modern Cardiac Surgery. Edited by D. Longmore. Baltimore, Maryland, University Park Press, 1978, pp. 271–275.

Melrose, D. G., Dreyer, B., Bentall, H. H., and Baker, J. B. E.: Elective cardiac arrest. Lancet, 2:21, 1955.

Najafi, H., Lal, R., Khalili, M., Serry, C., Rogers, A., and Haklin, M.: Left ventricular hemorrhagic necrosis. Experimental production and pathogenesis. Ann. Thorac. Surg., 12:400, 1971.

Najafi, H., Henson, D., Dye, W. S., Javid, H., Hunter, J. A., Callaghan, R., Eisenstein, R., and Julian, O. C.: Left ventricular hemorrhagic necrosis. Ann. Thorac. Surg., 7:550, 1969.

Nelson, R., Fey, K., Follette, D. M., et al.: The critical importance of intermittent infusion of cardioplegic solution during aortic cross clamping. Surg. Forum, 27:241, 1976.

Nordbeck, H., Bretschneider, H. J., Fuchs, C., Knoll, D., Kohl, F. V., Sakai, K., Spieckermann, P. G., and Stapenhorst, K.: Methode und Ergebnisse einer neuen Form des Kunstlichen Herzstillstandes im Tierexperiment und unter klinischen Bedingungen. Thoraxchirurgie, 22:582, 1974.

Olin, C. L., Bomfim, V., Bendz, R., Kaijser, L., Strom, S. J., and Sylven, C. H.: Myocardial protection during the aortic valve replacement: Comparison of different methods by intraoperative coronary sinus blood sampling and postoperative serial serum enzyme determinations. J. Thorac. Cardiovasc. Surg., 82:837, 1981.

Permutt, S., and Riley, R. L.: Hemodynamics of collapsible vessels with tone: The vascular waterfall. J. Appl. Physiol., 18:924, 1963.

Rahn, H., Reeves, R. B., and Howell, B. J.: Hydrogen ion regulation, temperature and evolution. Am. Rev. Respir. Dis., 112:165, 1975.

Robb-Nicholson, C., Currie, W. D., and Wechsler, A. S.: Effects of verapamil on myocardial tolerance to ischemic cardiac arrest. Circulation, 58(Suppl. 1):119, 1978.

Roe, B. B., Hutchinson, J. C., Fishman, N. H., Ullyot, D. J., and Smith, D. L.: Myocardial protection with cold, ischemic, potassium-induced cardioplegia. J. Thorac. Cardiovasc. Surg., 73:366, 1977.

Rosenfeldt, F. L., and Arnold, M.: Absence of myocardial damage during profound local cardiac hypothermia. In Proceedings Symposium on Cardioplegia: The First Quarter Century. London, 1980, pp. 158–160.

Rosenfeldt, F. L., and Watson, D. A.: Interference with local myocardial cooling by heat gain during aortic cross-clamping. Ann. Thorac. Surg., 27:13, 1979.

Rosenthal, T. B.: The effect of temperature on the pH of blood and plasma in vitro. J. Biol. Chem., 173:25, 1948.

Rowe, G. G., Castillo, C. A., Maxwell, G. M., and Crumpton, C. W.: Comparison of systemic and coronary hemodynamics in the normal human male and female. Circ. Res., 7:728, 1959.

Sabiston, D. C., Jr.: The coronary circulation. The William F. Rienhoff, Jr. Lecture. Johns Hopkins Med. J., 134:314, 1974.

Sabiston, D. C., Jr., and Gregg, D. E.: Effect of cardiac contraction on coronary blood flow. Circulation, 15:14, 1957.

Schachner, A., Schimert, G., Lajos, T. S., Lee, A. N., Montes, M., Chaudhry, A., Schaefer, P., Vladutin, A., and Siegel, J. H.: Selective intracavitary and coronary hypothermic cardioplegia for myocardial preservation. Arch. Surg., 111:1197, 1976.

Sealy, W. C., Young, W. G., Jr., Brown, I. W., Jr., Smith, W. W., and Lesage, A. M.: Profound hypothermia combined with extracorporeal circulation for open-heart surgery. Surgery, 48:432, 1960.

Sealy, W. C., Brown, I. W., Jr., Young, W. G., Jr., Stephen, C. R., Harris, J. S., and Merritt, D.: Hypothermia, low-flow extracorporeal circulation and controlled cardiac arrest for open-heart surgery. Surg. Gynecol. Obstet., 104:441, 1957.

Shen, A. C., and Jennings, R. B.: Myocardial calcium and magnesium in acute ischemic injury. Am. J. Pathol., 67:417, 1972.

Shragge, B. W., Digerness, S. B., and Blackstone, E. H.: Complete recovery of myocardial function following cold exposure. Circulation, 56(Suppl. 2):97, 1978.

Shumway, N. E., Lower, R. R., and Stofer, R. C.: Selective hypothermia of the heart in anoxic cardiac arrest. Surg. Gynecol. Obstet., 109:750, 1959.

Smith, P. K., and Cox, J. L.: Personal communication, December 1981.

Søndergaard, T., Berg, E., Staffeldt, I., and Szcezepanski, K.: Cardioplegic cardiac arrest in aortic surgery. J. Cardiovasc. Surg., 16:288, 1975.

Speicher, C. E., Ferrigan, L., Wolfson, S. K., Yalav, E. H., and Rawson, A. J.: Cold injury of myocardium and pericardium in cardiac hypothermia. Surg. Gynecol. Obstet., 114:659, 1962.

Taber, R. E., Morales, A. R., and Fine, G.: Myocardial necrosis and the postoperative low-cardiac-output syndrome. Ann. Thorac. Surg., 4:12, 1967.

Tyers, G. F. O.: Metabolic arrest of the heart. Ann. Thorac. Surg., 20:91, 1975.

Tyers, G. F. O., and Morgan, H. E.: Isolated heart perfusion techniques for rapid screening of myocardial preservation methods. Anoxia versus ischemia. Ann. Thorac. Surg., 20:56, 1975.

Tyers, G. F. O., Williams, E. H., Hughes, H. C., and Todd, G. J.: Effect of perfusate temperature on myocardial protection from ischemia. J. Thorac. Cardiovasc. Surg., 73:766, 1977a.

Tyers, G. F. O., Manley, N. J., Williams, G. H., Shaffer, C. W., Williams, D. R., and Kurusz, M.: Preliminary clinical experience with isotonic hypothermic potassium induced arrest. J. Thorac. Cardiovasc. Surg., 74:674, 1977b.

White, F. N.: A comparative physiological approach to hypothermia. (Editorial.) J. Thorac. Cardiovasc. Surg., 82:821, 1981.

Wildenthal, K., Mierzwiak, D. S., and Mitchell, J.: Acute effects of increased serum osmolality on left ventricular performance. Am. J. Physiol., 216:898, 1969.

Zimmerman, A. N. E., Daems, W., Hulsmann, W. C., Snijder, J., Wisse, E., and Durrer, D.: Morphological changes of heart muscle caused by successive perfusion with calcium-free and calcium-containing solutions (calcium paradox). Cardiovasc. Res., 1:201, 1967.

II PATHOLOGY OF CORONARY ATHEROSCLEROSIS

Zeev Vlodaver

Jesse E. Edwards

HISTORY*

The concept of calcification of the coronary arteries was introduced by Lorenzo Bellini (1643–1704) of Pisa. About the same time (1707), Giovanni Maria Lancisi mentioned calcification of coronary arteries as a cause of cardiac enlargement. In 1761, John Baptist Morgagni (1682–1771) of Venice was the first to regard arteriosclerosis as a lesion of the inner coats of the arteries. Thomas Hodgkin (1798–1866) of Tettenham and London, a capable clinician and an outstanding pathologist, described arteriosclerosis and classified the arterial lesions into three types—cartilaginous, pulpy, and purulent.

One of the leading contributors in the field of cardiology during the eighteenth century was Raymond Vieussens of Montpellier. In 1705, he advanced the idea that the coronary vessels have direct communication with the chambers of the heart, and he also described the position, structure, and pathologic changes of the heart. In 1708, Adam Christianus Thebesius conducted experiments in which he injected material into the coronary arteries to demonstrate their passage into the chambers of the heart.

Although several reports in the eighteenth century called attention to cases of chest pain without ascribing a name to the symptoms or postulating a cause for them, it was not until the work of William Heberden (1710–1801), published in 1802, that the clinical syndrome now known as angina pectoris was described and named and the cause suggested. Heberden attributed the painful syndrome to spasm of the heart.

Clinical observations by Edward Jenner of Berkeley, Gloucestershire, in 1799 and experimental work by Allan Burns of Glasgow in 1809 sustained the idea that angina pectoris results from myocardial ischemia. Later, in 1845, John Forbes of London described cases of angina pectoris in the absence of organic disease of the heart.

Acute infarction of the heart, undoubtedly with necrosis of tissue in a specimen, was observed and reported by Joseph Hodgson of Birmingham in 1815, and in 1827, Robert Adam of Dublin described findings that apparently represented a healed myocardial infarct in a patient with heart block. In 1850, Sir Richard Quain of London described localized infarction as corresponding to the region supplied by an extensively ossified coronary artery.

Classic descriptions of myocardial infarction and its relationship to obstructive coronary disease were presented by Carl Weigert of Silesia in 1880 and by Ernst Ziegler of Freiburg in 1887. Experimental ligations of the coronary arteries to produce infarction were performed in 1894 by William Townsend Porter and in 1899 by Walter Braumgartner, both of Cambridge, Massachusetts.

A clinicopathologic classification of coronary arterial disease was advanced by Ernst von Leyden (1832–1910), a prominent German clinician. The four different pictures of the disease that he reported were (1) sclerosis of the coronary arteries without symptoms; (2) thrombotic obstruction with acute myocardial infarction; (3) chronic type of coronary obliteration with patchy or extensive fibrosis of the myocardium; and (4) mixed form of chronic fibrosis associated with acute myocardial infarction.

The first case of coronary thrombosis diagnosed in the United States during the life of a patient was reported in 1896 by George Dock of Galveston and Ann Arbor. The first true and comprehensive description of the clinical diagnosis of coronary thrombosis, however, was published in 1912 by James B. Herrick of Chicago. Six years later, he also reported a case of coronary thrombosis studied by means of electrocardiography.

PRIMARY NATURE OF THE LESION

Established atheromatous lesions may be divided into the *simple* and *complex* forms. The latter include features of complicating lesions such as rupture of the fibrous tissue of an atheroma, intimal hemorrhage, and thrombosis. Secondary changes in thrombi may contribute to complex lesions.

The simple atheromatous lesion may be either the fibrous type or the lipoid type. The fibrous type is characterized by either eccentric or circumferential deposits in the intima of collagenous tissue (Fig. 50–15). Lightly staining foci may be found in collagen that is devoid of both foam cells and extracellular

---

*The references in this section are based on the work of Willius and Dry (1948).

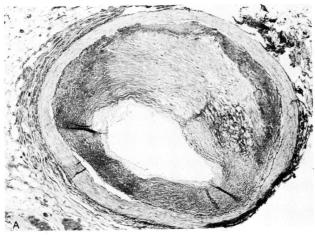

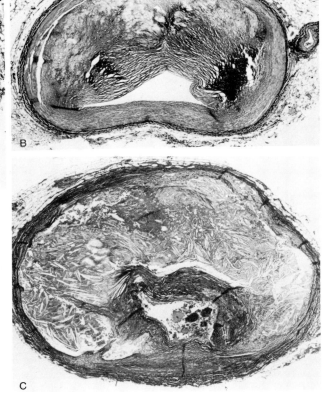

Figure 50–15. Simple types of coronary atherosclerosis. *a,* An eccentric fibrous lesion causes major thickening of the intima with eccentricity of the lumen. The latter has an ovoid shape. (Elastic tissue stain; × 13.) *b,* A lipoid type of atheroma is characterized by eccentric deposit of lipids (lightly stained areas). This deposit is separated from the eccentric ovoid lumen by a layer of fibrous tissue. The lipid accumulation and the fibrous tissue together are considered a parite. (Elastic tissue stain; × 11.) *c,* Another lipoid type of atheroma in which there is considerable deposit of lipids, some of which are crystallized. These are separated from the lumen by a layer of fibrous tissue. The lumen is eccentric and polymorphous in type. (Elastic tissue stain; × 19.)

pools of lipid. Because these foci are shown to contain lipids, Osborn (1963) named the process "collipid," a word coined from collagen and lipid.

The lipoid type of atheroma is more common than the fibrous type. In such an atheroma, there is an intimal deposit of lipids, including foam cells and, most prevalent, extracellular lipoid deposits (Fig. 50–16). Crystalline formation may occur (Fig. 50–16). A characteristic of the accumulation of lipid is its strong association with a fibrous wall on the lumen side of the accumulation. This association was designated "parite" by Osborn (1963). The simplest type of lipoid atheroma is that in which one parite is present. Many lesions, however, are more complex and are represented by a series of parites, suggesting an episodic character to progression in severity of atherosclerosis (Fig. 50–17).

Atherosclerosis develops focally. Atheromas usually occur focally along the length of the involved coronary artery; segments of normal artery are often present between severely obstructive atherosclerotic lesions. The focal nature of atherosclerosis is also emphasized in cross-sections of the arteries by the histologic appearance of involved segments. One arc of the intima may be uninvolved, whereas the remainder contains an atheroma. As a result of focal distribution, the narrowed lumen is eccentric and lies near the uninvolved arc.

The position and shape of the narrowed lumen depend on the distribution of the atheroma in the circumference of the intima. A circumferential lesion yields a central lumen. An eccentric atheroma causes an eccentric lumen, which may be ovoid or polymorphous in shape. In greatest width, the ovoid lumen may be as wide as the original lumen. The polymorphous lumen may be either circular or odd-shaped.

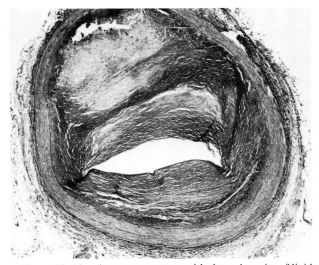

Figure 50–16. A coronary artery with three deposits of lipids, each in part or completely walled off by a layer of fibrous tissue. The result is an eccentric ovoid lumen. (Elastic tissue stain; × 10.)

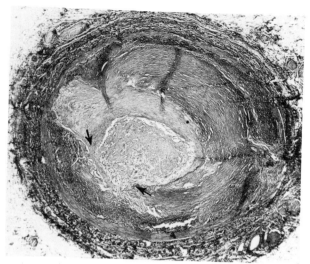

Figure 50–17. Photomicrograph of a coronary artery showing a fibrous type of atheroma yielding a central lumen. There has been a break (between arrows) of the fibrous tissue separating the lumen from the atheroma. Minor extravasation of blood occurs into the atheroma (lower part of the illustration). The lumen contains a recent thrombus. (Elastic tissue stain; × 15.)

The central lumen may show varying degrees of obstruction, but the eccentric lumen is always substantially narrowed.

COMPLICATING LESIONS

Calcification in Atheromas. This process occurs either in accumulations of extracellular lipid or in collagen of the intima and musculoelastic layer. It may be seen in atheromas causing severe stenosis and also in those causing minimal stenosis of the lumen. Calcification appears simply to be an indication that the lesion is old. Classically, calcification without significant luminal narrowing is observed in atheromas in older persons.

Hemorrhage into Atheromas. Hemorrhage into atheromas is a common phenomenon. There is a difference of opinion regarding the source of so-called intimal hemorrhages. One view is that the capillaries, which commonly appear in atheromas, rupture; another view is that primary fragmentation of the fibrous layer of the "parite" nearest the lumen occurs and blood escapes from the lumen into the lipid part of the "parite." The hematoma within the atheroma may become organized, leaving a vascular plexus in the wall beside the lumen. It is uncommon for the lumen to be narrowed by the hemorrhage. The irritative effect of an intramural hemorrhage, however, may perhaps cause spasm in the collateral vessels that bypass this arterial segment.

Coronary Thrombosis. Thrombosis occurring in a coronary artery may be mural but is usually occlusive. Underlying varying degrees of coronary atherosclerosis are present. Charactistically, thrombosis involves a short segment of the artery, often not more than 1 centimeter in length.

It may be the case that a thrombus may develop in an atherosclerotic but intact segment. Nevertheless, it is probably common, as judged from serial sections of involved segments, that the common underlying process for thrombosis is rupture of the fibrous tissue overlying a lipoid focus in the atheroma (Fig. 50–17).

As with all thrombi, coronary arterial thrombi are subject to one of two reactions, namely lysis by fibrinolytic enzymes and organization. Organization of coronary arterial thrombi qualitatively follows the same pattern as organization of thrombi in other arteries and in veins but is relatively slow because of the underlying disease of the artery. The end result is the presence of vascular connective tissue in the original lumen.

Although the vessels of the organized thrombus connect with the parent lumen, both proximally and distally, these vessels are usually narrow and, in the aggregate, do not carry any significant amount of blood (Fig. 50–18a,b). Uncommonly, the vessels of an organized thrombus are wide, and such vessels have been demonstrated to carry a significant amount of blood across the segment that earlier had been occluded by thrombus (Fig. 50–18c) (Zollikofer *et al.*, 1980).

Aneurysm. In spite of the common occurrence of medial atrophy in atherosclerotic coronary arteries, aneurysms rarely occur in these arteries. When such aneurysms do occur, they are usually saccular, and laminated thrombi are present within them. Generally, an effective lumen for the flow of blood remains. The main complication of coronary aneurysms of atherosclerotic origin lies in the possibility that portions of the thrombus may become dislodged and embolize, causing occlusion of the distal part of the parent artery or one of its branches.

DISTRIBUTION OF LESIONS

In subjects with clinical coronary disease, whether angina of stable or unstable type (Guthrie *et al.*, 1975) or acute myocardial infarction (Roberts and Jones, 1980), it is characteristic that obstructive coronary atherosclerosis is of severe degree and multifocal. From pathologic studies, it is common that segments of the right coronary, anterior descending, and circumflex arteries are each involved. In a study on angina, Guthrie and colleagues (1975) found that the main left coronary artery was involved in 30 per cent of cases, but in none was it the only site of significant disease.

From angiographic studies, the distribution of lesions is commonly found to be less extensive than that observed at autopsy. This difference may relate to the better prognosis in subjects with fewer arteries involved than in those with a greater number of diseased vessels (Hutter, 1980).

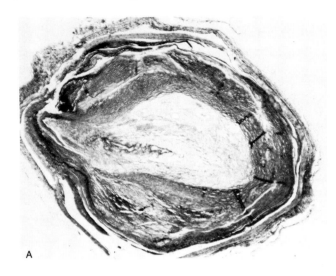

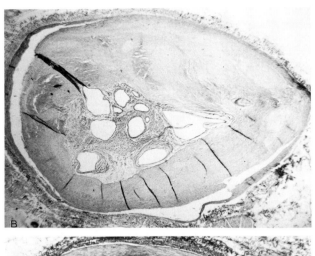

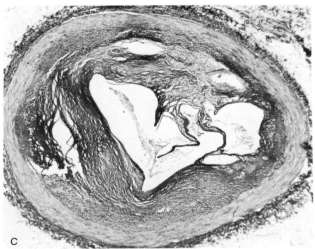

Figure 50–18. Coronary thrombosis with organization. *a*, A fibrous type of atheroma yields a central lumen that is occluded by a thrombus almost completely organized. The vessels in the thrombus are of restricted caliber. (Elastic tissue stain; × 10.) *b*, An organized thrombus is represented by a series of channels separated by fibrous tissue. (H & E stain; × 18.) *c*, An organized thrombus in which the recanalized channels are relatively wide, carrying a significant amount of blood. (Elastic tissue stain; × 17.)

It is commonly taught that the anterior descending artery is the site of severe involvement, that the severest degree of disease lies in the most proximal segment of an affected artery, and that a progressively decreasing degree of involvement occurs distally. None of these descriptions portrays the exact state of affairs. In our experience, the segment of the right coronary artery between the marginal and posterior descending branches (the intermediate segment) most commonly harbors the severely obstructive lesions of atherosclerosis. Another frequent site of obstruction is the proximal half of the anterior descending branch of the left coronary artery. The third most common site for severe disease is in the anterior segment of the right coronary artery, which lies between the ostium and the marginal branch (Vlodaver and Edwards, 1971b).

In the right coronary artery, at least, the concept of peripheral diminution of the severity of the disease does not hold. Even in the anterior descending artery, specific cases do not always conform. We studied the proximal and distal halves of the anterior descending arteries in cases of obstructive atherosclerotic disease. Significantly obstructive atherosclerotic lesions were localized to the proximal segment in 76 per cent of the specimens, involved both the proximal and distal

segments in 17 per cent, and involved only the distal segment in 7 per cent. The findings in the left circumflex artery conform in general to those in the anterior descending artery.

CORRELATION WITH ANGIOGRAPHY

The current trend toward surgical intervention in certain types of coronary artery disease relies on the coronary arteriogram to delineate the arterial lesions. The coronary arteriogram, however, even when obtained by postmortem injection, does not always correlate well with the gross and microscopic alterations found by dissection of the coronary arteries. The coronary arteriogram has generally been found to be less revealing of extensive disease than is the standard postmortem examination.

Two reasons have been put forward to explain this discrepancy: (1) the intravascular pressure of postmortem injection may distend a weakened sclerotic wall, and (2) the anatomic configuration of the arterial lumen may appear nearly normal in one projection of the coronary arteriogram, but in projections made at right angles to this view, the lumen may appear greatly obstructed. Our correlations of coronary arteriograms with pathologic observations support this explanation. In 29 per cent of sections of atherosclerotic coronary arteries that we studied, an ovoid ("slit-like") lumen occurred, whereas central and eccentric polymorphous lumens were found in 30 and 40 per cent of the sections, respectively. Among segments of coronary arteries with significantly obstructed lumens not identified by arteriography (false-negative), 68 per cent had ovoid lumens, and only 32 per cent had central or eccentric polymorphous lumens (Vlodaver *et al.*, 1973). Obviously, the ovoid lumen represents a trap for the arteriographer until an ideal projection can be found. We studied the position of atheromas with respect to the surface of the heart and found no consistent orientation. Thus, multiple projections are required to reduce the false-negative errors of coronary angiograms.

COLLATERAL CIRCULATION

The presence of obvious intercoronary collateral circulation is a hallmark of a severe and extensive atherosclerotic process. The basis for the formation of coronary collateral vessels is the presence of pre-existing coronary arterial anastomoses in the normal heart.

Baroldi and Scomazzoni (1967) described two types of coronary arterial anastomoses: (1) the homocoronary anastomosis, which connects various branches of the same coronary artery, and (2) the intercoronary anastomosis, which connects branches of two different coronary arteries. Grossly, the anastomotic vessels are of arteriolar size, but histologically, they resemble capillaries with an inner endothelial layer and thin medial and adventitial layers. Coronary arterial anastomotic vessels carry very little of the coronary blood flow in healthy hearts. Only with the development of obstructive lesions do they provide the basis for a significant amount of flow between vessels or segments of one vessel.

In order for collateral circulation to develop, severe coronary arterial narrowing causing obstruction of at least Grade 3+ must be present (Gensini and da Costa, 1969). According to various authors, complete occlusion of the coronary arteries, as visualized by angiography, is almost always accompanied by at least some collateral circulation to supply the segment distal to the occlusion (Abrams and Adams, 1969; Baltaxe *et al.*, 1973).

The development of collateral circulation may be considered as part of a process of revascularization of an area of ischemic myocardium; however, controversy exists about the functional role of these vessels and their ability to protect the myocardium against ischemia (Harris *et al.*, 1972; Miller *et al.*, 1972). By comparing the angiographic findings in two groups of patients with equally severe and extensive coronary arterial disease, one of which had functioning collateral vessels and the other none, Harris and associates (1972) and Miller and coworkers (1972) showed that

anastomotic vessels afforded no protection against myocardial ischemia, as measured by the treadmill stress test.

Similar conclusions were derived from studies on regional perfusion with thallium-201 scintigraphy (Berger *et al.*, 1980). With the use of intracoronary xenon-122, Cohn and colleagues (1980) found that the presence or absence of well-developed collateral systems had no effect on myocardial function at rest.

INVASIVE THERAPEUTIC PROCEDURES

This section will deal with the changes that occur in grafts used to bypass obstructive lesions of the native arteries, changes following coronary endarterectomy, and preliminary pathologic consideration of percutaneous arterioplasty.

Saphenous Vein Grafts

Approximately 15 per cent of saphenous vein grafts are noted to be occluded by 1 year after placement, and some occlude after that time. Three main lesions, either alone or in combination, are responsible for encroachment upon the lumen. These are thrombosis, intimal proliferation, and atherosclerosis. Medial changes in veins used as grafts vary. In many instances, the integrity of the media is maintained, whereas in some grafts fibrous replacement of medial elements of the vein occurs.

In the early postoperative period, a thin layer of platelets and fibrin is often deposited on the intimal surface of the graft (Fig. 50–19). In most instances, this is not progressive.

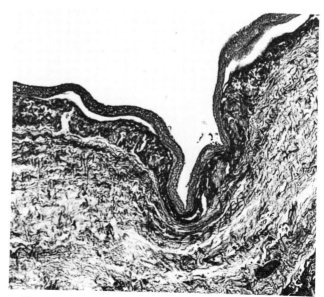

Figure 50–19. Segment of a saphenous vein graft in place for 2 days. A thin layer of fibrin and platelets lies on the intimal surface. (H & E stain; × 50.)

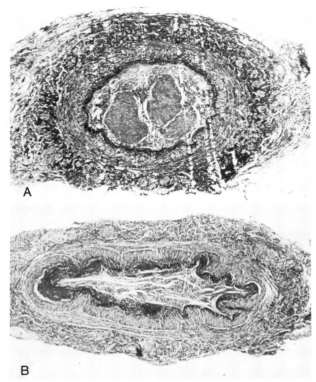

Figure 50–20. Saphenous vein grafts with thrombi. *a*, At 2 months postoperatively, the thrombus is incompletely organized. (Elastic tissue stain; × 14.) *b*, Three years postoperatively, the lumen contains an organized thrombus, which is represented by vascular connective tissue. (Elastic tissue stain; × 17.)

If occlusive thrombosis occurs, the sites of anastomosis appear to be the first areas involved, but the entire length of the graft may be so involved. Thrombosis is the usual basis for early postoperative occlusion of a graft. The thrombus undergoes the usual changes of organization and, finally, is represented by vascular connective tissue (Fig. 50–20).

All grafts in place for at least 1 month and not occluded by thrombosis show some features of the intimal proliferative lesion (Fig. 50–21*a*). In early stages, this lesion is characterized by the presence of fusiform cells, both fibroblasts and smooth muscle cells lying in a mucoid matrix having a high content of acid mucopolysaccharides (Vlodaver and Edwards, 1971a). In older lesions, collagenous fibers appear. The degree of encroachment upon the lumen varies. In exceptional cases, it may reach the stage of being occlusive. Such a state is hardly ever seen less than 3 months postoperatively.

The proliferative lesion seems poorly fused to the media of the vein, as judged by the observation that in some cases endothelium-lined spaces lie between the thickened intima and the venous media (Fig. 50–21*b*). In some grafts, thrombosis may occur on the surface of a nonobstructive intimal proliferative lesion and be obstructive. Segmental aneurysmal dilatation with thrombosis is an uncommon complication.

Atherosclerosis of grafts is a potentially late complication (Lie *et al.*, 1977). In our experience, it has usually not been observed less than 5 years postoperatively, although we have seen it 3 years postoperatively (Fig. 50–22). The lesion tends to have excessive amorphous lipoid deposits, and the fibrous wall separating the deposit from the lumen is thin. It is subject to the various complications of arterial atherosclerosis, including intimal hemorrhage and thrombosis (Fig. 50–23).

Endarterectomy

Endarterectomy in any artery is followed by the development of a new intima that has close similarity in its structure to the intimal proliferative lesions seen in saphenous veins used as grafts. In relatively small arteries, such as the coronary arteries, a relatively minor degree of new intimal formation may have a major effect on luminal narrowing.

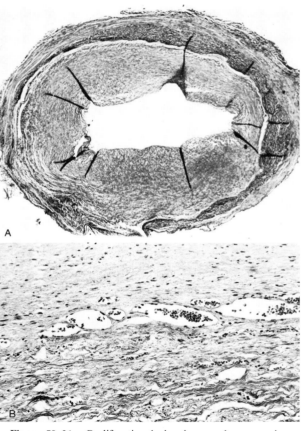

Figure 50–21. Proliferative lesion in a saphenous vein graft that had been in place for 3 years. *a*, The media shows irregular scarring. The intima is greatly thickened by a proliferative lesion, causing moderately severe narrowing of the lumen. (Elastic tissue stain; × 9.) *b*, The junction of the media (below) and the intimal proliferative lesion (above) shows a series of spaces lined by endothelium, suggesting that the intimal proliferative lesion had separated spontaneously from the underlying media. (H & E stain; × 150.)

Percutaneous Arterioplasty

Percutaneous transluminal coronary angioplasty offers an innovative alternative for some patients in whom medical therapy has been unsatisfactory in the control of ischemic episodes (Hamby and Katz, 1980). As judged from available studies, the basis for increasing flow by this procedure is separation of the diseased intima from the media and stretching of the media (Castaneda-Zuniga *et al.*, 1980). The effective basis is widening of the basic diameter of the artery, while the fundamental nature of the obstructive atheroma is not changed. There has been inadequate pathologic follow-up experience with this procedure for revelation of its long-range effects. An immediate problem is the potential of embolism of fragments of the intima separated from the media.

One potential late problem is thrombosis of the space between the separated intima and media. Another relates to the phenomenon that separation of

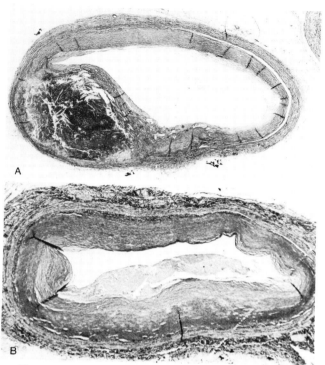

Figure 50–23. Saphenous vein grafts that had been in place for many years. *a,* Eight years postoperatively. In addition to a proliferative lesion of the intima, which causes mild narrowing of the lumen, is a focus of hemorrhage into an atheroma. (H & E stain; × 10.) *b,* Six years postoperatively. In addition to a proliferative lesion of the intima and irregular scarring of the media, there is a lightly staining layer (lower part of illustration) representing a site of atherosclerosis. The lumen contains a mural thrombus. (Elastic tissue stain; × 5.)

the intima from the media is essentially similar to endarterectomy, with the possibility of a reactive process filling in the newly created space.

SELECTED REFERENCES

Gensini, G. G., and da Costa, B. C. B.: The coronary collateral circulation in living man. Am. J. Cardiol., *24*:393, 1969.

This investigation is based on the study of coronary arteriograms in 100 patients selected at random and examined for the presence or absence of coronary collaterals. In 53 of those patients with a normal coronary arteriogram or with less than 50 per cent lumen reduction, *no* collaterals were found. Among the remaining 47 patients, each with more than 50 per cent lumen reduction of one or more major branches, 37 had collateral vessels. The presence of coronary collaterals is a reliable indication of severe coronary disease. The authors also describe several patterns of anastomotic pathways. Each illustrative case is accompanied by a diagram that makes its interpretation understandable.

Harris, C. N., Kaplan, M. A., Parker, D. P., Aronow, W. S., and Ellestad, M. H.: Anatomic and functional correlates of intercoronary collateral vessels. Am. J. Cardiol., *30*:611, 1972.

The authors studied 181 patients who had undergone coronary arteriography and treadmill stress testing for the evaluation of anginal pain. Only 21.5 per cent were found to have demonstrable intercoronary collateral vessels, and those were seen only when occlusion of the luminal diameter of at least one vessel exceeded

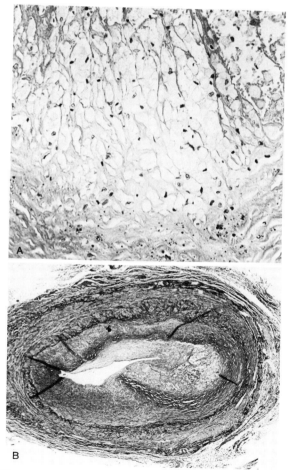

Figure 50–22. Saphenous vein graft with atherosclerosis 3 years postoperatively. *a,* A high-power view of a series of foam cells in the intima. (H & E stain; × 400.) *b,* The vein graft shows a circumferential layer of the proliferative lesion lying beneath the media, and internal to this is a focal eccentric superimposed lesion. This represents an atheroma. Recent hemorrhage was present in the latter lesion. (Elastic tissue stain; × 6.)

75 per cent. When the group with collateral vessels was compared with that without collateral vessels but with equal severity of disease, it was shown that collateral vessels offered no protection against the development of an ischemic ST segment response to treadmill stress testing.

Osborn, G. R.: The Incubation Period of Coronary Thrombosis. London, Butterworth, 1963.

In this excellent book, the author describes his experience with and presents his ideas on the structure of the coronary arteries, the development of atheromas, and the relationship of thrombi to the arterial lesion. This work is based on the study of 925 individuals of newborn, young normal, and old normal coronary arteries. In addition, in a group of 207 patients with coronary thrombosis, the arterial lesions were drawn in an attempt to identify processes taking place, and reconstruction of serial cross-sections was done in many of the cases. A description of the coronary arteries of children and young adults is well illustrated. The concepts of "parite," angular, and phasic activity in the development of the atheroma are introduced as new ways to understand the different stages of the lesion. The nature of the formation of thrombi as represented in a map diagram is an outstanding feature that makes this book exciting and very interesting.

Roberts, W. C., and Jones, A. A.: Quantification of coronary arterial narrowing at necropsy in acute transmural myocardial infarction analysis and comparison of findings in 27 patients and 22 controls. Circulation, 61:786, 1980.

In a previous histologic study of cross-sections of 5-mm. segments of the coronary artery system in patients with acute myocardial infarction, Roberts and Buja (Am. J. Med., 52:425, 1972) found that usually at least two to three major coronary arteries were more than 75 per cent narrowed by atherosclerotic plaques. This study is a quantitative approach to determine not only if a coronary artery was more than 75 per cent narrowed in cross-sectional areas at some point along its course, but also what percentage of its entire length was narrowed to lesser degrees. They examined 1403 5-mm. segments in 27 patients with acute myocardial infarction and found that 72 per cent of the lengths of the four major epicardial coronary arteries were narrowed more than 50 per cent of their cross-sectional area by atherosclerotic plaque (compared with 28 per cent in a control group). The degree of severe narrowing in the distal halves of the right, left anterior descending, and left circumflex arteries in the 27 patients with acute myocardial infarction was just as great as in the proximal halves of these arteries.

Vlodaver, Z., and Edwards, J. E.: Pathologic analysis in fatal cases following saphenous vein coronary arterial bypass. Chest, 64:555, 1973.

A pathologic study was done on 74 patients who had received a total of 124 saphenous vein grafts to bypass obstructive coronary arterial lesions. The periods of study after operation ranged from failure to survive the operation to 3½ years. Of significance was the high incidence of residual obstructive disease in the graft system (graft and distal artery) and in the nongrafted arteries. Obstruction was observed in 46 of the 124 vein grafts. The characteristic basis for occlusion of a graft 1 month or less after operation was thrombosis. In long-range grafts, occlusion was most commonly caused by fibrous intimal proliferation. The observations emphasize the high incidence of acute myocardial infarction among early postoperative deaths as well as thrombosis of the artery proximal to an anastomotic site. Postoperative acute myocardial infarction appears to play an important role as an underlying basis for low cardiac output. Late postoperative deaths (months or years) are commonly sudden and associated with obstructions in grafts and nongrafted arteries.

Willius, F. A., and Dry, T. J.: A History of the Heart and Circulation. Philadelphia, W. B. Saunders Company, 1948.

This book presents the historical developments of knowledge relating to the heart and circulation. In the first part, the authors present the material in a chronologic manner from 5000 B. C. to A. D. 1925. This period is divided into eras, recording the state of existing civilization in each era and emphasizing the advantages as well as the limitations of each period. The second section concerns special biographies of individuals contributing to the cardiovascular field. The third section chronologically summarizes specific subjects such as anatomy, arrhythmias, and diagnostic procedures. The authors succeed in tracing the influences of the past upon the present.

REFERENCES

Abrams, H. L., and Adams, D. F.: The coronary arteriogram: Structural and functional aspects. N. Engl. J. Med., 281:1276, 1969.

Baltaxe, H. A., Amplatz, K., and Levin, D. C.: Coronary Angiography. Springfield, Illinois, Charles C Thomas, 1973.

Baroldi, G., and Scomazzoni, G.: Coronary Circulation in the Normal and the Pathologic Heart. Washington, D. C., U. S. Government Printing Office, 1967.

Berger, B. C., Watson, D. D., Taylor, G. J., Burwell, L. R., Martin, R. P., and Beller, G. A.: Effect of coronary collateral circulation on regional myocardial perfusion assessed with quantitative thallium-201 scintigraphy. Am. J. Cardiol., 46:364, 1980.

Castaneda-Zuniga, W. R., Formanek, A., Tadavarthy, M., Vlodaver, Z., Edwards, J. E., Zollikofer, C., and Amplatz, K.: The mechanism of balloon angioplasty. Radiology, 135:565, 1980.

Cohn, P. F., Maddox, D. E., Holman, B. L., and See, J. R.: Effect of coronary collateral vessels on regional myocardial blood flow in patients with coronary artery disease. Am. J. Cardiol., 46:359, 1980.

Gensini, G. G., and da Costa, B. C. B.: The coronary collateral circulation in living man. Am. J. Cardiol., 24:393, 1969.

Guthrie, R. B., Vlodaver, Z., Nicoloff, D. M., and Edwards, J. E.: Pathology of stable and unstable angina pectoris. Circulation, 51:1059, 1975.

Hamby, R. I., and Katz, S.: Percutaneous transluminal coronary angioplasty: Its potential impact on surgery for coronary artery disease. Am. J. Cardiol., 45:1161, 1980.

Harris, C. N., Kaplan, M. A., Parker, D. P., Aronow, W. S., and Ellestad, M. H.: Anatomic and functional correlates of intercoronary collateral vessels. Am. J. Cardiol., 30:611, 1972.

Hutter, A. M., Jr.: Is there a left main equivalent? Circulation, 62:207, 1980.

Lie, J. T., Lawrie, G. M., and Morris, G. C., Jr.: Aortocoronary bypass saphenous vein graft atherosclerosis. Anatomic study of 99 vein grafts from normal and hyperlipoproteinemic patients up to 75 months postoperatively. Am. J. Cardiol., 40:906, 1977.

Miller, R. R., Mason, D. T., Salel, A., Zelis, R. F., Massumi, R. A., and Amsterdam, E. A.: Determinants and functional significance of the coronary collateral circulation in patients with coronary artery disease. (Abstract.) Am. J. Cardiol., 29:281, 1972.

Osborn, G. R.: The Incubation Period of Coronary Thrombosis. London, Butterworth, 1963.

Roberts, W. C., and Jones, A. A.: Quantification of coronary arterial narrowing at necropsy in acute transmural myocardial infarction. Analysis and comparison of findings in 27 patients and 22 controls. Circulation, 61:786, 1980.

Vlodaver, Z., and Edwards, J. E.: Pathologic analysis in fatal cases following saphenous vein coronary arterial bypass. Chest, 64:555, 1973.

Vlodaver, Z., and Edwards, J. E.: Pathologic changes in aortic-coronary arterial saphenous vein grafts. Circulation, 44:719, 1971a.

Vlodaver, Z., and Edwards, J. E.: Pathology of coronary atherosclerosis. Prog. Cardiovasc. Dis., 14:256, 1971b.

Vlodaver, Z., Frech, R., van Tassel, R. A., and Edwards, J. E.: Correlation of the antemortem coronary arteriogram and the postmortem specimen. Circulation, 47:162, 1973.

Willius, F. A., and Dry, T. J.: A History of the Heart and Circulation. Philadelphia, W. B. Saunders Company, 1948.

Zollikofer, C. L., Vlodaver, Z., Nath, H. P., Castaneda-Zuniga, W., Valdez-Davila, O., Amplatz, K., and Edwards, J. E.: Angiographic findings in recanalization of coronary arterial thrombi. Radiology, 134:303, 1980.

III   CORONARY ARTERIOGRAPHY

ROBERT H. PETER

HISTORY

Physicians have been studying coronary arteries by postmortem injection techniques for many years. These studies not only detailed pathologically specific anatomy and variations in anatomic patterns of the coronary circulation, but also provided an understanding of how obstruction to the coronary arteries related to pathologic findings in the myocardium (Schlesinger, 1940). The extensive coronary disease described by Zoll, Blumgart, and Schlesinger on the basis of many postmortem coronary artery barium injection studies performed in the 1940s gave little hope of developing surgical techniques that could relieve such obstruction (Blumgart *et al.*, 1940; Schlesinger and Zoll, 1941). Indeed, in the earlier attempts at myocardial revascularization—and in those of Beck and Leighminger (1954) and Vineberg (1952), which became the most widely accepted—surgery directly on the coronary arteries was not attempted. A missing link in both the surgical and medical approaches to treatment of the disease was the inability to study the coronary arteries in the living human.

In the mid 1950s, a practical pump-oxygenator made open heart surgery a reality and changed the outlook for many patients with acquired and congenital heart disease (Miller *et al.*, 1953). In 1957, Bailey performed the first coronary endarterectomy in this country, but operative mortality was high and clinical improvement limited (Bailey *et al.*, 1957). The limited success of this technique only served to emphasize further the need for angiographic visualization of the coronary arteries so that a continued direct and more feasible surgical approach to coronary disease could be found.

Attempts to examine the coronary arterial tree in living man continued to be fraught with problems. Radner (1948) visualized the coronary arteries by injecting contrast material into the ascending aorta via a transseptal puncture, but it was not until 1952 that DiGuglielmo and Guttadauro described the angiographic appearance of the coronary arteries in living man. In 1953, Seldinger introduced a method by which standard catheters could be introduced percutaneously into the femoral vessels without an arterial or venous cutdown. This made catheterization of the heart much less difficult and time-consuming. In the late 1950s, many investigators were working on obtaining better coronary artery opacification. Two methods were balloon occlusion of the ascending aorta during bolus injection of contrast material into the aortic root (Dotter and Frische, 1958) and causing temporary asystole with acetylcholine while the aortic root and coronary arteries were filled with contrast material (Lehman *et al.*, 1959). Another approach emphasized the type of catheter used. Catheters were specially designed to deliver a large bolus of contrast material into the aortic root near the coronary ostia (Paulen, 1964). Angiograms from these nonselective techniques were felt to provide satisfactory diagnostic data and were used in some laboratories into the late 1960s.

In October 1958, F. Mason Sones began deliberate attempts to inject contrast material directly into the sinuses of Valsalva. He was able to visualize the coronary arteries adequately in 90 per cent of 137 patients examined (Sones and Shirey, 1960). The much-feared serious ventricular arrhythmias did not occur. In addition, for the first time, intercoronary collateral vessels were clearly observed in living man. Within a few months. Sones developed and began using a specially designed tapered catheter for the selective opacification of the right and left coronary arteries in patients. At the eighth annual convention of the American College of Cardiology in May 1959 and 5 months later at the 32nd Scientific Sessions of the American Heart Association, Sones introduced the technique of selective coronary artery opacification. He was able to report on over 400 selective coronary arteriographic studies by 1960 (Sones and Shirey, 1960); 1020 by 1962 (Sones and Shirey, 1962); 8200 by 1967 (Sones, 1967); over 23,000 by 1972 (Sones, 1972); and 52,973 by 1978 (Sones, 1978). This technique soon proved to be the method of choice for visualizing the coronary arteries.

Other selective coronary arteriographic techniques have been developed since Sones presented his method. The percutaneous transfemoral approach of Ricketts and Abrams (1962) used separate preformed catheters for the right and left coronary arteries. Amplatz and associates (1967), Judkins (1967), and Bourassa and coworkers (1969) also designed preformed right and left coronary catheters for percutaneous transfemoral use. Schoonmaker and King (1974) described a percutaneous femoral technique using a single multipurpose catheter for selective coronary arteriography and left ventriculography. Some groups work with the transaxillary approach (Price and Rosch, 1973) and other specially formed catheters for both the brachial artery and the percutaneous transfemoral approach. However, the techniques originally described by Judkins and Sones are those most widely used and are popularly referred to as the Judkins technique and the Sones technique.

The innovation of selective coronary arteriography by Sones in 1959 and the perfection of the other techniques later allowed selection of patients with localized occlusions of the coronary arteries for the Vineberg procedure and coronary endarterectomy and, some 10 years later, for aortocoronary saphenous vein or internal mammary artery bypass graft surgery. In addition, selective coronary angiography was useful both in evaluating earlier surgical procedures developed to revascularize the heart (Vansant and Muller, 1960) and in assessing the patency of the saphenous vein and internal mammary coronary artery bypass grafts (Baltaxe, 1973). Patients who had undergone Beck's partial coronary sinus ligation procedure, Beck's pericardial poudrage, and internal mammary artery ligation were studied by Sones and Shirey (1960). No evidence of collateral vessels perfusing the myocardium could be found. Sones found angiographic evidence that some Vineberg procedures had been successful in that filling of the coronary arteries occurred after injection of contrast material into the left internal mammary artery implanted into the left ventricular myocardium years before. Although we also found "successful" Vineberg procedures, the limitation of these surgical procedures before the use of diagnostic coronary arteriography may be emphasized by two patients studied in our laboratory who had undergone the Vineberg procedure and were studied again several years later, at which time their implants provided blood flow only to the mediastinum and chest wall. Of particular interest, however, was the fact that both patients had normal selective coronary arteriograms.

These findings showed quite clearly the difficulty of interpreting the clinical significance of chest pain. Increasing numbers of patients with severe or suspected preinfarction "angina" have now been found angiographically to have normal coronary arteries or no significant coronary obstruction (Proudfit *et al.*, 1966; Scanlon *et al.*, 1973; Bruschke *et al.*, 1973). Therefore, two important contributions of the technique of selective coronary arteriography are the selection of those patients with occlusive coronary disease amenable to bypass surgery and the elimination as potential surgical candidates of those with chest pain who do not have obstructive coronary artery disease.

CORONARY ANATOMY

The physician who does selective coronary arteriography and the cardiac surgeon preparing to perform a bypass procedure must have detailed knowledge of the anatomy of both the normal and aberrant coronary arterial tree. Several excellent books on the coronary anatomy are available, most notably the earlier work of Gross (1921) and the books by Baroldi and Scomazzoni (1967) and James (1961a). The precise postmortem injection studies of these researchers complement and extend the findings of Schlesinger and Zoll (1941) and Blumgart and associates (1940) and add to the background in pathology and visual clarification of the common and uncommon anatomic patterns of the coronary arterial tree.

Right Coronary Artery

The right coronary artery, as seen in right and left anterior oblique projections by the angiographer, is shown in Figure 50–24. The right coronary artery arises from the middle of the right sinus of Valsalva. The right main coronary artery then passes beneath the right atrial appendage and courses posteriorly in the right atrioventricular groove until it reaches the crux, or the area where the right and the left atria and ventricles intersect. The first branch from the right coronary artery, the conus artery, passes anteriorly across the right ventricular outflow tract to the pulmonary conus. The conus branch, which is sometimes called a "third coronary artery," originates from a separate ostium near the right coronary ostium in about 50 per cent of cases (Schlesinger *et al.*, 1949). This vessel will frequently serve as a collateral to the left anterior descending artery when the latter vessel is occluded proximally (this had been referred to as the anatomic circle of Vieussens).

The second branch, the main atrial, is present in 55 per cent of cases. The main atrial branch divides

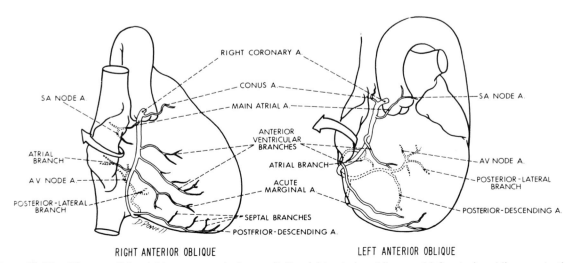

Figure 50–24. Diagram of the right coronary arteriogram in the right anterior oblique and left anterior oblique projections.

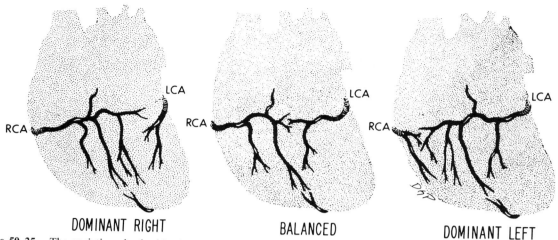

DOMINANT RIGHT   BALANCED   DOMINANT LEFT

Figure 50–25. The variations in the blood supply to the posterior diaphragmatic surface of the heart are viewed as the coronary angiographer would see these vessels in an anteroposterior projection.

into several atrial branches and the sinus node artery (James, 1961b). The next major branch is usually the acute marginal branch, a large vessel that courses down the anterior right ventricular wall toward the apex. It often serves as an important collateral pathway when the distal right or left anterior descending artery is occluded. One or more smaller branches spread through the anterior and anterolateral right ventricular muscle.

At the acute margin, the right main coronary artery turns posteriorly into the atrioventricular groove, giving rise to one or two usually small posterolateral right ventricular branches that course down the posterior aspect of the right ventricle. The main vessel then continues posteromedially to the crux of the heart, where it forms an inverted U turn. The atrioventricular (AV) nodal artery arises at the midpoint of the U turn, and the posterior descending artery continues down the posterior interventricular groove. In about one fifth of cases, the right coronary artery terminates at the crux. Many posterior septal perforating branches penetrate the inferior third of the interventricular septum and may serve as important collaterals of the septal perforating branches to the left anterior descending artery when that vessel is occluded proximally. In 90 per cent of hearts, however, the right coronary artery crosses the crux in the atrioventricular groove and extends for varying distances. Several posterolateral branches of this vessel spread over the left ventricle. In 20 per cent of cases, the right coronary artery extends all the way to the obtuse margin of the heart, supplying blood to the posterior portions of both the right and left ventricles (right dominant pattern).

In man, the artery supplying the AV node originates from the posterior descending artery at the crux, or from the atrioventricular branch crossing the crux, and therefore comes from the right posterior descending artery 90 per cent of the time (James, 1965). Conversely, in the remaining 10 per cent of cases, the left circumflex artery reaches the acute margin of the

right ventricle and, in so doing, crosses the crux and gives off the posterior descending artery and the AV nodal artery (left dominant pattern).

This relationship has led to the concept of right and left coronary "dominance" or "predominance." A "balanced" pattern occurs when branches of the left circumflex and right coronary arteries supply almost equal portions of the diaphragmatic surface of the heart (Fig. 50–25). In this pattern, since the right coronary artery anatomically crosses the crux about 90 per cent of the time, the AV nodal artery arises from the right coronary artery and has sometimes been included in the confusing designation of right coronary "dominance." (Since the right coronary artery does extend past the crux in 90 per cent of cases, some hearts, although showing a more "balanced" circulation, are usually designated right dominant.)

Left Coronary Artery

The left coronary artery, as seen in right and left anterior oblique projections by the angiographer in Figure 50–26, originates from the posterior aspect of the left sinus of Valsalva and extends for a varying distance until it bifurcates into the left anterior descending and left circumflex arteries. Occasionally, there is a trifurcation, and a large diagonal or left anterior ventricular branch will course down the middle surface of the left ventricular free wall. The left anterior descending artery may give off several small or large left and, occasionally, right ventricular branches as it travels down the anterior surface of the heart along the interventricular groove. This vessel usually curves around the apex of the heart and ends several millimeters after entering the posterior interventricular groove, but occasionally, it may terminate at the apex of the heart. In these instances, the right posterior descending artery will curl several millimeters around the apex of the heart and end on the

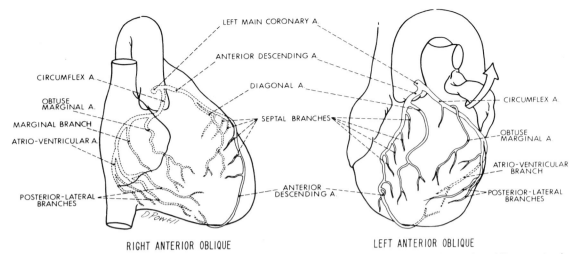

Figure 50–26. Diagram of the left coronary arteriogram in the right anterior oblique and left anterior oblique projections.

anterior interventricular groove. The left anterior descending artery is therefore characterized both by this relationship with the apex of the heart and by the many small and usually large first septal perforating branches that supply the superior two thirds of the interventricular septum. These vessels serve as important sources of collateral supply to the posterior descending branch of the right coronary artery when that vessel is obstructed.

The left circumflex artery extends laterally and to the left in the left anterior atrioventricular groove. At the obtuse margin of the heart, it bifurcates into one or more marginal arteries that course over the lateral aspect of the left ventricle and an atrioventricular artery that continues in the left atrioventricular groove around the posterior surface of the heart for a variable distance. It will give off one or more posterolateral and posterior left ventricular branches that course perpendicular to the atrioventricular groove toward the apex of the heart. In 90 per cent of cases, the atrioventricular branch ends before or at the crux. In 10 per cent, as mentioned previously, it extends to the acute margin of the heart on the right ventricular surface and supplies the posterior descending and AV nodal arteries; this is the so-called "left dominant or preponderant" pattern. A large left atrial circumflex artery is seen in about 30 per cent of patients and may give rise to the sinus node artery as well as provide an important source of collateral flow to the posterior right coronary circulation.

Special mention should be made concerning the blood supply to the left ventricular papillary muscles and the conduction tissue. The anterior papillary muscle derives its blood supply from the left anterior descending artery, from diagonal or anterior ventricular branches, and, occasionally, from marginal tributaries of the left circumflex artery. The posterior papillary muscle derives its blood supply from vessels that provide the predominant supply to the posterior surface of the heart. Therefore, posterior branches from both the circumflex and right coronary systems supply the posterior papillary muscle in 70 per cent

of hearts, whereas in 10 and 20 per cent the left circumflex and right coronary branches, respectively, predominate in supplying blood to the posterior diaphragmatic ventricular wall and posterior papillary muscle (James, 1965).

In man, the arterial supply to the AV node arises from the coronary vessel that gives off the posterior descending coronary artery or crosses the crux of the heart, usually (90 per cent) the right coronary artery. In the remainder, the node is supplied by the left circumflex artery. The AV nodal artery also supplies the main bundle and the origin of the bundle branches. The remainder of the bundle branches are supplied by the penetrating septal perforators of the left anterior descending artery. The posterior descending artery is a less important source of blood supply, unless the left anterior descending artery is occluded, with the posterior descending artery serving as a collateral vessel. These vessels also provide the major supply to the interventricular septum.

The sinoatrial nodal artery is supplied by the main atrial artery arising as the second branch of the right coronary artery in 55 per cent of humans. In the remaining 45 per cent, it arises from the left circumflex artery.

ANGIOGRAPHIC ANATOMY

With the advent of selective coronary arteriography, the different coronary artery patterns can now be identified in living man, both as still shots (serial roentgenograms) and in motion (cine film). A comprehensive and authoritative examination of the roentgenographic coronary anatomy has been described by Sewell (1966) and Gensini and associates (1967). Gensini and da Costa (1969) detailed the angiographic coronary collateral circulation in man.

Conventional right and left lateral, right anterior oblique (RAO), left anterior oblique (LAO), and anteroposterior views were utilized to examine the coronary arteries. With the availability of the C arm, U

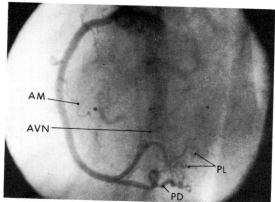

Figure 50–27. LAO view of a normal selective right coronary arteriogram. The acute marginal (AM), AV node (AVN), posterior descending (PD), and posterolateral (PL) arteries are shown.

arm, and parallelogram image intensification systems, cranial and caudal angulation of the image x-ray tubes allowed ease in obtaining additional views of the coronary arteries. These proved valuable in looking at areas that were not always well visualized in the conventional views (Lesperance *et al.*, 1974; Sos *et al.*, 1974).

The right coronary artery is most easily selectively catheterized utilizing the LAO projection. In this projection, the ostium is directly rightward and anterior. It should be remembered that it will not be easy to distinguish the direction of the catheter tip on the television screen if the tip is angled directly toward or away from the angiographer. For this reason, an anteroposterior or RAO view is more difficult to utilize for catheterization of the right coronary artery. The LAO and left lateral projections give the best views of the conus artery, the right muscular branches, and the marginal artery to the right of the main right coronary artery. The crux is easily seen in the LAO projection, with the posterior descending branch going down the posterior surface of the heart (Fig. 50–27). Since the posterior descending vessel sometimes appears "crumpled" like an accordion in this view, a 15-degree or less RAO or cranial RAO projection is

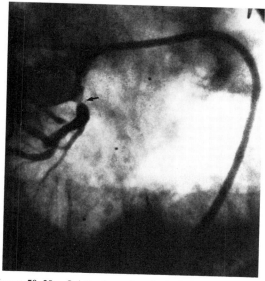

Figure 50–29. LAO view of a flush shot just under the left coronary orifice, showing a subtotal occlusion (arrow) in the proximal left main coronary.

preferred for good visualization of the crux and the posterior descending and distal posterolateral vessels (Fig. 50–28). An angle steeper than 15 degrees in the RAO projection frequently obscures the origins of the proximal vessels as they originate from the distal right

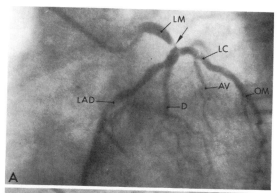

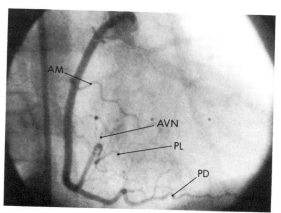

Figure 50–28. A 15-degree RAO view of the right coronary artery shown in Figure 50–27. The posterior descending artery is well visualized in this view.

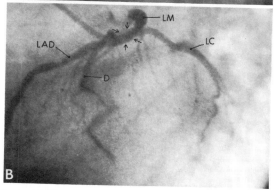

Figure 50–30. LAO view of a selective left coronary arteriogram showing left main (LM), left circumflex (LC), left anterior descending (LAD), diagonal (D), and obtuse marginal (OM) branches. *A,* A 30-degree LAO view reveals a severe obstructive lesion in the distal left main coronary artery (arrow). *B,* This is not appreciated (arrows) in the steeper left anterior oblique projection, because the left anterior descending artery overrides the left main coronary lesion.

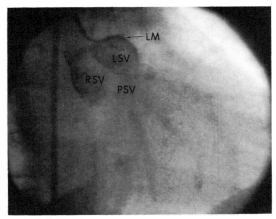

Figure 50–31. Selective contrast injection into a totally occluded left main coronary artery (LM). The right, left, and posterior sinuses of Valsalva (RSV, LSV, and PSV, respectively) are partially opacified. The patient underwent a successful internal mammary artery bypass procedure to his left anterior descending artery (see Figure 50–41.)

coronary artery and crux area, although the mid to distal portions of these vessels are well visualized. In the anteroposterior view, the vessels on the posterior surface of the heart are frequently obscured by the overlying spine.

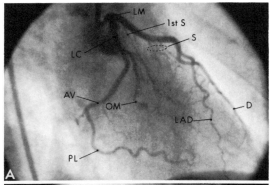

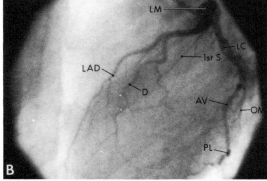

Figure 50–32. Selective left coronary arteriogram showing the major branches in RAO *(A)* and LAO *(B)* projections. The first septal perforator (1st S) is easily seen in both views, whereas the smaller septal perforating branches (S) are best viewed in the RAO projection. The atrioventricular branch (AV) of the left circumflex artery (LC) is best seen in the RAO view, whereas the diagonal (D) branch from the left anterior descending artery (LAD) is well seen in both projections. The obtuse marginal artery (OM) is small in this patient. The left main coronary artery (LM) is short compared with that illustrated in Figure 50–30.

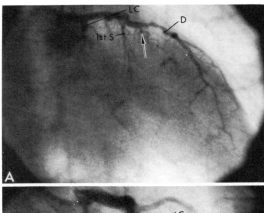

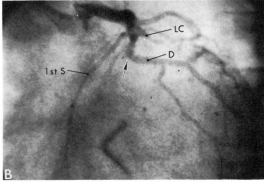

Figure 50–33. *A,* RAO view of a left coronary arteriogram showing a totally occluded left circumflex (LC) and left anterior descending artery. A large diagonal branch (D) could be misinterpreted as being the left anterior descending artery, which is totally occluded (arrow). *B,* LAO view of the same patient, with the large first septal perforator (1st S) giving a false appearance of the left anterior descending artery. The arrow points to the stump of the left anterior descending artery.

The left main coronary ostium and proximal left main coronary artery are best visualized in a 30-degree LAO view. The contrast material should be injected after placing the catheter just at but not in the coronary ostium (Fig. 50–29). In this way, very proximal lesions will not be obscured by a catheter placed past the lesion. The mid and distal segments are well visualized in 30-degree LAO and 30-degree RAO projections (Nath *et al.,* 1979). Proximal stenosis of the left main coronary artery carries a grim prognosis (Zeft *et al.,* 1974) and a severalfold increased risk of death in the Cardiac Catheterization Laboratory (Davis *et al.,* 1979). Adequate visualization of this vessel is mandatory (Fig. 50–30). This vessel is sometimes only 1 or 2 mm. in length, and selective injection of contrast medium into the left anterior descending artery may temporarily obstruct the left circumflex artery (or vice versa), simulating an anatomic occlusion. When either the left or right coronary artery is not seen, sinus of Valsalva opacification may reveal a severely or completely stenosed "stump" of the involved vessel (Fig. 50–31).

The left anterior descending artery is well seen in the LAO, LAO with cranial angulation, and RAO views (Fig. 50–32). When the left circumflex artery overrides the left anterior descending artery in the regular RAO views, caudal angulation usually separates the vessels. Elliott and coworkers (1981) thought

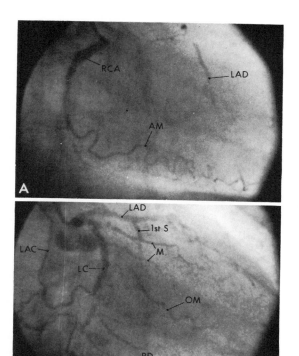

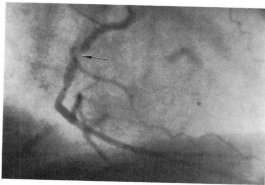

Figure 50–36. Selective right coronary arteriogram in the RAO projection showing a severe proximal localized stenosis that includes the origin of the acute marginal branch.

Figure 50–34. RAO views of a right coronary arteriogram *(A)* and a left coronary arteriogram *(B)* in a 42-year-old man with multiple total and almost total obstructions of both coronary arteries. Poor retrograde opacification of the left anterior descending artery (LAD) from the right coronary (RCA) injection and the (right) posterior descending artery (PD) from the left coronary (LC) injection. (LAC = left atrial circumflex artery; M = marginal branches from the left circumflex artery; OM = obtuse marginal branch.)

that the cranial RAO view was superior for visualizing the mid-left anterior descending artery and the origins of the septal perforators and diagonal branches. The very proximal portion of this vessel is foreshortened in the LAO projection and is better visualized in the cranial LAO and right lateral views. The curling of the distal portion around the apex of the heart and the presence of septal perforators breaking away at nearly 90-degree angles from the proximal and middle portions of this vessel help distinguish the left anterior descending artery from a nearby large diagonal branch. In the LAO projection, the first large septal perforator may be confused with the left anterior descending artery if the latter is totally occluded. An RAO view will distinguish the two vessels; the large septal perforator is clearly seen penetrating the septum at an acute angle from the left anterior descending stump, an angiographic aspect distinct from that of the normal left anterior descending artery (Fig. 50–33*A*). Similarly, a large diagonal branch may appear to be the left anterior descending artery in the RAO projection if the latter vessel is proximally and totally occluded. The LAO view will show the vessel in question to be a diagonal branch and not to follow the usual distribution of the left anterior descending artery (Fig. 50–33*B*).

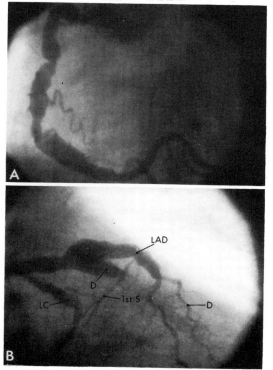

Figure 50–35. Arteriosclerotic aneurysms in the *(A)* right and *(B)* left coronary arteries in a 52-year-old man with angina.

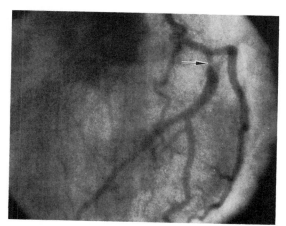

Figure 50–37. LAO view of a left coronary arteriogram showing a severe stenosis in the atrioventricular branch of the left circumflex artery.

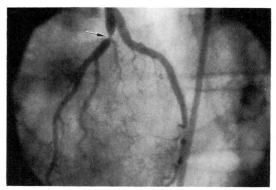

Figure 50–38. Severe localized stenosis in the left anterior descending artery at the origin of the first septal perforator.

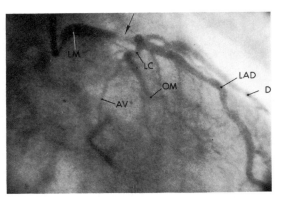

Figure 50–40. RAO view of a left coronary arteriogram in the same patient as in Figure 50–30 with severe stenosis of the left main coronary (arrow).

The left circumflex artery is best visualized in the cranial LAO, left lateral, or LAO projection (Fig. 50–32B). The marginal branch of the left circumflex artery is best seen in the RAO projection (Fig. 50–32A). A large or dominant AV branch of the circumflex artery (with the posterior descending and AV nodal arteries as offshoots) is best visualized in the LAO projection. Figures 50–34 to 50–43 present examples of different coronary artery lesions frequently seen during selective coronary arteriography as well as of opacified internal mammary and saphenous vein coronary bypass grafts.

CONGENITAL MALFORMATIONS

The congenital anomalies of the coronary arteries can be classified as those with anomalous origin (single coronary artery, origin of the left circumflex artery from the right coronary artery, origin of the right or left coronary artery from the pulmonary trunk), those

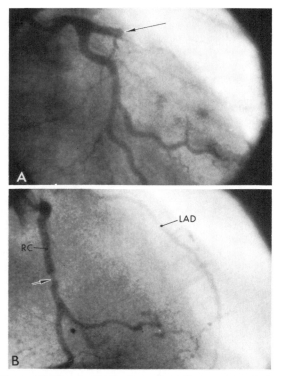

Figure 50–39. *A*, RAO view of a left coronary arteriogram showing a totally occluded left anterior descending artery (arrow) distal to the first septal perforator. *B*, RAO view of a right coronary arteriogram in the same patient showing collateral filling of the left anterior descending artery (LAD) from a right coronary artery (RC) that has a significant middle obstruction (arrow).

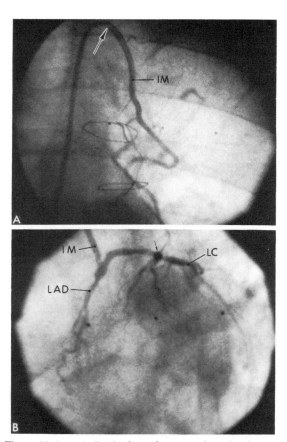

Figure 50–41. *A*, RAO view of contrast injection into the left internal mammary artery (IM). The arrow points to the tip of the catheter as it selectively enters the internal mammary artery. *B*, LAO view of the same patient with the left internal mammary bypass graft filling the left coronary artery (LC). This patient had a totally occluded left main coronary artery, indicated by the arrow. (This is the same patient as in Figure 50–31.)

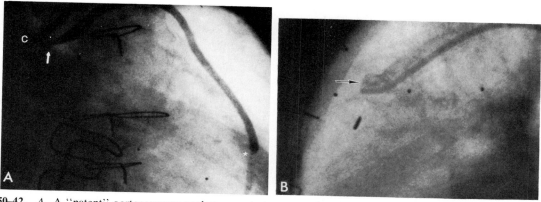

Figure 50–42. *A,* A "patent" aortocoronary saphenous vein bypass graft to the left anterior descending artery. The arrow points to a severe stenosis at the graft origin. Stenosis at the left anterior descending artery anastomosis is also seen (*). (C = catheter tip.) (This is the same patient as in Figures 50–29 and 50–61.) *B,* The arrow points to the stump of a totally occluded aortocoronary saphenous vein bypass graft.

with anomalous communication (to a cardiac chamber, the pulmonary trunk, or a cardiac vein), and those with congenital aneurysm of the coronary arteries (Edwards, 1960). Unusual coronary distribution is also seen in tetralogy of Fallot (Lurie, 1968) and in the transposition complexes (Elliott *et al.,* 1966).

Recent series on anomalous origin of the coronary arteries that arise from the same coronary sinus have pointed out that sudden death can occur in patients in whom the left main branch connecting the left anterior

descending and circumflex arteries originates from the right anterior sinus and passes between the aorta and the right ventricular infundibulum (Cheitlin *et al.,* 1974; Liberthson *et al.,* 1974). Liberthson and co-workers (1974) recommended selective opacification of the left coronary artery in the RAO projection to distinguish the more serious anomaly from the benign type in which this communicating vessel passes anterior the pulmonary outflow tract. Although we have found it difficult to separate the two types angiograph-

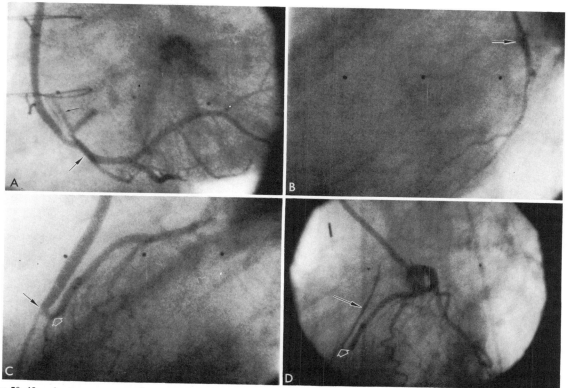

Figure 50–43. Aortocoronary saphenous vein bypass grafts to the *(A)* right coronary artery, *(B)* left circumflex artery, and *(C)* left anterior descending artery. The large arrows point to the junction of the graft and the artery. In *A,* some retrograde filling of the right coronary artery proximal to the graft is seen (small arrow). *D,* Selective left coronary arteriogram in same patient as shown in *C.* Note that the saphenous vein graft fills retrograde and was placed just distal to the severe stenoses (white arrow in *C* and *D*) in the left anterior descending artery.

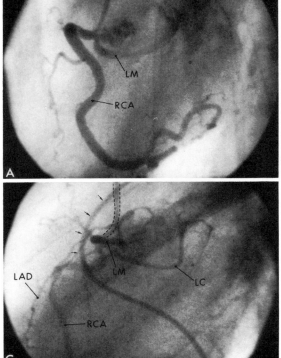

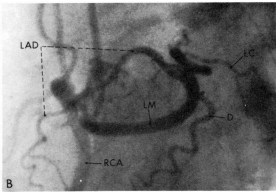

Figure 50–44. *A*, Single coronary artery arising from the right sinus of Valsalva. The left main coronary is partially filled in this LAO view. *B*, In the same patient, the proximal left anterior descending (LAD), left main (LM), right coronary (RCA), left circumflex (LC), and diagonal (D) arteries are all well seen in this LAO projection. What is not appreciated is whether the left main coronary artery passes behind or in front of the pulmonary artery (see text). In *C* (different patient), a left lateral view is used to show the anatomic course of the left main coronary artery. In this view, the pulmonary artery catheter (arrows) outlines the pulmonary outflow area well, and the injection of contrast material into the coronary artery shows the left main coronary artery coursing posteriorly behind the pulmonary artery. Simultaneous opacification of the main pulmonary artery through the right heart catheter can be done if necessary to outline the main pulmonary artery.

ically, we have found it helpful to place a catheter in the pulmonary artery and, during selective opacification of the coronary artery in a left lateral view, to inject a small bolus of contrast material into the pulmonary artery above the pulmonary valve (Fig. 50–44). Anomalous origin of the circumflex artery from the right coronary artery at its origin is a fairly common and benign lesion (Page *et al.*, 1974). It can, however, be mistakenly interpreted as a "nonvisualized" left circumflex coronary artery. Careful search with the coronary catheter in the right sinus should always be done if the left circumflex artery appears "totally occluded" and no late filling of that vessel is seen (Fig. 50–45).

Anomalous origin of the left coronary artery from the pulmonary artery can cause angina, myocardial infarction, and sudden death in both infants and adults (Perry and Scott, 1970). It is probably the most common serious anomalous origin of the coronary arteries, causing ischemia in the left coronary system and leading to papillary muscle dysfunction, mitral insufficiency, and heart failure. Angiographically, the left coronary ostium is absent and a very large left coronary artery fills in a retrograde fashion from the distal branches of a large right coronary artery and then empties into the pulmonary artery, forming a left-to-right shunt (Fig. 50–46).

Coronary arteriovenous fistulas are quite rare and may terminate in any one of the four cardiac chambers or in the pulmonary trunk. They frequently occur as a single coronary abnormality (Ramo *et al.*, 1968). Ninety per cent of coronary arteriovenous fistulas

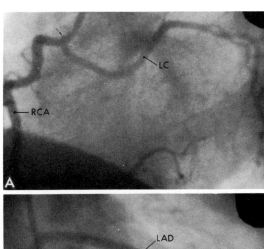

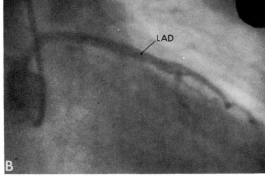

Figure 50–45. Left circumflex artery arising from the right coronary artery. *A*, LAO projection. The arrow points to the common coronary ostium. *B*, RAO view of a left coronary arteriogram in the same patient showing only the left anterior descending and diagonal branches. The absence of a left circumflex artery suggests either a total occlusion of that vessel or an anomalous origin from the right coronary artery.

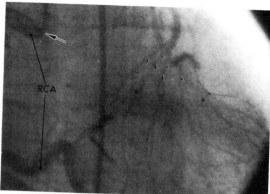

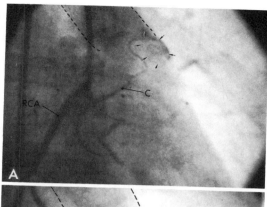

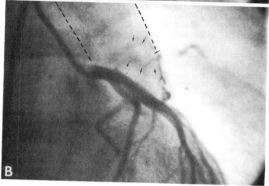

Figure 50–46. RAO projection of a selective right coronary arteriogram in a 34-year-old female with an anomalous left coronary artery arising from the pulmonary artery. The large arrow points to the catheter tip in the right coronary artery (RCA). The small arrows show many collateral vessels filling the left coronary artery retrograde.

Figure 50–47. RAO projection of *(A)* right and *(B)* left coronary arteriograms in an 18-year-old female clinically thought to have a small patent ductus arteriosus. An arteriovenous malformation (arrows) emptying into the pulmonary artery (dotted area) is seen. A small proximal left anterior artery branch is involved in the fistula from the left coronary artery, and the conus artery connects the right coronary artery to the fistula.

terminate in the right side of the heart; 55 per cent originate from the right coronary artery, 35 per cent from the left coronary artery, and 10 per cent from both coronary arteries (Upshaw, 1962). Some may be large enough to cause a significant left-to-right shunt and heart failure. Figure 50–47 shows a small conus artery and a branch from the left coronary artery forming an arteriovenous malformation that empties into the pulmonary artery.

Congenital aneurysms of the coronary arteries are unusual and should not be confused with aneurysm-like dilatation of a coronary artery secondary to the existence of a coronary arteriovenous fistula. The distinction between arteriosclerotic aneurysms of the coronary arteries and a congenital aneurysm is not clear, although the presence of obvious arteriosclerotic obstructive lesions would suggest that any aneurysmal changes are arteriosclerotic in origin (see Fig.

50–35). An isolated aneurysm of a single vessel with otherwise normal coronary arteries, as described by Ebert and associates (1971) and shown in Figure 50–48*A*, would suggest either a congenital aneurysm or perhaps an isolated inflammatory process. Scott

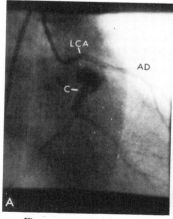

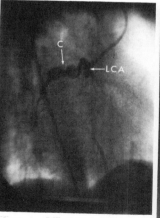

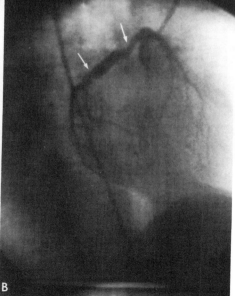

Figure 50–48. *A,* RAO and LAO views of left main coronary artery injection in a 31-year-old female with chest pain showing a normal left anterior descending artery (AD) and a large aneurysm of the circumflex artery (C). *B,* Lateral projection of the left coronary arteriogram 2 weeks after resection of the aneurysm and grafting with an interposition saphenous vein graft (between arrows). This graft was proved open and looked identical 9 years later. (From Ebert, P. A., *et al.*: Resecting and grafting of coronary artery aneurysm. Circulation, *43*:593, 1971.)

CINE VIEW

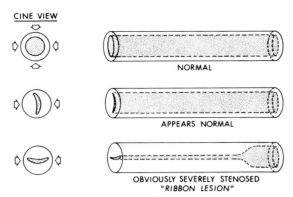

Figure 50–49. Diagrammatic representation of a ribbon lesion. A severe slit-like narrowing of a coronary artery may appear angiographically normal (middle drawing) if viewed in its widest diameter. The arrows point to the cineangiographic view of the cross-section of the vessel.

(1948), on the other hand, classified aneurysms as localized or diffuse, with the latter always considered congenital in origin.

There are some nonpathologic coronary anomalies that will be mentioned in the section entitled "Pitfalls of Coronary Arteriography"

CLASSIFICATION OF LESIONS

There is increasing evidence that an exact classification of angiographic severity of stenosis of coronary vessels can help determine long-term prognosis (Friesinger *et al.*, 1970; Webster *et al.*, 1974; Harris *et al.*, 1980). Usually, the classification records the number of major vessels involved and the severity of the stenosis. The number of obstructions in each major vessel, the collateral filling, and the status of distal vessels should also be recorded. The major vessels are usually defined as the left main coronary, left anterior descending, left circumflex, and right coronary arteries. A 50 per cent narrowing of the diameter of a vessel lumen has been considered clinically significant (Abrams and Adams, 1969). However, many believe that the best candidates for aortocoronary bypass surgery are those with a 75 per cent or greater obstruction (Report of the Inter-Society Commission for Heart Disease Resources, 1972). Although the subjective visual interpretation of the percentage of stenosis correlates well with the measured reduction, more precise quantitative assessment using digital computation may better define what a critical stenosis is with regard to the clinical severity (McMahon *et*

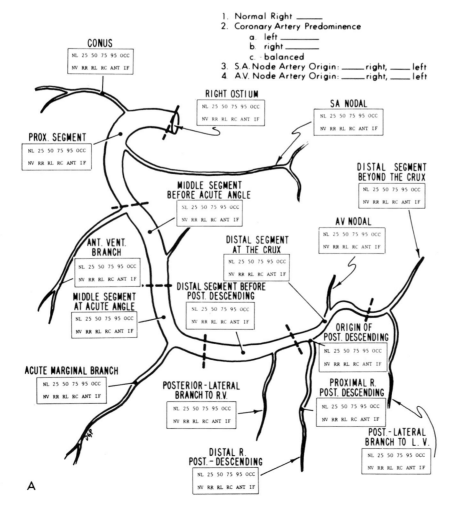

Figure 50–50. Diagram of *(A)* right and *(B)* left coronary arteries. The dotted line divides the vessels into segments for descriptive purposes. *C* illustrates the descriptive terms used to describe each segment as normal (NL) or having a 25, 50, 75, 95 per cent lesion or as being totally occluded (OCC). The bottom row relates the filling characteristics of the segment as nonvisualized (NV), retrograde right (RR), retrograde left (RL), retrograde circumflex (RC), antegrade (ANT), and inadequate fill (IF).

Illustration continued on opposite page

al., 1979). The "narrowest" diameter seen should be used for defining the severity of the lesion, since the slit-like lumen of a severely stenosed vessel in one view may appear normal in another view if the slit is shown in its widest diameter (Vlodaver *et al.*, 1973). This ribbon-like deformity is shown schematically in Figure 50–49.

The nonuniformity of lesion classification among reporting groups becomes readily apparent when a number of studies in which some type of lesion grading system is used are compared. Abrams and Adams (1969) reviewed several grading systems and proposed one of their own, which was relatively simple and could be put on punch cards for computer analysis. However, until a uniform method of classifying coronary lesions is accepted, data among groups cannot be accurately compared. Figure 50–50 *A* and *B* shows a diagram system currently used in our laboratory, which categorizes the information stored in a computer for recall and comparison (Peter *et al.*, 1980).

EQUIPPING THE CARDIOVASCULAR LABORATORY

The Inter-Society Commission for Heart Disease Resources (1971) has developed guidelines for a well-equipped cardiac catheterization laboratory in which selective coronary arteriography can be performed with either the Sones or the Judkins technique. Any cardiac catheterization procedure should be done under constant electrocardiographic monitoring as well as constant intravascular pressure recording. A well-equipped laboratory should include well-trained personnel, defibrillation equipment, an emergency cart, and cineangiographic or radiographic filming equipment with television-image intensification, which will give excellent pictures. A 10-ml. control syringe connected to a two- or three-way stopcock manifold is used by most coronary arteriographers. A rotating table that can be easily manipulated by the physician is often used. A C arm or similar type of cineangiographic unit is popular and can rotate more than 180 degrees around the table. Cineangiographic or radiographic filming equipment capable of visualizing coronary arteries with a lumen diameter of 100 to 200 microns is essential (Sones and Shirey, 1960). Most laboratories use 35-mm. film, with high-speed precision cameras filming at rates of 30 to 60 frames per second. Although 5- to 6-inch image intensifiers have been shown to visualize the coronary arteries adequately, the workers in many laboratories select a combination 6- to 9-inch image tube, which permits better visualization of the left ventricle, whereas the 6-inch mode provides more optimal visualization of the coronary arteries. In addition, a fixed overframing

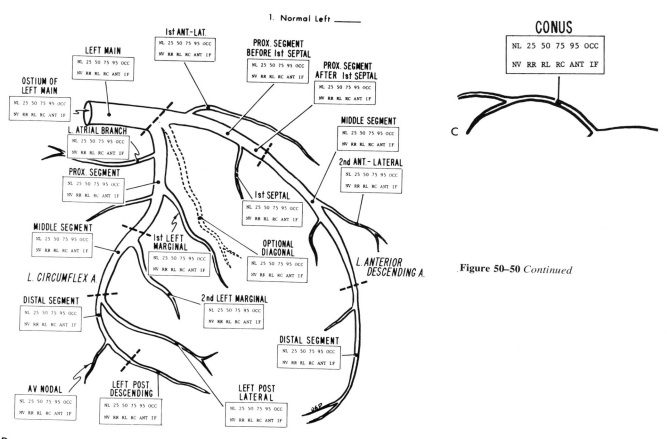

Figure 50–50 *Continued*

B

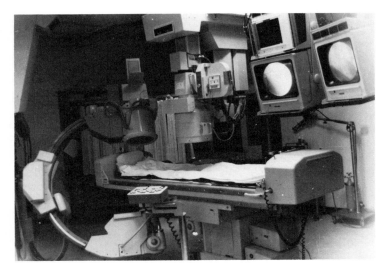

Figure 50–51. Biplane cineangiographic unit with 4-, 6-, and 9-inch tri-mode image intensifiers. The 35-mm. cameras operate at a film speed of 30 to 120 frames per second and are equipped with variable 70- to 150-cm. zoom lenses. The table top rotates to 180 degrees and has horizontal and vertical travel. The C arm is used as the lateral tube for biplane cineangiograms and is rotated for single-plane cineangiograms when routine views and cranial or caudal angulation are needed.

lens system, or the zoom lenses available more recently, can give even greater magnification with minimal distortion and less radiation to the angiographer for a comparable sized electrical image. Figure 50–51 shows a biplane cineangiographic unit with 4-, 6-, and 9-inch image tubes and zoom lenses. The C arm can be used as the lateral tube for biplane ventriculograms and then turned upright for the coronary shots, including all cephalic or caudal views.

BRACHIAL ARTERY CUTDOWN (THE SONES TECHNIQUE)

In 1959, a special woven Dacron catheter* was designed by F. Mason Sones for selective coronary arteriography. The Sones catheters presently used are 80 or 100 cm. long and have a tapered tip of 1.5 inches (Type I) or 1.0 inch (Type II) and a 7-French (F.) lumen tapered to a 5.5-F. tip that is open at the end and has four side openings within 7 mm. of its distal end. The outer diameters are 7, 7.5, and 8 F. The 7.5-F. catheter is called a "Positrol" coronary catheter and has a fine stainless steel wire mesh in its wall that permits better torque control. This catheter is shown in Figure 50–52. The Sones catheter can be used for the left ventriculogram and for selective study of the coronary arteries, aortocoronary saphenous vein bypass grafts, and internal mammary artery bypass grafts on the left side of the arterial cutdown.

Although there are many minor modifications of Sones' original technique, the following plan describes a usual procedure. If catheterization is to be performed in the morning, the patient is given nothing by mouth after midnight except for medications. If the patient is to be studied later in the day, a light breakfast of coffee and toast can be given. An appropriate premedication is usually administered 15 to 30

minutes before the procedure. We prefer 50 mg. of Benadryl administered intramuscularly.

Prior to catheterization, the procedure, including possible complications, is carefully explained to the patient, and signed informed consent is obtained.

The patient is brought to the laboratory and placed on the cardiac catheterization table. With sterile technique (mask, cap, gown, and gloves for the physician), the patient is draped with the right arm placed in a sleeve after the arm and the area of the antecubital fossa are surgically prepared. A brachial cutdown is then performed using an appropriate local anesthetic.

If right heart catheterization is also planned, this is done first. The patient is then intravenously heparinized with a 3000 to 5000 units of aqueous heparin through the right heart catheter or a vein. If right heart catheterization is not done, a venous needle should be placed in the patient's left arm, where medications can be given as necessary. Some physicians heparinize into the brachial artery used for the arterial cutdown.

The brachial artery is then exposed, and if Fick or dye curve cardiac outputs are planned, arterial samples can be withdrawn through an 18-gauge catheter needle placed in the brachial artery after a purse-

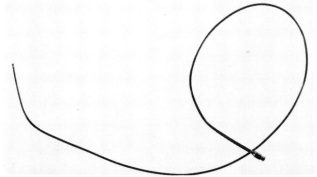

Figure 50–52. Sones catheter used for selective coronary arteriography.

---

*United States Catheter and Instrument Corp., Box 787, Glens Falls, New York.

string suture is placed in this vessel. The vessel can then be gently lifted with umbilical tape, and a small puncture of the artery can be spread easily with a pair of sharp scissor points. Hemostasis can be maintained by gently retracting the umbilical tape. A vessel dilator may be necessary to introduce the catheter into the vessel. Under fluoroscopic control, the catheter is advanced to the arch of the aorta, where pressure recordings are obtained. Occasionally, if the innominate or subclavian artery is tortuous, difficulty may be encountered in entering the root of the aorta. This problem can frequently be avoided by having the patient take a deep breath while the catheter is advanced. In this situation, it is often preferable to use an exposed guide wire to manipulate the catheter from the subclavian artery to the aortic root.

After appropriate pressures are recorded in the root of the aorta, the catheter can then be advanced into the left ventricle, where pressure readings and a left ventricular cineangiogram can be obtained, usually with the patient in the RAO and, if desired, also in the LAO position.

After the left ventriculogram, 0.5 mg. of atropine is given intravenously to counteract the bradycardia frequently seen during selective injection of contrast material into the coronary arteries. A vigorous cough by the patient will aid in clearing contrast material from the coronary arteries if bradycardia or asystole occurs at the end of the coronary injection. Additional atropine can be given when indicated. Although some physicians routinely give nitroglycerin prior to the procedure, we give nitroglycerin only if spasm of the coronary arteries is suspected from what is seen by the angiographer, if a patient has chest pain during the procedure, or if he is seen angiographically to have obstructive coronary disease. Nitroglycerin can dilate the normal coronary artery, sometimes making a "fixed" insignificant lesion appear more narrowed.

The catheter is then selectively placed into the left and right coronary arteries after a flush shot is taken of the left main coronary orifice in a shallow LAO projection, looking for a possible left main coronary artery lesion (see Fig. 50–29). Cineangiograms are obtained with the patient holding a deep breath as 3 to 8 ml. of contrast material* are injected. Multiple different RAO, LAO, cranial, and caudal views of each coronary artery can be done to provide adequate visualization of all coronary branches. Pressure can be monitored on the oscilloscope screen at all times, except during the injection of contrast material. When difficulty is encountered in locating a coronary ostium, injections of contrast material into the sinus of Valsalva will help identify its position. A videotape system is extremely helpful during a study, as it allows the arteriographer to be sure he has obtained visualization of the entire coronary arterial tree before terminating the study. A video disc system allows slow-motion replay, with freeze-framing giving excellent detail.

Upon removal of the catheter from the brachial artery, forward and backflow bleeding are permitted for a few seconds in order to flush any small thrombi from the vessel. Occasionally, a blunt instrument may be placed gently down the distal brachial artery if adequate backflow bleeding does not occur. A No. 4 Fogarty catheter* may have to be inserted to free the distal artery of clots. Some physicians routinely use Fogarty catheters in this manner in all patients. When adequate forward and backflow bleeding has occurred, the arteriotomy site is closed. For closure of the arteriotomy, 5-0 Tevdek† with a T1 (noncutting) needle can be used. Although some prefer to place a purse-string suture in the artery prior to catheter introduction, others use the same or a different method of arteriotomy closure after the catheter has been withdrawn. In order to facilitate hemostasis, gentle finger pressure over the artery after closure may be used if slight bleeding occurs. Occasionally, an additional mattress suture is needed to control bleeding after the arteriotomy is closed. If a good radial artery pulse is not felt, the vessel can be reopened and a Fogarty catheter introduced to remove the thrombus. The physician must be alert to thromboses that occur at the brachial artery cutdown site and cause ischemic symptoms in the patient's hand and arm. Although some physicians believe that the loss of the pulse causes little difficulty (Sones and Shirey, 1962), others feel strongly that the patient should, at some time within 24 hours of the procedure, have the vessel reopened and the clot cleared out with a Fogarty catheter (Campion et al., 1971). Our experience has shown no lasting ischemic complications with pulse loss, but we almost invariably re-explore the brachial artery via a Fogarty catheter within 24 hours of the pulse loss. The skin is then closed, and a light pressure dressing is placed over the area. The patient is sent back to his room with instructions to keep his arm bent 90 degrees at the elbow for about 2 hours and then to use his arm freely. The skin sutures are removed 6 days after cardiac catheterization.

Advantages and Disadvantages of the Sones Technique

The angiographer must be aware that the Sones catheter with side holes may record a normal-appearing aortic pressure when tightly wedged in the coronary artery if that portion of the catheter with the side holes is not wedged into the coronary artery. How much coronary perfusion occurs through the side holes of a wedged Sones catheter is not known, but slowing of the rate or ST-T changes are indications that inadequate coronary flow may be occurring. Since these catheters are frequently left in the coronary

---

*Hypaque 75 (Winthrop) or Renografin 76 (Squibb).

*Manufactured by Edwards Laboratories, 17221 Red Hill Avenue, Santa Ana, California.
†Manufactured by DeKnatel, Inc., Queens Village, New York.

artery after the injection and while the patient is being repositioned, wedging of the catheter may occur without being signaled by obvious pressure changes. Anytime that contrast material does not clear from the coronary artery, obstruction of the lumen by the wedged catheter is probable, and the catheter should be quickly removed from the coronary orifice.

There is increasing evidence that obtaining physiologic data (cardiac output, pressures, biplane ventricular volume data, ejection fraction) is mandatory during all coronary studies. The Sones technique does not lend itself to biplane cineangiographic studies without great difficulty, because the patient is studied from the arm. Furthermore, we have found that the left ventriculogram through a Sones catheter frequently results in a poorly opacified ventricle and that we have to change to a Gensini or pigtail catheter to do the left ventriculogram.

Although selective coronary cineangiography using the Sones technique can be done in a very short time (frequently "skin to skin" in well under 1 hour), there are cases in which the left coronary artery is extremely difficult to enter selectively. The angiographer must be very adept at catheter manipulation. For each ostium to be entered, the angiographer must make a loop with the end of the catheter and then skillfully place the tip correctly.

Sometimes the catheter will bend in the subclavian or innominate artery, as mentioned earlier. Attempts to manipulate the catheter only tend to make this type of catheter coil further. Under these circumstances, the standard catheter can be replaced with a left 4 Judkins catheter,* which is placed over a guide wire into the aortic root and then manipulated into the left coronary ostium after the guide wire has been removed, blood withdrawn, and the catheter flushed. Some other preformed catheters successfully used for the left coronary artery are brachial artery, multipurpose, and Headhunter catheters* passed over guide wires. In the rare cases in which there is difficulty entering the right coronary ostium, a Judkins right coronary catheter is helpful.

PERCUTANEOUS FEMORAL TECHNIQUE (THE JUDKINS TECHNIQUE)

In the percutaneous femoral approach, the most commonly used catheters are Judkins catheters, although the individual technique and type of catheter used may vary from Judkins' technique. Figure 50–53 shows the more commonly used preformed catheters for the percutaneous femoral technique. The Cordis multipurpose catheter and the Judkins right coronary catheter can also be used to selectively study aorto-coronary saphenous vein and internal mammary artery bypass grafts.

In 1967, Melvin P. Judkins reported on 100 consecutive patients who had undergone coronary arteriography via a percutaneous transfemoral technique. The actual introduction of the catheter was via the Seldinger (1953) technique. He had designed right and left coronary artery catheters that were used for selective injection into each of the coronary arteries. He initially had to make these preformed catheters himself, but they have long been commercially available in sizes 7 and 8 F., 100 cm. in length. These catheters have no side holes and are disposable. The left coronary artery catheter is available in sizes 4, 5, and 6, with the primary curve angle of the catheter varying from 100 to 90 to 80 degrees, respectively, and the secondary curve angle varying from 160 to 180 to 200 degrees, respectively. The No. 6 catheter is commonly used in patients with dilated aortic roots, whereas size 4 is the most frequently used catheter in patients who have normal-sized aortic roots. The right

---

*Manufactured by Cordis Corporation, Miami, Florida.

*Manufactured by Cordis Corporation, Miami, Florida.

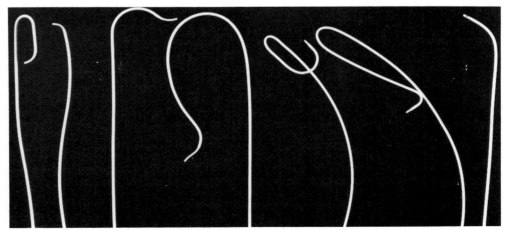

Figure 50–53.   Percutaneous femoral coronary catheters. From left to right are shown left and right coronary Judkins catheters, left and right Amplatz catheters, left and right coronary Bourossa catheters, and a Cordis multipurpose catheter, all of which can be used for selective coronary arteriography.

coronary artery catheter is also available in three sizes. The primary curve of the right coronary artery catheter is set at 95 degrees, with the secondary curve measuring 30 degrees. The secondary portion of the catheter varies in size from 4, 5, or 6 cm., a measurement that relates to the length of the secondary curve.

The procedures performed before cardiac catheterization, such as sedation and obtaining informed consent, are the same as those previously described for the brachial artery cutdown technique. Single-dose total-body heparinization is also being used by many to reduce thrombotic complications (Walker *et al.*, 1973), particularly if the pigtail catheter is used for the left ventriculogram. The catheters used are all introduced percutaneously via the Seldinger (1953) technique. Before coronary arteriography is performed, a left ventriculogram is obtained to evaluate left ventricular performance, using an appropriate left ventricular catheter (a Gensini or pigtail catheter* is adequate for this purpose). An 18-gauge thin-walled needle is inserted percutaneously into the femoral artery, and a 0.035-inch Teflon-coated guide wire is advanced through the needle just beyond the aortoiliac junction. While firm pressure is applied over the puncture site, the needle is removed, and the guide wire is wiped with a sponge soaked with heparinized saline solution. A size 8 Teflon introducer is inserted into the artery over the guide wire. After the introducer is removed and the wire is cleansed with heparinized saline, the left ventriculography catheter is slipped over the guide wire into the aorta. Three or four milliliters of blood are removed from the catheter, and heparinized saline is then flushed through the catheter. After this, the catheter is connected to a continuous pressure monitoring system. It can then be advanced under fluoroscopic guidance to the root of the aorta and across the aortic valve into the left ventricle for the left ventriculogram.

The left coronary artery catheter can be exchanged for a left ventriculogram catheter over Teflon-coated guide wire. The Teflon-coated guide wire is preferred since it is less adherent to the catheter and moves more easily. The guide wire is placed in the ascending aorta near the left subclavian artery. The catheter is then directed over the guide wire until about 2 cm. of floppy wire protrude from the tip of the catheter. The catheter is advanced into the upper root of the aorta but not near the left coronary ostia, and the wire is removed. Three or four milliliters of blood are then removed from the catheter and discarded. The catheter is well flushed with heparinized saline and connected to a continuous pressure monitoring system. Again, we sometimes administer 0.5 mg. of atropine intravenously prior to the coronary arteriography and repeat the dose if bradycardia occurs during coronary injections.

With the patient in a 30-degree LAO position, the catheter is advanced near the left coronary orifice and

a selective injection is made to visualize the left main coronary artery and ostium, as previously described for the brachial artery cutdown technique. Some angiographers remove the catheter after each injection, and others leave the catheter in place if it is not obstructing the orifice. Continuous pressure monitoring is reinstituted through the catheter tip at the completion of each injection. If damping of the pressure contour recorded from the coronary artery catheter is noted or if contrast material "hangs up" in the coronary artery after the injection, the coronary orifice has probably become obstructed by the catheter and the catheter should be removed immediately. If this occurs when the catheter is being placed in the ostium, the coronary artery injection should be done quickly and the catheter removed. If the heart rate slows or if premature ventricular contractions are noted, the arteriographer should also quickly withdraw the catheter. If the catheter is withdrawn too far, the tip will curl back into its natural position and reintroduction of the Teflon-coated guide wire will be necessary to straighten the catheter. This should be done after the catheter is pulled below the renal arteries. Occasionally, the contrast material will clear from the coronary artery slowly after the injection. The heart rate is usually slow and the arterial pressure low. The heart is ischemic and contracting poorly. Two or three hard coughs with a breath in between will raise intrathoracic pressure abruptly and help clear the contrast material quickly, reversing the bradycardia and hypotension (Conti, 1977).

After appropriate arteriograms are obtained in both the RAO and LAO positions, the catheter is pulled back to the descending aorta below the left subclavian artery, where it is exchanged for the right coronary artery catheter using the Teflon-coated guide wire. The right coronary artery catheter is then placed into the root of the aorta. With the patient in a 75-degree LAO position, the right coronary artery catheter can then be rotated slowly clockwise about 180 degrees and pulled back 1 or 2 cm. until it enters the right coronary orifice. Unlike the left coronary artery catheter, which easily falls into the coronary ostium in most instances, the right coronary artery catheter does require manipulation. Still, it is usually quite easy to enter the right coronary orifice and obtain multiple arteriograms in both oblique views.

After the coronary arteriograms have been obtained, the catheter can be removed, and the pressure is maintained in the femoral area for 10 minutes, which usually will stop any bleeding from the puncture site. The patient should be kept in bed for several hours, with the leg on the side of the groin used kept straight.

Advantages and Disadvantages of the Judkins Technique

There are several advantages to using this technique. First of all, it is simple and requires less

---

*Manufactured by Cordis Corporation, Miami, Florida.

technical skill. Although there is always concern about trauma to the left coronary orifice and possible dislodgement of an arteriosclerotic plaque that might occur during manipulation of the catheter in the aortic root, we have not encountered this problem in 12,000 coronary arteriograms. Nevertheless, the possibility of this happening still remains. The physician should be extremely careful when changing the catheters to avoid inadvertently introducing the guide wires into the coronary arteries. We feel that the coronary guide wire should not be advanced past the left subclavian artery when the catheter is being changed. However, once the catheter is 3 or 4 cm. from the tip of the guide wire, they both can be carefully advanced past the arch to the upper part of the ascending aorta.

Because of the femoral approach, biplane cineangiograms can be readily obtained, thereby permitting two simultaneous perpendicular views during each injection. Judkins (1968) stressed that cineangiography should be combined with direct serial radiography. However, we have found that biplane cineangiography alone gives excellent anatomic detail.

Occasionally, obstruction in the femoral or iliac artery is encountered when trying to introduce the guide wire. A straight guide wire can be replaced by a J-tip guide wire. If the J-tip guide wire cannot be advanced to the aorta after careful manipulation for 2 or 3 minutes, the guide wire and needle should be removed from the femoral artery and the other femoral artery entered. On the other hand, if the obstruction appears to be at the level of the aorta and all manipulatory efforts fail, the guide wire should then be removed and the brachial artery cutdown technique employed. It should be pointed out, however, that any patient with this degree of atherosclerotic disease in the large vessels of the lower trunk almost always has tortuosity and atherosclerotic changes in the subclavian and innominate vessels. Adequate coronary visualization may not be possible with either technique in these patients with advanced disease.

Perhaps the main disadvantage to the percutaneous femoral technique using Judkins catheters is also the main advantage—the procedure is quick and easy to perform. Unfortunately, the ease of doing the procedure induces many with inadequate experience to undertake it initially, resulting in high morbidity (Judkins and Gander, 1974). However, a multicenter study showed lower morbidity and mortality with the femoral approach when compared with the brachial approach (Davis et al., 1979).

INDICATIONS AND CONTRAINDICATIONS FOR SELECTIVE CORONARY ARTERIOGRAPHY

Selective coronary arteriography is assuming a more important role in the management of patients with suspected and proved obstructive coronary artery disease (Baltaxe and Levin, 1972). It is still the only method by which the presence of coronary lesions can be documented in living man. Patients studied with selective coronary arteriography seem to fall into two main categories: those whose diagnosis is uncertain (usually patients with chest pains that are atypical for angina or who have electrocardiographic abnormalities of recent onset in whom obstructive coronary artery disease is a possibility), and those who are being considered for coronary artery surgery or other types of heart surgery.

In any large group of patients reported who have undergone selective coronary arteriography, there are usually 20 to 30 per cent whose coronary arteriograms are normal (Proudfit et al., 1966; Friesinger et al., 1970). Some patients may present with chest pains not characteristic of angina, nonspecific electrocardiographic abnormalities, years of unsuccessful treatment with a variety of cardiac drugs, and symptoms that will be diagnosed clinically as preinfarction angina. Fifteen per cent of one series of 85 patients diagnosed as having preinfarction angina were "excluded" from a double-blind medical versus surgical treatment protocol because their coronary arteriograms were normal (Scanlon et al., 1973). Although it may be debated whether or not those with normal coronary arteriograms actually do have coronary artery "disease," they are certainly not candidates for coronary artery bypass surgery and have a good prognosis (Bemiller et al., 1973). On the other hand, some will have obstructive coronary artery disease truly unrecognized by what would be considered good angiograms because of occlusion of a small coronary branch or because the obstructive lesion is always obscured by another vessel in multiple cineangiographic views The latter problem has prompted some to suggest different patient positions during angiography (Nath et al., 1979); these positions have now become more routine with the advent of cineangiographic C-arm and U-arm systems that allow a variety of angled projections.

It should be pointed out that there will always be a group of patients with unexplained chest discomfort who will ultimately be diagnosed as having idiopathic hypertrophic subaortic stenosis (Peter et al., 1968), nonobstructive cardiomyopathy (Gault and Simon, 1968), ballooning mitral valves (Barlow et al., 1968), or coronary spasm. In our last 1000 patients who had normal coronary arteriograms, our routine practice of obtaining biplane left ventricular cineangiograms for optimal visualization of the mitral valve apparatus in all patients and of performing provocative tests with amyl nitrite and isoproterenol (Isuprel) for suspected hypertrophic obstructive cardiomyopathy and ergotamine for coronary spasm (Schroeder et al., 1977) has identified many patients with one of these disorders (Fig. 50–54).

Coronary arteriography is frequently considered for patients with incapacitating angina in whom all efforts at medical treatment have failed and for whom cardiac surgery is contemplated. Although there is some evidence that selective coronary arteriograms may be safely omitted in those patients who will need valve replacement but have no symptoms of ischemic

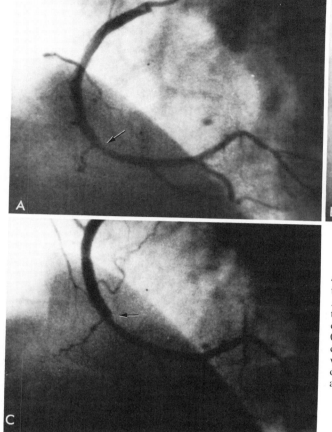

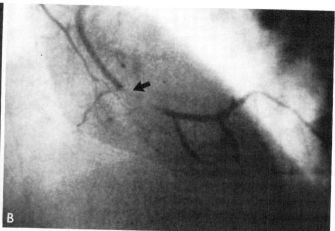

Figure 50–54. *A,* LAO view of the right coronary artery in 42-year-old man with classic exertional angina and a positive treadmill test showing ST-T depression in leads II, AVF, and III. A 50 per cent narrowing was noted (arrow) in the midportion of the right coronary artery. *B,* After 0.05, 0.1, and 0.15 mg. of ergotamine was given intravenously and 3 minutes apart (total dose 0.3 mg.), the patient experienced chest tightness, his ST-T segments dropped 2 mm. in lead II, and 2 cm. of his right coronary artery were obliterated (arrow). *C,* Ten seconds after 200 μg. of intracoronary nitroglycerin were given, the spasm (arrow), chest tightness, and depressed ST-T segments disappeared.

heart disease and are without coronary risk factors (Bonchek *et al.,* 1973), patients who will undergo aortic or mitral valve replacement are usually studied. Those who have cardiac decompensation presumably due to a left ventricular aneurysm for which surgical removal is a possibility should undergo arteriographic studies.

Sones (1972) has studied a small number of patients who are terrified of the possibility of sudden death because of a strong family history of coronary heart disease. He also feels that coronary arteriography should be routine in patients at the first appearance of anginal symptoms. This position is still debatable, but data collected in the last several years have shown that aortocoronary bypass surgery can prolong life in left main coronary artery and three-vessel disease, and this approach is becoming more prevalent. When we can evaluate the effect of surgical intervention on long-term morbidity and mortality, additional criteria for deciding when coronary arteriography is appropriate can be determined.

Patients who should not be studied are those who have severe congestive heart failure, digitalis toxicity, or chronic long-standing heart failure, unless a resectable ventricular aneurysm is suspected. The patient with multiple myocardial infarctions and chronic failure usually has a heart that is heavily scarred with a generalized poorly contracting ventricle. These pa-

tients with "ischemic cardiomyopathy" have a poor medical prognosis and at best an equally poor prognosis after an attempt at revascularization (Yatteau *et al.,* 1974). More recent studies in these patients with angina rather than congestive heart failure have shown a lower operative mortality (Zubiate *et al.,* 1977). Unless emergency coronary bypass surgery is contemplated, coronary arteriography and left ventriculography should not be performed within 4 to 6 weeks of an acute myocardial infarction. A debatable exception may be the patient in cardiogenic shock, a condition with extremely poor prognosis in which emergency cardiac surgery has had limited success (Mundt *et al.,* 1970). Without question, the most nondebatable contraindication to the procedure of selective coronary arteriography is the absence of a physician who has the skill, knowledge, common sense, and experience to do a first-rate study and to do it safely.

COMPLICATIONS

Brachial artery cutdown and percutaneous femoral techniques in selective coronary arteriography have been shown to be safe and reliable methods for obtaining necessary anatomic information about obstructive coronary lesions. As in any procedure requiring skill by the operator and in which the patient may have profound illness, complications occur despite meticulous adherence to technique by the well-trained physician. The low mortality rate of 0.3 to 0.5 per cent reported in large teaching hospitals where fellows and residents in training perform many of the selective coronary studies under the supervision of senior staff members indicates that an even lower mortality rate might well be obtained by any physician experienced in cardiac catheterization who does all of the studies himself. Figures for the private practice setting are not known, but there is compelling evidence that the highest morbidity and mortality rates are associated with those physicians doing the least number of cases (Adams et al. 1973). Sones (1972) stated that the risk of death attributable to the study should be less than 1/1000 (0.1 per cent). He reported three deaths in his first 1020 patients (0.29 per cent) (Sones and Shirey, 1962), five deaths in his next 7200 patients (0.8 per cent) (Sones, 1967), and 39 deaths (0.07 per cent) in 52,953 patients studied through 1976 (Sones, 1978).

The brachial artery cutdown technique of Sones and the percutaneous femoral technique of Judkins probably compare equally in terms of safety, despite the fact that more technical skill is required for the Sones technique. Critics of the hazards of the Judkins technique and the concomitant use of preformed catheters have been countered by low mortality rate associated with Judkins' own studies. He has argued that the fault lies in the quality of training of those using his technique and not in the technique itself (Judkins and Gander, 1974). We are in complete agreement with Judkins on this point. Many physicians with 6 months or less of training are doing cardiac catheterization procedures, including selective coronary arteriography in community hospitals with little or no evaluation of how well the studies are being performed and the data interpreted.

A summary of complications in 3312 selective coronary arteriograms via the brachial artery cutdown technique in 3264 patients was published in 1968 (Ross and Gorlin, 1968) as a cooperative study from seven laboratories. Eighty-one per cent of those patients examined were studied in the laboratory of F. Mason Sones, and the rest were studied in six other laboratories. Nevertheless, the findings were remarkable: There were three deaths (0.099 per cent), 10 myocardial infarctions (0.3 per cent), 26 episodes of ventricular fibrillation or tachycardia (0.8 per cent), and 15 brachial artery complications (0.5 per cent). Taken separately, the complications from Sones' laboratory were considerably less than those of the other six groups reporting—not an unexpected finding in view of the continuing vast experience of Sones and colleagues (1978). It is of interest that an early communication by Sones and Shirey (1962) mentioned a rate of occlusion at the brachial artery site of 6 to 7 per cent in 1020 patients (in between 60 and 70 patients). In a later communication (1978), Sones reported a 2.8 per cent brachial artery complication rate in 52,953 procedures. This certainly suggests that his increased experience has resulted not only in a decreased death rate but also a decreased arterial complication rate. A similar brachial artery thrombosis rate, in the vicinity of a 1 to 2 per cent, has been reported (Campion et al., 1971; Adams et al., 1973).

Sewell (1965) reported on procedures in 200 patients, with only one case of ventricular fibrillation and no deaths using the technique of Sones. Three patients lost the radial pulse, and one patient had a false aneurysm at the suture line of the brachial artery, which was repaired without difficulty.

The method of Judkins and colleagues has also been deemed safe. Judkins (1968) described one death in his first 600 cases (0.2 per cent). In 1972, Green and Judkins reported 20 complications using Judkin's technique in 445 consecutive cases, which included nine episodes of delayed femoral bleeding, five femoral thromboses, two embolic episodes, one episode of ventricular fibrillation, two myocardial infarctions, and one significant bradyarrhythmia. Two late deaths did not seem to be definitively related to the cardiac catheterization. A few case reports have described perforation or dissection of the left coronary artery during selective coronary arteriography using the Judkins technique (Morettin and Wallace, 1970; Haas et al., 1968). This danger may well be related to the difficulty in controlling the tip of the Judkins catheters while entering the main left coronary artery. Gentle manipulation of these catheters down the aortic root is frequently not enough to prevent them from literally jumping into the orifice of the left main coronary artery. Haas and coworkers (1968) have suggested that the catheter to be withdrawn several millimeters from the left main artery coronary after entry. Although this maneuver can be done, gentle retraction tends to flip the catheter out of the left coronary ostium and back into the aortic root.

Gau and associates (1970) examined a small number of patients using both the Sones and the Judkins techniques. Of 75 patients, 12 per cent had ventricular fibrillation; 1.3 per cent had myocardial infarction; 8.7 per cent had brachial artery thrombosis; and 3.8 per cent had femoral artery complications. There were no deaths. These investigators felt that the Judkins technique was the method of choice because of a higher success rate in obtaining coronary arteriograms and a lower peripheral vascular complication rate.

The true safety factor may never be known for any of these problems since only complications occurring during the catheterization procedure are measured. It is not possible to ascertain whether the patient who suffers an acute myocardial infarction 10 hours after a seemingly uncomplicated coronary arteriographic study did so because of the procedure. Furthermore, myocardial infarction and death also occur before the scheduled cardiac catheterization. Sones (1967) reported that during a 6-month period, 17 patients had been unable to keep their appointments for selective coronary arteriography because they had died. As in most procedural complications, the cause-and-effect relationship is not usually self-evident.

The most conclusive paper on complications using the femoral and brachial arteriography techniques

TABLE 50–8. COMPLICATION RATES FOR CORONARY ARTERIOGRAPHY*

| | LESS THAN 100 CASES/YEAR | | MORE THAN 400 CASES/YEAR | |
	Femoral Technique	Brachial Technique	Femoral Technique	Brachial Technique
Mortality rate	1.30%	0.38%	0.16%	0.06%
Myocardial infarction	1.90%	0.42%	0.19%	0.10%
Cerebral emboli	0.60%	0.10%	0.05%	0.00%

*Summary table compiled from Adams, D. F. *et al.*: The complications of coronary arteriography. Circulation, *48*:609, 1973. Morbid complications are several times more common in those laboratories in which less than 100 procedures per year are performed compared with those in which more than 400 arteriograms per year are done.

is still that of Adams and colleagues (1973), who examined 46,904 coronary arteriograms from 173 hospitals (significantly, questionnaires were never returned from 200 hospitals). They found an overall mortality rate of 0.45 per cent, with a death rate of 0.78 per cent with the femoral technique and 0.13 per cent with the brachial technique. The overall incidence of myocardial infarction was 0.61 per cent; ventricular fibrillation, 1.28 per cent; arterial thrombosis, 1.44 per cent; hemorrhage, 0.12 per cent; cerebral emboli, 0.23 per cent; and reaction to contrast material, 0.14 per cent.

However, it was clearly evident that those institutions in which less than 100 procedures per year were performed carried the main burden of the mortality and morbidity rates and that those in which the femoral technique and preformed catheters were used had a higher overall complication rate, except for local thrombosis, when compared with those in which the brachial technique was employed. Mortality rates as high as 7.7 per cent were reported in those hospitals in which 25 arteriograms were done in 2 years, with ranges of 2 to 3.5 per cent in those hospitals in which 100 procedures were performed over a 2-year period. The mortality rate for the femoral approach was consistently slightly higher than that for the brachial approach. This contrasted to the data from the two institutions in which the most procedures were done, where the mortality rate for the femoral (0.08 per cent) and brachial (0.06 per cent) approaches were many times lower and essentially equal. A summary of the complication rates from those laboratories in which less than 100 arteriograms per year were done and from those in which more than 400 procedures per year were performed is presented in Table 50–8. This summary highlights the conclusions of Adams and coworkers that coronary arteriography should not be a sporadic procedure performed by inexperienced physicians, that the risk of death or serious nonlethal complications such as myocardial infarction and cerebral embolus is increased in those laboratories in which a small number of studies are done, and that the femoral technique appeared to be slightly more hazardous than the brachial technique when all possible complications were considered. A more recent multicenter study on 7553 consecutive patients (Davis *et al.*, 1979) showed a higher death rate and myocardial infarction rate with the brachial approach when compared with the femoral approach (0.51 per cent vs. 0.14 per cent and 0.42 per cent vs. 0.22 per cent, respectively). The result did not apply when analysis was restricted to laboratories in which 80 per cent or more brachial procedures were performed.

PITFALLS OF CORONARY ARTERIOGRAPHY

Many problems that can arise in the performance of selective coronary catheterization and in interpretation of the results, mentioned earlier, are worth reemphasizing. Only superior physician acumen, training, and experience can assure safety to the patient. The physician who attempts occasional cardiac catheterizations needlessly endangers his patients. The morbidity and mortality in laboratories in which less than 50 studies per year are performed are strikingly high (Adams *et al.*, 1973). In addition, it is possible that these figures are even higher in those 200 institutions that did not choose to report their problems to Adams and colleagues in their revealing survey of complications in coronary arteriography.

Judkins and Gander (1974) strongly criticize those who use the Judkins technique for selective coronary arteriography without proper training. They recognize that the convenience of preformed catheters has unfortunately encouraged the marginally trained physician to attempt this procedure. Although the coronary ostium is usually easily reached, it is possible for the physician to introduce the catheter into "peculiar" positions that are actually outside a coronary vessel (Fig. 50–55). Air bubbles can be injected into the

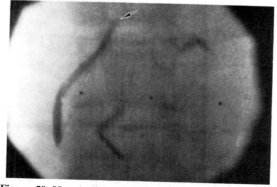

Figure 50–55. A dissection of the right coronary artery that was inadvertently produced by a Sones catheter during selective coronary arteriography. Contrast medium persists after a "test dose" as a subintimal hematoma (arrow). This patient suffered no permanent myocardial damage and was found to have a normal selective right coronary arteriogram 1 hour later after the contrast medium was reabsorbed.

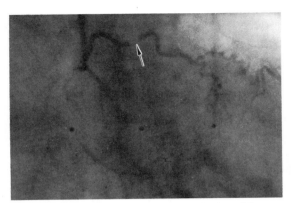

Figure 50–56. RAO projection of a selective right coronary arteriogram. Injection of a small air bubble (arrow) into the conus artery of a man with severe obstructive coronary artery disease. The distal right coronary artery and left anterior descending artery are seen.

coronary arteries if the control syringe is carelessly filled with contrast material (Fig. 50–56). A major pitfall in coronary arteriography as well as a contraindication to the procedure is, therefore, performance of the procedure by the inadequately trained physician. The same type of person is likely to misinterpret the arteriogram, fail to take enough pictures to obtain a satisfactory study, and inadequately handle difficult crises encountered in a cardiovascular laboratory.

Another major pitfall in selective coronary arteriography is interpretation. After injecting contrast material into the left coronary artery, the inexperienced angiographer may misinterpret a late-filling posterior cardiac vein as an "occluded" retrograde-filling posterior descending coronary artery. The veins draining the coronary capillaries have a distribution similar to that of the major arteries and fill late in the coronary injection sequence (Fig. 50–57). A "totally occluded" left circumflex artery interpreted by its absence in the left coronary injection may be nothing more than a normal but aberrant vessel that arises from the right

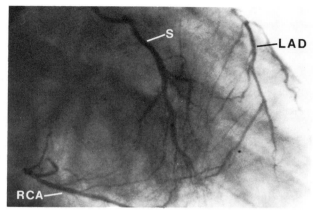

Figure 50–58. The coronary catheter fills a large septal perforator (S) arising near the right coronary sinus. Collaterals can be seen filling well a totally occluded left anterior descending artery (LAD) and right coronary artery (RCA). This man with severe angina had been refused bypass surgery 3 years previously because the totally occluded LAD and RCA were not seen during catheterization and were probably thought to be poor vessels for grafting. Since then, he has undergone aortocoronary bypass grafts to both occluded vessels, with relief of his angina.

coronary sinus (Fig. 50–45). The conus artery can serve as the main source of collateral flow to an occluded right or left anterior descending coronary artery (Levin *et al.*, 1981). Failure to visualize this vessel, which arises half the time from a separate

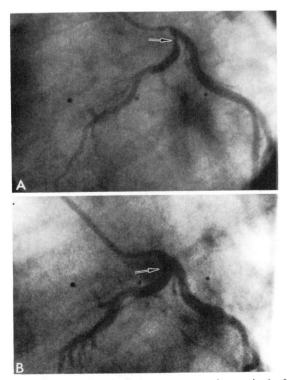

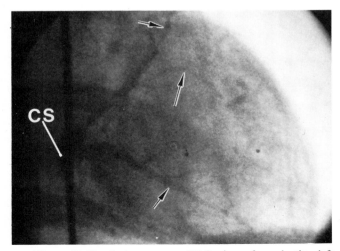

Figure 50–57. Late sequence RAO view of a selective left coronary arteriogram with the coronary veins (arrows) emptying into the coronary sinus (CS). These may be mistaken as late-filling distal coronary artery segments.

Figure 50–59. Selective left coronary arteriogram in the LAO projection. *A,* Catheter-induced spasm in the proximal left anterior descending artery giving the impression of a severe obstruction. The patient had no chest discomfort or electrocardiographic changes. *B,* A second left coronary injection 3 minutes after administration of nitroglycerin. The narrowed segment illustrated in *A* has resumed a normal appearance (arrow).

ostium in the right coronary sinus, could allow a vessel that has potential for bypass grafting to go undetected. We recently studied a man who had totally occluded left anterior descending and right coronary arteries, good left ventricular function, and no evident collateral filling of the occluded vessels. An aberrant large septal perforator was found off the right coronary sinus that filled these vessels via collaterals, showing good vessels for subsequent successful aortocoronary bypass surgery (Fig. 50–58).

Another problem of interpretation is caused by coronary spasm. Spasm usually occurs in the proximal right coronary artery at the site of the coronary catheter tip, although it can be seen in the middle portion of the right coronary artery and occasionally in the left coronary artery (Fig. 50–59). In addition, transient narrowing (myocardial bridging) can occur during systole, reflecting the anatomic route of the left anterior descending coronary artery, which occasionally dips into the myocardium as it passes down the anterior interventricular groove (Amplatz and Anderson, 1968). An example of myocardial bridging is shown in Figure 50–60. Either of these two observed phenomena could be mistaken for a fixed obstructive lesion.

Clinicopathologic correlations with angiographic findings have provided inconclusive evidence about the accuracy of the technique. Kemp and associates (1967) showed excellent correlation between selective coronary angiographic interpretations of an experi-

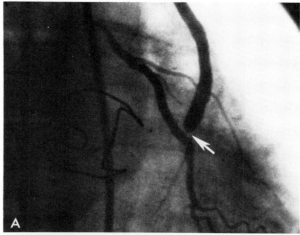
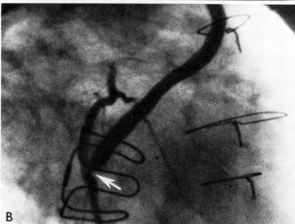

Figure 50–61. *A,* Severe narrowing at the insertion of a vein graft to the left circumflex artery seen in the anteroposterior view (arrow) was not apparent in *B,* a steep LAO projection (arrow). Note the Carpentier-Edwards porcine mitral prosthesis. This 35-year-old woman had the left main stenosis shown in Figure 50–29 and left anterior descending graft stenosis in Figure 50–42*A.*

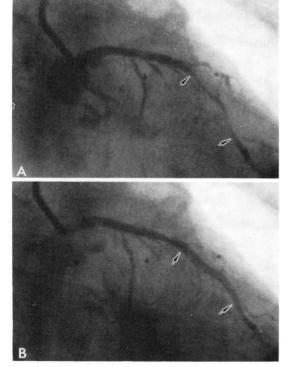

Figure 50–60. Myocardial bridging occurs when a coronary artery dips into the underlying myocardium and is compressed during ventricular systole, causing transient narrowing. The area of the muscle bridge is shown between the arrows in *(A)* systole and *(B)* diastole.

enced angiographer and postmortem pathologic findings in 29 patients. Gray and coworkers (1962) and Vlodaver and colleagues (1973) found the coronary angiographic interpretations far from satisfactory in their postmortem evaluations. Some of this limitation may have been caused by inadequate cine and serial roentgenographic equipment or by failure to obtain several different views of the coronary arteries (Fig. 50–61).

Eccentric plaques, sometimes called "ribbon" lesions, viewed in two dimensions, can appear normal if viewed from the flat side. These lesions are shown schematically in Figure 50–49. This type of lesion probably leads the coronary angiographer to underestimate the severity of the lesions. In addition, the reference areas for comparing narrowed sections of a vessel are the adjacent "normal" areas. If the whole vessel is already diseased and the lumen compromised, what appears as a minor irregularity in a certain portion of the vessel may be a severe narrowing (Vlodaver *et al.,* 1973). Visualization of the vessels in several planes will decrease misinterpretation of the eccentric plaque but not necessarily the evaluation of the vessel partially compromised in its entirety. As improved angiographic equipment and modifications of the different techniques of selective coronary arteriography are tested, better ways of visualizing smaller vessels should be developed.

CORONARY ARTERIOGRAPHY AND THERAPY

Until recently, the coronary arteriographer has used his skills for diagnosis only. Recently, two therapeutic interventions in the catheterization laboratory have allowed promising initial results that will have to be evaluated over the next several years before their true success and meaning are fully known.

PERCUTANEOUS TRANSLUMINAL CORONARY ANGIOPLASTY

In 1964, Dotter and Judkins described a technique for dilating femoral artery occlusions by passing a catheter with a 0.1-inch diameter and then one with a 0.2-inch diameter across the lesion. This technique for dilating a stenotic lesion was modified in 1974 by Andreas Gruentzig, who designed a balloon catheter that could be introduced percutaneously through a sheath and inflated and deflated as it was moved from the distal to the proximal portions of the femoral artery, dilating by compressing the arteriosclerotic narrowed areas in the vessel. By 1977, he had performed his dilatation procedure on 200 patients with femoral occlusive disease, with a 70 per cent 2-year patency rate.

In 1974, Gruentzig developed a double-lumen balloon catheter that allowed pressure to be monitored distal to the balloon and therefore distal to the lesion. In 1976, he reported on the successful dilatation of experimentally induced inflammatory coronary stenoses in 16 dogs (Gruentzig et al., 1976). The following year, he performed transluminal coronary dilatation on left anterior descending coronary artery lesions in three patients during aortocoronary bypass surgery. He showed that no debris was collected in a Millipore filter placed distal to the dilated lesion when blood was flushed out after compression of the lesion. By 1978, he had attempted percutaneous transluminal coronary angioplasty in 26 angina patients with 29 lesions (Gruentzig et al., 1978). Eighteen were clinically improved for up to 1 year, and 10 to 12 had shown an improvement in exercise thallium-imaging study. By 1979, he had successfully dilated lesions in 32 of 50 patients, a 64 per cent success rate (success was defined as a 20 per cent or greater increase in the luminal diameter), reducing gradients across the stenosed lesions from a mean of 58 mm. Hg to 19 mm. Hg (Gruentzig et al., 1979). Gruentzig's success rate after doing percutaneous transluminal coronary angioplasty for more than 3 years in over 300 patients is now 82 per cent. Seven per cent had emergency aortocoronary bypass surgery, and 3 per cent had a

myocardial infarction. During that period, there was a 14 per cent recurrence rate, with most of these patients undergoing a second dilatation.

By January 1981, there were over 1500 patients in the National Heart, Lung and Blood Institute Registry who had undergone this procedure, with an overall success rate of 62 per cent, a 5 per cent incidence of myocardial infarction, and a 1 per cent mortality rate. The long-term data on restenosis are not known in a large group of patients and are critical knowledge if efficacy is to be proved. There has been a need for immediate aortocoronary bypass surgery because of coronary dissection, a prolonged episode of chest pain in unsuccessful dilatation, and the evolution of a myocardial infarction. Because of these complications, a cardiac surgeon and full operating room back-up should be available. The procedure appears to be a promising alternative to aortocoronary bypass surgery, with an improving success rate.

The criteria presently accepted by most physicians doing the procedure and emphasized by Gruentzig are: (1) recent onset of angina refractory to medical treatment; (2) satisfactory left ventricular function; (3) evidence for a reversible wall motion abnormality using thallium or radionuclide exercise studies; and (4) a proximal, discrete, and concentric lesion not more than 15 mm. long in the right coronary artery, left anterior descending coronary artery, or left circumflex artery (see Fig. 50–63A). Most studies to date have involved patients with single coronary artery lesions; those having left main coronary artery stenosis show the highest mortality and, consequently, are not presently studied by most angiographers.

The technique for introducing the catheters is similar to the Judkins and Sones techniques previously mentioned. The guiding catheters are 8 or 9 F. and are virtually identical to the Sones coronary catheter for the brachial artery approach and Judkins coronary catheters for the femoral artery approach. With the patients anticoagulated with 5000 units of heparin and after administration of dipyridamole, aspirin, and/or low–molecular-weight dextran, the guiding catheter is placed at the orifice of the appropriate coronary artery. The arterial pressure proximal to the lesion is measured through the guiding catheter, and the pressure across the lesion can be measured through the side hole distal to the balloon in the angioplasty catheter (Fig. 50–62). The two presently used angioplasty catheters are one that has a diameter of 0.8 mm., a length of 20 mm., and a balloon with a 2-mm. diameter, and one with a diameter of 1.3 mm., a length of 20 mm., and a balloon with a 3-mm. diameter. Both catheters have two metal markers that delineate the boundaries for the proximal and distal ends of the balloon. The smaller-diameter angioplasty catheter can be used to dilate a very tight lesion, enhancing passage of the larger-diameter angioplasty catheter across the lesion. Each of these catheters has a small flexible wire at its tip, which aids in passing the catheter across the lesion and is thought to help prevent dissection of the arteriosclerotic plaque. A

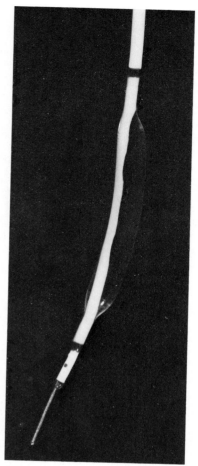

Figure 50–62. The double-lumen dilatation catheter allows continuous pressure measurements from the distal side holes and balloon inflation. Radiopaque markers identify the proximal and distal ends of the balloon. A soft, flexible guide wire is attached to the tip of the catheter to facilitate atraumatic entry of the catheter across the narrowing in the coronary artery.

double-lumen catheter with a removable stainless steel wire with a flexible tip has also been used for percutaneous transluminal coronary angioplasty (Simpson et al., 1981).

Careful monitoring of proximal and distal pressures and small injections of contrast material through the distal angioplasty catheter lumen and occasionally through the guiding catheter are important to insure proper placement of the catheter. The clearing of contrast material distal to the lesion is important, because any "hang-up" of contrast material could mean either that the vessel was occluded or that a dissection had occurred. When the catheter is thought to be properly placed, the balloon is inflated for 4 to 10 seconds. The balloon is filled with a solution of half contrast medium and half saline, which allows visualization when the balloon is inflated (Fig. 50–63C). Pressure of from 1 to 7 atmospheres can be applied with lower pressures used initially and being increased with each of several inflations, if necessary. A constriction in the inflated balloon delineates the lesion (Fig. 50–63B). These will usually decrease or

completely disappear as the lesion is compressed against the arterial wall (Fig. 50–63C). The gradient across the lesion will usually decrease dramatically, but is not always abolished completely (Fig. 50–64). Negative pressure should always be applied to the balloon when it is in the coronary artery, unless, of course, the balloon is inflated. The deflated angioplasty catheter can be withdrawn across the lesion under pressure monitoring, withdrawn into the guiding catheter, and then removed. Any final gradient can be measured at this time. After the angioplasty catheter is completely removed from the guiding catheter, selective injections of contrast material can be made into the coronary artery in appropriate views (Fig. 50–63D). Intracoronary nitroglycerin in 200- to 300-μg. boluses is often injected into the coronary artery prior to and after the angioplasty procedure. Calcium antagonists are usually given on the day of the procedure or longer to prevent coronary artery spasm; aspirin, dipyridamole, or sodium warfarin (Coumadin) has been given from several weeks to months after percutaneous transluminal coronary angioplasty to help prevent coronary thrombosis at the angioplasty site.

INTRACORONARY THROMBOLYSIS

It has been shown angiographically that a completely occluding coronary thrombus is frequently present in an acute evolving myocardial infarction (Reduto et al., 1981). Fresh thrombi are also found at the site of a high-degree atherosclerotic plaque in the majority of patients who undergo autopsy soon after a fatal acute myocardial infarction (Chandler et al., 1974) and in the coronary artery thought to be supplying an acute evolving myocardial infarction examined at the time of emergency aortocoronary bypass surgery (DeWood et al., 1980).

Recent studies in humans have shown that intracoronary thrombolysis and recanalization of occluded coronary arteries during acute myocardial infarction can be accomplished with the intracoronary infusion of streptokinase (Rentrop et al., 1981; Reduto et al., 1981; Mathey et al., 1981). Although the time course from onset of symptoms of acute myocardial infarction to reperfusion of the occluded coronary artery is important, the precise period of time when no salvageable myocardium remains after an occlusion in man is not known. This probably will vary with the number and degree of obstruction in other vessels, the maintained blood pressure, the medications being taken, and the extent of collateral circulation. Although little salvageable myocardium was present after 6 hours of acute coronary occlusion in dogs (Reimer et al., 1977), Reduto and associates (1981) showed a poor correlation between the onset of symptoms of acute myocardial infarction and reperfusion. Although there was no significant difference in ejection fraction from before infusion to discharge in 14 patients who showed no angiographic evidence of

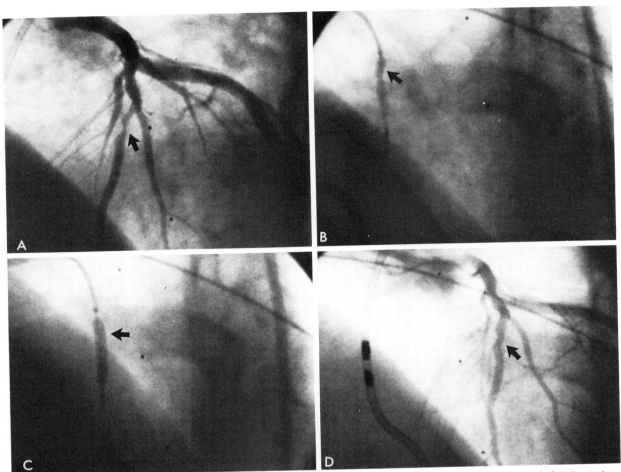

Figure 50–63. *A,* A high-grade lesion (arrow) in the proximal left anterior descending artery. *B,* The constriction (arrow) seen in the inflated balloon reveals where the catheter straddles the obstructing lesion. *C,* The well-filled and concentric balloon has compressed the arteriosclerotic plaque (arrow) against the arterial wall. *D,* The coronary artery fills well with minimal narrowing in the area previously stenosed (arrow).

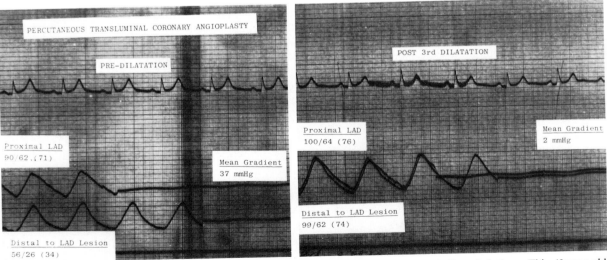

Figure 50–64. The pressure gradient across the lesion is shown prior to and after three balloon inflations. This 42-year-old man, whose percutaneous transluminal coronary angioplasty is shown in Figure 50–63, had a very abnormal exercise radionuclide angiogram prior to angioplasty that reverted to normal afterward.

perfusion after infusion of streptokinase, 18 patients who had a mean interval from the onset of chest pain to infusion of streptokinase of 9.2 ± 4 hours (range—2 to 18 hours) with reperfusion occurring from 7 to 45 minutes later, showed a greater than 10 per cent mean increase in ejection fraction by the time of discharge from the hospital.

Although most patients have been successfully reperfused using this technique, with a low morbidity and no mortality to date, they have all developed a myocardial infarction. Many questions have been raised regarding this approach in the management of patients with acute myocardial infarction, such as: How much time can elapse before reperfusion is no longer beneficial? Should treatment go a step further for the severely narrowed vessel that is now free of thrombus and open by performing balloon angioplasty or aortocoronary bypass grafting? Will all this alter infarction size, prolong life, or decrease the incidence of angina and reinfarction? These questions and many more should be answered in the next several years.

At present, the procedure in our institution involves patients with an evolving acute anterior or inferior myocardial infarction who can undergo cardiac catheterization within 6 hours of the onset of chest pain. Standard therapy for an acute myocardial infarction is given, and informed consent for the procedure is obtained. Patients excluded from attempted intracoronary thrombolysis are those with a history of multiple myocardial infarctions, chronic congestive heart failure, a history of gastrointestinal bleeding, an aortic aneurysm or aortic dissection, or a diastolic blood pressure above 110 mm. Hg, those who have had a recent stroke, those who have undergone a surgical procedure or major trauma within the last week, and those with an abnormal coagulation profile.

After biplane left ventriculography and visualization of both the right and left coronary arteries in multiple views, the coronary artery that is thought not to be the "involved" artery is studied first. The involved artery (left anterior descending coronary artery for an anterior infarction on the ECG and anterior wall asynergy on the ventriculogram, and right main coronary artery for an inferior infarction on the ECG and inferior wall asynergy on the ventriculogram) is then examined. If proximal total occlusion or evidence of thrombus is found (Fig. 50–65A), 200 to 500 μg. of nitroglycerin are injected into the occluded artery to look for spasm (Oliva and Breckenridge, 1977). If the lesion is unchanged angiographically in 2 minutes, 20,000 units of streptokinase are injected into the involved coronary artery over a 2- to 3-minute period. This is followed by a constant infusion of 2000 to 4000 units per minute through the coronary catheter up to a maximal total of 400,000 units. Some use a flexible-tip guide wire placed through the coronary catheter, attempting to disrupt the thrombus and/or allow better soaking of the thrombus with the streptokinase (Rentrop et al., 1981). A 3-F. Teflon-coated catheter can also be inserted through the standard coronary artery catheter and

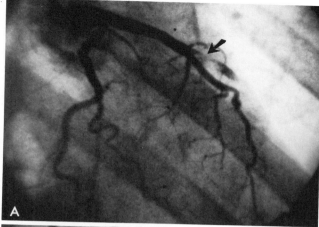

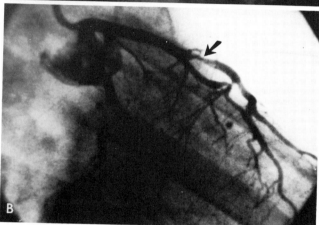

Figure 50–65. *A*, Totally occluded left anterior descending coronary artery (arrow) in a 38-year-old woman with 2 hours of chest pain and an evolving anterior wall infarction by ECG. *B*, After 30 minutes of intracoronary streptokinase infusion, the thrombosis disappeared, revealing a severe obstruction in a now well-opacified left anterior descending coronary artery (arrow).

positioned closer to the thrombus. It is not known whether the infusion of streptokinase through this small catheter has any advantage over infusion through the coronary artery catheter.

If recanalization is successful (Fig. 50–65B), a repeat ventriculogram is usually obtained. Most patients are recatheterized 24 hours later; some, however, will undergo percutaneous transluminal coronary angioplasty or aortocoronary bypass surgery, since a severely narrowed coronary artery remains. Before intracoronary thrombolysis could ever be recommended as a treatment of choice in the management of the acute myocardial infarction, it must be clearly shown to be potentially beneficial in preservation of the myocardium.

SELECTED REFERENCES

Abrams, H. L., and Adams, D. F.: The coronary arteriogram (second of two parts). Structural and functional aspects. N. Engl. J. Med., *281*:1336, 1969.

This complete treatise on the coronary arteriogram has 105 references and discusses anatomy, dynamics of coronary flow, technique of arteriography, indications, interpretation, applications, usefulness, and grading of the coronary arteriogram. The authors stress that the procedure is unique and that the balance between the risk involved and the information gained should be kept clearly in mind. The procedure should never be casually performed.

Adams, D. F., Fraser, D. B., and Abrams, H. L.: The complications of coronary arteriography. Circulation, 48:609, 1973.

This unique study of the complications of coronary arteriography over a 2-year period in 46,904 coronary arteriograms from 173 hospitals was analyzed in relationship to the technique employed (percutaneous femoral or brachial cutdown) and to the number of studies performed over that period of time. The overall mortality rate was 0.45 per cent, with the incidence of major complications being higher with the percutaneous femoral approach. However, the mortality rate in those institutions in which less than 100 arteriograms per year were performed was several times higher than in those in which more than 400 per year were done. In the two insitutions in which the largest number of femoral and brachial arteriograms were performed, the mortality rate was approximately the same—0.08 and 0.06 per cent, respectively.

Elliot, L. P., Green, C. E., Rogers, W. J., Mantle, J. A., Papapietro, S. E., Hood, W. P., and Russell, R. O., Jr.: Advantage of the cranial right anterior oblique view in diagnosing mid-left anterior descending and distal right coronary artery disease. Am. J. Cardiol., 48:754, 1981.

This most recent of several papers describing different views for delineating lesions during coronary arteriography provides references for all of the important studies and describes the advantage of using the cranial right anterior oblique view for examining the mid-left anterior descending and distal right coronary arteries. The authors uncovered lesions in 26 per cent of 300 consecutive patients that were not visualized by other views. This was also the most satisfactory view from a technical standpoint in examining very obese patients, in whom the diaphragms are high.

Friesinger, G. C., Page, E. E., and Ross, R. S.: Prognostic significance of coronary arteriography. Trans. Assoc. Am. Physicians, 83:78, 1970.

This study evaluates the prognosis in 224 patients who underwent selective coronary arteriography during a 7-year period and were followed for an average of 53 months. The patients' chest discomfort was classified, and a scoring technique was devised to grade the severity of arteriographic abnormalities. The coronary arteriographic study helped clarify the diagnosis in all patients, but particularly in those whose chest pain was not typical for angina pectoris. The prognosis was more accurately assessed by the severity of the arteriosclerotic changes than by any clinical parameter. Those patients with varying degrees of coronary stenosis had a predictable prognosis related to the severity of their disease. The predicted 5-year survival rate of 97 per cent in those without significant angiographic atherosclerosis was identical to that for the normal age-matched population. This study points out the necessity of establishing the diagnosis of ischemic heart disease when the diagnosis is in question. Essentially normal coronary arteriograms were found in many with the clinical diagnosis of ischemic heart disease.

Gensini, G. G., Buonanno, C., and Palacio, A.: Anatomy of the coronary circulation in living man. Coronary arteriography. Dis. Chest, 52:125, 1967.

This report of the angiographic coronary anatomy is based on 2500 coronary opacifications in 408 patients and shows the most common patterns of the human coronary arteries in several roentgenographic projections. As expected, no significant differences were found between the anatomy observed in living man and that described by others from postmortem studies. The thorough description of the

coronary anatomy is complemented by the cine frames and accompanying tracings of the coronary anatomy.

Gruentzig, A. R., Senning, Å, and Siegenthaler, W. E.: Nonoperative dilatation of coronary artery stenosis. N. Engl. J. Med., 301:61, 1979.

This is Gruentzig's first paper in the American literature in which he described the technique for percutaneous transluminal coronary angioplasty (PTCA). He described 32 successful balloon dilatations in 50 patients with coronary stenosis, reducing a coronary gradient of 58 mm. Hg to 19 mm. Hg and a mean stenosis of 84 per cent to 34 per cent. At that time, he felt that 10 to 15 per cent of patients would be candidates for the procedure. He suggested a randomized trial to examine the procedure's usefulness. Two years later, this had not been done.

Judkins, M. P.: Percutaneous transfemoral selective coronary arteriography. Radiol. Clin. North Am., 6:467, 1968.

Two years' experience with his technique of selective coronary arteriography is discussed by Dr. Judkins in this article. The catheter technique, including catheter design and configuration, selection of the proper catheters, technical tips, and the use of different types of guide wires, is described. Several excellent cine reproductions of the coronary arteries are shown.

Reduto, L., Smelling, R. W., Freund, G. L., and Gould, K. L.: Intracoronary infusion of streptokinase in patients with acute myocardial infarction. Effects of reperfusion on left ventricular performance. Am. J. Cardiol., 48:403, 1981.

This was the first of several papers describing the safety and efficacy of intracoronary thrombolysis during acute myocardial infarction that showed improvement in ventricular function in the group of patients in whom coronary thrombolysis was successful versus those in whom coronary thrombolysis was unsuccessful. Thirty-two consecutive patients with acute myocardial infarction were evaluated. Twenty-six had total occlusion of an infarct-related coronary artery, and six had severe proximal stenoses. Eighteen of the 26 with total occlusion were reperfused after intracoronary infusion of streptokinase. This study complemented other investigations that also showed that coronary arterial thrombosis is a frequent cause of an acute myocardial infarction and can be safely lysed by intracoronary streptokinase. The added information here is that reperfusion resulted in improved left ventricular performance over the next several days.

Schroeder, J. B., Bolen, J. L., Quint, R. A., Clark, D. A., Hayden, W. G., Higgins, C. R., and Wezler, L.: Provocation of coronary spasm with ergonovine maleate. New test with results in 57 patients undergoing coronary arteriography. Am. J. Cardiol., 40:487, 1977.

This is the first of several papers that showed that ergonovine given intravenously could produce segmental spasm, chest pain, and ST-segment changes consistent with Prinzmetal's angina. Fifty-seven patients had normal coronary arteries or insufficient occlusive disease to explain their symptoms. Forty-four did not demonstrate spasm in response to ergonovine, whereas coronary spasm was noted in 13. The spasm was easily reversed with sublingual nitroglycerin. Intracoronary nitroglycerin was given in later studies. Patients with spasm had chest pains, and 12 of the 13 had ST-segment elevation and one had ST-segment depression.

Sewell, W. H.: Coronary arteriography by the Sones technique—technical considerations. Am. J. Roentgenol., 95:673, 1965.

This is an excellent description of the technical aspects of the Sones technique. In this paper, there is also discussion of the indications for coronary arteriography, roentgenographic equipment, the surgical procedure for the arterial cutdown, use of vasodilators in the procedure, and the precautions and risks of the procedure. Several catheter maneuvers that might prove helpful in technically difficult cases are described.

Sones, F. M., Jr.: Cine coronary arteriography. Anesth. Analg., 46:499, 1967.

Although F. Mason Sones, Jr. was the first to perform selective coronary arteriography, which changed the whole concept of treatment for coronary artery disease, there are a few first-hand reports of his thoughts and concepts. A brief history of the coronary arteriographic procedure and the surgical procedures that arose form the ability to evaluate the coronary vessels in this manner are described in this article. The indications, observations, and complications of selective coronary arteriography are also discussed.

REFERENCES

Abrams, H. L., and Adams, D. F.: The coronary arteriogram (second of two parts). Structural and functional aspects. N. Engl. J. Med., 281:1336, 1969.

Adams, D. F., Fraser, D. B., and Abrams, H. L.: The complications of coronary arteriography. Circulation, 48:609, 1973.

Amplatz, K., and Anderson, R.: Angiographic appearance of myocardial bridging of the coronary artery. Invest. Radiol., 3:213, 1968.

Amplatz, K., Formanck, G., Stranger, P., and Wilson, W.: Mechanics of selective coronary artery catheterization via the femoral approach. Radiology, 89:1040, 1967.

Baily, C. P., May, A., and Lemmon, W. M.: Survival after coronary endarterectomy in man. J.A.M.A., 164:641, 1957.

Baltaxe, H. A.: Radiologic evaluation of coronary artery surgery. Circulation, 47:387, 1973.

Baltaxe, H. A., and Levin, D. C.: Coronary angiography. Its role in the management of the patient with angina pectoris. Circulation, 46:1161, 1972.

Barlow, J. B., Bosman, C. K., Popcock, W. A., and Marchand, D.: Late systolic murmurs and non-ejection ("mid-late") systolic clicks. An analysis of 90 patients. Br. Heart J., 30:203, 1968.

Baroldi, G., and Scomazzoni, G.: Coronary Circulation in the Normal and the Pathologic Heart. Washington, D.C., U.S. Government Printing Office, 1967.

Beck, C. S., and Leighminger, D. S.: Operations for coronary artery disease. J. Am. Heart Assoc., 156:1226, 1954.

Bemiller, C. R., Pepine, C. J., and Rogers, A.: Long term observation in patients with angina and normal coronary arteriograms. Circulation, 47:36, 1973.

Blumgart, H. L., Schlesinger, M. J., and Davis, D.: Studies on the relation of the clinical manifestations of angina pectoris, coronary thrombosis, and myocardial infarction to the pathologic findings. Am. Heart J., 19:1, 1940.

Bonchek, L. I., Anderson, R. P., and Rosch, J. R.: Should coronary arteriography be performed routinely before valve replacement? Am. J. Cardiol., 31:462, 1973.

Bourassa, M. G., Lesperance, J., and Campeau, L.: Selective coronary arteriography by the percutaneous femoral approach. Am. J. Roentgenol., 107:377, 1969.

Bruscke, A. V. G., Proudfit, W. L., and Sones, F. M., Jr.: Clinical course of patients with normal and slightly or moderately abnormal coronary arteriograms. A follow-up study on 500 patients. Circulation, 48:1151, 1973.

Bunnell, I. L., Greene, D. G., Tandon, R. N., and Arani, D. T.: The half-axial projection. A new look at the proximal left coronary artery. Circulation, 48:1151, 1973.

Campion, B. C., Frye, R. L., Pluth, J. R., Fairbourn, J. F., and Davis, G. D.: Arterial complications of retrograde brachial arterial catheterization: A prospective study. Mayo Clin. Proc., 46:489, 1971.

Chandler, A. B., Chapman, I., Erhardt, L. R., Roberts, W. C., Schwartz, C. J., Sinapius, D., Spain, D. M., Sherry, S., Ness, P. M., and Simon, T. L.: Coronary thrombosis in myocardial infarction. Am. J. Cardiol., 34:823, 1974.

Cheitlin, M. D., deCastro, C. M., and McAllister, H. A.: Sudden death as a complication of anomalous left coronary origin from the anterior sinus of Valsalva: A not-so-minor congenital anomaly. Circulation, 50:780, 1974.

Conti, C. R.: Coronary arteriography. Circulation, 55:227, 1977.

Davis, K., Kennedy, J. W., Kemp, H. G., Jr., Judkins, M. P., Gosselin, A. J., and Killip, T.: Complications of coronary arteriography from the collaborative study of coronary artery surgery (CASS). Circulation, 59:1105, 1979.

DeWood, M. A., Spores, J., Notske, R., et al.: Prevalence of total coronary occlusion during the early hours of transmural myocardial infarction. N. Engl. J. Med., 303:897, 1980.

DiGuglielmo, L., and Guttadauro, M.: A roentgenologic study of the coronary arteries in the living. Acta Radiol. (Suppl.), 97:5, 1952.

Dotter, C. T., and Frische, L. J.: Visualization of the coronary circulation by occlusion aortography: A practical method. Radiology, 71:502, 1958.

Dotter, C. T., and Judkins, M. P.: Transluminal treatment of arteriosclerotic obstruction: Description of a new technique and a preliminary report of its application. Circulation, 30:654, 1964.

Ebert, P. A., Peter, R. H., Gunnells, J. C., and Sabiston, D. C., Jr.: Resecting and grafting of coronary artery aneurysm. Circulation, 43:593, 1971.

Edwards, J. E.: Congenital malformation. F. Malformations of the coronary vessels. In Pathology of the Heart. 2nd Ed. Edited by S. E. Gould. Springfield, Illinois, Charles C Thomas, 1960.

Elliott, L. P., Amplatz, K., and Edwards, J. E.: Coronary arterial patterns in transposition complexes. Anatomic and angiographic studies. Am. J. Cardiol., 17:362, 1966.

Elliott, L. P., Green, C. E., Rogers, W. J., Mantle, J. A., Papapietro, S. E., Hood, W. P., and Russell, R. O., Jr.: Advantage of the cranial right anterior oblique view in diagnosing mid-left anterior descending and distal right coronary artery disease. Am. J. Cardiol., 48:754, 1981.

Friesinger, G. C., Page, E. E., and Ross, R. S.: Prognostic significance of coronary arteriography. Trans. Assoc. Am. Physicians, 83:78, 1970.

Gau, T., Oakley, C. M., Rahimtoola, S. H., Raphael, M. J., and Steiner, R. E.: Selective coronary arteriography. A review of 18 months' experience. Clin. Radiol., 21:275, 1970.

Gault, J. H., and Simon, R. L.: Clinical and laboratory findings in patients with nonobstructive intraventricular pressure differences. Circulation, 42:235, 1970.

Gensini, G. G., and daCosta, B. C. B.: The coronary collateral circulation in living man. Am. J. Cardiol., 24:393, 1969.

Gensini, G. G., Buonanno, C., and Palacio, A.: Anatomy of the coronary circulation in living man. Coronary arteriography. Dis. Chest, 52:125, 1967.

Gray, C. R., Hoffman, H. A., Hammond, W. S., Miller, K. L., and Oseasohn, R. O.: Correlation of arteriographic and pathologic findings in the coronary arteries in man. Circulation, 26:494, 1962.

Green, G. S., McKinnon, C. M., Rosch, J., and Judkins, M. P.: Complications of selective percutaneous transfemoral coronary arteriography and their prevention. Circulation, 45:552, 1972.

Gross, L.: The Blood Supply to the Heart. New York, Paul B. Hoeber, Inc., 1921.

Gruentzig, A. R., Senning, Å, and Siegenthaler, W. E.: Nonoperative dilatation of coronary artery stenosis. N. Engl. J. Med., 301:61, 1979.

Gruentzig, A. R., Turina, M. I., and Schneider, J. A.: Experimental percutaneous dilatation of coronary artery stenosis. Circulation, 53, 54 (Suppl. 2):81, 1976.

Gruentzig, A. R., Myler, K., Hanna, E. S., and Turina, M. I.: Coronary transluminal angioplasty. Circulation, 55, 56 (Suppl. 3):84, 1977.

Gruentzig, A. R., Myler, K., Stertzer, S., et al.: Coronary percutaneous transluminal angioplasty: Preliminary results, abstracted. Circulation, 58 (Suppl. 2):56, 1978.

Haas, J. M., Peterson, C. R., and Jones, R. C.: Subintimal dissection of the coronary arteries. A complication of selective coronary arteriography and the transfemoral percutaneous approach. Circulation, 38:678, 1968.

Harris, P. J., Behar, V. S., Conley, M. J., Harrell, F. E., Lee, K. L., Peter, R. H., Kong, Y., and Rosati, R. A.: The prognostic significance of 50% coronary stenosis in medically treated patients with coronary artery disease. Circulation, 62:240, 1980.

James, T. N.: Anatomy of the Coronary Arteries. New York, Paul B. Hoeber, Inc., 1961a.

James, T. N.: Anatomy of the coronary arteries in health and disease. Circulation, 32:1020, 1965.

James, T. N.: Anatomy of the human sinus node. Anat. Rec., 141:109, 1961b.

Judkins, M. P.: Percutaneous transfemoral selective coronary arteriography. Radiol. Clin. North Am., 6:467, 1968.

Judkins, M. P.: Selective coronary arteriography. Part I: A percutaneous transfemoral technique. Radiology, 89:815, 1967.

Judkins, M. P., and Gander, M. P.: Prevention of complications of coronary arteriography. Circulation, 49:599, 1974.

Kemp, H. G., Evens, H., Elliott, W. C., and Gorlin, R.: Diagnostic accuracy of selective coronary cinearteriography. Circulation, 36:526, 1967.

Lehman, J. S., Boyer, R. A., and Winter, F. S.: Coronary arteriography. Am. J. Roentgenol., 81:749, 1959.

Lesperance, J., Saltiel, J., Petitcherc, R., and Bourassa, M. G.: Angulated views in the sagittal plane for improved accuracy of cine-coronary angiography. Am. J. Roentgenol., 121:565, 1974.

Levin, D. C., Beckman, M. D., Garnick, J. D., Carey, P., and Bettman, M. A.: Frequency and clinical significance of failure to visualize the conus artery during coronary arteriography. Circulation, 63:833, 1981.

Liberthson, R. R., Dinsmore, R. E., Bharati, S., Rubenstein, J. J., Caulfield, J., Wheeler, E. D., Howthorne, J. W., and Lev, M.: Aberrant coronary artery origin from the aorta. Diagnosis and clinical significance. Circulation, 50:774, 1974.

Lurie, P. R.: Abnormalities and diseases of the coronary vessels. In Heart Disease in Infants, Children and Adolescents. Edited by A. J. Moss and F. Adams. Baltimore, Williams and Wilkins Co., 1968.

MacAlpen, R. N., Kattus, A. A., and Alvaro, A. B.: Angina pectoris at rest with preservation of exercise capacity. Prinzmetal's variant angina. Circulation, 47:946, 1973.

Mathey, D. G., Kuck, K. H., Tilsner, V., Krebber, H. J., and Bleifeld, W.: Nonsurgical coronary artery recanalization in acute transmural myocardial infarction. Circulation, 63:489, 1981.

McMahon, M. M., Brown, G. B., Cuckingnon, R., Rolett, E., Bolson, E., Frimer, M., and Dodge, H. T.: Quantitative coronary angiography: Measurement of the ''critical'' stenosis in patients with unstable angina and single-vessel disease without collaterals. Circulation, 60:106, 1979.

Miller, B. J., Gibbon, J. H., Jr., and Fineberg, C.: An improved mechanical heart-lung apparatus. Med. Clin. North Am., 37:1603, 1953.

Morettin, L. B., and Wallace, J. M.: Uneventful perforation of a coronary artery during selective arteriography. A case report. Am. J. Roentgenol., 100:14, 1970.

Mundt, E. D., Yurchak, P. M., Buckley, M. J., Leinback, R. C., Kantrowitz, A., and Austen, W. G.: Circulatory assistance and emergency direct coronary artery surgery for shock complicating acute myocardial infarction. N. Engl. J. Med., 283:1382, 1970.

Nath, P. H., Velasquez, G., Castaneda-Zuniga, W. R., Zollikofer, C., Formanek, A., and Amplatz, K.: An essential view in coronary arteriography. Circulation, 60:101, 1979.

Oliva, P. B., and Breckenridge, J. C.: Arteriographic evidence of coronary spasm in acute myocardial infarction. Circulation, 56:366, 1977.

Page, H. L., Engle, H. J., Campbell, W. B., and Thomas, C. S.: Anomalous origin of the left circumflex coronary: Recognition, angiographic demonstration and clinical significance. Circulation, 50:768, 1974.

Paulen, S.: Coronary angiography: A technical, anatomic, and clinical study. Acta Radiol. (Suppl.), 233:5, 1964.

Perry, L. W., and Scott, L. P.: Anomalous coronary artery from pulmonary artery. Report of 11 cases; review of indications for results of surgery. Circulation, 41:1043, 1970.

Peter, R. H., Gracey, J. G., and Beach, T. B.: Subaortic stenosis simulating coronary disease. Arch. Intern. Med., 121:564, 1968.

Peter, R. H., Harris, P. J., and Rosati, R. A.: A new approach to clinical decision-making in coronary artery disease: Observations on subsets within the Duke University Data Bank. Adv. Cardiol., 27:199, 1980.

Price, J. E., and Rosch, J.: Selective coronary arteriography by percutaneous left transaxillary approach using preshaped torque control catheters. Circulation, 48:1321, 1973.

Proudfit, W. L., Shirey, E. K., and Sones, F. M., Jr.: Selective cine coronary arteriography: Correlation with clinical findings in 1,000 patients. Circulation, 33:901, 1966.

Radner, S.: Thoracal aortography by catheterization from the radial artery: Preliminary report of new technique. Acta Radiol., 29:78, 1948.

Ramo, B. W., Peter, R. H., McIntosh, H. M., and Morris, J. J., Jr.: Muscular subaortic stenosis and coronary arteriovenous fistula. Report of an occurrence in the same patient. Arch. Intern. Med., 122:426, 1968.

Reduto, L., Smelling, R. W., Freund, G. L., and Gould, K. L.: Intracoronary infusion of streptokinase in patients with acute myocardial infarction: Effects of reperfusion on left ventricular performance. Am. J. Cardiol., 48:403, 1981.

Reimer, K. A., Lowe, J. E., Rasmussen, M. M., and Jennings, R. B.: The wavefront phenomenon of ischemic cell death. 1. Myocardial infarct size vs. duration of coronary occlusion in dogs. Circulation, 56:786, 1977.

Rentrop, P., Blanke, H., Karsch, K. R., Kaiser, M. D., Köstering, H., and Leitz, K.: Intracoronary thrombosis in acute myocardial infarction and unstable angina pectoris. Circulation, 63:307, 1981.

Report of the Inter-Society Commission for Heart Disease Resources: Optimal radiologic facilities for examination of the chest and the cardiovascular system. Circulation, 43A:135, 1971.

Report of the Inter-Society Commission for Heart Disease Resources: Optimal resources for coronary artery surgery. Committee on coronary artery surgery. Circulation, 46A:325, 1972.

Ricketts, H. J., and Abrams, H. L.: Percutaneous selective coronary cine arteriography. J.A.M.A., 181:620, 1962.

Ross, R. S., and Gorlin, R.: Coronary arteriography. Circulation, 37, 38 (Suppl. 3):67, 1968.

Scanlon, P. J., Rimgaudas, N., Moron, J. H., Talano, J. V., Firouz, A., and Pifarre, R.: Accelerated angina pectoris: Clinical, hemodynamic, arteriographic, and therapeutic experience in 85 patients. Circulation, 47:19, 1973.

Schlesinger, M. J.: Relation of anatomic to pathologic conditions of the coronary arteries. Arch. Pathol., 30:403, 1940.

Schlesinger, M. J., and Zoll, P. M.: Incidence and localization of coronary artery occlusions. Arch. Pathol., 32:178, 1941.

Schlesinger, M. J., Zoll, P. M., and Wessler, S.: The conus artery: A third coronary artery. Am. Heart J., 38:823, 1949.

Schoonmaker, F. W., and King, S. B., III: Coronary arteriography by the single catheter percutaneous femoral technique. Experience in 6,800 cases. Circulation, 50:735, 1974.

Schroeder, J. S., Bolen, J. L., Quint, R. A., Clark, D. A., Hayden, W. G., Higgins, C. R., and Wexler, L.: Provocation of coronary spasm with ergonovine maleate. New test with results in 57 patients undergoing coronary arteriography. Am. J. Cardiol., 40:487, 1977.

Scott, D. H.: Aneurysm of the coronary arteries. Am. Heart J., 36:403, 1948.

Seldinger, S. I.: Catheter replacement of the needle in percutaneous arteriography: A new technique. Acta Radiol., 39:368, 1953.

Sewell, W. H.: Coronary arteriography by the Sones technique—technical considerations. Am. J. Roentgenol., 95:673, 1965.

Sewell, W. H.: Roentgenographic anatomy of human coronary arteries. Am. J. Roentgenol., 97:359, 1966.

Simpson, J. B., Robert, N., Baim, D., and Harrison, D. C.: Clinical experience with a new catheter system for percutaneous transluminal coronary angioplasty. Am. J. Cardiol., 47:395, 1981.

Sones, F. M., Jr.: Cine coronary arteriography. Anesth. Anal., 46:499, 1967.

Sones, F. M., Jr.: Indications and value of coronary arteriography. Circulation, *46*:1155, 1972.

Sones, F. M., Jr.: Complications of coronary arteriography and left heart catheterization. Cleve. Clin. Q., *45*:21, 1978.

Sones, F. M., Jr., and Shirey, E. K.: Cine coronary arteriography. Mod. Concepts Cardiovasc. Dis., *31*:735, 1962.

Sones, F. M., Jr., and Shirey, E. K.: Collateral arterial channels in living human with coronary artery disease. Circulation, *22*:815, 1960.

Sos, T. A., Lee, J. Q., Levin, D. C., and Baltaxe, H. A.: A new lordotic projection for improved visualization of the left coronary artery and its branches. Am. J. Roentgenol., *121*:575, 1974.

Upshaw, C. B.: Congenital coronary arteriovenous fistula: Report of a case with an analysis of seventy-three reported cases. Am. Heart J., *63*:399, 1962.

Vansant, J. H., and Muller, W. H., Jr.: Surgical procedures to revascularize the heart. A review of the literature. Am. J. Surg., *100*:572, 1960.

Vineberg, A.: Treatment of coronary artery insufficiency by im-plantation of the internal mammary artery into the left ventricular myocardium. J. Thorac. Surg., *23*:42, 1952.

Vlodaver, Z., Frech, R., Von Tassel, R., and Edwards, J. E.: Correlation of the antemortem coronary arteriogram and the postmortem specimen. Circulation, *47*:162, 1973.

Walker, W. J., Mundal, S. L., Broderick, H. G., Prasod, B., Kim, J., and Ravi, J.: Systemic heparinization for femoral percutaneous coronary arteriography. N. Engl. J. Med., *288*:826, 1973.

Webster, J. S., Moberg, C., and Rencon, G.: Natural history of severe proximal coronary artery disease as documented by coronary cineangiography. Am. J. Cardiol., *33*:195, 1974.

Yatteau, R. F., Peter, R. H., Behar, V. S., Bartel, A. G., Rosati, R. A., and Kong, Y.: Ischemic cardiomyopathy, the myopathy of coronary artery disease. Am. J. Cardiol., *34*:520, 1974.

Zeft, H. J., Manley, J. C., Huston, J. H., Tector, A. J., Auer, J. E., and Johnson, W. D.: Left main coronary artery stenosis. Results of coronary bypass surgery. Circulation, *49*:68, 1974.

Zubiate, P., Kay, J. H., and Mendez, A. M.: Myocardial revascularization for the patient with drastic impairment of function of the left ventricle. J. Thorac. Cardiovasc. Surg., *73*:84, 1977.

IV CONGENITAL MALFORMATIONS OF THE CORONARY CIRCULATION

JAMES E. LOWE

DAVID C. SABISTON, JR.

Congenital coronary arterial malformations have long been recognized, but the frequency of such reports in the literature has increased greatly since the introduction of selective coronary arteriography by Sones in 1959. In a review of 224 patients with coronary malformations, Ogden (1970) proposed three basic classifications: (1) *major anomalies,* in which there is an abnormal communication between an artery and a cardiac chamber or abnormal origin of a major coronary artery from the pulmonary artery; (2) *minor anomalies,* in which there is variation of the origin of the vessels from the aorta, but the distal circulation is normal; and (3) *secondary anomalies,* in which the coronary arterial variation probably represents a circulatory response of the primary intracardiac pathologic defect. The distribution of coronary artery anomalies in these 224 patients is shown in Table 50–9.

Major anomalies that are amenable to surgical correction include congenital coronary fistulas, anomalous origin of either the left or right coronary artery from the pulmonary artery, congenital aneurysms of the coronary arteries, and congenital membranous obstruction of the ostium of the left main coronary artery. Minor anomalies, in which there is variation in the origin of the coronary arteries from the aorta with normal distal circulation, and secondary anomalies, associated with congenital heart defects, such as transposition of the great vessels, truncus arteriosus, and tetralogy of Fallot, seldom require surgical intervention. In this section, the clinical manifestations, evaluation, and surgical management of patients with major coronary anomalies, including congenital coronary artery fistulas, congenital origin of either the left or right coronary artery from the pulmonary artery, congenital coronary artery aneurysms, and membranous obstruction of the ostium of the left main coronary artery, are described.

Based on our experience and supported by that of others, it is recommended that most patients with major congenital coronary arterial malformations be considered candidates for surgical correction. In most instances, the natural history of these lesions is not associated with a normal life expectancy, with the possible exception of patients with congenital origin of the right coronary artery from the pulmonary artery. Since these malformations can now be safely corrected with gratifying long-term results, surgical intervention should be strongly recommended once a precise diagnosis has been established.

CORONARY ARTERY FISTULAS

Since Krause first described a coronary artery fistula in 1865, there have been nearly 300 additional

TABLE 50–9. CONGENITAL VARIATIONS OF THE CORONARY ARTERIES IN 224 PATIENTS†

CONGENITAL VARIATIONS	NO. OF CASES
Major coronary anomalies (75 cases)	
Coronary "arteriovenous" fistula*	31
Anomalous origin from the pulmonary artery	44
Left coronary artery	39
Right coronary artery	4
Both coronary arteries	1
Minor coronary variations (63 cases)	
High take-off	2
Multiple ostia	6
Anomalous circumflex artery origin	14
Anomalous anterior descending artery origin	11
Absent proximal ostium/single ostium in other aortic sinus	10
Absent proximal ostium/multiple ostia in other aortic sinus	10
Hypoplastic proximal coronary artery	5
Congenital proximal stenosis	2
Congenital distal stenosis	1
Coronary artery from the posterior aortic sinus	1
Ventricular origin of an accessory coronary artery	1
Second coronary anomalies (86 cases)	
Secondary coronary "arteriovenous" fistula	3
Variations in transposition of the great vessels	65
Variations in truncus arteriosus	6
Variations in tetralogy of Fallot	4
Ectasia of coronary arteries in supravalvular aortic stenosis	5
Mural coronary artery	3

*This category does not include cases of adult anomalous origin of the right or left coronary artery from the pulmonary artery.

†Adapted from Ogden, J. A.: Congenital anomalies of the coronary arteries. Am. J. Cardiol., *25*:474, 1970.

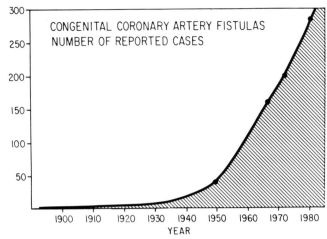

Figure 50–66. This graph shows a total of 286 patients with congenital coronary fistulas, including 28 in the present series from Duke University Medical Center. Increasing numbers are being recognized each year following the widespread use of cardiac catheterization and selective coronary arteriography in the evaluation of cardiac problems. (From Lowe, J. E., Oldham, H. N., Jr., and Sabiston, D. C., Jr.: Surgical management of congenital coronary artery fistulas. Ann. Surg., *194*:371, 1981.)

Clinical Manifestations

It is commonly believed that the majority of patients with coronary artery fistulas are asymptomatic. However, based on our experience with 28 patients and supported by a review of 258 others reported in the literature, 55 per cent are symptomatic at the time of presentation (Lowe *et al.*, 1981). Since the underlying pathophysiology is essentially that of a left-to-right cardiac shunt, it follows that the most common manifestation is that of congestive heart failure. Other common symptoms are angina pectoris, secondary to a steal of coronary arterial flow through the fistulous communication, and subacute bacterial endocarditis. Bacterial endocarditis, anemia, and glomerulonephritis in the same patient has been reported (Sabiston *et al.*, 1963). Infants and children with this lesion may demonstrate a failure to thrive. Less com-

patients with this malformation reported in the literature. Of particular interest is the finding that increasing numbers of patients with this anomaly are being recognized each year, resulting from the widespread use of cardiac catheterization and selective coronary arteriography in the evaluation of a variety of cardiac problems (Fig. 50–66).

Coronary artery fistulas are characterized by normal origin of the coronary artery from the aorta with a fistulous communication with the atria or ventricles or with the pulmonary artery, coronary sinus, or superior vena cava. These fistulas represent the most common of the congenital coronary malformations. Combining our series of 28 patients (Lowe *et al.*, 1981) with those previously reported in the literature now makes available a total of 286 patients for review. The right coronary artery is involved most frequently, and the abnormal communication most often is to the right ventricle followed in incidence by drainage into the right atrium and pulmonary artery. Left coronary artery fistulas are less common but may drain into the right ventricle, right atrium, or coronary sinus. On rare occasion, right or left coronary fistulas may communicate with the superior vena cava. The size of the fistulous communication may vary widely but generally becomes larger with the passage of time.

TABLE 50–10. MAJOR PRESENTING CLINICAL MANIFESTATIONS OF CORONARY ARTERY FISTULAS WHEN PRESENT AS SOLE CARDIAC ANOMALY*

	NO. OF CASES	PERCENTAGE OF TOTAL
Asymptomatic murmur	67	45
Dyspnea on exertion; fatigue	34	22
Congestive heart failure	21	14
Angina or nonspecific chest pain	10	7
Bacterial endocarditis	9	6
Frequent upper respiratory infections	9	6
Total	150	

*From Daniel, T. M., Graham, T. P., and Sabiston, D. C., Jr.: Coronary artery–right ventricular fistula with congestive heart failure: Surgical correction in the neonatal period. Surgery, *67*:985, 1970.

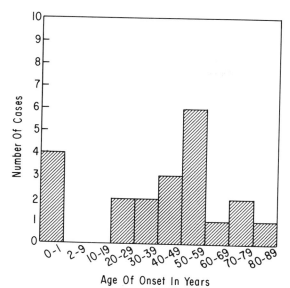

Figure 50–67. Age of onset of congestive heart failure in patients with an isolated coronary artery fistula. (From Daniel, T. M., Graham, T. P., and Sabiston, D. C., Jr.: Coronary artery–right ventricular fistula with congestive heart failure: Surgical correction in the neonatal period. Surgery, 67:985, 1970.)

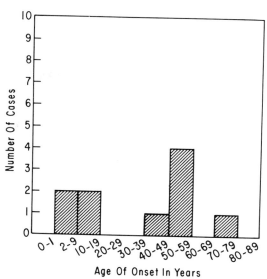

Figure 50–69. Age of onset of angina or chest pain in patients with an isolated coronary artery fistula. (From Daniel, T. M., Graham, T. P., and Sabiston, D. C., Jr.: Coronary artery–right ventricular fistula with congestive heart failure: Surgical correction in the neonatal period. Surgery, 67:985, 1970.)

monly, patients present with acute myocardial infarction, aneurysm formation with subsequent rupture or embolization, or symptoms secondary to pulmonary hypertension.

The major presenting features of coronary artery fistulas are listed in Table 50–10 (Daniel *et al.*, 1970). The age of onset of congestive heart failure among 21 patients who demonstrated this feature in a group of 150 studied is shown in Figure 50–67. In addition, the age of onset of dyspnea on exertion, the appearance of bacterial endocarditis, and the age of onset of

angina pectoris in this series are shown in Figures 50–68 to 50–70.

Congestive heart failure may actually appear quite early; the chest films and arteriogram of a 1-month-old infant with this complication are shown in Figures 50–71 and 50–72. The infant was managed by closure of the communication between the anterior descending coronary artery and the right ventricle, with an excellent clinical result. The postoperative aortogram is shown in Figure 50–73B (Daniel *et al.*, 1970).

Among those patients who are asymptomatic, the

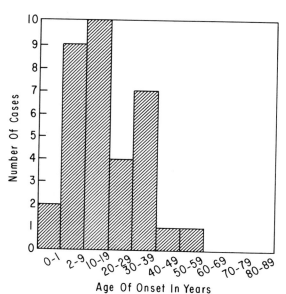

Figure 50–68. Age of onset of dyspnea on exertion or fatigue in patients with isolated coronary artery fistula. (From Daniel, T. M., Graham, T. P., and Sabiston, D. C., Jr.: Coronary artery–right ventricular fistula with congestive heart failure: Surgical correction in the neonatal period. Surgery, 67:985, 1970.)

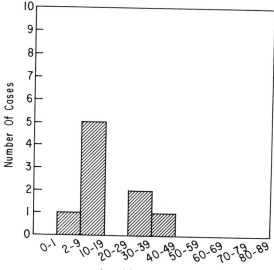

Figure 50–70. Age of onset of bacterial endocarditis in patients with an isolated coronary artery fistula. (From Daniel, T. M., Graham, T. P., and Sabiston, D. C., Jr.: Coronary artery–right ventricular fistula with congestive heart failure: Surgical correction in the neonatal period. Surgery, 67:985, 1970.)

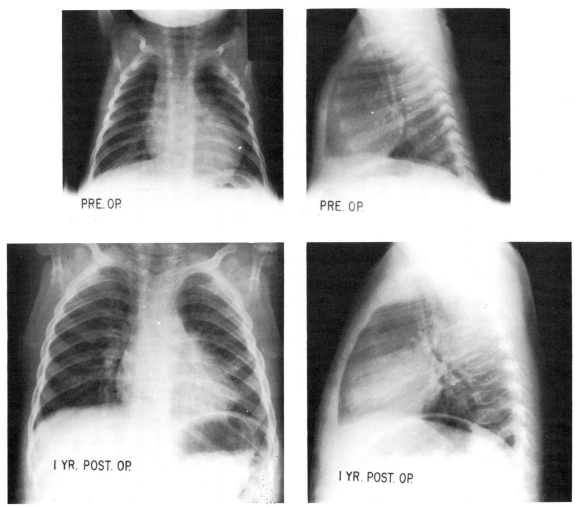

Figure 50–71. Preoperative chest films of an infant with a coronary artery fistula at 5 weeks of age. The interpretation included biventricular enlargement, left atrial enlargement, and increased pulmonary vasculature. Chest films 1 year after operation show decrease in cardiomegaly. (From Daniel, T. M., Graham, T. P., and Sabiston, D. C., Jr.: Coronary artery–right ventricular fistula with congestive heart failure: Surgical correction in the neonatal period. Surgery, *67*:985, 1970.)

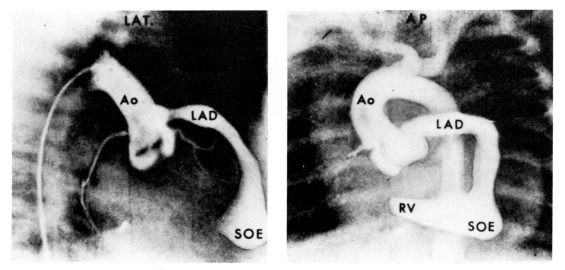

Figure 50–72. Ascending aortogram (lateral and anteroposterior views) in a 6-week-old infant who presented with severe congestive heart failure. The aortogram shows a left coronary artery–right ventricular fistula. (Ao = aorta; LAD = left anterior descending coronary; SOE = site of entry of the fistula into the right ventricle; RV = incompletely opacified right ventricle.) (From Daniel, T. M., Graham, T. P., and Sabiston, D. C., Jr.: Coronary artery–right ventricular fistula with congestive heart failure: Surgical correction in the neonatal period. Surgery, *67*:985, 1970.)

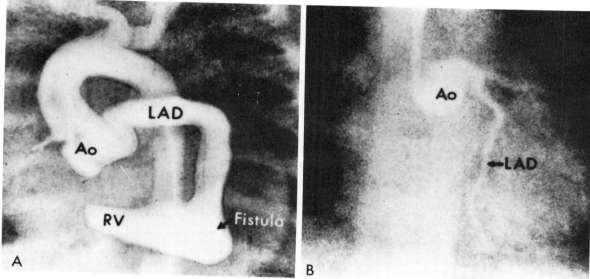

Figure 50–73. *A,* Preoperative aortogram of patient in Figure 50–72. *B,* Repeat aortogram 1 year following successful surgical obliteration of the fistula. The left anterior descending coronary artery has returned to normal size. (From Daniel, T. M., Graham, T. P., and Sabiston, D. C., Jr.: Coronary artery–right ventricular fistula with congestive heart failure: Surgical correction in the neonatal period. Surgery, *67*:985,1970.)

diagnosis is usually made following coronary angiography performed for evaluation of asymptomatic murmurs, mild cardiomegaly discovered on routine chest film, or persistent electrocardiographic abnormalities.

The main clinical manifestation of coronary artery fistulas is a continuous murmur over the site of the abnormal communication. This murmur may closely resemble that of a patent ductus arteriosus, and in fact, the first patient upon whom closure was performed was operated on by Bjork and Crafoord in 1947 for a presumed patent ductus. Because a patent ductus was not found, the pericardium was opened, and a coronary artery fistula draining into the pulmonary artery was identified and obliterated. The differential diagnosis of coronary artery fistulas, in addition to patent ductus arteriosus, includes congenital aortic-pulmonary fistula, sinus of Valsalva fistulas, ventricular septal defect with aortic insufficiency, pulmonary arteriovenous malformations, and fistulas of systemic vessels such as the subclavian and internal mammary arteries connecting to veins of the chest wall or to the lung.

Involved Coronary Artery and Site of Fistulous Communication. The right coronary artery is most often involved in the development of a congenital coronary artery fistula (56 per cent) (Table 50–11) and most commonly communicates with a chamber of the right heart (Table 50–12). Most frequently, the fistula involves the right ventricle (39 per cent), followed closely in incidence by drainage into the right atrium (33 per cent), including the coronary sinus and superior vena cava, or the pulmonary artery (20 per cent). Left coronary artery fistulas are less common but usually drain into the right ventricle or right atrium. Rarely, coronary artery fistulas may drain into the left atrium or left ventricle.

Evaluation

The successful surgical management of patients with congenital coronary artery fistulas is dependent on a thorough preoperative evaluation that precisely defines the anatomy and pathophysiology of the anomaly. The diagnosis therefore requires arteriographic demonstration of the involved coronary artery, the recipient cardiac chamber, and the exact site of communication. It should be emphasized that the clinical manifestations and the radiographic and electrocardiographic findings do not eliminate other lesions such as patent ductus arteriosus, sinus of Valsalva fistulas, or a ventricular septal defect with aortic insufficiency. In patients with a large fistula, injection of contrast

TABLE 50–11. CONGENITAL CORONARY ARTERY FISTULAS—INVOLVED CORONARY ARTERY IN 286 PATIENTS*

Right coronary artery	56%
Left coronary artery	36%
Both right and left coronary arteries	5%
Single coronary artery	3%

*From Lowe, J. E., Oldham, H. N., Jr., and Sabiston, D. C., Jr.: Surgical management of congenital coronary artery fistulas. Ann. Surg., *194*:371, 1981.

TABLE 50–12. CONGENITAL CORONARY ARTERY FISTULAS—SITE OF FISTULOUS COMMUNICATION IN 286 PATIENTS*

Right ventricle	39%
Right atrium (coronary sinus, superior vena cava)	33%
Pulmonary artery	20%
Left atrium	6%
Left ventricle	2%

*From Lowe, J. E., Oldham, H. N., Jr., and Sabiston, D. C., Jr.: Surgical management of congenital coronary artery fistulas. Ann. Surg., *194*:371, 1981.

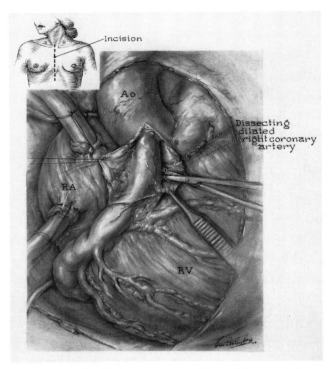

Figure 50–74. Right coronary–to–right atrial congenital coronary fistula as seen at operation in a 76-year-old female who presented with severe congestive heart failure. Through a median sternotomy, the patient was placed on cardiopulmonary bypass with separate venous return cannulas placed in the superior and inferior venae cavae. (From Lowe, J. E., and Sabiston, D. C., Jr.: Congenital coronary malformations. *In* Modern Technics in Surgery, Cardiac-Thoracic Surgery. Edited by L. Cohn. Mt. Kisco, New York, Futura Publishing Co., 1981, Chapter 35.)

medium into the aortic root may clearly delineate the lesion. In patients with a smaller fistula or fistulous communications from both coronary arteries, selective coronary arteriography is preferable and may be essential to establish the diagnosis.

Based on our experience and supported by that of others in the literature, it is recommended that nearly all patients with a major coronary artery fistula be considered candidates for surgical correction. In most instances, the natural history of these lesions is not associated with a normal life expectancy owing to the eventual development of congestive heart failure, angina, myocardial infarction, subacute bacterial endocarditis, aneurysm formation with rupture or embolization, or the development of pulmonary hypertension. It should be emphasized that the ideal time for elective surgical closure is prior to the development of symptoms and major pathologic changes in the heart, the coronary arteries, and the pulmonary circulation. As demonstrated by Liberthson and associates (1979), most patients with congenital coronary artery fistulas develop both symptoms and fistula-related complications with increasing age and are subject to increased morbidity and mortality when operation is performed later in life.

Surgical Management

Since patients with coronary artery fistulas have undergone a precise and detailed angiographic examination demonstrating the involved coronary artery, the recipient cardiac chamber, and the exact site of

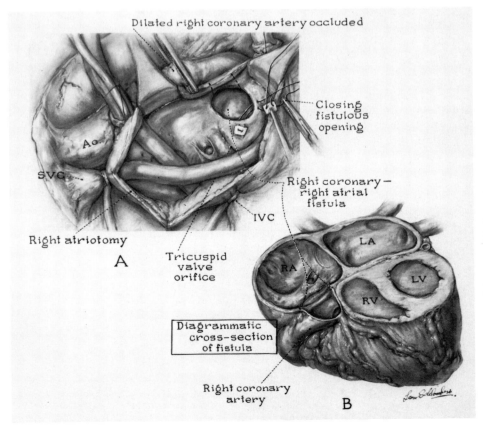

Figure 50–75. Tapes are secured around the superior and inferior venae cavae to eliminate venous return to the right atrium. The heart is then fibrillated and the right atrium opened. The large fistulous opening is identified and closed using interrupted nonabsorbable pledgeted sutures (*A*). The site of entry into the right coronary fistula is shown in *B*. (From Lowe, J. E., and Sabiston, D. C., Jr.: Congenital coronary malformations. *In* Modern Technics in Surgery, Cardiac-Thoracic Surgery. Edited by L. Cohn. Mt. Kisco, New York, Futura Publishing Co., 1981, Chapter 35.)

communication, it can often be anticipated preoperatively whether or not cardiopulmonary bypass will be required. Patients with a single communication that is easily dissected usually do not require bypass for suture obliteration. However, in patients with multiple communications or large, tortuous, draining channels, the fistula is best obliterated by opening the recipient cardiac chamber with the patient on bypass in order to completely close all fistulous tracts. Finally, if fistula obliteration in any way jeopardizes distal coronary arterial flow, a saphenous vein bypass graft should be placed under hypothermic potassium cardioplegic arrest. In any event, these procedures are always planned with a pump on stand-by.

After a median sternotomy or anterior thoracotomy is performed and a pericardial cradle is created, the fistulous communication is dissected and obliterated using multiple transfixion sutures of nonabsorbable material. If a cardiac chamber or the main pulmonary artery must be opened in order to close larger or multiple fistulous tracts, the patient is placed on cardiopulmonary bypass (Figs. 50–74 to 50–76). An arterial perfusion cannula is placed in the ascending aorta or femoral artery, and venous return cannulas are placed in the superior and inferior venae cavae. Tapes are placed around both the inferior and superior venae cavae. If the right atrium, right ventricle, or pulmonary artery is opened, the tapes are drawn tightly around the venous cannulas in order to prevent venous return to the right heart except for coronary sinus flow. The heart is then fibrillated, and the recipient cardiac chamber is opened. If the fistulous communication is with the left heart and obliteration requires opening of the left atrium or left ventricle or if saphenous vein bypass grafting is planned, the aorta is cross-clamped using cold potassium cardioplegic arrest and topical hypothermia. Following operative correction, intraoperative shunt curves are obtained to be certain that there is no residual left-to-right shunt.

In our experience with 22 patients treated surgically, 14 (64 per cent) underwent suture obliteration and did not require cardiopulmonary bypass. Six patients (27 per cent) required bypass in order to close multiple draining tracts from within a cardiac chamber (two from the right atrium and one from the right ventricle) or from within the main pulmonary artery (three patients). Two patients (9 per cent) required cardiopulmonary bypass in order to place saphenous vein interposition grafts since fistula obliteration jeopardized distal coronary arterial flow.

There were no operative or late deaths in this group of patients managed surgically. After a mean follow-up of 10 years, none of the patients had evidence of recurrent fistula formation, although one patient with a complex fistula of the circumflex coro-

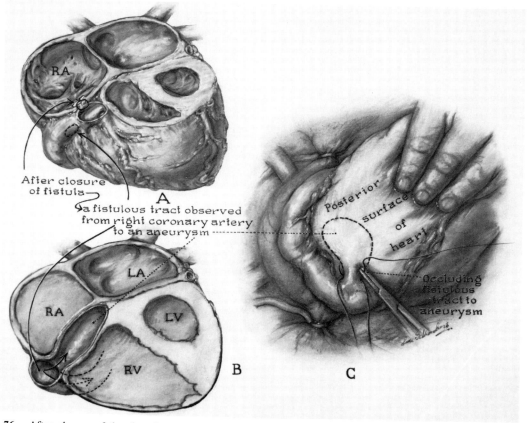

Figure 50–76. After closure of the site of entry into the right atrium, a second fistulous tract was found entering an aneurysm over the posterior surface of the heart (*A* and *B*). This fistulous tract was closed using multiple transfixion sutures (*C*). (From Lowe, J. E., and Sabiston, D. C., Jr.: Congenital coronary malformations. *In* Modern Technics in Surgery, Cardiac-Thoracic Surgery. Edited by L. Cohn. Mt. Kisco, New York, Futura Publishing Co., 1981, Chapter 35.)

nary artery to the right ventricle had a small residual shunt (Lowe *et al.*, 1981).

CONGENITAL ORIGIN OF THE LEFT CORONARY ARTERY FROM THE PULMONARY ARTERY

The first description of a left coronary artery originating from the pulmonary artery was made by Abbott in 1908. In 1911, Abrikossoff reported a 5-month-old infant who died of congestive heart failure and was found to have an aneurysm of the left ventricle at postmortem examination. Photomicrographs of the ventricle revealed infarction, including areas of calcification. In 1933, Bland and colleagues described the electrocardiographic changes in an infant with this malformation and demonstrated for the first time that a diagnosis could be established during life.

It is generally recognized that the prognosis of the vast majority of patients with origin of the left coronary artery from the pulmonary artery is quite poor. It has been estimated that 95 per cent of patients with this anomaly die within the first year of life unless surgical therapy is undertaken (Keith, 1959).

The pathophysiology of this malformation was poorly understood for many years, but evidence in the recent past has now made this aspect relatively straightforward. Numerous studies of postmortem specimens clearly reveal the presence of many collaterals originating from the right coronary artery and connecting to the left coronary artery. If the right coronary artery is injected in postmortem specimens, branches of the left coronary artery fill easily and in significant amounts (Case *et al.*, 1958). It has also been observed at the time of operation that occlusion of the left coronary artery at its anomalous origin from the pulmonary artery causes an increase in pressure within the artery, suggesting that flow originates from the right coronary artery via collaterals (Sabiston *et al.*, 1960a, 1960b). Of additional significance is the fact that blood withdrawn from the left coronary artery at operation has been found to be fully saturated with oxygen. Collectively, these findings are sound evidence that the direction of blood flow is from the right coronary artery via collaterals into the left coronary artery and then into the pulmonary artery. The resultant symptoms and clinical manifestations are secondary to left ventricular myocardial ischemia, which results either from inadequate right coronary artery–to–left coronary artery collateral flow or from a steal of adequate collateral flow into the low-pressure pulmonary arterial system.

Clinical Manifestations

The clinical manifestations of origin of the left coronary artery from the pulmonary artery become apparent in infancy in the majority of patients with this malformation. The infant usually appears normal at birth, since the pulmonary arterial pressure at this age is elevated and allows perfusion of the left coronary artery from the pulmonary artery. Nevertheless, symptoms may be present at birth, especially if there are associated cardiac malformations. Symptoms are most likely to occur during the first several months of life as left ventricular ischemia becomes more pronounced. Once symptoms appear, the course is usually one of progressive deterioration. Unless surgery is undertaken, progressively worsening left ventricular dysfunction occurs, which usually leads to death in infancy. Although the vast majority of patients with this malformation develop symptoms in infancy (95 per cent), a rare patient will survive to adult life with few, if any, symptoms. In 1927, Abbott reported a 64-year-old patient with this lesion, and in another collected review (Harthorne *et al.*, 1966), 28 adults were reported with this condition.

Symptoms. It was originally believed that symptoms resulted from poorly oxygenated blood from the pulmonary artery flowing into the left coronary arterial system. As described previously, however, a variety of studies have shown that blood flow is actually from the right coronary artery via collaterals into the left coronary artery and subsequently into the pulmonary artery. Symptoms result either from poor collateral flow from the right coronary artery or secondary to a steal phenomenon of blood passing through well-developed collaterals into the left coronary arterial system with drainage into the pulmonary artery. Because of the low pressures in the pulmonary artery, blood flow is selectively shunted into the pulmonary system instead of perfusing left ventricular myocardium. Two of the earliest and most characteristic symptoms are tachypnea and dyspnea. Coughing, wheezing, and cyanosis usually follow. One of the interesting findings that may be present has been described as the "angina of feeding," in which the infant shows evidence of pain during and immediately after feeding. As congestive heart failure worsens, cyanosis and pallor become apparent.

Physical Examination. The characteristic findings on physical examination include a rapid respiratory rate, tachycardia, and cardiac enlargement. Early in life, a murmur is not usually present, and congenital origin of the left coronary artery from the pulmonary artery is one of the few malformations that can cause congestive heart failure in infancy without a murmur. In older infants and children, mitral regurgitation develops secondary either to left ventricular dilatation (Burchell and Brown, 1962) or to chronic ischemia or infarction, which results in papillary muscle dysfunction. The liver is characteristically enlarged, and the spleen is palpable in a smaller number of patients. Occasionally, patients first present with signs of cardiovascular collapse and shock, similar to those manifested by adults with sudden coronary artery occlusion.

Evaluation

Chest Roentgenography. The chest film shows cardiomegaly, especially involving the left ventricle.

There is often evidence of congestive heart failure as well. Aneurysmal dilatation may be present as a result of marked thinning of the left ventricular wall. In many instances, the left border of the heart extends to the lateral rib margin. As a result of left ventricular failure, the pulmonary vascular markings are usually exaggerated.

Electrocardiography. Considerable emphasis has been placed on the changes that occur in the electrocardiogram leading to the establishment of a diagnosis. The first description of myocardial ischemia on the electrocardiogram of an infant with this condition was made by Bland and associates in 1933. Based on this work, congenital origin of the left coronary artery from the pulmonary artery has also been referred to as the Bland-White-Garland syndrome. Generally, it is possible to make a relatively confident diagnosis on the basis of electrocardiographic changes. Tachycardia is nearly always present. The T waves are characteristically inverted in the standard limb leads, and there may be slight ST-segment elevation in lead I. The T waves in the precordial leads, especially V_5 and V_6, are usually inverted, and deep Q waves are frequently present. The body surface potential distribution has also been helpful in diagnosis and in providing evidence of improved coronary blood flow following surgery (Flaherty *et al.*, 1967).

Angiocardiography. The right heart is usually normal. The pulmonary vasculature may show slight engorgement and enlargement. The most striking feature is enlargement of the left atrium and particularly of the left ventricle. The wall of the left ventricle may be quite thin, especially the anterolateral aspect near the apex. A true ventricular aneurysm with paradoxical pulsations may be present, and mitral insufficiency is relatively common. Contrast medium passing into the aorta demonstrates a single right coronary artery, although selective coronary arteriography is more reliable for precise demonstration of this feature.

Aortography. Injection of contrast medium into a catheter passed into the proximal aorta (or when possible directly into the right coronary ostium) demonstrates the classic findings. Contrast medium enters the right coronary artery as it originates from the aorta and passes through dilated collaterals that communicate with the left coronary artery. The contrast material can then be followed into the left circumflex and anterior descending coronary arteries, where it converges to enter the left main coronary artery, with ultimate drainage into the pulmonary artery. This finding is very impressive and conclusive, and large amounts of radiopaque contrast medium can be seen flowing freely into the pulmonary artery. Thus, retrograde flow of blood in the left coronary artery can be convincingly demonstrated in such a study, and this finding establishes an objective diagnosis (Fig. 50–77).

Cardiac Catheterization. Cardiac catheterization is also helpful in establishing the diagnosis. The right ventricular and pulmonary artery pressures may be elevated. Moreover, it is usually possible to demonstrate a left-to-right shunt at the pulmonary artery level by injection of contrast material. Although the

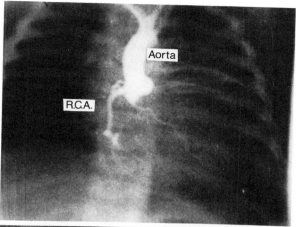

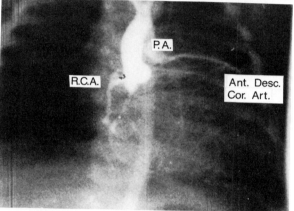

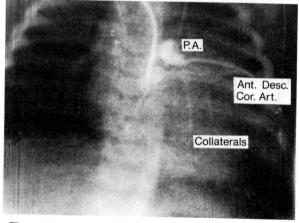

Figure 50–77. Several cine frames taken from a series illustrating coronary arterial filling during aortography. *A*, Filling of the right coronary artery as it arises normally from the aorta. Note that its size is somewhat greater than normal. *B*, Filling of the branches of the left coronary artery through collaterals from the right coronary artery. *C*, Filling of the pulmonary artery by retrograde flow from the left coronary artery. (From Sabiston, D. C., Jr., and Orme, S. K.: Congenital origin of the left coronary artery from the pulmonary artery. J. Cardiovasc. Surg., 9:543, 1968.)

oxygen saturation may at times show a significant increase from the right ventricle to the pulmonary artery, this is not always present, even when it can be demonstrated that the left coronary artery arises from the pulmonary artery.

The ejection fraction in patients with anomalous

origin of the left coronary artery has been determined in eight preoperative patients, in whom it ranged from 0.13 to 0.72. It is noteworthy that among those who died, the ejection fraction was less than 0.36, whereas in the survivors the figure was more than 0.55 (Menke *et al.*, 1972).

Pathology. The major pathologic features of this condition are apparent at the time of operation. The left ventricle is characteristically greatly dilated and the wall is thin. The left coronary artery is larger than normal, and numerous collateral vessels are apparent connecting the right and left coronary arteries. These are usually quite tortuous and thin-walled. The right coronary artery arises in its normal position and is also enlarged. Its branches tend to be more tortuous than usual as they give off various collateral vessels. With time, and especially in adults, the right coronary artery may become quite large and increasingly tortuous. Similarly, the left coronary artery may also become quite enlarged, up to 10 mm. or more in diameter at its origin. The left coronary artery arises from the left or posterior cusp of the pulmonary artery. The branches and course of the anterior descending and circumflex branches are usually otherwise normal. On section, the left ventricle may be markedly thin and in areas is totally replaced by scar tissue (Fig. 50–78). Varying degrees of subendocardial fibroelastosis may be present. Calcification is often present in the fibrotic portion of the left ventricle. Infarction of the ventricle may involve the papillary muscle, producing mitral insufficiency. If the left ventricle is dilated, the mitral ring may be sufficiently enlarged to prevent normal coaptation of the valve leaflets, which also results in mitral insufficiency.

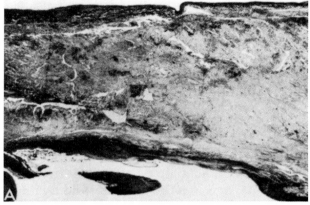

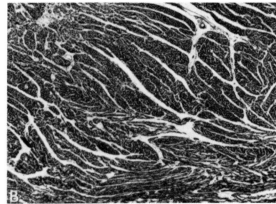

Figure 50–78. *A*, Histologic section of full thickness of left ventricle. Note that the left ventricular wall is almost totally replaced with scar tissue. The section represents the full thickness of the ventricle and is magnified 12 times, illustrating the extreme thinness of the left ventricle. *B*, Histologic section of right ventricular myocardium in the same patient showing normal cardiac muscle. (Published by Edizioni Minerva Medica, Turin, Italy, Nov.–Dec., 1968.)

Surgical Management

It is now recognized that the prognosis of origin of the left coronary artery from the pulmonary artery is generally poor once symptoms appear. Several surgical procedures were formerly advocated to improve the flow of blood in the left coronary artery, including a systemic-pulmonary anastomosis in an effort to increase both the oxygenation and pressure in the pulmonary artery; the production of a higher pressure in the left coronary artery by creating a coarctation of the pulmonary artery; and the creation of an increased blood supply to the left ventricle from the pericardium and other structures by means of irritants. Each of these operations has been attempted with disappointing results.

Since it has been demonstrated that blood flow in the left coronary artery is reversed or retrograde (blood flows from the normal right coronary artery through numerous dilated collateral vessels into the left coronary artery), an arteriovenous fistula is created, which deprives the left ventricular myocardium of a supply of blood that is badly needed. This phenomenon has been demonstrated by selective arteriography, in which the contrast medium can be

followed from the right coronary artery into the left coronary artery with ultimate drainage into the main pulmonary artery. Moreover, at the time of operation, blood aspirated from the left coronary artery and its branches is fully saturated with oxygen, indicating that it has a systemic arterial source. In addition, occlusion of the vessel at its origin causes a marked rise in the pressure within the left coronary artery. If the blood flow were actually from the pulmonary artery, a fall in the pressure would be expected. These observations led to the conclusion that ligation of the coronary artery would represent a logical procedure in the surgical treatment of this condition.

Two basic approaches are available in the surgical treatment of origin of the left coronary artery from the pulmonary artery. Simple ligation at the site of origin from the pulmonary artery is effective treatment if there are enough collaterals from the right coronary artery to adequately supply the left coronary arterial system. This approach is usually reserved for small infants, in whom the left coronary artery is too small for a direct anastomosis. Ligation prevents the steal of right coronary collateral flow into the low-pressure pulmonary artery system. The major disadvantage of this form of therapy is that the patient has a one coronary artery system. The long-term fate of even large collaterals from the right coronary artery is unknown, and atherosclerotic coronary artery disease later in life involving the right coronary artery would affect flow throughout the entire coronary arterial system. Simple ligation, however, may be lifesaving, and reconstruction of a two coronary artery system can be accomplished at a later time.

Rarely, a child may manifest severe symptoms during early life, with later remission of symptoms apparently due to the development of adequate collaterals (Ihenacho *et al.*, 1973). An infant with a left ventricular aneurysm in congestive heart failure has been reported; treatment consisted of resection of the aneurysm and ligation of the abnormal left coronary artery at its origin (Turina *et al.*, 1974). A combination procedure, resection of a left ventricular aneurysm and introduction of a saphenous vein graft from the

Figure 50–79. *A,* Congenital origin of the left coronary artery from the pulmonary artery. Through a left anterior third interspace thoracotomy, the left coronary artery is occluded at its site of origin with suture ligatures and then divided. *B,* The left subclavian artery is then anastomosed to the left coronary artery in end-to-end fashion using interrupted 7-0 nonabsorbable sutures. (From Lowe, J. E., and Sabiston, D. C., Jr.: Congenital coronary malformations. *In* Modern Technics in Surgery, Cardiac-Thoracic Surgery. Edited by L. Cohn. Mt. Kisco, New York, Futura Publishing Co., 1981, Chapter 35.)

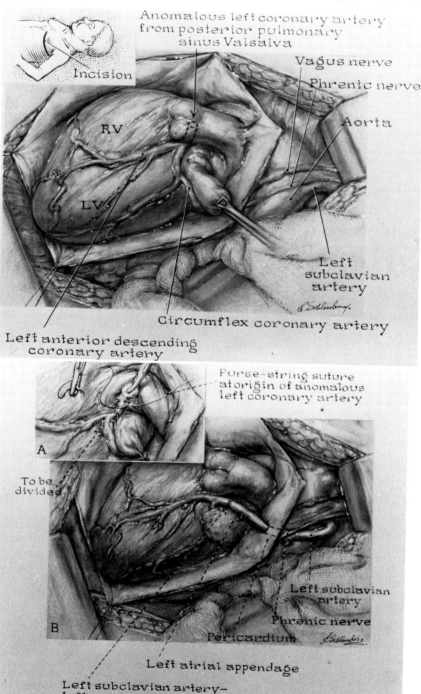

aorta to the anterior descending coronary artery, has also been reported in a young child with anomalous origin of the left coronary artery from the pulmonary artery (Flemma et al., 1975).

If collateral flow from the right coronary artery is inadequate or if the patient is an older infant, child, or adult with large enough vessels, the initial repair can be designed to reconstruct a two coronary artery system. At present, this is best accomplished by either ligation and saphenous vein bypass grafting or ligation and left or right subclavian artery–to–left coronary artery anastomosis. In younger children and infants, the latter form of therapy has technical advantages, since in this group, the subclavian artery is usually larger than autologous saphenous vein. Direct reimplantation of the left coronary artery to the aorta has also been reported (Grace et al., 1977).

Simple ligation is best accomplished through a left third interspace anterior thoracotomy. The pericardium is opened, with particular care being taken to avoid stretching or contusion of the phrenic nerve. Careful dissection near the posterior sinus of Valsalva of the pulmonary artery is necessary to assure that the origin is identified. The left coronary artery is then clamped at its site of origin, and if this is tolerated, it is permanently obliterated, using multiple transfixion sutures, and divided. Left subclavian artery–to–left coronary artery anastomosis is also performed through this incision, and the anastomosis is accomplished using interrupted sutures of 7-0 Prolene or Tycron (Fig. 50–79). If a two coronary artery system is to be reconstructed using saphenous vein, a median sternotomy is performed, and the procedure is usually done with cardiopulmonary bypass.

The best form of surgical treatment for this disorder is unknown. In those patients who survive beyond the age of 1 year, the proper form of treatment is controversial. Such patients have been successfully treated by ligation of the left coronary artery (Baue et al., 1967; Roche, 1967; Sabiston et al., 1968), and others have been treated by the anastomosis of the left coronary artery to the aorta either directly (Grace et al., 1977) or by means of a venous autograft or a prosthetic graft (Cooley et al., 1966). Although the single best form of surgical therapy for this disorder is unknown, simple ligation in the newborn with adequate right coronary artery collateral flow is generally recommended. In the older infant, child or the newborn with inadequate flow, our procedure of choice is ligation and immediate left or right subclavian artery–to–left coronary artery anastomosis. In the older child or adult, a two coronary artery system can be reconstructed using saphenous vein bypass grafting. It should be emphasized, however, that although our initial experience as well as that of others with left subclavian artery–to–left coronary artery anastomosis (Pinsky et al., 1973) and saphenous vein interposition grafting has been good (Lowe and Sabiston, 1981), the long-term results in significant numbers of patients are as yet unknown. In patients with adequate collateral flow from the right coronary artery to the left coronary system, immediate reconstruction assumes that vein graft or subclavian shunt flow is greater than intrinsic collateral flow. If this is not the case, the hemodynamics continue to favor collateral flow into the left coronary arterial system, which may result in subsequent vein graft or subclavian shunt failure (Anthony et al., 1975; Pinsky et al., 1976). Clinically, patients may continue to do well even with occluded vein grafts or subclavian shunts because of right coronary collateral flow.

CONGENITAL ORIGIN OF THE RIGHT CORONARY ARTERY FROM THE PULMONARY ARTERY

Brooks originally described this rare malformation in two cadavers studied in the anatomic dissection laboratory at the University of Dublin in 1886. Both lesions occurred in adults, neither of whom had evidence of heart disease. Brooks noted dilated collaterals from the left coronary artery feeding the right coronary artery and correctly postulated, based on this observation, that flow in the right coronary artery might actually be retrograde into the pulmonary artery.

Clinical Manifestations

The clinical manifestations of this condition are usually minimal or absent. In the 17 cases collected from the literature (reviewed by Tingelstad and associates [1972]), the abnormal artery was discovered in individuals whose ages ranged from 17 to 90 years. The malformation was thought to have been associated with death in only two instances. One of these was a 17-year-old female who died suddenly and in whom autopsy showed complete occlusion of the left coronary artery by thrombus with evidence of left ventricular infarction. The only other reported death occurred in a 55-year-old female who presented with angina and congestive heart failure. Three additional patients have been reported in whom the anomaly occurred in association with other congenital malformations.

Even though origin of the right coronary artery from the pulmonary artery is a rare anomaly with a benign natural history in most patients, it can lead to myocardial ischemia, congestive heart failure, and myocardial fibrosis. Since it can be safely corrected, once diagnosed, operative correction is indicated.

Evaluation

In the rare patient with this condition who comes to medical attention, the diagnosis is established by aortography and selective coronary arteriography. The left coronary artery is found to be dilated with large intercoronary collaterals feeding the right coronary artery. As Brooks correctly suggested, flow in the right coronary artery is retrograde, emptying into the pulmonary artery. In contrast to patients who have the more frequently occurring malformation of origin of the left coronary artery from the pulmonary artery, patients with origin of the right coronary artery from the pulmonary artery usually have no electrocardiographic or radiographic abnormalities. The diagnosis is therefore established only in those who undergo selective coronary arteriography.

Surgical Management

A very fascinating case has been reported of a 12-year-old male who was asymptomatic but had a to-and-fro systolic and diastolic murmur along the left sternal border in the third intercostal space. The chest films showed slight cardiac enlargement and normal pulmonary vasculature. Mild left ventricular hypertrophy was demonstrated on the scalar electrocardiogram. An aortogram demonstrated a dilated left coronary artery arising normally from the left sinus of Valsalva of the aorta, and the right coronary artery was filled through tortuous intercoronary anastomoses from the left coronary artery and drained into the main pulmonary artery. At operation, a narrow rim of tissue from the pulmonary artery was removed with the origin of the right coronary artery, and this was successfully reimplanted into the ascending aorta (Tingelstad *et al.*, 1972). This represents the ideal form of surgical management and has also been performed successfully by Bregman and colleagues (1976). Other alternatives include simple ligation at the site of anomalous origin (Rowe and Young, 1960), with or without saphenous vein bypass grafting.

CONGENITAL ORIGIN OF BOTH CORONARY ARTERIES FROM THE PULMONARY ARTERY

Five infants in whom both coronary arteries arose from the pulmonary artery have been reported in the literature. The survival time ranged from 9 hours to 5 months (Tedeschi and Helpern, 1954). There is also an interesting report of a child who lived to the age of 7 years with total coronary arterial circulation originating from the pulmonary artery (Feldt *et al.*, 1965); his prolonged survival was due to an interventricular septal defect with pulmonary hypertension and congenital mitral stenosis. The pressure in the pulmonary artery was sufficient to force blood into the myocardial capillary bed, and under these circumstances, the child lived for an amazingly long time. There have been no reports of surgical correction for this rare anomaly.

CONGENITAL ANEURYSMS OF THE CORONARY ARTERIES

In 1812, Bougon first reported an aneurysm of the coronary arteries. These lesions have been reported from infancy (Crocker *et al.*, 1957) to adult life. Congenital aneurysms of the coronary arteries are rare and constituted only 15 per cent of coronary artery aneurysms reported in 89 patients (Daoud *et al.*, 1963). Other causes of aneurysms of the coronary arteries include atherosclerosis, mycotic aneurysms, syphilis, rheumatic heart disease, and the recently recognized mucocutaneous lymph node syndrome.

These lesions are most often asymptomatic until complications occur. Complications include thrombosis or embolization with subsequent myocardial ischemia or infarction or actual rupture of the aneurysm. An intramural coronary aneurysm has also been reported and produced reversed flow during systole owing to bulging of the thin-walled chamber into the left ventricular cavity. The narrow neck of the aneurysm was successfully closed at surgery. An example of a congenital coronary artery aneurysm involving the left circumflex vessel is shown in Figure 50–80*A*. In this patient, a mural thrombus occurred in the aneurysm that embolized and produced acute myocardial infarction. The aneurysm was resected with insertion of a saphenous vein autograft (Fig 50–80*B* and *C*) (Ebert *et al.*, 1971). Surgical management of a coronary aneurysm is indicated if the aneurysm is symptomatic, especially if there is evidence of emboli arising from the aneurysm, producing myocardial ischemia in the distal coronary bed.

MEMBRANOUS OBSTRUCTION OF THE OSTIUM OF THE LEFT MAIN CORONARY ARTERY

Hypoplasia or atresia of the coronary arteries in infancy and childhood has been reported and usually causes severe impairment of ventricular function and sudden death. Congenital atresia of the left main coronary artery has been reported in nine patients, all of whom presented with signs and symptoms of myocardial ischemia, congestive heart failure, or both. Histopathologic studies in these patients showed that the left main coronary had been replaced by fibromuscular tissue and that the left coronary ostium was absent. These conditions are not surgically correctable. However, three patients have been reported with membranous obstruction at the ostium of the left main coronary artery, associated with a normal distal coronary artery. The first patient was a 6-month-old infant who died with myocardial infarction, and the diagnosis was established at the time of autopsy (Verney *et al.*, 1969). Recently, Josa and associates (1981) reported two cases diagnosed at the time of operation. One patient, a 2-year-old child, was being operated on for congenital aortic stenosis and was found to have a membrane markedly obstructing the ostium of the left main coronary artery. The second patient was an 8-year-old male with Type I truncus arteriosus, who also was found to have membranous obstruction of the ostium of the left main coronary artery at operation. Both of these patients demonstrated evidence of myocardial ischemia preoperatively, and following excision of the membrane at operation, the symptoms

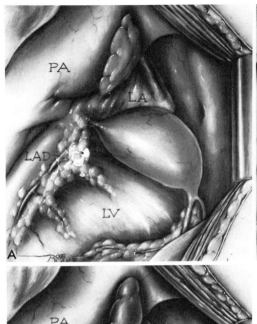

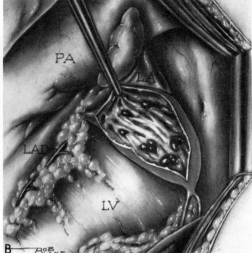

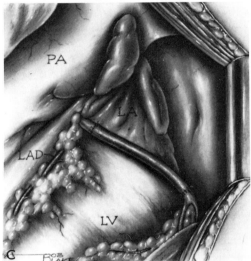

Figure 50–80. *A,* Congenital aneurysm of the left circumflex coronary artery as seen at operation in a 31-year-old female who presented with an acute myocardial infarction with subsequent disabling angina. (PA = pulmonary artery; LAD = left anterior descending coronary artery; LV = left ventricle; LA = left atrium.) *B,* Numerous small fresh thrombi are shown adherent to the rough, irregular surface of the aneurysm. The proximal opening into the aneurysm was a discrete, mildly dilated vessel of good quality and normal-appearing intima. The distal branches of the circumflex coronary artery are of normal size. *C,* The entire aneurysm was excised, and an interposition graft of saphenous vein was placed. There was only minimal discrepancy in the size of the saphenous vein graft and the ends of the circumflex coronary artery. A continuous 7-0 nonabsorbable suture was used at each anastomosis. (From Ebert, P. A., Peter, R. H., Gunnells, J. C., and Sabiston, D. C., Jr.: Resecting and grafting of coronary artery aneurysms. Circulation, *43:*593, 1971.)

were totally relieved. Grossly, the membranous structure appeared to be continuous with the aortic intima, and histologic studies revealed that its structure was similar to that of normal aortic root media. These two examples indicate the importance of careful evaluation of the origin and distribution of the coronary arteries in patients with congenital heart disease, especially when the signs and symptoms of ischemia and heart failure are disproportionate to the congenital lesion being evaluated (Josa *et al.,* 1981).

SELECTED REFERENCES

Abrikossoff, A.: Aneurysma des liken Herzventrikels mit abnqmer Abgangsstelle der linken Koronararterie von der Pulmonalis bei einem funfmonatlichen Kinde. Virchows Arch. (Pathol. Anat.), *203:*413, 1911.

The classic description of anomalous origin of the left coronary artery from the pulmonary artery is made in this historic paper. Both the gross and microscopic illustrations are excellent. The author describes in detail the clinical manifestations and postmortem findings.

Daniel, T. M., Graham, T. P., and Sabiston, D. C., Jr.: Coronary artery–right ventricular fistula with congestive heart failure: Surgical correction in the neonatal period. Surgery, *67:*985, 1970.

In this review, almost 200 patients with coronary arteriovenous fistulas are reported. The incidence of congestive heart failure was 14 per cent. Approximately half of all patients with isolated arteriovenous fistulas were symptomatic. The age of onset of dyspnea, congestive heart failure, bacterial endocarditis, and angina pectoris is reviewed.

Ebert, P. A., Peter, R. H., Gunnells, J. C., and Sabiston, D. C., Jr.: Resecting and grafting of coronary artery aneurysm. Circulation, *43:*593, 1971.

This paper describes an aneurysm of the circumflex coronary artery containing a thrombus that subsequently embolized and produced myocardial infarction. A review of the problem, the clinical manifestations, and management are discussed.

Feldt, R. H., Ongley, P. A., and Titus, J. L.: Total coronary arterial circulation from pulmonary artery with survival to age seven: Report of a case. Mayo Clin. Proc., *40:*539, 1965.

This paper presents the amazing report of a child who survived to the age of 7 years with a coronary circulation arising solely from the pulmonary artery. This case report is clearly a fascinating one and is an example of the marked compensatory power of the coronary circulation.

Lowe, J. E., and Sabiston, D. C., Jr.: Congenital coronary malformations. *In* Modern Technics in Surgery, Cardiac-Thoracic Surgery. Edited by L. Cohn. Mt. Kisco, New York, Futura Publishing Co., 1981, Chapter 35.

This review presents the surgical techniques used to correct congenital coronary artery fistulas, anomalous origin of the left or right coronary artery from the pulmonary artery, and congenital coronary artery aneurysms. The details of the preoperative evaluation, anesthetic management, and postoperative care are also reviewed.

Lowe, J. E., Oldham, H. N., Jr., and Sabiston, D. C., Jr.: Surgical management of congenital coronary artery fistulas. Ann. Surg., *194*:371, 1981.

This paper reports the clinical manifestations of 28 patients with congenital coronary artery fistulas seen at one institution and summarizes the results of surgical management in 22 patients. This is the largest single series of patients with congenital fistulas managed surgically. An additional 258 patients previously reported are also reviewed. The natural history and pathophysiology of coronary fistulas are discussed, and the rationale for early surgical intervention is presented.

Sabiston, D. C., Jr., and Orme, S. K.: Congenital origin of the left coronary artery from the pulmonary artery. J. Cardiovasc. Surg., *9*:543, 1968.

In this report, 23 patients with origin of the left coronary artery from the pulmonary artery are described. The youngest patient was 1 day of age and the oldest 31 years. The natural history, clinical findings, laboratory data, and ultimate course are presented.

REFERENCES

Abbott, M. E.: Congenital cardiac disease. *In* Modern Medicine. 3rd Ed. Edited by W. Osler. Philadelphia, Lea & Febiger, 1927.

Abbott, M. E.: Congenital cardiac disease. *In* Modern Medicine, Vol. 4. Edited by W. Osler. Philadelphia, Lea & Febiger, 1908.

Abrikossoff, A.: Aneurysma des liken Herzventrikels mit abnormer Abgangsstelle der linken Koronararterie von der Pulmonalis bei einem funfmonatlichen Kinde. Virchows Arch. (Pathol. Anat.), *203*:413, 1911.

Anthony, C. L., Jr., McAllister, H. A., Jr., and Cheitlin, M. D.: Spontaneous graft closure in anomalous origin of the left coronary artery. Chest, *68*:586, 1975.

Baue, A. E., Baum, S., Blakemore, W. S., and Zinsser, H. F.: A later stage of anomalous coronary circulation with origin of the left coronary artery from the pulmonary artery. Circulation, *36*:878, 1967.

Bjork, G., and Crafoord, C.: Arteriovenous aneurysm on the pulmonary artery simulating patent ductus arteriosus botalli. Thorax, *2*:65, 1947.

Bland, E. F., White, P. D., and Garland, J.: Congenital anomalies of coronary arteries: Report of an unusual case associated with cardiac hypertrophy. Am. Heart J., *8*:787, 1933.

Bougon: Bibl. Med., *37*:183, 1812. Cited by Packard, M., and Wechsler, H. F.: Aneurysm of the coronary arteries. Arch. Intern. Med., *43*:1, 1929.

Bregman, D., Brennan, J., Singer, A., Vinci, J., Parodi, E. N., Cassarella, W. J., and Edie, R. N.: Anomalous origin of the right coronary artery from the pulmonary artery. J. Thorac. Cardiovasc. Surg., *72*:626, 1976.

Brooks, H. St. J.: Two cases of an abnormal coronary artery of the heart arising from the pulmonary artery. J. Anat. Physiol., *20*:26, 1886.

Burchell, H. B., and Brown, A. L., Jr.: Anomalous origin of coronary artery from the pulmonary artery masquerading as mitral insufficiency. Am. Heart J., *63*:388, 1962.

Case, R. B., Morrow, A. G., Stainsby, W., and Nestor, J. O.: Anomalous origin of the left coronary artery: The physiologic defect and suggested surgical treatment. Circulation, *17*:1062, 1958.

Cooley, D. A., Hallman, G. L., and Bloodwell, R. D.: Definitive surgical treatment of anomalous origin of left coronary artery from pulmonary artery: Indications and results. J. Thorac. Cardiovasc. Surg., *52*:798, 1966.

Crocker, D. W., Sobin, S., and Thomas, W. C.: Aneurysms of the coronary arteries. Report of three cases in infants and review of the literature. Am. J. Pathol., *33*:819, 1957.

Daniel, T. M., Graham, T. P., and Sabiston, D. C., Jr.: Coronary artery–right ventricular fistula with congestive heart failure: Surgical correction in the neonatal period. Surgery, *67*:985, 1970.

Daoud, A. S., Pankin, D., Tulgan, H., and Florentin, R. A.: Aneurysms of the coronary artery. Am. J. Cardiol., *11*:228, 1963.

Ebert, P. A., Peter, R. H., Gunnells, J. C., and Sabiston, D. C., Jr.: Resecting and grafting of coronary artery aneurysm. Circulation, *43*:593, 1971.

Feldt, R. H., Ongley, P. A., and Titus, J. L.: Total coronary arterial circulation from pulmonary artery with survival to age seven: Report of a case. Mayo Clin. Proc., *40*:539, 1965.

Flaherty, J. T., Spach, M. S., Boineau, J. P., Canent, R. V., Jr., Barr, R. C., and Sabiston, D. C., Jr.: Cardiac potentials on body surface of infants with anomalous left coronary artery (myocardial infarction). Circulation, *36*:345, 1967.

Flemma, R. J., Marx, L., Litwin, S. B., and Gallen, W.: Left ventricular aneurysmectomy in infancy: Treatment of anomalous left coronary artery. Ann. Thorac. Surg., *19*:457, 1975.

Grace, R. R., Paolo, A., and Cooley, D. A.: Aortic implantation of anomalous left coronary artery arising from pulmonary artery. J. Cardiol., *39*:608, 1977.

Harthorne, J. W., Scannell, J. G., and Dinsmore, R. E.: Anomalous origin of the left coronary artery. Remediable cause of sudden death in adults. N. Engl. J. Med., *275*:660, 1966.

Ihenacho, H. N. C., Singh, S. P., Astley, R., and Parsons, C. G.: Case report. Anomalous left coronary artery. Report of an unusual case with spontaneous remission of symptoms. Br. Heart J., *35*:562, 1973.

Josa, M., Danielson, G. K., Weidman, W. H., and Edwards, W. D.: Congenital ostial membrane of left main coronary artery. J. Thorac. Cardiovasc. Surg., *81*:338, 1981.

Keith, J. D.: The anomalous origin of the left coronary artery from the pulmonary artery. Br. Heart J., *21*:149, 1959.

Krause, W.: Z. Rationelle Med., *24*, 1865.

Liberthson, R. R., Sagar, K., Behocoben, J. P., Weintraub, R. M., and Levine, F. H.: Congenital coronary arteriovenous fistula. Circulation, *59*:849, 1979.

Lowe, J. E., and Sabiston, D. C., Jr.: Congenital coronary malformations. *In* Modern Technics in Surgery, Cardiac-Thoracic Surgery. Edited by L. Cohn. Mt. Kisco, New York, Futura Publishing Co., 1981, Chapter 35.

Lowe, J. E., Oldham, H. N., Jr., and Sabiston, D. C., Jr.: Surgical management of congenital coronary artery fistulas. Ann. Surg., *194*:371, 1981.

Menke, J. A., Shaher, R. M., and Wolff, G. S.: Ejection fraction in anomalous origin of the left coronary artery from the pulmonary artery. Am. Heart J., *84*:325, 1972.

Ogden, J. A.: Congenital anomalies of the coronary arteries. Am. J. Cardiol., *25*:474, 1970.

Pinsky, W. W., Fagan, L. R., Mudd, J. F. G., and Willman, V. L.: Subclavian–coronary artery anastomosis in infancy for the Bland-White syndrome. J. Thorac. Cardiovasc. Surg., *72*:15, 1976.

Pinsky, W. W., Fagan, L. R., Kraeger, R. R., Mudd, J. F. G., and Willman, V. L.: Anomalous left coronary artery. J. Thorac. Cardiovasc. Surg., *65*:810, 1973.

Roche, A. H. G.: Anomalous origin of the left coronary artery from the pulmonary artery in the adult. Am. J. Cardiol., *20*:561, 1967.

Rowe, G. G., and Young, W. P.: Anomalous origin of the coronary arteries with special reference to surgical treatment. J. Thorac. Cardiovasc. Surg., *39*:777, 1960.

Sabiston, D. C., Jr., and Orme, S. K.: Congenital origin of the left coronary artery from the pulmonary artery. J. Cardiovasc. Surg., *9*:543, 1968.

Sabiston, D. C., Jr., Floyd, W. L., and McIntosh, H. D.: Anomalous origin of the left coronary artery from the pulmonary artery in adults. Arch. Surg., *97*:963, 1968.

Sabiston, D. C., Jr., Neill, C. A., and Taussig, H. B.: The direction of blood flow in anomalous left coronary artery arising from the pulmonary artery. Circulation, *22*:591, 1960a.

Sabiston, D. C., Jr., Pelargonio, S., and Taussig, H. B.: Myocardial infarction in infancy: The surgical management of a complication of congenital origin of the left coronary artery from the pulmonary artery. J. Thorac. Cardiovasc. Surg., *40*:321, 1960b.

Sabiston, D. C., Jr., Ross, R. S., Criley, J. M., Gaertner, R. A., Neill, C. A., and Taussig, H. B.: Surgical management of congenital lesions of the coronary circulation. Ann. Surg., *157*:908, 1963.

Sones, F. M., and Shirey, E. K.: Collateral arterial channels in living human with coronary artery disease. Circulation, *22*:815, 1960.

Tedeschi, C. G., and Helpern, M. M.: Heterotopic origin of both coronary arteries from the pulmonary artery. Review of literature and report of a case not complicated by associated defects. Pediatrics, *14*:53, 1954.

Tingelstad, J. B., Lower, R. R., and Eldredge, W. J.: Anomalous origin of the right coronary artery from the main pulmonary artery. Am. J. Cardiol., *30*:670, 1972.

Turina, M., Real, F., Meier, W., and Senning, Å.: Left ventricular aneurysmectomy in a 4-month-old infant. Alternative method of treatment of anomalous left coronary artery. J. Thorac. Cardiovasc. Surg., *67*:915, 1974.

Verney, R. N., Monnet, P., Arnaud, P., *et al.*: Infarctus du myocarde chez un nourrisson de cinq mois—ostium coronaire gauche punctiforme. Ann. Pédiatr. (Paris), *16*:260, 1969.

V SURGICAL MANAGEMENT OF CORONARY ARTERY DISEASE

1. Bypass Grafting for Coronary Artery Disease

Frank C. Spencer

HISTORICAL BACKGROUND

Coronary bypass surgery was developed between 1967 and 1968 at three major centers in the United States: the Cleveland Clinic in Cleveland, Ohio; the University of Wisconsin in Milwaukee; and New York University in New York City. Before this time, there had been a few isolated case reports of bypass grafting, but these had had little clinical impact.

The principal credit belongs to the pioneering efforts of Favaloro, Effler, and associates at the Cleveland Clinic, where, with the development of coronary angiography by F. Mason Sones, investigation of surgical treatment of coronary disease had been their primary objective for several years. Their observation of the usefulness of the saphenous vein for bypass grafting was the first clear indication of its widespread applicability. Johnson, in Milwaukee, quickly perceived the significance of this fact and made the quantum step of extending the procedure to the left coronary artery. The magnitude of this achievement is illustrated by the fact that before 1967 operative procedures on the left coronary artery had a mortality rate exceeding 50 per cent and had been virtually abandoned. By 1969, Johnson reported to the American Surgical Association successful operations on the left coronary artery in a series of 301 patients, with a mortality rate of 12 per cent. This report soundly launched the modern era of coronary bypass surgery,

which has grown in exponential proportions since that time. At least 100,000 such procedures were performed in the United States in 1981.

At New York University the concept of anastomosis of the internal mammary artery to the left anterior descending coronary artery using microsurgical technique was developed by Green and associates (1970) following earlier demonstration of the feasibility of this procedure in the laboratory (Spencer et al., 1964). One early report describing the use of the internal mammary artery had been published in 1967 by Kolessov in Russia, in which the operation was performed with a beating heart, an approach with little application.

In the decades before 1967, numerous indirect procedures had been evaluated. Virtually all were designed to enhance the growth of collateral circulation to the myocardium. Some were ingenious, others bizarre; all have now been discarded. The only procedure that offered some encouragement for several years was the Vineberg procedure of implantation of the internal mammary artery into the myocardium. The artery remains patent in the majority of instances, but the magnitude of flow through the implanted artery was disappointing in the majority of patients. Hence, it is rarely done today.

At present, the safety and immediate benefits of bypass grafting are well established. Probably varying somewhat with criteria used by different centers, 90

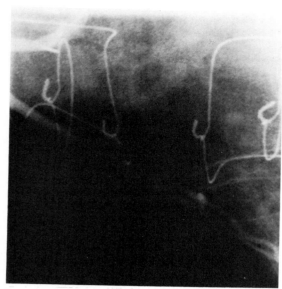

Figure 50–81. An angiogram performed 10 years following insertion of a saphenous vein bypass graft to the anterior descending coronary artery. The patient was studied again because of angina found to be due to atherosclerosis developing in the circumflex coronary artery. The graft appears normal, with adequate flow into the anterior descending coronary artery, both antegrade and retrograde.

to 95 per cent of patients with coronary disease can be operated on, with an operative mortality near 1 per cent in good-risk patients. In over 90 per cent of patients, operation is followed by dramatic improvement or disappearance of angina. Graft patency at 1 year should be near 90 per cent; occlusion apparently progresses thereafter at a rate near 3 per cent per year for the next 5 years (Grondin et al., 1979; Hamby et al., 1979). The deterioration of grafts is not uniform and is basically unpredictable. A graft in excellent condition on angiography 1 year after operation has an excellent likelihood of being patent 5 years later (Grondin, 1981) (Fig. 50–81). Degeneration of grafts is probably related to at least three factors: injury to the vein at operation; the degree of turbulent flow arising at the anastomosis; and the virulence of the basic atherosclerotic process.

The principal questions with coronary bypass are the durability of the bypass grafts and the progression of atherosclerosis. These two factors, of course, determine the influence of bypass grafting on longevity and protection from myocardial infarction. The influence on longevity in turn influences the decision for operation, with the deciding factor being either the findings on angiography (the extent of the disease and the impairment of ventricular function) or the severity of angina.

As will be discussed later in this section, the patency of vein grafts 5 years after operation seems to be in the range of 80 to 85 per cent, with occlusion occurring most frequently in the first year after operation and then occurring at a slower rate of 2 to 3 per cent per year. Probably the most significant factors influencing the rate of occlusion are the manner of

harvesting the vein and the storage at the time of the bypass procedure.

A disappointing fact is that little evidence has appeared that the atherosclerotic process can be controlled (Rifkind and Levy, 1978). Serial angiograms up to 6 years after operation have usually shown continued progression of atherosclerosis at a variable unpredictable rate (Grondin, 1981). With the data now available concerning 5-year survival from a number of reports summarized in this section, there is an increasing tendency to employ bypass grafting following angiographic demonstration of severe triple-vessel disease, even with minimal symptoms, especially if there is some impairment of ventricular function.

CORONARY ARTERY DISEASE

Frequency and Epidemiology

At a 2-day Consensus Conference at the National Institutes of Health in Bethesda, Maryland, in 1978, the frequency of coronary disease was reviewed in detail, with examination of the curious epidemiologic fact that the frequency of death from coronary disease in the United States gradually increased from about 1950 to 1966 and 1967, but subsequently gradually decreased so that the death rate in 1976 was near that in 1950. Why this decline occurred in the United States but not in many countries in the world was analyzed for 2 days with no clear conclusion being reached. This curious reversal in the death rate occurred before many modern methods of treatment were available, such as beta-blockade, bypass surgery, physical exercise, stringent dietary therapy, and avoidance of smoking.

Similarly, there has been a puzzling gradual increase in longevity of the United States population since around 1967, after it had remained at a plateau for the previous 10 to 15 years. Whether this was a result of the decrease in death from coronary disease and other diseases or whether it represented a basic biologic phenomenon of unknown origin could not be determined.

Nevertheless, atherosclerosis remains the most common serious disease in the Caucasian male, causing around 600,000 deaths annually in the United States. In worldwide epidemiologic studies, the United States has the second highest frequency of atherosclerosis in the world, exceeded only by Finland, whereas Japan has the lowest frequency (Stamler, 1978). The disease is seldom found in populations in which the average cholesterol concentration is below 200 mg. per 100 ml. In Japan, the average cholesterol level is said to be near 150 mg. per 100 ml.

At the 1978 Consensus Conference, the 1976 death statistics from the Bureau of Vital Statistics were analyzed in detail. In that year, there were 644,000 deaths from coronary disease, 360,000 males and 284,000 females. The variation in age distribution in males and females was quite striking, for only about 34,000 deaths occurred in females under 65 years of age, as compared with about 110,000 deaths in males under 65 years of age.

Analysis of deaths by decade was equally striking, showing that in both males and females the death rate per 100,000 population increased two to four times with each decade of life; for example, the number of deaths for males between 45 and 55 years old was 281 per 100,000, as compared with 66 per 100,000 for males between 35 and 44 years old—a fourfold difference. Similarly, for males between the ages of 55 and 65 years, the number of deaths was 756 per 100,000, a twofold increase over that for males between the ages of 45 and 55 years. This striking increase in the number of deaths with age probably indicates both the slowly progressive nature of coronary atherosclerosis and the inability of collateral circulation to compensate for the progressive obstruction.

Pathologic and Clinical Features

Coronary atherosclerosis usually develops in the proximal portion of the three major coronary arteries, within 5 cm. of their origin from the aorta. Fortunately, the distal segments are almost always patent. In addition, small endomyocardial branches are rarely involved, the principal disease being in the epicardial vessels.

The most commonly seen pattern with triple-vessel occlusive disease is stenosis or occlusion of the proximal right coronary artery, the anterior descending coronary artery, and the circumflex artery. The distal right coronary artery is often patent where it bifurcates into the posterior descending and the atrioventricular groove branches. The anterior descending artery is usually patent in its middle or distal third, and one or more marginal branches of the circumflex artery remain patent. This fortunate segmental localization of the disease, of course, is the basis for bypass grafting.

Several variations of this basic pattern have been recognized and are well illustrated in the monograph by Ochsner and Mills (1978), which describes more than six different pathologic variations encountered in their experiences with bypass grafting in over 1000 patients.

Separate from the degree of involvement of the coronary arteries is the degree to which the left ventricular muscle has been injured from previous infarctions. This is probably best expressed as ejection fraction, a comparison of the amount of blood estimated to be in the heart at the end of diastole with the amount remaining after systole. Normal ejection fraction is near 70 per cent, with moderate impairment of ventricular function represented by an ejection fraction of 40 to 45 per cent and severe impairment represented by an ejection fraction near 20 per cent. A less precise index is the left ventricular end-diastolic pressure, with the upper limit of normal being 12 mm.

Hg, moderate impairment represented by an elevation to 12 to 20 mm. Hg, and severe impairment represented by a level of 20 to 30 mm. Hg or higher. As several factors may transiently influence left ventricular function, such as medication or anesthesia, the influence of these must be evaluated in determining the significance of a single measurement of end-diastolic pressure.

The visual appearance of the contractility of the ventricle during ventriculography provides a reasonable estimate of the degree of impairment, ranging from normal to moderate impairment to severe impairment. Attempts have been made to define this subjective impression more precisely by specifying six different subsegments of the left ventricle and describing the degree of impairment in each. The ultimate function of the heart is expressed as cardiac output and cardiac work, with a normal cardiac index being near 3 liters/minute. This, however, is a relatively imprecise guide, because the cardiac index often declines significantly only in the later stages of the disease.

In general, it appears that the heart can function reasonably well until 30 to 40 per cent of the left ventricular muscle mass is lost. If more than 40 per cent of left ventricular muscle is lost from serial infarctions, chronic congestive heart failure gradually develops. With established chronic congestive failure the prognosis is grim, somewhat akin to that for metastatic malignancy. Cardiac transplantation, when clinically feasible on a widespread basis, is probably the only therapy that can be envisioned at present. In general, bypass grafting has been disappointing for such problems (Spencer et al., 1971).

Hence, the severity and the prognosis for coronary disease are primarily influenced by two factors, the number of vessels involved (one, two, or three) and the extent of impairment of ventricular function. For example, a patient with single-vessel disease and a normal myocardium has a 5-year survival rate that is virtually identical to that of the normal population, near 95 per cent. On the other end of the spectrum, a patient with triple-vessel disease and considerable impairment of ventricular function probably has a 5-year survival rate of less than 70 per cent, although extensive data are not available.

Nelson and associates (1975) emphasized the striking influence of ejection fraction on prognosis in their study of 144 patients over a period of 14 months. In the 92 patients with a normal ejection fraction (above 0.50), the mortality rate was 2 per cent. In the 52 patients with an ejection fraction less than 0.50, the mortality rate was 24 per cent; it rose to 42 per cent in the 24 patients with an ejection fraction less than 0.30. When patients with triple-vessel disease were analyzed, the influence of the ejection fraction was even more striking. Sixteen patients with triple-vessel disease and a normal ejection fraction had a mortality rate of 12 per cent, whereas 11 others with triple-vessel disease but with an ejection fraction less than 0.30 had a mortality rate of 56 per cent.

A great many other factors influence prognosis to a lesser degree. In a very detailed computerized study at Duke University, well over 40 different variables were found to have some influence, although most of these were minor. These numerous variations, however, indicate the difficulty in obtaining comparable data from different study groups (McNeer et al., 1974).

Pathophysiology

The fundamental physiologic defect, of course, is inadequate oxygen transport to the myocardium, manifested initially during periods of increased oxygen demand. Hence, the familiar characteristics of angina are that it appears during exercise, eating, or emotional stress but subsides with rest. Basically, it is a symptom arising from anaerobic metabolism. As such, it is similar to claudication of the calf muscles with occlusive disease of the arteries of the lower extremities. When occlusive coronary artery disease is more extensive, angina may appear at rest and last for longer periods. Such episodes may terminate in either myocardial infarction or death and, hence, are referred to as unstable angina, crescendo angina, or preinfarction angina. Again, comparing the clinical pattern with that of occlusive disease of the lower extremity, the patient with unstable angina is similar to the patient who has had intermittent claudication for some time and then acutely develops rest pain with cyanotic toes.

The patient with angina always has the unpredictable hazard of myocardial infarction or sudden death. A strange physiologic fact is that myocardial infarction often does not occur during periods of increased activity but during sedentary activity or even during sleep, indicating the influence of factors other than simply increased oxygen demand, probably vasomotor changes that influence coronary collateral circulation. When an infarction, perhaps a fatal one, occurs during sleep, a relatively small decrease in coronary blood flow to an area already severely ischemic probably precipitated the infarction. Often, when death occurs within 1 or 2 hours, an acute thrombus cannot be found by the pathologist. As the magnitude of decrease in regional coronary flow is probably small, it is plausible that a previous insertion of a bypass graft to the ischemic area might have prevented the infarction. Total coronary blood flow is 350 to 400 ml./min. (70 to 80 ml./100 gm. of left ventricle/min.). Hence, a bypass graft with a flow of 75 to 100 ml./min. significantly augments coronary flow.

It has also become increasingly apparent that death from coronary disease in many patients is due to an arrhythmia, not massive infarction. The most impressive data were published in 1980 from Seattle, describing 10 years' experience with cardiac resuscitation outside the hospital (Cobb et al., 1980a). Presently, about 300 patients with ventricular fibrillation have been resuscitated each year. Over the past several years, over 700 patients with ventricular fibrillation have survived and left the hospital. This remarkable experience has been accomplished with intensive training of laymen with techniques of cardiopulmonary resuscitation. Patients suddenly collapsing on the street often have resuscitation instituted within 3 to 4 minutes. Clearly, training laymen in cardiopulmonary resuscitation is most important, probably as important in high school education as the teaching of English or mathematics. This is particularly true because over *one half* of the patients did not have any signs of myocardial necrosis, although about 75 per cent had coronary disease and only 2 per cent did not have any form of cardiac disease. The fact that the majority of patients did not have a massive infarction lends emphasis to the urgency of immediate resuscitation. This is further magnified by the fact that over two thirds of the 700,000 deaths from cardiac disease that occur in this country each year occur outside the hospital. Prompt resuscitation is the only immediate prospect for effective treatment of these 400,000 deaths, over twice those due to all forms of cancer combined.

A grim fact is that the survivors who had an infarct did much better than those who did not have an infarct. A long-term follow-up, which is 98 per cent complete, found that patients discharged from the hospital following resuscitation had a mortality rate of 26 per cent in 1 year and 36 per cent in 2 years. Seventy-five per cent of the deaths were due to recurrence of the sudden death syndrome. If the patient had had a transmural infarction, there was only a 2 per cent rate of recurrent fibrillation, whereas in those who had not had an infarction, the rate was 20 per cent. This ominous fact clearly indicates the importance of long-term management. To date, neither antiarrhythmic therapy nor bypass surgery has had significant results, although bypass operations have not had an adequate trial. The most obvious approach is to monitor such patients frequently, probably with Holter monitoring and radionuclide imaging, to detect the presence of significant cardiac ischemia.

At present, the mortality rate from myocardial infarction is near 15 per cent, greatly decreased in the past decade by the use of coronary care units, where 24-hour monitoring permits the prompt detection and treatment of arrhythmias. After recovery from an infarction, a patient may follow any one of a number of patterns. He may become asymptomatic, may have recurrent angina, or may develop another infarction. The spectrum is wide, with some patients having difficulty immediately and others remaining almost symptom-free for 10 to 20 years. Ten to 15 per cent of patients who have had an infarction develop a ventricular aneurysm, which may require surgical therapy (this is discussed in another section of this chapter). Fortunately, congestive heart failure does not appear unless more than 40 per cent of the left ventricular muscle mass has been lost, as discussed previously.

Hence, the clinical spectrum of coronary disease

is a broad one, including the asymptomatic patient, even with extensive triple-vessel disease on the coronary angiogram, and the presence of mild angina, disabling angina, a myocardial infarction, a ventricular aneurysm, or congestive heart failure. This wide clinical spectrum, in turn, represents the balance between the rate of progression of atherosclerosis and the rate of growth of collateral circulation. For unknown reasons, both processes vary widely in individual patients. To date, neither process, the progression of atherosclerosis or the growth of collateral circulation, has been significantly influenced by any therapy yet available. Therefore, in many patients, a prudent course is to employ conservative treatment methods for 1 to 2 years, if possible, and to determine how rapidly the two opposing forces are developing.

The development of noninvasive radionuclide studies around 1975 provided techniques for serial measurement of ventricular function that were not possible before. These advances included the development of the electrocardiogram-gauged scintigraphic angiocardiogram (Green *et al.*, 1975) and, subsequently, the radioactive thallium scan. These studies evaluate myocardial function both at rest and during exercise. Three abnormalities have been found to develop in patients with coronary disease. When normal patients exercise, the ejection fraction remains unchanged or rises slightly, the left ventricular end-diastolic volume increases somewhat, and no abnormalities of left ventricular motion appear. When the patient with coronary disease exercises, however, there is a fall in the ejection fraction and a marked rise in left ventricular end-diastolic volume and regional abnormalities in left ventricular contraction appear. Rerych and associates (1980) performed detailed studies of 18 athletes during 6 months of intensive training for competitive swimming. The capacity of the heart to increase cardiac output was clearly defined with the remarkable demonstration that after athletic training the heart could increase its output from near 6 liters/minute at rest to over 30 liters/minute during intense exercise.

Kent and coworkers (1978) and Epstein and colleagues (1977) reported studies in 23 patients undergoing coronary revascularization. Before operation, the ejection fraction in these patients fell from 51 to 39 per cent with exercise, whereas in normal subjects, it increased to 71 per cent. Following operation, the ejection fraction rose slightly with exercise. Eighty-eight per cent of the 20 patients studied had patent grafts. Improvement also occurred in exercise-induced regional abnormalities of the left ventricular contraction.

In 1980, Hellman and associates reported studies in 36 patients before and after coronary bypass, comparing these with 15 normal male volunteers. In normal subjects, with exercise, the ejection fraction rose, end-diastolic volume increased 19 per cent, and there was no exercise-induced regional wall motion dysfunction. Before operation, in patients with coronary disease, with exercise, the ejection fraction fell from 66 to 53 per cent, end-diastolic volume increased 24 per cent (from 114 to 142 ml.), and 24 of the 36 patients developed abnormalities in regional wall contraction. Following operation, these abnormal responses were almost completely corrected.

The future of noninvasive radionuclide studies appears bright indeed. In a detailed presentation at the annual meeting of the American College of Surgeons in October 1981, Jones reported from Duke University detailed studies of patients before and after operation, showing that the degree of myocardial dysfunction induced during exercise provided a precise measurement of the physiologic handicap present in the patient with coronary disease, often contrasting markedly with the angiographic pattern of occlusive disease, probably as a result of variation in collateral circulation. Similarly, studies after operation indicated how adequately revascularization had eliminated these physiologic abnormalities.

Clinical Evaluation

Clinical evaluation of the patient with angina is done primarily with electrocardiography, radionuclide scanning, coronary angiography, and left ventriculography. The physical examination is not very helpful, because the results are normal in most patients, unless arrhythmias or mitral insufficiency from papillary muscle disease is present. Stress testing with the electrocardiogram is a useful screening procedure to select patients for further evaluation with radionuclide studies or angiography. In the future, the rapidly evolving technology of radionuclide studies will probably increase their importance in routine evaluation of patients, especially as these studies are noninvasive and less expensive than catheterization. At present, the cornerstones of evaluation are coronary angiography and ventriculography, developed primarily by Sones at the Cleveland Clinic in 1957 and 1958. These landmark achievements provided for the first time a sound basis for clinical therapy in patients with coronary disease.

A coronary artery is considered significantly obstructed if the diameter is narrowed more than 70 per cent on angiography. If angiography shows a patent artery distal to the obstruction, the feasibility of bypass grafting is certain. Often, however, a patent vessel cannot be seen on the angiogram but may be found at operation by exploration beyond the area of obstruction. This is particularly true of the distal anterior descending artery and to a lesser degree in the right coronary circulation. The ability to opacify the artery beyond the obstruction depends, of course, on the technique used at angiography as well as the degree of collateral circulation. At New York University, many patients have been seen with a patent artery distal to the site of obstruction, found only by dissection at operation. It is important to remember that the size of the patent artery distal to the obstruction as visualized on the angiogram is unreliable, as the artery may appear small and contracted from absence of normal arterial pressure and flow. Hence, the angiogram should not be used as a precise guide as to whether a patient is "operable" or not.

As mentioned earlier, the ventriculogram provides a crucial evaluation of ventricular function, showing the degree of injury that has already occurred. This, in turn, indicates both the hazard of operation and the likelihood of sustained benefit. Other different measurements of ventricular function—ejection fraction, end-diastolic pressure, and cardiac index—have already been discussed.

Medical and Surgical Treatment

How effective medical therapy is for coronary atherosclerosis remains uncertain. Many aspects can probably never be subjected to a precise randomized investigation. Data suggest considerable improvement in results in the last decade, although virtually no objective measurements were possible until arteriography became widely employed after 1960 to 1965. Hence, with a disease process that probably evolves over decades, the data base is small.

Cessation of smoking, control of hypertension, and modification of diet to resemble a Japanese diet, with emphasis on restriction of lipid intake, are the most logical forms of therapy. Nitrates, drugs for beta-blockade to decrease myocardial oxygen consumption, and, more recently, calcium antagonists (nifedipine) all provide symptomatic improvement, but data proving their benefit with regard to longevity are scanty. Only in recent months have randomized studies with beta-blockers demonstrated improved longevity in selected patients. Weight reduction and physical exercise are similarly plausible but unproved. The sad fact remains that reports from several angiographic studies in the past 2 to 3 years have all found that angiograms performed 5 years after coronary bypass usually demonstrate continued progression of atherosclerosis in the native coronary circulation, generally in the range of 8 to 11 per cent per year. How to control this process remains one of the foremost medical challenges for the future. A major benefit of bypass surgery, providing dramatic improvement in coronary blood flow but doing nothing to alter the underlying biochemical defect, is that the patient's condition is stabilized for a sufficient number of years to permit precise evaluation of different forms of medical therapy of the atherosclerotic process, probably with serial angiography or radionuclide studies.

With the many variables in patterns of coronary artery disease, the significance of cooperative studies, even though matched as carefully as possible, remains somewhat uncertain. One of the best studies was reported from Europe in 1980 (European Coronary Surgery Study group 1980). A randomized study was performed between 1973 and 1976 among a large number of centers in Europe, termed the European Coronary Surgery Group. Seven hundred and sixty-eight men were studied, selected with the following specifications: They were less than 65 years of age, with mild to moderate angina pectoris, good left ventricular function, and at least two-vessel disease. Three hundred and seventy-three patients were randomized to medical treatment and 395 to surgical treatment. In the patients with triple-vessel disease, the 5-year survival rate was 95 per cent in the surgically treated group, compared with 85 per cent in the medically treated group. In patients with left main coronary artery disease, comparable figures were 93 per cent and 62 per cent. Patients with severe angina that could not be controlled by medical therapy were excluded, as they were considered candidates for operation. Therefore, this group of patients includes one of the more benign forms of extensive coronary disease, i.e., that characterized by minimal angina and good ventricular function and occurring in individuals less than 65 years of age.

No significant difference was found in the survival rate for patients with two-vessel disease—88 per cent in the medically treated group and 92 per cent in the surgically treated group. A closer study of the patients with two-vessel disease revealed a striking difference related to where the obstruction was located in the anterior descending coronary artery. In 40 per cent of the patients, the proximal anterior descending artery was not obstructed and was associated with an extraordinarily good survival rate of 96 per cent. In the other 60 per cent of patients with obstruction of the proximal anterior descending coronary artery, the 5-year survival rate was only 82 per cent, similar to that for the patients with triple-vessel disease treated medically.

Only a limited comparison could be made with the findings of the VA Cooperative Study Group reported in 1978 (Read *et al.*, 1978). The operative mortality rate was much less in the European study, 3.5 per cent, compared with 5.6 per cent in the VA study. For patients with left main coronary artery disease, the difference was even greater—3 per cent in the European study, compared with 12 per cent in the VA study.

The VA Cooperative Study Group studied 686 men between 1972 and 1974 among 13 hospitals. These were patients with stable angina and adequate arteries for coronary bypass. As mentioned earlier, the operative mortality rate was 5.6 per cent. The graft patency was not very good, 69 per cent at 1 year, and all grafts occluded in 12 to 19 per cent of patients, clearly a mediocre surgical result (DeBakey and Lawrie, 1978). The survival rate at 4 years was 86 per cent in the surgically treated group and 83 per cent in the medically treated group.

This study, one of the first of its kind, was widely criticized because of the high operative mortality as well as the high rate of graft occlusion. Probably the most significant weakness was that in the participating hospitals, coronary bypass simply was not performed frequently enough to maintain a high quality of technical expertise, with an average of one operation being performed every 4 to 6 weeks. The most significant aspect of the study was that the 4-year survival rate of 83 per cent in the medically treated group was considerably better than anticipated. The surgical results are probably of little clinical significance, as they do not represent what was being achieved at experienced surgical centers at that time or, even more important, what has been achieved in the last 5 years in many surgical centers with modern techniques of myocardial preservation.

In a large collected series that compiled reports dealing with more than 3000 patients from 24 reported series, Green reported a 5-year survival rate near 70 to 75 per cent (Hurst *et al.,* 1978). Hurst and associates also quoted a report by Kouchoukos from Birmingham of three groups of patients with triple-vessel disease: At 46 months, the survival rate was 83 per cent for the surgically treated group; 53 per cent for those in whom operation was recommended and not performed, and 44 per cent for those considered inoperable because of diffuse vascular disease.

As repeatedly emphasized, the many variables with coronary artery disease indicate that comparable data can be obtained only by carefully matched subgroups (Kirklin *et al.,* 1979). The major variables include the number of arteries involved, the degree of impairment of left ventricular function, the size of the coronary arteries beyond the obstruction, and the extent of atherosclerosis in individual coronary arteries.

By far the most significant data about the natural history of coronary artery disease is emerging from the Coronary Artery Surgery Study (CASS), involving 15 participating institutions and coordinated by the National Heart, Lung and Blood Institute. The study now includes 24,959 patients who will be followed until June 1983. In a report prepared in 1981 (Mock *et al.,* 1982), data from 20,088 patients were analyzed regarding the course of the disease with medical therapy. Among this group, 14,284 patients had significant disease; 5804 did not. Significant obstruction of a coronary vessel was considered present if the diameter was narrowed more than 70 per cent in the three major vessels, more than 50 per cent in the left main coronary artery. The 4-year survival rate was 97 per cent for patients without coronary artery disease, 92 per cent for those with single-vessel disease, 84 per cent for those with double-vessel disease, 68 per cent for those with triple-vessel disease, and 60 per cent for those with left main coronary artery disease. The prognosis did not vary significantly between vessels considered "operable" and "inoperable."

Separately, left ventricular function was analyzed by a complex method, using the right anterior oblique projection during ventriculography and evaluating the segmental contraction of five different ventricular segments, with a score for each segment between 1 and 6, 1 being normal and 6 being the worst. Hence, a normal ventricle would have a score of 5, and the worst ventricle would have a score of 30.

The four major groups corresponded to a normal ejection fraction, an ejection fraction between 50 and 100 per cent, 35 to 49 per cent, and below 35 per cent. The 4-year survival rate was 92 per cent for those with a normal ventricle, 90 per cent for those with a decrease in ejection fraction to near 50 per cent (no significant difference), and 83 and 58 per cent, respectively, in the other two groups.

When the two major prognostic factors—number of vessels involved and ventricular performance—were analyzed together, the results were quite striking. The 4-year survival rate for patients with a normal left ventricle and triple-vessel disease was 79 per cent, a figure virtually identical to that found in the European Cooperative Study reported earlier. With severe impairment of ventricular function and an ejection fraction below 50 per cent, the prognosis was alarmingly ominous—67 per cent in patients with single-vessel disease, 61 per cent in those with double-vessel disease, and 42 per cent in those with triple-vessel disease, with the latter representing a mortality rate of 15 per cent per year. Hence, the patient with a severely impaired ventricle with single-vessel disease had a prognosis worse than the patient with triple-vessel disease and normal ventricular function. This most likely indicates that the most important factor influencing prognosis is ventricular function, probably representing the degree to which collateral circulation has compensated for the coronary artery obstruction. A significant area for future investigation would be to specifically operate on most patients with ventricular function decreased below 50 per cent, determining whether operation would improve this ominous mortality figure. The surgical results available thus far would suggest that the prognosis would be far better, as most 5-year survival rates, including patients with all types of ventricular function, range from around 87 or 88 per cent to 92 or 93 per cent.

Indications for Operation

At New York University between 1967 and 1978, the principal indication for operation was disabling angina not responding to conventional therapy. With this policy, the patients with the most severe disease were automatically selected for operation. It was a flexible, subjective guideline, depending on both the patient and the physician. "Disabling angina" is far different in a 40-year-old football coach than in a 70-year-old retired banker. The major exception to this policy was significant stenosis of the left main coronary artery, for which, as virtually everyone agrees, operation should be performed promptly, regardless of symptoms, because of the risk of sudden death. Abundant data show that survival, even within 2 or 3 years, is vastly improved with coronary bypass.

Since 1978, several reports indicate that surgically treated patients with triple-vessel disease, especially those with some impairment of left ventricular function, have a better survival at 5 years than those treated medically, regardless of symptoms. This has influenced us to cautiously extend operation to this group of patients, as well as those with double-vessel disease with persisting symptoms for over a year despite good medical therapy. In uncertain situations, 6 to 12 months of observation is useful, permitting the institution of dietary therapy and appropriate medical therapy. This period of observation will give some indication of the ability of the collateral circulation to compensate for the arterial obstruction.

Probably the largest group of patients seen as candidates for operation are either those with mild angina or those who have had a previous infarction but are now asymptomatic, in whom the angiogram shows extensive double- or triple-vessel disease with some impairment of myocardial function. Radionuclide scans, measuring the effect of exercise on myocardial ischemia and ventricular function, have been useful in some patients in deciding whether or not operation should be performed and, undoubtedly, will be used more widely in the future.

The patient with unstable angina, mentioned briefly earlier, should be promptly hospitalized in a coronary care unit, as the blood supply to an area of myocardium has been acutely decreased, probably from thrombosis of a significant tributary, to a point at which the circulation is barely adequate to prevent myocardial necrosis. With proper treatment in a coronary care unit, including rest, oxygen, beta-blockade, and other methods of support, most patients improve and do not require immediate operation. Those who do not respond, however, should be operated on promptly because of the risk of infarction. Furthermore, those patients who have already developed some myocardial necrosis but who have continuing angina despite intensive medical therapy should also be operated on promptly. With cold blood potassium cardioplegia, the risk of operation in these patients,

even with marginal collateral circulation, has decreased markedly.

Several years ago a widely publicized randomized study of patients with unstable angina, coordinated among several medical centers by the National Institutes of Health, did not show a major difference between patients treated surgically and those treated medically (Unstable angina pectoris, 1978). This was probably due to the fact that surgical mortality was significant, perhaps from inadequate myocardial preservation in the presence of limited collateral circulation. In addition, there was a striking crossover of patients requiring operation in the next 1 to 3 years because of persistence of symptoms, indicating the limitations of continued medical therapy in such patients with severe myocardial ischemia.

Once significant myocardial infarction has occurred, operation is best postponed for at least 4 to 6 weeks, unless postinfarction angina develops. Before cold blood cardioplegia was available for myocardial preservation, operation 2 to 3 weeks after an infarction was associated with a high mortality rate. With present methods of myocardial preservation, however, operative risk has decreased to less than 5 per cent. Therefore, continuing angina, representing possible extension of an infarction, is an urgent indication for operation (Fig. 50–82).

Similarly, with cold blood cardioplegia, patients with a recent infarction in whom there is rupture of the ventricular septum (Fig. 50–83) or a papillary muscle (Fig. 50–84), precipitating acute congestive heart failure, can also be operated on with a much lower operative mortality than in the past (Daggett et al., 1977).

Myocardial infarction per se is not generally accepted as an indication for operation, although a few

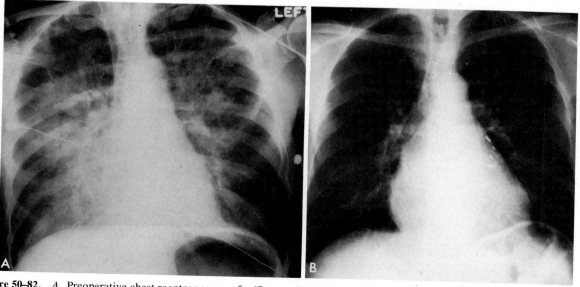

Figure 50–82. *A,* Preoperative chest roentgenogram of a 67-year-old patient who had had two myocardial infarctions in the preceding 10 days. A balloon pump had been used twice. A triple bypass was performed at the time that he was in pulmonary edema, 5 days after the second infarction. Blood cardioplegia was employed. *B,* Chest roentgenogram 8 months following operation. The patient still has mild congestive heart failure but has no angina and can function well to a limited degree.

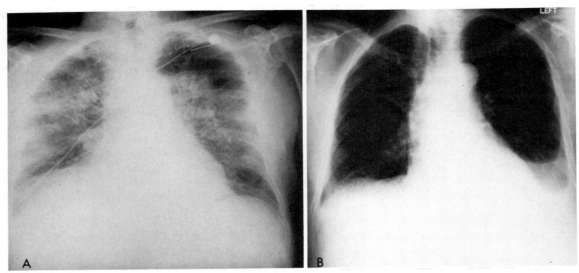

Figure 50–83. *A,* Chest roentgenogram of a patient 2 weeks following myocardial infarction and 5 days following rupture of the ventricular septum. The severe pulmonary congestion is obvious. This patient was also in oliguric renal failure, with a blood urea nitrogen of 60, despite inotropic therapy with dobutamine and dopamine. *B,* Chest roentgenogram prior to discharge from the hospital. At operation, using blood cardioplegia, an infarctectomy and a patch repair of the ruptured ventricular septum were done, which resulted in a complete recovery.

groups, particularly those led by Berg in Spokane, Washington, have employed emergency operation for infarction for several years, reporting experiences with 260 patients (Berg *et al.,* 1982). A highly coordinated team has been developed in Spokane. A patient with symptoms of acute infarction is treated much like a patient with a ruptured abdominal aneurysm, with immediate hospitalization, catheterization, and operation, with institution of bypass in most patients within less than 6 hours after the onset of infarction. The results are impressive, with a mortality rate of 2.3 per cent in those operated on within 6 hours and 1.2 per cent in the following year. How many patients would have recovered uneventfully without operation is uncertain. Less extensive experiences have been reported by Phillips and Zeff in Iowa, Mills in New Orleans, and others. In Phillips and Zeff and Mills' groups, operation was usually undertaken urgently when patients already hospitalized for an elective coronary bypass developed an acute infarction. Therefore, with all information already available, the patient could be readily operated on within a few hours.

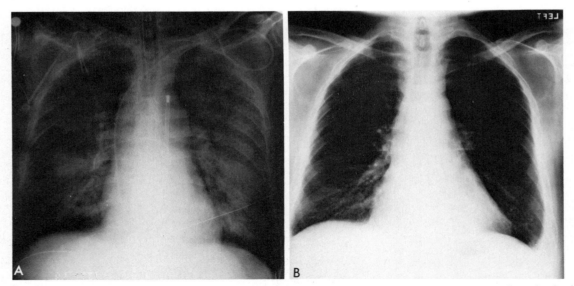

Figure 50–84. *A,* Chest roentgenogram of a 65-year-old patient transferred from another hospital in cardiogenic shock 1 week following a massive myocardial infarction, receiving infusions of dopamine and Levophed. He was comatose, intubated, and in renal failure. A balloon pump was inserted promptly. *B,* Chest roentgenogram prior to discharge from the hospital. At operation, a ruptured papillary muscle was found, and it was causing massive mitral insufficiency. The mitral valve was replaced, and the right coronary artery, which was totally obstructed, was bypassed. Blood cardioplegia was used. At catheterization 1 year later, the cardiac findings were normal, with a patent graft and a normal left atrial pressure.

Virtually everyone agrees that operation for an acute infarction is best done within 6 hours or less; otherwise, irreversible muscle injury has probably occurred. There is some hazard, although apparently much smaller than originally feared, of converting the infarction into a hemorrhagic infarction, akin to the cerebral complications of hemorrhagic cerebral infarction when carotid endarterectomy is performed several hours after an acute stroke.

Operation for left ventricular aneurysm is discussed in another section of this chapter.

Contraindications to Operation

The only absolute contraindication to operation at our institution is chronic congestive heart failure with pulmonary hypertension, hepatomegaly, and peripheral edema. In such instances, the myocardial ejection fraction is usually very low, often less than 0.20. Although such patients may survive operation, often requiring support with an intra-aortic balloon pump for a few days, there is little evidence that longevity is improved, for fatal congestive heart failure occurs in most patients within 1 to 3 years (Spencer et al., 1971).

An unusual group of patients are those with "intermittent pulmonary edema," patients who, for unknown reasons, acutely develop severe pulmonary edema requiring hospitalization for several days and who often have two to five such episodes within a year. Between these episodes, there are no symptoms of congestive heart failure. What precipitates these episodes has not been defined, but it is almost surely acute myocardial ischemia with elevation of end-diastolic pressure to levels of 30 mm. Hg or higher, resulting in pulmonary edema. Several such patients have been operated on at New York University in the past 3 to 4 years with excellent results.

A separate group of patients are those with depression of ejection fraction to near 0.20 or lower, those with the so-called "bad left ventricle." At one time, the erroneous concept widely prevailed that such patients should not be operated on because of both the operative risk and the fact that surviving patients were often worse rather than better. Contrary experiences were published by several groups. Our experiences were published by Isom and colleagues (1975).

In retrospect, the entire concept of operation being contraindicated was erroneous. Patients with severe impairment of left ventricular function will not tolerate a small myocardial infarction at operation resulting from ineffective myocardial preservation, whereas patients with good ventricular function may recover uneventfully despite infarction of 5 to 10 per cent of the left ventricular myocardium. With the development of much more effective cardioplegia with hypothermic potassium arrest, successful operations on such patients have been reported by several groups. Often, these patients need operation more urgently than those with a normal ventricle because their likelihood of recovery from a subsequent infarc-

tion is less than those with normal ventricular function (Jones et al., 1981).

In 1978, Jones reported experiences at Emory University in a group of 188 patients operated on for angina and congestive heart failure. All of the patients had angina and 20 per cent had congestive heart failure. The mean ejection fraction was 0.35, and it was 0.20 or less in 24 per cent of the patients. The operative mortality rate was impressively low, 2.1 per cent. The late mortality rate was 4.3 per cent, with relief of angina in 94 per cent of patients. Those with a history of congestive heart failure, however, had the same ominous late mortality rate, four times greater than that of the entire series. Because the average follow-up was only about 16 months, the sad fact that congestive heart failure is not significantly improved with operation is reaffirmed, even though the operative risk with potassium cardioplegia is low.

Advanced age has not been a contraindication, because operation has been performed successfully on a number of patients between 75 and 85 years of age. In general, our approach has been similar to that for abdominal aneurysms, performing operation for severe symptoms unless concomitant disease makes the operative risk prohibitive. Frequent associated diseases include diabetes, hypertension, stroke, emphysema, and renal disease. All of these increase the operative risk to some extent, but not to such a degree that operation is contraindicated.

It should be mentioned that not all groups agree with our broad definition of operability, which would permit over 95 per cent of patients to undergo bypass. Some patients are excluded because of ventricular function, others because of inability to visualize a patent vessel beyond the obstructed coronary artery on angiography or because the disease process is diffuse, involving multiple areas of the coronary arteries, rather than a single focal proximal stenosis. Recognition that the criteria of "inoperability" vary widely indicates the difficulty of comparing data from different institutions. Not only do the surgical opinions vary widely concerning operability, but in some institutions, the referring physician concludes that the patient is inoperable and, therefore, does not consult the surgeon. As a result, the surgeon is simply unaware of the fact that the patients he operates on are "preselected" beforehand.

As noted earlier, the two major factors influencing the operative risk are the degree of impairment of ventricular function and the extent of the coronary disease (single-, double- or triple-vessel disease with focal or multiple areas of involvement). Concomitant severe mitral insufficiency, resulting from papillary muscle disease, is often a grave sign of advanced ischemia. Occasionally, it can occur from isolated infarction or ischemia of a papillary muscle with excellent function in other areas of the ventricle. Although mitral valve replacement has been performed in some such patients, some type of anuloplasty, probably with the Carpentier ring, should suffice in the majority of cases. In 1980, Kay and associates reported excellent results in a group of 61 such patients operated on between 1970 and 1978, with an operative mortality rate of 8 per cent.

Ventriculography is also of value in determining the presence of a discrete aneurysm. Excision of a large saccular aneurysm, often 10 to 15 cm. in diameter, may dramatically improve congestive heart failure. On the other hand, excision of an aneurysm as small as 5 cm. has little demonstrable hemodynamic benefit. Excision of a flat, akinetic scar may actually be harmful if adjacent collateral circulation is injured. Determining whether or not a left ventricular aneurysm is present is often a crucial decision in the presence of severe congestive heart failure, because this is the only pathologic condition significantly improved by operation. Unfortunately, it is not always possible to distinguish between a large saccular aneurysm filled with clot and a flat, akinetic scar. Obviously, this is a grave decision. Excision of a large saccular aneurysm may produce a dramatic improvement in congestive heart failure, whereas identification and excision of a large akinetic scar at operation is usually followed by either lack of improvement or operative death.

Operative Technique

The three major considerations with coronary bypass are: (1) prevention of myocardial infarction with effective myocardial preservation; (2) the method of procurement and storage of the vein grafts used, usually the saphenous veins; and (3) a meticulous operative technique that constructs anastomoses with smooth intimal surfaces without stenoses. These are discussed in the following paragraphs.

Prevention of Myocardial Infarction. Prevention of myocardial infarction begins before operation by careful management with cardiac drugs, especially propranolol and nitrates. Formerly, propranolol was stopped several days before operation, occasionally resulting in a disastrous infarction. Now, propranolol is continued until the time of operation, attempting to avoid dosages larger than 400 mg./24 hours on the day preceding operation. Small amounts are also useful during and after operation to avoid tachycardia and other arrhythmias.

With unstable angina, an intravenous nitroglycerin infusion (25 to 50 μg./min.) may be useful to decrease preload. In hypertensive patients, afterload may be reduced by infusion of nitroprusside to decrease peripheral vascular resistance. Monitoring of such unstable patients is best done with a Swan-Ganz catheter to measure wedge pressure or pulmonary artery diastolic pressure. In extreme instances in which operation cannot be performed promptly, an intra-aortic balloon pump may be inserted. This will decrease cardiac work and also augment coronary blood flow by raising diastolic blood pressure.

The anesthetic technique employed similarly should avoid both hypertension and hypotension, with liberal use of nitroglycerin and sodium nitroprusside, as described above. At New York University, the Swan-Ganz catheter is almost routinely employed because an occasional patient will demonstrate an alarming increase in wedge pressure, rising from 10 to 20 or 30 mm. Hg and undetectable by arterial pressure or electrocardiographic changes, which can be reversed within 2 to 5 minutes by infusion of nitroglycerin. Otherwise, it is almost certain that a small subendocardial infarction will evolve.

The importance of a precise anesthetic technique can scarcely be overemphasized. Several years ago, we were astonished to find in a cooperative study among several institutions measuring CPK-MB* fraction before bypass that nearly 30 per cent of our patients had elevation of this enzyme before bypass was started, indicating some myocardial necrosis, even though their clinical course was uneventful. A change in anesthetic technique resulted in an astonishing tenfold decrease in these pre-bypass elevations in CPK-MB enzyme, now occurring in only 2 to 3 per cent of patients. Equally surprising was the fact that these subtle injuries induced during anesthesia were not reversible by subsequent bypass, perhaps because subendocardial edema occluded a small coronary arteriole long enough to produce necrosis.

Myocardial Preservation. One of the major advances in the 1970s was the development of hypothermic potassium cardioplegia, suggested several years ago by Gay and Ebert at Cornell University (1973), studied in detail at UCLA, and then in laboratories throughout the world, with international conferences devoted solely to this subject in 1979 and again in 1980. This has been a principal area of investigation in our laboratories for the past few years. Clearly, the technique of intermittent anoxic arrest, or ventricular fibrillation, used to still the heart since the beginning of open heart surgery in 1955, regularly produced a certain degree of myocardial injury, surprisingly well tolerated in children with normal coronary vessels but tolerated to a much lesser degree in elderly patients with advanced myocardial and coronary artery disease.

At present, there are both a large number of cardioplegic solutions and a wide range in the technique of application. To date, there is no uniform agreement about which technique is best. The method described in the following paragraphs is that currently employed at New York University and has been used for over 3 years in more than 3000 patients. In patients with normal coronary arteries, such as adults with valvular heart disease or children with congenital heart disease, periods of aortic occlusions as long as 3 or more hours are tolerated with astonishingly little harm. In the animal laboratory, virtually little myocardial injury can be demonstrated after 4 hours of aortic cross-clamping; serial measurements of myocardial ATP concentrations show virtually no change

---

*The myocardial component of the creatine phosphokinase enzyme.

(Cunningham *et al.*, 1979, 1982). In patients with coronary artery disease, however, the problem of uniform distribution of the cardioplegic agent exists, so that myocardial protection is less effective. At present, our technique seems adequate for 90 to 120 minutes in the majority of patients, although variations occur, probably because of the method of application of the technique rather than the composition of the solution.

At operation, a median sternotomy incision is used, avoiding opening the pleural cavities. Sufficient heparin is given to elevate the activated clotting time above 400 seconds, usually 400 units per kilogram, but occasionally, as much as 800 units per kilogram are required. During bypass, an additional 100 units per kilogram are given each hour. Following bypass, the initial dose of protamine is 2 mg. per kilogram, which will return the activated clotting time to the pre-bypass level in over half of the patients. If it does not return to normal levels, protamine is cautiously given in additional amounts of 0.5 mg. per kilogram until the activated clotting time is normal. Almost always, a total dose of 3 mg. of protamine per kilogram is sufficient.

Routinely, arterial cannulation is done with a cannula in the ascending aorta (Fig. 50–85), with any areas of atherosclerosis being carefully avoided. With the exception of patients with mitral valve disease, most bypasses have been performed with the single right atrial cannula, the Sarns No. 50. Some uncertainty still exists, however, as to whether this is better than the standard use of two venous cannulas.

The pump-oxygenator is a membrane oxygenator (Travenol) primed with 40 ml. per kilogram of balanced electrolyte solution, adding blood if necessary to keep the hematocrit above 20 per cent. Perfusion is at a flow rate near 2.5 liters/M.²/min., lowering the body temperature to about 20°C. Quite recently, flow rates near 2 liters/M.²/min. at 20°C. with a perfusion

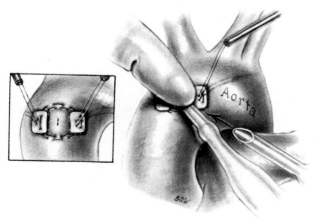

Figure 50–85. The arterial cannula is inserted into the ascending aorta through the center of two purse-string sutures with tourniquets opposite one another. The inset shows the method of placing the double row of purse-string sutures and their passage through pledgets of Teflon felt. (From Ochsner, J. L., and Mills, N. L.: Coronary Artery Surgery. Philadelphia, Lea and Febiger, 1978.)

pressure near 50 mm. Hg have been used to decrease bronchial blood flow, which will wash the potassium out of the coronary circulation.

In addition, for the past several months, oncotic pressure has been regularly measured with an oncometer, and it has been found that the hemodilution technique described usually decreases the oncotic pressure about 40 per cent, from 18 mm. Hg to around 10 mm. Hg, with the pressure gradually returning toward normal during bypass and thereafter. Enough data are not available to indicate what level of oncotic pressure may cause harmful intracellular edema. At present, levels below 8 mm. Hg are corrected by adding albumin to the perfusate.

At a body temperature of 25° to 30°C., the aorta is occluded and the heart is arrested and cooled by infusing 1200 to 1400 ml. of 10°C. blood containing 35 mEq. of potassium per liter, 1000 micrograms of nitroglycerin per liter, sufficient THAM (tromethamine) to adjust the pH to 7.60. The principal difference from the UCLA cardioplegic technique is that the calcium concentration is *not* lowered.

Infusion into the ascending aorta is done through a 15-gauge angiographic catheter inserted in the aorta. Aortic pressure is measured during infusion through a separate angiographic catheter inserted superiorly, avoiding levels greater than 80 to 90 mm. Hg during the initial infusion. During subsequent injections, about 300 to 500 ml. of blood every 30 minutes, blood is infused at a rate to produce a pressure near 60 to 70 mm. Hg. Higher perfusion pressure during subsequent injections can clearly cause myocardial injury.

After the heart is initially arrested, the myocardium is further cooled by pouring 2 to 4 liters of 4°C. Ringer's lactate solution into the pericardium, using the technique developed by Shumway at Stanford several years ago. Myocardial temperature is carefully measured with a thermistor in four areas of the myocardium, the anterior and inferior portions of both the right and left ventricles. Gradients as large as 8°C. may be found, indicating the maldistribution of the cardioplegic agent (Landymore *et al.*, 1981). Cold fluid is poured until the temperature of all areas is below 15°C. After this, a constant drip of iced Ringer's lactate solution is infused by the anesthesiologist through tubing anchored within the pericardial sac, placing one sponge behind the heart to separate it from the aorta and another inferiorly to protect it from the diaphragm and covering the right atrium with cottonoid sponges to prevent warming by the overhead lights. A small square of cottonoid is also placed between the aorta and the superior vena cava to cover the sinus node. A sump tube, inserted through a stab wound inferiorly, is placed over the diaphragm and behind the heart to aspirate fluid, so that the heart is bathed constantly with cold fluid, keeping the temperature below 15°C. Fluid is infused rapidly, often at a rate of about a liter every 10 minutes. A pool of the Ringer's lactate solution is regularly visible at the bottom of the pericardial well.

Considerable variation in opinion exists among

different members of our faculty regarding whether proximal aortic or distal coronary anastomoses should be performed first. No clear advantage of any method has emerged. If the distal coronary anastomoses are done first, about 50 ml. of cold hyperkalemic blood is injected down each vein graft to remove air from the graft before the suture line is tied and also to perfuse the area of myocardium grafted. This injection of individual grafts is repeated approximately every 30 minutes until these grafts are attached to the aorta. Blood is similarly reinfused into the aorta every 20 to 30 minutes in amounts of 400 to 500 ml. After each infusion of blood, at least a liter of iced Ringer's lactate solution is poured over the surface of the heart and the myocardial temperature checked in a manner similar to that done at the initiation of the cardiac arrest.

My preferred technique is to arrest the heart as soon as possible after bypass has been established and the temperature has been lowered to 30°C. Distal anastomoses are performed, serially injecting cold blood every 20 to 30 minutes, as described. The aortic clamp is then removed, and the proximal anastomoses are performed with the heart beating, again injecting blood down each graft every 20 minutes until it is attached to the aorta.

Another essential part of the cardioplegia technique is to keep the right atrium collapsed to avoid reflux of blood from the vena cava into the coronary sinus. As the temperature of the perfusate is 25°C., a momentary reflux of blood into the right atrium from the inferior vena cava, usually from inadvertent kinking of the venous cannula, can within 15 seconds cause retrograde reflux of blood through the coronary sinus, remove potassium from the heart, and induce visible fibrillatory activity in the right ventricle. One advantage of the double venous cannula system is that such reflux is much more easily avoided.

To recapitulate, the ideal technique is to promptly arrest and cool the heart as soon as possible after bypass is established. The heart is then kept arrested and cold (at a temperature below 15°C.) with a combination of continuous irrigation with cold electrolyte solution, injection of cold blood following each anastomosis, and injection of cold blood into the aorta every 20 to 30 minutes.

A left ventricular vent is ordinarily not used, but scrupulous care is taken to keep the right atrium decompressed. As mentioned previously, with this technique, the aorta may be safely occluded for more than 3 hours in patients with valvular disease (fortunately, very rarely necessary) and for at least 2 hours in patients with coronary artery disease.

Excellent results have been published by many groups with crystalloid cardioplegia for periods of aortic occlusion of 1 to 2 hours. To my knowledge, however, no report has described 3 hours of aortic cross-clamping with crystalloid cardioplegia similar to the ones in our experience with blood cardioplegia.

During the injection of the blood cardioplegic solution into the aorta, aortic insufficiency may be found, although not clinically evident before operation, with reflux of blood into the left ventricle. At times, digital compression may control the insufficiency. Otherwise, it is best to make a short aortotomy and infuse the cardioplegic solution directly into the coronary ostia, similar to the technique used during aortic valve replacement. In addition, a vent is inserted into the left ventricle, either through the apex or through the left atrium and across the mitral valve. Distention of the left ventricle must be scrupulously avoided. The potassium-arrested heart in diastole seems especially vulnerable to stretch injury.

When the aorta is unclamped, careful attention is necessary to be certain that distention of the left ventricle does not occur. Normally, blood is effectively aspirated from the left heart through the pulmonary circuit into the right atrium. If this does not occur because the mitral valve remains competent, the left ventricle should be vented promptly. Fibrillatory activity usually returns within 2 to 4 minutes, after which electrical defibrillation can soon be done. If potassium concentration is above 6 mEq. per liter, electrical pacing through a needle implanted in the right ventricular wall may be necessary for a short time.

Cardiac activity in the majority of patients returns promptly and uneventfully following unclamping. However, the time following release of the aortic clamp is when the heart is the most vulnerable to reperfusion edema, as it is being reperfused and rewarmed and beginning to perform cardiac work again, especially as bypass is slowed and stopped.

The first hour after bypass is probably the most hazardous for the development of myocardial edema, as the heart resumes its normal workload. Administration of protamine also may have some harmful effects, although it has never been possible to measure this precisely. Our most reliable monitors of cardiac function have been left atrial pressure, measured either directly or indirectly with a Swan-Ganz catheter from the pulmonary artery diastolic or wedge pressure, and serial measurements of cardiac output with a thermodilution technique, usually obtaining a cardiac index above 3. A cardiac index near 2 liters per minute or lower indicates a serious depression of cardiac output and the necessity for cardiac support, usually by insertion of a left ventricular vent and reinstitution of bypass for 30 to 60 minutes until cardiac function has improved. A persistent depression of cardiac index below 2 liters per minute is a firm indication for use of an intra-aortic balloon pump. Other useful indices of cardiac function are the electrocardiogram, the central venous pressure, and the amplitude of contraction of the ventricles.

Systolic blood pressure is maintained near 100 to 120 mm. Hg. Higher pressures are avoided to minimize afterload by infusion of sodium nitroprusside. Intravenous nitroglycerin is almost routinely given in small amounts, 25 to 50 μg./min. If inotropic support is necessary, small amounts of epinephrine, 2 μg./min., may be used. If additional inotropic support is necessary, dobutamine is the preferred agent and is usually administered in a dose in the range of 500 to 750 μg./min. Dopamine was previously employed but causes more tachycardia and vasodilatation; it is used if oliguria is present.

The availability of the oncometer in our unit in the past year to measure oncotic pressure has provided an additional quantitative measurement of hemodilution more precise than was previously possible. The benefits of this measurement seem significant, but sufficient data are not yet available.

Thermodilution cardiac outputs are easily measured through a Swan-Ganz catheter and constitute the monitoring technique of choice. If, for any reason, this is not possible, the older technique of serial monitoring of mixed venous oxygen tensions from blood samples withdrawn from a catheter in the pulmonary artery, a technique used since its development in 1958 (Boyd *et al.*, 1959), is quite satisfactory. Normally, the oxygen tension in the pulmonary artery is at least 30 mm. Hg. Levels in the range of 25 to 30 mm. Hg indicate some depression of oxygen transport and should be viewed with concern. Depression of mixed venous oxygen tension to the range of 20 to 25 mm. Hg is more ominous, and levels below 20 mm. Hg presage an impending fatality if they continue for several hours. In some ways, the mixed venous oxygen tension is a more precise measure of hemodynamic function than cardiac output, as it reflects how well cardiac output is meeting the oxygen needs of the body. Unless oxygen requirements of the body are increased by fever, shivering, or other mechanisms, cardiac output is simpler and easier to measure with thermodilution. The only situation in which mixed venous oxygen tensions are inaccurate is during administration of vasopressors or in other instances in which arteriovenous shunts are present.

In instances in which myocardial edema is severe, most commonly seen in patients with a recent infarction who undergo operation, administration of steroids seems reasonable, as well as the use of mannitol and albumin to keep the oncotic pressure above 14 mm. Hg. After bypass, cardiac compression of the pericardium is avoided by construction of a pericardial "apron," made by entering both pleural cavities, making longitudinal incisions in the pericardium bilaterally anterior to the phrenic nerve, and then detaching the pericardium from the diaphragm inferiorly. After this, the two pedicles of pericardium are approximated in the midline, constructing a pericardial "apron" that permits free drainage of blood into both pleural cavities and avoids any possibility of pericardial compression from the edematous heart. This has been a valuable technique in desperate situations with extreme edema.

Very rarely has the edema been so severe that it was not possible to close the sternum. In the few instances in which the sternum could not be closed, the sternum was stabilized with wire sutures, but the sternal edges were left 2 to 3 inches apart. Usually, within 24 to 48 hours, it was possible to return the

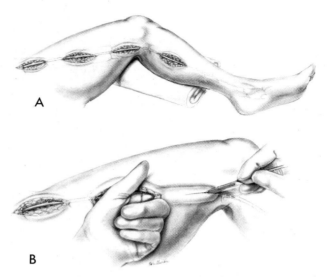

Figure 50–86. *A,* Multiple skin incisions with short skin bridges are used to avoid skin tension with closure. *B,* The index finger is used to develop a plane superficial to the vein, and the incision is made over the finger. (From Ochsner, J. L., and Mills, N. L.: Coronary Artery Surgery. Philadelphia, Lea and Febiger, 1978.)

patient to the operating room and close the sternum completely. Most such patients were being supported with left atrial–aortic bypass, which was also discontinued at that time (Rose *et al.*, in press).

Technique of Vein Procurement and Preservation. Data from many sources all indicate the great importance of a gentle, precise technique for removal of the saphenous vein and its preservation before insertion as a bypass graft (Fig. 50–86).

Both short-term patency and long-term patency are adversely influenced if the vein is injured by one of several mechanisms, such as stretching, spasm, endothelial disruption, or distention. Our preference is to initially explore the leg vein near the ankle and find veins between 4 and 6 mm. in diameter, either from the legs or the lower thighs, employing a longitudinal incision from the ankle upward, usually with a small skin bridge at the skin crease at the knee joint. In patients with varicosities, cephalic veins from the arms have been used. These seem satisfactory, although thinner, requiring the use of 7-0 Prolene. Long-term data are not available about whether these thin veins will ultimately dilate from arterial pressure. They have been reported to function well as femoropopliteal grafts. During dissection, the vein should be handled gently. Spasm is most easily produced by stretching. Initially, the vein is divided distally, and a small cannula is inserted. Papaverine in dilute amounts (120 mg. in 100 ml. of Plasmalyte with 1000 units of heparin) is then periodically injected during dissection to minimize spasm and stasis. Tributaries are ligated a short distance from the vein wall and secured distally with clips. Following removal, the vein is irrigated with the papaverine-heparin mixture to remove any remaining blood and to check for leaks. It is then stored in 25°C. Plasmalyte solution until it is to be used. Distention of the vein with high pressures is avoided, although pressures are usually not measured.

Previously, veins were filled with cold blood and stored in 5° and 10°C. Ringer's lactate solution. To our surprise, clinical and laboratory investigation found that the low temperature caused intense spasm of the vein with rupture of the endothelial lining, apparently from intense contraction of the internal elastic membrane. The platelets in the blood in the vein promptly aggregated onto areas of endothelial disruption, with initiation of a thrombotic process. These phenomena have been described in several reports from laboratory studies at New York University (Baumann *et al.*, 1981; Catinella *et al.*, 1981).

The incisions in the lower extremity are routinely closed with continuous sutures of Dexon. Closure is usually done following administration of protamine after bypass, but in some instances, the incisions are closed if bleeding is minimal before heparin is neutralized.

Grafting Technique. As noted previously, considerable variation exists among the operative techniques employed by different surgeons on our faculty at New York University regarding the sequence in which the grafts are attached to the aorta: attaching some or all of the grafts to the aorta initially, either before bypass is started or after bypass is begun, or alternately attaching all the grafts distally after the aorta is occluded and the heart arrested, then releasing the aortic clamp and serially attaching the grafts while the heart is being rewarmed. Comparison of results among the different techniques has shown no definite superiority of one over the others. My preferred technique has been described earlier.

The technique of coronary anastomosis, of course, must be very precise. Ocular magnification to 4 power is regularly used with binocular loupes (Fig. 50–87), developed at New York University (Spencer *et al.*, 1971) and now used throughout the world. The site of the arteriotomy (Fig. 50–88) is carefully selected by finding a "clear blue line" at least 1 cm. in length in the soft area of the artery, scrupulously avoiding incision of atherosclerotic plaques, which might lead to disruption of intima. The coronary artery is dissected anteriorly only enough to expose the "soft blue stripe" at the anterior surface. After the artery

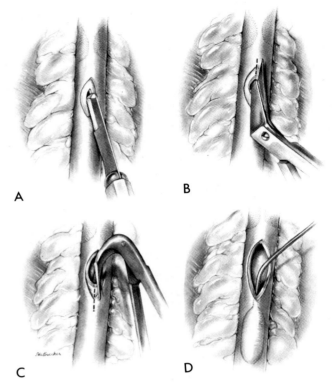

Figure 50–88. Arteriotomy. *A,* An incision is made first through the epicardium overlying the coronary artery and then through the entire thickness of the anterior wall with a miniblade. *B,* The arteriotomy is extended proximally with obtuse-angled Pott's scissors. *C,* The arteriotomy is extended distally with reverse acute-angle scissors. *D,* After completion of the arteriotomy, the lumen of the coronary artery is sized with calibrated obturators. (From Ochsner, J. L., and Mills, N. L.: Coronary Artery Surgery. Philadelphia, Lea and Febiger, 1978.)

is incised 8 to 10 mm., it is gently probed with calibrated metal dilators that are 1 to 3 mm. in diameter (Garrett dilator)* to confirm distal patency and the presence of a proximal stenosis. Anastomoses are regularly done with a single suture of 6-0 or 7-0 Prolene, locking the continuous suture at each angle of the anastomosis (Fig. 50–89) and then probing each orifice to confirm that a stenosis has not been produced from a "purse-string" effect. (Other types of anastomosis are illustrated in Figures 50–90 to 50–93.) Before the suture line is tied, blood is injected down the vein to displace any air. After the anastomosis is completed, additional blood is injected to perfuse the region of myocardium grafted.

The aortic anastomosis is a standard one, placing grafts to the left transversely on the anterior surface of the aorta, slightly to the left of the midline, removing a small isosceles triangle of aorta with a base about 4 mm. long, or using an aortic punch. Grafts to the right coronary artery are usually made to the right of the midline with a simple aortotomy about 8 mm. in length. Aortic anastomoses are done with continuous sutures of 6-0 Prolene.

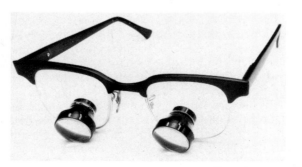

Figure 50–87. Binocular loupes that magnify to 4 power, with a focal length of 16 inches and a depth of field of 4 inches.

---

*The Pilling Company, Philadelphia, Pennsylvania.

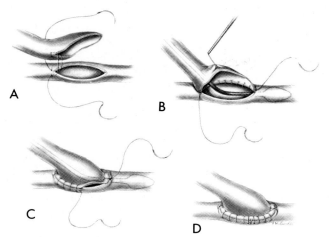

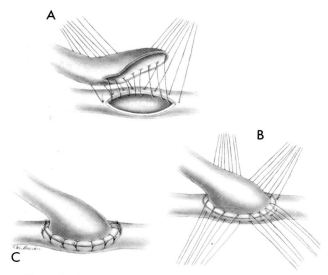

Figure 50–89. Continuous suture anastomosis. *A,* The anastomosis is begun with a double-ended mattress suture at the heel. *B,* One end of the suture is continued as an over-and-over stitch to the toe, where it is interrupted. A ball-point angle-tipped probe is used to place traction on the adventitia, thereby exposing the free edge of the saphenous vein graft. *C,* The other end of the original stitch is continued on the contralateral side to the midpoint of the arteriotomy. *D,* The second suture is continued as an over-and-over stitch from the toe to meet with the original stitch at the midpoint of the arteriotomy. (From Ochsner, J. L., and Mills, N. L.: Coronary Artery Surgery. Philadelphia, Lea and Febiger, 1978.)

Figure 50–91. Interrupted suture anastomosis. *A,* Half of the interrupted sutures are in place. *B,* All of the sutures are in place and pulled taut but not tied. They are divided into four quadrants, each of which contains four interrupted sutures. *C,* Anastomosis completed following the tying of each individual suture. (From Ochsner, J. L., and Mills, N. L.: Coronary Artery Surgery. Philadelphia, Lea and Febiger, 1978.)

Sequential anastomoses have become increasingly popular, using side-to-side anastomoses to different branches of a major coronary artery. The most common ones utilize two tributaries of a single large coronary artery, grafting the anterior descending coronary artery with an end-to-side anastomosis and its

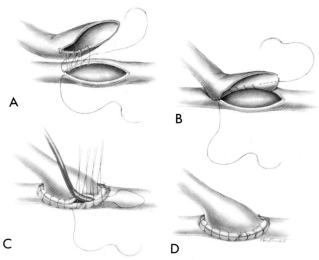

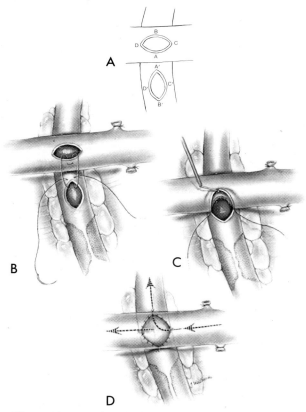

Figure 50–90. Combination continuous and interrupted suture anastomosis. *A,* The heel or proximal aspect of the anastomosis is begun as a horizontal mattress stitch, and four or five passes of the suture are performed before making the suture taut. *B,* The continuous suture has been made taut for one half of a side of the anastomosis. *C,* The proximal half of the anastomosis has been completed as a continuous over-and-over stitch. The distal half is completed with multiple interrupted sutures. A calibrated dilator is passed through the anastomosis prior to completion to assure patency. *D,* Completed anastomosis. (From Ochsner, J. L., and Mills, N. L.: Coronary Artery Surgery. Philadelphia, Lea and Febiger, 1978.)

Figure 50–92. Diamond anastomosis. *A,* Diagram demonstrating the method of alignment of the incisions in the bypass graft and coronary artery. *B,* The anastomosis is begun with a double-ended horizontal mattress suture placed at the midpoint of the venotomy and the apex of the arteriotomy. *C,* The anastomosis is continued halfway and then interrupted by tying to another suture. The second suture is a continuous anastomosis. *D,* Completed anastomosis and continuing through the graft to the primary anastomosis. (From Ochsner, J. L., and Mills, N. L.: Coronary Artery Surgery. Philadelphia, Lea and Febiger, 1978.)

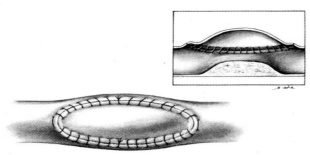

Figure 50–93. The arteriotomy is made through the stenotic lesion and into a sufficiently large lumen proximally and distally. A venous bypass graft is sutured end to side to the arteriotomy so that unobstructed flow is possible in both directions. (From Ochsner, J. L., and Mills, N. L.: Coronary Artery Surgery. Philadelphia, Lea and Febiger, 1978.)

diagonal branch with a side-to-side anastomosis. A similar procedure can be done with a single vein graft to the circumflex coronary artery, grafting two or three marginal branches. With the right coronary artery, a similar approach may be used to perform two anastomoses to the AV groove and the posterior descending branches of the right coronary artery.

For uncertain reasons, side-to-side anastomoses have been intermittently used for long periods of time but have never demonstrated clear superiority over end-to-side anastomoses. Theoretical arguments can be advanced both for and against multiple anastomoses from one graft. Sewell (1979) has presented some of the best long-term data supporting the advantages of side-to-side anastomoses. The high flow rate through the single graft would seem advantageous unless a thrombus developed at one of the anastomoses, which, in turn, might embolize to a distal anastomosis and occlude the entire graft. Long-term data are not yet available that demonstrate the superiority of side-to-side anastomoses, but these seem to be the simplest method of performing five or more anastomoses when indicated (Stiles, 1981).

Endarterectomy has been virtually abandoned by our group for several years, although it is reported to be useful by some centers. Our pessimism about its utility is due not only to the fact that a raw intimal surface is created, which may thrombose if the flow rate through the graft is not great enough, but also to doubt about long-term patency. Patency of an endarterectomized artery after 1 to 2 years is dubious because of the progressive cicatricial contraction of fibrous tissue, a phenomenon that led to abandonment of endarterectomy in the femoropopliteal system long ago in arteries smaller than 6 mm. in diameter.

Following bypass, flow rates are promptly measured with a flowmeter, preferably obtaining basal flows greater than 40 ml. per minute and peak flows greater than 80 to 100 ml. per minute. This, of course, depends on the size of the vessel grafted and the extent of distal disease. Normally, grafts are attached to vessels as small as 1.5 mm. in diameter if sufficient larger vessels are not available. With small vessels and limited runoff, the side-to-side type of anasto-

mosis seems attractive when feasible, as the higher flow rate through the parent graft should make the likelihood of long-term patency greater. Several reports have indicated a higher long-term patency if the initial basal flow rate is greater than 30 to 40 ml. per minute.

Before the incision is closed, the soft tissues are closed superiorly to cover the grafts, leaving the pericardium open inferiorly in the majority of patients. Routine coverage of the grafts with soft tissue is most important. In the rare instance of infection and disruption of the sternotomy, exposure of an uncovered graft will almost surely lead to thrombosis or rupture.

Following bypass, pacemaker wires are routinely left in the right ventricle and right atrium for control of postoperative arrhythmias. If a Swan-Ganz catheter is not left in the pulmonary artery, a plastic catheter is routinely left in the left atrium and another in the pulmonary artery, inserted through the right ventricle.

Arterial Grafts. The use of the internal mammary artery (Fig. 50–94) is discussed in the next section of this chapter. It was developed in our Department of Surgery in 1967 by Green and Tice. We have enthusiastically used this artery for grafts to the anterior descending coronary artery since that time because of the uniform high patency rates, near 95 per cent, 4 to 5 years after operation, as compared with vein patency rates near 80 per cent. In 1980, Loop and associates reported a patency rate of 81 per cent in 646 vein grafts studied 48 months after operation, whereas the patency rate of 88 internal mammary artery grafts for a similar period of time was 95 per cent. The internal mammary artery is not used if it is significantly smaller than the anterior descending coronary artery, and its use is also avoided in small patients, older patients with fragile sternums, or patients with severe emphysema in whom distended emphysematous lungs may cause kinking of the artery. For younger male patients with an obstructed anterior descending coronary artery, it is always the graft of choice.

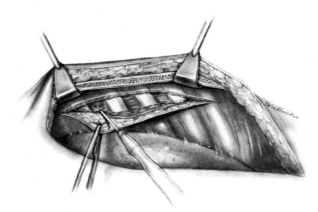

Figure 50–94. Mobilization of the internal mammary artery is begun over the third and fourth costal cartilages, using the "cold" electrocautery blade for dissection. Application of traction to the endothoracic fascia with tissue forceps helps to separate the structures from the chest wall. (From Ochsner, J. L., and Mills, N. L.: Coronary Artery Surgery. Philadelphia, Lea and Febiger, 1978.)

Postoperative Care

The central concerns of early postoperative care are cardiac function and adequacy of ventilation. Postoperative bleeding is not a frequent problem, with the usual amount of blood lost being near 500 ml. With excessive blood loss, determination of the activated clotting time will detect any residual heparin activity that can be corrected with additional protamine. Platelet transfusions may be indicated by low platelet counts or prolonged bleeding time. Fresh frozen plasma is given if there are signs of a coagulopathy with elevation of the prothrombin time and other coagulation abnormalities. A general rule is to almost always re-explore any patient who has bled as much as 1 liter following operation, even though his condition is satisfactory. A bleeding point may be found. This routine re-exploration has actually simplified convalescence, avoiding the problems of accumulation of clot within the mediastinum, with no discernible harmful effects from the repeat operation.

As discussed before, cardiac function is best measured by serial measurements of cardiac output and monitoring of left atrial pressure, either directly or from the pulmonary artery diastolic pressure or wedge pressure. Adequacy of blood volume can be judged by the response of left atrial pressure to infusion of fluid. Use of oxygen tension in mixed venous blood was discussed earlier, as well as the use of nitroglycerin, nitroprusside, and inotropic drugs. Ventilation is usually performed through an indwelling endotracheal tube for a few hours, but seldom for longer periods.

The precise diagnosis of a myocardial infarction remains debatable. The two most frequent criteria are Q waves on the electrocardiogram and the myocardial fraction of creatine phosphokinase (CPK-MB). Q waves are reported to develop on the electrocardiogram in a frequency of 3 to 4 per cent. Q waves, however, clearly do not always represent myocardial necrosis; exceptions are perhaps due to traction on the conduction bundles of the heart. Periodically, Q waves that are classic for infarction appear in the presence of normal CPK-MB enzyme.

On the other hand, the CPK-MB enzyme is not as specific as once thought. At present, there is considerable uncertainty as to its overall significance. This enzyme usually reaches its greatest concentration within 6 to 12 hours after myocardial injury. Certainly, a low value (400 to 500 units) indicates the absence of any myocardial injury, but a higher value (1000 units) apparently may occur from edema and not necrosis.

If there is uncertainty about the occurrence of a significant infarction, the ejection fraction can be measured with a radionuclide gated pool scan before the patient is discharged from the hospital.

Arrhythmias, although usually minor, occur frequently, so that the electrocardiogram should be monitored constantly. A variety of drugs may be useful, including an infusion of lidocaine (1 to 2 mg./min.), propranolol for tachycardia, or procainamide for premature ventricular contractions. Supplemental potassium therapy is given for hypokalemia. Other agents such as quinidine may be employed if necessary. Electrical pacing is almost routinely used for transient bradycardia.

With persistent arrhythmias, 24-hour Holter monitoring should be done before the patient leaves the hospital, because clinically silent arrhythmias of a serious nature may be detected only by this method. Subsequently, the Holter monitoring may be repeated every 3 to 6 months in the first year after operation if significant arrhythmias are present.

Although close observation is needed for the first 48 hours after operation, the majority of patients recover promptly and leave the hospital within 9 to 12 days after operation.

For the past 2 to 3 years, the incidence of some degree of myocardial necrosis following operation apparently has been quite small, in the range of 2 to 3 per cent. This is almost clinically asymptomatic, detectable only by the laboratory methods described. A persistent low cardiac output from extensive infarction has virtually disappeared with present techniques of myocardial preservation, except in patients with severe ischemia or a myocardial infarction immediately before operation.

Early Results Following Bypass Grafting

Operative Mortality. With present techniques, as described in the preceding paragraphs, the operative mortality rate is now consistently 1 per cent or less in good-risk patients, both at our own institution and among several large groups from different parts of the United States (Isom et al., 1978; Ochsner and Mills, 1978; Jones et al., 1980; Kirklin et al., 1979; Loop et al., 1979; Wukasch et al., 1979).

Operative risk is greater with significant impairment of ventricular function but has also improved markedly with potassium cardioplegia, seldom exceeding 5 to 8 per cent, even in patients with an ejection fraction of 0.20 or less (Jones et al., 1978).

Relief of Angina. The immediate relief of angina is the most dramatic feature of coronary bypass, with prompt and complete relief occurring in 60 to 80 per cent of patients and much improvement in most others; only 5 per cent of patients or less obtain little benefit. This dramatic result is responsible for the astronomically increasing frequency of bypass grafting since its introduction in 1967 and 1968. In 1973, about 25,000 bypass operations were performed in the United States. In 1981, over 100,000 were probably done, with the frequency steadily increasing as long-term benefits are better defined, and the operative mortality rate has decreased to near 1 per cent.

Long-Term Results Following Bypass Grafting

Patency of Vein Grafts; Progression of Atherosclerosis in Native Coronary Arteries; Changes in Left Ventricular Function. It is unfortunate that serial angiographic studies are done infrequently following operation, because they can provide valuable information concerning the patency and durability of vein grafts, the progression of atherosclerosis in the native coronary circulation, and changes in ventricular function. The data available are from selected groups of patients, because many asymptomatic patients will not consent to repeat angiography. Hence, patients studied often are those whose symptoms recur and are not comparable to asymptomatic patients. The two basic considerations, of course, are the patency of the vein grafts and the progression of coronary atherosclerosis.

Since the development of bypass grafting, data have uniformly shown that graft occlusion is most likely to occur in the first 12 months after operation, with a much smaller rate of occlusion thereafter. Closure occurring in the first 2 to 4 weeks after operation is surely due to different factors in operative technique. These are numerous, including the type of vein used for grafting; difference in diameter of the vein graft and the coronary artery; operative trauma to the vein graft in removal and storage; technical factors in performance of anastomoses; disruption in the intima of the coronary arteries, either from operative trauma or from endarterectomy; flow rates through the vein graft, depending on the size of the coronary artery grafted and the presence of distal disease; graft irregularities that predispose to turbulent flow of blood, such as kinking from an adhesion; and diffuse constriction from adhesions following a pericardiotomy syndrome. The most recently discovered factor in our experience is the fact that myocardial edema developing after removal of the aortic cross-clamp, in the presence of inadequate myocardial preservation, may increase coronary vascular resistance enough to decrease blood flow through the graft 50 to 70 per cent. This decrease in flow, which would precipitate thrombosis, can be partly reversed either by correction of the myocardial edema or by intra-aortic balloon pumping. These factors may cause occlusion of grafts in the first month after operation or may decrease flow enough to cause subsequent occlusion in the following year.

Several studies have shown that grafts usually thicken after operation, with proliferation of fibrous tissue around the internal elastic membrane, both in the media and in the intima. These changes are probably the normal physiologic response of the vein to arterial pressure; they are probably greater if structural features of the anastomoses produce turbulent flow. They were described in detail by Rossi and colleagues in 1965 in a study of arterial autografts applied as patch grafts to normal coronary arteries in dogs.

A decrease in diameter of the vein graft, varying somewhat but generally in the range of 20 to 30 per cent, has been found almost universally, probably as a consequence of both the fibromuscular hyperplasia and the fact that the vein graft is larger than the coronary artery, causing the flow of blood through the vein to be slower than through the artery. This de-crease in lumen diameter, probably a physiologic adaptation, usually does not progress to where the vein becomes smaller than the artery (Grondin, 1981; Hamby *et al.*, 1979). Grondin has also noted in serial studies that the process does not continue significantly after the first year after operation. Therefore, angiographic studies a year after operation may show a normal graft, diffuse narrowing of the graft, focal areas of stenosis, or other irregularities. Before 1975, graft patency at 1 month was in the range of 85 to 90 per cent, and at 1 year, it was 70 to 75 per cent. Patency rates in both categories have improved markedly in the past 8 years.

The best studies are those of Grondin and associates at the Montreal Heart Institute, who reported in 1979 and also in 1981 angiographic studies in 110 patients 6 years after operation, 94 of whom had undergone two previous angiographic studies. In this group of 94 patients, 13 of 170 grafts were occluded 2 weeks after operation, 13 more became occluded 1 year later, and 14 more became occluded in the subsequent 5 years. Hence, at 6 years, 130 of the 170 grafts remained patent, about 77 per cent. Studies of the same group of patients who had undergone operation earlier had found a much higher rate of occlusion, approaching 25 per cent between 1 month and 1 year after operation. This was reduced markedly by changes in methods of vein graft procurement and preservation. These studies are some of the best that indicate the great influence on long-term results of methods of vein graft procurement and preservation as well as other factors of operative technique. The fact that 10 of 144 grafts patent at 1 year occluded in the next 5 years, an occlusion rate near 2 to 3 per cent per year, is almost identical to that reported by other groups, representing probably a combination of deterioration in the vein graft and the progression of atherosclerosis in both the native coronary circulation and the vein graft.

In Grondin's report (1981) the subsequent course of 70 patients with 99 patent grafts who had a "perfect result" at 1 year was of particular interest. Among the 99 grafts, 20 had the same diameter as present when studied soon after operation, and *all* 20 were found to be patent 5 years later. Twenty-eight of the 99 grafts had a 10 to 20 per cent reduction in caliber; four of these 28 were occluded 5 years later. Fifty-one of the 99 grafts had a narrowing of 35 per cent or more; five of this group were occluded 5 years later. The numbers in the three groups were too small to be statistically significant but are most encouraging.

In 1981, Grondin stated that 97 per cent of grafts appearing normal on angiography 1 year after operation were patent 6 years later. Grafts with less than 50 per cent narrowing at 1 year had a 7-year patency rate of 84 per cent. Those with greater than 50 per cent narrowing, however, had a 7-year patency rate of only 37 per cent. It therefore seems that a graft that appears normal on angiography at 1 year has a very strong likelihood of remaining so 5 to 6 years later; a graft with some degenerative changes at 1 year also has an excellent chance of remaining patent, although it is not as great as the graft with a normal appearance (Fig. 50–81).

A particularly sobering finding was the progression of atherosclerosis in nongrafted coronary arteries. Fifty-six patients showed progression of coronary artery disease; 53 did not. This rate of progression of nearly 50 per cent clearly indicates the present limitation of medical therapy. Details of the type of therapy used in these patients are not available.

A separate interesting association was the fact that among the 56 patients with progression of atherosclerosis in the native coronary arteries, 17 had changes in the vein grafts, whereas only two of 53 patients without atherosclerotic progression had changes in the vein grafts, indicating that the atherosclerotic process was influencing both the native coronary circulation and the vein grafts.

The relative resistance of vein grafts to atherosclerosis, however, was clearly indicated by the fact that 85 per cent of the grafts (138 of 158) showed no angiographic signs of atherosclerosis at 6 years.

Finally, only three of 158 arteries showed atherosclerosis distal to the patent graft, refuting the concern that grafting may accelerate atherosclerosis in coronary arteries. Bypass grafting does, however, accelerate closure of a stenotic coronary artery proximal to the site of attachment to the vein graft. This finding has been noted by several groups. Apparently, it results from a decrease in flow of blood through the stenotic coronary artery because resistance to blood flow is less in the vein graft.

Several other groups have reported late angiographic findings, although none with the detailed serial studies reported by Grondin and associates. Because of the crucial importance of the long-term fate of vein grafts, results from seven of these reports are briefly mentioned in the following paragraphs.

In 1979, Hamby and coworkers stated that angiograms performed on 1197 grafts in 570 patients studied less than 2 weeks after operation revealed 90 per cent to be patent. A second angiogram performed in 85 of these patients, at an average time of 2½ years after operation, found that 92 per cent of the grafts patent at 2 weeks were still patent, an annual occlusion rate near 3 per cent. Progressive coronary artery disease was noted also, a rate near 12 per cent per year. Most grafts were narrowed and shortened, graft diameter decreasing in the range of 17 to 25 per cent, but the grafts still had a larger diameter than the coronary artery, with 71 per cent of grafts having a diameter about 1.5 times greater than that of the coronary artery.

In 1980, Fowler and associates described studies in 101 patients with 191 grafts who were operated on before 1976. Angiography 1 to 2 weeks after operation found a 94 per cent patency rate (174 of 187 vein grafts). One to 2 years later, 67 of these patients agreed to undergo repeat angiography; hence, the group studied was a selected one. The second angio-

graphic study found 101 of 108 vein grafts patent (94 per cent).

In 1978, Kouchoukos and colleagues reported studies at the University of Alabama in Birmingham. Four hundred and thirty-eight patients with 871 grafts were studied. Eighty per cent of the grafts were patent about 1 year after operation. Sixty-two patients of this group, with 134 grafts, were studied a second time, at an average of 42 months after operation. Of 116 grafts patent at the initial study, only 5 were occluded at the second study, representing an annual occlusion rate of 1.7 per cent.

The influence of distal endarterectomy was studied in 47 patients in whom grafts were placed into the right coronary artery in association with a distal endarterectomy. The graft patency rate was 62 per cent, as compared with 78 per cent for those not endarterectomized.

In 1979, Tyras and coworkers in St. Louis described a study of 181 patients from a group of 531 who had had bypass grafting 5 or more years earlier. Their study particularly focused on changes in ventricular function. Forty of the 181 patients had regained normal ventricular function, and 49 had retained normal ventricular function. Ventricular function had deteriorated in 20 per cent of patients. The remaining group had some abnormalities in ventricular function that either remained unchanged or improved to a limited degree. The graft patency rate varied between 65 per cent and 84 per cent among the five groups. Atherosclerosis progressed in the grafted coronary arteries to a similar degree among all five groups, ranging from 59 to 68 per cent. It was the same in coronary arteries with occluded grafts as in those with patent grafts. In ungrafted coronary arteries, progression of atherosclerosis ranged from 33 per cent in those with normal left ventricular function to 61 per cent in those with deteriorating left ventricular function. As observed by other groups, stenosis in a coronary artery often progressed to total occlusion after a bypass graft was inserted distally, the frequency varying with the severity of the stenosis beforehand. Seventy-four per cent of those with a preoperative stenosis of 90 per cent or more were totally occluded subsequently; 49 per cent with stenoses less than 90 per cent progressed to total occlusion. In ungrafted coronary arteries, only 1 per cent of vessels with preoperative stenosis less than 50 per cent progressed to total occlusion, whereas 44 per cent of those with stenosis greater than 90 per cent occluded.

In 1980, Loop and associates reported a patency rate of 81 per cent for 646 vein grafts in 471 patients studied more than 4 years after operation. By comparison, the patency rate of 88 internal mammary artery grafts studied for a comparable length of time was 94 per cent.

Finally, in 1977, Lawrie and coworkers reported on 596 vein grafts among 343 patients studied over a wide period of time, ranging from 1 to 84 months, with an average of 15 months. Hence, the group is a nonselected one, depending on when the angiogram was performed. However, 71 of 80 grafts studied 5 to 7 years after operation were patent, a patency rate of 89 per cent. The significance of these data is unclear, as patients with occluded grafts in the first 4 years after operation would automatically be excluded in calculating the 5-year patency rate.

The frequency of progression of atherosclerosis in ungrafted coronary arteries, 10 to 11 per cent per year in the few reports available, is an alarming indictment of the failure to date of available forms of therapy to stop the atherosclerotic process. This remains the greatest challenge with coronary artery disease. As stated earlier, bypass grafting, although dramatic, does not alter the underlying biochemical abnormality. A particular advantage of bypass grafting, separate from the benefits of relief of angina and improved longevity, is that it provides an objective measurement with an angiogram of the extent of atherosclerosis present at the time of operation. Repeat angiography years later can readily be done in controlled clinical studies to compare the effectiveness of different forms of medical therapy to alter the atherosclerotic process. Previously, such objective measurement has not been possible.

Recurrent Angina and Reoperation

Most groups report that following operation, angina is abolished in 60 to 65 per cent of patients and significantly relieved in another 30 per cent. During the next 5 years, there is a return of angina to some degree in 20 to 30 per cent of patients, although the frequency and severity vary widely among different reports (Isom *et al.*, 1978; Loop *et al.*, 1979; Jones *et al.*, 1980; DeBakey and Lawrie, 1978).

Some recurrence of angina would be expected, as vein grafts close at a rate of between 2 and 3 per cent per year after the first postoperative year, whereas atherosclerosis seems to progress at an average rate of about 10 per cent per year. The combination of progression of atherosclerosis and occlusion of vein grafts would naturally lead to recurrent angina. Hence, a patient who develops severe angina after a symptom-free interval of several years should have a repeat angiogram. Almost always, one of two things will be found: A vein graft has occluded, or atherosclerotic obstruction has progressed to a critical degree in arteries that were not grafted at the previous operation.

Fortunately, recurrent angina in most patients is mild and readily controlled with medical therapy. At New York University, we have found it necessary to reoperate on fewer than 100 patients in the past 13 years, during which time over 3000 bypass procedures have been performed (Culliford *et al.*, 1979). Similarly, Mills (1981), at the Ochsner Clinic in New Orleans, has found repeat operation necessary in only 56 patients in their total experience with over 3000 bypass procedures.

The largest experience with coronary bypass reoperation has been reported from the Cleveland Clinic

by Loop and associates. In 1981, they reported experiences with 500 repeat operations between 1967 and 1979. Repeat operation was necessary for progressive atherosclerosis in 51 per cent of the group, for graft failure in 29 per cent, and for a combination of these two factors in the others. The operative mortality rate was low, only 4 per cent. With an average follow-up of 42 months, angina was relieved in 86 per cent of the group. Repeat catheterization of 104 patients over a year after operation found a graft patency rate of 79 per cent with vein grafts and 97 per cent with internal mammary artery grafts. Hence, in this report the results achieved with the second operation were almost the same as those achieved with primary revascularization, a most encouraging finding.

When reoperation is necessary, with present techniques it can be performed with an operative risk less than 5 per cent, with an expected rate of improvement in the range of 75 to 80 per cent. The technical factors require considerable evaluation beforehand, depending on whether the obstructed artery was grafted before or not. If a previous graft has occluded, the capacity of the distal vascular bed to keep a second graft patent will depend on the size of the artery grafted, flow rate through the original graft, and other factors. Adhesion formation will, undoubtedly, be more severe after repeat operation.

Capacity to Return to Work Following Coronary Bypass

Several articles have been written about the ability of a patient to return to work after coronary bypass, with the socioeconomic implication that the operation is not "cost effective!" One study was from Canada; another dealt with Veterans Administration patients, many of whom were already partly retired on a pension.

The ability to return to work, of course, is influenced by cardiac function, but the most important factors are the motivation to return to work as well as the type of work, such as heavy physical labor versus a sedentary occupation. Isom and colleagues reported our total experiences at New York University in 1978, consisting of 1174 patients operated on between 1968 and 1975, with a 98 per cent follow-up. The majority of these patients were operated on for incapacitating angina, with threatened loss of employment. Most were anxious to return to work as soon as possible. In this group of patients, 64 per cent returned to full employment and 8 per cent to partial employment. About 15 to 20 per cent retired because of cardiac disease. Hence, most patients, as they were operated on because of inability to work, returned to work promptly. Actually, after the first 3 months after operation, following an uncomplicated recovery, no limitations of any kind are placed on patients after bypass.

In 1978, DeBakey and Lawrie noted that 80 per cent of their patients younger than 65 years of age were able to continue working more than 5 years after operation. In 1979, Loop and associates, reporting an 11-year experience with coronary bypass at the Cleveland Clinic, stated that 50 to 55 per cent of their patients were employed 5 years following operation. Therefore, contrary to the conclusions of some publications, the ability to return to normal physical activity, including working and participating in sports, is one of the major benefits of an effective coronary bypass procedure.

Changes in Left Ventricular Function

Many advances have been made with the safety and effectiveness of coronary bypass in the past 10 years. At one time, even the presence of significant impairment of ventricular function was considered a contraindication to bypass, although our experiences indicated that such patients had a much better survival after bypass than those who were not operated on (Isom et al., 1975). What apparently occurred with some early techniques was that the myocardial injury produced negated the benefit from the bypass grafts. In recent years, principally from the widespread use of potassium cardioplegia, several groups have reported operations on patients with low ejection fractions, 0.20 or lower, with a mortality rate of less than 10 per cent and significant improvement in angina. Unfortunately, however, there has rarely been a substantial improvement in ventricular function.

The experiences of Tyras and associates (1978) with 181 patients studied 5 years after operation has been described in the section "Long-term Patency of Venous Grafts." In 1979, Loop and coworkers reported a comparison of the ventriculogram before and after operation in a large number of patients. In 457 patients operated on between 1967 and 1970, the ventricular function appeared unchanged in 75 per cent, was better in 9 per cent, and was worse in 16 per cent. In 545 patients operated on in 1971, ventricular function was improved in 19 per cent, unchanged in 76 per cent, and worse in 5 per cent. In 1972, of 513 patients who underwent operation, ventricular function was improved in 24 per cent, unchanged in 70 per cent, and worse in 6 per cent. In the 537 patients operated on in 1973, ventricular function was improved in 24 per cent, unchanged in 70 per cent, and worse in 6 per cent.

When coronary bypass was first developed, it was hoped that operation might significantly improve ventricular function, especially in patients with congestive failure from extensive infarction of the left ventricle. Chronic congestive failure apparently develops when between 40 and 45 per cent of left ventricular muscle mass is not functioning. The question, of course, was whether the impaired function was due to irreversible injury from infarction or to inability of ischemic muscle to function, which would improve with bypass. Unfortunately, early experiences (Spencer et al., 1971) indicated that coronary bypass was contraindicated for congestive failure.

There was a high operative mortality, and survivors showed little benefit. Congestive failure apparently is due to loss of muscle function from infarction, not from ischemia. Intractable congestive failure, in the absence of a ventricular aneurysm, still remains a contraindication to bypass. In this unfortunate group of patients, cardiac transplantation is probably the only hope for even short-term improvement.

As described earlier in the section entitled "Contraindications to Operation," it is most important to recognize a separate group of patients, those with intermittent acute episodes of pulmonary edema, between which symptoms of congestive failure are not present. The exact mechanism precipitating these episodes has not been determined, but it is probably an acute episode of coronary insufficiency, elevating left ventricular end-diastolic pressure to ranges of 20 or 30 mm. Hg or more, with resulting pulmonary edema. Such acute episodes have been recognized in the operating room in anesthetized patients before bypass and have been promptly corrected by infusion of nitroglycerin. Several such patients have been operated on successfully by our group, with a low operative mortality and without further episodes of pulmonary edema in the subsequent 2 or 3 years. Hence, such patients fortunately are in a different category than those with chronic congestive failure.

A separate consideration is the changes in left ventricular function with exercise, measured by radionuclide studies (Spencer, 1980). Apparently, according to the limited data available, a complete bypass usually corrects these abnormalities completely. These data were discussed earlier in the section entitled "Pathophysiology."

Arrhythmias

In contrast to the effectiveness of bypass for relief of angina, arrhythmias have often remained unchanged, carrying with them the unpredictable hazard of sudden death. Arrhythmias are discussed in another chapter of this text and, therefore, will not be discussed here. Significant advances have been made in electrophysiologic mapping of ischemic zones of myocardium often near the border of a ventricular aneurysm. Excision of these areas has been effective in abolishing potentially lethal arrhythmias in a significant number of patients operated on in two or three institutions in the past few years (Harken et al., 1979).

The dramatic report by Cobb and associates (1980, 1980b) from Seattle about arrhythmias and sudden death was discussed in detail in the section "Pathophysiology."

Increase in Longevity with Coronary Bypass

Does coronary bypass prolong life? This, of course, is the major question that has been debated vigorously for several years, often with more emotion than logic. It is especially important in choosing therapy for the patient with few symptoms but with

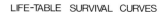

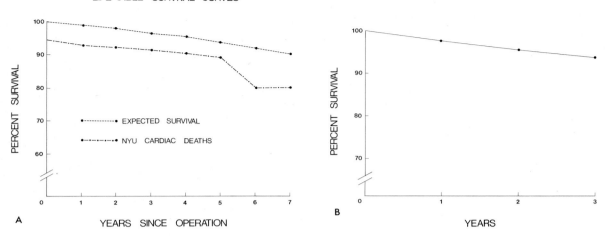

Figure 50–95. *A,* The 7-year actuarial survival of the first 1174 patients undergoing bypass at New York University Medical Center (1968 to 1975) compared with that of the matched general population. The average operative mortality rate was 5 per cent, declining to between 1 and 2 per cent during the later part of the study. The significant points are that the mortality rate between 1 and 4 years after operation was only 1.4 per cent per year, the same as that for the general population, and the mortality rate between 3 and 5 years after operation was identical to that between 1 and 3 years after operation. *B,* The 3-year survival for 249 patients undergoing three or more bypass grafts at New York University Medical Center between 1972 and 1974.

evidence of extensive disease on the coronary arteriogram.

The frequent occurrence of a fatal infarction during sleep or mild physical activity is a curious phenomenon that suggests that a relatively small decrease in regional blood flow may precipitate infarction in an area of severe ischemia. If death occurs in less than 4 to 6 hours, an autopsy may reveal a massive infarction with extensive occlusive disease, but no acute thrombosis of a major vessel that might have precipitated a large decrease in regional blood flow. In such instances, it seems highly probable that the decrease in blood flow that occurred was less than 100 ml./min., as total coronary blood flow at rest is less than 400 ml./min. in a heart of normal size. Hence, a bypass graft to the ischemic area that increased coronary blood flow 50 to 100 ml./min. might have prevented the fatal infarction. This hypothesis is further supported by the fact that late death following bypass is very rare if three bypass grafts remain patent.

The influence of operation on longevity in the first 1174 patients operated on at New York University between 1968 and 1975 was reported by Isom and colleagues in 1978. The follow-up was 98 per cent. Most of these patients had been operated on for disabling angina refractory to medical therapy. The series included the very first operations performed, starting in 1968, at which time operative mortality was higher and total revascularization uncommon. The circumflex artery was rarely grafted before 1971 or 1972. Hence, the group of patients is a selected one with severe disease. The patients had severe angina, often had incomplete revascularization, and had a less effective method of myocardial protection.

The average operative mortality rate for the entire group was 5 per cent, decreasing to between 2 and 3 per cent between 1972 and 1975. By actuarial methods, the first year survival rate, including operative deaths, was 88 per cent. It was astonishing that only 49 cardiac deaths occurred after discharge from the hospital in the entire group of over 1100 patients.

As shown in Figure 50–95, with an average operative mortality rate of 5 per cent, 95 of each group of 100 patients left the hospital. Eighty-eight of these 95 patients were alive 5 years later, a mortality rate near 1.5 per cent per year. A statistical comparison with a matched group of patients from life insurance tables, showing expected survival for a population group of similar age and sex, demonstrates virtually parallel curves, with survival resembling that of the normal population for the first 5 years after bypass. A separate interesting point is that the slope of the survival curve was unchanged for 4 years, indicating that there was not a greater death rate 3 to 5 years after operation as compared with 1 or 2 years. This similarity in death rates indicates that neither closure of bypass grafts nor progression of atherosclerosis had negated the effect of bypass grafting. Not shown in the illustration is the fact that survival rates for patients with single-, double-, and triple-vessel disease were slightly different, but not strikingly so. By contrast, several reports of experiences with patients treated with medical therapy have found a major difference in 5-year survival rates among patients with single-, double-, or triple-vessel disease. The abolition of the differences in survival among these groups after bypass grafting suggests a strong beneficial effect from grafting.

A separate fact found in the study was that cardiac death was virtually unknown in a patient with three functioning grafts.

Representative reports from several major cardiac centers are summarized in the following paragraphs.

In 1978, Hurst and associates extensively reviewed published experiences with coronary bypass grafting, finding that sufficient data were available to conclude that there was a significant improvement in longevity with bypass grafting. This report should be studied in detail. They analyzed four possible methods for evaluating the effects of coronary bypass surgery—retrospective matched studies, prospective matched studies, prospective randomized studies, and comparison of study groups by life tables—and indicated the limitations of each method. Their conclusion was that available evidence was sufficient to indicate a much wider application of bypass grafting.

Hurst and coworkers analyzed in detail the report by Greene and colleagues (1977), who found the combined 5-year survival rate in 3009 patients treated medically in 24 reported series to be near 75 per cent. Results from several surgical series were much better. One of the best of these was described by Kouchoukos (1980) from the University of Alabama in Birmingham. In patients with triple-vessel disease, the survival rate at 46 months was 83 per cent for the surgical group, 53 per cent for patients treated medically, and 44 per cent for patients considered inoperable. Similar to our experiences at New York University, Hurst and associates found that survival curves for surgically treated patients were nearly similar for single-, double-, and triple-vessel disease.

The Veterans Administration Cooperative Study performed between 1972 and 1974 (Read et al., 1978) was discussed previously in the section "Medical and Surgical Treatment."

In 1978, DeBakey and Lawrie stated that studies at the Baylor College of Medicine had found little deterioration in grafts 5 years after operation. In patients with good left ventricular function, the survival rate was 93 per cent, virtually identical to that of a similar general population of identical age and sex. Eighty per cent of patients younger than 65 years were working.

As noted earlier, in 1979 Loop and coworkers reported an 11-year evaluation of coronary bypass operations at the Cleveland Clinic. Four groups were analyzed, a 1967 to 1970 series and the 1971, 1972, and 1973 cohorts, respectively. The 5-year survival rates for the four groups were 90 per cent, 92 per cent, 93 per cent, and 92 per cent, respectively. The percentage of asymptomatic patients among the same groups was 66 per cent, 65 per cent, 69 per cent, and 67 per cent, respectively.

Also in 1979, Kirklin and associates analyzed available information about results with coronary bypass grafting, finding, in contrast to Hurst and coworkers, that available data did not permit a definite conclusion about a significant prolongation of life after coronary bypass grafting. He emphasized that many variations made statistical analysis extremely difficult. These included differences in age, race, sex, location of the stenosis in the arterial tree, degree of left ventricular damage, hypertension, obesity, smoking, variety of surgical techniques, and methods of myocardial preservation. For example, the in-hospital mortality rate in the Veterans Administration Study for patients with chronic stable angina from 1972 to 1974 was 5 per cent, 10 times that (0.4 per cent) in 1977 in patients in the same group. Their survival data (Fig. 50–96) were analyzed in relation to the extent of disease. A patient surviving operation after single-vessel disease had a 5-year survival rate of 94 per cent, identical to that of the United States' population. Similar patients with double-vessel disease had a 5-year survival rate of 88 per cent. With triple-vessel disease, the 5-year survival rate was around 89 per cent, about 6 per cent less than the 95 per cent survival rate for a matched general population. Findings with left main coronary artery disease were very similar. The 5-year survival rate in the Veterans Administration Cooperative Study of patients treated medically was only 72 per cent, far below that of about 95 per cent in the matched population.

At an international symposium in Athens in September 1980, Kouchoukos reported further data from the University of Alabama. Five hundred and thirteen patients with triple-vessel disease and a normal left ventricle were treated, 252 surgically and 261 medically. The 5-year survival rate was 95 per cent in the surgically treated group and 80 per cent in the medically treated group.

In 1980, at Emory University, Jones and associates reported experiences with 3479 operations. Patients with normal left ventricular function had an excellent 42-month survival rate, regardless of the extent of vessel disease—95 per cent for double-vessel disease and 94 per cent for triple-vessel disease.

The data from the European Cooperative Study, reported in 1980, were discussed earlier in the section entitled "Medical and Surgical Treatment."

Hence, the data from several sources from 1978 to 1981 are similar. The 5- to 6-year graft patency rate is near 80 per cent, and the 5-year survival rate is significantly greater in surgically treated patients with left main coronary artery or triple-vessel disease, even though they are asymptomatic when operated on.

Data for double-vessel disease with various degrees of impairment of left ventricular function show similar trends but are inconclusive. The location of the obstruction in the anterior descending coronary artery, proximal or distal, seems especially significant in this group. Serial radionuclide studies, performed over 6 to 24 months, to determine the changes in abnormalities of cardiac function that appear with exercise may provide the best data in the future to decide when operation should be done in the patient with significant disease but few symptoms. It is hoped that these studies eventually will be able to measure quantitatively the grams of left ventricular muscle that become ischemic with exercise or other forms of stress.

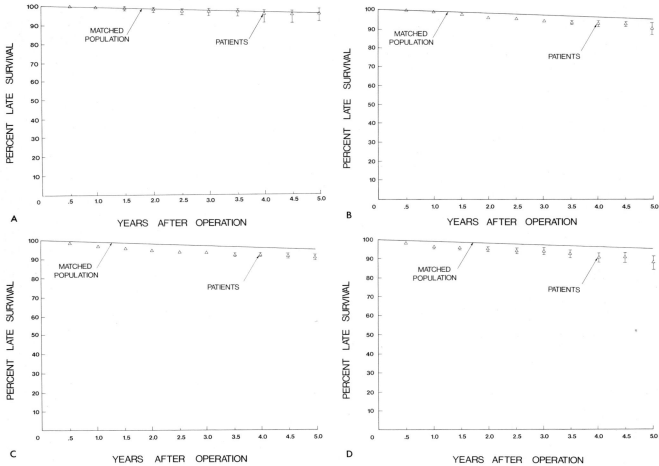

Figure 50–96. *A,* The actuarial survival of 182 patients surviving coronary bypass grafting for single-vessel disease. The vertical bar represents one standard error. Hence, the life expectancy of a patient with single-vessel disease after leaving the hospital is the same as that of the matched general population at 5 years. *B,* The five-year actuarial survival of 508 patients who survived coronary bypass grafting for double-vessel disease. The life expectancy at 5 years is about 5 per cent less than that of the matched general population. *C,* The 5-year actuarial survival of 863 patients surviving bypass grafting for triple-vessel disease. The life expectancy 5 years following operation is about 6 per cent less than that of the matched general population. *D,* The 5-year survival of 247 patients surviving operation for left main coronary artery disease. The 5-year life expectancy is about 7 per cent less than that of the matched general population.

SELECTED REFERENCES

Baumann, F. G., Catinella, F. P., Cunningham, J. N., Jr., and Spencer, F. C.: Vein contraction and smooth muscle cell extensions as causes of endothelial damage during graft preparation. Ann. Surg., *194*:199, 1981.

A striking phenomenon with removal of a saphenous vein is the development of spasm. This concentric contraction of the vessel, with contraction of the internal elastic membrane, may rupture the endothelial lining with exposure of the underlying vessel wall to elements in the blood. Hence, the graft is no longer a tube completely lined with endothelium and is more susceptible to thrombosis. This paper demonstrates with electron microscopy the mechanism of this phenomenon. It can be minimized by the use of papaverine at the time of removal of the saphenous vein.

Catinella, F. P., Cunningham, J. N., Jr., Srungaram, R. K., Baumann, F. G., Nathan, I. M., Glassman, E. A., Knopp, E. A., and Spencer, F. C.: Cold blood should not be used for vein preparation prior to coronary bypass grafting. J. Thorac. Cardiovasc. Surg., *82*:904, 1981.

There is an increasing amount of data that indicate that the method of handling the saphenous vein at the time of coronary bypass grafting is crucial, determining both early and long-term patency, possibly also the susceptibility of the vein to atherosclerosis. This paper indicates that cold blood is actually harmful, with the cold causing a contraction of the vein with disruption of the endothelium and the platelets in the blood then accumulating and initiating a thrombotic reaction. Moderately cold Plasmanate is superior.

Cobb, L. A., Werner, J. A., and Trobaugh, G. B.: Sudden cardiac death. I. A decade's experience with out-of-hospital resuscitation. Mod. Concepts Cardiovasc. Dis., *49*:31, 1980.

This remarkable paper from Seattle summarizing several years' experience with resuscitation of patients who develop cardiac arrest outside the hospital should be studied in detail. The data are especially significant because of the 600,000 deaths that occur annually in the United States, approximately two-thirds occur outside the hospital. The data are remarkable in that only one fifth of the patients resuscitated had a transmural infarction, and over half had no signs of myocardial necrosis whatsoever. About 75 per cent of the patients had triple-vessel disease, indicating that the event causing ventricular fibrillation was an arrhythmia, not an infarction. The implications for prompt cardiopulmonary resuscitation, as well as for the long-term monitoring for malignant arrhythmias, are clear.

European Coronary Surgery Study Group: Prospective randomised study of coronary artery bypass surgery in stable angina pectoris. Second interim report. Lancet, *2*:491, 1980.

The most important question with coronary bypass grafting is its influence on longevity. This randomized study is probably the best of its kind in the world. It was the first to conclusively show a significant difference in 5-year survival in patients with triple-vessel disease and good ventricular function. Patients with triple-vessel disease had a 5-year survival rate of 95 per cent after operation and one of 85 per cent after medical therapy.

Grondin, C. M., Campeau, L., Lespérance, J., Solymoss, B. C., Vouhé, P., Castonguay, Y. R., Meere, C., and Bourassa, M. G.: Atherosclerotic changes in coronary vein grafts six years after operation. Angiographic aspect in 110 patients. J. Thorac. Cardiovasc. Surg., 77:24, 1979.

This is a unique study of serial angiographic studies performed on 110 patients after operation, 1 year later, and again 6 years after operation. The study is unlike any other in the world, providing a valuable assessment of the changes in vein grafts over a period of time. It defines clearly that many changes occur in the first year, but that a graft appearing normal at 1 year has an excellent likelihood of remaining so in the next 5 years. Atherosclerosis continues to progress in the native coronary circulation. This paper is one of several that have indicated that vein graft patency 5 years after operation is between 70 and 85 per cent, probably influenced principally by the methods of handling the vein graft at the time of operation.

Harken, A. H., Josephson, M. E., and Horowitz, L. N.: Surgical endocardial resection for the treatment of malignant ventricular tachycardia. Ann. Surg., 190:456, 1979.

Coronary bypass has been dramatic for relief of angina but disappointing for influence on arrhythmias, especially following excision of a ventricular aneurysm. A remarkable development in the last 5 years has been the demonstration that foci within a centimeter of a ventricular aneurysm, usually zones of fibrotic endocardium, are the source of arrhythmias. Localization of these zones by electrophysiologic studies at operation, followed by their excision, has been a dramatic advance in the management of this disease. Pioneering studies have been done in this country by Dr. Harken's group in Philadelphia and Dr. Sabiston's group at Duke University.

Hellman, C. K., Kamath, M. L., Schmidt, D. H., Anholm, J., Blau, F., and Johnson, W. D.: Improvement in left ventricular function after myocardial revascularization. Assessment by first-pass rest and exercise nuclear angiography. J. Thorac. Cardiovasc. Surg., 79:645, 1980.

A question studied for a decade has been the influence of coronary bypass on ventricular function, with most studies showing little influence. The availability of radionuclide studies has made it possible to study ventricular function during and after excercise in more detail. This report is one of the first to demonstrate that abnormalities appear with exercise in patients with coronary disease and are corrected with operation.

Hurst, J. W., King, S. B., III, Logue, R. B., Hatcher, C. R., Jr., Jones, E. L., Craver, J. M., Douglas, J. S., Jr., Franch, R. H., Dorney, E. R., Cobbs, B. W., Jr., Robinson, P. H., Clements, S. D., Jr., Kaplan, J. A., and Bradford, J. M.: Value of coronary bypass surgery. Controversies in cardiology: Part I. Am. J. Cardiol., 42:308, 1978.

This extensive review of available data on coronary bypass surgery by Hurst and associates strongly endorsed coronary bypass surgery as providing a significant improvement in longevity. The paper stimulated a great deal of controversial discussion and is a valuable source of the data available at that time.

Isom, O. W., Spencer, F. C., Glassman, E., Cunningham, J. N., Jr., Teiko, P., Reed, G. E., and Boyd, A. D.: Does coronary bypass increase longevity? J. Thorac. Cardiovasc. Surg., 75:28, 1978.

This paper reports experiences at New York University with the first 1174 patients operated on between 1968 and 1975. The overall operative mortality rate was 5 per cent. In the subsequent 5 years, an additional 7 per cent of the patients died, an 88 per cent 5-year survival rate. This actuarial survival curve parallels that of a matched population of similar age and sex, and thus, this is one of the first papers to demonstrate the strong likelihood that bypass grafting greatly increased longevity.

Kirklin, J. W., Kouchoukos, N. T., Blackstone, E. H., and Oberman, A.: Research related to surgical treatment of coronary artery disease. Circulation, 60:1613, 1979.

This paper summarizes much of the current knowledge about coronary artery bypass and presents, as illustrated in this section, excellent data about the 5-year survival in single-, double-, and triple-vessel disease as compared with a matched population group.

Loop, F. D., Cosgrove, D. M., Kramer, J. R., Lytle, B. W., Taylor, P. C., Golding, L. A. R., and Groves, L. K.: Late clinical and arteriographic results in 500 coronary artery reoperations. J. Thorac. Cardiovasc. Surg., 81:675, 1981.

This report is the most extensive of its kind concerning the possibilities of reoperation after bypass. The data are excellent, demonstrating a low mortality rate and excellent results. About 50 per cent of the repeat operations were necessary for progressive atherosclerosis, 29 per cent for graft failure, and the others for a combination of the two factors.

Loop, F. D., Cosgrove, D. M., Lytle, B. W., Thurer, R. L., Simpfendorfer, C., Taylor, P. C., and Proudfit, W. L.: An eleven year evolution of coronary arterial surgery (1967–1978). Ann. Surg., 190:444, 1979.

This paper summarizes much of the extensive experience at the Cleveland Clinic over a period of several years. Graft patency rates for four different groups, each studied around 20 months after operation, ranged from 77 to 87 per cent. The 5-year survival rate for these four groups ranged from 89 to 92 per cent.

Mock, M. B., Ringqvist, I., Fisher, L. D., Davis, K. B., Chaitman, B. R., Kouchoukos, N. T., Kaiser, G. C., Alderman, E., Ryan, T. J., Russell, R. O., Jr., Mullin, S., Fray, D., Killip, T., III, and Participants in the Coronary Artery Surgery Study: Survival of medically treated patients in the Coronary Artery Surgery Study (CASS) Registry. Circulation, 66:562, 1982.

This study is a preliminary report from a long-term evaluation of the course of coronary artery disease in a group of 25,000 patients studied by cardiac catheterization in 15 different medical centers. The study was coordinated by the National Heart, Lung and Blood Institute of the National Institutes of Health. Final studies will be completed this year, but data available thus far, cited in the text, are the best yet for defining the natural history of the disease with present medical therapy. The most ominous form of the disease is a combination of severe depression of ventricular function with triple-vessel disease, which has a 4-year mortality rate near 60 per cent.

REFERENCES

Baumann, F. G., Catinella, F. P., Cunningham, J. N., Jr., and Spencer, F. C.: Vein contraction and smooth muscle cell extensions as causes of endothelial damage during graft preparation. Ann. Surg., 194:199, 1981.

Berg, R. J., Selinger, S. L., Leonard, J. J., Grunwald, R. P., and O'Grady, W. P.: Surgical Management of acute myocardial infarction. Cardiovasc. Clin. 12:61, 1982.

Boyd, A. D., Tremblay, R. E., Spencer, F. C., and Bahnson, H. T.: Estimation of cardiac output soon after intracardiac surgery with cardiopulmonary bypass. Ann. Surg., 150:613, 1959.

Catinella, F. P., Cunningham, J. N., Jr., Srungaram, R. K., Baumann, F. G., Nathan, I. M., Glassman, E. A., Knopp, E. A., and Spencer, F. C.: Cold blood should not be used for vein preparation prior to coronary bypass grafting. J. Thorac. Cardiovasc. Surg., 82:904, 1981.

Cobb, L. A., Werner, J. A., and Trobaugh, G. B.: Sudden cardiac death. I. A decade's experience with out-of-hospital resuscitation. Mod. Concepts Cardiovasc. Dis., 49:31, 1980a.

Cobb, L. A., Werner, J. A., and Trobaugh, G. B.: Sudden cardiac death. II. Outcome of resuscitation; management; and future directions. Mod. Concepts Cardiovasc. Dis., 49:37, 1980b.

Cukingnan, R. A., Carey, J. S., Wittig, J. H., and Brown, B. G.: Influence of complete coronary revascularization on relief of angina. J. Thorac. Cardiovasc. Surg., 79:188, 1980.

Culliford, A. T., Girdwood, R. W., Isom, O. W., Krauss, K. R., and Spencer, F. C.: Angina following myocardial revascularization. Does time of recurrence predict etiology and influence results of operation? J. Thorac. Cardiovasc. Surg., 77:889, 1979.

Cunningham, J. N., Jr., Adams, P. X., Knopp, E. A., Baumann, F. G., Snively, S. L., Gross, R. I., Nathan, I. M., and Spencer, F. C.: Preservation of ATP, ultrastructure, and ventricular function after aortic cross-clamping and reperfusion. Clinical use of blood potassium cardioplegia. J. Thorac. Cardiovasc. Surg., 78:708, 1979.

Cunningham, J. N., Jr., Catinella, F. P., and Spencer, F. C.: Blood cardioplegia—Experience with prolonged cross-clamping. In A Textbook of Clinical Cardioplegia. Edited by R. E. Engleman and S. Levitzky. Mt. Kisco, New York, Futura Publishing Co., 1982.

Daggett, W. M., Guyton, R. A., Mundth, E. D., Buckley, M. J., McEnany, M. T., Gold, H. K., Leinbach, R. C., and Austen, W. G.: Surgery for post-myocardial infarct ventricular septal defect. Ann. Surg., 186:260, 1977.

DeBakey, M. E., and Lawrie, G. M.: Aortocoronary-artery bypass. Assessment after 13 years. J.A.M.A., 239:837, 1978.

DeWood, M. A., Spores, J., Notske, R., Mouser, L. T., Burroughs, R., Golden, M. S., and Land, H. T.: Prevalence of total coronary occlusion during the early hours of transmural myocardial infarction. N. Engl. J. Med., 303:897, 1980.

Epstein, C. S., Kline, S. A., Levin, D. C., et al.: Left ventricular performance and graft patency after coronary artery–saphenous vein bypass surgery: Early and late follow-up. Am. Heart J., 93:547, 1977.

European Coronary Surgery Study Group: Prospective randomised study of coronary artery bypass surgery in stable angina pectoris. Second interim report. Lancet, 2:491, 1980.

Flemma, R. J., Mullen, D. C., Lepley, D., Jr., and Assa, J.: A comparative synchronous coronary surgery survival study. Ann. Thorac. Surg., 28:423, 1979.

Fowler, B. N., Jacobs, M. L., Zir, L., Dinsmore, R. E., Vezeridis, M. P., and Daggett, W. M.: Late graft patency and symptom relief after aorta-coronary bypass. J. Thorac. Cardiovasc. Surg., 79:288, 1980.

Gay, W. A., Jr., and Ebert, P. A.: Functional, metabolic, and morphologic effects of potassium-induced cardioplegia. Surgery, 74:284, 1973.

Green, G. E., Spencer, F. C., Tice, D. A., and Stertzer, S. H.: Arterial and venous microsurgical bypass grafts for coronary artery disease. J. Thorac. Cardiovasc. Surg., 60:491, 1970.

Green, M. V., Ostrow, H. G., Douglas, M. A., et al.: High temporal resolution ECG-gauged scintigraphic angiocardiography. J. Nucl. Med., 16:95, 1975.

Greene, D. G., Bunnell, I. L., Arani, D. T., et al.: Long-term survival after coronary bypass surgery. Buffalo General Hospital, State University of New York. Brochure for exhibit at American Heart Association Meeting, Miami, Florida, 1977.

Grondin, C. M.: Results of invasive studies to assess the first decade of coronary artery bypass operations. Presented at the American College of Surgeons Meeting, San Francisco, October 1981.

Grondin, C. M., Campeau, L., Lespérance, J., Solymoss, B. C., Vouhé, P., Castonguay, Y. R., Meere, C., and Bourassa, M. G.: Atherosclerotic changes in coronary vein grafts six years after operation. Angiographic aspect in 110 patients. J. Thorac. Cardiovasc. Surg., 77:24, 1979.

Hamby, R. I., Aintablian, A., Handler, M., Voleti, C., Weisz, D., Garvey, J. W., and Wisoff, G.: Aortocoronary saphenous vein bypass grafts. Long-term patency, morphology, and blood flow in patients with patent grafts early after surgery. Circulation, 60:901, 1979.

Harken, A. H., Josephson, M. E., and Horowitz, L. N.: Surgical endocardial resection for the treatment of malignant ventricular tachycardia. Ann. Surg., 190:456, 1979.

Hellman, C. K., Kamath, M. L., Schmidt, D. H., Anholm, J., Blau, F., and Johnson, W. D.: Improvement in left ventricular function after myocardial revascularization. Assessment by first-pass rest and exercise nuclear angiography. J. Thorac. Cardiovasc. Surg., 79:645, 1980.

Hurst, J. W., King, S. B., III, Logue, R. B., Hatcher, C. R., Jr., Jones, E. L., Craver, J. M., Douglas, J. S., Jr., Franch, R. H., Dorney, E. R., Cobbs, B. W., Jr., Robinson, P. H., Clements, S. D., Jr., Kaplan, J. A., and Bradford, J. M.: Value of coronary bypass surgery. Controversies in cardiology: Part I. Am. J. Cardiol., 42:308, 1978.

Isom, O. W., Spencer, F. C., Glassman, E., Cunningham, J. N., Jr., Teiko, P., Reed, G. E., and Boyd, A. D.: Does coronary bypass increase longevity? J. Thorac. Cardiovasc. Surg., 75:28, 1978.

Isom, O. W., Spencer, F. C., Glassman, E., Dembrow, J. M., and Pasternack, B. S.: Long-term survival following coronary bypass surgery in patients with significant impairment of left ventricular function. Circulation, 51(Suppl. 1):141, 1975.

Johnson, W. D., Flemma, R. J., Lepley, D., Jr., and Ellison, E. H.: Extended treatment of severe coronary artery disease: A total surgical approach. Ann. Surg., 170:460, 1969.

Jones, E. L., Craver, J. M., King, S. B., Douglas, J. S., Bradford, J. M., Brown, C. M., Bone, D. K., and Hatcher, C. R., Jr.: Clinical, anatomic and functional descriptors influencing morbidity, survival and adequacy of revascularization following coronary bypass. Ann. Surg., 192:390, 1980.

Jones, E. L., Craver, J. M., Kaplan, J. A., King, S. B., Douglas, J. S., Morgan, E. A., and Hatcher, C. R., Jr.: Criteria for operability and reduction of surgical mortality in patients with severe left ventricular ischemia and dysfunction. Ann. Thorac. Surg., 25:413, 1978.

Jones, E. L., Waites, T. F., Craver, J. M., Bradford, J. M., Douglas, J. S., King, S. B., Bone, D. K., Dorney, E. R., Clements, S. D., Thompkins, T., and Hatcher, C. R., Jr.: Coronary bypass for relief of persistent pain following acute myocardial infarction. Ann. Thorac. Surg., 32:33, 1981.

Kaiser, G. C., Barner, H. B., Tyras, D. H., Codd, J. E., Mudd, J. G., and Willman, V. L.: Myocardial revascularization: A rebuttal of the cooperative study. Ann. Surg., 188:331, 1978.

Kay, J. H., Zubiate, P., Mendez, M. A., Vanstrom, N., Yokoyama, T., and Gharavi, M. A.: Surgical treatment of mitral insufficiency secondary to coronary artery disease. J. Thorac. Cardiovasc. Surg., 79:12, 1980.

Kent, J. M., Borer, J. S., Green, M. V., et al.: Effects of coronary-artery bypass on global and regional left ventricular function during exercise. N. Engl. J. Med., 298:1434, 1978.

Kirklin, J. W., Kouchoukos, N. T., Blackstone, E. H., and Oberman, A.: Research related to surgical treatment of coronary artery disease. Circulation, 60:1613, 1979.

Kolessov, V. I.: Mammary artery–coronary artery anastomosis as a method of treatment for angina pectoris. J. Thorac. Cardiovasc. Surg., 54:535, 1967.

Kouchoukos, N. T.: Coronary artery bypass operations: Keeping records, reporting results, and establishing standards. Presented at American College of Surgeons Meeting, San Francisco, October 1981.

Kouchoukos, N. T.: Long-term results with medical and surgical treatment of three-vessel disease. Presented at the World Congress of Angiology, Athens, Greece, September 1980.

Kouchoukos, N. T., Oberman, A., and Karp, R. B.: Results of surgery for disabling angina pectoris. In Coronary Bypass Surgery. Edited by S. H. Rahimtoola. Philadelphia, F. A. Davis, 1977, p. 157.

Kouchoukos, N. T., Karp, R. B., Oberman, A., Russell, R. O., Jr., Alison, H. W., and Holt, J. H., Jr.: Long-term patency of saphenous veins for coronary bypass grafting. Circulation, 58(Suppl. 1):1, 1978.

Landymore, R. W., Tice, D., Trehan, N., and Spencer, F. C.: Does topical hypothermia prevent sublethal intraoperative injury during coronary artery bypass surgery? Presented at American Association for Thoracic Surgery Meeting, Washington, D.C., May 1981.

Lawrie, G. M., Morris, G. C., Jr., Chapman, D. W., Winters, W. L., and Lie, J. T.: Patterns of patency of 596 vein grafts up to seven years after aorta-coronary bypass. J. Thorac. Cardiovasc. Surg., 73:443, 1977.

Loop, F. D.: On reoperations. Ann. Thorac. Surg., 33:4, 1981.

Loop, F. D., Lytle, B. W., and Sheldon, W. C.: Hard and soft data on treatment of left main coronary lesions. Am. J. Cardiol., 45:524, 1980.

Loop, F. D., Cosgrove, D. M., Kramer, J. R., Lytle, B. W., Taylor, P. C., Golding, L. A. R., and Groves, L. K.: Late clinical and arteriographic results in 500 coronary artery reoperations. J. Thorac. Cardiovasc. Surg., 81:675, 1981.

Loop, F. D., Cosgrove, D. M., Lytle, B. W., Thurer, R. L., Simpfendorfer, C., Taylor, P. C., and Proudfit, W. L.: An eleven year evolution of coronary arterial surgery (1967–1978). Ann. Surg., 190:444, 1979.

McNeer, J. F., Starmer, C. F., Bartel, A. G., Behar, V. S., Kong, Y., Peter, R. H., and Rosati, R. A.: The nature of treatment selection in coronary artery disease. Experience with medical and surgical treatment of a chronic disease. Circulation, 49:606, 1974.

Miller, D. W., Jr., Ivey, T. D., Bailey, W. W., Johnson, D. D., and Hessel, E. A.: The practice of coronary artery bypass surgery in 1980. J. Thorac. Cardiovasc. Surg., 81:423, 1981.

Mills, N. L.: Re-operations for coronary artery disease: Indications, contra-indications, conduct of operation, and results. Presented at American College of Surgeons Meeting, San Francisco, October 1981.

Mock, M. B., Ringqvist, I., Fisher, L. D., Davis, K. B., Chaitman, B. R., Kouchoukos, N. T., Kaiser, G. C., Alderman, E., Ryan, T. J., Russell, R. O., Jr., Mullin, S., Fray, D., Killip, T., III, and Participants in the Coronary Artery Surgery Study. Survival of medically treated patients in the Coronary Artery Surgery Study (CASS) Registry. Circulation, 66:562, 1982.

Nelson, G. R., Cohn, P. F., and Gorlin, R.: Prognosis in medically treated coronary artery disease. Influence of ejection fraction compared to other parameters. Circulation, 52:408, 1975.

Ochsner, J. L., and Mills, N. L.: Coronary Artery Surgery. Philadelphia, Lea and Febiger, 1978.

Ochsner, J. L., Mills, N. L., and Bethea, M. C.: Operative technique of myocardial revascularization. World J. Surg., 2:767, 1978.

Principal Investigators of CASS and Associates: The National Heart, Lung, and Blood Institute Coronary Artery Surgery Study (CASS). Circulation, 63(Part II):I-1, 1981.

Read, R. C., Murphy, M. L., Hultgren, H. N., and Takaro, T.: Survival of men treated for chronic stable angina pectoris. A cooperative randomized study. J. Thorac. Cardiovasc. Surg., 75:1, 1978.

Rerych, S. K., Scholz, P. M., Sabiston, D. C., Jr., et al.: Effects of exercise training on left ventricular function in normal subjects: A longitudinal study by radionuclide angiography. Am. J. Cardiol., 45:244, 1980.

Rifkind, B. M., and Levy, R. I.: Testing the lipid hypothesis. Clinical trials. Arch. Surg., 113:80, 1978.

Rose, D. M., Colvin, S. B., Culliford, A. T., Adams, P. X., Cunningham, J. N., Jr., Isom, O. W., Glassman, E., and

Spencer, F. C.: Acute hemodynamic effects of a left heart assist device in patients with profound cardiac failure following cardiac surgery. Circulation, in press.

Rossi, N. P., Koepke, J. A., and Spencer, F. C.: Histologic changes in long-term autologous arterial patch grafts in coronary arteries. Surgery, 57:335, 1965.

Sewell, W. H.: Should we do Y and sequential grafts for coronary bypass? Ann. Thorac. Surg., 27:397, 1979.

Spencer, F. C.: Binocular loupes (microtelescopes) for coronary artery surgery. J. Thorac. Cardiovasc. Surg., 62:163, 1971.

Spencer, F. C.: The influence of coronary bypass on ventricular function. Consensus Meeting on Coronary Artery Bypass Surgery, Medical and Scientific Aspects, N.I.H., Bethesda, Maryland, December 1980.

Spencer, F. C., Yong, N. K., and Prachuabmoh, K.: Internal mammary–coronary artery anastomoses performed during cardiopulmonary bypass. Cardiovasc. Surg., 5:292, 1964.

Spencer, F. C., Green, G. E., Tice, D. A., Wallsh, E., Mills, N. L., and Glassman, E.: Coronary artery bypass grafts for congestive heart failure. A report of experiences with 40 patients. J. Thorac. Cardiovasc. Surg., 62:529, 1971.

Spencer, F. C., Isom, O. W., Glassman, E., Boyd, A. D., Engelman, R. M., Reed, G. E., Pasternack, B. S., and Dembrow, J. M.: The long-term influence of coronary bypass grafts on myocardial infarction and survival. Ann. Surg., 180:439, 1974.

Srungaram, R. K., Cunningham, J. N., Jr., Catinella, F. P., Knopp, E. A., Nathan, I. M., and Spencer, F. C.: Blood versus crystalloid cardioplegia: Which is superior for prolonged aortic cross-clamping? Surg. Forum, 32:288, 1981.

Stamler, J.: Dietary and serum lipids in the multifactorial etiology of atherosclerosis. Arch. Surg., 113:21, 1978.

Stiles, Q. R.: Use of a punch to obtain a consistently uniform venotomy for rapid coronary anastomoses. J. Thorac. Cardiovasc. Surg., 82:154, 1981.

Symposium: Current status of aortocoronary bypass surgery. Contemp. Surg., 19:113, 1981.

Tyras, D. H., Ahmad, N., Kaiser, G. C., Barner, H. B., Codd, J. E., and William, V. L.: Ventricular function and the native coronary circulation five years after myocardial revascularization. Ann. Thorac. Surg., 27:547, 1979.

Unstable angina pectoris: National Cooperative Study Group to compare surgical and medical treatment. II. In-hospital experience and initial follow-up results in patients with one, two and three vessel disease. Am. J. Cardiol., 42:839, 1978.

U. S. Department of Health, Education and Welfare: Proceedings of the Conference on the Decline in Coronary Heart Disease Mortality. NIH Publication 79-1610. Washington, D.C., U. S. Government Printing Office, May 1979.

Weisz, D., Hamby, R. I., Aintablian, A., Voleti, C., Fogel, R., and Wisoff, B. G.: Late coronary bypass graft flow: Quantitative assessment by roentgendensitometry. Ann. Thorac. Surg., 28:429, 1979.

Wukasch, D. C., Cooley, D. A., Hall, R. J., Reul, G. J., Jr., Sandiford, F. M., and Zillgitt, S. L.: Surgical versus medical treatment of coronary artery disease. Nine year follow-up of 9,061 patients. Am. J. Surg., 137:201, 1979.

2. Internal Mammary–Coronary Artery Anastomosis for Myocardial Ischemia

GEORGE E. GREEN

HISTORICAL ASPECTS

The internal mammary artery has been part of myocardial revascularization since the 1940s when Vineberg began laboratory studies on collateral circulation from the mammary artery implanted into the myocardium to surrounding coronary arterioles (Vineberg, 1946). Several investigators later reported successful suture anastomosis of the internal mammary artery to coronary arteries in the dog (Spencer et al., 1964). The common feature of these investigations was anastomosis to large proximal coronary trunks, but the diffuse nature of coronary arteriosclerosis precluded successful transfer of these experimental experiences to clinical application. A large clinical experience with Vineberg's internal mammary artery *implantation* was reported by Effler in 1965.

I began evaluation of internal mammary anastomosis to coronary arteries that were 1 mm. in diameter in 1965. Laboratory evaluation of techniques and 2-year follow-up of animals operated were completed, and clinical application was initiated in 1968 (Green *et al.,* 1968). This procedure was the first planned and sustained clinical application of bypass surgery of the left coronary artery. The first operations consisted of internal mammary artery–to–distal left anterior descending coronary artery anastomosis alone (February to May 1968). It was hoped that a single distal anastomosis would afford homogeneous augmentation of myocardial perfusion through the dilated arteriolar bed of ischemic heart disease (Blumgart *et al.,* 1959). Three of the first nine patients died within 30 days of operation; in each, myocardial infarction had occurred in areas that were not perfused by the single internal mammary artery anastomosis. In June 1968, internal mammary artery anastomosis was combined with single aorta–coronary saphenous vein bypass and, in November 1969, with multiple saphenous vein grafts. Thereafter, the hospital mortality rate remained below 5 per cent. Since 1971, the hospital mortality rate has been 1 per cent. Early concern about adequacy of flow from the internal mammary artery compared with that from saphenous vein grafts was resolved favorably by clinical investigation (Green, 1971; Green *et al.,* 1979).

When it became clear that patency rates of internal mammary artery anastomoses were significantly higher than those of saphenous vein grafts (Edwards *et al.,* 1970; Green, 1972; Loop *et al.,* 1973; Kay *et al.,* 1974), application of double internal mammary artery anastomoses was begun (Green, 1973). Limitations of double internal mammary artery anastomoses will be discussed in the following section.

ANATOMIC, HISTOLOGIC, AND PHYSIOLOGIC ASPECTS

Coronary arterial segments free of gross arteriosclerotic changes usually have an internal diameter (measured by calibrated probes [Figs. 50–97 and 50–98]) of 1 to 2 mm. If the internal mammary artery is to be anastomosed to such a segment, it should be 2 mm. in diameter. As the mammary artery is dissected from its subclavian origin to its epigastric termination, it gives off intercostal branches and becomes progressively smaller. At the level of the xiphoid process or sixth intercostal space, its internal diameter is usually less than 2 mm. At the level of the fifth intercostal space, its internal diameter is usually 2 mm. When the left mammary artery is mobilized from its origin to the fifth interspace, it will reach most segments of the left anterior descending coronary artery and many segments of the circumflex artery.

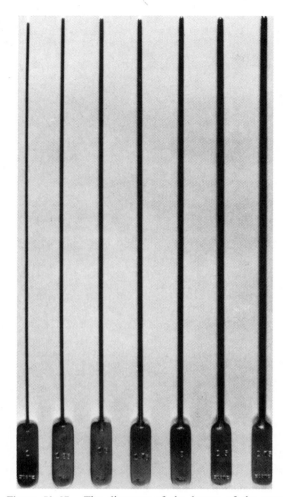

Figure 50–97. The diameter of the lumen of the coronary segment and of the mammary artery is determined by probes calibrated in 0.25-mm. dimensions. (From Green, G. E., *et al.*: Coronary bypass surgery. Five-year follow-up of a consecutive series of 140 patients. J. Thorac. Cardiovasc. Surg., 77:48, 1979.)

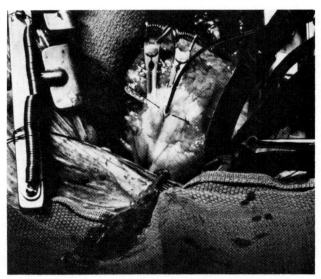

Figure 50–98. Arterial diameter is considered to be that of the largest probe easily accepted. (From Green, G. E.: Technique of internal mammary–coronary artery anastomosis. J. Thorac. Cardiovasc. Surg., 78:455, 1979.)

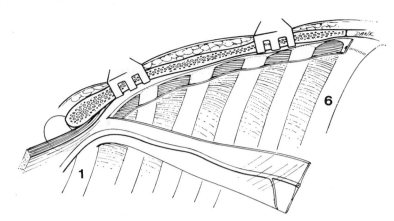

Figure 50–99. Mobilization of the internal mammary arterial pedicle is performed with the coagulation current of electrocautery. Margins of dissection are 1 cm. medial and 1 cm. lateral to the artery. Base of dissection is costal cartilage and external intercostal muscle. (From Green, G. E.: Rate of blood flow from the internal mammary artery. Surgery, *70*:809, 1971.)

However, with the sternum separated, a significantly longer length of the right mammary artery is required to reach distal left coronary artery segments. Lengths of the right mammary artery sufficient to reach distal left coronary artery segments or distal right or posterior descending coronary artery segments usually have a terminal diameter less than 2 mm. These are the limiting factors in double internal mammary artery anastomosis.

The internal mammary artery has been used as a free graft by mobilizing the pedicle, transecting it from its subclavian origin, and interposing it between the aorta and the coronary artery (Loop *et al.*, 1973). The friability of the internal mammary artery makes it less suitable for aortic anastomosis than a saphenous vein segment. Moreover, the reason for the superior long-term results of pedicled internal mammary artery grafts (Green, 1972; Kay *et al.*, 1974; Tector *et al.*, 1976; Loop *et al.*, 1977) is the stability of pedicled grafts compared with free grafts. The vasa vasorum of the pedicled internal mammary artery grafts are intact; the homeostasis of the artery and its endothelium remain intact. The vasa vasorum of free grafts are totally disrupted, and because of this, free grafts are subject to ischemic damage and sloughing of endothelium. Until vasa vasorum and endothelium have regenerated, the fibroblasts of the subintimal zone are in a hyperplastic state. This hyperplasia causes subintimal fibrosis and can cause stricture or total obstruction (Wyatt and Taylor, 1966; Chu-Jeng Chiu, 1976). Moreover, absence of endothelium predisposes to accelerated atherosclerosis—a liability shared by free grafts and endarterectomized segments (Rossiter *et al.*, 1974; Bulkley and Hutchins, 1977).

A disadvantage of the use of the internal artery is the time required for mobilization of the artery, during which other intrathoracic manipulation cannot be performed. It is therefore important that mobilization be done rapidly. Using the pure coagulation current of the electrocautery and the two anatomic planes, mammary artery mobilization can be done in 15 minutes (Fig. 50–99). The steps for mobilization

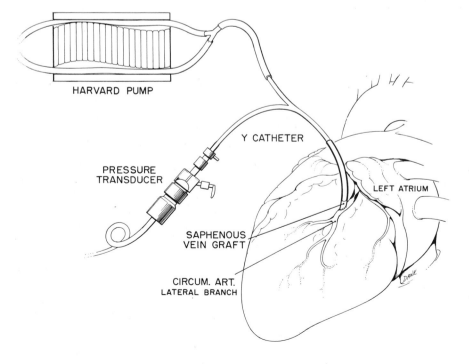

Figure 50–100. Flow capacities of various coronary segments were measured in 25 patients by infusion of blood into vein grafts and simultaneously measuring pressure. Capacity was defined as the flow at which coronary pressure equaled systemic pressure.

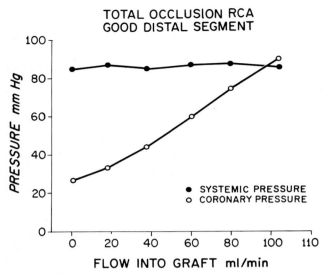

Figure 50–101. Flow capacity of normal distal segments was usually in the range of 100 ml. per minute.

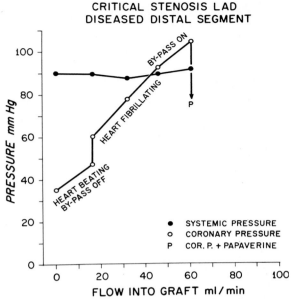

Figure 50–102. Flow capacity of diffusely diseased distal segments was usually in the range of 40 ml. per minute.

are as follow: the arterial pedicle should be separated from costal cartilages, leaving perichondrium on the pedicle; cartilage should be bared of perichondrium. After the pedicle is separated from costal cartilages, it should be separated from the external intercostal muscle; the internal intercostal muscle is left attached to the pedicle. This assures transection of arterial branches far from the parent artery. As do all arteries, the internal mammary artery has three conspicuous components—adventitia, media, and intima. The complex arterial structure makes it more friable than a vein, and in contrast to preparation of a saphenous vein segment, care must be taken to prevent traumatic separation of the arterial layers during mobilization and anastomosis.

After the pedicle has been separated from the chest wall, it is important to ascertain that flow from it is adequate. Operating room studies of capacity of various coronary vascular beds have shown that primary coronary trunks (i.e., those of the left anterior descending, right, or circumflex coronary artery) that are free of disease usually can accept more than 100 ml. of blood per minute, whereas diffusely diseased segments can accept only 20 to 40 ml. per minute (Figs. 50–100 to 50–102). Free flow should be measured from the cut end of the internal mammary artery, and the artery should be used for anastomosis only if its flow capacity is as large as the estimated capacity of the distal coronary bed. The artery will be suitable in 90 per cent of instances (Figs. 50–103 and 50–104).

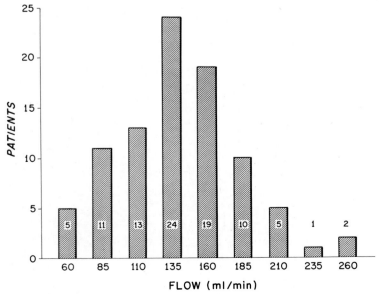

Figure 50–103. Flow was recorded from the transected end of the internal mammary artery in 89 consecutive patients just before mammary artery anastomosis.

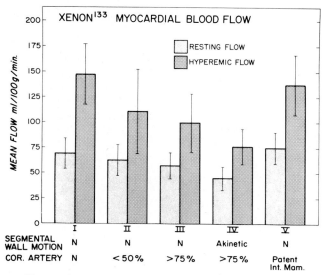

XENON^{133} MYOCARDIAL BLOOD FLOW

RESTING FLOW
HYPEREMIC FLOW

MEAN FLOW ml/100g/min.

SEGMENTAL WALL MOTION	I N	II N	III N	IV Akinetic	V N
COR. ARTERY	N	<50%	>75%	>75%	Patent Int. Mam.

Figure 50–104. Late postoperative measurement of resting and hyperemic blood flow with radioactive xenon demonstrates that the technique of measurement can quantitate varying degrees of coronary obstruction. The data further demonstrate that flow through mammary artery grafts is identical to flow through normal coronary arteries. (From Green, G. E., et al.: Coronary bypass surgery. Five-year follow-up of a consecutive series of 140 patients. J. Thorac. Cardiovasc. Surg., 77:48, 1979.)

SURGICAL TECHNIQUE

The following guidelines in surgical technique have been developed since 1968, during which time I have performed internal mammary artery anastomoses in more than 2000 patients. During the induction of anesthesia and until circulatory support with the heart-lung machine is instituted, systolic blood pressure should be kept down to a maximal range of 80 to 100 mm. Hg by the use of intravenous nitroglycerin.

A median sternotomy incision affords the best exposure. As soon as the sternotomy is completed, the pericardium should be opened and the pulmonary artery palpated. If the pulmonary artery is tense, despite maintenance of systolic blood pressure in the range of 80 to 100 mm. Hg, circulatory support with the heart-lung machine should be instituted. Excessive bleeding has not been encountered as a result of mobilizing the internal mammary artery after the institution of circulatory support, but myocardial infarction has occurred when pulmonary hypertension has not been used as an indication of the need for circulatory support. Favaloro's self-retaining sternal retractor is an important aid to exposure. Progressive rather than sudden traction on the sternum and chest wall should be made to prevent separation of cartilages from the ribs. Division of diaphragmatic muscular and fascial attachments from the posterior rectus sheath and costal arch facilitates maximal lateral traction on the sternum and chest wall. Exposure is improved by dividing the pleura and packing down the lung. Pleura and transverse thoracic muscle and fascia are divided

over the mammary artery in the fifth intercostal space to visualize the internal mammary artery. If the artery is smaller than 2 mm. in external diameter, no further dissection of it is made because it will be inadequate for anastomosis. If the external diameter is 2 mm. or larger, the pure coagulation current of the cautery is used to divide pleura, perichondrium, and internal intercostal muscle 1 cm. medial to and 1 cm. lateral to the mammary artery. The coagulating current is then turned down to the lowest intensity, which will divide thin tissue planes. With controlled traction on the internal mammary arterial pedicle, the perichondrium of the pedicle is separated from the underlying costal cartilages. Further traction facilitates separation of the internal intercostal muscle on the pedicle from the external intercostal muscle underlying the pedicle. The pedicle is completely mobilized to the top of the first rib. It is then mobilized distally to the sixth intercostal space. Heparin is administered at this time, and then the pedicle is clamped and divided. The bed of the pedicle on the chest wall is scrutinized, and any bleeding points are coagulated. The Favaloro retractor is removed.

By inspection and palpation, the site for coronary arteriotomy is determined, and the epicardium adjacent to it is marked with a stitch. Before the heart is decompressed, the optimal length for the pedicled graft is judged, and the pedicle is again divided (Fig. 50–105). As previously noted, definition of adequate flow from the internal mammary artery depends on the vascular bed to which it is to be sewn; however, if flow is less than 60 ml. per minute and cannot be increased to 60 ml. per minute by intra-arterial flushing with papaverine (30 mg. per 100 ml. of saline), it should not be used for coronary anastomosis.

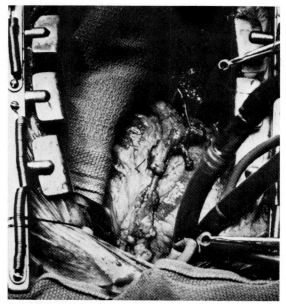

Figure 50–105. Length of the pedicle is tailored. (From Green, G. E.: Technique of internal mammary–coronary artery anastomosis. J. Thorac. Cardiovasc. Surg., 78:455, 1979.)

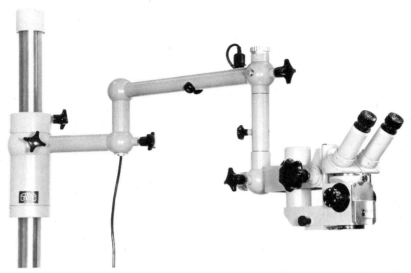

Figure 50–106. A Zeiss operation microscope used at 16× magnification facilitates the procedure. (From Green, G. E., Spencer, F. C., Tice, D. A., and Stertzer, S. H.: Arterial and venous microsurgical bypass grafts for coronary artery disease. J. Thorac. Cardiovasc. Surg., *60*:491, 1970.)

Heart-lung bypass is initiated, and the left ventricle is vented. Arteriotomy and anastomosis can be performed either in the fibrillating cool (28°C.) heart or in the totally arrested and ischemic heart. Exposure is usually superior when the heart has been arrested by clamping the aorta and administering cardioplegic solution. However, in the arrested ischemic heart, air replaces blood in the coronary arteries, and this air must be bled out before the suture securing the internal mammary–coronary artery anastomosis is tied if potential ischemic damage is to be prevented. An appropriate slit is made in the internal mammary artery, and suture anastomosis is performed. I prefer to utilize a continuous 7-0 monofilament suture, using the operating microscope at 16× magnification (Fig. 50–106). Other techniques have been used (Loop *et al.*, 1973; Kay *et al.*, 1974).

After completion of anastomosis, the mean perfusion pressure should be elevated to 100 mm. Hg to ascertain that the suture line is hemostatic. At that pressure, the pedicle is again scanned for bleeding points.

After discontinuation of heart-lung bypass, adequacy of anastomosis can be estimated by the presence of a strong retrograde pulse in the mammary artery when the pedicle is occluded proximally. Operating room studies with electromagnetic flowmeters have shown average flows of 50 ml. per minute (Green *et al.*, 1970). Postoperative studies with xenon-131 have shown flows equal to normal coronary flow (Fig. 50–104) (Green *et al.*, 1979).

Postoperative indicators of adequacy of revascularization are elimination of angina and elimination of ischemic electrocardiographic exercise changes. Postoperative arteriography is the best indicator of success. Patency of anastomosis has been reported in 95 per cent of cases by several authors (Edwards *et al.*, 1970; Green, 1972; Kay *et al.*, 1974; Loop *et al.*,

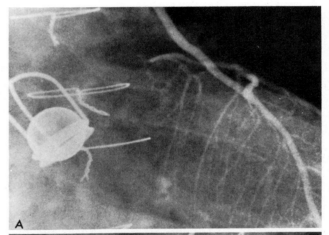

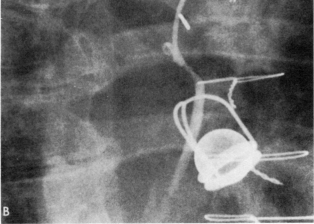

Figure 50–107. Eleven years following aortic valve replacement, internal mammary artery anastomosis to the left anterior descending artery, and a saphenous vein graft to the right coronary segment, angiography showed *(A)* a well-functioning internal mammary artery anastomosis and *(B)* a vein graft that had become stenotic just beyond the aortic anastomosis.

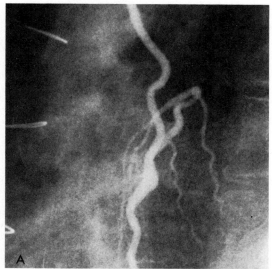

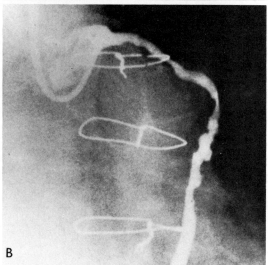

Figure 50–108. Eight years after internal mammary artery anastomosis to the left anterior descending artery and saphenous vein grafts to each of the two components of the circumflex artery, angiography showed *(A)* a well-functioning internal mammary artery anastomosis and *(B)* occlusion of one saphenous vein graft and severe atheromatous stenosis of the other saphenous vein graft.

1973). In addition to demonstration of patency, the arteriogram should show an internal mammary artery that is larger than the coronary vessel to which it is anastomosed. There should be no stenosis in the artery or at the site of the anastomosis. Transit of dye through the internal mammary artery should be brisk. Opacification of the coronary arterial system should be intense.

On sequential angiograms over a 13-year period, late alterations have not been detected in pedicled internal mammary arteries properly anastomosed to coronary artery segments (Figs. 50–107 and 50–108). Similar findings were reported by Tector and associates (1981). High patency and stability make internal mammary artery anastomosis an outstanding procedure in coronary revascularization.

Despite the advantages of internal mammary–

artery anastomosis, only 6 per cent of surgeons routinely use it (Miller *et al.,* 1977). It is technically more demanding than an aortocoronary saphenous vein graft.

SELECTED REFERENCES

Blumgart, H. L., Zoll, P. M., and Kurland, G.: Discussion of direct relief of coronary occlusion; the anatomic pathologic problem. Arch. Intern. Med., *104*:862, 1959.

Twenty years prior to this work, Blumgart and associates published the first of a series of postmortem studies of the alterations in coronary circulation caused by atherosclerosis. For more than two decades their findings were essentially the only angiographic data correlated with coronary artery disease. However, their conclusion about the planning of surgical intervention was erroneous. Planned reliance on the efficacy of collateral circulation will not yield optimal results.

Green, G. E.: Rate of flow from the internal mammary artery. Surgery, *70*:809, 1971.

When objections of the use of the internal mammary artery as a bypass graft were made on the grounds of limited flow, the limits of flow were methodically studied. It was found that flow capacity was inversely related to the length of the pedicle. Length of the pedicle is a limiting factor in using the internal mammary artery. However, with proper estimation of the flow that can be accepted by the coronary bed and proper selection of pedicle length, serial results of internal mammary artery bypass are unequaled in excellence.

Green, G. E., Som, M. L., and Wolff, W. I.: Experimental microvascular suture anastomosis. Circulation, *33*:1, 1966.

As a first step in establishing a program for coronary artery surgery, the patency rate of a series of measured vascular anastomoses was explored. As predicted by Jacobson, using the operating microscope at 16 to 25× magnifications, a patency rate better than 90 per cent was obtained. It is historically interesting that objections to the application of the operating microscope to cardiac surgery centered on the need for a very still field; now use of heart-lung bypass and cardiac arrest is common, but use of the operating microscope still is not.

Green, G. E., Stertzer, S. H., and Reppert, E. H.: Coronary arterial bypass grafts. Ann. Thorac. Surg., *5*:443, 1968.

This was the first and remains the only experimental study proving the feasibility of 1-mm. coronary arterial anastomosis with high long-term patency. It concludes with the first published report of bypass to the left coronary artery in humans.

Green, G. E., Kemp, H. G., Alan, S. E., Pierson, R. N., Friedman, M. I., and David, I.: Coronary bypass surgery. Five-year follow-up of a consecutive series of 140 patients. J. Thorac. Cardiovasc. Surg., *77*:48, 1979.

Late postoperative evaluation of flow through mammary artery grafts as measured by selective injection of xenon-133 showed both resting and hyperemic flow through the internal mammary artery grafts to be the same as resting and hyperemic flow through normal coronary arteries.

REFERENCES

Blumgart H. L., Zoll, P. M., and Kurland, G.: Discussion of direct relief of coronary occlusion: The anatomic pathologic problem. Arch. Intern. Med., *104*:862, 1959.
Bulkley, B. H., and Hutchins, G. M.: Accelerated atherosclerosis:

A morphologic study of 97 saphenous vein coronary artery bypass grafts. Circulation, 55:163, 1977.

Chiu, Chu-Jeng: Why do radial artery grafts for aorto-coronary bypass fail? A reappraisal. Ann. Thorac. Surg., 22:520, 1976.

Edwards, W. S., Jones, W. B., Dear, H. D., and Kerr, A. R.: Direct surgery for coronary artery disease: Technique for left anterior descending coronary artery bypass. J.A.M.A., 211:1182, 1970.

Effler, D. B., Sones, F. M., Groves, L. K., and Suarez, E.: Myocardial revascularization by Vineberg's internal mammary artery implant. J. Thorac. Cardiovasc. Surg., 50:527, 1965.

Geha, A. S., Krone, R. J., McCormick, J. R., et al.: Selection of coronary bypass: Anatomic, physiological, and angiographic consideration of vein and mammary artery grafts. J. Thorac. Cardiovasc. Surg., 70:414, 1975.

Green, G. E.: Technique of internal mammary–coronary artery anastomosis. J. Thorac. Cardiovasc. Surg., 78:455, 1979.

Green, G. E.: Discussion of aorta–to–coronary radial artery bypass grafts. Ann. Thorac. Surg., 16:118, 1973.

Green, G. E.: Internal mammary–coronary artery anastomosis: Three year experience with 165 patients. Ann. Thorac. Surg., 14:260, 1972.

Green, G. E.: Rate of flow from the internal mammary artery. Surgery, 70:809, 1971.

Green, G. E., Som, M. L., and Wolff, W. I.: Experimental microvascular suture anastomosis. Circulation, 33:1, 1966.

Green, G. E., Stertzer, S. H., and Reppert, E. H.: Coronary arterial bypass grafts. Ann. Thorac. Surg., 5:443, 1968.

Green, G. E., Spencer, F. C., Tice, D. A., and Stertzer, S. H.: Arterial and venous microsurgical grafts for coronary artery disease. J. Thorac. Cardiovasc. Surg., 60:491, 1970.

Green, G. E., Kemp, H. G., Alan, S. E., Pierson, R. N., Friedman, M. I., and David, I.: Coronary bypass surgery. Five-year follow-up of a consecutive series of 140 patients. J. Thorac. Cardiovasc. Surg., 77:48, 1979.

Kay, E. B., Naraghipour, H., Beg, R. A., DeManey, M., Tambe, A., and Zimmerman, H. A.: Long term follow-up of internal mammary artery bypass. Ann. Thorac. Surg., 18:269, 1974.

Loop, F. D., Irazzaval, M. J., Bredee, J. J., et al.: Internal mammary artery graft for ischemic heart disease: Effect of revascularization on clinical status and survival. Am. J. Cardiol., 39:516, 1977.

Loop, F. D., Spampinato, N., Cheanvechai, C., and Effler, D.: The free internal mammary artery bypass graft. Ann. Thorac. Surg., 15:53, 1973.

Miller, D. W., Hessell, E. L., II, Winterscheid, L. C., et al.: Current practice of coronary artery bypass surgery. J. Thorac. Cardiovasc. Surg., 73:75, 1977.

Rossiter, S. J., Brody, W. R., Kosek, J. C., et al.: Internal mammary artery versus autogenous vein for coronary artery bypass graft. Circulation, 50:1236, 1974.

Spencer, F. C., Yong, N. K., and Prachubrioh, K.: Internal mammary–coronary anastomosis performed during cardiopulmonary bypass. J. Cardiovasc. Surg., 5:292, 1964.

Tector, A. J., Davis, L., Gabriel, R., et al.: Experience with internal mammary artery grafts in 298 patients. Ann. Thorac. Surg., 22:515, 1976.

Tector, A. J., Terren, M. D., Schamahl, M., Janson, B., Kallies, J. R., and Johnson, G.: The internal mammary artery graft. Its longevity after coronary bypass. J.A.M.A., 246:281, 1981.

Vineberg, A. M.: Development of anastomosis between coronary vessels and transplanted internal mammary artery. Can. Med. Assoc. J., 55:117, 1946.

Wyatt, A. P., and Taylor, G. W.: Vein grafts. Changes in the endothelium of autogenous free vein grafts used as arterial replacements. Br. J. Surg., 53:943, 1966.

3. Prinzmetal's Variant Angina and Other Syndromes Associated with Coronary Artery Spasm

JAMES E. LOWE

In 1768, William Heberden presented a manuscript before the Royal College of Physicians of London entitled "Some Account of a Disorder of the Breast," in which he described chest pain associated with effort, eating, or anxiety. He termed this pain angina pectoris from the Greek word *anchein,* meaning "to choke." Subsequently, it has been shown that the pain of angina pectoris is associated with myocardial ischemia, although the neurophysiology of exactly how this pain is perceived remains unknown.

Since Heberden's original description of angina pectoris, several anginal syndromes have been described that have different clinical implications. Until relatively recently, it was thought that the underlying pathophysiology operative in these syndromes was related to various degrees of subtotal or totally obstructive atherosclerotic coronary artery disease and that clinically identifiable subgroups of patients had similar degrees of obstruction at certain anatomic sites that resulted in similar degrees of myocardial ischemic dysfunction. However, in 1959, Myron Prinzmetal reported 32 patients with a distinctly different type of anginal syndrome that could not be explained solely by the degree of atherosclerotic coronary artery disease thought to be present. Prinzmetal suggested that transient coronary artery spasm was occurring in this interesting subgroup. Subsequently, coronary artery spasm has been documented in increasing numbers of patients and is associated with a variety of clinical presentations, which will be discussed. Recognition of patients with coronary artery spasm and the selection of appropriate therapeutic interventions are two of the most current and significant problems challenging both cardiologists and cardiovascular surgeons.

CLASSIFICATION OF ANGINAL SYNDROMES

Since Heberden's original description of angina pectoris, it has been shown that there are various subgroups of patients with different types of angina that are important to identify because they have different clinical courses. *Stable angina* is the pain syndrome originally described by Heberden. It is associated with effort, anxiety, or eating. Although the frequency of attacks can increase over time, this type of angina usually remains predictable and stable over long periods. *Unstable angina* is a rapidly progressing pain syndrome that often results in myocardial infarction unless relieved by medical therapy or coronary artery bypass grafting. *Variant angina* is a distinctly different pain syndrome caused by coronary artery spasm, which can occur in normal coronary arteries or, more commonly, in coronary arteries with atherosclerotic lesions. Unlike stable and unstable angina, variant angina is not brought on by effort, eating, or anxiety. *Atypical angina* is a vague term that has a variety of meanings. To some, it represents chest pain secondary to coronary artery disease (with or without concomitant spasm) with a different kind of pain pattern, for example, pain radiating into the right chest or right arm; others have used the term to refer to chest pain that may not even be related to coronary disease. Finally, angina is observed in patients with congenital coronary arterial malformations such as coronary artery fistulas or anomalous origin of the left coronary artery from the pulmonary artery. In these patients, angina results not from atherosclerotic disease or spasm, but from a "steal" of normal coronary flow into the recipient cardiac chamber.

Each of these anginal syndromes is referred to by a variety of names. Stable angina is referred to as typical angina, classic angina, or Heberden's angina. It is also known as effort angina because of its association with exercise, eating, or anxiety, and recently, Maseri and associates (1978a) have termed it secondary angina because it appears to result secondary to fixed obstructive atherosclerotic coronary artery disease. Unstable angina is also known as preinfarction or crescendo angina because of its rapidly progressing nature. Stenosis of the left main coronary artery is one of the anatomic causes of this type of pain, and its clinical recognition is of obvious importance, because marked improvement in survival can be achieved by coronary artery bypass grafting. Variant angina is also known as Prinzmetal's angina, after Myron Prinzmetal, who first described its clinical manifestations in 1959, vasospastic angina, and angina decubitus, since it usually occurs at rest, and Maseri and colleagues (1978a) have termed it primary angina because it is caused by spasm of the coronary arteries and is not secondary to atherosclerotic disease alone. For clarification, the terminology used to describe these various anginal syndromes is summarized in Table 50–13.

PRINZMETAL'S VARIANT ANGINA

Stable angina, or classic Heberden's angina, is a distinct syndrome with two major clinical manifestations. First, the pain occurs when more work is demanded of the heart and is relieved by rest or the administration of nitroglycerin. Second, the electrocardiogram during an episode of pain often shows ST-segment depression in certain leads without reciprocal elevation. As mentioned previously, in 1959, Myron Prinzmetal reported 32 patients, 20 of whom were personally observed, with a distinctly different anginal syndrome. He referred to this syndrome as "a variant form of angina pectoris." Prinzmetal noted that this variant form of angina appeared to occur at rest or during ordinary activity and was not brought on by exercise, eating, or emotional stress. The pain was in the same location as that of classic angina, although the duration was usually longer and the pain more severe. Attacks often occurred at the same time each day or night, and the waxing and waning of the pain were of equal duration. Nitroglycerin would promptly relieve the pain of variant angina, but unlike classic angina, the electrocardiogram often showed ST-segment elevation mimicking changes observed in patients with acute myocardial infarction (Fig. 50–109). The ST-segment elevations were usually related to the

TABLE 50–13. ANGINAL SYNDROMES

STABLE ANGINA
    Heberden's angina
    Classic angina
    Typical angina
    Effort angina
    Secondary angina

UNSTABLE ANGINA
    Preinfarction angina
    Crescendo angina

VARIANT ANGINA
    Prinzmetal's angina
    Vasospastic angina
    Angina decubitus
    Primary angina

ATYPICAL ANGINA

ANGINA SECONDARY TO A STEAL PHENOMENON
    (Congenital coronary fistulas and anomalous origin of
    the left coronary artery from the pulmonary artery)

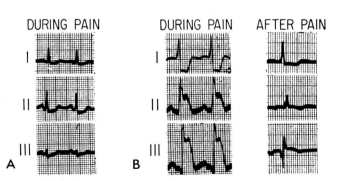

Figure 50–109. Comparison of electrocardiographic characteristics of classic angina pectoris and the variant form. *A*, Classic angina pectoris: ST segments show depression without reciprocal ST elevation. Electrocardiogram obtained after exercise. *B*, Variant form of angina pectoris: During spontaneous pain, ST segments show elevation in leads II and III with reciprocal ST depression in lead I. Immediately after pain, the electrocardiogram returns to normal or to pre-pain pattern. (From Prinzmetal, M., Kennamer, R., Merliss, R., Wada, T., and Bor, N.: Angina pectoris. I. A variant form of angina pectoris. Am. J. Med., 27:375, 1959.)

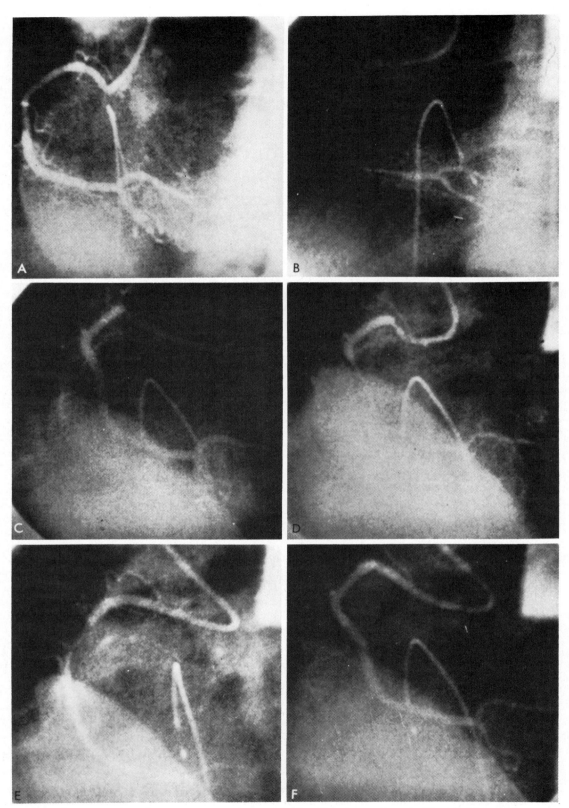

Figure 50–110. Documentation of coronary spasm during episodes of variant angina. *A,* Normal right coronary artery while the patient was pain-free, without electrocardiographic changes. *B,* During a spontaneous attack of angina, with electrocardiographic changes and spasm of a long segment of the midportion of the right coronary artery. *C,* During an injection while the patient was pain-free, showing a normal vessel (spasm could not be induced by the catheter or the contrast medium). *D,* Spasm of a long segment extending into the distal right coronary artery and posterior descending artery during the next attack of pain. *E,* During a subsequent but separate attack of angina, when a segmental area of spasm is noted. *F,* Within 2 minutes the angina subsided, and the vessel appeared normal.

Illustration continued on opposite page

distribution of one large coronary artery. Exercise testing of these patients could cause ST-segment depression but did not result in pain unless the patient also had angina secondary to fixed obstructive disease. Dysrhythmias were common during the pain of variant angina, and transient Q waves were occasionally observed. Prinzmetal further observed that infarction resulted in some patients weeks or months later in areas of previous ST-segment elevation. Finally, he noted that the pain of variant angina was often relieved by myocardial infarction, which was unlike the pain of stable angina, which often worsened following myocardial infarction. These precise and detailed observations remain the classic clinical criteria for establishing a diagnosis of variant angina today.

In addition to the observations described, Prinzmetal also noted that "it is not uncommon for both the variant and classic forms of angina pectoris to occur together in the same patient." The clinical significance of this observation is far-reaching and will be discussed in detail later. Subsequently, it has been well documented that coronary artery spasm occurs most commonly in patients with concomitant atherosclerotic coronary artery disease, but a number of patients have also been identified with variant angina and normal-appearing coronary arteries by arteriography. This subgroup of patients with "normal coronary arteries" and variant angina have been referred to as patients with a "variant of the variant" anginal syndrome of Prinzmetal (Cheng *et al.*, 1973; Guazzi *et al.*, 1976).

Of final significance in his classic manuscript, Prinzmetal postulated that "temporary increased tonus of a large coronary artery is suggested as the cause of pain in the variant form of angina." Arteriographic evidence of coronary artery spasm during an attack of Prinzmetal's variant angina was subsequently demonstrated by Phillip Oliva and associates in 1973 (Fig. 50–110).

Since Prinzmetal's initial observations reported in 1959 and following the conclusive demonstration of coronary artery spasm in patients with variant angina

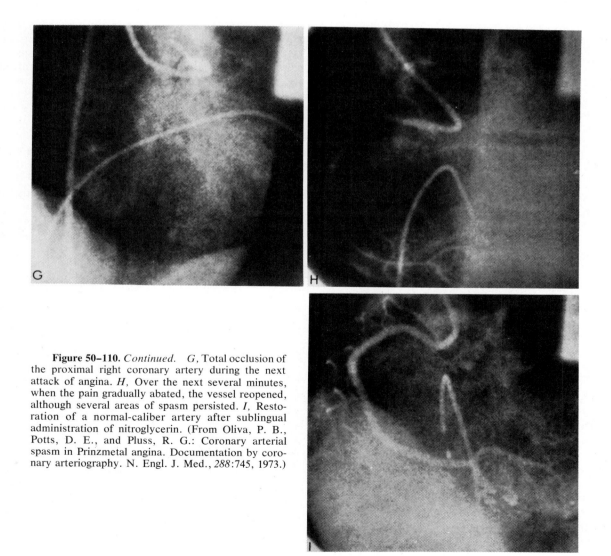

Figure 50–110. *Continued.* *G,* Total occlusion of the proximal right coronary artery during the next attack of angina. *H,* Over the next several minutes, when the pain gradually abated, the vessel reopened, although several areas of spasm persisted. *I,* Restoration of a normal-caliber artery after sublingual administration of nitroglycerin. (From Oliva, P. B., Potts, D. E., and Pluss, R. G.: Coronary arterial spasm in Prinzmetal angina. Documentation by coronary arteriography. N. Engl. J. Med., *288*:745, 1973.)

by Oliva and coworkers in 1973, a variety of other syndromes have been recognized in which coronary spasm is either responsible for the clinical manifestations or at least contributing to the clinical course of events. These will be discussed later.

Diagnosis and Incidence

It is generally accepted that coronary artery spasm may occur in both normal and diseased coronary arteries, but until recently, spasm was considered to be a rare phenomenon. The clinical significance of coronary artery spasm has been underrated by some because of its rarity during selective coronary arteriography (0.26 to 0.93 per cent) and the frequent absence of associated symptoms when spasm is documented (Demany et al., 1968; O'Reilly et al., 1970; Lavine et al., 1973). However, Chahine and associates (1975) reviewed 274 consecutive coronary angiograms obtained over a 1-year period and documented eight cases of spasm (3 per cent). This incidence, which was higher than that previously reported, was attributed to a systematic prospective search for the phenomenon and avoidance of vasodilators and premedication prior to arteriography. Although many cases of arteriographically demonstrated spasm are related to catheter tip irritation, Chahine has suggested that catheter-induced spasm may occur only in patients with a predisposition to spasm. Furthermore, spasm is often not specifically looked for because the majority of patients with spasm also have fixed obstructive coronary lesions, which are thought to explain their symptoms. Clinically, it is often difficult to obtain an electrocardiogram during an episode of spontaneous chest pain since attacks may be infrequent and often occur during sleep. Numerous provocation tests have been studied, but at present, only ergonovine appears to be diagnostically useful. Ergonovine is an ergot alkaloid and smooth muscle constrictor. Conti and colleagues (1979) and Oliva (1979) have observed that ergonovine produces spasm in nearly all patients with Prinzmetal's angina and is of diagnostic value if carefully administered during cardiac catheterization.

Once spasm is looked for, the observed incidence appears to increase dramatically. Maseri and coworkers (1978b) have reported that the incidence of variant angina in their experience increased from 2 per cent to more than 10 per cent of patients admitted for evaluation of anginal pain when systematic measures were applied for its detection. Furthermore, these authors have proposed that variant angina is only one manifestation of coronary artery spasm and that spasm contributes to practically all phases of ischemic heart disease.

Although the true incidence of variant angina remains unknown, it is becoming increasingly accepted that coronary artery spasm may be much more common than previously assumed and that spasm may contribute to the clinical manifestations of a variety of syndromes in addition to variant angina.

Natural History

Myocardial infarction and death from either infarction or ventricular arrhythmias are common in patients with documented variant angina. Bentivoglio and associates (1974) reviewed 90 cases reported between 1959 and 1972 for which long-term follow-up data were available. As pointed out by Raizner and Chahine (1980), this group of patients is most representative of the natural history of variant angina since, in 1972, the pathophysiology of the syndrome was not fully appreciated and appropriate therapy not yet in widespread use. Of these 90 patients, 22 (24 per cent) developed acute myocardial infarction within several months following onset of variant angina, and 13 patients (14 per cent) died suddenly. Catastrophic events, therefore, occurred in 38 per cent of the group, usually soon after onset of symptoms. Stenson and colleagues (1975) observed that variant angina that first presents following acute myocardial infarction has an even higher mortality rate (33 per cent). Although the current incidence of myocardial infarction and death in patients with variant angina has decreased, secondary to more aggressive medical and surgical therapy, patients with Prinzmetal's angina should be considered a high-risk subgroup of patients with ischemic heart disease. As a general rule, patients with variant angina and concomitant significant coronary artery disease are at greater risk than the less common group of patients with variant angina and normal coronary arteries (Selzer et al., 1976).

OTHER SYNDROMES ASSOCIATED WITH CORONARY ARTERY SPASM

In addition to Prinzmetal's variant angina, it is becoming increasingly apparent that coronary artery spasm may contribute to the clinical manifestations observed in a variety of ischemic heart disease syndromes (Table 50–14).

"Silent" Variant Angina. Since Prinzmetal's original description of the clinical characteristics of variant angina in 1959, a number of patients have been reported who are found to have ST-segment elevation and documented coronary artery spasm without chest

TABLE 50–14. SYNDROMES ASSOCIATED WITH CORONARY ARTERY SPASM

Prinzmetal's angina
"Silent" variant angina
Partial coronary artery spasm mimicking stable angina
Stable angina and coronary artery spasm
Preinfarction angina
Acute myocardial infarction
Sudden death
Nitrate withdrawal
Perioperative arrest following myocardial revascularization
Other vasospastic disorders
    Raynaud's phenomenon
    Migraine headaches
    Peripheral venous spasm

pain (Guazzi *et al.*, 1970; Lasser and de la Paz, 1973; Gorfinkel *et al.*, 1973; Prohkov *et al.*, 1974; Bodenheimer *et al.*, 1974). Clinically, these patients are obviously difficult to identify because their presenting symptoms are often vague and not directly referable to the heart or they may present with a catastrophic event such as acute myocardial infarction or a life-threatening arrhythmia. This interesting subgroup of patients with variant angina have been said to have "silent" variant angina (Prohkov *et al.*, 1974) since they have all of the hallmarks of Prinzmetal's angina with the important exception of no· accompanying chest pain.

Partial Spasm Mimicking Stable Angina. ST-segment elevation occurring with chest pain and documented coronary artery spasm are the classic clinical criteria for establishing a diagnosis of Prinzmetal's angina. However, Maseri and associates (1975) reported two patients and Chahine and coworkers (1975) reported a third patient with documented partial coronary artery spasm who had pain both at rest and with exercise. In contrast to Prinzmetal's angina, the episodes of pain were associated with ST-segment depression mimicking the electrocardiographic findings usually associated with classic angina secondary to fixed obstructive atherosclerotic coronary disease. Since the majority of patients with coronary artery spasm also have concomitant atherosclerotic disease, the importance of spasm in explaining a given patient's clinical course is perhaps often overlooked.

Coronary Artery Spasm and Stable Angina. A number of patients have been identified with variant angina at rest who have classic effort-induced angina with characteristic ST-segment depression in the same leads that demonstrated ST-segment elevation at rest (Maseri *et al.*, 1977). The identification of these patients is important in view of recent advances in the medical treatment of coronary artery spasm, so that appropriate treatment can be instituted to maximize control of the most important contributor to the chest pain syndrome. As will be discussed later, beta-blockers can exacerbate spasm in some patients and therefore may be contraindicated in those with both fixed obstructive disease and vasospastic disease in which spasm is the predominant feature.

Coronary Artery Spasm Resulting in Preinfarction Angina. It is generally accepted that patients with Prinzmetal's angina can develop a worsening pain syndrome and suffer subsequent myocardial infarction. Distinct from this group are patients with long-standing stable angina or those with recent onset of angina who have definite and severe atherosclerotic coronary disease and subsequently develop an accelerating pain syndrome that leads to infarction unless successful medical or surgical therapy is undertaken. A number of patients who have been observed to have stable, fixed obstructive disease by serial coronary angiograms subsequently progress to preinfarction angina. Linhart and colleagues (1972) and Bolooki and associates (1972) have reported patients with atherosclerotic coronary artery disease and preinfarc-

tion angina who were found to have ST-segment elevation with episodes of pain without evidence of subsequent myocardial infarction. These findings suggest that the addition of spasm to long-standing fixed obstructive disease resulted in preinfarction angina. The patients in both of these reports were successfully managed by coronary artery bypass grafting. These observations do not implicate spasm in all cases of preinfarction angina but are suggestive evidence that in some patients, the addition of spasm to fixed obstructive disease can explain the transition from stable to unstable or preinfarction angina.

Coronary Artery Spasm Resulting in Acute Myocardial Infarction. It is now well documented that coronary artery spasm can result in acute myocardial infarction in patients with variant angina and normal coronary arteries (King *et al.*, 1973; Johnson and Detwiler, 1977) as well as in patients without antecedent signs or symptoms of variant angina who have atherosclerotically diseased vessels (Oliva and Breckinridge, 1977). An intriguing study, reported by Oliva and Breckinridge in 1977, subjected 15 patients who presented with acute myocardial infarction to coronary arteriography within 6 hours following onset of infarction. Coronary angiograms were obtained prior to and following administration of nitroglycerin. Six of the 15 patients (40 per cent) were found to have coronary artery spasm superimposed on a high-grade atherosclerotic lesion. The involved coronary artery remained patent following the initial relief of spasm in two patients who were maintained on sublingual nitrates and heparin. The authors concluded that their results demonstrate the occurrence of spasm in significant numbers of patients with acute myocardial infarction, but they do not establish the importance of spasm in the pathophysiology of acute myocardial infarction or whether relief of spasm has a beneficial or harmful effect on myocardium rendered ischemic for a prolonged period prior to reperfusion. This very important study, however, underscores the necessity of further investigations into the role of spasm in patients with acute myocardial infarction, because of the possible therapeutic implications.

Coronary Artery Spasm Following Acute Myocardial Infarction. Stenson and associates (1975) identified an interesting group of nine patients out of a total of 57 patients who presented with acute myocardial infarction over a 1-year period. These nine patients (16 per cent) demonstrated episodes of angina occurring more than 24 hours after initial infarction, associated with transient ST-segment elevation. Seven of these patients (78 per cent) subsequently suffered a second myocardial infarction within 2 weeks to 4 1/2 months following their first infarction. Three of the nine patients died following reinfarction, an overall mortality rate of 33 per cent. All of these patients were found to have severe atherosclerotic coronary artery disease in addition to clinical evidence for coronary artery spasm. However, none had symptoms of variant angina prior to their first infarction. Thus, spasm appears to have become manifest in these patients following infarction and, furthermore, appears to have markedly increased subsequent morbidity and mortality.

Coronary Artery Spasm Resulting in Sudden Death. A number of patients who die suddenly have been found to have normal coronary arteries at postmortem examination. Presumably, they died of an arrhythmia of uncertain etiology or died secondary to vasospasm and severe ischemia or vasospasm initiating an arrhythmia. Cheng and coworkers (1973) described four patients with variant angina and normal coronary arteries at the time of catheterization. Since Prinzmetal originally postulated that spasm was most likely to occur in association with atherosclerotic lesions, Cheng suggested that spasm occurring in normal coronary arteries was a variant of Prinzmetal's angina and coined the term "a variant of the variant" angina to describe these patients. Interestingly, when one of these patients, a 60-year-old male with angina associated with ST-segment elevation, underwent coronary arteriography, no atherosclerotic disease was revealed. The patient subsequently developed ventricular fibrillation and expired. Postmortem examination confirmed that he had completely normal coronary arteries, strongly implicating coronary artery spasm as the cause of sudden death.

In further support of coronary artery spasm as the underlying mechanism contributing to certain instances of sudden death are numerous reports of ventricular fibrillation occurring in patients with documented coronary artery spasm. Prohkov and associates (1974) reported a patient who presented with ventricular fibrillation. He was successfully resuscitated and underwent coronary arteriography, which revealed total spasm of the right coronary artery, which completely resolved following the sublingual administration of nitroglycerin. Since the patient's coronary arteries were completely free of atherosclerotic lesions and since prior to ventricular fibrillation the patient had no symptoms suggestive of angina, the authors referred to this as "silent" variant angina and suggested that coronary artery spasm be considered a cause of the sudden death syndrome. Recently, Cipriano and colleagues (1981) reported the clinical course of 25 patients with coronary artery spasm documented by arteriography. Ventricular tachycardia occurred in seven patients (28 per cent) and led to death in one patient. Four of these seven patients had absent or minimal atherosclerotic coronary disease, and three had severe atherosclerotic disease in addition to spasm. Collectively, these reports are good evidence that spasm in both normal and diseased coronary arteries can result in life-threatening arrhythmias and the sudden death syndrome.

Coronary Artery Spasm and the Nitrate Withdrawal Syndrome. Lange and coworkers (1972) described the clinical, angiographic, and hemodynamic findings in nine patients who presented with nonatheromatous ischemic heart disease induced by chronic industrial exposure to nitroglycerin and subsequent withdrawal. This fascinating group represented nearly 5 per cent of a group of 200 workers with similar exposure. Five of these patients underwent coronary arteriography, which revealed reversible spasm with no underlying atherosclerotic coronary artery disease. Two patients died suddenly, most likely secondary to reflex coronary artery spasm following nitrate withdrawal. The authors suggested that long-term exposure to nitroglycerin resulted in chronic vasodilatation, which evoked a homeostatic vasoconstrictive response that resulted in severe spasm and ischemia following nitrate withdrawal.

Coronary Artery Spasm Resulting in Perioperative Arrest. Recently, Pichard and associates (1980) reported a patient who presented with both angina at rest and effort-induced angina. Prior to recent worsening of angina, the patient had an 8-year history of stable angina. Exercise testing revealed ST-segment elevation in leads AV_L and V_2 to V_4 in addition to a short run of ventricular tachycardia. Cardiac catheterization revealed a 70 per cent obstruction of the right coronary artery in its proximal third, with a 90 per cent obstruction in the left anterior descending artery proximal to the first septal perforator and a 50 per cent obstruction at the origin of a posterolateral circumflex branch. The left main coronary artery was normal, and the ejection fraction was 90 per cent. In view of his severe obstructive disease and recently worsening angina, the patient underwent uncomplicated internal mammary–to–left anterior descending coronary artery grafting and saphenous vein bypass grafting to the right coronary and posterolateral circumflex coronary arteries. He was easily separated from cardiopulmonary bypass in normal sinus rhythm and displayed evidence of good left ventricular contractility. However, as the chest was being closed, the patient developed rapid atrial fibrillation followed by ventricular arrhythmias and hypotension. He required multiple countershocks and reinstitution of cardiopulmonary bypass support.

The patient eventually was stabilized and again weaned from bypass uneventfully and transported to the intensive care unit. Two hours later, he again became hypotensive, with increasing left atrial pressures and associated ST-segment elevation on monitor leads. These changes progressed to rapid atrial fibrillation and recurrent ventricular tachycardia, which degenerated to ventricular fibrillation refractory to external countershock and intravenous lidocaine and procainamide. The chest was reopened; there was no evidence of tamponade, and all three grafts were found to be patent. With internal massage, the patient was stabilized again and the chest was closed, only to be reopened again 40 minutes later for resuscitation because of another episode of refractory ventricular fibrillation. The patient remained refractory to all resuscitative agents until papaverine (1 mg.) was injected into each graft and nitrol paste (2 per cent) was applied to the skin. Following this, he underwent successful cardioversion. An intra-aortic balloon pump was inserted, and the patient subsequently made an uneventful recovery. Serial postoperative electrocardiograms revealed no evidence of postoperative myocardial infarction. Thirteen days postoperatively, repeat cardiac catheterization revealed all three grafts to be patent. The native coronary circulation and ejection fraction were unchanged from findings prior to operation. However, when the internal mammary artery graft was injected with contrast medium, the patient developed ST-segment elevation without chest pain or arrhythmias. Repeat internal mammary artery visualization revealed severe, diffuse spasm of the entire left anterior descending coronary artery, which resolved following the administration of nitroglycerin. The patient was subsequently maintained on nitroglycerin and aspirin without further problems and returned to work 6 weeks following operation.

Retrospectively, it appears that this patient had fixed obstructive disease and manifested spasm when his angina worsened. Spasm persisted during the perioperative period and resulted in the harrowing course of clinical events reported. Based on these observations, the authors suggest that coronary artery spasm strongly be considered in the differential diagnosis of perioperative hemodynamic deterioration in patients following coronary artery bypass graft surgery, especially in the presence of ST-segment elevation or intractable ventricular arrhythmias. Recently, Buxton and associates (1981) reported an additional six patients who had similar problems immediately following myocardial revascularization. These reports suggest that coronary artery spasm following coronary artery bypass grafting may be more than a rare phenomenon.

Coronary Artery Spasm Associated with Other Vasospastic Disorders. There is some evidence, although not conclusive, that coronary artery spasm may be more common in patients with other vasospastic diseases such as Raynaud's phenomenon, progressive systemic sclerosis, peripheral venous spasm, and migraine headaches. Robertson and Oates (1978) described three patients with both variant angina and Raynaud's phenomenon. One patient underwent continuous electrocardiographic monitoring for 26 days and demonstrated 569 episodes of ST-segment elevation without chest pain ("silent" variant angina). None of these patients showed simultaneous chest pain with attacks of Raynaud's phenomenon, and although a cool environment could trigger signs of Raynaud's phenomenon, it was unrelated to episodes of variant angina. Spasm in normal coronary arteries resulting in myocardial infarction and sudden death has been associated with progressive systemic sclerosis in patients who previously had Raynaud's phenomenon (Bulkley *et al.*, 1978). Recently, Miller and colleagues (1981) studied 62 patients with variant angina and noted a statistically increased incidence of both Raynaud's phenomenon and migraine headaches compared with patients with atherosclerotic coronary disease without signs or symptoms of variant angina. This study, however, did not demonstrate that the prevalence of Raynaud's phenomenon in women with variant angina was statistically higher than in men with variant angina, although Raynaud's phenomenon

is five times more common in women than in men (Coffman and Cohen, 1981).

Of further interest is the report of Dagenais and associates (1970), who described a 15-year-old female with tetralogy of Fallot with severe peripheral venous spasm observed during cardiac catheterization. In association with venous spasm, the patient developed simultaneous chest pain and ST-segment elevation, which resolved at the same time that the venous spasm resolved.

Since Raynaud's phenomenon, migraine headaches, and peripheral venous spasm appear to be triggered at times by emotional stress, it has been suggested that further investigations into the etiology of variant angina should include study of the possibility of a central neurogenic trigger mechanism (Coffman and Cohen, 1981).

PATHOPHYSIOLOGY OF CORONARY ARTERY SPASM

It is well established that spasm can occur in both normal and atherosclerotically diseased coronary arteries and that spasm is an important component in a variety of ischemic heart disease syndromes other than Prinzmetal's variant angina. Furthermore, it has been shown that spasm can completely or partially occlude a coronary artery, involve one or more vessels, and be diffuse or segmental in nature (Conti *et al.*, 1979). Despite the wealth of clinical information available regarding Prinzmetal's angina and the apparent ubiquitous nature of spasm in other coronary syndromes, little is known about the exact pathogenesis of coronary spasm.

There are two general areas of investigation, however, which appear promising; one involves the study of neurogenic mechanisms and the other deals with humoral and metabolic factors affecting vascular smooth muscle tone. A number of clinical and animal studies can be cited to support either of these possibilities as being of primary importance in the pathogenesis of coronary spasm. It may eventually be established that both mechanisms are interrelated or that either can be of primary importance in specific groups of patients with spasm.

Neurogenic Mechanisms

There is considerable evidence suggesting that neurogenic stimulation originating either centrally or via the autonomic nervous system is of importance in the etiology of coronary artery spasm.

Central Nervous System. As described earlier, it has been reported that there may be an increased incidence of variant angina in patients with generalized vasospastic disorders such as Raynaud's phenomenon, progressive systemic sclerosis, peripheral venous spasm, and migraine headaches. Since these disorders can be triggered by emotional stress, it has been suggested that variant angina may also be initiated by consciously perceived stress (Coffman and Cohen, 1981). Melville and associates (1969) have shown that severe coronary constriction can result from electrical stimulation of the central nervous system in monkeys. Of additional interest are two reports of patients with subarachnoid hemorrhage who were observed to have transient and repeated episodes of ST-segment elevation with reciprocal ST-segment depression, presumably secondary to coronary artery spasm (Goldman et al., 1975; Toyama et al., 1979). However, Cipriano and coworkers (1979) have shown that ergonovine can cause coronary artery spasm in susceptible, totally denervated, transplanted human hearts. The fact that ergonovine can provoke spasm in totally denervated hearts suggests that the final trigger mechanism is either within intramyocardial autonomic receptors or that a humoral trigger mechanism is of primary importance.

Autonomic Nervous System. SYMPATHETIC INFLUENCES. An impressive network of autonomic nerve fibers supplying coronary arteries can be demonstrated by electron microscopic and histochemical studies. Both parasympathetic and sympathetic components of the autonomic nervous system have been implicated in coronary artery spasm.

Sympathetic nerves in large numbers correct with the smooth muscle cells of coronary arteries. Beta-adrenergic stimulation results in coronary arterial dilatation by both direct and indirect mechanisms. Stimulation of smooth muscle $beta_2$ receptors directly dilates coronary arteries. Stimulation of $beta_1$ receptors results in metabolically mediated dilatation due to an increase in heart rate and contractility. In contrast, alpha sympathetic receptor stimulation causes coronary arterial constriction. The balance between alpha and $beta_1$-$beta_2$ sympathetic discharge is thought to account for a component of normal coronary arteriolar resistance or "tone." Kelley and Feigl (1978) have shown in dogs that alpha receptor–induced coronary constriction can be produced by pretreatment with propranolol to block beta vasodilatory sympathetic responses, followed by the intracoronary injection of norepinephrine and simultaneous electrical stimulation of the left stellate ganglion. The increase in large vessel resistance was approximately 60 per cent of the total observed for the entire coronary bed, suggesting that sympathetically mediated coronary vasoconstriction affects distal small vessels and not just large epicardial vessels.

Of pertinence to patients with coronary artery spasm is the work of Ricci and associates (1979), who demonstrated that coronary artery spasm in eight patients was rapidly reversed by the intravenous administration of the alpha-adrenergic blocker phentolamine. In four additional patients with recurrent episodes of coronary spasm, the oral administration of the alpha-adrenergic blocker phenoxybenzamine prevented symptoms suggestive of spasm over a 1-year period of follow-up. Furthermore, certain patients with vasospastic angina have had attacks triggered by exposure to a cold environment. It has been suggested that the stress of cold exposure activates alpha sympathetic discharge, resulting in coronary artery spasm. To test this hypothesis, Mudge and coworkers (1976) subjected susceptible patients to exposure to cold following the intravenous administration of the alpha-adrenergic blocker phentolamine. The results showed that coronary vasoconstriction could be prevented in this group by pretreatment with phentolamine. Documenting increased alpha sympathetic tone in patients susceptible to spasm, however, has not been possible. Robertson and colleagues (1979) found normal levels of urinary and plasma catecholamines and metabolite levels of catecholamines in three patients with coronary artery spasm. In two patients, they obtained blood samples at the onset and termination of spontaneous episodes of ST-segment elevation and found no significant changes in catecholamine levels. They concluded that there was no evidence suggesting a generalized increase in sympathetic discharge in patients during episodes of coronary artery spasm. These data, however, do not discount the possibility that alpha–$beta_1$, $beta_2$ sympathetic imbalance could well be operative in patients with coronary artery spasm.

PARASYMPATHETIC INFLUENCES. In contrast to the dense network of sympathetic fibers supplying coronary arteries, parasympathetic fibers are found in much smaller numbers in the heart (Hillis and Braunwald, 1978). However, there is evidence that enhanced activity of the parasympathetic system can trigger spasm. The observation that patients with variant angina usually experience attacks of coronary artery spasm at rest supports this theory, since it is well established that parasympathetic activity is maximal at rest and suppressed during exercise.

Both sympathetic and parasympathetic fibers are found in parasympathetic vagal ganglia supplying innervation to the heart. Stimulation of the vagus (parasympathetic) nerve or the intracoronary injection of its neurotransmitter, acetylcholine, results in coronary vasodilatation (Berne et al., 1965; Feigl, 1969; Blumenthal et al., 1968; Levy and Zieske, 1969; Blesa and Ross, 1970; Hackett et al., 1972). However, in addition to causing direct vasodilatation, acetylcholine appears to cause release of norepinephrine from postganglionic sympathetic nerve endings in the heart (Blumenthal et al., 1968; Levy, 1971; Cabrera et al., 1966; Dempsey and Cooper, 1969; Burn, 1967). Normally, coronary blood flow is regulated primarily by metabolic requirements of the heart (an increase in myocardial oxygen consumption causes coronary vasodilatation), and neurogenic control is of lesser importance. Excess parasympathetic activity, however, decreases heart rate, blood pressure, and myocardial contractility, all of which lead to reduced myocardial oxygen consumption, thereby eliminating metabolic factors that normally control coronary vascular tone.

It has been postulated by Yasue and associates (1974) and Endo and coworkers (1976) that increased parasympathetic activity stimulates alpha sympathetic nerves in parasympathetic ganglia, which, in turn, can cause severe coronary artery spasm under resting conditions. In support of this concept, Yasue and colleagues (1974) studied 10 patients with Prinzmetal's angina and found that administration of the parasympathomimetic drug methacoline could induce spasm and that the parasympathetic blocker atropine could prevent attacks of spasm. Furthermore, epinephrine appeared to provoke attacks of spasm in certain patients if resting parasympathetic tone appeared increased and had little effect if resting parasympathetic tone was normal. Administration of the beta-adrenergic blocker propranolol could not prevent attacks, but administration of the alpha-adrenergic blocker phenoxybenzamine could prevent spasm. In view of these pharmacologic studies, the authors concluded that excessive parasympathetic activity may exist in patients prone to coronary artery spasm and that increased parasympathetic activity selectively causes stimulation of alpha sympathetic fibers in parasympathetic ganglia and that alpha-adrenergic stimulation is the final common pathway initiating coronary artery spasm. This work is supported by the clinical observation that attacks of variant angina usually occur in patients at rest when baseline parasympathetic tone is increased. Further support of this intriguing theory has been provided by the observations of Nowlin and associates (1965) and Murao and coworkers (1972), who have reported that attacks of variant angina in susceptible individuals are associated with the rapid eye movement (REM) period of sleep. It is known that REM sleep is triggered by acetylcholine, indicating increased parasympathetic activity, and is suppressed by atropine, which blocks acetylcholine release.

In summary, the aforementioned studies suggest that parasympathetic-sympathetic imbalance in the autonomic nervous sytem of patients with coronary artery spasm may be an important trigger mechanism (Fig. 50–111). Whether or not higher-level central nervous system imput relates to this imbalance is unknown. The single piece of evidence against neurogenic mechanisms is the fact that denervated hearts susceptible to spasm can still be provoked to demonstrate coronary artery spasm by administration of agents such as ergonovine (Clark *et al.,* 1977). However, since ergonovine appears to work by stimulation of alpha receptors in coronary arteries, the administration of ergonovine to totally denervated hearts with generation of spasm does not discount the neurogenic theories that postulate that the final pathway in the initiation of coronary artery spasm relates to alpha receptor activity in coronary arteries.

Humoral-Metabolic Mechanisms

Platelet–Prostaglandin–Vessel Wall Interactions. The role of prostaglandins in initiating and mediating a variety of physiologic responses is currently under intense investigation. Recently, it has been

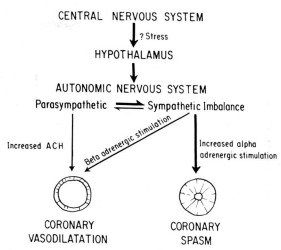

Figure 50–111. Schematic representation of postulated parasympathetic-sympathetic imbalances leading to increased alphasympathetic activity and coronary spasm. Heavy arrows indicate direction of the imbalance.

suggested that platelet-prostaglandin and coronary vessel wall interactions may be of critical importance in the pathophysiology of myocardial ischemia. It is generally accepted that platelet aggregation occurring on atherosclerotic plaques can initiate thrombosis, and there is recent evidence to suggest that platelets may also be involved in the initiation of coronary artery spasm. Platelets are known to release thromboxane A_2 as they aggregate. Thromboxane A_2 is a powerful endogenous vasoconstrictor as well as a stimulator for further platelet aggregation. Within vessel walls, a prostaglandin, prostacyclin (PGI_2), is normally synthesized, which has biologic actions directly opposing those of thromboxane A_2. Specifically, prostacyclin causes vasodilatation and inhibits platelet aggregation (Bunting *et al.,* 1976; Dusting *et al.,* 1978). It has been suggested that the relative balance between prostacyclin release and thromboxane release contributes to normal coronary vascular tone and the stimulation or inhibition of platelet aggregation (Moncada *et al.,* 1977; Dusting *et al.,* 1978; Boullin *et al.,* 1979). This precise homeostatic balance may be disrupted in coronary artery disease. It has been shown in both human and animal studies that atherosclerotic coronary arteries have a reduced ability to synthesize prostacyclin (Dembinska-Kiec *et al.,* 1977; D'Angelo *et al.,* 1978). Furthermore, platelets from patients who survive acute myocardial infarction have been shown to synthesize increased quantities of thromboxane A_2 (Szczeklik *et al.,* 1978). These studies suggest that in coronary artery disease, an imbalance between prostacyclin release and thromboxane release favors vasoconstriction and platelet aggregation. Although increased thromboxane release can cause vasoconstriction, it is unproved whether it is operative in producing coronary artery spasm. However, Lewy

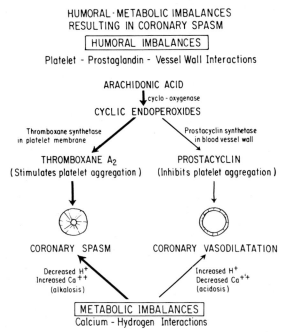

HUMORAL·METABOLIC IMBALANCES
RESULTING IN CORONARY SPASM

HUMORAL IMBALANCES

Platelet - Prostaglandin - Vessel Wall Interactions

ARACHIDONIC ACID
↓ cyclo - oxygenase
CYCLIC ENDOPEROXIDES

Thromboxane synthetase
in platelet membrane

Prostacyclin synthetase
in blood vessel wall

THROMBOXANE A₂
(Stimulates platelet aggregation)

PROSTACYCLIN
(Inhibits platelet aggregation)

CORONARY SPASM

CORONARY VASODILATATION

Decreased H⁺
Increased Ca⁺⁺
(alkalosis)

Increased H⁺
Decreased Ca⁺⁺
(acidosis)

METABOLIC IMBALANCES
Calcium - Hydrogen Interactions

Figure 50–112. Schematic representation of humoral-metabolic imbalances that have been postulated to initiate coronary spasm. Heavy arrows indicate direction of the imbalance. (Adapted from Conti, C. R., Pepine, C., and Curry, R. C.: Coronary artery spasm: An important mechanism in the pathophysiology of ischemic heart disease. Curr. Probl. Cardiol., *4*:1, 1979.)

and associates (1979) have reported marked elevation in levels of thromboxane B₂, the major metabolite of thromboxane A₂, in patients with Prinzmetal's angina. Whether thromboxane release initiated spasm or was secondary to spasm and platelet aggregation, however, is unknown.

Interestingly, synthesis of both thromboxane and prostacyclin begins with arachidonic acid, a free fatty acid. The metabolism of arachidonic acid and the possible relationship between platelets, prostaglandins, and vessel walls in initiating coronary artery spasm are depicted schematically in Figure 50–112.

Hydrogen Ion–Calcium Ion Imbalances. It is well accepted that contraction of vascular smooth muscle depends on the presence of calcium ions, which are necessary for the activation of myofibrillar ATPase (Bohr, 1973; Fleckenstein *et al.*, 1976). Physiologically, hydrogen ions have been shown to exert a highly potent calcium antagonist action by competition with calcium ions both for transport across cell membranes as well as for binding sites at the myofibrillar level (Fleckenstein *et al.*, 1976). It appears that vasoconstriction can occur if calcium ion concentration increases or hydrogen ion concentration decreases. In contrast, vasodilatation is produced by decreased transmembrane calcium flux or increased hydrogen ion concentration. Yasue and colleagues (1978) subjected nine patients with documented Prinzmetal's angina to infusion of 100 ml. of TRIS buffer over a 5-minute period, followed by hyperventilation for a second 5-minute period. Arterial pH increased from normal values to 7.65 using this protocol, and eight of the nine patients developed ST-segment elevation. With the onset of alkalosis and ST-segment elevation, simultaneous coronary angiograms revealed spasm. The patients were then pretreated with the calcium blocker diltiazem, and the same experimental protocol was performed again. Following pretreatment with diltiazem, alkalosis did not induce attacks of Prinzmetal's angina. Because hydrogen ion production decreases at rest, particularly during sleep, when metabolism slows, and since there is often an increase in the respiratory rate during REM sleep, alkalosis may result. Since it is known that Prinzmetal's angina is more likely to occur at rest and during periods of REM sleep, the authors suggest that hydrogen ion–calcium ion imbalances may trigger coronary artery spasm (Fig. 50–112).

MANAGEMENT OF PATIENTS WITH CORONARY ARTERY SPASM

As previously discussed, coronary artery spasm appears to be an important component in a variety of syndromes other than Prinzmetal's angina. In view of this, appropriate therapy must be carefully individualized. The majority of patients with coronary artery spasm also have atheromatous disease, and it is important to try to identify the relative contribution of each of these processes, so that successful treatment can be achieved. Furthermore, a rational approach to therapy must take into account that over time, the clinical manifestations of ischemia may at one point be secondary to spasm and later be due to worsening atherosclerotic disease with concomitant spasm. Appropriate therapy, therefore, involves both medical and surgical interventions (Table 50–15).

Medical Therapy

Nitroglycerin is highly effective in terminating acute attacks of coronary artery spasm and should be administered at the very onset of symptoms. Maintenance therapy is directed toward preventing recurrent attacks of spasm by the addition of long-acting nitrates. Patients should be cautioned regarding the

TABLE 50–15. THERAPY FOR CORONARY ARTERY SPASM

MEDICAL THERAPY
Calcium antagonists (nifedipine, verapamil, diltiazem, perhexiline maleate)
Nitrates
Nonsteroidal anti-inflammatory agents (aspirin, indomethacin, dipyridamole, sulfinpyrazone, ibuprofen)
Alpha-adrenergic blockers (phentolamine, phenoxybenzamine)
Beta-adrenergic blockers (select patients with atherosclerotic disease and spasm)

SURGICAL THERAPY (select patients only)
Coronary artery bypass grafting
Cardiac denervation

possible provocation of spasm by drugs such as Cafergot, an ergot alkaloid used to treat migraine headaches, and by environmental influences such as sudden exposure to cold. Although nitroglycerin and other nitrates are often effective, breakthrough attacks are common, and the majority of patients require more than just nitrate therapy for control.

Because most patients with coronary artery spasm also have concomitant atheromatous disease, beta-adrenergic blockers have been tried with variable success. Evidence can be cited, as summarized by Conti and associates (1979), which suggests that beta blockers are "effective, occasionally useful, ineffective or possibly harmful" in patients with attacks of coronary artery spasm. Theoretically, beta blockade can initiate spasm by allowing alpha-adrenergic sympathetic activity to predominate with subsequent vasoconstriction. However, in patients with ischemia due to fixed obstructive disease as well as intermittent spasm, beta blockers, such as propranolol, may definitely be an important adjunct to medical therapy. Obviously, therapy with beta blockers should be initiated slowly and under careful supervision.

As described earlier, there are isolated reports of the efficacy of alpha-adrenergic receptor blocking agents in preventing coronary artery spasm. Mudge and colleagues (1976) have shown that administration of the alpha-adrenergic blocker phentolamine can block reflex coronary constriction caused by exposure to cold. To date, however, there have been no large clinical trials investigating the efficacy of various alpha blockers. Since the final pathogenesis of spasm may well involve alpha-adrenergic receptors, it appears that alpha blockers deserve further clinical investigation, as recently suggested by Conti and coworkers (1979).

In view of humoral theories suggesting that platelet–vessel wall interactions are important in the pathogenesis of spasm, drugs such as aspirin, indomethacin, sulfinpyrazone, dipyridamole, and ibuprofen are currently being investigated. These drugs are nonsteroidal anti-inflammatory agents that appear to inhibit platelet aggregation as well as prevent the release of the potent vasoconstrictor thromboxane A_2 from platelet membranes.

At present, the most promising breakthrough in the treatment of Prinzmetal's angina and other syndromes involving coronary artery spasm is the addition of calcium antagonists (Fig. 50–113). These agents are powerful vasodilators, and initial reports indicate impressive clinical results in preventing coronary artery spasm. It has been shown that nitroglycerin causes vasodilatation by blocking calcium influx into smooth muscle cells of large epicardial coronary arteries and that adenosine preferentially dilates smaller intramyocardial coronary branches, also by blockade of calcium influx (Harder et al., 1979). Calcium antagonists, including nifedipine, verapamil, diltiazem, and perhexiline maleate, appear to dilate both large epicardial as well as small intramural coronary arteries. Although it is believed that the primary beneficial effect of these agents is via their potent

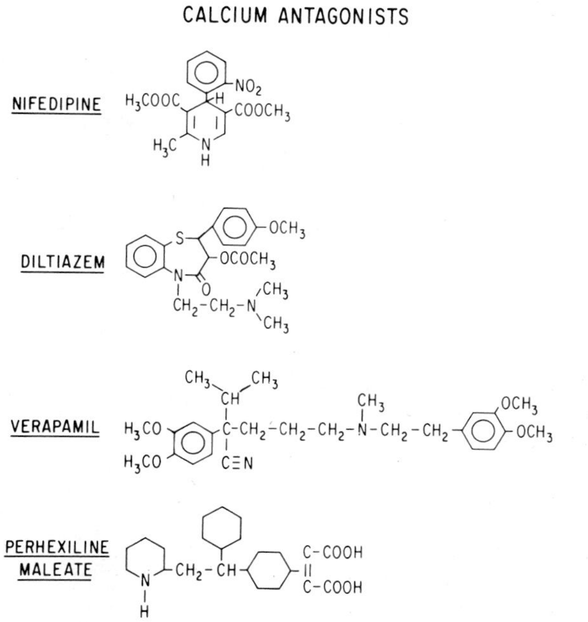

Figure 50–113. Structural formulas of the commonly used calcium antagonists.

vasodilatory actions, it has been shown that diltiazem and verapamil are also potent inhibitors of platelet aggregation (Shinjo et al., 1978).

Increasing numbers of patients are now being treated with calcium blockers, with impressive initial reports of their efficacy. Endo and associates (1975) reported 35 patients with variant angina (16 with spasm and atherosclerotic disease and 19 with spasm in normal coronary arteries). Twenty-six patients were treated medically, with one death and persistence of symptoms in most. The addition of nifedipine to the treatment regimen of the remaining 25 patients resulted in complete relief of symptoms in each case. Encouraging results with verapamil (Severi et al., 1979), diltiazem (Yasue et al., 1979), and perhexiline maleate (Conti et al., 1979; Raabe, 1979) have also been reported. In the majority of these reports, calcium antagonists have proved most efficacious when used concomitantly with long-acting nitrates. Although long-term follow-up must be awaited, the addition of calcium blockers to the medical therapy of coronary artery spasm appears to be a major contribution that will have an important impact on subsequent morbidity and mortality.

Surgical Therapy

It has been well established that coronary artery bypass grafting is very effective in relieving angina in patients with obstructive coronary artery disease and that prolongation of life results in specific subgroups such as those with left main coronary artery disease or severe three-vessel disease with impaired left ventricular function. Furthermore, numerous large series have been reported that document that these benefits

TABLE 50–16. RESULTS OF MEDICAL TREATMENT OF PRINZMETAL'S ANGINA*

| NUMBER OF PATIENTS | ATHEROMATOUS CORONARY DISEASE | | ASYMPTOMATIC OR IMPROVED | SAME OR WORSE | MYOCARDIAL INFARCTION | DIED |
	None	*One or More Arteries Involved*				
275	22%	78%	47%	47%	23%	6%

*Adapted from Raizner, A. E., and Chahine, R. A.: The treatment of Prinzmetal's variant angina with coronary bypass surgery. *In* Update II: The Heart — Bypass Surgery for Obstructive Coronary Disease. Edited by J. W. Hurst. New York, McGraw-Hill Book Company, 1980, Chapter 9.

can be achieved with very low operative morbidity and mortality. Surgical intervention in the management of patients with coronary artery spasm, however, is a more complex issue.

Since the initial report of Silverman and Flamm in 1971 about two patients with coronary disease and variant angina treated by bypass grafting, numerous small series have been reported with variable results. Conti and associates (1979) and Raizner and Chahine (1980) have reviewed the results of coronary artery bypass grafting in patients with variant angina with both normal and atherosclerotically diseased coronary arteries. As shown in Tables 50–16 to 50–19, these reviews have indicated that:

1. Coronary artery bypass grafting is generally contraindicated in patients with variant angina who do not have concomitant critical atherosclerotic disease.

2. Coronary artery bypass grafting may be an important adjunct to the medical treatment of patients with variant angina and concomitant atherosclerotic disease.

The addition of calcium blockers to the medical treatment of variant angina may well control spasm so effectively that patients with concomitant atherosclerotic disease may undergo bypass grafting with morbidity and mortality approaching that achieved in patients with obstructive disease alone. At present, however, the effect of calcium antagonist therapy on selection of patients for bypass grafting remains an unsettled issue. In general, patients with variant angina and normal coronary arteries should be treated medically, and those with critical obstructive disease and variant angina should be considered for operation only if they are refractory to medical therapy or, more ideally, if medical therapy is successful in relieving spasm but the patient remains symptomatic secondary to significant obstructive disease.

Although the importance of spasm in patients with atherosclerotic coronary artery disease and angina is becoming increasingly apparent, its role is often overlooked, and spasm may first be recognized in the perioperative period. A dramatic example of this is the case report of Pichard and associates (1980), which was cited earlier. This report and that of six additional patients described by Buxton and coworkers (1981) provide good evidence that coronary artery spasm occurring following coronary artery bypass grafting can result in cardiac arrest. A number of cardiovascular surgeons have had similar unreported experiences, and this phenomenon may be frequent enough to warrant further investigation. As suggested by Pichard and colleagues (1980), coronary artery spasm should be suspected perioperatively in the patient undergoing myocardial revascularization who displays ventricular arrhythmias or hemodynamic instability associated with ST-segment elevation. Prompt therapy with coronary vasodilators may be lifesaving.

As presented earlier, there is evidence to suggest that alpha-adrenergic–mediated neurogenic mechanisms may be responsible for the initiation of coronary artery spasm. Prompted by these observations, cardiac denervation in patients with variant angina has been reported (Grondin and Limet, 1977; Clark *et al.*, 1977), but the numbers of patients are too few at present to draw firm conclusions regarding possible therapeutic benefits.

TABLE 50–17. RESULTS OF CORONARY BYPASS GRAFTING IN PATIENTS WITH PRINZMETAL'S ANGINA AND ATHEROSCLEROTIC CORONARY ARTERY DISEASE*

NUMBER OF PATIENTS	ASYMPTOMATIC OR IMPROVED	SAME OR WORSE	MYOCARDIAL INFARCTION	DIED
90	73%	19%	12%	8%

*Adapted from Raizner, A. E., and Chahine, R. A.: The treatment of Prinzmetal's variant angina with coronary bypass surgery. *In* Update II: The Heart — Bypass Surgery for Obstructive Coronary Disease. Edited by J. W. Hurst. New York, McGraw-Hill Book Company, 1980, Chapter 9.

TABLE 50–18. RESULTS OF MEDICAL THERAPY IN PATIENTS WITH PRINZMETAL'S ANGINA AND "NORMAL" CORONARY ARTERIES*

NUMBER OF PATIENTS	ASYMPTOMATIC OR IMPROVED	SAME OR WORSE	MYOCARDIAL INFARCTION	DIED
41	66%	27%	7%	7%

*Adapted from Raizner, A. E., and Chahine, R. A.: The treatment of Prinzmetal's variant angina with coronary bypass surgery. *In* Update II: The Heart — Bypass Surgery for Obstructive Coronary Disease. Edited by J. W. Hurst. New York, McGraw-Hill Book Company, 1980, Chapter 9.

TABLE 50–19. RESULTS OF CORONARY ARTERY BYPASS GRAFTING IN PATIENTS WITH PRINZMETAL'S ANGINA AND "NORMAL" CORONARY ARTERIES*

NUMBER OF PATIENTS	ASYMPTOMATIC OR IMPROVED	SAME OR WORSE	MYOCARDIAL INFARCTION	DIED
8	50%	25%	13%	25%

*Adapted from Raizner, A. E., and Chahine, R. A.: The treatment of Prinzmetal's variant angina with coronary bypass surgery. *In* Update II: The Heart — Bypass Surgery for Obstructive Coronary Disease. Edited by J. W. Hurst. New York, McGraw-Hill Book Company, 1980, Chapter 9.

RESULTS OF THERAPY FOR VARIANT ANGINA

Conti and associates (1979) and Raizner and Chahine (1980) have reviewed in detail the results of medical and surgical therapy for variant angina. As shown in Tables 50–16 and 50–17, there is only a slight difference in mortality in patients with variant angina and coronary artery disease treated medically compared with those treated by coronary artery bypass grafting. These groups are not directly comparable, however, because, as can be seen in Table 50–16, 22 per cent of medically treated patients had no significant atherosclerotic coronary disease. However, there appears to be a definite decrease in symptoms in patients with variant angina and coronary disease who underwent successful coronary artery bypass grafting (73 per cent asymptomatic or improved compared with 47 per cent asymptomatic or improved with medical therapy).

Tables 50–18 and 50–19 compared medical and surgical results in the treatment of variant angina in patients without significant coronary artery disease. These data clearly indicate that coronary artery bypass grafting is contraindicated in this subgroup of patients and that medical therapy, although not ideal, is far superior. It should be emphasized that the data summarized in Tables 50–16 to 50–19 do not reflect the impact that calcium antagonists are expected to have in the treatment of coronary artery spasm. If spasm can be effectively controlled by these agents, selection of patients who would benefit from coronary artery bypass grafting or possible cardiac denervation procedures may become more objective. It is hoped that these agents will also decrease the incidence of perioperative myocardial infarction as well as operative mortality secondary to the persistence of spasm.

SELECTED REFERENCES

Conti, C. R., Pepine, C. J., and Curry, R. C.: Coronary artery spasm: An important mechanism in the pathophysiology of ischemic heart disease. Curr. Probl. Cardiol., *4*:1, 1979.

This monograph is an authoritative review of all facets of coronary artery spasm. The diagnosis, treatment, and pathophysiology of coronary artery spasm are discussed in detail, and the list of references is among the most complete ever assembled on the subject.

Maseri, A., Klassen, G. A., and Lesch, M.: Primary and Secondary Angina Pectoris. New York, Grune and Stratton, 1978.

A detailed discussion of the diagnosis, treatment, and pathophysiology of both vasospastic (primary) angina as well as angina secondary to atherosclerotic coronary disease is presented by recognized authorities. Professor Maseri and associates have contributed tremendously to our understanding of the clinical manifestations of coronary artery spasm and have accumulated convincing evidence that spasm may contribute to practically all aspects of ischemic heart disease.

Oliva, P. B., Potts, D. E., and Pluss, R. G.: Coronary arterial spasm in Prinzmetal angina. Documentation by coronary arteriography. N. Engl. J. Med., *288*:745, 1973.

This manuscript is among the first to convincingly document that the clinical and electrocardiographic manifestations of variant angina are secondary to transient episodes of coronary artery spasm. Furthermore, evidence is presented that the severity of coronary artery spasm can vary from one attack to another and that spasm can be diffuse or segmental in nature.

Prinzmetal, M., Kennamer, R., Merliss, R., Wada, T., and Bor, N.: Angina pectoris. I. A variant form of angina pectoris. Am. J. Med., *27*:375, 1959.

This classic article describes the clinical manifestations of 32 patients with a different kind of anginal syndrome referred to as variant angina. Unlike typical angina, the pain of variant angina is not associated with effort, eating, or anxiety. Prinzmetal correctly postulated that "temporary increased tonus of a large coronary artery" was occurring in these patients during episodes of chest pain. The clinical manifestations of variant angina, initially described by Prinzmetal, remain the criteria for establishing a diagnosis of vasospastic angina today. Appropriately, variant angina is commonly referred to as Prinzmetal's angina in recognition of this major contribution.

Raizner, A. E., and Chahine, R. A.: The treatment of Prinzmetal's variant angina with coronary bypass surgery. *In* Update II: The Heart—Bypass Surgery for Obstructive Coronary Disease. Edited by J. W. Hurst. New York, McGraw-Hill Book Company, 1980, Chapter 9.

This review summarizes the results of both medical and surgical therapy for Prinzmetal's angina. Convincing evidence is presented, indicating that patients with spasm and insignificant coronary artery disease are best treated medically and that select patients with spasm and significant atherosclerotic coronary disease are candidates for myocardial revascularization.

REFERENCES

Bentivoglio, L. G., Ablaza, S. G. G., and Greenberg, L. F.: Bypass surgery for Prinzmetal angina. Arch. Intern. Med., *134*:313, 1974.

Berne, R. M., Degust, H., and Levy, M. N.: Influence of the cardiac nerves on coronary resistance. Am. J. Physiol., *208*:763, 1965.

Blesa, M. I., and Ross, G.: Cholinergic mechanism on the heart and coronary circulation. Br. J. Pharmacol., *38*:93, 1970.

Blumenthal, M. R., Wang, H. H., Markee, S., and Wang, S. G.: Effects of acetylcholine on the heart. Am. J. Physiol., *214*:1280, 1968.

Bodenheimer, M., Lipski, J., Donoso, E., and Dack, S.: Prinzmetal's variant angina: A clinical and electrocardiographic study. Am. Heart J., *87*:304, 1974.

Bohr, D. F.: Vascular smooth muscle updated. Circ. Res., *32*:665, 1973.

Bolooki, H., Vargas, A., Gharamani, A., Sommer, L., Orvald, T., Jude, J., and Baccabella, K.: Aortocoronary bypass graft for preinfarction angina. Chest, *61*:312, 1972.

Boullin, D., Bunting, S., Blasp, W., Hunt, T., and Moncada, S.: Responses of human and baboon arteries to prostaglandin endoperoxides and biologically generated and synthetic prostacyclin: Their relevance to cerebral arterial spasm in man. Br. J. Clin. Pharmacol., *7*:139, 1979.

Bulkley, B., Klacsmann, P., and Hutchins, G.: Angina pectoris, myocardial infarction, and sudden death with normal coronary arteries: A clinicopathologic study of 9 patients with progressive systemic sclerosis. Am. Heart J., *95*:563, 1978.

Bunting, S., Gryglewski, R., Moncada, S., and Vane, J.: Arterial walls generate from prostaglandin endoperoxides a substance (prostaglandin X) which relaxes strips of mesenteric and coeliac arteries and inhibits platelet aggregation. Prostaglandins, *12*:897, 1976.

Burn, J. H.: Release of noradrenaline from the sympathetic postganglionic fiber. Br. Med. J., *2*:197, 1967.

Buxton, A. E., Goldberg, S., Harken, A., Hirshfield, J., Jr., and Kastor, J. A.: Coronary artery spasm immediately after myocardial revascularization: Recognition and management. N. Engl. J. Med., *304*:1249, 1981.

Cabrera, R., Cohen, A., Middleton, S., Utano, L., and Viveros, H.: The immediate source of noradrenaline released in the heart by acetylcholine. Br. J. Pharmacol., *27*:46, 1966.

Chahine, R., Raizner, A., Ishimori, T., Luchi, R., and McIntosh, H.: The incidence and clinical implications of coronary artery spasm. Circulation, *52*:972, 1975.

Cheng, T. O., Bashour, T., Kelser, G. A., Weiss, L., and Bacos, J.: Variant angina of Prinzmetal with normal coronary arteriograms. A variant of the variant. Circulation, *47*:476, 1973.

Cipriano, P., Koch, F., Rosenthal, S. J., and Schroeder, J. S.: Clinical course of patients following the demonstration of coronary artery spasm by angiography. Am. Heart J., *101*:127, 1981.

Cipriano, P., Guthaner, D., Orlick, A., Ricci, D., Wexler, L., and Silverman, J.: The effects of ergonovine maleate on coronary arterial size. Circulation, *59*:82, 1979.

Clark, D. A., Quint, R. A., Mitchell, R. L., and Angell, W. W.: Coronary artery spasm. Medical management, surgical denervation, and autotransplantation. J. Thorac. Cardiovasc. Surg., *73*:332, 1977.

Coffman, J. D., and Cohen, R. A.: Vasospasm—ubiquitous? N. Engl. J. Med., *304*:780, 1981.

Conti, C. R., Pepine, C. J., and Curry, R. C.: Coronary artery spasm: An important mechanism in the pathophysiology of ischemic heart disease. Curr. Probl. Cardiol., *4*:1, 1979.

Dagenais, G., Gundel, W., and Conti, C.: Peripheral venospasm associated with signs of transient myocardial ischemia. Am. Heart J., *80*:544, 1970.

D'Angelo, V., Ville, S., Mysliwiec, M., Donati, M. B., and de Gaetano, G.: Defective fibrinolytic and prostacyclin-like activity in human atheromatous plaques. Thromb. Haemost., *39*:535, 1978.

Demany, M., Tambe, A., and Zimmerman, H.: Coronary arterial spasm. Dis. Chest., *53*:714, 1968.

Dembinska-Kiec, A., Gryglewski, T., Zmuda, A., and Gryglewski, R. J.: The generation of prostacyclin by arteries and by the coronary vascular bed is reduced in experimental atherosclerosis in rabbits. Prostaglandins, *14*:1025, 1977.

Dempsey, P. J., and Cooper, T.: Ventricular cholinergic receptor systems: Interaction with adrenergic systems. J. Pharmacol. Exp. Ther., *167*:282, 1969.

Dusting, G., Chapple, D., Hughes, R., Moncada, S., and Vane, J.: Prostacyclin (PGI$_2$) induced coronary vasodilatation in anaesthetized dogs. Cardiovasc. Res., *12*:720, 1978.

Endo, M., Hirosawa, K., Kaneko, N., Hase, K., Inoue, Y., and Konno, S.: Prinzmetal's variant angina: Coronary arteriogram and left ventriculogram during angina attack induced by methacholine. N. Engl. J. Med., *294*:252, 1976.

Endo, M., Kanda, I., Hosoda, S., Hayashi, H., Hirosawa, K., and Konno, S.: Prinzmetal's variant form of angina pectoris. Circulation, *52*:33, 1975.

Feigl, E. O.: Parasympathetic control of coronary blood flow in dogs. Circ. Res., *25*:509, 1969.

Fleckenstein, A., Nakayama, K., Fleckenstein-Grün, G., and Byon, Y. K.: Interactions of hydrogen ions, calcium antagonistic drugs and cardiac glycosides with excitation-contraction coupling of vascular smooth muscle. *In* Ionic Actions on Vascular Smooth Muscle. Edited by E. Betz. Berlin, Springer-Verlag, 1976, p. 117.

Goldman, M., Rogers, E., and Rogers, M.: Subarachnoid hemorrhage. Association with unusual electrocardiographic changes. J.A.M.A., *234*:957, 1975.

Gorfinkel, H. J., Inglesby, T. V., Lansing, A. M., and Goodin, R. R.: ST-segment elevation, transient left-posterior hemiblock, and recurrent ventricular arrhythmias unassociated with pain. A variant of Prinzmetal's anginal syndrome. Ann. Intern. Med., *79*:795, 1973.

Grondin, C., and Limet, R.: Sympathetic denervation in association with coronary artery grafting in patients with Prinzmetal's angina. J. Thorac. Cardiovasc. Surg., *23*:111, 1977.

Guazzi, M., Fiorentini, C., Polese, A., and Magrini, F.: Continuous electrocardiographic recording in Prinzmetal's variant angina pectoris: A report of four cases. Br. Heart J., *32*:611, 1970.

Guazzi, M., Olivari, M., Polese, A., Fiorentini, C., and Magrini, F.: Repetitive myocardial ischemia of Prinzmetal type without angina pectoris. Am. J. Cardiol., *37*:923, 1976.

Hackett, J. G., Abboud, F. M., Mark, A. L., Schmid, P. B., Heistad, D. D.: Coronary vascular responses to stimulation of chemoreceptors and baroreceptors. Evidence for reflex activation of vagal cholinergic innervation. Circ. Res., *31*:8, 1972.

Harder, D., Belardinelli, L., Sperelakis, N., Rubio, R., and Berne, R.: Differential effects of adenosine and nitroglycerin on the action potentials of large and small coronary arteries. Circ. Res., *44*:176, 1979.

Heberden, W.: Some account of a disorder of the breast. Medical Transactions of the Royal College of Physicians of London, *2*:59, 1772.

Hillis, L., and Braunwald, E.: Coronary artery spasm. N. Engl. J. Med., *299*:695, 1978.

Johnson, A. D., and Detwiler, J. H.: Coronary spasm, variant angina, and recurrent myocardial infarctions. Circulation, *55*:947, 1977.

Kelley, K., and Feigl, E.: Segmental alpha-receptor mediated vasoconstriction in the canine coronary circulation. Circ. Res., *43*:908, 1978.

King, S., Mansour, K., Hatcher, C., Silverman, M., and Hart, N.: Coronary artery spasm producing Prinzmetal's angina in myocardial infarction in the absence of coronary atherosclerosis. Ann. Thorac. Surg., *16*:337, 1973.

Lange, R., Reid, M., Tresch, D., Keelan, M., Bernhard, V., and Coolidge, G.: Nonatheromatous ischemic heart disease following withdrawal from chronic industrial nitroglycerin exposure. Circulation, *46*:666, 1972.

Lasser, R. T., and de la Paz, N. D.: Repetitive transient myocardial ischemia, Prinzmetal type, without angina pectoris, presenting with Stokes-Adams attacks. Chest, *64*:350, 1973.

Lavine, P., Kimbiris, D., and Linhart, J.: Coronary artery spasm during selective coronary arteriography: A review of 8 years experience. (Abstract.) Circulation, *48* (Suppl. 4):89, 1973.

Levy, M. N.: Sympathetic-parasympathetic interactions in the heart. Circ. Res., *29*:437, 1971.

Levy, M. N., and Zieske, H.: Comparison of the cardiac effects of vagus nerve stimulation and of acetylcholine infusions. Am. J. Physiol., *216*:890, 1969.

Lewy, R., Smith, J., Silver, M., Saia, J., Walinsky, P., and Wiener, L.: Detection of thromboxane B$_2$ in the peripheral blood of patients with Prinzmetal's angina. Prostaglandins Med., *2*:243, 1979.

Linhart, J. W., Beller, B. M., and Talley, R. C.: Preinfarction angina: Clinical, hemodynamic and angiographic evaluation. Chest, *61*:312, 1972.

Maseri, A., Klassen, G. A., and Lesch, M. (Eds.): Primary and Secondary Angina Pectoris. New York, Grune and Stratton, 1978a.

Maseri, A., L'Abbate, A., Pesola, A., Ballestra, A. M., Marzilli, M., Severi, S., Maltinti, G., Denes, D. M., Parodi, O., and Biagini, A.: Coronary vasospasm in angina pectoris. Lancet, *1*:713, 1977.

Maseri, A., Severi, S., Nes, M. D., *et al.*: "Variant" angina: One aspect of a continuous spectrum of vasospastic myocardial ischemia. Am. J. Cardiol., *42*:1019, 1978b.

Melville, K., Garvey, H., Shister, E., *et al.*: Central nervous system stimulation and cardiac ischemic changes in monkeys. Ann. N.Y. Acad. Sci., *156*:241, 1969.

Miller, D., Waters, D. D., Warnica, W., *et al.*: Is variant angina the coronary manifestation of a generalized vasospastic disorder? N. Engl. J. Med., *304*:763, 1981.

Moncada, S., Higgs, E., and Vane, J.: Human arterial and venous tissues generate prostacyclin (prostaglandin X), a potent inhibitor of platelet aggregation. Lancet, *1*:18, 1977.

Mudge, G., Grossman, W., Miles, R., *et al.*: Reflex increase in coronary vascular resistance in patients with ischemic heart disease. N. Engl. J. Med., *295*:1333, 1976.

Murao, S., Harumi, K., Katayama, S., *et al.* All-night polygraphic studies of nocturnal angina pectoris. Jpn. Heart J., *13*:295, 1972.

Nowlin, J. B., Troyer, W. G., Collens, W. S., *et al.*: The association of nocturnal angina pectoris with dreaming. Ann. Intern. Med., *63*:1040, 1965.

Oliva, P. B.: Coronary artery spasm: An important mechanism in the pathophysiology of ischemic heart disease. (Editorial Comment). Curr. Probl. Cardiol., *4*:1, 1979.

Oliva, P. B., and Breckinridge, J.: Arteriographic evidence of coronary arterial spasm in acute myocardial infarction. Circulation, *56*:366, 1977.

Oliva, P. B., Potts, D. E., and Pluss, R. G.: Coronary peripheral spasm in Prinzmetal angina. Documentation by coronary arteriography. N. Engl. J. Med., *288*:745, 1973.

O'Reilly, R., Spellberg, R., and King, T.: Recognition of proximal right coronary artery spasm during coronary arteriography. Radiology, *95*:305, 1970.

Pichard, A. D., Ambrose, J., Mindrich, B., *et al.*: Coronary artery spasm and perioperative cardiac arrest. J. Thorac. Cardiovasc. Surg., *80*:249, 1980.

Prinzmetal, M., Kennamer, R., Merliss, R., Wada, T., and Bor, N.: Angina pectoris. I. A variant form of angina pectoris. Am. J. Med., *27*:375, 1959.

Prohkov, V. K., Mookherjee, S., Schiess, W., and Obeid, A. L.: Variant anginal syndrome, coronary artery spasm and ventricular fibrillation in absence of chest pain. Ann. Intern. Med., *81*:858, 1974.

Raabe, D.: Treatment of variant angina pectoris with perhexiline maleate. Chest, *75*:152, 1979.

Raizner, A. E., and Chahine, R. A.: The treatment of Prinzmetal's variant angina with coronary bypass surgery. In Update II:

The Heart—Bypass Surgery for Obstructive Coronary Disease. Edited by J. W. Hurst. New York, McGraw-Hill Book Company, 1980, Chapter 9.

Ricci, D., Orlick, A., Cipriano, P., Guthaner, D., and Harrison, D.: Altered adrenergic activity in coronary arterial spasm. Insight into mechanism based on study of coronary hemodynamics and the electrocardiogram. Am. J. Cardiol., *43*:1073, 1979.

Robertson, D., and Oates, J.: Variant angina and Raynaud's phenomenon. (Letter.) Lancet, *1*:452, 1978.

Robertson, D., Robertson, R., Nies, A., Oates, J., and Friesinger, G.: Variant angina pectoris: Investigation of indexes of sympathetic nervous system functioning. Am. J. Cardiol., *43*:1080, 1979.

Selzer, A., Langston, M., Ruggeroli, C., and Cohn, K.: Clinical syndrome of variant angina with normal coronary arteriogram. N. Engl. J. Med., *295*:1343, 1976.

Severi, S., Davies, T., L'Abbate, L., and Maseri, A.: Long-term prognosis of variant angina with medical management. Circulation, *60* (Suppl. 2):250, 1979.

Shinjo, A., Sasaki, Y., Inamasu, M., and Morita, T.: In vivo effect of the coronary vasodilator diltiazem on human and rabbit platelets. Thromb. Res., *13*:941, 1978.

Silverman, M., and Flamm, M.: Angina pectoris. Anatomic findings and prognostic implications. Ann. Intern. Med., *75*:339, 1971.

Stenson, R. E., Flamm, M. D., Zaret, B. L., and McGowan, R. L.: Transient ST-segment elevation with postmyocardial infarction angina: Prognostic significance. Am. Heart J., *89*:449, 1975.

Szczeklik, A., Gryglewski, R. J., Musial, J., Groxzinska, L., Serwonska, M., and Marcinkiewienicz, E.: Thromboxane generation and platelet aggregation in survivors of myocardial infarction. Thromb. Haemost., *40*:66, 1978.

Toyama, Y., Tanaka, H., Nuruki, K., and Shirao, T.: Prinzmetal's variant angina associated with subarachnoid hemorrhage: A case report. Angiology, *30*:211, 1979.

Yasue, H., Nagao, M., Omote, S., *et al.*: Coronary arterial spasm and Prinzmetal's variant form of angina induced by hyperventilation and TRIS-buffer infusion. Circulation, *58*:56, 1978.

Yasue, H., Omote, S., Takizawa, A., *et al.*: Exertional angina pectoris caused by coronary arterial spasm: Effects of various drugs. Am. J. Cardiol., *43*:647, 1979.

Yasue, H., Touyama, M., Shimamoto, M., Kato, H., Tanaka, S., and Akiyama, F.: Role of autonomic nervous system in the pathogenesis of Prinzmetal's variant form of angina. Circulation, *50*:534, 1974.

4. Repeat Coronary Artery Bypass Grafting for Myocardial Ischemia

Floyd D. Loop

INCIDENCE

New and progressive arterial obstructions, left ventricular impairment, and intimal lipid deposition in coronary artery bypass grafts are frequent but not inevitable manifestations of coronary atherosclerosis. Unfortunately, clinical and laboratory risk factors such as findings on the first arteriogram, hypertension, elevation of serum lipid levels, and smoking are not helpful in predicting who will experience further atherosclerotic changes (Bourassa *et al.*, 1978; Kramer

et al., 1981; Bruschke *et al.*, 1981). A 5 to 7 per cent annual recurrence of angina after myocardial revascularization is reported and related principally to early graft thrombosis, progressive arterial lesions in ungrafted coronary arteries, incomplete revascularization, and development of obstructive changes in vein grafts (Robert *et al.*, 1978; Campeau *et al.*, 1979; Hamby *et al.*, 1979). Thus, some patients face the prospect of another coronary artery operation.

The incidence of coronary artery reoperations is difficult to predict. On one hand, the sheer volume of bypass operations continues to escalate at approximately 15 to 20 per cent annually, and its application is estimated conservatively to reach some 600 operations per million population. However, certain procedural trends have occurred in the evolution of these operations and will affect the number of reoperations. The surfeit of patients with one-vessel disease selected for bypass surgery in the early years has decreased markedly in recent years. Improved myocardial protection and technical experience have resulted in more complete revascularization, with a doubling of the number of grafts per patient over the past decade. Graft performance has gradually improved, with higher early graft patency and a graft attrition rate of 1 to 2 per cent per year in the first 5 postoperative years. Today, grafting is frequently performed for the estimated 40 to 50 per cent coronary artery obstruction, a practice that was unconventional 5 years ago. Although there is an increasing number of surgical candidates and operations each year, the aforementioned factors potentially regulate the number of reoperations in later years. For example, more than half of our patients who underwent primary revascularization from 1967 to 1970 had one-vessel disease initially, and 17 per cent of them were reoperated on during the next 10 years. In contrast, one-vessel disease decreased to 18 per cent in our 1971 surgical series, and the frequency of reoperation fell to 10 per cent in the subsequent 10 years. Volume of cases and time of itself, leading to progressive changes in native vessels and grafts, indicate that several thousand coronary artery reoperations may be anticipated annually during the 1980s.

After coronary bypass surgery began in 1967, several years elapsed before publication of the first reports of reoperation. Adam and associates (1972) and Johnson and colleagues (1972) each reported approximately a 10 per cent operative mortality rate and higher morbidity in patients requiring second procedures, but the relief of angina was similar to the initial result. Higher risk in coronary artery reoperation is attributed to greater extent of coronary atherosclerosis, interim left ventricular damage, accidents during re-entry, technical difficulty caused by adhesions, and longer pump-oxygenator time. In the mid 1970s, other reports confirmed that reoperation was more hazardous, but the clinical results approached those achieved after the first operation (Skow et al., 1973; Benedict et al., 1974; Londe and Sugg, 1974; Macmanus et al., 1975; Winkle et al., 1975; Thomas et al., 1976; Stiles et al., 1976).

PREOPERATIVE ASSESSMENT

Reoperation candidates are not a homogeneous group. The complexities and the greater risk of reoperation have established a more conservative selection process. In contrast to selection for the first operation, severity of symptoms carries more weight for reoperation than functional anatomy. Some patients subjected to reoperation have undergone the first coronary artery bypass operation at a younger age, often in their late forties, which may indicate a predilection for more progressive atherosclerosis. The ratio of men to women, approximately 9:1 or 10:1, is unchanged. Concerning risk factors, the consensus is divided. Some reports indicate that there is a slightly higher prevalence of diabetes, but generally, hypertension and tobacco usage are nearly the same as before the first procedure. We have not found a higher incidence of hyperlipidemia in reoperation patients; however, Barboriak and associates (1978) found significantly higher levels of serum triglycerides in reoperation patients.

Assuming the patient is fit medically but has disabling angina pectoris, the angiographic findings in favor of reoperation are technically favorable coronary anatomy: specifically, adequate vessel size and good distal coronary arterial runoff. When the vessel in question is anatomically small or diffusely involved distally with atherosclerosis, it is less likely that a secondary graft will be clinically beneficial. Rarely do patients with two normally functioning grafts require reoperation. Angiographically, these indications are the most frequent reasons for additional surgery: (1) graft failure, (2) progressive atherosclerosis in grafted or ungrafted vessels, and (3) a combination of graft closure and progressive disease. Incomplete revascularization as an indication is rapidly disappearing, largely because of technical experience and more resolute angiography. The major angiographic indications are a 50 per cent or more stenosis in a previously unbypassed vessel or beyond a distal anastomosis, severe stenosis of a graft at either anastomosis, and graft occlusion with preservation of the native artery (Wukasch et al., 1977).

Our reoperations verified that more than half of the patients had one- or two-vessel disease at the first operation and more often patients received one or two grafts during the initial procedure. Progressive coronary atherosclerosis in previously ungrafted arteries is an indication in approximately half of the cases. Progression beyond a distal anastomosis occurs infrequently. In our experience, multiple-vessel disease occurred significantly more frequently in patients operated on for progressive arterial changes, and a third of the patients lost previously normal left ventricular function in the interval between operations.

Early graft failure results from technical errors such as twisting or kinking, tension, narrowing or "purse-stringing" of the anastomosis, grafts anastomosed to vessels with poor runoff, or intimal trauma inflicted during vein preparation. Later, graft obstruction may result from progressively poorer coronary artery runoff or from atherosclerosis in vein grafts.

Most reports in the 1970s have described reoperation experiences within intervals of 2 to 5 years. Evidence is emerging that this interval between operations will lengthen. A second wave of reoperation candidates is likely to follow successful medium-term results. Within the first 5-year interval, Culliford and colleagues (1979) observed that the early reappearance of angina is largely related to technical factors and that late onset angina is attributed to new native lesions. Our experience substantiates this conclusion in that angina recurred after a mean period of 17 months in patients operated on for graft closure, in contrast to 37 months for patients operated on for progressive atherosclerosis (Loop *et al.*, 1981). Reoperation for grafting only is advised mainly for relief of angina and is of no or little value for symptoms of congestive heart failure.

OPERATIVE MANAGEMENT

The previous operative notes and hospital records are read thoroughly to determine occurrence of technical difficulties, previous wound problems, and hospital course. Aspirin and aspirin-containing compounds are discontinued 7 to 10 days before surgery. Stability must be assured preoperatively. Propranolol and nitrates are continued, and the patient may require these medications intraoperatively. Anesthesia management plays a major role in maintenance of a low rate-pressure product perioperatively. A balloon flotation catheter may be inserted in patients with severe multiple-vessel disease, especially in those who have poor left ventricular function. The number of sternal wires inserted initially is noted to ensure complete removal before using the sternal saw.

A number of methods are suggested for sternal re-entry. Exposure of a femoral artery routinely as a safety measure is probably no longer necessary. Some surgeons prefer a heavy-duty pneumatic-powered oscillating saw, and others use this saw for the outer table of bone and divide the inner table with heavy scissors (Oyer and Shumway, 1974), a Lebsche knife, or an oscillating saw (Culliford and Spencer, 1979). The subxiphoid area is not probed, since the right ventricle is often closely adherent. To prevent tearing of the right ventricle or innominate vein by adhesions when the sternum is separated, the undersurface of both sternal halves must be dissected back 4 to 5 cm. before the retractor is inserted. Simultaneously, assistants remove an appropriate length of saphenous vein, preferably from one leg. If the internal mammary artery is used for a graft conduit, it is mobilized at this time.

According to one view, a primary closure of the pericardium results in a lower incidence of postoperative adhesion formation and a reduction of the postcardiotomy syndrome (Cunningham, *et al.*, 1975). Patients who are operated on many years after the initial procedure are less likely to have extensive or vascular adhesions than those who are reoperated on within the first few postoperative months. The pericardium over the right atrium can be found near the junction of the right atrium and the diaphragm or between the aorta and the right atrium. Only enough dissection to allow cannulation is performed. Pericardium adherent to previous cannulation sites is left undisturbed to avoid tearing the atrium. The trend

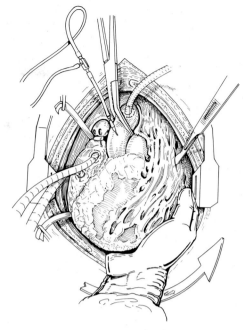

Figure 50–114. After a full or partial cannulation, left ventricular mobilization is begun along the diaphragmatic surface. Adhesions are divided with scissors up to the posterolateral margin. Frequently, the surgeon's right hand moves posterolaterally up to the pericardium anteriorly. This pericardium is incised longitudinally, and the pericardial incision is extended toward the cardiac apex. This maneuver frees the left ventricle and allows the anterior leaf of pericardium to be easily dissected from the antero-apical left ventricle.

today is toward use of a single atrial cannula and no vent or an aortic vent; however, some surgeons find more consistent decompression and more effective myocardial cooling with bicaval cannulation and, selectively, a left atrioventricular vent inserted through the right superior pulmonary vein. Left ventricular apex vents are obsolete. Left ventricular mobilization is performed on cardiopulmonary bypass with the heart either beating or arrested in a cold, flaccid state.

Mobilization of the left ventricle is begun by sharp dissection posteriorly along the diaphragmatic surface. When the posterolateral wall is reached, the surgeon's right hand moves laterally up to the pleuropericardial junction. With the left hand, an incision is made through the pericardium anteriorly and to the left of the decompressed heart (Fig. 50–114). Through this opening, the pericardium is incised longitudinally toward the cardiac apex and the left ventricle is mobilized.

Blood conservation is an important advance in all cardiac operations (Cosgrove *et al.*, 1979; Utley *et al.*, 1981), and particularly in reoperations, morbidity has been significantly affected by decreased blood usage. Blood may be withdrawn through the venous drainage cannula before cardiopulmonary bypass is instituted and stored for transfusion after protaminization. Nearly 20 per cent of the red cell volume can be protected from the effects of artificial oxygenation, and blood loss occurs at a lower hematocrit. Leg incisions should be closed promptly before institution of cardiopulmonary bypass. A regionally heparinized suction system is widely available for retrieval and collection of blood before heparinization and after protamine is administered; no blood is discarded to the wall suction. This collected blood is filtered, washed, and processed to yield packed red cells that are free of debris, heparin, or products of hemolysis. A nonhemic oxygenator prime is used routinely, and hemodilution to an intraoperative hematocrit level of 18 to 25 per cent is safe and well tolerated. Heparin levels may be monitored or activated clotting times used to monitor heparin and protamine dosage more precisely. All oxygenator contents are eventually returned to the patient. Postoperatively, shed mediastinal blood that is defibrinated by contact with the pleura and pericardium may be salvaged in a collection system, filtered, and transfused (Schaff *et al.*, 1978). In 10 years, blood usage has decreased fivefold, and the incidence of serum hepatitis has fallen concomitantly. Because of blood conservation techniques, no blood transfusions have been required for as many as 60 per cent of reoperation patients (Kobayashi *et al.*, 1978).

Most surgeons protect the myocardium by core cooling (22° to 28°C.) or topical cooling or both, combined with cold potassium cardioplegia injected into the ascending aorta. Inability to identify target vessels has been overcome largely by experience. Because of diffuse and extensive atherosclerosis, anastomoses in the distal half of coronary vessels are more frequent at reoperation than in the first procedure. A failed graft can be traced to its distal anastomosis and the second graft constructed beyond the first one (Fig. 50–115). A collapsed cord-like vein indicates that the graft closed soon after the first operation. We have found that the left internal mammary artery is an excellent substitute for failed saphenous vein grafts to the anterior descending artery,

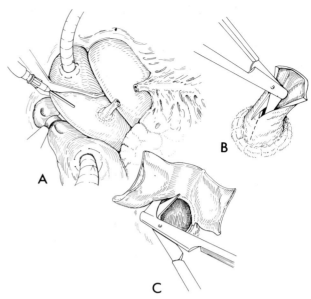

Figure 50–116. Sites of previous proximal graft anastomoses may be reused for attaching new grafts. This collage shows *(A)* division of the old, nonviable graft, *(B)* longitudinal division of the old graft back to the aortic opening, and *(C)* trimming the graft around the aortic opening.

especially for small coronary arteries (Loop *et al.*, 1976). Proximal anastomoses on the aorta are frequently difficult owing to inadequate aortic area, aortic atherosclerosis, or inaccessibility from previously constructed grafts. Occluded vein grafts can be divided a short distance from the aorta, incised back to the aortic anastomosis, and trimmed appropriately so that the aortic opening is used again for the new graft anastomosis (Fig. 50–116).

Before discontinuation of cardiopulmonary bypass, the posterior pericardium and any bleeding from

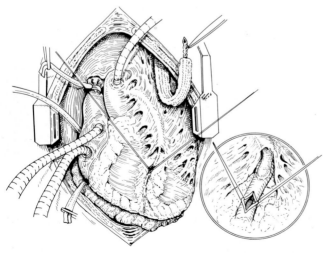

Figure 50–115. Regrafting after failure of the first graft is most frequently performed distal to the previous anastomosis. The coronary vessel is identified by tracing the old graft distally. In this line drawing, the left internal mammary artery pedicle has been prepared for regrafting the anterior descending artery.

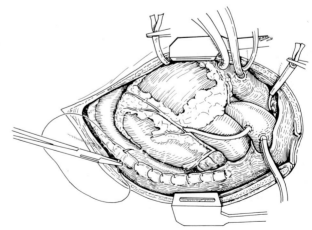

Figure 50–117. Frequent sites for hemorrhage are from adhesions posterolaterally and from the pericardial fat posterolaterally. The operator must gain hemostasis in these areas before discontinuation of cardiopulmonary support. Frequently, electrocautery suffices, but a running lock suture may be necessary while the patient remains on cardiopulmonary bypass. Attempts to secure this area after decannulation cause hemodynamic instability.

adhesions posterolaterally should be controlled by electrocautery or suture ligature (Fig. 50–117). An organized, methodical clean-up phase can be accomplished expeditiously; random cauterization and purposeless movements should be discouraged. After decannulation and secured hemostasis, a left atrial monitor line selectively, temporary atrial and ventricular pacing wires, and chest tubes are inserted. A heavy No. 6 stainless steel wire assures tight sternal closure and prevents dehiscence even when chronic ventilatory support is necessary postoperatively. Postoperative management, described in other chapters, is no different in the reoperation patient. Attention to afterload reduction, adequate volume replacement, and maintenance of normal hemodynamics usually result in early extubation and prompt recovery.

CLINICAL RESULTS OF CORONARY ARTERY REOPERATIONS

A cardiac mortality rate of 10 per cent or higher in the early years has been halved by greater experience technically in reoperation and improved myocardial protection (Keon et al., 1977; Irarrazaval et al., 1977; Krause et al., 1978; Stiles and Cunningham, 1981). The complication rate in reoperations remains approximately twice that after primary procedures. Recent reports indicate that morbidity, specifically perioperative myocardial infarction, low cardiac output, hemorrhage, infection, and respiratory insufficiency, has declined during the past 5 years. Improved myocardial protection has decreased perioperative infarction. Table 50–20 lists the clinical characteristics and results, including perioperative infarction rates for a normothermic series before 1977 and a 1977 to 1979 cardioplegia series (Loop et al., 1981).

There are few published reports of angiographic results after reoperation, and patency varies widely, but generally results are similar to those achieved after the first operation. In our experience of 104 patients recatheterized an average of 19 months after reoperation, we found that the catheterization was advised in nearly all patients because of angina. Yet

TABLE 50–20. MYOCARDIAL PROTECTION IN CORONARY ARTERY REOPERATION PATIENTS

VARIABLE	ISCHEMIC ARREST N = 387 1967–1977	CARDIOPLEGIA N = 113 1978–1979	
Median age (years)	54	54	
Extent of disease			
One vessel	5 (9.0%)	6 (5.3%)	
Two vessels	114 (29.5%)	32 (28.3%)	
Three vessels	238 (61.5%)	75 (66.4%)	
Normal left ventricle	222 (57.4%)	72 (63.7%)	
Grafts per patient	1.5	2.0	
Perioperative infarction	30 (7.8%)	3 (2.7%)	p = 0.055
Operative mortality	17 (4.4%)	3 (2.7%)	
Two-year survival rate	92.4%	95.3%	

the vein graft patency rate was 79 per cent and the internal mammary artery graft patency rate was 97 per cent. Grafts performed for graft failure had an 85 per cent patency rate, and grafts performed to arteries previously not grafted (progressive atherosclerosis) had an 83 per cent patency rate. Left ventricular status usually remains unchanged and there are fewer examples of improvement after reoperation. Patients with worse left ventricular function frequently have had a perioperative myocardial infarction.

Vein graft atherosclerosis accounts for an increasing number of reoperations. In our experience, intimal lipid deposition is a rare cause of graft narrowing before the third postoperative year. Bulkley and Hutchins (1977) have reported a subendothelial proliferation of smooth muscle cells within the first postoperative year; however, it is not known whether these changes are a precursor to advanced graft atherosclerosis. According to Spray and Roberts (1977), subendothelial fibrous tissue proliferation is variable in magnitude and location and infrequently causes severe graft narrowing. Although grafts studied by these investigators showed intimal changes, the degree and severity were variable along the length of the grafts and among separate grafts in the same patient. Campeau and associates (1978) noted in serial arteriograms that diffuse graft narrowing did not progress after the first year and did not appear to lead to late graft occlusion. However, grafts with localized stenoses frequently progressed to late occlusion. After 5 to 7 postoperative years, approximately 10 per cent of the grafts showed evidence of atherosclerotic changes. Grondin and coworkers (1970) have reported a higher incidence of progressive atherosclerosis in ungrafted arteries in patients with vein graft atherosclerosis. Late graft atherosclerosis has not been reported in internal mammary artery grafts (Fig. 50–118).

The common denominators for development of graft atherosclerosis appear to be an elevation of intravascular pressure (Stehbens, 1975), an increase in shear stress on the vascular wall, and, in many cases, hyperlipemia (Lie et al., 1977). Elevation in pressure may result in recurring endothelial damage, which is converted to intimal lesions by progressive fibrin deposition. In high-flow states, the endothelium may be "washed" of thrombi, whereas low-flow states may encourage thrombus formation and result in significant luminal narrowing. Focal graft stenosis that develops within the first postoperative year is nonatherosclerotic and caused by a reaction to traumatic handling or, rarely, fibrosis around a venous valve.

An atherosclerotic vein that retains antegrade flow has the propensity for embolization of atherosclerotic material into the native coronary circulation. At operation, these grafts should be clamped distally and handled gently. Inspection of atherosclerotic veins shows that although one major site of narrowing may be visible angiographically, the vein is usually lined with diffuse lipid deposits. Replacement of the atherosclerotic vein by a new vein segment is recommended

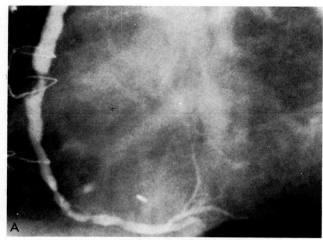

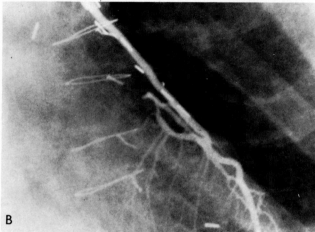

Figure 50–118. *A,* Severe diffuse atherosclerosis present in a right coronary artery graft performed 5 years previously. This graft was ligated proximally and distally and replaced with a new saphenous vein graft. *B,* This frame from the same patient shows smooth patency of a left internal mammary artery graft to the left anterior descending coronary artery. To date, we have seen numerous examples of vein graft atherosclerosis coexisting with a normal internal mammary artery graft in the same patient. Late internal mammary artery graft dysfunction is extremely rare.

rather than performance of interposition grafts. Finally, the new technique of balloon angioplasty has been successful in dilating graft stenoses near or in proximal or distal anastomoses, but dilatation of atheroslcerotic veins have met with mixed results (Ford *et al.,* 1980). Late results have not been reported.

The effect of reoperation on symptom status ranges from complete relief of angina in 30 to 75 per cent of patients to improvement in 50 to 94 per cent of patients within the first 2 years. Generally, follow-up has been short and often not complete. Earlier reports indicated a less favorable clinical response in patients reoperated on for graft closure. However, more recently the clinical status appears equal for all of the angiographic indication groups. At a mean follow-up of 42 months, we found that 59 per cent of our reoperation patients were free of angina, and at 63 months, 45 per cent were asymptomatic. Allen and colleagues (1978) assessed reoperative variables for

prognostic significance and found that vessel size greater than 2.0 mm. and isolated proximal plaque distribution correlated significantly with improved clinical status; i.e., outcome was less favorable when the patient had diffuse coronary atherosclerosis and poor left ventricular function. However, the few patients who have severe complications after reoperation that may result in chronic pain and anguish or those who experience psychosocial problems related to coronary heart disease do not have a clinical status that is reflected satisfactorily by statistics or functional classification.

SURVIVAL

Reul and colleagues (1979) reported a 90 per cent actuarial 5-year rate survival for 168 patients who underwent reoperation between 1968 and 1978. Of our first 1000 reoperation cases, intermediate-term follow-up has been completed for the first 750 patients. The 5-year survival rate was 89 per cent, which includes all early and late deaths from all causes. Patients who underwent reoperation for graft closure had a 91 per cent 5-year survival rate, whereas those reoperated on for progressive atherosclerosis in previously ungrafted arteries had an 87 per cent 5-year survival rate; among patients who were reoperated on for both graft closure and progressive atherosclerosis, 88 per cent were alive (Fig. 50–119). The survival rate varied from 95 per cent for patients with one-vessel disease to 87 per cent for patients with three-vessel disease. As expected, patients who had normal left ventricular contraction before reoperation had a higher survival rate (91 per cent) than patients with poor left ventricular function (81 per cent).

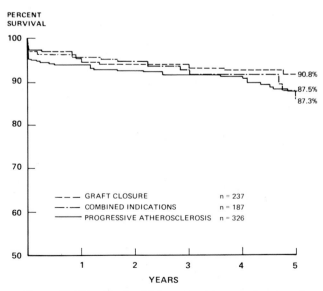

Figure 50–119. Kaplan-Meier actuarial survival curves from a coronary artery reoperation series of 750 patients who have been divided into angiographic indication groups. After a mean follow-up of 57 months, the 5-year survival rates were nearly the same, regardless of the reason for reoperation.

Comparative medical series do not exist, and it would be difficult to match patients for comparative purposes. At this stage in the evolution of reoperations for myocardial ischemia, it may be concluded that relief of symptoms is less after reoperation principally because of diffuse progressive atherosclerosis. Longevity has probably been improved, as evidenced by the nearly 90 per cent 5-year survival rate after reoperation. Revascularization as complete as possible at the first operation and a low graft attrition rate are the best means available to forestall reoperation.

SELECTED REFERENCES

Campeau, L., Lespérance, J., Hermann, J., Corbara, F., Grondin, C. M., and Bourassa, M. G.: Loss of the improvement of angina between 1 and 7 years after aortocoronary bypass surgery: Correlations with changes in vein grafts and in coronary arteries. Circulation, *60*(Suppl. 1):1, 1979.

Angina status was correlated with findings in serial coronary arteriograms 1 and 5 to 7 years postoperatively. Recurrence of angina in 36 per cent of patients over a 5-year period could be related to intrinsic changes in grafts and progression of coronary atherosclerosis, particularly in ungrafted coronary arteries. These changes were documented in 74 per cent of those with recurring angina in comparison with 18 per cent of patients whose improvement did not deteriorate.

Culliford, A. T., Girdwood, R. W., Isom, O. W., Krauss, K. R., and Spencer, F. C.: Angina following myocardial revascularization: Does time of recurrence predict etiology and influence results of operation? J. Thorac. Cardiovasc. Surg., *77*:889, 1979.

An excellent survey of reoperation experience that credits declining operative mortality to technique and improved myocardial protection. Early recurrence of symptoms correlated with technical factors and exuberant pericardial scarring. Late deterioration of clinical status most frequently was related to development of a new coronary lesion(s) or grafting proximal to a severe obstruction.

Grondin, C. M., Campeau, L., Lespérance, J., Solymoss, B. C., Vouhé, P., Castonguay, Y. R., Meere, C., and Bourassa, M. G.: Atherosclerotic changes in coronary vein grafts six years after operation: Angiographic aspects in 110 patients. J. Thorac. Cardiovasc. Surg., *77*:24, 1979.

Graft atherosclerosis is categorized by serial angiograms performed approximately 1 year and 6 years postoperatively. Thirteen per cent showed luminal changes, which were classified into five types: filling defect, smooth plaque, diaphragm, circumferential stenosis, and irregular contour. Approximately half of nongrafted arteries showed evidence of progressive coronary atherosclerosis. Histologic findings related to saphenous veins in the arterial position are discussed extensively.

Loop, F. D., Cosgrove, D. M., Kramer, J. R., Lytle, B. W., Taylor, P. C., Golding, L. A. R., and Groves, L. K.: Late clinical and arteriographic results in 500 coronary artery reoperations. J. Thorac. Cardiovasc. Surg., *81*:675, 1981.

This is a detailed report of reoperative revascularization from The Cleveland Clinic Foundation. Indication groups are compared with regard to clinical improvement, graft patency, and medium-term survival. Angina recurred relatively early in graft failure patients and nearly 2 years later in those affected with progressive coronary atherosclerosis. After an operative mortality rate of 4 per cent the actuarial 5-year survival rate was 89 per cent and was essentially equal among the indication groups.

REFERENCES

Adam, M., Geisler, G. F., Lambert, C. J., and Mitchel, B. F., Jr.: Reoperation following clinical failure of aorta-to-coronary artery bypass vein grafts. Ann. Thorac. Surg., *14*:272, 1972.

Allen, R. H., Stinson, E. B., Oyer, P. E., and Shumway, N. E.: Predictive variables in reoperation for coronary artery disease. J. Thorac. Cardiovasc. Surg., *75*:186, 1978.

Barboriak, J. J., Pintar, K., and Korns, M. E.: Atherosclerosis in aortocoronary vein grafts. Lancet, *2*:621, 1974.

Barboriak, J. J., Barboriak, D. P., Anderson, A. J., Rimm, A. A., Tristani, F. E., and Flemma, R. J.: Risk factors in patients undergoing a second aorta-coronary bypass procedure. J. Thorac. Cardiovasc. Surg., *76*:111, 1978.

Benedict, J. S., Buhl, T. L., and Henney, R. P.: Re-revascularization of the ischemic myocardium. Arch. Surg., *108*:40, 1974.

Bourassa, M. G., Lespérance, J., Corbara, F., Saltiel, J., and Campeau, L.: Progression of obstructive coronary artery disease 5 to 7 years after aortocoronary bypass surgery. Circulation, *58*(Suppl. 1):100, 1978.

Bruschke, A. V. G., Wijers, T. S., Kolsters, W., and Landmann, J.: The anatomic evolution of coronary artery disease demonstrated by coronary arteriography in 256 nonoperated patients. Circulation, *63*:527, 1981.

Bulkley, B. H., and Hutchins, G. M.: Accelerated "atherosclerosis": A morphologic study of 97 saphenous vein coronary artery bypass grafts. Circulation, *55*:163, 1977.

Campeau, L., Lespérance, J., Corbara, F., Hermann, J., Grondin, C. M., and Bourassa, M. G.: Aortocoronary saphenous vein bypass graft changes 5 to 7 years after surgery. Circulation, *58*(Suppl. 1):170, 1978.

Campeau, L., Lespérance, J., Hermann, J., Corbara, F., Grondin, C. M., and Bourassa, M. G.: Loss of the improvement of angina between 1 and 7 years after aortocoronary bypass surgery: Correlations with changes in vein grafts and in coronary arteries. Circulation, *60*(Suppl. 1):1, 1979.

Cosgrove, D. M., Thurer, R. L., Lytle, B. W., Gill, C. G., Peter, M., and Loop, F. D.: Blood conservation during myocardial revascularization. Ann. Thorac. Surg., *28*:184, 1979.

Culliford, A. T., and Spencer, F. C.: Guidelines for safely opening a previous sternotomy incision. J. Thorac. Cardiovasc. Surg., *78*:633, 1979.

Culliford, A. T., Girdwood, R. W., Isom, O. W., Krauss, K. R., and Spencer, F. C.: Angina following myocardial revascularization: Does time of recurrence predict etiology and influence results of operation? J. Thorac. Cardiovasc. Surg., *77*:889, 1979.

Cunningham, J. N., Jr., Spencer, F. C., Zeff, R., Williams, C. D., Cukingnan, R., and Mullin, M.: Influence of primary closure of the pericardium after open-heart surgery on the frequency of tamponade, postcardiotomy syndrome, and pulmonary complications. J. Thorac. Cardiovasc. Surg., *70*:119, 1975.

Ford, W. B., Wholey, M. H., Zikria, E. A., Miller, W. H., Samadani, S. R., Koimattur, A. G., and Sullivan, M. E.: Percutaneous transluminal angioplasty in the management of occlusive disease involving the coronary arteries and saphenous vein bypass grafts: Preliminary results. J. Thorac. Cardiovasc. Surg., *79*:1, 1980.

Grondin, C. M., Campeau, L., Lespérance, J., Solymoss, B. C., Vouhe, P., Castonguay, Y. R., Meere, C., and Bourassa, M. G.: Atherosclerotic changes in coronary vein grafts six years after operation: Angiographic aspect in 110 patients. J. Thorac. Cardiovasc. Surg., *77*:24, 1979.

Hamby, R. I., Aintablian, A., Handler, M., Voleti, C., Weisz, D., Garvey, J. W., and Wisoff, G.: Aortocoronary saphenous vein bypass grafts: Long-term patency, morphology and blood flow in patients with patent grafts early after surgery. Circulation, *60*:901, 1979.

Irarrazaval, M. J., Cosgrove, D. M., Loop, F. D., Ennix, C. L., Jr., Groves, L. K., and Taylor, P. C.: Reoperations for myocardial revascularization. J. Thorac. Cardiovasc. Surg., *73*:181, 1977.

Johnson, W. D., Hoffman, J. F., Jr., Flemma, R. J., and Tector, A. J.: Secondary surgical procedure for myocardial revascularization. J. Thorac. Cardiovasc. Surg., *64*:523, 1972.

Keon, W. J., Bédard, P., Akyurekli, Y., and Brais, M.: Experience with reoperation following coronary artery bypass grafting. Can. J. Surg., 20:142, 1977.

Kobayashi, T., Mendez, A. M., Zubiate, P., Vanstrom, N. R., Yokoyama, T., and Kay, J. H.: Repeat aortocoronary bypass grafting. Early and late results. Chest, 73:446, 1978.

Kramer, J. R., Matsuda, Y., Mulligan, J. C., Aronow, M., and Proudfit, W. L.: Progression of coronary atherosclerosis. Circulation, 63:519, 1981.

Krause, A. H., Jr., Page, U. S., Bigelow, J. C., Okies, J. E., and Dunlap, S. F.: Reoperation in symptomatic patients after direct coronary artery revascularization. J. Thorac. Cardiovasc. Surg., 75:499, 1978.

Lie, J. T., Lawrie, G. M., and Morris, G. C., Jr.: Aortocoronary bypass saphenous vein graft atherosclerosis: Anatomic study of 99 vein grafts from normal and hyperlipoproteinemic patients up to 75 months postoperatively. Am. J. Cardiol., 40:906, 1977.

Londe, S., and Sugg, W. L.: The challenge of reoperation in cardiac surgery. Ann. Thorac. Surg., 17:157, 1974.

Loop, F. D., Cosgrove, D. M., Kramer, J. R., Lytle, B. W., Taylor, P. C., Golding, L. A. R., and Groves, L. K.: Late clinical and arteriographic results in 500 coronary artery re-operations. J. Thorac. Cardiovasc. Surg., 81:675, 1981.

Loop, F. D., Carabajal, N. R., Taylor, P. C., and Irarrazaval, M. J.: Internal mammary artery bypass graft in reoperative myocardial revascularization. Am. J. Cardiol., 37:890, 1976.

Macmanus, Q., Okies, J. E., Phillips, S. J., and Starr, A.: Surgical considerations in patients undergoing repeat median sternotomy. J. Thorac. Cardiovasc. Surg., 69:138, 1975.

Oyer, P. E., and Shumway, N. E.: Again, via the median sternotomy. Arch. Surg., 109:604, 1974.

Reul, G. J., Jr., Cooley, D. A., Ott, D. A., Coelho, A., Chapa, L., and Eterovic, I.: Reoperation for recurrent coronary artery disease. Causes, indications and results in 168 patients. Arch. Surg., 114:1269, 1979.

Robert, E. W., Guthaner, D. F., Wexler, L., and Alderman, E. L.: Six-year clinical and angiographic follow-up of patients with previously documented complete revascularization. Circulation, 58(Suppl. 1):194, 1978.

Schaff, H. V., Hauer, J. M., Bell, W. R., Gardner, T. J., Donahoo, J. S., Gott, V. L., and Brawley, R. K.: Autotransfusion of shed mediastinal blood after cardiac surgery: A prospective study. J. Thorac. Cardiovasc. Surg., 75:632, 1978.

Skow, J. R., Carey, J. S., Plested, W. G., and Mulder, D. G.: Saphenous vein bypass as a secondary cardiac procedure. Arch. Surg., 107:34, 1973.

Spray, T. L., and Roberts, W. C.: Changes in saphenous veins used as aortocoronary bypass grafts. Am. Heart J., 94:500, 1977.

Stehbens, W. E.: The role of hemodynamics in the pathogenesis of atherosclerosis. Prog. Cardiovasc. Dis., 18:89, 1975.

Stiles, Q. R., and Cunningham, J. M.: Is re-revascularization clinically beneficial? Am. J. Surg., 141:656, 1981.

Stiles, Q. R., Lindesmith, G. G., Tucker, B. L., Hughes, R. K., and Meyer, B. W.: Experience with fifty repeat procedures for myocardial revascularization. J. Thorac. Cardiovasc. Surg., 72:849, 1976.

Thomas, C. S., Jr., Alford, W. C., Jr., Burrus, G. R., Frist, R. A., and Stoney, W. S.: Results of reoperation for failed aortocoronary bypass grafts. Arch. Surg., 111:1210, 1976.

Utley, J. R., Moores, W. Y., and Stephens, D. B.: Blood conservation techniques. Ann. Thorac. Surg., 31:482, 1981.

Winkle, R. A., Alderman, E. L., Shumway, N. E., and Harrison, D. C.: Results of reoperation for unsuccessful coronary artery bypass surgery. Circulation, 51, 52(Suppl. 1):61, 1975.

Wukasch, D. C., Toscano, M., Cooley, D. A., Reul, G. J., Jr., Sandiford, F. M., Kyger, E. R., and Hallman, G. L.: Reoperation following direct myocardial revascularization. Circulation, 56(Suppl. 2):3, 1977.

5.   Left Ventricular Aneurysm

ALDEN H. HARKEN

HISTORY

Early reports of cardiac aneurysms were confounded by the prosectors' failure to distinguish generalized cardiomegaly from aneurysm formation. Sternberg (1914) catalogued descriptions of cardiac enlargement by Baillow in 1538 and Lancisius in 1740. Schlichter and colleagues (1954) attribute the first reports of ventricular aneurysm to Dominicus Gusmanus Galeati (1751) and John Hunter (1757). Hunter's description specifically identified aneurysmal thinning of the left ventricular apex "... lined with a thrombus just the shape of the pouch in which it lay." In 1816, Cruveilhier first recognized that a ventricular aneurysm was myocardial fibrosis, but the pathogenesis of this fibrosis was unclear (Rokitansky, 1844). Toward the end of the nineteenth century, several cases of left ventricular aneurysm were convincingly suspected ante mortem (Voelcker, 1902), and Cohnheim and Shulthess-Rechberg traced the etiology of ventricular aneurysm to myocardial infarction. By 1914, Sternberg recognized the sequence of angina preceding myocardial infarction leading to ventricular aneurysm. He correctly diagnosed ventricular aneurysm based on the pathogenetic concept of coronary artery occlusion and even predicted the feasibility of radiologic confirmation.

In the early part of this century, x-rays greatly facilitated diagnosis, and Sezary and Alibert first visualized an aneurysm in 1922. Ten years later, mural calcification was noted radiologically. Subsequently, paradoxical systolic ventricular motion was appreciated fluoroscopically (Schwedel et al., 1950), and Dolly and coworkers demonstrated a ventricular aneurysm by angiography in 1951.

With the diagnosis established, Bailey initiated the surgical attack on left ventricular aneurysm in 1955 (Likoff and Bailey, 1955). Via the left chest, he applied a large clamp to the bulging, beating aneurysm and plicated the adjacent ventricle below this instrument. The development of cardiopulmonary bypass permitted Cooley and associates (1958) to establish the current open heart technique of aneurysmectomy. By 1973, Loop and colleagues had already established indications and were providing excellent surgical rehabilitation for a large group of patients with left ventricular aneurysms.

PATHOLOGY

Cardiac aneurysms most often occur as a result of myocardial ischemia and usually involve the left ventricle. Aneurysms of the right ventricle are uncommon and may be due to congenital dysplasia of the ventricle or may occur following trauma, and either type may be the site of dysrhythmias.

Ischemia of the Left Ventricle

The progressive imbalance of oxygen supply and demand leads to an ultimate failure of blood supply to support tissue viability, with consequent myocardial infarction. Three aspects of this pathologic process lead directly to the three clinical stigmata associated with left ventricular aneurysm.

First, as a thin layer of necrotic muscle and fibrous tissue replaces the contracting myocardium, paradoxical systolic motion "steals" left ventricular stroke volume, thus decreasing cardiac output (Alpert and Braunwald, 1980; Swan *et al.,* 1972). By LaPlace's law, wall tension increases as the ventricle dilates; thus, factors promoting even further global or regional ventricular dilatation increase rapidly.

Second, transmural or subendocardial infarction transforms the glimmering, smooth endocardium into a microscopically rough surface that encourages thrombus formation (Weiss, 1975). Endothelial injury promotes release of thromboxanes, which vigorously induce platelet release and aggregation (Didisheim and Foster, 1978). Evidence for platelet involvement is provided by elevations of circulating platelet factor four (PF-4), which is a marker of platelet activation (Handin *et al.,* 1978). Although conformational changes in the left ventricle (Fig. 50–120) may produce relative stasis that contributes to thrombus formation (Rosenthal and Braunwald, 1980), aneurysm formation is not essential to the development of endocardial clot (Cabin and Roberts, 1980).

Third, the thin wall of a left ventricular aneurysm and the adjacent jeopardized border are composed of a mixture of fibrous tissue, necrotic muscle, and viable myocardium (Schlichter *et al.,* 1954). The electrophysiologic properties of conduction and refractoriness in these tissues are quite logically different (Spear *et al.,* 1979). The conditions for re-entrant ventricular arrhythmias are satisfied when two or more electrically heterogeneous pathways (with respect to conduction and refractoriness) are connected proximally and distally (Wellens, 1975). An impulse must travel in only one direction along one of these pathways (unidirectional block). When this impulse arrives at the distal

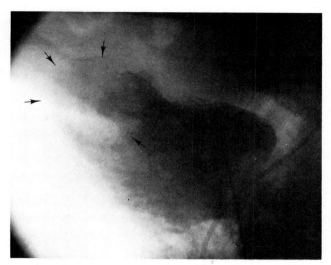

Figure 50–120. Contrast ventriculography showing an apical left ventricular aneurysm. Arrows delineate a large mural thrombus.

connection, it may return along the originally blocked pathway. If conduction of this impulse is sufficiently slow to permit repolarization of the origin, the impulse may re-enter the circuit (Fig. 50–121). Normal hearts contain a network of interarterial anastomotic channels that are 50 to 100 μ in diameter. In patients with coronary occlusive disease, these coronary collaterals become quite extensive (Gorlin, 1976). Subsequent myocardial infarction with multiple zones of pericollateral salvage produces a heterogeneously injured zone (Fig. 50–121**B**) that predisposes to re-entrant arrhythmias.

Other Causes

Schlichter and colleagues (1954) noted that the first description of aneurysmal dilatation of any cardiac chamber was of a right atrial aneurysm by Borrich in 1676. Left atrial aneurysms, although even less common, have been described both as "giant dog ears" (Galeati, 1757) and as aneurysms following mitral valvuloplasty (Fojo-Echevarria *et al.,* 1955). Right ventricular aneurysms do occur, but even these tend to be ischemic in origin (Stansel *et al.,* 1963). They may also be congenital. Iatrogenic "patch" or false pseudoaneurysms represent a complication of right ventricular closure following surgical repair of a congenital defect. Cardiac diverticular (Arnold, 1894) and congenital aneurysms (Klein, 1889) have been associated with hypoplasia of the aorta. Left ventricular aneurysm secondary to an aberrant coronary artery arising from the pulmonary artery has been diagnosed in a 2-month-old child (Schlichter *et al.,* 1954). Syphilitic ventricular aneurysm due to either gummatous myocarditis or luetic coronary ostial stenosis is referred to in the older literature (Basset-Smith, 1908; Bricout, 1912). Small mycotic aneurysms secondary to bacterial endocarditis have been identified (Schlichter *et al.,* 1954). False pseudoaneurysms

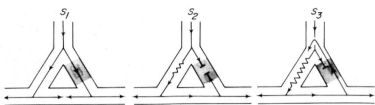

Figure 50–121. **A,** Schema for re-entrant arrhythmias induced by paced premature stimuli (S_1, S_2, and S_3). A heterogeneous area of myocardium capable of re-entry is depicted in each panel. With S_1, the depolarization wave front proceeds down both limbs of the potential circuit and extinguishes at the bottom. A second paced premature stimulus (S_2) proceeds down the left limb slowly (sawtoothed line), but its return up the right limb is blocked. A third premature stimulus (S_3) proceeds down the left limb even more slowly (slow conduction) and is blocked in the right limb (unidirectional block). Conduction down the left limb is sufficiently slow to permit repolarization of the pathologic (stippled area) right limb. The impulse may therefore return along the right limb and "re-enter" the circuit.

Illustration continued on opposite page

of both the right ventricle (Stansel *et al.,* 1963) and the left ventricle (Lyons and Perkins, 1958) due to traumatic disruption and containment rarely present. False left ventricular aneurysm secondary to ischemia, cardiac rupture, and containment is more common (Vlodaver *et al.,* 1975), and this lesion shares the hemodynamic and thromboembolic complications of a true aneurysm.

NATURAL HISTORY

The relationship between congestive heart failure, angiographic evidence of regional left ventricular dysfunction, and poor prognosis (regardless of medical or surgical therapy) is well established (Cohn and Braunwald, 1980). Indeed, of the myriad risk factors currently related to prognosis in ischemic heart disease, left ventricular function is unquestionably the dominant variable. Pathologic studies have classically presented a bleak outlook for patients with left ventricular aneurysm. In a group of 102 patients with pathologically proven aneurysms, only 27 per cent survived for 3 years and 12 per cent survived for 5 years (Schlichter *et al.,* 1954). Schattenberg and coworkers (1970) found a 76 per cent mortality rate in 39 months with a similar group of patients. Proudfit (1979) followed 74 patients with angiographically proven left ventricular aneurysms and observed a 5-year survival rate of 47 per cent and a 10-year survival rate of 18 per cent. Similarly, surgical results of aneurysmectomy are almost entirely dependent on the quantity of residual contracting ventricle (Cooperman *et al.,* 1975; Lee *et al.,* 1977).

In the classic study by Bruschke and colleagues (1973), 490 patients were studied angiographically and then treated medically, with a follow-up of 5 to 9 years. Again, survival depended primarily on the extent of coronary disease and left ventricular function. In the 10 years since publication of this report, medical therapy has improved immeasurably. No one is willing to accept these statistics as the currently achievable medical standard. For ethical, moral, perhaps legal, and certainly practical reasons, however, it will not be possible to improve on this study. Patients are necessarily culled out for surgery following angiographic documentation of left main coronary artery disease (Murphy *et al.,* 1977) or triple-vessel disease (European Coronary Surgery Study Group, 1979), even with regional ventricular dysfunction.

Grondin and coworkers (1979) have confirmed poor 10-year survival in symptomatic patients with left ventricular aneurysm. Conversely, this group has presented an actuarial survival rate of 90 per cent at 10 years for a small group of asymptomatic patients. One wonders why this group was catheterized. Prolongation of life as an isolated indication for surgery in patients with left ventricular aneurysm remains controversial. In symptomatic patients with medically intractable ventricular failure, angina, thromboemboli, and ventricular arrhythmias, the role of surgery is clearer.

DIAGNOSIS

Physical Examination. Multiple physical signs, such as enlargement of transverse cardiac fullness and forceful cardiac impulse concurrent with a weak peripheral pulse, have been noted as indicators of left ventricular aneurysm (Schlichter *et al.,* 1954). Libman (1932) stressed that a distinct pulsation independent of the apical impulse and associated with a gallop rhythm and a dull first heart sound was pathognomonic of an aneurysm. Today, an aneurysm may be suspected but never confirmed by physical examination.

Ventriculography. Regional contractility can be localized by superimposing the angiographic outlines of end-diastole (Herman *et al.,* 1967). Clearly, there is a spectrum of ventricular function from normal to gross paradox. Akinesis exists when a portion of the diastolic and systolic ventriculographic silhouettes share a common line. Dyskinesis is present when the end-systolic silhouette actually protrudes outside the end-diastolic outline. The nonischemic ventricle should exhibit synchronous and symmetric shortening of all segments (Sniderman *et al.,* 1973). Coronary artery disease typically produces regional rather than global damage. It is therefore mandatory to utilize biplane (at least two views) ventriculography (Cohn *et al.,* 1974).

With improvements in surgical techniques, it is now possible for almost anyone to survive surgery, but that does not mean that they will be functionally better postoperatively. For this reason, interventional angiography employing inotropic stimulation (Horn *et*

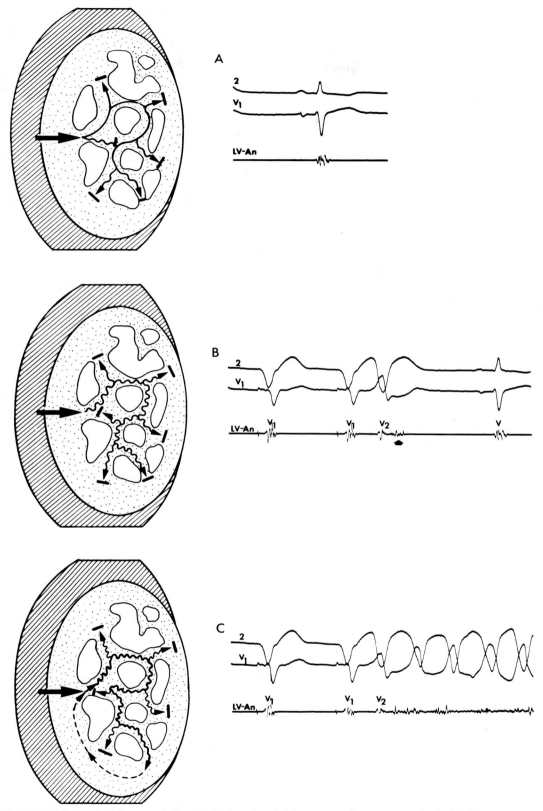

Figure 50–121. *Continued* **B,** Boineau and Cox (1963) introduced this concept of re-entrant arrhythmias. Heterogeneous myocardial ischemia and damage serve as a potential re-entrant circuit (as in Figure 50–121). *A,* The wave front enters the heterogeneous zone and is slowed, producing a fragmented afterpotential. *B,* Further heterogeneity and slower conduction produce a longer afterpotential. *C,* The ischemic zone is sufficiently complex to fragment and slow the wave front so that it may re-enter and sustain a re-entrant arrhythmia.

al., 1974), afterload reduction (Helfant et al., 1974), or postextrasystolic potentiation (Dyke et al., 1974) has been developed to assess regional "contractile reserve." In this fashion, the surgeon can glean some clue as to the functional response to aneurysmectomy and myocardial revascularization.

Echocardiography. Echocardiography provides a precise, noninvasive, almost universally available reflection of intracardiac structures. M-mode echocardiography emits a beam of ultrasound from a transducer placed on the patient's chest. Echoes arise from an interface in tissue density, such as blood to muscle. The spatial resolution ($\pm$ 1 to 2 mm.) and temporal resolution ($\pm$msec.) of the M mode are high, but the "tunnel vision" of the echo beam offers a narrow image of intracardiac structures (Parisi et al., 1980). Two-dimensional echocardiograms display a planar beam of echoes in a "slice-like" tomographic fashion. Regional left ventricular dysfunction (Fortuin and Pawsey, 1977) may distinguish true aneurysms and pseudoaneurysms (Gatewood and Nanda, 1980) with or without intraventricular clot.

Radionuclide Cineangiography. Real-time radionuclide cineangiography has proved to be of clinical value in the noninvasive evaluation of patients with coronary artery disease and its sequelae (Borer et al., 1977). The advocates of this technique note that it is safe, simple, and noninvasive and therefore comfortable for the patient, inexpensive when compared with cardiac catheterization, and accurate (Borer et al., 1980). The issue of accuracy has been examined by many groups, and the correlation between radionuclide cineangiography and contrast ventriculography has been good. In a study by Friedman and Cantor (1979), the radionuclide scintigram correctly identified all of 54 apical and anteroapical aneurysms and one inferior aneurysm. Scintigraphy missed one of six anterior aneurysms and two of three posterobasal aneurysms. Conversely, in 74 patients with angiograms negative for aneurysm, there were two false-positive radionuclide studies. The overall accuracy of gated heart scintigraphy was therefore 96 per cent. The relative "blind" zone appears to be the posterobasal region. Radionuclide cineangiography does have a role as a screening procedure in patients with suspected left ventricular aneurysm.

INDICATIONS FOR SURGERY

Left Ventricular Failure and Angina. The decrease in left ventricular function associated with myocardial infarction is logically related to the volume of muscle damage (Pfeffer et al., 1979). Owing to the virtual absence of oxygen reserve, contractility decreases significantly 4 to 6 seconds following the cessation of blood flow (Harden et al., 1979). In a normothermic, working heart, some cells begin to suffer irreversible damage following 20 minutes of ischemia (Jennings and Ganote, 1974). With continued ischemia, four sequential contraction abnormalities

result (Forrester et al., 1976): (1) *dyssynchrony*—dissociation of electrical and mechanical events in the same muscle region; (2) *hypokinesis*—reduced muscle shortening; (3) *akinesis*—absence of muscle shortening; and (4) *paradoxical motion*—systolic muscle bulging. By 6 to 8 hours, edema and cellular infiltration have increased left ventricular wall stiffness (decreased compliance), which actually improves function by decreasing paradoxical systolic wall motion (Vokonas et al., 1976). As pump function deteriorates, cardiac output, stroke volume, blood pressure, and contractility (dp/dt) are reduced (Pfeffer et al., 1979). Rackley and colleagues (1977) have correlated clinical measurements of left ventricular dysfunction with left ventricular angiography in man. A decrease in ejection fraction was detectable when 10 per cent of the ventricle contracted abnormally. An increase in left ventricular end-diastolic pressure and volume occurred when 15 per cent of the ventricle was involved. When 25 per cent of the ventricle contracted abnormally, patients exhibited congestive failure, and 40 per cent involvement was associated with shock.

Ultimately, myocardial ischemia results when oxygen demand exceeds supply, and wall motion abnormalities are seen universally in patients following clinical infarction (Wynne et al., 1977). The peri-ischemic "border zone" may contract weakly, whereas a compensatory increase in the force of contraction has been described in surrounding non-ischemic muscle (Katz, 1973). Braunwald and Sobel (1980) have identified the increase in wall tension associated with left ventricular dilatation as one of the primary determinants of myocardial oxygen consumption, and Harken and colleagues (1981), using a high-precision fluorophotographic technique, have demonstrated the exquisite sensitivity of the peri-ischemic border zone (thus infarct volume) to alterations in oxygen demand. According to LaPlace's law, wall tension (force/cm.) is the product of intraventricular pressure and radius. With an increase in either global or regional left ventricular dimensions, there is an obligatory increase in wall tension and a concurrent augmentation in muscle oxygen demand. Clinically, the largest cross-sectional wall tension at the equator of the ventricle is presented as circumferential wall stress (Mirsky, 1979) (dynes/cm.^{2} $\times$ 10^3):

LaPlace's law:

$$\text{Tension} = \text{pressure} \times \text{radius}$$

Mirsky's modification:

$$CWS = (P \cdot Y)(1 - Y^2/2X^2 - H/2Y + H^2/8X^2)/H$$

where H is wall thickness, P is left ventricular pressure (dynes/cm.^{2}), and X and Y are the horizontal and vertical axes (cm.) of the ventricle. Circumferential wall stress, and thus myocardial oxygen consumption, is a function of left ventricular dimensions. The rationale for surgical aneurysmectomy in congestive heart failure is firmly based on the principle that a smaller ventricular chamber will pump more efficiently while consuming less oxygen. LaPlace's law assists the surgeon.

Thromboemboli. Endocardial thrombosis frequently accompanies myocardial infarction (Handin *et al.,* 1978). Mural thrombus is identified (Fig. 50–120) at autopsy (Schlichter *et al.,* 1954) or operation (Rao *et al.,* 1974) in approximately half of the patients with a left ventricular aneurysm. In about half of these patients, systemic emboli are found (Schlichter *et al.,* 1954). Many emboli may be "silent" or not evident clinically. In a study of 500 patients, Davies and colleagues (1976), however, found that half of the emboli identified at autopsy were cerebral. Not all intraventricular clotting is obvious (Fig. 50–120). When thrombus is apparent, this constitutes a relative indication for surgery.

Tachyarrhythmias. The common denominator of both left ventricular aneurysm and ventricular irritability is myocardial ischemia. One does not necessitate the other, but they frequently coexist. When a rhythm originates in the ventricle, the pattern of ventricular activation is aberrant (wide QRS complex). The mechanism of premature ventricular contractions or ventricular tachycardia is enhanced automaticity, re-entry, or both (Harken *et al.,* 1980b). Automatic ventricular rhythms due to local myocardial irritability are common in the perioperative and peri-infarction periods. These rhythms are exacerbated by hypokalemia, catecholamines, or digitalis (Kastor *et al.,* 1981). A re-entrant rhythm may occur when two or more electrically heterogeneous (with respect to conduction and refractoriness) pathways are connected proximally and distally (Fig. 50–121). An impulse must travel in only one direction along one of these pathways (unidirectional block). When this impulse arrives at the distal connection, it may return by the initially blocked pathway. If conduction of the impulse is sufficiently slow to allow the originally blocked site to recover excitability, the impulse may re-enter the circuit. A re-entrant arrhythmia may be induced by a technique of specially timed paced beats termed programmed stimulation. This technique permits pharmacologic testing and eventual mapping of re-entrant rhythms such as ventricular tachycardia. Automatic arrhythmias cannot be induced and therefore cannot be tested or mapped. Surgery has recently proved to be a viable therapeutic option for re-entrant ventricular tachycardia. Currently, there is no evidence to support a surgical approach to automatic ventricular tachycardia and no reason to operate for isolated premature ventricular contractions.

Each year, one third of a million Americans die suddenly. The popularity of and education of civilians in cardiopulmonary resuscitation and emergency medical systems have increased the salvage in this catastrophe. Patients surviving episodes of recurrent ventricular tachycardia or sudden death are subjected to pharmacologic testing during programmed induction of their arrhythmia (Kastor *et al.,* 1981). If the rhythm cannot be suppressed with high-dose antiarrhythmic agents, these patients are considered candidates for surgical excision of the re-entrant circuit.

Ventricular Rupture. Although ventricular rupture occurs in 10 per cent of patients dying of acute myocardial infarction (Bjorck *et al.,* 1960), late rupture of a matured aneurysm almost never occurs (Vlodaver *et al.,* 1975). The incidence of cardiac rupture is high only during the acute phase of infarct evolution. During this phase, the pathophysiologic and technical risks associated with surgical intervention are prohibitively high. The avoidance of possible ventricular rupture for acute and certainly for chronic left ventricular aneurysms therefore does not routinely constitute an indication for surgery.

SURGICAL TECHNIQUE

Repair of a left ventricular aneurysm is accomplished through a standard median sternotomy. The aorta is cannulated, and a single venous cannula is sufficient, unless an associated ventricular septal defect is suspected. A postinfarction left ventricular aneurysm frequently presents with dense pericardial adhesions. Cardiopulmonary bypass decompresses the heart and facilitates "take-down" of the adhesions. The patient is cooled. The heart is allowed to cool until it fibrillates. The aorta is then cross-clamped to prevent left ventricular distention. With proper decompression, the aneurysmal zone should collapse, whereas viable left ventricle will remain firm. A linear incision is made in the collapsed aneurysm while cold potassium cardioplegic solution is infused into the aortic root. Cold saline solution is then poured directly into the left ventricle and over the epicardial surface. If coronary bypass or valve replacement is to be accomplished concurrently, the ventricular aneurysm is always opened first. This provides optimal ventricular decompression and permits thorough epicardial and endocardial cooling.

The entire ventricle is then inspected for mural thrombus. Thrombus should be removed and the underlying endocardium wiped clean with a sponge. The ventricular cavity is again irrigated with iced saline solution both to recool the myocardium and to wash out any residual flecks of thrombus. Coronary bypass grafting or valve surgery is performed at this time in a cool, flaccid, decompressed heart.

The aneurysmal edge is trimmed back, leaving a 1-cm. fibrous rim. The aneurysm is closed with 0 monofilament suture material in a horizontal mattress fashion over long felt buttresses (Fig. 50–122). Felt strips that are at least 1 cm. wide will facilitate closure. Separate sutures are started at either end, brought to the middle, and tied. Prior to tying this row, the ventricle is filled with blood by inflating the lungs. The atrial appendage should be inverted. A second row of 0 monofilament sutures are placed in an over-and-over fashion at both ends and tied over a felt

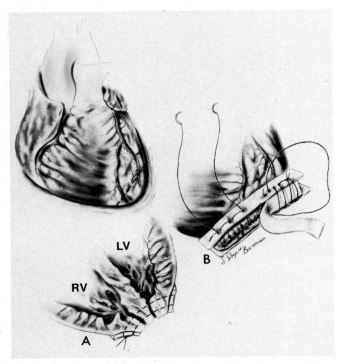

Figure 50–122. *A,* Repair of the aneurysmectomy following excision involves reapproximation of the fibrous rims of the aneurysm. In closing an antero-apical or posterior aneurysm, the left anterior descending or posterior descending coronary artery is typically occluded and may therefore be included in the repair with impunity. *B,* The aneurysm is closed with 0 monofilament suture in a horizontal mattress fashion over long felt strips. Separate sutures are placed at either end, brought to the middle, and tied. A secondary row of 0 monofilament suture is placed in an over-and-over fashion at both ends and tied over a felt buttress in the middle. When closed in this way, the ventriculotomy is less likely to bleed. Seemingly minor traction on the felt buttresses, however, can tear the heart at the lateral junction between the ventricle and the suture line. This typically occurs on the right ventricular side in older patients.

buttress in the middle (Fig. 50–122). Closed in this fashion, the ventriculotomy will never bleed. Seemingly minor traction on these felt buttresses, however, can tear the heart at the lateral junction between the ventricle and the suture line. This typically occurs on the right ventricular side in older patients. Repair of this ominous complication requires recooling and decompression of the heart. Sutures placed (even with pledgets) into a firm, beating ventricle are prone to tear.

Variations

Inferior aneurysms are more difficult to expose but should be repaired in an identical fashion. Some landmarks are worthy of attention, however. The aneurysm may run right up to the mitral valve posteriorly. The mitral anulus is a firm anchor for one end of the closure, and inclusion of the mitral anulus typically does not distort the mitral valve and does not lead to mitral regurgitation. The posterior de-

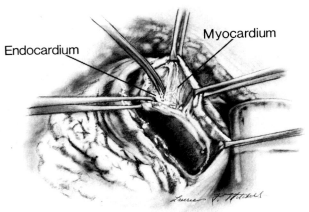

Figure 50–123. Endocardial excision for ventricular tachycardia. The aneurysm has been resected. The endocardium (free wall or septum) is then pulled back and excised 2 or 3 cm. from the aneurysmectomy edge in the zone identified by electrophysiologic mapping.

scending coronary artery is characteristically occluded in the presence of an inferior aneurysm. The posterior descending coronary artery and its adjacent vein may therefore be included in the aneurysm repair with impunity. Occasionally, the posterior papillary muscle has clearly been infarcted and replaced by firm scar. This does not necessarily mean that it no longer serves as adequate support for the mitral valve. The blood supply to the papillary muscle is derived both from up its center and from the lateral wall (Estes *et al.,* 1966).

If the indication for surgery is recurrent sustained ventricular tachycardia, the left ventricular endocardium should be mapped on opening the aneurysm (Harken *et al.,* 1980a). After locating the area of earliest activation, this endocardial zone is peeled back beyond the aneurysmal edge into grossly viable myocardium (Fig. 50–123) (Horowitz *et al.,* 1980).

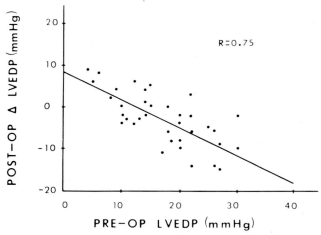

Figure 50–124. Linear regression analysis revealing the relationship between the preoperative left ventricular end-diastolic pressure (pre-op LVEDP) to the postoperative reduction (post-op Δ LVEDP). Patients with the highest preoperative end-diastolic pressures improved the most with surgery.

RESULTS OF SURGERY

The rapid evolution of both medical and surgical therapy for patients with ischemic cardiac disease has confounded attempts to characterize and compare results. It is impractical and perhaps even unethical to randomize patients prospectively following catheterization demonstrating left ventricular aneurysm and differing ventricular dysfunction, noncomparable coronary artery disease, variable associated valvular lesions, and myriad concurrent risk factors. Until recently, medical management of patients with postinfarction aneurysms was associated with an appalling prognosis. In Schlichter and associates' autopsy series (1954), three quarters of patients with documented ventricular aneurysm died in 3 years, and only 12 per cent were alive 5 years after the precipitating myocardial infarction. Medical therapy is now much better. Prospective follow-up studies of angiographically proven surgical candidates treated medically (the only convincing control population) do not exist. Some comparative information is available. However, examination of aneurysmectomy results is simplified by categorizing the patients with respect to the indication for surgery.

Enthusiasm for aneurysm resection in patients with angina with congestive failure (Cooperman *et al.*, 1975) or without congestive failure (Lefemine *et al.*, 1977) is based on subjective clinical improvement and a reduction in expected late mortality compared with earlier natural history studies (Borer *et al.*, 1980). The presence of a left ventricular aneurysm necessarily burdens nonaneurysmal myocardial fibers, increasing systolic shortening and thus myocardial oxygen uptake. When an aneurysm involves more than 25 per cent of the ventricular surface, myocardial fiber shortening limits are exceeded. The ventricle dilates and stiffens, stroke volume decreases, end-diastolic pressure increases, and congestive heart failure with or without ischemia ensues (Klein *et al.*, 1967). That aneurysmectomy reverses this process at least partially is evident.

Some groups (Bjorck *et al.*, 1960; Spencer *et al.*, 1971), however, have reported disappointing symptomatic relief and marginal influence on expected long-term survival. Conversely, Froehlich and colleagues (1980) examined 18 patients, 13 of whom had concurrent angina and congestive failure and 11 of whom underwent aneurysm resection. Only 50 per cent of the noncontractile area visualized on contrast ventriculography was resected surgically. There was a startling discrepancy between substantial symptomatic relief and marginal objective functional improvement. Patients improved from New York Heart Association Functional Class 3.6 prior to surgery to 2.3 (p < 0.005) following aneurysmectomy. Only four patients in this series had either an increase in ejection fraction or a greater than 10 per cent reduction in end-diastolic volume. There were no operative deaths. In contrast, other groups (Cullhed *et al.*, 1975) have documented a decrease in both end-diastolic and end-systolic heart volume postoperatively, with an increase in left ventricular ejection fraction. In our own series (Martin *et al.*, 1982) of 62 patients examined with preoperative and postoperative cardiac catheterization, there was gratifying symptomatic relief associated with an increase in ejection fraction from 28 to 39 per cent (p < 0.001) and a decrease in left ventricular end-diastolic pressure (LVEDP) from 17 to 14 mm. Hg (p < 0.005) (Fig. 50–124).

Again, it is difficult to compare aneurysmectomy and endocardial excision for ventricular tachycardia with rapidly evolving medical therapy. In round numbers, however, in patients with left ventricular dysfunction and ventricular tachycardia not controllable with drugs, an 80 per cent mortality rate may be anticipated during the first year (Kastor *et al.*, 1981). When ventricular tachycardia is suppressible with drugs, one third to one half of patients can be expected to survive the first year. With surgical aneurysmectomy and endocardial excision, 80 per cent of patients are expected to survive the first year (Harken *et al.*, 1980a; Kastor *et al.*, 1981).

SELECTED REFERENCES

Boineau, J. P., and Cox, J. L.: Slow ventricular activation in acute myocardial infarction: A source of re-entrant premature ventricular contractions. Circulation, *48*:702, 1973.

This study was the first to suggest that a heterogeneous pattern of myocardial ischemia led to zones of slow conduction predisposing to re-entrant ventricular arrhythmias. The discussion lucidly explains automatic and re-entrant arrhythmias and relates them to fragmentation of intramyocardial potentials.

Borer, J. S., Jacobstein, J. G., Bacharach, S. L., and Green, M. V.: Detection of left ventricular aneurysm and evaluation of effects of surgical repair: The role of radionuclide cineangiography. Am. J. Cardiol., *45*:1103, 1980.

A concise pathophysiologic approach to the selection of patients for left ventricular aneurysmectomy is presented, suggesting a role for radionuclide angiography.

Harken, A. H., Horowitz, L. N., and Josephson, M. E.: Comparison of standard aneurysmectomy and aneurysmectomy with directed endocardial resection for the treatment of recurrent sustained ventricular tachycardia. J. Thorac. Cardiovasc. Surg., *80*:527, 1980.

A retrospective, nonrandomized comparison of 19 patients treated with standard aneurysmectomy and 30 patients treated with aneurysmectomy plus directed endocardial excision for ventricular tachycardia. The operative mortality rate in the group who underwent standard aneurysmectomy was 42 per cent, and 79 per cent of patients (15/19) still had spontaneous ventricular tachycardia postoperatively. The operative mortality rate in the electrophysiologically directed group was 6.7 per cent (2/30), and 10 per cent (3/30) had inducible ventricular tachycardia with postoperative programmed stimulation.

Kastor, J. A., Horowitz, L .N., Harken, A. H., and Josephson, M. E.: Clinical electrophysiology of ventricular tachycardia. N. Engl. J. Med., *304*:1004, 1981.

An exhaustive review of the relationship between left ventricular scar and electrophysiologic abnormalities.

Klein, M. D., Herman, M. V., and Gorlin, R.: A hemodynamic study of left ventricular aneurysm. Circulation, *35*:614, 1967.

Left ventricular volume and extent of scar in patients with left ventricular aneurysms are correlated with stroke volume, wall tension, and, therefore, myocardial oxygen uptake using logical physical principles. The pathophysiology of left ventricular aneurysm and concurrent dysfunction is discussed.

Martin, J. L., Untereker, W. J., Harken, A. H., Horowitz, L. N., and Josephson, M. E.: Aneurysmectomy and endocardial resection for ventricular tachycardia: Favorable hemodynamic and antiarrhythmic results in patients with global left ventricular dysfunction. Am. Heart J., *103*:960, 1982.

Sixty-two patients were catheterized before and after aneurysmectomy and endocardial excision for recurrent ventricular tachycardia and left ventricular failure. Ejection fraction increased from 28 ± 8 per cent to 39 ± 10 per cent ($p < 0.001$), and left ventricular end-diastolic pressure (LVEDP) decreased from 17 ± 8 mm. Hg to 14 ± 5 mm. Hg ($p < 0.005$). Aneurysmectomy does objectively improve left ventricular function.

Schlichter, J., Hellerstein, H. K., and Katz, L. N.: Aneurysm of the heart: A corrective study of 102 proved cases. Medicine, *33*:43, 1954.

A classic clinicopathologic correlation of 102 confirmed cases of left ventricular aneurysm. The history, diagnosis, pathology, and prognosis are reviewed in detail. The authors indicate that three quarters of patients are dead in 3 years and that there is a 12 per cent 5-year survival rate.

REFERENCES

Abrams, D. L., Edelist, A., Luria, M. H., and Miller, A. J.: Ventricular aneurysm: A reappraisal based on a study of 65 consecutive autopsied cases. Circulation, *27*:164, 1963.

Alpert, J. S., and Braunwald, E.: Pathological and clinical manifestations of acute myocardial infarction. *In* Heart Disease: A Textbook of Cardiovascular Medicine. Edited by E. Braunwald. Philadelphia, W. B. Saunders Company, 1980, p. 1309.

Arnold, J.: Ueber angeborene Divertikel des Herzens. Virchows Arch. (Pathol. Anat.), *137*:318, 1894.

Basset-Smith, P. W.: Aneurysm of the heart due to syphilitic gummata. Br. Med. J., *2*:1060, 1908.

Bjorck, G., Morgensen, L., Nyquist, O., Orinius, E., and Sjogren, A.: Studies of myocardial rupture with cardiac tamponade in acute myocardial infarction. Concours Med., *82*:2637, 1960.

Boineau, J. P., and Cox, J. L.: Slow ventricular activation in acute myocardial infarction: A source of re-entrant premature ventricular contractions. Circulation, *48*:702, 1973.

Borer, J. S., Jacobstein, J. G., Bacharach, S. L., and Green, M. V.: Detection of left ventricular aneurysm and evaluation of effects of surgical repair: The role of radionuclide cineangiography. Am. J. Cardiol., *45*:1103, 1980.

Borer, J. S., Bacharach, S. L., Green, M. V., Kent, K. M., Epstein, S. E., and Johnston, G. S.: Real time radionuclide cineangiography in the noninvasive evaluation of global and regional left ventricular function at rest and during exercise in patients with coronary artery disease. N. Engl. J. Med., *296*:839, 1977.

Borrich, O.: Acta Societatis Med. Hafniensis. Barthol. Observ., *48*:150, 1676.

Braunwald, E., and Sobel, B. E.: Coronary blood flow and myocardial ischemia. *In*: Heart Disease: A Textbook of Cardiovascular Medicine. Edited by E. Braunwald. Philadelphia, W. B. Saunders Company, 1980, p. 1279.

Bricout, C.: Syphilis du coeur. Thèse. Paris, 1912, p. 45.

Bruschke, A. V. G., Proudfit, W. L., and Sones, F. M.: Progress study of 490 consecutive non-surgical cases of coronary disease followed 5 to 9 years. II. Ventriculographic and other correlation. Circulation, *47*:1154, 1973.

Cabin, H. S., and Roberts, W. C.: True left ventricular aneurysm and healed myocardial infarction. Am. J. Cardiol., *45*:754, 1980.

Cohn, P. F., and Braunwald, E.: Chronic coronary artery disease. *In* Heart Disease: A Textbook of Cardiovascular Medicine. Edited by E. Braunwald. Philadelphia, W. B. Saunders Company, 1980, p. 1387.

Cohn, P. F., Gorlin, R., Adams, D. F., Chahine, R. A., Vokonas, P. S., and Herman, M. V.: Comparison of biplane and single-plane left ventriculography in patients with coronary artery disease. Am. J. Cardiol., *33*:1, 1974.

Cohnheim, J., and Shulthess-Rechberg, G.: Ueber die Folgen der Kranzarterienuer Schilessung fur das Herz. Virchows Arch., *85*:503, 1881.

Cooley, D. A., Collins, H. A., Morris, G. C., and Chapman, D. W.: Ventricular aneurysm after myocardial infarction. Surgical excision with use of temporary cardiopulmonary bypass. J.A.M.A., *167*:557, 1958.

Cooperman, M., Stinson, E. B., Griepp, R. B., and Shumway, N. E.: Survival and function after left ventricular aneurysmectomy. J. Thorac. Cardiovasc. Surg., *69*:321, 1975.

Cruveilhier, J.: Essai sur l'anatomie pathologique en general, et sur les transformations et productions organiques en particulier. Nouvelle Bibliotheque Med., *2*:72, 1827.

Cullhed, I., Delius, W., Bjork, L., Hallen, A., and Nordgren, L.: Resection of left ventricular aneurysm—late results. Acta Med. Scand., *197*:241, 1975.

Davies, M. J., Woolf, N., and Robertson, W. B.: Pathology of acute myocardial infarction with particular reference to occlusive coronary thrombi. Br. Heart J., *38*:659, 1976.

Didisheim, P., and Foster, V.: Actions and clinical status of platelet suppressive agents. Semin. Hematol., *15*:55, 1978.

Dimond, E. G., Kittle, F., and Voth, D. W.: Extreme hypertrophy of the left atrial appendage. The case of the giant dog ear. Am. J. Cardiol., *5*:122, 1960.

Dolly, C. H., Dotter, C. T., and Steinberg, H.: Ventricular aneurysm in a 29-year-old man studied angiocardiographically. Am. Heart J., *42*:894, 1951.

Dyke, S. H., Cohn, P. F., Gorlin, E., and Sonnenblick, E. H.: Detection of residual myocardial function in coronary artery disease using post-extrasystolic potentiation. Circulation, *50*:694, 1974.

Estes, E. H., Dalton, F. M., Entman, M. L., Dixon, H. B., and Hackel, D. B.: The anatomy and blood supply of the papillary muscles of the left ventricle. Am. Heart J., *71*:356, 1966.

European Coronary Surgery Study Group: Coronary artery bypass surgery in stable angina pectoris: Survival at two years. Lancet, *1*:889, 1979.

Fojo-Echevarria, P., Muniz-Sotolongo, J. C., and Aixala, R.: Aneurysma de la auticula izquierda como sequela de comisurotomia. Revista Cubana de Cardiologia, *16*:377, 1955.

Forrester, J. S., Wyatt, H. L., DaLuz, P. L., Tyberg, J. V., Diamond, G. A., and Swan, H. J. C.: Functional significance of regional ischemic contraction abnormalities. Circulation, *54*:64, 1976.

Fortuin, N. J., and Pawsey, C. G. K.: The evaluation of left ventricular function by echocardiography. Am. J. Med., *63*:1, 1977.

Friedman, M. L., and Cantor, R. E.: Reliability of gated heart scintigrams for detection of left ventricular aneurysm: Concise communication. J. Nucl. Med., *20*:720, 1979.

Froehlich, R. T., Falsetti, H. L., Doty, D. B., and Marcus, M. L.: Prospective study of surgery for left ventricular aneurysm. Am. J. Cardiol., *45*:923, 1980.

Galeati, D. G.: DeBononiensi scientiarum et atrium instituto atque academia commentarii. De Morbis Duobus, *4*:25, 1757.

Gatewood, R., and Nanda, N.: Differentiation of left ventricular pseudoaneurysm from true aneurysm with two dimensional echocardiography. Am. J. Cardiol., *46*:869, 1980.

Gorlin, R.: Coronary collaterals. *In* Coronary Artery Disease. Philadelphia, W. B. Saunders Company, 1976, p. 59.

Grondin, P., Kretz, J. G., Bical, O., Donzeau-Gouge, P., Petitclerc, R., and Campeau, L.: Natural history of saccular aneurysms of the left ventricle. J. Thorac. Cardiovasc. Surg., *77*:57, 1979.

Handin, R. I., McDonough, M., and Lesch, M.: Elevation of platelet factor four in acute myocardial infarction: Measurement of radioimmunoassay. J. Lab. Clin. Med., 91:340, 1978.

Harden, W. R., Barlow, C. H., Simson, M. J., and Harken, A. H.: Temporal relation between the onset of cell anoxia and ischemic contractile failure. Am. J. Cardiol., 44:741, 1979.

Harken, A. H., Horowitz, L. N., and Josephson, M. E.: Comparison of standard aneurysmectomy and aneurysmectomy with directed endocardial resection for the treatment of recurrent sustained ventricular tachycardia. J. Thorac. Cardiovasc. Surg., 80:527, 1980a.

Harken, A. H., Horowitz, L. N., and Josephson, M. E.: The surgical treatment of ventricular tachycardia. Ann. Thorac. Surg., 30:499, 1980b.

Harken, A. H., Simson, M. B., Weststein, L. W., Haselgrove, J., Harden, W. R., and Barlow, C. H.: Early ischemia following complete coronary ligation in the rabbit, dog, pig and monkey. Am. J. Physiol., 241:202, 1981.

Helfant, R. H., Pine, R., Meister, S. G., Feldman, M. S., Trout, R. G., and Banka, V. S.: Nitroglycerine to unmask reversible asynergy: Correlation with post-coronary bypass ventriculography. Circulation, 50:108, 1974.

Herman, M. V., Heinle, R. A., Klein, M. D., and Gorlin, R.: Localized disorders in myocardial contraction: Asynergy and its role in congestive heart failure. N. Engl. J. Med., 277:222, 1967.

Horn, H. R., Teichholz, L. E., Cohn, P. F., Herman, M .V., and Gorlin, R.: Augmentation of left ventricular contraction pattern in coronary artery disease by inotropic catecholamine: The epinephrine ventriculogram. Circulation, 49:1063, 1974.

Horowitz, L. N., Harken, A. H., Kastor, J. A., and Josephson, M. E.: Ventricular resection guided by epicardial and endocardial mapping for the treatment of recurrent ventricular tachycardia. N. Engl. J. Med., 302:589, 1980.

Hunter, J.: An account of the dissection of morbid bodys. A manuscript copy in the Library of the Royal College of Surgeons, No. 32, p. 30–32, 1757.

Jennings, R. B., and Ganote, C. E.: Structural change in myocardium during acute ischemia. Circ. Res.,35(Suppl. 3):156, 1974.

Kastor, J. A., Horowitz, L. N., Harken, A. H., and Josephson, M. E.: Clinical electrophysiology of ventricular tachycardia. N. Engl. J. Med., 304:1004, 1981.

Katz, A. M.: Effects of ischemia on the contractile processes of heart muscle. Am. J. Cardiol., 32:456, 1973.

Klein, G. I.: Zur Aetiologie der aneurysmen der pars membranacea septi ventriculorum cordis und deren ruptur. Virchows Arch. (Pathol. Anat.), 118:57, 1889.

Klein, M. D., Herman, M. V., and Gorlin, R.: A hemodynamic study of left ventricular aneurysm. Circulation, 35:614, 1967.

Kouchoukos, N. T., Doty, D. B., Buettner, L. E., and Kirklin, J. W.: Treatment of post-infarction cardiac failure by myocardial excision and revascularization. Circulation, 45(Suppl. 1):72, 1972.

Lee, D. C., Johnson, R. A., Boucher, C. A., Wexler, L. F., and McEnany, M. T.: Angiographic predictors of survival following left ventricular aneurysmectomy. Circulation, 56(Suppl. 2):12, 1977.

Lefemine, A. R., Govindarajan, R., Ramaswamy, K., Black, H., Madoff, I., and Sanella, N.: Left ventricular wall resection for aneurysm and akinesia due to coronary artery disease: Fifty consecutive patients. Ann. Thorac. Surg., 23:461, 1977.

Libman, E.: Affections of the coronary arteries. Interst. Postgrad. Med. Assoc. North Am., 2:405, 1932.

Likoff, W., and Bailey, C. P.: Ventriculoplasty: Excision of myocardial aneurysm. J.A.M.A., 158:915, 1955.

Loop, F. D., Effler, D. B., Navia, J. A., Sheldon, W. C., and Groves, L. K.: Aneurysms of the left ventricle: Survival and results of a ten year experience. Ann. Surg., 178:399, 1973.

Lyons, C., and Perkins, R.: Resection of a left ventricular aneurysm secondary to a cardiac stab wound. Ann. Surg., 147:256, 1958.

Martin, J., Untereker, W. J., Harken, A. H., Horowitz, L. N., and Josephson, M. E.: Aneurysmectomy and endocardial resection for ventricular tachycardia: Favorable hemodynamic and antiarrhythmic results in patients with global left ventricular dysfunction. Am. Heart J., 103:960, 1982.

Mirsky, I.: Elastic properties of the myocardium: A quantitative

approach with physiological and clinical applications. In Handbook of Physiology. Vol. I, The Heart. Edited by R. M. Berne. Bethesda, Maryland, American Physiological Society, 1979, p. 501.

Murphy, M. L., Hultgren, H. N., Detre, K., Thomsen, J., and Takaro, T.: Treatment of chronic stable angina. N. Engl. J. Med., 297:621, 1977.

Parisi, A. F., Moynihan, P. F., Ray, B. J., and Pietro, D. A.: Two dimensional echocardiography. J. Cardiovasc. Med., 5:39, 1980.

Pfeffer, M. A., Pfeffer, J. M., Fishbein, M. C., Fletcher, P. J., Spadaro, J., Kloner, R. A., and Braunwald, W.: Myocardial infarct size and ventricular function in rats. Circ. Res., 44:503, 1979.

Proudfit, W. L.: Personal communication. Cited in Grondin, P., Kretz, J. G., Bical, O., Donzeau-Gouge, P., Petitclerc, R., and Campeau, L.: Natural history of saccular aneurysms of the left ventricle. J. Thorac. Cardiovasc. Surg., 77:57, 1979.

Rackley, C. E., Russell, R. O., Jr., Mantle, J. A., and Rogers, W. J.: Modern approach to the patient with acute myocardial infarction. Curr. Probl. Cardiol., 1:49, 1977.

Rao, G., Zikria, E. A., Miller, W. H., Samadani, S. R., and Ford, W. B.: Experience with sixty consecutive ventricular aneurysm resections. Circulation, 49(Suppl. 2):149, 1974.

Rokitansky, C.: Handbuch der Pathologischen Anatomie. Vol. II. Vienna, Braumuller and Seidel, 1844, p. 449.

Rosenthal, D. S., and Braunwald, E.: Hematologic oncologic disorders and heart disease. In Heart Disease: A Textbook of Cardiovascular Medicine. Edited by E. Braunwald. Philadelphia, W. B. Saunders Company, 1980, p. 1771.

Schattenberg, T. T., Giuliana, E. R., Campion, B. C., and Danielson, G. K., Jr.: Post-infarction ventricular aneurysm. Mayo Clin. Proc., 45:13, 1970.

Schlichter, J., Hellerstein, H. K., and Katz, L. N.: Aneurysm of the heart: A correlative study of 102 proved cases. Medicine, 33:43, 1954.

Schwedel, J. B., Samet, P., and Mednick, H.: Electrokymographic studies of abnormal left ventricular pulsations. Am. Heart J., 40:410, 1950.

Sezary, A., and Alibert, T.: Aneurysm in wall of heart. Bull. Mem. Soc. Med. Hosp. Paris, 46:172, 1922.

Sniderman, A. D., Marpole, D., and Fallen, E. L.: Regional contraction patterns in the normal and ischemic left ventricle in man. Am. J. Cardiol., 31:484, 1973.

Spear, J. F., Horowitz, L. N., Hodess, A. B., MacVaugh, H., and Moore, E. N.: Cellular electrophysiology of human myocardial infarction. I. Abnormalities of cellular activation. Circulation, 59:247, 1979.

Spencer, F. C., Green, G. E., Tice, D. A., Walsh, E., Mills, N. L., and Glassman, E.: Coronary artery bypass grafts for congestive heart failure: A report of experience with 40 patients. J. Thorac. Cardiovasc. Surg., 62:529, 1971.

Stansel, J. C., Jr., Julian, O. C., and Dye, W. S.: Right ventricular aneurysm. J. Thorac. Cardiovasc. Surg., 46:66, 1963.

Sternberg, M.: Das chronische partielle herzaneurysma. Vienna and Leipzig, Franz Deuticke, 1914.

Swan, H. J. C., Forrester, J. S., Diamond, G., Chatterjee, K., and Parmley, W. W.: Hemodynamic spectrum of myocardial infarction and cardiogenic shock. Circulation, 45:1097, 1972.

Vlodaver, Z., Coe, J. I., and Edwards, J. E.: True and false left ventricular aneurysms: Propensity for the latter to rupture. Circulation, 51:567, 1975.

Voelcker, A. F.: Aneurysm of the heart. Trans. Pathol. Soc. (Lond.), 53:409, 1902.

Vokonas, P. S., Pirzada, F. A., and Hood, W. B., Jr.: Experimental myocardial infarction. XII. Dynamic changes in segmental mechanical behavior of infarcted and non-infarcted myocardium. Am. J. Cardiol., 37:853, 1976.

Weiss, H. J.: Platelet physiology and abnormalities of platelet function. N. Engl. J. Med., 293:531, 1975.

Wellens, H. J. J.: Observations on the pathophysiology of ventricular tachycardia in man. Arch. Intern. Med., 135:473, 1975.

Wynne, J., Birnholz, J., Fineberg, H., and Alpert, J. S.: Assessment of regional left ventricular wall motion in acute myocardial infarction by two-dimensional echocardiography. Circulation, 56(Suppl. 2):152, 1977.

6.   Assisted Circulation

ELDRED D. MUNDTH

HISTORICAL CONSIDERATIONS

There are few areas of special study in the health sciences that better exemplify the effectiveness and success of a multidisciplinary approach, including physiology, bioengineering, clinical medicine, and surgery, than the development of clinically safe and effective assisted circulation devices. The evolution of the concept of prolonged assisted circulation for support of the failing heart and circulation occurred simultaneously with the development of cardiopulmonary bypass devices for use in open-heart surgery. Early in the nineteenth century, Legallois (1813) proposed the possibility of paracorporeal circulatory support, and in 1882, von Schroder suggested the concept of a bubble oxygenator. As early as 1885 von Frey and Gruber and Jacobi (1890) had proposed designs of heart-lung bypass machines. However, it required the discovery of heparin by Howell and Holt in 1918 and the definition of blood groups by Landsteiner in 1900 for a clinically practicable system. With the development of the roller pump by DeBakey in 1934, Dennis (1951) and Gibbon (1954) were able to incorporate the appropriate technology and sound physiologic principles into a clinically effective cardiopulmonary bypass system.

Early investigators envisaged prolonged cardiopulmonary bypass for support of the failing heart and circulation, but it became readily apparent that successful cardiopulmonary bypass, with subsequent full recovery of cardiovascular function, could rarely be continued for periods longer than 4 to 6 hours. Damage to the formed elements in blood and functional deterioration of vital organs were shown to be progressive as a function of time. Lee and associates (1961) demonstrated that damage to the formed elements of blood and alterations in tissue microcirculation were, in part, a result of denaturation of plasma lipoproteins and changes in physical characteristics of cell membranes occurring with prolonged exposure of blood to a blood-gas interface in an oxygenator. Many and coworkers (1967) and German and associates (1972) assessed the effects on renal function of nonpulsatile perfusion, as used in most cardiopulmonary bypass pump devices, and found progressive deterioration in function resulting from inadequate capillary perfusion, progressive metabolic abnormalities, and interstitial edema.

Despite the physiologic limitations of prolonged assisted circulation using cardiopulmonary bypass, there continued to be interest in developing an effective method for short- and long-term assisted circulation to support the failing heart. Stuckey and col-

leagues (1957) employed brief periods of partial cardiopulmonary bypass utilizing a bubble oxygenator to achieve circulatory assistance in three patients in cardiogenic shock following acute myocardial infarction, with one subsequent survivor. As was true in the early and even subsequent clinical experience, in which physiologic categorization of patients has improved, it has been difficult to prove that circulatory assistance resulted directly in survival of the patient.

Aware of the time limitation of partial cardiopulmonary bypass using a blood-gas interface oxygenator in the circuit, Connolly and associates (1958) proposed venoarterial bypass for cardiogenic shock, hoping to achieve significant hemodynamic benefit to the failing heart without severely depressing peripheral arterial oxygen saturation (Fig. 50–125). Although venoarterial partial bypass could relieve right ventricular failure and reduce left ventricular volume work, it did not relieve left ventricular pressure work significantly unless bypass became nearly total. In more recent years, the development of an effective membrane oxygenator that eliminated the blood-gas interface allowed the potential for near-total cardiopulmonary bypass with preservation of arterial oxygen saturation (Fig. 50–126). Because of the invasiveness of the system, the need for constant monitoring, and progressive destruction of the formed elements of blood, this approach has not achieved the clinical applicabil-

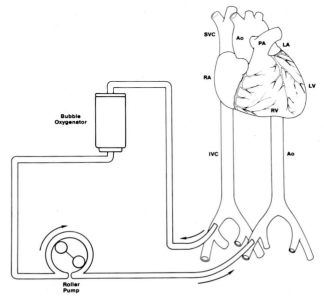

Figure 50–125. Venoarterial bypass mechanical circulatory assist system utilizing partial cardiopulmonary bypass and a liquid-gas interface oxygenator (see Table 50–21).

The Coronary Circulation / **1491**

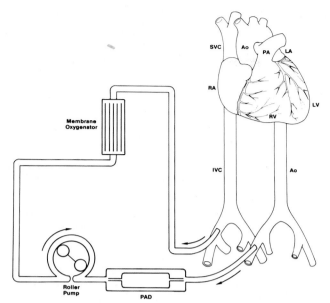

Figure 50–126. Venoarterial bypass circulatory assist system utilizing partial cardiopulmonary bypass with a membrane oxygenator (see Table 50–21).

ity and success of less invasive counterpulsation assist systems. Table 50–21 lists circulatory assist systems in chronologic order, outlining their physiologic advantages and disadvantages and providing commentary on their clinical applicability.

Clauss and associates (1961), working as an effective surgical, physiologic, and bioengineering team, developed the concept of arterial counterpulsation. This assist system was based on withdrawal of arterial blood from an indwelling cannula during ventricular systole and pulsatile return of the blood to the arterial system during diastole, with control and phasing accomplished by electrocardiographic gating (Fig. 50–127; Table 50–21). Arterial counterpulsation, when properly phased, reduced left ventricular pressure work in the range of 20 to 40 per cent, as reported by Soroff and coworkers (1963) and Rosensweig and Chatterjee (1968). Nacklas and Siedband (1967) and, later, Sugg and associates (1969) were able to demonstrate that arterial counterpulsation could significantly reduce infarct size in the experimental animal if instituted soon after coronary artery occlusion. However, clinical use of the system was not particularly effective in patients with cardiogenic shock and was not associated with improved survival (Sugg *et al.*, 1970). It was noted in the laboratory and clinically that when arterial counterpulsation was attempted in the presence of severe hypotension, it was difficult to achieve rapid withdrawal of blood during systole, particularly when tachycardia was present. The necessary rapid withdrawal of arterial blood frequently collapsed the artery, preventing adequate volume withdrawal and causing severe mechanical trauma to the blood and subsequent hemolysis.

The decade of the 1960s witnessed rapid development of circulatory assistance technology, and the founding of the Artificial Heart Program by the National Institutes of Health in 1964 gave great impetus to the programs. Dennis and colleagues (1962) and Senning and associates (1962) developed a system of left heart bypass that eliminated the need for an oxygenator and physiologically achieved reduced left ventricular myocardial oxygen consumption by decreasing pressure work in addition to volume work (Fig. 50–128; Table 50–21). This technique required transatrial septal puncture by a relatively large-bore cannula to accomplish left atrial–arterial bypass and was significantly invasive as well as requiring a roller pump for bypass. Left heart bypass had to be virtually complete to diminish myocardial oxygen consumption by more than 20 per cent. Left ventricular preload was significantly reduced, resulting in decreased left ventricular wall tension, although little change was noted in left ventricular tension-time index or myocardial contractility (Chiu *et al.*, 1969).

A relatively simple but ingenious device to achieve arterial diastolic counterpulsation was introduced by Moulopoulos and coworkers in 1962. The intra-aortic balloon (IAB) was introduced mounted on a catheter via the trans–femoral artery route and was placed in the descending thoracic aorta (Fig. 50–129; Table 50–21). Gas-driven volume displacement of the balloon electronically gated to the electrocardiogram achieved effective arterial counterpulsation.

The development of this minimally invasive, physiologically effective assisted circulation device was further pioneered by Kantrowitz and associates (1968), Laird and coworkers (1968), Buckley and associates (1970), and Bregman and colleagues (1970). The principle of arterial diastolic counterpulsation for circulatory assistance and the use of the intra-aortic balloon pump device in particular have continued to be the primary modes of clinical application of assisted circulation over the past two decades. Other types of assist systems have been developed and have been shown to be effective, but they are not superior to the aforementioned modes of assisted circulation in physiologic effectiveness, ease and safety of use, or scope of clinical applicability.

The concept of direct mechanical compression of the failing heart for circulatory assistance was developed by Anstadt and coworkers (1966) and was found to be effective hemodynamically in laboratory animals over relatively short periods of time (Fig. 50–130; Table 50–21). It has the disadvantage of being invasive, requiring thoracotomy, and, potentially traumatic to the heart, requiring placement of a compression cap over the ventricular apex. A somewhat analogous approach, developed by Donald and associates (1972) utilized an intraventricular volume displacement balloon inserted via the ventricular apex (Fig. 50–131; Table 50–21). Synchronous inflation of the balloon during ventricular systole gated by the electrocardiogram achieved an increase in left ventricular stroke volume and a 40 to 60 per cent increase in cardiac output and reduced left ventricular filling pressures by 35 to 45 per cent in experimental animals

TABLE 50–21. CIRCULATORY ASSIST SYSTEMS: CHRONOLOGY, PHYSIOLOGIC ADVANTAGES AND DISADVANTAGES, AND CLINICAL APPLICABILITY

CIRCULATORY ASSIST SYSTEM	DEGREE OF INVASIVENESS	PHYSIOLOGIC MECHANISM	PHYSIOLOGIC EFFECTIVENESS			CLINICAL APPLICABILITY	POTENTIAL DRAWBACKS AND COMPLICATIONS
			Left Ventricular Afterload Reduction	Left Ventricular Preload Reduction	Cardiac Index Augmentation		
Cardiopulmonary partial bypass	++ Requires femoral arterial and venous cannulation	Venoarterial partial bypass with blood-gas interface oxygenator	± ↓ When bypass near complete	++ ↓ Proportional to degree of partial bypass	+++ ↑ Proportional to degree of partial bypass	1. Limited applicability because of invasiveness and potential drawbacks	1. Blood element destruction with hemolysis, ↓ platelets, ↓ WBCs 2. Requires full heparinization
Cardiopulmonary partial bypass with membrane oxygenator	++ Requires femoral arterial and venous cannulation	Venoarterial partial bypass with membrane oxygenator	± ↓ When bypass near complete	++ ↓ Proportional to degree of partial bypass	+++ ↑ Proportional to degree of partial bypass	1. Limited applicability because of invasiveness and potential drawbacks	1. Requires full heparinization 2. Nonpulsatile assist unless pulsatile assist device used
Arterial counterpulsation	++ Requires bilateral femoral artery cannulation	Arterio-arterial diastolic counterpulsation	++ ↓ 20 to 40%	++ ↓ Proportional to degree of afterload reduction	+ ↑ Depends on stroke volume of counterpulsation	1. Limited applicability currently as less invasive and more effective IABP system used to achieve similar physiologic results	1. Ineffective with severe hypotension and cardiogenic shock 2. Hemolysis and damage to blood elements 3. Invasiveness
Left heart partial bypass	++ Requires cannulation of femoral artery and jugular vein with transseptal passage of cannula to left atrium	Left atrial–arterial partial bypass	+ ↓ Requires near-total bypass to reduce Mv_{O_2} by $\geq 20\%$	++ ↓ Proportional to degree of bypass	+++ ↑ Proportional to degree of bypass	1. Limited applicability currently owing to invasiveness and potential drawbacks	1. Blood element damage 2. Requires full heparinization 3. Invasiveness 4. Requires perforation of interatrial septum with cannula? subsequent residual ASD
Intra-aortic balloon pump (IABP)	+ Requires femoral artery cutdown and cannulation, percutaneous technique now available without cutdown	Intra-aortic volume displacement achieving diastolic counterpulsation	++ ↓ 20 to 30%	++ ↓ 20 to 30%	++ ↑ 20 to 40%	Extensive clinical applicability in management of: 1. Refractory acute myocardial ischemia 2. Complications of myocardial infarction (CS, VSD, MR) 3. Postoperative cardiogenic shock (CS)	1. Distal arterial insufficiency 2. Infection with prolonged use 3. Assist system only—must have some effective left ventricular function

Method	Invasiveness	Mechanism	Afterload/aortic pressure effect	Preload/CO effect	LV stroke volume/CO effect	Clinical status	Disadvantages
Anstadt cup	+++ Requires thoracotomy for placement of cup around left ventricular apex	Direct mechanical compression of left ventricle	± Assists left ventricle during systole, increasing peak aortic pressure	± If left ventricular systolic emptying approaches normal end-diastolic volume	↑ With left ventricular systolic emptying, left ventricular stroke volume and cardiac output ↑	and low cardiac output syndrome 4. Prophylactic preoperative use for left main coronary artery disease, severe left ventricular dysfunction 1. Experimental study only	1. Trauma to myocardium 2. Technically difficult to achieve effective compression 3. Invasiveness
Intraventricular balloon	+++ Requires thoracotomy and introduction of balloon through left ventricular apex	Systolic volume displacement within left ventricular chamber	± Peak aortic pressure ↑ with ↑ peak left ventricular pressure	++ ↓ 20 to 30% in experimental animals	++ ↑ Augmentation of left ventricular stroke volume	1. Experimental study only	1. Invasiveness 2. Trauma to left ventricle
Left ventricular assist device (LVAD)	+++ Requires thoracotomy and introduction of left atrial or left ventricular apical cannula plus aortic anastomosis	Left ventricular–aortic or left atrial–aortic bypass	+++ ↓ With left ventricular–aortic bypass; + ↓ with left atrial–aortic bypass	+++ ↓	+++ ↑ System capable of maintaining adequate CO even with no left ventricular contribution	1. Proven clinical effectiveness for circulatory support or postoperative CS when IABP is inadequate. Ultimate effectiveness dependent on potential "recoverability" of left ventricular function	1. Invasiveness 2. Requires cannulation of left ventricular apex or left atrium 3. Requires operative removal* 4. Potential thromboembolic complications
External diastolic counterpulsation	Minimal	Diastolic arterial counterpulsation by external tissue compression of lower extremities	+ ↓ Afterload ↓ by abrupt systolic decompression of lower extremities and ↓ systemic arterial resistance	± Venous return ↑	++ ↑ 15 to 20%	1. Clinically helpful for mild left ventricular dysfunction after MI but overall less effective than IABP	1. May ↑ left ventricular preload by ↑ venous return 2. Uncomfortable for patient after several hours
Body acceleration synchronous with heartbeat (BASH)	Minimal	Kinetic energy transposed into ↑ systolic emptying of left ventricle	± Peak systemic arterial pressure ↑ most instances	+ ↓	++ ↑	1. Limited clinical trial and evaluation currently	1. Uncomfortable for patient after several hours 2. Complex equipment required

*The Litwak LVAD employs percutaneous cannulas that may be occluded and discontinued following left heart assist using obturators.

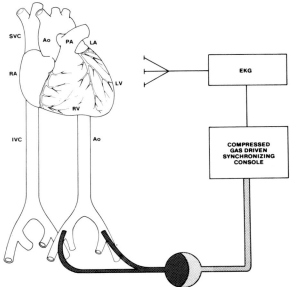

Figure 50–127. Arterioarterial counterpulsation circulatory assist system. Negative-pressure phase withdraws arterial blood during ventricular systole and positive-pressure phase pulses during diastole to achieve diastolic counterpulsation (see Table 50–21).

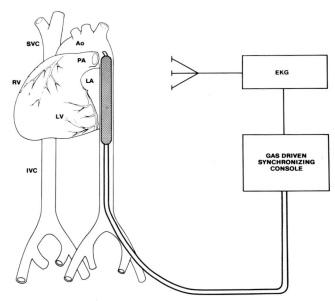

Figure 50–129. Intra-aortic balloon pump counterpulsation circulatory assist system. Balloon deflation occurs in ventricular systole, with inflation occurring during diastole, achieving diastolic counterpulsation (see Table 50–21).

in cardiogenic shock (Satava and McGoon, 1974). This system, however, also has the disadvantage of invasiveness, requiring a thoracotomy for insertion and removal. The effects of prolonged use and the potential for endocardial trauma have not yet been fully evaluated.

The technologic advances during the 1960s in assisted circulation and the development of clinically successful cardiac transplantation together furthered interest in the artificial heart program. With the development of improved biocompatible surfaces and efficient, compact, implantable pumping chambers, development of an effective, clinically applicable, totally implantable left ventricular assist device was made possible (Filler *et al.*, 1967; DeBakey, 1971; Pierce *et al.*, 1974; Norman *et al.*, 1979; Litwak *et*

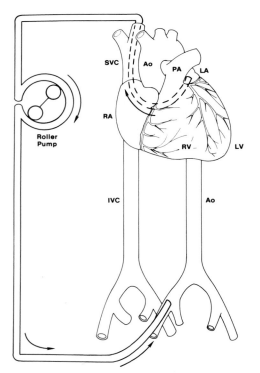

Figure 50–128. Left atrial-arterial partial bypass circulatory assist system not requiring an oxygenator. Left atrial blood withdrawal is achieved by transatrial septal cannulation (see Table 50–21).

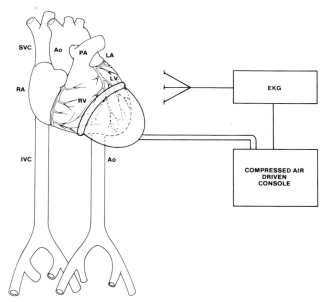

Figure 50–130. Anstadt cup circulatory assist system consisting of pneumatic cup encircling the ventricular apex. Direct mechanical ventricular systolic augmentation is achieved by compression of the ventricle (see Table 50–21).

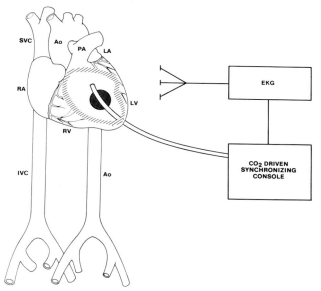

Figure 50–131. Intraventricular balloon circulatory assist system employing intracavitary ventricular volume displacement to achieve systolic pressure augmentation (see Table 50–21).

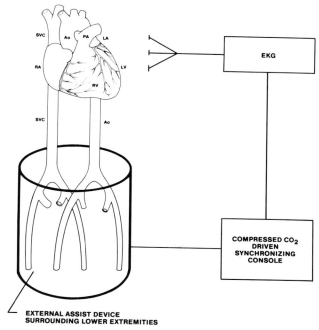

EXTERNAL ASSIST DEVICE
SURROUNDING LOWER EXTREMITIES

Figure 50–133. External counterpulsation assist device. Extramural mechanical compression of the lower extremities during diastole with deflation during ventricular systole achieves diastolic counterpulsation assistance (see Table 50–21).

al., 1973; Deutsch, 1979). These devices, although hemodynamically more effective in supporting left ventricular function than counterpulsation devices, are considerably more invasive and currently relatively limited to use in investigative clinical trials (Fig. 50–132; Table 50–21). In current clinical practice, the left ventricular assist device is generally reserved for use in patients who have failed to wean from cardiopulmonary bypass following open heart surgical procedures and in those patients in whom intra-aortic balloon counterpulsation has not been sufficiently effective to maintain circulation.

The concept of arterial counterpulsation by arterial volume displacement using an external device was developed by Dennis and coworkers (1963), Osborn

and colleagues (1964), and Soroff and associates (1965). This system utilizes a sealed chamber surrounding the lower extremities and is activated by alternating negative-pressure decompression and positive-pressure compression phased to achieve diastolic arterial counterpulsation (Fig. 50–133; Table 50–21). Although this procedure is noninvasive, prolonged periods of external counterpulsation can be uncomfortable to the patient. Although cardiac output can be effectively increased and left ventricular afterload reduced (Mueller *et al.*, 1974), venous return is aug-

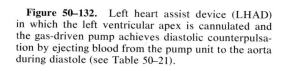

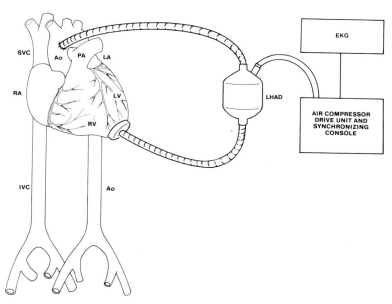

Figure 50–132. Left heart assist device (LHAD) in which the left ventricular apex is cannulated and the gas-driven pump achieves diastolic counterpulsation by ejecting blood from the pump unit to the aorta during diastole (see Table 50–21).

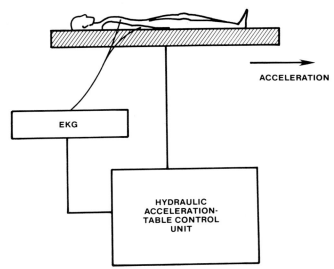

Figure 50–134. Body acceleration synchronized with heart rate (BASH) circulatory assistance system. Sudden cephalad acceleration during ventricular systole increases ventricular systolic ejection (see Table 50–21).

mented, thereby increasing left ventricular preload. Thus, left ventricular stroke work and myocardial oxygen demand can be significantly reduced, although not to the same extent as can be achieved with intra-aortic balloon counterpulsation.

Arntzenius and associates (1970) developed another form of noninvasive assisted circulation in the form of body acceleration synchronous with heartbeat (BASH). This system involves rapid movement of a special table on which the patient lies, displacing intra-aortic blood away from the left ventricle by the mechanism of sudden acceleration (Fig. 50–134; Table 50–21). The effectiveness of this unique method of assisted circulation has not been tested extensively.

PHYSIOLOGIC CONSIDERATIONS

The metabolic demands of the myocardium under varying workloads in the nondiseased heart are readily met by the normal coronary circulation. The coronary circulation normally is an autoregulatory system, with increasing myocardial perfusion demands being met by increased coronary circulation within the normal physiologic range of arterial perfusion pressure. Dis-

ease states such as coronary arterial occlusive disease and intrinsic myocardial disease or imposed conditions such as occur in cardiac surgical procedures may result in a failure of autoregulatory control and a consequent imbalance between myocardial metabolic demands and myocardial perfusion.

Myocardial ischemia results when there is an imbalance between myocardial oxygen demand and oxygen delivery (Fig. 50–135). The immediate physiologic effect of myocardial ischemia is a reduction in myofibrillar contractility, resulting in a decrease in the force and velocity of left ventricular wall motion. The reduction in myocardial contractility associated with myocardial ischemia is caused, in part, by reduction of high-energy phosphate stores, including creatine phosphate (CP) and adenosine triphosphate (ATP). As a consequence, myocardial ischemia leads to a decrease in the velocity and extent of myofibrillar shortening and subsequent myofibrillar lengthening in the resting state to achieve the same active tension (Frank-Starling mechanism). Thus, with increasing myocardial ischemia, there is an associated increase in left ventricular end-diastolic volume and left ventricular end-diastolic pressure. The corresponding increase in left ventricular wall stress (law of LaPlace) results in an increased oxygen demand and consumption, if oxygen delivery can meet the demand. Particularly in circumstances in which there is significant coronary artery occlusive disease or ischemia of the left ventricle following cardiopulmonary bypass and cardiac surgical procedures in which aortic cross-clamping is required, oxygen delivery may be inadequate to meet the demand. A vicious circle of events may develop, with progressive myocardial ischemia and left ventricular functional impairment (Fig. 50–136).

The important studies of Sarnoff and associates (1958) concerning the hemodynamic determinants of myocardial oxygen consumption formed the physiologic basis for the design of effective circulatory assist devices. These studies indicated that the principal determinant of myocardial oxygen consumption was left ventricular pressure work (Fig. 50–137) and that it could be directly related to the tension-time index (Fig. 50–138). Volume work (left ventricular stroke work), left ventricular preload, and heart rate were found to be significant but relatively lesser contributing factors to myocardial oxygen demand. Corrobo-

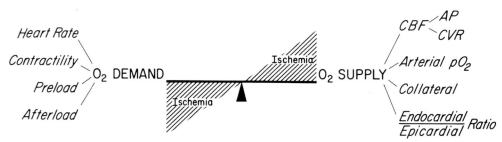

Figure 50–135. Physiologic balance between myocardial oxygen demand and supply indicating influencing factors. Imbalance between excessive myocardial oxygen demand or lessened myocardial oxygen supply results in myocardial ischemia.

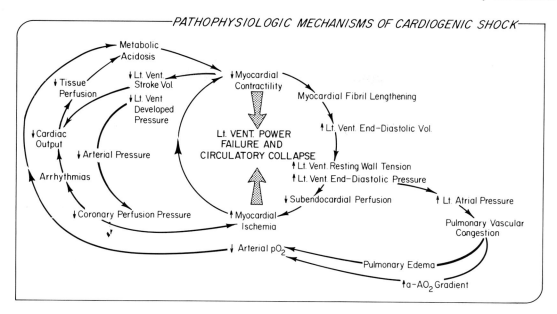

PATHOPHYSIOLOGIC MECHANISMS OF CARDIOGENIC SHOCK

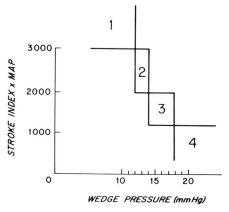

Figure 50–136. *A,* Vicious circle of hemodynamic, circulatory, and metabolic events that take part in development of left ventricular power failure and cardiogenic shock secondary to acute myocardial infarction. *B,* Schema for classification of patients into four hemodynamic categories. With a wedge pressure of 18 mm. Hg or more and a mean arterial pressure (**MAP**) × stroke index product of 1200 or less, a patient would be in Category 4.

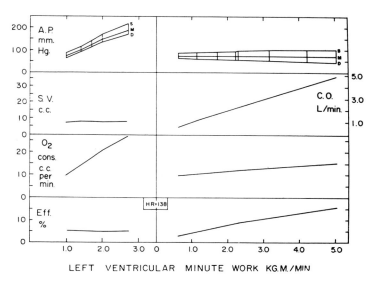

LEFT VENTRICULAR MINUTE WORK KG.M./MIN

Figure 50–137. Relationship of myocardial oxygen utilization and pressure versus volume work. Increasing left ventricular pressure work results in a near-linear increase in myocardial oxygen consumption, whereas increasing volume work results in a lesser increase. (From Sarnoff, S. J., *et al.:* Hemodynamic determinants of oxygen consumption of the heart with special reference to the tension-time index. Am. J. Physiol., *192*:148, 1958.)

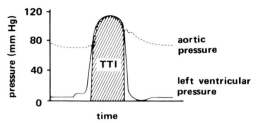

Figure 50–138. Tension-time index. The oxygen consumption of the heart is roughly proportional to the area under the ejection phase of the left ventricular pressure curve, which represents the tension-time index (TTI). (From Katz, A. M.: Physiology of the Heart. New York, Raven Press, 1977.)

rating these findings were the studies of Graham and colleagues (1968), indicating that myocardial oxygen demand is dependent primarily on two physiologic variables: (1) left ventricular peak wall stress and (2) the intrinsic contractile state of the muscle, neither of which is directly correlated with ventricular stroke work or performance. Since myocardial contractility is already depressed with myocardial ischemia, a further therapeutic attempt to reduce contractility in order to decrease myocardial oxygen demand would have an adverse effect on ventricular performance. Thus, reduction of myocardial oxygen demand is better accomplished by reduction of peak ventricular wall stress or left ventricular afterload while maintaining or improving contractility.

Optimal therapeutic management of myocardial ischemia thus involves (1) reduction of myocardial oxygen consumption, (2) augmentation of coronary blood flow, and (3) improvement in ventricular performance. Although positive inotropic agents such as isoproterenol, dopamine, dobutamine, epinephrine, and norepinephrine can increase myocardial contractility, cardiac output, and mean arterial pressure, they do so at the expense of increasing myocardial oxygen consumption, often under conditions in which oxygen delivery cannot be readily enhanced. Maroko and associates (1971) demonstrated that isoproterenol increased myocardial contractility in experimental myocardial infarction, but at the expense of increasing the extent of infarction. Similarly, alpha-adrenergic agents such as norepinephrine increased the extent of muscle injury, despite an increase in mean arterial pressure and mean coronary perfusion pressure. Any intervention resulting in increased myocardial oxygen demand by augmentation of contractility, left ventricular afterload, or heart rate may increase the severity of myocardial ischemia, despite temporary hemodynamic benefit. Thus, the physiologic approach to management of myocardial ischemia must be directed toward (1) reduction of left ventricular afterload and left ventricular wall tension, (2) augmentation of myocardial perfusion with normal distribution of flow, and (3) maintenance of physiologically adequate systemic cardiac output.

Left ventricular impedance, defined as instant left ventricular pressure divided by instant aortic flow, was found by Urschel and associates (1970) to be inversely proportional to left ventricular stroke volume and performance. Thus, lowering impedance by afterload reduction not only reduces left ventricular wall stress and oxygen consumption but also reduces ventricular size and volume. This is associated with an increase in stroke volume and ejection fraction, enhancing ventricular performance. Reduction of myocardial oxygen consumption pharmacologically by either reduction of myocardial contractility with beta-adrenergic blockade and/or decrease in left ventricular afterload with vasodilators can be effective in reducing myocardial ischemia, as shown by Forrester and coworkers (1975) and Maroko and colleagues (1971, 1976). Myocardial ischemia, without infarction and severe ventricular functional impairment, can, in most cases, be resolved with pharmacologic interventions that result in effective reduction of myocardial oxygen demand. This is usually accomplished pharmacologically by a combination of afterload and preload reduction and by decreasing heart rate and myocardial contractility. The commonly used pharmacologic agents used clinically are intravenous sodium nitroprusside, nitroglycerin, and propranolol. However, when there is significant muscle injury and associated severe impairment of left ventricular function, pharmacologic reduction in myocardial oxygen consumption may be difficult to achieve while still preserving an adequate cardiac output and arterial pressure.

Mechanical circulatory assistance that effectively achieves ventricular afterload reduction and augmentation of cardiac output can accomplish the physiologic objectives of reduction in myocardial oxygen consumption (Mv_{O_2}) and support of the failing circulation concurrent with resolution of myocardial ischemia (Powell et al., 1970). The various forms of cardiopulmonary and left heart bypass previously discussed can reduce left ventricular afterload and Mv_{O_2} while augmenting systemic flow, but near-total bypass is required to gain very significant effects (Pennock et al., 1976; Wakabayashi et al., 1975). With left atrial–arterial bypass, reduction of Mv_{O_2} is primarily a consequence of a decrease in preload with a curvilinear relationship between Mv_{O_2} reduction and percentage of total bypass. Left ventricular bypass, as achieved with a left ventricular assist device, reduces Mv_{O_2} in a direct linear relationship by progressive reduction in peak left ventricular pressure (afterload) rather than indirectly by reduction of preload as with left atrial–arterial bypass (Laks et al., 1977). Thus, with partial bypass systems of mechanical circulatory assistance, the system that achieves a greater reduction in afterload and left ventricular tension-time index has been shown to be most effective in resolving ischemia (Pennock et al., 1979).

Intra-aortic balloon counterpulsation, a less invasive form of mechanical circulatory assistance, has been shown to be effective in achieving the three physiologic objectives required in the management of myocardial ischemia refractory to pharmacologic intervention. The experimental study of Powell and associates (1970) demonstrated that intra-aortic balloon pump (IABP) counterpulsation significantly increased coronary blood flow in the failing ischemic

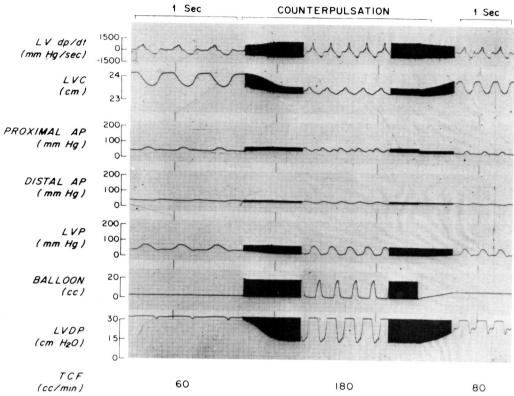

Figure 50–139. The effect of IABP on cardiac hemodynamics in an experimental failing left ventricle preparation. IABP significantly reduced left ventricular end-diastolic pressure and left ventricular volume (circumference) and increased total coronary flow and left ventricular dp/dt. (LVC = left ventricular circumference; LV dp/dt = first derivative of the slope of left ventricular pressure development; AP = aortic pressure; LVP = left ventricular pressure; TCF = total coronary blood flow.) (From Powell, W. J., et al.: Effects of intra-aortic balloon counterpulsation on cardiac performance, oxygen consumption and coronary blood flow in dogs. Circ. Res., 26:753, 1970. By permission of The American Heart Association, Inc.)

ventricle and, as a result of reducing left ventricular afterload, decreased left ventricular end-diastolic pressure and volume and achieved physiological unloading of the left ventricle (Fig. 50–139). This study further demonstrated that IABP counterpulsation in the normotensive, nonischemic heart resulted in no significant change in coronary blood flow or left ventricular performance but was capable of reducing left ventricular peak systolic pressure and left ventricular end-diastolic pressure independent of changes in coronary flow.

It is questionable whether IABP counterpulsation can increase regional coronary blood flow to an ischemic region (Swank et al., 1978) or improve subendocardial perfusion in the ischemic zone more than transiently (Cox et al., 1975). Improvement in coronary flow and in both subendocardial and subepicardial perfusion has been demonstrated in the peri-ischemic zone but not in distant nonischemic myocardium (Shaw et al., 1974; Jett et al., 1980). Although Willerson and coworkers (1976) demonstrated a 20 per cent increase in coronary blood flow to an ischemic myocardial zone after instituting IABP in an experimental preparation, the measurements were taken only acutely after the ischemic period. Cox and associates (1975) found that the initial improvement in ischemic zone coronary blood flow and subendo-

cardial perfusion was not maintained with IABP, noting a subsequent reduction in subendocardial flow. Subsequently, Jett and colleagues (1980) have shown that a combination of IABP with pharmacologic agents such as hyperosmolar mannitol or isosorbide dinitrate and propranolol further augmented coronary blood flow to an ischemic myocardial region to a greater extent than when any of the agents were used alone. These pharmacologic agents also increased nonischemic myocardial blood flow, suggesting that combined mechanical circulatory support and pharmacologic management in the treatment of myocardial ischemia is better than either method alone. As a corollary to the studies indicating little long-term improvement in ischemic zone coronary blood flow with IABP, there is little evidence of improvement in myocardial performance with IABP in the immediate ischemic zone (Kerber et al., 1976; Sasayama et al., 1979). In the latter experimental study, however, it was shown that IABP counterpulsation selectively improved peri-ischemic zone function by returning previously reduced myocardial segment active shortening toward pre-ischemia control values. In a clinical study using multigated nuclear cardiac scanning of two groups of patients with acute ischemia (unstable angina) or acute infarction, Nichols and colleagues (1978) demonstrated that IABP counterpulsation enhanced segmental myocardial contractility in an ischemic zone but not in an infarcted region. The improvement in ventricular function with IABP in patients with acute myocardial infarction was found to occur as a result of reduction in end-diastolic and end-systolic volumes and not as a result of improved function of the infarcted segment.

The potential for circulatory assistance in reducing the extent of injury in acute myocardial infarction has been widely investigated. The experimental studies of Roberts and associates (1978), Sugg and coworkers (1969), and Maroko and colleagues (1972) have suggested that IABP counterpulsation instituted as late as 3 hours after coronary artery occlusion significantly reduced expected infarct size. Other studies (Laas et al., 1980; Ergin et al., 1976; Haston and McNamara, 1979) have not substantiated a significant effect on infarct size using IABP in the experimental model. The clinical studies of Leinbach and associates (1973a) and Parmley and coworkers (1974) suggested that the combination of circulatory assistance and pharmacologic afterload reduction plus the use of propranolol could reduce the expected infarct size in patients with evolving acute myocardial infarction, particularly in patients without total occlusion of the coronary artery in the distribution of the infarct. However, a recent randomized controlled trial of IABP counterpulsation in early myocardial infarction complicated by left ventricular failure indicated no significant modification of infarct size, mortality, or morbidity (O'Rourke et al., 1981). The exact time interval between acute coronary arterial occlusion and completion of infarction during which mechanical circulatory assistance can be effective in reducing the extent of muscle necrosis has not been clearly defined. In clinical practice, it would be rare to have the opportunity to institute circulatory assistance within 4 hours of the onset of pain. With established infarction (more than 4 hours after the onset of persistent pain) or with left ventricular failure progressing, circulatory assistance probably does not alter the established infarct, but it may prevent further extension of infarction to jeopardized ischemic myocardium by reducing left ventricular workload and augmenting coronary blood flow to adjacent areas.

Life-threatening ventricular arrhythmias associated with acute myocardial ischemia or infarction may be controlled by circulatory assistance if that mode is the only intervention that is effective in controlling ischemia. Experimental studies by Fleming and associates (1968) demonstrated that counterpulsation improved salvage in ventricular fibrillation following acute occlusion of the left anterior descending coronary artery. Clinical experience with IABP in the management of refractory ventricular tachyarrhythmias has been small but encouraging (Mundth et al., 1973a) (Fig. 50–140). Reduction of left ventricular workload and improvement in myocardial oxygenation would appear to be the mechanisms for the effectiveness of circulatory assistance in the management of ventricular irritability.

The use of mechanical circulatory assistance for

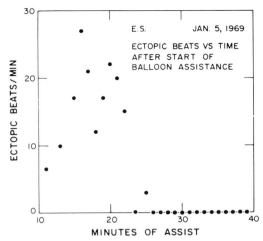

Figure 50–140. Dramatic reduction in the frequency of premature ventricular contractions by institution of IABP in a patient with acute myocardial infarction and medically refractory ventricular irritability.

circulatory support in shock states not associated with primary ischemic left ventricular failure has been reviewed by Beckman and colleagues (1973). Lovett and associates (1971) demonstrated a myocardial depressant factor in terminal septic shock that ultimately resulted in left ventricular failure. Circulatory assistance may be of value in supporting circulation at this stage of septic shock (Dunn et al., 1974), although in earlier phases septic shock is usually associated with a high cardiac output state.

INDICATIONS FOR USE OF ASSISTED CIRCULATION AND CLINICAL RESULTS

Indications for the clinical use of assisted circulation have changed significantly over the past 5 years. As therapeutic goals and the effectiveness of circulatory assistance devices have become better defined, indications for their clinical use have also become more clearly delineated. During the developmental 5-year period from 1970 to 1975, the primary indication for mechanical circulatory assistance was cardiogenic shock complicating acute myocardial infarction. Associated with the increasingly successful results of managing cardiogenic shock by circulatory assistance and early surgical intervention (Mundth et al., 1975b) has been an increased awareness of the mechanisms of development and pathophysiology of cardiogenic shock. This has resulted in earlier recognition, effective treatment, and a gradual reduction in the incidence of post–myocardial infarction cardiogenic shock (Bolooki, 1977). An independent national market survey in 1978 indicated that intraoperative use of IABP for weaning patients from cardiopulmonary bypass due to intraoperative cardiogenic shock had displaced postinfarction cardiogenic shock as the leading indication for IABP counterpulsation (Table 50–22). In an analysis of the extensive clinical experience with IABP at the Massachusetts General Hospital, McEnany and associates (1978) found that

TABLE 50–22. INDICATIONS, CLINICAL USE, AND RESULTS OF
INTRA-AORTIC BALLOON COUNTERPULSATION: RESULTS OF A NATIONAL SURVEY*

INDICATION FOR IABP	NUMBER OF PATIENTS TREATED	HOSPITAL SURVIVAL	
		Number of Patients	*Per cent*
Shock following cardiac surgery	374	250	67%
Postinfarction cardiogenic shock	215	76	35%
Unstable angina	136	129	95%
Intractable left ventricular failure	52	21	40%
Ventricular arrhythmias	21	8	38%
Total	798	484	61%

*From Medtronic, Inc., Marketing Research Report 3/78. (Sampling from previous 6 months' experience from 91 respondents.)

whereas prior to 1974 78 per cent of the indications for IABP was for postinfarction cardiogenic shock, only 26 per cent of patients had IABP for postinfarction cardiogenic shock from 1974 to 1976. Overall, the leading indications for institution of IABP were for support of the failing myocardium following cardiopulmonary bypass (30 per cent), control of refractory myocardial ischemia (23 per cent), and management of postinfarction cardiogenic shock (20 per cent). Similar relative indications have been reported by Macoviak and colleagues (1979) and Bolooki (1977).

Indications for assisted circulation vary also as to the type of assist device used. Of the 10 circulatory assist devices outlined in Table 50–21, only three devices have had very extensive clinical use. The predominant clinical experience has been with intraaortic balloon pump (IABP) assistance, with less experience using the modalities of external diastolic counterpulsation (EDCP) and left ventricular assist devices (LVAD). The relatively complex invasive nature of left ventricular assistance has largely precluded its use to support the failing left ventricle after cardiopulmonary bypass when IABP has not been sufficiently effective (McGee *et al.*, 1980). EDCP has been used primarily in clinical studies evaluating its effectiveness in the management of acute myocardial infarction with mild to moderate left ventricular dysfunction (Amsterdam *et al.*, 1978). With exclusion of these more specialized modes of assisted circulation,

TABLE 50–23. CURRENT INDICATIONS FOR ASSISTED CIRCULATION USING INTRA-AORTIC BALLOON COUNTERPULSATION

1. Left ventricular power failure following cardiac surgery
2. Myocardial ischemia refractory to medical therapy (unstable angina)
3. Complications of acute myocardial infarction
   a. Left ventricular power failure with cardiogenic shock
   b. Rupture of interventricular septum with left-to-right shunt
   c. Rupture of papillary muscle with acute mitral regurgitation
   d. Recurrent angina (ischemia) with threatened extension
   e. Refractory ventricular tachyarrhythmias
4. Prophylaxis (preoperative)
   a. Severe left main coronary artery disease
   b. Severe left ventricular dysfunction
5. Infarct reduction in early evolving acute myocardial infarction
6. Other (primary noncardiac procedures)
   a. Prophylactic use in patients with suspected severe coronary artery disease undergoing major general surgical procedure

the primary current indications for intra-aortic balloon counterpulsation are as shown in Table 50–23.

Left Ventricular Power Failure (Low Cardiac Output Syndrome) Following Cardiac Surgery

Although the use of cold potassium cardioplegia during cardiac surgical procedures has greatly enhanced effective myocardial preservation and significantly decreased the incidence of postoperative low output syndrome, the increasing scope and complexity of procedures in high-risk patients currently have provided a significant number of patients who cannot be readily weaned from cardiopulmonary bypass. In some instances, although the patient is weaned successfully from cardiopulmonary bypass, there may be a persistent low cardiac output syndrome postoperatively, requiring effective management if a successful outcome is to be achieved in both the short term and the long term.

Postoperative left ventricular power failure usually occurs as a result of multiple factors, including (1) the preoperative hemodynamic status of the left ventricle, (2) the presence or absence of unstable myocardial ischemia preoperatively, (3) the incidence of complications during induction of anesthesia, (4) the duration of aortic cross-clamping (global myocardial ischemia period), (5) the effectiveness of cardioplegia, (6) the degree of completeness and technical success of the surgical procedure, (7) the physiologic adequacy of cardiopulmonary bypass and metabolic management, and, undoubtedly, other unknown factors. The reversibility of postoperative left ventricular power failure appears to depend on whether a potentially reversible acute ischemic injury has occurred (Buckley *et al.*, 1973a) and on prompt, effective intervention using pharmacologic and circulatory assist support (Phillips and Bregman, 1977). Mechanical circulatory assistance provides the beneficial effect of both supporting the circulation and reducing left ventricular workload until myocardial functional recovery can occur.

There have been few survivors among patients with preoperative severe left or right ventricular dysfunction, i.e., ejection fraction less than 20 per cent, who develop postoperative ventricular power failure associated with a dilated, largely fibrotic ventricle, whether based on chronic coronary artery disease or valvular disease. The greatest success has been obtained in patients with left ventricular hypertrophy and an identifiable intraoperative ischemic event (Buckley *et al.*, 1973a, McEnany *et al.*, 1978; Scanlon *et al.*, 1976). In the last study, the authors found that the survival rate using IABP for postoperative left ventricular power failure was 86 per cent in patients with identifiable perioperative infarction and normal preoperative left ventricular function. However, the survival rate was only 30 per cent in patients with significant preoperative left ventricular dysfunction. Similarly, Sturm and associates (1980) reported better survival rates for IABP treatment of postoperative low output syndrome in patients with coronary artery disease alone as compared with patients with valvular disease or combined valvular and coronary artery disease.

In most reported series, the prompt use of IABP assistance for postoperative cardiogenic shock has resulted in successful weaning from cardiopulmonary bypass in 75 to 85 per cent of patients, with a hospital survival rate of approximately 55 per cent (Buckley *et al.*, 1973a; Parker *et al.*, 1974; Scanlon *et al.*, 1976; Sturm *et al.*, 1980; Macoviak *et al.*, 1979; Kaplan *et al.*, 1979; Kaiser *et al.*, 1976; Golding *et al.*, 1980; Bolooki, 1977). The reported incidence of postoperative left ventricular power failure requiring assisted circulation (IABP) has been in the range of 2 to 6 per cent in the collected series reviewed. The overall survival rate of approximately 55 per cent is impressive, considering the expected near 100 per cent mortality rate of patients who fail to wean from cardiopulmonary bypass despite inotropic support. Despite the desperate state of this group of patients immediately following surgery, late follow-up of hospital survivors demonstrated a 2-year cardiac actuarial survival rate of 96 per cent, with excellent symptomatic relief and functional status (Golding *et al.*, 1980). This clinical experience clearly emphasizes the potential reversibility of profound left ventricular functional impairment when circulatory support is instituted promptly, providing maintenance of physiologically adequate circulation simultaneously with reduction of left ventricular workload.

With this considerable clinical experience, prognostic indices for survival and procedural protocols have been developed. Norman and coworkers (1977) described three clinical categories of patients requiring postcardiotomy IABP support that correlated well with prognosis. Physiologic and clinical parameters analyzed during IABP assistance were left ventricular function curves, systemic vascular resistance (SVR), and urine output. Class A patients (cardiac index [CI] > 2.1 L./min./M.^{2} and SVR < 2100 dynes sec. cm.$^{-5}$) had an 80 per cent survival rate, whereas Class C patients (CI < 2.1 L./min./M.^{2} with SVR > 2100 dynes sec. cm.$^{-5}$ or CI < 1.2 L./min./M.^{2} regardless of SVR) all expired despite continued IABP assistance if they remained in Class C for greater than 12 hours. Bolooki (1977) similarly analyzed his experience with postcardiotomy IABP and described correlations be-

TABLE 50–24. CRITERIA FOR ELECTIVE INTRA-AORTIC BALLOON PUMPING IN CARDIAC SURGERY*

DEFINITE
Severe preoperative left ventricular dysfunction:
Cardiac index (CI) < 1.8 L./min./M.^{2}, ejection fraction (EF) < 30%, and left ventricular end-diastolic pressure (LVEDP) > 22 mm. Hg

RELATIVE
Association of moderate left ventricular dysfunction (CI < 2.0 L./min./M.^{2}; EF < 40%; LVEDP > 18 mm. Hg) with:
A. Severe aortic stenosis (gradient > 90 mm. Hg)
B. Acute myocardial infarction or its complications
C. Intermediate coronary syndrome with hypertension due to left main and right coronary artery lesions.
D. Valvular heart disease and multiple coronary obstructive lesions

*From Bolooki, H., *et al.*: J. Thorac. Cardiovasc. Surg., *72*: 756, 1976.

tween cardiac pathology, preoperative hemodynamics, the incidence of postoperative left ventricular power failure requiring IABP, and mortality. On the basis of these studies, Bolooki and associates (1976) recommended elective (prophylactic) IABP preoperatively for patients in certain clinical categories (Table 50–24). The prophylactic elective use of IABP preoperatively remains somewhat controversial in some of these clinical categories, and it is not clear that preoperative IABP will necessarily decrease the incidence of postoperative hemodynamic problems. It has been well documented, however, that prompt institution of assisted circulation intraoperatively is important to successful management of left ventricular power failure following cardiopulmonary bypass (Phillips and Bregman, 1977).

Recently, Sturm and colleagues (1981) have shown a significant improvement in the management of postcardiotomy low output syndrome by combining pharmacologic management with IABP and careful volume (preload) adjustment. Intravenous infusion of nitroprusside (0.5 to 5.0 gm./kg./min.) and dopamine (7.5 μg./kg./min.) in 10 patients during IABP for postcardiotomy low output syndrome resulted in a significant increase in cardiac index from a mean of 1.6 to 2.5 L./min./M.^{2} (p < 0.01) and a fall in SVR from 2774 to 1439 dynes sec. cm.$^{-5}$ (p < 0.02). Thus, Class C patients were successfully moved to a Class A category, and all were weaned from IABP and pharmacologic support. Seven of the 10 patients were hospital survivors. Despite the effectiveness of IABP and pharmacologic support in the management of intraoperative left ventricular power failure, approximately 15 per cent of patients cannot be weaned from cardiopulmonary bypass. It is this group of patients who, currently, can be considered for a left heart assist device.

A retrospective study of 14,168 patients undergoing cardiac surgery over approximately a 4-year period at the Texas Heart Institute (McGee *et al.*, 1980) indicated that 2.3 per cent (326 patients) required IABP and pharmacologic support in attempted weaning from cardiopulmonary bypass, with 0.7 per cent (94 patients) failing to respond. Of these, 21 patients underwent implantation and use of an abdominal left ventricular assist device (ALVAD), which was subsequently successfully weaned and removed from three patients who recovered. Litwak and colleagues (1978) reported successful weaning and removal of a left heart assist device (LHAD) in 13 of 18 patients in whom it was employed for severe postcardiotomy left ventricular power failure, with subsequent long-term survival of five patients (28 per cent). Other clinical successes have been reported by Pierce and associates (1978), Bernhard and coworkers (1979), and Wolner and Turina (reported by Norman and Bregman [1978]). Thus, current clinical experience would indicate there is a rationale for use of an LVAD in refractory cardiogenic shock in selected patients (Pae and Pierce, 1981). The potential for cardiac transplantation in the event of persistent LVAD dependence has been demonstrated by Reemtsma and colleagues (1978). Unquestionably, further testing and development of reliable selection criteria for clinical use of LVADs will be essential and undoubtedly accomplished over the next several years.

Myocardial Ischemia Refractory to Medical Therapy (Unstable Angina)

Although preinfarction angina is a term that can be applied only retrospectively, numerous clinical studies have indicated that there is an identifiable syndrome of unstable angina associated with an increased incidence of subsequent acute myocardial infarction and death (Beamish and Storrie, 1960; Gazes et al., 1973). Agreement on a precise definition of unstable angina has been difficult to achieve, but currently, most would agree with the clinical definition proposed by the National Randomized Study Group that unstable angina pectoris consists of (1) one or more prolonged episodes of chest pain at rest, (2) documented ST/T-wave electrocardiographic changes of ischemia during one or more episodes of pain, and (3) acute myocardial infarction excluded by assessing serial electrocardiographic tracings and CPK myocardial band isoenzymes (Hutter et al., 1977; Russell et al., 1978).

Medical treatment for the patient with unstable angina should be instituted promptly in a coronary care unit setting with appropriate monitoring (Krauss et al., 1972). Pharmacologic management is directed toward (1) afterload reduction using sodium nitroprusside and nitrates and (2) beta-adrenergic blockade with propranolol to decrease myocardial oxygen demand. In the majority of cases, myocardial ischemia can be interrupted and the patient stabilized (Krauss et al., 1972; Bertolasi et al., 1976; Selden et al., 1975; Russell et al., 1978). The medically stabilized patient has then undergone elective coronary angiographic study and elective coronary bypass surgery if operable anatomy was found, with overall excellent early and long-term results (Hultgren et al., 1977; Langou et al., 1978; Olinger et al., 1978; Russell et al., 1978). Emergency myocardial revascularization for unstable angina, which was recommended by some in the past, now is largely avoided because of the substantial operative mortality and excessive incidence of perioperative infarction (Dumesnil et al., 1972; Lambert et al., 1972; Sustaita et al., 1972; Flemma et al., 1972).

Despite the medical therapy just outlined, a certain number of patients with unstable angina will remain refractory to treatment and continue to have unstable myocardial ischemia. Assisted circulation in these patients using IABP has been an effective adjunct in addition to pharmacologic management in resolving acute myocardial ischemia, allowing safe angiographic study and early revascularization surgery (Gold et al., 1973; Mundth et al., 1975a; Steele et al., 1976; Levine et al., 1978; Weintraub et al., 1979; Langou et al., 1978; Harris et al., 1980). Clinical studies by Gold and associates (1973) demonstrated that acute myocardial ischemia refractory to medical treatment could be promptly and effectively resolved with intra-aortic balloon counterpulsation (Figs. 50–141 and 50–142). This was manifested by abolishment of pain, reversal (normalization) of electrocardiographic ST/T-wave changes of ischemia, and improvement in abnormal left ventricular hemodynamics. In 1978, Nichols and coworkers, using multigated nuclear cardiac scanning, were able to demonstrate significant improvement in ischemic zone segmental wall contraction with IABP counterpulsation, indicating functional reversibility of the myocardium with resolution of ischemia. Similarly, Aroesty and colleagues (1979) were able to show a significant decrease in left ventricular systolic and end-diastolic pressures and volumes without change in cardiac index with use of IABP in unstable angina patients. Previous studies from their laboratory (Weintraub and Aroesty, 1976) had shown improvement with IABP in ejection fraction, left ventricular end-diastolic volume, circumferential fiber shortening, and segmental contraction. In addition, Steele and associates (1976), using a radionuclide technique, demonstrated that the combination of IABP and isosorbide dinitrate in unstable angina patients resulted in a decrease in left ventricular stroke volume index (SVI) and left ventricular end-diastolic volume (LVEDV) associated with an increase in left ventricular ejection fraction. Despite the potentially tenuous status of this group of patients, the combination of IABP and pharmacologic management, angiographic study, and early myocardial revascularization has resulted in an operative mortality rate in the range of 1.7 to 5.3 per cent and a perioperative infarction incidence of only 2.2 to 6.6 per cent (Weintraub et al., 1979; Levine et al., 1978; Langou et al., 1978).

Long-term follow-up of patients with unstable angina refractory to medical therapy undergoing intra-aortic balloon counterpulsation and operation has indicated excellent functional results and a low late mortality. Weintraub and associates (1979) reported that of 59 hospital survivors, only one late death occurred in a mean follow-up period of 31 months. More than 90 per cent of patients were classified in

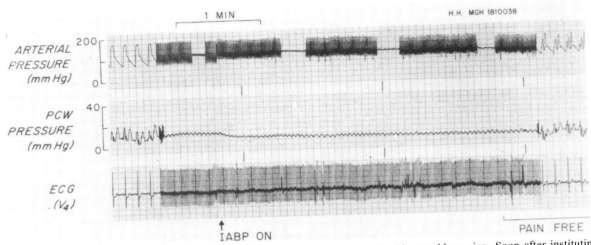

Figure 50–141. Reversal of acute myocardial ischemia with IABP in a patient with unstable angina. Soon after instituting IABP assistance, the depressed ST segments in lead V₄ of the electrocardiogram became isoelectric in association with cessation of pain. Concomitant with reversal of myocardial ischemia the pulmonary capillary wedge pressure (PCW) was reduced from 14 mm. Hg to 5 mm. Hg, reflecting "unloading of the left ventricle." Excellent diastolic counterpulsation was achieved by IABP, as can be noted in the right portion of the arterial pressure tracing, with a reduction of 20 mm. Hg in peak left ventricular pressure. (From Gold, H. K., *et al.*: Intraaortic balloon pumping for control of recurrent myocardial ischemia. Circulation, *47*:1197, 1973. By permission of The American Heart Association, Inc.)

NYHA functional Class I or II. Gold and coworkers (1976) reported no late deaths in an average follow-up period of 18 months postoperatively, with uniformly excellent functional results. In a more recent update of this series, Levine and colleagues (1978) reported four late deaths (4.5 per cent) after an average follow-up of 38 months. Of the remaining surviving patients, there was only one symptomatic infarction, and 93 per cent had no significant angina.

In the group of patients with continuing pain from unstable angina, interruption of myocardial ischemia with circulatory assistance appears to be the safest and most successful method of approach to their management, with subsequent urgent coronary angiographic study and coronary bypass surgery.

Complications of Acute Myocardial Infarction

Although the overall mortality from acute myocardial infarction has been significantly reduced over the past two decades, the mortality associated with left ventricular power failure (Scheidt *et al.*, 1970; Gunnar *et al.*, 1974) and acute mechanical complications of myocardial infarction, including rupture of the interventricular septum (Sanders *et al.*, 1956; Donahoo *et al.*, 1975), papillary muscle rupture (Sanders *et al.*, 1957), or rupture of the ventricular wall (Friedman, 1973; Naeim *et al.*, 1972), remains substantial. Medical therapy incorporating the use of vasodilators and/or beta-adrenergic blocking agents to reduce left ventricular afterload and myocardial oxygen requirements has helped to improve survival, particularly in those patients in whom left ventricular function is not yet profoundly impaired (Gold *et al.*, 1972; Shell and Sobel, 1974; Forrester *et al.*, 1975). However, with profound left ventricular power failure and cardiogenic shock, the expected mortality rate remains 90 per cent or greater, despite medical therapy (Gunnar and Loeb, 1972; Smith *et al.*, 1967; Russell *et al.*, 1970; Mundth *et al.*, 1972).

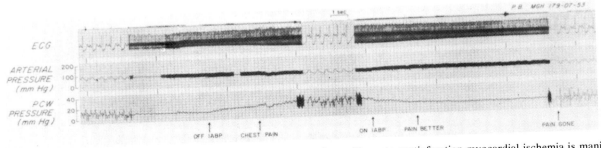

Figure 50–142. The effect of temporary cessation of IABP in a patient with acute postinfarction myocardial ischemia is manifested by a prompt rise in pulmonary capillary wedge pressure (PCW) without change in mean arterial pressure, indicating deterioration of left ventricular function. The patient experienced chest pain associated with a significant deepening of depressed ST segments in lead V₄ of the electrocardiogram. Reinstitution of IABP resulted in prompt return of these parameters to baseline with complete resolution of pain. (From Gold, H. K., *et al.*: Intraaortic balloon pumping for control of recurrent myocardial ischemia. Circulation, *47*:1197, 1973. By permission of The American Heart Association, Inc.)

Postinfarction Cardiogenic Shock

In recent years, the development of effective modalities of mechanical circulatory assistance has significantly improved salvage in patients with postinfarction cardiogenic shock, particularly when combined with pharmacologic therapy or with urgent revascularization surgery (Mundth *et al.*, 1975b; Bolooki, 1977; Bardet *et al.*, 1977b; Johnson *et al.*, 1977; DeWood *et al.*, 1980). The basis for this combined therapeutic approach is related to the known pathophysiology of postinfarction left ventricular power failure. The clinicopathologic studies of Page and associates (1971) demonstrated that in patients dying of postinfarction cardiogenic shock, there was 40 per cent or greater loss of the left ventricular wall from a combination of acute infarction and residual scar from previous infarction. Histologic examination revealed irregular and scattered areas of myocardial necrosis of varying ages, indicative of progressive extension of the original acute infarction. Recent extension of myocardial necrosis was found to be more extensive in the peri-infarction zone adjacent to the original acute infarction, where myocardial perfusion was most severely jeopardized by virtue of occlusive coronary artery disease involving major coronary arterial branches to that distribution.

These findings strongly suggested that postinfarction left ventricular power failure leading to cardiogenic shock often evolves as a result of a "vicious circle" of hemodynamic events as a consequence of progressive extension of the original acute infarct rather than as a result of a sudden catastrophic event (Fig. 50–136*A*). In experimental studies of acute myocardial infarction, Cox and colleagues (1968) had confirmed the validity of this concept by demonstrating progressive myocardial necrosis in the peri-infarction zone of initially ischemic myocardium up to 1 week after the original infarct. Hood (1970) and Schelbert and coworkers (1971) demonstrated a significant decrease in contractility in the ischemic peri-infarction zone, which, however, was capable of responding to inotropic stimulus until cell death occurred in that segment. Maroko and associates (1971) also demonstrated that contractility of ischemic peri-infarction zone myocardium could be enhanced by inotropic drugs but at the expense of increasing myocardial oxygen requirements, which led to extension of the infarct as a function of time. As a result of infarction and increased left ventricular wall tension, diffuse subendocardial ischemia may ensue, with a resulting deterioration in left ventricular function, and may contribute to the vicious circle of hemodynamic deterioration (Schaper and Pasyk, 1976). Since myocardial cellular function and viability depend on a favorable balance between oxygen and metabolic substrate supply and demand, therapeutic intervention intended to interrupt the ischemic process and possibly achieve salvage requires both reduction in myocardial oxygen consumption and improvement in oxygen delivery concomitant with maintenance of adequate cardiac output.

IABP counterpulsation has been shown to be capable of achieving these therapeutic goals, with reversal of the shock syndrome in approximately 75 per cent of patients (Table 50–25) (Kantrowitz *et al.*, 1969; Dunkman *et al.*, 1972; Mueller *et al.*, 1972; Bregman *et al.*, 1971; Johnson *et al.*, 1977; Bolooki, 1977; Ehrich *et al.*, 1977; Hagemeijer *et al.*, 1977; Bardet *et al.*, 1977a; DeWood *et al.*, 1980). Careful hemodynamic categorization of the postinfarction patient with left ventricular power failure is imperative to objectively assess results of therapy (Leinbach *et al.*, 1973b; Scheidt *et al.*, 1970; Bolooki, 1977; Norman *et al.*, 1977; Lorente *et al.*, 1980). The most important hemodynamic parameters determining prognosis were found to be cardiac index, left ventricular preload, and systemic vascular resistance. Patients in cardiogenic shock Category 4 (Leinbach *et al.*, 1973b) (Fig. 50–136*B*), Class C (Norman *et al.*, 1977), or Class E or F (Bolooki, 1977) have an expected mortality rate of virtually 100 per cent with medical treatment alone and only a moderate improvement in survival when the combination of IABP plus medical therapy is used. The hospital survival rate of patients in profound cardiogenic shock treated with the combination of IABP plus medical therapy alone has been less than 25 per cent, with a long-term survival rate (1 year) of 12 per cent (Dunkman *et al.*, 1972). With less profound degrees of left ventricular failure, the salvage rate of patients treated by IABP has been substantially better. DeWood and associates (1980) reported a hospital survival rate of 48 per cent, with a 6- to 24-month survival rate of 29 per cent. O'Rourke and coworkers (1979) reported a hospital survival rate of 34 per cent, with a survival rate of 10 per cent at 4 years in patients categorized as having postinfarction left ventricular failure. Similarly, Johnson and colleagues (1977) reported a hospital survival rate of 44 per cent and one

TABLE 50–25. PHYSIOLOGIC EFFECTS OF IABP ASSISTANCE IN ISCHEMIC LEFT VENTRICULAR POWER FAILURE AFTER INFARCT

AUTHORS	NUMBER OF PATIENTS	PEAK LVP	TOTAL SYSTEMIC RESISTANCE	PCW	CI	SWI	UO
Dunkman *et al.* (1972)	40	23%	—	22%	44%	—	—
Bardet *et al.* (1977a)	42	—	—	27%	45%	—	>400%
Ehrich *et al.* (1977)	16	—	33%	25%	53%	50%	—

LVP = left ventricular pressure
PCW = pulmonary capillary wedge pressure
SWI = left ventricular stroke work index
UO = (hourly) urinary output

TABLE 50–26. CLINICAL, ANGIOGRAPHIC, AND HEMODYNAMIC CRITERIA FOR PATIENT SELECTION FOR URGENT SURGICAL INTERVENTION IN POSTINFARCTION CARDIOGENIC SHOCK

I. *Clinical Criteria*
  1. Duration of cardiogenic shock < 24 hours from onset until institution of IABP assistance
  2. Reversal of cardiogenic shock with IABP assistance plus pharmacologic therapy or evidence of progressive hemodynamic improvement
  3. Absence of history of chronic low output state associated with end-stage disease

II. *Angiographic Criteria*
  1. Evidence of some vascularity and ventricular wall motion in area of or immediately adjacent to infarcted segment(s)
  2. Adequate coronary vessels distally for bypass with good peripheral run-off.

III. *Hemodynamic Criteria* (IABP hemodynamic dependence with temporary interruption of IABP)
  1. Cardiac index < 2 L./min./M.^{2}
  2. Pulmonary capillary wedge pressure > 20 mm. Hg
  3. Mean aortic blood pressure < 60 mm. Hg
  4. Recurrent myocardial ischemia (angina and/or ECG ST-segment changes of ischemia)

of 39 per cent at 6 months after discharge. It is clear that this group of patients, particularly those with profound cardiogenic shock, is at high risk for subsequent lethal cardiac events even if hospital survival is achieved.

Although the combination of IABP plus pharmacologic therapy has been shown to be very effective in achieving dramatic hemodynamic improvement during support, even in patients with severe left ventricular power failure, the statistics reviewed in the preceding paragraphs made it apparent that further definitive therapy often was necessary to improve oxygen delivery to the ischemic myocardium (Mundth, 1977; Mundth *et al.*, 1973b, 1975b; Leinbach *et al.*, 1973b; Dilley *et al.*, 1973). The criteria by which the decision can be reached concerning the indication for urgent revascularization surgery have continuously evolved with accumulated experience. Hemodynamic factors, IABP dependence, and angiographic and clinical factors require careful analysis for an appropriate, well-guided decision (Table 50–26) (Mundth, 1976; Bolooki, 1977; Lorente *et al.*, 1980; Bardet *et al.*, 1977a; Leinbach *et al.*, 1973b). If the patient demonstrates lack of progressive improvement and IABP dependence either hemodynamically or by recurrent myocardial ischemia with temporary cessation of assistance and is judged to be an operable candidate, surgery should be undertaken expeditiously to achieve best results (Mundth, 1976; Bolooki, 1977; O'Rourke *et al.*, 1979; Johnson *et al.*, 1977; Hill *et al.*, 1974; DeWood *et al.*, 1980). In the last study, DeWood and associates (1980) found that although the hospital mortality of patients treated for cardiogenic shock secondary to acute myocardial infarction with IABP plus medical therapy alone was not significantly different from that of patients treated with IABP plus surgical revascularization, there was a statistically significant improvement in long-term survival in the surgically treated group when treated within 18 hours after onset of symptoms (75 per cent versus 29 per cent). The operative mortality rate of the group of patients operated on less than 16 hours after onset of symptoms was found to be significantly less than in those operated upon more than 18 hours after onset of symptoms (25 per cent versus 71 per cent). It is my opinion, however, that if there is evidence of progressive improvement with IABP plus pharmacologic therapy, particularly in the absence of mechanical defects, immediate surgical intervention may be deferred with an excellent likelihood that the patient will continue to improve, be weaned from circulatory assistance, and subsequently undergo more elective coronary artery revascularization. Recent experience has indicated a significantly higher salvage rate with this approach. The lack of hemodynamic improvement and demonstrated IABP dependence with repeated testing at intervals are critical to the decision concerning urgent surgical intervention.

In a relatively large experience of managing 120 patients with postinfarction cardiogenic shock at the Massachusetts General Hospital (Mundth, 1977), 14 per cent of the patients were weaned from IABP, and 76 per cent of these survived. Eighty-six per cent of the patients remained hemodynamically IABP-dependent, and 75 per cent underwent urgent angiographic study. All patients not undergoing urgent angiographic study died. Sixty-six per cent of the studied patients were considered operable, and of these, 88 per cent underwent urgent surgery, with 47 per cent surviving. All of the patients judged inoperable and those who were considered operable but did not undergo surgery died, despite continued IABP plus pharmacologic therapy. Recent reports have indicated a similar expected salvage rate of approximately 50 per cent in patients with cardiogenic shock refractory to medical therapy who are treated by a combination of IABP and surgery (Mundth and Austen, 1978; Bardet *et al.*, 1977b; DeWood *et al.*, 1980; Johnson *et al.*, 1977; Bolooki, 1977).

Although the results of urgent surgical intervention for postinfarction cardiogenic shock for mechanical complications are somewhat better than for left ventricular power failure alone, the difference does not appear to be significant (Mundth and Austen, 1978) (Tables 50–27 and 50–28). Circulatory assistance using IABP has proved to be an effective adjunct in the management of mechanical complications of acute myocardial infarction (Mundth, 1977). With in-

TABLE 50–27. RESULTS OF COMBINED IABP AND REVASCULARIZATION SURGERY FOR MANAGEMENT OF "PURE" POSTINFARCTION LEFT VENTRICULAR POWER FAILURE

NUMBER OF PATIENTS	ASSOCIATED INFARCTECTOMY	SURVIVAL	LATE DEATHS (AFTER 6 MONTHS TO 8 YEARS)
60	51%	29 (50%)	4

TABLE 50–28. RESULTS OF COMBINED IABP AND DEFINITIVE SURGERY FOR POSTINFARCTION VSD AND RUPTURED PAPILLARY MUSCLE

	NUMBER OF PATIENTS	SURVIVAL
VSD	20	11 (55%)
Ruptured papillary muscle	30	17 (57%)

tra-aortic balloon pump assistance in patients with postinfarction VSD and acute left ventricular failure, the left-to-right shunt may be reduced as much as 30 per cent, the left-sided filling pressure may be reduced by 30 per cent, and the cardiac index may be improved by 20 per cent. Similar hemodynamic improvement in cardiac index, left-sided filling pressures, and reduction in the amplitude of pulmonary capillary wedge V waves has been observed with IABP support of patients with acute mitral regurgitation secondary to postinfarction papillary muscle rupture (Gold et al., 1973). IABP plus pharmacologic management has allowed for hemodynamic stabilization of patients with postinfarction mechanical complications as well as for complete and safe angiographic study. Unless prompt, near-complete hemodynamic stabilization occurs with IABP plus pharmacologic therapy, urgent surgical intervention is indicated for mechanical complications of acute myocardial infarction, with an expected survival rate of over 50 per cent (Loisance et al., 1980; Daggett et al., 1977; Buckley et al., 1973b).

Long-term follow-up of patients with postinfarction cardiogenic shock treated by circulatory assistance and surgery has indicated overall excellent late survival and functional status (Mundth and Austen, 1978; Pierri et al., 1980). In the latter study (Pierri et al., 1980), of 34 patients undergoing coronary bypass surgery within 24 hours of instituting IABP for cardiogenic shock, 47 per cent were alive approximately 2 years after surgery. Exercise testing in 13 late survivors indicated substantial exercise capacity with minimal residual symptomatology. Most of these patients had returned to work. The early and late survival and the excellent functional status maintained in these patients support the rationale of aggressive intervention utilizing circulatory assistance and urgent surgery in carefully selected patients with cardiogenic shock complicating acute myocardial infarction.

Postinfarction Agina Refractory to Medical Therapy

Recurrent pain of myocardial ischemia in the recovery phase of acute myocardial infarction may presage extension of the infarction with subsequent hemodynamic deterioration and an increase in mortality. Early reports of urgent coronary bypass surgery for patients with an established acute infarct and recurrent ischemia indicated a substantial operative risk (Hill et al., 1971). Subsequent experience (Sustaita et al., 1972) of coronary bypass surgery initiated soon after the development of recurrent ischemia was

encouraging. The significant risk of invasive diagnostic study and operative intervention in this group of patients stimulated the use of IABP, which was shown to resolve myocardial ischemia effectively and to allow successful urgent myocardial revascularization (Gold et al., 1973; Mundth, 1976; Bardet et al., 1977a; Levine et al., 1978). In the last study, Levine and associates (1978) reported that in 33 patients, IABP interrupted postinfarction angina in 81 per cent and significantly reduced the severity and intensity of ischemic attacks in the remaining patients. The operative mortality rate was 9.1 per cent, and the incidence of perioperative myocardial infarction was 2.2 per cent. Late survival and functional status have been excellent, with 70 per cent of patients fully active and 93 per cent with no significant angina. Bardet and associates (1977b) similarly reported excellent results, with an operative mortality rate of 6 per cent. Brundage and coworkers (1980) reported similar results for urgent surgery without IABP assistance for postinfarction angina refractory to medical therapy in 22 patients but did note a perioperative infarction rate of 13.6 per cent. It is my opinion that IABP serves as an important and relatively safe adjunct in the management of patients with postinfarction refractory angina in terms of reducing both operative mortality and morbidity, i.e., perioperative infarction.

Postinfarction Ventricular Arrhythmias Refractory to Medical Therapy

Occasionally, ventricular tachyarrhythmias refractory to all conventional modes of medical therapy may persist following acute myocardial infarction, posing a dangerous threat to life. Resection of a left ventricular aneurysm has been successful in a number of instances in the chronic phase following myocardial infarction, when refractory recurrent episodes of ventricular tachyarrhythmias have been associated with left ventricular aneurysm (Magdison, 1969; Gudarshar et al., 1971; Donaldson et al., 1976; Ricks et al., 1977), and coronary artery revascularization has been effective in many instances in the absence of a well-defined ventricular aneurysm (Ecker et al., 1971; Graham et al., 1973; Mundth et al., 1973a; Yashar et al., 1977).

Not uncommonly, patients with recurrent episodes of ventricular tachyarrhythmia in the acute postinfarction state also demonstrate significant hemodynamic instability and may develop left ventricular power failure. The operative risk in this group of patients is high but has been dramatically reduced by the use of IABP assistance as an adjunct in management (Hanson et al., 1980). In their study, Hanson and associates (1980) reviewed 22 patients with medically refractory ventricular irritability after acute myocardial infarction in whom IABP was instituted in the acute phase. Ventricular irritability was completely resolved by IABP in 55 per cent of patients and improved in a total of 86 per cent. Hemodynamic improvement occurred in all patients, with evidence of ischemia resolved in 100 per cent. Fifteen patients who remained IABP-dependent underwent urgent surgical revascularization and/or infarctectomy, with a 47 per cent survival rate and no late deaths after an average follow-up of 46 months. The survival rate was 100 per cent in patients who were weaned from IABP without urgent surgery being required, although there were two late deaths in this group without revascularization (29 per cent). Increased survival was seen in those patients who had identifiable acute ischemia, absence of ventricular aneurysm, and complete control of ventricular irritability with IABP plus pharmacologic therapy and in those patients with less extensive coronary artery disease.

Application of newer techniques of epicardial-endocardial mapping location and surgical ablation of the irritable focus or re-entry pathway, as developed by Harken and associates (1979), Gallagher and coworkers (1975), and Guiraudon and colleagues (1978), may further improve results. Unquestionably, circulatory assistance will play a major role in the management of patients with post–acute infarction ventricular irritability, even with the newer and apparently more effective modalities of surgical therapy.

Myocardial Infarct Reduction

The use of mechanical circulatory assistance early in the course of evolving acute myocardial infarction has been studied by numerous investigators (Leinbach *et al.*, 1978; Parmley *et al.*, 1974; Amsterdam, 1980; Gowda *et al.*, 1978) to determine the potential of reducing expected infarct size. As yet, there is no clear-cut evidence that any intervention, including circulatory assistance, can significantly reduce expected infarct size, even in the early evolving phase of acute myocardial infarction. The major problems that investigators must face are the lack of any single or even multiple techniques for accurate infarct size quantification and the logistic problems inherent in instituting definitive interventions in the early acute phase of evolving acute myocardial infarction. Reversal of myocardial ischemia, evidenced by elimination of pain and decrease in the amplitude of electrocardiographic ST-segment abnormalities, has been shown with early intervention in the course of acute myocardial infarction using IABP (Leinbach *et al.*, 1978). In this noncontrolled study, 11 patients with less than 6-hour-old anterior myocardial infarction underwent IABP, with five patients responding promptly, with an 84 per cent fall in ST-segment elevation. In contrast, six patients responded poorly, with a 40 per cent decrease in ST-elevation within 1 hour. A positive response correlated directly to angiographic demonstration of subtotal occlusive disease of the left anterior descending coronary artery. A poor response was noted in all six patients in whom there was complete occlusion of the left anterior descending coronary artery.

Amsterdam (1980), in a nationwide cooperative study of 258 patients undergoing 4 or more hours of external pressure circulatory assistance (EPCA) within 24 hours after admission for acute myocardial infarction, showed a significant decrease in hospital mortality and morbidity in these patients compared with a control group not treated by EPCA. The hospital mortality rates were 6.5 and 14.7 per cent, respectively, and morbidity, as manifested by recurrent angina, progressive heart failure, occurrence of ventricular fibrillation, change in heart size, and clinical cardiac functional status at discharge, was significantly less in the treated group. However, Gowda and coworkers (1978) were unable to show a significant effect of EPCA on estimated infarct size with monitoring plasma creatine kinase time-activity curves and serial electrocardiograms in 39 patients with evolving acute myocardial infarction. Available experimental data also tend to confirm these latter findings. Whether circulatory assistance plus pharmacologic intervention can actually diminish the total amount of muscle necrosis and decrease the extent of an acute myocardial infarction has not yet been proved, but this question surely provides impetus for further careful study and evaluation.

Preoperative (Prophylactic) Use of Circulatory Assistance

The use of elective preoperative prophylactic intra-aortic balloon pump assistance to decrease operative mortality and morbidity in certain higher-risk cardiac surgical procedures has gained considerable advocacy over recent years. Preoperative elective circulatory support utilizing the intra-aortic balloon pump has been recommended in several categories (Table 50–29).

There still remains considerable controversy regarding the need for preoperative prophylactic IABP, and this is based on the significant disparity in operative mortality and morbidity for similar conditions reported by different groups. Observed operative mortality and morbidity are not only related to the pathophysiology of the disease process but also, unquestionably, are strongly linked to the skill of the operating surgeons, the anesthetic management, the effectiveness of myocardial preservation intraoperatively, and the skill and effectiveness of early postoperative management. It seems clear to me that IABP circulatory assistance is indicated preoperatively in

TABLE 50–29. RECOMMENDED USES FOR ELECTIVE PREOPERATIVE (PROPHYLACTIC) IABP

1. Left main coronary artery disease
2. Severe left ventricular dysfunction (left ventricular ejection fraction < 30%)
3. Unstable or recent crescendo angina (responsive to medical therapy)
4. Combined valvular and coronary artery disease with significant left ventricular dysfunction
5. Major noncardiac operations in patients with known severe coronary artery disease

the management of patients with complications of acute myocardial infarction and in patients with unstable myocardial ischemia refractory to medical treatment.

Patients with significant left main coronary artery disease have a somewhat higher operative mortality and morbidity as reported in most series. Although some investigators have reported dramatic improvement in operative results by instituting elective preoperative IABP (Cooper *et al.*, 1977; Gunstensen *et al.*, 1976), others (Kaplan *et al.*, 1979) have reported equally good results with surgery without circulatory assistance. It is my opinion that elective preoperative IABP for left main coronary artery disease is not uniformly indicated, with the exceptions of the following subgroups: (1) unstable or crescendo angina associated with left main coronary artery disease, even if responsive to medical therapy; (2) total right coronary artery occlusion with significant left main coronary artery disease and jeopardized collaterals; (3) severe left ventricular dysfunction (ejection fraction < 35 per cent) associated with left main coronary artery disease; or (4) significant complications during catheterization, with angina or electrocardiographic changes of ischemia.

Severe left ventricular dysfunction with an ejection fraction of less than 30 per cent constitutes an indication for preoperative prophylactic IABP for many surgeons (Feola *et al.*, 1977; Bolooki *et al.*, 1976; Gunstensen *et al.*, 1976). Although IABP circulatory support may be required for weaning from cardiopulmonary bypass in some patients with marginal left ventricular function preoperatively, it is not clear that preoperative circulatory support would influence the course of events. If unstable myocardial ischemia is present, there is a much greater rationale for the use of prophylactic IABP. With the increasing emphasis on the importance of intraoperative myocardial preservation, there has been less need overall for circulatory support, even in patients with poor left ventricular function.

Circulatory support has been used very effectively in patients with known severe coronary artery disease who must undergo major noncardiac surgical procedures in which the risk of intraoperative myocardial infarction is high (Bonchek and Olinger, 1979; Foster *et al.*, 1976). A particularly effective use of prophylactic IABP in this setting has been in the patient with unstable angina and bilateral significant carotid artery disease. Prophylactic IABP assistance with initial unilateral carotid endarterectomy followed by combined contralateral carotid endarterectomy and coronary bypass surgery 3 days later with continued balloon pump assistance has effectively managed these patients, with no mortality or morbidity (Goel *et al.*, 1981).

Since the complication rate of circulatory assistance using IABP is not trivial, it is important to carefully define pathophysiologic conditions and select individual patients appropriate for elective prophylactic preoperative circulatory support.

COMPLICATIONS OF MECHANICAL CIRCULATORY ASSISTANCE

As is true with any invasive modality of medical treatment, there are significant potential complications of mechanical circulatory assist devices. Obviously, there are complications related to the specific circulatory assist device used, but there are many similarities, and consequently, this discussion will be limited primarily to those complications related to the use of the intra-aortic balloon pump, the most frequently used device clinically.

Complications of intra-aortic balloon counterpulsation and their relative frequency are noted in Table 50–30 (McEnany *et al.*, 1978; McCabe *et al.*, 1978; Beckman *et al.*, 1977; Lefemine *et al.*, 1977; Isner *et al.*, 1980; Jarmolowski and Poirier, 1980; Tyras and Willman, 1978). The incidence of major complications resulting in significant morbidity is approximately 8 per cent, with minor complications occurring in approximately 13 per cent (McEnany *et al.*, 1978). IABP-related mortality is less than 1 per cent.

The incidence of vascular lower limb ischemic problems has been reported to be as high as 36 per cent, 85 per cent of which required femorofemoral cross-over grafting (Alpert *et al.*, 1976). More recent experience by Alpert and associates indicated a reduction in significant balloon catheter–induced vascular complications to 16 per cent, 68 per cent of which required thrombectomy, angioplastic repair, or femorofemoral cross-over grafting. McEnany and co-workers (1978) and Lefemine and colleagues (1977) have reported significant vascular complications in 9 and 10 per cent of patients, respectively. Unquestionably, considerable care and experience are required for safe insertion and positioning of the intra-aortic balloon. Forceful insertion should never be attempted. Routes other than the transfemoral one must be considered in patients with poor lower extremity pulses or when a difficult insertion is encountered. In reviewing 45 patients at necropsy who had had prior balloon

TABLE 50–30. COMPLICATIONS OF INTRA-AORTIC BALLOON COUNTERPULSATION

COMPLICATION	FREQUENCY
1. Vascular insufficiency of catheterized limb	10–15%
2. Infection	4%
3. Hemorrhage (local)	4%
4. Wound drainage (sterile)	2%
5. Inappropriate position	1–2%
6. Inability to pass balloon catheter	< age 70: 10–15%
	> age 70: 50%
7. Embolism	Rare
8. Aortic dissection	Rare
9. Thrombocytopenia	Usually mild
10. Balloon leak with gas embolization	Rare
11. Free perforation of aorta, iliac artery	Rare
12. Paraplegia secondary to aortic dissection	Rare
13. Small bowel infarction secondary to superior mesenteric artery thrombosis	Rare
14. Renal failure	Rare

insertion, Isner and associates (1980) found complications in 36 per cent, of which only 20 per cent had been diagnosed or suspected before death. The major complications were vascular, consisting of dissection, arterial perforation, arterial thrombi, and emboli. The authors appropriately concluded that most of the observed complications were consequences of insertion of the device, not consequences of it being in place.

Where lower limb circulation is marginal prior to or after insertion of the intra-aortic balloon, repeated close observation, including distal Doppler pulse monitoring is essential. If ischemia develops, either the balloon must be promptly removed or a cross-over femorofemoral graft performed.

Complications related to the wound at the site of insertion, including hemorrhage, hematoma, infection, and sterile drainage, are related to the technique of insertion. Recent experience with percutaneous insertion has greatly decreased the incidence of these complications and has represented a significant advance (Bemis *et al.*, 1981).

FUTURE CONSIDERATIONS

Recent developments in the technique of introduction of the intra-aortic balloon catheter have led to significantly fewer major complications and an increased success rate for insertion (Bemis *et al.*, 1981; Gueldner and Lawrence, 1975; Phillips and Zeff, 1975). Percutaneous insertion of a balloon catheter of newer design utilizing a guide-wire introducer technique appears to have increased the incidence of successful insertion and lessened both vascular and wound complications (Bregman and Casarella, 1980; Subramanian *et al.*, 1980; Bemis *et al.*, 1981). A modified balloon catheter with a central lumen allowing passage over a guide wire, dye-constrast angiography at the catheter tip, and catheter-tip pressure monitoring has represented a significant design improvement but does not allow percutaneous insertion (Lundell *et al.*, 1981). Percutaneous insertion of the IABP catheter also has facilitated more prompt institution of circulatory assistance in patients with critical conditions, regardless of the location and availability of a surgical team. Of particular advantage has been the ability to expeditiously insert a percutaneous IABP catheter in the cardiac catheterization laboratory in a situation in which a patient develops myocardial ischemia or hemodynamic problems during study. Clearly, prompt institution of circulatory assistance in this setting may avert myocardial injury.

Continued research and development of improved mechanical circulatory assistance devices are required to achieve an ideal device. Some of the criteria for an ideal mechanical circulatory assistance device are as follows:

1. Hemodynamic effectiveness
   a. Reduction in myocardial oxygen consumption by reduction of left ventricular preload and afterload
   b. Augmentation of cardiac output
   c. Augmentation of coronary blood flow
2. Minimal invasiveness and comfortable for the patient
3. Safety—minimal potential complications related to insertion or application or to continued operation
4. Ease of application and operation
5. Transportability
6. Effectiveness and safety for prolonged usage
7. Lack of requirement for continuous heparinization
8. Reasonable cost

Recent design advances (percutaneous IABP balloon catheter and central lumen catheter) have significantly improved the ease of application, increased the potential availability of circulatory assistance, and reduced the potential complication rate. Careful patient selection for circulatory assistance, improved physiologic monitoring, and appropriate combined pharmacologic management of patients have improved salvage and significantly reduced morbidity. Unquestionably, continued improvement and progress can be expected in the future.

Prolonged circulatory support and perhaps, eventually, total artificial heart function may well be the major objectives of future progress in the field of circulatory assistance. The continued productive, close interdisciplinary cooperative effort among physicians, surgeons, biophysicists, and bioengineers may well achieve this goal within the next two decades.

REFERENCES

Alpert, J., Bhaktan, E., Gielchinsky, I., Gilbert, L., Brener, B. J., Brief, D. K., and Parsonnet, V.: Vascular complications of intra-aortic balloon pumping. Arch. Surg., *111*:1190, 1976.

Amsterdam, E. A.: Clinical assessment of external pressure circulatory assistance in acute myocardial infarction. Report of a cooperative clinical trial. Am. J. Cardiol., *45*:349, 1980.

Amsterdam, E. A., DeMaria, A. N., Lee, G., Miller, R. R., and Mason, D. T.: Mechanical circulatory assist in acute ischemic heart disease. Adv. Cardiol., *23*:142, 1978.

Anstadt, G. L., Schiff, P., and Baue, A. E.: Prolonged circulatory support by direct mechanical ventricular assistance. Trans. Am. Soc. Artif. Intern. Organs, *12*:72, 1966.

Arntzenius, A. C., Koops, S., Rodrigo, F. A., Elsbach, H., and Brummelen, A. G. W.: Circulatory effects of body acceleration given synchronously with the heart beat (BASH): Ballistocardiography and cardiovascular therapy. Bibl. Cardiol., *26*:180, 1970.

Aroesty, J. M., Weintraub, R. M., Paulin, S., and O'Grady, G. P.: Medically refractory unstable angina pectoris. II. Hemodynamic and angiographic effects of intraaortic balloon counterpulsation. Am. J. Cardiol., *43*:883, 1979.

Bardet, J., Masquet, C., Kahn, J. C., Gourgon, R., Bourdarias, J. P., Mathivat, A., and Bouvrain, Y.: Clinical and hemodynamic results of intraaortic balloon counterpulsation and surgery for cardiogenic shock. Am. Heart J., *93*:280, 1977a.

Bardet, J., Rigand, M., Kahn, J. C., Huret, J. F., Gandjbakhch, I., and Bourdarias, J. P.: Treatment of post-myocardial infarction angina by intra-aortic balloon pumping and emergency revascularization. J. Thorac. Cardiovasc. Surg., *74*:299, 1977b.

Beamish, R., and Storrie, V.: Impending myocardial infarction. Circulation, *21*:1107, 1960.

Beckman, C. B., Geha, A. S., Hammond, G. L., and Baue, A.: Results and complications of intraaortic balloon counterpulsation. Ann. Thorac. Surg., 24:550, 1977.

Beckman, C. B., Dietzman, R. H., Romero, L. H., Shatney, C. A., Nicoloff, D. M., and Lillchei, R. C.: Hemodynamic evaluation of external counterpulsation in surgical patients. Surgery, 74:846, 1973.

Bemis, C. E., Mundth, E. D., Mintz, G. S., Hakki, A. H., Iskandrian, A. S., Kimbiris, D., Goel, I. P., and Riddle, M.: Comparison of techniques for intraaortic balloon insertion. Am. J. Cardiol., 47:417, 1981.

Bernhard, W. F., Berger, R. L., Stetz, J. P., et al.: Temporary left ventricular bypass: Factors affecting patient survival. Circulation, 60(Suppl. 2):131, 1979.

Bertolasi, C. A., Tronge, J. E., Riccitelli, M. A., Villamayor, R. M., and Zuffardi, E.: Natural history of unstable angina with medical or surgical therapy. Chest, 70:596, 1976.

Bolooki, H.: Indications for use of intra-aortic balloon pump: Cardiogenic shock. In Clinical Application of Intra-Aortic Balloon Pump. Mount Kisco, New York, Futura Publishing Co., 1977, p. 353.

Bolooki, H., Williams, W., Thurer, R. J., Vargars, A., Kaiser, G. A., Mack, F., and Ghahramani, A. R.: Clinical and hemodynamic criteria for use of the intra-aortic balloon pump in patients requiring cardiac surgery. J. Thorac. Cardiovasc. Surg., 72:756, 1976.

Bonchek, L. I., and Olinger, G. N.: Intra-aortic balloon counterpulsation for cardiac support during noncardiac operations. J. Thorac. Cardiovasc. Surg., 78:147, 1979.

Bregman, D., and Casarella, W. J.: Percutaneous intraaortic balloon pumping: Initial clinical experience. Ann. Thorac. Surg., 29:153, 1980.

Bregman, D., Kripke, D. C., and Goetz, R. H.: The effect of synchronous unidirectional intraaortic balloon pumping on hemodynamics and coronary blood flow in cardiogenic shock. Trans. Am. Soc. Artif. Intern. Organs, 16:439, 1970.

Bregman, D., Kripke, D. C., Cohen, M. N., Laniado, S., and Goetz, R. H.: Clinical experience with the unidirectional dual-chambered intraaortic balloon assist. Circulation, 43(Suppl. 1):82, 1971.

Brundage, B. H., Ullyst, D. J., Winokur, S., Chatterjee, K., Ports, T. A., and Turly, K.: The role of aortic balloon pumping in postinfarction angina. A different perspective. Circulation, 62(Suppl. 1):119, 1980.

Buckley, M. J., Craver, J. M., Gold, H. K., Mundth, E. D., Daggett, W. M., and Austen, W. G.: Intraaortic balloon pump assist for cardiogenic shock after cardiopulmonary bypass. Circulation, 48(Suppl. 3):90, 1973a.

Buckley, M. J., Leinbach, R. C., Kastor, J. A., Laird, J. D., Kantrowitz, A. R., Madras, P. N., Sanders, C. A., and Austen, W. G.: Hemodynamic evaluation of intraaortic balloon pumping in man. Circulation, 46(Suppl. 2):130, 1970.

Buckley, M. J., Mundth, E. D., Daggett, W. M., et al.: Surgical management of ventricular septal defects and mitral regurgitation complicating acute myocardial infarction. Ann. Thorac. Surg., 16:598, 1973b.

Chiu, C. J., Dennis, C., and Harris, B.: Response of myocardial fiber length to left heart bypass. J. Surg. Res., 9:241, 1969.

Clauss, R. H., Birtwell, W. C., Albertal, G., Luzer, S., Taylor, W. J., Fosberg, A. M., and Harken, D. E.: Assisted circulation. I. The arterial counterpulsator. J. Thorac. Cardiovasc. Surg., 41:447, 1961.

Connolly, J. E., Bacaner, M. B., Bruns, E. L., Lowenstein, J. J., and Storli, E.: Mechanical support of the circulation in acute heart failure. Surgery, 44:225, 1958.

Cooper, G. N., Singh, A. K., Vargas, L. L., and Karlson, K. E.: Pre-op intraaortic balloon assist in high risk revascularization patients. Am. J. Surg., 133:463, 1977.

Cox, J. L., McLaughlin, V. W., Flowers, N. C., et al.: The ischemic zone surrounding acute myocardial infarction. Its morphology as detected by dehydrogenase staining. Am. Heart J., 76:650, 1968.

Cox, J. L., Pass, H. I., Anderson, R. W., Wechsler, A. S., Oldham, H. N., and Sabiston, D. C., Jr.: Augmentation of coronary collateral blood flow in acute myocardial infarction. Surg. Forum, 26:238, 1975.

Daggett, W. M., Guyton, R. A., Mundth, E. D., Buckley, M. J.,

McEnany, M. T., Gold, H. K., Leinbach, R. C., and Austen, W. G.: Surgery for post myocardial infarct ventricular septal defect. Ann. Surg., 186:260, 1977.

DeBakey, M. E.: A simple continuous flow blood transfusion instrument. New Orleans Med. Surg. J., 87:386, 1934.

DeBakey, M. E.: Left ventricular bypass pump for cardiac assistance: Clinical experience. Am. J. Cardiol., 27:3, 1971.

Dennis, C.: Development of a pump oxygenator to replace the heart and lungs; an apparatus applicable to human patients and application to one man. Ann. Surg., 134:709, 1951.

Dennis, C., Hall, D. P., Moreno, J. R., and Senning, Å.: Reduction of the oxygen utilization of the heart by left heart bypass. Circ. Res., 10:298, 1962.

Dennis, C., Moreno, J. R., Hall, D. P., Grosy, C., Ross, S. M., Wesolowski, S. A., and Senning, Å.: Studies on external counterpulsation as a potential measure for acute left heart failure. Trans. Am. Soc. Artif. Intern. Organs, 9:186, 1963.

Deutsch, M.: The ellipsoid left ventricular assist device: Experimental and clinical results. In Assisted Circulation. Edited by F. Unger. Berlin, Springer-Verlag, 1979, p. 127.

DeWood, A. M., Notske, R. N., Hensley, G. R., Shields, J. P., O'Grady, W. P., Spores, J., Goldman, M., and Ganji, J. H.: Intraaortic balloon counterpulsation with or without reperfusion for myocardial infarction shock. Circulation, 61:1105, 1980.

Dilley, R. B., Ross, J., Jr., and Bernstein, E. F.: Serial hemodynamics during intra-aortic balloon counterpulsation for cardiogenic shock. Circulation, 48(Suppl. 3):99, 1973.

Donahoo, J. S., Brawley, R. K., Taylor, D., et al.: Factors influencing survival following post-infarction ventricular septal defects. Ann. Thorac. Surg., 19:648, 1975.

Donald, D. E., Bove, A. A., and McGoon, D. C.: Sustained circulation by a left ventricular balloon pump after severe myocardial damage in dogs. J. Thorac. Cardiovasc. Surg., 63:681, 1972.

Donaldson, R. M., Honey, M., Balcon, R., Banim, S. O., Sturridge, M. F., and Wright, J. E. C.: Surgical treatment of post-infarction left ventricular aneurysm in 32 patients. Br. Heart J., 38:1223, 1976.

Dumesnil, J. G., Gau, G., and Callahan, J.: Emergency myocardial revascularization with saphenous vein bypass graft. Am. J. Cardiol., 29:260, 1972.

Dunkman, W. B., Leinbach, R. C., Buckley, M. J., Mundth, E. D., Kantrowitz, A. R., Austen, W. G., and Sanders, C. A.: Clinical and hemodynamic results of intra-aortic balloon pumping and surgery for cardiogenic shock. Circulation, 46:465, 1972.

Dunn, J. M., Kirsh, M. M., Harness, J., Lee, R., Strakes, J., and Sloan, H.: The role of assisted circulation in the management of endotoxic shock. Ann. Thorac. Surg., 17:574, 1974.

Ecker, R. R., Mullins, C. B., Grammer, J. C., Rea, W. J., and Atkins, J. M.: Control of intractable ventricular tachycardia by coronary revascularization. Circulation, 44:666, 1971.

Ehrich, D. A., Biddle, J. L., Kronenberg, M. W., and Yu, P. N.: The hemodynamic response to intra-aortic balloon counterpulsation in patients with cardiogenic shock complicating acute myocardial infarction. Am. Heart J., 93:274, 1977.

Ergin, M. A., Dastgir, G., Butt, K. M. H., and Stuckey, J. H.: Prolonged epicardial mapping of myocardial infarction. The effects of propranolol and intra-aortic balloon pumping following coronary artery occlusion. J. Thorac. Cardiovasc. Surg., 72:892, 1976.

Feola, M., et al.: Improved survival after coronary artery bypass surgery in patients with poor LV function: Role of intraaortic balloon counterpulsation. Am. J. Cardiol., 39:1021, 1977.

Filler, R. M., Bernhard, W. F., Robinson, T., Bankole, M. A., and LaFarge, C. G.: An implantable left ventricular–aortic assist device. J. Thorac. Cardiovasc. Surg., 54:795, 1967.

Fleming, W. H., Schultz, J., and Malm, J. R.: Synchronized counterpulsation in the management of ventricular fibrillation following coronary artery ligation. J. Thorac. Cardiovasc. Surg., 56:253, 1968.

Flemma, R. J., Johnson, D., Tector, A. J., et al.: Surgical treatment of preinfarction angina. Arch. Intern. Med., 129:828, 1972.

Forrester, J. S., Chatterjee, K., and Jobin, G.: A new conceptual approach to the therapy of acute myocardial infarction. Adv. Cardiol., 16:111, 1975.

Foster, E. D., Olsson, C. A., Rutenberg, A. M., and Berger, R. L.: Mechanical circulatory assistance with intraaortic balloon counterpulsation for major abdominal surgery. Ann. Surg., 183:73, 1976.

Friedman, H. S.: Cardiac rupture following myocardial infarction: A review. Cardiol. Digest, 8:10, 1973.

Gagemeyer, F., Laird, J. D., Haalebos, M. M. P., and Hugenholtz, P. G.: Effectiveness of intraaortic balloon pumping without cardiac surgery for patients with severe heart failure secondary to a recent myocardial infarction. Am. J. Cardiol., 40:951, 1977.

Gallagher, J. J., Oldham, H. N., Wallace, A. G., Peter, R. H., and Kasell, J.: Ventricular aneurysm with ventricular tachycardia. Report of a case with epicardial mapping and successful resection. Am. J. Cardiol., 35:696, 1975.

Gazes, P. C., Mobley, E. M., Faris, H. M., Duncan, R. C., and Humphrey, G. B.: Preinfarctional (unstable) angina—a prospective study—ten year follow-up. Circulation, 48:331, 1973.

German, J. C., Chalmers, G. S., Hirai, J., Mukherjee, N. D., Wakabayashi, A., and Connelly, J. E.: Comparison of nonpulsatile and pulsatile extracorporeal circulation on renal tissue perfusion. Chest, 61:65, 1972.

Gibbon, J. H., Jr.: Application of a mechanical heart and lung apparatus to cardiac surgery. Minn. Med., 37:171, 1954.

Goel, I. P., Rodigas, P. C., Wolferth, C. C., and Mundth, E. D.: The surgical correction of severe bilateral carotid artery stenosis and unstable angina. A staged approach utilizing circulatory assistance. J. Cardiovasc. Surg., 22:459, 1981.

Gold, H. K., Leinbach, R. C., and Sanders, C. A.: Use of sublingual nitroglycerin in congestive failure following acute myocardial infarction. Circulation, 46:839, 1972.

Gold, H. K., Leinbach, R. C., Buckley, M. J., Mundth, E. D., Daggett, W. M., and Austen, W. G.: Refractory angina pectoris: Follow-up after intraaortic balloon pumping and surgery. Circulation, 54(Suppl. 3):41, 1976.

Gold, H. K., Leinbach, R. C., Sanders, C. A., Buckley, M. J., Mundth, E. D., and Austen, W. G.: Intraaortic balloon pumping for control of recurrent myocardial ischemia. Circulation, 47:1197, 1973.

Gold, H. K., Leinbach, R. C., Sanders, C. A., et al.: Intraaortic balloon pumping for ventricular septal defect or mitral regurgitation complicating acute myocardial infarction. Circulation, 47:1191, 1973.

Golding, L. A. R., Loop, F. D., Mohan, P., Cosgrove, D. M., Taylor, P. C., and Phillips, D. F.: Late survival following use of intraaortic balloon pump in revascularization operations. Ann. Thorac. Surg., 30:48, 1980.

Gowda, S. K., Gillespie, T. A., Byrne, J. D., Ambas, H. D., Sobel, B. E., and Roberts, R.: Effects of external counterpulsation on enzymatically estimated infarct size and ventricular arrhythmia. Br. Heart J., 40:308, 1978.

Graham, A. F., Miller, D. C., Stinson, E. B., Daily, P. O., Fogarty, T. J., and Harrison, D. C.: Surgical treatment of refractory life-threatening ventricular tachycardia. Am. J. Cardiol., 32:909, 1973.

Graham, T. P., Jr., Covell, J. W., Sonnenblick, E. H., et al.: Control of myocardial oxygen consumption: Relative influence of contractile state and tension development. J. Clin. Invest., 47:375, 1968.

Gudarshar, S. T., Blakemore, W. S., and Zinsser, H. F.: Ventricular aneurysmectomy for the treatment of recurrent ventricular tachyarrhythmia. Am. J. Cardiol., 27:690, 1971.

Gueldner, T. C., and Lawrence, G. H.: Intraaortic balloon assist through cannulation of the ascending aorta. Ann. Thorac. Surg., 19:88, 1975.

Guiraudon, G., Fontaine, G., and Frank, R.: Encircling endocardial ventriculotomy: A new surgical treatment for life-threatening ventricular arrhythmias resistant to medical treatment following myocardial infarction. Ann. Thorac. Surg., 26:438, 1978.

Gunnar, R. M., and Loeb, H. S.: Use of drugs in cardiogenic shock due to acute myocardial infarction. Circulation, 45:1111, 1972.

Gunnar, R. M., Loeb, H. S., and Rahimtoola, S. H.: Hemodynamic studies in shock with myocardial infarction. In Shock in Myocardial Infarction. Edited by R. M. Gunnar, H. S. Loeb, and S. H. Rahimtoola. New York, Grune and Stratton, 1974, pp. 113–130.

Gunstensen, J., Goldman, B. S., Scully, H. E., Huckell, V. F., and Adelman, A. G.: Evolving indications for preoperative intraaortic balloon pump assistance. Ann. Thorac. Surg., 22:535, 1976.

Hagemeijer, F., Laird, J. D., Haalebos, M. M., and Hugenholtz, P. G.: Effectiveness of intraaortic balloon pumping without cardiac surgery for patients with severe heart failure secondary to a recent myocardial infarction. Am. J. Cardiol., 40:951, 1977.

Hanson, E. C., Levine, F. H., Kay, H. R., Leinbach, R. C., Gold, H. K., Daggett, W. M., Austen, W. G., and Buckley, M. J.: Control of postinfarction ventricular irritability with the intraaortic balloon pump. Circulation, 62(Suppl. 1):130, 1980.

Harken, A. H., Josephson, M. E., and Horwitz, L. N.: Surgical endocardial resection for the treatment of malignant ventricular tachycardia. Ann. Surg., 190:456, 1979.

Harris, P. L., Woollard, K., Bartoli, A., and Makey, A. R.: The management of impending myocardial infarction using coronary artery bypass grafting and an intra-aortic balloon pump. J. Cardiovasc. Surg., 21:405, 1980.

Haston, H. H., and McNamara, J. J.: The effects of intraaortic balloon counterpulsation on myocardial infarct size. Ann. Thorac. Surg., 28:335, 1979.

Hill, J. D., Kerth, W. J., DeLeval, M. R., et al.: Myocardial infarction and preinfarction. Results of emergency myocardial revascularization. J. Cardiovasc. Surg., 15:205, 1974.

Hill, J. D., Kerth, W. J., Kelly, J. J., Selzer, A., Armstrong, W., Popper, R. W., Langston, M. F., and Cohn, K. E.: Emergency aortocoronary bypass for impending or extending myocardial infarction. Circulation, 43(Suppl. 1):105, 1971.

Hood, W. B., Jr.: Experimental myocardial infarction. III. Recovery of left ventricular function in the healing phase. Contribution of increased fiber shortening in non-infarcted myocardium. Am. Heart J., 79:531, 1970.

Howell, W. H., and Holt, E.: Two new factors in blood coagulation: Heparin and proantithrombin. Am. J. Physiol., 47:388, 1918.

Hultgren, H. N., Pfeifer, J. F., Angell, W. W., Lipton, M. J., and Biligoly, J.: Unstable angina: A comparison of medical and surgical management. Am. J. Cardiol., 39:734, 1977.

Hutter, A. M., Jr., Russell, R. O., Jr., Resnekov, L., et al.: Unstable angina pectoris—national randomized study of surgical vs. medical therapy. Results in 1, 2 and 3 vessel disease. Circulation, 56(Suppl.):60, 1977.

Isner, J. M., Cohen, S. R., Virmani, R., Lawrinson, W., and Roberts, W. C.: Complications of the intraaortic balloon counterpulsation device: Clinical and morphologic observations in 45 necropsy patients. Am. J. Cardiol., 45:260, 1980.

Jacobi, C.: Apparat zur Durchblutung isolierter überlebender Organe. Arch. Exp. Pathol., 26:388, 1890.

Jarmolowski, C. R., and Poirier, R. L.: Small bowel infarction complicating intra-aortic balloon counterpulsation via the ascending aorta. J. Thorac. Cardiovasc. Surg., 79:735, 1980.

Jett, G. K., Dengle, S. K., Barnett, P. A., Platt, M. R., Willerson, J. T., Watson, J. T., and Eberhart, R. C.: Intraaortic balloon counterpulsation: Its influence alone and combined with various pharmacological agents on regional myocardial blood flow during experimental acute coronary occlusion. Ann. Thorac. Surg., 31:144, 1980.

Johnson, S. A., Scanlon, P. J., Loeb, H., Moran, J. M., Pifarre, R., and Gunnar, R. M.: Treatment of cardiogenic shock in myocardial infarction by intraaortic balloon counterpulsation and surgery. Am. J. Med., 62:687, 1977.

Kaiser, G. C., Marco, J. D., Barnes, H. B., Codd, J. E., Laks, H., and Willman, V. L.: Intraaortic balloon assistance. Ann. Thorac. Surg., 21:487, 1976.

Kantrowitz, A., Krakauer, J. S., Rosenbaum, A., Butner, A. N., Freed, P. S., and Jaron, D.: Phase-shift balloon pumping in medically refractory cardiogenic shock. Results in 27 patients. Arch. Surg., 99:739, 1969.

Kantrowitz, A., Tjonneland, S., Krakauer, J. S., Phillips, S. J., Freed, P. S., and Butner, A. N.: Mechanical intraaortic cardiac assistance in cardiogenic shock. Hemodynamic effects. Arch. Surg., 97:1000, 1968.

Kaplan, J. A., Craver, J. M., Jones, E. L., and Sumpter, R.: The role of the intraaortic balloon in cardiac anesthesia and surgery. Am. Heart J., 98:580, 1979.

Katz, A. M.: Physiology of the Heart. New York, Raven Press, 1977.

Kerber, R. E., Marcus, M. L., Ehrhardt, J., and Abboud, F. M.: Effect of intra-aortic balloon counterpulsation on the motion and perfusion of acutely ischemic myocardium. An experimental echocardiographic study. Circulation, 53:853, 1976.

Krauss, K. R., Hutter, A. M., Jr., and DeSanctis, R. W.: Acute coronary insufficiency. Arch. Intern. Med., 129:808, 1972.

Laas, J., Campbell, C. D., Takanashi, Y., Pick, R., and Repogle, R. L.: Failure of intra-aortic balloon pumping to reduce experimental myocardial infarct size in swine. J. Thorac. Cardiovasc. Surg., 80:85, 1980.

Laird, J. D., Madras, P. N., Jones, R. T., Kantrowitz, A. R., Kothari, M. L., Buckley, M. J., and Austen, W. G.: Theoretical and experimental analysis of the intraaortic balloon pump. Trans. Am. Soc. Artif. Intern. Organs, 14:338, 1968.

Laks, H., Ott, R. A., Standeven, J. W., Hahn, J. W., Blair, O. M., and Willman, V. L.: The effect of left atrium-to-aortic assistance on infarct size. Circulation, 56(Suppl. 2):38, 1977.

Lambert, C. J., Mitchel, B. F., Adam, M., et al., Emergency myocardial revascularization for impending myocardial infarctions. Chest, 61:479, 1972.

Langou, R. A., Geha, A. S., Hammond, G. L., and Cohen, L. S.: Surgical approach for patients with unstable angina pectoris: Role of the response to initial medical therapy and intraaortic balloon pumping in perioperative complications after aortocoronary bypass grafting. Am. J. Cardiol., 42:629, 1978.

Lee, W. H., Jr., Krumhaar, E., Forkalsrud, E. W., Schjeide, O. A., and Maloney, J. V., Jr.: Denaturation of plasma proteins as a cause of morbidity and death after intracardiac operations. Surgery, 50:29, 1961.

Lefemine, A. A., Kosowsky, B., Madoff, I., Block, H., and Lewis, M.: Results and complications of intraaortic balloon pumping in surgical and medical patients. Am. J. Cardiol., 40:416, 19

Legallois, J. J. C.: Experiments on the Principle of Life a Particularly on the Principle of the Motions of the Heart a on the Seat of this Principle, Including the Report Made to First Class of the Institute. Translated by N. C. and J. G. Nancrede. Philadelphia, 1813.

Leinbach, R. C., Gold, H. K., Buckley, M. J., Austen, W. G., and Sanders, C. A.: Reduction of myocardial injury during acute infarction by early application of intraaortic balloon pumping and propranolol. Circulation, 48(Suppl. 4):100, 1973a.

Leinbach, R. C., Gold, H. K., Harper, R. W., Buckley, M. J., and Austen, W. G.: Early intraaortic balloon pumping for anterior myocardial infarction without shock. Circulation, 58:204, 1978.

Leinbach, R. C., Gold, H. K., Dinsmore, R. E., Mundth, E. D., Buckley, M. J., Austen, W. G., and Sanders, C. A.: The role of angiography in cardiogenic shock. Circulation, 47, 48(Suppl. 3):95, 1973b.

Levine, F. H., Gold, H. K., Leinbach, R. C., Daggett, W. M., Austen, W. G., and Buckley, M. J.: Management of acute myocardial ischemia with intraaortic balloon pumping and coronary bypass surgery. Circulation, 58(Suppl. 1):69, 1978.

Litwak, R. S., Koffsky, R. M., Jurado, R. A., Lukban, S. B., Saha, C. K., Vrandecic, M., Mindich, B., Mitchell, B., King, P., and Kaminsk, L.: Support of severely impaired cardiac performance with left-heart assist device following intracardiac operation. Heart Lung, 7:62, 1978.

Litwak, R. S., Lajam, F., Koffsky, R. M., Silvay, G., Shiang, H., Geller, S. A., and Pedersen, F. S.: Obturated permanent left atrial and aortic cannulae for assisted circulation after cardiac surgery. Trans. Am. Soc. Artif. Intern. Organs, 19:243, 1973.

Loisance, D. Y., Cachera, J. P., Paulain, H., Aubry, P., Juvin, A. M., and Galez, J. J.: Ventricular septal defect after acute myocardial infarction. Early repair. J. Thorac. Cardiovasc. Surg., 80:61, 1980.

Lorente, P., Gourgon, R., Beaufils, P., Masquet, C., Rosengarten, M., Azancot, F., and Slama, R.: Multivariates statistical evaluation of intraaortic counterpulsation in pump failure complicating acute myocardial infarction. Am. J. Cardiol., 46:124, 1980.

Lovett, W. L., Wangensteen, S. L., Gleen, T. M., and Lefer, A. M.: Presence of a myocardial depressant factor in patients in circulatory shock. Surgery, 70:223, 1971.

Lundell, D. C., Hammond, G. L., Geha, A. S., Laks, H., and Wolfson, S.: Randomized comparison of the modified wire-guided and standard intraaortic balloon catheters. J. Thorac. Cardiovasc. Surg., 81:297, 1981.

Macoviak, J., Stephenson, L. W., Edmunds, L. H., Jr., Harken, A., and MacVaugh, H.: The intraaortic balloon pump: An analysis of five years experience. Ann. Thorac. Surg., 29:451, 1979.

Magdison, O.: Resection of post-myocardial infarction ventricular aneurysms for cardiac arrhythmias. Chest, 56:211, 1969.

Many, M., Birtwell, W. C., Giron, F., Wise, H., Soroff, H. S., and Deterling, R. A., Jr.: The effects of pulse wave pattern on renal function. Trans. Am. Soc. Artif. Intern. Organs, 13:157, 1967.

Maroko, P. R., and Braunwald, E.: Effects of metabolic and pharmacologic interventions on myocardial infarct size following coronary occlusion. Circulation, 53(Suppl. 3):162, 1976.

Maroko, P. R., Bernstein, E. F., Libby, P., et al.: Effects of intraaortic balloon counterpulsation on the severity of myocardial ischemic injury following acute coronary occlusion. Circulation, 45:1150, 1972.

Maroko, P. R., Kjekshues, J. K., Sobel, B. E., et al.: Factors influencing infarct size following experimental coronary artery occlusion. Circulation, 43:67, 1971.

McCabe, J. C., Abel, R. M., Subramanian, V. A., and Gay, W. A., Jr.: Complications of intra-aortic balloon insertion and counterpulsation. Circulation, 57:769, 1978.

McEnany, M. T., Kay, H. R., Buckley, M. J., Daggett, W. M., Erdmann, A. J., Mundth, E. D., Rao, R. S., DeToeuf, J., and Austen, W. G.: Clinical experience with intraaortic balloon pump support in 728 patients. Circulation, 58(Suppl. 1):124, 1978.

McGee, M. G., Zillgit, S. L., Trono, R., Turner, S. A., Davis, G. L., Fuqua, J. M., Edelman, S. K., and Norman, J. C.: Retrospective analyses of the need for mechanical circulatory support (intraaortic balloon pump/abdominal left ventricular assist device or partial artificial heart) after cardiopulmonary bypass. A 44 month study of 14,168 patients. Am. J. Cardiol., 46:135, 1980.

Moulopoulos, S. D., Topaz, S., and Kolff, W. J.: Diastolic balloon pumping (with carbon dioxide) in the aorta: Mechanical assistance to the failing circulation. Am. Heart J., 63:669, 1962.

Mueller, H., Evans, R., and Ayres, S.: External counterpulsation— a non-invasive form of cardiac assistance. Am. J. Cardiol., 33:158, 1974.

Mueller, H., Ayres, S. M., Giannelli, S., Jr., Conklin, E. F., Mazzara, J. T., and Grace, W. J.: Effect of isoproterenol, 1-norepinephrine, and intraaortic counterpulsation on hemodynamics and myocardial metabolism in shock following acute myocardial infarction. Circulation, 45:335, 1972.

Mundth, E. D.: Mechanical and surgical interventions for the reduction of myocardial ischemia. Circulation, 53(Suppl. 1):176, 1976.

Mundth, E. D.: Surgical treatment of cardiogenic shock and of acute mechanical complications following myocardial infarction. In Coronary Bypass Surgery. Edited by S. H. Rahimtoola. Philadelphia, F. A. Davis Co., 1977, pp. 241–264.

Mundth, E. D., and Austen, W. G.: Surgical treatment of acute cardiac ischemia. In Proceedings of VIII World Congress of Cardiology. Edited by D. Hayase and S. Murao. Amsterdam, Oxford, Princeton, Excerpta Medica, 1978, pp. 359–365.

Mundth, E. D., Buckley, M. J., Daggett, W. M., et al.: Surgery for complications of acute myocardial infarction. Circulation, 45:1279, 1972.

Mundth, E. D., Buckley, M. J., Daggett, W. M., McEnany, M., Gold, H. K., Leinbach, R. C., and Austen, W. G.: Surgical intervention for pre-infarction angina. Adv. Cardiol., 15:59, 1975a.

Mundth, E. D., Buckley, M. J., DeSanctis, R. W., Daggett, W. M., and Austen, W. G.: Surgical treatment of ventricular irritability. J. Thorac. Cardiovasc. Surg., 66:943, 1973a.

Mundth, E. D., Buckley, M. J., Daggett, W. M., McEnany, M. T., Leinbach, R. C., Gold, H. K., and Austen, W. G.: Intraaortic balloon pump assistance and early surgery in cardiogenic shock. Adv. Cardiol., 15:159, 1975b.

Mundth, E. D., Buckley, M. J., Leinbach, R. C., Gold, H. K., Daggett, W. M., and Austen, W. G.: Surgical intervention for the complications of acute myocardial ischemia. Ann. Surg., 178:379, 1973b.

Nachlas, M. M., and Siedband, M. P.: The influence of diastolic augmentation on infarct size following coronary artery ligation. J. Thorac. Cardiovasc. Surg., 53:698, 1967.

Naeim, F., De LaMaza, L. M., and Robbins, S. L.: Cardiac rupture during myocardial infarction. A review of 44 cases. Circulation, 45:1231, 1972.

Nichols, A. B., Pohost, G. M., Gold, H. K., Leinbach, R. C., Beller, G. A., McKusick, K. A., Strauss, H. W., and Buckley, M. J.: Left ventricular function during intra-aortic balloon pumping assessed by multigate cardiac blood pool imaging. Circulation, 58(Suppl. 1):176, 1978.

Norman, J. C., and Bregman, D.: Mechanical circulation support: Evolving perspectives. Trans. Am. Soc. Artif. Intern. Organs, 24:782, 1978.

Norman, J. C., Cooley, D. A., Igo, S. R., Hibbs, C. W., Johnson, M. D., Bennett, J. G., Fuqua, J. M., Trono, R., and Edmonds, C. H.: Prognostic indices for survival during postcardiotomy intra-aortic balloon pumping methods of scoring and classification, with implication for left ventricular assist device utilization. J. Thorac. Cardiovasc. Surg., 74:709, 1977.

Norman, J. C., Fuqua, J. M., Trono, R., Hibbs, C. W., Edmonds, C. H., Igo, S., Brewer, M. A., Holut, D. A., and Cooley, D. A.: An intracorporeal (abdominal) left ventricular assist device: Initial clinical trials. In Assisted Circulation. Edited by F. Unger. Berlin, Springer-Verlag, 1979, p. 107.

Olinger, G. N., Boncheck, L. I., Keelan, M. H., Jr., Tresch, R. S., Bamrah, V., and Tristani, F. H.: Unstable angina: The case for operation. Am. J. Cardiol., 42:634, 1978.

O'Rourke, M. R., Sammel, N. C., and Chang, V. P.: Arterial counterpulsation in severe refractory heart failure complicating acute myocardial infarction. Br. Heart J., 41:308, 1979.

O'Rourke, M. F., Norris, R. N., Campbell, T. J., Chang, V. P., and Sammel, N. C.: Randomized controlled trial of intraaortic balloon counterpulsation in early myocardial infarction with acute heart failure. Am. J. Cardiol., 47:815, 1981.

Osborn, J. J., Russi, M., Salel, A., Bramson, M. L., and Gerbate, R.: Circulatory assistance by external pulsed pressures. Am. J. Med. Electron., 3:87, 1964.

Pae, W. E., and Pierce, W. S.: Temporary left ventricular assistance in acute myocardial infarction and cardiogenic shock. Rationale and criteria for utilization. Chest, 79:692, 1981.

Page, D. L., Caulfield, J. B., Kastor, J. A., DeSanctis, R. W., and Sanders, C. A.: Myocardial changes associated with cardiogenic shock. N. Engl. J. Med., 285:133, 1971.

Parker, F. B., Jr., Neville, J. F., Hanson, E. L., and Webb, W. R.: Intraaortic balloon counterpulsation and cardiac surgery. Ann. Thorac. Surg., 17:144, 1974.

Parmley, W. W., Chatterjee, K., Charuzi, V., and Swan, H. J. C.: Hemodynamic effects of non-invasion systolic unloading (nitroprusside) and diastolic augmentation (external counterpulsation) in patients with acute myocardial infarction. Am. J. Cardiol., 33:819, 1974.

Pennock, J. L., Pierce, W. S., and Waldhausen, J. A.: Quantitative evaluation of left ventricular bypass in reducing myocardial ischemia. Surgery, 79:523, 1976.

Pennock, J. L., Pae, W. E., Jr., Pierce, W. S., and Waldhausen, J. A.: Reduction of myocardial infarct size: Comparison between left atrial and left ventricular bypass. Circulation, 59:275, 1979.

Phillips, P. A., and Bregman, D.: Intraoperative application of intraaortic balloon counterpulsation determined by clinical monitoring of the endocardial viability ratio. Ann. Thorac. Surg., 23:45, 1977.

Phillips, S. J., and Zeff, R. H.: Letter to the editor on Gueldner and Lawrence. Ann. Thorac. Surg., 20:367, 1975.

Pierce, W. S., Brighton, J. A., O'Bannon, W., et al.: Complete left ventricular bypass with a paracorporeal pump: Design and evaluation. Ann. Surg., 180:418, 1974.

Pierce, W. S., Donachy, J. H., Landis, D. L., Brighton, J. H., Rosenberg, G., Migliore, J. J., Prophet, G. A., White, W. J., and Waldhausen, J. A.: Prolonged mechanical support of the left ventricle. Circulation, 58(Suppl. 1):133, 1978.

Pierri, M. K., Zema, M., Kingfield, P., McCabe, J., Hoover, E., Gay, W., and Subramanian, V.: Exercise tolerance in late survivors of balloon pumping and surgery for cardiogenic shock. Circulation, 62(Suppl. 1):138, 1980.

Powell, W. J., Jr., Daggett, W. M., Magro, A. E., Bianco, J. A., Buckley, M. J., Sanders, C. A., Kantrowitz, A. R., and Austen, W. G.: Effects of intra-aortic balloon counterpulsation on cardiac performance, oxygen consumption, and coronary blood flow in dogs. Circ. Res., 26:753, 1970.

Reemtsma, K., Drusin, R., Edie, R., Bregman, D., and Dobelle, W. H.: Cardiac transplantation for patients requiring mechanical circulatory support. N. Engl. J. Med., 298:61, 1978.

Ricks, W. B., Winkle, R. A., Shumway, N. E., and Harrison, D. C.: Surgical management of the life-threatening ventricular arrhythmias in patients with coronary artery disease. Circulation, 56:38, 1977.

Roberts, A. J., Alonso, D. R., Combes, J. R., Jacobstein, J. G., Post, M. R., Cahill, P. T., Ho, S. T., Abel, R. M., Subramanian, V. A., and Gay, W. A.: Role of delayed intraaortic balloon pumping in treatment of experimental myocardial infarction. Am. J. Cardiol., 141:1202, 1978.

Rosensweig, J., and Chatterjee, S.: Restoration of normal cardiac metabolism and hemodynamics after coronary occlusion. Ann. Thorac. Surg., 6:146, 1968.

Rosensweig, J., Chatterjee, S., and Merino, F.: Treatment of acute myocardial infarction by counterpulsation. Experimental rationale and clinical experience. J. Thorac. Cardiovasc. Surg., 59:243, 1970.

Russell, R. O., Jr., Rackley, C. E., Pombo, J., et al.: Effects of increasing left ventricular filling pressure in patients with acute myocardial infarction. J. Clin. Invest., 49:1539, 1970.

Russell, R. O., Jr., Resnekov, L., Wolk, M., Rosati, R. A., Conti, C. R., Becker, L. C., Hutler, A. M., Jr., Biddle, T. L., Schroeder, J., Kaplan, G. M., Frommer, P. L., and collaborators: Unstable angina pectoris: National cooperative study group to compare surgical and medical therapy. Am. J. Cardiol., 42:839, 1978.

Sanders, R. J., Kern, W. H., and Blount, S. G.: Perforation of the interventricular septum complicating myocardial infarction. Am. Heart J., 51:736, 1956.

Sanders, R. J., Neuberger, K. J., and Ravin, A.: Rupture of papillary muscles: Occurrence of rupture of posterior muscle in posterior myocardial infarction. Dis. Chest, 31:316, 1957.

Sarnoff, S. J., Braunwald, E., Welch, G. H., Case, R. B., Stainsby, W. N., and Macruz, R.: Hemodynamic determinants of oxygen consumption of the heart with special reference to the tension-time index. Am. J. Physiol., 192:148, 1958.

Sasayama, S., Osakoda, G., Takahashi, M., Hamashim, H., Hirose, K., Nishimura, E., and Kawai, C.: Effect of intraaortic balloon counterpulsation on regional myocardial function during acute coronary occlusion in the dog. Am. J. Cardiol., 43:59, 1979.

Satava, R. M., and McGoon, D. C.: Cardiac assist with an intraventricular balloon. J. Thorac. Cardiovasc. Surg., 67:780, 1974.

Scanlon, P. J., O'Connell, J., Johnson, S. A., Moran, J. M., Grennar, R., and Pifarre, R.: Balloon counterpulsation following surgery for ischemic heart disease. Circulation, 54(Suppl. 3):90, 1976.

Schaper, W., and Pasyk, S.: Influence of collateral flow on the ischemic tolerance of the heart following acute and subacute coronary occlusion. Circulation, 53(Suppl. 1):57, 1976.

Scheidt, S., Aschein, R., and Killep, J.: Shock after acute myocardial infarction. A clinical and hemodynamic profile. Am. J. Cardiol., 26:556, 1970.

Schelbert, H. R., Covell, J. W., Burns, J. W., et al.: Observations on factors affecting local forces in the left ventricular wall during acute myocardial ischemia. Circ. Res., 29:306, 1971.

Selden, R., Neill, W. A., Ritzmann, L. W., Okies, J. E., and Anderson, R. P.: Medical versus surgical therapy for acute coronary insufficiency. N. Engl. J. Med., 293:1329, 1975.

Senning, Å., Dennis, C., Moreno, J. R., and Hall, D. P.: Atrial septal puncture without thoracotomy for total left heart bypass. Acta Chir. Scand., 132:267, 1962.

Shaw, J., Taylor, D. R., and Pitt, B.: Effects of intraaortic balloon counterpulsation on regional coronary blood flow in experimental myocardial infarction. Am. J. Cardiol., 34:552, 1974.

Shell, W. E., and Sobel, B. E.: Protection of jeopardized ischemic myocardium by reduction of ventricular afterload. N. Engl. J. Med., *291*:481, 1974.

Smith, H. J., Oriol, A., March, J., *et al.*: Hemodynamic studies in cardiogenic shock: Treatment with isoproterenol and metaraminol. Circulation, *35*:1084, 1967.

Soroff, H. S., Birtwell, W. C., Giron, F., Collins, J. A., and Deterling, R. A.: Support of the systemic circulation and left ventricular assist by synchronous pulsation of extramural pressure. Surg. Forum, *16*:148, 1965.

Soroff, H. S., Levine, H. J., Sacks, B. F., Birtwell, W. C., and Deterling, R. A.: Assisted circulation: II. Effects of counterpulsation on left ventricular oxygen consumption and hemodynamics. Circulation, *27*:722, 1963.

Soroff, H. S., Cloutier, C. T., Birtwell, W. C., Banos, J. S., Brilla, A. H., Begley, L. A., and Messer, J. V.: Clinical evaluation of external counterpulsation in cardiogenic shock. Circulation, *45, 46*(Suppl. 2):75, 1972.

Steele, P., Pappas, G., Vogel, R., Jenkins, M., and Battock, D.: Isosorbide dinitrate and intra-aortic balloon pumping in pre-infarction angina. Effects on central circulatory dynamics. Chest, *69*:712, 1976.

Stuckey, J. H., Newman, M. M., Dennis, C., Berg, E. H., Goodman, S. E., Fries, C. C., Karlson, K. F., Blumenfeld, M., Weitzner, S. W., Binder, L. S., and Winston, A.: The use of the heart-lung machine in selected cases of acute myocardial infarction. Surg. Forum, *8*:342, 1957.

Sturm, J. T., McGee, M. G., Fuhrman, T. M., Davis, G. C., Turner, S. A., Edelman, S. K., and Norman, J. C.: Treatment of postoperative low output syndrome with intraaortic balloon pumping. Experience with 419 patients. Am. J. Cardiol., *45*:1033, 1980.

Sturm, J. T., Fuhrman, T. M., Sterling, R., Turner, S. A., Igo, S. R., and Norman, J. C.: Combined use of dopamine and nitroprusside therapy in conjunction with intraaortic balloon pumping for the treatment of postcardiotomy low-output syndrome. J. Thorac. Cardiovasc. Surg., *82*:13, 1981.

Subramanian, V. A., Goldstein, J. E., Sos, T. A., McCabe, J. C., Hoover, E. A., and Gay, W. A., Jr.: Preliminary clinical experience with percutaneous intraaortic balloon pumping. Circulation, *62*(Suppl. 1):123, 1980.

Sugg, W. L., Webb, W. R., and Ecker, R. R.: Reduction of extent of myocardial infarction by counterpulsation. Ann. Thorac. Surg., *7*:310, 1969.

Sugg, W. L., Rea, M. J., Webb, W. R., and Ecker, R. R.: Cardiac assistance (counterpulsation in 10 patients). Clinical and hemodynamic observations. Ann. Thorac. Surg., *9*:1, 1970.

Sustaita, H., Chatterjee, K., Matloff, J. M., Marty, A. J., Swan, H. J. C., and Fields, J.: Emergency bypass surgery in impending and complicated acute myocardial infarction. Arch. Surg., *105*:30, 1972.

Swank, M., Singh, H. N., Flemma, R. J., Mulen, D. C., and Lepley, D., Jr.: Effect of intra-aortic balloon pumping on nutrient coronary flow in normal and ischemic myocardium. J. Thorac. Cardiovasc. Surg., *76*:538, 1978.

Tyras, D. H., and Willman, V. L.: Paraplegia following intra-aortic balloon assistance. Ann. Thorac. Surg., *25*:164, 1978.

Urschel, C. W., Eber, L., Forrester, J., Matloff, J., Cargreni, R., and Sonnenblick, E.: Alteration of mechanical performance of the ventricle by intraaortic balloon counterpulsation. Am. J. Cardiol., *25*:546, 1970.

von Frey, M., and Gruber, M.: Untersuchungen über den Stoffwechsel isolierter Organe. Ein Respirations appara fur isolierte organe. Virchows Arch. Physio., *9*:519, 1885.

Wakabayashi, A., Kubo, T., Gilman, P., Zuber, W. F., and Connolly, J. E.: Oxygen consumption of the normal and failing heart during left heart bypass. J. Thorac. Cardiovasc. Surg., *70*:9, 1975.

Weintraub, R. M., and Aroesty, J. M.: The role of intraaortic balloon pumping and surgery in the treatment of preinfarction angina. Chest, *69*:707, 1976.

Weintraub, R. M., Aroesty, J. M., Paulin, S., Levine, F. H., Markis, J. E., LaRaia, P. J., Cohen, S. F., and Kurland, G. F.: Medically refractory unstable angina pectoris. Long-term follow-up of patients undergoing intra-aortic balloon counterpulsation and operation. Am. J. Cardiol., *43*:877, 1979.

Willerson, J. T., Watson, J. T., and Platt, M. R.: Effect of hypertonic mannitol and intraaortic counterpulsation on regional myocardial blood flow and ventricular performance in dogs during myocardial ischemia. Am. J. Cardiol., *37*:514, 1976.

Yashar, J., Yashar, J. J., Witoszka, M., Kitzes, D. C., and Simeone, F. A.: The treatment of patients with recurrent ventricular fibrillation. Am. J. Surg., *133*:453, 1977.

7.   Partial Ileal Bypass for Control of Hyperlipidemia and Atherosclerosis

HENRY BUCHWALD

RICHARD B. MOORE

RICHARD L. VARCO

The primary effort of the cardiovascular surgeon today is directed toward management of the complications of atherosclerosis. Coronary artery bypass procedures, resection of ventricular aneurysms, certain valve replacements, and cardiac transplantation are operations designed to benefit individuals with coronary atherosclerosis. Prosthetic and venous peripheral bypass operations, prosthetic replacement of aortic aneurysms, and endarterectomies are all concerned with amelioration of atherosclerotic disease. These procedures are, at best, palliative. Yet, the surgeon tends to concern himself little with the basic disease problem.

Atherosclerosis is not equivalent to aging but is a *disease*. Indeed, it is a rarity in some areas of the world. However, it is uncommon in industrialized countries for man to be free of atherosclerotic disease (Keys, 1970). Moreover, it is endemic in the United States and the countries of Western Europe. Approximately 650,000 coronary deaths occur yearly in the United States alone. Diseases of the heart, cerebrovascular accidents, and generalized arteriosclerosis

TABLE 50–31. CAUSES OF DEATH, WITH RELATIVE RANK, DEATH RATE, AND PER CENT OF TOTAL, FROM THE VITAL STATISTICS OF THE UNITED STATES, 1977

RANK	CAUSE OF DEATH	DEATH RATE*	PER CENT OF TOTAL
	All causes	816.3	100.0
1	Diseases of the heart	303.4	37.8
2	Cancer	168.4	20.4
3	Stroke	75.3	9.6
4	Accidents	45.4	5.4
5	Influenza and pneumonia	21.4	2.7
6	Diabetes mellitus	14.1	1.7
7	Cirrhosis of the liver	14.0	1.6
8	Arteriosclerosis	12.0	1.5
9	Suicide	12.6	1.5
10	Diseases of infancy	13.0	1.2
11	Homicide	8.6	1.1
12	Emphysema	7.1	0.9
13	Congenital anomalies	6.8	0.7
14	Nephritis and nephrosis	3.7	0.5
15	Septicemia and pyemia	3.2	0.4
	Other and ill-defined	107.3	13.1

*Per 100,000 population

account for 49 per cent of the total deaths in the United States (Table 50–31). Although the mortality rate for overall cardiovascular diseases has declined 21.4 per cent from 1968 to 1976 (Stern, 1979), the overall incidence rate has not declined. Over 10 million Americans alive today have a history of a heart attack and/or angina pectoris, and over 1 million Americans will have a myocardial infarction this year. The American Heart Association estimated that cardiovascular diseases cost the people of this country 46.2 billion dollars in 1981 (American Heart Association, 1981). Since the greater majority of myocardial infarction victims survive the initial insult and only end-stage peripheral vascular disease results in death, clearly the pain, incapacitation, emotional impact, economic hardship, and career deprivation from atherosclerotic cardiovascular disease create problems of substantial magnitude for those who would treat these afflictions.

It is increasingly evident to students of atherosclerosis that this disease has its origins in childhood and perhaps often in the preconception germ plasm (Boas and Adlersberg, 1945; Boas et al., 1948; Adlersberg et al., 1949; Adlersberg, 1951). Plaque lesions of hemodynamic significance are present in American men in their early twenties. Possibly the most telling statistics are those from the autopsies of young American men killed in the Korean and Viet Nam conflicts. In the Korean study (Enos et al., 1953), it was reported that 77.3 per cent of these men, with an average age of 22.1 years, had coronary atherosclerosis and that 15.3 per cent had greater than 50 per cent luminal narrowing of one or more vessels. In the Viet Nam study (McNamara et al., 1971), disease was judged by postmortem arteriography, in addition to gross pathologic examination. These data showed evidence of coronary atherosclerosis in 45 per cent of the autopsies, with a 5 per cent rate of severe coronary involvement. Although the figures in these studies vary significantly, the common finding is ominous.

HISTORICAL NOTES

Atherosclerosis is an ancient disease. An autopsy performed by G. Elliot Smith (1933) on the mummy of the Pharoah Memephtah, the nemesis of Moses in the Bible, revealed a piece of the aorta that remained after the preparative evisceration. This was sent to S. G. Shattock (1908) in London, who confirmed by studying microscopic sections of the centuries-old tissue that typical advanced lesions of atherosclerosis with extensive deposits of calcium phosphate were present. Ruffer (1911), of the Cairo Medical School, published an extensive review of the prevalence of atherosclerotic lesions in mummies embalmed from approximately 1580 B.C. to 525 A.D. (Fig. 50–143). Leonardo da Vinci (Heydenreich, 1954) was the first man known to accurately describe and draw the lesions of atherosclerosis; he also suggested that sudden death might be due to thickening and narrowing of "the blood vessels which supply the musculature of the heart, with resultant failure of blood flow to the heart."

Retrospective and prospective studies of atherosclerotic risk in man over the past 40 years have incriminated certain atherosclerotic risk factors (Dawber et al., 1957; Katz et al., 1958): family history, hyperlipidemia (primarily hypercholesterolemia), hypertension, cigarette smoking, and, to a lesser degree, obesity and other independent variables. In this section, we will identify the role of the hyperlipidemias. Cornfield (1962) showed that the risk of a definitive atherosclerotic event (e.g., myocardial infarction) is an exponential function of the plasma cholesterol concentration, with these exponents ranging from 3 to 6. Thus, a doubling of the circulating cholesterol content increases the atherosclerotic risk rate from 8-fold to 64-fold.

Doree (1909), in a classic article of comparative biochemistry, described cholesterol as the phylogenetically dominant sterol. Bergman (1958), also influenced by darwinian theory, designated it the "fittest" sterol. The first to demonstrate that cholesterol was a constituent of the atherosclerotic plaque was probably Vogel (1847). Joslin (1926–1927) postulated that the premature development of arteriosclerosis in diabetics was related to the excess of fat and cholesterol found in the blood of these patients. There have been case reports of advanced atherosclerosis in children with hyperlipidemia secondary to the nephrotic syndrome (Schwartz and Kohn, 1935; Gofman et al., 1950). Familial hypercholesterolemia, described as being due to a dominant gene with incomplete penetrance, is the most obvious clinical example of the relationship of atherosclerosis to hypercholesterolemia (Wilkinson et al., 1948; Adlersberg et al., 1949).

Today's generally accepted tenet that the level of

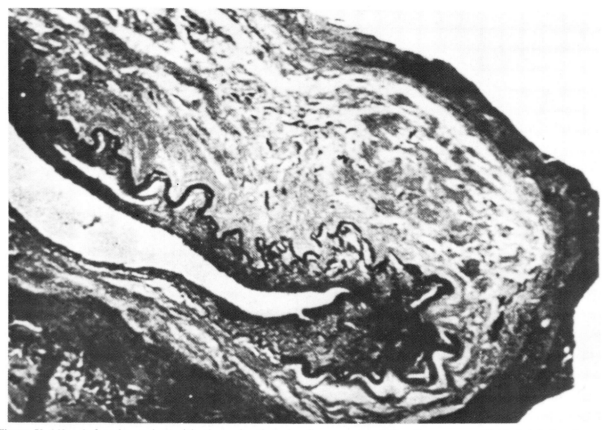

Figure 50–143. A far-advanced arterial atherosclerotic lesion from an ancient Egyptian mummy (Heidenhain's iron-hematoxylin stain; × 260). (Photograph taken from a slide, University of Minnesota rare references library.)

circulating cholesterol is a major indicator of atherosclerotic risk has evolved from epidemiologic studies over the past 40 years. In 1934, Rosenthal concluded, "In no race for which a high cholesterol intake (in the form of eggs, butter and milk) and fat intake are recorded is atherosclerosis absent. . . where the neutral fat intake is low, atherosclerosis is not prevalent." After reviewing 787 articles on the subject, Katz and associates (1958) concluded that in addition to the dietary neutral fat content and the presence of atherosclerosis, a third component in this computation of correlation is the circulating cholesterol concentration. Such retrospective analyses have been confirmed by prospective data from population studies at Framingham (Dawber *et al.*, 1957), Albany (Doyle *et al.*, 1957), and Los Angeles (Chapman *et al.*, 1957).

More recently, the role of cholesterol in atherogenesis has been further defined. Plasma total cholesterol is the sum of the cholesterol in the three major plasma lipoprotein classes—very-low-density lipoprotein (VLDL), low-density lipoprotein (LDL), and high-density lipoprotein (HDL). LDL cholesterol is directly related to the risk of coronary heart disease, and HDL cholesterol has been shown to be inversely related to this risk; multivariant analysis has shown that these two lipoprotein fractions exert an independent effect on the risk of coronary heart disease (Gordon *et al.*, 1977; Castelli *et al.*, 1977). The precise

mechanism relating cholesterol to the pathologic process of atherosclerosis remains unclear, however. The LDL cholesterol can be considered a chemical agent capable, as a function of its concentration in the plasma and/or in combination with injurious elements (e.g., hemodynamic stress, carbon monoxide, catecholamines), of injuring the endothelium and infiltrating the intima to induce proliferation of smooth muscle cells and the initiation of the plaque lesion (Davignon, 1978). The work of Brown and Goldstein (1975, 1976) has further broadened our understanding of the role of LDL cholesterol. They have shown in human fibroblasts and in surface cells of the human aorta the existence of a cell-surface receptor that binds and degrades plasma LDL. Individuals with heterozygous familial hypercholesterolemia have a reduced number of these receptors, and subjects with the homozygous form of this disease have virtually none.

CLASSIFICATION OF THE HYPERLIPIDEMIAS

In the past, the designations of familial hypercholesterolemia, familial hypertriglyceridemia, and familial xanthomatosis were used to describe severe and hereditary forms of hyperlipidemia. Acquired hypercholesterolemia and hypertriglyceridemia indicated less "florid" manifestations of this spectrum of con-

Type	Cholesterol	Triglycerides	Chylomicrons	LDL	VLDL	Other
I	Normal	Increased	Increased	Decreased	Normal or Slightly Increased	HDL Decreased
II$_a$	Increased	Normal	Normal	Increased	Normal	
II$_b$	Usually Increased	Increased	Normal	Increased	Increased	
III	Increased	Increased	Normal	Sf 0-12 Decreased Sf 12-20 Increased	Sf 100-400 Increased	"Floating" Beta Present
IV	Normal or Increased	Increased	Normal	Normal or Decreased	Increased	HDL may be Decreased
V	Increased	Increased	Increased	Usually Decreased	Increased	HDL may be Decreased

Figure 50–144. Chart representation of the current classification system of the hyperlipoproteinemias by Fredrickson and associates (1967).

ditions. Fredrickson and associates (1967) more effectively categorized such lipid elevations as functions of lipoprotein abnormalities. Their schema was subsequently revised by others, as well as by themselves (Beaumont et al., 1970). Its current format provides a standard nomenclature and is widely accepted today for discussions of the hyperlipidemias. In this schema, the hyperlipoproteinemias are divided into five types (Fig. 50–144):

Type I—a hyperchylomicronemia due to a lipoprotein lipase deficiency and the resultant inability to clear the circulating chylomicrons derived from intestinally absorbed fatty acids and cholesterol.

Type II—defined as hyperbetalipoproteinemia and further subdivided into Type IIA (without concomitant hyperprebetalipoproteinemia) and Type IIB (with associated hyperprebetalipoproteinemia). Hyperbetalipoproteinemia is characterized by an increased concentration of low-density lipoproteins (density 1.006 to 1.063 gm./ml., Sf 0 to 20, beta mobility on electrophoresis). These low-density lipoproteins are rich in cholesterol content. By definition, the ratio of the plasma concentrations of cholesterol to triglyceride in Type IIA hyperlipoproteinemia is greater than 1.5. The Type IIA individual is most synonymous with the patient previously classified as having primary hypercholesterolemia. In Type IIB, in addition to an increase in the low-density lipoproteins and the plasma cholesterol concentration, there is an increased plasma triglyceride level in association with an increased concentration of the triglyceride-rich very-low-density lipoproteins (density around 0.94 to 1.006 gm./ml., Sf 20 to 400, prebeta mobility on electrophoresis). The Type II patterns result from an hereditary dominant gene with incomplete penetrance. When this gene is inherited from a single parent, the

individual is heterozygous for the trait, and if the gene is inherited from both parents, the person is, of course, homozygous. The heterozygous Type IIA hypercholesterolemic patient generally has a plasma cholesterol concentration between 300 and 400 mg. per 100 ml. and often manifests overt atherosclerotic coronary artery disease in early adulthood. The homozygous individual, with cholesterol concentrations between 400 and 1000 mg. per 100 ml., if he reaches adulthood, rarely escapes being severely handicapped by coronary atherosclerosis prior to his third decade.

Type III—an uncommon hyperlipoproteinemia resulting from a block in the metabolism of very-low-density lipoproteins to low-density lipoproteins. Thus, an abnormal or "intermediate" form of lipoprotein circulates in the plasma. This is characterized as a "floating beta," identifiable on electrophoresis by a broad beta band extending from the beta position into the prebeta position. Both the plasma cholesterol and triglyceride concentrations are elevated, with the cholesterol-to-triglyceride ratio generally being about 1.0 (with a range of 0.3 to greater than 2.0).

Type IV—a hyperprebetalipoproteinemia due to either excess production or inadequate clearance of very-low-density lipoproteins. It is characterized by an elevated triglyceride concentration, increased concentration of very-low-density lipoproteins, an essentially normal cholesterol level, normal concentrations of low-density lipoproteins, and increased staining intensity of the prebeta band on electrophoresis. Type IV and Type II hyperlipoproteinemias account for the majority of the lipoprotein abnormalities in the general population. The Type IV pattern may be more characteristically associated with a later onset of atherosclerotic disease and a more diffuse and peripheral distribution of plaque lesions in comparison with the

TABLE 50–32. A CLASSIFICATION OF THE HYPERLIPIDEMIAS BY PEDIGREE ANALYSIS*

DISORDER	CHOLESTEROL	TRIGLYCERIDE	MODE OF INHERITANCE
Sporadic hypertriglyceridemia	Normal	Elevated	Nongenetic
Polygenic hypercholesterolemia	Elevated	Normal to elevated	Polygenic
Familial hypercholesterolemia	Elevated	Normal	Autosomal dominant
Familial hypertriglyceridemia	Normal	Elevated	Autosomal dominant
Familial combined hyperlipidemia	Elevated	Elevated	Autosomal dominant

*Adapted from the work of Goldstein and associates (1973).

Type II (especially Type IIA) pattern of earlier disease with predominance of coronary arterial involvement.

Type V—a rare type of hyperlipoproteinemia characterized by the combined presence of a hyperchylomicronemia, increased levels of very-low-density lipoproteins, essentially normal levels of low-density lipoproteins, increased staining of the prebeta band and the presence of chylomicrons on electrophoresis, and increased plasma cholesterol and triglyceride concentrations. The cholesterol-to-triglyceride ratio is usually greater than 0.15 but less than 0.6.

An alternative classification system, based on the plasma lipid levels in the patient and his relatives, has been proposed by Goldstein and coworkers (1973). The proportion of relatives having elevated plasma cholesterol and/or triglyceride levels and the proximity of their relationship to the patient having the hyperlipidemia serve as the bases for classification into one of five categories (Table 50–32). Sporadic hypertriglyceridemia reflects exogenous factors and is considered to be nongenetic. Polygenic hypercholesterolemia is manifested primarily as an elevated plasma cholesterol level but may also include an elevated plasma triglyceride level, presumably reflecting a combination of genetic and environmental influences. The monogenetic forms of hyperlipidemia are (1) familial hypercholesterolemia—elevation of plasma cholesterol alone; (2) familial hypertriglyceridemia—elevation of plasma triglycerides alone; and (3) familial combined hyperlipidemia—elevation of both plasma cholesterol and triglycerides. The use of this classification system should be helpful to the clinician in genetic counseling and could be of benefit in the selection of appropriate therapeutic measures for hyperlipidemic patients.

CLINICAL TRIALS OF PLASMA LIPID REDUCTION

The lipid hypothesis of atherogenesis states that atherosclerosis is a disease of multiple causes in which altered lipid metabolism, primarily manifested as hypercholesterolemia, plays a crucial and operant role.

A very large body of evidence from several different scientific disciplines has convincingly demonstrated the significant positive association between elevated plasma cholesterol levels (mainly LDL cholesterol) and the incidence of atherosclerotic cardiovascular disease in man. However, the corollary to this hypothesis—Does a reduction in plasma cholesterol result in a decrease in the incidence of atherosclerosis and its clinical manifestations?—has yet to be conclusively demonstrated.

The natural history of atherosclerotic cardiovascular disease has been arbitrarily divided into a prolonged preclinical stage and an overt clinical period. Therapy directed toward altering the course of the disease has, likewise, been divided into primary intervention and secondary intervention treatment. Clinical trials of the corollary of the lipid hypothesis are similarly divided into primary and secondary intervention trials. Since the mid 1950s, more than 20 major clinical lipid modification trials have been initiated. The "first-generation" trials were all negative or inconclusive. The current six "second-generation" clinical trials have either demonstrated no significant benefit with respect to risk of atherosclerosis from cholesterol reduction or are still in progress. A summary of these "second-generation" randomized clinical intervention trials is presented in Table 50–33, which lists the time of period of the study; the number, sex, and age range of subjects; the length of the follow-up period; the treatment modality used for plasma cholesterol reduction; and the average plasma cholesterol reduction observed in the completed studies or postulated to occur in the studies currently being conducted.

The Coronary Drug Project was the first of this group and was initiated in 1966 and completed in 1974 (Coronary Drug Project Research Group, 1975). This was a secondary intervention trial that showed no beneficial effect on the progression of coronary heart disease with the use of either clofibrate or nicotinic acid therapy. The degree of plasma total cholesterol reduction was, however, only 6.5 per cent with clofibrate and 9.9 per cent with nicotinic acid.

The Minnesota Coronary Survey, a primary in-

TABLE 50–33. THE SIX "SECOND-GENERATION" CLINICAL TRIALS
OF THE LIPID-ATHEROSCLEROSIS HYPOTHESIS

STUDY	NUMBER OF SUBJECTS	SEX	AGE (YEARS)	FOLLOW-UP PERIOD (YEARS)	LIPID-LOWERING THERAPY	CHOLESTEROL EFFECT (%)
Primary Prevention Trials						
Minnesota Coronary Survey (1967–1973)	9449	M & F	21–100	1–5	Diet	−14
MRFIT (1972–1982)	12,000	M	35–57	6	Diet	−10
Coronary Primary Prevention Trial, CPPT (1971–1982)	4000	M	35–59	7	Cholestyramine	−24
WHO Cooperative Clofibrate Trial (1965–1976)	15,745	M	30–55	5.3	Clofibrate	−9
Secondary Prevention Trials						
Coronary Drug Study (1966–1974)	8341	M	30–64	6.2	Clofibrate or Nicotinic acid	−6.5 −9.9
Surgical Control of The Hyperlipidemias (1973–	1000	M & F	30–64	5	Partial ileal bypass surgery	−40

tervention trial completed in 1973, also failed to show definitive beneficial effects (morbidity or mortality), with an average plasma cholesterol reduction of 14 per cent with dietary modification therapy (Frantz *et al.,* 1975).

The European World Health Organization cooperative clofibrate trial, a primary intervention trial conducted from 1965 to 1976, showed no reduction in coronary heart disease mortality, with an average plasma cholesterol lowering of 9 per cent. However, this trial did report a lower incidence of nonfatal myocardial infarctions in the clofibrate-treated group compared with the control group. On the other hand, there was an increase in mortality from noncardiovascular diseases in the treated group (Report from the Committee of Principal Investigators, 1978). A further report (Report from the Committee of Principal Investigators, 1980) on the mortality of these subjects, an average of 4.3 years after the end of the trial, showed 25 per cent more deaths in the clofibrate-treated group than in the control group. In addition, there was a higher overall mortality from all causes in the treated group compared with the high-cholesterol controls; no particular disease accounted for this excess, and there was no excess mortality due to accidents or violence. There was also a significant excess in mortality from all causes and from diseases other than coronary heart disease in the clofibrate-treated group when compared with the low plasma cholesterol control group. Obviously, this study has raised the question of a long-term toxic effect of clofibrate.

The Multiple Risk Factor Intervention Trial (MRFIT) is a current primary intervention trial employing modest (less than 10 per cent) plasma cholesterol reduction as one of three intervention modalities, with the other two being blood pressure control and cessation of cigarette smoking (Kuller *et al.,* 1980).

At present, there are basically only two intervention trials, one primary and one secondary, using a unifactorial approach. The Coronary Primary Prevention Trial (CPPT) of the Lipid Research Clinics (LRC) Program is using the bile-acid sequestrant cholestyramine for cholesterol reduction (The Lipid Research Clinics Program, 1979). This trial was scheduled to be completed in 1982 and was designed for an average 24 per cent reduction in plasma total cholesterol level. It is doubtful if this degree of cholesterol reduction will actually be achieved because of the problems of long-term adherence to drug therapy.

The Program on the Surgical Control of the Hyperlipidemias (POSCH) is a secondary intervention trial using partial ileal bypass surgery to effect plasma cholesterol reduction. In this study, 1000 subjects, aged 30 to 64 years, not hypertensive, not obese, and not diabetic, who have had only one documented myocardial infarction, will be randomly assigned to a surgical or control group. The follow-up period will be a minimum of 5 years after entry into the trial. In addition to the determination of cardiovascular mortality and morbidity, this study will document the anatomic extent of atherosclerotic disease using peripheral and coronary arteriography prior to randomization and at two subsequent intervals. This trial was designed for an average cholesterol reduction of 40 per cent in the surgically treated group. A major advantage of using partial ileal bypass surgery as the treatment modality in such a clinical trial is that the effects on body lipids and cholesterol metabolism are obligatory. This benefit minimizes or eliminates the problem of subject compliance. A recently published preliminary analysis of the plasma lipid and lipoprotein changes following partial ileal bypass in this trial (Moore *et al.,* 1980) showed that there was an average reduction of 31 per cent in plasma total cholesterol and an average reduction of 49 per cent in the atherogenic LDL cholesterol at 1 year after operative intervention. Thus, POSCH is providing maximal reduction of the major atherogenic risk factors with a negligible subject noncompliance rate, and it is the only lipid-hypothesis clinical intervention trial employing serial arteriographic assessment.

THERAPY FOR THE HYPERLIPOPROTEINEMIAS

Rationale

Although definitive evidence is, as yet, still lacking to support the necessity for lipid reduction in the management and prevention of atherosclerotic cardiovascular disease, it is eminently logical to assume that lowering the atherogenic plasma lipid components would reduce the risk of atherosclerosis. Certain regression studies in experimental animals, as well as limited studies in man (Baltaxe et al., 1969; Blankenhorn et al., 1978) support this reasoning. Today, the majority of clinicians have adopted the concept that it is prudent to attempt atherosclerosis risk modification by plasma lipid reduction while awaiting the results of the current clinical trials, as long as the means utilized for lipid reduction are effective and safe.

Diet and Drug Antihyperlipidemic Therapy

Based on retrospective and prospective studies of the influence of various diets on the circulating cholesterol concentration, the most effective dietary regimen for lowering the cholesterol level includes a diet low in saturated fats, with a relative increase in the proportion of polyunsaturated fatty acids and with a low daily dietary cholesterol intake (McGandy et al., 1967). The following general rules seem sound: Total fats, less than 30 per cent of total calories; a polyunsaturated/saturated fatty acid ratio of at least 1.5; and the daily intake of cholesterol less than 300 mg. Lowering of triglyceride concentration by diet is often accomplished by weight reduction. Secondarily, a dietary carbohydrate reduction, particularly of the free sugars, can prove beneficial (Kuo, 1969).

After an extensive review of the literature on cholesterol modification by diet, we have summarized the 16 most widely mentioned studies.* These studies examined 2516 patients, nearly evenly divided into 1370 free-living individuals and 1146 confined individuals. This distinction is relevant since adherence, and possibly response, to a dietary program is often a function of whether food selection, preparation, and availability are institutionalized or occur in the community at large (Brown and Green, 1962; Lewis et al., 1970). The range of mean percentage circulating cholesterol level change from the pretreatment baseline varied from +6.0 to -22.0 per cent for the free-living subjects and from -8.1 to -18.4 per cent for the confined subjects.

The average follow-up period was 32.44 months in these 16 studies, or 1,305,804 patient-months' experience. The average circulating cholesterol level reduction in these studies was 12.68 per cent. In those studies with control groups, a universal decrease of about 6 per cent occurred in the plasma cholesterol of the controls. This finding implies that inclusion into a study program of at-risk individuals, especially those having had a myocardial infarction, induces some voluntary life-pattern changes, possibly dietary, in all individuals, both those who are given specific therapeutic recommendations and those who are not. If we subtract the control group plasma cholesterol reduction from the gross test group average cholesterol reduction (12.68 per cent minus 6 per cent), a net cholesterol lowering of 6 to 7 per cent resulted from these dietary programs.

No comparable studies exist from which we can derive an equivalent appraisal of dietary influence on triglyceride reduction.

We have also recently reviewed the literature on drugs currently utilized for lipid modification. From our study, we conclude that data on long-term triglyceride lowering are sketchy at best. In that review, the mean reductions of circulating cholesterol levels for the more common drugs utilized in hyperlipidemia management include 22 per cent for cholestyramine.* Cholestyramine is not absorbed from the gut, and no adverse systemic side effects have been reported. Its bile acid–binding action can cause constipation when the resin is given in therapeutic amounts. To date, this powdered substance is available only for suspension in a liquid medium.

The average range of the plasma cholesterol response to clofibrate was a 15 to 20 per cent lowering.† As previously stated, in the Coronary Drug Project, clofibrate reduced the plasma cholesterol by only 6.5 per cent, and in the World Health Organization Trial, it reduced the plasma cholesterol by 9 per cent. For clofibrate, the evidence is quite explicit for escape from effective therapy in the face of adequate drug dosage (Hunninghake et al., 1969). Lipid level rebound well above the pretreatment baseline after discontinuation of clofibrate management has been

---

*Jolliffe et al., 1961; Green et al., 1963; Leren, 1968; National Diet Heart Study, 1968; Report of a Research Committee to the Medical Research Council, 1968; Rinzler, 1968; Strisower et al., 1968a; Dayton and Pierce, 1969; Turpeinen et al., 1969; Bierenbaum et al., 1970; Evans et al., 1972.

---

*Berkowitz, 1963; Blacket et al., 1964; Hashim and Van Itallie, 1965; Bressler et al., 1966; Casdorph, 1967; Connor, 1968; Fallon and Woods, 1968; Goodman and Noble, 1968; Khachadurian and Demirjian, 1968; Jepson et al., 1969; Grundy et al., 1971; Howard and Hyams, 1971; Levy, 1972.

†Jolliffe et al., 1961; Best and Duncan, 1966; Jepson et al., 1969; Levy et al., 1969; Heffernan et al., 1969; Hunninghake et al., 1969; Nordøy and Gjone, 1970; Five-Year Study, Newcastle, 1971; Report of a Research Committee of the Scottish Society of Physicians, 1971; Krasno and Kidera, 1972.

documented (Levy et al., 1969). The side effects of clofibrate are few, yet abnormal liver function (Symposium on Atromid, 1963) and myositis (Langer and Levy, 1968) have developed with its use. The manufacturer warns that clofibrate can potentiate warfarin anticoagulants and causes nausea in about 5 per cent of individuals on this medication. The potential lethal toxicity of clofibrate demonstrated in the World Health Organization Trial has been discussed.

For nicotinic acid, effective therapeutic dosage yielded, on the average, a 23 per cent plasma cholesterol level reduction (Berge et al., 1961; Parsons, 1961a, 1961b; Heffernan et al., 1969; Nordøy and Gjone, 1970; Vikrot et al., 1971; Charman et al., 1972). However, in a randomized trial, the Coronary Drug Project, the cholesterol reduction achieved was a minimal 9.9 per cent. The mechanisms by which nicotinic acid affects circulating cholesterol levels are not fully understood. The use of nicotinic acid has been limited by its predictable and rather potent side effects. Flushing of the skin occurs initially in nearly all patients started on therapy and persists in 10 to 15 per cent of all individuals who remain on this agent (Eder, 1965). Other known side effects of nicotinic acid include erythematous rash, pruritis, hyperpigmentation, gastrointestinal disturbances, hyperglycemia, and postural hypotension. More serious reactions are an induced hyperuricemia and impairment of liver function, including jaundice (Berge et al., 1961; Parsons, 1961a, 1961b; Drugs, 1963; Eder, 1965).

Probucol (a substituted dithioacetal) has recently been introduced as a lipid-lowering agent in adults. The mechanism of action is postulated to be a block in the early stages of cholesterol biosynthesis. Approximately 10 per cent of the patients receiving the recommended dose of 500 mg. twice a day reported mild side effects consisting of diarrhea, flatulence, abdominal pain, and nausea; however, patient acceptance and adherence to the drug appear to be good. Initial results have shown a 10 to 20 per cent reduction in plasma cholesterol in familial hypercholesterolemic subjects and in individuals whose average plasma cholesterol is about 250 mg./100 ml. (Muellies et al., 1980; Riesen et al., 1980; Samuel, 1980). Both LDL and HDL cholesterol are reduced but VLDL cholesterol and serum triglycerides remain at their original levels. Since the risk of coronary heart disease has been shown to be inversely associated with the plasma HDL cholesterol, the use of a drug that reduces this lipoprotein may not be beneficial over a long period of time.

New drugs are continuously being proposed for the management of the hyperlipidemias. Clinicians should be wary of recourse to agents before their actions are well studied and their reactions characterized. Estrogen therapy has now been abandoned; it caused feminization in men (Russ et al., 1955) and intravascular clotting (Jeffcoate et al., 1968), and its use was associated with an increased frequency of sudden death (Stamler et al., 1963). Although the

early reports on the use of dextrothyroxine were promising, other effects of this agent have argued against its greater use. Dextrothyroxine can potentiate angina pectoris and arrhythmias, induce hypermetabolism, and lead to functional hyperthyroidism (Boyd and Oliver, 1960; Steinberg, 1962; Eisalo et al., 1963; Eder, 1965; Mishkel, 1967). Indeed, because of these consequences the code in the national Coronary Drug Study was broken for dextrothyroxine, and it was removed from the protocol (Special Communication, 1970, 1972).

Surgical Approach to the Hyperlipidemias— Partial Ileal Bypass

History

We performed the first human partial ileal bypass operation specifically for cholesterol reduction on May 29, 1963. Currently, other institutions in the United States and in Europe have programs testing this method of cholesterol lowering.* At this time, we have performed over 350 partial ileal bypass operations. Since this method of lowering lipids is a surgical procedure, it has encountered resistance from the nonsurgical medical community. Nevertheless, in recent years, this reluctance is slowly giving way, and we are beginning to see partial ileal bypass candidates at a rate of about one per week.

Understanding the Procedure—Metabolic Studies and Cholesterol Dynamics

From 1962 to 1964, the first experiments designed to develop the rationale for partial ileal bypass management of the hyperlipidemias were performed at the University of Minnesota (Buchwald and Gebhard, 1964, 1968; Gebhard and Buchwald, 1970; Buchwald et al., 1974b). Studies in white New Zealand rabbits, in pigs, and, by retrospective analysis, in patients who had undergone ileal resections for causes other than carcinoma (e.g., incarcerated hernia) showed that both the cholesterol absorption from the intestinal tract and the whole blood cholesterol concentration were markedly and significantly (statistically) reduced, without concomitant weight loss, following diversion or loss of substantial lengths of bowel. Additional studies demonstrated that although the entire small intestine is capable of cholesterol absorption, with normal bowel continuity preferential cholesterol uptake occurs in the distal half of the small bowel. Transit time in the small intestine strongly influences quantitative cholesterol absorption.

The data with respect to absorption sites for bile

---

*Fritz and Walker, 1966; Lewis et al., 1968; Strisower et al., 1968b; Swan and McGowan, 1968; Helsinger and Rootwelt, 1969; Rowe et al., 1969; Miettinen, 1970; Sodal et al., 1970; Clot et al., 1971; Balfour and Kim, 1974; Streuter, 1970; Morgan and Moore, 1970.

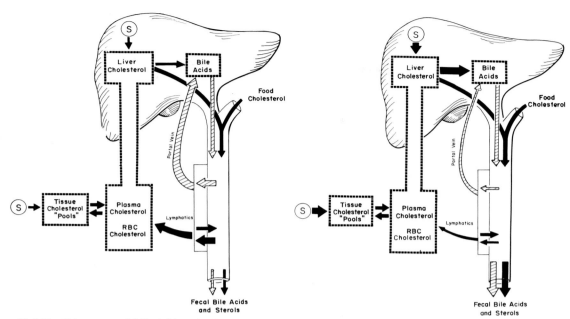

Figure 50–145. Prior to partial ileal bypass (diagram on the left), the major portion of the exogenous cholesterol and bile and mucosal secreted cholesterol is absorbed from the distal small intestine; similarly, the majority of secreted bile acids are reabsorbed by the ileum. After the operation (diagram on the right), there is a marked decrease in intestinal absorption and an increase in fecal excretion of both cholesterol and bile acids. There is also an increase in cholesterol synthesis (S). The net effect is a reduction in the circulating cholesterol concentration and the miscible body cholesterol pool.

acids are not as clear as the experimental findings for cholesterol absorption, and often they have been contradictory. We have demonstrated that bypass of the distal third of the small bowel interferes with the enterohepatic bile acid cycle and results in a loss of bile acids in the feces at a rate at least three times normal (Buchwald and Gebhard, 1968). Thus, the partial ileal bypass operation alters body cholesterol homeostasis by (1) a direct drain on the body cholesterol pool and (2) an indirect drain on the cholesterol pool through forced conversion of cholesterol to its metabolic end-product bile acids in order to maintain the stressed bile acid reservoir (Fig. 50–145).

An animal model of a reproducible 50 per cent myocardial infarction attack rate has been developed in the rabbit by maintenance of a diet high in cholesterol content for prolonged periods of time (Buchwald, 1965b). Using this model, it has been demonstrated both for adult rabbits (Buchwald, 1965a) and infant rabbits (Buchwald et al., 1972) that partial ileal bypass will prevent hypercholesterolemia and atherosclerosis despite consumption of a severely atherogenic (2 per cent cholesterol) diet for 4 months. In rabbits with established hypercholesterolemia and atherosclerosis, the operation returns their whole blood cholesterol values to below normal and reduces cholesterol xanthomata accumulations, even though they remain on the 2 per cent cholesterol diet. In addition, partial ileal bypass will arrest and reverse their atherosclerotic process. The plaque lesions evolve from a proliferative to a scarring or healing phase with quantitatively less cholesterol content. For the infant rabbit, loss of absorption from the bypassed segment does

not interfere with structural growth or normal body weight gain. Finally, adaptive mechanisms do not, in time, lead to increased cholesterol or bile salt absorption.

Investigators have confirmed these findings in other animal species—the dog (Scott et al., 1966) and the rhesus monkey (Shepard et al., 1968). Scott and associates have also shown that partial ileal bypass achieved twice the circulating cholesterol reduction that cholestyramine (1.5 mg./kg. daily) did in the rhesus monkey (Younger et al., 1969). With all animals on the same atherogenic regimen, the average serum cholesterol concentration was 803 mg./100 ml. for the nontreated monkeys, 418 mg./100 ml. for the cholestyramine-treated animals, and 175 mg./100 ml. for the animals who underwent partial ileal bypass. In addition, significant differences in protection were afforded against the development of atherosclerotic plaque lesions by comparison of the aortas of the monkeys treated by partial ileal bypass, the cholestyramine-treated animals, and the nontreated hypercholesterolemic animals. In studies with the white Carneau pigeon (Gomes et al., 1971), birds with naturally occurring atherosclerosis, partial ileal bypass decreased the aortic atherosclerosis involvement, without interfering with avian growth and weight gain. This study also demonstrated atherosclerotic plaque regression following partial ileal bypass.

These laboratory experiments have been complemented by human cholesterol dynamics studies utilizing radioisotope methods (Moore et al., 1969, 1970): Cholesterol absorption is reduced 60 per cent following partial ileal bypass. This state of reduced absorp-

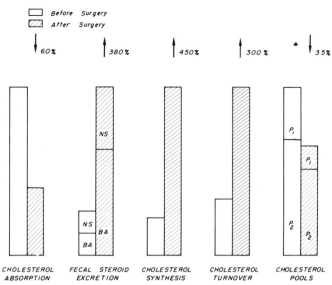

Figure 50–146. Summary of changes in cholesterol dynamics following partial ileal bypass (NS = neutral steroids; BA = bile acids; P₁ = freely miscible cholesterol pool; P₂ = less freely miscible cholesterol pool). (From Buchwald, H., *et al.*: *Circulation*, *49*(Suppl. 1):1, 1974, and Buchwald, H., *et al.*: *Ann. Surg.*, *180*:384, 1974. By permission of The American Heart Association, Inc.)

tion capacity has been maintained for at least 10 years. Complementary data in human subjects show a 3.8-fold increase in total fecal steroid excretion, with a much greater increase in bile acids (4.9-fold) than in neutral steroids (2.7-fold). This state of increased steroid excretion has also been maintained for 10 years of follow-up. Compensatory cholesterol and bile-acid absorptive adaptation by the functioning small intestine apparently does not occur. Thus, the effect of partial ileal bypass on the cholesterol and the bile-acid enterohepatic cycles appear to endure.

Other homeostatic mechanisms in man do respond to the increased loss of cholesterol and bile acids by increasing cholesterol synthesis. Indeed, a 5.7-fold increase in cholesterol synthesis rate has been shown to occur following partial ileal bypass, and this effect, too, has been maintained. Concomitantly, the cholesterol turnover rate has been demonstrated to increase markedly. The total exchangeable cholesterol pool, on the other hand, is reduced by about one-third at 1 year after partial ileal bypass. This lowering is reflected in both the freely miscible cholesterol pool (plasma, red blood cells, liver, intestinal mucosa) and the less freely miscible cholesterol pool (depot fat, muscle, organs). The less freely miscible cholesterol pool includes cholesterol in the arterial walls. Therefore, loss of cholesterol from this pool can reflect a loss of cholesterol from atherosclerotic plaques.

Cholesterol dynamics are graphically summarized in Figure 50–146.

Operative Technique

Usually, the abdomen is entered through a right lower quadrant transverse incision about 2 cm. below the umbilicus (Fig. 50–147). When an additional procedure (e.g., cholecystectomy) is planned, we prefer to use an upper transverse abdominal incision. After abdominal exploration, the entire small intestine is measured along the mesenteric border with a piece of calibrated umbilical tape. This intestinal length, as measured between the ileocecal valve and the ligament of Treitz and under general anesthesia, will vary from 400 to 700 cm. The bowel is then transected at a site 200 cm. from the ileocecal valve, or at a site 250 cm. from the valve if the total small bowel length is greater than 600 cm., allowing 25 cm. for the duodenum. The distal end of the divided ileum is closed. The proximal end is anastomosed end to side to the cecum into the anterior taenia some 6 cm. above the inverted appendiceal stump (the appendix, if present, is removed). The cecum has been retained to maximize the colonic water-absorbing surface. The anastomosis is distal to the ileocecal valve to minimize ileal absorption of cholesterol and bile acids. The closed end of the bypassed distal bowel is sutured to the anterior taenia of the cecum, between the anastomosis and the appendiceal stump, to prevent intussusception. The small divisional mesenteric defect and the large rotational mesenteric defect are carefully closed to prevent internal herniation. The abdomen is thoroughly irrigated and closed in layers, using nonabsorbable sutures for the fascia. No drains are used. Postoperative in-hospital convalescence averages about 6 days.

Effect on Plasma Lipids and Lipoproteins (Pre-POSCH)

Cholesterol Concentrations. The plasma cholesterol content is a fraction of the freely miscible cholesterol pool and represents a small percentage of the total exchangeable pool. It is, nevertheless, indicative of body cholesterol balance. The plasma cholesterol content is also the cholesterol environment of the arteries and the source most accessible for easy measurement.

In our experience, the circulating cholesterol concentration is reduced an average of 41 per cent from the preoperative and postdietary baseline after partial ileal bypass (Buchwald *et al.*, 1974c, 1974d). In combination with type-specific dietary management, a 53 per cent lowering of the cholesterol level, on the average, has been achieved in Type IIA individuals (Buchwald *et al.*, 1968) (Fig. 50–148). Parenthetically, certain Type IIA patients are likely to be refractory to dietary therapy alone or to drugs, singly or in combination. In addition to its effectiveness in the type IIA individual, partial ileal bypass lowers the cholesterol concentration in all of the types of hyperlipidemia. These results have not been compromised by effect escape in our experience, which now extends for more than 20 years postoperatively (Fig. 50–149).

The cholesterol-lowering effect of the operation is neither uniform nor precisely predictable for each person. The lowering of cholesterol from the preoperative postdietary baseline has varied from 5 to 79 per cent (Fig. 50–150). But in the series reported by

ILEAL BYPASS
PROCEDURE

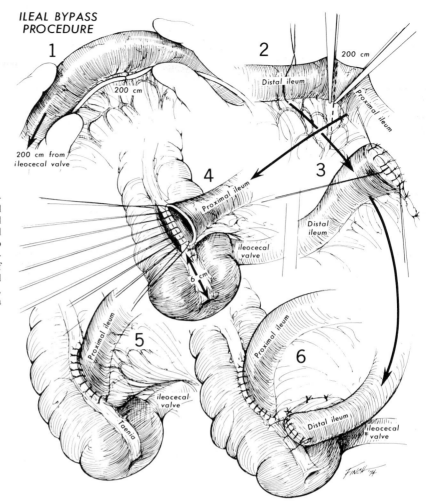

Figure 50–147. Operative technique of partial ileal bypass: (1) measurement of the bowel along the mesenteric border; (2) division of bowel between marking sutures; (3) closure of distal end of the division, with the middle and the two corner sutures left uncut; (4) end-to-side anastomosis of proximal bowel to the anterior taenia of the cecum; (5) completion of anastomosis; and (6) suturing of closed end of bypassed segment, utilizing the uncut sutures, to the anterior taenia and closure of mesenteric defects.

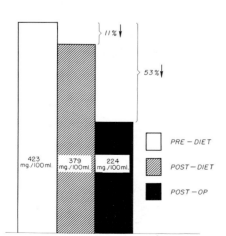

Figure 50–148. Lowering of the circulating cholesterol level following type-specific diet and partial ileal bypass management, in 24 Type IIA individuals. (From Buchwald, H., *et al.*: Surgical treatment of hyperlipidemia. Circulation, *49*:(Suppl. 1):1, 1974. By permission of The American Heart Association, Inc.)

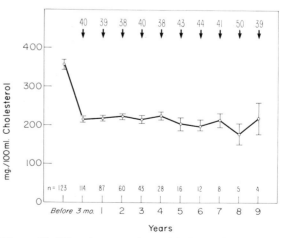

Figure 50–149. Average plasma cholesterol concentrations (± 1 S.E.) for up to 9 years following partial ileal bypass; the preoperative baseline was obtained after at least 3 months of type-specific dietary therapy. The number of patients available at each time interval is denoted as n. (From Buchwald, H., *et al.*: Ten years clinical experience with partial ileal bypass in management of the hyperlipidemias. Ann. Surg., *180*:384, 1974.)

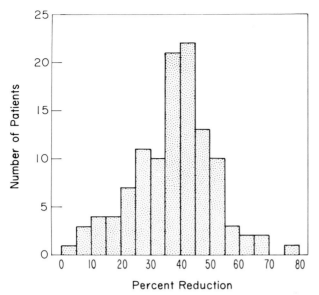

Figure 50–150. Frequency distribution of percentage of circulating cholesterol level reduction 1 year after partial ileal bypass. (From Buchwald, H., et al.: Ten years clinical experience with partial ileal bypass in management of the hyperlipidemias. Ann. Surg., *180*:384, 1974.)

investigative groups elsewhere in the United States and in Europe, the mean cholesterol concentration reduction after dietary therapy has been virtually identical to our finding—40 per cent.*

To date, the least impressive responses have been in Type IIA homozygous young people. Yet, Balfour and Kim (1974) reported two homozygous children followed for 3 years who had sustained cholesterol reductions of 42 per cent and 33 per cent.

We will now examine more closely the cholesterol response as a function of lipoprotein typing performed prior to operation. The term "mixed type" will be employed to describe those individuals with electrophoretic staining patterns characteristic for both Type II and Type IV (Fredrickson Type V), and Type IIX will be used for those individuals imprecisely classifiable because they were operated on prior to the publication of the Fredrickson classification system. One year postoperatively, the plasma cholesterol reductions from the postdietary preoperative baseline were as follows: Type IIA—34.8 per cent; Type IIB—41.3 per cent; Type IIX—32.0 per cent; Type III—47.5 per cent; Type IV—45.6 per cent; and mixed type—41.1 per cent (Fig. 50–151).

The average cholesterol concentration of middle-aged men in the United States is about 250 mg./100 ml.; the average preoperative cholesterol concentration reported for individuals who have undergone

partial ileal bypass has been over 330 mg./100 ml. Following partial ileal bypass, more than 80 per cent of these subjects have circulating cholesterol levels below 250 mg./100 ml., and better than 50 per cent have levels below 200 mg./100 ml. (Fig. 50–152).

In Figure 50–153, we have compared the cumulative average circulating cholesterol reductions for diet, clofibrate, cholestyramine, nicotinic acid, and partial ileal bypass.

Triglyceride Concentration. Published data on the effect of partial ileal bypass on triglyceride levels are not as extensive as those for cholesterol. Partial ileal bypass, however, has demonstrated effectiveness in lowering triglyceride levels following maximal type-specific dietary therapy (Buchwald *et al.*, 1974c, 1974d). The largest reductions have been achieved in the Type IV individuals (those with primary hypertriglyceridemia). For the Type IV individual, the average triglyceride concentration reduction by partial ileal bypass from the postdietary preoperative baseline has been 53 per cent in our experience (Fig. 50–154). A small paradoxical increase in triglyceride levels has been noted in the Type IIA patients, those hypercholesterolemic individuals with low or normal preoperative triglyceride concentrations. Nevertheless, despite this increase, the average triglyceride level has remained within the accepted normal range. A satisfactory explanation for this phenomenon in the Type IIA patients is currently unavailable, but it may be related to the bile-acid loss engendered by the bypass operation. A similar finding has been reported following the use of cholestyramine (Grundy *et al.*, 1971).

Lipoprotein Concentrations. The published information is meager with respect to changes in the circulating lipoprotein concentrations and the synthesis of lipoproteins following partial ileal bypass. Reports have indicated a reduction in circulating low-density lipoproteins following this operation (Lewis *et al.*, 1968; Strisower *et al.*, 1968b).

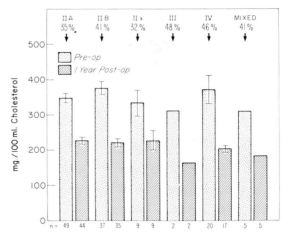

Figure 50–151. Average plasma cholesterol level response by lipoprotein type (± 1 S.E.) 1 year postoperatively. (Type IIX = no triglyceride values before operation.) (From Buchwald, H., et al.: Ten years clinical experience with partial ileal bypass in management of the hyperlipidemias. Ann. Surg., *180*:384, 1974.)

---

*Fritz and Walker, 1966; Lewis *et al.*, 1968; Strisower *et al.*, 1968b; Swan and McGowan, 1968; Helsinger and Rootwelt, 1969; Rowe *et al.*, 1969; Miettinen, 1970; Sodal *et al.*, 1970; Clot *et al.*, 1971; Streuter, 1970; Morgan and Moore, 1970.

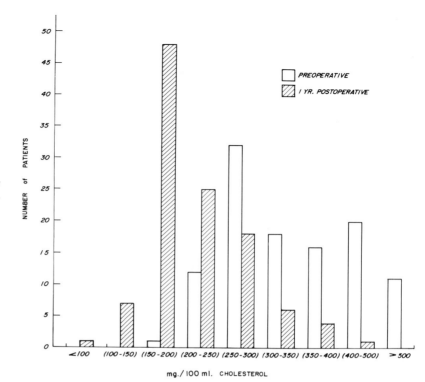

Figure 50–152. Patient distribution by plasma cholesterol levels in 50 mg. per 100 ml. increments, preoperatively and postoperatively.

Effect on Plasma Lipids and Lipoproteins in the POSCH Study

A preliminary report on the effect of partial ileal bypass on the plasma lipids and lipoproteins in 28 male survivors of a first myocardial infarction in the POSCH trial (Moore *et al.*, 1980) showed that at 1 year after operation, there were significant ($p < 0.01$) average reductions in plasma total cholesterol (31 per cent) and LDL cholesterol (49 per cent) and nonsignificant ($p > 0.05$) changes in plasma triglycerides (+ 9.6 per cent), VLDL cholesterol (− 14 per cent), and HDL cholesterol (− 3 per cent).

A more recent analysis of the plasma lipids and lipoproteins in this trial extends follow-up to 3 years and includes 165 operated patients (Table 50–34). During this 3-year period of follow-up, there were significant and sustained reductions in both plasma

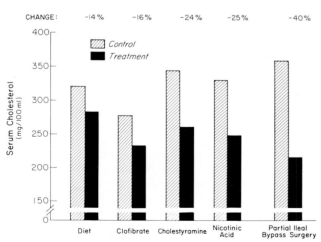

Figure 50–153. Comparison of cumulative average plasma cholesterol reduction for diet, clofibrate, cholestyramine, nicotinic acid, and partial ileal bypass; the diet and drug responses are compared with their respective control groups, and the partial ileal bypass response is measured against the preoperative postdietary baseline.

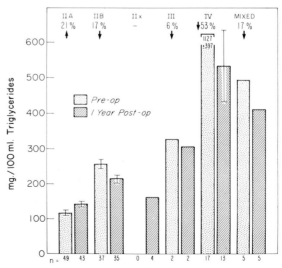

Figure 50–154. Average triglyceride level response by lipoprotein type (± 1 S.E.) 1 year postoperatively. (Type IIX = no triglyceride values before operation.) (From Buchwald, H., *et al.*: Ten years clinical experience with partial ileal bypass in management of the hyperlipidemias. Ann. Surg., *180*:384, 1974.)

TABLE 50–34. SUMMARY OF CURRENT LIPID CHANGES IN THE PARTIAL ILEAL BYPASS PATIENTS IN THE PROGRAM ON THE SURGICAL CONTROL OF THE HYPERLIPIDEMIAS (POSCH) OVER 3 YEARS

	BEFORE AV ± SD (mg./100 ml.)	% CHANGE AFTER PARTIAL ILEAL BYPASS			
		3 mos.	*1 yr.*	*2 yrs.*	*3 yrs.*
(Number of patients)	(165)	(148)	(118)	(83)	(43)
Cholesterol	258 ± 17	−34.9	−29.7	−29.0	−31.2
LDL cholesterol	186 ± 38	−47.2	−42.3	−42.9	−43.5
HDL cholesterol	40.9 ± 10.0	+ 2.6	+ 7.4	+ 3.1	+ 1.0
Triglycerides	201 ± 95	− 5.6	+ 4.2	+12.6	+ 2.7
VLDL cholesterol	30.5 ± 17.8	− 9.5	− 3.6	+11.2	− 2.5
HDL/LDL	0.220 ± 0.012	+94.2	+85.9	+80.4	+78.9

total cholesterol (ranging from 35 per cent at 3 months to 31 per cent at 3 years) and LDL cholesterol (ranging from 47 per cent at 3 months to 43.5 per cent at 3 years). There was no significant average effect on plasma triglycerides or VLDL cholesterol levels in the overall group of subjects, which included both normotriglyceridemic and hypertriglyceridemic patients. In the 140 normotriglyceridemic subjects, there was a slight, but not statistically significant, increase in plasma triglycerides and VLDL cholesterol, and in the 40 hypertriglyceridemic subjects (Types IIB and IV), there were variable individual responses, with an overall average reduction (not statistically significant) in plasma triglycerides and VLDL cholesterol. HDL cholesterol levels tended to increase after partial ileal bypass surgery; when the surgically treated group was compared with the control group, in which there was an average decrease in HDL cholesterol over time, there was a significant (p < 0.05) difference between the two groups (10.4 per cent at 1 year; 9.3 per cent at 3 years). Following partial ileal bypass surgery, there was a marked increase in the ratio of HDL cholesterol to LDL cholesterol (ranging from 94 per cent at 3 months to 79 per cent at 3 years).

These results definitively show that partial ileal bypass results in a marked reduction in the plasma total cholesterol and the major atherogenic plasma lipoprotein (LDL), with an increase in the presumably protective plasma lipoprotein (HDL) and the HDL/LDL ratio.

In-Hospital Statistics: Mortality and Complications

We believe that the partial ileal bypass procedure can be performed with an in-hospital, or operative, mortality of less than 1 per cent, the presence of coexisting coronary artery disease in many of these patients notwithstanding. Wound infections, pulmonary emboli, or other serious postoperative complications that resulted in prolonging hospitalization beyond 1 week have occurred in only 2 per cent of these patients (Buchwald et al., 1974c, 1974d).

To date, in the Minnesota series, no instance of intussusception of the proximal end of the bypassed segment or obstruction secondary to an internal hernia created by inadequate closure of the rotational mesenteric defect has occurred. These complications seem to be avoidable.

Side Effects of Partial Ileal Bypass

Diarrhea is the one annoying side effect experienced by the majority of individuals after partial ileal bypass.* Commonly, it is not persistent. Within a year or so, approximately 90 per cent of patients have less than five bowel movements daily, while taking no bowel-controlling medications. Patients generally also report an increase in the firmness and consistency of stools with time. Only two patients (out of 350) in our experience have requested operative restoration of bowel continuity because of intractable diarrhea.

It has been stated that the terminal ileum is uniquely capable of absorbing vitamin B_{12} (combination of intrinsic and extrinsic factors) and that only vitamin B_{12} had the distinction of a singular site for absorption from the gut (Booth and Mollin, 1959). Following partial ileal bypass, vitamin B_{12} absorption is either severely impaired or totally lost (Buchwald, 1964). After several years, however, absorptive adaptation for vitamin B_{12} occurs in about one half of these patients (Nygaard et al., 1970; Coyle et al., 1977). Nevertheless, we believe it prudent to prescribe parenteral vitamin B_{12} supplementation, 1000 μg. intramuscularly every 2 months, for all partial ileal bypass patients. We continue this regimen indefinitely.

Although variable in occurrence, gastric hypersecretion following massive intestinal resection or the jejunoileal bypass for obesity has been documented (Frederick et al., 1965; Osborne et al., 1966). However, laboratory and clinical study of gastric volume and acid output, before and after partial ileal bypass, in a random group of our patients has demonstrated no similar hypersecretory effect (Buchwald and Varco, 1971; Buchwald et al., 1974a).

Contrary to the often encountered experience with jejunoileal bypass for obesity is the fact that no change in the serum electrolytes follows partial ileal bypass. Specifically, the serum potassium, calcium, and magnesium values remain within normal limits (Buchwald et al., 1969). We have found no recorded need for electrolyte supplements following partial ileal bypass. Nutrient malabsorption has not been described following partial ileal bypass; no essential long-term weight loss occurs (Buchwald et al., 1974c).

---

*Strisower et al., 1968b; Swan and McGowan, 1968; Helsinger and Rootwelt, 1969; Sodal et al., 1970; Buchwald et al., 1974c, 1974d; Brown, H. B., 1970; Miettinen, T. A., 1970; Streuter, 1970.

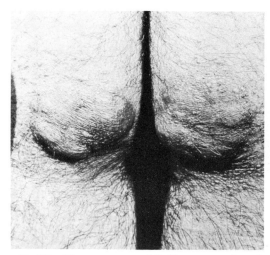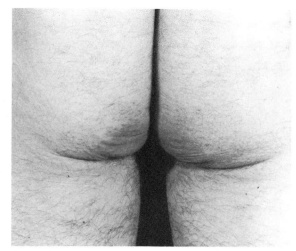

Figure 50–155. Disappearance of lipid contents from buttock xanthomata 1 year after partial ileal bypass (*left* preoperative appearance; *right,* postoperative appearance).

Arthritic phenomena or an increased rate of nephrolithiasis as described following jejunoileal bypass has not been found after partial ileal bypass. Lithogenic bile and the formation of gallstones have not been causatively related to partial ileal bypass in our experience. Finally, and of considerable importance in distinguishing partial ileal bypass from jejunoileal bypass for obesity, hepatic fatty infiltration or fibrosis has not occurred following partial ileal bypass, clinically or experimentally (Schwartz *et al.,* 1971).

Postoperative Clinical Observations

Xanthomata. Various investigators have reported a postoperative decrease in size or even disappearance of periorbital xanthelasma, subcutaneous xanthomata (Fig. 50–155), and tendon xanthomata, especially of the plantar extensor tendons (Helsinger and Rootwelt, 1969; Buchwald, 1970; Buchwald *et al.,* 1974c, 1974d). By analogy, a reduction in size of xanthomatous lesions should indicate that other tissue stores of lipid have been mobilized and excreted from the body. During a period of rapid mobilization, lipid transport may occur at the expense of a reduction in circulating lipid concentrations.

Angina Pectoris. Many individuals afflicted with angina pectoris have testified to a reduction in the frequency of their attacks or the complete disappearance of these symptoms during comparable effort after partial ileal bypass (Fritz and Walker, 1966; Swan and McGowan, 1968; Sodal *et al.,* 1970; Buchwald *et al.,* 1974c; Streuter, 1970). A survey of 101 patients by personal interviews (Buchwald *et al.,* 1974d) showed that of the 41 individuals who were angina pectoris–negative prior to the partial ileal bypass operation, none developed these symptoms subsequently. Of the 60 preoperative angina pectoris–positive patients, 7 per cent stated that they were worse; 27 per cent had no change; 23 per cent reported moderate improvement, as determined by a reduction in their use of

nitroglycerin; 18 per cent stated that they had marked improvement, as determined by their reduced use of nitroglycerin and their increased exercise capacity; and 25 per cent stated that they had complete remission of angina. Thus, 66 per cent of the patients with angina pectoris prior to operation experienced improvement postoperatively (Fig. 50–156). In certain of these patients, although not in all, there has been a concomitant improvement in exercise tolerance, free of the development of ischemic ST/T-wave changes, on the time- and grade-controlled treadmill exercise electrocardiogram. Although difficult to quantify, these findings may be indicative of an improvement in circulatory hemodynamics or tissue oxygen availability.

In vitro experiments utilizing rabbit blood demonstrate that oxygen extraction from blood with a high cholesterol content is significantly less than from blood with a low cholesterol content (Steinbach *et al.,* 1974). It seems that a barrier to oxygen diffusion

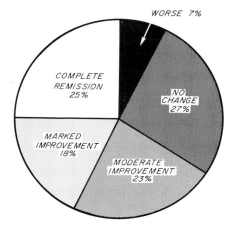

Total Improvement : 66%

Figure 50–156. Changes in angina pectoris following partial ileal bypass in 60 patients with angina at the time of their operation.

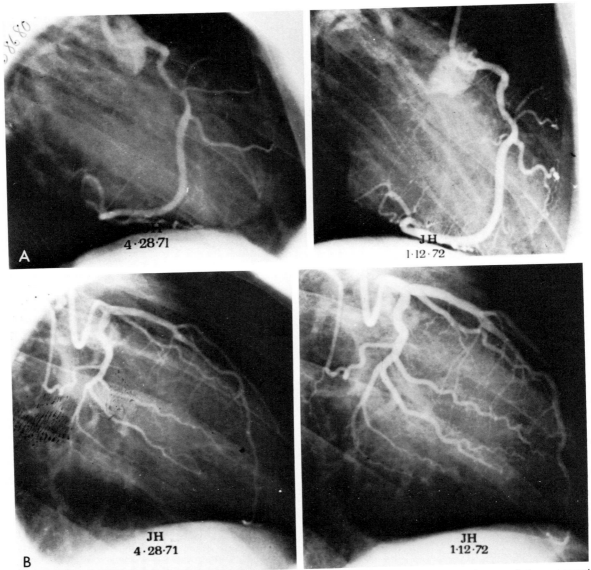

Figure 50–157. *A,* Right coronary arteriograms showing plaque regression following partial ileal bypass (*left,* preoperative film; *right,* film 1 year postoperatively). *B,* Left coronary arteriograms of the same patient preoperatively (*left*) and 1 year postoperatively (*right*).

resides within the red blood cell membrane when its cholesterol content is increased sufficiently because of hypercholesterolemia. The effect of this diffusion block is to shift the oxygen-hemoglobin dissociation curve to the left.

Serial Arteriography. Serial evaluation of coronary atherosclerotic plaque changes by serial arteriography yields data that are inconclusive (Baltaxe *et al.,* 1969; Rowe *et al.,* 1969; Knight *et al.,* 1972). A randomized control population for objective statistical comparison has not been available. One study (Knight *et al.,* 1972) indicates an apparent nonprogressive rate of coronary artery disease in 55 per cent of patients followed for up to 3 years. Apparent coronary arteriographic evidence of plaque regression was noted in three partial ileal bypass patients at 1 to 2 years postoperatively (Fig. 50–157).

Other Metabolic Operations Resulting in Lipid Lowering

The jejunoileal bypass operation for morbid exogenous obesity, as a rule, markedly lowers the plasma cholesterol and the plasma triglyceride concentrations (Payne *et al.,* 1963; Lewis *et al.,* 1962). Recently, we have compiled the differences in plasma lipids following jejunoileal bypass and gastric bypass for morbid obesity (Rucker *et al.,* 1981): there is a comparable reduction in triglycerides after both procedures (35 per cent), but the effect on the plasma cholesterol is markedly different, with only a 14 per cent reduction of plasma cholesterol 1 year after gastric bypass in contrast to a 42 per cent lowering after the jejunoileal bypass. Thus, for those obese individuals who also suffer from hyperlipidemia, jejunoileal bypass can have a salutary effect on their hyperlipidemia and, possibly, on their atherosclerosis.

End-to-side portacaval anastomosis also has been used clinically in the management of Type IIA homozygous hyperlipoproteinemic patients (Starzl *et al.*, 1973; Stein *et al.*, 1975; Cywes *et al.*, 1976) and in at least one heterozygous individual (Mieny, 1980). Recently, this innovative method has received only minimal attention; the procedure and modifications thereof deserve further careful laboratory study and supervised clinical trial.

Quite predictably, other intestinal, circulatory, or endocrine operations will be tried for lowering plasma lipids, especially if current clinical trials of the lipid-atherosclerosis hypothesis verify its postulates. Indeed, if the degree of benefit is exponentially proportional to the lipid lowering, a multiplicity of biochemical attacks on the involved metabolic pathways are sure to follow.

CONCLUSION

Partial ileal bypass is not proposed as the treatment of choice for that segment of the population with hyperlipidemic disease. It may be the treatment of choice for certain patients with hyperlipidemia. The available data clearly show that diet and drug therapy, singly or in combination, rarely achieve the lipid reductions reached by partial ileal bypass. Contrary to the results of drug therapy, the cholesterol-lowering effect of partial ileal bypass is universally lasting. Patients may or may not adhere to diet, may or may not take pills, but once the operation has been performed, its therapeutic effects are obligatory.

SELECTED REFERENCES

Buchwald, H., Moore, R. B., and Varco, R. L.: Surgical treatment of hyperlipidemia. Circulation, 49(Suppl. 1):1, 1974.

This three-part monograph, subtitled "Apologia, The Laboratory Experience, and Clinical Status of the Partial Ileal Bypass Operation," summarizes our thoughts and work in this field. It offers the reader the only appraisal by surgeons of diet and drug therapy of the hyperlipidemias, as well as an overview of the world experimental and clinical partial ileal bypass literature through 1974. This effort is written in the scientific journal format, as distinguished from textbook style. It details our methodology and offers tabulations of the data. The references provided include all of our publications on this subject, as well as the related publications of others, to the time of this report. It may be useful to the student interested in the laboratory experiments and the study of clinical cholesterol dynamics.

Fredrickson, D. S., Levy, R. I., and Lees, R. S.: Fat transport in lipoproteins: An integrated approach to mechanisms and disorders. N. Engl. J. Med., 276:32, 94, 148, 215, 273, 1967.

This five-part paper established the basis for the current typing nomenclature for the hyperlipoproteinemias. It broke the tradition of referring to lipid disorders as a function of the circulating lipid concentrations and placed them into a schema based on the carrier lipoproteins.

Katz, L. N., Stamler, J., and Pick, R.: Nutrition and Atherosclerosis. Philadelphia, Lea & Febiger, 1958.

This is a classic summary of the retrospective epidemiologic literature, resulting in the equating of the incidence rate of atherosclerosis, the saturated fat content of the diet, and the plasma cholesterol concentration in population groups throughout the world.

Moore, R. B., Buchwald, H., Varco, R. L., and the participants in the Program on Surgical Control of the Hyperlipidemias (POSCH): The effect of partial ileal bypass on plasma lipoproteins. Circulation, 62:469, 1980.

This article is a preliminary report of the sequential lipid findings in partial ileal bypass patients in the current Program on the Surgical Control of the Hyperlipidemias (POSCH). In addition to the lipid findings in this trial, an overall summary of the trial methods, parameters of analysis, and projections is given.

Younger, R. K., Shepard, G. H., Butts, W. H., and Scott, H. W., Jr.: Comparison of the protective effects of cholestyramine and ileal bypass in Rhesus monkeys on an atherogenic regimen. Surg. Forum, 20:101, 1969.

This is the only published experiment comparing the relative efficacy of cholestyramine and the partial ileal bypass operation in the reduction of circulating cholesterol levels and on the development of atherosclerotic plaque lesions. This paper clearly demonstrates that partial ileal bypass is twice as effective as cholestyramine in accomplishing these ends.

REFERENCES

Aldersberg, D.: Hypercholesterolemia with predisposition to atherosclerosis: Inborn error of lipid metabolism. Am. J. Med., 11:600, 1951.

Aldersberg, D., Parets, A. D., and Boas, E. P.: Genetics of atherosclerosis: Studies of families with xanthoma and unselected patients with coronary artery disease under the age of 50 years. J.A.M.A., 141:246, 1949.

American Heart Association: Heart Facts 1981. Dallas, Texas, American Heart Association Communications Division, 1981.

Balfour, J. F., and Kim, R.: Homozygous type II hyperlipoproteinemia treatment, partial ileal bypass in two children. J.A.M.A., 227:1145, 1974.

Baltaxe, H., Amplatz, K., Varco, R. L., and Buchwald, H.: Coronary arteriography in hypercholesterolemic patients. Am. J. Roentgenol., 105:784, 1969.

Beaumont, J. L., Carlson, L. A., Cooper, G. R., Fejfar, Z., Fredrickson, D. S., and Stasser, T.: Classification of hyperlipidemias and hyperlipoproteinemias. Bull. WHO, 43:891, 1970.

Berge, K. G., Achor, R. W. P., Christensen, N. A., Mason, H. L., and Barker, N. W.: Hypercholesteremia and nicotinic acid: A long-term study. Am. J. Med., 31:24, 1961.

Bergman, W.: Evolutionary aspects of the sterols. *In* Cholesterol. Edited by R. P. Cook. New York, Academic Press, 1958, p. 435.

Berkowitz, D.: Selective blood lipid reductions by newer pharmacological agents. Am. J. Cardiol., 12:834, 1963.

Best, M. M., and Duncan, C. H.: Effects of clofibrate and dextrothyroxine singly and in combination on serum lipids. Arch. Intern. Med., 118:97, 1966.

Bierenbaum, M. L., Fleischman, A. I., Green, D. P., Raichelson, R. I., Hayton, T., Watson, P. B., and Caldwell, A. B.: The five-year experience of modified fat diets on younger men with coronary heart disease. Circulation, 42:943, 1970.

Blacket, R. B., Woodhill, J., and Brown, W. D.: The effect of cholestyramine ("MK 135") on the serum cholesterol level in man. Med. J. Aust., 2:15, 1964.

Blankenhorn, D. H., Brooks, S. H., Slezer, M. S., and Barndt, R., Jr.: The rate of atherosclerosis change during treatment of hyperlipoproteinemia. Circulation, 57:355, 1978.

Boas, E. P., and Adlersberg, D.: Familial hypercholesterolemia (xanthomatosis) and atherosclerosis. J. Mt. Sinai Hosp. N.Y., *12*:84, 1945.

Boas, E. P., Parets, A. D., and Adlersberg, D.: Hereditary disturbance of cholesterol metabolism: Factor in genesis of atherosclerosis. Am. Heart J., *35*:611, 1948.

Booth, C. C., and Mollin, D. L.: The site of absorption of B_{12} in man. Lancet, *1*:18, 1959.

Boyd, G. S., and Oliver, M. F.: Effect of certain thyroxine analogues on the serum lipids in human subjects. J. Endocrinol., *21*:33, 1960.

Bressler, R., Nowlin, J., and Bogdonoff, M. D.: Treatment of hypercholesterolemia and hypertriglyceridemia by anion exchange resin. South. Med. J., *59*:1097, 1966.

Brown, H. B.: Personal communication, 1970.

Brown, H. B., and Green, J. G.: Diets suitable for reduction of serum cholesterol levels. The Cleveland Clinic Dietary Research Project. Cleve. Clin. Q., *29*:101, 1962.

Brown, M. S., and Goldstein, J. L.: Receptor-mediated control of cholesterol metabolism. Science, *191*:150, 1976.

Buchwald, H.: Alterations in the cutaneous lesions of the hyperlipidemias following partial ileal bypass. Dermatol. Dig., *9*:65, 1970.

Buchwald, H.: The effect of ileal bypass on atherosclerosis and hypercholesterolemia in the rabbit. Surgery, *58*:22, 1965a.

Buchwald, H.: Myocardial infarction in rabbits induced solely by a hypercholesterolemic diet. J. Atheroscler. Res., *5*:407, 1965b.

Buchwald, H.: Vitamin B_{12} absorption deficiency following bypass of the ileum. Am. J. Dig. Dis., *9*:755, 1964.

Buchwald, H., and Gebhard, R. L.: Effect of intestinal bypass on cholesterol absorption and blood levels in the rabbit. Am. J. Physiol., *207*:567, 1964.

Buchwald, H., and Gebhard, R. L.: Localization of bile salt absorption in vivo in the rabbit. Ann. Surg., *167*:191, 1968.

Buchwald, H., and Varco, R. L.: Human gastric secretory studies following distal small bowel bypass. Curr. Top. Surg. Res., *3*:409, 1971.

Buchwald, H., Coyle, J. J., and Varco, R. L.: Effect of small bowel bypass on gastric secretory function: Postintestinal exclusion hypersecretion, a phenomenon in search of a syndrome. Surgery, *75*:821, 1974a.

Buchwald, H., Gebhard, R. L., and Varco, R. L.: Relative secretion of cholesterol-4-^{14}C in the bile and upper and lower small intestinal washings of the bile fistula rabbit. Surgery, *75*:266, 1974b.

Buchwald, H., Moore, R. B., and Frantz, I. D., Jr.: Serum uric acid, carotene and vitamin A, proteins, sugar, and electrolytes before and after partial ileal bypass for hyperlipidemia. Circulation, *40*(Suppl. 3):4, 1969.

Buchwald, H., Moore, R. B., and Varco, R. L.: Surgical treatment of hyperlipidemia. Circulation, *49*(Suppl. 1):1, 1974c.

Buchwald, H., Moore, R. B., and Varco, R. L.: Ten years clinical experience with partial ileal bypass in management of the hyperlipidemias. Ann. Surg., *180*:384, 1974d.

Buchwald, H., Moore, R. B., Bertish, J., and Varco, R. L.: Effect of ileal bypass on cholesterol levels, atherosclerosis and growth in the infant rabbit. Ann. Surg., *175*:311, 1972.

Buchwald, H., Moore, R. B., Lee, G. B., Frantz, I. D., Jr., and Varco, R. L.: Combined dietary, surgical, and bile salt binding resin therapy in the treatment of hypercholesterolemia. Arch. Surg., *97*:275, 1968.

Casdorph, H. R.: Hypercholesterolemia—treatment with cholestyramine, a bile acid sequestering resin. Calif. Med., *106*:293, 1967.

Castelli, W. P., Doyle, J. T., Gordon, T., Hames, C. G., Hjortland, M. C., Holley, S. B., Kagan, A., and Zukel, W.: HDL cholesterol and other lipids in coronary heart disease. The cooperative lipoprotein phenotyping study. Circulation, *55*:767, 1977.

Chapman, J. M., Goerke, L. S., Dixon, W., Loveland, D. B., and Phillips, E.: The clinical status of a population group in Los Angeles under observation for two to three years. Am. J. Public Health, *47*(Suppl. 2):33, 1957.

Charman, R. C., Matthews, L. B., and Braeuler, C.: Nicotinic acid in the treatment of hypercholesterolemia. Angiology, *23*:29, 1972.

Clot, J. P., Rouffy, J., Loeper, J., and Mercadier, M.: Dérivation iléal, thérapeutique, chirurgicale des hypercholesterolemies pures majeures (à propos de deux observations). Chirurgie, *97*:57, 1971.

Connor, W. E.: Measures to reduce the serum lipid levels in coronary heart disease. Med. Clin. North Am., *52*:1249, 1968.

Cornfield, J.: Joint dependence of risk of coronary heart disease on serum cholesterol and systolic blood pressure: Discriminant function analysis. Fed. Proc., *21*:58, 1962.

Coronary Drug Project Research Group: Clofibrate and niacin in coronary heart disease. J.A.M.A., *231*:360, 1975.

Coyle, J. J., Varco, R. L., and Buchwald, H.: Vitamin B_{12} absorption following human intestinal bypass surgery. Am. J. Dig. Dis., *22*:1069, 1977.

Cywes, S., Davis, M. R. Q., Louw, J. H., et al.: Portacaval shunt in two patients with homozygous type II hyperlipoproteinaemia. South Afr. Med. J., *50*:239, 1976.

Davignon, J.: The lipid hypothesis: Pathophysiological basis. Arch. Surg., *113*:28, 1978.

Dawber, T. R., Moore, F. E., and Mann, G. V.: Coronary heart disease in the Framingham study. Am. J. Public Health, *47*(Suppl. 2):4, 1957.

Dayton, S., and Pierce, M. L.: Diet high in unsaturated fat. Minn. Med., *52*:1237, 1969.

Doree, C.: The occurrence and distribution of cholesterol and allied bodies in the animal kingdom. Biochem. J., *4*:72, 1909.

Doyle, J. T., Heslin, A. S., Hilleboe, H. E., Formel, P. F., and Korns, R. F.: A prospective study of degenerative cardiovascular disease in Albany: Report of three years' experience. I. Ischemic heart disease. Am. J. Public Health, *47*(Suppl. 2):25, 1957.

Drugs which lower the blood lipids. Med. Lett. Drugs Ther., *5*:81, 1963.

Eder, H. A.: Drugs used in the prevention and treatment of atherosclerosis. *In* The Pharmacological Basis of Therapeutics. 3rd Ed. Edited by L. S. Goodman and A. Gilman. New York, The Macmillan Company, 1965.

Eisalo, A., Ahrenberg, P., and Nikkila, E. A.: Treatment of hyperlipidemia with d-thyroxine. Acta Med. Scand., *173*:639, 1963.

Enos, W. F., Holmes, R. H., and Beyer, J.: Coronary disease among United States soldiers killed in action in Korea: Preliminary report. J.A.M.A., *152*:1090, 1953.

Evans, D. W., Turner, S. M., and Ghosh, P.: Feasibility of long-term plasma-cholesterol reduction by diet. Lancet, *1*:172, 1972.

Fallon, H. J., and Woods, J. W.: Response of hyperlipoproteinemia to cholestyramine resin. J.A.M.A., *204*:1161, 1968.

Five-year Study by a Group of Physicians of the Newcastle-upon-Tyne Region: Trial of clofibrate in the treatment of ischaemic heart disease. Br. Med. J., *4*:767, 1971.

Frantz, I. D., Jr., Dawson, E. A., Kuba, K., Brewer, E. R., Gatewood, L. D., and Bartsch, G. E.: The Minnesota Coronary Survey: Effect of diet on cardiovascular events and deaths. Circulation, *52*:4, 1975.

Frederick, P. L., Sizer, J. S., and Osborne, M. P.: Relation of massive bowel resection to gastric secretion. N. Engl. J. Med., *272*:509, 1965.

Fredrickson, D. S., Levy, R. I., and Lees, R. S.: Fat transport in lipoproteins: An integrated approach to mechanisms and disorders. N. Engl. J. Med., *276*:32, 94, 148, 215, 273, 1967.

Fritz, S. H., and Walker, W. J.: Ileal bypass in the control of intractable hypercholesterolemia. Am. Surg., *32*:691, 1966.

Gebhard, R. L., and Buchwald, H.: Cholesterol absorption after reversal of the upper and lower halves of the small intestine. Surgery, *67*:474, 1970.

Gofman, J. W., Jones, H. B., Lindgren, F. T., Lyon, T. P., Elliot, H. A., and Strisower, B.: Blood lipids and human atherosclerosis. Circulation, *2*:161, 1950.

Goldstein, J. L., and Brown, M. S.: Lipoprotein receptors, cholesterol metabolism and atherosclerosis. Arch. Pathol., *99*:181, 1975.

Goldstein, J. L., Schrott, H. G., Hazzard, W. R., Bierman, E. L., and Motulsky, A. G.: Genetic analysis of lipid levels in 176 families and delineation of a new inherited disorder, combined hyperlipidemia. J. Clin. Invest., 52:1544, 1973.

Gomes, M. M., Kottke, B. A., Bernatz, P., and Titus, J. L.: Effect of ileal bypass on aortic atherosclerosis of white Carneau pigeons. Surgery, 70:353, 1971.

Goodman, D. S., and Noble, R. P.: Turnover of plasma cholesterol in man. J. Clin. Invest., 47:231, 1968.

Gordon, T., Castelli, W. P., Hjortland, M. C., Kannel, W. B., and Dawber, T. R.: High density lipoprotein as a protective factor against coronary heart disease. Framingham Study. Am. J. Med., 62:707, 1977.

Green, J. G., Brown, H. B., Meredith, A. P., and Page, I. H.: Use of fat-modified foods for serum cholesterol reduction. J.A.M.A., 183:5, 1963.

Grundy, S. M., Ahrens, E. H., Jr., and Salen, G.: Interruption of the enterohepatic circulation of bile acids in man: Comparative effects of cholestyramine and ileal exclusion on cholesterol metabolism. J. Lab. Clin. Med., 78:94, 1971.

Hashim, S. A., and Van Itallie, T. B.: Cholestyramine resin therapy for hypercholesteremia. J.A.M.A., 192:289, 1965.

Heffernan, A., Hickey, N., Mulcahy, R., and Fitzgerald, O.: The chemotherapy of hypercholesterolaemia. Acta Cardiol., 24:47, 1969.

Helsinger, N., Jr., and Rootwelt, K.: Partial ileal bypass for surgical treatment of hypercholesterolemia. Nord. Med., 82:1409, 1969.

Heydenreich, L. H.: Leonardo da Vinci. New York and Basel, Macmillan-Holbein, 1954, Vols. I and II.

Howard, A. N., and Hyams, D. E.: Combined use of clofibrate and cholestyramine or DEAE Sephadex in hypercholesterolemia. Br. Med. J., 3:25, 1971.

Hunninghake, D. B., Tucker, D. R., and Azarnoff, D. L.: Long-term effects of clofibrate (Atromid-S) on serum lipids in man. Circulation, 39:675, 1969.

Jeffcoate, T. N. A., Miller, J., Roos, R. F., and Tindall, V. R.: Puerperal thromboembolism in relation to the inhibition of lactation by oestrogen therapy. Br. Med. J., 4:19, 1968.

Jepson, E. M., Fahmy, M. F. I., Torrens, P. E., and Billimoria, J. D.: Treatment of essential hyperlipidaemia. Lancet, 2:1315, 1969.

Jolliffe, N., Maslansky, E., Rudensey, F., Simon, M., and Faulkner, A.: Dietary control of serum cholesterol in clinical practice. Circulation, 24:1415, 1961.

Joslin, E. P.: Arteriosclerosis and diabetes. Ann. Clin. Med., 5:1061, 1926–1927.

Katz, L. N., Stamler, J., and Pick, R.: Nutrition and Atherosclerosis. Philadelphia, Lea & Febiger, 1958.

Keys, A.: Coronary heart disease in seven countries. Circulation, 41(Suppl. 1):1, 1970.

Khachadurian, A. K., and Demirjian, Z. N.: Cholestyramine therapy in patients homozygous for familial hypercholesterolemia. J. Atheroscler. Res., 8:177, 1968.

Knight, L., Scheibel, R., Amplatz, K., Varco, R. L., and Buchwald, H.: Radiographic appraisal of the Minnesota partial ileal bypass study. Surg. Forum, 23:141, 1972.

Krasno, L. R., and Kidera, G. J.: Clofibrate in coronary heart disease: Effect on morbidity and mortality. J.A.M.A., 219:845, 1972.

Kuller, L., Neaton, J., Caggiula, A., Flavo-Gerhard, L.: Primary prevention of heart attacks: The multiple risk factor intervention trial. Am. J. Epidemiol., 112:185, 1980.

Kuo, P. T.: Dietary treatment of hyperlipidemia. Mod. Treat., 6:1328, 1969.

Langer, T., and Levy, R. I.: Acute muscular syndrome associated with administration of clofibrate. N. Engl. J. Med., 279:856, 1968.

Leren, P.: The effect of plasma cholesterol-lowering diet in male survivors of myocardial infarction. Bull. N.Y. Acad. Med., 44:1012, 1968.

Levy, R. L.: Dietary and drug treatment of primary hyperlipoproteinemia. Ann. Intern. Med., 77:267, 1972.

Levy, R. L., Quarfardt, S. H., and Brown, W. V.: The efficacy of clofibrate (CPIB) in familial hyperlipoproteinemias. Adv. Exp. Med. Biol., 4:377, 1969.

Lewis, L. A., Brown, H. B., and Page, I. H.: Ten years' dietary treatment of primary hyperlipidemia. Geriatrics, 25:64, 1970.

Lewis, L. A., Brown, H. B., and Page, I. H.: Ten years' treatment of hyperlipidemia. Circulation, 38:128, 1968.

Lewis, L. A., Turnbull, R. B., and Page, I. H.: Short-circuiting of the small intestine. J.A.M.A., 182:77, 1962.

McGandy, R. B., Hegsted, D. M., and Stare, F. J.: Dietary fats, carbohydrates and atherosclerotic vascular disease. N. Engl. J. Med., 277:186, 242, 1967.

McNamara, J. J., Molot, M. A., Stremple, J. F., and Cutting, R. T.: Coronary artery disease in combat casualties in V J.A.M.A., 216:1185, 1971.

Mieny, K.: Personal communication, 1980.

Miettinen, T. A.: Personal communication, 1970.

Miettinen, T. A.: Commentary. In Proceedings of the Second International Symposium on Atherosclerosis. Edited by R. J. Jones. New York, Springer-Verlag, 1970.

Mishkel, M. A.: Diagnosis and management of the patient with xanthomatosis: An experience with thirty-five cases. Q. J. Med., 36:107, 1967.

Moore, R. B., Frantz, I. D., Jr., and Buchwald, H.: Changes in cholesterol pool size, turnover rate, and fecal bile acid and sterol excretion after partial ileal bypass in hypercholesterolemic patients. Surgery, 65:98, 1969.

Moore, R. B., Frantz, I. D., Jr., Varco, R. L., and Buchwald, H.: Cholesterol dynamics after partial ileal bypass. In Proceedings of the Second International Symposium on Atherosclerosis. Edited by R. J. Jones. New York, Springer-Verlag, 1970.

Moore, R. B., Buchwald, H., Varco, R. L., and the participants in the Program on the Surgical Control of the Hyperlipidemias (POSCH): The effect of partial ileal bypass on plasma lipoproteins. Circulation, 62:469, 1980.

Morgan, J., and Moore, R. D.: Personal communication, 1970.

Muellies, P. S., Gartside, P. S., Gladfelter, L., Vink, P., Guy, G., Schonfeld, G., and Glueck, C. J.: Effects of probucol on plasma cholesterol, high and low density lipoprotein cholesterol and apolipoproteins A₁ and A₂ in adults with primary familial hypercholesterolemia. Metabolism, 29:956, 1980.

National Diet Heart Study: Circulation, 37(Suppl. 1):1, 1968.

Nordøy, A., and Gjone, E.: Treatment of essential hypercholesterolemia with clofibrate and nicotinic acid. Acta Med. Scand., 188:487, 1970.

Nygaard, K., Helsinger, N., and Rootwelt, K.: Adaptation of vitamin B₁₂ absorption after ileal bypass. Scand. J. Gastroenterol., 5:349, 1970.

Osborne, M. P., Frederick, P. L., Sizer, J. S., Blair, D., Cole, P., and Thum, W.: Mechanism of gastric hypersecretion following massive intestinal resection: Clinical and experimental observations. Ann. Surg., 164:622, 1966.

Parsons, W. B., Jr.: Studies of nicotinic acid use in hypercholesteremia: Changes in hepatic function, carbohydrate tolerance, and uric acid metabolism. Arch. Intern. Med., 107:653, 1961a.

Parsons, W. B., Jr.: Treatment of hypercholesterolemia by nicotinic acid: Progress report with review of studies regarding mechanism of action. Arch. Intern. Med., 107:639, 1961b.

Payne, J. H., DeWind, L. T., and Commons, R. R.: Metabolic observations in patients with jejunocolic shunts. Am. J. Surg., 106:273, 1963.

Report from the Committee of Principal Investigators: A cooperative trial in the primary prevention of ischemic heart disease using clofibrate. Br. Heart J., 40:1069, 1978.

Report from the Committee of Principal Investigators: WHO cooperative trial on primary prevention of ischaemic heart disease using clofibrate to lower serum cholesterol: Mortality follow-up. Lancet, 2:379, 1980.

Report of a Research Committee to the Medical Research Council: Controlled trial of soya bean oil in myocardial infarction. Lancet, 2:693, 1968.

Report of a Research Committee of the Scottish Society of Physicians: Ischaemic heart disease: A secondary prevention trial using clofibrate. Br. Med. J., 4:775, 1971.

Riesen, W. F., Keller, M., and Mardasini, R.: Probucol in hypercholesterolemia. A double blind study. Atherosclerosis, 36:201, 1980.

Rinzler, S. H.: Primary prevention of coronary heart disease by diet. Bull. N.Y. Acad. Med., 44:936, 1968.

Rosenthal, S. R.: Studies in atherosclerosis: Chemical, experimental and morphological; roles of cholesterol metabolism, blood pressure and structure of aorta; fat angle of aorta (F.A.A.), and infiltration—expression theory of lipoid deposit. Arch. Pathol., 18:473, 1934.

Rowe, G. G., Young, W., and Wasserburger, R. H.: The effect of reduced serum cholesterol on human coronary atherosclerosis. Circulation, 40(Suppl. 3):22, 1969.

Rucker, R. D., Jr., Goldenberg, F., Varco, R. L., and Buchwald, H.: Lipid effects of obesity operations. J. Surg. Res., 30:229, 1981.

Ruffer, M. A.: On arterial lesions found in Egyptian mummies. J. Pathol. Bacteriol., 15:453, 1911.

Russ, E. M., Eder, H. A., and Barr, D. P.: Influence of gonadal hormones on protein-lipid relationships in human plasma. Am. J. Med., 19:4, 1955.

Samuel, P.: Appraisal and reappraisal of cardiac therapy. Drug treatment of hyperlipidemia. Am. Heart J., 100:573, 1980.

Schwartz, H., and Kohn, J. L.: Lipoid nephrosis: Clinical and pathologic study based on 15 years' observation with special reference to prognosis. Am. J. Dis. Child., 49:579, 1935.

Schwartz, M. Z., Varco, R. L., and Buchwald, H.: Liver function and morphology following distal ileal excision in the rabbit. Surg. Forum, 22:355, 1971.

Scott, H. W., Jr., Stephenson, S. E., Jr., Younger, R., Carlisle, R. B., and Turney, S. W.: Prevention of experimental atherosclerosis by ileal bypass: Twenty-percent cholesterol diet and I-131 induced hypothyroidism in dogs. Ann. Surg., 163:795, 1966.

Shattock, S. G.: A report on the pathological condition of the aorta of King Memephtah, traditionally regarded as the pharaoh of the Exodus. Proc. R. Soc. Med. Lond., 2:122, 1908.

Shepard, G. H., Wimberly, J. E., Younger, R. K., Stephenson, S. E., Jr., and Scott, H. W., Jr.: Effects of bypass of the distal third of the small intestine on experimental hypercholesterolemia and atherosclerosis in Rhesus monkeys. Surg. Forum, 19:302, 1968.

Smith, G. E.: Cited by Long, E. R.: The development of our knowledge of arteriosclerosis. In Arteriosclerosis. Edited by E. V. Cowdry. New York, The Macmillan Co., 1933.

Sodal, G., Gjertsen, K. T., and Schrumpf, A.: Surgical treatment of hypercholesterolemia. Acta Chir. Scand., 136:671, 1970.

Special Communication: Coronary Drug Project. Findings leading to further modifications of its protocol with respect to d-thyroxine. J.A.M.A., 220:996, 1972.

Special Communication: Coronary Drug Project. Initial findings leading to modifications of its research protocol. J.A.M.A., 214:1303, 1970.

Stamler, J., Pick, R., Katz, L. N., Pick, A., Kaplan, B. M.,

Berkson, D. M., and Century, D.: Effectiveness of estrogens for therapy of myocardial infarction in middle-age men. J.A.M.A., 183:632, 1963.

Starzl, T. E., Chase, H. P., Putnam, C. W., and Porter, K. A.: Portacaval shunt in hyperlipoproteinaemia. Lancet, 2:940, 1973.

Stein, E. A., Mieny, C., Spitz, L., et al.: Portacaval shunt in four patients with homozygous hypercholesterolemia. Lancet, 1:832, 1975.

Steinbach, J. H., Blackshear, P. L., Jr., Varco, R. L., and Buchwald, H.: High blood cholesterol reduces in vitro blood oxygen delivery. J. Surg. Res., 16:134, 1974.

Steinberg, D.: Chemotherapeutic control of serum lipid levels. Trans. N.Y. Acad. Sci., 24:704, 1962.

Stern, M. P.: The recent decline in ischemic heart disease mortality. Ann. Intern. Med., 91:630, 1979.

Streuter, M.: Personal communication, 1970.

Strisower, E. H., Adamson, G., and Strisower, B.: Treatment of hyperlipidemias. Am. J. Med., 45:488, 1968a.

Strisower, E. H., Kradjian, R., Nichols, A. V., Coggiola, E., and Tsai, J.: Effect of ileal bypass on serum lipoproteins in essential hypercholesterolemia. J. Atheroscler. Res., 8:525, 1968b.

Swan, D. M., and McGowan, J. M.: Ileal bypass in hypercholesterolemia associated with heart disease. Am. J. Surg., 116:81, 1968.

Symposium on Atromid: Proceedings of a conference held in Buxton (England) June 5–6, 1963. J. Atheroscler. Res., 3:341, 1963.

The Lipid Research Clinics Program: Coronary Primary Prevention Trial: Design and implementation. J. Chronic Dis., 32:609, 1979.

Turpeinen, O., Miettinen, M., Karvonen, M. J., Roine, P., Pekkarinen, M., Lehtosuo, E. J., and Alivirta, P.: Blood lipids and primary coronary events. Minn. Med., 52:1247, 1969.

United States Department of Health, Education, and Welfare, National Center for Health Statistics. Vital Statistics of the United States. Rockville, Maryland, U.S. Government Printing Office, 1979.

Vikrot, O., Beslin, R., and Oldfelt, C. O.: Influence of nicotinic acid on individual plasma phospholipids in hypercholesterolemia. Acta Med. Scand., 190:133, 1971.

Vogel, J.: The Pathological Anatomy of the Human Body. Philadelphia, Lea and Blanchard, 1847.

Wilkinson, C. F., Jr., Hand, C. A., and Fliegelman, M. T.: Essential familial cholesterolemia. Ann. Intern. Med., 29:671, 1948.

Younger, R. K., Shepard, G. H., Butts, W. H., and Scott, H. W., Jr.: Comparison of the protective effects of cholestyramine and ileal bypass in Rhesus monkeys on an atherogenic regimen. Surg. Forum, 20:101, 1969.

VI   DIETARY AND PHARMACOLOGIC MANAGEMENT OF ATHEROSCLEROSIS

JAMES C. A. FUCHS

Despite the encouraging decrease in the mortality rate from ischemic heart disease (Levy, 1981; Stern, 1981), atherosclerosis remains a leading cause of death and morbidity in the United States. The prevalence of this condition is so significant that considerable resources have been expended to obtain objective information about its origin, development, and treatment. As these data have accrued, certain topics emerge as important issues for understanding the disease and for treating or preventing its consequences. Prominent among these subjects are the role of nutrition in the origin and evolution of atherosclerosis and the place of pharmacologic therapy for patients with this disorder. The available information will be reviewed in this section in an effort to clarify the methods of dietary and pharmacologic management and the indications for their use in the treatment of vascular atherosclerosis.

Over the past 30 years, the use of vascular surgical procedures to compensate for arterial disease has risen considerably. During this time, evidence has accumulated to establish that atherosclerosis evolves over a considerable period before symptoms occur (Bourassa *et al.*, 1973; Griffith *et al.*, 1973) and has the potential to progress, even after surgical intervention (Henderson and Rowe, 1973; Imparato *et al.*, 1972). This is reinforced by the follow-up of patients with coronary artery bypass grafts and by frequent angiography and noninvasive assessment of patients with vascular disease. Any patient with atherosclerosis must be considered to have the potential for enlargement of present lesions or development of the disease in a previously normal site.

Extremely important issues are whether this process can be arrested and if regression can occur. There is ample evidence that the pathologic changes of atherosclerosis can be reduced or even cleared in experimental animals (Henahan, 1981; Malinow, 1980) by diet (Avoy *et al.*, 1965), drugs (Malinow *et al.*, 1978), or operation (Subbiah *et al.*, 1978). Evidence is accumulating that such changes may occur in humans as well (Blankenhorn, 1981; Malinow, 1981; Rafflenbeul *et al.*, 1979). Although it appears that some lesions are resistant to regression (DePalma *et al.*, 1977), the possibility that this disease might be lessened underscores the importance of understanding the factors that are involved in its development. Surgeons performing vascular procedures in patients with atherosclerosis should be familiar with this information in order to give patients appropriate instruction in matters that may influence the course of their disease.

ATHEROSCLEROSIS

Pathology

Anatomic pathologists in the eighteenth and nineteenth centuries provided thorough descriptions of atherosclerosis, and for a considerable length of time, investigation was limited to this discipline (Fig. 50–158). In 1755, Albrecht von Haller emphasized the soft character of the lesion, and the Greek term for gruel, *athere,* was incorporated into the phase "atherosclerosis" by Marchand in 1904. Rokitansky and Virchow described the appearance and distribution of atherosclerotic lesions, and each pathologist hypothesized an origin of the process (Cowdry, 1933).

Although gross vascular lesions appeared to be the result of aging, significant discrepancies were found in the age-related incidence of this disease. More comprehensive examination revealed early lesions in a young, otherwise healthy population (Strong and Guzman, 1980). On the other hand, the disease may be minimal in some elderly individuals, thereby emphasizing that it is not an inevitable consequence

of aging. In fact, its early appearance and variable course speak for a prolonged pathogenesis in selected individuals. As a consequence, enthusiasm arose for a search for underlying etiologic factors, an appeal that has led to extensive epidemiologic surveys.

The distribution of lesions within the vascular tree has been established by anatomic studies (McGill, 1968; Schwartz and Mitchell, 1962). Raised yellow lesions or plaques, often with ulcerated or thrombosed surfaces, are familiar pathologic entities to the cardiovascular surgeon, as they regularly present during procedures on the carotid, coronary, aortic, femoral and tibial vessels. In man, the disease is limited primarily to the tunica intima of the artery and to the adjacent portion of media. It is just this localization that permits removal of the atheromatous portions of arteries by the surgical procedure of endarterectomy, with retention of enough normal vessel for sufficient structural integrity.

Histologic study of atherosclerotic lesions has provided a wealth of pertinent information. Four microscopic features in particular merit consideration (Fig. 50–159).

Tissue proliferation appears to be present in all lesions. The stimulus for this process remains unclear, but extensive investigation suggests that this basic reaction involves differentiation and duplication of intrinsic smooth muscle cells (Ross, 1981, Wissler, 1968). As well as cellular proliferation, increased amounts of collagen and ground substance are associated with this response (Wolinsky, 1973). The resulting tissue build-up is largely responsible for the intrusion of the atherosclerotic plaque on the vascular lumen.

Tissue disruption, particularly of the elastic fibers, occurs in atherosclerotic disease. The structural disintegration of the vessel wall produces a loss of tensile strength and elasticity that may contribute to the vascular dilatation seen in atherosclerotic vessels.

Lipid infiltration, both intracellular (Smith and Slater, 1973) and extracellular (Adams, 1973), remains a keystone of the histopathology of atherosclerosis. The cholesterol clefts of the plaques were among the earliest identified components of this disease (Cowdry, 1933). In fact, free cholesterol and esterified cholesterol are the major lipid constituents of the plaque (Smith and Slater, 1973). The observations that lipid content increases with the severity of disease and that submicroscopic lipid in the form of immunologically intact lipoproteins is present in early lesions (Adams, 1973) have implicated these compounds in the etiology of the atherosclerosis (Abdulla *et al.*, 1967).

Tissue reaction adjacent to areas of atherosclerosis takes the form of platelet build-up and thrombosis at the blood-plaque interface or of infiltration by inflammatory cells in the periplaque region. The presence of thrombus on a plaque may be secondary to ulceration of the endothelial surface. However, opinions vary as to whether the ulceration stimulates the thrombus or occurs as a result of endothelial injury secondary to layering of coagulated blood products

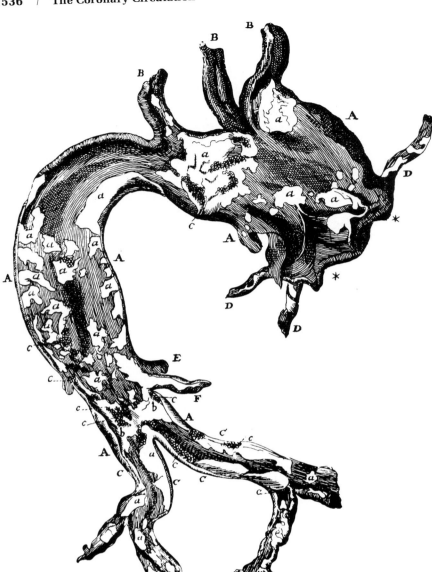

Figure 50–158. The aorta of Johann Wepfer who died in 1695 (Cowdry, 1933). This descriptive portrayal reveals the knowledge of diffuse vascular involvement that was available to the early anatomic pathologist.

(Kinlough-Rathbone and Mustard, 1981). Injected lipids will incite an inflammatory response (Abdulla *et al.*, 1967), and accumulation of these agents may be responsible for the cellular inflammation accompanying this disease. These two features—intravascular thrombus and perivascular inflammation with fibrosis—are frequently problems encountered by surgeons during the exposure and opening of atherosclerotic vessels.

Pathogenesis

The aforementioned pathologic changes have been important elements in the construction of hypotheses explaining the etiology and course of atherosclerosis. Theories of atherogenesis must take into account such diverse factors as hypertensive pressure, hemodynamic shear stress, vascular permeability, platelet and thrombus encrustation, alterations in lipid content, changes in biochemical metabolism, protein accumulations within diseased arterial tissue, endothelial and smooth muscle cell replication, mutagenic agents, hypoxia, and inflammation. The necessity to explain so many complicated factors has encouraged numerous hypotheses for the pathogenesis of arterial atherosclerosis. Although each explanation for the etiology and progression of arterial lesions is usually presented as a self-contained concept, there is considerable overlap in the elements of these theories. For practical purposes, these multiple hypotheses can be classed into three groups: (1) response to injury, (2) reaction to serum lipids, and (3) mutagenic transformation of vascular tissue into freely replicating tumor-like colonies of cells.

The Injury Hypothesis. The pragmatic approach of explaining atherosclerosis with an injury hypothesis began as early as 1852 with Rokitansky. Modified over

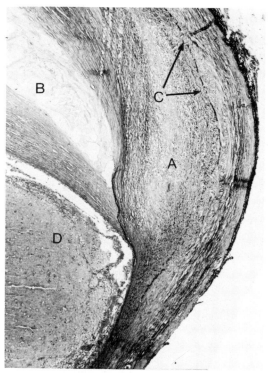

Figure 50–159. Atherosclerosis involving the right coronary artery of a 41-year-old man with Type II hyperlipidemia. Tissue proliferation within the intimal region *(A)* intrudes into the lumen, and the cholesterol clefts of lipid deposition are present *(B)*. The intrinsic structures of elastic fibers are disrupted *(C)*, and thrombosis has occurred within the lumen *(D)*.

the years by increasingly sophisticated concepts of different sources of injury and knowledge of the tissue response to such noxious forces, this hypothesis remains the subject of much recent investigation (Bomberger *et al.*, 1981; Fry, 1976; Ross, 1981; Ross and Glomset, 1976; Schwartz *et al.*, 1981). In simplistic terms, this approach starts with an endothelial injury—in the form of hypertensive pressure, hemodynamic shearing forces, thrombosis, humoral stimuli, chemical irritation, immunologic trauma, hypoxia, or lipid build-up. The injury alters endothelial integrity or permeability and elicits a multiphasic response that leads to the mature atherosclerotic lesion or plaque. The important proliferative response, basic to all lesions, occurs in the medial and subintimal smooth muscle cells (Wissler, 1968). Platelets adherent to the site of endothelial injury or desquamation have been found to release growth factors that appear to initiate this critical process (Ross and Vogel, 1978). Thus, the complex interaction of platelets, clotting factors, and thrombus is involved to some degree in this explanation of atherogenesis (Ross, 1981) (Fig. 50–160). This response of smooth muscle cell replication produces the histologic picture of intimal hyperplasia that is so often seen postoperatively after vascular grafting procedures (McCann *et al.*, 1979; Ross and Glomset, 1976) and endarterectomy (Imparato *et al.*, 1972). Smooth muscle cell proliferation may regress if its initiating factors are reversed, or it may evolve into

the mature lesions of occlusive arterial disease (Fig. 50–160).

As an atherosclerotic plaque matures or progresses, there is a fibrous transformation of the vascular wall. Collagen synthesis is enhanced in these areas (McCullagh and Ehrhart, 1974), and glycopeptides accumulate (Richardson *et al.*, 1980). The net result of such changes is a thickened and scarred arterial wall that induces local hypoxia by interrupting normal diffusion and transport of oxygen through the vasa vasorum (Adams and Bayliss, 1969). Hypoxic alterations in cellular metabolism can be demonstrated in plaques (Gainer and Chisolm, 1974) and may be responsible for necrosis and inflammation so commonly seen in mature lesions.

The Lipid Hypothesis. The lipid hypothesis has many features in common with the process just described. However, the emphasis in this explanation is on the pivotal role of lipids or lipoproteins in the initiation and development of atherosclerosis. Such substances can begin and maintain the early stages of atherosclerosis (Ross and Harker, 1976). The relation to the injury hypothesis is demonstrated by the fact that certain lipoproteins stimulate replication of smooth muscle cells and are in turn broken down into component lipids by intracellular enzymes (Deduve, 1974).

Serum lipids and lipoproteins can be demonstrated in the regions of developing plaques in amounts corresponding to the severity of the disease (Kao and Wissler, 1965; Smith and Slater, 1973). With advanced

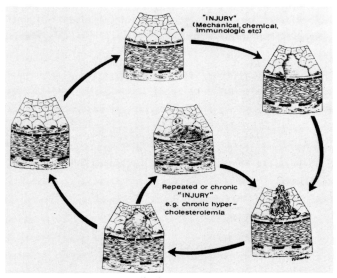

Figure 50–160. Proposed description of vascular cellular response to injury. Injury from any noxious stimulus leads to desquamation of endothelial cells. Platelets adhere to the denuded surface and release substances that stimulate proliferation of myointimal and medial smooth muscle cells. With no further injury, this process can resolve, leaving a slightly thickened intima lined with endothelium. On repeated injury, the proliferating smooth muscle cells undergo further degeneration and accumulate the intracellular and extracellular lipids and ground substance associated with mature atherosclerotic lesions. (From Ross, R., and Glomset, J. A.: Pathogenesis of atherosclerosis. N. Engl. J. Med., *295*:369, 420, 1976.)

lesions, the lipid accumulation is predominantly cholesterol, particularly in its esterified form (Lofland *et al.*, 1968). The massive deposition of cholesterol has lent support to the importance of this agent in atherogenesis (Frantz and Moore, 1969; McGill, 1979). Distinct changes in arterial wall metabolism have been documented in atherosclerosis, favoring the production of certain cholesteryl esters (Dayton and Hashimoto, 1970; Smith, 1977). These products of altered metabolism are small in quantity compared with imbibed serum lipids, yet they are known to elicit distinct cellular responses (Abdulla *et al.*, 1967). The fibrosis and inflammation found in atherosclerotic plaques may be a response to the build-up of toxic products of altered metabolism. Such reactions can lead to fully mature fibrous plaques. The lipid theory considers mature atherosclerosis to be the direct result of serum lipids, in particular cholesterol and low-density lipoproteins. The relationship of these entities to diet and lipid metabolism and their implication to the treatment of atherosclerosis will be discussed later.

The Monoclonal Hypothesis. The monoclonal hypothesis takes a novel view of atherogenesis. This theory regards each arterial plaque as a benign tumor arising from a single smooth muscle cell (Benditt, 1977). Proof of this concept lies in the monotypic nature of enzyme patterns in plaque tissue from heterozygous individuals as contrasted to the bimorphic values seen in undiseased arterial wall (Person *et al.*, 1977). The initiating factor for smooth muscle cell transformation is considered a mutagen, and progression of the replication is brought about by conditions that stimulate cell proliferation. The maturing process, resulting in fibrosis, necrosis, calcification, and thrombosis, is the same as in other hypotheses.

In overview, there are marked similarities in these three approaches and significant overlap appears in the detailed explanations for atherogenesis. This duplication arises from the fact that certain features of atherosclerosis are so consistent that they must be part of any comprehensive hypothesis. In addition, these explanations must take into account the major factors that large-scale epidemiologic surveys have found to be associated with atherosclerotic vascular disease.

Epidemiology

For the past 30 years, extensive studies have been conducted on worldwide populations in order to determine the features associated with atherosclerotic vascular disease (Keys, 1980; Wright and Frederickson, 1973). A mass of information has been accumulated through retrospective and ongoing prospective analyses. These have revealed a universal difference in the incidence of atherosclerosis, as manifested by coronary heart disease. For example, a 10-fold difference in the incidence of coronary disease exists between middle-aged men in parts of Northern Europe and men of the same age group in the Mediterranean area (Blackburn, 1970).

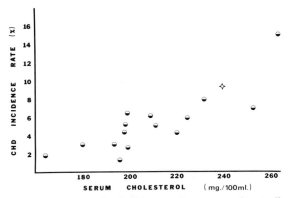

Figure 50–161. The incidence of coronary heart disease (CHD) in national populations compared with the mean level of serum cholesterol. The relationship is a linear one. The United States, represented by a star, is exceeded only by Finland in incidence of this disease (Keys, 1970).

The United States population remains among the top three national populations in terms of coronary disease incidence and mortality (Fig. 50–161). The alarming statistics show that the North American man has a 20 per cent chance of developing this disorder before the age of 60 (Wright and Frederickson, 1973). Six leading study centers have combined their data in the Pooling Project of the American Heart Association Council on Epidemiology (1978). Prospective studies following 12,381 men who were free of coronary disease at entry into the study have been performed for 98,741 person-years, with the goal of determining the factors, both major and minor, that will predict the risk of developing atherosclerosis or the future course of established disease. As a result, three major risk factors have emerged as significant contributions to the disease in North America (Fig. 50–162):

1. *Hypertension* has been found to be associated with a greater incidence of coronary atherosclerosis in most populations surveyed (Stamler, 1967). The increased incidence with high pressure is severalfold and is characterized by heightened susceptibility to

RISK FACTORS

MAJOR

HYPERTENSION
HYPERCHOLESTEROLEMIA
CIGARETTE SMOKING

MINOR

OBESITY
DIABETES MELLITUS
HYPERTRIGLYCERIDEMIA
SEDENTARY LIVING
STRESS
FAMILY HISTORY

Figure 50–162. Risk factors for atherosclerosis. Epidemiologic surveys have defined major factors that have a strong correlation with vascular disease and minor ones that are associated less positively. This particular set of features applies to the population surveyed in the United States.

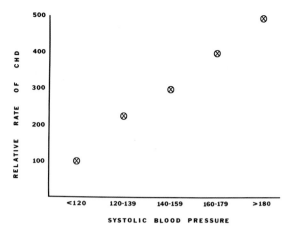

Figure 50–163. Relative risk of developing coronary heart disease (CHD) in the Framingham, Massachusetts population (Stamler, 1967) compared with the systolic blood pressure on entry into the study. This linear relationship has been found to apply to the diastolic pressure as well.

peripheral vascular and cerebral involvement (Kannel et al., 1965a, 1965b). The relationship between hypertension and coronary artery disease is continuous, with each increment of pressure increasing the risk (Fig. 50–163). The exception to this relationship is seen only in those few populations who live where conditions exist to decrease the prevalence of hypercholesterolemic hyperlipidemia (Stamler, 1967).

2. *Hypercholesterolemia* remains the most significant single factor correlated with atherosclerosis. The epidemiologic evidence linking serum lipids and atherosclerosis lends strong support to the lipid hypothesis of atherogenesis. The initial data for this concept stemmed from clinical observations that certain diseases such as hypothyroidism, the nephrotic syndrome, diabetes mellitus, and familial xanthomatosis were associated with persistent hypercholesterolemia. In these situations, premature atherosclerosis was a frequent component of the clinical presentation. The argument that elevated serum lipids contribute to the development of atherosclerosis has gained considera-

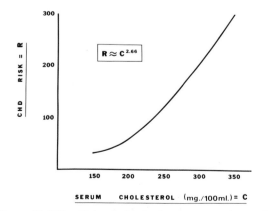

Figure 50–164. Risk of developing coronary heart disease (CHD) compared with the serum level of total cholesterol. Biostatistical analysis has revealed an exponential relationship between these entities (Cornfield, 1962).

ble support by prospective population surveys (Keys, 1980; Pooling Project Research Group, 1978). It has become apparent that a patient's risk of developing the disease is exponentially related to his serum cholesterol level (Cornfield, 1962) (Fig. 50–164). The incidence of coronary disease in a specific population varies with the mean serum cholesterol level (Fig. 50–161). This is the one constant risk factor that holds true regardless of the population examined. The data are unequivocal; the higher the serum cholesterol level, the greater the incidence of coronary atherosclerosis (McGill, 1979; Shebelle et al., 1981). Even greater specificity for the predictive value of serum cholesterol is obtained when the lipid is put in terms of lipoprotein fractions. In particular, low-density lipoprotein (LDL) cholesterol has been found to be a significant and independent risk factor positively related to coronary disease in both men and women well into the seventh or eighth decade of life (Gordon et al., 1977).

3. Although *cigarette smoking* has not been found to have a positive correlation worldwide with coronary artery disease (Keys, 1970), its relationship to mortality from atherosclerosis is remarkably constant (Hammond and Garfinkel, 1969). For each age and sex group, mortality increases with the degree of cigarette smoking. Studies document a positive relationship between the number of cigarettes smoked and the extent and character of aortic atherosclerosis and cerebral vascular involvement (Hammond and Garfinkel, 1969; Strong et al., 1969). Men smoking more than one pack of cigarettes per day have more than three times the risk of coronary events compared with nonsmokers (Pooling Project Research Group, 1978). The data are especially strong relating cigarette smoking to the course of atherosclerosis in the United States.

Apart from hypertension, hypercholesterolemia, and cigarette smoking, the remaining minor risk factors have been more variable in their correlation with atherosclerotic disease. Categorized as minor risk factors are diabetes mellitus, obesity, hypertriglyceridemia, hyperuricemia, sedentary life style, psychosocial tensions, and a positive family history (Fig. 50–162). Although these are common features in patients with atherosclerosis, they are classified as minor by the fact that they cannot be separated from the other factors as independent predictors for the disease (Stout, 1981).

Information obtained from the study of pathogenesis and risk factors provides a solid rationale for the treatment or prevention of atherosclerotic arterial disease. Although the former is hypothetical and the latter may be more circumstantial than causal, they nonetheless suggest means for management of this complicated problem. Two such features that are amenable to medical control are lipid metabolism and platelet function. Each explanation for atherogenesis is couched in terms of these two topics, and they form the basis for the dietary and pharmacologic management of this disease.

LIPID METABOLISM

Lipids are classified as organic substances that are soluble only in certain nonaqueous solvents. Within living tissue, they form the basic structure of membranes, act as storage or carrier agents of metabolic fuel, or convey properties of biologic activity in the form of hormones or vitamins. A brief description of the structure and metabolism of certain lipids is essential to understand the mechanisms behind the therapy of atherosclerosis.

Cholesterol, a sterol-structured neutral lipid, was first identified as a human tissue constituent in the eighteenth century, when it was extracted from gallstones. It was soon found in the circulating blood and was isolated from atherosclerotic plaques by Vogel in 1835. From that time, this lipid has been implicated in the process of atherosclerosis. Serum cholesterol has three possible origins (Fig. 50–165): (1) It is *synthesized* in the liver or intestine, utilizing acetate as a basic building unit. One of the enzymes of this metabolic pathway, hydroxymethylglutaryl (HMG)-CoA reductase, is an essential rate-limiting factor inhibited by elevated serum cholesterol, drugs, and intestinal levels of bile acids (Goldstein and Brown, 1977; Siperstein and Guest, 1960) (Fig. 50–166). (2) Cholesterol is *absorbed* from the diet in a variable fashion, depending on bile acids, dietary fat, and intestinal enzyme activity (Kaplan *et al.,* 1963). (3) It can be *mobilized* from tissue pools (Chobanian *et al.,* 1962). The final measured result—serum cholesterol—is thus the product of interrelated and balanced metabolic pathways.

A major portion of cholesterol in the serum is in the form of esters of fatty acids (Fig. 50–167). The lecithin-cholesterol acyltransferase (LCAT) (Glomset, 1968) enzyme system mediates this change in the serum. A similar pathway may be involved in the tissue of the blood vessel (Abdulla *et al.,* 1969), but direct acylation through fatty acyl CoA (Proudlock and Day, 1972) is more likely. The latter enzyme system favors the production of monosaturated fatty

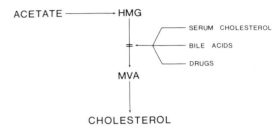

Figure 50–166. Pathway of endogenous cholesterol synthesis. Acetate is used to form beta-hydroxymethylglutarate (HMG). The enzyme system (HMG-CoA reductase) involved in the conversion of this to mevalonate (MVA) is inhibited by elevated serum cholesterol levels and by certain pharmacologic agents. Inhibition at this early stage of synthesis avoids the build-up of toxic metabolites as other pathways are available to the HMG. Mevalonate fragments combine to form long-chain structures that are converted to sterols.

acids, which are plentiful in the lipid accumulation of atherosclerosis.

Triglycerides or triacyl esters of glycerol are the basic units of energy storage in body fat deposits. They are synthesized by the liver, intestine, or adipose tissue by metabolic pathways that generally require alpha-glycerophosphate as a precursor. A similar course is followed in the production of phospholipids (Fig. 50–168). The free fatty acids for this reaction are synthesized de novo in the liver (Wakil, 1970), absorbed from the breakdown of dietary triglycerides, or arise from mobilization of storage pools of triglycerides. The release of fatty acids from body storage is markedly sensitive to hormones of broad physiologic activity, such as catecholamines, prostaglandins (Carlson and Hallberg, 1968), and insulin (Randle *et al.,* 1963). This complex interrelation of basic biochemical reactions makes it difficult to determine the exact role of serum triglycerides in atherosclerotic arterial disease.

Phospholipids are another group of lipids closely associated with the metabolism of cholesterol and triglycerides. The glycerophospholipids have the basic structure of glycerol with fatty acids esterified in positions 1 and 2 and a phosphoric acid at position 3. The latter is then linked to various compounds such

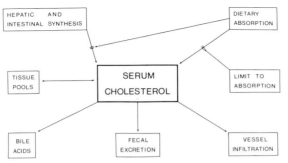

Figure 50–165. A scheme of the features contributing to the level of serum cholesterol. The input sources are endogenous synthesis in the liver and intestine, dietary absorption, and mobilization from the body stores. There is a limit to absorption, and elevated serum levels will inhibit hepatic synthesis. The circulating cholesterol can be excreted in the stool in a free or bile acid form or can be shunted into the tissue pools. As low-density lipoprotein, serum cholesterol is found within normal arterial tissue.

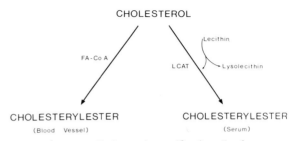

Figure 50–167. Cholesterol esterification. In the serum, the lecithin-cholesterol acyltransferase system (LCAT) mediates the transfer of the more unsaturated fatty acid chain from the two position of lecithin to the hydroxy position of cholesterol. This system favors the production of cholesteryllinoleate, the major component of low density lipoproteins. In tissues, another enzyme low-density system mediates the acylation of cholesterol with the production of more saturated cholesterylesters such as cholesteryloleate.

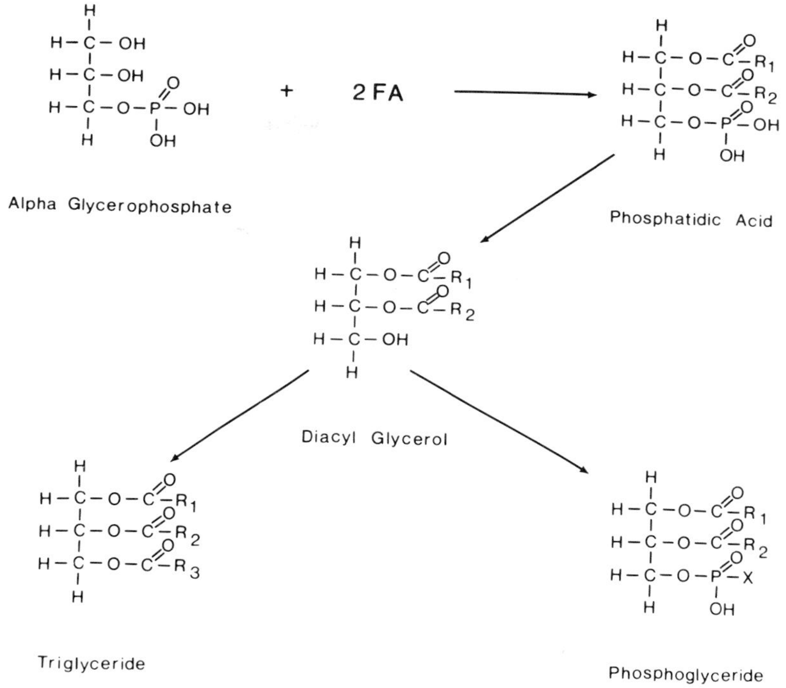

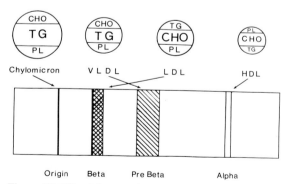

Figure 50–168. Triglyceride synthesis. The acylation of glycerol with fatty acid (FA) occurs in the liver and intestines. Factors that increase the serum free fatty acids or stimulate the enzymes involved will favor synthesis of triglycerides. Polar lipids or phosphoglycerides will follow a similar pathway.

as choline, ethanolamine, or an alcohol to form substances that are major constituents of all organic membranes. Their synthesis is intimately related to that of triacylglycerol (Fig. 50–168), and phosphatidylcholine or lecithin plays an important part in the esterification of serum cholesterol (Fig. 50–167). More significant perhaps are the functions that these polar substances perform in the dispersion of nonsoluble lipids in the serum or in the intestinal lumen. This characteristic is particularly essential to lipoproteins, the circulating form of lipids.

Because of their insolubility, the lipids just described do not exist as free entities in the serum. Instead they are transported in the form of lipoproteins—macromolecular combinations of all three lipids—and variable lipoprotein polypeptides (Scanu, 1973). In human serum, these large lipoprotein complexes have been separated into four distinct groups by ultracentrifugation or electrophoresis (Fig. 50–169).

Chylomicrons are triglyceride-rich conglomerates of lipids that are absorbed into the bloodstream following a meal. Most of the constituents are derived from exogenous diet and are dispersed to various areas of the body (liver, blood vessels, adipose tissue), where they are metabolized. This clearing process is mediated through lipoprotein lipases and is accelerated by heparin. Such lipolytic enzyme activity is found in vascular endothelium and in the apoprotein components of some of the lipoproteins (Sigurdsson et al., 1975). The fragments of metabolized chylomicrons are taken up by the liver, where they may be combined with apoproteins to form triglyceride-rich *very-low-density lipoprotein* (VLDL).

The half-life of VLDL far exceeds that of chylomicrons, and an increase in their synthesis will produce prolonged hypertriglyceridemia. Carbohydrate

ingestion (Lees and Frederickson, 1965), especially in the form of sucrose excess (Yudkin and Roddy, 1964), stimulates this production, possibly through elevated levels of insulin (Ford et al., 1967) (Fig. 50–170). On the other hand, fatty acid mobilization brought on by starvation or stress-induced elevations of catecholamines will also increase hepatic synthesis of VLDL (Carlson and Hallberg, 1968). Ingested ethanol produces hypertriglyceridemia but through a mechanism different from that of carbohydrate induction (Kudzma and Schonfeld, 1971). The regulation of hepatic synthesis of VLDL is thus a multifactorial process subject to endogenous and exogenous influences.

Figure 50–169. Lipoproteins. These entities are arranged in order of increasing density from left to right: chylomicrons, very low-density lipoproteins (VLDL), low-density lipoproteins (LDL), and high-density lipoproteins (HDL). The lipid content, with the predominant fractions being in larger letters, is made up of triglycerides (TG), cholesterol (CHO), and phospholipids (PL). When placed in an electromagnetic field, the chylomicrons remain at the origin. The LDL migrate in the area of beta-globulins and are called beta-lipoproteins. The VLDL precede the beta and are named pre-beta. The high-density lipoproteins migrate in the zone of alpha-globulins and are indicated as alpha-lipoproteins.

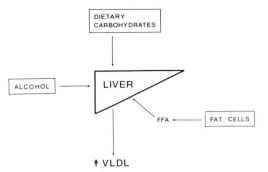

Figure 50–170. VLDL synthesis. These lipoproteins are synthesized predominantly in the liver with a combination of apoprotein and lipid constituents. Alcohol, serum free fatty acids (FFA), and dietary carbohydrates all stimulate this process.

As they circulate, VLDL molecules are in turn hydrolyzed by lipases to form smaller *intermediate-density lipoproteins* (IDL). Some of these entities are cleared by the liver, but the majority are further degraded to *low-density lipoprotein* (LDL) (Sigurdsson et al., 1975). LDL, which contains a large component of cholesterol esters, has the important function of transporting cholesterol to peripheral tissues (Fig. 50–171). LDL normally carries one half to two thirds of human plasma cholesterol (Gotto et al., 1979). Because of its small size, it appears to be transported across the endothelium through microvascular pores at a high rate (Stender and Zilversmit, 1981). In addition, there are specific receptors on cell membranes to facilitate cellular entry (Goldstein and Brown, 1977). Absence of such receptors may lead to failure of inhibition of intracellular cholesterol synthesis or may decrease LDL catabolism, thus resulting in hyperlipidemia characterized by elevated LDL and intracellular cholesterol.

Peripheral cells are unable to catabolize cholesterol. Instead, this substance must be transported back to the liver for further metabolism. *High-density li-*

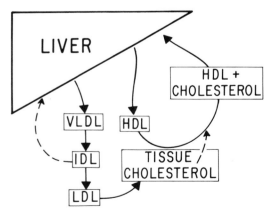

Figure 50–171. Scheme of lipoprotein metabolism. VLDL synthesized by the liver undergoes lipolysis of tissue lipases. The IDL formed is predominantly transformed to LDL by further degradation of triglycerides. (A small portion of IDL is cleared by the liver.) Cholesterol-rich LDL transports cholesterol into cells. Excess tissue cholesterol cannot be catabolized and is cleared by HDL and returned to the liver for further metabolism.

poproteins (HDL) appear to perform this function (Fig. 50–171). These small, dense units are one-half protein by weight. Originally found as discs, they appear to enlarge and become spherical as they accumulate cholesterol esters. The esterification of tissue cholesterol may be mediated by the apoprotein moiety of HDL, which has LCAT (Fig. 50–167) enzyme activity.

This process of mobilization and accumulation of tissue cholesterol is thought possibly to account for the inverse relation of HDL cholesterol level and atherosclerosis (Hamel, 1979). Another postulated mechanism is that HDL may block LDL uptake at tissue receptor sites (Carew et al., 1976). Whatever the case, there is a strong negative association of HDL with atherosclerosis, and future therapy may involve agents or regimens that can increase this plasma lipoprotein.

As knowledge of apoprotein constituents has expanded, the topic appears more complicated than the simplistic scheme presented above. Each group of lipoproteins has several types of apoprotein, thereby making it a heterogeneous collection rather than a distinct molecular entity. The apoproteins have enzymatic activities that determine lipoprotein activity and metabolism. In addition, the apoproteins are not peculiar to particular lipoprotein groups, and they can be exchanged during stages of lipoprotein interconversion.

Because of the importance of apoproteins in lipid metabolism, classification of lipoproteins may some day be in terms of dominant apoprotein rather than density or separation characteristics. For the time being, however, attempts at therapy involve steps to alter the distribution and balance of major lipoprotein fractions—VLDL, LDL, and HDL. In certain aspects, this approach is applicable to so-called "normolipidemic" individuals as well as to those with clinically recognized hyperlipidemia.

Appreciation of the importance of lipoproteins and their association with specific clinical situations has been a major advance in medical care. The thorough investigations of Frederickson and associates (1967) classified abnormal lipoprotein patterns of large populations into the familiar Types I to V. Most important is the fact that specific clinical presentations could be correlated with the individual classification type. With background knowledge of lipids and lipoproteins, a rational means of therapy can be designed to correct derangement in lipoprotein homeostasis (DePalma et al., 1970; Lees and Wilson, 1971).

This metabolic approach to disease is too recent to allow full assessment of its efficacy. Serum lipoprotein patterns can definitely be altered, but the major issue of whether the associated manifestations will be permanently changed remains unclear. This is exactly the case with atherosclerosis. A high incidence of atherosclerotic vascular disease is found in hyperlipoproteinemia Types II, III, and IV (Brown and Daudiss, 1973). Epidemiologic evidence emphasizing the importance of lipoprotein levels lends powerful support to the concept of treating atherosclerosis through manipulation of serum lipoprotein fractions. Should this therapy prove to be of value for hyperlipidemic populations, it may be applicable to patients without fully developed hyperlipidemias but who are at high risk for atherosclerosis.

PLATELET FUNCTIONS

Platelets appear to play a role in the course of atherosclerotic vascular disease. The possible involvement of platelet factors in the initiation and progression of early atherosclerotic lesions has been mentioned previously (Ross, 1981; Ross and Vogel, 1978). In addition, they may be associated with accumulation of particulate material on the surface of arterial lesions. Such deposits may embolize, lead to subsequent thrombosis, or contribute to vasoconstriction. These blood particles thus appear important in the development of intra-arterial plaques as well as contributing to thromboembolic complications of mature lesions.

Normally, platelets circulate as flat discs with a mean survival time of 9 to 10 days. When confronted with a thrombogenic surface such as denuded endothelium, these particles adhere, release factors that stimulate further platelet aggregation, and lead to coagulation. In addition, platelets form thromboxane A_2 through arachidonate metabolism, a substance that stimulates further platelet adherence and intense vasospasm. Another product of arachidonate metabolism, prostacyclin, acts as a potent vasodilator and inhibits platelet aggregation. This substance is produced by endothelial cells and may account for the antithrombotic effect of this tissue (Moncada et al., 1976). Manipulation of platelet function offers the potential for control of atherogenesis as well as the possible prevention of acute complications arising in the course of clinical atherosclerosis. The means to accomplish these goals and results of preliminary trials will be discussed in the following section.

THERAPY

When a patient presents with atherosclerosis and a demonstrable lipid abnormality, the rationale for dietary and pharmacologic therapy is firmly based on clinicopathologic, epidemiologic, and experimental study data. On the other hand, many patients do not have such serum lipid alterations, and thus, nonoperative management is based on different principles. The value of medical therapy for atherosclerotic patients has been questioned, especially in "normolipidemic" individuals (Mann, 1977). Even more unproved is the unrestricted use of diet or drugs designed to alter platelet function. However, in certain situations, this approach appears advantageous in altering the clinical course of atherosclerotic vascular disease (Garton, 1980; Gent et al., 1980; Persantine-Aspirin Reinfarction Study Research Group, 1980). To advo-cate the application of these principles to normal persons who are "at risk" for the development of atherosclerosis later is certainly questionable. It would be unethical to subject an apparently normal person to an unestablished treatment program that is potentially hazardous. This is especially true in the case of pharmacologic agents, all of which have toxic side effects. However, many of the "general" means of therapy and "dietary" recommendations are already established public health tenets which become even more important in light of their relationship to atherosclerosis.

General Therapy

The basic approach to atherosclerosis therapy involves manipulation of the risk factors found to be strongly associated with the disease. Most of these fall within the scope of general medical care. Such issues as cessation of cigarette smoking, control of hypertension, changes of patterns of activity and stress, weight loss, and the regulation of diabetes mellitus have been recommended for years. They involve basic changes in life style that require an extensive follow-up period for successful application. Such a therapeutic course is best controlled by a doctor who can work out an extensive day-to-day program and follow its progress with the patient.

Diet Therapy

Dietary treatment requires a commitment of instructional time that is often unavailable to active clinicians. Nonetheless, basic advice should be given to each patient, and provisions should be made for follow-up analysis after intensive instruction by a dietitian. If a program can be initiated while a patient is hospitalized, the simultaneous presentation of dietary instructions with palatable, modified meals will enhance acceptance of these principles. Practical instructions and literature are available to help the patient with the day-to-day problems arising in a program of this nature (Eshleman and Soderquist, 1973; Frederickson et al., 1970).

There are five features to be considered in determining dietary recommendations that may alter the factors associated with arterial atherosclerosis.

1. *Caloric content* is important, especially if obesity is present. This condition is very common in patients who show elevations of serum VLDL, as in Type III and Type IV hyperlipidemia. The presence of increased serum free fatty acids, from either excessive mobilization (Carlson and Hallberg, 1968) or decreased clearance, appears to stimulate hepatic VLDL synthesis (Eaton et al., 1969) (Fig. 50–170). Obesity, with excessive adipose tissue, enhances turnover of serum free fatty acid (Nestel and Whyte, 1968). The fat cell in obese subjects appears to be

insulin-resistant, thereby clearing serum VLDL at a decreased rate (Salans *et al.*, 1968). Loss of adipose tissue through caloric restriction and weight reduction reverses these abnormal features and will often result in a marked reduction of VLDL and serum triglycerides.

2. *Carbohydrate restriction,* particularly in the form of sucrose-rich sweet concentrates, also has a beneficial effect on the serum VLDL (Hulley *et al.*, 1972; Kuo, 1967). Oral carbohydrates enhance the endogenous synthesis and transport of triglycerides through a mechanism related to glucose-insulin balance (Lees and Frederickson, 1965). The fact that weight reduction usually accompanies carbohydrate restriction makes the intrinsic value of this mechanism difficult to evaluate. Nonetheless, a low carbohydrate intake is a basic feature of the dietary therapy for Types III and IV hyperlipidemia.

3. The contribution of dietary *cholesterol* to hypercholesterolemia is an unsettled issue. Serum cholesterol levels in man can be manipulated through changes in the oral intake of this substance (Shebelle *et al.*, 1981). However, the complicating features of limited dietary absorption and feedback control of cholesterol synthesis enter into this relationship (Grundy *et al.*, 1969; Kaplan *et al.*, 1963) (Fig. 50–165).

Whatever the degree of intestinal absorption in man may be, dietary cholesterol above 300 mg. per day appears to elevate the serum levels (Connor and Connor, 1972). Since the average American diet contains between 600 mg. and 1 gm., restriction in cholesterol content to 300 mg. per day is usually recommended. In spite of the popular emphasis on this dietary constituent, the other components described here are likely to be of equal importance.

The ubiquitous correlation of dietary cholesterol and vascular diseases stems primarily from the fact that almost every animal model of atherosclerosis relies on a large oral dose of cholesterol. Particularly striking is the work in nonhuman primates, where a cholesterol-rich diet will produce atherosclerotic lesions that are reversible on return to a diet low in that substance (Avoy *et al.*, 1965; Malinow, 1980). Epidemiologic studies reaffirm that serum cholesterol can be altered with diet and is related to the course of vascular disease in man (McGill, 1979; Shebelle *et al.*, 1981).

4. Dietary *fat* restriction was one of the earliest therapeutic maneuvers for control of hyperlipidemia. It is evident that the degree of saturation of the fatty acid chains of ingested triglycerides is as important as the quantity of fats in the diet (Ahrens *et al.*, 1957). The American diet has 40 per cent of its caloric content in fats, with a ratio of polyunsaturated to saturated fats of 1 to 2. Lowering of serum lipids and lipoproteins has been produced by either increasing the ratio of unsaturated to saturated fats (Wilson *et al.*, 1971) or reducing the total intake of dietary fats (Bierenbaum *et al.*, 1973; Ernst *et al.*, 1980). The mechanism whereby saturated fats elevate and unsaturated fats decrease the serum cholesterol level involves either the fecal excretion of sterols or the balance between body pools and serum cholesterol levels (Connor and Connor, 1971).

Since fatty acids are precursors of prostaglandins and thromboxanes, dietary fat may be implicated in platelet functions. Although there is little documentation of this phenomenon in man, early experimental data (ten Hoor *et al.*, 1980) suggest that dietary manipulation of ingested fats may someday be available to control platelet activity in a manner that will discourage the development or complications of atherosclerosis.

5. Ingestion of *alcohol* leads to elevated serum triglycerides. This seems to be related to a distinct stimulatory effect of ethanol on hepatic fatty acid synthesis (Kudzma and Schonfeld, 1971) (Fig. 50–170) and can occur with consumption within the range of "social drinking" (Connor and Connor, 1971). This is particularly the case when alcohol adds extra unnecessary calories that lead to obesity and hyperlipidemia. Recently appreciated is the positive correlation between ethanol consumption and serum HDL levels (Hulley and Gordon, 1981). Studies reveal this to be a dose-related phenomenon within the low and moderate daily alcohol consumption range. This may account for the reported inverse relationship between daily moderate alcohol consumption and complications of atherosclerotic disease (Hennekens *et al.*, 1979).

Since these dietary components have potential for influencing the course of atherosclerosis, it is not surprising that multiple prospective intervention trials and retrospective epidemiologic surveys have been undertaken to establish a solid link between diet and arterial disease (Stamler, 1979). The first major study, the National Diet Heart Study, was set up on a controlled, double-blind basis in a free-living population. Such a plan proved feasible, and it demonstrated a 14 per cent reduction in serum cholesterol levels in those receiving the experimental diet which was low in saturated fats and cholesterol (National Diet Heart Study Research Group, 1968).

These principles have been applied on a large scale to groups of patients with existing atherosclerotic disease (Bierenbaum *et al.*, 1973; Carew *et al.*, 1976; Dayton and Pearce, 1969; Ernst *et al.*, 1980; Leren, 1970). Under these circumstances, modifications of fat and cholesterol intake have succeeded in lowering the serum cholesterol and LDL value, usually in the range of 14 to 17 per cent (Frederickson *et al.*, 1970; Leren, 1970). At the same time, favorable results are beginning to appear in the form of reduction of atherosclerotic events such as myocardial infarction (Leren, 1970; Miettinen *et al.*, 1972) and peripheral vascular complications (Dayton and Pearce, 1969). The difficulty of obtaining parallel control groups and the prolonged clinical course of atherosclerosis have engendered criticism of these conditions (Mann, 1977). On the other hand, the recent 20-year follow-up of epidemiologic surveys strongly underscores the importance of dietary constituents and the value of

DIET FACTORS

	Average	A. H. A.
Cholesterol (mg/day)	> 500	< 300
Fats (% calories)	40	40
Saturated Fats* (S)	15	<10
Polyunsaturated Fats* (P)	5	15
P:S Ratio	0.3	> 1.5

(* per cent daily caloric intake)

Figure 50–172. Diet factors. The composition of an average American diet as compared with that recommended by the American Heart Association (AHA). The primary points of difference in the "prudent" diet of the AHA are a lowering of daily cholesterol to below 300 mg., reduction of total fats to 30 per cent and of saturated fats to below 10 per cent of total calories, and increase in polyunsaturated/saturated fat ratio to greater than 1.5.

modification in terms of coronary heart disease (Shebelle et al., 1981; Turpeinen, 1979).

A safety question has recently arisen, as some epidemiologic surveys have suggested that low serum cholesterol levels are associated with an increased noncoronary death rate, especially from bowel cancer (Pearce and Dayton, 1971; Peterson et al., 1981). This particular issue has been considered tentative by experienced investigators (Grundy, 1981), and the American Heart Association feels secure in recommending a diet to lower serum cholesterol (American Heart Association Committee Report, 1978) (Fig. 50–172). For patients with hyperlipidemia, including children (Committee on Nutrition, 1972), such diets are strongly recommended, and their use has been expanded to the population in general (Wright and Frederickson, 1973).

Adults with specific lipoprotein abnormalities require more intensive control of diet. Those with an elevated LDL, or *Type II hyperlipidemia,* should be maintained on a diet that is reduced in cholesterol content and in which unsaturated fats are used to replace saturated animal fats. With such a diet, the total serum cholesterol and LDL content can be reduced as much as 15 per cent (Ernst et al., 1980; Wilson et al., 1971). The other common lipoprotein disorder, elevated VLDL, or *Type IV hyperlipidemia,* requires a basic treatment program consisting of weight loss and a reduction of the oral intake of carbohydrates and alcohol. As the weight falls to normal levels, calories can be supplied by the addition of polyunsaturated fats. With patient cooperation, this dietary regimen is very successful and is often the only means of therapy required (Kuo, 1967).

Antilipid Drug Therapy

Results of diet therapy alone have consistently revealed a limit to its efficacy from the standpoint of lipid alterations. Maximum lowering of serum cholesterol and LDL is in the range of 12 to 15 per cent (Bierenbaum et al., 1973; Ernst et al., 1980; Leren, 1970; National Diet Heart Study Research Group, 1968; Wilson et al., 1971). Poor patient compliance often requires institution of additional treatment measures. The decision to begin drug therapy is usually made after diet has failed to control serious, documented hyperlipidemia. There is general agreement that antilipemics should be limited to these situations, as serious toxic sequelae have occurred in the past with pharmacologic agents.

Patients with elevation of LDL, or *Type II hyperlipidemia,* are at greater risk for atherosclerotic disease (Gordon et al., 1977). The type of drug therapy selected depends on the degree of hypercholesterolemia. For severe cases, usually familial in origin, in which the serum cholesterol is usually above 300 mg./100 ml., a *bile acid–binding resin* is selected. These agents, either *cholestyramine* or *colestipol,* are nonabsorbable resins with attached quaternary amine groups. When taken orally, their charged sites are bound to chloride. Internally, this exchanges with bile acids, which remain bound to the resin and are excreted in the stool. The resulting interruption of the enterohepatic circulation stimulates de novo bile acid synthesis from body cholesterol. Most patients respond with a lowering of LDL levels to 20 to 25 per cent below the levels achieved by diet alone (Steinberg and Grundy, 1978). Administered as a total daily dose of 16 to 20 gm., this drug remains entirely within the gut and therefore has no systemic side effects. However, it is constipating and may adsorb other concurrently administered drugs.

At lower levels of hypercholesterolemia, other drugs may be selected. Clofibrate, which will be discussed later, has a modest depressant effect on LDL, perhaps because of its interference in synthesis of VLDL, a precursor of LDL. *Niacin* or *nicotinic acid* is effective in lowering both VLDL and LDL levels, with serum reduction in the range of 20 to 40 per cent (Committee on Nutrition, 1972). It appears to limit the mobilization of free fatty acids from adipose tissue (Carlson et al., 1968), thereby reducing hepatic synthesis of VLDL (Fig. 50–170). Lowering of serum cholesterol occurs through interference of the conversion of VLDL to LDL (Carlson et al., 1968) and decreased endogenous synthesis at the HMG-CoA reductase level (Miller and Hamilton, 1964) (Fig. 50–166).

The side effects of nicotinic acid are marked. Gastrointestinal irritation is sufficient to preclude its use in patients with peptic ulcer disease. Abnormalities in liver function are frequent, and prolonged use has produced histologic liver damage and cholangitis (Berenson and Cho, 1974). Probably, the most limiting feature of nicotinic acid is that in the usual dose of 3 to 6 gm. per day, the unpleasant sensations of cutaneous flushing and itching are so severe that patients are unwilling to continue its use. These experiences can be reduced by gradual increase of daily doses to the therapeutic range.

Dextrothyroxine, the D-isomer of the naturally occurring hormone L-thyroxine, has hypocholesterolemic activity and will lower the serum LDL as much as 20 per cent in euthyroid patients (Schneeberg *et al.*, 1962). Therapeutic doses may produce mild hyperthyroid-like symptoms, and beta-blocking agents can be administered simultaneously to reduce hormonal side effects (Krikler *et al.*, 1971). Of particular concern is the finding of increased mortality when this agent is used in patients with previous myocardial infarction (Coronary Drug Project, 1972). The use of dextrothyroxine is contraindicated in patients with coronary artery disease, thereby limiting its application in most adult patients with diffuse atherosclerosis. This drug appears to augment the catabolism and excretion of endogenous cholesterol (Simons and Myant, 1974). The starting doses are 1 to 2 mg. per day with a gradual increase of 1 mg. every 2 to 4 weeks until there is a reduction of serum cholesterol. The usual daily dose reached is 4 to 8 mg.

A recent drug, *probucol*, appears to lower LDL by as yet undetermined means. Given in doses of 1 gm. per day, this agent may inhibit the initial steps of cholesterol synthesis or enhance fecal sterol excretion. Significant cardiac toxicity has been demonstrated in animals on markedly severe atherogenic diets, suggesting that this is not an innocuous drug. Its use will probably be in cases of mild hypercholesterolemia that are not responsive to diet therapy or as an additional drug for more severe cholesterolemia.

The other common lipid abnormality associated with atherosclerosis is *Type IV hyperlipidemia* with elevation of serum VLDL. Although this disorder is often extremely responsive to weight loss and diet, there remain many situations in which drug intervention may be indicated. The agent most commonly selected is *clofibrate*. This drug, which has been used for over 15 years, is markedly successful in the reduction of serum lipids, with triglyceride lowering of 50 per cent and cholesterol reduction of 20 per cent being reported (Berkowitz, 1973). After oral ingestion, this drug is well absorbed and is strongly bound to serum albumin. Free fatty acids in the serum decrease with clofibrate, possibly because of inhibition of albumin anionic binding sites (Barrett and Thorp, 1968), and this may account for diminished VLDL synthesis in the liver. Release of albumin-bound thyroxine has been suggested to be the basis of the action of this drug (Thorp *et al.,* 1968). The reduction of serum levels of cholesterol with clofibrate is thought to be due to inhibition of HMG-CoA reductase in the endogenous synthesis of this compound (Aspirin Myocardial Infarction Study Research Group, 1980) (Fig. 50–166) or to reduction of the transformation of VLDL to LDL. The net result of clofibrate administration is reduction of total body cholesterol levels. Some of this may occur through increased biliary excretion, possibly accounting for the increased gallstone formation seen with its use (Coronary Drug Project Research Group, 1977; Cooperative Trial in the Primary Prevention of Ischemic Heart Disease Using Clofibrate, 1978).

Given as a daily adult dose of 2 gm., clofibrate may produce gastrointestinal distress and skin rashes. More rarely encountered are leukopenia and genitourinary dysfunction. Three to 5 per cent of patients will have a peculiar muscle stiffness associated with elevated serum creatine phosphokinase (CPK), although this usually resolves with dosage reduction. Coumarin-type anticoagulants are potentiated by this drug and require reduction in dose when it is administered. Animal toxicity studies have revealed hepatic tumorigenicity with clofibrate, although this has not been established in human subjects. The large-scale population studies utilizing the drug have raised sufficient problems to recommend its use only in patients with unresponsive and persistent hyperlipidemia.

Clofibrate has been the experimental drug in two of the largest multicenter cooperative trials designed to assess the use of pharmacologic agents in long-term prevention of coronary heart disease (Coronary Drug Project, 1975; Cooperative Trial in the Primary Prevention of Ischemic Heart Disease Using Clofibrate, 1978). The Coronary Drug Project compared results in 1000 post–myocardial infarction patients with those in 3000 control subjects on placebo. No substantially significant improvement in myocardial infarction events was established, despite the 10 per cent decrease in serum cholesterol and the 22 per cent reduction of triglycerides (Coronary Drug Project, 1975). Drug-treated patients did show a higher incidence of cholelithiasis and biliary tract disease with their associated complications (Coronary Drug Project Research Group, 1977).

The more recently completed WHO coordinated cooperative trial in three cities compared 5000 drug-treated healthy volunteers with 5000 volunteers who were given placebo. Both groups consisted of individuals with serum cholesterol values in the upper third of those who volunteered. Another 5000 individuals from the group with lower third serum cholesterol values were given placebo and used as a second set of controls. After 5 years, the drug-treated subjects had a 9 per cent decrease in serum cholesterol and demonstrated a 25 per cent decrease in nonfatal myocardial infarctions. The incidence of fatal infarctions was unchanged by the drug. The rate of ischemic heart disease remained low in the control groups with the initially lower serum cholesterol values. A very alarming result in the clofibrate-treated subjects was an increased death rate from noncardiovascular diseases, with half of the deaths being due to malignancies. This has stimulated the FDA to issue a statement that clofibrate should not be used for community-wide prevention of ischemic heart disease and should be limited to patients with documented lipid disorders.

Multicenter drug trials have also been used in patients with severe hyperlipidemia. Of frequent use in this respect are the bile acid–binding resins (Kuo *et al.*, 1979). These drugs have been successful in lowering serum cholesterol 25 per cent, and aside from the gastrointestinal symptoms mentioned earlier, they do not yet appear to have such severe side effects as clofibrate. Initial results in patients with Type II hyperlipidemia suggest that this approach will lower coronary mortality rates (Dorr *et al.*, 1978) and may actually stabilize intra-arterial disease in those patients who usually have an exuberantly progressive clinical picture (Kuo *et al.*, 1979). More complete information on the value of this approach will be available with the final reports of the Lipid Research Primary Prevention Trials that will be published after the patient follow-ups are completed in mid 1983. In the meantime, it appears reasonable to recommend antilipid drug therapy for patients with documented primary hyperlipidemia that is unresponsive to other means of treatment.

Antiplatelet Drug Therapy

The other potential drug therapy for atherosclerosis, antiplatelet agents, deals mostly with prevention of thromboembolic complications of existing arterial lesions (Packham and Mustard, 1980). Some benefit may exist in terms of altering the process of atherogenesis if the mechanisms discussed previously are operable (Ross and Glomset, 1976). Although there is some epidemiologic support for the prophylactic value of these drugs (Boston Collaborative Drug Surveillance Group, 1974), there are insufficient data to recommend the use of these agents in primary prevention of atherosclerosis. On the other hand, multiple trials have been undertaken to assess their value in the secondary prevention of cardiovascular events.

Platelet function can be altered through several pharmacologic means. Primary among these is the inhibition of arachidonate metabolism in order to inhibit thromboxane A_2 synthesis by platelets. *Aspirin* will irreversibly acetylate platelet cyclo-oxygenase and thereby limit the endoperoxides available for conversion to thromboxane A_2 (Burch *et al.*, 1978). Since endoperoxides are also necessary for endothelial production of the potent antiaggregant prostacyclin, an appropriate dose of aspirin must be selected so as not to inhibit endothelial cyclo-oxygenase. Six hundred to 1200 mg. per day is generally accepted as an appropriate total dose, and this drug can be administered once or twice a day.

Sulfinpyrazone in a total daily dose of 800 mg. appears to produce reversible inhibition of cyclo-oxygenase and should be given on a frequent dosing schedule (Ali and McDonald, 1978). Despite the inconvenience of the multiple daily doses, this agent will avoid some of the undesirable side effects of aspirin (Canadian Cooperative Study Groups, 1978) and does appear to have more favorable effects on platelet survival and endothelial stability (Harker *et al.*, 1978).

Dipyridamole inhibits phosphodiesterase and thereby increases the platelet content of cyclic adenosine monophosphate (AMP). Increased levels of cyclic AMP within platelets appear to stabilize these particles and will decrease their adhesion, aggregation, and release of granules. Theoretically, this would be favorable in limiting smooth muscle cell replication during atherogenesis as well as in avoiding the throm-

boembolic complications of intravascular lesions. The total daily dose ranges from 200 to 300 mg., usually administered three to four times a day. Because it works differently from aspirin, dipyridamole is frequently given in conjunction with that drug to achieve a wider interference of platelet function.

Numerous studies have been performed worldwide to assess the value of antiplatelet agents in patients with coronary artery and cerebrovascular disease in whom relief from thromboembolic complications would offer a real clinical advantage. In treated patients with previous myocardial infarctions, there has been a trend toward reduced mortality and a slightly significant reduction of recurrent nonfatal infarctions (Garton, 1980). The small benefit seen with the use of aspirin and the incidence of drug-related complications have led some investigators to state that this drug should not be recommended for routine use in patients surviving myocardial infarction (Anturane Reinfarction Trial Research Group, 1980). The concomitant use of dipyridamole did not produce significantly different effects from aspirin alone. Sulfinpyrazone was used alone and appeared to be related to a highly significant reduction of the risk of sudden death during the initial 6 months following myocardial infarction (Anturane Reinfarction Trial Research Group, 1980). This finding suggests that another mechanism of action may exist for this drug rather than its antiplatelet activities.

The two major studies of patients with transient ischemic attacks (TIAs) and carotid artery disease have shown favorable results with the use of aspirin (Fields *et al.*, 1980). In one group, there appeared to be preferential protection from further stroke in the males utilizing this drug (Canadian Cooperative Study Groups, 1978). These data have been consistent and suggest that aspirin will reduce the risk of further TIAs and the incidence of subsequent stroke. Such benefits apply to patients when aspirin is used as primary medical therapy or as a postendarterectomy adjuvant.

At least 17 large-scale trials are in progress to establish the role of antiplatelet therapy in patients with coronary artery disease, extracranial cerebrovascular symptoms, arterial bypass grafts, and diabetic retinopathy. In addition, the drugs are being used in some groups of ostensibly normal subjects to see if they may have prophylactic value. As information is returned from these investigations, the rational use of drugs to suppress platelet function should become apparent. In the meantime, the use of such agents is reasonable when patients are at real risk from the thromboembolic complications of atherosclerotic vascular disease.

The issues of diet therapy and drug therapy for atherosclerosis have yet to be firmly settled. Clinical trials are encouraging enough to allow safe recommendation of diet modification to the general population and to suggest the use of drugs in specific cases of lipidemia or of risk from thromboembolic complications of vascular disease. If physicians follow this lead and advise appropriate treatment, the value of this therapeutic rationale will be decided more promptly. The importance of such information is so obviously immense that it is worthy of the cooperation of every physician dealing with atherosclerosis.

SELECTED REFERENCES

Berkowitz, D.: Management of the hyperlipidemic patient. Med. Clin. North Am., *57*:881, 1973.

This succinct account of the medical management of hyperlipidemia is recommended as a practical introduction to the problems of diagnosis and management of these metabolic disorders.

Braunwald, E., Friedewald, W. T., and Furberg, C. D. (Eds.): Proceedings of the workshop on platelet-active drugs in the secondary prevention of cardiovascular events. Circulation, *62*(Suppl. 5):1, 1980.

This monograph summarizes the important basic details and clinical studies dealing with the role of platelets in thrombosis and atherogenesis. In particular, the results of patient trials are described along with the current state of ongoing studies dealing with this important topic.

Frederickson, D. S., Levy, R. I., and Lees, R. S.: Fat transport in lipoproteins—an integrated approach to mechanism and disorders. N. Engl. J. Med., *276*:34, 94, 148, 215, 273, 1967.

The pioneering work of these authors established the basic clinical presentations of hyperlipidemia. Since diagnosis and treatment of lipid disorders rely on their classification system, these initial articles are noteworthy medical contributions.

Goldstein, J. L., and Brown, M. S.: The low density lipoprotein pathway and its relationship to atherosclerosis. Ann. Rev. Biochem., *46*:897, 1977.

These investigators have developed an important hypothesis to explain the biochemical defect leading to Type II hyperlipidemia. Based on cellular receptors for LDL, this concept offers a valuable insight into the relationship of lipoproteins and the tissue responses leading to atherosclerosis.

Jackson, R. L., Morrisett, J. D., and Gotto, A. M., Jr.: Lipoprotein structure and metabolism. Physiol. Rev., *56*:259, 1976.

This comprehensive work gives a thorough explanation of the composition and structure of lipoproteins as well as their complex metabolic interconversions. The important topic of apoprotein structure and function is also discussed.

Keys, A.: Seven Countries, A Multivariate Analysis of Death and Coronary Heart Disease. Cambridge, Massachusetts, Harvard University Press, 1980.

This book summarizes the work of this author in worldwide epidemiologic review. It contains basic data dealing with possible etiologic factors in atherosclerotic disease.

Levy, R. I.: Declining mortality in coronary heart disease. Arteriosclerosis, *1*:312, 1981.

This is a precise review of the intriguing epidemiologic observation of the recent decrease in cardiovascular mortality. Possible explanations are offered for this development.

Levy, R. I., Rifkind, B., Dennis, B., and Ernst, N. (Eds.): Nutrition, Lipids and Coronary Heart Disease. New York, Raven Press, 1979.

This book contains chapters written by authorities on the subject of nutrition and atherosclerosis. It offers a thorough review of these topics from the standpoint of historical background, epidemiology, pathogenesis, biochemistry, and review of clinical studies.

Malinow, M. R.: Regression of atherosclerosis in humans: Fact or myth? Circulation, *64*:1, 1981.

This editorial nicely summarizes the data dealing with this important concept.

McGill, H. L., Jr.: The relationship of dietary cholesterol to serum cholesterol concentration and to atherosclerosis in man. Am. J. Clin. Nutr., *32*:2664, 1979.

An extremely comprehensive overview of the relation of cholesterol to atherosclerosis is offered by this author. He summarizes the historical, epidemiologic, experimental, and clinical investigations dealing with this important topic.

Ross, R: Atherosclerosis: A problem of the biology of arterial wall cells and their interactions with blood components. Arteriosclerosis, *1*:293, 1981.

This excellent review is a thorough explanation of the initial cellular responses seen in early atherosclerosis. It offers a comprehensive description of atherogenesis that incorporates features from all of the leading hypotheses dealing with the development and progression of this disease.

Wright, I. S., and Frederickson, D. T. (Eds.): Cardiovascular Diseases: Guidelines of Prevention and Cure. Washington, D.C., U.S. Government Printing Office, 1973.

This single volume condenses a massive amount of data concerning the contributing factors, etiology, and pathogenesis of cardiovascular disease. The NIH-appointed committee responsible for this impressive achievement is composed of the leading figures working with these health problems. The lengthy lists of references supply detailed information for those seeking an in-depth analysis of the data supporting the concept of preventive therapy for cardiovascular disease.

REFERENCES

Abdulla, Y. H., Adams, C. W. M., and Bayliss, O. B.: The location of lecithin-cholesterol transacylase activity in the atherosclerotic arterial wall. J. Atheroscler. Res., *10*:229, 1969.

Abdulla, Y. H., Adams, C. W. M., and Morgan, R. S.: Connective-tissue reactions to implantation of purified sterol, sterol esters, phosphoglycerides, glycerides and free fatty acids. J. Pathol. Bacteriol., *94*:63, 1967.

Adams, C. W. M.: Tissue changes and lipid entry in developing atheroma. *In* Atherogenesis: Initiating Factors. New York, Association of Scientific Publishers, 1973.

Adams, C. W. M., and Bayliss, O. B.: The relationship between diffuse intimal thickening, medial enzyme failure, and intimal lipid deposition in various human arteries. J. Atheroscler. Res., *10*:327, 1969.

Ahrens, E. H., Jr., Hirsch, J., Insull, W., Tsaltas, T. T., Bloomstrand, R., and Peterson, M. L.: The influence of dietary fats on serum lipids in man. Lancet, *1*:943, 1957.

Ali, M., and McDonald, J. W. D.: Reversible and irreversible inhibition of platelet cyclo-oxygenase and serotonin release by nonsteroidal antiinflammatory drugs. Thromb. Res., *13*:1057, 1978.

American Heart Association Committee Report: Diet and coronary heart disease. Circulation, *58*:762A, 1978.

Anturane Reinfarction Trial Research Group: Sulfinpyrazone in the prevention of sudden death· after myocardial infarction. N. Engl. J. Med., *302*:250, 1980.

Armstrong, M. L., Warner, E. D., and Connor, W. E.: Regression of coronary atherosclerosis in Rhesus monkeys. Circ. Res., *27*:59, 1970.

Aspirin Myocardial Infarction Study Research Group: A randomized, controlled trial of aspirin in persons recovered from myocardial infarction. J.A.M.A., *243*:661, 1980.

Avoy, D. R., Swyryd, E. A., and Gould, R. G.: Effects of alpha-parachlorophenoxyisobutyryl ethyl ester (CPIB) with and without androsterone on cholesterol biosynthesis in rat liver. J. Lipid Res., 6:369, 1965.

Barrett, A. M., and Thorp, J. M.: Studies on the mode of action of clofibrate. Br. J. Pharmacol. Chemother., 32:381, 1968.

Benditt, E. P.: Implications of the monoclonal character of human atherosclerotic plaques. Am. J. Pathol., 86:693, 1977.

Berenson, G. S., and Cho, Y. W.: Provocative antilipidemic therapy in the management of peripheral arterial insufficiency. In Vasodilators: Evaluation and Clinical Pharmacology. Edited by Y. W. Cho and R. D. Allison. Pittsburgh, Instrument Society of America, 1974.

Berkowitz, D.: Management of the hyperlipidemic patient. Med. Clin. North Am., 57:881, 1973.

Bierenbaum, M. I., Fleischman, A. I., Raichelson, R. I., Hayton, T., and Watson, P. B.: Ten-year experience of modified-fat diets on younger men with coronary heart disease. Lancet, 1:1404, 1973.

Blackburn, H.: Current developments in North America. The Pooling Project Report. Council on Epidemiology. In Atherosclerosis: Proceedings of the Second International Symposium. Edited by R. J. Jones. New York, Springer-Verlag, 1970.

Blankenhorn, D. H.: Will atheroma regress with diet and exercise? Am. J. Surg., 141:644, 1981.

Bomberger, R. A., Zarins, C. K., and Glagov, S.: Subarterial stenosis enhances distal atherosclerosis. J. Surg. Res., 30:205, 1981.

Boston Collaborative Drug Surveillance Group: Regular aspirin intake and acute myocardial infarction. Br. Med. J., 1:440, 1974.

Bourassa, M. G., Goulet, C., and Lespérance, J.: Progression of coronary arterial disease after aortocoronary bypass grafts. Circulation, 47, 48(Suppl. 3):127, 1973.

Braunwald, E., Friedewald, W. T., and Furberg, C. D. (Eds.): Proceedings of the workshop on platelet-active drugs in the secondary prevention of cardiovascular events. Circulation, 62(Suppl. 5):1, 1980.

Brown, D. F., and Daudiss, K.: Hyperlipoproteinemia prevalence in a free-living population in Albany, New York. Circulation, 47:558, 1973.

Burch, J. W., Stanford, N., and Majeruo, P. W.: Inhibition of platelet prostaglandin synthetase by oral aspirin. J. Clin. Invest., 61:314, 1978.

Canadian Cooperative Study Groups: A randomized trial of aspirin and sulfinpyrazone in threatened stroke. N. Engl. J. Med., 299:53, 1978.

Carew, T. E., Hayes, S. B., Koschinsky, T., and Steinberg, D.: A mechanism by which high density lipoproteins may slow the atherogenic process. Lancet, 1:1315, 1976.

Carlson, L. A., and Hallberg, D.: Basal lipolysis and effects of norepinephrine and prostaglandin E_1 on lipolysis in human subcutaneous and omental adipose tissue. J. Lab. Clin. Med., 71:368, 1968.

Carlson, L. A., Oro, L., and Ostman, J.: Effect of nicotinic acid on plasma lipids in patients with hyperlipoproteinemia during the first week of treatment. J. Atheroscler. Res., 8:667, 1968.

Chobanian, A. V., Hollander, W., Sullivan, M., and Colombo, M.: Body cholesterol metabolism in man. I. The equilibrium of serum and tissue cholesterol. J. Clin. Invest., 41:1732, 1962.

Committee on Nutrition: Childhood diet and coronary heart disease. Pediatrics, 49:305, 1972.

Connor, W. E., and Connor, S. L.: Dietary factors in the treatment of hyperlipidemic disorders. In Treatment of Hyperlipidemic States. Edited by H. Casdorph. Springfield, Illinois, Charles C Thomas, 1971.

Connor, W. E., and Connor, S. L.: The key role of nutritional factors in the prevention of coronary heart disease. Prev. Med., 1:49, 1972.

Cooperative Trial in the Primary Prevention of Ischemic Heart Disease Using Clofibrate. Br. Heart J., 40:1069, 1978.

Cornfield, J.: Joint dependence of risk of coronary heart disease on serum cholesterol and systolic blood pressure: A discriminant function analysis. Fed. Proc., 21(Suppl 2):58, 1962.

Coronary Drug Project: Clofibrate and niacin in coronary heart disease. J.A.M.A., 231:306, 1975.

Coronary Drug Project: Findings leading to further modification of its protocol with respect to dextrothyroxine. J.A.M.A., 220:996, 1972.

Coronary Drug Project Research Group: Gallbladder disease as a side effect of drugs influencing lipid metabolism. N. Engl. J. Med., 296:1185, 1977.

Cowdry, E. V. (Ed.): Arteriosclerosis. New York, Macmillan Co., Inc., 1933.

Dayton, S., and Hashimoto, S.: Origin of cholesteryl oleate and other esterified lipids of rabbit atheroma. Atherosclerosis, 12:371, 1970.

Dayton, S., and Pearce, M. L.: Prevention of coronary heart disease and other complications of atherosclerosis by modified diet. Am. J. Med., 46:751, 1969.

Deduve, C.: The participation of lysosomes in the transformation of smooth muscle cells to foamy cells in the aorta of cholesterol-fed rabbits. Acta Cardiol. (Suppl.), 20:9, 1974.

DePalma, R. G., Hubay, C. A., Botti, R., and Peterka, J. L.: Treatment of surgical patients with atherosclerosis and hyperlipidemia. Surg. Gynecol. Obstet., 131:313, 1970.

DePalma, R. G., Koletsky, S., Bellon, E. M., and Insull, R., Jr.: Failure of regression of atherosclerosis in dogs with moderate cholesterolemia. Atherosclerosis, 27:297, 1977.

Dorr, A. E., Gundersen, K., Schneider, J. C., Jr., Spencer, T. W., and Martin, W. B.: Colestipol hydrochloride in hypercholesterolemia patients—effect on serum cholesterol and mortality. J. Chron. Dis., 31:5, 1978.

Eaton, R. P., Berman, M., and Steinberg, D.: Kinetic studies of plasma free fatty acid and triglyceride metabolism in man. J. Clin. Invest., 48:1560, 1969.

Ernst, N., Bowan, P., Fisher, M., Shaefer, E. J., and Levy, R. I.: Changes in plasma lipids and lipoproteins after a modified fat diet. Lancet, 1:111, 1980.

Eshleman, R., and Soderquist, K. (Eds.): The American Heart Association Cookbook. New York, David McKay, Co., Inc., 1973.

Fields, W. S., Lemak, N. A., Frankowski, R. F., Hardy, R. J., and Bigelow, R. H.: Controlled trial of aspirin in cerebral ischemia. Circulation, 62(Suppl. 5):90, 1980.

Ford, S., Jr., Bozian, R. C., and Knowles, H. C., Jr.: Interaction of obesity, insulin and glucose levels in hypertriglyceridemia. Clin. Res., 15:428, 1967.

Frantz, I. D., Jr., and Moore, R. B.: The sterol hypothesis in atherogenesis. Am. J. Med., 46:684, 1969.

Frederickson, D. S., Levy, R. I., and Lees, R. S.: Fat transport in lipoproteins—an integrated approach to mechanisms and disorders. N. Engl. J. Med., 276:34, 94, 148, 215, 273, 1967.

Frederickson, D. S., Levy, R. I., Jones, E., Bonnell, M., and Ernst, N.: The Dietary Management of Hyperlipoproteinemia: A Handbook for Physicians. Washington, D.C., U.S. Government Printing Office, 1970.

Fry, D. L.: Hemodynamic forces in atherosclerosis. In Cerebrovascular Diseases, Tenth Princeton Conference. Edited by P. Steinberg. New York, Raven Press, 1976.

Gainer, J. L., and Chisolm, G. M., III: Oxygen diffusion and atherosclerosis. Atherosclerosis, 19:135, 1974.

Garton, E.: A perspective on platelet-suppressant drug treatment in coronary artery and cerebrovascular disease. Circulation, 62(Suppl. 8):121, 1980.

Gent, M., Barnett, H. J. M., Sachett, D. L., and Taylor, D. W.: A randomized trial of aspirin and sulfinpyrazone in patients with threatened stroke. Circulation, 62(Suppl. 5):97, 1980.

Glomset, J. A.: The plasma lecithin-cholesterol acyltransferase reaction. J. Lipid Res., 9:155, 1968.

Goldstein, J. L., and Brown, M. S.: The low density lipoprotein pathway and its relation to atherosclerosis. Ann. Rev. Biochem., 46:897, 1977.

Gordon, T., Castelli, W. P., Hjortland, M. C., Kannel, W. B., and Dawber, T. R.: Predicting coronary heart disease in middle-aged and older persons. The Framington study. J.A.M.A., 238:497, 1977.

Gotto, A. M., Jr., Sheperd, J., Scott, L. W., and Manis, E.: Primary hyperlipoproteinemia and dietary management. In Nutrition, Lipids and Coronary Heart Disease. Edited by R. I. Levy, B. Rifkind, B. Dennis, and N. Ernst. New York, Raven Press, 1979.

Griffith, L. S. C., Achuff, S. C., Conti, C. R., Humphries, J. O., Brawley, R. K., Gott, V. L., and Ross, R. S.: Changes in intrinsic coronary circulation and segmental ventricular motion after saphenous-vein coronary bypass graft surgery. N. Engl. J. Med., 288:589, 1973.

Grundy, S. M.: The relationship between low cholesterol levels and cancer symptoms: Nutrition and heart disease. The 1981 Perspective, New York City, June 17, 1981.

Grundy, S. M., Ahrens, E. H., Jr., and Davignon, J.: The interaction of cholesterol absorption and cholesterol synthesis in man. J. Lipid Res., 10:304, 1969.

Hamel, R. J.: High density lipoproteins, cholesterol transport, and coronary heart disease. Circulation, 60:1, 1979.

Hammond, E. C., and Garfinkel, L.: Coronary heart disease, stroke and aortic aneurysm—factors in the etiology. Arch. Environ. Health, 19:167, 1969.

Harker, L., Wall, R. T., Harlan, J. M., and Ross, R.: Sulfinpyrazone prevention of homocysteine-induced endothelial cell injury and arteriosclerosis. Clin. Res., 26:554A, 1978.

Henahan, J.: Regression of atherosclerosis: Preliminary but encouraging news. J.A.M.A., 246:2309, 1981.

Henderson, R. R., and Rowe, G. G.: The progression of coronary atherosclerotic disease as assessed by cine-coronary arteriography. Am. Heart J., 86:165, 1973.

Hennekens, C. H., Willett, W., Rosner, B., Cole, D. S., and Mayrent, S. L.: Effects of beer, wine, and liquor in coronary deaths. J.A.M.A., 242:1973, 1979.

Hulley, S. B., and Gordon, S.: Alcohol and high-density lipoprotein cholesterol, causal inference from diverse study designs. Circulation, 64(Suppl. 3):57, 1981.

Hulley, S. B., Wilson, W. S., Burrows, M. I., and Nichaman, M. Z.: Lipid and lipoprotein response of hypertriglyceridemic outpatients to a low carbohydrate modification of the AHA fat controlled diet. Lancet, 2:551, 1972.

Imparato, A. M., Bracco, A., Kim, G. E., and Zeff, R.: Intimal and neointimal fibrous proliferation causing failure of arterial reconstructions. Surgery, 72:1007, 1972.

Jackson, R. L., Morrisett, J. D., and Gotto, A. M., Jr.: Lipoprotein structure and metabolism. Physiol. Rev., 56:259, 1976.

Kannel, W. B., Dawber, T. R., Cohen, M. E., and McNamara, P. M.: Vascular disease of the brain, epidemiologic aspects—the Framingham study. Am. J. Publ. Health, 55:1355, 1965a.

Kannel, W. B., Dawber, T. R., Skinner, J. J, McNamara, P. M., and Shurtleff, D.: Epidemiological aspects of intermittent claudication—the Framingham study. Circulation, 32(Suppl. 2):121, 1965b.

Kao, V. C. Y., and Wissler, R. W.: A study of the immunohistochemical localization of serum lipoproteins and other plasma proteins in human atherosclerotic lesions. Exp. Mol. Pathol., 4:465, 1965.

Kaplan, J. A., Cox, G. E., and Taylor, C. B.: Cholesterol metabolism in man. Studies on absorption. Arch. Pathol., 76:359, 1963.

Keys, A. (Ed.): Coronary heart disease in seven countries. Circulation, 41(Suppl. 1):1, 1970.

Keys, A.: Seven Countries, A Multivariate Analysis of Death and Coronary Heart Disease. Cambridge, Massachusetts, Harvard University Press, 1980.

Kinlough-Rathbone, R. L., and Mustard, J. F.: Atherosclerosis, current concepts. Am. J. Surg., 141:638, 1981.

Krikler, D. M., Lefevre, D., and Lewis, B.: Dextrothyroxine with propranolol in treatment of hypercholesterolemia. Lancet, 1:934, 1971.

Kudzma, D. J., and Schonfeld, G.: Alcoholic hyperlipidemia: Induction by alcohol but not by carbohydrate. J. Lab. Clin. Med., 77:384, 1971.

Kuo, P. T.: Hyperglyceridemia in coronary artery disease and its management. J.A.M.A., 201:87, 1967.

Kuo, P. T., Hayase, K., Kosis, J. B., and Moreyra, A. E.: Use of combined diet and colestipol in long term (7–7½ years) treatment of patients with Type II hyperlipidemia. Circulation, 59:199, 1979.

Lees, R. S., and Frederickson, D. S.: Carbohydrate induction of hyperlipidemia in normal man. Circ. Res., 13:327, 1965.

Lees, R. S., and Wilson, D. E.: The treatment of hyperlipidemia. N. Engl. J. Med., 284:186, 1971.

Leren, P.: The Oslo diet-heart study. Circulation, 42:935, 1970.

Levy, R. I.: Declining mortality in coronary heart disease. Arteriosclerosis, 1:312, 1981.

Levy, R. I., Rifkind, B., Dennis, B., and Ernst, N. (Eds.): Nutrition, Lipids and Coronary Heart Disease. New York, Raven Press, 1979.

Lofland, H. B., Jr., St. Clair, R. W., Clarkson, T. B., Bullock, B. C., and Lehner, N. D. M.: Atherosclerosis in Cebus monkeys. II. Arterial metabolism. Exp. Mol. Pathol., 9:57, 1968.

Malinow, M. R.: Regression of atherosclerosis in humans: Fact or myth? Circulation, 64:1, 1981.

Malinow, M. R.: Atherosclerosis, regression in nonhuman primates. Circ. Res., 46:311, 1980.

Malinow, M. R., McLaughlin, P., McNulty, W. P., Naito, H. K., and Levin, L. A.: Treatment of established atherosclerosis during cholesterol feeding in monkeys. Atherosclerosis, 31:185, 1978.

Mann, G. V.: Diet-heart: End of an era. N. Engl. J. Med., 297:644, 1977.

McCann, R. L., Larson, R. M., Mitchener, J. S., Fuchs, J. C. A., and Hagen, P.-O.: Intimal thickening and hyperlipidemia in experimental primate vascular autografts. Ann. Surg., 189:62, 1979.

McCullagh, K. G., and Ehrhart, L. A.: Increased arterial collagen synthesis in experimental canine atherosclerosis. Atherosclerosis, 19:13, 1974.

McGill, H. C., Jr.: Introduction to the geographic pathology of atherosclerosis. Lab. Invest., 18:465, 1968.

McGill, H. C., Jr.: The relationship of dietary cholesterol to serum cholesterol concentration and to atherosclerosis in man. Am. J. Clin. Nutr., 32:2664, 1979.

Miettinen, M., Turpeinen, O., Karvonen, M. J., Elosuo, R., and Paavilainen, E.: Effect of cholesterol-lowering diet on mortality from coronary heart disease and other causes—a twelve year clinical trial in men and women. Lancet, 2:835, 1972.

Miller, D. N., and Hamilton, J. G.: Nicotinic acid and derivatives. In Lipid Pharmacology. Edited by R. Paoletti. New York, Academic Press, Inc., 1964.

Moncada, S., Gryglewski, R., Bunting, S., and Vane, J. R.: An enzyme isolated from arteries transforms prostaglandin endoperoxides to an unstable substance that inhibits platelet aggregation. Nature, 263:663, 1976.

National Diet Heart Study Research Group: The National Diet Heart Study final report. Circulation, 37(Suppl. 1):1, 1968.

Nestel, P. J., and Whyte, H. M.: Plasma free fatty acid and triglyceride turnover in obesity. Metabolism, 17:1122, 1968.

Packham, M. A., and Mustard, J. F.: Pharmacology of platelet-affecting drugs. Circulation, 62(Suppl. 5):26, 1980.

Pearce, M. L., and Dayton, S.: Incidence of cancer in men on a diet high in polyunsaturated fat. Lancet, 1:464, 1971.

Persantine-Aspirin Reinfarction Study Research Group: The persantine-aspirin reinfarction study. Circulation, 62(Suppl. 5):85, 1980.

Person, T. A., Kramer, E. C., Solez, K., and Hepinstall, R. H.: The human atherosclerotic plaque. Am. J. Pathol., 86:657, 1977.

Peterson, B., Trell, E., and Sternby, N. H.: Low cholesterol levels as risk factor for noncoronary death in middle aged men. J.A.M.A., 245:2056, 1981.

Pooling Project Research Group: Relationship of blood pressure, serum cholesterol, smoking habit, relative weight and EKG abnormalities to incidence of major coronary events. J. Chron. Dis., 31:201, 1978.

Proudlock, J. W., and Day, A. J.: Cholesterol esterifying enzymes of atherosclerotic rabbit intima. Biochim. Biophys. Acta, 260:716, 1972.

Rafflenbeul, W., Smith, L. R., Rogers, W. J., Mantle, J. A., Rackley, C. E., and Russell, R. O., Jr.: Quantitative coronary arteriography: Coronary anatomy of patients with unstable angina pectoris reexamined 1 year after optimal medical therapy. Am. J. Cardiol., 43:699, 1979.

Randle, P. J., Garland, P. B., Hales, C. N., and Newsholme, E.

A.: The glucose fatty acid cycle: Its role in insulin sensitivity and the metabolic disturbances of diabetes mellitus. Lancet, *1*:785, 1963.

Richardson, M., Ihnatowycz, I., and Moore, S.: Glycosaminoglycan distribution in rabbit aortic wall following balloon catheter deendothelialization. An ultrastructural study. Lab. Invest., *43*:509, 1980.

Ross, R.: Atherosclerosis: A problem of the biology of arterial wall cells and their interactions with blood components. Arteriosclerosis, *1*:293, 1981.

Ross, R., and Glomset, J. A.: Pathogenesis of atherosclerosis. N. Engl. J. Med., *295*:369, 420, 1976.

Ross, R., and Harker, L.: Hyperlipidemia and atherosclerosis. Science, *193*:1094, 1976.

Ross, R., and Vogel, A.: The platelet derived growth factor. Cell, *14*:203, 1978.

Salans, L. B., Knittle, J. L., and Hirsch, J.: The role of adipose cell size and adipose tissue insulin sensitivity in the carbohydrate intolerance of human obesity. J. Clin. Invest., *47*:153, 1968.

Scanu, A. M.: The structure of human serum low and high density lipoproteins. *In* Atherogenesis: Initiating Factors. New York, Associated Scientific Publishers, 1973.

Schneeberg, N. G., Herman, E., Menduke, H., and Altschuler, N. K.: Reduction of serum cholesterol by sodium dextrothyroxine in euthyroid subjects. Ann. Intern. Med., *56*:265, 1962.

Schwartz, C. J., and Mitchell, J. R. A.: Observations on localization of arterial plaques. Circ. Res., *11*:63, 1962.

Schwartz, S. M., Gajdusek, C. M., and Selden, S. C., III: Vascular wall growth control: The role of endothelium. Arteriosclerosis, *1*:107, 1981.

Shebelle, R. B., Shyrock, A. M., Paul, O., Lepper, M., Stamler, J., Lin, S., and Raynor, W. J., Jr.: Diet, serum cholesterol, and death from coronary heart disease. N. Engl. J. Med., *304*:65, 1981.

Sigurdsson, G., Nicole, A., and Lewis, B.: Conversion of very low density lipoprotein to low density lipoprotein. J. Clin. Invest., *56*:1481, 1975.

Simons, L. A., and Myant, N. B.: The effect of D-thyroxine on the metabolism of cholesterol in familial hyperbetalipoproteinemia. Atherosclerosis, *19*:103, 1974.

Siperstein, M. D., and Guest, M. J.: Studies on the site of the feedback control of cholesterol synthesis. J. Clin. Invest., *39*:642, 1960.

Smith, E. B.: Molecular interactions in human atherosclerotic plaques. Am. J. Pathol., *86*:665, 1977.

Smith, E. B., and Slater, R. S.: Lipids and low-density lipoproteins in intima in relation to its morphological characteristics. *In* Atherogenesis: Initiating Factors (A Symposium Held at the Ciba Foundation, July 5, 6, 1972. Edited by Ruth Porter and Julie Knight) Symposium on Mechanisms in the Development of Early Atheroma, Ciba Foundation Symposium New Series 12. New York, Associated Scientific Publishers, 1973.

Stamler, J.: The coronary risk factors. *In* Preventive Cardiology. New York, Grune and Stratton, Inc., 1967.

Stamler, J.: Population studies. *In* Nutrition, Lipids and Coronary Heart Disease. Edited by R. Levy, B. Rifkind, B. Dennis, and N. Ernst. New York, Raven Press, 1979.

Steinberg, D., and Grundy, S. M.: Management of hyperlipidemia. Diet and Drugs. Arch. Surg., *113*:55, 1978.

Stender, S., and Zilversmit, D. B.: Transfer of plasma lipoprotein components and of plasma proteins into aortas of cholesterol-fed rabbits. Arteriosclerosis, *1*:38, 1981.

Stern, M. P.: Ischemic heart disease: An epidemic on the wane? Am. J. Surg., *141*:646, 1981.

Stout, R. W.: Blood glucose and atherosclerosis. Arteriosclerosis, *1*:227, 1981.

Strong, J. P., and Guzman, M. A.: Decrease in coronary atherosclerosis in New Orleans. Lab. Invest., *43*:297, 1980.

Strong, J. P., Richards, M. L., McGill, H. C., Jr., Eggen, D. A., and McMurry, M. T.: On the association of cigarette smoking with coronary and aortic atherosclerosis. J. Atheroscler. Res., *10*:303, 1969.

Subbiah, M. T. R., Dicke, B. A., Kottbe, B. A., Carlo, I. A., and Dinh, D. M.: Regression of naturally occurring atherosclerotic lesions in pigeon aorta by intestinal bypass surgery. Atherosclerosis, *31*:117, 1978.

ten Hoor, F., de Deckere, E. A. M., Holdeman, E., Hornstra, G., and Quadt, J. F. A.: Dietary manipulations of prostaglandin and thromboxane synthesis in heart, aorta and blood platelets of the rat. Adv. Prostaglandin Thromboxane Res., *8*:1771, 1980.

Thorp, J. M., Cotton, R. C., and Oliver, M. F.: Role of the endocrine system in the regulation of plasma lipids and fibrinogen with particular reference to the effects of "Atromid S." Progr. Biochem. Pharmacol., *4*:64, 1968.

Turpeinen, O.: Effects of cholesterol-lowering diet on mortality from coronary heart disease and other causes. Circulation, *59*:1, 1979.

Vlodaver, Z., and Edwards, J. E.: Pathologic changes in aortic-coronary arterial saphenous vein grafts. Circulation, *44*:719, 1971.

Wakil, S. J.: Fatty acid metabolism. *In* Lipid Metabolism. Edited by S. J. Wakil. New York, Academic Press, Inc., 1970.

Wilson, W. S., Hulley, S. B., Burrows, M. I., and Nichaman, M. Z.: Several lipid and lipoprotein responses to the American Heart Association fat controlled diet. Am. J. Med., *51*:491, 1971.

Wissler, R. W.: The arterial medial cell smooth muscle or multifunctional mesenchyme. J. Atheroscler. Res., *8*:201, 1968.

Wolinsky, H.: Mesenchymal response of the blood vessel wall, a potential avenue for understanding and treating atherosclerosis. Circ. Res., *32*:543, 1973.

Wright, I. S., and Frederickson, D. T. (eds.): Atherosclerosis and epidemiology study groups: Primary prevention of atherosclerotic disease. *In* Cardiovascular Diseases: Guidelines for Prevention and Care. Washington, D.C., U.S. Government Printing Office, 1973.

Yudkin, J., and Roddy, J.: Levels of dietary sucrose in patients with occlusive atherosclerotic disease. Lancet, *2*:6, 1964.

Chapter 51

The Surgical Management of Cardiac Arrhythmias

JAMES L. COX

The recent development of new methods for the experimental and clinical evaluation of cardiac arrhythmias has led to a better understanding of their pathogenesis and to a more scientific approach to their treatment. The diagnosis and treatment of cardiac arrhythmias have resided and continue to remain primarily within the realm of medical management. During the past decade, however, surgical therapy has proved to be an invaluable addition to the antiarrhythmia armamentarium. The success of surgical procedures for the treatment of Wolff-Parkinson-White (WPW) syndrome, AV node re-entry, "concealed" accessory atrioventricular connections, ectopic atrial foci, and, more recently, several different types of ventricular tachyarrhythmias portends a greater future role for the cardiac surgeon in this field.

Surgical procedures for arrhythmias are confined presently to only a few medical centers that are properly equipped to evaluate and treat these problems. However, once the newer surgical techniques are perfected, it is unlikely that their application will uniformly require the sophisticated intraoperative electrical studies that are being performed at present. Moreover, our experience with the surgical approach for Wolff-Parkinson-White syndrome and for ventricular tachycardia associated with coronary artery disease clearly indicates that the number of patients requiring operation is directly related to the clinical awareness of the problem and to the degree of success of the applicable surgical procedure. Therefore, it seems apparent that within the next decade, all cardiac surgeons will be expected to become more familiar with the normal and abnormal aspects of cardiac electrophysiology.

BASIC ELECTROPHYSIOLOGIC CONCEPTS

The introduction of the microelectrode by Draper and Weidmann in 1957 led to general acceptance of the theory that normal cardiac cells generate upstrokes by a rapid, voltage-dependent, transient inflow of sodium ions ("rapid channel"). The resultant trans- membrane action potential recorded by a microelectrode from normal myocardial cells has five distinctive phases (Fig. 51–1). Phase 0 represents the sharp upstroke recorded during depolarization of the cell, when sodium ions pass rapidly into the cell. Phases 1 and 2 occur immediately after completion of cellular depolarization, during which time the cell is absolutely refractory to further depolarization. During phase 3, the cell begins to repolarize as sodium ions transfer out of the cell and potassium ions flow inward to reestablish the resting transmembrane potential (phase 4). In 1967, Reuter demonstrated a slow inward current of calcium ions during the plateau (phase 2) of the transmembrane action potential. Because the kinetics of activation, inactivation, and reactivation of sinoatrial (SA) node and atrioventricular (AV) node cells and of certain abnormal cells with low resting

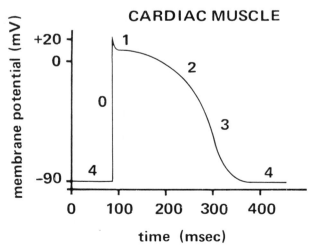

Figure 51–1. The cardiac action potential (shown here for Purkinje fiber) lasts for more than 300 msec. and consists of five phases. Phase 0 (upstroke) corresponds to depolarization in skeletal muscle, and phase 3 (repolarization) corresponds to repolarization in that tissue. Phases 1 (early repolarization) and 2 (plateau) have no clear counterpart in skeletal muscle, whereas phase 4 (diastole) corresponds to the resting potential. (From Katz, A. M.: The arrhythmias, II: Abnormal impulse formation and re-entry, premature systoles, pre-excitation. *In* Physiology of the Heart. New York, Raven Press, 1977.)

transmembrane potentials are considerably slower than those for the inward sodium current, the "slow channel" of calcium ion influx is considered to be a major factor in the activation of these cells. SA nodal cells probably operate with a mixed dependence on rapid and slow currents (Strauss *et al.*, 1977). Although spontaneous phase 4 depolarization (characteristic of pacemaker cells) is due in part to deactivation of a fast potassium current (McAllister *et al.*, 1975), the sensitivity of SA node cells to slow-channel blocking agents (Zipes and Fisher, 1974) suggests that the background inward current may be the slow calcium current rather than a sodium current. While these ionic currents form the basis for normal cardiac impulse generation and conduction, pathologic changes in myocardial cells may lead to a detrimental interplay between the rapid and slow currents and thereby to the two basic types of cardiac rhythm disturbances, ectopic (automatic) arrhythmias and re-entrant arrhythmias.

The appearance of automaticity in pathologic myocardial cells is believed to develop on the same electrochemical basis that gives rise to spontaneous activity in normal pacemaker cells. Injured cells exhibit spontaneous phase 4 depolarization, which may result in atrial or ventricular premature systoles or, if repetitive, in atrial or ventricular tachycardia.

The physiologic basis for re-entrant arrhythmias is somewhat more complex in that several different types of re-entry may occur, depending on the type of anatomic-electrophysiologic abnormality present. The simplest type of re-entry is that of a "circus movement," first described by Mines in 1914 (Fig. 51–2). In this type of re-entrant arrhythmia, it is essential that a unidirectional block develop at some point in a contiguous conducting circuit. If the course of the circuit is sufficiently long (or the refractory period sufficiently short) to allow previously depolarized tissue to repolarize before the electrical wave front traverses the circuit, the wave front will always be preceded by excitable tissue, and the arrhythmia may continue indefinitely. This type of re-entrant mechanism (usually called "macro-re-entry") is responsible for the reciprocating tachycardia of Wolff-Parkinson-White syndrome, certain types of atrial flutter, and, occasionally, unusual types of ventricular tachycardia in which the re-entrant circuit involves various branches of the His-Purkinje system.

Re-entrant arrhythmias associated with ischemic heart disease most commonly result from micro-re-entrant circuits in which two conditions are essential for the development of sustained re-entry: (1) unidirectional block and (2) slow conduction. Unidirectional block plays the same role in micro-re-entry as it does in macro-re-entry, i.e., it dictates that the wave front of depolarization be propagated in only one direction around the circuit. Although some asymmetry of conduction exists in normal myocardial tissue owing to differences in the passive or active properties of cells, local unidirectional block is an extreme form of asymmetry of conduction. This asymmetry is exaggerated by conditions that depress excitability, such as high local extracellular potassium concentrations that exist in ischemic myocardium. In addition, myocardial fibrosis, which reduces the ability of an electrical impulse to be propagated by increasing the resistance, can cause unidirectional block when the fibrosis is distributed asymmetrically.

Because of the comparatively long distances traversed by an electrical impulse in macro-re-entrant circuits (e.g., in Wolff-Parkinson-White syndrome), slow conduction in a portion of these circuits is not

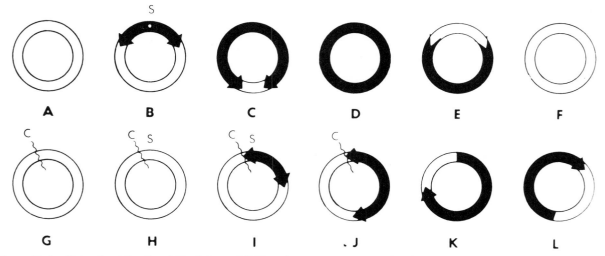

Figure 51–2. Role of unidirectional block in establishing circus movement. Application of a stimulus to a ring of excitable tissue (unshaded area) in the absence of block *(B)* initiates an impulse (shaded area) that depolarizes the entire ring *(D)*. Mutual cancellation of the impulses moving in opposite directions *(C)* allows the tissue to repolarize completely *(E,F)*. However, if unidirectional block is established by temporary clamping of the tissue (C in *G–J*), the impulse propagated in the clockwise direction can continue to travel around the ring *(K,L)*, thereby establishing a circus movement. (From Katz, A. M.: The arrhythmias, II: Abnormal impulse formation and re-entry, premature systoles, pre-excitation. *In* Physiology of the Heart. New York, Raven Press, 1977.)

an absolute requisite for the development of sustained re-entry. However, in micro-re-entrant circuits, the actual distance traversed by the electrical impulse may be so short (e.g., perhaps involving only a few cells) that sustained re-entry cannot occur unless conduction velocity is decreased in some portion of the circuit. Four physiologically interdependent factors influence conduction velocity in myocardial tissue: (1) action potential amplitude, (2) rate of depolarization of the action potential, (3) threshold, and (4) electrical resistance. In regions of ischemia, myocardial cells become partially depolarized because some of the intracellular potassium is replaced with sodium. This results in partial inactivation of the rapid sodium channels and, therefore, decreases both action potential amplitude and the rate of depolarization. Such partially depolarized tissues can conduct a propagated action potential, although extremely slowly and usually with decrement. These conductive properties, which give rise to slowly propagated waves of depolarization, exhibit the features of the slow inward current carried mainly by calcium ions. For these reasons, calcium-mediated slow responses are regarded as playing an important, if not exclusive, role in the genesis of micro-re-entrant arrhythmias (Katz, 1977). The conditions necessary for the development of sustained micro-re-entrant arrhythmias may occur in an ischemic limb of distal Purkinje fibers or in an ischemic strand of myocardial muscle (Fig. 51–3).

Clinical differentiation between refractory ectopic and re-entrant arrhythmias is important because, with few exceptions, surgical therapy is less effective in the treatment of ectopic arrhythmias. However, the ability to discriminate between these two types of arrhythmias clinically is limited. Current practice involves the use of rapid "burst" pacing or programmed premature stimulation. With the latter technique, regular pacing stimuli (S_1) are introduced at a given cycle length, and a premature stimulus (S_2) is delivered in late diastole. The premature stimulus is then introduced progressively earlier until it no longer elicits a depolarization, thus delineating the refractory period of the tissue being stimulated. If the arrhythmia is not induced by this single premature impulse delivered at different intervals throughout electrical diastole, double premature stimuli (S_2, S_3) are introduced, with S_3 being delivered at progressive intervals beginning 50 to 100 msec. longer than the effective refractory period of the tissue. This sequence is repeated until the arrhythmia is initiated. The same programmed single, double, and triple stimuli may then be delivered to terminate the arrhythmia. Clinically, arrhythmias that respond to programmed premature stimulation are considered to be re-entrant arrhythmias, and those that do not respond are classified as ectopic (automatic) arrhythmias. Although this clinical classification is strictly empiric, it is useful in that it provides: (1) a means of assessing medical management, (2) a rationale for the use of pacemaker devices, and (3) some assurance that the arrhythmia can be invoked for investigative purposes at the time of surgery.

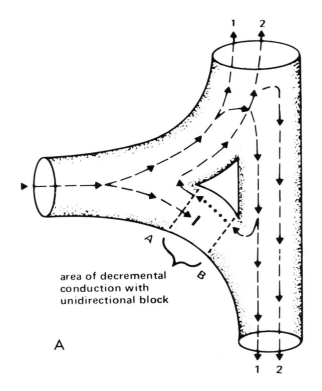

area of decremental conduction with unidirectional block

A

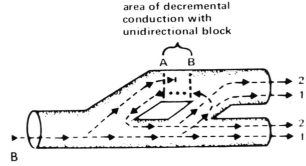

area of decremental conduction with unidirectional block

B

Figure 51–3. Re-entry at the point of impingement of a Purkinje fiber on the ventricular myocardium *(A)* and within a strand of cardiac muscle *(B)*. In both situations, a region of decremental conduction with unidirectional block (A–B) blocks antegrade conduction of the normal impulse (1) but allows this impulse to traverse the depressed region in the retrograde direction (dotted line) after a delay. This retrograde impulse re-enters the myocardium proximal to the region of decremental conduction after the proximal tissue has recovered from the normal impulse, thereby allowing the retrograde impulse to initiate a premature systole (2). (From Katz, A. M.: The arrhythmias, II: Abnormal impulse formation and re-entry, premature systoles, pre-excitation. *In* Physiology of the Heart. New York, Raven Press, 1977.)

ANATOMY OF THE CARDIAC CONDUCTION SYSTEM AND RELATED STRUCTURES

The SA mode is a small subepicardial group of highly specialized cells located in the sulcus terminalis just lateral to the junction of the superior vena cava and the right atrium (Anderson and Becker, 1978). The cells are arranged around a central SA node artery that may arise from either the right or left coronary system and may pass either anterior or posterior to the superior vena cava. Studies suggest that the SA node consists of three distinct regions, each responsive to a separate group of neural and circulatory stimuli (Boineau *et al.,* 1977). The inter-relationship of these three regions determines the ultimate output of the SA node. Under normal conditions, these cells are the only ones in the heart capable of spontaneous phase 4 depolarization, thus establishing the SA node as the site of origin of the normal cardiac impulse.

The existence of specialized conduction pathways between the SA node and the AV node has been a subject of controversy for many years. Most authorities now agree, however, that although an electrical impulse emanating from the SA node travels to the AV node preferentially via the crista terminalis and the limbus of the fossa ovalis, these muscle bundles do not represent specialized, insulated conduction tracts comparable to the ventricular bundle branches. Although electrical impulses travel more rapidly through these thick atrial muscle bundles, surgical transection will not block internodal conduction.

The atrioventricular junctional area is the most complex anatomic portion of the cardiac conduction system. From a functional standpoint, the AV node should be considered as the area in which there occurs a normal delay in atrioventricular conduction. This area corresponds anatomically to a group of atrioventricular junctional cells that are histologically distinct from working myocardium (Anderson and Becker, 1976). As an atrial impulse approaches the AV node area, it traverses a "transition zone" of specialized cells located anteriorly in the base of the atrial septum slightly to the right of and cephalad to the central fibrous body. This transition zone surrounds the atrial aspect of the "compact AV node," where the major conduction delay occurs. The lower, longitudinal portion of the compact AV node penetrates the central fibrous body immediately posterior to the membranous portion of the intra-atrial septum to become the bundle of His. The AV node, its transitional zone, and its penetrating bundle are all contained within the triangle of Koch, an anatomically discrete region bounded by the tendon of Tadaro, tricuspid valve anulus, and thebesian valve of the coronary sinus (Fig. 51-4). There is little danger of surgical damage to AV conduction if this triangle is avoided in all procedures.

As just mentioned, once the penetrating portion of the AV node traverses the central fibrous body, it becomes the bundle of His. The anatomy in this area is complicated by the fact that the junction of the right heart chambers occupies a different spatial plane from the junction of the left heart chambers, the anulus of the tricuspid valve being situated more toward the ventricular apex than that of the mitral valve (Anderson and Becker, 1979). The bundle of His travels along the posteroinferior rim of the membranous portion of the interventricular septum. The right bundle branch proceeds subendocardially toward the base of

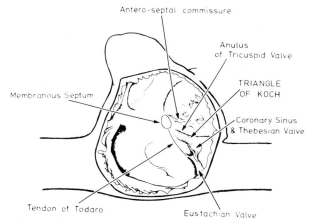

Figure 51–4. Landmarks of the triangle of Koch. (From Anderson, R. H., and Becker, A. E.: Cardiac anatomy for the surgeon. *In* Lewis Practice of Surgery. Hagerstown, Maryland, Harper and Row, 1979.)

the medial papillary muscle and descends toward the ventricular apex, partly crossing the cavity of the ventricle in the moderator band. At the lower level of the membranous interventricular septum, the His bundle gives off a broad band of fasciculi, forming the left bundle branch that extends down the left side of the septum for a distance of 1 to 2 cm., where it divides into a smaller anterior and a larger posterior radiation. The medial aspects of each of these radiations usually become intermeshed distally to form three anastomosing nets of fibers—anterior, middle, and posterior. When the left side of the ventricular septum is viewed through the aortic valve, the danger area from the standpoint of the conduction tissue is immediately subjacent to the right coronary-noncoronary commissure.

The distal branches of the conduction system terminate in an intermediate zone between the Purkinje cells and the myocardium, where the cells gradually lose their Purkinje characteristics and take on the characteristics of working ventricular myocardium.

Of particular importance to the cardiac surgeon dealing with conduction abnormalities are the relationships of the various structures and potential spaces composing the junction of the atrial septum, the ventricular septum, the atrioventricular grooves, and the fibrous skeleton of the heart. The cardiac skeleton is strongest at the central fibrous body where the anuli of the mitral, tricuspid, and aortic valves meet (Fig. 51-5). Since the tricuspid anulus is more apical in position than the mitral anulus, the anterior part of the central fibrous body extends into the ventricles beneath the attachment of the tricuspid valve and forms the interventricular component of the membranous septum between the aortic outflow tract and the right atrium. Likewise, immediately posterior to the membranous septum, the right atrial wall is in potential communication with the inlet portion of the left ventricle.

The mitral and aortic valve anuli contribute sig-

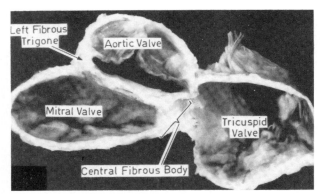

Figure 51–5. Dissection showing the fibrous cardiac skeleton after it has been removed from the ventricles. (From Anderson, R. H., and Becker, A. E.: Cardiac anatomy for the surgeon. *In* Lewis' Practice of Surgery, Hagerstown, Maryland, Harper and Row, 1979.)

nificantly to the structural integrity of the fibrous skeleton and are further strengthened at their left junction to form the left fibrous trigone. The left anterior portion of the central fibrous body is designated as the right fibrous trigone. The AV groove between these two trigones represents the site of continuity between the anterior leaflet of the mitral valve and the aortic valve anulus and is the only area in the AV groove where atrial muscle is not in juxtaposition to ventricular muscle. For this reason, accessory atrioventricular pathways are not found between the left and right fibrous trigones.

The potential space overlying the inlet septum (Fig. 51–6) has been demonstrated to harbor all posterior septal accessory pathways in Wolff-Parkinson-White syndrome (Sealy and Gallagher, 1980). The floor of this pyramidal space is formed by the upper posterior interventricular septum. The superior and lateral limits are formed by the divergent right and left atrial walls, and the posterior aspect is covered with epicardium reflected from the atrium to the ventricle over the AV groove fat pad. The space contains the terminal portion of the coronary sinus,

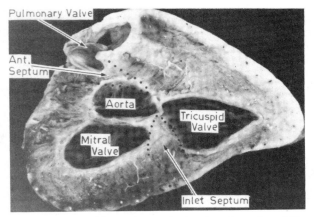

Figure 51–6. The atrioventricular junction viewed from above and from the right following removal of the atrial chambers. (From Anderson, R. H., and Becker, A. E.: Cardiac anatomy for the surgeon. *In* Lewis Practice of Surgery. Hagerstown, Maryland, Harper and Row, 1979.)

the AV node artery, and the fat pad. Its complex anatomy represents a continuing challenge to the surgeon attempting to ablate an accessory AV connection passing through this space.

PATIENT SELECTION

The proper selection of patients for the surgical treatment of cardiac arrhythmias is based on several variables, including the patient's age and general condition, the nature of the presenting arrhythmia, its response to medical treatment, and the presence of associated anomalies that may require additional surgical correction. Patients with intractable supraventricular arrhythmias due to one of the pre-excitation syndromes are generally relatively low-risk surgical candidates, with the exception of those patients with associated Ebstein's anomaly or coronary artery disease. In contradistinction, those patients who present with intractable ventricular arrhythmias have either an associated cardiomyopathy or coronary artery disease, usually with a ventricular aneurysm. Moreover, surgery for the latter patients is commonly performed as a last resort and frequently under urgent or emergency conditions. Regardless of their clinical status, however, all patients who are to be subjected to cardiac surgery for intractable arrhythmias should undergo a thorough preoperative catheter electrophysiologic study.

SUPRAVENTRICULAR ARRHYTHMIAS

Preoperative Electrophysiologic Evaluation

Atrial flutter, atrial fibrillation, junctional tachycardia, chaotic atrial tachycardia, and most cases of sick sinus syndrome can be diagnosed by routine, noninvasive electrocardiography. However, refractory supraventricular tachycardia due to an accessory atrioventricular connection (Wolff-Parkinson-White syndrome), enhanced AV node conduction, AV node re-entry, Mahaim fibers, or "concealed" accessory connections that conduct only retrograde require more sophisticated electrophysiologic evaluation. Patients with these suspected abnormalities undergo a multifaceted study in which catheters are positioned in the high right atrium, low right atrium, coronary sinus (quadrapolar catheter), and right ventricular apex and along the bundle of His (Fig. 51–7).

The initial His bundle recordings are most helpful in determining whether or not an accessory pathway is present (Fig. 51–8). Normally, the His electrode records atrial activity at the onset of the P wave and ventricular activity at the onset of the QRS complex of the standard electrocardiogram (Fig. 51–8A). If an accessory connection is present that bypasses the AV node, the A-H and A-V intervals are shortened, but the H-V interval is normal (Fig. 51–8B). This anomaly is classified clinically as "enhanced AV node conduction," and if it is refractory to medical therapy,

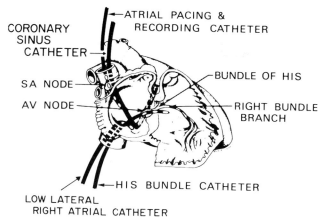

Figure 51–7. Position of intracardiac electrode catheters during preoperative electrophysiologic study. Note that there are two right atrial electrodes, one located near the region of the SA node and one located in the low lateral portion of the right atrium. The coronary sinus catheter is quadripolar, thus allowing four separate sites of the posterior left atrium to be recorded simultaneously. A right ventricular catheter electrode is usually positioned into the right ventricular apex.

it requires elective cryoablation of both the accessory pathway and the His bundle, since they cannot be separated anatomically at the time of surgery. In the presence of a Mahaim fiber connecting the His bundle to the septal myocardium, the A-H interval is normal,

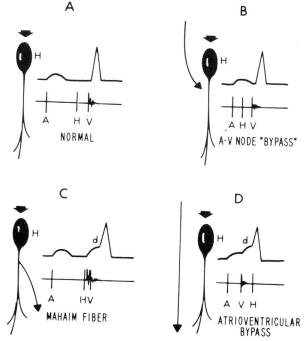

Figure 51–8. Types of accessory pathways. The electrocardiogram, His bundle electrogram, and schematic diagram of the conducting pathways associated with a normal conduction system *(A)*, an atrioventricular node "bypass" *(B)*, a Mahaim fiber *(C)*, and a complete atrioventricular bypass *(D)* are shown. (A = atrial electrogram; H = His bundle electrogram; V = ventricular electrogram; d = delta wave.) (From Gallagher, J. J., *et al.*: The Wolff-Parkinson-White syndrome and the pre-excitation dysrhythmias: Medical and surgical management. Med. Clin. North Am., *60*:101, 1976.)

since the electrical impulse is unaffected until after it exists the AV node (Fig. 51–8*C*). However, the H-V interval is shortened since the impulse can travel via the Mahaim fiber to the myocardium, resulting in pre-excitation and a delta wave. When a complete atrioventricular bypass tract exists (Kent bundle in Wolff-Parkinson-White syndrome), the electrical impulse travels both antegrade down the normal conduction system (normal A-H interval) and antegrade down the Kent bundle (markedly shortened A-V interval). This results in pre-excitation of the ventricular myocardium at the insertion of the Kent bundle, producing the short P-R interval, delta wave, and wide QRS complex characteristic of Wolff-Parkinson-White syndrome (Fig. 51–8*D*).

If stable antegrade pre-excitation does not exist, it may be difficult to differentiate between AV node re-entry and Wolff-Parkinson-White syndrome. In these cases, the patient undergoes programmed stimulation of the atrium in an effort to induce a reciprocating tachycardia. Once a stable tachycardia (PAT) is induced, a premature ventricular complex (PVC) is introduced immediately after activation of the His bundle. If the atrium is pre-excited by the PVC, an accessory pathway capable of retrograde conduction *must* be present, since retrograde conduction up the His bundle is impossible because of its state of refractoriness. Inability to pre-excite the atrium by introducing a "PVC in PAT" is strong evidence for the presence of AV node re-entry. If the patient has refractory PAT due to AV node re-entry, elective cryoablation of the bundle of His is the only effective surgical treatment.

Once an accessory AV connection has been documented, an effort is made to determine its location. This step is most important to the surgeon because the surgical approach to left free-wall, right free-wall, and septal pathways is different. In addition, AV connections occasionally become nonfunctional at the time of surgery (owing to trauma or anesthesia), thereby precluding intraoperative localization of the site of the accessory pathway. Left free-wall pathways are identified in two ways: (1) during induced reciprocating tachycardia or ventricular pacing, the quadripolar coronary sinus catheter (which is in contact with the left atrial wall) records atrial activity traveling retrograde across the accessory pathway earlier than do the right atrial catheters; and (2) by inducing left bundle branch block during reciprocating tachycardia, the V-A interval is prolonged 25 msec. or more in the presence of a left free-wall pathway. This prolongation with left bundle branch block occurs because normally during reciprocating tachycardia the impulse travels down the His bundle, left bundle branch, and left ventricular myocardium and retrograde up the left-sided accessory pathway to reach the atrium. However, with left bundle branch block, the impulse must travel down the *right* bundle branch, across the septum to the left ventricular myocardium, and then up the accessory pathway to the atrium. The longer route results in significant prolongation of the V-A interval (Fig. 51–9). The opposite findings occur in the pres-

EFFECT OF BBB ON RT UTILIZING A LEFT FREE-WALL AP.

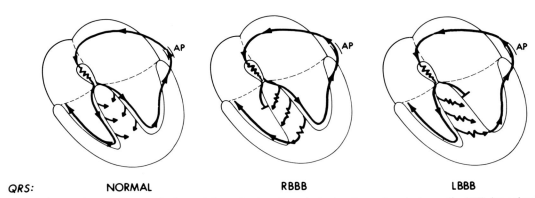

QRS: NORMAL   RBBB   LBBB

Figure 51–9. Prolongation of the ventricular-atrial conduction time during reciprocating tachycardia (RT) by selectively induced bundle branch block (BBB). In the presence of a left free-wall accessory pathway (AP), the V-A interval is prolonged by induction of left bundle branch block (LBBB) during reciprocating tachycardia. Right bundle branch block (RBBB) has no effect on the V-A interval in the presence of a left free-wall AP. (Courtesy of Dr. Mark Josephson.)

ence of a free-wall right ventricular accessory pathway. Induced right bundle branch block during reciprocating tachycardia results in prolongation of the V-A interval for 25 msec. or more.

Septal pathways are suspected if the V-A interval is not prolonged (i.e., prolonged less than 25 msec.) with either right bundle branch block or left bundle branch block. In addition, the proximal electrode on the quadripolar coronary sinus catheter is normally positioned at the coronary sinus orifice, and in the presence of a septal pathway, it records the earliest atrial activity during reciprocating tachycardia. In addition to the aforementioned recordings, a study of the functional properties of the accessory pathway and associated arrhythmias is accomplished by performing straight pacing as well as refractory period determinations from the right atrium, the left atrium (i.e., the coronary sinus), the right ventricle, and, rarely, the left ventricle. This allows assessment of the conduction and refractoriness of the normal conduction system and the accessory pathway in both the antegrade direction and the retrograde direction.

Wolff-Parkinson-White Syndrome

The description of Wolff-Parkinson-White syndrome as a distinct clinical entity (Wolff *et al.*, 1930) prompted much controversy regarding the etiology of the observed electrocardiographic abnormalities. The combination of a short P-R interval, delta wave, and widened QRS complex was attributed by various authors to fusion beats, hyperexcitable myocardium in the upper ventricular septum, accelerated AV node conduction, longitudinal dissociation in the His bundle, and accessory AV connections in or around the AV node but within the septum. Thus, direct surgical treatment of Wolff-Parkinson-White syndrome became feasible only after the conclusive demonstration that an abnormal anatomic connection existed between the atrium and the ventricle and that this

connection was capable of conducting electrical impulses. Holzmann and Scherf (1932) first suggested that the short P-R interval and delta wave might result from early excitation of the ventricle by an impulse that passed via an accessory AV pathway. Their theory was supported anatomically by the earlier studies of Kent (1893), who described muscular bridges connecting the right atrium and the right ventricle in a variety of mammalian species. In 1958, Truex and associates demonstrated similar muscular bridges between the atrium and the ventricle in human hearts up to the age of 6 months. In 1967, Durrer and Roos (1968) employed intraoperative epicardial mapping techniques to provide the first direct electrophysiologic evidence of ventricular pre-excitation occurring via an accessory AV connection in a patient with Wolff-Parkinson-White syndrome. Later that year, Burchell and colleagues confirmed Durrer's findings and were able to abolish ventricular pre-excitation temporarily by injecting procaine into the AV groove at the site of earliest ventricular excitation (Burchell *et al.*, 1967). Final demonstration of the presence of functional accessory AV connections and their importance in the genesis of Wolff-Parkinson-White syndrome occurred in 1968, when Sealy surgically divided the accessory AV pathway in a patient with type B Wolff-Parkinson-White syndrome (Cobb *et al.*, 1968). The procedure resulted in a normal P-R interval and QRS complex with disappearance of the delta wave and permanently abolished the ventricular pre-excitation and recurrent supraventricular tachyarrhythmia.

The surgical procedure for interruption of an accessory AV connection in Wolff-Parkinson-White syndrome consists of two steps: (1) localization of the accessory pathway by intraoperative electrical mapping techniques and (2) division of the accessory pathway. After a median sternotomy is performed, fixed epicardial electrodes are sutured to both the atrium and the ventricle for purposes of pacing and recording. Generally, the electrodes are positioned as

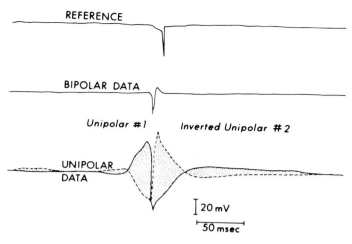

REFERENCE

BIPOLAR DATA

Unipolar #1   *Inverted Unipolar #2*

UNIPOLAR
DATA

⌶ 20 mV

⌐ 50 msec ⌐

Figure 51–10. Determination of local activation. Tracings from above down include a bipolar ventricular reference (Reference) recorded together with bipolar and unipolar electrograms from two closely spaced electrodes. One of the unipolar electrograms, shown with a dotted outline, has been electrically inverted. The stippled areas between the two electrograms demonstrate the forces that cancel each other out. The bipolar spike corresponds to the rapid intrinsic deflection in the unipolar electrogram. (From Gallagher, J. J., *et al.*: The technique of intraoperative electrophysiologic mapping. Am. J. Cardiol., 1982.)

close as possible to the suspected site of the accessory pathway.

Intraoperative Electrophysiologic Mapping. In 1915, Lewis and Rothschild first attempted to map the sequence of epicardial activation of the ventricular myocardium by recording the "intrinsic deflection" of unipolar tracings as a measure of local activation. Because of the recognition that the downstroke of the unipolar electrogram did not coincide with local depolarization, it became customary to record a differential (bipolar) electrogram from two closely spaced (less than or equal to 1 mm.) epicardial electrodes. The intrinsic deflection in an epicardial unipolar electrogram corresponds to activation of the subepicardial muscle immediately beneath the exploring electrode, but the electrogram is influenced by electrical activity from the whole heart. Two unipolar electrograms recorded from epicardial electrodes located 1 mm. apart are shown in Figure 51–10. Both electrograms show initial slow activity, reflecting activation from more distant parts of the heart. The rapid intrinsic deflection occurs with activation immediately beneath each electrode, and finally, slow activity returns, reflecting again more distant activity. These two adjacent unipolar electrograms differ only in the detail of the tracing recorded at the moment of local activation. If one of the unipolar electrograms is electrically inverted, the resultant tracings can be algebraically summated, and the two electrograms will cancel each other except where differences occur, resulting in a differential, or bipolar, electrogram. The bipolar electrogram thus recorded from these two epicardial leads appears as a rapid deflection, representing the slight difference in the two intrinsic deflections recorded by each of the unipolar leads.

The actual amplitude recorded by an electrode at any instant relates to the cross-sectional area of myocardial fibers "viewed" by the solid angle subtending the recording electrode. Unipolar electrograms recorded from normal human myocardium vary in amplitude from 20 to 60 mv. on the ventricle and 2 to 10 mv. on the atrium. Bipolar derivatives of closely spaced unipolar electrodes record amplitudes approximately one half of this value. Unipolar recordings

such as those shown in Figure 51–10 are generally recorded at frequency settings of 0.1 to 1200 Hz. The low-frequency response tends to make the unipolar electrogram unstable; the bipolar derivative of two adjacent electrodes, however, recorded at filter frequencies of 5 to 1200 Hz., provides a sharp deflection ideally suited to trigger a digital timer.

A schematic representation of a typical mapping system is shown in Figure 51–11. The mapping and recording areas are physically separated but linked by slaved monitoring oscilloscopes and a two-way communication system. Once the reference electrodes are secured, data sampling is achieved by use of a handheld electrode that can be positioned over any area of the heart. Standard surface electrocardiographic leads are relayed, together with the reference and data channels, by field-effect amplifiers (input impedance 10^{11} ohms) to high-gain differential amplifiers. The overall frequency response of the system should be 0.1 to 1200 Hz. Data are usually tape recorded, and a print-out of the data is obtained, permitting direct examination of the analogue signals. A digital timer displays on-line timing differences between the reference and data signals on a beat-by-beat basis. The recorded data are related to the heart by the use of a grid composed of 53 points. This allows a preliminary scan of the heart to be made with reasonable reproducibility. Once the area of interest is identified, point-by-point continuous scanning of the area can be performed, directly relating the data to surface landmarks. The sequence of surface activation can be depicted as isochronous lines drawn by hand or plotted by computer program (Davidow and Brown, 1975; Barr *et al.*, 1980).

The normal sequence of epicardial activation recorded in this manner is shown in Figure 51–12. The earliest epicardial breakthrough usually occurs over the area trabecularis on the anterior right ventricle 18 to 25 msec. after the onset of the surface QRS complex. The general sequence of activation that follows is that of radial spread toward the apex and base, with latest activation occurring at the base of the heart 70 to 80 msec. after the onset of the QRS complex. Multiple areas of epicardial breakthrough are fre-

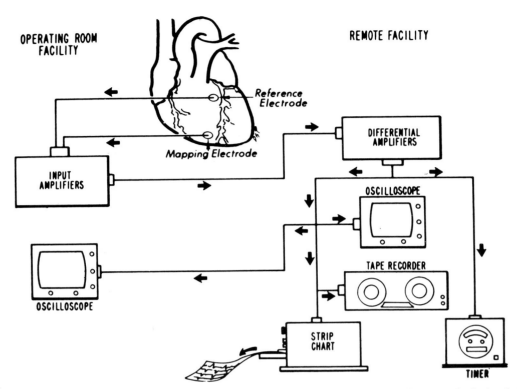

Figure 51–11. System for cardiac mapping. A typical mapping system for use in the operating room is depicted. Data recorded from a reference and a mapping electrode are relayed by buffer amplifiers in the operating room to a remote facility. The activation data are then relayed by differential amplifiers to a digital timer with simultaneous display on an oscilloscope operating in parallel with an oscilloscope in the operating room. All data are permanently stored on magnetic tape and can be intermittently displayed in graphic form by a strip chart recorder.

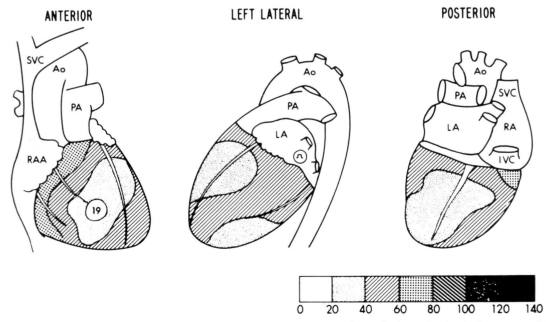

Figure 51–12. Normal sequence of epicardial activation. A normal sequence of ventricular activation is demonstrated. Isochrones are drawn every 10 msec. and connect areas activating at the same time. All time intervals shown are referenced to the onset of the QRS complex. Earliest epicardial activation is initiated 20 msec. after the onset of the QRS complex and is located on the low anterior right ventricle. Latest activation occurs in the basal region of the heart.

quently noted, usually occurring over the middle portion of the left anterior and posterior paraseptal regions and occasionally occurring over the left anterior septum near the base (Gallagher *et al.*, 1978c; Wyndham *et al.*, 1979; Abendroth *et al.*, 1980).

In patients with Wolff-Parkinson-White syndrome, the intraoperative mapping technique is performed as follows: If the patient is in a normal sinus rhythm with stable antegrade pre-excitation, the initial electrophysiologic mapping is performed using a ventricular reference. This map localizes the site (or sites) of earliest ventricular activation, thereby establishing the location of the ventricular insertion of the accessory pathway. In patients in whom stable antegrade pre-excitation is not present at the beginning of the mapping study, the atrium is paced in a region near the suspected site of the accessory pathway to elicit pre-excitation (Fig. 51–13). However, atrial pacing under these circumstances may obscure the possible detection of other accessory pathways by promoting preferential conduction across the nearest accessory AV connection. If stable antegrade pre-excitation cannot be elicited, the accessory pathway can be localized by retrograde (atrial) mapping during reciprocating tachycardia or ventricular pacing (Fig. 51–14). Many patients do not exhibit a stable reciprocating tachycardia during surgery, whereas others may not tolerate the hemodynamic consequences associated with this arrhythmia. In this situation, retrograde (atrial) mapping during ventricular pacing near the suspected site of the accessory pathway will localize the accessory tract. This technique, however, may also obscure

more remote accessory AV connections. It is sometimes necessary to institute cardiopulmonary bypass in these patients to provide hemodynamic stability while performing retrograde mapping.

Although the preceding steps allow localization of the accessory pathway in the majority of patients, occasionally special problems may be encountered. In the presence of a septal accessory pathway, the point of earliest epicardial excitation occurs at a site remote from the actual location of the accessory AV pathway. Therefore, a surgical incision at the site of the earliest ventricular activation will not modify the pre-excitation. Fortunately, certain features of the epicardial map may suggest the presence of a septal pathway. If unipolar epicardial data are recorded near the site of earliest excitation with free-wall AV connections, the earliest ventricular activation occurs before or simultaneous with the onset of the delta wave. In patients with septal pathways, the earliest epicardial activation occurs after the onset of the surface delta wave (Fig. 51–15). Identification of the presence of a septal pathway necessitates instituting total cardiopulmonary bypass with antegrade and retrograde intracardiac mapping. Local intracardiac endocardial mapping is performed in the same manner as that described for epicardial mapping.

Atrial fibrillation also constitutes a special problem, since no stable antegrade pre-excitation can be established and retrograde (atrial) mapping is impossible. This problem is circumvented by recording variable activation times between the ventricular reference electrode and any given ventricular site. By

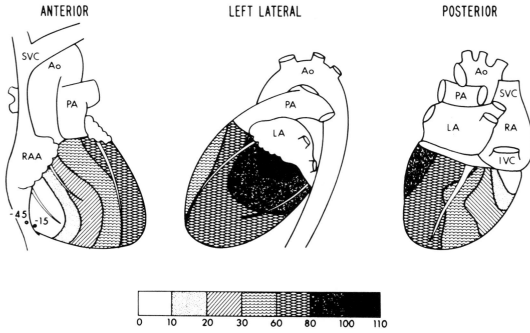

Figure 51–13. Epicardial map of the ventricle in a patient with right lateral pre-excitation. The earliest area of pre-excitation occurs at the right lateral AV groove 15 msec. before the onset of the surface delta wave. The adjacent atrium activates 30 msec. prior to the appearance of ventricular pre-excitation. Activation spreads tangentially across the anterior and posterior right ventricle, with the latest area of activation on the lateral base of the left ventricle.

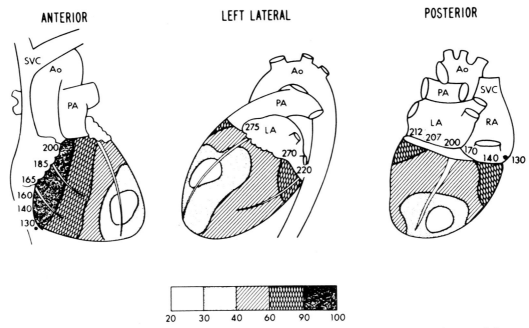

Figure 51–14. Epicardial map performed during reciprocating tachycardia. Ventricular activation is essentially normal, with two early epicardial breakthrough sites present over the low anterior septum and the posterior right ventricular apex. There is some evidence of conduction delay along the basal portion of the right ventricle owing to the presence of an incomplete right bundle branch block. The ventriculoatrial activation times are indicated by the numerals along the atrial margin of the AV groove. Note that earliest retrograde atrial activation occurs at the low lateral right atrial border, corresponding closely to the demonstrated site of ventricular pre-excitation in Figure 51–13.

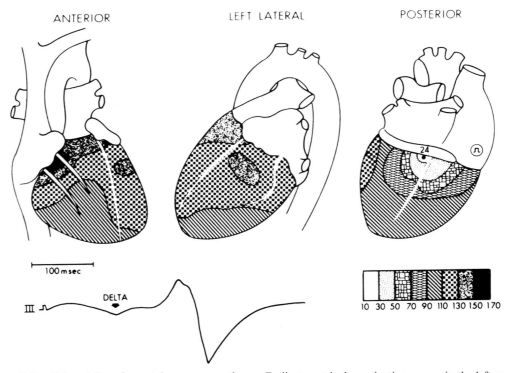

Figure 51–15. Epicardial mapping of a septal accessory pathway. Earliest ventricular activation occurs in the left crux of the heart, with the onset of activation 24 msec. *after* the appearance of the surface delta wave, characteristic of a septal accessory pathway.

noting only those beats with early activation times (and manifest pre-excitation), an epicardial map can be constructed.

Surgical Technique for Division of an Accessory AV Connection. Accessory AV connections may occur at any point around the anulus fibrosus on either side of the heart. However, from a surgical standpoint their locations are classified as (1) right free-wall, (2) left free-wall, (3) anterior septal, and (4) posterior septal.

A median sternotomy is performed regardless of the suspected position of the accessory AV pathway prior to surgery. Once the atrial and ventricular insertions of the accessory pathway have been identified, cardiopulmonary bypass is instituted. If the pathway is located on the right side, the superior vena cava is cannulated via the right atrial appendage and the inferior vena cava is cannulated via the deep femoral vein to allow better visualization of the right anulus fibrosus.

Accessory pathways on the *right free wall* are approached initially by incising the epicardium as it reflects off the right atrium to cover the AV groove structures. A plane of dissection is established between the external right atrial wall and the AV groove fat pad in the region of the accessory AV connection. This dissection is usually performed with the patient in a normal sinus rhythm and stable antegrade pre-excitation, so that if the dissection results in division of the accessory AV connection, confirmation is established by instantaneous disappearance of the delta wave. External dissection of the right free-wall pathways is especially important in patients with associated Ebstein's anomaly. In those patients, there is a "folding over" of the junction of atrial and ventricular muscle that may protect an accessory atrioventricular connection near the anulus from surgical division. It is essential that this junction of atrial and ventricular muscle be unfolded in patients with Ebstein's anomaly if the right free-wall accessory connections are to be divided successfully.

If stable antegrade pre-excitation persists during the external dissection of right free-wall pathways, a right atriotomy is performed. The area of the anulus corresponding to the site of pre-excitation is identified. An incision is made through the atrial wall approximately 2 mm. above the anulus of the tricuspid valve, exposing the fat pad surrounding the right coronary artery and vein. Generally, the incision is extended 1 cm. to each side of the presumed location of the accessory pathway. The fat pad containing the coronary vessels is separated from the top of the external wall of the atrium and the ventricle all the way to the epicardium. All fibrous bands and even small vessels are divided if they enter the atrium or the ventricle (Fig. 51–16). If necessary, it is possible to extend the incision from the anterior aspect of the membranous septum (Fig. 51–17*A*) clockwise completely around the free wall of the right anulus fibrosus to the posterior aspect of the membranous septum (Fig. 51–17*A'*). There is a slight risk of injuring the bundle of His near the posterior region of the membranous

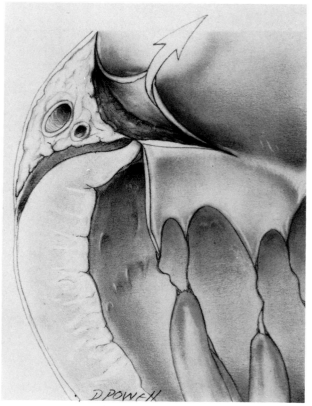

Figure 51–16. This diagram illustrates the appropriate plane of dissection to be established beneath the AV groove fat pad for surgical ablation of an accessory atrioventricular pathway. Note that the endocardial incision is made slightly above the valve anulus and that a plane of dissection is established between the external atrial wall and the fat pad. Next, a plane of dissection is established between the external portion of the upper ventricle and the AV groove fat pad.

septum, but the danger is minimal since at this level the His bundle has either entered the membranous septum or joined the left ventricle. The extension of this incision anteromedially to the anterior aspect of the membranous septum is occasionally necessary in order to divide *anterior septal* pathways passing through the fat pad between the right fibrous trigone and the site of insertion of the right coronary artery into the AV groove. This fat pad lies just anterior to the membranous septum between the pericardial reflection of the ascending aorta and the medial wall of the right atrium (Fig. 51–17*B*). After completion of the incision, the atrial muscle is closed with a running 3-0 Prolene suture.

Exposure of *left free-wall* pathways is accomplished via a left atriotomy in the manner routinely used to expose the mitral valve. Potassium cardioplegia is used in these patients to provide better visibility of the entire mitral valve anulus. A monofilament suture is passed through the mitral anulus at the epicardial site of the accessory pathway to identify the corresponding endocardial point on the mitral anulus. If the tract is located anteriorly on the free wall, the incision is begun at the left fibrous trigone

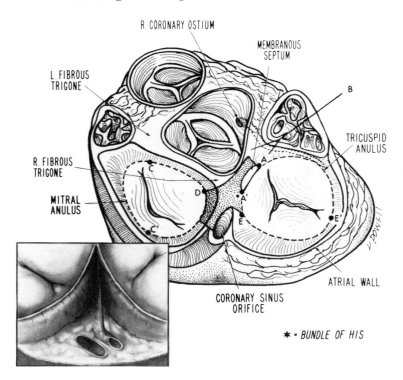

Figure 51–17. Extent of various incisions employed to interrupt atrioventricular pathways (see text for discussion). Septal pathways may be located anywhere within the heavily stippled area. *Inset,* Dissection of the pyramidal space above the posterior ventricular septum to interrupt septal accessory pathways (see text for discussion).

(Fig 51–17*C*) and is extended counterclockwise to beyond the midportion of the anulus of the free wall (Fig. 51–17*C'*). If the pathway is on the posterior free wall, the incision is begun at the right fibrous trigone (Fig. 51–17*D*) and is extended clockwise to beyond the midportion of the free wall of the anulus (Fig. 51–17*C'*). Recently, both of these incisions have been made more generous owing to the possibility of multiple accessory pathways. If necessary, a single incision can be made from the left fibrous trigone (Fig. 51–17*C*) counterclockwise to the right fibrous trigone (Fig. 51–17*D*).

The most difficult accessory AV connections to interrupt surgically are those located posteriorly in the region of the crux (*posterior septal* pathways). These pathways may pass on either side of the ventricular septum within 1 cm. of the posterior descending coronary artery. A right atriotomy is performed, and the right atrial endocardium is incised above the anulus fibrosus beginning just posterior to the His bundle and continuing posteriorly to the free wall of the tricuspid ring. The fat pad surrounding the coronary vessels and in the pyramidal space above the posterior ventricular septum is dissected away to expose the top of the ventricular septal musculature and the posteromedial aspect of the left atrium (Fig. 51–17, inset). With left-sided posterior septal pathways, it occasionally has been necessary to open the left atrium and make an incision above the mitral valve anulus from the right fibrous trigone (Fig. 51–17*D*) to the lateral midportion of the anulus (Fig. 51–17*C'*). By reflecting the coronary sinus, the AV node artery, and the surrounding fat pad away from the entire inlet portion of the upper posterior ventric-

ular septum (Fig. 51–6), most of these posterior septal pathways can be ablated without injury to the normal conduction system.

Two significant problems have persisted with the surgical treatment of posterior septal pathways, however. The first has been a somewhat higher incidence of initial surgical failure requiring early reoperation. The second problem, which is much more common with dissection in the pyramidal space overlying the ventricular septum, is inadvertent interruption of the bundle of His. Since dissection in the posterior pyramidal space is performed during cardioplegic arrest of the heart, surgical injury of the bundle of His is not recognized until the aortic cross-clamp is released and the patient is rewarmed. In an effort to avoid injury to the bundle of His, we have recently been performing all of the dissection of the anterior portion of the pyramidal space during atrial pacing prior to inducing cardioplegic arrest. Once the dissection is completed in the region near the His bundle and normal AV conduction is seen to be maintained, the heart is arrested cardioplegically and the remainder of the pyramidal space is dissected, as described previously. The problem of initial failure of surgical division of posterior septal pathways is suspected to derive from the fact that only a microscopic residual fiber of the accessory pathway need remain after dissection to result in persistence of abnormal AV conduction and pre-excitation. As a result, we have recently begun placing cryolesions in the extreme left posterior recess of the pyramidal space overlying the posterior superior process of the left ventricle. In addition, following completion of dissection in the posterior aspect of the pyramidal space, cryolesions are applied posteriorly

TABLE 51–1. RESULTS OF SURGERY IN 200 CONSECUTIVE PATIENTS WITH WOLFF-PARKINSON-WHITE SYNDROME*

LOCATIONS OF KENT BUNDLE	NUMBER OF KENT BUNDLES	KENT BUNDLES SUCCESSFULLY DIVIDED	ELECTIVE HIS BLOCK	FORCED HIS BLOCK	MORTALITY
Left free wall	101	93	7	0	3
Right free wall	41	39	0	0	0
Anterior septum	21	17	0	1	1
Posterior septum	56	42	4	9	1
Total	219	191	11	10	5

*From Gallagher, J. J., et al.: Results of surgery for pre-excitation in 200 cases. Presented at the 54th Scientific Sessions, American Heart Association, November 1981.

to the AV groove fat pad from within the pyramidal space. These multiple cryolesions are applied in an effort to ablate all remaining microscopic connections between the atrium and the ventricle in the posterior pyramidal space.

Recent clinicopathologic studies have shown that accessory AV connections may be located in or near the epicardium overlying the AV groove, thereby skirting the anulus fibrosus entirely. Detailed intra-operative mapping of the AV groove usually identifies the subepicardial location of these pathways. Large "QS" deflections appear in the electrogram recorded at the site of earliest ventricular pre-excitation, in contrast to the "rS" configuration of the more common type of connection. In these patients, cryoablation has been employed successfully to interrupt the accessory AV pathway. The local area is first cooled with a cryoprobe to 0°C. If evidence of pre-excitation disappears and then reappears on rewarming, the area is ablated by subsequent freezing at −60°C. for 2 minutes. If cooling fails to modify the pre-excitation, the accessory pathway is approached by conventional dissection, as described earlier.

Results. Since 1968, when Wolff-Parkinson-White syndrome was first treated successfully surgically, 341 patients with this syndrome have been evaluated at our institution (Gallagher *et al.* 1981). Twelve of these patients were treated medically; 18 patients received antitachycardia pacemakers; and 200 of the patients underwent surgery (Table 51–1). Surgical division of the accessory atrioventricular pathway was successful in 98 per cent of right free-wall pathways, 92 per cent of left free-wall pathways, and 77 per cent of septal pathways. In the last 100 patients who have undergone surgery, there have been 45 patients who had posterior septal pathways, 41 (91 per cent) of which have been divided successfully.

Occasionally, it is necessary to interrupt the normal pathway for AV conduction in patients with Wolff-Parkinson-White syndrome. This procedure may be prompted by an inability to divide the accessory pathway or by associated cardiac problems that make prolonged cardiopulmonary bypass inadvisable. Although interruption of the His bundle effectively abolishes reciprocating tachycardia, it requires insertion of a permanent ventricular pacemaker. In addi-

tion, it offers no protection against tachyarrhythmias in patients with atrial fibrillation and rapid antegrade conduction across the accessory pathway, unless the atrial fibrillation developed secondary to the reciprocating tachycardia.

Intractable Supraventricular Tachyarrhythmias Not Associated with Wolff-Parkinson-White Syndrome

Refractory supraventricular tachycardia may occur on the basis of a variety of abnormalities exclusive of Wolff-Parkinson-White syndrome and include (1) paroxysmal supraventricular tachycardia (PSVT) due to AV node re-entry or to the presence of a "concealed" accessory AV connection capable of conducting in the retrograde (ventriculoatrial) direction only; (2) refractory atrial flutter/fibrillation with a rapid ventricular response; (3) accessory AV node bypass tracts connecting the atrial muscle directly to the bundle of His; (4) Mahaim fibers connecting the AV node to the ventricular septum (nodoventricular fibers) or connecting the His bundle to the ventricular septum (fasciculoventricular fibers); and (5) ectopic atrial foci. Patients who have paroxysmal supraventricular tachycardia due to a concealed accessory AV connection that conducts in the retrograde direction only are approached surgically in the same manner as a patient with Wolff-Parkinson-White syndrome. Since the accessory atrioventricular connection in these patients is incapable of conducting in the antegrade (atrioventricular) direction, no delta wave is present on the electrocardiogram during normal sinus rhythm. At the time of surgery, ventricular epicardial mapping is of no value. Retrograde atrial mapping is performed during the tachycardia or during ventricular pacing to identify the site of atrial insertion of the accessory pathway, which is then divided surgically according to the methods described earlier.

At present, the only surgical therapy available for patients with AV node re-entry, refractory atrial flutter/fibrillation, AV node bypass tracts, Mahaim fibers, or ectopic atrial foci is elective cryoablation of the bundle of His.

Surgical Technique for Interruption of the Bundle of His. Patients who are selected for elective cryoab-

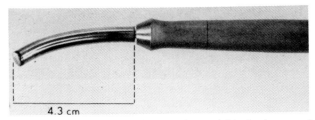

Figure 51–18. Hand-held cryoprobe used for elective cryoablation of the bundle of His. The cryoprobe has a 5-mm. diameter tip that can be cooled to −60°C. by expanding nitrous oxide.

lation of the bundle of His undergo a standard median sternotomy and are cannulated for cardiopulmonary bypass using separate cannulas for the superior and inferior venae cavae. An epicardial pacing electrode is sutured onto the right atrium, and normothermic cardiopulmonary bypass is instituted. A right atriotomy is performed, and a hand-held exploring electrode is positioned over the suspected site of the His bundle just posterior to the membranous portion of the interatrial septum during atrial pacing. Once a definite His complex is recorded by the hand-held electrode, the electrode is replaced with a cryoprobe (Fig. 51–18), the tip of which can be cooled with internally expanding nitrous oxide. The temperature of the cryoprobe is decreased to 0°C., at which time atrioventricular conduction should cease. The tissue is then allowed to rewarm to normothermia, at which time AV conduction returns. This process of temporary cooling and rewarming confirms that the tip of the cryoprobe is in the appropriate position overlying the His bundle. The temperature of the probe is then decreased to −60°C. for 2 minutes, resulting in cryoablation of the His bundle and permanent atrio-

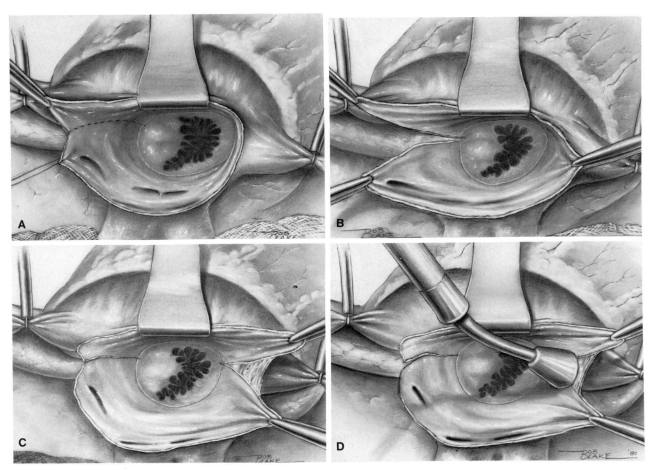

Figure 51–19. Left atrial isolation procedure. *A,* Following a standard left atriotomy incision, the interatrial septum is retracted gently, and the atriotomy is extended anteriorly (dashed line) across Bachmann's bundle to the level of the mitral valve anulus just to the left of the right fibrous trigone. *B,* The anterior extension of the standard left atriotomy has been completed. The base of the aorta and its juxtaposition with the anterior leaflet of the mitral valve are demonstrated. Note that the anterior atriotomy extends across the mitral valve anulus. The main body of the left atrium has been separated anteriorly from the remainder of the heart. *C,* The transmural left atriotomy is extended posteriorly to the level of the coronary sinus. The remaining portion of the incision is made through the endocardium and extends across the mitral valve anulus posteriorly just to the left of the interatrial septum. At this point, electrical activity continues to be propagated in a 1:1 fashion between the right and left atria because of the presence of interatrial muscular connections accompanying the coronary sinus. *D,* A cryoprobe is positioned over the endocardial aspect of the posterior atriotomy, and its temperature is decreased to −60°C. for 2 minutes. This cryolesion ablates the endocardial interatrial fibers accompanying the coronary sinus. A similar cryolesion is created on the epicardial aspect of the atrioventricular groove on the opposite side of the coronary sinus to ablate all remaining interatrial epicardial connections. The left atriotomy is closed with a continuous 4-0 nonabsorbable suture.

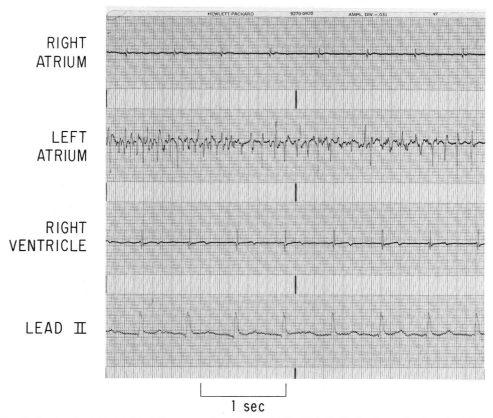

POSTOPERATIVE
LEFT ATRIAL FIBRILLATION

RIGHT ATRIUM

LEFT ATRIUM

RIGHT VENTRICLE

LEAD II

1 sec

Figure 51–20. Following the left atrial isolation procedure, induced left atrial fibrillation is confined to the left atrium. Postoperative right atrial, left atrial, right ventricular, and lead II electrograms recorded during left atrial fibrillation demonstrate that the fibrillation is not conducted to the remainder of the heart, which remains in a "normal sinus rhythm" with normal atrioventricular conduction.

ventricular conduction block. Thirty-one patients have undergone elective cryoablation of the bundle of His for a variety of refractory supraventricular tachyarrhythmias, with a success rate of 89 per cent (Sealy et al., 1981).

Two newer surgical approaches are being developed in an attempt to avoid the necessity for creating permanent atrioventricular block in some of these patients. We have developed a technique for isolating the left atrium from the remainder of the heart for the treatment of ectopic atrial foci arising in the left atrium (Fig. 51–19) (Williams et al., 1980). The left atrial isolation procedure is also capable of confining atrial fibrillation to the left atrium (Fig. 51–20) and may prove beneficial as an adjunctive procedure in patients undergoing mitral valve replacement who have associated chronic atrial fibrillation. For the treatment of AV node re-entrant tachycardia, methods are also being evaluated in which multiple, discrete cryolesions are placed over the input pathways to the AV node in an effort to ablate the AV node re-entrant circuit without permanently abolishing normal atrioventricular conduction (Holman et al., 1982). The feasibility of such an approach is based on the results reported by Pritchett and associates (1979) in which surgical dissection in the AV node region abolished AV node re-entrant tachycardia but preserved normal atrioventricular conduction with no change in the patient's status during a 4-year follow-up period.

VENTRICULAR ARRHYTHMIAS

Among the most common and certainly the most lethal of arrhythmias are those arising in the ventricles. Although the medical treatment of ventricular arrhythmias, particularly those associated with ischemic heart disease, has improved enormously in the past decade, there remains a rather large group of patients in whom the ventricular arrhythmias are refractory to medical treatment. The term "ventricular arrhythmias" is usually thought of as being associated with ischemic heart disease, but there are many types of ventricular arrhythmias unrelated to coronary heart disease. Most of the ventricular arrhythmias unassociated with coronary disease are remarkably intractable to medical therapy. As a result, much emphasis has been placed recently on the surgical therapy of these arrhythmias.

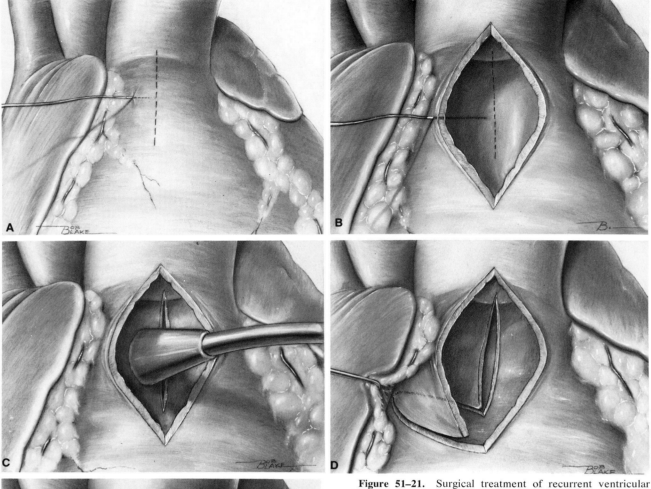

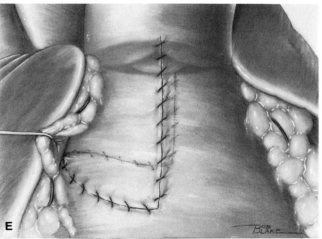

Figure 51–21. Surgical treatment of recurrent ventricular tachycardia in a 16-year-old female with nonischemic cardiomyopathy secondary to Coxsackie myocarditis. Initial intraoperative electrophysiologic mapping indicated that the ventricular tachycardia arose from the free wall of the pulmonary outflow tract near the AV groove and just proximal to the level of the pulmonic valve anulus. An intramural needle electrode was inserted at that epicardial site and was passed transmurally so that its tip was positioned in the interventricular septum between the crista supraventricularis and the pulmonic valve anulus. Intramural electrograms were recorded from electrode contacts located every millimeter along the needle shaft. Earliest ventricular activation during ventricular tachycardia occurred at the electrode contact point at the tip of the needle shaft, indicating that the ventricular tachycardia was originating in the supracristal portion of the interventricular septum.

A, A longitudinal incision was made on the free wall of the pulmonary outflow tract, beginning just distal to the level of the pulmonic valve anulus and extending proximally, as depicted by the dashed line. This free-wall incision did not alter the ventricular tachycardia.

B, The pulmonary outflow tract has been opened, and the needle electrode is seen to lie intramurally in the supracristal portion of the interventricular septum. A counterincision was made on the posterior wall of the pulmonary outflow tract, beginning just distal to the pulmonic valve anulus and extending proximally to the level of the crista supraventricularis (dashed line). This incision was transmural, and the aortic root could be visualized through this posterior incision. This counterincision did not alter the ventricular tachycardia.

C, A cryoprobe was positioned over the site of earliest activation during ventricular tachycardia, and the myocardium was frozen at −60°C. for 2 minutes. This cryolesion resulted in cessation of the ventricular tachycardia.

D, The proximal ends of the anterior and posterior ventriculotomies were then connected by a transmural semicircular incision around the left side of the pulmonary outflow tract, as depicted. This resulted in total isolation of the segment of the pulmonary outflow tract that contained the arrhythmogenic myocardium.

E, The incisions were closed with a continuous 3-0 nonabsorbable suture, as depicted. The patient has remained free of ventricular tachycardia for 4 years following this surgical procedure.

Ventricular Tachyarrhythmias in the Absence of Coronary Artery Disease

Idiopathic ventricular tachycardia refers to an arrhythmia in patients in whom the only clinical manifestation of cardiac disease is the arrhythmia. Both the macroscopic appearance of the heart at operation and the pathologic data acquired at the time of autopsy in such patients fail to show any evidence of primary cardiac disease. The only abnormality noted has been global dilatation of the heart secondary to functional post-tachycardia heart failure. If these patients require surgery, they first undergo intraoperative electrophysiologic mapping during ventricular tachycardia in an effort to localize the apparent site of origin of the arrhythmia. Surgical approaches have included simple ventriculotomy, exclusion procedures, and cryoablation, but the results have been poor, primarily because many of these arrhythmias arise within the ventricular septum (Guiraudon *et al.*, 1981).

A small group of patients have been shown to have ventricular tachycardia due to *nonischemic cardiomyopathy*. This group comprises patients with angiographic and catheter data indicating some type of abnormal myocardial contractility associated with recurrent ventricular tachycardia. These patients usually show a diffuse dilatation of both ventricles with widespread patchy myocardial fibrosis. These tachyarrhythmias frequently arise in the right ventricle, and our approach to such patients has been to employ a combination of surgical isolation and cryoablation of the apparent site of origin of the arrhythmia. One of our patients, a 16-year-old female with Coxsackie myocarditis, was documented to have intermittent ventricular tachycardia for 7 years following her initial viral infection. Preoperative electrophysiologic studies indicated that the ventricular tachycardia was arising from the pulmonary infundibulum near the level of the pulmonic valve anulus. However, the intraoperative electrophysiologic studies demonstrated the tachycardia to be arising in the high right ventricular septum between the crista supraventricularis and the pulmonic valve anulus. A combination of surgical isolation and cryoablation of the apparent site of origin of the ventricular tachycardia (Fig. 51–21) resulted in cessation of the arrhythmia. The patient has remained free of ventricular tachycardia for 4 years and has required no antiarrhythmic medication.

Fontaine and associates (1979) have described a previously unrecognized form of cardiomyopathy localized to the right ventricle to which they have applied the term *arrhythmogenic right ventricular dysplasia*. This syndrome appears to be a congenital cardiomyopathy characterized by transmural infiltration of adipose tissue resulting in weakness and aneurysmal bulging of the infundibulum, apex, and/or posterior basilar region of the right ventricle. The syndrome is characterized clinically by intractable ventricular tachycardia originating from one or all of the three pathologic areas of the right ventricle (Fig. 51–22). Since the origin of the tachycardia is in the

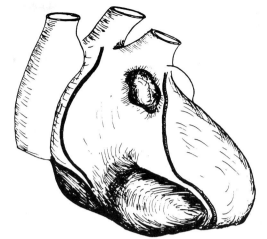

Figure 51–22. Diagrammatic sketch of the three areas of pathologic involvement in arrhythmogenic right ventricular dysplasia. (Courtesy of Dr. G. Guiraudon.)

right ventricle, the standard electrocardiogram shows a pattern consistent with left bundle branch block during the tachycardia. Right ventricular angiography should be performed in all patients who exhibit ventricular tachycardia with a left bundle branch block pattern. In patients with arrhythmogenic right ventricular dysplasia, the right ventricle appears enlarged, ventricular bulges or frank aneurysms are seen in the infundibulum, the apex, and/or the basal portion of the inferior wall, and right ventricular contractility is usually markedly decreased. Hypertrophic muscular bands in the infundibulum and anterior right ventricular wall result in apparent pseudodiverticula, the so-called "feathering" appearance of the right ventricular outflow tract (Fig. 51–23).

Guiraudon and colleagues (1981) have employed simple ventriculotomies, aneurysm excision, or a combination of ventriculotomy and excision in a group of 12 patients, with one operative death and a 25 per cent recurrence of ventricular tachycardia postoperatively. Our current approach to such patients employs a transmural encircling ventriculotomy that effectively isolates the arrhythmogenic myocardium from the remainder of the heart. The operation depicted in Figure 51–24 was performed on a 69-year-old male with arrhythmogenic right ventricular dysplasia who was in continuous ventricular tachycardia for 28 days prior to his operation. Preoperative electrophysiologic studies revealed the tachycardia to be originating from the posterior basilar region of the right ventricle. Preoperative right ventricular angiography demonstrated feathering of the right ventricular outflow tract (Fig. 51–23) and aneurysmal bulging of the infundibulum, apex, and posterior basilar region of the right ventricle. Intraoperative electrophysiologic studies revealed the tachycardia to be arising in the posterior basilar region of the right ventricle adjacent to an area on the anterior right ventricle measuring 2 × 3 cm. that was electrically silent. In such cases, one must recognize the possibility that the actual site of origin of the ventricular tachycardia

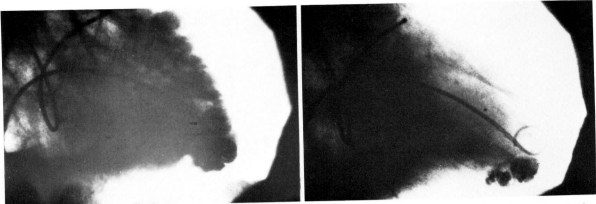

Figure 51–23. Right ventricular angiocardiogram during diastole *(left panel)* and systole *(right panel)* of a patient with arrhythmogenic right ventricular dysplasia. Note the uneven appearance of the anterior portion of the right ventricular outflow tract during systole, the saccular aneurysm near the right ventricular apex, and bulging of the posterior-basilar region of the right ventricle during systole. This right ventricular angiogram was performed on a 69-year-old male who experienced incessant ventricular tachycardia arising from the posterior-basilar region of the right ventricle for 4 weeks prior to surgery. His surgical procedure is depicted in Figure 51–24.

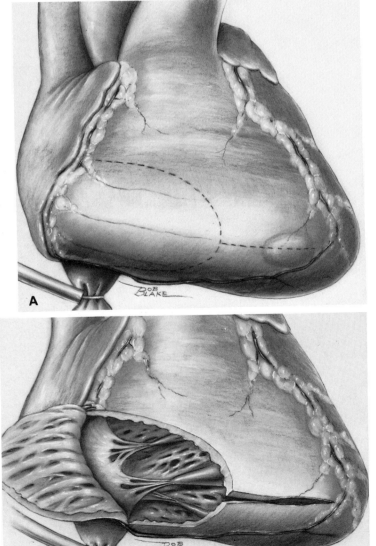

Figure 51–24. *A*, Appearance of the right ventricle in a patient with arrhythmogenic right ventricular dysplasia. Note the three coronary arteries coursing from the atrioventricular groove across the surface of the right ventricle. The acute margin of the right ventricle corresponded to the location of the middle coronary artery depicted in this drawing. An area approximately 2 × 3 cm. near the upper coronary artery was electrically silent. Epicardial mapping during ventricular tachycardia demonstrated the earliest site of activation to be located near the lower edge of this electrically silent region just below the midsegment of the middle coronary artery on the posterior-basilar region of the right ventricle. A transmural ventriculotomy was placed around the electrically silent area and included the apparent site of origin of the ventricular tachycardia on the posterior-basilar region of the heart (dashed line). The two ends of this incision were based at the AV groove, where cryolesions were applied to insure isolation of the arrhythmogenic region of myocardium from the remainder of the heart. In addition, a second transmural incision was made from the apex of the semicircular incision to the apex of the right ventricle to include the small saccular aneurysm in that region.

B, The isolated pedicle of right ventricular myocardium containing the electrically silent area and the apparent site of origin of the ventricular tachycardia has been reflected to demonstrate the internal anatomy of the right ventricle. Note the extension of the incision to the right ventricular apex to open the small aneurysm located in that region.

Illustration continued on opposite page

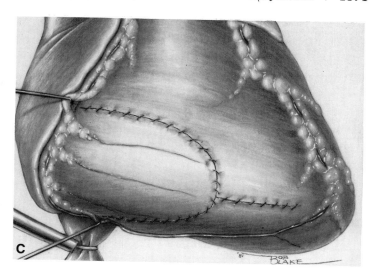

Figure 51–24 *Continued.* *C,* The transmural encircling ventriculotomy around the arrhythmogenic region of the right ventricle and the simple ventriculotomy through the right ventricular apical aneurysm have been closed with a continuous 3-0 nonabsorbable suture. Following completion of this procedure for arrhythmogenic right ventricular dysplasia, the isolated pedicle was paced at a rapid rate, but the paced impulses were not conducted to the remainder of the heart. In addition, the remainder of the right ventricle was then paced rapidly, but those paced impulses were not conducted into the isolated pedicle, confirming total isolation of the arrhythmogenic right ventricular myocardium from the remainder of the heart.

may be in the electrically silent region and that it appears to arise from the border of the silent region only because a certain critical mass of synchronously depolarized myocardium is essential to produce an electrogram large enough to be detected by the exploring electrode. Since the three pathologically abnormal regions of the right ventricle in arrhythmogenic right ventricular dysplasia may exhibit electrical silence on epicardial mapping, every attempt should be made to isolate the entire pathologic area giving rise to the tachycardia from the remainder of the heart. The surgically isolated "pedicle" shown in Figure 51–24*B* is based on a vascular supply originating from the right coronary artery. The incision is begun in the atrioventricular groove at the level of the tricuspid anulus and is extended around the arrhythmogenic region of myocardium and returned to the level of the tricuspid anulus inferiorly. At both ends of the incision, a cryolesion is placed to assure complete separation of all ventricular myocardial fibers on either side of the incision. In the operation depicted in Figure 51–24, a separate incision was extended to the right ventricular apex because of the presence of a discrete aneurysm (Fig. 51–23). In making such an incision in the right ventricle, care is taken to avoid the base of the papillary muscles, but should it be necessary, the incision can be extended around the base of a papillary muscle. The incision is closed in two layers with a continuous suture. The patient whose operation is depicted in Figure 51–24 has remained free of ventricular arrhythmias for 40 months following surgery and has received no antiarrhythmic medication.

Uhl's syndrome is a rare congenital cardiomyopathy that, from the anatomic point of view, may be considered to be a more complete form of arrhythmogenic right ventricular dysplasia. The right ventricle is extremely dilated, but the tricuspid valve remains in a normal position, thus differentiating it from Ebstein's anomaly. The main characteristic of Uhl's syndrome is the complete absence of myocardium in the right ventricular free wall, resulting in the endo-

cardial and epicardial layers being in direct contact without interposition of myocardial fibers. Since Uhl's description of this cardiomyopathy in 1952, the descriptive term "parchment heart" has been applied to the abnormality. Although Uhl's syndrome usually leads to rapid cardiac failure in the first months or years of life, an adult form of this condition occurs in which associated ventricular tachycardia is the dominant feature.

In 1957, Jervell and Lange-Nielsen described a clinical entity consisting of a *long Q-T interval*, congenital deafness, and syncopal attacks due to ventricular fibrillation following emotional or physical stresses. The absence of congenital deafness characterizes the otherwise identical Romano-Ward syndrome (Romano *et al.*, 1963; Ward, 1964). The prolongation of the Q-T interval in both of these syndromes has been considered to be congenital in origin, and both syndromes are recognized to contribute to sudden death in children (Fraser and Froggatt, 1966; Schwartz *et al.* 1975). However, in 1978, Schwartz and Wolf demonstrated that certain patients who sustained acute myocardial infarctions subsequently developed Q-T interval prolongation and thereafter experienced a significantly higher rate of sudden death. Although the pathogenesis of the long Q-T syndrome is poorly understood, James and associates (1978) demonstrated the presence of focal neuritis and neural degeneration within the specialized conduction system and the ventricular myocardium. They suggested the possibility that a chronic viral infection or some noninfectious degenerative process of the cardiac nerves might be responsible for the prolongation of the Q-T interval and the associated fatal ventricular arrhythmias.

Ventricular tachycardia that occurs in association with the long Q-T syndrome is frequently of a distinct type called *torsades de pointes.* This term is derived from the appearance of the ventricular tachycardia on a standard electrocardiogram, on which the polarity of the tachycardia is inconstant (Fig. 51–25). The electrocardiographic features of torsades de pointes

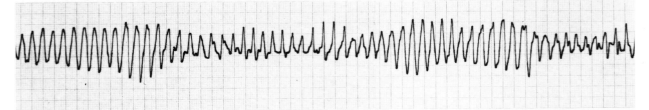

Figure 51–25. Torsade de pointes. This type of ventricular tachycardia, which is usually associated with the long Q-T syndrome, is characterized by rhythmic changes in the polarity of successive QRS complexes.

are unique and may be described as follows (Dessertenne, 1966; Krikler and Curry, 1976; Kulbertus, 1978): (1) the episodes are generally initiated by a ventricular ectopic beat following late after the preceding sinus complex; (2) the successive QRS complexes during tachycardia show an "undulating series of rotations" (Wellens et al., 1975) of the electrical axis; and (3) the episodes most frequently cease spontaneously. In addition, the arrhythmia is usually preceded by variations in the T wave during the last several beats prior to development of the tachycardia. One of the most frequent causes of torsades de pointes is the administration of medications that prolong ventricular repolarization, particularly quinidine (Kulbertus, 1980).

These observations support the concept that torsades de pointes represents an abnormality in myocardial repolarization, as opposed to most other types of ventricular tachycardia, which are thought to be abnormalities in myocardial depolarization. As a result, the surgical treatment of recurrent ventricular tachycardia associated with the long Q-T syndrome has centered around efforts to modify cardiac innervation. The classic studies of Yanowitz and coworkers (1966) showed that unilateral alterations in sympathetic tone altered not only the shape of the T wave but also its duration (Q-T interval). Their study in animals showed that resection of the right stellate ganglion or stimulation of the left stellate ganglion resulted in prolonged Q-T intervals and increased T-wave amplitude. Conversely, resection of the left stellate ganglion or stimulation of the right stellate ganglion produced increased T-wave negativity without measurable changes in the Q-T interval. These findings and those of others (Schwartz et al., 1975) have led to the hypothesis that the electrocardiographic changes following unilateral alterations of sympathetic tone provide a functional explanation for the electrocardiographic abnormalities seen in patients with lesions of the central nervous system as well as in patients with the long Q-T syndrome. Left stellate ganglion resection has been reported to abolish symptoms in approximately 20 patients with the long Q-T syndrome (Moss and McDonald, 1971; Schwartz et al., 1975; Smith and Gallagher, 1979; Malliani et al., 1980). However, our experience with left stellate ganglion resection for the treatment of torsades de pointes associated with the long Q-T syndrome has been characterized by early success and late failure (Benson and Cox, 1982).

Ventricular Tachyarrhythmias Associated with Coronary Artery Disease

The most common ventricular arrhythmias are those that occur in association with ischemic heart disease. Meticulous follow-up studies document that serious ventricular arrhythmias of this type are harbingers of sudden cardiac death within the first year after an acute myocardial infarction (Ruberman et al., 1977). Survival seems to be improved by antiarrhythmic drugs, but the arrhythmias persist in many patients despite all combinations of pharmacologic therapy available. Many surgical techniques have been used in the past in an attempt to alleviate ventricular arrhythmias associated with coronary artery disease. To determine whether surgery is indicated and the optimal surgical approach, it is necessary to understand the mechanisms of ventricular tachyarrhythmias associated with ischemic heart disease.

Cardiac rhythm reflects a balance or stable behavior resulting from a complex system of interacting anatomic and electrophysiologic variables. These components include normal or abnormal conduction pathways, homogeneous versus heterogeneous excitability, conduction, recovery, and exaggerated automaticity. Tachycardia represents an imbalance or unstable electrophysiologic state due to the interaction among one or more abnormal variables. Current concepts of the mechanisms of ventricular tachycardia associated with ischemic heart disease include re-entry, enhanced or abnormal automaticity, and triggered automaticity. Although the latter two mechanisms are believed to account for certain arrhythmias, re-entry has been most convincingly documented in patients.

Older generalized concepts of the re-entrant pathway were confined to relatively simple substrates, such as Purkinje-myocardial junction models, when, in fact, they may be as complex as the heterogeneous three-dimensional structure of actual myocardial infarcts. In 1968, we reported the presence of an "ischemic zone" surrounding experimental acute myocardial infarctions (Cox et al., 1968). Subsequent studies have modified our initial concept of this border zone, but its importance in the genesis of ischemic ventricular tachyarrhythmias is well documented (Cox et al., 1969; Han et al., 1970; Durrer et al., 1971; Boineau and Cox, 1973; Waldo and Kaiser, 1973; Scherlag et al., 1974; El-Sherif et al., 1977). Such studies in animal models and, more recently, in man

(Wittig and Boineau, 1975; Fontaine *et al.*, 1977; Horowitz *et al.*, 1980) suggest that most re-entrant ventricular tachycardias in ischemic heart disease are primarily myocardial, micro-re-entrant (confined to a relatively small area of contiguous myocardium) rather than macro-re-entrant (pathways involving broad Purkinje-myocardial loops), and more complex geometrically than previously thought. Re-entrant ischemic ventricular arrhythmias result from a complex interplay between (1) a nonuniform (heterogeneous) state of repolarization, (2) slow desynchronized conduction over abnormal myocardial pathways created by fibrotic or ischemic discontinuity, and (3) ventricular ectopy. Premature beats interacting with nonuniform (heterogeneous) recovery result in regional differences in conduction of the impulse (Han and Moe, 1964; Boineau and Farlow, 1975; Boineau *et al.*, 1980). Some regions fail to excite, and others excite but propagate slowly, whereas immediately adjacent regions excite normally. Later, the same impulse invades regions not excited initially as they finally repolarize. Even later, these delayed impulses re-excite or re-enter the areas first excited by the premature beat and, therefore, first to repolarize. This type of re-entry typically results in short cardiac cycles and fast rates, i.e., ventricular fibrillation or flutter. Ventricular tachycardia is determined by a longer re-entrant cycle time, which necessitates either complex dissociation and extreme slowing of the re-entrant wave within a small area (micro-re-entry) or circus-like conduction over a long pathway (macro-re-entry). Slow, desynchronized conduction is a hallmark of myocardial injury or fibrosis (Durrer *et al.*, 1971; Daniel *et al.*, 1971). Conduction velocity depends on the synchrony of the activation process. Fibrosis is nonuniform at the borders of infarcts and produces complex interdigitations between normal myocardium and scar (Boineau and Cox, 1973, 1982). On approaching such an area, synchronous wave fronts may become desynchronized, fragmenting into many individual wavelets. Slow conduction accompanies the dysynchronization (Durrer *et al.*, 1971). Slow, desynchronized conduction can also be produced by applying tension or compression forces to the myocardium. Tension forces existing at the margins of aneurysms or infarcts may extend or radiate through the myocardium, resulting in desynchronization of activation or ectopy (Gallagher *et al.*, 1975; Cobbs and King, 1977; Sanders *et al.*, 1979). This mechanism may be similar to the myocardial compression re-entry model of Schmitt and Erlanger (1928) and probably explains why standard left ventricular aneurysm resection occasionally results in relief of associated ventricular tachycardia. Since resection of the aneurysm alters overall left ventricular geometry, it would also be expected to alter the tension forces existing at the margin of the aneurysm and radiating through the adjacent myocardium. Whether these mechanical forces act through the induction of ischemia or directly is unknown.

Differentiation between slow, desynchronized conduction (e.g., most types of ischemic tachyar-

rhythmias) and inhomogeneous repolarization (e.g., torsades de pointes) as the *primary* cause of the ventricular arrhythmia is essential. Slow, desynchronized conduction can be approached by direct myocardial surgery, and inhomogeneous repolarization cannot. Slow conduction is typically associated with focal myocardial pathologic entities such as infarction that can be recognized electrocardiographically and by segmental abnormal wall motion during contraction. Although future electrophysiologic studies may implicate local repolarization abnormalities that correlate with abnormal segmental relaxation, presently there is no firm basis for performing *direct* myocardial surgery if the principal mechanism is inhomogeneous repolarization and there is no evidence of activation delay or basis for slow conduction, such as myocardial fibrosis, infarction, abnormal wall tension, or a regional wall motion (contraction) abnormality.

Indirect Surgical Procedures. It has been recognized for many years that enhanced sympathetic activity predisposes the heart to ventricular arrhythmias, whereas reduced activity decreases this tendency. As a result, thoracic sympathectomy has been employed in patients with malignant ventricular arrhythmias both with and without coronary artery disease in an effort to take advantage of this experimental observation. With the advent of direct coronary artery revascularization on a large scale in the past decade, there have been several reports indicating that coronary artery bypass grafting may alleviate arrhythmias associated with coronary artery disease in some patients. In addition, isolated left ventricular aneurysm or infarct resection or resection in combination with coronary artery bypass grafting has proved to be successful in certain patients with ventricular arrhythmias associated with coronary artery disease. In a recent review of the literature, 179 patients were reported to have undergone these indirect surgical procedures for the treatment of recurrent ventricular arrhythmias associated with coronary artery disease (Table 51–2) (Boineau and Cox, 1982). The overall operative mortality rate was 26 per cent, and the failure rate was 16 per cent. The overall success rate of 58 per cent was remarkably consistent, regardless of the type of procedure employed to control the arrhythmia. These results probably represent the best experiences of surgeons involved in the treatment of this difficult problem, since it is likely that many failures have not been reported. Therefore, it seems reasonable that for any given patient with intractable ventricular arrhythmia associated with coronary artery disease, these indirect surgical procedures can be expected to be successful in approximately 50 per cent of them.

Within this group of 179 patients, there is a subgroup of patients who have not had previous myocardial infarctions and who experienced ventricular tachycardia only during episodes of angina pectoris or during physical exertion such as treadmill exercising. We have now collected approximately 45 patients who fall into this subgroup (Cox *et al.*, 1982b). All of these patients have undergone coronary angiog-

TABLE 51-2. RESULTS IN 179 PATIENTS TREATED WITH ONE OF THE INDIRECT SURGICAL PROCEDURES FOR REFRACTORY ISCHEMIC VENTRICULAR TACHYCARDIA*

PROCEDURE		PATIENTS	OPERATIVE MORTALITY RATE	FAILURE RATE	SUCCESS RATE
Sympathectomy		12	25%	17%	58%
CABG		45	22%	22%	56%
Resection		95	24%	17%	59%
CABG and Resection		27	41%	4%	55%
	Total	179	*Average* 26%	16%	58%

*From Ungerleider, R. M., *et al.*: Encircling endocardial ventriculotomy (EEV) for refractory ischemic ventricular tachycardia. I. Electrophysiologic effects. J. Thorac. Cardiovasc. Surg., *83*:840, 1982.
CABG = coronary artery bypass graft
Resection = myocardial infarctectomy or standard left ventricular aneurysmectomy

raphy and subsequent aortocoronary bypass grafting (both usually as an emergency procedure), with two operative deaths and with no recurrence of ventricular tachycardia in any of the patients. With the exception of this subgroup of patients, the indirect surgical approach to ischemic ventricular tachyarrhythmias should be considered obsolete.

Direct Surgical Procedures. The direct surgical treatment of any arrhythmia may be successful by either of two means—isolation or ablation (Camm *et al.*, 1979; Boineau and Cox, 1982; Ungerleider *et al.*, 1982a, 1982b, 1982c). An isolation procedure alleviates the detrimental effects of an arrhythmia by limiting its exit conduction pathways, but it does not alter the presence, frequency, or electrophysiologic characteristics of the arrhythmia. By confining an arrhythmia to a relatively localized region of the heart, it may continue to occur unabated, but since the abnormal electrical activity cannot escape the confines imposed by the surgical procedure, the remainder of the heart is unaffected. Examples of surgical isolation procedures are elective cryoablation of the bundle of His in patients with refractory supraventricular tachyarrhythmias (SVT) in which the SVT is confined to the atria (Sealy *et al.*, 1981), left atrial isolation for the treatment of ectopic SVT arising in the left atrium (Williams *et al.*, 1980), and isolation of arrhythmogenic regions of ventricular myocardium giving rise to nonischemic re-entrant arrhythmias associated with cardiomyopathies and arrhythmogenic right ventricular dysplasia (Cox and Gallagher, in press).

An ablative procedure destroys the arrhythmia by surgical resection (Wittig and Boineau, 1975), by thermoablation of the arrhythmogenic region (Wittig and Boineau, 1975; Gallagher *et al.*, 1978a; Camm *et al.*, 1979), or by interruption of re-entrant circuits responsible for the arrhythmia (Wittig and Boineau, 1975; Spurrell *et al.*, 1975; Guiraudon *et al.*, 1978). Surgical division of the Kent bundle for the treatment of Wolff-Parkinson-White syndrome is the most commonly employed ablative procedure in which the actual re-entrant circuit is purposely interrupted. The encircling endocardial ventriculotomy, the endocardial resection procedure, and endocardial cryoablation, all of which will be discussed in subsequent

sections, are examples of ablative procedures that are directed toward alleviating ischemic ventricular tachyarrhythmias by destroying or removing the entire area of arrhythmogenic myocardium.

Preoperative Electrophysiologic Evaluation. Patients with ischemic ventricular tachyarrhythmias who are considered candidates for surgical therapy undergo a preoperative electrophysiologic evaluation employing intracardiac catheter electrodes similar to that described for the preoperative evaluation of supraventricular tachyarrhythmia (see Fig. 51–7). In most patients, an electrode is also positioned in the left ventricle. The major objectives of the preoperative electrophysiologic study are (1) to document that the arrhythmia is ventricular tachycardia and not aberrantly conducted supraventricular tachycardia, (2) to demonstrate that programmed premature stimulation is capable of initiating and terminating the ventricular arrhythmia, thus indicating its re-entrant pathogenesis, and (3) to localize the origin of the ventricular tachycardia to the region of the myocardial infarction or left ventricular aneurysm, as determined by standard electrocardiography and left ventricular angiography. It is essential to document during this preoperative study that the electrically induced ventricular tachyarrhythmia has the same electrocardiographic characteristics that the patient's spontaneous ventricular arrhythmia exhibited prior to the study.

Intraoperative Electrophysiologic Evaluation. Following exposure of the heart and cannulation for cardiopulmonary bypass, a pacing and sensing electrode is sutured into the epicardial surface of the left ventricle near the base of the patient's aneurysm or infarction. Isochronous epicardial electrophysiologic mapping is performed during sinus rhythm to document that all electrophysiologic abnormalities are confined to the region of known myocardial injury. The sinus rhythm epicardial map usually shows fragmentation of the epicardial electrogram over the area of myocardial injury associated with delayed activation potentials (postexcitation phenomenon), Q waves, and slow ventricular activation (Durrer *et al.*, 1964; Gallagher *et al.*, 1974). If necessary, transmural multipoint needle electrodes may be placed through the wall of the left ventricle for intramural and endocardial mapping to determine if the observed alterations in epicardial activation are due to disturbances in the specialized conduction system and/or the myocardium (Durrer *et al.*, 1964).

Programmed premature stimulation of the left ventricle is then employed to induce ventricular tachycardia. Although the ability to induce and terminate ventricular tachycardia by programmed premature stimulation preoperatively is a prerequisite for selecting patients as candidates for surgery, the induction of ventricular tachycardia in the operating room may be extremely difficult. Since data points are recorded individually, several hundred cycles of ventricular tachycardia must be available for analysis to complete a sequence of epicardial activation. However, many factors necessary for the induction of sustained reentrant ventricular tachycardia may be altered in the operating room, precluding induction of tachycardia. These include the effects of anesthesia, myocardial temperature loss with exposure to room air, change in the level of circulating catecholamines, and changes in ventricular volume and wall tension due to alterations in preload and/or afterload (Gallagher *et al.*, 1982a). We have found that although institution of cardiopulmonary bypass may be a necessity during ventricular tachycardia mapping because of hemodynamic instability, it also allows the temperature of the myocardium to be raised as high as 38.5°C., a maneuver that usually makes it easier to maintain the patient in a stable ventricular tachycardia. It should be emphasized that it is absolutely essential to document that the ventricular tachycardia induced in the operating room is identical to the spontaneous tachycardia experienced by the patient preoperatively. At times, ventricular tachycardia may be induced that is extremely rapid, deteriorating into ventricular fibrillation after a limited number of cycles. In this setting, it has become commonplace to administer procainamide to permit a slower and more stable ventricular tachycardia to be induced, but it remains to be proved that the ventricular tachycardia induced under such conditions can be assumed to be the same as that initially present. When ventricular tachycardia cannot be readily induced in the operating room, more aggressive pacing techniques are employed, and as a result, a number of "nonclinical" ventricular tachyarrhythmias may be elicited.

Even if one is rewarded with a stable ventricular tachycardia intraoperatively, there may be difficulties encountered in the analysis of data recorded during the mapping procedure. These include problems relating to the three-dimensional nature of the heart and to the determination of an absolute reference point to which to relate the data. Our concept of ischemic reentrant ventricular tachycardia is that the source, or proximal end, of the re-entrant pathway may be located during sinus rhythm and corresponds to the site of most pronounced delayed conduction. The point of earliest activity during ventricular tachycardia represents the distal end of the connecting re-entrant pathway and is defined by mapping during ventricular

tachycardia. Since ischemic ventricular tachycardia is considered to be micro-re-entrant in most cases, the proximal and distal ends of the re-entrant circuit should be close to each other. Although one would like to assume that the ventricles are relatively homogeneous structures with uniform propagation in all directions, the ventricles are composed of a specialized conduction system capable of rapid conduction as well as ordinary myocardium, which conducts more slowly. Further inhomogeneity results from varied effects of the cause of ventricular tachycardia on the spread of impulses in the specialized conduction system and in the myocardium. These factors, in concert with the three-dimensional geometry of the heart, lead to a number of distortions that may further hamper proper interpretation of the isochronous map. A propagating wave front may secondarily invade the specialized conduction system, resulting in relatively early activation of a distant site. The same conditions that result in conduction delay during sinus rhythm and that serve as a substrate for re-entry can also result in distortion of propagation of ventricular tachycardia from the site of origin owing to differential spread of activation, depending on the relative proximity of normal myocardial tissue to specialized conducting tissues. Since a three-dimensional substrate must be considered, a distinct possibility exists that an activation front could travel a reasonable distance from its true site of origin before reaching a recording electrode. With this consideration in mind, one must distinguish between the true site of origin of the tachycardia and the earliest activity recorded during tachycardia. In order to result in a discernable deflection on the recording instrument being used, a propagating wave front must reach a sufficient volume of excitable tissue. One can easily envision ventricular tachycardia arising in a relatively scarred area with the earliest recognizable deflection being recorded in more healthy tissue some distance away.

Because of the frequent difficulties in inducing stable ventricular tachycardia intraoperatively and the inherent difficulties in interpreting two-dimensional data recorded from a three-dimensional structure, a computerized mapping system has been developed at our institution so that multiple epicardial, intramural, and endocardial sites can be recorded simultaneously (Smith *et al.*, 1977; Gallagher *et al.*, 1978b; Ideker *et al.*, 1979, 1980). The epicardial isochronous maps during normal sinus rhythm and during ventricular tachycardia are recorded by a sock electrode (Fig. 51–26) that contains multiple epicardial electrodes embedded in an elastic nylon mesh that holds the electrodes in contact with the epicardial surface. The earliest and latest activated regions recorded during normal sinus rhythm and ventricular tachycardia determine the sites of subsequent insertion of multiple transmural plunge needle electrodes (Fig. 51–27). These electrodes record endocardial, intramural, and epicardial electrograms from contact points located 1 mm. apart along the needle shaft (Kasell and Gallagher, 1977). The data are digitized and analyzed on

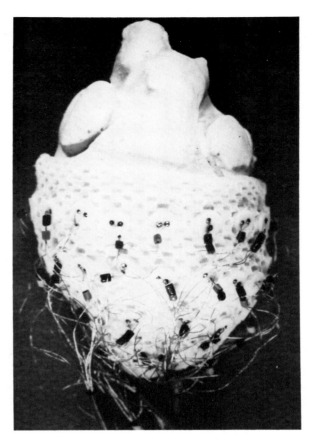

Figure 51–26. *A* "sock electrode" shown in position over a clay model of a canine heart. The material used is a flexible nylon mesh that is contoured to fit the heart and can be slipped over the ventricles and positioned in a matter of seconds. Within the nylon mesh, 27 pairs of electrodes are imbedded such that the global epicardial activation sequence can be obtained from a single beat. (Courtesy of Dr. R. E. Ideker.)

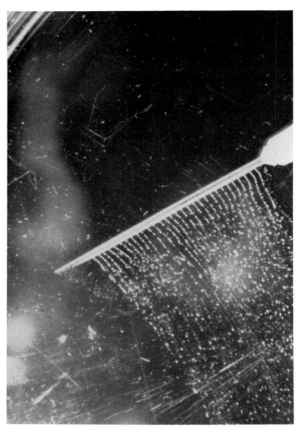

Figure 51–27. Plunge needle electrode used for recording intramural electrograms. A 0.22-gauge needle shaft is constructed such that electrode contacts are located every millimeter along the electrode shaft, allowing unipolar or bipolar intramural electrograms to be recorded. In this photograph, the multipoint needle electrode has been immersed in an electrolyte solution, and electrical current is being passed through each contact point to demonstrate their spacing along the needle shaft. (Courtesy of Dr. J. J. Gallagher.)

line by computer. This system allows a complete epicardial isochronous map to be obtained from a single beat of tachycardia, thus eliminating the problem of nonsustained ventricular tachycardia in the operating room. The computer is programmed to construct an isochronous epicardial map within 8 minutes after the data have been recorded (Fig. 51–28). The area of origin of the repetitive wave fronts during ventricular tachycardia is used as the marker that indicates the exit site nearest the reentrant circuit. If the ventricular tachycardia is due to micro-re-entry, the site of origin will be sought close to areas of delay and the critical dysrhythmic circuit. In patients with single confluent infarction, the site of origin of ventricular tachycardia is typically associated with the border zone of the infarct. Frequently, the earliest site of origin is noted to be intramural as opposed to endocardial or epicardial (Boineau and Cox, 1982).

Surgical treatment is most effective in patients with well-defined regions of pathology such as discrete infarcts or aneurysms. In these patients, because of the focal anatomic landmark and its association with the dysrhythmic circuit, surgery is more likely to alter the dysrhythmic areas. In patients without evident local pathology, successful intervention will depend on the electrocardiographic pattern during premature ventricular contractions, ventricular tachycardia, and sinus rhythm, the preoperative electrophysiologic data, and mapping at surgery. In certain patients, the dysrhythmic circuit may not be associated with the more obvious area of infarction. This can be suspected preoperatively from the disparity between the site of the infarct and the origin of the ventricular tachycardia as indicated by the electrocardiographic pattern or from differences in the electrocardiographic pattern of premature ventricular contractions and ventricular tachycardia indicating different regions of origin.

Encircling Endocardial Ventriculotomy. Prior to the present state of development of intraoperative mapping techniques, Guiraudon and Fontaine attempted to extrapolate their method of simple ventriculotomy used for nonischemic ventricular arrhythmias to the setting of ventricular tachycardia associated with coronary artery disease (Fontaine *et al.*, 1977). However, the operative findings and the clinical results differed markedly from those obtained when simple ventriculotomy was performed in the setting of a nonischemic cardiomyopathy. Thus, in a group of 13 operated patients with ventricular tachycardia secondary to ischemic heart disease, the intra-operative epicardial map during sinus rhythm showed delayed potentials in only one patient. The epicardial map during ventricular tachycardia was uninterpretable in 11 of the 13 patients. Simple ventriculotomy was successful in only one of the remaining two patients.

Guiraudon subsequently developed a technique of encircling endocardial ventriculotomy (EEV) for the treatment of ischemic ventricular arrhythmias (Guiraudon et al., 1978). As originally described, the EEV requires opening the left ventricle through the previous myocardial infarction or aneurysm. If the latter is present, a standard aneurysmectomy is performed, leaving a 1-cm. cuff of fibrous-tissue aneurysm wall with which to close the ventricle after completion of the procedure. The border between endocardial fibrosis at the base of the aneurysm and surrounding normal myocardium is identified. An incision perpendicular to the plane of the left ventricular wall is placed just outside the border of endocardial fibrosis and is continued around the entire base of the aneurysm. The depth of the incision on the left ventricular free wall is such that only a narrow bridge of subepicardium, the epicardium, and the overlying coronary vessels are spared. The incision is made approximately 1 cm. deep on the septal side of the aneurysm. The EEV is most easily performed in the presence of anterior left ventricular aneurysms, with or without involvement of the ventricular septum (Fig. 51–29).

In our experience, ventricular tachycardia associated with these aneurysms usually arises along the margins of the ventricular septal fibrosis or at the junction of the septal fibrosis and the left ventricular free wall anteriorly or posteriorly. If the ventricular septal portion of the EEV extends transmurally into the right ventricular cavity, the incision is simply buttressed at that point with a pledgeted 3-0 nonabsorbable suture. No ventricular septal defects or adverse sequelae have been experienced as a result of the septal portion of the incision.

The surgical approach to ventricular tachycardia arising posteriorly is much more difficult, especially if the aneurysm is small or if a myocardial infarction with no aneurysm exists. In the latter situation, the ventriculotomy must be made parallel to and within 1 cm. of the posterior ventricular septum in order to avoid the posterior papillary muscle (Cox et al., 1982a) (Fig. 51–30). In addition, the incision should be started as near the base of the left ventricle as possible, since the extension of the posterior papillary muscle from the left ventricular free wall is more narrow toward the mitral valve anulus. If the posterior ventriculotomy is placed too far laterally or apically, the posterior papillary muscle will be divided longitudinally, resulting in irreparable damage to the mitral valve apparatus. In addition, adequate visualization of the posterior septum and of the endocardium of the posterior ventricular free wall is virtually impossible through such an incision. In our experience, endocar-

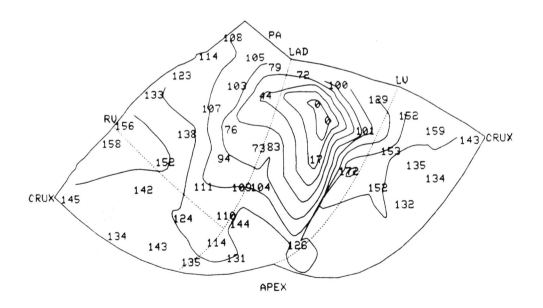

PROCEDURE GARRET.PRE   ACTIVATION TIME MAP
BEAT NUMBER   1
TIME ZERO IS EARLIEST LAT IN BEAT
ISOCHRONE INTERVAL = 20 MSEC

Figure 51–28. Isochronous epicardial electrophysiologic map constructed by a specially designed computer program (see text for discussion). This map was recorded intraoperatively from a patient who had sustained blunt injury to the chest resulting in total occlusion of the left anterior descending coronary artery with subsequent development of a large anterior septal left ventricular aneurysm and intractable ventricular tachycardia. This isochronous map recorded during ventricular tachycardia demonstrates the apparent site of origin of the tachycardia to be just left of the left anterior descending coronary artery at the base of the anterior left ventricular aneurysm.

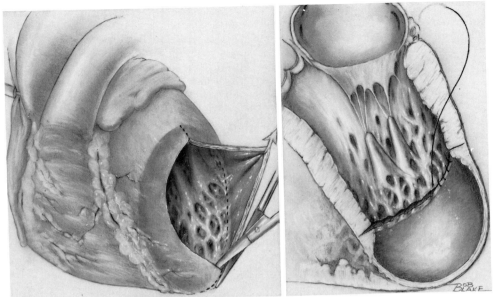

Figure 51–29. Encircling endocardial ventriculotomy (EEV), as described by Guiraudon in 1978. The left ventricle is entered through the center of an aneurysm. The border of endocardial fibrosis is visualized as it abuts normal endocardium. It is between fibrotic subendocardium and adjacent normal myocardium that re-entry circuits have been shown to originate. The EEV entails making an incision with a scapel in normal myocardium along the border of endocardial fibrosis (dashed line). The panel on the right demonstrates how the EEV incision should extend through all layers of the heart, sparing only a thin bridge of subepicardium that preserves the coronary vessels. On the septum, the incision should extend for a depth of 1 cm. Prior to closing the ventricle, the EEV incision is repaired with a running suture. Standard aneurysmectomy can be performed if appropriate. Intraoperative electrophysiologic mapping is not mandatory for performance of this procedure.

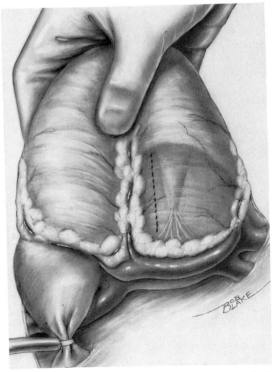

Figure 51–30. Proper placement of a posterior ventriculotomy (dashed line) for safe and effective exposure of the endocardium of a posterior-basilar myocardial infarction.

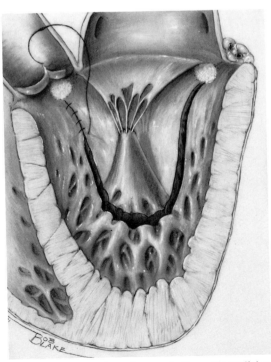

Figure 51–31. Location of an encircling endocardial ventriculotomy (EEV) positioned around the endocardial fibrosis associated with a posterior myocardial infarction. Since the EEV cannot be extended safely to the level of the mitral and aortic valve anuli, endocardial cryolesions (white circles) are placed at either end of the EEV to complete the "encirclement" of the fibrotic area.

dial fibrosis associated with posterior myocardial infarctions or aneurysms has invariably involved the high posterior septum up to the level of the aortic valve anulus. In most cases, the fibrosis has also extended to the level of the mitral valve anulus and around at least a portion of the base of the posterior papillary muscle. Although the EEV can be extended around the base of the posterior papillary muscle without causing mitral valve regurgitation (Guiraudon et al., 1978), it cannot be extended safely to the level of the aortic or mitral valve anulus. We extend the EEV to within 0.5 cm. of each valve anulus and then place an endocardial cryolesion between each end of the incision and the valve anulus to complete the "encirclement" of the endocardial fibrosis (Fig. 51–31). Following completion of the encircling endocardial ventriculotomy, closure is done with a continuous 3-0 nonabsorbable suture, and the ventricle is closed in the routine fashion.

Guiraudon and colleagues (1978) have suggested that the encircling endocardial ventriculotomy either isolates arrhythmogenic myocardium from the remainder of the heart or ablates ventricular tachycardia by surgical division of at least one limb of the re-entrant circuit responsible for the arrhythmia. Although our studies have demonstrated that the EEV is capable of isolating arrhythmogenic myocardium under certain experimental conditions (Ungerleider et al., 1982a), neither isolated, nonpropagated dysrhythmic activity nor local parasystole has been demonstrated clinically following the procedure. That the incision itself may divide a re-entrant circuit has been neither confirmed nor refuted either experimentally or clinically. Our experimental studies have shown that the EEV causes a profound decrease in regional blood flow in the encircled myocardium, especially the subendocardium (Ungerleider et al., 1982b). This surgically induced regional ischemia results in ablation of much of the normal and abnormal intramural electrical activity in the encompassed myocardium (Ungerleider et al., 1982a). These findings suggest that the EEV alters local conduction characteristics in the region of arrhythmogenesis such that the conditions necessary for regional re-entry are ablated (Cox et al., 1982a). Although such a mechanism of action is quite effective from an electrophysiologic standpoint, the decreased regional myocardial blood flow results in a concomitant depression of the regional myocardial function of any nonfibrosed tissue that is encircled (Ungerleider et al., 1982c). The alteration in regional function may be of little consequence if the associated aneurysm or infarction is small, but if the encompassed region of myocardium is large, left ventricular power failure can result from the procedure, as evidenced by the fact that the majority of operative deaths following an EEV have resulted from left ventricular power failure (Guiraudon et al., 1980; Arciniegas et al., 1980).

Endocardial Resection Procedure. In 1979, Harken and Josephson introduced the endocardial resection procedure for the treatment of ischemic ventricular tachyarrhythmias (Josephson et al., 1979; Harken et al., 1979). Following identification of the region of arrhythmogenesis, cold potassium cardioplegia is instituted, and undermining of the endocardial fibrosis is performed in the area of arrhythmogenesis from which the earliest activity was recorded during ventricular tachycardia. The edge of the aneurysm is grasped with clamps, and the endocardium is undermined with scissors (Fig. 51–32). In this fashion, an 8 to 25 cm.² piece of endocardium extending 2 to 3

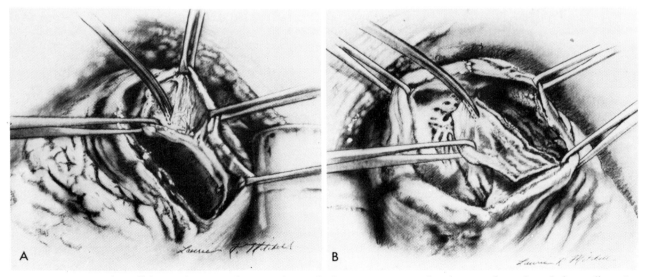

Figure 51–32. Endocardial resection procedure. *A,* A standard aneurysmectomy has been performed, and the earliest site of ventricular activation has been identified by endocardial mapping during ventricular tachycardia. The fibrous endocardial layer in the offending area is underlined sharply and resected. *B,* The endocardial resection is carried 2 to 3 cm. laterally and up into the ventricle on all sides of the earliest site of activation during ventricular tachycardia as determined by endocardial mapping. (From Harken, A. H., Horowitz, L. N., and Josephson, M. E.: Endocardial resection for recurrent sustained ventricular tachycardia. *In* Modern Technics in Surgery, Cardiac/Thoracic Surgery. Edited by L. H. Cohn. Mount Kisco, New York, Futura Publishing Company, 1981, Chapter 37, p. 6.)

cm. beyond the edge of the aneurysm is removed. In each case, this involves removal of 25 to 40 per cent of the circumference of the base of the aneurysm. In patients without left ventricular aneurysms but with myocardial infarctions, a ventriculotomy is placed through the center of the infarction, and endocardial resection of local areas of the infarction or of the posterior septum is accomplished. The area of tissue removed in these patients is usually less than 10 cm.². The majority of endocardial resections reported by Harken and Josephson were from the ventricular septum, either anteriorly or posteriorly. The remaining patients had endocardial resections from the infero-posterior free wall or the left ventricular free-wall border of either an anteroapical or an anterolateral aneurysm. Following the endocardial resection, the ventriculotomy or aneurysmectomy is closed.

In order to perform the local endocardial resection procedure, it is necessary to obtain an intraoperative isochronous endocardial map that is capable of localizing the arrhythmogenic area to at least one quadrant of the base of the infarction or aneurysm. Such extensive intraoperative mapping may require a considerable amount of cardiopulmonary bypass time if a computerized system such as that described previously is not available. However, if sustained ventricular tachycardia can be induced in the operating room to allow sufficient time for appropriate mapping procedures to be performed, the endocardial resection procedure is an excellent technique for alleviating these tachyarrhythmias. The exact mechanism of action of the endocardial resection procedure is unknown, but it is likely that the entire micro-re-entrant circuit responsible for the ventricular tachycardia is resected with the surgical specimen. The only apparent disadvantages of the endocardial resection procedure are (1) the necessity for extensive intraoperative electrophysiologic mapping, (2) the questionable structural integrity of closure of the left ventricular aneurysmectomy incision in the region of endocardial resection, and (3) the potential for an increase in the postoperative recurrence rate of ventricular tachycar-

dia owing to the localized nature of the resection and the possibility that ventricular tachycardia could arise from other sites around the border of the endocardial fibrosis. For the most part, the disadvantages cause no problem since most patients can be maintained in stable ventricular tachycardia long enough for the mapping procedures to be performed, the integrity of left ventricular closure following the procedure has not posed a problem thus far, and the recurrence rate of ventricular tachycardia following the procedure has been low (Josephson *et al.*, 1981).

Indications for and Results of Encircling Endocardial Ventriculotomy and the Endocardial Resection Procedure. Both the EEV of Guiraudon and the ERP of Harken and Josephson have proved to be superior to the previously employed indirect surgical procedures for the treatment of refractory ischemic ventricular tachycardia (Table 51–3). A total of 47 patients are known to have undergone the EEV, with a 17 per cent operative mortality rate, four late deaths (9 per cent), two of which were related to the EEV, and no known late recurrences (Guiraudon *et al.*, 1980, 1981; Arciniegas *et al.*, 1980; Cox *et al.*, 1982a; Shardey, 1981). Of 76 patients known to have undergone the ERP, there have been seven operative deaths (9 per cent), nine late deaths (13 per cent), and four late recurrences (6 per cent) (Josephson *et al.*, 1981; Shardey, 1981; Cox *et al.*, 1982a). Thus, of the 123 patients who have undergone one of the direct procedures, 108 (88 per cent) have survived the procedure, there have been two late deaths related to the surgery (2 per cent), and there has been only one patient with recurrent refractory tachycardia postoperatively (1 per cent). Therefore, 85 per cent of the patients undergoing either an EEV or an ERP have had successful surgical results.

Special intraoperative problems may arise that necessitate an alteration in the planned surgical procedure for the treatment of ischemic ventricular tachyarrhythmias. The most common of these problems is that ventricular tachycardia frequently does not last long enough intraoperatively to allow accurate locali-

TABLE 51–3. RESULTS OF INDIRECT AND DIRECT SURGICAL PROCEDURES FOR THE TREATMENT OF REFRACTORY ISCHEMIC VENTRICULAR TACHYCARDIA§

PROCEDURE	NUMBER OF PATIENTS	OPERATIVE MORTALITY	LATE MORTALITY	POSTOPERATIVE RECURRENCE WITHOUT DRUG THERAPY	REFRACTORY POSTOPERATIVELY WITH DRUG THERAPY	OVERALL SUCCESS RATE‡
Indirect	179	47 (26%)	?	29 (16%)	29 (16%)	103 (58%)
EEV	47	8 (17%)	4 (9%)*	3 (7%)	0%	37 (79%)
ERP	76	7 (9%)	10 (13%)†	4 (5%)	1 (1%)	68 (89%)

EEV = encircling endocardial ventriculatomy
ERP = endocardial resection procedure

*Two late deaths related to EEV.
†No late deaths related to ERP.
‡Overall success rate includes the total number of patients (column 1) minus the operative deaths (column 2), late deaths related to surgery or recurrent ventricular tachycardia, and postoperative recurrences with medical therapy.
§From Cox, J. L., *et al.*: Encircling endocardial ventriculotomy (EEV) for refractory ischemic ventricular tachycardia. IV. Clinical indications, surgical technique, mechanism of action, and results. J, Thorac. Cardiovasc. Surg., *83*:865, 1982.

zation of the arrhythmogenic site. If the area of endocardial fibrosis in such cases is reasonably small and preoperative left ventricular function is not severely depressed, an encircling endocardial ventriculotomy is recommended. If the patient has a large ventricular aneurysm and extensive endocardial fibrosis with poor left ventricular function, we perform a standard left ventricular aneurysmectomy and then resect *all* of the remaining endocardial fibrosis except that extending onto the papillary muscles. The same approach is recommended in institutions in which an emergency operation is required and no equipment exists for intraoperative electrophysiologic mapping.

The second common problem relates to the surgical treatment of ventricular tachycardia associated with posterior left ventricular aneurysms or infarctions. Either the EEV or the ERP may be employed in such cases, but if the posterior papillary muscle is intimately involved with the arrhythmia and its endocardium is fibrosed, we place an EEV around the base of the papillary muscle and extend it to within 0.5 cm. of both the aortic valve anulus and mitral valve anulus, if necessary. An endocardial cryolesion is then applied between either end of the incision and the respective valve anulus, as mentioned previously. If the arrhythmogenic region is high on the posterior septum and can be localized by endocardial mapping, an ERP is performed in that location. Since the endocardial resection cannot be safely extended to involve the aortic valve anulus, we have found it necessary after resection to place an endocardial cryolesion beyond the border of resection at the level of the aortic valve anulus to ablate the arrhythmia. This frequently results in temporary or permanent heart block because of the proximity of the bundle of His.

The specific surgical approach to the treatment of refractory ventricular tachycardia associated with coronary artery disease must be tailored to meet the needs of the individual anatomic-electrophysiologic problem. The newer endocardial surgical techniques are promising in that they direct attention to the border zone and to the septal areas of the left ventricle. They are predicated, however, on the presence of a localized area of pathology, i.e., endocardial fibrosis or aneurysm, and not diffuse myocardial disease as a substrate for the ventricular arrhythmias. In addition, these techniques prolong the duration and the complexity of the operative interventions. The long-term sequelae of these operations remain to be defined with regard to hemodynamic function, structural integrity, and electrophysiologic stability of the ventricle. Moreover, they do not alter the uncertain natural history of a dynamic disease process such as coronary artery disease. Finally, these interventions focus on the existence of a substrate of ventricular arrhythmia that is largely static and thus amenable to modification or ablation. This emphasis minimizes the role that dynamic variables such as spasm, reperfusion, stretch, and circulating catecholamines play in the genesis of ventricular arrhythmias (Lown and DeSilva, 1978).

Early and late mortality associated with surgical attempts to correct ventricular arrhythmias related to ischemic heart disease may improve as better techniques for myocardial preservation are developed. In all likelihood, survival will be a function of the underlying hemodynamic condition and the time of operation relative to the ischemic event. One series, however, shows that in properly selected patients, early surgical intervention may significantly improve the survival of patients suffering from intractable arrhythmias following myocardial infarction (Wald *et al.*, 1979).

FUTURE DIRECTIONS OF SURGERY FOR CARDIAC ARRHYTHMIAS

At present, there are three basic means of treating intractable arrhythmias: (1) drug therapy, (2) pacing, and (3) surgery. The availability of newer antiarrhythmic agents (Zipes and Troup, 1978) may diminish the need for surgical treatment in the future. However, as noted by Gallagher and Cox (1979), much of the pioneering work in the surgical treatment of ventricular arrhythmias has occurred in France and England, where there is ready access to all the potent antiarrhythmic agents. This fact suggests that if the newer surgical techniques for ventricular arrhythmias prove to be as effective as those introduced for the treatment of the pre-excitation syndromes, they may be preferable to the vagaries of drug therapy.

With few exceptions, the role of cardiac pacing for the treatment of arrhythmias remains investigative. A significant contribution in this field has been made by Waldo and associates (1976), who have employed rapid atrial pacing with "atrial entrainment" for the control of supraventricular arrhythmias following cardiac surgery. The use of automatic defibrillating devices for the control of recurrent ventricular tachycardia is an ingenious concept, but one that would appear to be limited in scope. Our experience with refractory ventricular tachyarrhythmias with or without associated coronary artery disease has shown that many of the patients with this condition are in continuous ventricular tachycardia and that programmed stimulation may break the tachycardia only for a few seconds. Pacing devices would appear to be of no value in such patients.

SELECTED REFERENCES

Anderson, R. H., and Becker, A. E.: Cardiac anatomy for the surgeon. *In* Lewis' Practice of Surgery. Edited by G. K. Danielson. Hagerstown, Maryland, Harper and Row, 1979, Chapter 16.

This chapter is an excellent, concise description of the anatomy of the heart pertinent to the cardiac surgeon. Most of the diagrams are drawn in the view in which they appear during cardiac surgery. The anatomy of the atrioventricular junctional area and of the normal cardiac conduction system is described particularly well.

Boineau, J. P., and Cox, J. L.: Slow ventricular activation in acute myocardial infarction. A source of re-entrant premature ventricular contractions. Circulation, *48*:702, 1973.

In this paper, the authors demonstrate that ventricular arrhythmias associated with ischemic myocardium may occur on a re-entrant basis and that such intramyocardial re-entrant arrhythmias originate in the border zone of a myocardial infarction. The accepted theory of ischemic re-entrant ventricular arrhythmias is discussed in detail. Guiraudon formulated his encircling endocardial ventriculotomy on the basis of this study.

Cobb, F. R., Blumenschein, S. D., Sealy, W. C., Boineau, J. P., Wagner, G. S., and Wallace, A. G.: Successful surgical interruption of the bundle of Kent in a patient with Wolff-Parkinson-White syndrome. Circulation, *38*:1018, 1968.

This is the first description of the successful surgical treatment of the Wolff-Parkinson-White syndrome. Although current surgical techniques differ significantly from those described in this original article, this paper represents a milestone in the surgical treatment of cardiac arrhythmias.

Cox, J. L., McLaughlin, V. W., Flowers, N. C., and Horan, L. G.: The ischemic zone surrounding acute myocardial infarction. Its morphology as detected by dehydrogenase staining. Am. Heart J., *76*:650, 1968.

This article offers the first pathologic description of the so-called "twilight zone" of intermediate cellular injury located at the periphery of an acute myocardial infarction. Although subsequent, more sophisticated pathologic studies have questioned the existence of such an intermediate zone of ischemic injury, much of the pharmacologic and mechanical (i.e., intra-aortic balloon pumping) therapy introduced for the treatment of myocardial ischemic injury in the past decade has been based on the presence of such a zone. In addition, most investigators feel that this "twilight zone" is the site of origin of re-entrant ventricular tachyarrhythmias associated with coronary artery disease.

Guiraudon, G., Fontaine, G., Frank, R., Escande, G., Etievent, P., and Cabrol, C.: Encircling endocardial ventriculotomy: A new surgical treatment for life-threatening ventricular tachycardias resistant to medical treatment following myocardial infarction. Ann. Thorac. Surg., *26*:438, 1978.

In this article, Guiraudon describes the first five patients to undergo an encircling endocardial ventriculotomy for the treatment of ischemic ventricular tachyarrhythmias. In this series, there were no operative deaths, and antiarrhythmic therapy was discontinued postoperatively, with no recurrence of the ventricular tachycardia during a follow-up of 6 to 24 months. This article represents the first scientific approach to the direct surgical treatment of ischemic ventricular tachyarrhythmias. With this paper, these pioneers ushered in a new era in the treatment of this problem.

Josephson, M. E., Harken, A. H., and Horowitz, L. N.: Endocardial excision: A new surgical technique for the treatment of recurrent ventricular tachycardia. Circulation, *60*:1430, 1979.

In this paper, the authors describe the endocardial resection procedure based on extensive intraoperative electrophysiologic studies for the treatment of ischemic ventricular tachycardia. Initially, this technique was viewed as an alternative to Guiraudon's encircling endocardial ventriculotomy, but subsequent clinical experience with the endocardial resection procedure has established it as the current procedure of choice for the treatment of refractory ischemic ventricular tachycardia. These authors have made many significant contributions to the field of surgery for ventricular tachycardia, and this article describes their scientific approach to an extremely difficult problem in critically ill patients.

REFERENCES

Abendroth, R. R., Ostermeyer, J., Breithardt, G., Seipel, L., and Bircks, W.: Reproducibility of local activation times during intraoperative epicardial mapping. Circulation, *62*:75, 1980.

Anderson, R. H., and Becker, A. E. Anatomy of conducting tissue revisited. Br. Heart J., *40*(Suppl.):2, 1978.

Anderson, R. H., and Becker, A. E.: Cardiac anatomy for the surgeon. *In* Lewis' Practice of Surgery. Edited by G. K. Danielson. Hagerstown, Maryland, Harper and Row, 1979, Chapter 16.

Anderson, R. H., and Becker, A. E.: Morphology of the human atrioventricular junction area. *In* The Conduction System of the Heart: Structure, Function and Clinical Implications. Edited by H. J. J. Wellens, K. I. Lie, M. J. Janse, H. F. Leiden, and B. V. Stenfert-Kroese. Philadelphia, Lea & Febiger, 1976, p. 264.

Arciniegas, J. G., Klein, H., Karp, R. B., Kouchoukos, N. T., James, T. N., Kirklin, J. W., and Waldo, A. L.: Surgical treatment of life-threatening ventricular tachyarrhythmias. (Abstract.) Circulation, *62*(Suppl. 3):42, 1980.

Barr, R. C., Gallie, T. M., and Spock, M. S.: Automated production of contour maps for electrophysiology. III. Construction of contour maps. Comput. Biomed. Res., *13*:171, 1980.

Benson, D. W., Jr., and Cox, J. L.: Surgical treatment of cardiac arrhythmias. *In* Cardiac Arrhythmias in the Neonate, Infant and Child. 2nd ed. Edited by N. K. Roberts and H. Gelband. New York, Appleton-Century-Crofts, 1982, pp. 341–366.

Boineau, J. P., and Cox, J. L.: Rationale for a direct surgical approach to control ventricular arrhythmias. Am. J. Cardiol., *49*:381, 1982.

Boineau, J. P., and Cox, J. L.: Slow ventricular activation in acute myocardial infarction. A source of re-entrant premature ventricular contractions. Circulation, *48*:702, 1973.

Boineau, J. P., and Farlow, W.: The use of a computer model to understand mechanisms of ventricular fibrillation. Circulation, *52*(Suppl. 2):162, 1975.

Boineau, J. P., Mooney, C., Hudson, R., Hughes, D., Erdin, R., and Wylds, A.: Observations on re-entrant excitation pathways and refractory period distribution in spontaneous and experimental atrial flutter in the dog. *In* Re-entrant Arrhythmias. Edited by H. E. Kulbertus. Baltimore, Maryland, University Park Press, 1977, pp. 79–98.

Boineau, J. P., Schuessler, R. B., Mooney, C. R., Miller, C. B., Wylds, A. C., Hudson, R. D., Borremans, J. M., and Brockus, C. W.: Natural and evoked atrial flutter due to circus movement in dogs. Am. J. Cardiol., *45*:1167, 1980.

Burchell, H. B., Frye, R. L., Anderson, M. W., *et al.*: Atrial-ventricular and ventricular-atrial excitation in Wolff-Parkinson-White syndrome (type B): Temporary ablation at surgery. Circulation, *36*:663, 1967.

Camm, J., and Rees, G.: Is the surgical solution to the treatment of tachycardias justified? Thorax, *34*:434, 1979.

Camm, J., Ward, D. E., Cory-Pearce, R., Reese, G. M., and Spurrell, R. A. J.: The successful cryosurgical treatment of paroxysmal ventricular tachycardia. Chest, *75*:621, 1979.

Cobb, F. R., Blumenschein, S. D., Sealy, W. C., Boineau, J. P., Wagner, G. S., and Wallace, A. G.: Successful surgical interruption of the bundle of Kent in a patient with Wolff-Parkinson-White syndrome. Circulation, *38*:1018, 1968.

Cobbs, B. W., Jr., and King, S. B.: Ventricular buckling: A factor in the abnormal ventriculogram and peculiar hemodynamics associated with mitral valve prolapse. Am. Heart J., *93*:741, 1977.

Cox, J. L., and Gallagher, J. J.: Transmural encircling ventriculotomy (TEV) and cryosurgery for intractable ventricular tachycardia arising in the right ventricle. Circulation, in press.

Cox, J. L., Gallagher, J. J., and Ungerleider, R. M.: Encircling endocardial ventriculotomy (EEV) for refractory ischemic ventricular tachycardia. IV. Clinical indications, surgical technique, mechanism of action, and results. J. Thorac. Cardiovasc. Surg., *83*:865, 1982a.

Cox, J. L., Daniel, T. M., Sabiston, D. C., Jr., and Boineau, J. P.: Desynchronized activation in myocardial infarction—a re-entry basis for ventricular arrhythmias. (Abstract.) Circulation, *39*(Suppl. 3):63, 1969.

Cox, J. L., Lowe, J. E., Morris, J. J., and Hackshaw, B.: The surgical treatment of angina-induced or exercise-induced ventricular tachycardia. Unpublished data, 1982b.

Cox, J. L., McLaughlin, V. W., Flowers, N. C., and Horan, L.

G.: The ischemic zone surrounding acute myocardial infarction. Its morphology as detected by dehydrogenase staining. Am. Heart J., 76:650, 1968.

Daniel, T. M., Boineau, J. P., and Sabiston, D. C., Jr.: Comparison of human ventricular activation with a canine model and chronic myocardial infarction. Circulation, 44:74, 1971.

Davidow, L. S., and Brown, P. B.: A contour mapping algorithm suitable for small computers. In Technology in Neuroscience. Edited by P. B. Brown. New York, John Wiley and Sons, 1975, p. 321.

Dessertenne, F.: La tachycardie ventriculaire à deux foyers opposés variables. Arch. Mal. Coeur, 59:263, 1966.

Draper, M. H., and Weidmann, S.: Cardiac resting and action potentials recorded with an intracellular electrode. J. Physiol., 115:74, 1957.

Durrer, D., and Roos, J. T.: Epicardial excitation of the ventricles in a patient with Wolff-Parkinson-White syndrome. Circulation, 38:1018, 1968.

Durrer, D., Van Lier, A. A. W., and Buller, J.: Epicardial and intramural excitation in chronic myocardial infarction. Am. Heart J., 68:765, 1964.

Durrer, D., van Dam, R. T., Freud, G. E., and Janse, M. J.: Re-entry and ventricular arrhythmias in local ischemia and infarction of the intact dog heart. Proc. K. Ned. Akad. Wet. (Biol. Med.), 74:321, 1971.

El-Sherif, N., Scherlag, B. J., Lazzara, R., and Hopen, R. R.: Re-entrant ventricular arrhythmias in the late myocardial infarction period. I. Conduction characteristics of the infarction zone. Circulation, 55:686, 1977.

Fontaine, G., Guiraudon, G., and Frank, R.: Management of chronic ventricular tachycardia. In Innovations in Diagnosis and Management of Cardiac Arrhythmias. Edited by O. S. Narula. Baltimore, Williams and Wilkins, 1979.

Fontaine, G., Guiraudon, G., Frank, R., Vedel, J., Grosgogeat, Y., Cabrol, C., and Facquet, J.: Stimulation studies and epicardial mapping in ventricular tachycardia: Study of mechanisms and selection for surgery. In Re-entrant Arrhythmias. Edited by H. E. Kulbertus. Baltimore, Maryland, University Park Press, 1977, pp. 334–350.

Fraser, G. R., and Froggatt, P.: Unexpected cot deaths. Lancet, 2:56, 1966.

Gallagher, J. J., and Cox, J. L.: Status of surgery for ventricular arrhythmias. (Editorial.) Circulation, 60:1440, 1979.

Gallagher, J. J., Anderson, R. W., Kasell, J., Rice, J. R., Pritchett, E. L. C., Gault, J. H., Harrison, L., and Wallace, A. G.: Cryoablation of drug-resistant ventricular tachycardia in a patient with a variant of scleroderma. Circulation, 57:190, 1978a.

Gallagher, J. J., Ideker, R. E., Smith, W. M., Kasell, J., Harrison, L., and Wallace, A. G.: Epicardial mapping of ventricular arrhythmias by digital computer. In Management of Ventricular Tachycardia—Role of Mexiletine. Edited by E. Sandoe, D. J. Julian, and J. W. Bell. Amsterdam, Excerpta Medica, 1978b, pp. 17–38.

Gallagher, J. J., Kasell, J. H., Cox, J. L., and Smith, W. M.: The technique of intraoperative electrophysiologic mapping. Am. J. Cardiol., 49:221, 1982.

Gallagher, J. J., Kasell, J., Sealy, W. C., Pritchett, E. L. C., and Wallace, A. G.: Epicardial mapping in the Wolff-Parkinson-White syndrome. Circulation, 57:854, 1978c.

Gallagher, J. J., Oldham, H. N., Jr., Wallace, A. G., Peter, R. H., and Kasell, J.: Ventricular aneurysm with ventricular tachycardia. Report of a case with epicardial mapping and successful resection. Am. J. Cardiol., 35:696, 1975.

Gallagher, J. J., Sealy, W. C., Cox, J. L., and Kasell, J. H.: Results of surgery for pre-excitation in 200 cases. Presented at the 54th Scientific Sessions, American Heart Association, November 1981.

Gallagher, J. J., Ticzon, A. R., Wallace, A. G., and Kasell, J.: Activation studies following experimental hemiblock in the dog. Circ. Res., 35:752, 1974.

Gallagher, J. J., et al.: The Wolff-Parkinson-White syndrome and the pre-excitation dysrhythmias: Medical and surgical management. Med. Clin. North Amer., 60:101, 1976.

Guiraudon, G., Fontaine, G., Frank, R., Escande, G., Etievent,

P., and Cabrol, C.: Encircling endocardial ventriculotomy: A new surgical treatment of life-threatening ventricular tachycardias resistant to medical treatment following myocardial infarction. Ann. Thorac. Surg., 26:438, 1978.

Guiraudon, G., Fontaine, G., Frank, R., Grosgogeat, Y., and Cabrol, C.: Encircling endocardial ventriculotomy: Late follow-up results. (Abstract.) Circulation, 62(Suppl. 3):320, 1980.

Guiraudon, G., Fontaine, G., Frank, R., Leandri, R., Barra, J., and Cabrol, C.: Surgical treatment of ventricular tachycardia guided by ventricular mapping in 23 patients without coronary artery disease. Presented at the 17th Annual Meeting of the Society of Thoracic Surgery, January 1981.

Han, J., Gael, B. G., and Hansen, C. S.: Re-entrant beats induced in the ventricle during coronary occlusion. Am. Heart J., 80:778, 1970.

Han, J., and Moe, G. K.: Non-uniform recovery of excitability in ventricular muscle. Circ. Res., 14:44, 1964.

Harken, A. H., Horowitz, L. N., and Josephson, M. E.: Endocardial resection for recurrent sustained ventricular tachycardia. In Modern Technics in Surgery, Cardiac/Thoracic Surgery. Edited by L. H. Cohn. Mount Kisco, New York, Futura Publishing Co., 1981, Chapter 37.

Harken, A. H., Josephson, M. E., and Horowitz, L. N.: Surgical endocardial resection for the treatment of malignant ventricular tachycardia. Ann. Surg., 190:456, 1979.

Holman, W., Ikeshita, M., Lease, J., Smith, P., Ferguson, T., and Cox, J.: Elective prolongation of atrioventricular conduction by multiple discrete cryolesions: A new technique for the treatment of paroxysmal supraventricular tachycardia. J. Thorac. Cardiovasc. Surg., 84:554, 1982.

Holzmann, M., and Scherf, D.: Über Elektrokardiogramme mit Verkuryter Vorhof-Krammer-Distanz und Positiven P-Zacken. Z. Klin. Med., 121:404, 1932.

Horowitz, L. N., Josephson, M. E., and Harken, A. H.: Epicardial and endocardial activation during sustained ventricular tachycardia in man. Circulation, 61:1227, 1980.

Ideker, R. E., Klein, G. J., Smith, W. M., Harrison, L., Kasell, J., Wallace, A. G., and Gallagher, J. J.: Epicardial activation sequences during the onset of ventricular tachycardia and ventricular fibrillation. In Sudden Death. Edited by H. E. Kulbertus. Lancaster, England, MTP Press Ltd., 1980, pp. 165–185.

Ideker, R. E., Smith, W. M., Wallace, A. G., Kasell, J., Harrison, L. A., Klein, G. J., Kinicki, R. E., and Gallagher, J. J.: A computerized method for the rapid display of ventricular activation during the intraoperative study of arrhythmias. Circulation, 59:449, 1979.

James, T. N., Froggatt, P., Atkinson, W. J., Jr., Lurie, P. R., McNamara, D. G., Miller, W. W., Schloss, G. T., Carroll, J. F., and North, R. L.: De subitaneis mortibus XXX: Observations on the pathophysiology of the long Q-T syndromes with special reference to the neuropathology of the heart. Circulation, 57:1221, 1978.

Jervell, A., and Lange-Nielsen, F.: Congenital deaf-mutism, functional heart disease with prolongation of the Q-T interval, and sudden death. Am. Heart J., 54:59, 1957.

Josephson, M. E., Harken, A. H., and Horowitz, L. N.: Endocardial excision—a new surgical technique for the treatment of recurrent ventricular tachycardia. Circulation, 60:1430, 1979.

Josephson, M. E., Horowitz, L. N., and Harken, A. H.: Surgery for recurrent sustained ventricular tachycardia associated with coronary artery disease: The role of subendocardial resection. Submitted to New York Academy of Sciences, 1981.

Kasell, J., and Gallagher, J. J.: Construction of multi-polar needle electrode for activation study of the heart. Am. J. Physiol., 233:H312, 1977.

Katz, A. M.: The arrhythmias. II: Abnormal impulse formation and re-entry, premature systoles, pre-excitation. In Physiology of the Heart. New York, Raven Press, 1977, pp. 331.

Kent, A. F. S.: Researches on structure and function of mammalian heart. J. Physiol., 14:233, 1893.

Krikler, D. M., and Curry, P. V. L.: Torsades de pointes: An atypical ventricular tachycardia. Br. Heart J., 38:117, 1976.

Kulbertus, H. E.: La torsades de pointes. Rev. Med. Liege, 33:63, 1978.

Kulbertus, H. E.: The arrhythmogenic effects of anti-arrhythmic agents. *In* Selected Topics in Cardiac Arrhythmias. Edited by B. Befeler. Mount Kisco, New York, Futura Publishing Company, 1980, pp. 113.

Lewis, T., and Rothschild, M. A.: The excitatory process in the dog's heart. II. Ventricles. Philos. Trans. R. Soc. Lond., *206*:181, 1915.

Lown, B., and DeSilva, R. A.: Roles of psychologic stress and autonomic nervous system changes in provocation of ventricular premature complexes. Am. J. Cardiol., *41*:979, 1978.

Malliani, A., Schwartz, P. J., and Zanchetti, A.: Neural mechanisms and life-threatening arrhythmias. Am. Heart J., *100*:705, 1980.

McAllister, R. E., Noble, D., and Tsien, R. W.: Reconstruction of the electrical activity of cardiac Purkinje fibers. J. Physiol., *251*:1, 1975.

Moss, A. J., and McDonald, J.: Unilateral cervicothoracic sympathetic ganglionectomy for the treatment of long Q-T interval syndrome. N. Engl. J. Med., *285*:903, 1971.

Pritchett, E. L. C., Anderson, R. W., Benditt, B. G., Kasell, J., Harrison, L., Wallace, A. G., Sealy, W. C., and Gallagher, J. L.: Re-entry within the A-V node: Surgical cure with preservation of atrioventricular conduction. Circulation, *60*:440, 1979.

Reuter, H.: The dependence of slow inward current in Purkinje fibers on the extracellular calcium concentration. J. Physiol., *192*:479, 1967.

Romano, C., Gemme, G., and Pongiglione, R.: Aritmie Cardiache Rare Dell'eta Pediatrica. Clin. Pediatr., *45*:656, 1963.

Ruberman, W., Weinblatt, E., Goldberg, J., Frank, C., and Shapiro, S.: Ventricular premature beats and mortality after myocardial infarction. N. Engl. J. Med., *297*:750, 1977.

Sanders, R., Myerburg, R. J., Gelband, H., and Bassett, A. L.: Dissimilar length-tension relations of canine ventricular muscle and false tendon: Electrophysiologic alterations accompanying defamation. J. Mol. Cell. Cardiol., *11*:209, 1979.

Scherlag, B. J., El-Sherif, N., Hopen, R. R., and Lazzara, R.: Characterization and localization of ventricular arrhythmias resulting from myocardial ischemia and infarction. Circ. Res., *35*:372, 1974.

Schmitt, F. O., and Erlanger, J.: Directional differences in the conduction of the impulse through heart muscle and their possible relation to extrasystolic and fibrillatory contractions. Am. J. Physiol., *87*:326, 1928.

Schwartz, P. J., and Wolf, S.: Q-T interval prolongation as a predictor of sudden death in patiens with myocardial infarction. Circulation, *57*:1074, 1978.

Schwartz, P. J., Periti, M., and Malliani, A.: The long Q-T syndrome. Fund. Clin. Cardiol., *89*:378, 1975.

Sealy, W. C., and Gallagher, J. J.: The surgical approach to the septal area of the heart based on the experiences with 45 patients with Kent bundle. J. Thorac. Cardiovasc. Surg., *79*:542, 1980.

Sealy, W. C., Gallagher, J. J., and Kasell, J. H.: His bundle interruption for control of inappropriate ventricular responses to atrial arrhythmias. Ann. Thorac. Surg., *32*:429, 1981.

Shardey, G.: Personal communication, *32*:429, 1981.

Smith, W., and Gallagher, J. J.: Q-T prolongation syndromes. Practical Cardiology, *5*:118, 1979.

Smith, W. M., Ideker, R. E., Kinicki, R. E., Harrison, L. A., Wallace, A. G., and Gallagher, J. J.: A computer system for the on-line study of ventricular arrhythmias. *In* Computers in Cardiology. Long Beach, IEE, 1977, pp. 311–316.

Spurrell, R. A. J., Yates, A. K., Thorburn, C. W., Sowton, G. E., and Deuchar, D. C.: Surgical treatment of ventricular tachycardia after epicardial mapping studies. Br. Heart J., *37*:115, 1975.

Strauss, H. C., Prystowsky, E. N., and Scheinman, N. M.: Sinoatrial and atrial electrogenesis. Prog. Cardiovasc. Dis., *19*:385, 1977.

Truex, R. C., Bishof, J. K., and Hoffman, E. L.: Accessory atrial ventricular muscle bundles of developing human heart. Anat. Rec., *131*:45, 1958.

Uhl, H. S.: A previously undescribed malformation of the heart: Almost total absence of the myocardium of the right ventricle. Bull. Johns Hopkins Hosp., *91*:197, 1952.

Ungerleider, R. M., Holman, W. L., Stanley, T. E., III, Lofland, G. K., Williams, J. M., Ideker, R. E., Smith, P. K., Quick, G., and Cox, J. L.: Encircling endocardial ventriculotomy (EEV) for refractory ischemic ventricular tachycardia. I. Electrophysiologic effects. J. Thorac. Cardiovasc. Surg., *83*:840, 1982a.

Ungerleider, R. M., Holman, W. L., Stanley, T. E., III, Lofland, G. K., Williams, J. M., Smith, P. K., Quick, G., and Cox, J. L.: Encircling endocardial ventriculotomy (EEV) for refractory ischemic ventricular tachycardia. II. Effects on regional myocardial blood flow. J. Thorac. Cardiovasc. Surg., *83*:850, 1982b.

Ungerleider, R. M., Holman, W. L., Calcagno, D., Williams, J. M., Lofland, G. K., Smith, P. K., Stanley, T. E., III, Quick, G., and Cox, J. L.: Encircling endocardial ventriculotomy (EEV) for refractory ischemic ventricular tachycardia. III. Effects on regional left ventricular function. J. Thorac. Cardiovasc. Surg., *83*:857, 1982c.

Wald, R. W., Waxman, M. B., Corey, P. M., Gunstensen, J., and Goldman, B. S.: Management of intractable ventricular tachyarrhythmias after myocardial infarction. Am. J. Cardiol., *44*:329, 1979.

Waldo, A. L., and Kaiser, G. A.: A study of ventricular arrhythmias associated with acute myocardial infarction in the canine heart. Circulation, *47*:1222, 1973.

Waldo, A. L., MacLean, W. A. H., Karp, R. B., Kouchoukos, N. T., and James, T. N.: Continuous rapid atrial pacing to control recurrent or sustained supraventricular tachycardias following open heart surgery. Circulation, *54*:245, 1976.

Ward, O. C.: New familial cardiac syndrome in children. J. Irish Med. Assoc., *54*:103, 1964.

Wellens, H. J. J., Duren, D. R., Liem, K., and Lie, K. I.: Effects of digitalis in patients with paroxysmal atrioventricular nodal tachycardia. Circulation, *52*:779, 1975.

Williams, J. M., Ungerleider, R. M., Lofland, G. K., and Cox, J. L.: Left atrial isolation: New technique for the treatment of supraventricular arrhythmias. J. Thorac. Cardiovasc. Surg., *80*:373, 1980.

Wittig, J. H., and Boineau, J. P.: Surgical treatment of ventricular arrhythmias using epicardial transmural and endocardial mapping. Ann. Thorac. Surg., *20*:117, 1975.

Wolff, L., Parkinson, J., and White, P. D.: Bundle branch block with short PR interval in healthy young people prone to paroxysmal tachycardia. Am. Heart J., *5*:685, 1930.

Wyndham, C. R., Meeran, M. K., Smith, T., Saxena, A., Engelman, F. M., Levitski, S., and Rosen, K. M.: Epicardial activation of the intact human heart without conduction defects. Circulation, *59*:161, 1979.

Yanowitz, F., Preston, J. B., and Abildskov, J. A.: Functional distribution of right and left stellate innervation to the ventricles. Circ. Res., *18*:416, 1966.

Zipes, D. P., and Fisher, J. C.: Effects of agents which inhibit the slow channel on sinus node automaticity and atrioventricular induction in the dog. Circ. Res., *34*:184, 1974.

Zipes, D. P., and Troup, P. J.: New anti-arrhythmic agents: amiodarone, aprindine, disopyramide, ethmozin, mexiletine, tocainide, verapamil. Am. J. Cardiol., *41*:1005, 1978.

Chapter 52

Tumors of the Heart

DAVID C. SABISTON, JR.
BRACK G. HATTLER, JR.

Primary neoplasms of the heart are uncommon and constitute one of the rarer forms of cardiac disease. The clinical spectrum of these tumors encompasses those that are rapidly progressive and usually fatal and those neoplasms, primarily myxomas, that are curable.

Although cardiac tumors have been recognized since the sixteenth century (Columbus, 1562), it was not until 1934 that Barnes and associates reported the first *clinical* diagnosis in a patient with a primary cardiac neoplasm. This later proved to be a primary sarcoma. With the advent of angiocardiography, the first clinical demonstration of an intracardiac myxoma was made in 1951 (Goldberg *et al.*, 1952), and the first successful removal of a left atrial myxoma using extracorporeal circulation was performed in 1954 (Crafoord, 1955). Bigelow and colleagues (1955) employed total-body hypothermia for removal of such a lesion.

In reviewing primary tumors of the pericardium and heart, Fine (1968) recorded an incidence of 0.028 per cent in 157,512 autopsied cases. Metastatic lesions are most frequent, followed by benign tumors, and least common are primary malignant neoplasms (Prichard, 1951; Yater, 1931).

BENIGN NEOPLASMS

Approximately 70 per cent of all primary neoplasms of the heart are benign and potentially curable by surgical excision (Table 52–1) (McAllister and Fenoglio, 1978). With the exception of myxomas, which constitute approximately half of these lesions, lipomas, angiomas, fibromas, hamartomas, and teratomas are usually discovered as incidental findings at autopsy (Clay and Shorter, 1957; Griffiths, 1962; McCue *et al.*, 1955). Clinically, these tumors may present rarely with complete heart block and obstruction of the right or left ventricular outflow tract (Clay and Shorter, 1957; Grant and Camp, 1932; McCue *et al.*, 1955). Surgical removal of these lesions has been reported (Williams *et al.*, 1972).

Although cardiac neoplasms are rare and usually benign in infancy, rhabdomyoma is the most common

lesion in the pediatric age group and has been reported in stillborn infants (Bigelow *et al.*, 1954). Approximately 85 per cent are found in children under the age of 15 (Batchelor and Maun, 1945), and more than 50 per cent of cases occur in association with tuberous sclerosis (Goyer and Bowden, 1962). Lesions are seen as single or multiple homogeneous masses of yellow- to grey-colored tissue varying from 1 to 25 mm. in

TABLE 52–1. NEOPLASMS OF THE HEART AND PERICARDIUM*

TYPE	NUMBER	PERCENTAGE
Benign		
Myxoma	130	29.3
Lipoma	45	10.1
Papillary fibroelastoma	42	9.5
Rhabdomyoma	36	8.1
Fibroma	17	3.8
Hemangioma	15	3.4
Teratoma	14	3.2
Mesothelioma of the AV node	12	2.7
Granular cell tumor	3	0.7
Neurofibroma	3	0.7
Lymphangioma	2	0.5
Subtotal	319	72
Malignant		
Angiosarcoma	39	8.8
Rhabdomyosarcoma	26	5.8
Mesothelioma	19	4.2
Fibrosarcoma	14	3.2
Malignant lymphoma	7	1.6
Extraskeletal osteosarcoma	5	1.1
Neurogenic sarcoma	4	0.9
Malignant teratoma	4	0.9
Thymoma	4	0.9
Leiomyosarcoma	1	0.2
Liposarcoma	1	0.2
Synovial sarcoma	1	0.2
Subtotal	125	28
Total	444	100

*From McAllister, H. A., Jr., and Fenoglio, J. J., Jr.: Tumors of the cardiovascular system. *In* Atlas of Tumor Pathology, Sec. Series, Fasc. 15. Washington, D.C., Armed Forces Institute of Pathology, 1978.

size. These nodular tumors can be found anywhere in the heart and may present as intramural lesions displacing normal myocardial cells or as intracavitary masses. Frequent involvement of the ventricular septum has been noted, but metastases have not been reported with these tumors. Histologically, the nodules appear as collections of vacuolated spaces with intermittent central nuclei and a narrow rim of cytoplasm. Processes radiate from the center toward the outer membrane, producing the pathognomonic spider cell (Landing and Farber, 1956). When fixed in alcohol, these vacuoles are found to contain glycogen. Three different views concerning the etiology of the myocardial lesions have been expressed: (1) They represent localized areas of glycogen storage disease (Batchelor and Maun, 1945). However, unlike the glycogen in glycogen storage disease, that found in rhabdomyoma is readily removed by aqueous fixatives (Hueper, 1941). (2) Anomalous development of the Purkinje cells is suggested by areas of myofibril degeneration that have been observed in these lesions (Farber, 1931). (3) Rhabdomyomas are hamartomas of the myocardium. This concept is supported by a frequent association with tuberous sclerosis, a condition in which involvement of numerous organs with hamartomas is seen (Hudson, 1965).

Symptoms arise from the obstructive effects of large intracavitary lesions or from widespread replacement of the myocardium, leading to early death from heart failure or sudden lethal arrhythmias. Typically, a patient presents with a history of seizures, mental retardation, skin lesions, and various signs and symptoms of heart failure and intermittent cardiac arrhythmias. However, 50 per cent of patients do not demonstrate the stigmata of tuberous sclerosis. Rhabdomyoma should therefore be considered in infants with an abnormal electrocardiogram and/or symptoms of heart failure for which a ready explanation is not apparent. Angiocardiography at the time of cardiac catheterization is essential in establishing the diagnosis. These benign tumors have now been surgically removed from various chambers of the heart with good results (Golding and Reed, 1967; Kilman *et al.*, 1973; Shaher *et al.*, 1972).

MYXOMAS

About half of all primary cardiac neoplasms are myxomas (Heath, 1968; Prichard, 1951). These lesions constitute the most significant of all cardiac tumors, not only because of their relative frequency, but also because once diagnosed, the probability is one of total cure following surgical removal. Although the exact incidence of myxomas is not known, an active cardiology service can expect to encounter several each year. It has been estimated that one in 350 patients with a diagnosis of mitral valve disease actually suffers from myxoma (Effert and Domanig, 1959). These neoplasms present on the left side of the interatrial septum in about 75 per cent of cases, and the remain-

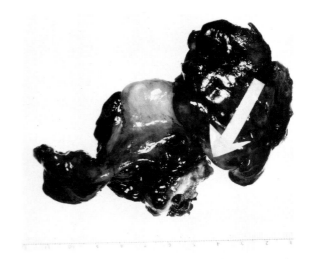

Figure 52–1. A left atrial myxoma. The arrow points to the area of the pedicle where the tumor was removed.

der are found mainly in the right atrium. However, myxomatous tumors have been reported in all chambers of the heart and may have multiple origins (Anderson *et al.*, 1970; Gerbode *et al.*, 1967; Gottsegen *et al.*, 1963). Cardiac myxomas occur most frequently in the third to sixth decades of life (Thomas *et al.*, 1967), although they have been reported in patients aged 3 months to 85 years (Fatti and Reid, 1958; Mahaim, 1945). They are more common in females, and a familial tendency has been noted (Heydorn *et al.*, 1973; Krause *et al.*, 1971).

Myxomas are lobulated single masses resting on a pedicle attached to the fossa ovalis. Their origin from primitive endothelial or subendothelial cells, found more abundantly in the region of the fossa ovalis than elsewhere in the heart, has been suggested from electron microscopic observations (Glasser *et al.*, 1971). Myxomas are true neoplasms. Usually benign in biologic potential, they may demonstrate malignant propensities, with rapid and invasive growth (Bahl *et al.*, 1969; Gerbode *et al.*, 1967; Kabbani and Cooley, 1973; Kelly and Bhagwat, 1972; Read *et al.*, 1974; Walton *et al.*, 1972). These tumors are extremely friable, polypoid masses of pale, soft, gelatinous tissue (Fig. 52–1). Areas of calcification and hemorrhage are frequently encountered. Microscopically, the tumor consists of fibroblasts, multinucleated cells, and round or polygonal cells within a polysaccharide-rich, myxoid stroma. Plasma cells, lymphocytes, and hemosiderin-laden macrophages may be seen scattered throughout a network of loose connective tissue (Fig. 52–2). Blood vessels are prominent at the tumor base, whereas peripherally the tumor is relatively avascular and is lined by endothelium.

Clinical Manifestations

A variety of signs and symptoms may alert the physician to an unusual form of heart disease and

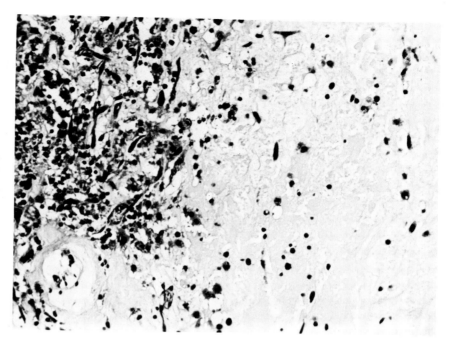

Figure 52–2. Histologic section of a left atrial myxoma. (U. S. Army photograph.)

suggest the presence of a cardiac neoplasm. Clinical syndromes produced by these tumors include: (1) pericardial tamponade or pericardial constriction, (2) cardiomyopathy, (3) intracavitary or valvular obstruction, (4) conduction defects and other rhythm disorders, (5) embolism, and (6) paraneoplastic syndromes.

Myxomas of the heart are the most common lesion, and a wide range of signs and symptoms may occur with this condition. Small tumors may remain asymptomatic. Patients with atrial myxomas usually present with symptoms of peripheral embolization, atrioventricular valvular obstruction, or a systemic illness (Hattler *et al.*, 1970; Selzer *et al.*, 1972; Vidne *et al.*, 1971). Following embolization of friable myxomatous material, a diagnosis of myxoma is made by histologic examination of the surgical specimen removed at thrombectomy. Pulmonary embolization may occur in right-sided lesions. Embolic episodes in young patients or in older patients with normal sinus rhythm should arouse suspicion of this tumor (Pridie, 1972). In 1959, MacGregor and Cullen were the first to report systemic symptoms, including recurrent fever, weight loss, arthralgia, anemia, increased erythrocyte sedimentation rate, and elevated globulins. In the differential diagnosis, a number of possibilities should be considered, including subacute bacterial endocarditis, collagen vascular disease, acute rheumatic fever, and myocarditis. Atypical cases of suspected bacterial endocarditis with negative blood cultures and patients with ''mitral stenosis'' without a history of rheumatic fever or a previous murmur— especially if the symptoms are intermittent and the time course variable—should suggest myxoma. The physical findings are completely reversed after removal of the tumor (Goodwin, 1963; Hattler *et al.*, 1970). The hypergammaglobulinemia probably represents a reaction to the tumor and not gammaglobulin

production by the tumor itself. Absence of immunofluorescence after specific anti-immunoglobulin staining of the tumor strengthens this concept (Glasser *et al.*, 1971). Systemic constitutional reactions and an elevation in immunoglobulins may represent an immune reaction to the neoplasm. The ability of the patient's tumor cells to stimulate proliferative reactivity with his own lymphocytes in culture suggests that immune sensitization has taken place (Hattler, 1974).

One of the most common clinical features of atrial myxomas is associated with atrioventricular valvular obstruction. With left atrial tumors, symptoms of valvular obstruction may be attributed to mitral stenosis (Winters *et al.*, 1961). An early diastolic sound is frequently heard in myxomas that has the timing of an opening snap but is of a lower-pitched quality and has been called a ''tumor plop'' (Harvey, 1968). These findings may vary with positional change. Right atrial myxomas are most often confused with constrictive pericarditis, Ebstein's anomaly, or tricuspid stenosis. The murmur of isolated tricuspid stenosis, however, should arouse suspicion of a right atrial myxoma, for isolated tricuspid stenosis is rare. In general, therefore, a high index of suspicion by the clinician confronted with a patient with unusual signs of valvular disease or bizarre and fluctuating systemic manifestations should lead to further diagnostic tests.

Noninvasive Screening Tests

Echocardiography. Echocardiography has become a very important method in establishing an objective diagnosis of cardiac neoplasms and has led to an increased accuracy in the preoperative diagnosis (Bulkley and Hutchins, 1979). Standard M-mode echocardiography demonstrates a left

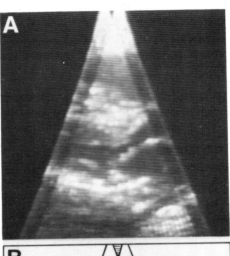

EKG

AML

Figure 52–3. M-mode echocardiogram of the anterior mitral valve leaflet (AML) in a patient with a left atrial myxoma. The leaflet opens anteriorly in early diastole and is followed an instant later by the large tumor mass (arrow). (Courtesy of Joseph A. Kisslo, M.D., Duke University Medical Center.)

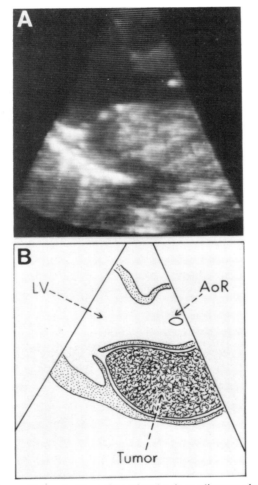

Figure 52–4. *A*, Two-dimensional echocardiogram showing a large left atrial myxoma obstructing the mitral valve, with resultant symptoms mimicking rheumatic mitral stenosis. *B*, Diagrammatic illustration of *A*. (LV = left ventricle; AoR = aorta.) (Courtesy of Joseph A. Kisslo, M.D., Duke University Medical Center.)

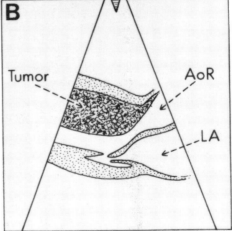

Figure 52–5. Myxoma that presented with syncope and chest pain. *A*, Two-dimensional echocardiogram showing a left ventricular myxoma that presented with syncope and chest pain. The original clinical diagnosis was idiopathic hypertrophic subaortic stenosis. *B*, Diagrammatic illustration of *A*. (LA = left atrium; AoR = aorta.) (Courtesy of Joseph A. Kisslo, M.D., Duke University Medical Center.)

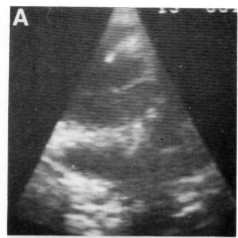

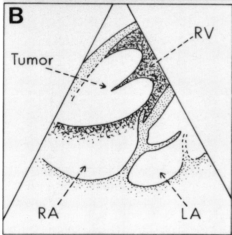

Figure 52–6. *A,* Two-dimensional echocardiogram of a primary lymphoma obliterating the right ventricular cavity. Surgical resection and adjuvant chemotherapy produced complete remission. *B,* Diagrammatic illustration of *A.* (RV = right ventricle; RA = right atrium; LA = left atrium.) (Courtesy of Joseph A. Kisslo, M.D., Duke University Medical Center.)

atrial myxoma as a mass of reflected echoes behind, but separate from, the anterior mitral valve leaflet, which moves during the cardiac cycle (Fig. 52–3). With various beam projections, tumors in each of the cardiac chambers have been accurately visualized. However, intracavitary tumors are more echogenic than intramural neoplasms owing to their intra-

cardiac mobility. Increased accuracy can be obtained by using two-dimensional echocardiography (Lappe *et al.,* 1978), by means of which the size and shape of the tumor and its motion can be quantitated. Moreover, cardiac function can be assessed, and all chambers can be visualized simultaneously. The technique has become so accurate that it may itself provide sufficient information to proceed with surgical correction without the necessity for angiocardiography (Figs. 52–4 to 52–6).

Limitations of echocardiographic techniques in the diagnosis of left atrial masses have been emphasized. For example, patients with proven atrial myxomas by angiocardiography have been reported to have had echocardiograms that were normal (Come *et al.,* 1981). This fact needs to be kept in mind in terms of establishment of an *absolute* diagnosis, and especially in being certain that the patients who have signs and symptoms suggestive of atrial myxomas do not categorically have these lesions excluded by echocardiographic techniques alone. However, in a recent study of 19 patients with left atrial masses, the presence of the lesion was detected in each instance by two-dimensional echocardiography (DePace *et al.,* 1981). Pericardial metastases can also be determined by cross-sectional echocardiography. This examination was performed in a series of 69 patients with pericardial effusion, and the etiology of the effusion was malignant infiltration of the pericardium in nine patients, chronic renal failure in 10, postcardiac surgery in 31, viral pericarditis in three, and tuberculous pericarditis in two and was of undetermined origin in 14 (Chandraratna and Aronow, 1981). An example of the detection of a pericardial metastasis by cross-sectional echocardiography is shown in Figure 52–7.

Phonocardiography (Fig. 52–8). In patients with myxomas, the intensity of the first heart sound is almost uniformly increased (Zitnik and Giuliani, 1970; Glasser *et al.,* 1971; Nasser *et al.,* 1972). During early diastole, a low-frequency sound or "tumor plop" can be identified in the majority of left atrial myxomas and is probably due to sudden stretching of the tumor on its pedicle as it gravitates toward the left ventricle. The late occurrence of this sound (0.08 to 0.12 second after A2) will differentiate it from tight mitral stenosis and suggest myxoma. A diastolic murmur is usually noted. Rapid changes in the intensity of the diastolic

Figure 52–7. Cross-sectional echocardiogram in the long-axis view in a patient with surgically proved pericardial metastases. A large, irregular mass (T) is seen to protrude into the pericardial effusion (PE). The mass probably represents pericardial metastases. (LVW = left ventricular wall.) (From Chandraratna, P. A. N., and Aronow, W. S.; Detection of pericardial masses by cross-sectional echocardiography. Circulation, *63*:197, 1981.)

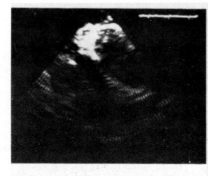

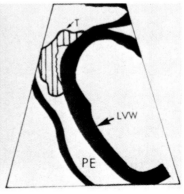

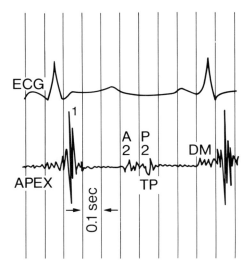

Figure 52–8. Simultaneous lead II electrocardiogram (ECG) and apex phonocardiogram tracings from a patient with a left atrial myxoma. An intense first heart sound and "tumor plop" sound (TP) are demonstrated. (DM = diastolic murmur; bandpass filter, 100–500 c.p.s.)

murmur can occur and are secondary to spontaneous or positional rearrangement of the tumor–mitral orifice geometry. Since left atrial myxomas may initially be considered to be rheumatic mitral stenosis, attention to subtle differences is important (Adams *et al.*, 1961).

Miscellaneous Tests. Electrocardiographic findings are usually nonspecific. The incidence of atrial fibrillation has been found to be less than 15 per cent in patients with myxomas. Large right atrial P waves may be seen in patients with right atrial tumors.

Films of the chest may reveal calcification in the area of the myxoma that may be difficult to differentiate from mitral anular or valvular calcification. The presence of severe pulmonary venous congestion with a normal-sized heart (suggesting acute atrioventricular obstruction) should alert the physician to the possibility of a left atrial tumor.

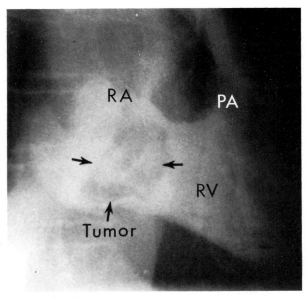

Figure 52–10. Angiocardiogram of a right atrial myxoma producing superior vena caval obstruction. (RA = right atrium; RV = right ventricle; PA = pulmonary artery.) (From Silverman, N. A., and Sabiston, D. C., Jr.: Cardiac Neoplasms. *In* Textbook of Surgery. 12th Ed. Edited by D. C. Sabiston, Jr. Philadelphia, W. B. Saunders Company, 1981.)

Angiocardiography

The most objective assessment of a myxoma is obtained by angiocardiography, and with this technique, the neoplasm can usually be demonstrated to move back and forth across the mitral or tricuspid anulus. Left atrial tumors are seen following the injection of dye into the left atrium or pulmonary artery (levophase) (Fig. 52–9) (Cipriano *et al.*, 1981). A left atrial approach, however, may be unwise since the transseptal puncture is usually performed in the area of the fossa ovalis, from which the friable myxomas often arise. Injection of contrast material into the superior vena cava will allow visualization of right atrial tumors. An example of a right atrial myxoma is

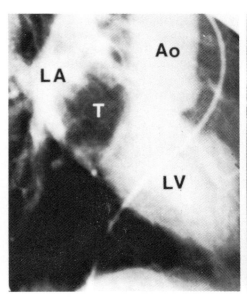

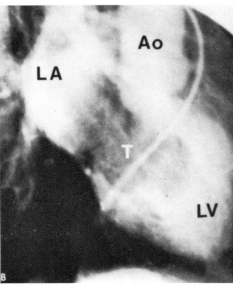

Figure 52–9. Left atrial myxoma. *A.* Levophase of a pulmonary angiogram in the lateral view during ventricular systole in an adult patient, which shows a large filling defect in the left atrium due to a myxoma. *B,* During ventricular diastole, the tumor is demonstrated to prolapse through the mitral valve into the left ventricle. The myxoma was successfully removed by surgery. (Ao = aorta; LA = left atrium; LV = left ventricle; T = tumor.) (From Cipriano, P. R., Martin, R. P., and Wexler, L.: Cardiac Neoplasms. *In* Surgical Radiology. Edited by J. G. Teplick and M. E. Haskin. Philadelphia, W. B. Saunders Company, 1981.)

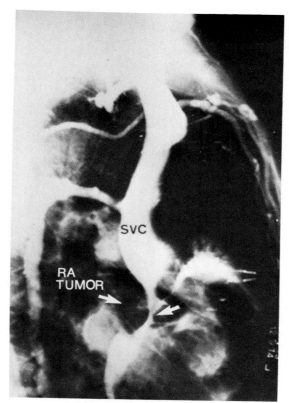

Figure 52–11. Right atrial tumor obstructing the caval atrial junction with retrograde filling of the azygos vein. (From Torstveit, J. R., *et al.*: Primary plasmacytoma of the atrium: Report of a case with successful surgical management. J. Thorac. Cardiovasc. Surg., *74*:563, 1977.)

shown in Figure 52–10, and a right atrial plasmacytoma is illustrated in Figure 52–11 (Torstveit *et al.*, 1977).

Cardiac Catheterization

The hemodynamic changes that may be present can be documented by cardiac catheterization, and the degree of atrioventricular valvular obstruction can be determined, although this is often not necessary. A diastolic gradient that varies with position should bring to mind an atrial myxoma. Cardiac catheterization without angiography frequently fails to establish a diagnosis (Hattler *et al.*, 1970). Analysis of pressure recordings may reveal tracings inconsistent with mitral stenosis and suggest an atrial tumor (Blackmon and Winterscheid, 1967; Glasser *et al.*, 1971; Ognibene and Nelson, 1967).

Computed Tomography

In the recent past, computed tomography has evolved as a new method for diagnosing neoplasms of the heart (Huggins *et al.*, 1980; Lackner *et al.*, 1978). An example of an unsuspected metastasis of liposarcoma of the heart is shown in Figure 52–12 (Godwin *et al.*, 1981). Further computed tomographic study

with intravenous administration of contrast medium provided excellent delineation of the tumor. Compared with two-dimensional echocardiography and angiocardiography, computed tomographic examination was superior in showing the myocardial and intrapericardial extension of the neoplasm, but it did not show movement of the lesion during the cardiac cycle.

Management

Once the diagnosis of myxoma has been made, operation should be performed as soon as feasible, since embolism or sudden death is a continuous threat. Although closed heart procedures with hypothermia were formerly used for removal of intracardiac neoplasms, this approach is now essentially of historic interest only. Intracardiac neoplasms are best managed by excision under direct vision with the use of extracorporeal circulation. During operation, embolization is a hazard until all of the neoplasm is removed. The potential for recurrence of myxoma has been adequately demonstrated, as, indeed, have distant metastases (Bahl *et al.*, 1969; Gerbode *et al.*, 1967; Kabbani and Cooley, 1973; Read *et al.*, 1974; Walton *et al.*, 1972). Therefore, an adequate margin of the tumor pedicle should be excised at the time of operation.

The surgical approach for excision of these neoplasms is a median sternotomy (or a right anterolateral thoracotomy through the fourth interspace). The latter approach can be used especially in younger women, in whom the cosmetic aspect is significant. The patient is then placed on cardiopulmonary bypass with moderate systemic hypothermia. The ascending aorta is cross-clamped, and potassium cardioplegic arrest is induced. The myxoma is then removed through the appropriate atriotomy (Fig. 52–13) (Silverman and Sabiston, 1981). If any question arises concerning the margin of tumor resection, a full-thickness section of interatrial septum should be excised together with the myxoma and its pedicle, with closure of the interatrial defect. The mitral valve is kept incompetent by catheter placement during removal of a left atrial myxoma. Air is carefully removed from the heart before normal cardiac rhythm is allowed to return. In a series of 15 consecutive primary myxomas of the heart treated at Duke University Medical Center, there has been no surgical mortality and no late recurrence (Silverman, 1980).

Although initially considered benign neoplasms (Firor *et al.*, 1966; Malm *et al.*, 1958), myxomas have recently received greater attention with stress upon their malignant potential, with metastases reported in the spine and the pelvis (Read *et al.*, 1974). Their rapid regrowth following resection, including a core of atrial septum, underscores the possible need for an even more aggressive approach when these tumors are first encountered. A "recurrence" may, in fact, represent a second tumor originating from primitive endothelial cells found in and around the fossa ovalis. Should this suspicion be confirmed by recurrence, in

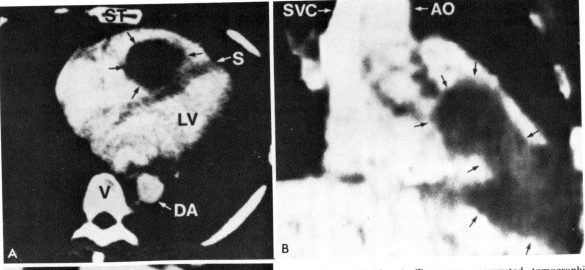

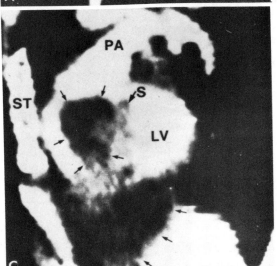

Figure 52–12. *A,* Transverse computed tomographic (CT) scan through the right and left ventricles (RV and LV) during IV infusion of 76 percent diatrizoate. The patient's right side is projected at the left side of the illustration, as in a conventional radiograph of the chest. The sternum (ST) and vertebral body (V) are marked for orientation. Contrast material fills the ventricles and descending aorta (DA). The large low-density tumor (arrows) occupies the cavity of the right ventricle and lies alongside the interventricular septum (S). *B,* Reformatted CT image made from contiguous transverse CT slices taken during infusion of contrast medium. The plane of reformatting passes through the right ventricle, corresponding to the right anterior oblique projection of an angiocardiogram. The low-density tumor (arrows) forms a pedunculated mass in the cavity with invasion through the myocardium of the apex of the right ventricle into the pericardial sac. The lowermost arrows indicate the intrapericardial component of the tumor. (SVC = superior vena cava; AO = ascending aorta.) *C,* Reformatted CT image made from contiguous transverse CT slices taken during infusion of contrast material. The plane of reformatting passes through both ventricles, corresponding to the left anterior oblique projection of an angiocardiogram, but the plane is also angled along the axis extending from the right ventricular apex to the outflow tract, roughly corresponding to a half axial projection. The pedunculated low-density tumor (arrows) is again visualized in the right ventricular cavity and extending through the apex into the pericardial sac (lowermost arrows). (ST = sternum; PA = pulmonary artery; S = interventricular septum; LV = left ventricular cavity.) (From Godwin, J. D., *et al.*: Computed tomography: A new method for diagnosing tumor of the heart. Circulation, *63*:448, 1981.)

spite of complete surgical resections, including the fossa ovalis, a more definitive future procedure may be the primary excision of the tumor and most of the atrial septum. Prognosis following surgical excision is usually excellent (Firor *et al.*, 1966; Hattler *et al.*, 1970). Regression of all preoperative symptoms with complete cure for follow-up periods up to 15 years has been documented. In an interesting report, a patient with a left atrial myxoma and subacute bacterial endocarditis due to *Streptococcus viridans* had a saddle embolus to the terminal aorta while undergoing antibiotic treatment. Microscopic examination of the tumor embolus removed from the aorta showed a myxomatous tumor with bacterial colonies present on the surface of and within the neoplasm. Although an echocardiogram obtained prior to development of the aortic embolus showed evidence of a left atrial myxoma on three occasions, a repeat echocardiogram

after aortic embolectomy was normal, as was an additional echocardiogram obtained 8 months later. The authors concluded that the infection present in the left atrial myxoma produced a "spontaneous cure" (Schweiger *et al.*, 1980). Nevertheless, two additional possibilities exist, the first being that the entire atrial myxoma embolized and the second being that the postembolic echocardiogram failed to reveal the presence of a continuing myxoma.

MALIGNANT NEOPLASMS

Cardiac sarcomas rank next in frequency to myxomas and represent the most common primary *malignant* tumor of the heart. Of 329 primary cardiac neoplasms recorded by Mahaim (1945), 87 (26 per cent) were sarcomas. More than 200 patients with

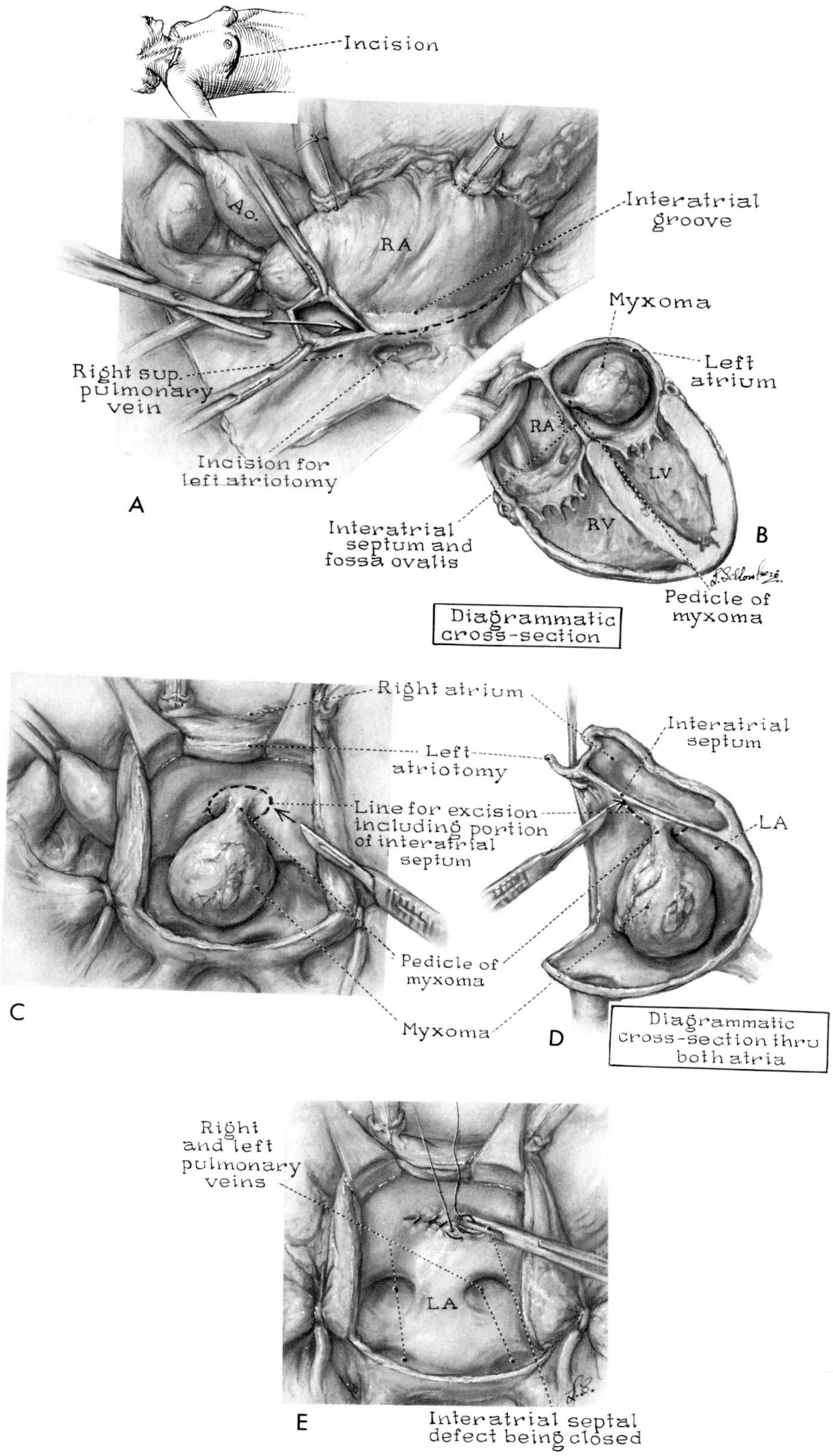

Figure 52–13. Surgical technique for removal of a left atrial myxoma. *A,* The aorta is clamped, and potassium cardioplegic arrest is induced. The left atrial myxoma is approached through a left atriotomy. *B,* The myxoma is exposed, and a portion of the atrial septum is excised at the attachment of the pedicle. *C,* The atrial defect created by excision of the tumor attachment is closed primarily. With large defects, a patch may be necessary for the atrial repair. *D,* If the tumor has a large, broad-based attachment to the atrial septum, the neoplasm is better exposed via a right atrial approach. The fossa ovalis is more easily exposed through a right atriotomy, and the base of the tumor can be readily excised. (From Silverman, N. A., and Sabiston, D. C., Jr.: Cardiac Neoplasms. *In* Textbook of Surgery. 12th Ed. Edited by D. C. Sabiston, Jr. Philadelphia, W. B. Saunders Company, 1981.)

myocardial sarcomas have now been reported (Fine, 1968). Metastases from these lesions occur in about 80 per cent of cases and involve the lung and mediastinum most frequently and, less commonly, those organs supplied by the systemic circulation. Among the various types of sarcomas, rhabdomyosarcomas occur most frequently (approximately 15 per cent), with lymphosarcomas, fibrosarcomas, myxosarcomas, and a variety of malignant vascular tumors composing the rest (Fine, 1968; Somers and Lothe, 1960). It is always necessary to exclude sarcoma elsewhere before accepting it as a primary tumor of the heart.

These tumors are seen in persons of all ages but occur most frequently between the third and fifth decades of life. A slight predilection for men (1.5:1) has been noted (Fine, 1968). The atria are more frequently involved than the ventricles, with tumors most often found in the right atrium.

The growth pattern of a sarcoma may take the form of exophytic masses, contributing to an irregular cardiac contour, often with extension into the surrounding mediastinum. In this setting, bloody pericardial effusions are frequently found. A second form of growth is that seen with intramural spread of the neoplasm. Here, conduction abnormalities, complete heart block, and cardiac failure may predominate, and the differential diagnosis will include the various cardiomyopathies. Finally, these tumors may present largely as intracavitary growths, sometimes detectable by angiocardiography. In contrast to the myxomas, however, the tumor pedicles are usually broad-based but can produce symptoms by obstructing blood flow or following the embolization of tumor cells (Goodwin, 1968). Therefore, clinical findings will depend largely on the growth characteristics of the cancer and will include signs and symptoms of ball valve obstruction of the tricuspid valve or superior vena caval obstruction. Although cytologic features of pericardial fluid may be diagnostic, exploratory operations are often performed to assess the nature and extent of the tumor and its potential curability. Realistically, however, prognosis with the tumors is usually dismal, and widespread infiltration with distant metastases is the rule. Although potential cures with early surgical excision have been noted, death usually occurs within the first year following the onset of symptoms (Fine, 1968).

Mesothelioma is the most significant tumor of the pericardium. It is a malignant lesion, and in Mahaim's collected series of 84 pericardial neoplasms, 45 were malignant, and over 50 per cent of these were mesotheliomas (Mahaim, 1945). Two types of cells are derived from the mesothelial lining of the pericardium—epithelial cells and spindle-like cells (Stout and Murray, 1942). These two types of cells give rise to three types of tumors: (1) *epithelial*, in which papillary, cylindric, or glandular structures predominate, (2) *fibrous*, which are composed of spindle cells in various arrangements, and (3) *mixed*, containing both spindle-cell and epithelial types in various proportions (Dawe *et al.*, 1953). Diffuse thickening of the pericardium is usually noted with these neoplasms and may lead to complete obliteration of the pericardial cavity. Extension into the underlying heart or surrounding mediastinum can be demonstrated, with metastases occurring most frequently to the regional lymph nodes and lung. These tumors have been reported almost exclusively in young adults. The clinical findings are those of pericarditis, and tamponade results from hemorrhagic pericardial effusions. Vena caval obstruction secondary to invasive growth may occur. A definitive diagnosis can be established by cytologic examination of pericardial fluid, but surgical biopsy

may be necessary. Temporary improvement may follow the removal of pericardial fluid or constricting lesions. Definitive surgical excision is not generally possible (Fine, 1968; Nissen, 1947), and death usually ensues within the first year following the onset of signs and symptoms.

METASTATIC NEOPLASMS

Essentially all primary neoplasms throughout the body have been described as metastasizing to the heart and pericardium. The heart is involved more frequently by true metastatic deposits that reach the myocardium by hematogenous routes and less commonly by lymphatic spread (Scott and Garvin, 1939). Direct extension from intrathoracic tumors often involves the pericardium. With an increase in bronchogenic carcinoma, this type of metastatic spread is the most common. The incidence of metastases to the heart and pericardium varies from 2 to 21 per cent of necropsies for malignant disease and between 0.24 and 6.4 per cent among 58,600 unselected autopsies (Fine, 1968). In all studies, metastatic tumors occur many times more frequently than primary lesions and have been found to have a frequency of from 13 to 39 times that of benign lesions (Harris, 1960). Although any malignant tumor possesses the potential to metastasize to the heart and pericardium, carcinoma of the lung and breast, leukemia (including Hodgkin's disease), and malignant melanoma are encountered most frequently (Fine, 1968). Of patients with one of this group of neoplasms, 25 to 50 per cent are found to have cardiac or pericardial involvement at autopsy. Metastases to the heart and pericardium are usually seen with concomitant metastases to other organs (Herbut and Maisel, 1942). The ventricles are more commonly involved than the atria, but no predilection for one ventricle over the other has been described (Willis, 1952). Macroscopically, metastases appear in the heart or pericardium as multiple nodules, but their growth may be diffuse.

Cardiac metastases usually remain undetected, but secondary involvement is most likely to be diagnosed when the pericardium is involved. Under these circumstances, signs of pericardial effusion are likely to develop. When tapped, the effusion is frequently bloody. A diagnosis can be made by cytologic examination of the fluid and may be suspected in a patient with a known malignancy from the irregular contour of the cardiac silhouette on the chest film. With involvement of the heart, lesions may continue to grow without symptoms, unless critical areas are involved. Bisel and associates (1953) have reported that approximately 10 per cent of patients with metastatic involvement of the heart have symptoms related to the cardiac pathology. Arrhythmias of supraventricular and ventricular origin are a common clinical manifestation of metastatic cardiac tumors. Complete heart block has been described less frequently but may be caused by local infiltrates of bronchogenic carcinoma, reticulum cell sarcoma, and melanoma (Yater, 1931). Congestive heart failure and cardiac arrhythmias in a patient with a known primary malignant neoplasm should raise a suspicion of myocardial metastases.

At times, the only means of establishing an objective diagnosis is by direct cardiac biopsy. Treatment is usually palliative. Creation of a pericardial window or wide excision of the pericardium will help prevent fluid reaccumulation and may be indicated in the patient with constrictive pericarditis secondary to diffuse pericardial spread.

Carcinoid tumors may involve the heart indirectly without actual anatomic invasion. These tumors originate in the gastrointestinal tract from argentaffin cells in the crypts of Lieberkühn. They are most commonly found in the appendix and terminal ileum (MacDonald, 1956). These tumors secrete serotonin, or 5-hydroxytryptamine, which is inactivated in the liver, lungs, and brain, organs rich in monoamine oxidase. In the presence of hepatic metastasis, normal breakdown of the tumor product does not occur, and symptoms of the malignant carcinoid syndrome appear (Lembeck, 1953). These include intermittent flushing, telangiectasis, bronchospasm, diarrhea, and malabsorption, each representing a pharmacologic effect of serotonin. Cardiac involvement is found in patients with metastatic liver disease and may be due to the excessive amounts of serotonin reaching the right heart without inactivation by an already compromised liver. Attempts to produce cardiac disease in animals with injections of serotonin, however, have been unsuccessful (Roberts and Sjoerdsma, 1964). Collections of fibrous tissue are seen in the endocardium and valvular cusps, involving mainly the tricuspid and pulmonic valves. The left side of the heart is protected by the inactivation of serotonin by pulmonary monoamine oxidase. Rarely, the mitral and aortic valves can be involved in patients with right-to-left shunts (McKusick, 1956). Typically, patients present with symptoms of right-sided heart failure, in addition to the other features characteristic of the malignant carcinoid syndrome. Treatment is usually confined to the medical therapy of heart failure in addition to possible chemotherapy directed at the carcinoid. In patients whose right-sided failure is poorly controlled by medical means, operation may be indicated. Replacement of the tricuspid valve and pulmonary valvotomy have been performed as means of extending the time of survival and improving the quality of life in these patients (Aroesty et al., 1966; Carpena et al., 1973). A rationale for this procedure, in spite of the presence of a malignant tumor, rests with the frequently prolonged survivals recorded in patients with malignant carcinoid tumors.

In the recent past, surgical resection of solitary metastases to the right atrium and right ventricle of malignant renal tumors has been successfully achieved (Keir and Keen, 1978; Paul et al., 1975; Rote et al., 1977). In addition, the use of extracorporeal circulation has been found useful in the removal of direct extension of these renal neoplasms extending from the inferior vena cava into the right atrium. It has been recognized that some of these neoplastic extensions into the inferior vena cava and right atrium can embolize to the lungs, with the resulting pulmonary embolism causing cardiac decompensation.

SELECTED REFERENCES

Come, P. C., Riley, M. F., Markis, J. E., and Malagold, M.: Limitations of echocardiographic techniques in evaluation of left atrial masses. Am. J. Cardiol., 48:947, 1981.

In this paper, attention is directed toward the limitations of echocardiographic techniques in the evaluation of left atrial masses; data are presented that demonstrate that even large left atrial tumors within the body of the left atrium may not be apparent or may be underestimated in size by currently available ultrasonic techniques.

DePace, N. L., Soulen, R. L., Kotler, M. N., and Mintz, G. S.: Two dimensional echocardiographic detection of intraatrial masses. Am. J. Cardiol., 48:954, 1981.

This is a review of the role of two-dimensional echocardiographic detection of masses in the left atrium. Ten patients had rheumatic mitral stenosis with a left atrial thrombus; seven had a left atrial myxoma; one had a right atrial angiosarcoma; and the final patient had a left atrial leiomyosarcoma. M-mode echocardiography detected six of the seven myxomas, one thrombus, and neither of the other two tumors. However, two-dimensional echocardiography demonstrated the mass in all 19 patients, indicating its superiority.

McAllister, H. A., Jr.: Primary tumors and cysts of the heart and pericardium. Curr. Probl. Cardiol., 4:1, 1979.

This monograph comprehensively reviews the vast experience of the Armed Forces Institute of Pathology with 430 primary cardiac tumors. The numerous tables and figures are pertinent and clearly illustrate the gross and histologic characteristics of these neoplasms. Excellent clinical correlations are also presented.

Silverman, N. A.: Primary cardiac tumors. Ann. Surg., 191:127, 1980.

This is a review of primary cardiac neoplasms with emphasis on modern diagnosis and treatment. Sixteen consecutive patients with primary neoplasms managed surgically from one center are reported, with no perioperative deaths and no late recurrences.

REFERENCES

Adams, C. W., Collins, H. D., Dummiti, E. S., and Allen, J. H.: Intracardiac myxomas and thrombi; clinical manifestations, pathology and treatment. Am. J. Cardiol., 8:176, 1961.

Anderson, S. T., Pitt, A., Zimmet, R., Kay, H. B., and Morris, K. N.: A case of bi-atrial myxomas with successful surgical removal. J. Thorac. Cardiovasc. Surg., 59:768, 1970.

Aroesty, J. M., DeWeese, J. A., Hoffman, M. J., and Yu, P. N.: Carcinoid heart disease. Successful repair of the valvular lesions under cardiopulmonary bypass. Circulation, 34:105, 1966.

Bahl, O. P., Oliver, G. C., Ferguson, T. B., Schad, N., and Parker, B. M.: Recurrent left atrial myxoma: Report of a case. Circulation, 40:673, 1969.

Barnes, A. R., Beaver, D. C., and Snell, A. M.: Primary sarcoma of the heart: Report of a case with electrocardiographic and pathological studies. Am. Heart J., 9:480, 1934.

Batchelor, T. M., and Maun, U. M. E.: Congenital glycogenic tumors of the heart. Arch. Pathol., 39:67, 1945.

Bigelow, W. G., Dolan, F. G., and Campbell, F. W.: The effect of hypothermia on the risk of surgery. Soc. Intern. Chir., 16th Congress, 1955.

Bigelow, N. H., Klinger, S., and Wright, A. W.: Primary tumors of the heart in infancy and early childhood. Cancer, 7:549, 1954.

Bisel, H. F., Wroblewski, F., and La Due, J. S.: Incidence and clinical manifestations of cardiac metastases. J.A.M.A., 153:712, 1953.

Blackmon, J. R., and Winterscheid, L. D.: Atrial myxoma, a curable systemic disease. Abstract of the 40th Scientific Sessions. Circulation, 35,36(Suppl. 2):70, 1967.

Bulkley, B. H., and Hutchins, G. M.: Atrial myxomas: A fifty year review. Am. Heart J., 97:639, 1979.

Carpena, C., Kay, J. H., Mendez, A. M., Redington, J. V., Zubiate, P., and Zucker, R.: Carcinoid heart disease. Surgery for tricuspid and pulmonary valve lesions. Am. J. Cardiol., 32:229, 1973.

Chandraratna, P. A. N., and Aronow, W. S.: Detection of pericardial masses by cross-sectional echocardiography. Circulation, 63:197, 1981.

Cipriano, P. R., Martin, R. P., and Wexler, L.: Cardiac neoplasms. In Surgical Radiology. Edited by J. G. Teplick and M. E. Haskin. Philadelphia, W. B. Saunders Company, 1981.

Clay, R. D., and Shorter, R. D.: Intramural fibroma of the heart. J. Pathol. Bacteriol., 74:163, 1957.

Columbus, M. R.: De Re Anatomica, Libri XV. Paris, 1562, p. 482.

Come, P. C., Riley, M. F., Markis, J. E., and Malagold, M.: Limitations of echocardiographic techniques in evaluation of left atrial masses. Am. J. Cardiol., 48:947, 1981.

Crafoord, C.: Case report. In International Symposium of Cardiovascular Surgery. Detroit, Henry Ford Hospital, 1955.

Dawe, C. S., Wood, D. A., and Mitchell, S.: Diffuse fibrous mesothelioma of the pericardium. Cancer, 6:794, 1953.

DePace, N. L., Soulen, R. L., Kotler, M. N., and Mintz, G. S.: Two dimensional echocardiographic detection of intraatrial masses. Am. J. Cardiol., 48:954, 1981.

Effert, S., and Domanig, E.: Diagnosis of intra-auricular and large thrombi with the aid of ultrasonic echography. Dtsch. Med. Wochenschr., 84:6, 1959.

Farber, S.: Congenital rhabdomyoma of the heart. Am. J. Pathol., 7:105, 1931.

Fatti, L., and Reid, F. P.: Excision of atrial myxoma. Br. Med. J., 2:531, 1958.

Fine, G.: Neoplasms of the pericardium and heart. In Pathology of the Heart and Blood Vessels. Edited by S. E. Gould. Springfield, Illinois, Charles C Thomas, 1968.

Firor, W. B., Aldridge, H. E., and Bigelow, W. G.: A follow-up study of three patients after removal of left atrial myxoma five to ten years previously. J. Thorac. Cardiovasc. Surg., 51:515, 1966.

Gerbode, F., Kerth, W. J., and Hill, J. D.: Surgical management of tumors of the heart. Surgery, 61:94, 1967.

Glasser, S. P., Bedynek, J. L., Hall, R. J., Hopeman, A. R., Treasure, R. L., McAllister, H. A., Esterly, J. A., and Manion, W. C.: Left atrial myxoma: Report of a case including hemodynamic, surgical, histologic and histochemical characteristics. Am. J. Med., 50:113, 1971.

Godwin, J. D., Axel, L., Adams, J. R., Schiller, N. B., Simpson, P. C., Jr., and Gertz, E. W.: Computed tomography: A new method for diagnosing tumor of the heart. Circulation, 63:448, 1981.

Goldberg, H. P., Glenn, F., Dotter, C. T., and Steinberg, I.: Myxoma of left atrium: Diagnosis made during life with operative and postmortem findings. Circulation, 6:762, 1952.

Golding, R., and Reed, G.: Rhabdomyoma of the heart. N. Engl. J. Med., 276:957, 1967.

Goodwin, J. F.: Diagnosis of left atrial myxoma. Lancet, 1:464, 1963.

Goodwin, J. F.: The spectrum of cardiac tumors. Am. J. Cardiol., 21:304, 1968.

Gottsegen, G., Wesseley, J., Arvay, A., and Temesvari, A.: Right ventricular myxoma simulating pulmonary stenosis. Circulation, 27:95, 1963.

Goyer, R. A., and Bowden, D. H.: Endocardial fibroelastosis associated with glycogen tumors of the heart and tuberous sclerosis. Am. Heart J., 64:539, 1962.

Grant, R. T., and Camp, P. D.: A case of complete heart block due to an arterial angioma. Heart, 16:137, 1932.

Griffiths, G. C.: Primary tumors of the heart. Clin. Radiol., 13:183, 1962.

Harris, H. R.: Angiosarcoma of the heart. J. Clin. Pathol., 13:205, 1960.

Harvey, W. P.: Clinical aspects of cardiac tumors. Am. J. Cardiol., 21:328, 1968.

Hattler, B. G., Jr.: Unpublished observations, 1974.

Hattler, B. G., Jr., Fuchs, J. C. A., Casson, R., and Sabiston, D. C., Jr.: Atrial myxoma: An evaluation of clinical and laboratory manifestations. Ann. Thorac. Surg., 10:65, 1970.

Heath, D.: Pathology of cardiac tumors. Am. J. Cardiol., 21:315, 1968.

Herbut, P. A., and Maisel, A. L.: Secondary tumors of the heart. Arch. Pathol., 34:358, 1942.

Heydorn, W. H., Gomez, A. C., Kleid, J. J., and Haas, J. M.: Atrial myxoma in siblings. J. Thorac. Cardiovasc. Surg., 65:484, 1973.

Hudson, R. E. B.: Cardiovascular Pathology. Vol. 2. Baltimore, Williams and Wilkins, 1965, pp. 1581–1586.

Hueper, W. C.: Rhabdomyomatosis in the heart of a guinea pig. Am. J. Pathol., 17:121, 1941.

Huggins, T. J., Huggins, M. J., Schnapf, D. J., Brott, W. H., Sinnott, R. C., and Shawl, F. A.: Left atrial myxoma: Computed tomography as a diagnostic modality. J. Comput. Asst. Tomogr., 4:253, 1980.

Kabbani, S. S., and Cooley, D. A.: Atrial myxoma—surgical considerations. J. Thorac. Cardiovasc. Surg., 65:731, 1973.

Keir, P., and Keen, G.: Secondary leiomyosarcoma of the right ventricle. A surgical report. Br. Heart J., 40:328, 1978.

Kelly, M., and Bhagwat, A. G.: Ultrastructural features of a recurrent endothelial myxoma of the left atrium. Arch. Pathol., 93:219, 1972.

Kilman, J. W., Craenen, J., and Hosier, D. M.: Replacement of entire right atrial wall in an infant with a cardiac rhabdomyoma. J. Pediatr. Surg., 8:317, 1973.

Krause, S., Adler, L. N., Reddy, P. S., and Magovern, G. J.: Intracardiac myxoma in siblings. Chest, 60:404, 1971.

Lackner, K., Heuser, L., Friedman, G., and Thurn, P.: Computer-kardiotomographie bei Tumoren des linken Vorhofes. Forstch. Roentgenstr., 129:735, 1978.

Landing, B. H., and Farber, S.: Tumors of the cardiovascular system. In Atlas of Tumour Pathology, Sec. III, Fasc. VII. Washington, D.C., U. S. War Department, 1956, p. 13.

Lappe, D. L., Bulkley, B. H., and Weiss, J. L.: Two-dimensional echocardiographic diagnosis of left atrial myxoma. Chest, 74:55, 1978.

Lembeck, F.: 5-Hydroxytryptamine in a carcinoid tumor. Nature, 172:910, 1953.

MacDonald, R. A.: Study of 356 carcinoids of the gastrointestinal tract: Report of four new cases of carcinoid syndrome. Am. J. Med., 21:867, 1956.

MacGregor, G. A., and Cullen, R. A.: Syndrome of fever, anaemia, and high sedimentation rate with an atrial myxoma. Br. Med. J., 2:991, 1959.

Mahaim, I.: Les Tumeurs et les Polypes du Coeur. Étude Anatomo-clinique. Paris, Masson et Cie, 1945, p. 180.

Malm, J. R., Henry, J. G., and Deterling, R. A., Jr.: Clinical and pathological study of benign intracardiac tumors: Report of successful removal of a myxoma of the left atrium. Circulation, 18:745, 1958.

McAllister, H. A., Jr.: Primary tumors and cysts of the heart and pericardium. Curr. Probl. Cardiol., 4:1, 1979.

McAllister, H. A., Jr., and Fenoglio, J. J., Jr.: Tumors of the cardiovascular system. In Atlas of Tumor Pathology, Sec. Series, Fasc. 15. Washington, D.C., Armed Forces Institute of Pathology, 1978.

McCue, C. M., Henninger, G. R., Davis, E., and Roy, J.: Congenital subaortic stenosis by fibroma of left ventricle. Pediatrics, 16:372, 1955.

McKusick, V. A.: Carcinoid cardiovascular disease. Bull. Johns Hopkins Hosp., *98*:13, 1956.

Nasser, W. K., Davis, R. H., Dillon, J. C., Tavel, M. E., Helmen, C. H., Feigenbaum, H., and Fisch, C.: Atrial myxoma. II. Phonocardiographic, echocardiographic, hemodynamic, and angiographic features in nine cases. Am. Heart J., *83*:810, 1972.

Nissen, R.: Intrapericardial sarcoma. J. Int. Coll. Surg., *19*:588, 1947.

Ognibene, A. J., and Nelson, W. P.: Atrial myxomas: Comments on hemodynamic alterations. Dis. Chest, *52*:699, 1967.

Paul, J. G., Rhodes, D. B., and Skow, J. R.: Renal cell carcinoma presenting as right atrial tumor with successful removal using cardiopulmonary bypass. Ann. Surg., *181*:471, 1975.

Prichard, R. W.: Tumors of the heart: Review of the subject and report of one hundred and fifty cases. Arch. Pathol., *51*:98, 1951.

Pridie, R. B.: Left atrial myxomas in childhood: Presentation with emboli—diagnosis by ultrasonics. Thorax, *27*:759, 1972.

Read, R. C., White, H. J., Murphy, M. L., Williams, D., Sun, C. N., and Flanagan, W. H.: The malignant potentiality of left atrial myxoma. J. Thorac. Cardiovasc. Surg., *68*:857, 1974.

Roberts, W. C., and Sjoerdsma, A.: The cardiac disease associated with the carcinoid syndrome (carcinoid heart disease). Am. J. Med., *36*:5, 1964.

Rote, A. R., Flint, L. D., and Ellis, F. H., Jr.: Intracaval recurrence of pheochromocytoma extending into right atrium. Surgical management using extracorporeal circulation. N. Engl. J. Med., *296*:1269, 1977.

Schweiger, M. J., Hafer, J. G., Jr., Brown, R., and Gianelly, R. E.: Spontaneous cure of infected left atrial myxoma following embolization. Am. Heart J., *99*:630, 1980.

Scott, R. W., and Garvin, C. F.: Tumors of the heart and pericardium. Am. Heart J., *17*:431, 1939.

Selzer, A., Sakai, F. J., and Popper, R. W.: Protean clinical manifestations of primary tumors of the heart. Am. J. Med., *52*:9, 1972.

Shaher, R. M., Farina, M., Allay, R., Hansen, P., and Bishop, M.: Congenital subaortic stenosis in infancy caused by rhabdomy- oma of the left ventricle. J. Thorac. Cardiovasc. Surg., *63*:157, 1972.

Silverman, N. A.: Primary cardiac tumors. Ann. Surg., *191*:127, 1980.

Silverman, N. A., and Sabiston, D. C., Jr.: Cardiac neoplasms. *In* Davis-Christopher Textbook of Surgery. 12th Ed. Edited by D. C. Sabiston, Jr. Philadelphia, W. B. Saunders Company, 1981.

Somers, K., and Lothe, L.: Primary lymphosarcoma of the heart. Review of the literature and report of 3 cases. Cancer, *13*:449, 1960.

Stout, A. P., and Murray, M. R.: Localized pleural mesothelioma. Investigation of its characteristics and histogenesis. Arch. Pathol., *34*:951, 1942.

Thomas, K. E., Winchell, C. P., and Varco, R. L.: Diagnostic and surgical aspects of left atrial tumors. J. Thorac. Cardiovasc. Surg., *53*:535, 1967.

Torstveit, J. R., Bennett, W. A., Hinchcliffe, W. A., and Cornell, W. P.: Primary plasmacytoma of the atrium: Report of a case with successful surgical management. J. Thorac. Cardiovasc. Surg., *74*:563, 1977.

Vidne, B., Atsmon, A., Aygen, M., and Levy, M. J.: Right atrial myxoma. Case report and review of the literature. Isr. J. Med. Sci., *7*:1196, 1971.

Walton, J. A., Kahn, D. R., and Willis, P. W., III: Recurrence of a left myxoma. Am. J. Cardiol., *29*:872, 1972.

Williams, W. G., Trusler, G. A., Fowler, R. S., Scott, M. E., and Mustard, W. T.: Left ventricular myocardial fibroma: A case report and review of cardiac tumors in children. J. Pediatr. Surg., *7*:324, 1972.

Willis, R. A.: Spread of Tumors in the Human Body. 2nd Ed. London, Butterworth, 1952.

Winters, W. L., Mark, G. E., and Soloff, L. A.: Left atrial pressure curve in left atrial myxoma. Arch. Intern. Med., *107*:384, 1961.

Yater, W. M.: Tumors of the heart and pericardium. Arch. Intern. Med., *48*:627, 1931.

Zitnik, R. S., and Giuliani, E. R.: Clinical recognition of atrial myxoma. Am. Heart J., *80*:689, 1970.

Chapter 53

Heart and Lung Transplantation

Bruce A. Reitz

Eugene Dong

William A. Baumgartner

Norman E. Shumway

Transplantation has progressed enormously in the last two decades. Renal allografting has been an accepted and highly successful therapy for end-stage renal disease. Although many important contributions have been made by thoracic surgeons interested in transplantation, the real therapeutic potential for heart or lung transplants, or combined procedures, remains to be established. At present, heart transplantation is established as therapeutic for highly selected patients; until recently, lung transplantation had not been successful and was virtually abandoned as a clinical procedure.

In this chapter, we will present the important historical developments, experimental and clinical, and the present status of heart, lung, and combined transplantation procedures. The emphasis will be on surgical technique, postoperative management of immunosuppression and complications, and expected results.

HEART TRANSPLANTATION

More than 15 years have passed since the first human cardiac transplantation was performed in December 1967 (Barnard, 1967). Although heralded with enthusiasm and the performance of approximately 150 transplant procedures over the next 2 years, early experience was largely unsuccessful (Meere et al., 1971; Kantrowitz et al., 1969; Cooley et al., 1969b). Indeed, throughout most of the subsequent decade, clinical heart transplantation programs were limited to a few centers, where persistent effort led to an evolutionary development of procedures and improved results (Baumgartner et al., 1979; Cooper et al., 1980; Calne, 1980; English et al., 1980; Hastillo et al., 1980; Reemtsma et al., 1978). Heart transplantation is now attracting renewed interest.

As of January 1, 1982, at least 664 patients have undergone cardiac transplantation throughout the world, with slightly more than a third of these procedures being performed at Stanford Medical Center (246 cardiac transplant procedures in 225 patients).

The 1-year survival rate in this program since 1974 has been 64 per cent, and 85 of these patients were living, with the longest survivor living more than 12 years after the transplant.

Experimental Background

It is important to realize that clinical cardiac transplantation is based on decades of laboratory investigation dating back to the early part of the twentieth century. Key problems addressed in the experimental laboratory included (1) design of a simplified and routinely successful surgical technique, (2) development of techniques for organ preservation during interruption of the coronary circulation, (3) documentation of satisfactory postoperative function of the anatomically denervated and transplanted heart, both early and late, (4) investigation of sensitive and accurate methods for the diagnosis and treatment of graft rejection, and (5) identification and control of the morphologic consequences of chronic immune reaction of the host to the transplanted heart.

Cardiac transplantation originated with Carrel and Guthrie (1905), who reported successful heterotopic cardiac transplant procedures in dogs. Following this pioneer work, there was nearly a 30-year hiatus in reported experimental transplantation. The efforts of subsequent investigators, beginning with Mann and associates (1933), were directed primarily toward modification and simplification of the techniques of heterotopic cardiac transplantation. Demikhov (1950), by means of ingenious operative methods not involving the use of cardiopulmonary bypass, was able to effect total circulatory support in experimental animals for short periods. These remarkable results were obtained in the early 1950s, when techniques for effective myocardial preservation and cardiopulmonary bypass were still to be developed.

The first fully successful orthotopic cardiac transplantations were described by Lower and Shumway in 1960. Essential features of this now standard technique included retainment of the recipient's right and left atrial cuffs in situ and use of topical hypothermia for myocardial preservation. Nearly routine long-term survival was obtained. Subsequently, other investigators using the same techniques confirmed the feasibility of orthotopic cardiac transplantation and also obtained prolonged survival (Kondo et al., 1965).

The efficacy of simple hypothermia for myocardial preservation during cardiac transplantation warranted further study prior to its use in clinical heart transplantation. It was shown to provide satisfactory myocardial protection for periods of up to 7 hours prior to reimplantation (Lower et al., 1962; Copeland et al., 1973; Watson, 1977).

The earliest experiences in experimental heart transplantation demonstrated that the transplanted heart, like other solid organ grafts, elicits an immune response from the host that, if not controlled, results in destruction of the graft. In 1962, it was shown that rejection of the canine heart was manifested by decreases in generalized QRS voltage, as measured by standard electrocardiograms (Lower et al., 1966; Semb et al., 1971). It was also found that both atrial and ventricular arrhythmias commonly occurred during episodes of graft rejection. These early observations provided an important noninvasive diagnostic index that remained useful for the treatment of patients in whom conventional immunosuppression was used.

Inability to control the immune response to the cardiac allograft precludes long-term survival. Reemtsma and associates (1962) achieved prolonged survival of recipients of cardiac allografts by using methotrexate and then azathioprine. Survival of canine recipients of orthotopic cardiac grafts for periods of up to 42 days was obtained by Blumenstock and coworkers (1963), who used methotrexate for immunosuppression. Further immunosuppressive protocols in experimental laboratories (Lower et al., 1965a; Kondo et al., 1974b) relied on prednisone, azathioprine, and antithymocyte antiserum raised in various species. Greater than 1 year survival in an outbred canine population was achieved using the principle of intermittent treatment based on identification of rejection episodes.

Cyclosporin A, a new immunosuppressive agent, has been extensively evaluated. This drug, a fungal metabolite, provides possibly superior immunosuppression for organ transplantation by virtue of its potency in suppression of graft rejection without the myeloproliferative toxicity of conventional agents such as azathioprine or cyclophosphamide. It is one of a series of cyclic oligopeptides first isolated from at least two fungal species (Petcher et al., 1976; Ruegger et al., 1976; Dreyfuss et al., 1976) and observed to have potential immunosuppressive qualities by Borel and colleagues in 1976. Kostakis and associates (1977) subsequently provided initial evidence for the potential usefulness of cyclosporin A in organ grafting by showing substantially prolonged survival of heterotopic cardiac allografts in rats after administration of the agent. Calne and others (Calne et al.,

1978b; Jamieson et al., 1979) shortly thereafter confirmed the ability of cyclosporin A to prolong survival of other organ grafts in other species, including primates. In 1978, Calne began a clinical trial in which cyclosporin A was used for renal, hepatic, and pancreatic allografts (Calne et al., 1981). Following the encouraging initial results in this series, trials were established in a number of other centers (Starzl et al., 1981; Tutschka, 1982) for evaluation of the efficacy of this drug. Initial investigational work with cyclosporin A at Stanford was begun in 1978 in two species, rats and primates. Early results indicated that cyclosporin A alone might be inadequate to maintain cardiac allografts free of any histologic evidence of rejection; all rhesus monkeys treated with the drug at high doses showed histologic evidence of allograft rejection by 30 days. It was concluded that a combination of cyclosporin A with low-dose corticosteroids and possibly antihuman thymocyte globulin (Pennock et al., 1981) might constitute the best initial immunosuppressive regimen with which to institute a clinical trial, which then began in December 1980.

Operative Technique for Experimental Transplantation

Using the canine model, the root of the great vessels and atrium can be exposed through a left thoracotomy incision (Fig. 53–1). Following ligation of the azygos vein, the superior and inferior venae cavae are looped with umbilical tapes. The pericardium is opened parallel to the phrenic nerve and tacked to the surrounding wound edges to form a pericardial well. Following heparinization, peripheral venous and arterial cannulation is done. With the onset of cardiopulmonary bypass, the great vessels are clamped and the heart is removed in the standard manner. At this point, an infusion of cold hyperkalemic cardioplegic solution is employed for initial arrest of the graft. The dog heart is excised, preserving adequate cuffs of both great vessels as well as atria and protecting the sinoatrial node. The heart is submerged in cold saline solution prior to reimplantation.

The right atrial wall is first sutured, starting at the inferior vena cava–septal junction. Upon completion, the pericardial cradle on the right side is released, and the heart is dropped down into the right chest, resulting in exposure of the septa of both the donor and recipient. A running suture through the septum then closes the entire right atrium. The left atrial free wall is sutured, and the heart is brought back into the pericardial cradle, which is again tacked up to the thoracotomy edges. A left atrial catheter is inserted through the appendage, and cold saline solution is infused to maintain hypothermia and to displace trapped air. The great vessel anastomoses are then completed using monofilament sutures. The venous tapes are removed, the aortic clamp released, and the heart resuscitated. After defibrillation, the heart gradually assumes support of the circulation. Pacing wires can

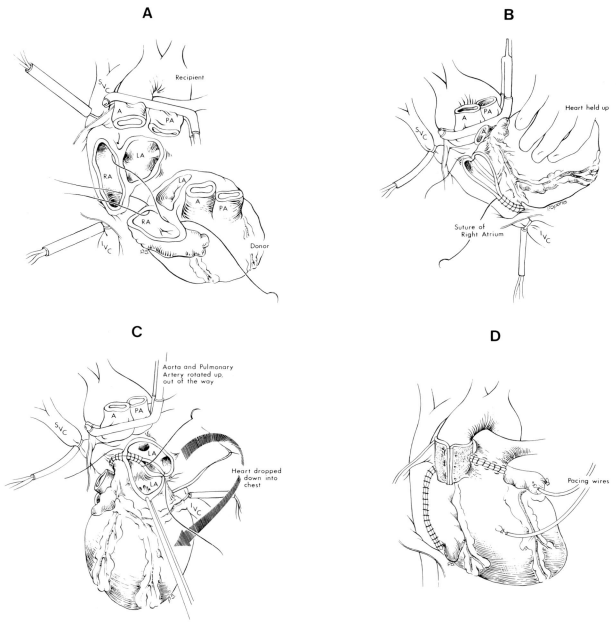

Figure 53–1. Operative technique in canine cardiac transplantation. *A*, Anastomosis of right atrium. *B*, Completion of right atrial anastomosis. *C*, Anastomosis of the left atrium. *D*, Completion of transplantation operation with Teflon wrap-around aortic anastomosis.

be applied. The duration of cardiac ischemia is approximately 1 hour. Regular decannulation, reversal of heparinization, and chest closure are performed.

Recipient Selection

Strict criteria for the selection of appropriate cardiac recipients are essential to the success of clinical heart transplantation at the present time. Most patients currently referred for cardiac transplantation have terminal cardiac disease due to a primary cardi-

omyopathy or ischemic heart disease with global left ventricular dysfunction (Table 53–1). Advanced functional disability is usually present when a prognosis for less than 6 months' survival can be made with reasonable certainty (Hunt and Stinson, 1981). As an example of the kind of selectivity used in choosing appropriate patients, only 38 of 260 referred patients during 1980 were eventually accepted as suitable candidates for transplantation at Stanford.

Initial evaluation includes a routine history and physical examination, as well as hematologic, roentgenographic, and biochemical studies. All patients

TABLE 53–1. STANFORD CARDIAC TRANSPLANTATION RECIPIENTS CATEGORIZED BY PREOPERATIVE DIAGNOSIS (JANUARY 1982)

	NUMBER OF PATIENTS
Coronary artery disease	105
Idiopathic cardiomyopathy	102
Post-traumatic aneurysm	1
Valve disease with cardiomyopathy	11
Congenital heart disease	4
Cardiac tumor	1
Coronary artery emboli	1
Total	225

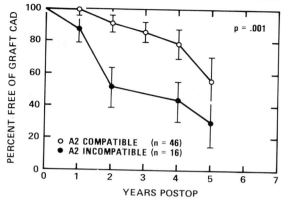

Figure 53–2. Incidence of graft atherosclerosis as a function of HLA typing at the HLA-A$_2$ locus.

undergo cardiac catheterization and coronary angiography. A repeat right-heart catheterization may be performed to accurately quantify pulmonary vascular resistance. Elevation of pulmonary vascular resistance above 6 to 8 Wood units is an absolute contraindication for orthotopic cardiac transplantation. A normal donor right ventricle will acutely fail when presented with this level of resistance (Taquini *et al.*, 1960). Such patients may be considered for either heterotopic heart transplantation or combined heart-lung transplantation. Another exclusionary criterion is advanced age. Retrospective analysis of the Stanford experience indicates that patients older than 50 years of age have significantly inferior survival rates compared with patients younger than 50 years of age (1-year survival rate of 37 per cent versus 60 to 70 per cent) (Dong and Shumway, 1977; Griepp *et al.*, 1971c). Other contraindications include (1) the presence of any active systemic infection, (2) a positive lymphocyte crossmatch, (3) insulin-dependent diabetes mellitus, (4) severe, irreversible hepatic or renal dysfunction, the etiology of which is considered separate from cardiac failure, (5) recent and unresolved pulmonary infarction, (6) severe peripheral or cerebral vascular disease considered highly likely to limit or preclude survival and rehabilitation, (7) active peptic ulcer disease, and (8) history of a behavior pattern, such as drug or alcohol use, or psychiatric illness that might preclude compliance with the lifelong medical regimen required after transplantation (Christopherson and Lunde, 1971).

Histocompatibility Typing

Matching of donors and recipients of cardiac transplantation by histocompatibility typing on the basis of classic HLA-A and HLA-B loci has not proved to be of practical benefit (Stinson *et al.*, 1971) with the exception of HLA-A2 (Hunt and Stinson, 1981). Because patients mismatched for this antigen appear to exhibit an increased incidence of accelerated graft atherosclerosis (Fig. 53–2), an attempt is presently made to avoid a mismatch of this antigen. Of more importance for donor-recipient matching is standard ABO blood group compatibility and a nega-

tive crossmatch of recipient serum against donor lymphocytes to exclude the presence of preformed antibodies.

Evaluation and Management of Cardiac Donors

Donor heart procurement became legally feasible with the adoption of guidelines for pronouncement of cerebral death such as those of the Ad Hoc Committee of the Harvard Medical School in 1968. Other suitable criteria for brain death have also been proposed and adopted (Mohandas and Chou, 1971). Passage of the Uniform Anatomical Gift Act in 1970 provided for the possibility of organ donation before death and reflected increasing public awareness regarding organ transplantation.

The most frequent neurologic catastrophe resulting in irreversible brain death has been nonpenetrating head trauma. The pertinent characteristics of donors evaluated for potential cardiac transplantation are summarized in Table 53–2. Cardiac donors are limited to younger individuals, usually less than 35 years of age. Retrospective analysis of donor age revealed a

TABLE 53–2. PERTINENT CHARACTERISTICS OF 230 STANFORD CARDIAC TRANSPLANTATION DONORS

ETIOLOGY OF BRAIN DEATH		ON SITE	DISTANT
Cranial trauma			
Vehicular		85	44
GSW		19	6
Other		20	7
CVA		37	9
Anoxic brain death		7	2
Other		3	1
	Total	171	69
AGE	Mean	23	
	Range	12–51	
SEX	Men	187	
	Women	53	

significant correlation between the development of coronary atherosclerosis in the graft and the age of the donor (Baumgartner *et al.*, 1979).

Maintenance of cardiovascular stability in the potential heart donor requires meticulous attention. Extreme fluctuations in arterial blood pressure occur with elevated intracranial pressure, and severe hypotension usually accompanies tonsillar herniation and brain stem compression. Diabetes insipidus often results and produces a profound diuresis. Thus, intensive care and strict attention to fluid and electrolyte balance, with vigorous supportive measures, are required (Griepp *et al.*, 1971b).

Distant heart procurement is now used by most centers performing cardiac transplantation (Watson *et al.*, 1979; Thomas *et al.*, 1978). Donor hearts are arrested by hypothermic, hyperkalemic aortic root perfusion, excised, and transferred during storage in cold saline solution within an ice chest. Ischemic times of up to 4.5 hours have been reported, with good graft function. Light and electron microscopic examination of ventricular biopsies obtained from distantly procured grafts has shown no significant structural damage (Billingham *et al.*, 1980). Actuarial analysis comparing patient survival is not significantly different when comparing the site of graft removal. Presently, more than two thirds of all hearts transplanted are obtained at sites other than the transplant center.

This method of procurement, although requiring careful planning and coordination with both donor and recipient transplant teams, has distinct advantages. There is expansion of the donor pool, leading to increased transplantation activity. This is reflected in a lower death rate in recipients awaiting transplantation (11 per cent versus 33 per cent prior to the use of distant donor heart procurement). The donor's family, referring physician, and local coroner all prefer that the body not be moved, and graft procurement can be coordinated with renal transplant groups.

Operative Technique for Clinical Transplantation

The operative procedure developed in the laboratory was applied with minimal changes from the original description (Lower and Shumway, 1960). The donor heart is excised through a midline sternotomy incision after intrapericardial dissection of the superior and inferior venae cavae, the ascending aorta, and the main pulmonary artery at its bifurcation. Upon completion of the preparatory dissection, heparin (300 units per kilogram) is administered intravenously to the donor. A single bolus of 500 ml. of a hyperkalemic cardioplegic solution is infused into the aortic root, leading to arrest of the heart in diastole. Following this, the superior vena cava is doubly ligated and divided immediately below the entrance of the azygos vein, followed by division of the inferior vena cava, pulmonary veins, pulmonary artery, and aorta.

Cannulation of the recipient for cardiopulmonary bypass is similar to the standard techniques for most open heart surgical procedures. The arterial cannula is inserted as distally as possible in the ascending aorta. The atrial cannulas are both placed in a lateral position in the high right atrium near the junction of the superior vena cava and the right atrium. After institution of cardiopulmonary bypass, snares placed around the superior and inferior venae cavae exclude the atrial cannulas, the ascending aorta is cross-clamped, and both great vessels are then divided at the level of the commissures of the semilunar valves. The aorta and main pulmonary artery are separated by division of the visceral pericardium to provide maximal exposure and mobility. The atria are transected immediately above their atrioventricular grooves, but posterior to the level of the atrial appendages, since these structures constitute potential sites of postoperative thrombus formation.

Vascular anastomoses are illustrated in Figure 53–3. Following removal of the aortic clamp, an appropriate period of continued cardiopulmonary bypass support allows for complete resuscitation of the graft. Prior to discontinuation of cardiopulmonary bypass, an infusion of isoproterenol is initiated at a rate of 1 to 2 μg. per minute. The rate of infusion is titrated to increase heart rate to approximately 110 beats per minute; this chronotropic effect, as well as the inotropic effect of isoproterenol, increases the cardiac output and facilitates early postoperative recovery. Two temporary pacing wires are placed on the donor right atrium; these are subsequently used for recording daily electromyograms for measurement of electrocardiographic voltage or for atrial pacing, as necessary.

Postoperative Management

Immediate postoperative monitoring and care differ little from those of most patients recovering from cardiac surgery. Ventilatory support is provided for approximately 24 hours; extubation is accomplished as soon as possible. Patients are monitored in reverse isolation, with frequent cultures of urine, sputum, or other appropriate sources. Daily electrocardiograms for measurement of QRS voltage and daily chest roentgenograms are obtained.

The "conventional" regimen for postoperative immunosuppression consists of corticosteroid, azathioprine, and antihuman thymocyte globulin of rabbit origin (RATG). Immunosuppression is initiated immediately before operation. Upon confirmation of donor availability, the recipient is treated with a loading dose of azathioprine (4 mg./kg. given orally) and one dose of RATG (2.5 mg. of IgG per kg.), which is given intramuscularly. Methylprednisolone is administered intravenously immediately following operation and is continued in intermittent doses over the next 36 hours to a total dose of approximately 10 mg./kg. Thereafter, maintenance therapy with oral prednisone is begun at an initial dose of 1.5 mg./kg. daily (given in two divided doses) and is gradually

Figure 53–3. Operative technique for human cardiac transplantation. *A,* Cannulation technique is similar to routine cardiac procedures involving central cannulation. Tapes have been placed around the superior and inferior venae cavae, and the aorta has been cross-clamped to exclude the heart from the circulation. The recipient's heart has been excised at the atrioventricular groove. The superior vena cava of the donor's heart has been ligated. The left atrial anastomosis has been started. *B,* The left atrial anastomosis has been completed. The incision in the right atrium of the donor heart is curved away from the superior vena cava and the adjacent SA node. The right atrial anastomosis is begun at the inferior border of the atrial septum. *C,* The right atrial anastomosis is completed. A perfusion catheter has been inserted into the left atrium through which cold (4°C.) normal saline is infused to further cool the left ventricular cavity as well as displace air. The aortic anastomosis is being completed. *D,* The aortic cross-clamp has been released following completion of the aortic anastomosis. The perfusion catheter has been removed from the left atrium, and the pulmonary anastomosis is completed with the heart fibrillating. *E,* The bypass cannulas have been removed. Pacing wires have been inserted on the right atrium of the donor heart. (Reproduced with permission from Baumgartner, W. A., *et al.:* Cardiac homotransplantation. Curr. Probl. Surg., *16*:1, 1979. Copyright © 1979 by Year Book Medical Publishers, Inc., Chicago.)

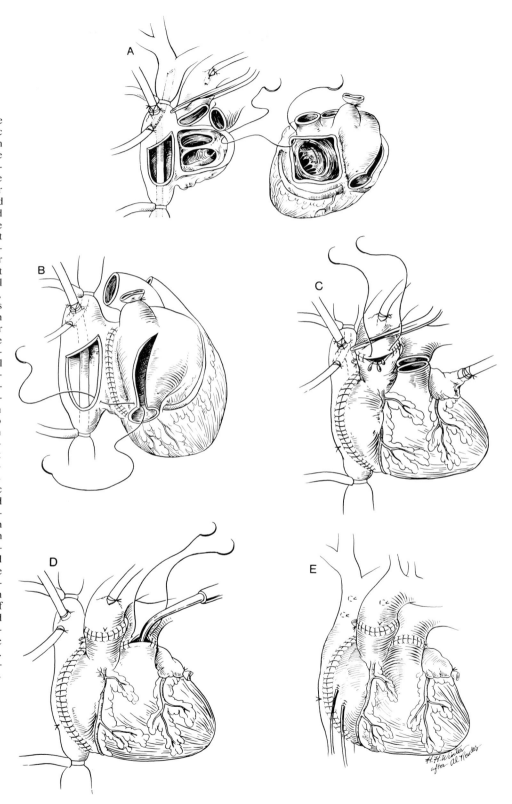

reduced to a level of 1 mg./kg. daily by the end of the second postoperative month. Maintenance prednisone dosage is gradually tapered to an end point of 0.2 to 0.3 mg./kg. per day by the end of the first year. Long-term maintenance immunosuppression consists of prednisone in the lowest dose necessary to prevent rejection and azathioprine in the highest dose compatible with preservation of bone marrow and hepatic function. Administration of RATG is initiated preoperatively, and the subsequent early postoperative course of this agent consists of alternating daily intravenous or intramuscular doses for the first 2 postoperative weeks, with dosage determined by *in vitro* E-rosette inhibition titer, maintaining the percentage of circulating T lymphocytes at less than 10 per cent.

The present immunosuppressive regimen based on cyclosporin A consists of a preoperative oral dose of 18 mg./kg. The drug is tapered to a maintenance dose in the range of 8 to 10 mg./kg./day by 2 weeks after the transplant. Azathioprine is not given with this regimen. Corticosteroid doses in patients treated with cyclosporin A consist of similar intravenous doses of methylprednisolone in the perioperative period, followed by oral maintenance prednisone at a dose of 1 mg./kg./day tapered to a dose of 0.2 to 0.25 mg./kg./day by the end of the fourth postoperative week. Further decreases to levels near 0.1 mg./kg./day are achieved by 6 months. This "corticosteroid-sparing" effect would appear to constitute one of the major benefits associated with the use of cyclosporin A. Rabbit antihuman thymocyte globulin administration is very abbreviated or is eliminated with this regimen, with a maximum of three doses in the immediate postoperative period.

Monitoring of Allograft Rejection

Clinical Signs. The clinical diagnosis of acute rejection, using "conventional immunosuppression," is based on signs and symptoms indicative of graft dysfunction (Griepp *et al.*, 1971a). During episodes of rejection classified histologically as mild or moderate, most patients experience no symptoms. Development of an abnormal diastolic gallop rhythm, indicative of decreased ventricular compliance, is common during moderately severe graft rejection. Episodes of severe graft rejection, however, are often associated with weakness, fatigue, malaise, and, occasionally, symptoms of orthostatic hypotension. Signs of congestive heart failure (manifested by elevated venous pressure, hepatomegaly, and dependent edema) appear at a late stage of rejection.

Standard 12-lead electrocardiograms are obtained daily during the early postoperative period. A fairly sensitive although nonspecific sign of rejection of the orthotopically placed cardiac graft is a generalized decrease in the total QRS voltage obtained by measuring peak-to-peak deflections of leads I, II, III, V_1, and V_6. A decrease of 20 per cent or more from a baseline voltage established for that particular patient is considered significant (Scheuer *et al.*, 1969). It

should be noted, however, that electrocardiographic voltage may be influenced by other factors unassociated with acute rejection. These include pericardial fluid, generalized edema, consolidative processes within the lung parenchyma, and a separate systemic disease resulting in inactivity (e.g., infection). Additional electrocardiographic findings that suggest graft rejection and constitute an indication for biopsy include premature atrial contractions, atrial flutter or fibrillation, and a rightward shift in the mean frontal plane axis.

Transvenous Endomyocardial Biopsy. Transvenous endomyocardial biopsy has come to play a crucial role in the diagnosis of allograft rejection. This is a modified cardiac catheterization procedure performed with local anesthesia utilizing the Seldinger technique for cannulation of the right internal jugular vein with subsequent passage of a flexible bioptome into the interior of the right ventricle (Caves *et al.*, 1973) (Fig. 53–4). Three to four 2- × 3-mm. biopsy specimens are obtained with routine histologic preparation. More than 3500 biopsy procedures have been performed at our center without mortality or serious morbidity. Routine biopsy is performed at weekly intervals during the first few months following transplantation or at any time upon suspicion of rejection, as well as after treatment of rejection for assessment of response. Routine endomyocardial biopsy may provide the initial evidence for an otherwise unsuspected episode of acute rejection. Assessment of the histologic response to specific treatment by repeat graft biopsy has been found to be important in order to document reversal and resolution of an active rejection process and

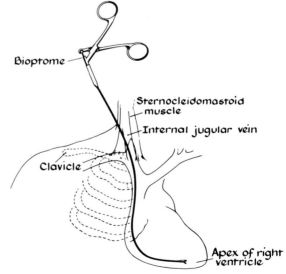

Figure 53–4. A flexible bioptome, 50 cm. in length and 2 mm. in diameter, is introduced by percutaneous Seldinger technique into the right internal jugular vein just above the clavicle. It is advanced under fluoroscopic control to the apex of the right ventricle, where the endomyocardial biopsy specimen is obtained. (Reproduced with permission from Baumgartner, W. A., *et al.*: Cardiac homotransplantation. Curr. Probl. Surg., *16*:1, 1979. Copyright © 1979 by Year Book Medical Publishers, Inc., Chicago.)

TABLE 53–3. HISTOLOGIC CHARACTERISTICS IN MILD, MODERATE, AND SEVERE REJECTION

HISTOLOGIC FINDINGS IN REJECTION	MILD	MODERATE	SEVERE
Myocardial interstitial edema	+	++	+++
Mononuclear cell infiltrate in myocardium	+	++	+++
Mononuclear pyroninophilic cell infiltrate in endocardium	+	+	++
Perivascular cuffing	+	+	++
Polymorphonuclear infiltrate in myocardium	–	–	+
Hemorrhage in myocardium	–	–	+
Myocytolysis	–	+	++

thereby obviate the need for additional corticosteroid doses.

Histologic findings observed on biopsy during acute rejection include interstitial edema, perivascular and interstitial infiltration with mononuclear cells, endocardial thickening and infiltration with mononuclear cells that stain positively with methyl green–pyronine, myocyte necrosis, and interstitial hemorrhage and infiltration with polymorphonuclear cells. These pathologic features observed in acute rejection (classified as mild, moderate, or severe) are summarized in Table 53–3. Representative histopathologic findings are illustrated in Figure 53–5.

Immunologic Monitoring. Although the cellular details of organ-graft rejection remain poorly understood, progress has been made in the early diagnosis of rejection by immunologic methods. Two assays in particular have been useful. The first of these involves the early postoperative measurement of the half-life of circulating rabbit globulin by a modified Farr technique (Bieber *et al.*, 1977). This radioimmune assay is performed three times weekly in order to quantitate serum levels and define removal kinetics. A second immunologic method that has proved useful in the monitoring of rejection involves determination of circulating levels of T lymphocytes, as measured by sheep red blood cell E-rosette formation (Bentwich *et al.*, 1973). It has been demonstrated that fluctuations in the levels of circulating T lymphocytes reflect the immune status of cardiac transplant patients since there is a close correlation between the postoperative data of a significant (+3 SD) rise in the T-cell fraction of peripheral blood lymphocytes and the time of onset of rejection as diagnosed by graft biopsy (p < 0.001) (Bieber *et al.*, 1977). This correlation has been found to be reliable only during the first postoperative month, following which rates of "false-positive" rises in T-lymphocyte fractions have made this assay invalid. With "conventional" immunosuppression, the fraction of circulating T cells is depressed to a level of less than 10 per cent of normal during the first 2 postoperative weeks by the administration of RATG. If the circulating T cells rise during the initial month following transplantation, RATG therapy is reinstituted and biopsy is performed. If biopsies remain negative, no further immunosuppressive medications are administered. In this way, it is sometimes possible to reverse very early rejection episodes with RATG alone and thereby reduce the total corticosteroid dose received by the patient.

In patients receiving cyclosporin A, many of the clinical and immunologic signs of allograft rejection are invalid. Histopathologic findings are notable for an absence of interstitial edema, even in the presence of other severe pathologic changes. This finding may provide an explanation for the observation that acute rejection in patients treated with cyclosporin A has not been associated with generalized decreases in electrocardiographic voltage nor with the appearance of diastolic filling sounds indicative of diminished ventricular compliance. Elevation of circulating T-lymphocyte levels has likewise not provided a reliable index of rejection in those patients treated with cyclosporin A. In all of these patients, circulating T-lymphocyte levels have diminished to approximately 1 per cent of normal during the first 4 postoperative days under the influence of a short course of RATG. Subsequent increases in circulating T-lymphocyte levels have occurred in all patients after variable periods of time, but in distinct contrast to conventionally treated patients, such rises in T-lymphocyte levels do not correlate with subsequent allograft rejection. It has been observed, however, that patients in whom T-lymphocyte values remain depressed for a prolonged period after operation (greater than 2 weeks) continue to be free of any evidence of rejection.

The preceding considerations indicate that among previously established indices of acute cardiac allograft rejection, at present only endomyocardial graft biopsy provides a reliable means of diagnosis in patients immunosuppressed with cyclosporin A. Furthermore, preliminary experience has shown that histologic findings characteristic of acute rejection in cyclosporin A–treated patients may be distributed focally rather than diffusely, as in conventionally treated patients (Oyer *et al.*, 1982). Serum levels of cyclosporin A are measured either by a radioimmune assay or by a high-pressure liquid chromatography technique, and maintenance doses, including those during the early postoperative period, are adjusted on the basis of these levels, with a goal of maintaining serum trough levels in the range of 100 to 300 nanograms/milliliter, although optimal levels remain to be defined. We believe that rational manipulation of cyclosporin A dosage requires monitoring of serum drug levels because of a wide variability in serum levels and immune responses observed among patients on identical dose schedules.

Treatment of Acute Rejection

The treatment of biopsy-proven graft rejection has remained standard over the past several years, irrespective of the type of maintenance immunosuppression (Oyer *et al.*, 1979). The principal antire-

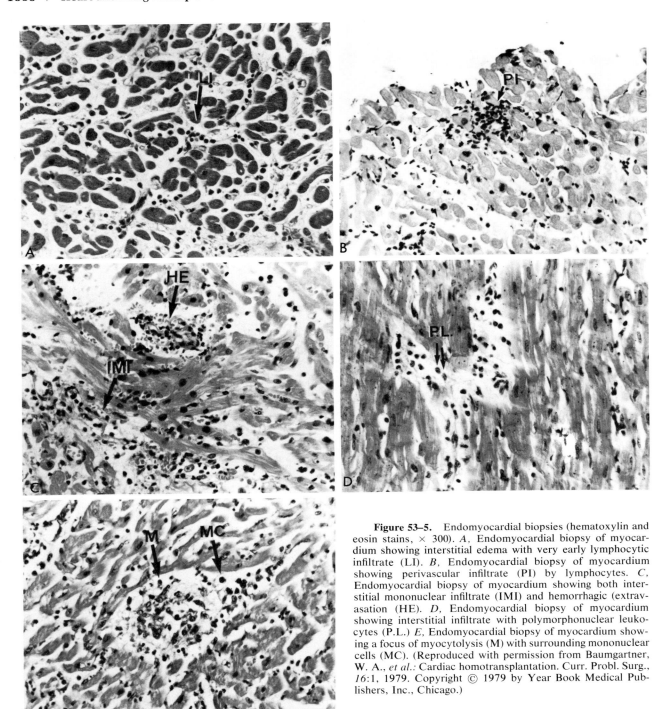

Figure 53–5. Endomyocardial biopsies (hematoxylin and eosin stains, × 300). *A,* Endomyocardial biopsy of myocardium showing interstitial edema with very early lymphocytic infiltrate (LI). *B,* Endomyocardial biopsy of myocardium showing perivascular infiltrate (PI) by lymphocytes. *C,* Endomyocardial biopsy of myocardium showing both interstitial mononuclear infiltrate (IMI) and hemorrhagic (extravasation (HE). *D,* Endomyocardial biopsy of myocardium showing interstitial infiltrate with polymorphonuclear leukocytes (P.L.) *E,* Endomyocardial biopsy of myocardium showing a focus of myocytolysis (M) with surrounding mononuclear cells (MC). (Reproduced with permission from Baumgartner, W. A., *et al.*: Cardiac homotransplantation. Curr. Probl. Surg., *16*:1, 1979. Copyright © 1979 by Year Book Medical Publishers, Inc., Chicago.)

jection agent is methylprednisolone, which is usually given intravenously as a 1-gram bolus injection each day for 3 days. With conventional immunosuppression, a full course of six doses of RATG is reinstituted. The patient's oral prednisone dosage is also increased to 100 mg. daily, with subsequent tapering by 2.5 to 5.0 mg. per day. With cyclosporin A, early experience indicates intravenous methylprednisolone to be adequate by itself. Serial biopsies are obtained at 4- to 7-day intervals during periods of rejection and serve to modulate subsequent treatment. Occasionally, in patients receiving cyclosporin A, with rejection of only moderate histologic severity, elevation of oral prednisone dosage alone to a level of 1.5 mg./kg./day, with subsequent tapering to the pre-rejection dosage, may be effective. In all cases, however, the adequacy of treatment is evaluated objectively by serial graft biopsy.

Morbidity and Mortality

Since all currently available methods for the prevention or reversal of graft rejection result in generalized immunosuppression, infection remains a major source of both morbidity and mortality for the cardiac transplant recipient (Mason *et al.*, 1976). This is true during the early 3-month postoperative interval as well as for the long term. Over half of the early deaths were directly attributable to infection, many in patients who had recently received treatment for rejection. The second leading cause of early postoperative death has been uncontrollable acute rejection, with a third important cause of death being acute failure of the right ventricle, a result of increased pulmonary vascular resistance. The primary causes of death observed in patients who survive the first 3 postoperative months include infection, graft atherosclerosis, acute rejection, and malignancy (Table 53–4).

Etiologic agents responsible for infections are varied and include all bacteria as well as viruses, fungi, and unusual parasites (Krick *et al.*, 1975; Copeland *et al.*, 1981). The target organ most affected is the lung. With "conventional" immunosuppression, almost all patients have had one or more potentially life-threatening infections following transplantation. Early experience with cyclosporin A indicates a favorable decrease in the number of infectious complications. Early and aggressive diagnosis and treatment of infectious complications are a cornerstone of the successful management of such patients (Mason *et al.*, 1976). Daily chest roentgenograms and sputum cultures are important during the initial month after transplantation (Blank *et al.*, 1973). The detection of pulmonary abnormalities mandates aggressive diagnostic maneuvers, including tracheal aspiration or direct lung aspiration by a fluoroscopically guided needle. Broad-spectrum antibiotic coverage is then commenced, or appropriate other treatment is instituted, as dictated by culture results or clinical course. Suspicion of central nervous system involvement warrants immediate computed tomographic brain scan and lumbar puncture (Hotson and Pedley, 1976; Britt *et al.*, 1981).

TABLE 53–4. PRIMARY CAUSE OF DEATH IN 139 PATIENTS AFTER CARDIAC TRANSPLANTATION (STANFORD SERIES, JANUARY 1968 TO JANUARY 1982)

CAUSE OF DEATH	EARLY (0–3 months)	LATE (>3 months)	TOTAL
Infection	37 (66%)	44 (53%)	81 (58%)
Acute rejection	12 (21%)	11 (14%)	23 (17%)
Graft atherosclerosis		14 (17%)	14 (10%)
Malignancy		8 (10%)	8 (6%)
Pulmonary hypertension	5 (9%)	0	5 (4%)
CVA	2 (4%)	1 (1%)	3 (2%)
Suicide		1 (1%)	1 (1%)
Pulmonary embolus		2 (2%)	2 (1%)
Unknown		2 (2%)	2 (1%)
Total	56 (40%)	83 (60%)	139 (100%)

Cardiac transplant patients, like immunosuppressed recipients of other human organ grafts (Matas *et al.*, 1976; Sheil, 1977), are subject to a substantially higher risk of de novo malignancy. In 124 cardiac recipients at risk 3 months or longer after transplantation and treated by "conventional" immunosuppression, 10 lymphomas and one case of leukemia have occurred. Six lymphomas and the single case of leukemia occurred during the course following initial transplantation, and four lymphomas developed among 10 patients at risk almost 3 months after retransplantation. Altogether, four patients, all with lymphoma at a single site, have been successfully treated (two with local cranial radiation therapy and two by segmental pulmonary resection for an isolated pulmonary nodule). The linearized time-related incidence of lymphoproliferative disease in these patients is 2.6 per cent per patient year; it is approximately twice this in younger patients, whose presenting etiology was idiopathic cardiomyopathy. It is unknown whether age per se or underlying pathogenetic features of idiopathic cardiomyopathy are the primary determinant.

Malignant lymphoproliferative disease has also occurred in three of the first 27 consecutive patients undergoing isolated heart transplantation with cyclosporin A immunosuppression (at 3, 5, and 6 months postoperatively). This incidence is not significantly different from that reported for other large series of transplant patients treated with cyclosporin A (Calne *et al.*, 1979). The accumulation of additional experience is necessary for thorough clarification of the incidence and predisposing factors of malignancies in patients treated with cyclosporin A.

Graft Atherosclerosis

Coronary artery disease in the transplanted allograft, with its attendant sequelae, represents the second most common cause of late death in cardiac transplant recipients (Kosek *et al.*, 1971; Bieber *et al.*, 1981). The hypothetical pathophysiology of this accelerated form of atherosclerosis is direct endothelial injury caused by low-grade, immune-mediated injury to vascular endothelium (Griepp *et al.*, 1977). Prior to 1970, the incidence of graft atherosclerosis was nearly 100 per cent at 3 years postoperatively. At that time, a prophylactic regimen using dipyridamole (Persantine), a low-cholesterol diet, and exercise was initiated. Since establishing this protocol, development of post-transplant graft atherosclerosis has decreased to 38 per cent at 5 years following operation, as assessed by annual coronary angiography.

Accelerated graft atherosclerosis occurs with the same frequency in all recipients, regardless of preoperative diagnosis (Pennock *et al.*, 1982). Several features that do appear to correlate with the development of this complication include HLA-A$_2$ incompatibility, hypertriglyceridemia, and a donor age greater than 35 years. Presently, control of these variables is partially achieved by matching at the HLA-A$_2$ locus, diet control, and use of donors less than 35 years of age. Because of the diffuse nature of the coronary artery disease, conventional bypass grafting alone is inappropriate, and retransplantation is required. Perhaps more efficacious immunosuppressive regimens with more complete control of the host immune response will further reduce the incidence of this late complication.

Corticosteroid Side Effects

The necessity for indefinite administration of corticosteroids to cardiac allograft recipients has resulted in varying degrees of morbidity (Kaplan et al., 1970). More common complications include mild myopathy, osteoporosis, weight gain, personality changes, and increased susceptibility to infection. Aseptic necrosis of the femur may require total hip replacement (Burton et al., 1978). In contrast with experience in the field of renal transplantation, attempts to decrease the frequency of corticosteroid complications in cardiac recipients by alternate-day steroid therapy have been unsuccessful because of an increased frequency of acute rejection episodes. In general, major operative procedures required for the treatment of late postoperative complications have been well tolerated (Reitz et al., 1977).

Retransplantation

Retransplantation remains an important alternative for transplant recipients with graft failure secondary to recurrent rejection episodes or the development of severe atherosclerosis (Copeland et al., 1977; Watson et al., 1980) (Table 53–5). Retransplantation has been performed 21 times in 19 patients in the Stanford series of 225 patients (two patients thus undergoing retransplantation twice).

Five patients have undergone retransplantation because of uncontrolled early postoperative acute allograft rejection. Three survived beyond 3 months postoperatively, and two were long-term survivors.

TABLE 53–5. CHARACTERISTICS OF PATIENTS UNDERGOING CARDIAC RETRANSPLANTATION (STANFORD SERIES, JANUARY 1968 to JANUARY 1981)

	NUMBER OF PATIENTS	SURVIVAL >3 MONTHS (%)
1. First retransplant		
Immediate graft failure	2	0
Acute rejection	5	3 (60%)
Graft atherosclerosis	12	6 (50%)
2. Second retransplant		
Immediate graft failure	1	1 (100%)
Graft atherosclerosis	1	0

One patient underwent retransplantation because of acute donor right ventricular failure secondary to pulmonary hypertension but died soon thereafter for the same reason.

Another 12 patients have undergone retransplantation on an elective basis because of identification by serial coronary arteriography of advanced graft atherosclerosis between 2.2 and 6 years after the initial procedure (Silverman et al., 1974; Griepp et al., 1972). Six of these patients (50 per cent) achieved long-term survival, one by virtue of immediate retransplantation again (the third graft) necessitated by acute donor heart failure. Graft replacement must realistically be a feature in any active clinical transplantation program.

Heterotopic Cardiac Transplantation

The use of auxiliary hearts in the intrathoracic position was extensively investigated by Demikhov during the 1950s. He described 24 variations of his technique for the implantation of an auxiliary intrathoracic heart. Since then, numerous investigators have developed various techniques for parallel assistance of the circulation (Reemtsma, 1964).

In 1975, Barnard (Barnard and Losman, 1975) reported two patients who had undergone left ventricular bypass with a cardiac homograft placed in the right side of the chest by a technique developed in his experimental laboratory (Losman and Barnard, 1977). By this method, the left atrial anastomosis was first constructed between the recipient's left atrium, below the intra-arterial groove on the right side of the heart, and the posterior left atrium of the donor heart. The donor-to-recipient aortic connection was made in end-to-side fashion, and the pulmonary artery of the donor heart was sutured to the recipient's right atrial appendage to decompress the right side of the donor heart, which received the coronary sinus return. The vena caval orifices were simply oversewn. Subsequently, in other patients undergoing transplantation by "piggy-back" hearts, both the right and left ventricles were bypassed by performing donor-to-recipient right atrial anastomoses, as well as pulmonary arterial anastomoses, utilizing Dacron graft material (Fig. 53–6). This series now includes 30 patients who show excellent symptomatic improvement, with survival comparable to that seen with orthotopic transplantation (Barnard et al., 1981).

The primary indication for heterotopic heart transplantation has been excessively elevated pulmonary vascular resistance in the recipient, which absolutely contraindicates orthotopic cardiac transplantation. With heterotopic transplantation, the recipient's enlarged and chronically adapted right ventricle continues to function in the delivery of blood to the lungs. Moreover, it has been reported that the recipient's own heart can provide additional circulatory assistance during episodes of acute donor heart rejection (Barnard et al., 1977).

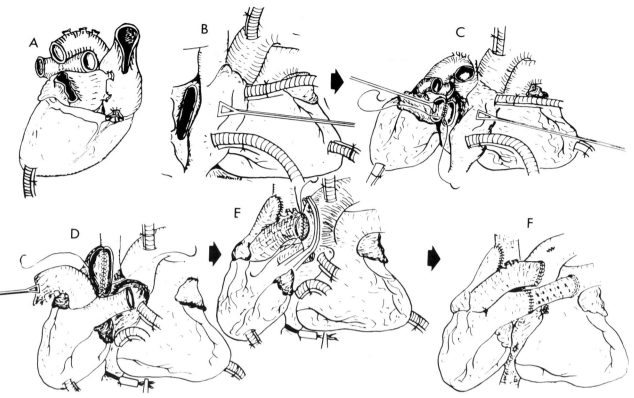

Figure 53–6. The heterotopic cardiac transplant. *A,* Posterior view of the donor after preparation for anastomosis. *B,* Left atriotomy. *C,* Left atrial anastomosis. *D,* Right atrial anastomosis. *E,* Aortic anastomosis. *F,* Completed anastomosis with a pulmonary-to-pulmonary arterial graft. (Reproduced with permission from Barnard, C. N., and Wolpowitz, A.: Heterotopic versus orthotopic heart transplantation. Transplant. Proc., *11:*309, 1979.)

Another indication for the procedure occurred in our series. It was required by the severity of the recipient's illness and a disparity in size of the organs, with the donor being much smaller than the recipient. Because of the small size of the donor heart, it was placed in the heterotopic position. The patient remains asymptomatic more than 1 year after the transplant, and studies show that the recipient's heart does not eject blood from the left ventricle; the aortic valve is continuously closed throughout the cardiac cycle.

Physiology and Function of the Transplanted Heart

That the transplanted heart can support a virtually normal functional existence has been clearly demonstrated, both in the laboratory and in the clinical setting (Kahn *et al.,* 1971; Beck *et al.,* 1971). Early experiments indicated that transplanted hearts devoid of innervation could adequately support normal activities (Dong *et al.,* 1964; Shumway *et al.,* 1966). Although resting hemodynamics are normal in most instances, the transplanted heart responds atypically to exercise and to certain cardioactive drugs, effects that are thought to be due primarily to the lack of direct neural control of the allograft (Shaver *et al.,* 1969; Campeau *et al.,* 1970).

Cardiac catheterization studies performed 1 or more years postoperatively have documented normal or near-normal function of the transplanted heart under conditions of rest (Stinson *et al.,* 1972; Schroeder, 1979). Mild sinus tachycardia without respiratory variation is generally present, representing the "intrinsic" heart rate resulting from autonomic denervation. Cardiac output is in the lower range of normal or slightly subnormal. Intracardiac pressures at rest are normal, and pulmonary vascular resistance, although elevated preoperatively in nearly all recipients, is usually normal upon subsequent study 1 year or later postoperatively. Response of the transplanted heart to exercise is characteristic of the denervated state, consisting of a gradual increase in heart rate and cardiac output, both of which eventually reach near-normal levels for the amount of work performed during a sustained exercise period. However, for any given workload, as measured in terms of oxygen consumption, the absolute level of cardiac output achieved is usually slightly subnormal, and elevation of arterial blood lactate levels is evident, especially with sustained, heavy workloads (Clark *et al.,* 1973; Savin *et al.,* 1980).

Responses of cardiac transplant recipients to graded, symptom-limited treadmill exercise, as compared with those of normal subjects, are characterized by mildly decreased chronotropic reserve, earlier onset of anaerobiosis, decreased work time, and, as noted, elevated postexercise blood lactate levels. These observations are consistent with mild limitation of oxygen supplied to the exercising periphery, but overall impairment is not severe (Savin et al., 1980). Levels of circulating norepinephrine rise markedly and produce enhancement of left ventricular contractile state under conditions of heavy workloads (Pope et al., 1980).

Electrophysiologic studies have documented that intrinsic pacemaker and conduction system functions in the transplanted heart are normal, as assessed by sinus node responses to pacing, conduction intervals (AH and AB), and atrioventricular nodal refractory periods (Cannom et al., 1973; Harrison et al., 1978). Appropriate responses to adrenergic drugs such as norepinephrine and isoproterenol have documented the presence and activity of beta-adrenergic receptors in the myocardium (Cannom et al., 1975). Although partial reinnervation has been demonstrated in a few canine allografts, numerous studies of human cardiac recipients, extending to 11 years following transplantation, have failed to demonstrate postoperative reinnervation.

These studies of exercise responses have indicated that the transplanted human heart, although utilizing atypical adaptive mechanisms for increasing systemic flow during exercise, is functionally competent to support physical rehabilitation.

Survivor's Quality of Life

Patients selected for cardiac transplantation have severe cardiac disability and life expectancy measured in weeks or months. Worldwide experience during the early years of clinical cardiac transplantation showed that, in isolated cases, patients could regain a normal cardiac function and enjoy prolonged survival and virtually complete rehabilitation. These patients proved the remarkable potentialities of biologic heart replacement. More than a decade of additional clinical cardiac transplantation experience has established this procedure as a therapeutic modality for selected patients. Actuarial survival rates for cardiac transplantation recipients are divided into two groups, based on the date of operation (Fig. 53–7). Also shown are similar survival data for 70 patients selected for transplantation during this same period who died before a suitable donor could be found. The average time of survival of these patients was 46 days, with a range of 1 to 393 days. Although these patients do not strictly constitute a control group for recipients undergoing transplantation (since, in fact, all of the latter must have survived until the time of operation), they do illustrate the severity of cardiac disease present in patients selected for heart replacement. The 1-year survival rate has increased from 41 per cent before 1974 to 64 per cent currently (79 per cent since cyclosporin A).

Equally important is the degree of rehabilitation obtained. Of the 116 patients who survived for at least

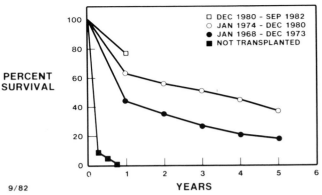

STANFORD CARDIAC TRANSPLANTATION

9/82

Figure 53–7. Actuarial survival curves of 225 cardiac transplantation recipients divided into two groups according to the date of operation and 20 patients who were selected for transplantation but who died before a donor became available.

3 months after the operation, 85 per cent returned to their previous occupations or similar activities. Although some patients have mild to moderate limitations, due most often to complications of corticosteroid therapy, there have been virtually no instances of disability attributed to primary cardiac insufficiency.

Conclusion

Experience with cardiac transplantation will continue to achieve improved survival. With new types of immunosuppression (notably cyclosporin A at present), we anticipate increased survival, decreased morbidity, decreased hospital stay after transplantation and, therefore, decreased costs, and widening of selection criteria. The coming decade will see wider application of this therapy.

LUNG TRANSPLANTATION

Although experimental and human heart transplantation were both accomplished significantly later than unilateral lung transplantation, it is recognized that the clinical results in heart transplantation have been far more satisfactory than the results accomplished in clinical lung transplantation. Workers in this field have characterized the application of organ transplantation to the solution of advanced disease of the lungs as "disappointing" (Blumenstock, 1977), whereas cardiac transplantation is considered "therapeutic" (Baumgartner et al., 1979).

There is little doubt, however, that there is a continued need for a successful approach to terminal lung parenchymal and vascular disease in view of the increasing numbers of the population who continue to smoke and/or are exposed to respiratory environmental toxins or suffer acute respiratory

TABLE 53–6. HUMAN LUNG TRANSPLANT CASES IN ORDER OF POST-OPERATIVE SURVIVAL

CASE NUMBER*	OPERATION DATE (YEAR/MONTH/DAY)	ORIGINAL DISEASE†	ORGAN TRANS-PLANTED‡	SURVIVAL (DAYS)	ORGAN CAUSE OF DEATH	REJECTION§	COPD**	RESPIRATORY INSUFFICIENCY	INFECTION	ISCHEMIC TIME (MINUTES)
07	67/01/05	Toxic	LL	0	Lung	N	N	Y	—	80
11	68/05/14	CA	LL	0	Lung	N	N	Y	N	270
34	72/07/07	CLD	—	0	Cardiac	N	N	N	N	—
04	64/09/13	CA	RL	0	Lung	N	N	Y	N	>1000
32	67/09/28	COPD, CA	LL	1	Lung	N	Y	Y	N	—
36	73/12/04	COPD	LL	2	Lung	N	Y	Y	N	—
10	67/11/05	Trauma	RL	2	Lung	N	N	Y	—	60
22	69/09/01	COPD	LL	4	Lung	N	Y	Y	—	—
33	71/12/12	Toxic	—	5	Lung	N	N	?	N	—
15	68/11/08	COPD	LL	6	Lung	Y	Y	Y	—	—
31	67/03/30	COPD	RL	6	Lung	N	Y	Y	N	15
05	65/09/25	Silicosis	LL	7	Lung	Y	N	Y	Y	—
02	63/07/06	CLD	LL	8	Lung	Y	Y	Y	Y	120
35	73/05/14	CLD	—	9	Gastric	N	N	N	N	90
37	75/08/22	Trauma	LL	10	Bronchus	N	N	—	Y	—
19	69/03/26	COPD	LL	10	Lung	A	Y	Y	N	75
20	69/04/09	COPD	LL	10	Lung	A	Y	Y	Y	75
24	70/03/17	COPD	RLLL	11	Lung	A	Y	Y	Y	120
21	69/06/01	TB, COPD	LL	11	Lung	A	Y	Y	Y	66
12	68/05/15	Toxic	LL	13	Lung	—	N	Y	N	120
18	69/03/06	CA	RL	14	Lung	A	N	Y	N	80
30	72/05/06	COPD	LL	15	Lung	N	Y	N	N	—
25	70/04/19	TB, COPD	RL	15	Bronchus	B	Y	N	N	80
01	63/06/11	CA	LL	18	Renal	B	N	N	N	90
38	77/05/13	Trauma	RL	18	Bronchus	N	N	N	N	135
13	68/08/31	COPD	LL	26	Lung	A	Y	Y	Y	50
17	69/01/18	CLD	LL	29	Lung	A	N	Y	N	180
27	71/03/20	CLD	LL	30	Lung	N	N	Y	Y	—
26	71/03/26	Fibrosis	RL	60	Bronchus	N	N	N	Y	59
29	72/01/07	COPD	RL	180	Bronchus	N	Y	N	N	—
16	68/11/14	Silicosis	RL	300	Lung	Y	N	Y	Y	50

*From Veith, F. J., and Koerner, S. K.: Lung transplantation, 1977. World J. Surg., *1*:177, 1977.

†CA = cancer of the lung; CLD = chronic lung disease; COPD = chronic obstructive lung disease; TB = tuberculosis

‡LL = left lung; RL = right lung

§N = no rejection reported; Y = rejection reported; A = no rejection reported originally, but "alveolar phase" suggested on re-examination (see text); B = "alveolar phase," but cause of death extrapulmonary; — = no information

**Y = contralateral lung emphysema present after transplant

failure from a variety of other causes. The mortality rate from pulmonary disease was 14.5 per 100,000 Americans in 1971. By 1979, the mortality rate had increased to 22.7 per 100,000 (Vital Statistics of the United States, 1980). Besides the morbidity of the lung disease itself, Hardy (1976) pointed out that patients with respiratory disease may be denied other needed surgical procedures because of the high morbidity associated with surgery in such patients.

Since Blumenstock's first comprehensive summary of the field in 1967, subsequent reviewers have expressed cautious optimism to the effect that the various problems leading to the disastrous results would soon be solved (Veith and Koerner, 1977). Each reviewer has been disappointed. This situation has now been changed with the successful physiologic and clinical results obtained by Reitz and associates (1982) in patients in whom both diseased lungs and the heart were replaced en bloc. The cumulative survival of the patients has already exceeded the cumulative survival of all previous patients who underwent clinical unilateral lung transplants (Table 53–6). In light of this accomplishment, the body of surgical science relevant to lung transplantation accumulated over approximately 30 years may be reviewed with a sense of renewed importance.

Historical Review

As would be expected, the initial studies of lung transplantation were concerned with developing suitable techniques to accomplish a successful transfer. The earliest lung transplant recorded was by Guthrie (1907) of a kitten lung to the carotid system of an adult cat utilizing the vascular techniques developed by Carrel and Guthrie (1905).

The first successful lung autotransplant was performed in 1950 by Juvenelle and associates (1951). The surgeons performed a pneumonectomy and replanted that lung by individual anastomosis of the bronchus and the pulmonary artery and veins. Their postoperative studies demonstrated vascular perfusion of both lungs on the eighteenth postoperative day by angiocardiography and good oxygen uptake by bronchospirometry when the dog was sacrificed in the thirty-fifth postoperative month.

Between 1950 and 1952, there were reports of orthotopic lung allografts from several different groups of surgeons, with each group apparently developing their surgical techniques independently. The most significant technical advance was described by Metras (1950), Hardin and associates (1952), and Neptune and colleagues (1952) and involved the retention of a cuff of left atrium about the *donor* pulmonary veins so that the anastomosis would be between the donor left atrium and the recipient left atrium. This singular concept reduced but, of course, did not eliminate the dangers of obstruction of the pulmonary venous ingress due to thrombosis and/or iatrogenic stenosis of the small and delicate pulmonary veins.

A report of five complete transplants by Davis and coworkers (1952b) preceded those of Neptune and Hardin, but their technique included ligating the pulmonary artery and vein leading to the middle lobe of the donor lung in order to reduce the number of anastomoses. Thus, it would not appear that this method was an advance suitable for clinical application.

Even earlier, Demikhov described techniques of pulmonary lobe and lung transplantation, but his work escaped the attention of the Western world until published in translation in 1962. In 1950, Staudacher and associates reported a technique using Vitallium tubes for the vascular connections in studying allografted and autografted pulmonary lobes in dogs.

The papers of Hardin and coworkers and Neptune and colleagues hold additional interest beyond their descriptions of the surgical technique. Both groups found that corticosteroids would extend the life of their animal, however limited it was, indicating the future usefulness of this class of drugs in lung transplants, as has been demonstrated in kidney and heart transplantation.

In light of the so-called "reimplantation" response to be described subsequently, Hardin and associates (1952) noted, in confirmation of Davis' work, that alveolar edema fluid appeared from 1 to 5 days after surgery and that if the animal survived, the alveoli cleared.

In addition, in light of subsequent clinical experience with bronchial problems, to be more fully discussed later, Neptune and colleagues (1952) observed, in one of two animals treated with ACTH, that the bronchial anastomosis "revealed evidence of some slough of the mucosa of the transplanted lung near the suture line, but this had healed with only a minimum of scar contracture." In the other animal, they reported that "the main bronchus and the beginning of the branch bronchi had apparently developed a slough of the mucosa and part of the submucosa, and the resulting granulation and contracture produced complete stenosis." They did not observe this problem with lung autografts, which suggests that it is related in some way to the immune response and immunosuppression.

Occasional long-term survival of immunosuppressed canine lung allografts was reported by Blumenstock and Kahn in 1961 in their own experience. Blumenstock (1967) has summarized the experience of others with a wide variety of protocols.

In 1963, Hardy and associates reported the first clinical attempt at lung allotransplant, with the patient succumbing to renal failure on the eighteenth day after the transplant. There was no evidence of allograft rejection.

From 1963 to 1978, there were 38 human lobar, whole lung, and/or heart-lung transplants performed, with three patients surviving from 2 to 10 months.

In 1981, using cyclosporin A as the primary immunosuppressive agent and developing an atrial-caval technique, Reitz and colleagues reported the survival of heart lung transplants in small primates to greater than 8 months.

Finally, in March and May 1981, Reitz and coworkers performed two consecutive human heart-lung transplants, with both patients surviving to leave the hospital. They have lived at least 20 and 18 months after transplantation, respectively.

Lung Transplantation in Animals

Operative Techniques. The fundamental surgical principles for lung transplantation have been recognized, as outlined previously. Careful attention to proper technique of anastomosis of the atrium and pulmonary vessels has reduced postoperative stenotic and thrombotic complications. It is agreed that among the complications attributed to restriction of flow is pulmonary vascular hypertension. Furthermore, it appears that there is no fundamental physiologic contraindication to unilateral lung transplantation arising from denervation, temporary lymphatic obstruction, or diversion of total vascular flow through one adequate pulmonary vascular bed, as is reflected in reports of long-term survival and function following lung autotransplantation (Benfield and Coon, 1967; Veith and Richards, 1969a).

The common features for operation in the canine model are as follows: Both donor and recipient animals are anesthetized simultaneously. A left thoracotomy is made through the fifth intercostal space. (In the case of one-stage bilateral lung allotransplantation, the right lung is transplanted first. We shall describe only the sequence for unilateral left lung transplantation.) The inferior pulmonary ligament is divided. The pericardium is divided over the main pulmonary artery, and the left pulmonary artery is dissected circumferentially. By traction on the left lower lobe, the plane between the left main bronchus and the left atrium is developed. Appropriate clamps are placed on the left pulmonary artery in such a manner as to provide adequate length and circumference. Similarly, clamps are next placed across the bronchus, which is then divided. It has been recommended that the donor bronchus be short to avoid ischemic problems, inasmuch as the bronchial vessels are transected and/or ligated at this stage (Pinkser *et al.,* 1979)., The left atrium is then clamped, and the recipient pulmonary *veins* are transected. Subsequent division of the tissue between the orifices of the veins results in a single generous orifice, which will be circumferentially anastomosed to the atrial cuff of the donor lung.

The donor lung is removed following the same sequence. Of course, rather than transecting the pulmonary veins, the left atrium is transected in the donor.

The arterial anastomosis is completed first. It has

been recommended that an everting mattress stitch be used to obtain intima-to-intima contact, reducing thrombotic complications coincident with exposure of myocardium.

Two different suggestions have been advanced to handle post-transplant bronchial complications: One is to telescope the donor bronchus into the recipient bronchus (Veith and Richards, 1970), and the other is to restore bronchial circulation by direct anastomosis (Mills *et al.*, 1970).

The pulmonary artery connection is then completed and the flow restored.

Hypothermic flushing of the lungs with a Sacks-type solution (Sacks *et al.*, 1973) and inflation of the lungs have been found to be means sufficient to achieve preservation up to 24 hours (Crane *et al.*, 1975).

"Reimplantation" Response. With both unilateral and one-stage bilateral lung transplants, it has been noted that there is a period of transitory diminished pulmonary function, indicated by decreased arterial saturation, increased pH, and normal P_{CO_2} (Reemtsma *et al.*, 1963). Chest x-ray examinations correlate with pathologic examinations, which uniformly reveal pulmonary edema maximizing on the third day and regressing after the seventh day (Siegelman *et al.*, 1971). Because this phenomenon is observed in lung reimplants, it may safely be inferred that the early roentgenographic appearance may not be due to the rejection phenomenon, from which it must be distinguished since the therapeutic modalities to be applied are different.

The phenomenon has been attributed variously to interruption of the lymphatics, denervation, interruption of the bronchial supply, and ischemia (Eraslan *et al.*, 1964; Pearson *et al.*, 1970; Trummer and Christiansen, 1965). These factors have also been implicated in the dysfunction seen following transplantation of the heart and the kidney. The issue is to weigh the importance of these factors. It would appear that ischemia followed by increased capillary permeability and increased capillary resistance is the most important factor. This is supported by the early study of Davis and associates (1952b) showing pulmonary edema following 1 hour of temporary pulmonary artery ligation and subsequent restoration of flow. The time course is quite similar to the time course reported with lung implantation. This phenomenon occurred in the presence of putatively intact nerves, lymphatic channels, and bronchial vessels.

Allograft Survival. The early observations have defined the pathologic sequence of events in the unmodified recipient. Inflammatory and round cell infiltration appeared within 2 days around the blood vessels and bronchi (Hardin *et al.*, 1952). Alveolar edema fluid appeared from 1 to 5 days (Davis *et al.*, 1952a). After the fourth day, necrosis of the alveolar walls and hemorrhage and destruction of pulmonary tissue occur. Interestingly, it has been observed that the bronchial anastomosis showed advanced fibroplasia, although there may be patches of mucosal ulceration (Neptune *et al.*, 1952).

The clinical appearance of the animals begins to deteriorate on or about the second day, beginning with a cough, the bringing up of frothy sputum, and listlessness. Chest films show progressive opacification of the transplanted lung. The animals succumb, even with just one lung transplanted, between the fifth and twelfth day (Blumenstock and Kahn, 1961).

In animals with one-stage bilateral lung allotransplants, survival ranges from 4 to 12 days. As might be expected, the most advanced pathologic alteration, hemorrhagic necrosis of pulmonary tissue, is not seen, because the animal succumbs to respiratory insufficiency before the stage is attained (Kondo *et al.*, 1974a).

Following immunosuppressive therapy, the animals show a broad spectrum of pathologic alterations or nonalterations, as the case may be. Depending on the time and success of the therapy, light and electron microscopy may reveal essentially normal tissue to far-advanced cellular infiltrate correlated with depressed respiratory function. In long-term surviving animals, the alveolar lining cells were frequently replaced with atypical cells presumed to be Type 2 pneumocytes. The bronchus may be occluded by mucous plugs, and the alveolar surface may be covered with "hyaline membrane" or obliterated by organized tissue. The alveolar walls and perivascular area are thickened by fibrosis. Interestingly, obliterative intimal thickening (accelerated arteriosclerosis), commonly observed in both renal and cardiac blood vessels after long-term survival, has not been reported in pulmonary artery vessels (Kondo *et al.*, 1974a).

Attention has been drawn to a so-called "alveolar" phase of lung rejection, characterized by alveolar fluid and little perivascular cuffing (Veith *et al.*, 1972). This histologic feature has not been observed with the more effective immunosuppression achieved with cyclosporin A (Veith *et al.*, 1981).

A number of immunosuppressive drugs and immunologically based techniques have been used to attempt to prevent lung rejection in outbred animal populations. These include azathioprine, methotrexate, alone and in combination with marrow transplantation, cyclophosphamide, corticosteroids, antilymphocyte serum, cyclosporin A, and donor pretreatment with concanavalin A, or cyclophosphamide and prednisone (Barnes and Flax, 1964; Blumenstock, 1967; Goldberg *et al.*, 1977; Veith *et al.*, 1981.)

Occasional long-term survival has been reported in many of the studies. There have been major difficulties in interpreting for extrapolation to clinical application. First, most studies have consisted of replacement of just one lung. Thus, the test of function sufficient to maintain life on the transplanted lung alone has not been generally met. The consequence is that tests of these data using an end point of "survival" are subject to great uncertainty as to sufficiency. Second, as part of the plan of study, many animals were sacrificed or succumbed to untreated infection, situations that obviously would not obtain clinically. Third, and most important, until recently, investigators have not used protocols based on the diagnosis of rejection episodes with intermittent therapy on a background of immunosuppression, a concept that has been accepted clinically and experimentally with transplants of other organs (Lower *et al.*, 1965b).

In connection with this last point, it should be noted that a major problem in taking this approach has been the lack of development of tests that reliably diagnose rejection of the lung *in vivo* and that differentiate between radiographic infiltrates associated with rejection and those associated with infection (Koerner *et al.*, 1976). Bronchoalveolar lavage may be just such a tool for unilateral lung transplantation (Achterrath *et al.*, 1975). Cardiac biopsy appears to be quite advantageous as an indicator for episodic rejection therapy in lung transplant with the heart.

Bronchial Anastomotic Problems. Since the earliest animal lung transplants, there has been concern about healing in the area of the anastomosis of the bronchus, since the transplantation process necessarily interrrupts the bronchial arterial supply from the aorta. Injection of the bronchial artery with bismuth, thus permanently interrupting the blood supply, led to ulceration and necrosis of the main stem bronchus and the proximal millimeter or two of the lobar bronchus (Ellis *et al.*, 1951). Experiments in which the effects of reconstructing the bronchial supply in immunosuppressed canine lung allografts were studied showed nicely that such animals had significantly fewer bronchial complications than did the animals that did not have the reconstruction. In addition, those animals that had bronchial ulcerations had significantly more incidents of pneumonia than those with no bronchial ulceration (Mills *et al.*, 1970). Furthermore, experiments with division and resuturing of the left main bronchus indicate that the mucosa is less likely to show ulceration when the division is close to the lobar bronchus than when the division is closer to the carina. These observations suggest that collateral flow from pulmonary artery–bronchial artery channels is relatively inadequate for the proximal portions of the left main stem bronchus (Pinkser *et al.*, 1979).

On the other hand, it has been demonstrated by arteriography that bronchial blood flow is re-established quite early in lung autografts and that there does not appear to be a correlation between bronchial mucosal ulceration and the contemporaneous appearance of bronchial collaterals (Blank *et al.*, 1966; Siegelman *et al.*, 1977). Furthermore, a technique of telescoping the donor bronchus into the recipient bronchus apparently decreases the incidence of bronchial complications. This technique, of course, does not augment the blood flow to the bronchus (Veith and Richards, 1970). Finally, although there is superficial ulceration of the mucosa and subsequent squamous metaplasia in the region of the bronchus anastomosis in the lung autotransplant, animals survived for long periods of time without reports of failure in this region (Blumenstock and Kahn, 1961).

In weighing the importance of the factors that play a role in postoperative bronchial anastomotic problems, the twin factors of rejection and immunosuppression must also be considered. In preliminary studies with cyclosporin A in unilateral canine lung transplant, it has been reported that prolonged survival has been obtained with "good" bronchial healing (Veith *et al.*, 1981).

Apparent good healing of the tracheal anastomosis in animal and human heart-lung transplants has been observed without attempts to reconstruct the bronchial supply from the aorta. It should be realized that there are abundant channels of natural anastomoses between the *coronary* circulation and the *bronchial* circulation that are not disturbed and may contribute to the promotion of tracheal healing in heart-lung transplantation (see the later section on heart-lung transplantation).

Preservation. There is an obligatory period of time during which the lung will be ischemic during transplantation. There has been a considerable effort to define the limits of such ischemia for the purposes of achieving safe immediate transfer and for possible storage to permit better histocompatibility matching and improved donor availability from a larger geographic area (Toledo-Pereyra *et al.*, 1977).

The physiologic effects of warm ischemia are twofold. First, after restoration of flow, pulmonary edema and increased vascular resistance are noted. The degree of both is related to the length of the period of ischemia. If severe enough, the animal will succumb despite the presence of an intact contralateral lung. Second, in the event that the animal survives the immediate insult, there may be permanent loss of pulmonary tissue. It has been noted that there is gradual recovery that reaches a maximum some 3 weeks after the insult. Subsequently, there may be decreased ventilatory capacity and increased vascular resistance (Garzon *et al.*, 1977).

As with the protocols testing the effects of immunosuppression, the interpretation of lung preservation techniques has been uncertain when the protocol does not call for immediate postoperative support by the transplanted lung(s) following the experimental stress. The two most satisfactory techniques are (1) one-stage bilateral lung transplantation (Alican *et al.*, 1973) and (2) one-lung allotransplant with immediate contralateral pulmonary artery ligation (Veith and Richards, 1969b).

The normothermic tolerance of ischemia for the lung appears to range between 1 and 2 hours in the deflated state. The tolerance is apparently extended to 3 hours if the lung is ventilated and to 4 hours if the lung is inflated in the unilateral lung transplant with pulmonary artery ligation model.

There are two basic methods of organ preservation—metabolic inhibition and organ perfusion. Metabolic inhibition is achieved by hypothermia, and perfusion is achieved with certain types of hyperosmotic electrolyte solutions approximating intracellular concentrations (Sacks *et al.*, 1973; Collins *et al.*, 1969). Subsequent normothermic ischemia to 3 hours is tolerated in the bilateral lung transplant model if the donor organs are flushed first with a hyperosmotic intracellular electrolyte solution. This time was extended to 5 hours of storage when the temperature was maintained at 4°C. in the same experimental model. Twenty-four hours of preservation was achieved using the unilateral lung model with Sacks' solution (Crane *et al.*, 1975).

Use of various compositions for the solutions has been reviewed (Toledo-Pereyra and Condie, 1978), and they remain to be shown to be more effective than Sacks' solution. On the other hand, Ringer's solution has been shown to be detrimental.

Work with metabolic maintenance using pulsatile and nonpulsatile perfusion continues at this stage for even longer storage.

Lung Transplantation in Man

The cases of human lung transplants were collected and published in 1970 (Wildevuur and Benfield, 1970), 1974 (Veith and Koerner, 1974), and 1978 (Veith, 1978). These reports are important chapters in the development of a safe and efficacious surgical approach to the treatment of advanced, otherwise untreatable lung disease and provide a standard against which to judge the efficacy of the currently proposed approach of combined heart-lung transplantation or further attempts at unilateral lung transplantation with cyclosporin A. In the sections that follow, recipient selection, donor management, extracorporeal membrane oxygenator support, operative techniques, postoperative management and complications, and correlations with mortality will be reviewed. The analysis is based on the published data concerning 31 unilateral or bilateral whole-lung transplants without the heart, as tabulated in Table 53–6.

There have been 42 human lung allografts performed between 1963 and 1981. Of these, 31 have been unilateral or bilateral lung allografts, seven heart and lung allografts, and three lobe allografts. Eight lung allografts were performed between 1963 and 1967; 11 were performed in 1968 and 1969; 10 were performed between 1970 and 1973; then only one each were done in 1975 and 1977. The length of survival for the three longest-surviving patients who underwent lung transplant only, and the only ones *over* 30 days, were 10 months (patient operated on in 1968), 2 months (patient operated on in 1971), and 6 months (patient operated on in 1972).

Recipient Selection. The factors for selecting a recipient for lung transplantation may be divided into two categories; (1) the severity of the lung disease and (2) nature of the disease itself. The typical patient selected for lung transplantation had chronic bilateral disease necessitating repeated or continuous hospitalization. Factors of chronicity, severity, and progression of disease should be weighed in the decision to transplant the lung so as to avoid the situation of unexpected recovery from the underlying disease (Benfield, 1977). The only patients in this series with

relatively short histories of pulmonary disease had histories of possible paraquat exposure.

Five patients known to have lung cancer were subjected to lung transplantation. It has now been well documented that immunosuppression is associated with an increased incidence of malignancy and is considered a *complication* of organ transplantation. Some of the malignancies in other organ transplants have been transplanted inadvertently from the donor. Reduction of immunosuppression has been successful in treating this complication. However, when the source of the malignancy is the recipient, it is predictable that the results of such treatment will not be as satisfactory. The preoperative presence of a malignancy should now be considered a *contraindication* to transplantation (Penn *et al.*, 1971).

Two patients had chronic obstructive lung disease associated with tuberculosis; one was reported to be active. Active infections are also considered to be *contraindications* to organ transplantation today. Of four patients in this series with reported pretransplant infection in the contralateral lung, three died with pneumonia. The dangers of infection are great in transplantation, despite the fact that it may be successfully treated. Of 22 patients surviving for 6 days or longer, 12 died with infection. Therefore, eight developed infections despite the absence of culturable microorganisms *ab initio*.

Ten patients had "chronic obstructive lung disease," five patients had "chronic lung disease," two had silicosis, one had fibrosing alveolitis, three had toxic pneumonitis, and three had lung disease related to trauma. One of the last two had injury due to smoke inhalation.

The question has been raised as to the role of unilateral lung transplantation for chronic obstructive lung disease (COPD). It has been suggested that, after transplantation, the remaining emphysematous lung increases in volume and receives much ventilation, while, because it presents a high pulmonary vascular resistance, the pulmonary blood flow is shunted to the transplanted lung, creating a ventilation-perfusion imbalance. The high vascular resistance and static compliance of the remaining lung predispose it to further hypoperfusion and hyperinflation (Stevens *et al.*, 1970). That this shunting is not obligatory is demonstrated by the 6-month survival of one patient with emphysema treated with a one-lung allograft (Veith *et al.*, 1973). On the other hand, of the five longest-surviving lung transplant patients, the lung disease of four was of the restrictive variety. Further comment on this subject is found in the section entitled "Conclusion."

Donor Management. All whole-lung transplants have come from cadavers, and it appears that all future whole-lung transplants will be from the same source. The considerations for maintaining the cardiopulmonary status of the donor while preparing for lung transplant are described in the sections on donor management for heart-lung and heart transplantation. There is a paucity of information describing the experience of successfully managing donors for lung transplantation alone.

From a review of the ischemic times that are available for 20 human lung transplants, it appears that at least 75 minutes of room-temperature ischemia and 3 hours of cold ischemia are compatible with survival beyond the immediate postoperative period.

The initial successes with heart-lung transplantation should rekindle interest in developing more sensitive measures of adequacy of function than mere survival for testing methods of lung preservation, because ischemia may be the major determinant of postoperative nonrejection acute respiratory distress syndrome (ARDS).

Extracorporeal Membrane Oxygenation. Developments in this field are reciprocally related to lung transplantation. On the one hand, use of extracorporeal membrane oxygenation in acute situations may result in certain patients becoming machine-dependent and require transplant to wean the patient off the machine. On the other hand, it may be useful in the aforementioned acute respiratory distress syndrome following lung transplantation. Both have been tried (Thomas *et al.*, 1978; Nelums *et al.*, 1980). It is clear that the use of extracorporeal membrane oxygenation in the case reported by Nelums and associates (1980) can be classified as successful. The field is advancing rapidly. The availability of such supportive management should be investigated at the inception of any lung transplant program but will not be discussed further here.

Operative Technique. In bilateral disease, one is faced first with a choice of which lung to transplant. It should be pointed out that the three longest survivors all had the right lung transplanted. One rationale for the choice of transplanting the right lung has been that cannulating the patient for cardiopulmonary bypass is easier if it should be necessary. Temporary clamping of the ipsilateral pulmonary artery will demonstrate whether bypass will be necessary.

To date, the donor and recipient have been operated on simultaneously. Heparin, 3 mg./kg., is administered. Flushing with Sacks' solution has been used in heart-lung transplantation with success. As has been mentioned, warm ischemia to 75 minutes has been tolerated in the human experience.

The anastomosis of the pulmonary veins may be either at the vein level or at the atrial level in the human. Both have been used. Obviously, the pulmonary veins are more generously sized than in the dog or lower primates. Nevertheless, it appears that using the atrial anastomotic level is quicker. In the patient with the longest survival, the bronchus anastomosis was at a level that was close to the origin of the upper lobe bronchus. Continuous and interrupted sutures have been used on the bronchus. Some surgeons take the vascular clamp off before completing the bronchus suture line. Care to remove trapped air must be exercised to avoid arterial air embolism (Fig. 53–8).

Postoperative Management. The management of unilateral lung transplants involves three different

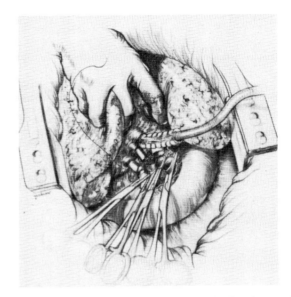

Figure 53–8. Operative technique used in first human lung transplant. (From Hardy, J. D., *et al.:* Lung homotransplantation in man: Report of initial case. J.A.M.A., *186*:1065, 1963. © 1963, American Medical Association.)

phases: (1) maintenance of lung function in the immediate postoperative period; (2) provision of baseline immunosuppression and diagnosis and treatment of acute rejection episodes; and (3) diagnosis and treatment of infectious complications.

Postoperative maintenance of lung function has been a major problem in unilateral lung transplantation. Of 12 patients dying before the end of the first week following transplantation, 10 were reported to have respiratory insufficiency. In these 10, the respiratory insufficiency was not related to either pneumonia or rejection. Two factors may be considered. First, there is an almost obligatory diminution of transplanted lung function for a variable period of time after the insult of ischemia during transplantation. Second, the contralateral lung contributes little if any physiologic function and may be detrimental with ventilatory-perfusion imbalances. Thus, the patient will be supported in the postoperative period by one, only partially functional lung. If the margin of safety for these patients is to be improved, it would appear that additional pulmonary function must be provided. We speak of *margin of safety,* for it is evident that some patients have survived the immediate postoperative period using the techniques available between 1963 and 1977. The additional margin may be provided by the temporary use of extracorporeal membrane oxygenation or bilateral lung (with heart) transplantation.

We are at a time of change with respect to immunosuppression for lung transplantation. All but one lung transplant patient prior to those who underwent the heart-lung transplants reported in this chapter have been treated with a variety of so-called "conventional" immunosuppressive drugs, including azathioprine, corticosteroids, actinomycin, and antilymphocyte sera. The general pattern was to start out with azathioprine at a dose of about 200 mg. per day, prednisone at a dose of 100 mg. per day, and antilymphocyte sera intramuscularly in volumes determined by the *in vitro* potency tests of the particular preparation. These drugs would be diminished according to the local protocol and varied with the appearance of drug toxicity or signs of rejection.

The treatment of lung rejection episodes may well have been hampered by the acknowledged lack of secure means of diagnosing lung rejection in the intact human recipient. The reports of diagnosis have necessarily been anecdotal. In case 16 (10 months' survival) (Derom *et al.,* 1971), the surgeons determined rejection on the basis of "general malaise, increasing fever, and a reticular image of the transplanted lung on chest x-ray," which responded to increased prednisolone, 300 mg. on the first day. However, later, the surgeons report that they treated "pronounced general malaise, persistent coughing, expectoration of fairly viscous mucopurulent secretions, dyspnea, and dropping of arterial Po_2" as rejection, but the patient died with rejection and bronchopneumonia in the transplanted lung.

In case 30 (6 months' survival) (Veith *et al.,* 1973a), the surgeons reported that apparent multiple episodes of rejection were characterized by

. . . dyspnea, an increase in body temperature (102–104 F.), the appearance of an infiltrate on chest roentgenograms, a decrease in the arterial oxygen tension to 52–62 mm. Hg and a need for increased inspired oxygen concentrations in the absence of any significant change in the number or character of organisms present on culture or smear of the tracheal secretions. All the manifestations in each [episode] were completely reversed by supplementing the patient's immunosuppressive therapy with 1 gm. doses of methylprednisolone. . . .

In case 26 (2 months' survival) (Hugh-Jones *et al.,* 1971), the surgeons reported with respect to the diagnosis of rejection that

Our interpretation is based mainly on the combination of changes in the clinical grade and the rosette test, total white cell and lymphocyte count, temperature, and arterial oxygen tension breathing air . . . together with other information such as chest signs, haematology, sputum culture, biochemistry, and daily radiographs.

The introduction of a new immunosuppressant, cyclosporin A, and the early good results reported in human and lower primate heart-lung transplants (Reitz *et al.,* 1980) do not change the necessity for reliable methods of monitoring the rejection process. In heart transplants, it has been observed that the electrocardiographic and histologic manifestations are altered (Oyer *et al.,* 1982). The diminution of edema in rejection in the presence of cyclosporin A is correlated with the apparent absence of voltage changes on the electrocardiogram. This phenomenon is predictable, based on electrophysiologic principles. If lung rejection in the presence of cyclosporin A is also associated with less edema, radiographic abnormalities may be even less reliable indicators of rejection than they are

currently. This possibility re-emphasizes the clinical utility and significant advantage of *cardiac* biopsy as a monitor of both heart and lung rejection in combined heart-lung transplantation.

The point that should not be overlooked with respect to rejection of the lung is the simple fact that it is reversible, as has been demonstrated before in kidney, liver, and heart transplantation.

Infection has been a major consideration in immunosuppressed patients in general and in organ transplantation in particular. Of the 19 lung transplant patients who survived for longer than a week, 10 died with pneumonia or signs of other infections. As with the treatment of rejection, it is clear from the collected experience that infection in the lung transplant patient is a condition that may be successfully treated. The elimination from consideration for lung transplants of patients with documented pre-existing infection should reduce the incidence of fatal postoperative infections. However, it certainly will not eliminate infection-related deaths. The major problem for lung transplant surgeons, besides obtaining the ideal immunosuppressant, is the differentiation of pneumonic infiltrates—postischemic pulmonary edema, infective pneumonic processes, and lung rejection (Veith *et al.,* 1973a). Once this is accomplished, the therapeutic course may be determined. Based on the heart and kidney transplant experience, it may be safely stated that powerful antimicrobial agents are available and that, in most instances, if the nature of the infection is determined early enough and differentiated from rejection, they may be used with success.

Complications. Acute respiratory distress syndrome, rejection, and infection are all treatable complications of lung transplantation and have been discussed earlier under postoperative management. There are two additional issues to be discussed: (1) late bronchial anastomotic complications and (2) respiratory distress associated with desquamation of pneumocytes.

The site of the bronchial anastomosis has been quite troublesome in the 31 whole-lung transplants that have been performed. Of the 21 patients who died between the operation and the fourteenth postoperative day, only one developed a bronchopleural fistula, dying on the tenth postoperative day, with several other contributing problems. On the other hand, of the 10 patients surviving for more than 2 weeks, the death of four patients was directly attributable to bronchial complications, including broncho-pulmonary artery fistula, bronchial artery hemorrhage, ulceration of the bronchial mucosa with aspirated pneumonia, and necrotic dehiscence of membranous bronchus.

These bronchial anastomotic complications may be related to the interruption of the bronchial blood supply, and the suggestions for avoiding the problem, without notable success, have included reanastomosis of the bronchial arteries, bolstering the suture line with vascularized tissue, and setting the line of anastomosis close to the upper lobe bronchus, reducing the area to be nourished by donor pulmonary-bronchial collateral channels (Pinkser *et al.*, 1979; Mills *et al.*, 1970; Veith and Richards, 1970). Another argument for transplanting the heart and both lungs may be the retention of coronary-bronchial collaterals to nourish the trachea, carina, and bronchus. These collaterals have been shown to be extensive after heart-lung transplants. (See the discussion in the following section on heart-lung transplantation.)

The last complication to discuss is respiratory insufficiency between the tenth and thirtieth postoperative day. There were 14 patients in the series who succumbed in this period. Nine patients were considered to have died with respiratory insufficiency as a major factor contributing to death. In all nine, initial histologic examination of the lung demonstrated no rejection, as indicated by the absence of cells of the lymphocytic series. On a subsequent review, it was asserted that there was a characteristic pattern within the alveoli of edema fluid, fibrillar strands of fibrin, and sloughed pulmonary pneumocytes (Veith *et al.*, 1972). The etiology of this finding is unproved. It has been suggested that there is an immunological basis for the desquamation. If so, it would have to be due to circulating antibodies, since, by definition, there were no lymphocytes present. It should be noted that this pattern had not been seen before the tenth postoperative day nor after the thirtieth postoperative day. An alternative hypothesis to an immunologic basis for the phenomenon is that the desquamation is the end result of lung ischemia during the operation manifesting itself over an intermediate time course. Whatever the cause, filling of the alveoli with cellular debris and edema apparently caused sufficient respiratory embarrassment to result in death.

Survival and Outlook. The three longest survivors after unilateral lung transplant lived for 2, 6, and 10 months after operation. Only the 10 months' survivor had been discharged from inpatient care at 6 months, but he returned 2 months later with a fracture and remained in the hospital until his death.

In all three patients, physiologic studies indicated that the transplanted lung improved arterial oxygenation and carbon dioxide removal and decreased the work of respiration. Isotopic perfusion studies indicated that in two patients, virtually all the blood was directed through the transplanted lung, whereas in the third patient, the "bulk" of the pulmonary blood flow was so directed. Ventilation studies indicated that ventilation was virtually nil in the unoperated lung in two patients, whereas in the third, the scan was reported as indicating that the transplanted lung was ventilated more rapidly and more evenly than the emphysematous lung. Xenon wash-out from the emphysematous lung was distinctly delayed.

As for exercise tolerance, one patient was noted to be able to "walk briskly up steps and about a quarter of a mile (400 M.) without breathlessness."

In summary, it appears that unilateral lung transplant in the two patients with restrictive lung disease achieved the best physiologic results. In the patient with chronic obstructive lung disease, the transplantation achieved palliation but not to the extent that the patient could leave the hospital.

Conclusion

The application of the techniques of organ transplantation to the treatment of severe lung disease is being reconsidered after a long period of introspection because of the introduction of newer immunosuppressive agents and early success with combined heart-lung transplantation. We suggest that the issue to be considered is not whether lung transplants should or should not be done, but whether it is to be one or two lungs that will be transplanted as the course of choice.

The first considerations that we have reviewed here are technical and anatomic. In unilateral lung transplants, there are no direct means of assessing rejection in the same direct manner as cardiac biopsy in heart-lung transplants. Following unilateral lung transplants, the bronchial anastomosis is subject to a high incidence of complications, which studies seem to strongly indicate are due to the interruption of the bronchial blood supply. In combined heart-lung transplants, there is apparently the early maintenance of collateral blood supply from cardiac collaterals until direct bronchial arterial regeneration can occur. With unilateral lung transplantation, there is an apparent need for additional respiratory support in the period following transplant owing to temporary transplanted lung dysfunction in the presence of, for all intents and purposes, a diseased nonfunctioning contralateral lung. With combined heart-lung transplants, the second lung, although also temporarily dysfunctional, provides additional respiratory surface area during this critical period.

It is clear that the investment of resources by the institution in providing for transplants either of the lung alone or of the heart and lung together will be similar, if not identical. Cardiopulmonary bypass has been used to accomplish unilateral lung transplantation and has been on "stand-by" on other occasions. It would appear, however, that operative costs contribute relatively small increments to the economic costs of transplantation either of the lung or of the heart and lungs. Furthermore, it would appear that the resources of the family and the patient, emotional and financial, would be similarly taxed in either case.

It is apparent, too, that suitable donor lungs are scarce, although as physicians we should not bemoan that fact for there is tragedy with every suitable donor. Nevertheless, they are available. It would be a rare circumstance in which the lungs would be suitable and the heart not suitable for transplant.

Perhaps the more important considerations are those of utilizing scarce resources for maximal benefit, balancing cost and risk. The lung disease that requires transplantation as the mode of treatment is necessarily bilateral. The physiologic results obtained with unilateral transplants are, at best, modest when the contralateral lung remains either causing some physiologic embarrassment or, in any event, not contributing in a positive way to the respiratory needs of the patient. It would appear that removing both recipient lungs and using both donor lungs and heart would achieve (1) the maximal physiologic benefit, (2) a means for more accurate monitoring of allograft rejection by cardiac biopsy, and (3) removal of all abnormal lung tissue.

We noted at the outset that past reviewers of the lung transplantation literature have expressed hope that the identification of past problems and diligent experimental observation would change the outlook for the application of the art and science of organ transplantation for severe, otherwise untreatable lung disease. We believe that the wait has been rewarded and that the outlook has already changed for the better.

COMBINED HEART AND LUNG TRANSPLANTATION

The technical ability to perform combined heart-lung transplantation and prevent rejection of the allograft postoperatively could offer a new lifesaving procedure to patients with a variety of devastating diseases, including some patients who presently are disqualified from cardiac transplantation because of high pulmonary vascular resistance. Other patients with developmental abnormalities of the lung, congenital heart disease with resulting pulmonary vascular disease, or various diffuse pulmonary diseases also may be candidates for this procedure if it is shown to be therapeutically effective.

Experimental Heart-Lung Transplantation

Perhaps the earliest experimental attempts at orthotopic replacement of the heart and lungs together was the work of the Russian surgeon Demikhov, which was performed in the 1940s but reported in the West in 1962. Without the aid of hypothermia or cardiopulmonary bypass, he devised a method for systematically dividing inflow and outflow from the heart and lung block, with separate anastomoses of the right and left bronchi, resulting in replacement of the heart and both lungs. Two of 67 dogs survived for as long as 5 days postoperatively. In a report entitled "Complete Homologous Heart Transplantation," Neptune and associates (1953) reported a technique for en bloc replacement of the heart and lungs using hypothermia and circulatory arrest. Webb and Howard (1957) and Lower and associates (1961) used cardiopulmonary bypass for the procedure, and the latter group obtained a 6-day survivor.

In the majority of studies, technical difficulties with the operation itself precluded survival (Cooper, 1969). However, even following a technically successful operation, long-term survival was impossible be-

cause of respiratory insufficiency caused by interruption of pulmonary innervation in the dog. In a study by Nakae and associates (1967) comparing respiratory patterns in cats, dogs, and monkeys following cardiopulmonary denervation, normal respiratory control was markedly altered in the dog. Bilateral denervation produced increased tidal volumes but slowed respiratory rate with long periods of apnea. It appears that pulmonary stretch receptors within the lung are important in modulating the pattern of respiration in dogs. However, primates had normal respiratory patterns following denervation, and this was later substantiated by the results of Castaneda and associates (1972a). They performed complete cardiopulmonary autotransplantation in baboons, with survival of five of 25 animals for at least 6 months and up to periods greater than 2 years. These animals first showed that en bloc heart-lung transplants were compatible with long survival when performed in primates; normal cardiopulmonary function was demonstrated in several animals over 2 years after the transplant (Castaneda *et al.*, 1972b).

Experiments by Reitz and colleagues (1980) confirmed long-term survival after heart-lung transplantation in monkeys, both autotransplants and allotransplants. With cyclosporin A for immunosuppression, animals receiving heart-lung allografts have lived for more than 2½ years with excellent function.

Operative Technique

In all of the previously mentioned studies and reports, except for that of Longmore and associates (1969), heart-lung transplantation was performed through a lateral thoracotomy, with separate anastomoses of the ascending aorta, trachea, and both venae cavae. Recently, a simplified operative method was reported (Reitz *et al.*, 1981b) that incorporates the recipient's right atrium into a single inflow anastomosis to the heart and lung, eliminating separate vena caval anastomoses. The donor right atrium is handled as described for isolated cardiac transplantation, preserving the sinus node in the donor organ. This facilitates the operation in man, where the intrathoracic component of the inferior vena cava is short.

The operative technique is shown in Figure 53–9. After a standard median sternotomy incision, a complete anterior pericardiectomy is performed. Cannulation for cardiopulmonary bypass in the recipient is all within the thorax. The recipient's heart and lungs are removed as shown, with division of the ascending aorta just above the aortic valve, the right atrium at the atrioventricular groove, and the trachea just above the carina. Special care throughout the dissection is required to preserve both the right and left phrenic nerves, the vagus nerves on the esophagus, and the recurrent laryngeal nerve at the aortic arch. The donor's heart and lungs are removed with a good length of both superior and inferior vena cava; the superior vena cava is ligated, and the right atrium is

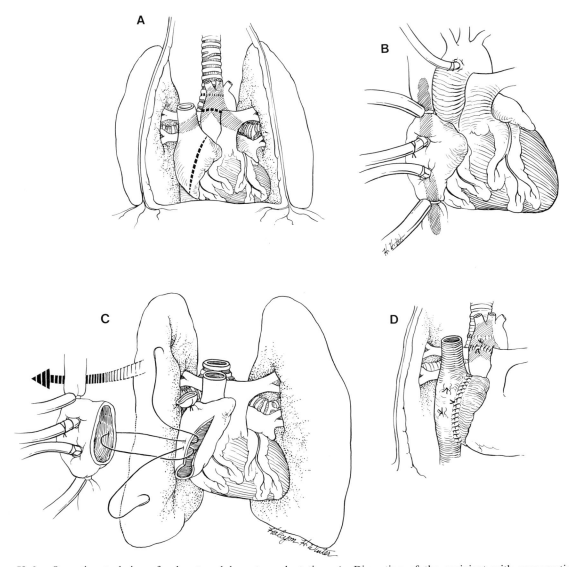

Figure 53–9. Operative technique for heart and lung transplantation. *A,* Dissection of the recipient with preservation of the phrenic nerves on pedicles. Anticipated lines of transection are shown. *B,* Cannulation of the recipient for cardiopulmonary bypass. *C,* Appearance of the empty thorax after removal of the heart and lungs. The recipient's right atrium is retained, including a portion of the interatrial septum. The reimplantation is shown, emphasizing the right atrial anastomosis. *D,* Final appearance of the transplant procedure with completed anastomoses and repair of cannulation sites. (From Rietz, B. A., *et al.:* Simplified method for heart and lung transplantation. J. Surg. Res., *31*:1, 1981.)

opened from the inferior vena cava toward the right atrial appendage. The trachea is joined with a running suture of polypropylene material, adjusting for size discrepancy at the membranous portion of the trachea. A similar anastomosis of the ascending aorta follows, with the right atrial anastomosis done last. After removal of the aortic cross-clamp, the heart and lungs are resuscitated, and bypass can be discontinued after a short period. Both pleural spaces are drained, and chest closure is performed.

Allograft Rejection

Very little information is available about the pattern of allograft rejection in combined heart-lung transplants. In the study by Lower and associates (1961), one dog lived for 6 days and had a mild lymphocytic infiltrate in both organs. The only long-surviving heart-lung allografts are in several monkeys who have received cyclosporin A for immunosuppression and who survived for more than 2 years after transplant in our laboratory (Reitz *et al.*, 1980). In these animals, transvenous endomyocardial biopsies have corresponded to normal chest roentgenograms. An allograft in a rhesus monkey that died of metastatic lymphoma 5 months after transplant had a normal myocardium and only mild interstitial thickening of alveoli without lymphocytic perivascular cuffing. In a further study of heart-lung transplantation in monkeys in which 20 animals received cyclosporin A alone or in combination with either azathioprine or a corticosteroid, there was extremely close concordance between the degree of rejection found in the heart and lungs at the time of death. A close concordance between onset and degree of histologic rejection in both organs would allow close monitoring of the cardiac allograft as a sensible method for determining the status of rejection or results of treatment with immunosuppressive drugs in the combined graft.

The most efficacious use of cyclosporin A, whether alone or in combination with another agent, is unknown for heart-lung transplantation at this time. Since cyclosporin A by itself seems inadequate for heart, kidney, and liver transplantation in animals and man, combination of the drug with other agents also seems necessary for this application.

Bronchial or Tracheal Anastomotic Healing

Healing has been a major concern in transplantation of the lung. Anatomic factors such as the length of the bronchial segment of the graft have affected healing, probably by the degree of vascularity. When corticosteroids are used for immunosuppression, delayed healing results; allograft rejection may also be an important factor. Because of the relatively long segment of tracheobronchial tree used in combined heart-lung transplants, there has been obvious concern. This concern led Barnard and associates (1981) to perform separate right and left bronchial anastomoses in the hilum of both lungs in the one clinical procedure they performed in 1971. Among survivors of heart-lung transplant procedures, both monkeys and human beings, no complications attributable to this anastomosis have occurred in our experience. Specifically, there has been no necrosis, rupture, or late stenosis. Arteriograms in animals and patients have shown neovascularity of the trachea and bronchus in the donor organs both from bronchial arteries coming across the suture line from the trachea and from collaterals arising from the coronary artery atrial branches (Fig. 53–10).

Previous Clinical Heart-Lung Transplantation

Prior to 1981, three patients were reported to have received combined heart-lung transplants. The first of these patients was a 2-month-old infant with complete atrioventricular canal defect and pulmonary edema. The procedure was performed in 1968 and reported by Cooley and associates (1969a). It was performed through a midline sternotomy incision, using cardiopulmonary bypass, and by making separate vena caval anastomoses, a tracheal anastomosis, and aortic anastomosis. Spontaneous respiratory movements resumed immediately after operation, but continued mediastinal hemorrhage required a re-exploration to control bleeding. Following this, the lungs became progressively more edematous, and the child died of pulmonary insufficiency 14 hours postoperatively. The second patient was operated on by Lillehei (1970). The patient was a 43-year-old man with advanced emphysema, pulmonary hypertension, and right heart failure. The operative technique was similar to that described in the first case, and the patient made a good immediate recovery. Extubation was accomplished on the third postoperative day, but by the fifth day, chest roentgenograms showed bilateral interstitial infiltrate. This extended despite efforts to treat both rejection and infection. At autopsy, there were findings compatible with a severe Pseudomonas pneumonia and also possible rejection. The third patient underwent combined heart-lung transplantation

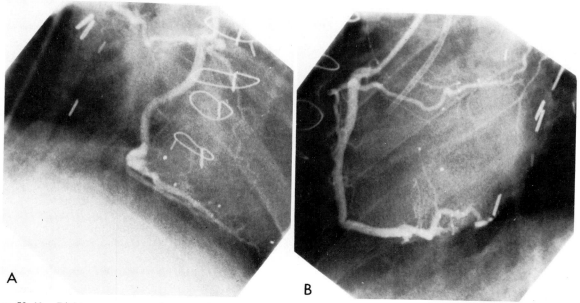

Figure 53–10. Right coronary arteriogram of patient obtained 11 months after transplant. A large atrial branch now passes posteriorly into the right hilar region, filling bronchial arterial vessels. *A,* Right anterior oblique projection. *B,* Left anterior oblique projection.

in 1971 in South Africa, the operation being performed by Barnard and associates (1981). The patient was a 49-year-old man with chronic obstructive lung disease who had been chronically ill for a number of years. Their operation was different from those described in the first two patients in that separate right and left main stem bronchial anastomoses were performed. However, a right bronchial leak 12 days postoperatively eventually required a right pneumonectomy, and the patient succumbed to infection on the twenty-third postoperative day. There was no significant rejection in the heart or lung at autopsy. These early experiences with combined heart-lung transplantation parallel the results after unilateral lung transplantation in man described previously.

Recent Experience with Heart-Lung Transplantation

A clinical trial of combined heart-lung transplantation has recently begun at Stanford Medical Center. After successful laboratory experimentation with both autotransplantation and allotransplantation in primates and with increasing experience using cyclosporin A for standard cardiac transplantation, a trial of this procedure in patients with severe pulmonary vascular disease was undertaken. Patients considered as active recipients had either primary pulmonary hypertension or pulmonary hypertension secondary to congenital heart disease (Eisenmenger's syndrome). They were chosen as recipients because of severe illness with a pattern of clinical deterioration that suggested life expectancy of less than 6 months. By December 1981, five patients had undergone heart-lung transplantation.

Recipient Selection

Several categories of potential patients might benefit from combined heart and lung transplantation. These would include patients with primary cardiac disease with secondary pulmonary vascular disease, as in uncorrected congenital heart disease with increased pulmonary blood flow. Other patients with anatomic developmental abnormalities of the pulmonary arteries such as severe pulmonary atresia might also be treated in this way. Other patients with diffuse bilateral lung disease with or without secondary right heart failure may also be potential candidates. This group would include a large number of patients with chronic obstructive lung disease or others with rare interstitial fibrosis or primary pulmonary hypertension. In patients with severe emphysema and secondary changes in thoracic volumes, transplantation with donor organs of normal volumes may be impractical. Patients with pulmonary vascular disease are a relatively favorable group for consideration. Although unilateral lung transplantation might be considered in these patients, isolated unilateral lung transplantation

would result in ventilation-perfusion imbalance, with preferential perfusion of the transplant. Since long survival of animals with unilateral transplantation and contralateral pulmonary artery ligation has been reported, this would not be incompatible with survival but would require that the majority of the cardiac output traverse the transplant vascular bed.

Other requirements are similar to those of cardiac transplant recipients. Younger patients without systemic illness and without severe secondary organ dysfunction that is considered to be irreversible should be considered. Contraindications include any active infection, diabetes mellitus, or extensive previous cardiac surgery. It is important that patients be psychologically stable with a good family support structure and able to reliably follow a complex medical regimen.

The first five patients to undergo combined heart-lung transplantation at our institution were three women and two men, ranging in age from 29 to 45 years old. Two patients had the diagnosis of primary pulmonary hypertension, and three had congenital heart disease with pulmonary vascular disease (Reitz *et al.*, 1982).

Donor Selection and Management

Donors suitable for lung transplantation will occur less frequently than those for renal or cardiac transplantation. Brain death may be accompanied by neurogenic pulmonary edema or may be secondary to severe cranial trauma with attendant thoracic trauma, and prolonged ventilatory support may predispose to nosocomial pneumonia or tracheobronchial infection. Probably only one fourth of cadaver donors would have lungs suitable for transplantation. We believe additional requirements for combined heart-lung transplant donors include a close size match to approximate lung volumes, satisfactory gas exchange with an arterial PO_2 of greater than 400 torr on 100 per cent oxygen, good lung compliance with low peak inspiratory pressures at normal tidal volumes, and absence of pulmonary infection. The chest roentgenogram of a 21-year-old man who suffered brain death in a motorcycle accident is shown in Figure 53–11. Satisfactory graft function was evident even after 55 hours of ventilatory support prior to transplantation.

Clinical Perioperative Management

The details of operative technique have been described earlier. Anesthetic techniques do not differ significantly from those employed for standard cardiac operations. Monitoring includes central venous pressure and radial arterial pressure lines. Extreme care is used, including a sterile oral endotracheal tube, to insure that the airway is maintained as clear as possible. Median sternotomy and routine cannulation for cardiopulmonary bypass within the thorax are em-

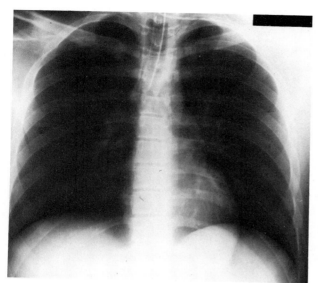

Figure 53–11. Portable anteroposterior chest roentgenogram of a 21-year-old man who suffered brain death following cranial trauma. Appearance of the chest just prior to use as a cardiopulmonary transplant donor.

ployed. Removal of the recipient's heart and lungs is facilitated by first performing cardiectomy and then removing the lungs en bloc, leaving most of the posterior pericardium intact over the esophagus and aorta. This tends to minimize the dissection of multiple collateral blood vessels in the posterior mediastinum, which are especially prominent in cyanotic patients. The trachea is accessible just to the right and posterior to the aorta.

Removal of the heart-lung graft from the donor is performed from a standard median sternotomy incision. Complete anterior pericardiectomy is performed. Long segments of superior and inferior vena cava and the aorta are dissected free. Heparin is administered (300 units per kilogram), and temporary inflow occlusion leads to a fall in systemic pressure. The aorta is then cross-clamped, and cold cardioplegic solution is instilled into the aortic root. The inferior vena cava is transected so that the cardioplegic solution can drain freely from the coronary sinus. Simultaneously, a similar cold electrolyte solution is flushed through the pulmonary artery and the tip of the left atrial appendage is amputated to allow egress of blood and fluid from the lungs. Continued ventilation during in situ perfusion facilitates the flow of the solution through all segments of the pulmonary vascular bed. The vena cava, aorta, and trachea are transected. A culture is taken from the exposed trachea, which is then clamped, and the entire graft is immersed in cold saline solution. The trachea is then cut one complete cartilaginous ring above the carina and reimplantation performed. At the conclusion of the operation, a low dose of isoproterenol is used for chronotropic response. The patient is transferred directly to a reverse isolation room in the intensive care unit.

The general features of the immediate postoperative management are similar to those routinely em-

ployed in cardiac surgical patients. Endotracheal suctioning for maintenance of a clear airway is performed without hesitation, with precautions taken to insure absolute sterility. The patient is allowed to awaken from anesthesia and is weaned from the respirator, with extubation accomplished after a 4-hour period of spontaneous breathing with the endotracheal tube in place. Surveillance for infection, allograft rejection, and immunosuppression is routine. The measures used for prevention and detection of infectious complications are similar to those used in cardiac transplant patients.

Surveillance for rejection includes twice daily clinical examination, daily electrocardiogram, measurement of arterial blood gases during the first few postoperative days, and serial transvenous endomyocardial biopsy on a weekly basis (or more frequently if dictated by clinical findings). Immunologic monitoring is helpful if the patient receives antihuman thymocyte globulin; cyclosporin A serum levels are helpful in monitoring this drug. A graphic summary of the in-hospital transplantation course of a 45-year-old woman receiving a heart-lung transplant for primary pulmonary hypertension is shown in Figure 53–12. Transvenous endomyocardial biopsies showing rejec-

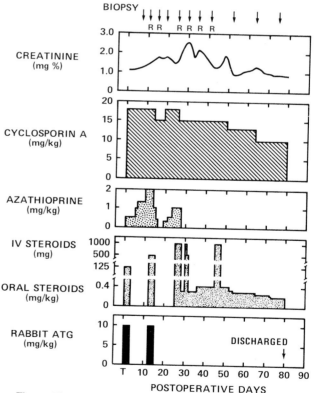

Figure 53–12. Graphic summary of in-hospital transplantation course of the patient shown in Figure 53–10. The timing of transvenous endomyocardial biopsy is indicated by the arrows at the top. Biopsies that had findings of acute rejection are marked by "R." The serum creatinine and immunosuppressive agents are illustrated as a function of time after transplant. (From Reitz, B. A., *et al.*: Heart-lung transplantation: Successful therapy for patients with pulmonary vascular disease. N. Engl. J. Med., *306*:557, 1982.)

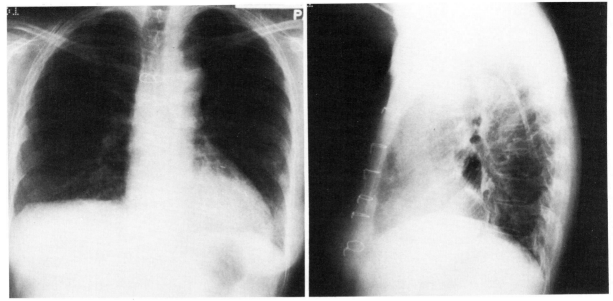

Figure 53–13. Post-transplant chest roentgenograms of a 45-year-old woman 8 months following combined heart and lung transplantation. (From Reitz, B. A., *et al.*: Heart-lung transplantation: Successful therapy for patients with pulmonary vascular disease. N. Engl. J. Med., *306*:557, 1982.)

tion were obtained on the tenth and twenty-fifth postoperative days, and treatment for rejection was begun using intravenous methylprednisolone and additional antihuman thymocyte globulin. Subsequent to these two episodes of rejection, this patient has not had any other rejection while on a maintenance dose of cyclosporin and low-dose prednisone and is fully active, with normal cardiopulmonary function, more than 20 months after transplant. A representative late chest roentgenogram of this patient is shown in Figure 53–13.

Lung Transplant Reimplantation Response

Experimental lung transplantation investigations have suggested a transient reversible defect in pulmonary gas exchange, compliance, and vascular resistance, coinciding with roentgenographic pulmonary edema early postoperatively. The time course of this phenomenon has varied from 3 to 21 days postoperatively and has been termed "reimplantation response," as described previously (Siegelman *et al.*, 1971). Multiple causes may contribute to this observed event. Serial measurements of left ventricular filling pressures are normal in animals, suggesting that pulmonary edema is due to a pulmonary capillary-leak syndrome and the accumulation of interstitial edema. The "reimplantation response" is also observed routinely in experimental heart-lung transplants, after both autotransplantation and allotransplantation (Reitz *et al.*, 1980). This phenomenon has also been observed routinely in patients receiving heart-lung transplants. It regresses spontaneously after approximately 3 weeks.

Therapeutic intervention during the period of transient pulmonary edema is limited but crucial. Most important is the maintenance of a low circulating blood volume by vigorous diuresis. Any tendency toward overhydration or expanded blood volume will magnify changes in interstitial edema. It is important to rule out a coexistence of significant allograft rejection by transvenous endomyocardial biopsy, since rejection injury in addition to "reimplantation response" may result in significant pulmonary insufficiency. If transient renal failure results in oliguria, strong consideration should be given to ultrafiltration hemodialysis in order to remove excess fluid being mobilized from tissues and ascites present preoperatively. Adequate nutrition with maintenance of the serum albumin in a normal range also helps reduce the accumulation of interstitial edema.

Complications of Immunosuppression

All transplant recipients receiving immunosuppression are at an increased risk of infection. These infectious complications often involve opportunistic and unusual organisms, including viruses, fungi, and unusual bacteria. For the most part, morbidity and mortality following combined heart-lung transplantation are expected to parallel those that occur after cardiac transplantation. Development of atherosclerosis in the transplanted heart, continued susceptibility to opportunistic infections, and other complications secondary to chronic corticosteroid administration may occur in these patients. Because the primary immunosuppressive drug is cyclosporin A, late complications associated with this drug (yet to be established) also may occur. The lung equivalent of cardiac allograft atherosclerosis is still unknown. Lung transplant recipients have not survived long enough as yet to develop this complication. Whether this may result in pulmonary vascular disease and recurrent pulmonary hypertension or late pulmonary fibrosis interfering with gas exchange remains to be learned. Up to 10 months after transplant, normal pulmonary function at rest and at exercise has been demonstrated (Reitz et al., 1982).

Physiology and Functional Capacity

Many interesting and important questions about lung disease physiology can be studied in patients who receive combined heart-lung transplants. By necessity, transplantation results in immediate loss of three important systems: (1) integration with the autonomic nervous system, (2) the bronchial arterial circulation, and (3) the connection of pulmonary lymphatics to the lymphatic circulation. Of particular interest will be studies of neuroregulation of ventilation, airway reactivity after denervation, and the regulation of the pulmonary arterial bed after denervation. Serial evaluation of cardiopulmonary functional capacity will be crucial in determining the therapeutic potential for this procedure.

Conclusion

Although successful combined heart-lung transplantation has only recently been achieved, preliminary laboratory experience, better immunosuppression provided by cyclosporin A, and extensive experience with cardiac transplant patients suggest that it may become a feasible and therapeutic procedure for selected patients. If results approach those presently achieved with cardiac transplantation without inordinate late complications, it holds the promise of extending life and improving the quality of life where no mechanical substitute is likely to be available for many years.

SELECTED REFERENCES

Baumgartner, W. A., Reitz, B. A., Oyer, P. E., Stinson, E. B., and Shumway, N. E.: Cardiac transplantation. Curr. Probl. Surg., 16:1, 1979.

This monograph represents a comprehensive review and discussion of all aspects of cardiac transplantation. It deals exclusively with cardiac transplantation and conventional immunosuppression.

Calne, R. Y.: Immunosuppression for organ grafting—observations on cyclosporin A. Immunol. Rev., 46:113, 1979.

This paper summarizes the experience with cyclosporin A in a number of animal models as well as its clinical application. The description of the drug itself, its mode of action, and side effects are also elucidated.

Carrel, A., and Guthrie, C. C.: The transplantation of veins and organs. Am. J. Med., 11:1101, 1905.

This reference, which describes a heterotopic heart transplant, is frequently cited as the beginning of the field. Unfortunately, details of the actual vascular arrangements are not described, and "survival" was exceedingly short.

REFERENCES

Achterrath, U., Blümcke, S., Koerner, S. K., Yipintsoi, T., Siegelman, S. S., Chandler, P., Hagstrom, J. W. C., Torres, M., Cobbah, J. E., Fujii, P., and Veith, F. J.: Alveolar lavage cytology in transplanted lungs. I. Staining methods and findings in dogs with autografts and allografts without immunosuppression. J. Thorac. Cardiovasc. Surg., 69:510, 1975.

Alican, F., Isin, E., and Cockrell, J. V.: One-stage allotransplantation of both lungs in the dog. Ann. Surg., 177:193, 1973.

Barnard, C. N.: The operation. S. Afr. Med. J., 41:1271, 1967.

Barnard, C. N.: The present status of heart transplantation. S. Afr. Med. J., 49:213, 1975.

Barnard, C. N., and Cooper, D. K. C.: Clinical transplantation of the heart: A review of 13 years' personal experience. J. R. Soc. Med., 74:670, 1981.

Barnard, C. N., and Losman, J. G.: Left ventricular bypass. S. Afr. Med. J., 49:303, 1975.

Barnard, C. N., and Wolpowitz, A.: Heterotopic versus orthotopic heart transplantation. Transplant. Proc., 11:309, 1979.

Barnard, C. N., Barnard, M. S., Cooper, D. K. C., Curchio, C. A., Hassoulas, J., Novitsky, D., and Wolpowitz, A.: The present status of heterotopic cardiac transplantation. J. Thorac. Cardiovasc. Surg., 81:433, 1981.

Barnard, C. N., Losman, J. G., Curcio, C. A., et al.: The advantage of heterotopic cardiac transplantation over orthotopic cardiac transplantation in the management of severe acute rejection. J. Thorac. Cardiovasc. Surg., 74:918, 1977.

Barnes, B. A., and Flax, M. H.: Experimental pulmonary homografts in the dog. II. Modification of the homograft response by BW 57-322. Transplantation, 2:343, 1964.

Baumgartner, W. A., Reitz, B. A., Oyer, P. E., Stinson, E. B., and Shumway, N. E.: Cardiac homotransplantation. Curr. Probl. Surg., 16:1, 1979.

Beck, W., Barnard, C. N., and Schrire, V.: Hemodynamic studies in two long-term survivors of heart transplantation. J. Thorac. Cardiovasc. Surg., 62:315, 1971.

Beecher, H. K., et al.: A definition of irreversible coma. (Report of the Ad Hoc Committee of the Harvard Medical School to examine the definition of brain death.) J.A.M.A., 205:85, 1968.

Benfield, J. R.: Invited commentary. World J. Surg., 1:182, 1977.

Benfield, J. R., and Coon, B. S.: The role of the left atrial anastomosis in pulmonary reimplantation. J. Thorac. Cardiovasc. Surg., 53:626, 1967.

Bentwich, Z., Douglas, S. D., Skultelsky, E., et al.: Sheep red cell binding to human lymphocytes treated with neuraminidase; enhancement of T-cell binding and identification of a subpopulation of B cells. J. Exp. Med., 137:1532, 1973.

Bieber, C. P., Griepp, R. B., Oyer, P. E., et al.: Relationships of rabbit ATG serum clearance rates to circulatory T-cell levels, rejection onset, and survival in cardiac transplantation. Transplant. Proc., 9:1031, 1977.

Bieber, C. P., Jamieson, S. W., Reitz, B. A., Oyer, P. E., Shumway, N. E., and Stinson, E. B.: Complications in long-term survivors of cardiac transplantation. Transplant. Proc., 13:207, 1981.

Billingham, M. E., Baumgartner, W. A., Watson, D. C., et al.: Distant heart procurement for human transplantation: Ultrastructural studies. Circulation, 62:1, 1980.

Blank, N., Castellino, R. A., and Shah, V.: Radiographic aspects of pulmonary infection in patients with altered immunity. Radiol. Clin. North Am., 11:175, 1973.

Blank, N., Lower, R. R., and Adams, D. F.: Bronchial dynamics and the reconstitution of bronchial artery supply in the autotransplanted lung. Invest. Radiol., 1:363, 1966.

Blumenstock, D. A.: Invited commentary. World J. Surg., 1:183, 1977.

Blumenstock, D. A.: Transplantation of the lung. Transplantation, 5:917, 1967.

Blumenstock, D. A., and Kahn, D. R.: Replantation and transplantation of the canine lung. J. Surg. Res., 1:40, 1961.

Blumenstock, D. A., et al.: Prolonged survival of orthotopic homotransplants of the heart in animals treated with methotrexate. J. Thorac. Cardiovasc. Surg., 46:616, 1963.

Borel, J., Feurer, C., Gubler, H. U., and Stahelin, H.: Biological effects of cyclosporin A: A new lymphocytic agent. Agents Actions, 6:468, 1976.

Britt, R. H., Enzman, D. R., and Remington, J. S.: Intracranial infection in cardiac transplant recipients. Ann. Neurol., 9:107, 1981.

Burton, D. S., Mochizuki, R. M., and Helpern, A. A.: Total hip arthroplasty in the cardiac transplant patient. Clin. Orthop., 130:186, 1978.

Calne, R. Y.: Immunosuppression for organ grafting—observations on cyclosporin A. Immunol. Rev., 46:113, 1979.

Calne, R. Y.: Transplant surgery: Current status. Br. J. Surg., 67:765, 1980.

Calne, R. Y., et al.: Cyclosporin-A initially as the only immunosuppressant in 34 recipients of cadaveric organs: 32 kidneys, 2 pancreases, and 2 livers. Lancet, 2:1033, 1979.

Calne, R. Y., White, D. J. G., Thiru, S., et al.: Cyclosporin A in patients receiving renal allografts from cadaver donors. Lancet, 2:1323, 1978a.

Calne, R. Y., Rolles, K., White, D. J. G., et al.: Cyclosporin A in clinical organ grafting. Transplant. Proc., 13:349, 1981.

Calne, R. Y., White, D. J. G., Rolles, K., et al.: Prolonged survival of pig orthotopic heart grafts treated with cyclosporin-A. Lancet, 1:1183, 1978b.

Campeau, L., Pospisil, L., Grondin, P., Dyrda, I., and Lepage, G.: Cardiac catheterization findings at rest and after exercise in patients following cardiac transplantation. Am. J. Cardiol., 25:523, 1970.

Cannom, D. S., Graham, A. F., and Harrison, D. C.: Electrophysiologic studies in the denervated transplanted human heart. Response to atrial pacing and atropine. Circ. Res., 32:268, 1973.

Cannom, D. S., Rider, A. K., Stinson, E. B., and Harrison, D. C.: Electrophysiologic studies in the denervated transplanted human heart. II. Response to norepinephrine, isoproterenol and propranolol. Am. J. Cardiol., 36:856, 1975.

Carrel, A., and Guthrie, C. C.: The transplantation of veins and organs. Am. J. Med., 11:1101, 1905.

Castaneda, A. R., Arnar, O., Schmidt-Habelmann, P., Moller, J. H., and Zamora, R.: Cardiopulmonary autotransplantation in primates. J. Cardiovasc. Surg., 37:523, 1972a.

Castaneda, A. R., Zamora, R., Schmidt-Habelmann, P., Hornung, J., Murphy, W., Ponto, D., and Moller, J. H.: Cardiopulmonary autotransplantation in primates (baboons). Late functional results. Surgery, 72:1064, 1972b.

Caves, P. K., Stinson, E. B., Graham, A. E., et al.: Percutaneous transvenous endomyocardial biopsy. J.A.M.A., 225:289, 1973.

Christopherson, L. K., and Lunde, D. T.: Selection of cardiac transplant recipients and their subsequent psychosocial adjustment. Semin. Psychiatry, 3:36, 1971.

Clark, D. A., Schroeder, J. S., Griepp, R. B., et al.: Cardiac transplantation in man, review of first three years experience. Am. J. Med., 54:563, 1973.

Collins, G. M., Bravo-Shugarman, M., and Terasaki, P. I.: Kidney preservation using a new perfusate. Lancet, 2:1219, 1969.

Cooley, D. A., Bloodwell, R. D., Hallman, G. L., Nora, J. J., Harrison, G. M., and Leachman, R. D.: Organ transplantation for advanced cardiopulmonary disease. Ann. Thorac. Surg., 8:300, 1969a.

Cooley, D. A., Nora, J. J., Trentin, J. J., Hallman, G. L., Bloodwell, R. D., and Leachman, R. D.: Clinical experience in transplantation of the human heart: Report of 10 cases. Transplant. Proc., 1:703, 1969b.

Cooper, D. K. C.: Transplantation of the heart and both lungs. I. Historical review. Thorax, 24:383, 1969.

Cooper, D. K. C., Charles, R. G., Fraser, R. C., Beck, W., and Barnard, C. N.: Long-term survival after orthotopic and heterotopic cardiac transplantation. Br. Med. J., 281:1093, 1980.

Copeland, J., Wieden, M., Feinberg, W., Salomon, N., Hager, D., and Galgiani, J.: Legionnaires' disease following cardiac transplantation. Chest, 79:669, 1981.

Copeland, J. G., Jones, M., Spragg, R., and Stinson, E. B.: In vitro preservation of canine hearts for 24 to 28 hours followed by successful orthotopic transplantation. Ann. Surg., 178:687, 1973.

Copeland, J. G., Griepp, R. B., Bieber, C. P., Billingham, M.,

Schroeder, J. S., Hunt, S., Mason, J., Stinson, E. B., and Shumway, N. E.: Successful retransplantation of the human heart. J. Thorac. Cardiovasc. Surg., 73:242, 1977.

Crane, R., Torres, M., Hagstrom, J. W. C., Koerner, S. K., and Veith, F. J.: Twenty four hour preservation and transplantation of the lung without functional impairment. Surg. Forum, 26:111, 1975.

Davis, H. A., O'Connor, J. P., Coloviras, G. J., and Strawn, D. A.: Homotransplantation of lung. Arch. Surg., 64:745, 1952a.

Davis, H. A., Gordon, W. B., Hayes, E. W., Jr., and Wasley, M. T.: The effects upon the lung of varying periods of temporary occlusion of the pulmonary artery. Arch. Surg., 64:464, 1952b.

Demikhov, V. P.: Experimental Transplantation of Vital Organs. New York, Consultants Bureau, 1962.

Demikov, V. P. (assisted by Goryainov, V. M.): Byull Eksp. Biol. Med., Vol. 4, 1950.

Derom, F., Barbier, F., Ringoir, S., Versieck, J., Rolly, G., Berzsenyi, G., Vermeire, P., and Vrints, L.: Ten-month survival after lung homotransplantation in man. J. Thorac. Cardiovasc. Surg., 61:835, 1971.

Dong, E., Jr., and Shumway, N. E.: Current results of human heart transplantation. World J. Surg., 1:157, 1977.

Dong, E., Hurley, E. J., Lower, R. R., and Shumway, N. E.: Performance of the heart two years after autotransplantation. Surgery, 56:270, 1964.

Dreyfuss, M., Harri, E., Hofman, H., et al.: Cyclosporin A and C: New metabolites from Trichoderma polysporum. Eur. J. Appl. Microbiol., 3:125, 1976.

Ellis, F. H., Jr., Grindlay, J. D., and Edwards, J. E.: The bronchial arteries. I. Experimental occlusions. Surgery, 30:810, 1951.

English, T. A. H., Cooper, D. K. C., and Cory-Pearce, R.: Recent experience with heart transplantation. Br. Med. J., 281:699, 1980.

Eraslan, S., Turner, M. D., and Hardy, J. D.: Lymphatic regeneration following lung reimplantation in dogs. Surgery, 56:970, 1964.

Garzon, A. A., Goldstein, S., Okadigwe, C. I., Paley, N. B., and Minkowitz, S.: Hypothermic lung preservation functions, six or more years later. Ann. Surg., 186:711, 1977.

Goldberg, M., Luk, S. C., Greyson, N. D., and Greenaway, A.: Canine lung allotransplantation: Donor pretreatment. Ann. Thorac. Surg., 24:462, 1977.

Griepp, R. B., Stinson, E. B., Dong, E., Jr., and Shumway, N. E.: Acute rejection of the allografted human heart. Ann. Thorac. Surg., 12:113, 1971a.

Griepp, R. B., Stinson, E. B., Clark, D. A., Dong, E., Jr., and Shumway, N. E.: The cardiac donor. Surg. Gynecol. Obstet., 133:792, 1971b.

Griepp, R. B., Wexler, L., Stinson, E. B., et al.: Coronary arteriography following cardiac transplantation. J.A.M.A., 221:147, 1972.

Griepp, R. B., Stinson, E. B., Bieber, C. P., Reitz, B. A., Copeland, J. G., Oyer, P. E., and Shumway, N. E.: Control of graft arteriosclerosis in human heart transplant recipients. Surgery, 81:262, 1977.

Griepp, R. B., Stinson, E. B., Dong, E., Jr., Clark, D. A., and Shumway, N. E.: Determinants of operative risk in human heart transplantation. Am. J. Surg., 122:192, 1971c.

Guthrie, C. C.: The surgery of blood vessels. Bull. Johns Hopkins Hosp., 18:25, 1907.

Hardin, C. A., Kittle, C. F., and Schafer, P. W.: Preliminary observations on homologous lung transplants in dogs. Surg. Forum, 3:374, 1952.

Hardy, J. D.: Lung transplantation. In Gibbon's Surgery of the Chest. 3rd Ed. Edited by D. C. Sabiston, Jr. and F. C. Spencer. Philadelphia, W. B. Saunders Company, 1976.

Hardy, J. D., Webb, W. R., Dalton, M. L., and Walker, G. R.: Lung homotransplantation in man: Report of initial case. J.A.M.A., 186:1065, 1963.

Harrison, D. C., Mason, J. W., Schroeder, J. S., and Stinson, E. B.: Effects of cardiac denervation on cardiac arrhythmias and electrophysiology. Br. Heart J., 40:17, 1978.

Hastillo, A., Hess, M. L., Richardson, D. W., and Lower, R. R.: Cardiac transplantation—1980: the Medical College of Virginia program. South. Med. J., 73:909, 1980.

Hotson, J. R., and Pedley, T. A.: The neurological complications of cardiac transplantation. Brain, 99:673, 1976.

Hugh-Jones, P., Macarthur, A. M., Cullum, P. A., Mason, S. A., Crosbie, W. A., Hutchison, D. C. S., Winterton, M. C., Smith, A. P., Mason, B., and Smith, L. A.: Lung transplantation in a patient with fibrosing alveolitis. Br. Med. J., 3:391, 1971.

Hunt, S. A., and Stinson, E. B.: Cardiac transplantation. Ann. Rev. Med., 32:213, 1981.

Jamieson, S. W., Burton, N. A., Bieber, C. P., et al.: Cardiac allograft survival in primates treated with cyclosporin A. Lancet, 1:545, 1979.

Juvenelle, A. A., Citret, C., Wiles, C. E., and Stewart, J. D.: Pneumonectomy with reimplantation of the lung in the dog for physiologic study. J. Thorac. Surg., 21:111, 1951.

Kahn, D. R., Carr, E. A., and Kersh, M. M.: Long-term function after human heart transplantation. J.A.M.A., 218:1699, 1971.

Kantrowitz, A., Yasunari, K., Carstensen, H. F., Sujansky, E., Haller, J. D., Krakauer, J. S., Neches, W., and Sherman, J. L., Jr.: Clinical and experimental observations in heart transplantation. Transplant. Proc., 1:727, 1969.

Kaplan, J., Aguirre, H., Eberhard, R., and Adriazola, N.: Complications of prolonged cortisone therapy. Laval Med., 41:292, 1970.

Koerner, S. K., Hagstrom, J. W. C., and Veith, F. J.: Transbronchial biopsy for the diagnosis of lung transplant rejection: Comparison with needle and open lung biopsy techniques in canine lung allografts. Am. Rev. Respir. Dis., 114:575, 1976.

Kondo, Y., Grodel, F., and Kantrowitz, A.: Heart transplantation in puppies: Long survival without immunosuppressive therapy. Circulation, 31, 32(Suppl. 1):181, 1965.

Kondo, Y., Cockrell, J. V., Kuwahara, O., and Hardy, J. D.: Histopathology of one-stage bilateral lung allografts. Ann. Surg., 180:753, 1974a.

Kondo, Y., Grogan, J. B., Cockrell, J. V., Kuramochi, T., Smith, G. V., and Hardy, J. D.: Comparison of the efficacy of immunosuppressive regimens on orthotopic heart allografts. J. Thorac. Cardiovasc. Surg., 67:612, 1974b.

Kosek, J. C., Bieber, C. P., and Lower, R. R.: Heart graft arteriosclerosis. Transplant. Proc., 3:512, 1971.

Kostakis, A. J., White, D. J. G., and Calne, R. Y.: Prolongation of rat heart allograft survival by cyclosporin A. IRCS Med. Sci., 5:280, 1977.

Krick, J. A., Stinson, E. B., and Remington, J. S.: Nocardia infection in heart transplant patients. Ann. Intern. Med., 82:128, 1975.

Lillehei, C. W.: Discussion of Wildevuur, C. R. H., and Benfield, J. R.: A review of 23 human lung transplantations by 20 surgeons. Ann. Thorac. Surg., 9:489, 1970.

Longmore, D. B., Cooper, D. K. C., Hall, R. W., Sekabunga, J., and Welch, W.: Transplantation of the heart and both lungs. II. Experimental cardiopulmonary transplantation. Thorax, 24:391, 1969.

Losman, J. G., and Barnard, C. N.: Hemodynamic evaluation of left ventricular bypass with a homologous cardiac graft. J. Thorac. Cardiovasc. Surg., 74:695, 1977.

Lower, R. R., and Shumway, N. E.: Studies on orthotopic transplantation of the canine heart. Surg. Forum, 11:18, 1960.

Lower, R. R., Dong, E., Jr., and Glazener, F. S.: Electrocardiograms of dogs with heart homografts. Circulation, 33:455, 1966.

Lower, R. R., Dong, E., Jr., and Shumway, N. E.: Long-term survival of cardiac homografts. Surgery, 58:110, 1965a.

Lower, R. R., Dong, E., Jr., and Shumway, N. E.: Suppression of rejection crises in the cardiac homograft. Ann. Thorac. Surg., 1:645, 1965b.

Lower, R. R., Stofer, R. C., Hurley, E. J., and Shumway, N. E.: Complete homograft replacement of the heart and both lungs. Surgery, 50:842, 1961.

Lower, R. R., Stofer, R. C., Hurley, E. J., Dong, E., Jr., Cohn, R. B., and Shumway, N. E.: Successful homotransplantation of the canine heart after anoxic preservation for seven hours. Am. J. Surg., 104:302, 1962.

Mann, F. C., Priestly, J. R., Markowitz, J., and Yates, W. M.: Transplantation of the intact mammalian heart. Arch. Surg., 26:219, 1933.

Mason, J. W., Stinson, E. B., Hunt, S. A., Schroeder, J. S., and Rider, A. K.: Infections after cardiac transplantation: Relation to rejection therapy. Ann. Intern. Med., 85:69, 1976.

Matas, A. J., Hertel, B. F., Rossi, J., Simmons, R. L., and Najarian, J. S.: Post-transplant malignant lymphoma—distinctive morphologic features related to its pathogenesis. Am. J. Med., 61:716, 1976.

Meere, C., Grondin, C. M., Castonguay, Y., Lepage, G., and Grondin, P.: Clinical experience with cardiac transplantation: Retrospective considerations. Cardiovasc. Clin., 2:277, 1971.

Metras, H.: Preliminary report of lung grafts in the dog. C. R. Acad. Sci. (Paris), 231:1176, 1950. Cited in Transplantation. Edited by J. S. Najarian and R. L. Simmons. Philadelphia, Lea & Febiger, 1972.

Mills, N. L., Boyd, A. D., and Gheranpong, C.: The significance of bronchial circulation in lung transplantation. J. Thorac. Cardiovasc. Surg., 60:866, 1970.

Mohandas, A., and Chou, S. N.: Brain death: A clinical and pathological study. J. Neurosurg., 32:211, 1971.

Nakae, S., Webb, W. R., Theodorides, T., and Sugg, W. L.: Respiratory function following cardiopulmonary denervation in dog, cat and monkey. Surg. Gynecol. Obstet, 125:1285, 1967.

Nelums, J. M. B., Rebuck, A. S., Cooper, J. D., Goldberg, M., Halloran, P. F., and Hellend, H.: Human lung transplantation. Chest, 78:569, 1980.

Neptune, W. B., Redondo, H., and Bailey, C. P.: Experimental lung transplantation. Surg. Forum, 3:379, 1952.

Neptune, W. B., Cookson, B. A., Bailey, C. P., Appler, R., and Rajkowski, F.: Complete homologous heart transplantation. Arch. Surg., 66:174, 1953.

Oyer, P. E., et al.: Preliminary results of cyclosporin A in clinical cardiac transplantation. In Proceedings of the International Symposium on Cyclosporin A. Edited by R. Calne and D. White. Elsevier North-Holland, 1982.

Oyer, P. E., Stinson, E. B., Bieber, C. P., Reitz, B. A., Raney, A. A., Baumgartner, W. A., and Shumway, N. E.: Diagnosis and treatment of acute cardiac allograft rejection. Transplant. Proc., 11:296, 1979.

Pearson, F. G., Goldberg, M., Stone, R. M., and Colapinto, R. F.: Bronchial arterial circulation restored after reimplantation of canine lung. Can. J. Surg., 13:243, 1970.

Penn, I.: Development of cancer as a complication of clinical transplantation. Transplant. Proc., 9:1121, 1977.

Penn, I., Halgrimson, C. G., and Starzl, T. E.: De novo malignant tumors in organ transplant recipients. Transplant. Proc., 3:773, 1971.

Pennock, J. L., Reitz, B. A., Bieber, C. P., Jamieson, S. W., et al.: Cardiac allograft survival in cynomolgus monkeys treated with cyclosporin A in combination with conventional immunosuppression. Transplant. Proc., 13:390, 1981.

Pennock, J. L., Oyer, P. E., Reitz, B. A., et al.: Cardiac transplantation in perspective for the future: Survival, complications, rehabilitation, and costs. J. Thorac. Cardiovasc. Surg., 83:168, 1982.

Petcher, T. J., Weber, H. P., and Ruegger, A.: Crystal and molecular structure of an iodo-derivative of the cyclic undecapeptide cyclosporin A. Helv. Chim. Acta, 59:1480, 1976.

Pinkser, K. L., Koerner, S. K., Kamholz, S. L., Hagstrom, J. W. C., and Veith, F. J.: Effect of donor bronchial length on healing. J. Thorac. Cardiovasc. Surg., 77:669, 1979.

Pope, S. E., Stinson, E. B., Daughters, G. T., Schroeder, J. S., Ingels, N. B., and Alderman, E. L.: Exercise response of the denervated heart in long-term cardiac transplant recipients. Am. J. Cardiol., 46:213, 1980.

Reemtsma, K.: The heart as a test organ in transplantation studies. Ann. N.Y. Acad. Sci., 120:778, 1964.

Reemtsma, K., Drusin, R., Edie, R., Bergman, D., Dobelle, W., and Hardy, M.: Cardiac transplantation for patients requiring mechanical circulatory support. N. Engl. J. Med., 298:670, 1978.

Reemtsma, K., Williamson, W. E., Jr., Iglesias, F., Pena, E., Sayegh, S. F., and Creech, O., Jr.: Studies in homologous canine heart transplantation: Prolongation of survival with a folic acid antagonist. Surgery, 52:127, 1962.

Reemtsma, K., Rogers, R. E., Lucas, J. F., Schmidt, F. E., and Davis, F. H., Jr.: Studies of pulmonary function in transplantation of the canine lung. J. Thorac. Cardiovasc. Surg., 46:589, 1963.

Reitz, B. A., Baumgartner, W. A., Oyer, P. E., and Stinson, E. B.: Abdominal aortic aneurysmectomy in long-term cardiac transplant survivors. Arch. Surg., 112:1057, 1977.

Reitz, B. A., Bieber, C. P., Raney, A. A., Pennock, J. L., Jamieson, S. W., Oyer, P. E., and Stinson, E. B.: Orthotopic heart and combined heart and lung transplantation with cyclosporin-A immune suppression. Transplant. Proc., 13:393, 1981a.

Reitz, B. A., Burton, N. A., Jamieson, S. W., Bieber, C. P., Pennock, J. L., Stinson, E. B., and Shumway, N. E.: Heart and lung transplantation, autotransplantation and allotransplantation in primates with extended survival. J. Thorac. Cardiovasc. Surg., 80:360, 1980.

Reitz, B. A., Wallwork, J. L., Hunt, S. A., Pennock, J. L., Billingham, M. E., Oyer, P. E., Stinson, E. B., and Shumway, N. E.: Heart-lung transplantation: Successful therapy for patients with pulmonary vascular disease. N. Engl. J. Med., 306:557, 1982.

Reitz, B. A., Pennock, J. L., and Shumway, N. E.: Simplified method for heart and lung transplantation. J. Surg. Res., 31:1, 1981b.

Ruegger, A., Kuhm, M., Lichiti, H., et al.: Cyclosporin A, ein immunosuppressiv wirksemer peptidmetabolit aus Trichoderma polysporum. Helv. Chim. Acta, 59:1075, 1976.

Sacks, S. A., Petritisch, P. H., and Kaufman, J. J.: Canine kidney preservation using a new perfusate. Lancet, 1:1024, 1973.

Savin, W. M., Haskell, W. L., Schroeder, J. S., and Stinson, E. B.: Cardiorespiratory responses of cardiac transplant patients to graded, symptom-limited exercise. Circulation, 62:55, 1980.

Scheuer, J., Shaver, J. A., Harris, B. C., Leonard, J. J., and Bahnson, H. E.: Electrocardiographic findings in cardiac transplantation. Circulation, 40:289, 1969.

Schroeder, J. S.: Hemodynamic performance of the human transplanted heart. Transplant. Proc., 11:304, 1979.

Semb, B. K. H., Abraham, D. M., and Barnard, C. N.: Electrocardiographic changes during the unmodified rejection of heterotopic canine heart allografts. Scand. J. Thorac. Cardiovasc. Surg., 5:120, 1971.

Shaver, J. A., Leon, D. F., Gray, G., III, Leonard, J. J., and Bahnson, H. T.: Hemodynamic observations after cardiac transplantation. N. Engl. J. Med., 281:822, 1969.

Sheil, A. C. R.: Cancer in renal allograft recipients in Australia and New Zealand. Transplant. Proc., 1:1133, 1977.

Shumway, N. E., Lower, R. R., and Stofer, R. C.: Transplantation of the heart. Adv. Surg., 2:265, 1966.

Siegelman, S. S., Sinha, S. B. P., and Veith, F. J.: Pulmonary reimplantation response. Ann. Surg., 177:30, 1971.

Siegelman, S. S., Hagstrom, J. W. C., Koerner, S. K., and Veith, F. J.: Restoration of bronchial artery circulation after canine lung allotransplantation. J. Thorac. Cardiovasc. Surg., 73:30, 1977.

Silverman, J. F., Lipton, M. J., Graham, A., Harris, S., and Weller, L.: Coronary arteriography in long-term human cardiac transplantation survivors. Circulation, 50:838, 1974.

Starzl, T. E., Iwatsuki, S., Klintmalm, G., et al.: Liver transplantation 1980, with particular reference to cyclosporin A. Transplant. Proc., 13:281, 1981.

Staudacher, V. E., Bellinazzo, P., and Pulin, A.: Chirurgia (Milano), 5:223, 1950. Cited by Blumenstock, D.: Transplantation of the lung. Transplantation, 5:917, 1967.

Stevens, P. M., Johnson, P. C., Bell, R. L., Beall, A. C., Jr., and Jenkins, D. E.: Regional ventilation and perfusion after lung transplantation in patients with emphysema. N. Engl. J. Med., 282:245, 1970.

Stinson, E. B., Payne, R., Griepp, R. B., Schroeder, J. S., Dong, E., Jr., and Shumway, N. E.: Correlation of histocompatibility matching with graft rejection and survival after cardiac transplantation in man. Lancet, 2:459, 1971.

Stinson, E. B., Griepp, R. B., Schroeder, J. S., et al.: Hemodynamic observations one and two years after cardiac transplantation in man. Circulation, 45:1183, 1972.

Taquini, A. C., Fermoso, J. D., and Aramendia, P.: Behavior of the right ventricle following acute constriction of the pulmonary artery. Circ. Res., 8:315, 1960.

Thomas, F. J., Blaisdell, F. W., and Veith, F. J.: Unpublished data. Cited in Veith, F. J.: Lung transplantation. Surg. Clin. North Am., 58:357, 1978.

Thomas, F. T., Szentpetery, S. S., Mammana, R. E., Wolfgang, T. C., and Lower, R. R.: Long-distance transportation of human hearts for transplantation. Ann. Thorac. Surg., 26:346, 1978.

Toledo-Pereyra, L. H., and Condie, R. M.: Lung transplantation, hypothermic storage for 24 hours in a colloid hyperosmolar solution. J. Thorac. Cardiovasc. Surg., 76:846, 1978.

Toledo-Pereyra, L. H., Hau, T., Simmons, R. L., and Najarian, J. S.: Lung preservation techniques (collective review). Ann. Thorac. Surg., 3:487, 1977.

Trummer, M. J., and Christiansen, K. H.: Radiographic and functional changes following autotransplantation of the lung. J. Thorac. Cardiovasc. Surg., 49:1006, 1965.

Tutschka, P. J.: Cyclosporin A in bone marrow transplantation. In Proceedings of the International Symposium on Cyclosporin A. Edited by R. Calne and D. White. Elsevier North-Holland, 1982.

Veith, F. J.: Lung transplantation. Surg. Clin. North Am., 58:357, 1978.

Veith, F. J., and Koerner, S. K.: The present status of lung transplantation. Arch. Surg., 109:734, 1974.

Veith, F. J., and Koerner, S. K.: Lung transplantation, 1977. World J. Surg., 1:177, 1977.

Veith, F. J., and Richards, K.: Mechanism and prevention of fixed high vascular resistance in autografted and allografted lungs. Science, 163:699, 1969a.

Veith, F. J., and Richards, K.: Improved technic for canine lung transplantation. Ann. Surg., 171:553, 1970.

Veith, F. J., and Richards, K.: Lung transplantation with simultaneous contralateral pulmonary artery ligation. Surg. Gynecol. Obstet., 129:768, 1969b.

Veith, F. J., Hagstrom, J. W. C., et al.: Alveolar manifestations of rejection: An important cause of the poor results with human lung transplantation. Ann. Surg., 175:336, 1972.

Veith, F. J., Koerner, S. K., Siegelman, S. S., Kawakami, M., Kaufman, S., Attai, L. A., Hagstrom, J. W. C., and Gliedman, M. L.: Diagnosis and reversal of rejection in experimental and clinical lung allografts. Ann. Thorac. Surg., 16:172, 1973a.

Veith, F. J., Koerner, S. K., Siegelman, S. S., Torres, M., Bardfeld, P. A., Attai, L. A., Boley, S. J., Takaro, T., and Gliedman, M. L.: Single lung transplantation in experimental and human emphysema. Ann. Surg., 178:463, 1973b.

Veith, F. J., Norin, A. J., Montefusco, C. M., Pinsker, K. L., Kamholz, S. L., Gliedman, M. L., and Emeson, E.: Cyclosporin-A in experimental lung transplantation. Transplantation, 32:474, 1981.

Vital Statistics of the United States. Washington, D.C., Health, Education and Welfare, Public Health Service, National Center for Health Statistics, 1980.

Watson, D. C., Jr.: Consistent survival after prolonged donor heart preservation. Transplant. Proc., 9:297, 1977.

Watson, D. C., Reitz, B. A., Baumgartner, W. A., Raney, A. A., Oyer, P. E., Stinson, E. B., and Shumway, N. E.: Distant heart procurement for transplantation. Surgery, 86:56, 1979.

Watson, D. C., Reitz, B. A., Oyer, P. E., Stinson, E. B., and Shumway, N. E.: Sequential orthotopic heart transplantation in man. Transplantation, 30:401, 1980.

Webb, W. R., and Howard, H. S.: Cardiopulmonary transplantation. Surg. Forum, 8:313, 1957.

Wildevuur, C. R. H., and Benfield, J. R.: A review of 23 human lung transplantations by 20 surgeons. Ann. Thorac. Surg., 9:489, 1970.

Chapter 54

The Total Artificial Heart

WILLIAM C. DeVRIES

Heart disease in the United States takes its toll of over one million lives each year. Hopes that preventive measures may soon reduce this number are balanced by many therapeutic procedures being developed to prevent death from previously existing disease. Since the mid 1960s, approximately $160 million in federal funds have been used for research in the development of the total artificial heart. Significant advances in biomaterials and pump and energy systems as well as animal experimentations have led to the current clinical reality of total artificial heart implantation in man.

HISTORY

In 1813, Legallois first postulated continuous perfusion of oxygenated blood to support the circulation and suggested replacement of hearts in animals. He noted that "if the place of the heart could be supplied by injection — and if for the regular continuance of this injection, there could be furnished a quantity of arterial blood, whether natural, or artificially formed, supposing such a formation possible — then life might be indefinitely maintained in any portion."

In 1868, Ludwig and Schmidt oxygenated blood extracorporeally by swirling venous blood in a flask. A simple continuous-flow bubble-oxygenator was first demonstrated by Von Schroder in 1882. Von Frey, in 1884, and Jacobi, in 1890, developed early designs for pump-oxygenators.

In 1904, Herrick described the first antemortem diagnosis of coronary artery insufficiency. Since this time, scientists have been struggling with many means of supporting the failing myocardium. Two significant milestones in the development of successful blood pumps were the discovery of the different blood groups in 1900 by Landsteiner and the discovery of heparin by McLean in 1916. Soon after his first solo transatlantic flight in 1927, Charles A. Lindbergh was stimulated by his sister-in-law, who was critically ill with valvular heart disease, to study the possible modes of cardiac support. Lindbergh sought the advice of Dr. Alexis Carrel in developing a pump-oxygenator, and in 1935, Lindbergh demonstrated the feasibility of total body perfusion:

We can perhaps dream of removing diseased organs from the body and placing them in the Lindbergh pump as the patients are placed in a hospital. There the organs could be treated far more energetically than within the organism and, if cured, replanted in the patient.

As early as 1934, Dr. Michael DeBakey designed a simple roller pump and suggested its use as an augmenting device for the transport of blood. In 1937, Dr. John Gibbon, a surgical fellow, developed early working models of the heart-lung machine, and in the 1950s, he was the first to use it clinically.

In the early 1950s, investigators such as Kantrowitz, Shumtcher, DeBakey, Kolff, and Birtwell began working with the concept of mechanical devices to assist a failing heart rather than merely to bypass the heart during the periods of intracardiac operations. As early as 1953, Kantrowitz found that augmenting the arterial diastolic pressure and augmenting coronary perfusion by retardation of the systolic pressure could increase coronary flow up to 50 per cent. In 1958, Kantrowitz immobilized the left hemidiaphragm of a dog and sutured it around the distal thoracic aorta. By synchronized electrical stimulation to the phenic nerve in this dog, he was able to augment aortic diastolic pressures. In 1961, Clauss used an external pump actuator system and arterial cannulation to reduce systolic pressure and augment diastolic arterial pressure in dogs by synchronized withdrawal and infusion of blood through the femoral artery. In 1962, Moulopoulos and Kolff constructed an inflatable latex balloon that was inserted in the descending aorta of a dog through the femoral artery and thus introduced the modern concept of intra-aortic balloon pumping. Intra-aortic counterpulsation was first clinically used by Kantrowitz in 1967. In his series, 16 patients in cardiogenic shock were supported with an intra-aortic balloon pump. Three died during the interruption of counterpulsation. Of the 13 patients who recovered from the cardiogenic shock, seven were long-term survivors. Since its early beginnings, the intra-aortic balloon pump has become a household word in medical centers in which patients with failing hearts are cared for, as well as in many centers in which cardiac surgery is performed, and has saved countless numbers of patients who would have otherwise died. The first clinically working cardiopulmonary bypass machine, developed by Gibbon in the early 1950s, has opened the doors for the correction of many cardiac disease states and has also saved millions of lives.

As early as 1961, Edmunds described the possibility of maintaining systemic circulation at levels of 100 mm. Hg by left atrial–to–systemic bypass pumping. This system was later applied to six patients, to one for as long as 2 hours. One patient with a ruptured aortic aneurysm survived for 35 days. In these patients, left heart bypass was used after closed chest cardiopulmonary resuscitation had been ineffective. In 1961, Dr. Clarence Dennis described the clinical application of transjugular cannulation of the left atrium to left ventricular bypass support. This technique was applied to one patient with cardiac failure for a period of 12 hours. In 1963, Liotta described application of a pneumatically powered auxiliary left ventricle in three patients with postoperative left heart failure. This device was not successful in permitting the survival of any of these patients. Later, Kennedy described the use of open chest left heart bypass for intractable ventricular fibrillation in two patients who had undergone cardiac surgery using cardiopulmonary bypass. Several years later, Spencer used an open chest left heart bypass, with some degree of success, in a patient who could not be withdrawn from cardiopulmonary bypass following cardiac surgery. In 1975, Litwak anastomosed mandrel-fitted conduits to the ascending aorta from the left atrium at the conclusion of surgery in patients who could not be withdrawn from cardiopulmonary bypass. A roller pump–type assist was instituted in 14 patients, and the condition of nine could be stabilized. Six of these patients were eventually discharged from the hospital, and four have been long-term survivors. In 1971, DeBakey reported two successful clinical cases in which the patients were pumped with left ventricular assist devices for 4 to 10 days.

Within the last 5 years, well over 170 patients have been supported with bypass ventricles in Houston (Norman), Boston (Barnhardt), Salt Lake City (Peters), Hershey (Pierce), Vienna (Unger), Zurich (Senning), Japan (Taguchi), and New York (Spencer). The clinical outcome has been generally disappointing. Approximately 66 patients have been weaned from their devices, and 36 were reported to have left the hospital, with even fewer long-term survivors (Table 54–1).

The current left ventricular assist devices pump blood either via the left atrium to the aorta (Taguchi, Pierce, Litwak, Laks) or via the left ventricular apex to the aorta (Peters, Bernstein, Radvany, Norman) with a roller pump or an auxiliary ventricle placed in extracorporeal circulation in the intrathoracic, extrathoracic, or intra-abdominal position.

The major problems with these clinical left ven-

TABLE 54–1. EXPERIENCE WITH TEMPORARY LEFT VENTRICULAR ASSISTANCE (MARCH 1981)*

	PATIENTS	WEANED	LONG-TERM SURVIVORS
ROLLER PUMP			
Houston (DeBakey)	1	1	1
New York (Litwak)	15	10	5
Hiroshima (Taguchi)	20	11	7
St. Louis (Laks)	3	2	1
New York (Spencer)	15	6	4
Utah (Peters)	8	2	1
CENTRIFUGAL PUMP			
Cleveland (Golding)	12	3	2
St. Louis (Pennington)	13	4	2
SAC-TYPE PUMP			
Houston (DeBakey)	10	2	2
Houston (Norman)	22	3	1
Boston (Bernhard)	17	6	3
Hershey (Pierce)	17	6	1
Vienna (Wolmer)	10	6	1
Zurich (Turina)	6	4	2
Tokyo (Atsumi)	1	0	0
Total	170	66	33

*Reported by the National Heart, Lung and Blood Institute Working Council on the Report on the Artificial Heart, March 1981.

tricular mechanical pump cases have been (1) right ventricular failure, which limits left ventricular filling and bypass pumping, (2) massive hemorrhage, (3) infection, and (4) patient multisystem failure. The guidelines for utilizing the assist device in some of these cases were so stringent that many of the patients were bypassed in a near-terminal state.

The first total artificial heart replacement in an animal was successfully performed by Akutsu and Kolff in 1957 on a dog that survived approximately 90 minutes at the Cleveland Clinic. From this beginning, investigators at other centers have designed and implemented successful heart transplantation experiments in calves and sheep.

In 1969, Denton Cooley was faced with a 47-year-old man with irreversible cardiac decompensation. The patient was taken to the operating room for a ventricular aneurysmectomy. The patient could not be weaned from cardiopulmonary bypass, and his native heart was removed. Total pneumatically driven right and left ventricles were implanted. This orthotopic cardiac prosthesis was used to keep the patient alive for approximately 64 hours after implantation. At that time, a cardiac transplant was performed. This heart transplant functioned for 32 hours, at which time the patient died of overwhelming pneumonia.

In July 1981, Cooley was faced with a young Dutchman who had cardiac arrest in the intensive care unit several hours after undergoing a triple-vessel coronary artery bypass graft operation. He was returned to the operating room, and a pneumatic artificial heart, developed by Akutsu, was implanted. The patient survived for several days until heart transplantation could be performed. The artificial heart was removed, and the transplant was implanted. The patient survived for 10 additional days before succumbing. In both cases, the artificial heart was used an in intermediary device until cardiac implantation could be performed.

DESCRIPTION OF THE UNIVERSITY OF UTAH TOTAL ARTIFICIAL HEART AND DRIVING SYSTEM

The Utah total artificial heart is one that has been developed through approximately 20 years by scientists associated with the University of Utah group. The current pump has been designed by Dr. Robert K. Jarvik. The ventricles are constructed of a smooth blood surface fabricated by Biomer (segmented polyurethane). It is pneumatically powered, consisting of two separate ventricles with air chambers (Figs. 54–1 and 54–2). Air is intermittently pulsed (at adjustable rates of 40 to 120 per minute) in and out of the air chamber, activating the diaphragm. The ventricles are fashioned so that the blood surface is attached to the housing in a continuous layer. The two ventricles displace a total of 680 ml. Each ventricle has a stroke volume of 120 ml. The overall shape is spherical, with anatomic transitions to the great vessels and atria. Four clinical grade pyrolytic carbon disc valves are used to achieve unidirectional flow. Connections to the natural atria are achieved by atrial cuffs fabricated of Dacron felt connected to the total artificial heart by "quick connect systems" consisting of coated rigid polycarbonated segments. The connections to the great vessels consist of Dacron vascular prosthetic grafts (Fig. 54–2).

The drive lines consist of ½-inch reinforced polyurethane tubing exiting the body in the left periumbilical area. These lines are covered at the skin level with uniquely constructed velour skin buttons to en-

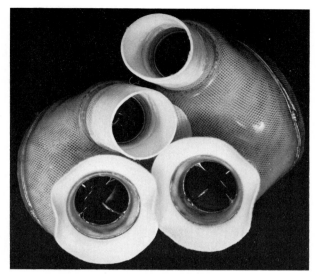

Figure 54–2. Utah total artificial heart.

hance tissue ingrowth around the skin in spite of the frequent external movement by the patients. These tubes will connect to two 6-foot long ⅝-inch polyurethane tubes into the drive system (Fig. 54–3). These drive tubes will be further secured to the patient's body by a specially adapted abdominal belt. This prevents any tension from the tube being converted to the exiting drive lines. All connections will be tightly fixed to prevent disconnection.

The Utah pneumatic heart driver is connected to a source of compressed air, vacuum, and electricity. The compressed air may be adapted from the routine hospital outlets or from portable cylinders of N_2 or air. Portable cylinders the size of two scuba tanks could support the patient for approximately 4 to 6

JARVIK ELLIPTICAL ARTIFICIAL HEART VENTRICLE

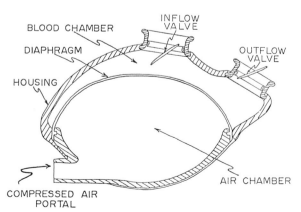

Figure 54–1. Cutaway of pneumatic ventricle.

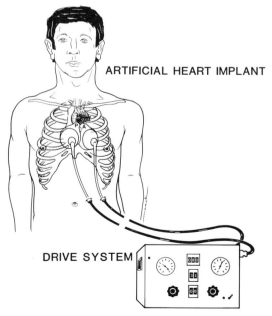

Figure 54–3. Artificial heart and drive system.

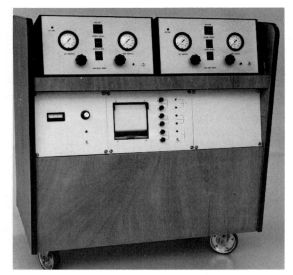

Figure 54–4. Utah heart drive system.

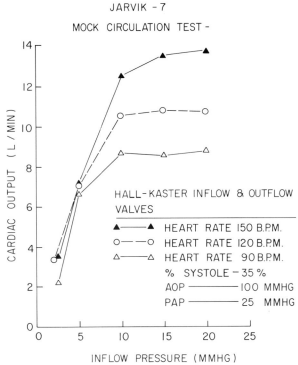

Figure 54–6. Starling curves for the artificial heart.

hours. The vacuum line is optional. The electrical system is backed up by rechargeable batteries in order to compensate immediately for interruption of electricity. The driving system may be simply regulated as to beats per minute and independent strength to the right ventricle as well as to the left ventricle (Fig. 54–4). The entire driving system with back-up facilities for air and electricity can be made into a portable cart about the size of an adult wheelchair.

Currently being tested is a portable drive system weighing less than 8 pounds and measuring approximately the size of a small camera case. This system has rechargeable batteries capable of up to 3 hours' operation and is completely portable. Several animals have been exercised while using this portable system, with excellent results (Fig. 54–5).

Physiologically, the pump has been tested by numerous *in vivo* as well as extensive *in vitro* studies. The heart obeys Starling's length-tension relationships, with cardiac outputs of 13 liters per minute capable at inflow pressures of 18 mm. Hg. This device is totally autoregulated on inflow pressures (and therefore volumes) because of the vented end-diastolic pressures. If inflow pressures are low, the resulting stroke volume is low. If inflow pressures are higher,

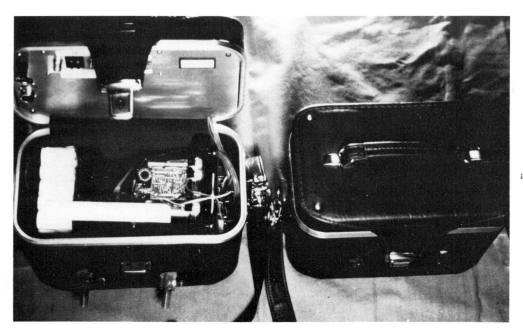

Figure 54–5. Utah portable drive system.

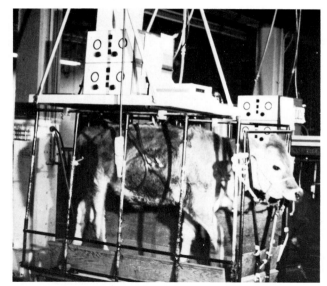

Figure 54–7. "Tennyson," a calf with an artificial heart, 221 days after implantation—a world record!

TABLE 54–2. COMPLICATIONS OF THE TOTAL ARTIFICIAL HEART

1. Hemorrhage
2. Infection
3. Pneumothorax
4. Emboli
5. Device failure
   Driver
   Pump
   Valves
6. Hemolysis

the resulting stroke volume is greater. Complete autoregulation is thus only dependent on inflow volumes and resulting stroke volumes (Fig. 54–6).

Numerous mock circulation tests have shown that the Utah total artificial heart ventricles as well as driving systems are extremely durable and reliable mechanically. Currently, Jarvik-7 hearts and drivers have been tested under physiologic stresses in an *in vitro* system for over 2 years (108,079,500 cycles) without physiologic deterioration.

Since 1968, approximately 250 total artificial hearts have been implanted at the University of Utah in either growing calves or sheep. Mean survival times have increased from 10 hours in 1969 to over 75 days currently. Recently, our group had one calf live for 221 days (Fig. 54–7).

Causes of termination have been diverse (Table 54–2). Many calves have outgrown the mechanical heart. (The adult cow requires a cardiac output of greater than 16 liters per minute. The total artificial heart will not consistently supply this great output.) Some animals have developed a fibrous connective tissue (pannus) around the inflow ports, causing relative tricuspid or mitral stenosis. (It is believed that this scarring is a unique characteristic of the calf.) Infection of the prosthesis has not been a common problem since the use of specifically designed skin buttons has decreased infection around the pump lines. Mechanical failure is an unusual occurrence that leads to termination.

Damage to the cellular components of the blood was once considered a limiting factor in the survival of calves with a total artificial heart. Improvements in heart design, materials, fabrication techniques, and postoperative management have resulted in animals in an excellent state of health for prolonged periods of time with hematologic, chemical, and coagulation assays well within normal limits. At 10 to 14 days, the hematocrits reach the lowest level (approximately 24 per cent) and then begin a gradual increase until an approximate level of 31 to 34 per cent is reached (normals: 37.6 ± 4.3). Blood transfusions are usually given only during the initial 24 postoperative hours (Fig. 54–8).

The interaction of the artificial heart and the blood does cause mild alterations in the kinetics of the platelets and fibrinogen. However, the calves appear to compensate for these changes and are maintained in healthy conditions for extended periods.

Figure 54–8. Destruction of blood cells during pumping with the artificial heart (n = 34).

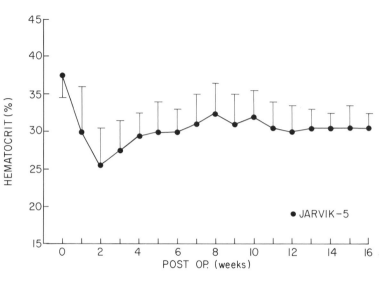

TABLE 54–3. SUGGESTED PROTOCOL FOR A PATIENT WHO IS UNABLE TO BE WEANED FROM CARDIOPULMONARY BYPASS

1. Drugs: Dopamine, nitroprusside, epinephrine, Levophed

2. Intra-aortic balloon pump (IABP)

3. Hemodynamics:
   CPB less than 0.8 L./M.^{2}
   LAP greater than 25 mm. Hg
   CI less than 1.8 L./M.^{2}
   AVO$_2$ greater than 7.0
   BP less than 80 mm. Hg

4. Implantation of total artificial heart (TAH)

PATIENT SELECTION

Before considering the group of patients in whom this device should be used, it is important to be able to define the success ratio for any device. It is important to emphasize that this is an *experimental device* and that any implied therapeutic efficacy will have to be determined after patient trials. Before tethering a patient to a pneumatic artificial heart, one must be sure that the artificial heart drive system is a reliable, simple, and effective physiologic support mechanism. Before implanting an artificial heart in a patient, a group must be able to demonstrate successful animal experimentation data showing good average life expectancy of the animals, as well as some long-term survivors.

There are three main groups of patients who may benefit from the total artificial heart in the United States. The first group is a small number of patients who have undergone corrective cardiac surgery and are unable to be weaned from the heart-lung bypass (Table 54–3). This group of patients will have many pharmacologic support mechanisms as well as an intra-aortic balloon pump in place. Several groups applying left ventricular assist devices have stated that approximately 1800 patients in this group in the United States may require a left ventricular assist device or a total artificial heart in order to maintain life after failing to be weaned from the pump with pharmacologic support and an intra-aortic balloon pump in place (Table 54–4). It is mandatory that these patients provide informed consent, having been given details of all the risks and benefits before the original corrective surgery is performed. It should be emphasized that this particular group of patients are faced with few ethical problems because the artificial heart is an attractive alternative to death.

The next group of patients are the ones with end-

TABLE 54–4. CURRENT POST-PUMP SUPPORT MECHANISMS IN THE UNITED STATES OF AMERICA

125,000	(estimated) require *CPB*/year
30,000	require *pharmacologic support*
7500	require additional *IABP*
1875	require additional *LVAD* or *TAH*

stage, intractable cardiac failure. It has been estimated that there are approximately 5000 to 15,000 deaths a year in this group in the United States. This group would be available to be completely informed about the procedure and to give informed consent before the surgery and would understand that the device would be implanted before he or she underwent the procedure. This group does require careful ethical consideration in that each patient will have to accept the fact that the device may shorten rather than lengthen his life. Many people believe that patients should not be considered from this group until human clinical efficacy is demonstrated in the unweanable cardiopulmonary bypass patient group.

Cardiac transplantation has been successful in this group of patients with end-stage cardiac failure. Currently, approximately 30 transplants are performed yearly in the United States because of limited donors. The 1-year survival rate is estimated to be approximately 70 per cent, with a 50 per cent 5-year survival rate. Because of the shortage of donors, transplants are not effective treatment modalities for emergency patients such as those who are unweanable from cardiopulmonary bypass or who are in cardiogenic shock. The total artificial heart, however, may serve well as an interim device. Still, there are many patients who die of heart disease who are not transplant candidates because of age or existing diseases. These patients may well have to choose the artificial heart. There are a considerable number of patients who expire while awaiting cardiac transplantation (up to 30 per cent of patients on the waiting list). The total artificial heart may be an excellent device to sustain life until an appropriate donor match may be obtained. The surgical implantation of the artificial heart does not destroy the natural atrial pulmonary artery or the aorta's anatomy for a later transplantation (Fig. 54–9).

The third group consists of patients dying of acute cardiogenic shock. It is estimated that between 10,000 and 30,000 of these patients die per year in the United States. At present, the difficulty with this group is the

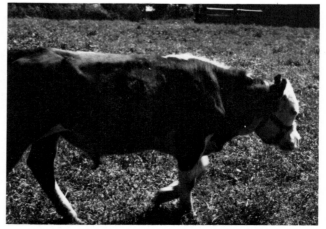

Figure 54–9. "Fernando." This calf lived for 90 days with his natural heart, 44 days with a total artificial heart, and, shown here, 372 days after a living related cardiac transplant, demonstrating the feasibility of using the artificial heart as a "stopgap" method.

TABLE 54–5. POSSIBLE TAH CANDIDATES (USA)

1. Unweanable from CPB	2000/year
2. Cardiomyopathy	5000–10,000/year
3. Acute cardiogenic shock	10,000–20,000/year

lack of ability to get informed consent from the patient. This is especially important when dealing with an experimental device whose clinical efficacy has not yet been determined. (See Table 54–5.)

As the total artificial heart, short- and long-term left and right ventricular assist devices, and cardiac transplantation are used more clinically, we will, in the very near future, learn which clinical conditions are appropriate indications for each modality. Left ventricular assist devices should be used in cases of *reversible* myocardial insufficiency to support the circulation until healing occurs. Some patients who are thought now to be unweanable from cardiopulmonary bypass or who are in cardiogenic shock may respond successfully to the assist pumps and not require the extirpation necessary with the total artificial heart. The clinical problem is to determine which subgroups of patients have irreversible damage and which do not. The question of whether a left ventricular assist device may be used initially to see if the patient's heart is capable of hemodynamic recovery and then implanting the total artificial heart if the natural heart does not recover has been raised. Another pertinent question may also be asked: "Does the failure of one experimental device indicate the placement of another experimental device?"

The common clinical failures of the left ventricular assist devices are shock, hypoperfusion, disseminated intravascular coagulation, infection, acute tubular necrosis, pulmonary insufficiency, and bleeding. Any one of these complications would rule out the implantation of a total artificial heart. This point is pertinent when the possibility of success with a total artificial heart used initially may be greater than that with a left ventricular assist device. Most of the investigators in the field of left ventricular assist devices will admit that the chances of a total artificial heart functioning after failure of the left ventricular assist device is extremely slight and that, at this time, it is not a viable patient treatment alternative (Tables 54–6 and 54–7).

TABLE 54–6. COMPARISON OF THE TOTAL ARTIFICIAL HEART CARDIAC TRANSPLANTATION

ADVANTAGES	DISADVANTAGES
1. No donor problem	1. Experimental
2. No immunosuppression	2. Tether
3. Emergency—shelf item	3. Infection
4. Relatively low cost	4. Hemolysis
5. Age not contraindication	5. Emboli
6. Pulmonary hypertension not contraindicated	6. Bleeding

TABLE 54–7. CONDITIONS FOR WHICH THE ARTIFICIAL HEART IS MORE EFFECTIVE THAN THE LEFT VENTRICULAR ASSIST DEVICE

1. Acute post infarction ventricular septal defect (VSD)
2. Fibrotic left ventricle after aneurysmectomy
3. Left ventricular rupture; acute myocardial infarction
4. Mitral valve disruption
5. Irresponsive fibrillation
6. Some complex congenital defects
7. Some cardiac tumors; trauma

COSTS

It is estimated that the cost of an artificial heart for the first year will be approximately $60,000. At estimates of 10,000 implants per year, the cost of a long-term implantable artificial heart program is approximately $600 million per year in the United States. The current renal dialysis program cost is approximately $1 billion per year. Cardiac pacemakers cost approximately $250,000 per year. These cost factors raise several ethical considerations in the implementation of the total artificial heart program.

FUTURE CONSIDERATIONS

The electrohydraulic heart has stimulated intense interest worldwide. This type of implantable artificial heart would allow clinicians to discard the pneumatic tether lines and pave the way for a totally implantable device. The power requirements for a total artificial heart are over a million times those of a pacemaker, and currently available energy convertors cannot be made small enough for implantation. Nuclear sources capable of delivering the required 15 watts of power are not only prohibitively expensive but also present a hazard to the public. There is no question that the development of fully implantable artificial hearts is on the horizon.

Many ethical considerations exist in making the decision to implant the total artificial heart, and it is hoped that these will be eliminated with clinical expertise. The replacement of the "site of the soul, the seat of love" with a pump may soon be a common practical clinical reality.

SELECTED REFERENCES

Cooley, D. A., Akutsu, T., Norman, J. C., Serrato, M. A., and Frazier, O. H.: Total artificial heart in two-staged cardiac transplantation. Cardiovasc. Dis. Bull. Texas Heart Institute, *8*:305, 1981.

In this paper, the authors draw attention to the use of a two-staged procedure for cardiac transplantation, with implantation of a total artificial heart (TAH) as the first stage to maintain the patient's life until preparation can be made for a cardiac allograft. The first patient was a 47-year-old male whose life was sustained for 64 hours with a TAH and another 32 hours by a cardiac allograft, indicating that the TAH had clinical applicability. In that patient, the major complications described were early hemolysis, probably due to the fabric (Dacron) internal lining of the ventricle, and marginal function of the pumping chambers caused by the incompetence of the Wada-Cutter hingeless valves.

In this report, the authors add another patient, a 36-year-old male with ischemic myocardial insufficiency, who underwent a triple-vessel aortocoronary bypass followed by ventricular fibrillation refractory to cardioversion. The patient was returned to the operating room and placed on partial cardiopulmonary bypass with implantation of a total artificial heart. A cardiac donor was located in another state and was transported by chartered jet aircraft with life support systems intact. The donor heart was removed and placed into the recipient, with removal of the total artificial heart. The patient succumbed 7 days after cardiac allografting of multiple organ failure, including septicemia. The authors continue to conclude that this two-stage approach may be a viable method of management in this situation.

DeBakey, M. E.: Mechanical circulatory support: Current status. Am. J. Cardiol., 27:1, 1971.

In this article, a world leader in the field of mechanical support of the circulation reviews the present status of this important subject.

Norman, J. C.: ALVAD 1979: Precedence, potentials, prospects and problems. Cardiovasc. Dis. Bull. Texas Heart Institute, 6:384, 1979.

In this review, the author summarizes his groups' experience with an intracorporeal partial artificial heart or abdominal left ventricular assist device (ALVAD). These devices were conceived in the 1960s and followed by an extended period of modifications, improvement, and bovine testing and were used clinically in the mid 1970s. The clinical indications to date have included use in weaning from cardiopulmonary bypass, in providing circulatory support in irretrievable postinfarction cardiogenic shock, in supporting patients with severe cardiac failure awaiting cardiac transplantation, and in preoperative or prophylactic techniques of decreasing mortality in cardiac surgical procedures currently of unacceptably high risk.

Pierce, W. S., Phillips, W. M., Rosenberg, G., Donachy, J. H., and Landis, D. L.: Total heart replacement with modified sac-type ventricles. *In* Circulatory Assistance and the Artificial Heart. USA-USSR Joint Symposium, Tbilisi, USSR, September 20–22, 1979. Edited by W. S. Pierce. NIH Publication 80-2032, July 1980.

In this paper, the authors summarize a 3-year experience with development and evaluation of an artificial heart consisting of two modified sac-type ventricles using a pneumatic power system and automatic control. The modified sac ventricles are composed of a flexible seam-free polyurethane sac positioned with a polysulfone housing. The sac motion is controlled by a diaphragm interposed between the sac and the air cap of the housing. The ventricles have undergone extensive *in vitro* evaluation, including hemodynamic characterization and flow visualization studies. Each ventricle pumps 13 L./min. against an arterial pressure of 100 mm. Hg with an inlet pressure of 15 mm. Hg when Bjork-Shiley valves are employed. The artificial heart has been implanted in 12 calves. The longest period of continuous pumping has been 140 days, and the average period of pumping has been 70 days (excluding one operative death). The automatic control system has functioned well in each calf. The control system requires no implanted pressure transducer and balances the output of the two ventricles. Furthermore, the cardiac output is automatically increased with exercise. Important problems requiring further attention include (1) elevations in central venous pressure observed in some calves, (2) sepsis secondary to percutaneous lines and frequent venipuncture, (3) disproportion between the required cardiac output of the growing calf and the relatively limited output of the artificial heart, and (4) polyurethane sac damage, including flexion failure and calcification.

REFERENCES

Berser, R. L., Merin, G., Carr, J., Sossman, H. A., and Bernhard, W. F.: Successful use of a left ventricular assist device in cardiogenic shock from massive postoperative myocardial infarction. J. Thorac. Cardiovasc. Surg., 78:626, 1979.

Cooley, D. A., Liotta, D., and Hallman, G. L.: Orthotopic cardiac prosthesis for two-staged cardiac replacement. Am. J. Cardiol., 24:730, 1969.

Cooley, D. A., Akutsu, T., Norman, J. C., Serrato, M. A., and Frazier, O. H.: Total artificial heart in two-staged cardiac transplantation. Cardiovasc. Dis. Bull. Texas Heart Institute, 8:305, 1981.

DeBakey, M. E.: Mechanical circulatory support: Current status. Am. J. Cardiol., 27:1, 1971.

DeVries, W. C., Kwan-Gett, C. S., and Kolff, W. J.: Consumptive coagulopathy, shock and the artificial heart. Trans. Am. Soc. Artif. Intern. Organs, 16:29, 1970.

Golding, L. R., Loop, F. D., Sandberg, G. W., Jacobs, G., and Lewis, R. C.: Left ventricular assist device support: Twenty-one-month survival. Cleve. Clin. Q., 48:373, 1981.

Hastings, W. L., Aaron, J. L., Deneris, J., Kessler, T. R., Pons, A. B., Razzeca, K., Olsen, D. B., and Kolff, W. J.: A retrospective study of eight calves surviving five months on the pneumatic total artificial heart. Trans. Am. Soc. Artif. Intern. Organs, 27:71, 1981.

Jarvik, R. K.: Recent successes with total replacement of the heart. *In* Quantitative Cardiovascular Studies: Clinical and Research Applications of Engineering Principles. Edited by N. H. C. Hwang, D. R. Gross, and D. J. Patel. Baltimore, University Park Press, 1979, p. 751.

Jarvik, R. K., Isaacson, M. S., Nielsen, S. D., Orth, J., Hiddema, P., and Landstra, M.: Toward a portable human total artificial heart, utilizing a miniature electrohydraulic energy convertor. J. Artif. Organs, 3(Suppl.):320, 1979.

Jarvik, R. K., Olsen, D. B., Lawson, J., Fukumasu, H., Kessler, T., and Kolff, W. J.: Recent advances with the total artificial heart. N. Engl. J. Med., 298:404, 1978.

Kolff, W. J., Akutsu, T., Dreyer, B., *et al.*: Artificial heart in the chest and use of the polyurethane for making hearts, valves and aortas. Trans. Am. Soc. Artif. Intern. Organs, 5:228, 1959.

Norman, J. C.: ALVAD 1979: Precedence, potentials, prospects and problems. Cardiovasc. Dis. Bull. Texas Heart Institute, 6:384, 1979.

Olsen, D. B.: The total artificial heart—a research tool or potential clinical reality? *In* Assisted Circulation. Edited by F. Unser. New York, Springer-Verlag, 1979, p. 283.

Olsen, D. B., Nielsen, M., Lawson, J., Nielsen, S., Stanley, T., and Kolff, W. J.: Total artificial heart performance in the calf. Am. J. Cardiol., 37:160, 1976.

Olsen, D. B., DeVries, W. C., Oyer, P., Reitz, B., Murashita, J., Kolff, W. J., Diatoh, N., and Jarvik, R.: Artificial heart implantation, later cardiac transplantation in the calf. Trans. Am. Soc. Artif. Intern. Organs, 27:132, 1981.

Olsen, D. B., DeVries, W. C., Murashita, J., Oyer, P., Reitz, B., Blaylock, R., Gaykowski, R., and Kolff, W. J.: Long-term total body preservation while awaiting a suitable cardiac donor. J. Artif. Organs, 5:53, 1981.

Pierce, W. S., Parr, G. V. S., Myers, J. L., Donachy, J. H., Rosenberg, G., Landis, D. L., and Bull, A. P.: Clinical effectiveness of mechanical ventricular bypass in treating postoperative heart failure. Second USA-USSR Symposium on Circulatory Assistance and the Artificial Heart. Houston, Texas, September 1981.

Pierce, W. S., Phillips, W. M., Rosenberg, G., Donachy, J. H., and Landis, D. L.: Total heart replacement with modified sac-type ventricles. *In* Circulatory Assistance and the Artificial Heart. USA-USSR Joint Symposium, Tbilisi, USSR, September 20–22, 1979. Edited by W. S. Pierce. NIH Publication No. 80–2032, July 1980.

Index

Page numbers in *italics* indicate illustrations. Page numbers followed by t indicate tables.

Angiography (Continued)
in coronary arteriovenous fistulas, 1388–
1389, *1389*
in coronary atherosclerosis, 1428–1429
in Ebstein's anomaly, 1206
in malformations of left coronary artery,
1387–1388, *1388*
in mitral stenosis, 1229
in pulmonary atresia with intact
ventricular septum, 1173, *1173, 1174*
in thoracic outlet syndrome, 446, *446*
internal mammary artery in, 1386, *1386*
Judkins technique in. See *Judkins
technique, in angiography.*
laboratory equipment for, 1391–1392,
1392
left anterior descending coronary artery
in, 1384–1385, *1384*
left circumflex artery in, *1385*, 1386, *1386*
left coronary artery in, *1383*, 1384, *1384*
percutaneous femoral technique in. See
Judkins technique, in angiography.
right coronary artery in, 1383, *1383*
selective coronary, complications of,
1397–1399, 1399t
brachial artery thrombosis in, 1398
bradyarrhythmias in, 1398–1399
contraindications to, 1396–1397, *1397*
coronary spasm in, 1401, *1401*
indications for, 1396–1397
interpretation of, 1400–1401
pitfalls of, 1399–1401, *1399, 1400,
1401*
Sones technique in. See *Sones technique,
in angiography.*
thromboembolism in, 1274
Angioplasty, percutaneous transluminal
coronary, 1402–1403
development of, 1402
indications for, 1402
results of, 1402
technique of, 1402–1403, *1403, 1404*
Anomalous pulmonary venous drainage,
dye-dilution studies in, 886, *887*
Anstadt cup, historical aspects of, 1491,
1493t, *1494*
physiologic advantages and disadvantages
of, 1493t
Antibiotic(s). See also specific drug.
adverse reactions to, 85
bacterial resistance to, 85
bactericidal versus bacteriostatic, 83–84
classification of, by mechanism of action,
81, 81t
for prosthetic valve endocarditis, 1258,
1259t
historical aspects of, 80
in cardiac and thoracic surgery, 80–95
bactericidal versus bacteriostatic, 83–84
dosages for, 82
drug selection in, 83
duration of therapy, 82
routes of administration of, 82
multiple drug therapy and toxicity, 84
overuse of, 84–85
pharmacology of, in impaired renal
function, 170t
prophylactic use of, 94–95
for pacemaker insertion, 1339
in postoperative period, 178–180, *179*
in tracheal reconstruction, 263
Anticholinergic(s). See also specific drug.
in preoperative therapy, 100–101
Anticoagulant drug(s), characteristics of,
1274–1275

Anticoagulant therapy, following mitral
valve replacement, 1243
for pulmonary embolisms, 639–640
for thromboembolism of vascular
prostheses, 1273
long-term, 1274–1275
with heparin, 1274. See also *Heparin.*
with warfarin, 1275
Antidiuretic hormone, secretion of, in lung
carcinoma, 459
Antihuman thymocyte globulin,
immunosuppression with, in heart
transplantations, 1602, 1604
Antihyperlipidemic drug(s), for
hyperlipidemia, 1521–1522
Antilipemic drug(s), for atherosclerosis,
1545–1547
Antilymphocyte serum, for myasthenia
gravis, 859–860
Antiplatelet drug(s), for atherosclerosis,
1547
results of, 1547–1548
mechanism of action of, 1275, *1275*
types of, 1275
Antitachycardia pacing. See *Pacemaking,
antitachycardia.*
Anuloplasty, Carpentier ring, for acquired
tricuspid disease, 1217–1218, *1217,
1218*
DeVega, for reversible tricuspid
insufficiency, *1216*, 1217
mitral valve, technique of, 1248–1250,
1249
Anti-reflux repair, Belsey Mark IV. See
Belsey Mark IV anti-reflux repair.
Aorta, 926–990. See also under *Aortic.*
aneurysms of, surgical treatment of, 970–
976. See also *Aneurysm(s), thoracic.*
arch of. See *Aortic arch.*
ascending, cannulation of, in
cardiopulmonary bypass, 910–911,
911, 911t
in coronary artery bypass, 1435,
1435
atresia of, 940–941
branches of, occlusive disease of, 988–
990
clinical manifestations of, 988
diagnosis of, 988–989
pathology of, 988
surgical treatment of, 989–990, *989*
coarctation of, 940–946
clinical manifestations of, 941
diagnosis of, 941–942, *942*
heparinized vascular shunts for, 985–
986
pathology of, 940–941, *940*
physiology of, 943
prognosis in, 942–943
surgical treatment of, 944–946, *944,
945*
complications of, 946
necrotizing arteritis following, 946
patient selection in, 943
prostheses in, 945
results of, 946
ventricular septal defects and, 1068
management of, 1080
cross-clamping of, time limits of, 979
dissection of. See *Aortic dissection.*
grafts and prostheses for, composition of,
928
historical aspects of, 927–928
incompetence of, in ventricular septal
defects, 1072

Aorta (Continued)
injuries to, clinical manifestations of,
300, *300*
diagnosis of, 300, *300*
etiology of, 299, *299*
management of, 300–301
interrupted, 940–941
penetrating wounds of, 305–310
clinical manifestations of, 306–307
diagnosis of, 307, *308*
etiology of, 305
management of, 307–310, *309*
anesthesia in, 308
median sternotomy in, 308–310, *309*
site of, 305–306
stenosis of. See *Aortic stenosis.*
transposition of. See *Transposition of
great arteries.*
trauma to, heparinized vascular shunts
for, 981–983, *982*
Aortic anulus, small, management of, in
aortic valve replacement, 1295–1296,
1296, 1297, 1298
Aortic arch, aneurysms of, surgical
treatment of, 972, *975*
anomalies of, 928–933
clinical manifestations of, 931
diagnosis of, 931–932, *932*
embryology of, 929–930, *929*
in transposition of great arteries, 1128
pathology of, 930–931, *930, 931*
results of, 933
surgical treatment of, 932–933
double, *930*
interrupted, in truncus arteriosus, 1104
laterality of, in transposition of great
arteries, 1128
Aortic bypass, heparinized vascular shunt
for, 977, *977*
Aortic dissection, 956–966
classification of, 959–960
clinical manifestations of, 957
complications of, 957t
diagnosis of, 957–959, *958, 959*
angiography in, 958, *958*
aortography in, 958, *959*
computed tomography in, 958–959
incidence and etiology of, 956
medical treatment of, 960–961, 960t
pathogenesis of, 956
pathology of, 956–957, *957*
pathophysiology of, 959
prognosis in, 959
surgical treatment of, 961–965
complications of, 965
indications for, 961–962, *962*
results of, 965–968
technique in, 962–965, *963, 964*
Aortic insufficiency, left heart
catheterization in, 879
Aortic pressure, in aortic regurgitation,
1286–1287
in aortic stenosis, 1286
Aortic regurgitation, clinical manifestations
of, 1287
following aortic stenosis repair, 1114
hemodynamic alterations in, 1286–1287
left heart catheterization in, 1287
pathology of, 1287, *1287*
postoperative management in, 1289–1291
neurologic status in, 1291
pulmonary support in, 1290–1291
renal support in, 1291
surgical treatment of, anesthetic
techniques in, 1288

Keflin. See *Sodium cephalothin (Keflin)*.
"Kerley's lines," in mitral stenosis, 1228
Kidney failure. See *Renal failure*.
Kidney function. See *Renal function*.
Kim-Ray-Greenfield filter, complications
  of, 1273, 1273t
  for ligation of inferior vena cava, 646–
  647, *648, 649*
Kistner tracheostomy tube, characteristics
  of, 191, *191*
Konno procedure, for management of small
  aortic anulus, 1296, *1298*

Lanz tracheostomy tube, characteristics of,
  187t, *188*
Laplace's law, in physiologic dynamics of
  pneumothorax, 363, *363*
Laryngotracheal cleft, surgical correction
  of, 718
Laryngotrachiectomy, tracheal
  reconstruction and, 271, *272*
Larynx, carcinoma of, spread to trachea,
  251
  postintubation injuries to, 254, *254*
  subglottic, stenosis of, surgical repair of,
  267–269, *268*
Lasix. See *Furosemide (Lasix)*.
Latissimus dorsi pedicled graft, in chest
  wall reconstruction, 349–350, *350, 352,
  353*
LDL. See *Lipoprotein(s), low-density*.
Lead(s), pacemaker. See *Pacemaker(s),
  leads and electrodes of*.
Left anterior descending coronary artery,
  angiographic visualization of, 1384–1385,
  1384
Left atrial pressure, in mitral stenosis,
  1226–1227
Left circumflex artery, anatomy of, 1382,
  1382
  angiographic visualization of, *1385, 1386,
  1386*
Left heart catheterization. See
  Catherization, left heart.
Left heart partial bypass, historical aspects
  of, 1491, 1492t, *1494*
  physiologic advantages and disadvantages
  of, 1492t
Left subclavian artery-to-left coronary
  artery anastomosis, for congenital origin
  of left coronary artery from pulmonary
  artery, *1419*, 1420
Left ventricular aneurysm(s). See
  Aneurysm(s), left ventricular.
Left ventricular assist device(s). See also
  Heart(s), total artificial.
  complications of, 1635
  for myocardial ischemia, 1498
  historical aspects of, 1493t, 1494–1495,
  1495, 1630
  indications for, 1501
  physiologic advantages and disadvantages
  of, 1493t
  results with, 1630, 1630t
Left ventricular failure, pulmonary blood
  flow and, 27–28, *27*
Left ventricular outflow tract, evaluation
  of, in transposition of great arteries,
  1157–1158, *1158*
  obstruction of, in transposition of great
  arteries, 1127–1128
Left ventricular power failure. See *Low
  cardiac output syndrome*.

Left-to-right shunting. See *Shunt(ing), left-
  to-right*.
Leiomyoma, esophageal, diagnosis of, 755,
  755
  incidence and clinical manifestations
  of, 755
  surgical treatment of, 755–756
  pulmonary or bronchial, clinical
  manifestations of, 519
  histology of, 519, *520*
  treatment of, 519
Lenegre's disease, cardiac conduction
  dysfunction in, 1335
Letterer-Siwe disease, congenital cystic
  lesions of lung and, 681, *682*
Leukocyte(s), damage to, in
  cardiopulmonary bypass, 921
Levophed. See *Norepinephrine (Levophed)*.
Lev's disease, cardiac conduction
  dysfunction in, 1335
Lidocaine hydrochloride (Xylocaine),
  dosages of, pediatric, 288t
  for bronchoscopy, 62
  for cardiopulmonary arrest, 232
  for premature ventricular contractions,
  177
  for topical anesthesia, in tracheal
  intubation, 183
  pharmacology of, in impaired renal
  function, 170t
Lincomycin, pharmacology of, in impaired
  renal function, 170t
Lipid(s), metabolism of, 1540–1543
  cholesterol in, 1540, *1540*
  chylomicrons in, 1541
  phospholipids in, 1540–1541, *1541*
  triglycerides in, 1540, *1541*
  very-low-density lipoproteins in, 1541–
  1542, *1542*
Lipoid granuloma, 579
Lipoma(s), pleural, 399
  pulmonary or bronchial, 518–519, *519*
Lipoprotein(s), characteristics of, *1541*
  high-density, cholesterol transport by,
  1542, *1542*
  in atherosclerosis, 1517
  low-density, biosynthesis of, 1542, *1542*
  in type II hyperlipidemia, 1518, 1518t
  plasma levels of, effects of partial ileal
  bypass on, 1526
  very-low-density (VLDL), in lipid
  metabolism, 1541–1542, *1542*
Lithium power cells, for pacemakers, 1312–
  1315
  voltages of, 1312, 1312t
Liver function, in infants, 289
Lobectomy. See also *Lung resection*.
  for histoplasmosis, 557
  for pulmonary arteriovenous
  malformation, 695
  for pulmonary sequestration, 687–688,
  690
  left lower, for lung carcinoma, *480–482*
  left upper, for lung carcinoma, *478–479*
  prophylactic antibiotic therapy for, 94
  right lower, for lung carcinoma, *476–477*
  right upper, for lung carcinoma, *468–475*
  sleeve, historical aspects of, 498–499
  indications for, 499
  postoperative care and complications
  in, 502–503
  preoperative evaluation in, 499
  pulmonary function preservation in,
  502–503
  results in, 503–504, 504t

Lobectomy (Continued)
  sleeve, techniques in, 499–502, *500*
  technique of, bronchial closure in, *585,
  586, 586*
  lower left, *596, 597, 598, 599*
  middle and lower right, *587, 588, 589,
  590, 591*
  upper left, *587, 592, 593, 594, 595, 599*
  upper right, *582–586, 583, 584, 585*
Loeffler's syndrome, *Ascaris lumbricoides*
  in, 573
Low cardiac output syndrome, cardiac
  index in, 157–158, *159*
  diagnosis and treatment of, 157–158, *158,
  159*
  etiology of, 158, 159t
  following cardiac surgery, 126–127, 1501–
  1503
  etiology of, 1501
  intra-aortic balloon counterpulsation
  for, 1502
  medical treatment of, 1502
  prognosis in, 1501–1502
Lung(s). See also *Pulmonary*.
  abscess of. See *Lung abscess(es)*.
  adenocarcinoma of, characteristics of,
  457
  adenomatous hamartoma of infancy in,
  522
  agenesis and hypoplasia of, 676–678
  conditions associated with, 676–678,
  677
  diaphragmatic hernia and, 678
  histology of, 678
  incidence of, 676
  alveolar cell carcinoma of, 457–458
  anatomic variations in, 672–673, *672, 673*
  azygos lobe of, *672, 672*
  benign tumors of. See also specific type.
  classification of, 516, 516t
  clinical manifestations of, 516
  diagnosis of, 516–517
  of epithelial origin, 517
  of mesodermal origin, 517–521
  of unknown origin, 521–522
  blastoma of, 522
  blood flow in, 25–30. See also *Blood
  flow, pulmonary*.
  bronchiolar carcinoma of, 457–458
  bronchogenic carcinoma of, pulmonary
  osteoarthropathy in, *463*
  bronchogenic cyst of, 681–684. See also
  Cyst(s), bronchogenic.
  bronchogram of, normal, *540*
  carcinoma of, alveolar cell, 457–458
  antidiuretic hormone secretion in, 459
  Bacille-Calmette-Guérin for, 494, 530
  carcinoembryonic antigen in, 529
  chemotherapy for, 493
  chest pain in, 458
  corticotropin secretion in, 459–460
  diagnosis of, 461–466, *460, 461, 462,
  463*
  aspiration needle biopsy in, *464,
  465–466, 465*
  bronchoscopy in, 464
  chest films in, *460, 461, 461, 462,
  463*
  computed tomography in, 462, 464
  mediastinoscopy in, 466
  radioactive scanning in, 461–462
  scalene node biopsy in, 466
  supraclavicular thoracotomy in, 466,
  466
  differential diagnosis of, 467

Myocardium *(Continued)*
intraoperative protection of, intermittent coronary perfusion in, 1360
minimizing operative injury in, 1361
topical cardiac hypothermia in, 1360
membrane action potential of, 1552–1553, *1552*
normal blood flow to, 1356
oxygen consumption of, myocardial wall tension in, 894–895
oxygen demand of, 1496, *1496, 1497, 1498, 1498*
oxygen transport in, in coronary artery disease, 1427–1428
Myomectomy, Morrow's, for idiopathic hypertrophic subaortic stenosis, 1300–1301, *1300, 1301*
Myotomy, cricopharyngeal, technique of, 741, 743, *743*
Myotonia dystrophica, esophageal motility disorders in, 750
Myxoma(s), cardiac, 1586–1592
angiocardiography in, 1590–1591, *1590, 1591*
cardiac catheterization for, 1591
clinical manifestations of, 1586–1587
computed tomography for, 1591, *1592*
differential diagnosis of, 1587
echocardiography for, 1587, *1588, 1589, 1589*
electrocardiography in, 1590
locations and incidence of, 1586
pathology of, 1586, *1586, 1587*
phonocardiography for, 1589–1590, *1590*
surgical management of, 1591–1592, *1593*
"tumor plop" in, 1587

Nafcillin, for prosthetic valve endocarditis, 1259t
use of, 88
Narcotic(s). See also specific drug.
anesthesia with, 102
Neck, penetrating wounds of, clinical manifestations of, 302
diagnosis of, 302
management of, 302, *303, 304,* 305, *305, 306, 307*
Neomycin, irrigation with, for postpneumonectomy empyema, 387
use of, 90
Neoplasm(s). See also specific type.
benign bronchial. See *Bronchi, benign tumors of.*
cardiac, benign, 1585–1586, 1585t, 1586t
historical aspects of, 1585
malignant, 1592–1594
metastatic, 1594–1595
cardiac conduction system dysfunction in, 1336
chest wall, diagnosis of, 347
surgical treatment of, 347–348, *348, 353*
diaphragmatic, 835, *835*
esophageal. See *Esophagus, malignant tumors of.*
mediastinal, 413–424. See also *Mediastinum, neoplasms of* and specific neoplasm.
pericardial, 995

Neoplasm(s) *(Continued)*
pleural, 398–402
pulmonary. See *Lung(s), neoplasms of* and specific neoplasm.
rib, 343–356
sternal, 343–356
tracheal, 249–252
Neostigmine (Prostigmin), for myasthenia gravis, 858
in diagnosis of myasthenia gravis, 853
Neo-Synephrine. See *Phenylephrine (Neo-Synephrine).*
Nerve conduction velocity, measurement of, by electromyography, 444–445, *444, 445, 446*
ulnar, normal values of, 445–446
Nervous system, autonomic, in pathophysiology of coronary artery spasms, 1466–1467
central, cardiopulmonary bypass complications and, 173–175
in infants, 280–281
in pathophysiology of coronary artery spasms, 1465–1466
Neurilemmoma(s), mediastinal, 415
pulmonary or bronchial, 519–521, *520*
Neuroblastoma(s), mediastinal, pathology and management of, 417, *417*
Neurofibroma(s), mediastinal, clinical manifestations of, 415, *416*
histology of, 415
pulmonary or bronchial, 519–521
Neuroma, pulmonary or bronchial, 519–521
Neuromyopathy, in lung carcinoma, 460
Neurovascular compression syndrome(s). See also *Thoracic outlet syndrome.*
etiology of, 439, 439t
Niacin, for atherosclerosis, 1545
Nicotinic acid, for atherosclerosis, 1545
adverse effects of, 1545
for hyperlipidemia, 1522
Nifedipine, for coronary artery spasms, 1469, *1469*
Nissen fundoplication. See *Fundoplication, Nissen.*
Nitrofurantoin (Furadantin), pharmacology of, in impaired renal function, 170t
Nitrogen, absorption atelectasis and, 35–36, *37*
atmospheric, effect on arterial blood oxygenation, 35–36, *36*
Nitroglycerin, for coronary artery spasms, 1468–1469
in coronary artery bypass, 1434
in intracoronary thrombolysis, 1405
ointment, pharmacology of, 160t
pharmacology of, 160, 160t
withdrawal syndrome, coronary artery spasms and, 1464
Nitroprusside, for low cardiac output syndrome following cardiac surgery, 1502
pharmacology of, 160, 160t
Nitrous oxide, anesthesia with, 102
diffusion through tissues, 40–41
Nitrous oxide test, in diagnosis of left-to-right shunts, 887–888, *888*
Nocardia asteroides, morphology of, 551–552, *552*
Nocardia brasiliensis, morphology of, 551–552, *552*
Nocardia madurae, morphology of, 551–552, *552*

Nocardiosis, pulmonary, clinical manifestations of, 552, *552*
complications of, 552–553
etiology of, 550–552
treatment of, 552–553
Nonthrombogenic material(s), characteristics of, 1275–1276
Norepinephrine (Levophed), dosage and pharmacology of, 161t
for cardiac contractility abnormalities, 161
levels of, in response to cardiopulmonary bypass, *916,* 917–918
Norpace. See *Disopyramide phosphate (Norpace).*
North American blastomycosis. See *Blastomycosis, North American.*
Nutrition, in infants, 289
Nystatin (Mycostatin), following mitral valve replacement, 1243

Old tuberculin, in tuberculosis skin tests, 609
Omental pedicled graft, in chest wall reconstruction, 349, *349*
One-lung anesthesia. See *Anesthesia, one-lung.*
Open heart surgery. See *Cardiac surgery.*
Oropharyngeal dysphagia, clinical manifestations and etiology of, 740, *741*
Osmolarity, of cardioplegia solutions, 1365
Osserman classification, of myasthenia gravis, 850, 851t
Osteoarthropathy, pulmonary, in bronchogenic carcinoma, *463*
Osteochondroma, bronchial, 518
Osteotomy, sternal, for pectus excavatum, 325, *327*
Ostium primum, atrioventricular canal defects and, 1051–1054, 1051t
Ostium primum defect(s), 1017–1021
clinical manifestations and diagnosis of, 1018
left-to-right shunting in, 1018
mitral insufficiency in, 1018
surgical repair of, 1020
pathology of, 1017–1018
pathophysiology of, 1018
postoperative care in, 1021
surgical treatment of, air embolism prevention in, 1020–1021
heart block in, 1020
patient selection in, 1018
technique of, 1018–1021, *1019, 1020*
Ostium secundum defect. See *Atrial septal defect(s).*
Oxacillin, pharmacology of, in impaired renal function, 170t
use of, 88
Oxygen, consumption of, typical values of, 2t
diffusion through tissues, 40–42, *41, 42*
in arterial blood, atmospheric nitrogen and, 35–36, *36*
factors affecting, 35
intrapulmonary shunt and, 35, *36*
process of, 34, *34*
typical values of, 2t
in infants and children, 14t
in oxyhemoglobin (HbO_2) dissociation curve, 9–10, *9*

Stricture(s) *(Continued)*
  peptic, surgical treament of, fundic patch
      technique in, 822–824, *822, 823*
    historical aspects of, 809–810
    Nissen fundoplication in, 818, *819, 820*
    results of, 818–821, 821t
  reflux esophageal, 752–753, *752,* 753t,
      754
    treatment of, 753
  tracheal, idiopathic, 252–253
    postintubation, 255–258, *256, 257, 258*
    tuberculous, 252
St. Thomas' cardioplegia solution,
    composition of, 1368, 1368t
Subaortic stenosis, idiopathic hypertrophic,
    1296–1301
  clinical manifestations of, 1298
  definition of, 1296
  diagnosis of, 1298–1299, *1298, 1299*
  hemodynamic studies in, 1298–1299,
      1298, 1299
  mitral valve abnormalities in, 1299,
      1299
  Morrow's ventriculomyotomy and
      myomectomy in, 1300–1301, *1300,
      1301*
  pathophysiology of, 1296–1298
  treatment of, 1299–1301, *1300, 1301*
Subclavian artery, aneurysm of, in thoracic
    outlet syndrome, 440, *441*
  compression by, surgical treatment of,
      932
  injury of, management of, 302, *303, 304,
      305, 305, 306, 307*
Subclavian vein, transvenous electrode
    placement through, 1342–1343, *1342,
    1343*
Subclavian-pulmonary anastomosis, for
    tetralogy of Fallot, 1087–1088, *1087,
    1088, 1089*
Subxiphoid thoracic incision(s), procedures
    performed through, 152
  technique of, 152
Suctioning, of bronchopulmonary secretions
    from tracheal tube, technique of, 190
Sulfadiazine, for pulmonary nocardiosis,
    552
Sulfinpyrazone, antiplatelet action of, 1275
  for atherosclerosis, 1547
  for pulmonary embolisms, 641
Sulfisoxazole (Gantrisin), for pulmonary
    nocardiosis, 552
  pharmacology of, in impaired renal
      function, 170t
Sulfonamide(s), adverse effects of, 86
  indications for, 86
  pharmacology of, 85–86
Superior sulcus, carcinoma of, 506–514
  chest film of, *462*
  clinical manifestations of, 507–508, *507*
  combined preoperative irradiation and
      extended resection for, 509–514,
      509t, *510, 511,* 511t, *512, 513*
    survival rates in, 510, *510*
  diagnosis of, 507–508, *508*
  histology of, radiation therapy and,
      510, *511,* 511t
  historical aspects of, 506–507
  pathology of, 509
  surgical resection of, 512–514, *512, 513*
    contraindications to, 514
    neurologic defects following, 513–
        514
  treatment of,
      509–514

Superior vena cava. See also *Inferior vena
    cava.*
  left, surgical management of, 1014
  obstruction of. See *Superior vena caval
      syndrome.*
  persistent left, anatomy of, 1046–1047,
      1046
    associated anomalies of, 1047
    cardiac catheterization of, 1047, *1047*
    clinical manifestations of, 1047
    surgical treatment of, 1047, *1048*
    with failure of coronary sinus
        development, *1046,* 1047
Superior vena caval syndrome, clinical
    manifestations of, 412
  diagnosis of, 412, *412*
  etiology of, 412
  following cavopulmonary anastomosis,
      1193
  in bronchogenic carcinoma, *462*
  management of, 412
Superior vena cava–pulmonary
    anastomosis, for tetralogy of Fallot,
    1088–1089, *1090*
Supraclavicular thoracic incision(s),
    procedures performed through, 152
  technique of, 152–153, *153*
Supraventricular tachyarrhythmia. See
    Tachyarrhythmia, supraventricular.
Surgery. See *Cardiac surgery* and *Thoracic
    surgery.*
Swallowing, process of, 776–777
Swan-Ganz catheterization, technique of,
    873–874, *874*
Sympathectomy, thoracic, for ventricular
    arrhythmias associated with coronary
    artery disease, 1573–1574
Sympathomimetic agent(s), in management
    of cardiogenic shock, 124
Synchronized intermittent mandatory
    ventilation (SIMV), definition of, 197
  in infants and children, 218
  technique of, 204
Syphilis, aortic valve disease in, 1282–1283
  in etiology of thoracic aneurysms, 967–
      968, *968*
Systemic–to–pulmonary artery shunt, for
    tricuspid atresia, 1191
  in transposition of great arteries. 1161,
      1161
Systemic venous system, embryology of,
    1029–1030, *1030*

Tachyarrhythmia(s), in left ventricular
    aneurysms, 1485
  intractable supraventricular, etiology of,
      1565
    surgical interruption of bundle of His
        in, 1565–1567, *1566, 1567*
  pacemaking for, 1327–1328
  supraventricular, atrial pacing for, 178
    cardioversion for, 178
    postoperative, diagnosis of, 177, *177*
      digitalis toxicity and, 178
      etiology and treatment of, 177–178
  ventricular, arrhythmogenic right
      ventricular dysplasia and, 1569,
      1569, 1570, 1571, 1571
    associated with coronary artery
        disease, coronary artery bypass
        for, 1573–1574
      encircling endocardial ventriculot-
          omy for, 1576–1579, *1578*

Tachyarrhythmia(s) *(Continued)*
  ventricular, associated with coronary
      artery disease, endocardial
      resection procedure for, 1579–
      1580, *1579*
    intraoperative electrophysiologic
        evaluation in, 1574–1576, *1576,
        1577*
    isolation or cryoablation for, 1574
    pathophysiology of, 1572–1573
    preoperative electrophysiologic
        evaluation in, 1574
    surgical management of, 1572–1581
    thoracic sympathectomy for, 1573–
        1574
      in absence of coronary artery
          disease, surgical management
          of, 1569–1572
      torsades de pointes, 1571–1572,
          1572
    Uhl's syndrome and, 1571
Tachycardia, as complication of angiogra-
    phy, 1398–1399
  atrial, atrial pacing for, 178
  burst pacing for, 1331
  idiopathic ventricular, characteristics of,
      1569
  pacemaking for, 1329–1334. See also
      Pacemaking, antitachycardia.
  reciprocating, cardiac mapping in, *1562*
  ventricular, nonischemic cardiomyopathy
      and, *1568,* 1569
Taenia echinococcus, life cycle of, 571, *571*
Talc, iodized, chemical pleurodesis with, 379
Tamponade, cardiac. See *Cardiac
    tamponade.*
  pericardial, in hypovolemic shock, 115, *116*
TAPVC. See *Total anomalous
    pulmonary venous connection (TAPVC).*
Teflon, vascular prostheses of,
    characteristics of, 1272t
Temperature, body. See *Body temperature.*
Tensilon (edrophonium), in diagnosis of
    myasthenia gravis, 852–853
Teratoma, bronchial or pulmonary, 522
  mediastinal, characteristics of, 418
Tetracaine hydrochloride (Pontocaine), for
    bronchoscopy, 65
Tetracycline, chemical pleurodesis with, 379
  contraindications to, 87
  indications for, 87
  pharmacology of, 87
    in impaired renal function, 170t
Tetralogy of Fallot, 1083–1097
  anatomy of, 1083–1084
  clinical manifestations of, 1084
  coeur en sabot, 1084, *1085*
  definition of, 1084
  diagnosis of, angiocardiogram in, 1085,
      1085, 1086
    blood studies in, 1085
    cardiac catheterization in, 1085
    electrocardiogram in, 1085
    physical examination in, 1084
    roentgenograms in, 1084–1085, *1085*
  historical aspects of, 1083
  surgical treatment of, 1086–1092
    Blalock-Taussig anastomosis in, 1086–
        1087, *1087*
    cardiac output following, 1092
    cardiac tamponade following, 1092
    hemodynamic results of, 1093–1094
    indications for, 1085–1086
    open correction in, 1089–1092, *1090,
        1091, 1092, 1093*